cpt® CODING ESSENTIALS

Neurology and Neurosurgery | 2020

CPT® Coding Essentials Neurology and Neurosurgery 2020

Fee schedules, relative value units, conversion factors and/or related components are not assigned by the AMA, are not part of CPT, and the AMA is not recommending their use. Neither DecisionHealth nor the AMA directly or indirectly practices medicine or dispenses medical services. The AMA and DecisionHealth assume no liability for data contained or not contained herein. The AMA and DecisionHealth disclaim responsibility for any consequences or liability attributable to or related to any use, nonuse or interpretation of information contained in this product.

This publication does not replace the AMA's Current Procedural Terminology codebook or other appropriate coding authority. The coding information in this publication should be used only as a guide.

Disclaimer

This publication is sold with the understanding that neither DecisionHealth nor the American Medical Association is engaged in rendering legal, medical, accounting, or other professional services in specific situations. Although prepared for professionals, this publication should not be used as a substitute for professional services in specific situations. If legal or medical advice is required, the services of a professional should be sought.

Printed in the United States of America

ISBN: 978-1-62202-911-2
OP260420

Additional copies of this book or other AMA products may be ordered by calling 800-621-8335 or visiting the AMA Store at amastore.com. Refer to product number OP260420.

AMA publication and product updates, errata, and addendum can be found at *amaproductupdates.org*.

Published by DecisionHealth, a division of Simplify Compliance
100 Winners Circle, Suite 300
Brentwood, TN 37027
www.codingbooks.com

Contents

Codes List

The CPT surgery and ancillary codes and code ranges that appear in this book are listed below.

Surgery Codes

10140-10160
10180
11042-11047
11104-11105
13160
20200-20205
20526
20550-20551
20552-20553
20660
20930-20931
20936-20938
20939
22010-22015
22206-22208
22210-22216
22220-22226
22310-22315
22318-22319
22325-22328
22513-22515
22532-22534
22551-22552
22554
22558
22585
22600-22614
22630-22632
22633-22634
22830
22840
22842-22844
22845-22847
22849
22850
22852
22853-22854
22855
22859
22867-22868
27096
27279
35301
36000
36215-36218
36222-36223
36224
36225-36226
36227
36228
36415-36416
37215-37216
51784-51785
61020-61026
61070
61105-61107
61108
61140
61150-61151
61154-61156
61210
61215
61304-61305
61312-61313
61314-61315
61316
61320-61321
61322-61323
61343
61345
61450
61458-61460
61500
61501
61510-61512
61514-61516
61517
61518-61519
61520
61521
61522-61524
61526-61530
61531-61533
61534
61535-61536
61537-61540
61541
61545
61546-61548
61566-61567
61580-61581
61582-61583
61584-61585
61590
61591
61592
61595
61597
61598
61600-61601
61605-61606
61607-61608
61615-61616
61618-61619
61623
61624-61626
61630-61635
61640-61642
61645
61650-61651
61680-61686
61690-61692
61697-61698
61700-61702
61703
61705
61708
61710
61711
61720-61735
61750-61751
61760
61781-61782
61783
61790-61791
61796-61797
61798-61799
61800
61863-61864
61867-61868
61880
61885-61888
62000-62010
62100
62120-62121
62140-62141
62142
62143
62145
62146-62147
62148
62160
62161-62162
62164
62165
62190-62192
62194
62200
62201
62220-62223
62225
62230
62252
62256-62258
62263-62264
62267
62270-62272
62273
62280-62282
62284
62287
62290-62291
62292
62302-62305
62320-62323
62324-62327
62328-62329
62350-62351
62355
62360-62362
62365

62367-62370
62380
63001-63011
63012
63015-63017
63020-63035
63040-63044
63045-63048
63050-63051
63055-63057
63064-63066
63075-63076
63077-63078
63081-63082
63085-63086
63087-63088
63090-63091
63101-63103
63172-63173
63185-63190
63198-63199
63200
63250-63252
63265-63268
63270-63273
63275-63278
63280-63283
63285-63287
63290
63300
63301-63302
63303
63304
63305-63306
63307
63308
63620-63621
63650-63655
63661-63662
63663-63664
63685-63688
63707-63709
63710
63740-63741
63744-63746
64400-64405
64415-64416
64417-64418
64420-64421
64425
64445-64446
64447-64448
64449
64450
64451
64479-64480
64483-64484
64490-64492
64493-64495
64505
64520
64553
64555
64566
64568
64569-64570
64575
64585
64590-64595
64600-64610
64611
64612
64615
64616
64617
64625
64633-64636
64640
64642-64643
64644-64645
64646-64647
64650-64653
64681
64708-64712
64713
64714
64718-64719
64721
64722
64727
64771-64772
64788-64792
64795
64910-64911
69990

Ancillary Codes

70015
70250-70260
70360
70450-70470
70486-70488
70496
70498
70540-70543
70544-70546
70547-70549
70551-70553
70557-70559
71045-71048
72020
72040-72052
72070-72074
72080
72081-72084
72100-72114
72120
72125-72127
72128-72130
72131-72133
72141-72142
72146-72147
72148-72149
72156-72158
72170-72190
72195-72197
72240-72270
72275
72295
73020-73030
73120-73130
73221-73223
73501-73503
73521-73523
73560-73565
73620-73630
73700-73702
73721-73723
74018-74022
74176-74178
74230
75705
75710
75774
75894
75898
76000
76120
76125
76376-76377
76536
76700-76705
76770-76775
76800
76881-76882
76937
76942
76998
77002
77003
77011
77012
78600-78601
78605-78606
78608
78610
78630-78635
78645
78650
78814
78815
80047-80048
80053
80061
80069
80076
80156-80157
80164-80165
80168
80173
80175
80177
80178
80183
80184
80185-80186
80188
80235
80305-80307
80339-80341
80349
80350-80352
81000-81003
81271
81274
81448
82043-82044
82306
82550-82554
82565
82570
82575
82607-82608
82728
82746-82747
82947-82948
82962
83036-83037
83090
83540
83550
83735

83970
84100-84105
84156
84165
84436-84439
84443
84450
84460
84520
84550
85025-85027
85576
85610-85611
85651-85652
86038-86039
86140
86235
86592-86593
86618
86780
88302-88309
88312-88313
88314
88319
88341-88344
88356
90662
90674
90685-90686
90791-90792
90832-90838
90867-90869
90901
90935-90937
90945-90947
90960-90962
90966
90967-90970
92060
92083
92133-92134
92250
92507-92508
92522
92537
92538
92540
92541
92542
92546
92547
92548-92549
92585-92586
92610
93000-93010
93040-93042
93224-93227
93228-93229
93268-93272
93306
93660
93880-93882
93886-93888
93890
93892-93893
93922-93923
93925-93926
93970-93971
94010
94660
94760-94762
95700
95705-95710
95711-95716
95717-95720
95721-95726
95806
95808-95811
95812-95813
95816-95822
95829
95830
95860-95864
95865
95867-95868
95869
95870
95873
95874
95885-95886
95887
95907-95913
95921-95922
95923
95924
95925-95927
95928-95929
95930
95933
95937
95938
95939
95940-95941
95943
95954
95955
95957
95958
95961-95962
95970-95972
95976-95977
95983-95984
95990-95991
95992
96105
96116
96121
96127
96132
96133
96136
96137
96138
96139
96146
96164-96171
96360-96361
96365-96368
96372
96374-96376
96413-96417
96450
96542
97032
97110
97112
97116
97124
97140
97161-97164
97530
97597-97598
97750
97810-97814
99151-99153
99183
0075T-0076T
0106T-0110T
0213T-0215T
0216T-0218T
0274T-0275T

Introduction

Unlike other specialty coding books on the market, *CPT® Coding Essentials for Neurology and Neurosurgery 2020* combines neurological-specific procedural coding and reimbursement information with verbatim guidelines and parenthetical information from the Current Procedural Terminology (CPT®) codebook. In addition, *CPT® Coding Essentials for Neurology and Neurosurgery 2020* enhances that CPT-specific information by displaying pertinent diagnostic codes, procedural descriptions, illustrations, relative value units (RVUs), and more on the same page as the CPT code being explained. This one book provides neurological coding and billing knowledge that otherwise might take years of experience or multiple resources to accumulate. It sets a foundation for neurology and neurosurgery coders and subspecialty coding experts that facilitates correct code assignment.

This book includes reporting rules for CPT code submission as written and enforced by the Centers for Medicare & Medicaid Services (CMS). *CPT® Coding Essentials for Neurology and Neurosurgery 2020* is not intended to equip coders with information to make medical decisions or to determine diagnoses or treatments; rather, it is intended to aid correct code selection that is supported by physician or other qualified health care professional (QHP) documentation. This reference work does not replace the need for a CPT codebook.

About the CPT® Coding Essentials Editorial Team and Content Selection

The *CPT® Coding Essentials* series is developed by a team of veteran clinical technical editors and certified medical coders. When developing the content of this book, the team members consider all annual new, revised, and deleted medical codes. They adhere to authoritative medical research; medical policies; and official guidelines, conventions; and rules to determine the final content presented within this book. In addition, the team monitors utilization and denial trends when selecting the codes highlighted in *CPT® Coding Essentials for Neurology and Neurosurgery.*

The main section of the book is titled "CPT® Procedural Coding." This section is organized for ease of use and simple lookup by displaying CPT codes in numeric order. Each code-detail page of this section presents a single code or multiple codes representing a code family concept.

The procedures featured here are those commonly performed by a neurologist or neurosurgeon, but more difficult to understand or miscoded in claims reporting. This book does not provide a comprehensive list of all services performed in the specialty, nor all sites within impacted body systems. Similarly, the CPT to ICD-10-CM crosswalks are intended to illustrate those conditions that would most commonly present relative to the procedure and the specialist. The crosswalks are not designed to be an exhaustive list of all possible conditions for each procedure, nor medical necessity reasons for coverage.

The "CPT Procedural Coding" section is complemented by other sections that review neurological and neurosurgical terminology and anatomy, ICD-10-CM conventions and coding, ICD-10-CM documentation tips, and the ICD-10-PCS coding and format. The appendices contain data from the CMS National Correct Coding Initiative, multiple ICD-10-CM compliant neurological condition documentation checklists, and evaluation and management (E/M) documentation guidelines.

Sections Contained Within This Book

What follows is a section-by-section explanation of *CPT® Coding Essentials for Neurology and Neurosurgery 2020.*

Terminology, Abbreviations, and Basic Anatomy

This section provides a quick reference tool for coders who may come across unfamiliar terminology in medical record documentation. This review of basic terminology displays lists of alphabetized Greek and Latin root words, prefixes, and suffixes associated with neurology and neurosurgery.

The combination of root words with prefixes and suffixes is the basis of medical terminology and enables readers to deduce the meaning of new words by understanding the components. For example, *neuro* is a root word for *nerve,* and *–algia* is a suffix for *pain*; thus, *neuralgia* describes nerve pain.

Also included in this section are a glossary of neurological and neurosurgical-specific terms and a list of acronyms and abbreviations. Keep in mind that these glossary definitions are neurology-specific. The same word may have a different meaning in a different specialty. In some cases, a parenthetical phrase after the term may provide the reader with a common acronym or synonym for that term. Pay particular attention to the use of capitalization in the abbreviation and acronym list, as the same letters sometimes have varied meaning in clinical nomenclature, depending on capitalization.

Introduction to ICD-10-CM and ICD-10-PCS

For coders who want a review, *CPT® Coding Essentials for Neurology and Neurosurgery 2020* recaps the development of the ICD-10-CM and ICD-10-PCS code sets and outlines important concepts pertaining to both.

Lists of common ICD-10-CM diagnoses and conditions for each selected CPT code or code range may be found within the "CPT Procedural Coding" section.

The ICD-10-CM content provided within this book complements your use of the *ICD-10-CM 2020* codebook. This section provides a chapter-by-chapter overview of ICD-10-CM that includes common new diagnoses and their codes, as well as identification of new or substantially changed chapter-specific guidelines for 2020.

ICD-10-PCS is not used for reporting physician services; however, an understanding of ICD-10-PCS is essential to physician practices because physician inpatient surgical documentation is used by hospitals for the abstraction of ICD-10-PCS codes for hospital billing. An overview of this structure is reviewed in this section.

ICD-10-CM Anatomy and Physiology

Advanced understanding of the nervous system, anatomy, and pathophysiology is essential to accurate coding for neurology and neurosurgery. A detailed study of the neurological anatomy and physiology gives beginner or intermediate coders the information boost they may need to abstract the medical record accurately.

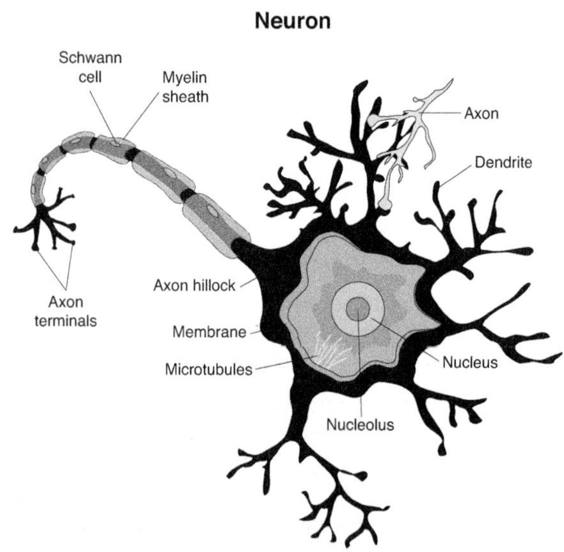

The anatomy and physiology explanations are accompanied by labeled and detailed illustrations for neurology, beginning at the cellular level and extending to the functions and interactions of the various body parts and tissues. This section also includes discussion of common disorders affecting the nervous system, their pathophysiology, as well as coding exercises to assess mastery of the documentation topic.

ICD-10-CM Documentation

Accurate, complete coding of diseases, disorders, injuries, conditions, and even signs and symptoms using ICD-10-CM codes requires extensive patient encounter documentation. This section highlights commonly encountered conditions that require a high level of specificity for documentation and reporting.

The documentation information is presented in an easy-to-understand bulleted format that enables the physician, other QHP, and/or coder to identify quickly the specificity of documentation required for accurate ICD-10-CM code abstraction. This section also includes coding exercises to assess mastery of the documentation topic.

CPT® Procedural Coding

"CPT Procedural Coding" is the main section of this book and displays pertinent coding and reimbursement data for each targeted CPT code or code family on code-detail pages. The following is presented within each surgical code detail page:

- CPT code and verbatim description with icons (when required)
- Parentheticals (when they exist)
- Official CPT coding guidelines
- Plain English descriptions
- Illustrations
- ICD-10-CM diagnostic codes
- AMA *CPT® Assistant* newsletter references
- CMS Pub 100 references
- CMS base units or relative value units
- CMS global periods
- CMS modifier edits

Category III codes and codes from diagnostic (ancillary) sections will contain a truncated version of the code-detail page content, as diagnostic tests are too broad for all data elements contained in the code-detail pages.

CPT Coding Guidelines

The guidelines and parenthetical instructions included in the CPT codebook provide coders with insight into how the CPT Editorial Panel and CPT Advisory Committee intend the codes to be used. This information is critical to correct code selection, and until now, has been unavailable in books other than official AMA CPT codebooks.

Section guidelines for the pertinent sections of the CPT code set (Anesthesia, Surgery, Radiology, Pathology, and Medicine) appear before the code-detail pages associated with the respective CPT section. Guidelines that appear elsewhere within a CPT code set section are displayed on the code-detail page, whenever appropriate. The reproduction of coding guidelines and parenthetical information in *CPT® Coding Essentials for Neurology and Neurosurgery 2020* is verbatim from the AMA CPT codebook.

CPT Codes and Descriptions

CPT codes are listed in numerical order and include surgery, radiology, pathology and laboratory, medicine, and Category III codes pertinent to neurology and neurosurgery.

The CPT code set has been developed as stand-alone descriptions of medical services. However, not all descriptions of CPT codes are presented in their complete form within the code set. In some cases, one or more abbreviated code descriptions (known as *child codes*) appear indented and without an initial capital letter. Such codes refer back to a common portion of the preceding code description (known as a *parent code*) that includes a semi-colon (;) and includes all of the text prior to the semi-colon. An example of this parent–child code system is as follows:

62280	Injection/infusion of neurolytic substance (eg, alcohol, phenol, iced saline solutions), with or without other therapeutic substance; subarachnoid
62281	epidural, cervical or thoracic
62282	epidural, lumbar, sacral (caudal)

The full descriptions for indented codes 62281 and 62282 are:

62281	Injection/infusion of neurolytic substance (eg, alcohol, phenol, iced saline solutions), with or without other therapeutic substance; epidural, cervical or thoracic
62282	Injection/infusion of neurolytic substance (eg, alcohol, phenol, iced saline solutions), with or without other therapeutic substance; epidural, lumbar, sacral (caudal)

When a group of similar codes is found on a code-detailed page in *CPT® Essentials*, a full description of each code will be displayed.

Icons

Icons on the code-detail page may affect ICD or CPT codes. The male (♂) and female (♀) edit icons are applied to ICD codes. New or revised CPT codes are identified with a bullet (●) or triangle (▲), respectively. The plus sign (+) identifies add-on codes. Addon codes may never be reported alone, but are always reported in addition to the main procedure, and should never be reported with modifier 51, *Multiple Procedures*.

A bullet with the numeral 7 within it (❼) is displayed next to ICD-10-CM codes that require a seventh character. Consult the ICD-10-CM codebook for appropriate seventh characters.

The bolt symbol (⚡) identifies CPT codes for vaccines pending FDA approval.

The star symbol (★) identifies CPT codes that may be used to report telemedicine services when appended by modifier 95.

The right/left arrows symbol (⇄) identifies where the full range of lateral codes would be appropriate. To conserve space in the *CPT® Coding Essentials* series, we have chosen to use this icon to denote laterality.

The cell phone icon (📱) denotes the *CPT® QuickRef*, a mobile app created by the AMA and available from the App Store and Google Play. The icon indicates that additional dynamic information can be accessed within the app (in-app purchases required).

Parenthetical Information

The CPT code set sometimes provides guidance in the form of a parenthetical note. For example:

(For injection procedure at C1-C2, use 61055)

Code-detail pages include parenthetical instructions specific to both the code and the section within which the code is placed within the CPT code set. Not all codes and/or sections have associated parenthetical notes.

CPT® Assistant References

CPT® Assistant is a monthly newsletter published by the AMA to provide supplemental guidance to the CPT codebook. If a CPT code is the subject of discussion in a past issue of *CPT® Assistant*, the volume and page numbers are noted beneath the code to direct readers to the relevant newsletter archives to keep abreast of compliant coding rules.

Plain English Description

A simple description of what is included in the service represented by each CPT code is provided as a guide for coders to select the correct CPT code while reading the medical record. Not all approaches or methodologies are described in the Plain English Description; rather, the most common approaches or methodologies are provided. In some cases, the description provides an overview to more than one code, as some code-detail pages have multiple codes listed.

Illustrations

Streamlined line drawings demonstrate the anatomical site of the procedure, illustrating the basics of the procedure to assist in code selection. In some cases, not all codes on the code-detail page and not all approaches or methodologies are captured in the single illustration.

Diagnostic Code Crosswalk

ICD-10-CM codes commonly associated with the service represented on the code-detail page are listed with their official code descriptions. These crosswalk codes were selected by trained coding professionals based on their knowledge and experience. The most common and medically related ICD-10-CM codes appropriate to the procedure or services represented on the code-detail pages are provided within space constraints. The intent is not to provide a list of codes that are deemed medically necessary or relate to payment policies.

While most codes support the medical necessity of the procedure performed, medical necessity rules vary by payer, and the acceptability of these diagnoses for medical necessity purposes cannot be guaranteed.

When a seventh character is required for a code, a bullet with the numeral 7 within it (❼) alerts the coder. Sometimes, a seventh character is appended to a code with only three, four, or five characters. In those cases, "X" placeholders are to be appended to the codes so that only the seventh character must be added. For example, the following ICD-10-CM diagnosis code:

T88.4	Failed or difficult intubation requires a seventh character; therefore, it is displayed with six characters in this manner:
❼ T88.4XX	Failed or difficult intubation

Within ICD-10-CM, many diagnoses have different codes based on laterality (for example, right plantar nerve, left plantar nerve, unspecified plantar nerve). Due to space constraints, not every laterality code is listed. Rather, a representative code is listed along with an icon indicating that other laterality code versions are available.

The provided crosswalks are not meant to replace your ICD-10-CM codebook. Please consult your manual for all seventh characters needed to complete listed codes and additional laterality choices, as well as ICD-10-CM coding conventions essential to proper use.

Pub 100

CMS Pub 100 (Publication 100-04, "Medicare Claims Processing Manual") is an online resource of federal coding regulations that often relate to CPT coding. If a CPT code or its associated procedure is the topic of discussion in a CMS Pub 100 entry, the Pub 100 reference is noted so that coders may access it at www.cms.gov/regulations-and-guidance/guidance/manuals/internet-onlymanuals-IOMs.html.

Payment Grids

Information in the payment grids that appear on the code-detail pages comes from CMS. These grids identify the base units used to compute allowable amounts for anesthesia services or the relative value of providing a specific professional service in relation to the value of other services, the number of postoperative follow-up days associated with each CPT code, and other reimbursement edits. All data displayed in the payment grids are relevant to physicians participating in Medicare.

Global Period

During the follow-up, or global surgery period, any routine care associated with the original service is bundled into the original service. This means that, for example, an E/M visit to check the surgical wound would not be billable if it occurs during the global surgery period.

Possible global periods under Medicare are 0, 10, and 90 days. "XXX" indicates that the global period concept does not apply to the service.

Relative Value Units (RVUs)

RVU data show the breakout of work, practice expense (PE), and malpractice expense (MP) associated with a code, and provides a breakout for the service depending on whether it was performed in the physician's office or in a facility not belonging to the physician. Understandably, the physician payment for a surgical procedure is reduced if a procedure is hosted by a facility, as the facility would expect payment to cover its share of costs. A physician who performs the surgery in his or her own office is not subject to the same cost-sharing. This cost difference is shown in the PE column.

The payment information provided is sometimes used to set rates or anticipate payments. Payment information may be affected by modifiers appended to the CPT code.

Modifiers

Sometimes, modifiers developed by the AMA and CMS may be appended to CPT codes to indicate that the services represented by the codes have been altered in some way. For example, modifier 26 reports the professional component (PC) of a service that has both a professional and a technical component (TC). A patient who undergoes an ultrasound might have a technician perform the ultrasound itself, while the physician interprets the ultrasound results to determine a diagnosis. The technician's service would be reported with the same ultrasound CPT code as the physician, but the physician would use modifier 26 to indicate the PC only, and the technician would report modifier TC, which is a Healthcare Common Procedure Coding System (HCPCS; pronounced as "hick-picks") Level II modifier identifying the service as the technical portion only. If the physician performs the ultrasound and interprets the results, no modifier is required.

When such circumstances affect the code, users may find the payment information provided for the full code, the professional services–only code, and the technical component–only code.

Many modifiers affect payment for services or with whom payment is shared when multiple providers or procedures are involved in a single surgical encounter. CMS provides definitions for the payments, based on the number listed in the modifier's field.

Modifier 50 (Bilateral Procedure)

This modifier indicates which payment-adjustment rule for bilateral procedures applies to the service.

0 150% payment adjustment for bilateral procedures does not apply. If a procedure is reported with modifier 50 or with modifiers RT and LT, Medicare bases payment for the two sides on the lower of (a) the total actual charge for both sides or (b) 100% of the fee-schedule amount for a single code. For example, the fee-schedule amount for code XXXXX is $125. The physician reports code XXXXX-LT with an actual charge of $100 and XXXXX-RT with an actual charge of $100.

Payment would be based on the fee-schedule amount ($125) because it is lower than the total actual charges for the left and right sides ($200). The bilateral adjustment is inappropriate for codes in this category (a) due to physiology or anatomy or (b) because the code descriptor specifically states that it is a unilateral procedure and there is an existing code for the bilateral procedure.

1 150% payment adjustment for bilateral procedures applies. If a code is billed with the bilateral modifier or is reported twice on the same day by any other means (such as with RT and LT modifiers or with a "2" in the units field), payment is based for these codes when reported as bilateral procedures on the lower of (a) the total actual charge for both sides or (b) 150% of the fee-schedule amount for a single code. If a code is reported as a bilateral procedure and is reported with other procedure codes on the same day, the bilateral adjustment is applied before any applicable multiple procedure rules are applied.

2 150% payment adjustment for bilateral procedure does not apply. RVUs are already based on the procedure being performed as a bilateral procedure. If a procedure is reported with modifier 50, or is reported twice on the same day by any other means (such as with RT and LT modifiers with a "2" in the units field), payment is based for both sides on the lower of (a) the total actual charges by the physician for both sides, or (b) 100% of the fee-schedule amount for a single code. For example, the fee-schedule amount for code YYYYY is $125. The physician reports code

YYYYY-LT with an actual charge of $100 and YYYYY-RT with an actual charge of $100.

Payment would be based on the fee-schedule amount ($125) because it is lower than the total actual charges for the left and right sides ($200). The RVUs are based on a bilateral procedure because (a) the code descriptor specifically states that the procedure is bilateral, (b) the code descriptor states that the procedure may be performed either unilaterally or bilaterally, or (c) the procedure is usually performed as a bilateral procedure.

3 The usual payment adjustment for bilateral procedures does not apply. If a procedure is reported with modifier 50, or is reported for both sides on the same day by any other means (such as with RT and LT modifiers or with a "2" in the units field), Medicare bases payment for each side or organ or site of a paired organ on the lower of (a) the actual charge for each side or (b) 100% of the fee-schedule amount for each side. If a procedure is reported as a bilateral procedure and with other procedure codes on the same day, the fee-schedule amount for a bilateral procedure is determined before any applicable multiple procedure rules are applied. Services in this category are generally radiology procedures or other diagnostic tests that are not subject to the special payment rules for other bilateral procedures.

9 Concept does not apply.

Modifier 51 (Multiple Procedures)

This modifier indicates which payment-adjustment rule for multiple procedures applies to the service.

0 No payment-adjustment rules for multiple procedures apply. If the procedure is reported on the same day as another procedure, payment is based on the lower of (a) the actual charge or (b) the fee schedule amount for the procedure.

1 This indicator is only applied to codes with a procedure status of "D." If a procedure is reported on the same day as another procedure with an indicator of "1," "2," or "3," Medicare ranks the procedures by the fee-schedule amount, and the appropriate reduction to this code is applied (100%, 50%, 25%, 25%, 25%, and by report). Carriers and Medicare Administrative Contractors (MACs) base payment on the lower of (a) the actual charge or (b) the fee-schedule amount reduced by the appropriate percentage.

2 Standard payment-adjustment rules for multiple procedures apply. If the procedure is reported on the same day as another procedure with an indicator of "1," "2," or "3," carriers and MACs rank the procedures by the fee-schedule amount and apply the appropriate reduction to this code (100%, 50%, 50%, 50%, 50%, and by report). MACs base payment on the lower of (a) the actual charge or (b) the fee-schedule amount reduced by the appropriate percentage.

3 Special rules for multiple endoscopic procedures apply if a procedure is billed with another endoscopy in the same family (ie, another endoscopy that has the same base procedure). The base procedure for each code with this indicator is identified in field 31G of Form CMS-1500 or its electronic equivalent claim. The multiple endoscopy rules apply to a family before ranking the family with other procedures performed on the same day (for example, if multiple endoscopies in the same family are reported on the same day as endoscopies in another family or on the same day as a non-endoscopic procedure). If an endoscopic procedure is reported with only its base procedure, the base procedure is not separately paid. Payment for the base procedure is included in the payment for the other endoscopy.

4 Diagnostic imaging services are subject to multiple procedure payment reduction (MPPR) methodology. Technical component (TC) of diagnostic imaging services are subject to a 50% reduction of the second and subsequent imaging services furnished by the same physician (or by multiple physicians in the same group practice using the same group national provider identifier [NPI]) to the same beneficiary on the same day, effective for services July 1, 2010, and after. Physician component (PC) of diagnostic imaging services are subject to a 25% payment reduction of the second and subsequent imaging services effective Jan. 1, 2012.

5 Selected therapy services are subject to MPPR methodology. Therapy services are subject to 20% of the PE component for certain therapy services furnished in office or other non-institutional settings, and a 25% reduction of the PE component for certain therapy services furnished in institutional settings. Therapy services are subject to 50% reduction of the PE component for certain therapy services furnished in both institutional and non-institutional settings.

6 Diagnostic services are subject to the MPPR methodology. Full payment is made for the TC service with the highest payment under the Medicare physician fee schedule (MPFS). Payment is made at 75% for subsequent TC services furnished by the same physician (or by multiple physicians in the same group practice using the same group NPI) to the same beneficiary on the same day.

7 Diagnostic ophthalmology services are subject to the MPPR methodology. Full payment is made for the TC service with the highest payment under the MPFS. Payment is made at 80% for subsequent TC services furnished by the same physician (or by multiple physicians in the same group practice using the same group NPI) to the same beneficiary on the same day.

9 Concept does not apply.

Modifier 62 (Two Surgeons)

This modifier indicates services for which two surgeons, each in a different specialty, may be paid.

0 Co-surgeons not permitted for this procedure.

1 Co-surgeons could be paid. Supporting documentation is required to establish medical necessity of two surgeons for the procedure.

2 Co-surgeons permitted. No documentation is required if two specialty requirements are met.

9 Concept does not apply.

Modifier 66 (Surgical Team)

This modifier indicates services for which a surgical team may be paid.

0 Team surgeons not permitted for this procedure.

1 Team surgeons could be paid. Supporting documentation is required to establish medical necessity of a team; paid by report.

2 Team surgeons permitted; paid by report.

9 Concept does not apply.

Modifier 80 (Assistant Surgeon)

This modifier indicates services for which an assistant at surgery is never paid.

0 Payment restriction for assistants at surgery applies to this procedure unless supporting documentation is submitted to establish medical necessity.

1 Statutory payment restriction for assistants at surgery applies to this procedure. Assistants at surgery may not be paid.

2 Payment restriction for assistants at surgery does not apply to this procedure. Assistants at surgery may be paid.

9 Concept does not apply.

Because many of the services represented by CPT codes in the Radiology, Pathology, and Medicine sections of the CPT code set are diagnostic in nature, crosswalks to the ICD-10-CM code set are too numerous to list. Instead, a narrative description of the service is followed by RVU, modifier, and global information. The official CPT parenthetical information associated with the CPT code is included as well.

The following page presents a guide to the information contained within a code-detail page.

HCPCS Level II Codes

The HCPCS Level II code set is a collection of codes that are used to report health care procedures, supplies, and services. HCPCS Level I codes are CPT codes, developed and copyrighted by the AMA. HCPCS Level II codes include alphanumeric codes developed by CMS to report services, procedures, and supplies that are not reported with CPT codes. These codes include: ambulance services; durable medical equipment; prosthetics, orthotics, and supplies (DMEPOS); drugs; and quality-measure reporting. HCPCS Level II codes also include two-character modifiers used to identify anatomic sites, describe the provider of care or supplies, or describe specific clinical findings.

Modifiers

HCPCS Level II and CPT modifiers appropriate to neurology and neurosurgery coding are included in this chapter. A modifier provides the means to report or indicate that a service reported with a CPT or HCPCS Level II code has been altered by some specific circumstance but unchanged in its definition or code. The service may have been greater, or lesser, or may have been performed by multiple physicians who will share in reimbursement for the service. Modifiers also enable health care professionals to effectively respond to payment policy requirements established by other entities, and often affect reimbursement.

Modifiers may be part of the CPT code set or part of the HCPCS Level II code set. Both types are included in this chapter. CMS rules specific to the assignment of modifiers are presented in numeric (CPT modifiers) or alphanumeric order (HCPCS Level II modifiers).

In addition to modifiers developed by the AMA and by CMS, a set of modifiers has been developed by the American Society of Anesthesiologists (ASA) to describe the well-being of the patient undergoing anesthesia. The modifier section of this book also describes the ASA physical status modifiers P1 through P6.

Appendices

What follows is an explanation the appendices contained within *CPT® Coding Essentials for Neurology and Neurosurgery.*

Appendix A: National Correct Coding Initiative Edits

The National Correct Coding Initiative (CCI) was developed by CMS to restrict the reporting of inappropriate code combinations and reduce inappropriate payments to providers. The CCI edits essentially identify when a lesser code should be bundled into the parent code and not separately reported, and when two codes are mutually exclusive. In either case, only one of the codes is eligible for reimbursement. In other cases, it is only appropriate to report both codes concurrently if modifier 59 is appended to identify that one of the codes reported is a distinct procedural service.

Each of the CCI edits presented in this appendix includes a superscript that identifies how the edit should be applied. With a superscript of 0 (12001^{0}), the two codes may never be reported together. With a superscript of 1 (12001^{1}), a modifier may be applied and both codes reported, if appropriate. A superscript of 9 (12001^{9}) indicates that the modifier issue is not applicable to this code pairing, and the two codes should not be reported together. Remember, the modifier can only be used when the paired codes represent distinct procedural services. The modifier would be appended to the lesser of the two codes, as defined by their RVUs.

The CCI edits for each of the anesthesia and pain management CPT codes found in this guide are included in this appendix, listed in numeric order for simple lookup. CCI edits are updated quarterly. Those listed in this guide are effective Jan. 1, 2020, through March 31, 2020. Future quarterly CCI edits can be found at https://www.cms.gov/Medicare/Coding/NationalCorrectCodInitEd/Version_Update_Changes.html.

Appendix B: Clinical Documentation Checklist

One of the biggest challenges of ICD-10-CM coding is ensuring that the clinical documentation from providers is sufficient.

The Clinical Documentation Checklists were developed to be used as a communication tool between coder and physician, or as a document that can be reproduced as a template for documentation by the physician. Essentially, the checklist identifies those documentation details required for complete and accurate code selection. For example, in ICD-10-CM, secondary diabetes is divided into diabetes due to underlying condition (E08) and diabetes induced by drugs or chemicals (E09). Furthermore, another category, other specified diabetes mellitus (E13), has been added. This category is selected for patients who have postsurgical or postpancreatectomy diabetes, or when the cause of secondary diabetes is not documented. Type 1 is reported with E10 codes, and type 2 with E11 codes.

Master code or code family for this code-detail page. All information on this page links to or crosswalks to this code(s).

Official CPT code description(s) for the master code(s) enable coders to double-check their code selections.

Citations for *CPT® Assistant* are provided so coders know when to seek further information from this authoritative reference.

RVUs are national Medicare relative value units, or a breakdown of the costs of medical care based on CPT code. Physician work, practice expense, malpractice expense, and total expense differ for facility and nonfacility, so both are listed. RVUs may be used to predict or set fees for physician payment. RVUs shown are for physicians participating in the Medicare program.

Parenthetical instructions that are part of the official CPT codebook give crucial direction to prevent coding errors.

Plain English Descriptions of the procedure or service explain what the master code represents, enabling the coder to verify code selections against the medical record.

From the CMS database, key CPT code modifiers affecting relative values when they indicate multiple procedures or multiple providers, as in co-surgery, team surgery, or assistant surgery are listed here.

The Medicare global period indicates the number of postoperative days during which any routine care associated with the original service is bundled into the original service. Possible global periods are 0, 10, and 90 days.

Simple line illustrations bring clarity and understanding to complex procedures.

Common diagnoses associated with the procedure are linked to the ICD-10-CM code set. Icons identify when a seventh character is required, and Xs have been added to codes as placeholders to prevent errors when assigning the seventh character. Diagnoses that are limited to one sex are noted with an icon. Diagnoses that apply to multiple sides/regions of the body are noted with an icon.

Citations for the CMS' Pub 100 billing guidance is provided so coders know when to seek further information from this two authoritative references.

CPT® Coding Essentials for Neurology and Neurosurgery 2020

36415

36415 Collection of venous blood by venipuncture

(Do not report modifier 63 in conjunction with 36415)

[A]MA Coding Guideline
[V]enous Procedures

[Ve]nipuncture, needle or catheter for diagnostic [st]udy or intravenous therapy, percutaneous. [Th]ese codes are also used to report the therapy [as] specified. For collection of a specimen from an established catheter, use 36592. For collection of a specimen from a completely implantable venous [de]vice, use 36591.

[Vascula]r Introduction and Injection [Procedu]res

[Ser]vices for injection procedures include [any] local anesthesia, introduction of [needle o]r catheter, injection of contrast media [wi]thout automatic power injection, and/or [any] pre- and postinjection care specifically [related to] the injection procedure.

[Selective] vascular catheterization should be coded [to include] introduction and all lesser order selective [catheteriz]ation used in the approach (eg, the [descriptio]n for a selective right middle cerebral artery catheterization includes the introduction and placement catheterization of the right common and internal carotid arteries).

Additional second and/or third order arterial catheterization within the same family of arteries or veins supplied by a single first order vessel should be expressed by 36012, 36218, or 36248.

Additional first order or higher catheterization in vascular families supplied by a first order vessel different from a previously selected and coded family should be separately coded using the conventions described above.

Surgical Procedures on Arteries and Veins

Primary vascular procedure listings include establishing both inflow and outflow by whatever procedures necessary. Also included is that portion of the operative arteriogram performed by the surgeon, as indicated. Sympathectomy, when done, is included in the listed aortic procedures. For unlisted vascular procedure, use 37799.

Please see the Surgery Guidelines section for the following guidelines:

- *Surgical Procedures on the Cardiovascular System*

AMA Coding Notes
Vascular Introduction and Injection Procedures

(For radiological supervision and interpretation, see Radiology)

(For injection procedures in conjunction with cardiac catheterization, see 93452-93461, 93563-93568)

(For chemotherapy of malignant disease, see 96401-96549)

AMA *CPT Assistant*

36415: Jun 96: 10, Mar 98: 10, Oct 99: 11, Aug 00: 2, Feb 07: 10, Jul 07: 1, Dec 08: 7, May 14: 4

Plain English Description

In 36415, an appropriate vein is selected, usually one of the larger antecubital veins such as the median cubital, basilic, or cephalic veins. A tourniquet is placed above the planned puncture site. The site is disinfected with an alcohol pad. A needle is attached to a hub and the vein is punctured. A Vacutainer tube is attached to the hub and the blood specimen is collected. The Vacutainer tube is removed. Depending on the specific blood tests required, multiple Vacutainers may be filled from the same puncture site. In 36416, a blood sample is obtained by capillary puncture usually performed on the fingertip, ear lobe, heel or toe. Heel and toe sites are typically used only on neonates and infants. The planned puncture site is cleaned with an alcohol pad. A lancet is used to puncture the skin. A drop of blood is allowed to form at the puncture site and is then touched with a capillary tube to collect the specimen.

Collection of venous blood by venipuncture

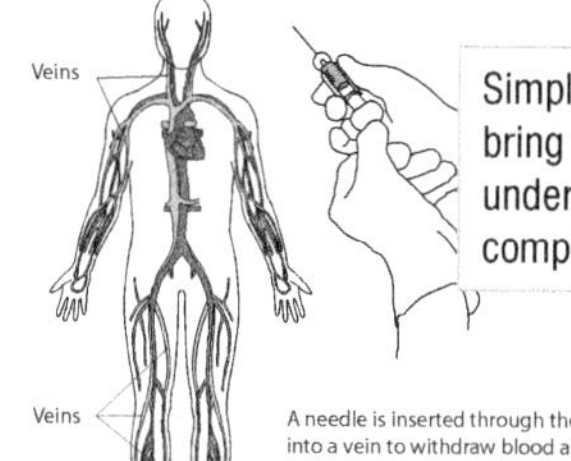

ICD-10-CM Diagnostic Codes

There are too many ICD-10-CM codes to list. Refer to ICD-10-CM code book for associated diagnostic codes.

CCI Edits

Refer to Appendix A for CCI edits.

Pub 100

36415: Pub 100-04, 12, 30.6.12, Pub 100-04, 16, 60.1.4

Facility RVUs

Code	Work	PE Facility	MP	To[tal] Fa[cility]
36415	0.00	0.00	0.00	

Non-facility RVUs

Code	Work	PE Non-Facility	MP	Tot[al] Fa[cility]
36415	0.00	0.00	0.00	0.00

Modifiers (PAR)

Code	Mod 50	Mod 51	Mod 62	Mod 66	Mod 8[0]
36415	9	9	9	9	

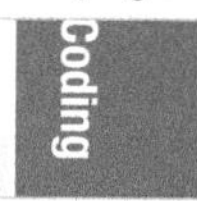

Global Period

Code	Days
36415	XXX

● New ▲ Revised ✚ Add On ⊘Modifier 51 Exempt ★Telemedicine ▢CPT QuickRef FDA Pending ⇄ Laterality Seventh Character ♂Male ♀Female

485

Appendix C: Documentation Guidelines for Evaluation and Management (E/M) Services

As the author and owner of E/M codes found in the CPT code set, the AMA has developed detailed guidelines on how to determine which code is appropriate to report, based on the medical record for the encounter. These guidelines look at the quality and quantity of the data in the record:

- History
- Examination
- Medical decision making
- Counseling
- Coordination of care
- Nature of the presenting problem
- Length of the visit

In 1995, CMS published its own documentation guidelines (DGs). Recognizing that the 1995 DGs did not appropriately reflect the work performed in some specialties, CMS published a second set of DGs in 1997. Both sets are still in use. The 1995 DGs are appropriate for multisystem examinations (eg, internal medicine physician). The 1997 DGs are appropriate for in-depth, single-system examinations (eg, retinal specialist).

For Medicare and Medicaid, either the 1995 or 1997 DGs is to be followed, depending on the preference of the provider or coder. The CPT guidelines, while largely incorporated into the 1995 and 1997 DGs, still have unique features accepted by some private payers. Unabridged copies of all three sets of DGs are presented in Appendix C.

Terminology, Abbreviations, and Basic Anatomy

This chapter can be used as a reference tool if there is confusion when reading medical record documentation or when a more extensive understanding of medical terminology is needed. The following chapter includes terms, abbreviations, symbols, prefixes, suffixes, and anatomical illustrations that will help clarify some of the more difficult issues, and give a firmer understanding of information that is in medical record documentation.

Medical Terminology

Majority of medical terms are composed of Greek and Latin word parts and can be broken down into different elements. One element is the root word. The root word is the foundation of the medical term and contains the fundamental meaning. All medical terms have one or more roots.

Examples:

hydr = water

lith = stone

path = disease

Combining forms (or vowel, usually "o") links the root word to the suffix or to another root word. This combining vowel does not have a meaning on its own; it only joins one part of a word to another.

Prefixes and suffixes are two of the other elements used in medical terminology and consist of one or more syllables placed before or after root words to show various kinds of relationships. Prefixes come before the root word and suffixes come after the root word and consist of one or more letters grouped together. They are never used independently; however, they can modify the meaning of the other word parts.

Examples:

Prefixes:

micro = small

peri = surrounding

Suffixes:

algia = pain

an = pertaining to

The following are lists of roots, prefixes, and suffixes typically seen in Neurology/Neurosurgery:

Root Words/Combining Forms

abdomin/o	abdomen
acous/o	hearing
acr/o	extremities, top, extreme point
aden/o	gland
adip/o	fat
andr/o	male
angi/o	blood vessel
ankyl/o	stiff, bent, crooked
anter/o	front
arteri/o	artery
arthr/o	joint
ather/o	yellowish, fatty plaque
audi/o	hearing
aur/o	ear
aut/o	self
axill/o	armpit
bi/o	life
blast/o	developing cell
blephar/o	eyelid
brachi/o	arm
brady	slow
bronch/o	bronchial tubes
carcin/o	cancer
cardi/o	heart
cerebr/o	brain
cheil/o	lip
chol/o	gall, bile
cholangi/o	bile duct
chondr/o	cartilage
cis/o	to cut
coron/o	heart
cost/o	ribs
crani/o	skull
cry/o	cold
cutane/o	skin
cyan/o	blue
cyst/o	urinary bladder
cyt/o	cell
dacry/o	tear duct, tear
derm/o	skin
dermat/o	skin
dipl/o	double, two
dips/o	thirst
dist/o	distant, far
dyn/o	pain
ech/o	sound
encephal/o	brain
enter/o	intestine

erythr/o	red
erythem/o	red
estesi/o	sensation
eti/o	cause of disease
gastr/o	stomach
gloss/o	tongue
gluc/o	sugar
glyc/o	sugar
gynec/o	female, woman
hemat/o	blood
hepat/o	liver
hidr/o	sweat
hist/o	tissue
home/o	sameness
inguin/o	groin
isch/o	to hold back, restrict
kal/o	potassium
kerat/o	horny tissue, hard
labi/o	lip
lapar/o	abdomen, abdominal
laryng/o	larynx
lei/o	smooth
leuk/o	white
lingu/o	tongue
lith/o	stone
lord/o	swayback, curvature in lumbar region
mamm/o	breast
mast/o	breast
melan/o	black
ment/o	mind
morph/o	shape, form
my/o	muscle
myc/o	fungus
myel/o	spinal cord
myring/o	eardrum
natr/o	sodium
necr/o	death
nephr/o	kidney
neur/o	nerve
noct/o	night
odont/o	tooth
odyn/o	pain
olig/o	few, scanty
omphal/o	naval, umbilicus
onc/o	tumor
onych/o	nail
opt/o	eye
ophthalm/o	eye
or/o	mouth
orth/o	straight
oste/o	bone
ot/o	ear
pachy/o	thick
path/o	disease
phag/o	to eat, swallow
phleb/o	vein
phon/o	voice
phot/o	light
phren/o	diaphragm
plas/o	formation, development
pleur/o	of or pertaining to the ribs
pneumon/o	lungs
poli/o	gray matter
proct/o	rectum and anus
pulmon/o	lungs
psych/o	mind
py/o	pus
quadr/o	four
ren/o	kidney
rhin/o	nose
rhytid/o	wrinkle
rhiz/o	nerve root
sial/o	salivary gland
sarc/o	flesh
scler/o	hardening
sect/o	to cut
sinistr/o	left side
somat/o	body; bodily
spasm/o	spasm
spir/o	breathing
spondyl/o	vertebra
squam/o	scale-like
staphyl/o	clusters
steat/o	fat
sten/o	narrowing
strept/o	twisted chains
terat/o	monster
thec/o	sheath
thorac/o	chest
thromb/o	clot
tympan/o	eardrum
ung/o	nail
varic/o	twisted
vas/o	vessel
vascul/o	blood vessel
ven/o	vein
viscer/o	internal organs
xanth/o	yellow
xer/o	dry

Prefixes

a(d)-	towards
a(n)-	without
ab-	from
ab(s)-	away from
ad-	towards
allo-	other, another
ambi-	both
amphi-	on both sides, around
ana-	up to, back, again, movement from
aniso-	different, unequal
ante-	before, forwards
anti-	against, opposite
ap-, apo-	from, back, again
auto-	self
bi(s)-	twice, double
bio-	life
brachy-	short
cardi-	heart
cata-	down
circum-	around
con-	together
contra-	against
cyto-	cell
de-	from, away from, down from
deca-	ten
di(s)-	two
dia-	through, complete
di(a)s-	separation
diplo-	double
dolicho-	long
dur-	hard, firm
dys-	bad, abnormal
e-, ec-, ek-	out, from out of
ecto-	outside, external
em-	in
en-	into
endo-	into
ent-	within
epi-	on, up, against, high
eso-	will carry
eu-	well, abundant, prosperous
eury-	broad, wide
ex-, exo-	out, from out of
extra-	outside, beyond, in addition
haplo-	single
hapto-	bind to
hemi-	half
hept-	seven
hetero-	different
idio-	self; oneself
in-	into, to
infra-	below, underneath
inter-	among, between
intra-	within, inside, during
intro-	inward, during
isch-	restriction
iso-	equal, same
juxta-	adjacent to
kata-	down, down from
macro-	large
magno-	large
medi-	middle
mega-	large
megalo-	very large
meso-	middle
meta-	beyond, between
micro-	small
neo-	new
non-	not
ob-	before, against
octa-	eight
octo-	eight
oligo-	few
pachy-	thick
pan-	all
para-	beside, to the side of, wrong
pent-	five
per-	by, through, throughout
peri-	around, round-about
pleo-	more than usual
poly-	many
post-	behind, after
pre-	before, in front, very
pros-	besides
prox-	besides
pseudo-	false, fake
quar(r)-	four
re, red-	back, again
retro-	backwards, behind
sangui-	pertaining to blood
semi-	half
sex-	six
sept-	seven
sub-	under, beneath
super-	above, in addition, over
supra-	above, on the upper side
syn-	together, with
sys-	together, with
tachy-	fast
tetra-	four
thio-	sulfur

trans-	across, beyond
tri-	three
uni-	one
ultra-	beyond, besides, over

Suffixes

-ad	toward
-algia	pain
-ase	enzyme
-asthenia	weakness
-centesis	surgical puncture to remove fluid
-cide	killing
-c(o)ele	cavity, hollow
-crit	to separate
-desis	to bind, tie together
-dynia	pain
-ectasis	expansion; dilation
-ectomy	removal of, cut out
-emia	blood condition
-esis	condition
-eurysm	widening
-form	shaped like
-ia	pathological state
-iasis	infestation, pathological state
-ile	little version
-illa	little version
-illus	little version
-in	a substance, chemical, chemical compound
-ism	condition indicated by root/prefix
-itis	inflammation
-ity	makes a noun of quality
-ium	structure; tissue
-logy	study of, reasoning about
-lysis	breakdown; destruction; loosening
-malacia	softening
-megaly	large
-mimetic	mimic; copy
-noid	mind, spirit
-oid	resembling, image of
-ogen	precursor
-ol	alcohol
-ole	little version
-oma	tumor (usually)
-osis	full of
-ostomy	artificial opening
-pathy	disease of, suffering
-penia	lack; deficiency
-pexy	fix in place
-plasty	re-shaping
-ptosis	falling; prolapse
-ptysis	spitting
-rhage	burst out
-rrhaphy	suturing
-rhea	discharge, flowing out
-rhexis	rupture; shredding
-sis	state of; condition
-stalsis	contraction
-stasis	stop; standstill
-staxis	dripping; trickling
-stenosis	tightening; stricture
-stitial	pertaining to; standing; or positioned
-stomy	artificial opening
-thorax	chest; pleural cavity
-thrix	hair
-tomy	cut; incise
-ule	little version
-um	thing (makes a noun, typically concrete)

Neurology/Neurosurgery Terms

The following definitions are medical terms commonly seen while coding/billing for Neurology/Neurosurgery:

Acupressure – A therapy developed by the ancient Chinese and used in eastern cultures for thousands of years. Practitioners apply varying physical pressure, through touch, to specific body sites in order to channel and stimulate energy flow.

Acupuncture – An ancient Chinese practice, using needles inserted into specific sites in the body, along "meridians," to stimulate body systems. This therapy is used for a wide variety of purposes including relaxation, pain relief, and treating illness and disease.

Acute Pain – The physiological response to trauma, injury, surgery or illness. It is generally time limited from days to weeks.

Adjuvant – Generally used to describe an "add-on" or additional therapy.

Adjuvant Analgesic – Generally used to describe drugs that have a primary use other than pain control but have secondary pain-relieving qualities.

Algology – The science and study of pain.

Allodynia – Pain due to a stimulus that does not normally provoke pain. The original definition adopted by the IASP committee was pain due to non-noxious stimulus to the normal skin. Allodynia involves a change in the quality of a sensation, tactile, thermal, or of any other kind. The usual response to a stimulus was not painful, but the present response is.

Analgesia – Absence of pain in response to stimulation that would normally be painful.

Analgesia – A painkiller; any drug or substance with a pain-relieving effect (as opposed to an anesthetic which temporarily eliminates sensation).

Anesthesia – The absence of sensation, either in a region of skin, a region of the body, or as a total loss of consciousness. "Local" anesthesia affects (numbs) a specific area of the body and "general" anesthesia results in unconsciousness.

Anesthesia Dolorosa – Where pain is present in an area that is anesthetic.

Anesthetic – An agent or agents that produce regional anesthesia (certain part of the body) or general anesthesia (loss of consciousness).

Anterior – A term used by medical professionals meaning at the front of, or close to the front of the body. (*See* Posterior)

Anticonvulsants – Group of drugs used to prevent seizures, also used as adjuvant analgesics in chronic pain treatment to alter transmission of the pain signal.

Arthralgia – Pain in a joint, usually due to arthritis.

Biofeedback – A non-drug technique used to treat a wide variety of pain conditions. A non-invasive electronic device is used to monitor various biologic responses (such as heart rate). Information is gathered, and then used to teach the patient various control techniques.

Causalgia – A syndrome of sustained burning pain, allodynia, and hyperpathia after a nerve injury, often combined with vasomotor and sudomotor dysfunction and later trophic changes.

Central Pain – Pain associated with a lesion of the central nervous system.

Chronic – Long term or ongoing.

Chronic Pain – An ongoing or persistent pain syndrome; generally lasting more than six months.

Complex Regional Pain Syndrome – Chronic pain condition that can affect any area of the body, subdivided into two types. Type 1 is typically triggered by an injury, often minor, that does not directly involve the nerves. It may also be triggered by an illness or have no known cause. Type 2, more commonly referred to as causalgia, is the result of an injury to a nerve. Both types are characterized by neuropathic pain that can be severe or even disabling. In addition, the affected body site, which is usually an extremity, may show evidence of sympathetic nervous system changes such as abnormal circulation, temperature, and sweating. Loss of function of the extremity, muscle atrophy, and hair and skin changes may also eventually occur.

Contraindicated – A term frequently used in pain management to mean that a medication or treatment is not to be used in a specific patient because it may cause serious side effects or reactions.

Cutaneous – Generally referring to the skin and/or the tissues directly underneath the skin.

Cutaneous Intervention – A variety of treatments through the skin used to promote healing or pain relief, including heat, cold, massage, acupressure, ultrasound, hydrotherapy, TENS, and vibration.

Deafferentation Pain – Pain due to loss of sensory input into the central nervous system (as can occur with avulsion of the brachial plexus), or other types of peripheral nerve lesions. Can also be due to pathologic lesions of the central nervous system.

Dermatome – A term related to very specific sections of the body that are associated with the distribution of the large nerves coming from the spine. Dermatomes are helpful in locating which area in the spine is malfunctioning.

Dysesthesia – An abnormal, unpleasant sensation that can be spontaneous or evoked.

Edema – Swelling; generally, an abnormal accumulation of body fluids, often accompanying inflammation.

Endorphin – A substance the body manufactures that acts like morphine in the brain and central nervous system. This natural pain-relieving agent can be stimulated by exercise.

Epidural Space – A space located between the spinal cord and the vertebral column in the spine.

Epidural Steroid Injection – An injection of steroid medication into the epidural space of the spine; used in some forms of back pain.

Epidurogram – An x-ray test using contrast dye to confirm epidural catheter placement and obtain information about the epidural space.

Fibromyalgia – A muscle and connective tissue disorder characterized by symptoms of pain, tenderness, and stiffness of tendons, muscles, and surrounding soft tissue.

Fibrosis – Scarring of tissue; abnormal formation of fibrous tissue.

General Anesthesia – During surgery, using a mixture of medications and gas in a gradual titration under the direction of a trained anesthetist or anesthesiologist to induce sleep and maintain a state of unconsciousness.

Hyperalgesia – An increased response to a stimulus that is normally painful.

Hyperesthesia – Increased sensitivity to any stimulation.

Hyperpathia – Abnormally exaggerated subjective response to painful stimuli. May occur with hyperesthesia, hyperalgesia, or dysesthesia. The pain is often explosive in character.

Hypoalgesia – Diminished sensation to noxious stimulation.

Hypoesthesia – Abnormally decreased sensitivity, particularly to touch in its absence.

Intramuscular (IM) – An injection of medication or fluids into a muscle.

Intravenous (IV) – An injection of medication or fluids into a vein.

Migraine Aura, Persistent, without Cerebral Infarction – A rare complication of a migraine characterized by the presence of a migraine aura lasting more than one week without radiographic evidence of cerebral infarction.

Migraine, Chronic – 15 or more migraine headache days per month.

Migraine, Episodic – Occasional episodes of experiencing migraines, without being deemed chronic.

Migraine, Hemiplegic – Migraine with aura accompanied by muscle/motor weakness. Hemiplegic migraines are further differentiated as familial or sporadic. A familial hemiplegic migraine is one in which the patient has at least one first- or second-degree family member who has also been diagnosed with hemiplegic type migraines. Sporadic hemiplegic migraine is one in which the patient does not have any first- or second-degree family members who have also been diagnosed with hemiplegic type migraines.

Migraine with Aura – Migraine accompanied by visual, sensor, or speech disorders.

Migraine without Aura – The most common type of migraine. Symptoms typically include unilateral headache, pulsating pain, moderate to severe in intensity, aggravated by physical activity, associated with nausea/vomiting, sensitivity to light (photophobia) and/or sound (phonophobia), duration typically 4-72 hours.

Myopathy – Any abnormal disease or condition of muscle tissue, often involving pain.

Myotome – Sections of the body that are associated with a muscle or muscle group the insertion sites at either end of the muscle fibers.

Nervous System – The organs and tissues of the body made up of specialized neural cells that provide communication to other parts of the body by transmitting electrical signals. The brain and spinal cord are components of the central nervous system, and the nerves outside those structures make up the peripheral nervous system.

Neuralgia – Pain in the distribution of a specific nerve or nerves.

Neuritis – Acute and/or chronic inflammation of nerves.

Neuropathic Pain – Pain syndrome in which the predominant mechanism is aberrant somatosensory processing. May be restricted to pain originating in peripheral nerves and nerve roots.

Neuropathy – A functional disturbance or pathological change in the peripheral nervous system, sometimes limited to noninflammatory lesions as opposed to neuritis.

Nociceptor – A receptor for pain, preferentially sensitive to a noxious stimulus or to a stimulus that would become noxious if continued. Pain is a perception that takes place at higher levels of the central nervous system.

Non-Steroidal Anti-inflammatory Drug (NSAID) – A specific class of drugs that reduces inflammation and swelling in and around the site of injury or irritation. These drugs (such as ibuprofen) are widely used in acute pain management and for chronic inflammatory conditions such as arthritis.

Noxious Stimulus – Stimulus that is potentially or actually damaging to body tissue.

Opioid – A narcotic that acts on opioid receptors and induces pain-relieving effects used to help treat pain.

Pain – Sensation of discomfort, distress, or agony, resulting from the stimulation of specialized nerve endings. Pain serves as a protective mechanism inducing the sufferer to remove or withdraw from the cause.

Pain Threshold – Threshold is the least experience of pain that a subject can recognize.

Pain Tolerance Level – The greatest level of pain that a patient is able to tolerate.

Paresthesia – An abnormal sensation, such as burning, or prickling, that may be spontaneous or in response to a stimulus.

Patient-Controlled Analgesia (PCA) – An intravenous drug delivery system, generally used after surgery, that allows patients to control the amount of pain medicine they receive, by pushing a button that causes the system to administer a dose of medicine. Patients are taught to administer pain medication depending on the level of pain. This method has been shown to provide effective pain relief using less medication.

Physiological Dependence – A condition that occurs with many drugs whereby the body becomes accustomed to having the chemical. Often confused with addiction or psychological dependence, this condition is common and not associated with drug abuse. The hallmark of physiological dependence is the need to avoid abrupt discontinuation of the drug, which will cause a predictable withdrawal syndrome. Discontinuation of the drug can be easily accomplished by slowly tapering the under the direction of the physician.

Posterior – Close to, or at the back of the body. Also called "dorsal."

Pseudoaddiction – A desperate drug seeking behavior pattern seen in pain patients who are not getting adequate pain relief and not stemming from true drug addiction. For example, a patient is given a pain pill that only lasts for four hours, but is only allowed to take it every six hours.

Psychosomatic – A term used to describe a physical disorder or symptom thought to be caused partly or entirely by psychological problems.

Radiculalgia – Pain along the distribution of one or more sensory nerve roots.

Radiculitis – Inflammation of one or more nerve roots.

Radiculopathy – A usually painful disturbance of function or pathologic change in one or more spinal nerve roots.

Referred Pain – Pain that is felt in a place different from the place of origin. For example, pain from pressure in the liver is often felt in the right upper chest or shoulder.

Somatosensory – Pertaining to sensations that can be experienced in all parts of the body, such as pressure or warmth, as opposed to a single sense organ, such as taste or smell.

Sonogram – The picture produced by using high frequency sound waves to view tissues inside the body for diagnostic purposes.

Titration – Increasing or decreasing a medication in an incremental manner, to reach a desired level. This method is used to allow the body to adjust, or to find an effective dose. Titration is used with anti-depressants, steroids, opioids and other drugs.

Tolerance – A physiological phenomenon that develops with long term opioid use where the body requires increasing amounts of the drug to achieve the same level of effect. There are several theories that may explain tolerance including the body becoming a more effective metabolizer of the medication, and the body making less receptor sites for a drug after long exposure.

Transcutaneous Electrical Nerve Stimulation (TENS) – A cutaneous intervention that relieves pain by sending electrical stimulation to nerve fibers and interfering with pain signal transmission. This method employs electrodes placed on the skin in various locations, using various degrees of intensity to achieve pain relief.

Transdermal – The application or administration of a drug into the body through the skin.

Trigger Point – A hypersensitive area in muscle or connective tissue with pain locally as well as referred pain and tenderness.

Withdrawal – A syndrome that occurs when opioids and some other drugs are abruptly discontinued, or a condition marked by a pattern of behavior observed in schizophrenia and depression, characterized by a pathological retreat from interpersonal content and social involvement and leading to pre-occupation.

Abbreviations/Acronyms

The following abbreviations and acronyms are commonly seen in documentation for Neurology/Neurosurgery:

A	without, lack of, Apathy (lack of feeling); apnea (without breath); aphasia (without speech); anemia (lack of blood)
A & P	anterior and posterior; auscultation and percussion
Ab	antibody
ab	away from, Abductor, (leading away from); aboral (away from mouth)
Abd	abdomen
ABG	arterial blood gases
ABP	arterial blood pressure
Ac	before meals
ACT	anticoagulant therapy; active motion
ACTH	adrenocorticotropic hormone
Ad	to, toward, near to, Adductor, (leading toward); adhesion, (sticking to); adnexa (structures joined to); adrenal (near the kidney)
ADH	antidiuretic hormone
ADL	activities of daily living
Ad lib	as desired
AFB	acid-fast bacilli
AKA	above knee amputation
Allo	other, another
ALP	alkaline phosphatase
AMA	against medical advice
AMB	ambulatory
Ambi	both, Ambidextrous, (ability to use hands equally); ambilateral (both sides)
AMI	acute myocardial infarction
a(n)	without
Ana	up, back, again, excessive
Ante	Before, forward, in front of
Anti	against, opposed to, reversed
AP	apical pulse
Apo	from, away from
AU	both ears
BBS	bilateral breath sounds
BG	blood glucose
BI	brain injury
bi	twice, double
BID	twice a day
bilat	bilateral
B/K	below knee
BMR	basal metabolic rate
BP	blood pressure
Brachy	slow
BRP	bathroom privileges
BS	bowel sounds
BSA	body surface area
BT	bowel tones
bx	biopsy
C	Celsius (centigrade)
c (C)	with
C&S	culture and sensitivity
c/o	complaint of
Ca	calcium, cancer, carcinoma
CA	cardiac arrest
CAT	computerized tomography scan
Cata	down, according to, complete
CBC	complete blood count
CBR	complete bed rest
CC	chief complaint
Circum	Around, about, surrounding
CMS	circulation, motion, sensation
CO	cardiac output
Com	With, together
Con	With, together
Contra	Against, opposite
CO2	carbon dioxide
CP	chest pain, cleft palate
CPAP	continuous positive airway pressure
CPR	cardiopulmonary resuscitation
CRPS	complex regional pain syndrome
CRT	capillary refill time
CSF	cerebrospinal fluid, colony stimulating factors
CT	chest tube, computed tomography
CVA	cerebral vascular accident, costovertebral angle
CVP	central venous pressure
CX	circumflex
Cx'd	cancelled

CXR	chest x-ray
D5W	Dextrose 5% in water
D5LR	Dextrose 5% with lactated ringers
DAT	diet as tolerated
DBP	diastolic blood pressure
DC (dc)	discontinue
DEX (DXT)	blood sugar
De	Away from, remove
deca	ten
Di	Twice, double
Dia	Through, apart, across, completely
Diplo	double
Dis	Reversal, apart from, separation
DKA	diabetic ketoacidosis
DM	diabetes mellitus
DNA	deoxyribonucleic acid
DNR	do not resuscitate
DTR	deep tendon reflex
DVT	deep vein thrombosis
Dx	diagnosis
Dys	Bad, difficult, disordered
E, ex	Out, away from
EBV	Epstein-Barr Virus
Ec	Out from
ECF	extracellular fluid, extended care facility
ECG (EKG)	electrocardiogram/electrocardiograph
Ecto	On outer side, situated on
EENT	eye, ear, nose and throat
Em, en	Empyema (pus in); encephalon (in the head)
EMG	electromyogram
Endo	Within
Ent	within
Epi	Upon, on
ERCP	endoscopic retrograde cholangiopancreatography
ET	endotracheal tube
Exo	Outside, on outer side, outer layer
Extra	Outside
F & R	force and rhythm
FBS	fasting blood sugar
FD	fatal dose, focal distance
FDA	Food & Drug Administration
Fx	fracture
FUO	fever of unknown origin
FVD	fluid volume deficit
HA	headache
Haplo	single

Hapto	bind to
Hb	hemoglobin
HCO3	bicarbonate
HCT	hematocrit
HDL	high density lipoprotein
HEENT	head, eye, ear, nose and throat
Hemi	Half,
hept	seven
hetero	different
hex	six
Hgb	hemoglobin
HM	heart murmur
h/o	history of
homo	same
HPI	history of present illness
HRT	hormone replacement therapy
HS	hour of sleep
HTN (BP)	hypertension
Hx	history
Hyper	Under, below, deficient
I & O	intake and output
IBC	iron binding capacity
ICF	intermediate care facility
ICP	intracranial pressure
ICS	intercostal space
ICT	inflammation of connective tissue
ICU	intensive care unit
IDDM	insulin dependent diabetes mellitus
IM	Intramuscular
Im, in	In, Into
Imp	impression
IMV	intermittent mandatory ventilation
Infra	Below
Inter	Between
Intra	Within
Intro	Into, within
Iso	equal, same
IV	intravenous
JAMA	Journal of the American Medical Association
Juxta	adjacent to
JVP	jugular venous pressure
K	potassium
Kata	down, down from
KCl	potassium chloride
KI	potassium iodide
KVO	keep vein open

LLQ	left lower quadrant
LP	lumbar puncture
LUQ	left upper quadrant
Lytes	electrolytes
Macro	large
Magno	large
MAP	mean arterial pressure
MAR	medication administration record
MDI	multiple daily vitamin
Medi	middle
Mega	large
Megalo	very large
Meso	middle
Meta	Beyond, after, change
MI	myocardial infarction
Micro	small
MLC	midline catheter
MM	mucous membrane
MoAbs	monoclonal antibodies
MRDD	mental retarded/developmentally disabled
MRI	magnetic resonance imaging
MS	multiple sclerosis, morphine sulfate
Na	sodium
NaCl	sodium chloride
NAD	no apparent distress
NED	no evidence of disease
Neg	negative
Neo	new
NIDDM	noninsulin dependent diabetes mellitus
NKA	no known allergies
NKDA	no known drug allergies, non-ketotic diabetic acidosis
NKMA	no known medication allergies
noc	night
non	not
NPO	nothing by mouth
NS (NIS)	normal saline
NSAID	nonsteroidal anti-inflammatory drug
NS	normal saline
NSR	normal sinus rhythm
NTD	neural tube defect
NV	nausea & vomiting
NYD	not yet diagnosed
O_2	oxygen
Ob	before, against
Octa	eight
Octo	eight
Oligo	few
OOB	out of bed
Opistho	Behind, backward
ORIF	open reduction internal fixation
OS	left eye
OT	occupational therapy
OU	both eyes
P	after
P	pulse
Pachy	thick
Pan	all
Para	Beside, beyond, near to
PCA	patient controlled analgesia
PCN	packed cell volume
PDR	physician's desk reference
PE	physical examination
Peri	around
PERL	pupils equal, react to light
PERRLA	pupils equal, round, react to light, accommodation
PET	positron emission tomography
PH	past history
PI	present illness
PICC	peripherally inserted central venous catheter
Pleo	more than usual
PMI	point of maximal impulse
PMH	past medical history
PO	by mouth
Poly	many
Post	after, behind
post op	post-operative
PRBC	packed red blood cells
Pre	before, in front of
pre op	pre-operative
prep	preparation
PRN	as needed
Pro	before, in front of
pros	besides
prox	besides
Pseudo	false, fake
PT	prothrombin time
P.T.	physical therapy
PTT	partial thromboplastin time
PVD	peripheral vascular disease
Q	every
QD	everyday
QH	every hour

Q2H	every 2 hours
QID	four times a day
qns	quantity not sufficient
QOD	every other day
Qs	quantity sufficient, quantity required
quar(r)	four
R	respirations
RAD	reactive airway disease
RAI	radioactive iodine
RAIU	radioactive iodine uptake
RBC	red blood cells
RDW	red cell distribution width
Re	back, again, contrary
REEDA	redness, edema, ecchymosis, drainage, approximation
Retro	backward, located behind
RLQ	right lower quadrant
RM	respiratory movement
RO	rule out
ROM	range of motion
ROS	review of systems
RT or R	right
RUQ	right upper quadrant
Rx	prescription, pharmacy
S(s)	without
S/S	signs & symptoms
SAB	spontaneous abortion
SB	spina bifida
Semi	half
SNF	skilled nursing facility
SOB	shortness of breath
SOBOE	shortness of breath on exertion
SOP	standard operating procedure
SR	sinus rhythm
SS	social services
STAT	immediately
STM	short term memory
Sub	under
super	above, upper, excessive (excessive number); supermedial (above middle)
supra	above, upper, excessive
SVR	systemic vascular resistance
sym	together, with
syn	together, with
sys	together, with
Sx	symptoms
T	temperature

T3	triiodothyronine
T4	thyroxine
TBSA	total body surface area
TEP	transesophageal puncture
Tetra	four
THR	total hip replacement
TIBC	total iron binding capacity
TID	three times a day
TIL	tumor infiltrating lymphocytes
TKR	total knee replacement
TNF	tumor necrosis factor
TNM	tumor, node, metastases
TNTC	too numerous to mention
TP	tuberculin precipitation
TPN	total parenteral nutrition
TPR	temperature, pulse, respiration
Trans	across, through, beyond
Tri	three
Tx	treatment, traction
UA	urinalysis
UAO	upper airway obstruction
UBW	usual body weight
UGA	under general anesthesia
UGI	upper gastrointestinal
Ultra	beyond, in excess
Uni	one
up ad lib	up as desired
URI	upper respiratory infection
US	ultrasonic, ultrasound
USA	unstable angina
UTI	urinary tract infection
VA	visual acuity
VBP	venous blood pressure
VENT	ventral
VF/Vfib	ventricular fibrillation
VLDL	very low density lipoprotein
VP	venous pressure, venipuncture
VPB	ventricular premature beats
VPC	ventricular premature contractions
VS	vital signs
VT/Vtach	ventricular tachycardia
W	vessel wall
W/C	wheelchair
WBC	white blood cell
WD	well developed
WHO	World Health Organization

WN	well nourished
WNL	within normal limits
X	times

Anatomy

Anatomy is the science of the structure of the body. This section will address systemic, regional, and clinical anatomy as it applies to coding in the Anesthesia setting. Anatomical terms have distinct meanings and are a major part of medical terminology.

Anatomical Positions

Often in medical records, anatomical positional terms are used to identify specific areas of body parts and body positions. The following list is commonly used terms that may be found in medical documentation:

- Superior = Nearer to head
- Inferior (caudal) = Nearer to feet
- Anterior (ventral) = Nearer to front
- Proximal = Nearer to trunk or point of origin (e.g., of a limb)
- Distal = Farther from trunk or point of origin (e.g., of a limb)
- Superficial = Nearer to or on surface
- Deep = Farther from surface
- Posterior (dorsal) = Nearer to back
- Medial = Nearer to median plane
- Lateral = Farther from median plane

Anatomical Planes

Anatomical descriptions are based on four anatomical planes that pass through the body in the anatomical position:

- Median plane (midsagittal plane) is the vertical plane passing longitudinally through the body, dividing it into right and left halves
- Paramedian (parasagittal) plane is a sagittal plane that divides the body into unequal right and left regions.
- Coronal (frontal) planes are vertical planes passing through the body at right angles to the median plane, dividing it into anterior (front) and posterior (back) portions
- Horizontal planes are transverse planes passing through the body at right angles to the median and coronal planes; a horizontal plane divides the body into superior (upper) and inferior (lower) parts (it is helpful to give a reference point such as a horizontal plane through the umbilicus).

Anatomical Movement Terms

Various terms are used to describe movements of the body. Movements take place at joints where two or more bones or cartilages articulate with one another. They are described as pairs of opposites.

Flexion Bending of a part or decreasing the angle between body parts.

Extension Straightening a part or increasing the angle between body parts.

Abduction Moving away from the median plane of the body in the coronal plane.

Adduction Moving toward the median plane of the body in the coronal plane. In the digits (fingers and toes), abduction means spreading them, and adduction refers to drawing them together.

Rotation Moving a part of the body around its long axis. Medial rotation turns the anterior surface medially and lateral rotation turns this surface laterally.

Circumduction The circular movement of the limbs, or parts of them, combining in sequence the movements of flexion, extension, abduction, and adduction.

Pronation A medial rotation of the forearm and hand so that the palm faces posteriorly.

Supination A lateral rotation of the forearm and hand so that the palm faces anteriorly, as in the anatomical position.

Eversion Turning sole of foot outward.

Inversion Turning sole of foot inward.

Protrusion (protraction) To move the jaw anteriorly.

Retrusion (retraction) To move the jaw posteriorly.

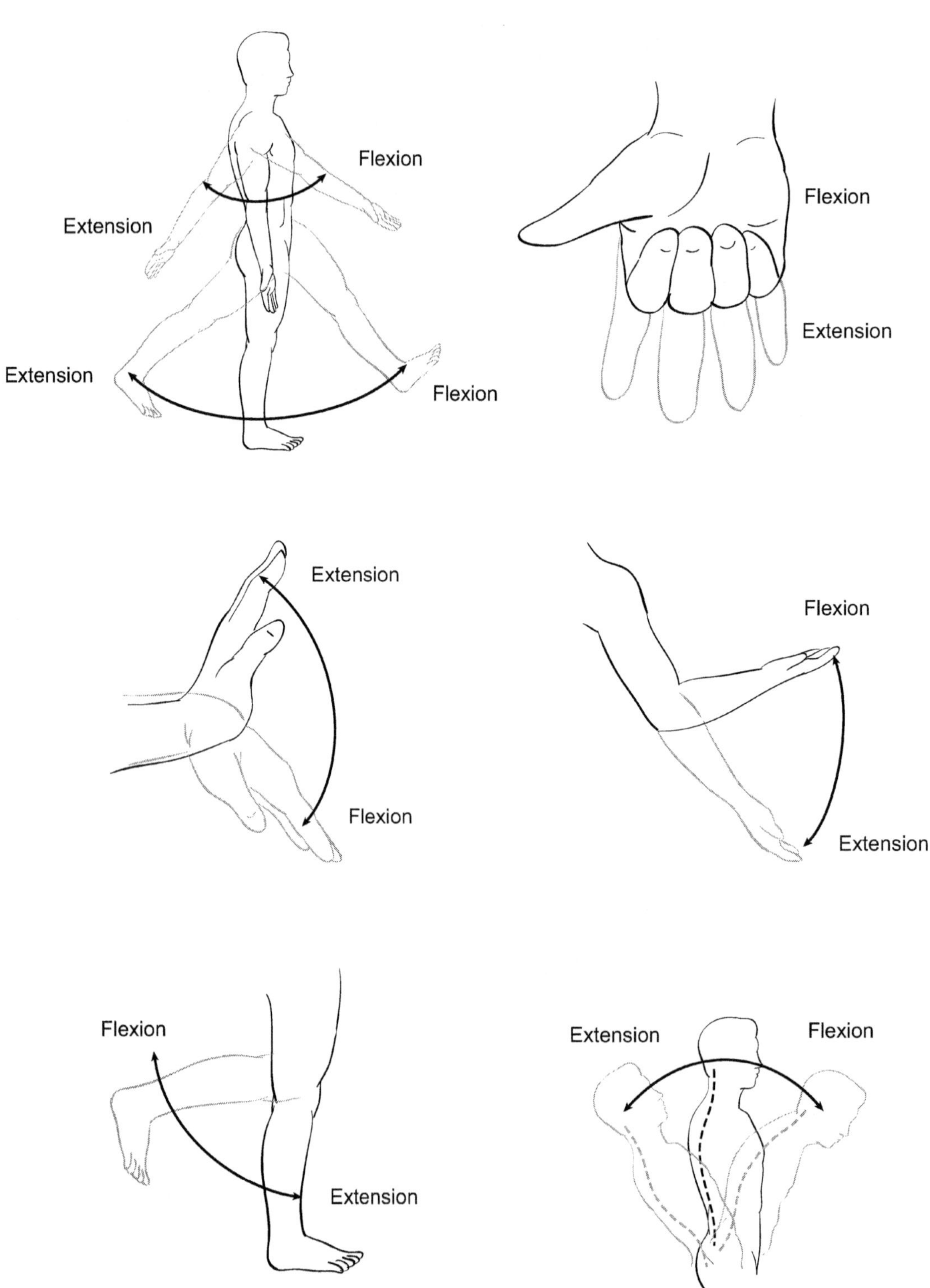
Flexion
Extension
Extension
Flexion
Flexion
Extension
Extension
Flexion
Flexion
Extension
Flexion
Extension
Extension
Flexion

Male Figure
(Anterior View)

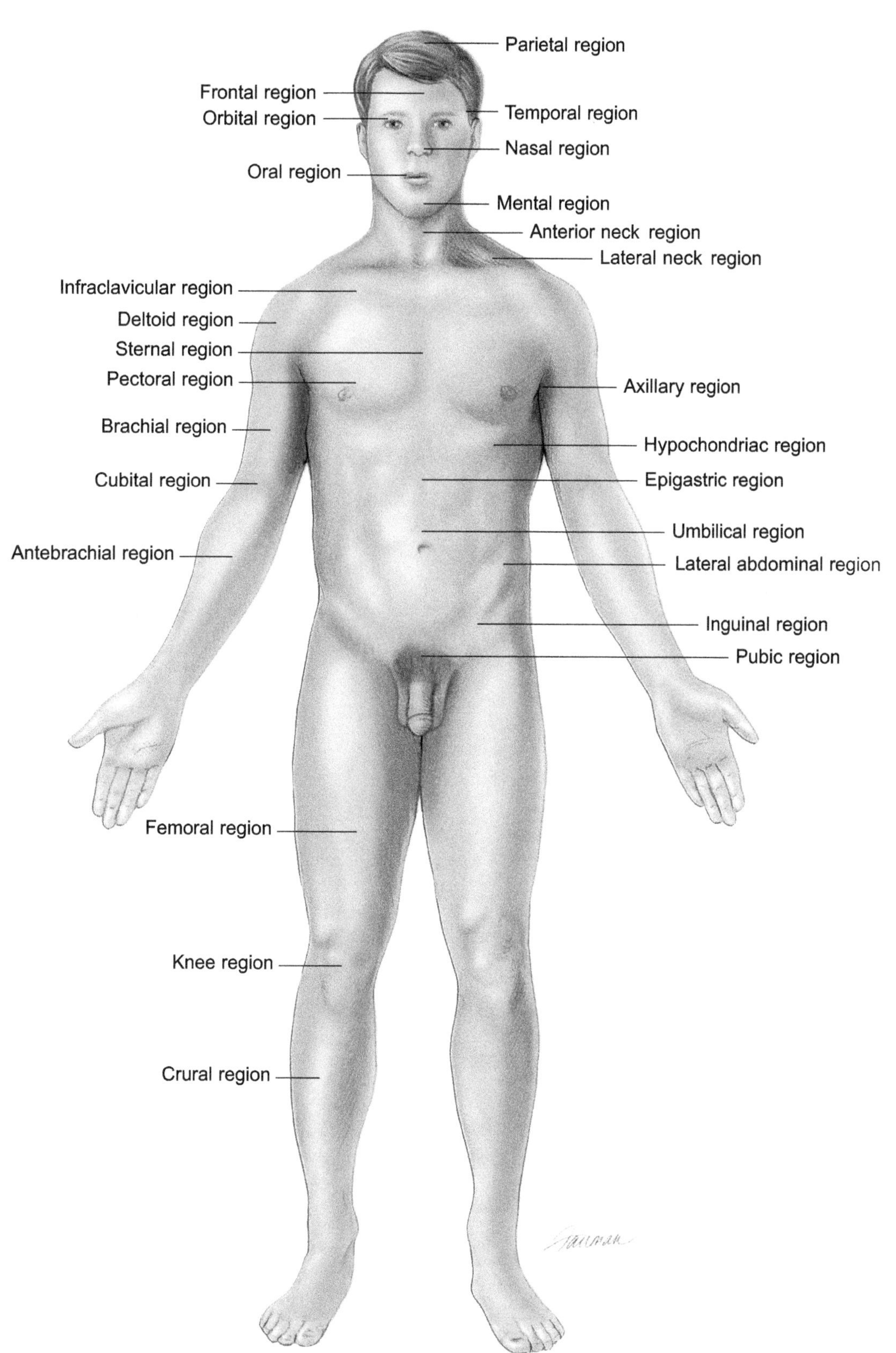

Female Figure
(Anterior View)

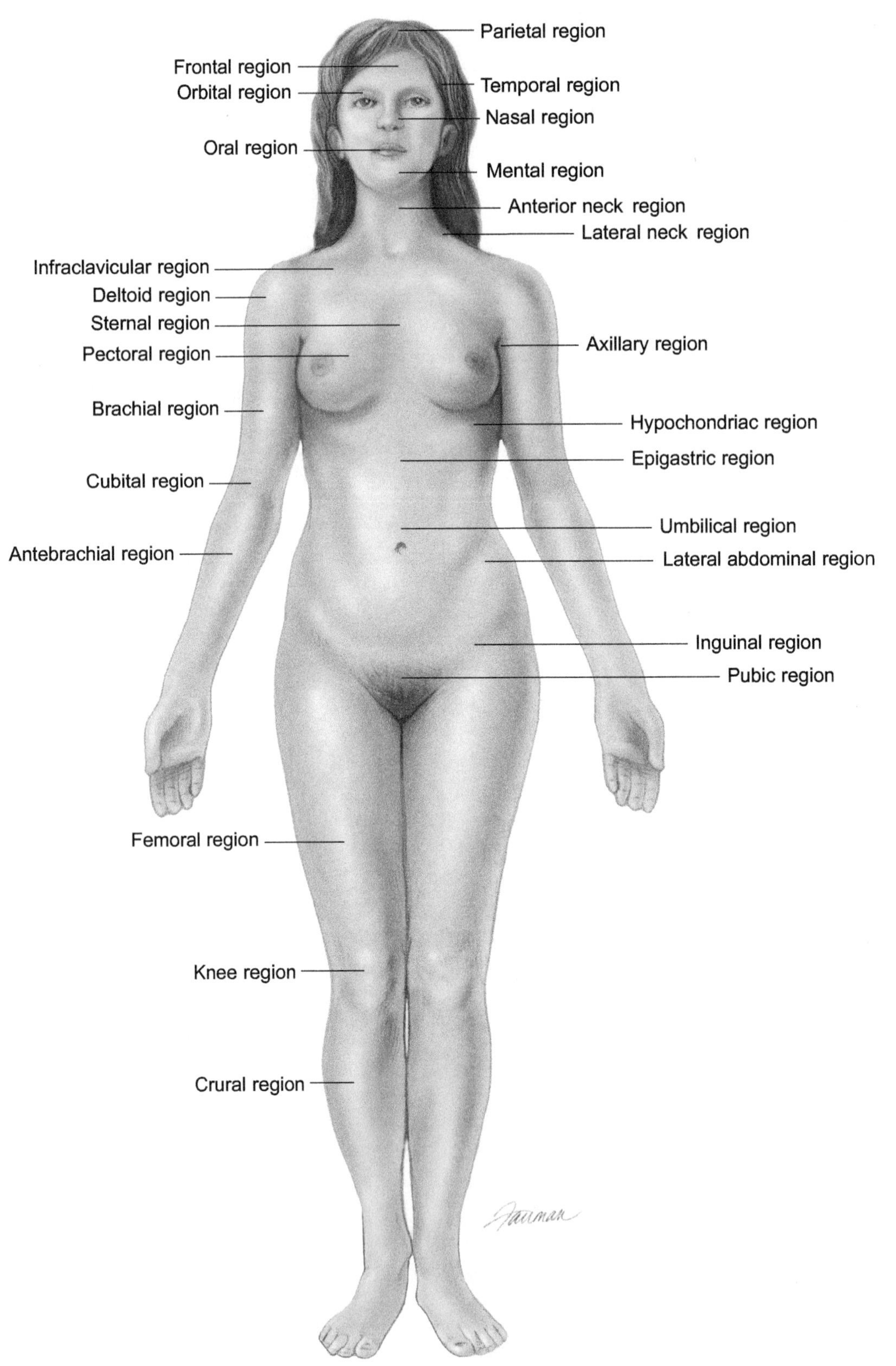

Female Breast

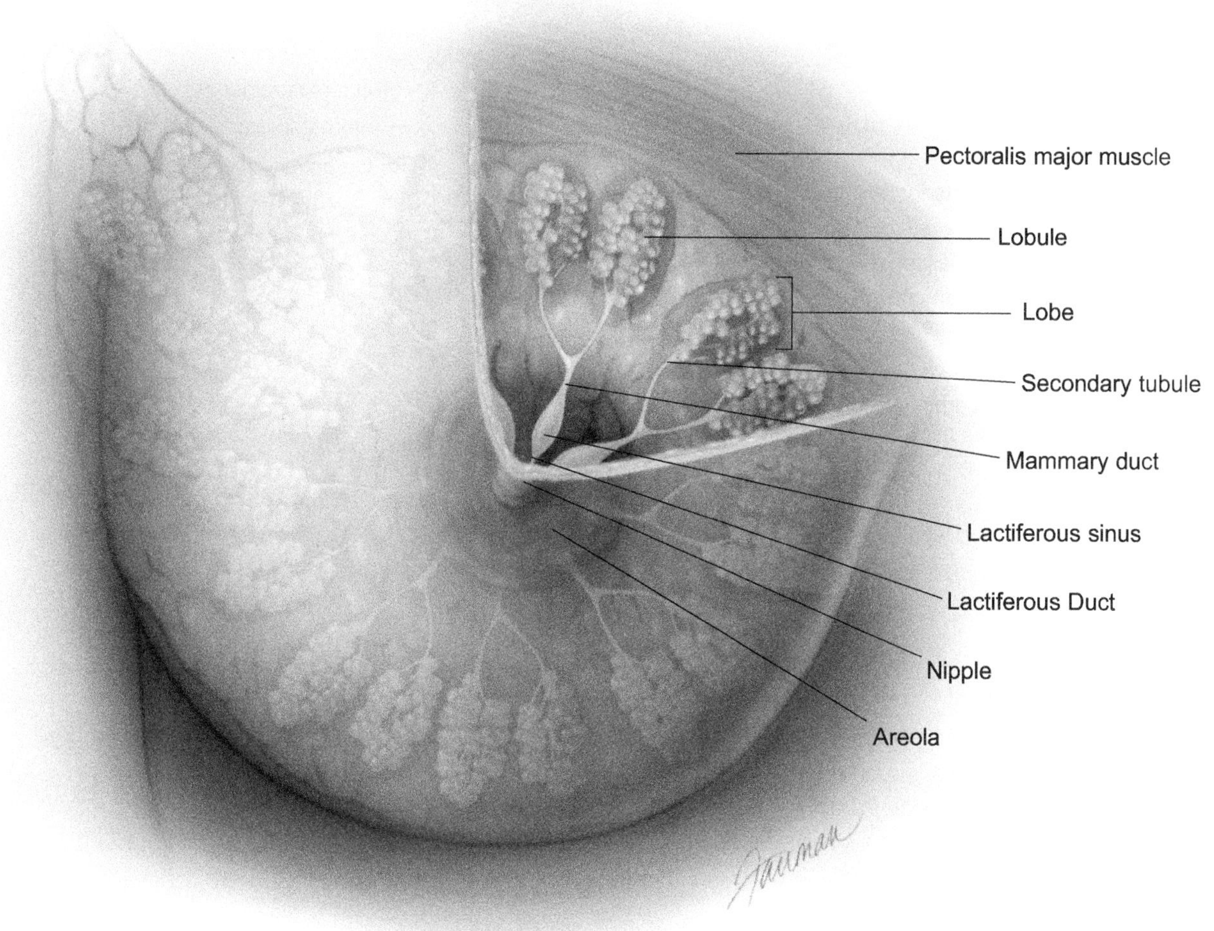

Muscular System
(Anterior View)

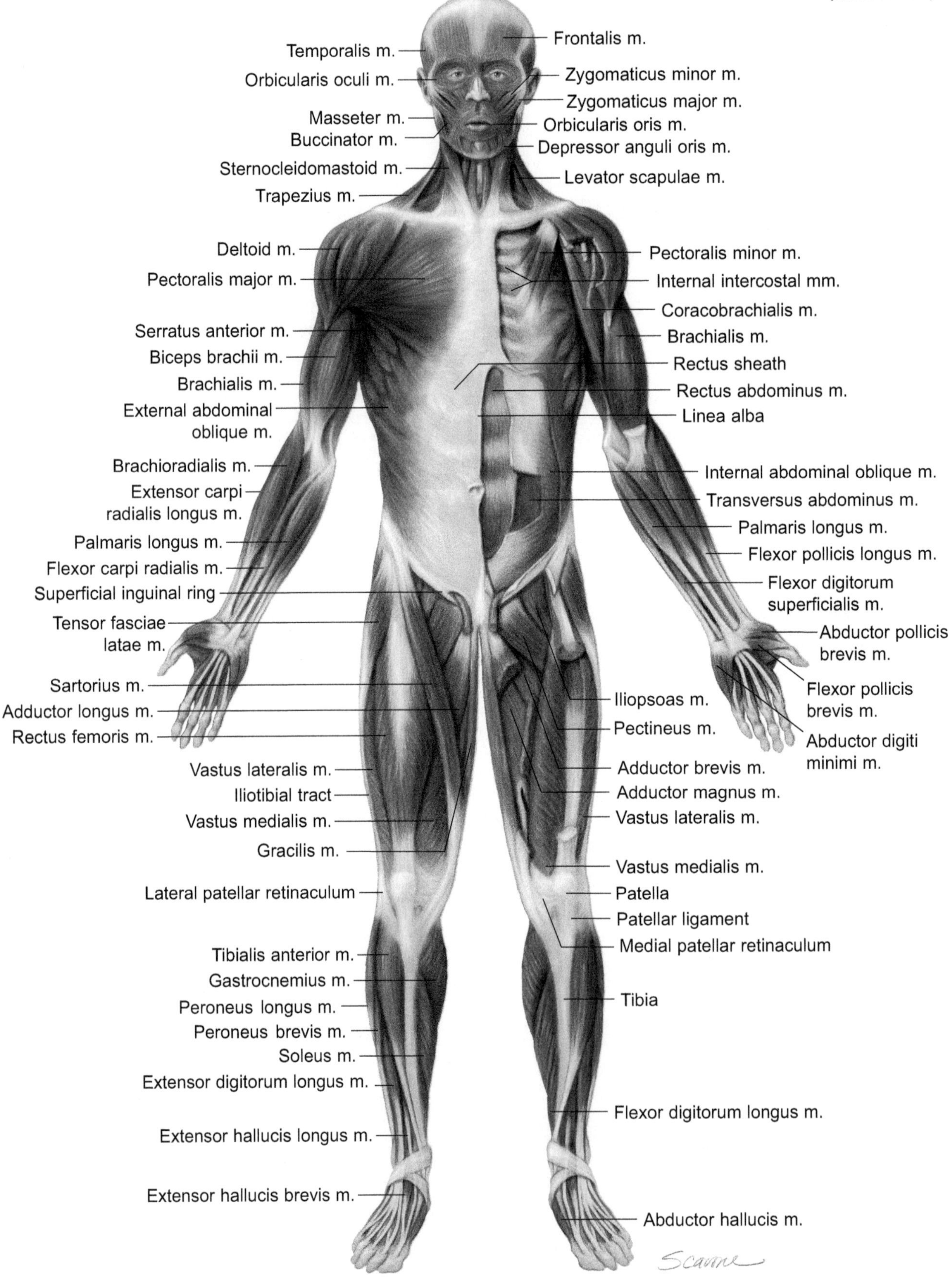

Temporalis m.
Orbicularis oculi m.
Masseter m.
Buccinator m.
Sternocleidomastoid m.
Trapezius m.
Deltoid m.
Pectoralis major m.
Serratus anterior m.
Biceps brachii m.
Brachialis m.
External abdominal oblique m.
Brachioradialis m.
Extensor carpi radialis longus m.
Palmaris longus m.
Flexor carpi radialis m.
Superficial inguinal ring
Tensor fasciae latae m.
Sartorius m.
Adductor longus m.
Rectus femoris m.
Vastus lateralis m.
Iliotibial tract
Vastus medialis m.
Gracilis m.
Lateral patellar retinaculum
Tibialis anterior m.
Gastrocnemius m.
Peroneus longus m.
Peroneus brevis m.
Soleus m.
Extensor digitorum longus m.
Extensor hallucis longus m.
Extensor hallucis brevis m.

Frontalis m.
Zygomaticus minor m.
Zygomaticus major m.
Orbicularis oris m.
Depressor anguli oris m.
Levator scapulae m.
Pectoralis minor m.
Internal intercostal mm.
Coracobrachialis m.
Brachialis m.
Rectus sheath
Rectus abdominus m.
Linea alba
Internal abdominal oblique m.
Transversus abdominus m.
Palmaris longus m.
Flexor pollicis longus m.
Flexor digitorum superficialis m.
Abductor pollicis brevis m.
Flexor pollicis brevis m.
Abductor digiti minimi m.
Iliopsoas m.
Pectineus m.
Adductor brevis m.
Adductor magnus m.
Vastus lateralis m.
Vastus medialis m.
Patella
Patellar ligament
Medial patellar retinaculum
Tibia
Flexor digitorum longus m.
Abductor hallucis m.

Muscular System
(Posterior View)

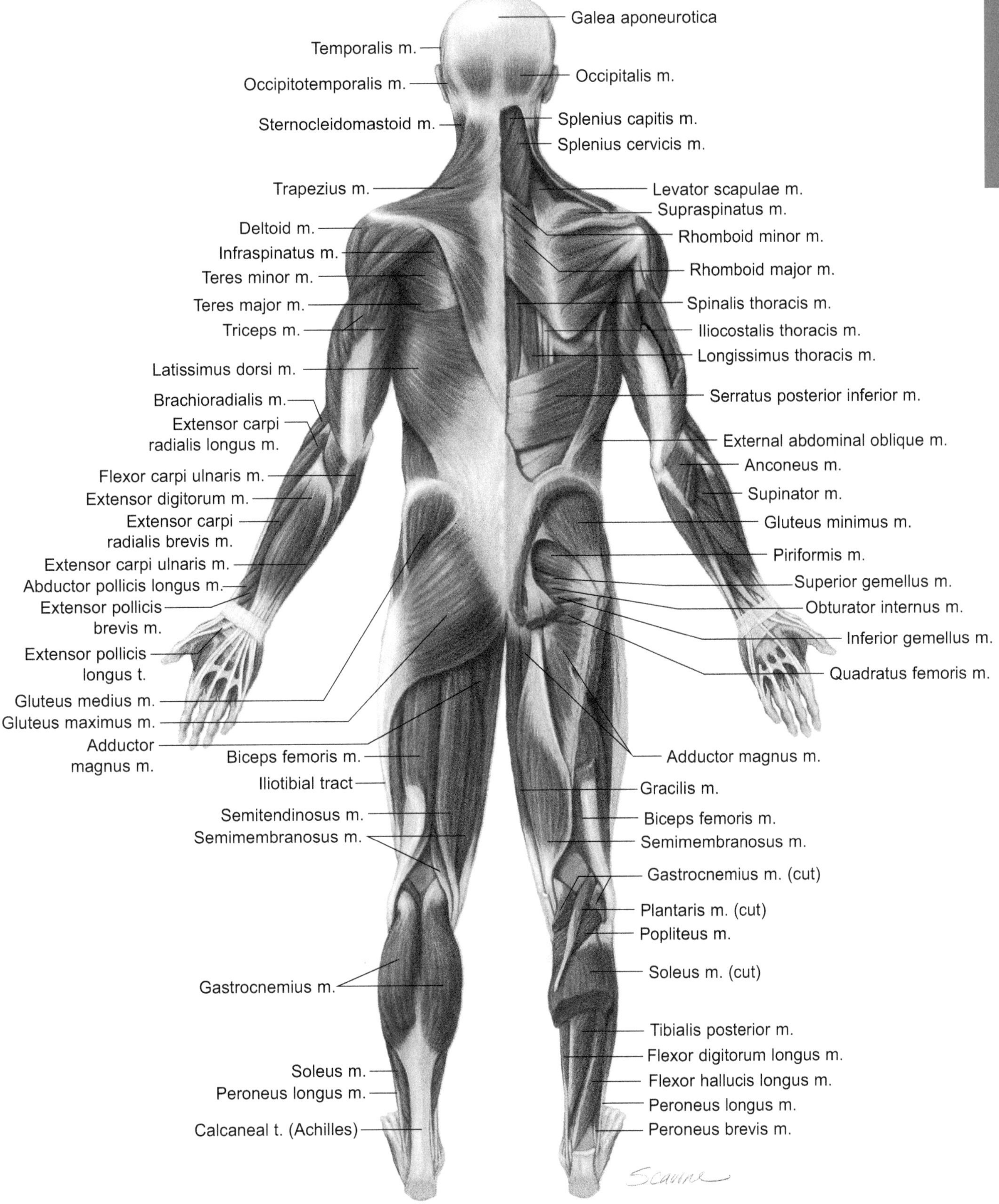

Galea aponeurotica
Temporalis m.
Occipitotemporalis m.
Occipitalis m.
Sternocleidomastoid m.
Splenius capitis m.
Splenius cervicis m.
Trapezius m.
Levator scapulae m.
Supraspinatus m.
Deltoid m.
Rhomboid minor m.
Infraspinatus m.
Teres minor m.
Rhomboid major m.
Teres major m.
Spinalis thoracis m.
Triceps m.
Iliocostalis thoracis m.
Longissimus thoracis m.
Latissimus dorsi m.
Brachioradialis m.
Serratus posterior inferior m.
Extensor carpi radialis longus m.
External abdominal oblique m.
Flexor carpi ulnaris m.
Anconeus m.
Extensor digitorum m.
Supinator m.
Extensor carpi radialis brevis m.
Gluteus minimus m.
Piriformis m.
Extensor carpi ulnaris m.
Abductor pollicis longus m.
Superior gemellus m.
Extensor pollicis brevis m.
Obturator internus m.
Inferior gemellus m.
Extensor pollicis longus t.
Quadratus femoris m.
Gluteus medius m.
Gluteus maximus m.
Adductor magnus m.
Biceps femoris m.
Adductor magnus m.
Iliotibial tract
Gracilis m.
Semitendinosus m.
Biceps femoris m.
Semimembranosus m.
Semimembranosus m.
Gastrocnemius m. (cut)
Plantaris m. (cut)
Popliteus m.
Gastrocnemius m.
Soleus m. (cut)
Tibialis posterior m.
Flexor digitorum longus m.
Soleus m.
Flexor hallucis longus m.
Peroneus longus m.
Peroneus longus m.
Calcaneal t. (Achilles)
Peroneus brevis m.

Shoulder and Elbow

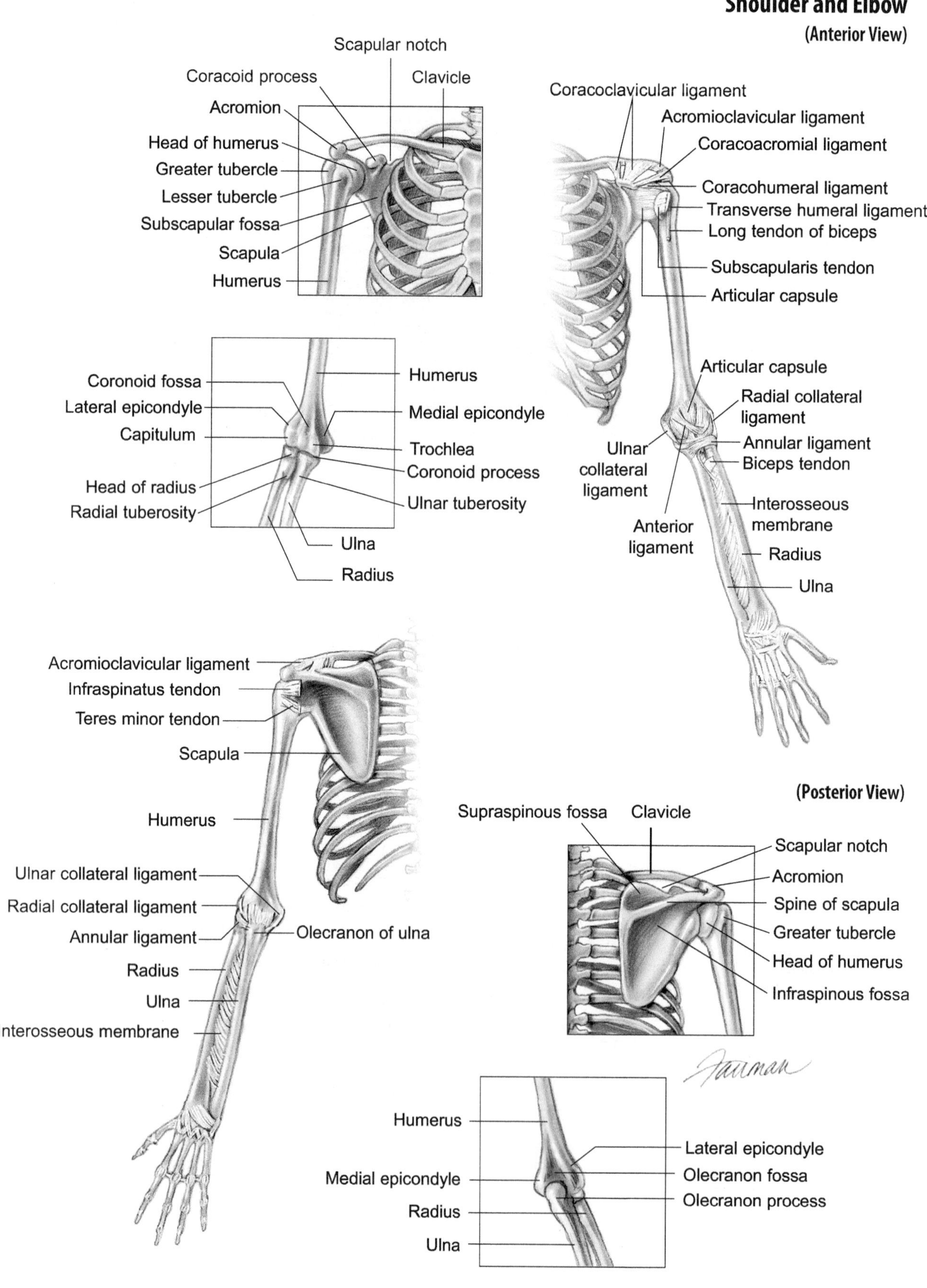

Skeletal System

(Anterior View)

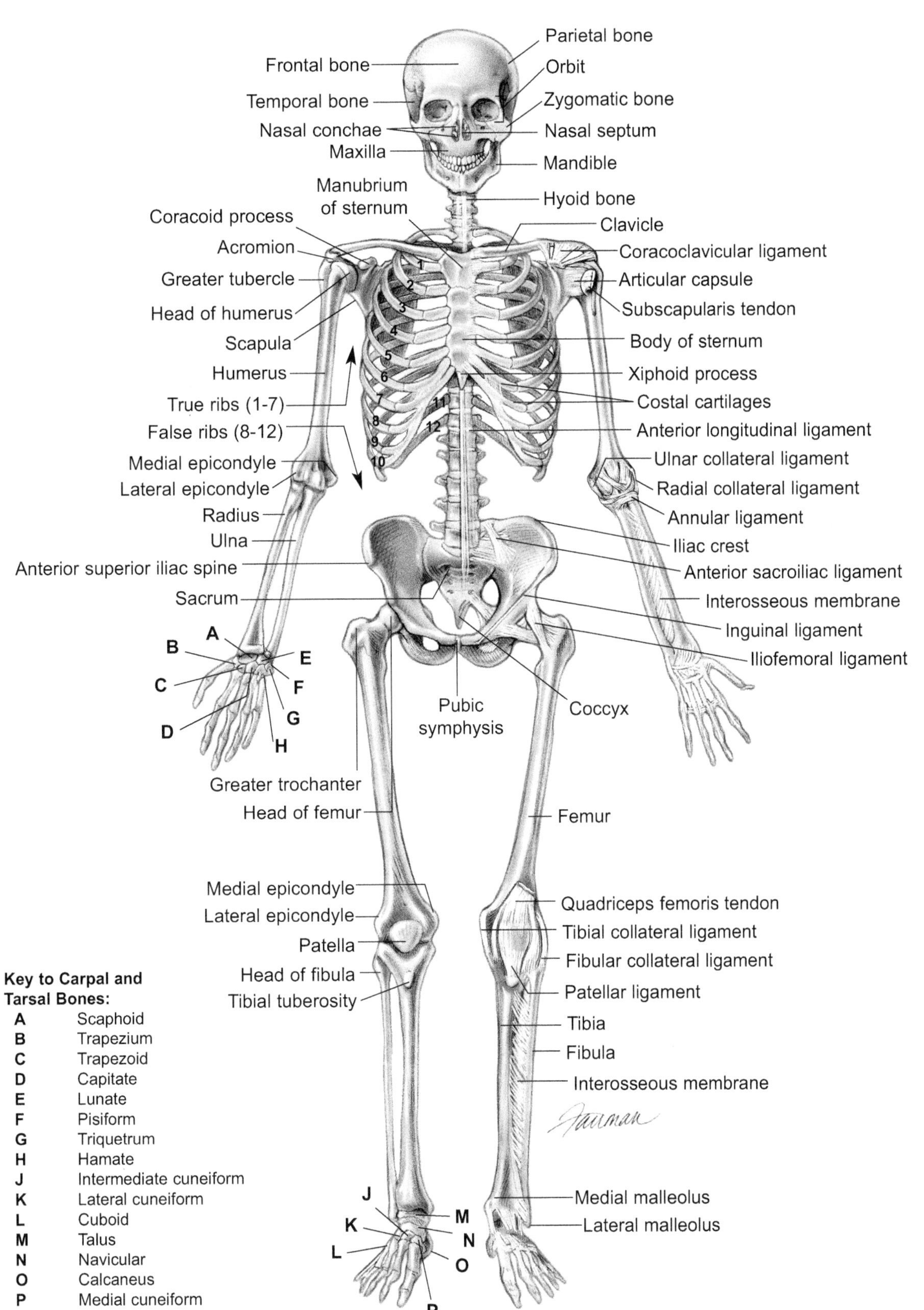

Skeletal System

(Posterior View)

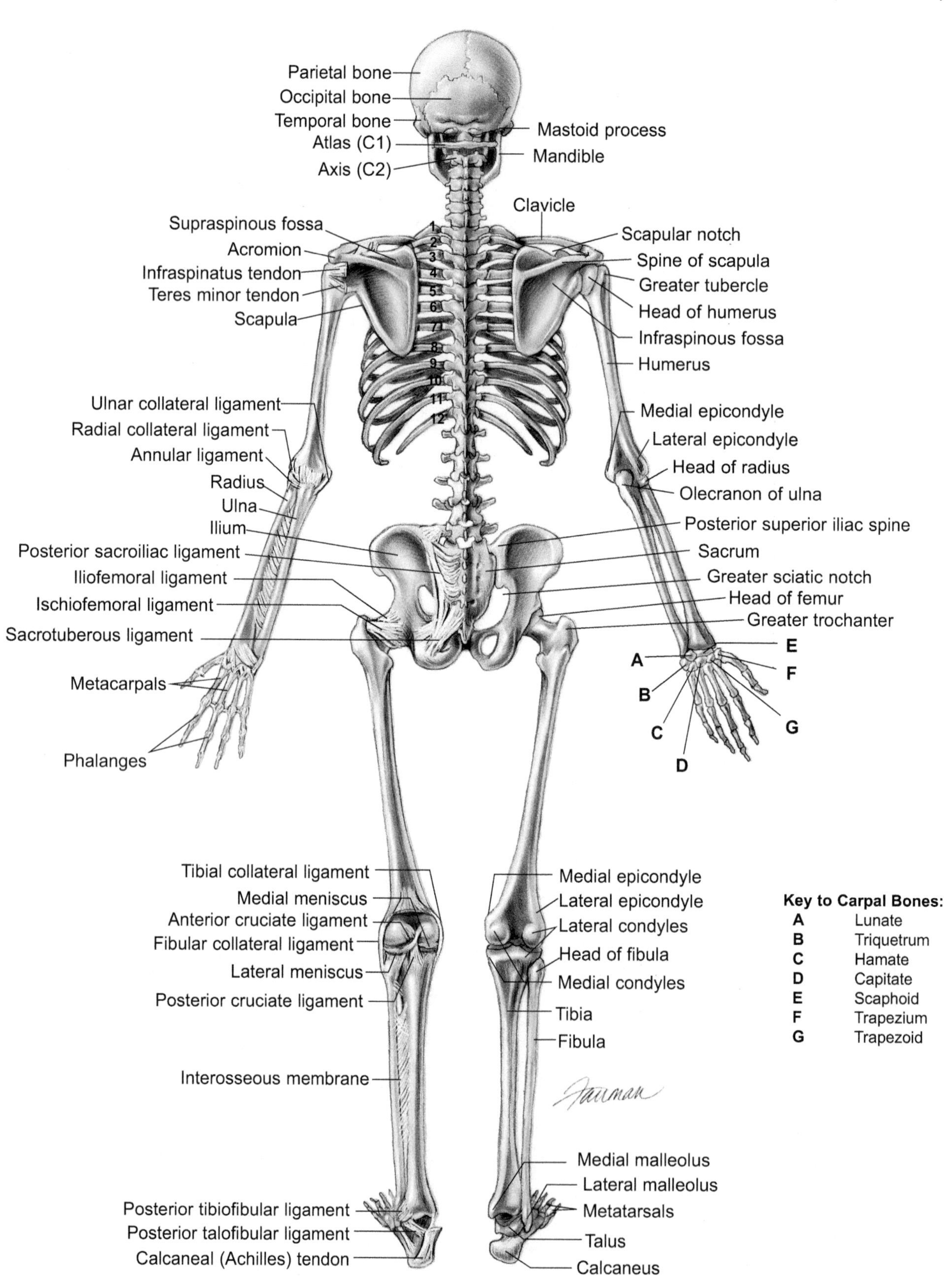

Skeletal System

(Vertebral Column – Left Lateral View)

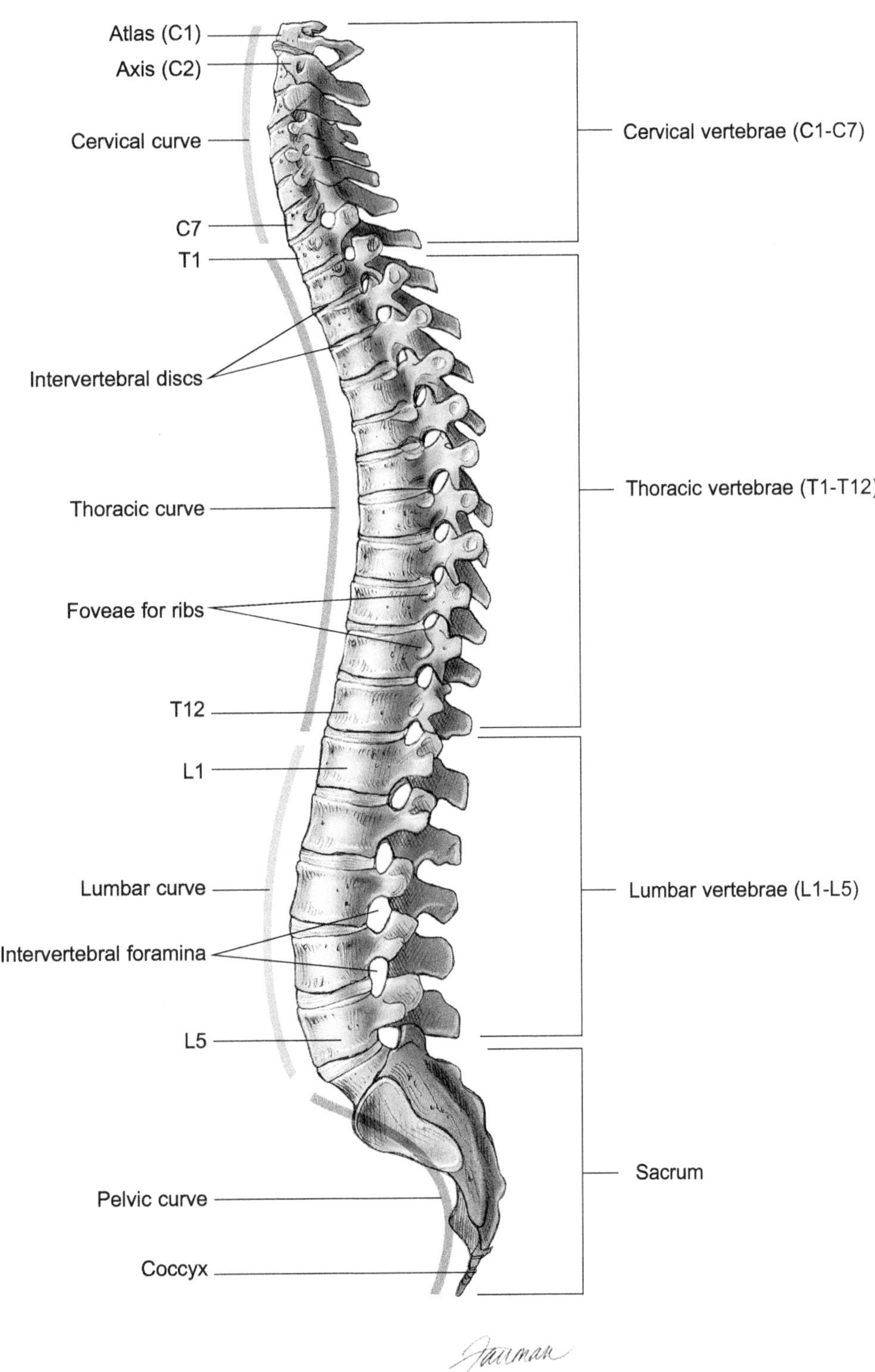

Respiratory System

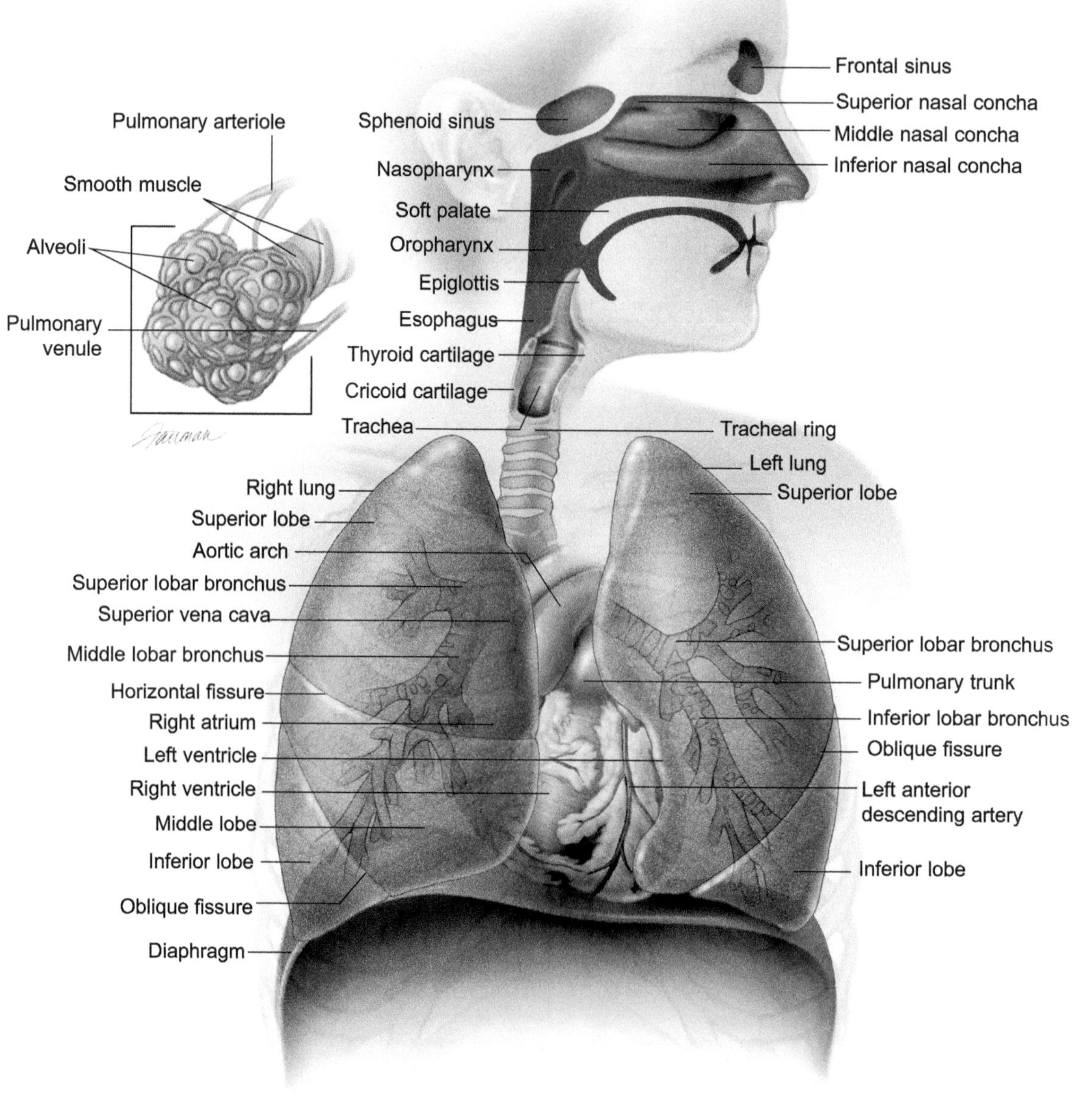

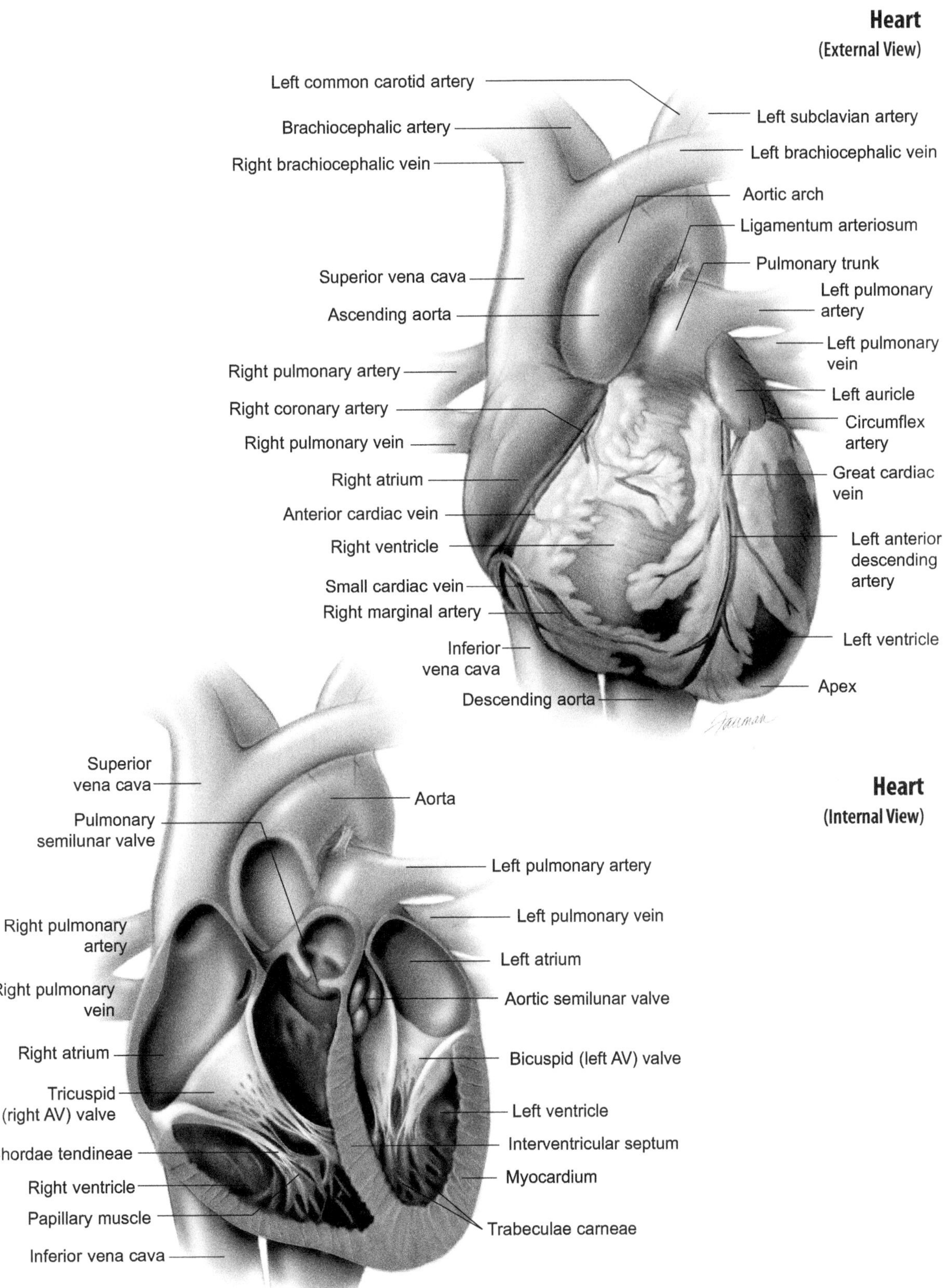
Heart
(External View)
Left common carotid artery
Brachiocephalic artery
Right brachiocephalic vein
Left subclavian artery
Left brachiocephalic vein
Aortic arch
Ligamentum arteriosum
Pulmonary trunk
Superior vena cava
Ascending aorta
Left pulmonary artery
Left pulmonary vein
Right pulmonary artery
Left auricle
Right coronary artery
Circumflex artery
Right pulmonary vein
Great cardiac vein
Right atrium
Anterior cardiac vein
Right ventricle
Left anterior descending artery
Small cardiac vein
Right marginal artery
Left ventricle
Inferior vena cava
Apex
Descending aorta
Heart
(Internal View)
Superior vena cava
Aorta
Pulmonary semilunar valve
Left pulmonary artery
Right pulmonary artery
Left pulmonary vein
Left atrium
Right pulmonary vein
Aortic semilunar valve
Right atrium
Bicuspid (left AV) valve
Tricuspid (right AV) valve
Left ventricle
Chordae tendineae
Interventricular septum
Right ventricle
Myocardium
Papillary muscle
Trabeculae carneae
Inferior vena cava

Vascular System

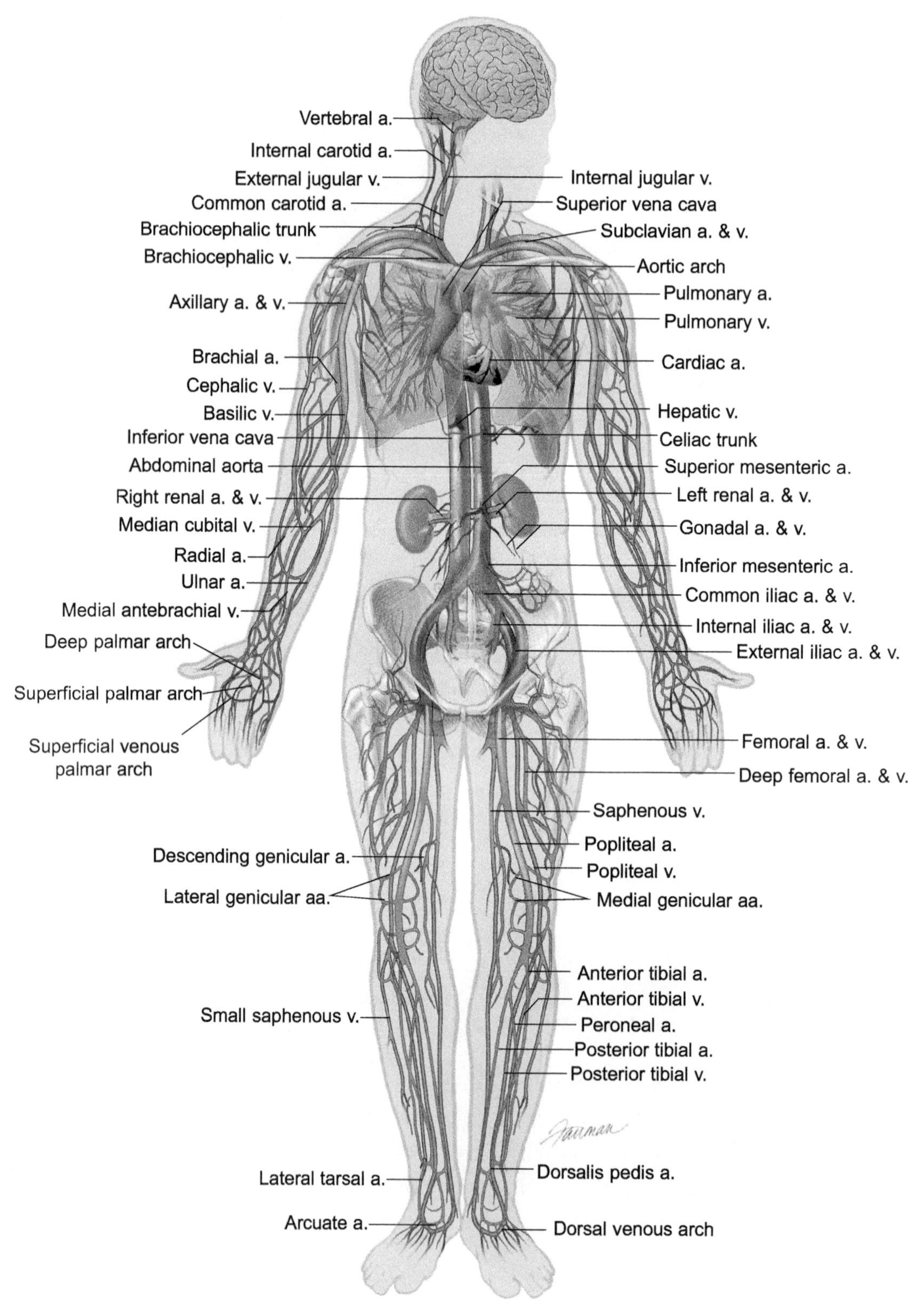

Digestive System

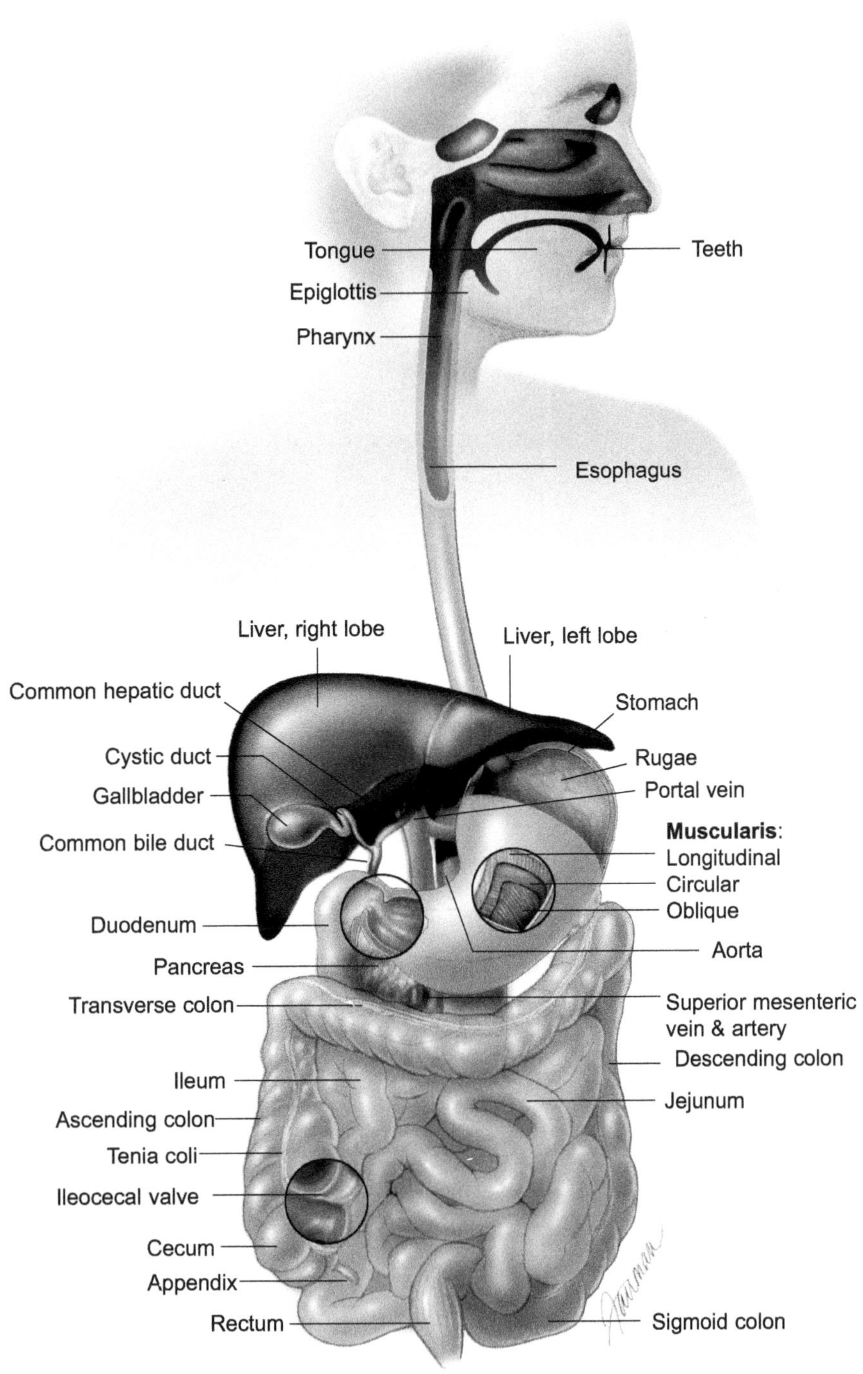

Urinary System

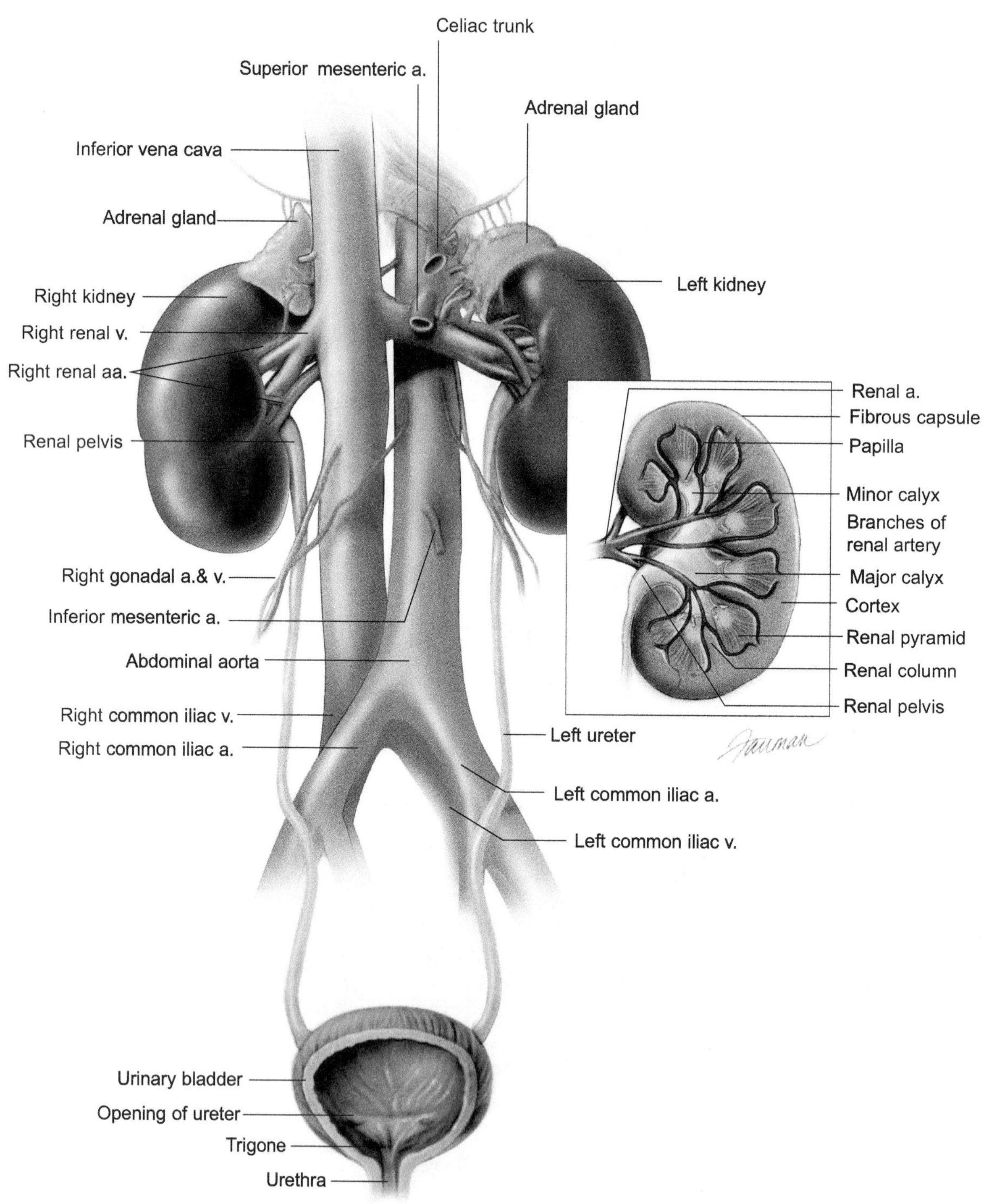

Male Genital System

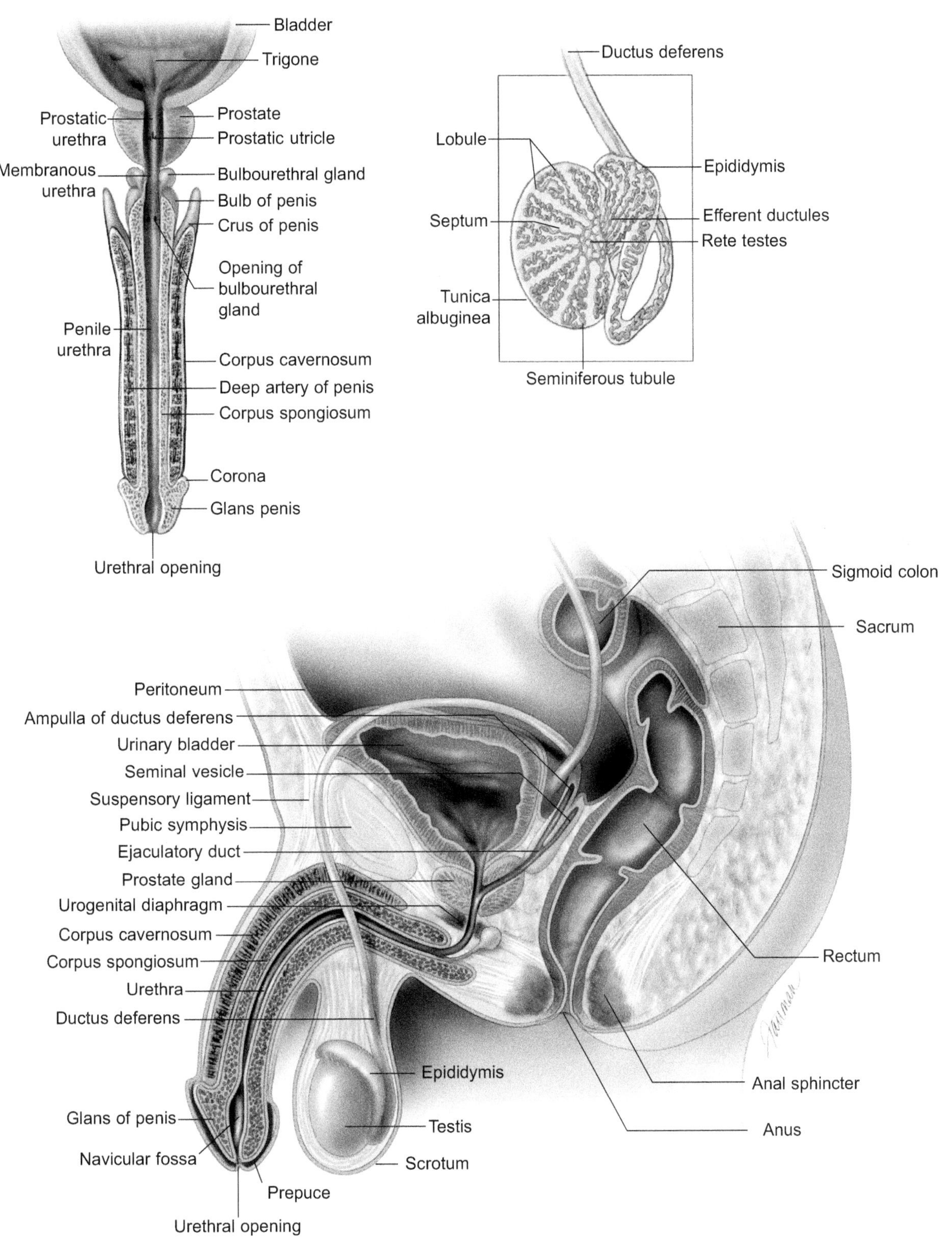

Female Genital System

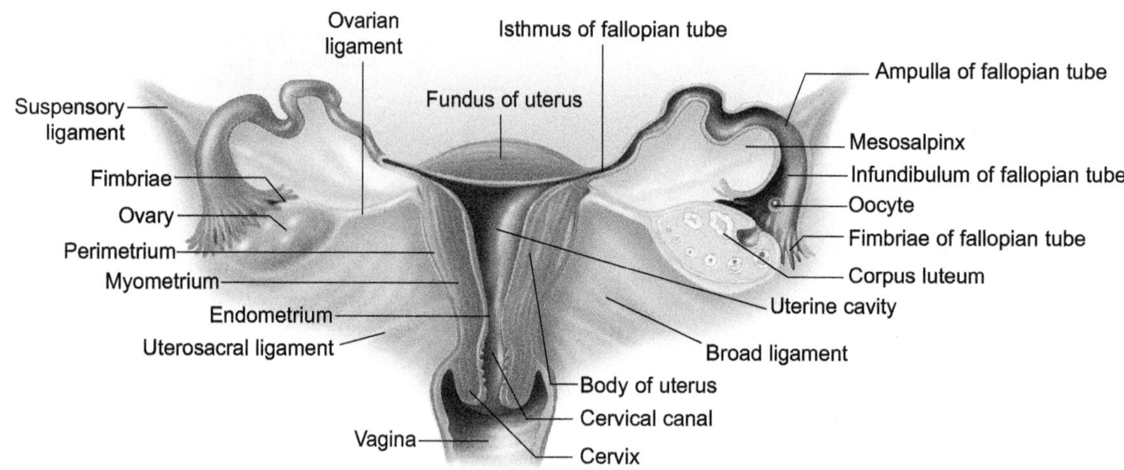

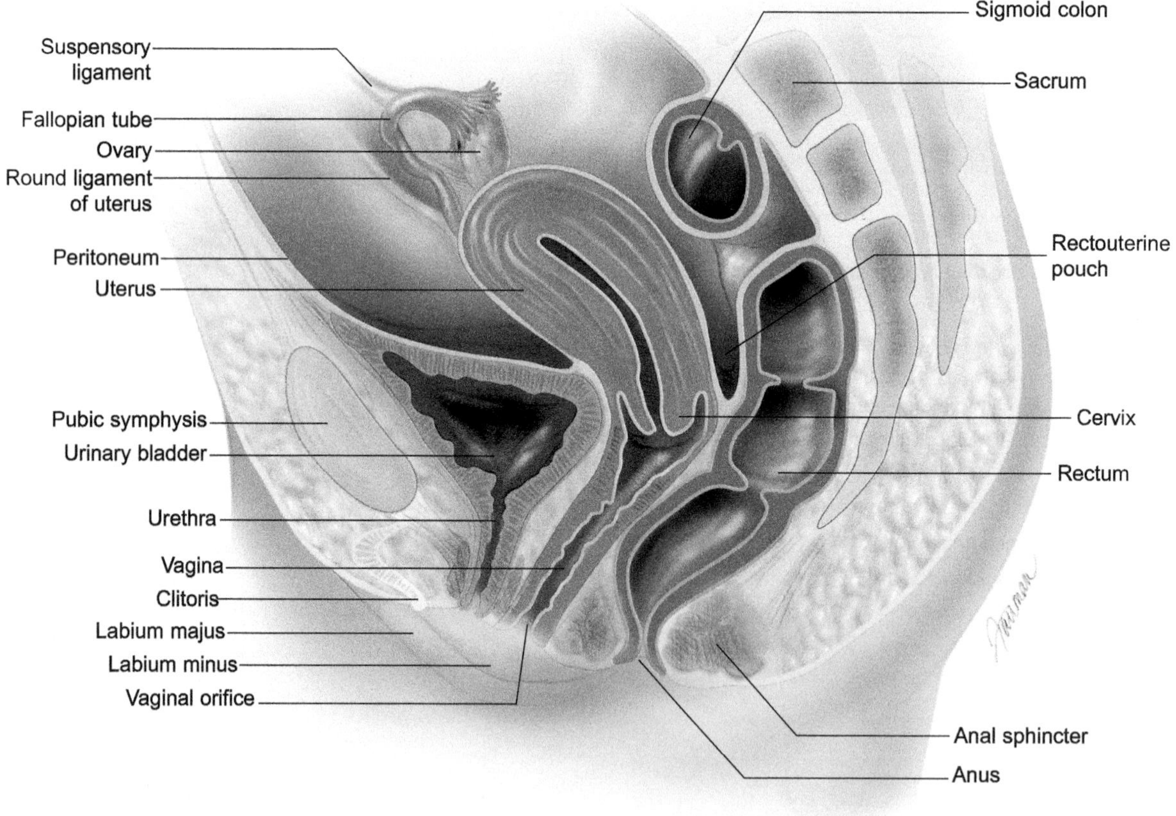

Nervous System

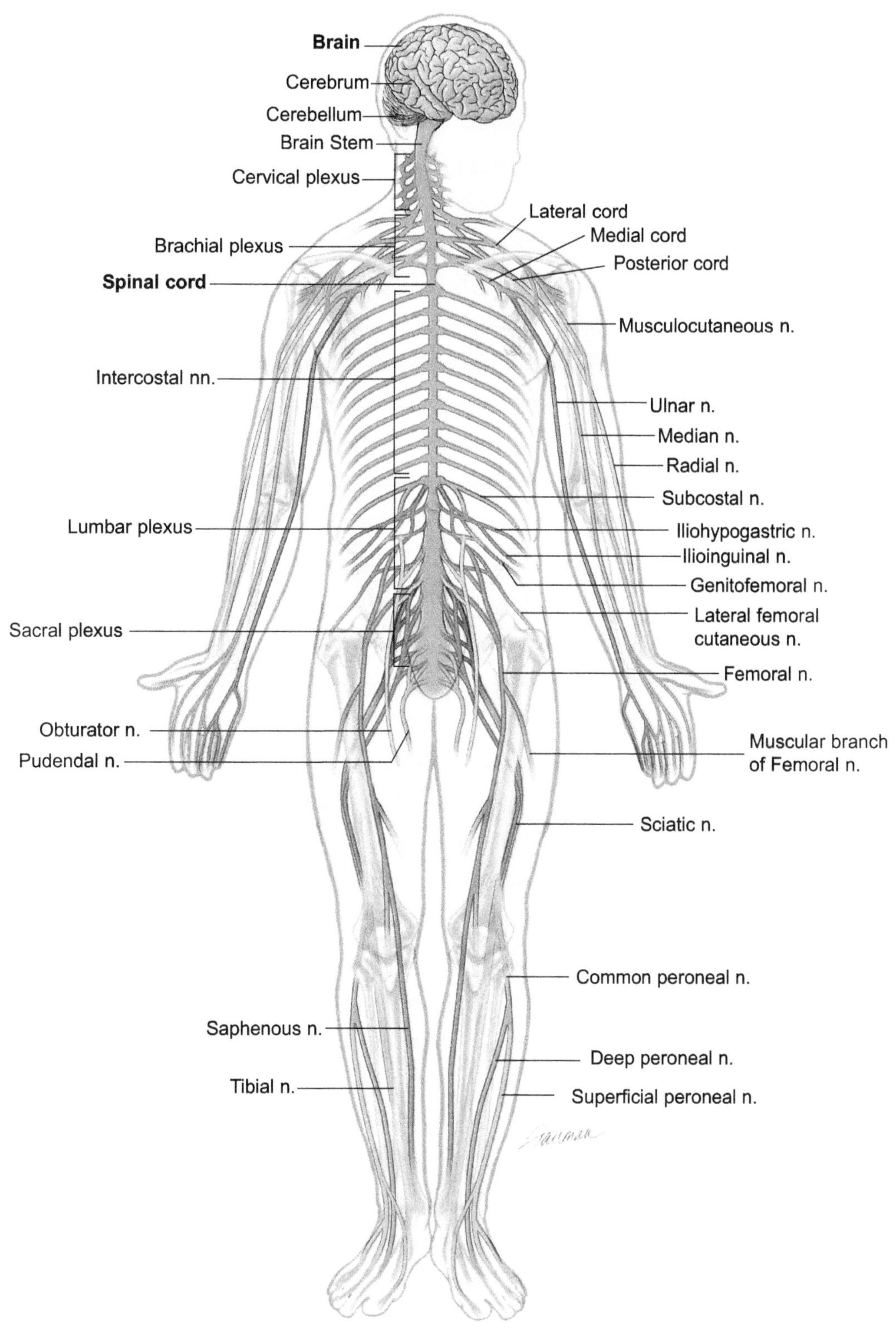

Introduction to ICD-10-CM and ICD-10-PCS Coding

ICD-10

The International Classification of Diseases (ICD) is designed to promote international comparability in the collection, processing, classification, and presentation of mortality statistics. This includes providing a format for reporting causes of death on the death certificate. The reported conditions are translated into medical codes through use of the classification structure and the selection and modification rules contained in the applicable revision of the ICD, published by the World Health Organization (WHO). These coding rules improve the usefulness of mortality statistics by giving preference to certain categories, consolidating conditions, and systematically selecting a single cause of death from a reported sequence of conditions.

ICD-10 is used to code and classify mortality data from death certificates, having replaced ICD-9 for this purpose as of January 1, 1999. The ICD-10 is copyrighted by the WHO, which owns and publishes the classification. WHO has authorized the development of an adaptation of ICD-10 for use in the United States for U.S. government purposes.

Development of ICD-10-CM

The National Center for Health Statistics (NCHS) is the Federal agency responsible for use of the *International Statistical Classification of Diseases and Related Health Problems,* 10th revision (ICD-10) in the United States. The NCHS has developed ICD-10-CM, a clinical modification of the classification for morbidity purposes. As agreed, all modifications must conform to WHO conventions for the ICD. ICD-10-CM was developed following a thorough evaluation by a Technical Advisory Panel and extensive additional consultation with physicians, clinical coders, and others, including public comment, to assure clinical accuracy and utility.

On August 22, 2008, Health and Human Services (HHS) published a proposed rule to adopt ICD-10-CM (and ICD-10-PCS) to replace ICD-9-CM in HIPAA transactions. On January 16, 2009, the final rule on adoption of ICD-10-CM and ICD-10-PCS was published. The final initial implementation date was October 1, 2015.

The ICD-10-CM Coordination and Maintenance Committee

Annual modifications are made through the ICD-10-CM Coordination and Maintenance Committee. The Committee is made up of representatives from two Federal Government agencies, the National Center for Health Statistics (NCHS) and the Centers for Medicare and Medicaid Services (CMS). The Committee holds meetings twice a year which are open to the public. Modification proposals submitted to the Committee for consideration are presented at the meetings for public discussion. Approved modification proposals are incorporated into the official government version and become effective for use October.

ICD-10-CM Official Guidelines for Coding and Reporting

The structure and format of the Guidelines for Coding and Reporting are as follows:

- Section I. Conventions, general coding guidelines and chapter-specific guidelines
- Section II. Selection of principal diagnosis
- Section III. Reporting additional diagnoses
- Section IV. Diagnostic coding and reporting guidelines for outpatient services
- Appendix I. Present on admission reporting guidelines

Section I – Conventions, General Coding Guidelines, and Chapter-Specific Guidelines

Section I of the Guidelines is divided into three general areas:

- A. Conventions of the ICD-10-CM
- B. General Coding Guidelines
- C. Chapter-Specific Coding Guidelines

Conventions

The conventions for the ICD-10-CM are the general rules for its use independent of the guidelines. These conventions are incorporated within the Alphabetic Index and the Tabular List as instructional notes, which take precedence over general guidelines.

The Alphabetic Index and Tabular List

The ICD-10-CM is divided into the Alphabetic Index of terms and their corresponding code, and the Tabular List, a chronological list of codes divided into chapters based on body system or condition. The Alphabetic Index contains the Index of Diseases and Injury, the Index of External Causes of Injury, the Table of Neoplasms, and the Table of Drugs and Chemicals.

Format and Structure

The ICD-10-CM Tabular List contains categories, subcategories, and codes made up of characters that are either a letter or a number. All categories are 3 characters. A three-character category with no further subdivision is equivalent to a code. Subcategories are either 4 or 5 characters. Valid codes may consist of 3, 4, 5, 6 or 7 characters. Each level of subdivision after a category is a subcategory. The final level of subdivision is the valid code. Codes that have applicable 7th characters are still referred to as codes, not subcategories. A code that requires an applicable 7th character is considered invalid without the 7th character.

When locating a code in ICD-10-CM, it is important to note that the 7th characters do not appear in the Alphabetic Index. The Tabular List must be checked to determine whether a 7th character should be assigned, and if so, which one to select.

7th Characters

Certain categories have applicable 7th characters. The meanings of the 7th character are dependent on the chapters, and in some cases the categories, in which they are used. The applicable 7th characters and their definitions are found under each category or subcategory to which they apply in the Tabular List. When 7th character designations are listed under a category or subcategory, the 7th character is required for all codes in that category or subcategory. Failing to assign a 7th character results in an invalid diagnosis code that will not be recognized by payers. Because the 7th character must always be in the 7th place in the data field, codes that are not 6 characters in length require the use of the placeholder 'X' to fill the empty characters. There are a number of chapters that make use of 7th characters including:

- Chapter 7 – Diseases of the Eye and Adnexa (H00-H59). The 7th character is used for glaucoma codes to designate the stage of the glaucoma.
- Chapter 13 – Diseases of the Musculoskeletal System and Connective Tissue (M00-M99). A 7th character is required for chronic gout codes to identify the condition as with or without tophus. The 7th character is also used for stress fractures and pathological fractures due to osteoporosis, neoplastic or other disease to identify the episode of care (initial, subsequent, sequela). For subsequent encounters, the 7th character also provides information on healing (routine, delayed, with nonunion, with malunion).
- Chapter 15 – Pregnancy, Childbirth, and the Puerperium (O00-O9A). The 7th character identifies the fetus for those conditions that may affect one or more fetuses in a multiple gestation pregnancy. The 7th character identifies the specific fetus as fetus 1, fetus 2, fetus 3, and so on – NOT the number of fetuses.
- Chapter 18 – Symptoms, Signs and Abnormal Clinical/ Laboratory Findings, NOS (R00-R99). There are sub-categories for coma that identify elements from the coma scale and the 7th character provides information on when the coma scale assessment was performed.
- Chapter 19 – Injury, Poisoning and Certain Other Consequences of External Causes (S00-T88). The 7th character is used to identify the episode of care (initial, subsequent, sequela). For fractures, it identifies the episode of care, the status of the fracture as open or closed, and fracture healing for subsequent encounters as routine, delayed, non-union, or malunion.
- Chapter 20 – External Causes of Morbidity (V01-Y99). The 7th character is used to identify the episode of care (initial, subsequent, sequela).

Examples of codes with applicable 7th characters:

- M48.46XA Fatigue fracture of vertebra, lumbar region, initial encounter for fracture
- M80.051D Age-related osteoporosis with current pathological fracture, right femur, subsequent encounter for fracture with routine healing
- O33.4XX0 Maternal care for disproportion of mixed maternal and fetal origin, fetus not applicable or unspecified. Note: 7th character 0 is used for single gestation
- O36.5932 Maternal care for other known or suspected poor fetal growth, third trimester, fetus 2
- S52.121A Displaced fracture of head of right radius, initial encounter for closed fracture
- T88.2XXS Shock due to anesthesia, sequela
- W11.XXXA Fall on and from ladder, initial encounter

Note the use of the placeholder 'X' for those codes that are less than 6 characters in the examples above.

Excludes Notes

There are two types of excludes notes in ICD-10-CM which are designated as Excludes1 and Excludes2. The definitions of the two types differ, but both types indicate that the excluded codes are independent of each other. A type 1 Excludes note, identified in the Tabular as ***Excludes1***, is a pure excludes. It means that the condition referenced is "NOT CODED HERE." For an Excludes1 the two codes are never reported together because the two conditions cannot occur together, such as a congenital and acquired form of the same condition. An exception to the Excludes1 definition is the circumstance when the two conditions are unrelated to each other. If it is not clear whether the two conditions involving an Excludes1 note are related or not, query the provider. For example, code F45.8, Other somatoform disorders, has an Excludes1 note for "sleep related teeth grinding (G47.63)," because "teeth grinding" is an inclusion term under F45.8. Only one of these two codes should be assigned for teeth grinding. However, psychogenic dysmenorrhea is also an inclusion term under F45.8, and a patient could have both this condition and sleep related teeth grinding. In this case, the two conditions are clearly unrelated to each other, and so it would be appropriate to report F45.8 and G47.63 together.

A type 2 Excludes note, identified in the Tabular as ***Excludes2***, indicates that the excluded condition is "NOT INCLUDED HERE." This means that the excluded condition is not part of the condition represented by the code, but the patient may have both conditions at the same time and the two codes may be reported together when the patient has both conditions.

General Coding Guidelines

Locating a code in the ICD-10-CM

To select a code in the classification that corresponds to a diagnosis or reason for visit documented in a medical record, first locate the term in the Alphabetic Index, and then verify the code in the Tabular List. Read and be guided by instructional notations that appear in both the Alphabetic Index and the Tabular List.

It is essential to use both the Alphabetic Index and Tabular List when locating and assigning a code. The Alphabetic Index does not always provide the full code. Selection of the full code, including laterality and any applicable 7th character can only be done in the Tabular List. A dash (-) at the end of an Alphabetic

Index entry indicates that additional characters are required. Even if a dash is not included at the Alphabetic Index entry, it is necessary to refer to the Tabular List to verify that no 7th character is required.

Each unique ICD-10-CM diagnosis code may be reported only once for an encounter. This applies to bilateral conditions when there are no distinct codes identifying laterality or two different conditions classified to the same ICD-10-CM diagnosis code.

Laterality

Some ICD-10-CM codes indicate laterality, specifying whether the condition occurs on the left, right or is bilateral. If no bilateral code is provided and the condition is bilateral, assign separate codes for both the left and right side. If the side is not identified in the medical record, assign the code for the unspecified side.

The assignment of a diagnosis code is based on the provider's (i.e., physician or other qualified healthcare practitioner legally accountable for establishing the patient's diagnosis) diagnostic statement that the condition exists with a few exceptions such as reporting body mass index and social determinants for health issues. The provider's statement that the patient has a particular condition is sufficient. Code assignment is not based on clinical criteria used by the provider to establish the diagnosis.

Chapter-Specific Coding Guidelines

The information that follows provides an overview of each chapter and highlights some of the more significant aspects of the guidelines. Using this overview is a good starting point for learning about ICD-10-CM; however, this resource must be combined with more intensive training using the Official Guidelines for Coding and Reporting and the current code set in order to attain the proficiency needed to assign ICD-10-CM codes accurately to the highest level of specificity.

Chapter 1 – Certain Infectious and Parasitic Diseases (A00-B99)

Infectious and parasitic diseases are those that are generally recognized as communicable or transmissible. Examples of diseases in Chapter 1 include: human immunodeficiency virus, scarlet fever, sepsis due to infectious organisms, meningococcal infection, and genitourinary tract infections. It should be noted that not all infectious and parasitic diseases are found in Chapter 1. Localized infections are found in the body system chapters. Examples of localized infections found in other chapters include strep throat, pneumonia, influenza, and otitis media.

Chapter Guidelines

Guidelines in Chapter 1 relate to coding of infections that are classified in chapters other than Chapter 1 and for infections resistant to antibiotics. Note that only severe sepsis and septic shock require additional codes from Chapter 18 – Symptoms, Signs, and Abnormal Clinical Findings NOS. Exceptions include sepsis complicating pregnancy, childbirth and the puerperium and congenital/newborn sepsis which are found in Chapters 15 and 16 respectively. In order to report sepsis, severe sepsis, and septic shock accurately, both the guidelines and coding instructions in the Tabular List must be followed.

Some infections are classified in chapters based on the body system that is affected rather than in Chapter 1. For infections that are classified in other chapters that do not identify the infectious organism, it is necessary to assign an additional code from the following categories in Chapter 1:

- B95 Streptococcus, Staphylococcus, and Enterococcus as the cause of diseases classified elsewhere
- B96 Other bacterial agents as the cause of diseases classified elsewhere
- B97 Viral agents as the cause of diseases classified elsewhere

Codes for infections classified to other chapters that require an additional code from Chapter 1 are easily identified by the instructional note, "Use additional code (B95-B97) to identify infectious agent."

In addition to the extensive guidelines related to MRSA infections, there are also guidelines for reporting bacterial infections that are resistant to current antibiotics. An additional code from category Z16 is required for all bacterial infections documented as antibiotic resistant for which the infection code does not also capture the drug resistance.

Chapter 2 – Neoplasms (C00-D49)

Codes for all neoplasms are located in Chapter 2. Neoplasms are classified primarily by site and then by behavior (benign, carcinoma in-situ, malignant, uncertain behavior, and unspecified). In some cases, the morphology (histologic type) is also included in the code descriptor. Many neoplasm codes have more specific site designations and laterality (right, left) is a component of codes for paired organs and the extremities. In addition, there are more malignant neoplasm codes that capture morphology.

Chapter Guidelines

Careful review of the guidelines related to neoplasms, conditions associated with malignancy, and adverse effects of treatment for malignancies is required. The guidelines provide instructions for coding primary malignancies that are contiguous sites versus primary malignancies of two sites where two codes are required. Another coding challenge related to neoplasms is determining when the code for personal history should be used rather than the malignant neoplasm code. For blood cancers, this is further complicated because it is necessary to determine whether the code for "in remission" or "personal history" should be assigned.

Primary malignancies that overlap two or more sites that are next to each other (contiguous) are classified to subcategory/code .8 except in instances where there is a combination code that is specifically indexed elsewhere. When there are two primary sites that are not contiguous, a code is assigned for each specific site. For example, a large (primary) malignant mass in the right breast (female) that extends from the upper outer quadrant to the lower outer quadrant would be reported with code C50.811 Malignant neoplasm of overlapping sites of right female breast. However, if there are two distinct lesions in the right breast (female), a 0.5 cm lesion in the upper outer quadrant and a noncontiguous 1 cm lesion in the lower outer quadrant, two codes would be required, C50.411 for the 0.5 cm lesion in the upper outer quadrant and C50.511 for the 1 cm lesion in the lower outer quadrant.

Malignant neoplasms of ectopic tissue are coded to the site of origin. For example, ectopic pancreatic malignancy involving the stomach is assigned code C25.9 Malignant neoplasm of pancreas, unspecified.

There are guidelines for anemia associated with malignancy and for anemia associated with treatment. When an admission or encounter is for the management of anemia associated with a malignant neoplasm, the code for the malignancy is sequenced first followed by the appropriate anemia code, such as D63.0 Anemia in neoplastic disease. For anemia associated with chemotherapy or immunotherapy, when the treatment is for the anemia only, the anemia code is sequenced first followed by the appropriate code for the neoplasm and code T45.1X5- Adverse effect of antineoplastic and immunosuppressive drugs. For anemia associated with an adverse effect of radiotherapy, the anemia should be sequenced first, followed by the code for the neoplasm and code Y84.2 Radiological procedure and radiotherapy as the cause of abnormal reaction in the patient.

Code C80.0 Disseminated malignant neoplasm, unspecified is reported only when the patient has advanced metastatic disease with no known primary or secondary sites specified. It should not be used in place of assigning codes for the primary site and all known secondary sites. Cancer unspecified is reported with code C80.1 Malignant (primary) neoplasm, unspecified. This code should be used only when no determination can be made as to the primary site of the malignancy. This code would rarely be used in the inpatient setting.

The guidelines provide detailed information on sequencing of neoplasm codes for various scenarios, such as sequencing for an encounter for a malignant neoplasm during pregnancy. Be sure to review the Official Guidelines for Coding and Reporting for this chapter before assigning a code.

Coding for a current malignancy versus a personal history of malignancy is dependent on two factors. First, it must be determined whether the malignancy has been excised or eradicated. Next, it must be determined whether any additional treatment is being directed to the site of the primary malignancy.

Primary malignancy excised/or eradicated?	Still receiving treatment directed at primary site?	Code Assignment
No	Yes	Use the malignant neoplasm code
Yes	Yes	Use the malignant neoplasm code
Yes	No	Use a code from category Z85 Personal history of primary or secondary malignant neoplasm

There are also guidelines related to coding for leukemia in remission versus coding for personal history of leukemia. These guidelines also apply to multiple myeloma and malignant plasma cell neoplasms. Categories with codes for "in remission" include:

- C90 Multiple myeloma and malignant plasma cell neoplasms
- C91 Lymphoid leukemia
- C92 Myeloid leukemia
- C93 Monocytic leukemia
- C94 Other leukemias of specified cell type

Coding for these neoplasms requires first determining, based on the documentation, whether or not the patient is in remission. If the documentation is unclear as to whether the patient has achieved remission, the physician should be queried.

Coding is further complicated because it must also be determined whether a patient who has achieved and maintained remission is now "cured," in which case the applicable code for personal history of leukemia or personal history of other malignant neoplasms of lymphoid, hematopoietic and related tissues should be assigned. If the documentation is not clear, the physician should be queried. Categories that report a history of these neoplasms include:

- Z85.6 Personal history of leukemia
- Z85.79 Personal history of other malignant neoplasms of lymphoid, hematopoietic and related tissues

Multiple myeloma, malignant plasma cell neoplasm, leukemia eradicated?	Still receiving treatment for the neoplasm?	Documentation that patient is currently in remission or has maintained remission and is now "cured"?	Code Assignment
No	Yes	No	Use the malignant neoplasm code with fifth character '0' for not having achieved remission or fifth character '2' for in relapse
Yes	No	In remission	Use the malignant neoplasm code with fifth character '1' for in remission
Yes	No	Maintained remission/cured	Use a code from category Z85 Personal history of primary or secondary malignant neoplasm

Chapter 3 – Diseases of the Blood and Blood-Forming Organs and Certain Disorders Involving the Immune Mechanism (D50-D89)

Diseases of the blood and blood-forming organs include disorders involving the bone marrow, lymphatic tissue, platelets, and coagulation factors. Certain disorders involving the immune mechanism such as immunodeficiency disorders (except HIV/AIDS) are also classified to Chapter 3.

Chapter Guidelines

There are no chapter-specific guidelines for Chapter 3. However, Chapter 2 guidelines should be reviewed for anemia associated with a malignancy or with treatment of a malignancy.

Chapter 4 – Endocrine, Nutritional, and Metabolic Diseases (E00-E89)

Chapter 4 covers diseases and conditions of the endocrine glands which include the pituitary, thyroid, parathyroids, adrenals, pancreas, ovaries/testes, pineal gland, and thymus; malnutrition and other nutritional deficiencies; overweight and obesity; and metabolic disorders such as lactose intolerance, hyperlipidemia, dehydration, and electrolyte imbalances. One of the most frequently treated conditions, diabetes mellitus, is found in this chapter.

Diabetes Mellitus

Diabetes mellitus, one of the most common diseases treated by physicians, is classified in Chapter 4 and since complications of diabetes can affect one or more body systems, all physician specialties must be familiar with diabetes coding. Two significant concepts to note in diabetes coding include 1) the code categories, and 2) most codes are combination codes that capture the type of diabetes, the body system affected as well as the specific manifestations/complications. However, some categories include instructional notes to assign additional codes from other chapters for added specificity. Diabetes mellitus code categories include:

- E08 Diabetes mellitus due to an underlying condition. Examples of underlying conditions include:
  - Congenital rubella
  - Cushing's syndrome
  - Cystic fibrosis
  - Malignant neoplasm
  - Malnutrition
  - Pancreatitis and other diseases of the pancreas
- E09 Drug or chemical induced diabetes mellitus
- E10 Type 1 diabetes mellitus
- E11 Type 2 diabetes mellitus
- E13 Other specified diabetes mellitus. This category includes diabetes mellitus:
  - Due to genetic defects of beta-cell function
  - Due to genetic defects in insulin action
  - Postpancreatectomy
  - Postprocedural
  - Secondary diabetes not elsewhere classified

Combination codes capture information about the body system affected and specific complications/manifestations affecting that body system. Specific information regarding some types of complications may be captured in a single code:

- Ketoacidosis which is further differentiated as with or without coma
- Kidney complications with specific codes for diabetic nephropathy, diabetic chronic kidney disease, and other diabetic kidney complications
- Ophthalmic complications with specific codes for diabetic retinopathy including severity (nonproliferative - mild, moderate, severe; proliferative; unspecified) and whether there is any associated macular edema or retinal detachment; diabetic cataract; and other ophthalmic complications
- Diabetic neurological complications with specific codes for amyotrophy, autonomic (poly)neuropathy, mononeuropathy, polyneuropathy, other specified neurological complication
- Diabetic circulatory complications with specific codes for peripheral angiopathy differentiated as with gangrene or without gangrene
- Diabetic arthropathy with specific codes for neuropathic arthropathy and other arthropathy
- Diabetic skin complication with specific codes for dermatitis, foot ulcer, other skin ulcer, and other skin complication
- Diabetic oral complications with specific codes for periodontal disease and other oral complications
- Hypoglycemia which is further differentiated as with or without coma

"Uncontrolled" and "not stated as uncontrolled" are not components of the diabetes codes. Uncontrolled' diabetes may mean either with hyperglycemia or hypoglycemia per the Alphabetic Index. Terms such as 'poorly controlled', 'out of control', or 'inadequately controlled' default to the specified type of diabetes with hyperglycemia. Therefore, diabetes with hyperglycemia should be based only on the documentation to avoid reporting cases of uncontrolled diabetes meant with hypoglycemia incorrectly.

Chapter Guidelines

All chapter-specific guidelines for Chapter 4 relate to coding diabetes mellitus. Some of the guidelines are discussed below.

Diabetics may have no complications, a single complication or multiple complications related to their diabetes. For diabetics with multiple complications it is necessary to report as many codes within a particular category (E08-E13) as are necessary to describe all the complications of the diabetes mellitus. Sequencing is based on the reason for the encounter. In addition, as many codes from each subcategory as are necessary to completely identify all of the associated conditions that the patient has should be assigned. For example, if an ophthalmologist is evaluating a patient with type 1 diabetes who has mild nonproliferative diabetic retinopathy without macular edema and diabetic cataracts, two codes from the subcategory for type 1 diabetes with ophthalmic complications must be assigned, code E10.329 for mild nonproliferative retinopathy without macular edema and code E10.36 to capture the diabetic cataracts.

The physician should always be queried when the type of diabetes is not documented. However, the guidelines do provide instructions for reporting diabetes when the type is not documented. Guidelines state that when the type of diabetes mellitus is not documented in the medical record the default is E11 Type 2 diabetes mellitus. In addition, when the type of diabetes is not documented but there is documentation of long-term insulin or hypoglycemic drug use, a code from category E11 Type 2 diabetes mellitus is assigned along with code Z79.4 Long-term (current) use of insulin or Z79.84, Long term (current) use of oral hypoglycemic drugs.

Diabetes mellitus in pregnancy and gestational diabetes are reported with codes from Chapter 15 Pregnancy, Childbirth, and the Puerperium as the first listed diagnosis. For pre-existing diabetes mellitus, an additional code from Chapter 4 is reported to identify the specific type and any systemic complications or manifestations.

Complications of insulin pump malfunction may involve either overdosing or underdosing of insulin. Underdosing of insulin or other medications is captured by the addition of a column and codes in the Table of Drugs and Chemicals specifically for underdosing. Underdosing of insulin due to insulin pump failure requires a minimum of three codes. The principal or first-listed diagnosis code is the code for the mechanical complication which is found in subcategory T85.6-. Fifth, sixth and seventh characters are required to capture the specific type of mechanical breakdown or failure (fifth character), the type of device which in this case is an insulin pump (sixth character '4'), and the episode of care (seventh character). The second code T38.3X6- captures underdosing of insulin and oral hypoglycemic [antidiabetic] drugs. A seventh character is required to capture the episode of care. Then additional codes are assigned to identify the type of diabetes mellitus and any associated complications due to the underdosing.

Secondary diabetes mellitus is always caused by another condition or event. Categories for secondary diabetes mellitus include: E08 Diabetes mellitus due to underlying condition, E09 Drug and chemical induced diabetes mellitus, and E13 Other specified diabetes mellitus. For patients with secondary diabetes who routinely use insulin or hypoglycemic drugs, code Z79.4 Long-term (current) use of insulin or Z79.84, Long term (current) use of oral hypoglycemic drugs should be reported. Code Z79.4 is not reported for temporary use of insulin to bring a patient's blood sugar under control during an encounter. Coding and sequencing for secondary diabetes requires review of the guidelines as well as the instructions found in the tabular. For example, a diagnosis of diabetes due to partial pancreatectomy with postpancreatectomy hypoinsulinemia requires three codes. Code E89.1 Postprocedural hypoinsulinemia is the principal or first-listed diagnosis followed by a code or codes from category E13 that identifies the type of diabetes as "other specified" and the complications or manifestations, and lastly code Z90.411 is reported for the acquired partial absence of the pancreas.

Chapter 5 – Mental and Behavioral Disorders (F01-F99)

Mental disorders are alterations in thinking, mood, or behavior associated with distress and impaired functioning. Many mental disorders are organic in origin, where disease or injury causes the mental or behavioral condition. Examples of conditions classified in Chapter 5 include: schizophrenia, mood (affective) disorders such as major depression, anxiety and other nonpsychotic mental disorders, personality disorders, and intellectual disabilities.

Chapter Guidelines

Detailed guidelines are provided for coding certain conditions classified in Chapter 5, including pain disorders with related psychological factors, and mental and behavioral disorders due to psychoactive substance use, abuse, and dependence.

Pain related to psychological disorders may be due exclusively to the psychological disorder, or may be due to another cause that is exacerbated by the psychological factors. Documentation of any psychological component associated with acute or chronic pain is essential for correct code assignment. Pain exclusively related to psychological factors is reported with code F45.41, which is the only code that is assigned. Acute or chronic pain disorders with related psychological factors are reported with code F45.42 Pain disorder with related psychological factors and a second code from category G89 Pain not elsewhere classified for documented acute or chronic pain disorder.

Mental and behavioral disorders due to psychoactive substance use are reported with codes in categories F10-F19. Both the guidelines and tabular instructions must be followed to code mental and behavioral disorders due to psychoactive substance use correctly. As with all other diagnoses, the codes for psychoactive substance use, abuse, and dependence may only be assigned based on provider documentation and only if the condition meets the definition of a reportable diagnosis. In addition, psychoactive substance use codes are reported only when the condition is associated with a mental or behavioral disorder and a relationship between the substance use and the mental or behavioral disorder is documented by the physician.

The codes for mental and behavioral disorders caused by psychoactive substance use are specific as to substance; selecting the correct code requires an understanding of the differences between use, abuse, and dependence. Physicians may use the terms use, abuse and/or dependence interchangeably; however only one code should be reported for each behavioral disorder documented when the documentation refers to use, abuse and dependence of a specific substance. When these terms are used together or interchangeably in the documentation the guidelines are as follows:

- If both use and abuse are documented, assign only the code for abuse
- If both use and dependence are documented, assign only the code for dependence
- If use, abuse and dependence are all documented, assign only the code for dependence
- If both abuse and dependence are documented, assign only the code for dependence

Coding guidelines also provide instruction on correct reporting of psychoactive substance dependence described as "in remission." Selection of "in remission" codes in categories F10-F19 requires the physician's clinical judgment. Codes for "in remission" are assigned only with supporting provider documentation. If the documentation is not clear, the physician should be queried.

Chapter 6 – Diseases of Nervous System (G00-G99)

Diseases of the Nervous System include disorders of the brain and spinal cord (the central nervous system) such as cerebral degeneration or Parkinson's disease, and diseases of the peripheral nervous system, such as polyneuropathy, myasthenia gravis, and muscular dystrophy. Codes for some of the more commonly treated pain diagnoses are also found in Chapter 6 including: migraine and other headache syndromes (categories G43-G44); causalgia (complex regional pain syndrome II) (CRPS II) (G56.4-, G57.7-); complex regional pain syndrome I (CRPS I) (G90.5-); neuralgia and other nerve, nerve root and plexus disorders (categories G50-G59); and pain, not elsewhere classified (category G89).

Chapter Guidelines

Chapter-specific coding guidelines for the nervous system and sense organs cover dominant/nondominant side for hemiplegia and monoplegia, and pain conditions reported with code G89 Pain not elsewhere classified.

Codes for hemiplegia and hemiparesis (category G81) and monoplegia of the lower limb (G83.1-), upper limb (G83.2-), and unspecified limb (G83.3-) are specific to the side affected and whether that side is dominant or non-dominant. Conditions in these categories/subcategories are classified as:

- Unspecified side
- Right dominant side
- Left dominant side
- Right non-dominant side
- Left non-dominant side

When documentation does not specify the condition as affecting the dominant or non-dominant side the guidelines provide specific instructions on how dominant and non-dominant should be determined. For ambidextrous patients, the default is dominant. If the left side is affected, the default is non-dominant. If the right side is affected, the default is dominant.

There are extensive guidelines for reporting pain codes in category G89, including sequencing rules and when to report a code from category G89 as an additional code. It should be noted that pain not specified as acute or chronic, post-thoracotomy, postprocedural, or neoplasm-related is not reported with a code from category G89. Codes from category G89 are also not assigned when the underlying or definitive diagnosis is known, unless the reason for the encounter is pain management rather than management of the underlying condition. For example, when a patient experiencing acute pain due to vertebral fracture is admitted for spinal fusion to treat the vertebral fracture, the code for the vertebral fracture is assigned as the principal diagnosis, but no pain code is assigned. When pain control or pain management is the reason for the admission/encounter, a code from category G89 is assigned and in this case the G89 code is listed as the principal or first-listed diagnosis. For example, when a patient with nerve impingement and severe back pain is seen for a spinal canal steroid injection, the appropriate pain code is assigned as the principal or first-listed diagnosis. However, when an admission or encounter is for treatment of the underlying condition and a neurostimulator is also inserted for pain control during the same episode of care, the underlying condition is reported as the principal diagnosis and a code from category G89 is reported as a secondary diagnosis. Pain codes from category G89 may be used in conjunction with site-specific pain codes that identify the site of pain (including codes from chapter 18) when the code provides additional diagnostic information such as describing whether the pain is acute or chronic. In addition to the general guidelines for assignment of codes in category G89, there are also specific guidelines for postoperative pain, chronic pain, neoplasm related pain and chronic pain syndrome.

Postoperative pain may be acute or chronic. There are four codes for postoperative pain: G89.12 Acute post-thoracotomy pain, G89.18 Other acute post-procedural pain, G89.22 Chronic post-thoracotomy pain, and G89.28 Other chronic post-procedural pain. Coding of postoperative pain is driven by the provider's documentation. One important thing to remember is that routine or expected postoperative pain occurring immediately after surgery is not coded. When the provider's documentation does support reporting a code for post-thoracotomy or other postoperative pain, but the pain is not specified as acute or chronic, the code for the acute form is the default. Only postoperative pain that is not associated with a specific postoperative complication is assigned a postoperative pain code in category G89. Postoperative pain associated with a specific postoperative complication such as painful wire sutures is coded to Chapter 19, Injury, Poisoning, and Certain Other Consequences of External Causes with an additional code from category G89 to identify acute or chronic pain.

Chronic pain is reported with codes in subcategory G89.2- and includes: G89.21 Chronic pain due to trauma, G89.22 Chronic post-thoracotomy pain, G89.28 Other chronic post-procedural pain, and G89.29 Other chronic pain. There is no time frame defining when pain becomes chronic pain. The provider's documentation directs the use of these codes. It is important to note that central pain syndrome (G89.0) and chronic pain syndrome (G89.4) are not the same as "chronic pain," so these codes should only be used when the provider has specifically documented these conditions.

Code G89.3 is assigned when the patient's pain is documented as being related to, associated with, or due to cancer, primary or secondary malignancy, or tumor. Code G89.3 is assigned regardless of whether the pain is documented as acute or chronic. Sequencing of code G89.3 is dependent on the reason for the admission/encounter. When the reason for the admission/encounter is documented as pain control/pain management, code G89.3 is assigned as the principal or first-listed code with the underlying neoplasm reported as an additional diagnosis. When the admission/encounter is for management of the neoplasm and the pain associated with the neoplasm is also documented, the neoplasm code is assigned as the principal or first-listed diagnosis and code G89.3 may be assigned as an additional diagnosis. It is not necessary to assign an additional code for the site of the pain.

Chapter 7 – Diseases of Eye and Adnexa (H00-H59)

Chapter 7 classifies diseases of the eye and the adnexa. The adnexa includes structures surrounding the eye, such as the tear (lacrimal) ducts and glands, the extraocular muscles, and the eyelids. Coding diseases of the eye and adnexa can be difficult due to the complex anatomic structures of the ocular system. Laterality is required for most eye conditions. For conditions affecting the eyelid, there are also specific codes for the upper and lower eyelids.

Not all eye conditions are found in Chapter 7. For example, some diseases that are coded to other chapters have associated eye manifestations, such as eye disorders associated with infectious diseases (Chapter 1) and diabetes (Chapter 4). There are also combination codes for conditions and common symptoms or manifestations. Most notable are combination codes for diabetes mellitus with eye conditions (E08.3-, E09.3-, E10.3-, E11.3-, E13.3-). Because the diabetes code captures the manifestation, these conditions do not require additional manifestation codes from Chapter 7.

Chapter Guidelines

All guidelines for Chapter 7 relate to assignment of codes for glaucoma. Glaucoma codes (category H40) are specific to type and, in most cases, laterality (right, left, bilateral) is a component of the code. For some types of glaucoma, the glaucoma stage is also a component of the code. Glaucoma stage is reported using a 7th character extension as follows:

- 0 – Stage unspecified
- 1 – Mild stage
- 2 – Moderate stage
- 3 – Severe stage
- 4 – Indeterminate stage

Indeterminate stage glaucoma identified by the 7th character 4 is assigned only when the stage of the glaucoma cannot be clinically determined. If the glaucoma stage is not documented, 7th character 0, stage unspecified, must be assigned.

Because laterality is a component of most glaucoma codes, it is possible to identify the specific stage for each eye when the type of glaucoma is the same, but the stages are different. When the patient has bilateral glaucoma that is the same type and same stage in both eyes, and there is a bilateral code, a single code is reported with the seventh character for the stage. When laterality is not a component of the code (H40.10-, H40.20-) and the patient has the same stage of glaucoma bilaterally, only one code for the type of glaucoma with the appropriate 7th character for stage is assigned. When the patient has bilateral glaucoma but different types or different stages in each eye and the classification distinguishes laterality, two codes are assigned to identify appropriate type and stage for each eye rather than the code for bilateral glaucoma. When there is not a code that distinguishes laterality (H40.10-, H40.20-) two codes are also reported, one for each type of glaucoma with the appropriate seventh character for stage. Should the glaucoma stage evolve during an admission, the code for the highest stage documented is assigned.

Chapter 8 – Diseases of the Ear and Mastoid Process (H60-H95)

Chapter 8 classifies diseases and conditions of the ear and mastoid process by site, starting with diseases of the external ear, followed by diseases of the middle ear and mastoid, then diseases of the inner ear. Several diseases with associated ear manifestations are classified in other chapters, such as otitis media in influenza (J09.X9, J10.83, J11.83), measles (B05.3), scarlet fever (A38.0), and tuberculosis (A18.6).

Chapter Guidelines

Currently, there are no chapter-specific guidelines for diseases of the ear and mastoid process.

Chapter 9 – Diseases of the Circulatory System (I00-I99)

This chapter conditions affecting the heart muscle and coronary arteries, diseases of the pulmonary artery and conditions affecting the pulmonary circulation, inflammatory disease processes such as pericarditis, valve disorders, arrhythmias and other conditions affecting the conductive system of the heart, heart failure, cerebrovascular diseases, and diseases of the peripheral vascular system.

Hypertension

Essential hypertension is reported with code I10 Essential hypertension and is not designated as benign, malignant, or unspecified. The classification presumes a causal relationship between hypertension and heart involvement and between hypertension and kidney involvement, as the two conditions are linked by the term "with" in the Alphabetic Index.

For hypertension and conditions not specifically linked by relational terms such as "with," "associated with" or "due to" in the classification, provider documentation must link the conditions in order to code them as related.

There are categories for hypertensive heart disease (I11), hypertensive chronic kidney disease (I12), hypertensive heart and chronic kidney disease (I13), and secondary hypertension (I15).

Myocardial Infarction

The period of time for initial treatment of acute myocardial infarction (AMI) is 4 weeks. Codes for the initial treatment should be used only for an AMI that is equal to or less than 4 weeks old (category I21). If care related to the AMI is required beyond 4 weeks, an aftercare code is reported. Codes for subsequent episode of care for AMI (category I22) are used only when the patient suffers a new AMI during the initial 4-week treatment period of a previous AMI. In addition, codes for initial treatment of acute type 1 ST elevation myocardial infarction (STEMI) are more specific to site requiring identification of the affected coronary artery. Type 1 anterior wall AMI is classified as involving the left main coronary artery (I21.01), left anterior descending artery (I21.02), and other coronary artery of anterior wall (I21.09). A type 1 AMI of the inferior wall is classified as involving the right coronary artery (I21.11) or other coronary artery of the inferior wall (I21.19). Codes for other specified sites for type 1 STEMI include an AMI involving the left circumflex coronary artery (I21.21) or other specified site (I21.29). There is also a code for an initial type 1 STEMI of an unspecified site (I21.3). Type 1 NSTEMI (I21.4) is not specific to site. A subsequent type 1 STEMI within 4 weeks of the first AMI is classified as involving the anterior wall (I22.0), inferior wall (I22.1), or other sites (I22.8). There is also a code for a subsequent STEMI of an unspecified site (I22.9). No site designation is required for a subsequent type 1 NSTEMI (I22.2).

ICD-10-CM provides codes for different types of myocardial infarction. Type 1 myocardial infarctions are assigned to codes I21.1-I21.4. Type 2 myocardial infarction, and myocardial infarction due to demand ischemia or secondary to ischemic balance, is assigned to code I21.A1, Myocardial infarction type 2 with a code for the underlying cause. Assign code I21.A1 when a type 2 AMI code is described as NSTEMI or STEMI. Acute myocardial infarctions type 3, 4a, 4b, 4c, and 5 are assigned to code I21.A9, Other myocardial infarction type. If the type of AMI is not documented, code I21.9 Acute myocardial infarction, unspecified would be assigned.

Coronary Atherosclerosis

Codes for coronary atherosclerosis (I25.1-, I25.7-, I25.81-) continue to be classified by vessel type, but codes also capture the presence or absence of angina pectoris. When angina is present the codes capture the type of angina (unstable, with documented spasm, other forms of angina, unspecified angina).

Nontraumatic Subarachnoid/Intracerebral Hemorrhage

These codes are specific to site. For nontraumatic subarachnoid hemorrhage (category I60), the specific artery must be identified, and laterality is also a component of the code. For example, code I60.11 reports nontraumatic subarachnoid hemorrhage from right middle cerebral hemorrhage. Nontraumatic intracerebral hemorrhage (category I61) is specific to site as well with the following site designations: subcortical hemisphere, cortical hemisphere, brain stem, cerebellum, intraventricular, multiple localized, other specified, and unspecified site.

Cerebral Infarction

Codes for cerebral infarction (category I63) are specific to type (thrombotic, embolic, unspecified occlusion or stenosis), site, and laterality. The site designations require identification of the specific precerebral or cerebral artery.

Chapter Guidelines

Guidelines for coding diseases of the circulatory system cover five conditions which include hypertension, acute myocardial infarction, atherosclerotic coronary artery disease and angina, intraoperative and postprocedural cerebrovascular accident, and sequelae of cerebrovascular disease.

As was stated earlier, hypertension is not classified as benign, malignant, or unspecified. Hypertension without associated heart or kidney disease is reported with the code I10 Essential hypertension.

There are combination codes for atherosclerotic coronary artery disease with angina pectoris. Documentation of the two conditions are reported with codes from subcategories I25.11- Atherosclerotic heart disease of native coronary artery with angina pectoris, and I25.7- Atherosclerosis of coronary artery bypass grafts and coronary artery of transplanted heart with angina pectoris. It is not necessary to assign a separate code for angina pectoris when both conditions are documented because the combination code captures both conditions. A causal relationship between the atherosclerosis and angina is assumed unless documentation specifically indicates that the angina is due to a condition other than atherosclerosis.

Intraoperative and postprocedural complications and disorders of the circulatory system are found in category I97. Codes from category I97 for intraoperative or postprocedural cerebrovascular accident are found in subcategory I97.8-. Guidelines state that a cause and effect relationship between a cerebrovascular accident (CVA) and a procedure cannot be assumed. The physician must document that a cause and effect relationship exists. Documentation must clearly identify the condition as an intraoperative or postoperative event. The condition must also be clearly documented as an infarction or hemorrhage. Intraoperative and postoperative cerebrovascular infarction (I97.81-, I97.82-) are classified in the circulatory system chapter while intraoperative and postoperative cerebrovascular hemorrhage (G97.3-, G97.5-) are classified in the nervous system chapter.

Category I69 Sequelae of cerebrovascular disease is used to report conditions classifiable to categories I60-I67 as the causes of late effects, specifically neurological deficits, which are classified elsewhere. Sequelae/late effects are conditions that persist after the initial onset of the conditions classifiable to categories I60-I67. The neurologic deficits may be present at the onset of the cerebrovascular disease or may arise at any time after the onset. If the patient has a current CVA and deficits from an old CVA, codes from category I69 and categories I60-I67 may be reported together. For a cerebral infarction without residual neurological deficits, code Z86.73 Personal history of transient ischemic attack (TIA) is reported instead of a code from category I69 to identify the history of the cerebrovascular disease

Acute myocardial infarction (AMI) is reported with codes that identify type 1 AMI as ST elevation myocardial infarction (STEMI) and non ST elevation myocardial infarction (NSTEMI). Initial acute type 1 myocardial infarction is assigned a code from category I21 for STEMI/NSTEMI not documented as subsequent or not occurring within 28 days of a previous myocardial infarction. All encounters for care of the AMI during the first four weeks (equal to or less than 4 full weeks/28 days), are assigned a code from category I21. Encounters related to the myocardial infarction after 4 full weeks of care are reported with the appropriate aftercare code. Old or healed myocardial infarctions are assigned code I25.2 Old myocardial infarction. Code I21.9 Acute myocardial infarction, unspecified is the default for unspecified acute myocardial infarction or unspecified type. If only type 1 STEMI or transmural MI without the site is documented, assign code I21.3 ST elevation (STEMI) myocardial infarction of unspecified site.

Subsequent AMI occurring within 28 days of a previous type 1 or unspecified AMI is assigned a code from category I22 for a new STEMI/NSTEMI documented as occurring within 4 weeks (28 days) of a previous myocardial infarction. The subsequent AMI may involve the same site as the initial AMI or a different site. Codes in category I22 are never reported alone. A code from category I21 must be reported in conjunction with the code from I22. Codes from categories I21 and I22 are sequenced based on the circumstances of the encounter.

Do not assign code I22 for subsequent myocardial infarctions other than type 1 or unspecified. For subsequent type 2 AMI assign only code I21.A1. For subsequent type 4 or type 5 AMI, assign only code I21.A9.

Chapter 10 – Diseases of the Respiratory System (J00-J99)

Diseases of the respiratory system include conditions affecting the nose and sinuses, throat, tonsils, larynx and trachea, bronchi, and lungs. Chapter 10 is organized by the general type of disease or condition and by site with diseases affecting primarily the upper respiratory system or the lower respiratory system in separate sections.

Chapter Guidelines

The respiratory system guidelines cover chronic obstructive pulmonary disease (COPD) and asthma, acute respiratory failure, influenza due to avian influenza virus, and ventilator associated pneumonia.

Codes for COPD in category J44 differentiate between uncomplicated cases and those with an acute exacerbation. For coding purposes an acute exacerbation is defined as a worsening or decompensation of a chronic condition. An acute exacerbation is not the same as an infection superimposed on a chronic condition, though an exacerbation may be triggered by an infection.

Guidelines for reporting acute respiratory failure (J96.0-) and acute and chronic respiratory failure (J96.2-) relate to sequencing of these codes. Depending on the documentation these codes may be either the principal or first-listed diagnosis or a secondary diagnosis. Careful review of the provider documentation and a clear understanding of the guidelines including the definition of principal diagnosis are required to sequence these codes correctly.

There are three code categories for reporting influenza which are as follows: J09 Influenza due to certain identified influenza viruses, J10 Influenza due to other identified influenza virus, and J11 Influenza due to unidentified influenza virus. All codes in category J09 report influenza due to identified novel influenza A virus with various complications or manifestations such as pneumonia, other respiratory conditions, gastrointestinal manifestations or other manifestations. Identified novel influenza A viruses include avian (bird) influenza, influenza A/H5N1, influenza of other animal origin (not bird or swine), and swine influenza. Codes from category J09 are reported only for confirmed cases of avian influenza and the other specific types of influenza identified in the code description. This is an exception to the inpatient guideline related to uncertain diagnoses. Confirmation does not require a positive laboratory finding. Documentation by the provider that the patient has avian influenza or influenza due other identified novel influenza A virus is sufficient to report a code from category J09. Documentation of "suspected," "possible," or "probable" avian influenza or other novel influenza A virus is reported with a code from category J10.

Ventilator associated pneumonia (VAP) is listed in category J95 Intraoperative and postprocedural complications and disorders of respiratory system not elsewhere classified, and is reported with code J95.851. As with all procedural and postprocedural complications, the provider must document the relationship between the conditions, in this case VAP, and the procedure. An additional code should be assigned to identify the organism. Codes for pneumonia classified in categories J12-J18 are not assigned additionally for VAP. However, when a patient is admitted with a different type of pneumonia and subsequently develops VAP, the appropriate code from J12-J18 is reported as the principal diagnosis and code J95.851 is reported as an additional diagnosis

Chapter 11 – Diseases of the Digestive System (K00-K95)

Diseases of the digestive system include conditions affecting the esophagus, stomach, small and large intestines, liver, and gallbladder. Some of the most frequently diagnosed digestive system diseases and conditions, such as cholecystitis and cholelithiasis, have specific elements incorporated into the codes. For example, cholecystitis is classified as acute, chronic, or acute and chronic regardless of whether the cholecystitis occurs alone or with cholelithiasis. Combination codes for cholelithiasis with cholecystitis identify the site of the calculus as being in the gallbladder and/or bile duct and the specific type of cholecystitis. Combination codes also report cholelithiasis of the bile duct with cholangitis. There are other digestive system conditions that require an acute or chronic designation as well as more combination codes that capture diseases of the gallbladder and associated complications.

Chapter Guidelines

Currently there are no guidelines for the digestive system.

Chapter 12 – Diseases of the Skin and Subcutaneous Tissue (L00-L99)

Diseases of the skin and subcutaneous tissue include diseases affecting the epidermis, dermis and hypodermis, subcutaneous tissue, nails, sebaceous glands, sweat glands, and hair and hair follicles. Common conditions of the skin and subcutaneous tissue include boils, cellulitis, abscess, pressure ulcers, lymphadenitis, and pilonidal cysts.

Chapter Guidelines

All guidelines related to coding of diseases of the skin and subcutaneous tissue relate to pressure ulcers and non-pressure chronic ulcers. Codes from category L89 Pressure ulcer are combination codes that identify the site of the pressure ulcer as well as the stage of the ulcer. For patients with multiple pressure ulcers, multiple codes should be assigned to capture all pressure ulcer sites.

Pressure ulcer stages are based on severity. Severity is designated as:

- Stage 1 – Pressure ulcer skin changes limited to persistent focal edema
- Stage 2 – Pressure ulcer with abrasion, blister, partial thickness skin loss involving epidermis and/or dermis
- Stage 3 – Pressure ulcer with full thickness skin loss involving damage or necrosis of subcutaneous tissue

- Stage 4 – Pressure ulcer with necrosis of soft tissues through to underlying muscle, tendon, or bone
- Unstageable – Pressure ulcer stage cannot be clinically determined
- Unspecified – Pressure ulcer stage is not documented

Assignment of the pressure ulcer stage code should be guided by clinical documentation of the stage or documentation of the terms found in the Alphabetic Index. For clinical terms describing the stage that are not found in the Alphabetic Index and when there is no documentation of the stage, the provider should be queried. Assignment of the code for unstageable pressure ulcer (L89.--0) should be based on the clinical documentation. These codes are used for pressure ulcers whose stage cannot be clinically determined (e.g., the ulcer is covered by eschar or has been treated with a skin or muscle graft) and pressure ulcers that are documented as deep tissue injury, but not documented as due to trauma. Unstageable pressure ulcers should not be confused with the codes for unspecified stage (L89.--9). When there is no documentation regarding the stage of the pressure ulcer, the appropriate code for unspecified stage (L89.--9) is assigned.

The depth of non-pressure chronic ulcers and the stage of pressure ulcers may be coded from documentation provided by a clinician other than the patient's provider, such as a wound care nurse. The actual diagnosis must be made by the patient's provider. Code assignment for the specific type and site of the ulcer must be based on information in the provider's documentation.

Patients admitted with pressure ulcers documented as healing should be assigned the appropriate pressure ulcer stage code based on the documentation in the medical record. If the documentation does not provide information about the stage of the healing pressure ulcer, a code for unspecified stage is assigned. If the documentation is unclear as to whether the patient has a current (new) pressure ulcer or if the patient is being treated for a healing pressure ulcer, query the provider. No code is assigned if the documentation states that the pressure ulcer is completely healed.

If a patient is admitted with a pressure ulcer at one stage and it progresses to a higher stage, two separate codes should be assigned: one code for the site and stage of the ulcer on admission and a second code for the same ulcer site and the highest stage reported during the stay. For ulcers that were present on admission but healed at the time of discharge, assign the code for the site and stage of the pressure ulcer at the time of admission.

Non-pressure ulcers described as healing should be assigned the appropriate non-pressure ulcer code based on the documentation in the medical record. If the documentation does not provide information about the severity of the healing non-pressure ulcer, assign the appropriate code for unspecified severity. For ulcers that were present on admission but healed at the time of discharge, assign the code for the site and severity of the non-pressure ulcer at the time of admission.

If the patient is admitted with a non-pressure ulcer at one severity level and it progresses to a higher severity level, two separate codes should be assigned: one code for the site and severity level of the ulcer on admission and a second code for the same ulcer site and the highest severity level reported during the stay.

Chapter 13 – Diseases of the Musculoskeletal System and Connective Tissue (M00-M99)

Coding of musculoskeletal system and connective tissue conditions requires both precise site specificity and laterality. For example, conditions affecting the cervical spine require identification of the site as occipito-atlanto-axial, mid-cervical or cervicothoracic. Laterality is also included for most musculoskeletal and connective tissue conditions affecting the extremities. For some conditions only right and left are provided, but for other conditions that frequently affect both sides, codes for bilateral are also listed. For example, osteoarthritis of the hips has designations for bilateral primary osteoarthritis (M16.0), bilateral osteoarthritis resulting from hip dysplasia (M16.2), bilateral post-traumatic osteoarthritis (M16.4), and other bilateral secondary osteoarthritis of the hip (M16.6). In addition, there are 7th characters for some code categories.

7th Characters

In Chapter 13, 7th characters are required for chronic gout to identify the presence or absence of tophus (tophi). Tophi are solid deposits of monosodium urate (MSU) crystals that form in the joints, cartilage, bones, and elsewhere in the body. Chronic gout is reported with codes in category M1A. The required 7th characters identify chronic gout as without tophus (0) or with tophus (1).

Fatigue and compression fractures of the vertebra, stress fractures, and pathological fractures due to osteoporosis, neoplastic or other disease also require 7th characters to identify the episode of care. For fatigue fractures of the vertebra (M48.4-) and collapsed vertebra (M48.5-) the 7th character designates episode of care as: initial encounter for fracture (A), subsequent encounter for fracture with routine healing (D), subsequent encounter for fracture with delayed healing (G), and sequela (S). For age-related osteoporosis with current pathological fracture (M80.0-), other osteoporosis with current pathological fracture (M80.1-), stress fracture (M84.3-), pathological fracture not elsewhere classified (M84.4-), pathological fracture in neoplastic disease (M84.5-), and pathological fracture in other disease (M84.6-), 7th character designations include those listed for fatigue and compression fractures of the vertebra, and also include two additional 7th characters for subsequent encounter with nonunion (K) or malunion (P). The table below explains and defines the 7th characters used for fractures classified in Chapter 13.

Character	Definition	Explanation
A	Initial encounter for fracture	Use 'A' for as long as the patient is receiving active treatment for the pathologic fracture. Examples of active treatment are: surgical treatment, emergency department encounter, evaluation and treatment by a new physician
D	Subsequent encounter with routine fracture healing	For encounters after the patient has completed active treatment and when the fracture is healing normally
G	Subsequent encounter for fracture with delayed healing	For encounters when the physician has documented that healing is delayed or is not occurring as rapidly as normally expected
K	Subsequent encounter for fracture with nonunion	For encounters when the physician has documented that there is nonunion of the fracture or that the fracture has failed to heal. This is a serious fracture complication that requires additional intervention and treatment by the physician
P	Subsequent encounter for fracture with malunion	For encounters when the physician has documented that the fracture has healed in an abnormal or nonanatomic position. This is a serious fracture complication that requires additional intervention and treatment by the physician
S	Sequela	Use for complications or conditions that arise as a direct result of the pathological fracture, such as a leg length discrepancy following pathological fracture of the femur. The specific type of sequela is sequenced first followed by the pathological fracture code.

Chapter Guidelines

Chapter specific guidelines are provided for musculoskeletal system and connective tissue coding related to the following: site and laterality, acute traumatic versus chronic or recurrent musculoskeletal conditions, osteoporosis, and pathological fractures. Guidelines related to coding of pathological fractures relate to the use of 7th characters which are discussed above.

Most codes in Chapter 13 have site and laterality designations. Site represents either the bone, joint or muscle involved. For some conditions where more than one bone, joint, or muscle is commonly involved, such as osteoarthritis, there is a "multiple sites" code available. For categories where no multiple site code is provided and more than one bone, joint or muscle is involved, it is necessary to report multiple codes to indicate the different sites involved. Because some conditions involving the bones occur at the upper and/or lower ends at the joint, it is sometimes difficult to determine whether the code for the bone or joint should be reported. The guidelines indicate that when a condition involves the upper or lower ends of the bones, the site code assigned should be designated as the bone, not the joint.

Many musculoskeletal conditions are a result of a previous injury or trauma to a site, or are recurrent conditions. Musculoskeletal conditions are classified either in Chapter 13, Diseases of the Musculoskeletal System and Connective tissue or in Chapter 19, Injury, Poisoning, and Certain Other Consequences of External Causes. The table below identifies where various conditions/injuries are classified.

Condition	Chapter
Healed injury	Chapter 13
Recurrent bone, joint, or muscle condition	Chapter 13
Chronic or other recurrent conditions	Chapter 13
Current acute injury	Chapter 19

Osteoporosis is a systemic condition, meaning that all bones of the musculoskeletal system are affected. Therefore, site is not a component of the codes under category M81 Osteoporosis without current pathological fracture. The site codes under M80 Osteoporosis with current pathological fracture identify the site of the fracture not the osteoporosis. A code from category M80, not a traumatic fracture code, should be used for any patient with known osteoporosis who suffers a fracture, even if the patient had a minor fall or trauma, if that fall or trauma would not usually break a normal, healthy bone. For a patient with a history of osteoporosis fractures, status code Z87.31, Personal history of osteoporosis fracture should follow the code from category M81.

Chapter 14 – Diseases of the Genitourinary System (N00-N99)

The Genitourinary System includes the organs and anatomical structures involved with reproduction and urinary excretion in both males and females. Female genitourinary disorders include pelvic inflammatory diseases, vaginitis, salpingitis and oophoritis. Common male genitourinary disorders include prostatitis, benign prostatic hyperplasia, premature ejaculation, and erectile dysfunction.

Chapter Guidelines

All coding guidelines relate to coding of chronic kidney disease. The guidelines cover stages of chronic kidney disease (CKD), CKD and kidney transplant status, and CKD with other conditions.

Chapter 15 – Pregnancy, Childbirth and the Puerperium (O00-O9A)

The majority of codes for complications that occur during pregnancy require identification of the trimester.

Trimester

The trimester is captured by the fourth, fifth, or sixth character. The fourth, fifth, or sixth character also captures the episode of care for complications that can occur at any point in the pregnancy, during childbirth, or postpartum, such as eclampsia (O15). Some complications of pregnancy that typically occur or are treated only in a single trimester such as ectopic pregnancy (O00) do not identify the trimester. In addition, complications that occur only during childbirth or the puerperium contain that information in the code description, such as obstructed labor due to generally contracted pelvis (O65.1) or puerperal sepsis (O85).

7th Character

A 7th character identifying the fetus is required for certain categories. Some complications of pregnancy and childbirth occur more frequently in multiple gestation pregnancies. These complications may affect one or more fetuses and require a 7th character to identify the fetus or fetuses affected by the complication. The following categories/subcategories require identification of the fetus:

- O31 Complications specific to multiple gestation
- O32 Maternal care for malpresentation of fetus
- O33.3 Maternal care for disproportion due to outlet contraction of pelvis
- O33.4 Maternal care for disproportion of mixed maternal and fetal origin
- O33.5 Maternal care for disproportion due to unusually large fetus
- O33.6 Maternal care for disproportion due to hydrocephalic fetus
- O35 Maternal care for known or suspected fetal abnormality and damage
- O36 Maternal care for other fetal problems
- O40 Polyhydramnios
- O41 Other disorders of amniotic fluid and membranes
- O60.1 Preterm labor with preterm delivery
- O60.2 Term delivery with preterm labor
- O64 Obstructed labor due to malposition and malpresentation of fetus
- O69 Labor and delivery complicated by umbilical cord complications

The 7th character identifies the fetus to which the complication code applies. For a single gestation, when the documentation is insufficient, or when it is clinically impossible to identify the fetus, the 7th character '0' for not applicable/unspecified is assigned. For multiple gestations, each fetus should be identified with a number as fetus 1, fetus 2, fetus 3, etc. The fetus or fetuses affected by the condition should then be clearly identified using the number assigned to the fetus. For example, a triplet gestation in the third trimester with fetus 1 having no complications, fetus 2 in a separate amniotic sac having polyhydramnios, and fetus 3 having hydrocephalus with maternal pelvic disproportion would require reporting of the complications as follows: Fetus 1 – No codes; Fetus 2 – O40.3XX2, Polyhydramnios, third trimester, fetus 2; Fetus 3 – O33.6XX3, Maternal care for disproportion due to hydrocephalic fetus, fetus 3. An additional code identifying the triplet pregnancy would also be reported. Applicable 7th characters are:

- 0 – not applicable or unspecified
- 1 – fetus 1
- 2 – fetus 2
- 3 – fetus 3
- 4 – fetus 4
- 5 – fetus 5
- 9 – other fetus

Chapter Guidelines

Chapter 15 guidelines include information covering general rules and sequencing of codes and coding rules for specific conditions. Only guidelines related to trimester, pre-existing conditions versus conditions due to pregnancy, and gestational diabetes are discussed here. Consult the Official Guidelines for Coding and Reporting for the complete Chapter 15 guidelines.

Most codes for conditions and complications of pregnancy have a final character indicating the trimester. Assignment of the final character for trimester is based on the provider's documentation which may identify the trimester or the number of weeks of gestation for the current encounter. Trimesters are calculated using the first day of the last menstrual period and are as follows:

- First trimester – less than 14 weeks 0 days
- Second trimester – 14 weeks 0 days to less than 28 weeks 0 days
- Third trimester – 28 weeks 0 days to delivery

There are codes for unspecified trimester; however, these codes should be used only when the documentation is insufficient to determine the trimester and it is not possible to obtain clarification from the provider. If a delivery occurs during the admission and there is an "in childbirth" option for the complication, the code for "in childbirth" is assigned.

When an obstetric patient is admitted and delivers during that admission, the condition that prompted the admission should be sequenced as the principal diagnosis. If multiple conditions prompted the admission, sequence the one most related to the delivery as the principal diagnosis. A code for any complication of the delivery should be assigned as an additional diagnosis.

For inpatient services, when an inpatient admission encompasses more than one trimester, the code is assigned based on when the condition developed not when the discharge occurred. For example, if the condition developed during the second trimester and the patient was discharged during the third trimester, the code for the second trimester is assigned. If the condition being treated developed prior to the current admission/encounter or was a pre-existing condition, the trimester character at the time of the admission/encounter is used.

Certain categories in Chapter 15 distinguish between conditions that existed prior to pregnancy (pre-existing) and those that are a direct result of the pregnancy. Two examples are hypertension (O10, O11, O13) and diabetes mellitus (O24). The physician must provide clear documentation as to whether the condition existed prior to pregnancy or whether it developed during the pregnancy or as a result of the pregnancy. Categories that do not distinguish between pre-existing conditions and pregnancy related conditions may be used for either. If a puerperal complication develops during the delivery encounter and a specific code for the puerperal complication exists, the code for the puerperal complication may be reported with codes related to complications of pregnancy and childbirth.

Gestational diabetes can occur during the second and third trimesters in women without a pre-pregnancy diagnosis of diabetes mellitus. Gestational diabetes may cause complications similar to those in patients with pre-existing diabetes mellitus.

Gestational diabetes is classified in category O24 along with pre-existing diabetes mellitus. Subcategory O24.4- Gestational diabetes mellitus, cannot be used with any other codes in category O24. Codes in subcategory O24.4- are combination codes that identify the condition as well as how it is being controlled. In order to assign the most specific code, the provider must document whether the gestational diabetes is being controlled by diet or insulin. If documentation indicates the gestational diabetes is being controlled with both diet and insulin, only the code for insulin-controlled is assigned. Code Z79.4 for long-term insulin use is not reported with codes in subcategory O24.4-. Codes for gestational diabetes are not used to report an abnormal glucose tolerance test which is reported with code O99.81 Abnormal glucose complicating pregnancy, childbirth, and the puerperium.

Chapter 16 – Newborn (Perinatal) Guidelines (P00-P96)

Perinatal conditions have their origin in the period beginning before birth and extending through the first 28 days after birth. Codes from this chapter are used only on the newborn medical record, never on the maternal medical record. These conditions must originate during this period but for some conditions morbidity may not be manifested or diagnosed until later. As long as the documentation supports the origin of the condition during the perinatal period, codes for perinatal conditions may be reported. Examples of conditions included in this chapter are maternal conditions that have affected or are suspected to have affected the fetus or newborn, prematurity, light for dates, birth injuries, and other conditions originating in the perinatal period and affecting specific body systems.

Chapter Guidelines

The principal diagnosis for the birth record is always a code from Chapter 21, category Z38 Liveborn according to place of birth and type of delivery. Additional diagnoses are assigned for all clinically significant conditions identified on the newborn examination. Other guidelines relate to prematurity, fetal growth retardation, low birth weight and immaturity status.

In determining prematurity, different providers may utilize different criteria. A code for prematurity should not be assigned unless specifically documented by the physician. Two code categories are provided for reporting prematurity and fetal growth retardation, P05 Disorders of newborn related to slow fetal growth and fetal malnutrition and P07 Disorders of newborn related to short gestation and low birth weight, not elsewhere classified. Assignment of codes in categories P05 and P07 should be based on the recorded birth weight and estimated gestational age.

To identify those instances when a healthy newborn is evaluated for a suspected condition that is determined after study not to be present, assign a code from category Z05, Observation and evaluation of newborns and infants for suspected conditions ruled out. Do not use a code from category Z05 when the patient has identified signs or symptoms of a suspected problem; in such cases code the sign or symptom. A code from category Z05 may also be assigned as a principal or first-listed code for readmissions or encounters when the code from category Z38 code no longer applies. Codes from category Z05 are for use only for healthy newborns and infants for which no condition after study is found to be present. On a birth record, a code from category Z05 is to be used as a secondary code after the code from category Z38, Liveborn infants according to place of birth and type of delivery.

Chapter 17 – Congenital Malformations, Deformations, and Chromosomal Abnormalities (Q00-Q99)

Congenital anomalies are conditions that are present at birth. Congenital anomalies include both congenital malformations, such as spina bifida, atrial and ventricular septal heart defects, undescended testes, and chromosomal abnormalities such as trisomy 21 also known as Down's syndrome. Chapter 17 is organized with congenital anomalies, malformations, or deformations grouped together by body system followed by other congenital conditions such as syndromes that affect multiple systems with the last block of codes being chromosomal abnormalities.

Codes for congenital malformations, deformations and chromosomal abnormalities require specificity. For example, codes for encephalocele (category Q01) are specific to site and must be documented as frontal, nasofrontal, occipital, or of other specific sites. Cleft lip and cleft palate (categories Q35-Q37) require documentation of the site of the opening in the palate as the hard or soft palate and the location of the cleft lip as unilateral, in the median, or bilateral.

Chapter Guidelines

When a malformation, deformation, or chromosomal abnormality is documented, the appropriate code from categories Q00-Q99 is assigned. A malformation, deformation, or chromosomal abnormality may be the principal or first-listed diagnosis or it may be a secondary diagnosis. For the birth, admission the principal diagnosis is always a code from category Z38 and any congenital anomalies documented in the birth record are reported additionally. In some instances, there may not be a specific diagnosis code for the malformation, deformation, or chromosomal abnormality. In this case the code for other specified is used and additional codes are assigned for any manifestations that are present. However, when there is a specific code available to report the congenital anomaly, manifestations that are an inherent component of the anomaly should not be coded separately. Additional codes may be reported for manifestations that are not an inherent component of the anomaly. Although present at birth the congenital malformation, deformation, or chromosomal abnormality may not be diagnosed until later in life and it is appropriate to assign a code from Chapter 17 when the physician documentation supports a diagnosis of a congenital anomaly. If the congenital malformation or deformity has been corrected, a personal history code should be used to identify the history of the malformation or deformity.

Chapter 18 – Symptoms, Signs, and Abnormal Clinical and Laboratory Findings, Not Elsewhere Classified (R00-R99)

Codes for symptoms, signs, abnormal results of laboratory or other investigative procedures, and ill-defined conditions without a diagnosis classified elsewhere are classified in Chapter 18. There are 7 code blocks that identify symptoms and signs for specific body systems followed by a code block for general symptoms and signs. The last 5 code blocks report abnormal findings for laboratory tests, imaging and function studies, and tumor markers. Examples of signs and symptoms related to specific body systems include: shortness of breath (R06.02), epigastric pain (R10.13), cyanosis (R23.0), ataxia (R27.0), and dysuria (R30.0). Examples of general signs and symptoms include: fever (R50.9), chronic fatigue (R53.82), abnormal weight loss (R63.4), systemic inflammatory response syndrome (SIRS) of non-infectious origin (R65.1-), and severe sepsis (R65.2-). Examples of abnormal findings include: red blood cell abnormalities (R71.-), proteinuria (R80-), abnormal cytological findings in specimens from cervix uteri (R87.61-), and inconclusive mammogram (R92.2).

Combination Codes

A number of codes identify both the definitive diagnosis and common symptoms of that diagnosis. When using these combination codes, an additional code should not be assigned for the symptom. For example, R18.8 Other ascites is not reported with the combination code K70.31 Alcoholic cirrhosis of the liver with ascites because code K70.31 identifies both the definitive diagnosis (alcoholic cirrhosis) and a common symptom of the condition (ascites).

Coma Scale

One significant ICD-10-CM coding concept relates the coma scale codes (R40.2-). Coma scale codes can be used by trauma registries in conjunction with traumatic brain injury codes, acute cerebrovascular disease, and sequela of cerebrovascular disease codes or to assess the status of the central nervous system. These codes can also be used for other non-trauma conditions, such as monitoring patients in the intensive care unit regardless of medical condition. The coma scale codes are sequenced after the diagnosis code(s).

The coma scale consists of three elements, eye opening (R40.21-), verbal response (R40.22-), and motor response (R40.23-) and a code from each subcategory must be assigned to complete the coma scale. If all three elements are documented, codes for the individual scores should be assigned. In addition, a 7th character indicates when the scale was recorded and the 7th character should match for all three codes. The 7th characters identify the time/place as follows:

- 0 – Unspecified time
- 1 – In the field (EMT/ambulance)
- 2 – At arrival in emergency department
- 3 – At hospital admission
- 4 – 24 hours or more after hospital admission

If all three elements are not known but the total Glasgow coma scale is documented, the code for the total Glasgow coma score is assigned. The Glasgow score is classified as follows:

- Glasgow score 13-15
- Glasgow score 9-12
- Glasgow score 3-8
- Other coma without documented Glasgow coma scale score or with partial score reported

Chapter Guidelines

There are a number of general guidelines for the use of symptom codes and combination codes that include symptoms as well as some specific guidelines related to repeated falls, the coma scale (discussed above), and systemic inflammatory response syndrome (SIRS) due to non-infectious process. There are also some guidelines referencing signs and symptoms in Section II Selection of Principal Diagnosis. For example, the first guideline related to the use of symptom codes indicates that these codes are acceptable for reporting purposes when a related definitive diagnosis has not been established (confirmed) by the provider. It may also be appropriate to report a sign or symptom code with a definitive diagnosis. However, this is dependent upon whether or not the symptom is routinely associated with the definitive diagnosis/disease process. When the sign or symptom is not routinely associated with the definitive diagnosis, the codes for signs and symptoms may be reported additionally. The definitive diagnosis should be sequenced before the symptom code. When the sign or symptom is routinely associated with the disease process, the sign or symptom code is not reported additionally unless instructions in the Tabular indicate otherwise.

There is a code for repeated falls (R29.6) and another code for history of falling (Z91.81). The code for repeated falls is assigned when a patient has recently fallen and the reason for the fall is being investigated. The code for history of falling is assigned when a patient has fallen in the past and is at risk for future falls. Both codes may be assigned when the patient has had a recent fall that is being investigated and also has a history of falling.

Guidelines related to SIRS due to a non-infectious process (R65.1-) relate to sequencing of codes. Also discussed is the need to verify whether any documented acute organ dysfunction is associated with the SIRS or due to the underlying condition that caused the SIRS or another related condition as this affects code assignment.

Chapter 19 – Injury, Poisoning, and Certain Other Consequences of External Causes (S00-T88)

Codes for injury, poisoning and certain other consequences of external causes are found in Chapter 19. One of the important characteristics to note is that injuries are organized first by body site and then by type of injury. Another is that laterality is included in the code descriptor. The vast majority of injuries to paired organs and the extremities identify the injury as the right or left. In addition, most injuries are specific to site. For example, codes for an open wound of the thorax (category S21), are specific to the right back wall, left back wall, right front wall or left front wall. For open wounds of the abdominal wall (S31.1-, S31.6-), the site must be identified as right upper quadrant, left upper quadrant, epigastric region, right lower quadrant, or left lower quadrant. Also, the vast majority of codes require a 7th character to identify episode of care. Episode of care designations have been discussed previously and many of the same designations are used in Chapter 13. However, there are some additional 7th characters for episode of care that are used only in this chapter for fractures of the long bones. Additionally, the codes for poisoning, adverse effects and toxic effects are combination codes that capture both the drug and the external cause. The Table of Drugs and Chemicals includes an underdosing column.

Application of 7th Characters

Most categories in the injury and poisoning chapter require assignment of a 7th character to identify the episode of care. For most categories there are three (3) 7th character values to select from: 'A' for initial encounter; 'B' for subsequent encounter and 'S' for sequela. Categories for fractures are an exception with fractures having 6 to 16 7th character values in order to capture additional information about the fracture including, whether the fracture is open or closed and whether the healing phase is routine or complicated by delayed healing, nonunion, or malunion. Detailed guidelines are provided related to selection of the 7th character value. Related guidelines and some examples of encounters representative of the three episodes of care 7th character values found in the majority of categories are as follows:

A Initial encounter. Initial encounter is defined as the period when the patient is receiving active treatment for the injury, poisoning, or other consequences of an external cause. An 'A' may be assigned on more than one claim. For example, if a patient is seen in the emergency department (ED) for a head injury that is first evaluated by the ED physician who requests a CT scan that is read by a radiologist and a consultation by a neurologist, the 7th character 'A' is used by all three physicians and also reported on the ED claim. If the patient required admission to an acute care hospital, the 7th character 'A' would be reported for the entire acute care hospital stay because the 7th character extension 'A' is used for the entire period that the patient receives active treatment for the injury.

D Subsequent encounter. This is an encounter after the patient has completed the active phase of treatment and is receiving routine care for the injury or poisoning during the period of healing or recovery. Unlike aftercare following medical or surgical services for other conditions which are reported with codes from Chapter 21, Factors Influencing Health Status and Contact with Health Services (Z00-Z99), aftercare for injuries and poisonings is captured by the 7th character D. For example, a patient with an ankle sprain may return to the office to have joint stability re-evaluated to ensure that the injury is healing properly. In this case, the 7th character 'D' would be assigned.

S Sequela. The 7th character extension 'S' is assigned for complications or conditions that arise as a direct result of an injury. An example of a sequela is a scar resulting from a burn.

Fracture Coding

Two things of note related to fracture coding include the 7th character extensions which differ from the 7th character extensions for other injuries, and the incorporation of information from certain fracture classification systems in the code descriptors. In fact, for open fractures of the long bones, correct assignment of the 7th character requires an understanding of the Gustilo classification system. For most fractures the 7th character extensions are the same as those detailed in Chapter 13 for pathological fractures. The designations are again summarized here and are as follows:

7th Character	Description
A	Initial encounter for closed fracture
B	Initial encounter for open fracture type
D	Subsequent encounter for fracture with routine healing
G	Subsequent encounter for fracture with delayed healing
K	Subsequent encounter for fracture with nonunion
P	Subsequent encounter for fracture with malunion
S	Sequela

For fractures of the shafts of the long bones, the 7th characters further describe the fracture as open or closed. When documentation does not indicate whether the fracture is open or closed, the default is closed. For open fractures, the 7th character also captures the severity of the injury using the Gustilo classification. The Gustilo classification applies to open fractures of the long bones including the humerus, radius, ulna, femur, tibia, and fibula. The Gustilo open fracture classification groups open fractures into three main categories designated as Type I, Type II and Type III with Type III injuries being further divided into Type IIIA, Type IIIB, and Type IIIC subcategories. The categories are defined by characteristics that include the mechanism of injury, extent of soft tissue damage, and degree of bone injury or involvement. The table below identifies key features of Gustilo fracture types. When the Gustilo classification type is not specified for an open fracture, the 7th character for open fracture type I or II should be assigned.

Type	Wound/ Contamination	Soft Tissue Damage	Type of Injury	Most Common Fracture Type(s)
Gustilo Type I	< 1 cm/Wound bed clean	Minimal	Low-energy	Simple transverse, short oblique, minimally comminuted
Gustilo Type II	> 1 cm/ Minimal or no contamination	Moderate	Low-energy	Simple transverse, short oblique, minimally comminuted

Type	Wound/ Contamination	Soft Tissue Damage	Type of Injury	Most Common Fracture Type(s)
Gustilo Type III	> 1 cm/ Contaminated wound	Extensive Type IIIA – Adequate soft tissue coverage open wound; No flap coverage required; Type IIIB Extensive soft tissue loss; Flap coverage required; Type IIIC Major arterial injury; Extensive repair; May require vascular surgeon for limb salvage	High-energy	Unstable fracture with multiple bone fragments including the following: Open segmental fracture regardless of wound size; Gun-shot wounds with bone involvement; Open fractures with any type of neurovascular involvement; •Severely contaminated open fractures; •Traumatic amputations; •Open fractures with delayed treatment (over 8 hours)

The applicable 7th character extensions for fractures of the shafts of the long bones are as follows:

7th Character	Description
A	Initial encounter for closed fracture
B	Initial encounter for open fracture type I or II
C	Initial encounter for open fracture type IIIA, IIIB, or IIIC
D	Subsequent encounter for closed fracture with routine healing
E	Subsequent encounter for open fracture type I or II with routine healing
F	Subsequent encounter for open fracture type IIIA, IIIB, or IIIC with routine healing
G	Subsequent encounter for closed fracture with delayed healing
H	Subsequent encounter for open fracture type I or II with delayed healing
J	Subsequent encounter for open fracture type IIIA, IIIB, or IIIC with delayed healing
K	Subsequent encounter for closed fracture with nonunion
M	Subsequent encounter for open fracture type I or II with nonunion
N	Subsequent encounter for open fracture type IIIA, IIIB, or IIIC with nonunion
P	Subsequent encounter for closed fracture with malunion
Q	Subsequent encounter for open fracture type I or II with malunion
R	Subsequent encounter for open fracture type IIIA, IIIB, or IIIC with malunion
S	Sequela

Chapter Guidelines

There are detailed guidelines for reporting of injury, poisoning and certain other consequences of external causes. The following topics are covered in the chapter-specific guidelines: application of 7th characters; coding of injuries, traumatic fractures, burns and corrosions; adverse effects, poisoning, underdosing and toxic effects; adult and child abuse, neglect and other maltreatment; and complications of care.

The principles for coding traumatic fractures are the same as coding of other injuries. Applicable 7th characters for fractures have already been discussed. Two additional guidelines of note provide default codes when certain information is not provided. A fracture not indicated as open or closed is coded as closed. A fracture not indicated as displaced or nondisplaced is coded as displaced.

Burns are classified first as corrosion or thermal burns and then by depth and extent. Corrosions are burns due to chemicals. Thermal burns are burns that come from a heat source but exclude sunburns. Examples of heat sources include: fire, hot appliance, electricity, and radiation.

The guidelines are the same for both corrosions and thermal burns with one exception: corrosions require identification of the chemical substance. The chemical substance that caused the corrosion is the first-listed diagnosis and is found in the Table of Drugs and Chemicals. Codes for drugs and chemicals are combination codes that identify the substance and the external cause or intent, so an external cause of injury code is not required. However, external cause codes should be assigned for the place of occurrence, activity, and external cause status when this information is available. The correct code for an accidental corrosion is found in the column for poisoning, accidental (unintentional).

Codes for adverse effects, poisoning, underdosing and toxic effects are combination codes that include both the substance taken and the intent. If the intent of the poisoning is unknown or unspecified, code the intent as accidental intent. The undetermined intent is only for use if the documentation in the record specifies that the intent cannot be determined. No additional external cause code is reported with these codes. Underdosing is defined as taking less of a medication than is prescribed by the provider or the manufacturer's instructions. Underdosing codes are never assigned as the principal or first-listed code. The code for the relapse or exacerbation of the medical condition for which the drug was prescribed is listed as the principal or first-listed code and the underdosing code is listed secondarily. An additional code from subcategories Z91.12- or Z91.13-, Z91.14- should also be assigned to identify the intent of the noncompliance if known. For example, code Z91.120 would be assigned for intentional underdosing due to financial hardship.

Complications of surgical and medical care not elsewhere classified are reported with codes from categories T80-T88. However, intraoperative and post-procedural complications are reported with codes from the body system chapters. For example, ventilator associated pneumonia is considered a procedural or post-procedural complication and is reported with code J95.851 Ventilator associated pneumonia from Chapter 10 – Diseases of the Respiratory System. Complication of care code assignment is based on the provider's documentation of the relationship between the condition and the care or procedure. Not all conditions that occur following medical or surgical treatment are classified as complications. Only conditions for which the provider has documented a cause-and-effect relationship between the care and the complication should be classified as complications of care. If the documentation is unclear, query the provider. Some complications of care codes include the external cause in the code. These codes include the nature of the complication as well as the type of procedure that caused the complication. An additional external cause code indicating the type of procedure is not necessary for these codes.

Pain due to medical devices, implants, or grafts requires two codes, one from the T-codes to identify the device causing the pain, such as T84.84- Pain due to internal orthopedic prosthetic devices, implants, and grafts and one from category G89 to identify acute or chronic pain due to presence of the device, implant, or graft.

Transplant complications are reported with codes from category T86. These codes should be used for both complications and rejection of transplanted organs. A transplant complication code is assigned only when the complication affects the function of the transplanted organ. Two codes are required to describe a transplant complication, one from category T86 and a secondary code that identifies the specific complication. Patients who have undergone a kidney transplant may have some form of chronic kidney disease (CKD) because the transplant may not fully restore kidney function. CKD is not considered to be a transplant complication unless the provider documents a transplant complication such as transplant failure or rejection. If the documentation is unclear, the provider should be queried. Other complications (other than CKD) that affect function of the kidney are assigned a code from subcategory T86.1- Complications of transplanted kidney and a secondary code that identifies the complication.

Chapter 20 – External Causes of Morbidity (V00-Y99)

Codes for external causes of morbidity are found in Chapter 20. External cause codes classify environmental events and other circumstances as the cause of injury and other adverse effects.

Codes in this chapter are always reported as a secondary code with the nature of the condition or injury reported as the first-listed diagnosis. Codes for external causes of morbidity relate to all aspects of external cause coding including: cause, intent, place of occurrence, and activity at the time of the injury or other health condition.

External cause codes are most frequently reported with codes in Chapter 19, Injury, Poisoning and Certain Other Consequences of External Causes (S00-T88). There are conditions in other chapters that may also be due to an external cause. For example, when a condition, such as a myocardial infarction, is specifically stated as due to or precipitated by strenuous activity, such as shoveling snow, then external cause codes should be reported to identify the activity, place and external cause status. As was discussed previously, separate reporting of external cause codes is not necessary for poisoning, adverse effects, or underdosing of drugs and other substances (T36-T50), or for toxic effect of nonmedicinal substances (T51-T65), since the external cause is captured in a combination code from Chapter 19.

External Cause Coding and Third Party Payer Requirements

While not all third party payers require reporting of external cause codes, they are a valuable source of information to public health departments and other state agencies regarding the causes of death, injury, poisoning and adverse effects. In fact, more than half of all states have mandated that hospitals collect external cause data using statewide hospital discharge data systems. Another third of all states routinely collect external cause data even though it is not mandated. There are also 15 states that have mandated statewide hospital emergency department data systems requiring collection of external cause data.

These codes provide a framework for systematically collecting patient health-related information on the external cause of death, injury, poisoning and adverse effects. These codes define the manner of the death or injury, the mechanism, the place of occurrence of the event, the activity, and the status of the person at the time death or injury occurred. Manner refers to whether the cause of death or injury was unintentional/accidental, self-inflicted, assault, or undetermined. Mechanism describes how the injury occurred such as a motor vehicle accident, fall, contact with a sharp object or power tool, or being caught between moving objects. Place identifies where the injury occurred, such as a personal residence, playground, street, or place of employment. Activity indicates the activity of the person at the time the injury occurred such as swimming, running, bathing, or cooking. External cause status is used to indicate the status of the person at the time death or injury occurred such as work done for pay, military activity, or volunteer activity.

7th Characters

Most external cause codes require a 7th character to identify the episode of care. The 7th characters used in Chapter 20 are A, D and S. These external cause codes have the same definitions as they do for most injury codes found in Chapter 19. Initial encounter is defined as the period when the patient is receiving active treatment for the injury, poisoning, or other consequences of an external cause and is reported with 7th character 'A'. Subsequent encounters are identified with 7th character 'D'. This is an encounter after the active phase of treatment and when the patient is receiving routine care for the injury or poisoning during the period of healing or recovery. Sequela is identified by 7th character 'S' which is assigned for complications or conditions that arise as a direct result of an injury.

Chapter Guidelines

As with other chapter guidelines, the guidelines for Chapter 20 External Causes of Morbidity are provided so that there is standardization in the assignment of these codes. External cause codes are always secondary codes, and these codes can be used in any health care setting. An overview of the guidelines is provided here. For the complete guidelines related to external causes, the Official Guidelines for the Code Set should be consulted.

The general external cause coding guidelines relate to all external cause codes including those that describe the cause, the intent, the place of occurrence, the activity of the patient, and the patient's status at the time of the injury. External cause codes may be used with any code in ranges A00.0-T88.9 or Z00-Z99 when the health condition is due to an external cause. The most common health conditions related to external causes are those for injuries in categories S00-T88. It is appropriate to assign external cause codes to infections and diseases in categories A00-R99 and Z00-Z99 that are the result of an external cause, such as a heart attack resulting from strenuous activity.

External cause codes are assigned for the entire length of treatment for the condition resulting from the external cause. The appropriate 7th character must be assigned to identify the encounter as the initial encounter, subsequent encounter, or sequela. For conditions due to an external cause, the full range of external cause codes are used to completely describe the cause, intent, place of occurrence, activity of patient at time of event, and patient's status. No external cause code is required if the external cause and intent are captured by a code from another chapter. For example, codes for poisoning, adverse effect and underdosing of drugs, medicaments, and biological substances in categories T36-T50 and toxic effects of substances chiefly nonmedicinal as to source in categories T51-T65 capture both the external cause and the intent.

When applicable, place of occurrence (Y92), activity (Y93), and external cause status (Y99) codes are sequenced after the main external cause codes. Regardless of the number of external cause codes assigned, there is generally only one place of occurrence code, one activity code, and one external cause status code assigned. However, if a new injury should occur during hospitalization, it is allowable in such rare instances to assign an additional place of occurrence code. Codes from these categories are only assigned at the initial encounter for treatment so these codes do not make use of 7th characters. If the place, activity, or external cause status is not documented, no code is assigned. These codes do not apply to poisonings, adverse effects, misadventures, or sequela.

If the intent (accident, self-harm, assault) of the cause of an injury or other condition is unknown or unspecified, code the intent as accidental. All transport accident categories assume accidental intent. A code for undetermined intent is assigned only when the documentation in the medical record specifies that the intent cannot be determined.

The external cause of sequelae are reported using the code for the external cause with the 7th character extension 'S' for sequela. An external cause code is assigned for any condition described as a late effect or sequela resulting from a previous injury.

Chapter 21 – Factors Influencing Health Status and Contact with Health Services (Z00-Z99)

The codes for factors influencing health and contact with health services represent reasons for encounters. These codes are located in Chapter 21 and the initial alpha character is Z so they are referred to as Z-codes. While code descriptions in Chapter 21, such as Z00.110 Health examination of newborn under 8 days old may appear to be a description of a service or procedure, codes in this chapter are not procedure codes. These codes represent the reason for the encounter, service, or visit. The procedure must be reported with the appropriate procedure code.

Chapter Guidelines

There are extensive chapter-specific coding guidelines for factors influencing health status and contact with health services. The guidelines identify broad categories of Z-codes, such as status Z-codes and history Z-codes. Each of these broad categories contains categories and subcategories of Z-codes for similar types of patient visits/encounters with similar reporting rules. Z-codes may be used in any health care setting and most Z-codes may be either a principal/first-listed or secondary code depending on the circumstances of the encounter. However, certain Z-codes, such as Z02 Encounter for administrative examination, may only be used as a first-listed or principal diagnosis. An overview of the guidelines for the broad categories of Z-codes is provided here. Consult the Official Guidelines for the complete guidelines for Chapter 21.

Contact/Exposure – There are two categories of contact/ exposure codes which may be reported as either a first-listed or secondary diagnosis although they are more commonly reported as a secondary diagnosis. Category Z20 indicates contact with, and suspected exposure to communicable diseases. These codes are reported for patients who do not show signs or symptoms of a disease but are suspected to have been exposed to it either by a close personal contact with an infected individual or by currently being in or having been in an area where the disease is epidemic. Category Z77 indicates contact with or suspected exposure to substances that are known to be hazardous to health. Code Z77.22 Exposure to tobacco smoke (second hand smoke) is included in this category.

Inoculations and Vaccinations – Inoculations and vaccinations may also be either the first-listed or a secondary diagnosis. There is a single code Z23 Encounter for immunization for reporting inoculations and vaccinations. A procedure code is required to capture the administration of the immunization of vaccination and to identify the specific immunization/vaccination provided.

Status – Status codes indicate that a patient is either a carrier of a disease or has the sequelae or residual of a past disease or condition. Codes for the presence of prosthetic or mechanical devices resulting from past treatment are categorized as status codes. Status codes should not be confused with history codes which indicate that a patient no longer has the condition. Status codes are not used with diagnosis codes that provide the same information as the status code. For example, code Z94.1 Heart transplant status should not be used with a code from subcategory T86.2- Complications of heart transplant because codes in subcategory T86.2- already identify the patient as a heart transplant recipient.

History (of) – There are two types of history Z-codes, personal and family. Personal history codes explain a patient's past medical condition that no longer exists and is not receiving any treatment, but that has the potential for recurrence, and therefore may require continued monitoring. Family history codes are for use when a patient has a family member who has had a particular disease that causes the patient to be at higher risk of also contracting the disease.

Screening – Screening is testing for disease or disease precursors in seemingly well individuals so that early detection and treatment can be provided for those who test positive for the disease (e.g. screening mammogram). The testing of a person to rule out or confirm a suspected diagnosis because the patient has some sign or symptom is a diagnostic examination not a screening and a sign or symptoms code is used to explain the reason for the visit.

Observation – There are three observation categories (Z03-Z05) for use in very limited circumstances when a person is being observed for a suspected condition that has been ruled out. The observation codes are to be used as principal diagnosis only. The only exception to this is when the principal diagnosis is required to be a code from category Z38, Liveborn infants according to place of birth and type of delivery. Then a code from category Z05, Encounter for observation and evaluation of newborn for suspected diseases and conditions ruled out, is sequenced after the Z38 code. Additional codes may be used in addition to the observation code, but only if they are unrelated to the suspected condition being observed.

Aftercare – Aftercare visit codes cover situations when the initial treatment of a disease has been performed and the patient requires continued care during the healing or recovery phase, or for the long-term consequences of the disease. Aftercare for injuries is not reported with Z-codes. The injury code is reported with the appropriate 7th character for subsequent care. Aftercare Z-codes/categories include Z42-Z49 and Z51. Z51 includes other aftercare and medical care.

Follow-up – The follow-up Z-codes are used to explain continuing surveillance following completed treatment of a disease, condition, or injury. They imply that the condition has been fully treated and no longer exists. Do not confuse follow-up codes with aftercare codes or injury codes with 7th character 'S'. Follow-up Z-codes/categories include: Z08-Z09 and Z39.

Donor – Codes in category Z52 Donors of organs and tissues are used for living individuals who are donating blood or other body tissue. These codes are only for individuals donating for other individuals, not for self-donations. The only exception to this rule is blood donation. There are codes for autologous blood donation in subcategory Z52.01-. Codes in category Z52 are not used to identify cadaveric donations.

Counseling – Counseling Z-codes are used when a patient or family member receives assistance in the aftermath of an illness or injury or when support is required in coping with family or social problems. They are not used in conjunction with a diagnosis code when the counseling component of care is considered integral to standard treatment. Counseling Z-codes/categories include: Z30.0-, Z31.5, Z31.6-, Z32.2-Z32.3, Z69-Z71, and Z76.81.

Encounters for Obstetrical and Reproductive Services – Routine prenatal visits and postpartum care are reported with Z-codes. Codes in category Z34 Encounter for supervision of normal pregnancy are always the first-listed diagnosis and are not to be used with any other code from the OB chapter. Codes in category Z3A Weeks of gestation may be assigned to provide additional information about the pregnancy. Codes in category Z37 Outcome of delivery should be included on all maternal delivery records. Outcome of delivery codes are always secondary codes and are never used on the newborn record. Examples of other conditions reported with Z-codes include family planning, and procreative management and counseling. Codes in category Z3A, Weeks of gestation, may be assigned to provide additional information about the pregnancy. Category Z3A codes should not be assigned for pregnancies with abortive outcomes (categories O00-O08), elective termination of pregnancy (code Z33.32), nor for postpartum conditions, as category Z3A is not applicable to these conditions. The date of the admission should be used to determine weeks of gestation for inpatient admissions that encompass more than one gestational week.

Newborns and Infants – There are a limited number of Z-codes for newborns and infants. Category Z38 Liveborn infants according to place of birth and type of delivery is always the principle diagnosis on the birth record. Subcategory Z00.11- Newborn health examination reports routine examination of the newborn. A 6th character is required that identifies the age of the newborn as under 8 days old (0) or 8-28 days old (1).

Routine and Administrative Examinations – An example of a routine examination is a general check-up. An example of an examination for administrative purposes is a pre-employment physical. These Z-codes are not to be used if the examination is for diagnosis of a suspected condition or for treatment purposes. In such cases the diagnosis code is used. During a routine exam, should a diagnosis or condition be discovered, it should be coded as an additional code. Some of the codes for routine health examinations distinguish between "with" and "without" abnormal findings. An examination with abnormal findings refers to a condition/diagnosis that is newly identified or a change in severity of a chronic condition (such as uncontrolled hypertension, or an acute exacerbation of chronic obstructive pulmonary disease) during a routine physical examination. Code assignment depends on the information that is known at the time the encounter is being coded. For example, if no abnormal findings were found during the examination, but the encounter is being coded before the test results are back, it is acceptable to assign the code for "without abnormal findings" diagnosis. When assigning a code for "with abnormal findings," additional codes should be assigned to identify the specific abnormal findings. Z-codes/categories for routine and administrative examinations include: Z00-Z02 (except Z02.9) and Z32.0-.

Miscellaneous Z-Codes – The miscellaneous Z-codes capture a number of other health care encounters that do not fall into one of the other categories. Certain of these codes identify the reason for the encounter; others are for use as additional codes that provide useful information on circumstances that may affect a patient's care and treatment. Miscellaneous Z-codes/categories are as follows: Z28 (except Z28.3), Z29, Z40-Z41 (except Z41.9) Z53, Z55-Z60, Z62-Z65, Z72-Z75 (except Z74.01 and only when the documentation specifies that the patient has an associated problem), Z76.0, Z76.3, Z76.5, Z91.1-, Z91.83, Z91.84-, and Z91.89.

Introduction to ICD-10-PCS

ICD-10-PCS is a procedure coding system used to report inpatient procedures beginning October 1, 2015. As inpatient procedures associated with changing technology and medical advances are developed, the structure of ICD-10-PCS allows them to be easily incorporated as unique codes. This is possible because during the development phase, four attributes were identified as key components for the structure of the coding system – completeness, expandability, multiaxial, and standardized terminology. These components are defined as follows:

Completeness

Completeness refers to the ability to assign a unique code for all substantially different procedures, including unique codes for procedures that can be performed using different approaches.

Expandability

Expandability means the ability to add new unique codes to the coding system in the section and body system where they should reside.

Multiaxial

Multiaxial signifies the ability to assign codes using independent characters around each individual axis or component of the procedure. For example, if a new surgical approach is used for one of the root operations on a specific body part, a value for the new surgical approach can be added to the approach character without a need to add or change other code characters.

Standardized Terminology

ICD-10-PCS includes definitions of the terminology used. While the meaning of specific words varies in common usage, ICD-10-PCS does not include multiple meanings for the same term, and each term is assigned a specific meaning. For example, the term "excision" is defined in most medical dictionaries as surgical removal of part or all of a structure or organ. However, in ICD-10-PCS excision is defined as "cutting out or off, without replacement, a portion of a body part." If all of a body part is surgically removed without replacement, the procedure is defined as 'resection' in ICD-10-PCS.

General Development Principles

In the development of ICD-10-PCS, several general principles were followed:

Diagnostic Information is Not Included in Procedure Description

When procedures are performed for specific diseases or disorders, the disease or disorder is not contained in the procedure code. There are no codes for procedures exclusive to aneurysms, cleft lip, strictures, neoplasms, hernias, etc. The diagnosis codes, not the procedure codes, specify the disease or disorder.

Limited Use of Not Elsewhere Classified (NEC) Option

Because all significant components of a procedure are specified, there is generally no need for an NEC code option. However, limited NEC options are incorporated into ICD-10-PCS where necessary. For example, new devices are frequently developed, and therefore it is necessary to provide an "Other Device" option for use until the new device can be explicitly added to the coding system.

Level of Specificity

All procedures currently performed can be specified in ICD-10-PCS. The frequency with which a procedure is performed was not a consideration in the development of the system. Rather, a unique code is available for variations of a procedure that can be performed.

ICD-10-PCS Structure

ICD-10-PCS has a seven-character alphanumeric code structure. Each character contains up to 34 possible values. Each value represents a specific option for the general character definition (e.g., stomach is one of the values for the body part character). The ten digits 0-9 and the 24 letters A-H, J-N and P-Z may be used in each character. The letters O and I are not used in order to avoid confusion with the digits 0 and 1.

Procedures are divided into sections that identify the general type of procedure (e.g., medical and surgical, obstetrics, imaging). The first character of the procedure code always specifies the section. The sections are shown in Table 1.

Table 1: ICD-10-PCS Sections

0	Medical and Surgical
1	Obstetrics
2	Placement
3	Administration
4	Measurement and Monitoring
5	Extracorporeal or Systemic Assistance and Performance
6	Extracorporeal or Systemic Therapies
7	Osteopathic
8	Other Procedures
9	Chiropractic
B	Imaging
C	Nuclear Medicine
D	Radiation Therapy
F	Physical Rehabilitation and Diagnostic Audiology
G	Mental Health
H	Substance Abuse Treatment
X	New Technology

The second through seventh characters mean the same thing within each section, but may mean different things in other sections. In all sections, the third character specifies the general type of procedure performed, or root operation (e.g., resection, transfusion, fluoroscopy), while the other characters give additional information such as the body part and approach. In ICD-10-PCS, the term "procedure" refers to the complete specification of the seven characters.

ICD-10-PCS Format

The ICD-10-PCS is made up of three separate parts:

- Tables
- Index

The Index allows codes to be located by an alphabetic lookup. The index entry refers to a specific location in the Tables. The Tables must be used in order to construct a complete and valid code.

Tables in ICD-10-PCS

Each page in the Tables is composed of rows that specify the valid combinations of code values. ***Table 2*** is an excerpt from the ICD-10-PCS tables. In the system, the upper portion of each table specifies the values for the first three characters of the codes in that table. In the administration section, the first three characters are the section, the body system and the root operation.

In ICD-10-PCS, the values 3E0 specify the section Administration (3), the body system Physiological Systems/Anatomical Region (E), and the root operation Introduction (0). As shown in Table 2, the root operation (i.e., introduction) is accompanied by its definition. The lower portion of the table specifies all the valid combinations of the remaining characters four through seven. The four columns in the table specify the last four characters. In the administration section they are labeled Body System, Approach, Substance and Qualifier, respectively. Each row in the table specifies the valid combination of values for characters four through seven. The Tables contain only those combinations of values that result in a valid procedure code.

Table 2: Excerpt from the ICD-10-PCS tables

<table>
<tr><td colspan="4">3 Administration
E Physiological Systems/Anatomical Regions
0 Introduction: Putting in or on a therapeutic, diagnostic, nutritional, physiological, or prophylactic substance except blood or blood products</td></tr>
<tr><td>Character 4</td><td>Character 5</td><td>Character 6</td><td>Character 7</td></tr>
<tr><td>T Peripheral Nerves and Plexi
X Cranial Nerves</td><td>3 Percutaneous</td><td>3 Anti-inflammatory
B Anesthetic Agent
T Destructive Agent</td><td>Z No Qualifier</td></tr>
</table>

There are 6 code options for the table above:

3E0T33Z	Introduction (injection) anti-inflammatory peripheral nerves and plexi
3E0T3BZ	Introduction (injection) anesthetic agent peripheral nerves and plexi
3E0T3TZ	Introduction (injection) destructive agent peripheral nerves and plexi
3E0X33Z	Introduction (injection) anti-inflammatory peripheral cranial nerves
3E0X3BZ	Introduction (injection) anesthetic agent cranial nerves
3E0X3TZ	Introduction (injection) destructive agent cranial nerves

ICD-10-CM Anatomy and Physiology

Nervous System

Chapter Objectives

After studying this chapter, you should be able to:

- Describe the function of the nervous system
- Classify nervous system organs into central and peripheral divisions
- Explain the functions of neuroglia and neurons
- Describe the different types of neuroglial cells
- Identify the two principle tissues types in the nervous system
- Identify the two principle divisions of the nervous system
- Identify central nervous system organs
- Identify three principle areas of the brain
- Identify the protective coverings of the brain and spinal cord
- Identify the two principle divisions of the peripheral nervous system
- Identify peripheral nervous system organs
- Describe nervous system functions
- Explain how nerve impulses are initiated and transmitted
- Describe a reflex arc
- Define the terms irritability and conductivity as they pertain to transmission of nerve impulses
- Describe a variety of diseases and disease processes affecting the nervous system
- Identify how these diseases and disease processes affect and alter nervous system function
- Assign ICD-10-CM codes to diseases, injuries, and other conditions affecting the nervous system
- Define the following terms: central nervous system, peripheral nervous system, neuron, neuroglia, nerve root, nerve, ganglion, nerve reflex, meninges, dura mater, pia mater, arachnoid, encephalon, intracranial, extracranial, extradural, subdural, intraspinal

Overview

The nervous system is the control, regulatory, and communication center of the body. Important functions that the nervous system performs are the maintenance of homeostasis, the stimulation of movement, and the ability to analyze and respond to the world around each person. The nervous system senses both changes within the body, also referred to as the internal environment, and changes around the body, also referred to as the external environment. It then interprets these changes, integrates them, decides on a course of action, and then elicits a response by sending impulses through the body.

The nervous system is divided into two portions – the central nervous system or CNS, and the peripheral nervous system or PNS. The nervous system is composed of four principle organs. These include the brain, spinal cord, nerves, and ganglia. The brain and spinal cord are part of the central nervous system and the nerves and ganglia are part of the peripheral nervous system. The peripheral nervous system has two divisions – the somatic nervous system and the autonomic nervous system.

The somatic nervous system contains nerve fibers that connect the central nervous system with skeletal muscles and skin. The autonomic nervous system contains nerve fibers that connect the central nervous system with cardiac muscle, smooth muscle, and glands.

Cells

The nervous system is composed of two cell types, neurons and neuroglia.

Neurons

Neurons, also called nerve cells, are the cells that conduct impulses from one part of the body to another. These cells have three distinct portions: a cell body, dendrites, and an axon. The dendrites pick up a stimulus and transmit that stimulus to the cell body. The axon picks up the stimulus from the cell body and conducts it away from the cell body to another neuron or another organ of the body.

Neurons are subdivided based on their function into sensory neurons and motor neurons. Sensory neurons carry impulses from receptors in the skin and sense organs to the spinal cord and brain. Motor neurons, also called efferent neurons, carry impulses from the brain and spinal cord to muscles or glands.

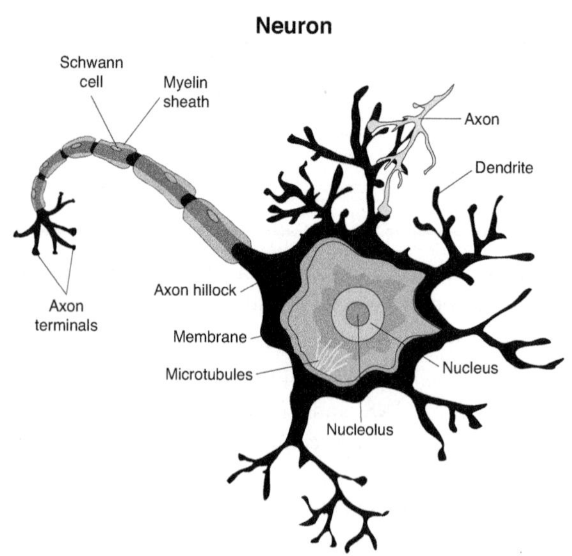

Neuroglia

Neuroglia, also called glial cells, form the connective tissue of the nervous system. These cells combine to form a thick tissue that supports the nerve cells and nerve tissue. In the central nervous system there are four primary types of glial cells, including oligodendrocytes, astrocytes, microglia, and ependymal cells. In the peripheral nervous system, connective tissue cells that serve the same function as oligodendrocytes are called Schwann cells.

Neuroglia are of special interest to the medical coder because they are a common source of tumors of the nervous system. Two common types of central nervous system connective tissue tumors are astrocytomas and gliomas. Schwannomas or neurilemomas are connective tissue tumors found in the peripheral nervous system.

Oligodendrocytes

Oligodendrocytes in the central nervous system are connective tissue cells that form rows of semirigid tissue between neurons in the brain and spinal cord. The oligodendrocytes produce a thick, fatty sheath called the myelin sheath that covers the neurons of the central nervous system. These myelinated nerve fibers in the brain and spinal column make up the white matter in the central nervous system.

Astrocytes

Astrocytes are star-shaped cells that wrap around nerve cells to form a supporting network around the neurons in the brain and spinal cord. They also attach neurons to blood vessels.

Microglia

Microglia are specialized neuroglia that protect the nervous system from disease by engulfing pathogens and clearing away debris. This process is known as phagocytosis.

Schwann cells

The axons of some neurons in the peripheral nervous system are also covered with a myelin sheath formed by flattened Schwann cells. Each Schwann cell produces a portion of the myelin sheath by wrapping itself around the axon and encircling a portion of axon multiple times. The cytoplasm is forced into the inside layer of the Schwann cell forming the myelin sheath. The cell membrane of the Schwann cell wraps itself around the neuron forming a delicate, continuous sheath called the neurilemma that encloses the myelin and assists in the regeneration of injured axons. Other axons are not covered by Schwann cells and these are called unmyelinated axons.

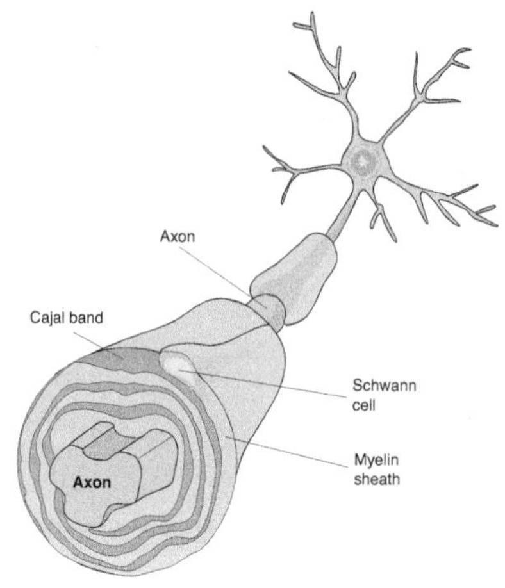

Tissues

Nervous system organs are composed of two principle tissues, nervous and connective tissue. The brain, spinal cord, and nerves are composed of nervous tissue. Nervous tissue is composed of neurons that generate and conduct impulses. The connective tissue is composed of neuroglia. Nervous system connective tissue is a nonconductive tissue that supports and insulates the nervous tissue.

Neural tissue is generally neatly arranged together with the axons of a group of neurons all pointed in the same direction. Myelinated axons which are white in color form the white matter of the brain. Nerve cell bodies and dendrites or unmyelinated axons form the gray matter.

Organs

The nervous system is divided into two parts, the central nervous system (CNS) and the peripheral nervous system (PNS). The CNS is comprised of the brain and spinal cord. The PNS consists of nerves, nerve plexuses, and ganglia.

Brain

The brain is the control center of the body, and along with the endocrine system, it is responsible for maintaining homeostasis. Studying the regions of the brain can be quite confusing as there are a number of ways of dividing brain structures. Some references divide the brain into three principle regions, the forebrain (containing the cerebrum, thalamus, hypothalamus, and pituitary gland), midbrain, and hindbrain (containing the cerebellum, medulla oblongata, and pons). Other references discuss the major structures which include the cerebrum, cerebellum and brainstem (which contains the medulla oblongata, pons, and midbrain). Still others refer to the prosencephalon (forebrain), mesencephalon (midbrain) and rhombencephalon (hindbrain). The prosencephalon is then further subdivided into the telencephalon (region containing the cerebrum) and diencephalon (region containing the thalamus, hypothalamus, and pituitary gland). In this section, the following structures will be described: cerebrum, thalamus, hypothalamus, cerebellum, and brainstem.

Brain

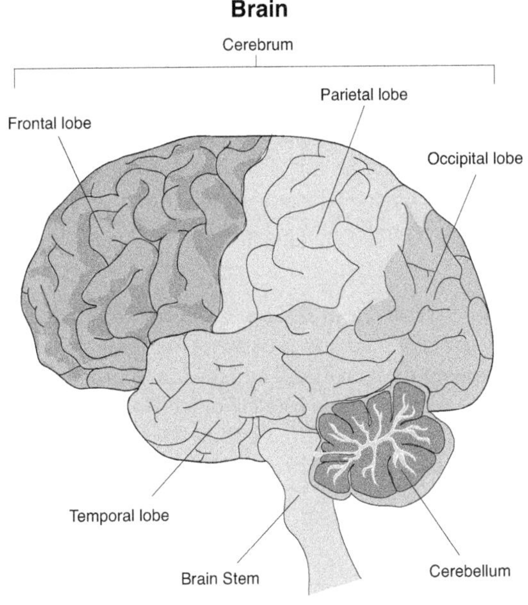

Cerebrum

The cerebrum is the largest portion of the brain. The surface is composed of gray matter which is referred to as the cerebral cortex. The cortex consists of six layers of nerve cell bodies and contains millions of cells. Under the cortex is the cerebral white matter which is composed of the myelinated axons of millions of nerve cells.

As the brain forms during embryonic development, the cortex is much larger than the white matter. As the brain grows, the cortex rolls and folds upon itself creating upfolds called gyri or convolutions, deep downfolds called fissures, and shallow downfolds called sulci. The most prominent fissure is called

the longitudinal fissure because it almost completely separates the brain into two halves called the right and left hemispheres. They are connected by a large bundle of transverse nerve cell fibers called the corpus callosum. The right and left cerebral hemispheres are each divided into four lobes which include the frontal lobe, parietal lobe, temporal lobe, and occipital lobe.

The myelinated nerve fibers of the white matter are arranged to transmit impulses in three directions. They are named based on the direction of the nerve impulses they transmit. Association fibers transmit impulses from one part of the cerebral cortex to another within the same hemisphere. Commissural fibers transmit impulses from one hemisphere to another. Projection fibers transmit impulses from the cerebrum to other parts of the brain and spinal cord.

The functions of the cerebrum are numerous and complex but they can be divided into three general functions that include motor functions, which govern muscle movement; sensory functions, which interpret sensory input; and association functions, which are concerned with emotional and intellectual processes.

Brain cells within the cerebrum generate electrical potentials called brain waves. These brain waves pass through the skull and can be detected with sensors called electrodes. Brain waves can be recorded and graphed using an electroencephalograph. The recording is called an electroencephalogram or EEG.

An EEG is used in a clinical setting for many different purposes:

- to diagnose conditions such as epilepsy or narcolepsy
- to determine the cause of nontraumatic loss of consciousness or dementia
- to determine the extent of brain injury following trauma
- to help determine whether a behavior or condition is the result of a physiological condition of the brain, spinal cord, or nerves or whether it is a mental health condition

Thalamus

The thalamus is a large oval structure that lies above the midbrain. One function of the thalamus is to relay all sensory impulses excluding those for smell to the cerebral cortex. A second function is to interpret and produce conscious recognition of pain. It also controls sleep and awake states.

Hypothalamus

The hypothalamus is located below the thalamus. Even though it is relatively small in size, it controls many body activities related to homeostasis. Key functions of the hypothalamus include:

- Controlling and integrating functions of the autonomic nervous system, such as:
  - Heartbeat
  - Movement of food through the digestive tract
  - Contraction of the urinary bladder
- Receiving and interpreting sensory impulses from the viscera
- Monitoring and working with the endocrine system to maintain homeostasis
- Controlling body temperature
- Responding to changes in mental states such as fear by initiating changes in heart rate, respiratory rate, etc.
- Regulating food intake by stimulating the hunger and satiety sensations
- Regulating fluid intake by stimulating the thirst sensation
- Regulating biorhythms that control wake and sleep Patterns

Cerebellum

The cerebellum is located below the posterior aspect of the cerebrum and is separated from it by the transverse fissure. Like the cerebrum, the cerebellum has two hemispheres that are separated by a structure called the vermis. The cerebellum is composed of both gray matter and white matter and attached to the brain stem by paired bundles of fibers called the cerebellar peduncles. The cerebellum is the motor area of the brain and controls unconscious movements in the skeletal muscles that are required for coordination, posture, and balance.

Injury to the cerebellum caused by trauma or disease is characterized by certain symptoms such as lack of muscle coordination, also referred to as ataxia. To examine a patient for ataxia, the physician may ask the patient to hold the arms out to the side and then touch the index finger to the nose. Ataxia involving the speech muscles may be indicated by a change in speech pattern. Cerebellar damage may also affect gait causing the patient to stagger or exhibit other abnormal walking movements.

Thalamus and Brainstem

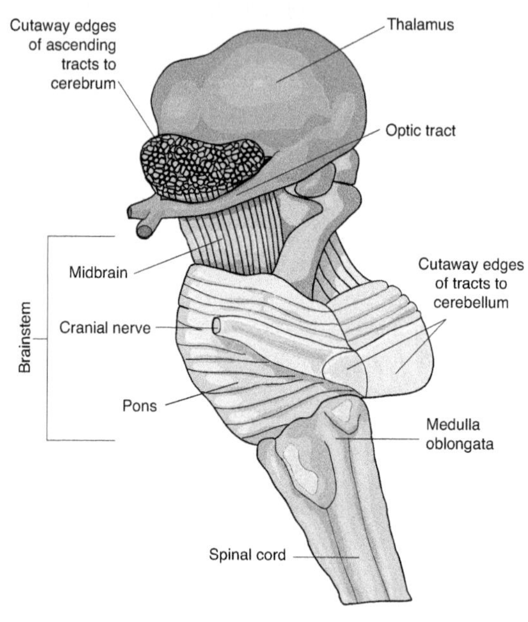

Brain Stem

The brain stem consists of the following structures:

- Medulla oblongata
- Pons
- Midbrain

Medulla oblongata

The medulla oblongata is the most inferior portion of the brain and also forms the upper portion of the spinal cord. One primary function of the medulla is the conduction of nerve impulses between the spinal cord and brain. Two sets of structures in the medulla form the principle conduction pathways. These include the two pyramids on the ventral aspect of the medulla and two nuclei on the dorsal aspect. The two pyramids are composed of motor tracts running from the cortex to the spinal cord. At the junction of the two pyramids are nerve fibers. Some nerve fibers that originate in one side cross to the opposite side, which is why motor areas in the right cerebral cortex control voluntary movement on the left side of the body and those in the left cerebral cortex control voluntary movement on the right side of the body. The two nuclei, called the nucleus gracilis and nucleus cuneatus, receive sensory impulses from the ascending tract of the spinal cord. The nuclei then relay these impulses to the opposite side of the medulla. Impulses received on one side of the body are processed on the opposite side of the brain.

Four pairs of cranial nerves also originate in the medulla oblongata. These include the glossopharyngeal (cranial nerve IX), the vagus nerve (X), the accessory nerve (XI), and the hypoglossal nerve (XII).

Three vital reflex centers are also located in the medulla. The cardiac center regulates heartbeat; the respiratory center adjusts the rate and depth of breathing; and the vasoconstrictor center regulates the diameter of the blood vessels.

Given the vital activities performed by the medulla, it is not surprising that trauma to this area can be fatal. Non-fatal injuries may cause cranial nerve malfunctions, paralysis or loss of sensation, or respiratory irregularities.

Pons

The pons lies above the medulla and anterior to the cerebellum. Pons means bridge and just as its name implies it serves as a bridge between the spinal cord and the brain. It also connects the various parts of the brain with each other. Four cranial nerves originate in the pons. These include the trigeminal nerve (cranial nerve V), abducens (VI), facial nerve (VII), and vestibulocochlear nerve (VIII).

Midbrain

The midbrain is a short, constricted structure that connects the pons and the cerebellum. Two cranial nerves originate in the midbrain, the oculomotor nerve (III) and the trochlear nerve (IV).

Spinal Cord

The spinal cord begins as a continuation of the medulla extending from the foramen magnum to the level of the second lumbar vertebra. The diameter of the spinal cord is enlarged in two regions where spinal nerves that supply the extremities are contained. The first enlarged area is in the cervical region and contains nerves that supply the upper extremities. It extends from the fourth cervical vertebra to the first thoracic vertebra. The second enlarged area is in the lumbar region and contains nerves that supply the lower extremities. This enlarged area is widest at the T12-L1 interspace. The spinal cord then tapers, ending in the conus medullaris at the second lumbar vertebra. Spinal nerves arise from the conus medullaris. These spinal nerves which look like coarse strands of hair do not leave the vertebral canal immediately. They run through the subarachnoid space and exit at the interspaces between the lumbar vertebrae. This bundle of nerve roots in the lumbosacral region is also referred to as the cauda equine, which is Latin for horse's tail.

Spinal column with spinal nerves

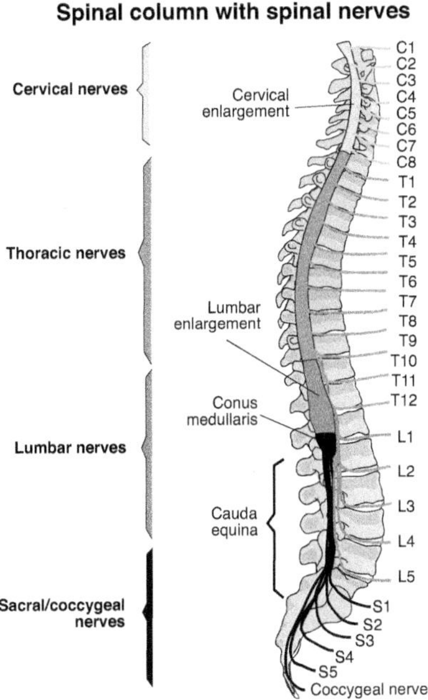

Brain ventricles and CSF flow

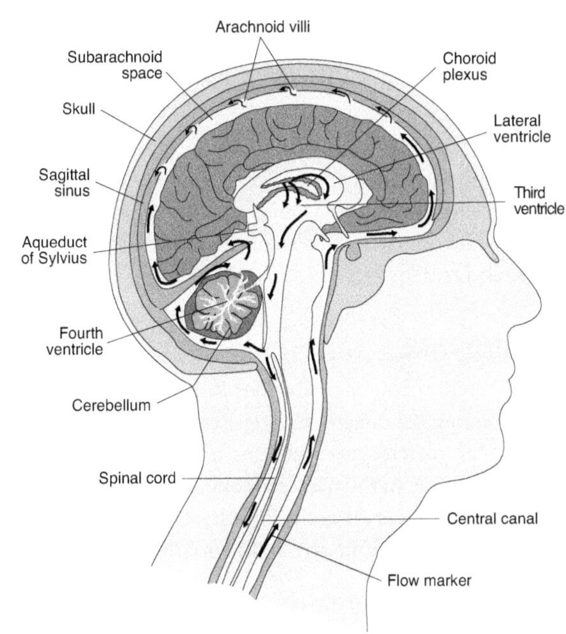

The term cauda or tail is one that medical coders should recognize as the directional term caudad is frequently seen in operative, radiology, and other medical reports. Caudad means toward the tail or situated in relation to a specific reference point. In contrast, the term cephalad is a directional term meaning toward the head.

Meninges

The brain and spinal cord are delicate vital structures that are protected by three membranes called the meninges. The outer membrane is composed of a tough fibrous tissue called the dura mater. The middle membrane is a delicate fibrous tissue called the arachnoid. The inner membrane, called the pia mater, is a transparent layer containing blood vessels and is adherent to the surfaces of the brain and spinal cord.

The medical coder should be familiar with the meninges because they are referenced when coding certain types of injuries, such as a subdural or subarachnoid hemorrhage, and infection or inflammation, such as viral or bacterial meningitis.

Cerebrospinal Fluid

The central nervous system is further protected by cerebrospinal fluid contained in the space between the arachnoid membrane and pia mater. This space is also called the subarachnoid space. The cerebrospinal fluid circulates around the brain and spinal cord and through the ventricles of the brain. The ventricles are cavities within the brain that communicate with each other and with the central canal of the spinal cord. Cerebrospinal fluid is continuously formed within the ventricles and then drains into the subarachnoid spaces.

Obstruction of the flow of cerebrospinal fluid can cause hydrocephalus which may be congenital or acquired.

Peripheral Nervous System

The peripheral nervous system (PNS) is essentially all neural tissue that lies outside of the brain and spinal cord. The PNS is subdivided into somatic and autonomic systems.

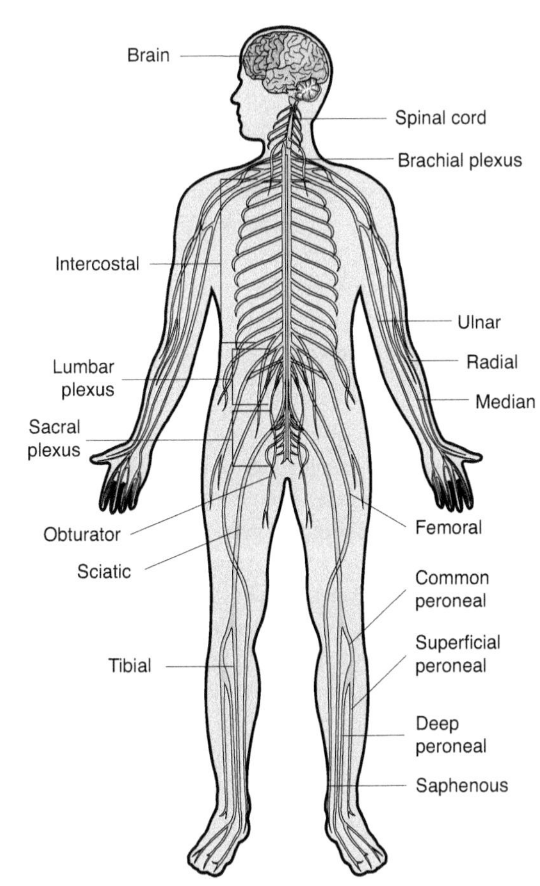

Somatic Nervous System

The somatic nervous system is composed of motor fibers that run from the CNS to the skeletal muscles and sensory fibers that run from the skeletal muscles, skin, and viscera to the CNS. The somatic nervous system consists of 12 pairs of cranial nerves that originate from the brain and 31 pairs of spinal nerves that originate from the spinal cord. Cranial nerves are distributed primarily to the head, neck, and viscera of the thorax and abdomen, while spinal nerves are primarily distributed to the arms, legs, and trunk.

Cranial Nerves

Ten of the 12 cranial nerves originate from the brain stem. The two exceptions are the olfactory nerves (cranial nerve I) and optic nerves (II). The olfactory nerves consist of numerous olfactory filaments originating in the nasal mucosa that convey impulses to the brain. The optic nerves are really extensions of the forebrain and convey impulses from the retina to the forebrain. Some cranial nerves are referred to as mixed nerves in that they contain both sensory and motor fibers. Some contain only sensory fibers while others consist primarily of motor fibers.

Spinal Nerves

The spinal nerves are named for the region of the vertebral column from which they emerge. There are 8 pairs of cervical nerves, 12 pairs of thoracic nerves, 5 pairs of lumbar nerves, 5 pairs of sacral nerves, and 1 pair of coccygeal nerves. Each spinal nerve is a mixed nerve that is indirectly attached to the spinal cord by two short roots. The dorsal root, also referred to as the posterior or sensory root, contains afferent nerve fibers that conduct impulses into the spinal cord. The ventral root, also referred to as the anterior or motor root, contains axons of motor neurons that conduct impulses away from the spinal cord. Before leaving the spinal canal via the intervertebral foramen, the two roots combine to form the spinal nerve. After the spinal nerve leaves the spinal canal it divides into dorsal (posterior), ventral (anterior), and visceral branches. The dorsal and ventral branches are part of the somatic nervous system while the visceral branches are part of the autonomic nervous system.

Nerve Plexus

Only the ventral branches of spinal nerves T2-T12 are distributed directly to the skin and muscle. The other spinal nerves combine to form plexuses which are complex networks of nerve fibers. The cervical plexus is formed by spinal nerves C1-C4; the brachial plexus is formed by spinal nerves C5-T1; the lumbar plexus is formed by spinal nerves L1-L4; the sacral plexus is formed by spinal nerves L5-S3; and the coccygeal plexus by spinal nerves S4-C1. Nerves that emerge from these plexuses are generally named for the regions they supply. Each of these nerves is subdivided into branches that are usually named for the specific structures they supply.

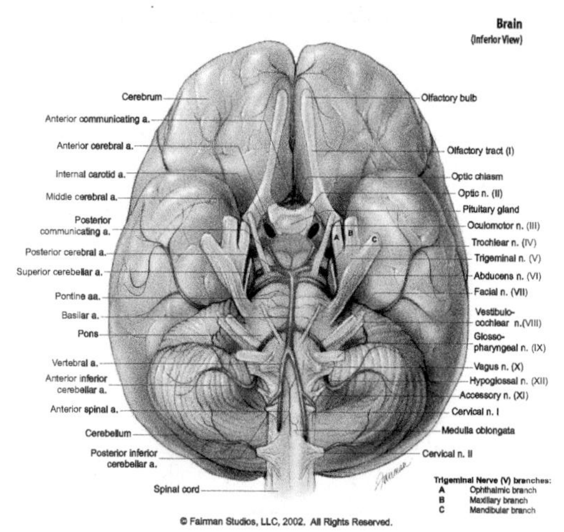

Spinal nerves/nerve plexus

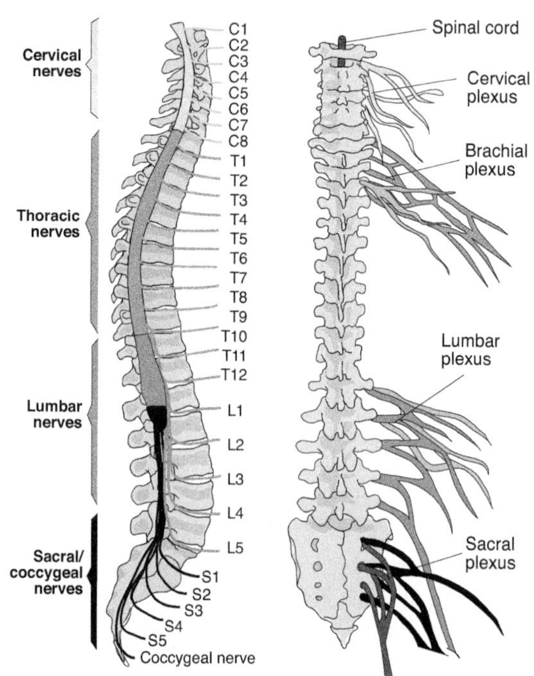

Autonomic Nervous System

The autonomic nervous system controls the smooth muscle, cardiac muscle, and glands. It functions automatically and involuntarily and is regulated by centers in the brain, including the cerebral cortex, hypothalamus, and the medulla oblongata. The autonomic nervous system affects visceral functions and consists entirely of motor fibers that transmit impulses from the CNS to smooth muscle, cardiac muscle, and glandular epithelium.

Examples of visceral functions affected by the autonomic nervous system include:

- Dilation and constriction of blood vessels
- Control of the force and rate of heartbeats

- Relaxation of bladder to allow urination
- Regulation of gastric peristalsis
- Regulation of glandular secretions

The autonomic nervous system is subdivided into parasympathetic and sympathetic functions. Generally, the parasympathetic division works to restore and conserve energy while the sympathetic division expends just enough energy to maintain homeostasis. However, in a situation of extreme threat, the sympathetic division dominates the parasympathetic producing the "fight or flight" response.

Autonomic Nerve Pathways

The autonomic nerve pathways always consist of two neurons. The cell body of the first neuron, also called the preganglionic neuron, is contained in the brain or spinal cord. The axon of the first neuron, also called preganglionic fiber, passes out of the CNS as part of a cranial or spinal nerve. It then separates from the somatic nerve and runs to an autonomic ganglion. There it synapses with the second neuron, also called the postganglionic neuron. The postganglionic axon or fiber then transmits the impulse to the smooth muscle, cardiac muscle, or glandular epithelium.

Function

As was stated earlier, the nervous system is the control, regulatory, and communication center of the body. Nervous system tissue is defined by two distinctive characteristics. The first is its ability to carry electrical messages called nerve impulses to and from the CNS. The second is the very limited ability of nervous tissue to regenerate.

The nervous system has three general overlapping functions: sensory, integrative, and motor.

Sensory

Sensory input is gathered by millions of sensory receptors that detect changes occurring inside and outside the body. These sensory receptors monitor external stimuli such as temperature, light, and sound, as well as internal stimuli such as blood pressure, pH, and carbon dioxide concentration.

Integration

The sensory input is then converted into nerve impulses which are electrical signals that are transmitted to the central nervous system. These nerve impulses create sensations, produce thoughts, or add to memory. Conscious and unconscious decisions are then made in the central nervous system, which is the integrative function of the nervous system.

Motor

Once the central nervous system has integrated the sensory input, the nervous system initiates a response by sending signals to tissues, organs, or glands which elicit a response such as muscle contraction or gland secretion. Tissues, organs, and glands are called effectors because they cause an effect in response to directions received from the central nervous system. This response is referred to as motor output or motor function.

Nerve Impulses

Nerve cells respond to stimuli and convert them into nerve impulses. This is called irritability. Once the stimuli are converted into a nerve impulse, the nerve cells have the ability to transmit that impulse to another nerve cell or to another tissue. This is called conductivity.

Irritability

Any stimulus that is strong enough to initiate transmission of a nerve impulse is referred to as a threshold impulse. A stimulus that is too weak to initiate a response is called a subthreshold stimulus. However, a series of subthreshold stimuli that are applied quickly to a neuron can have a cumulative effect that may initiate a nerve impulse. This is called summation of inadequate stimuli. The speed with which an impulse is transmitted depends on the size, type, and condition of the nerve fiber. Myelinated fibers with larger diameters transmit nerve impulses faster than mid-sized and small fibers or unmyelinated fibers. Sensory and motor fibers that detect and respond to potentially dangerous situations in the outside environment are generally larger in diameter than those that control or respond to less critical stimuli.

Conductivity

Conductivity is the ability of the nerve cell to transmit an impulse to another nerve cell or another tissue via a conduction pathway. The reflex arc is the most basic type of conduction pathway. There are five basic components to a reflex arc that are required to transmit an impulse.

1. A receptor consisting of the distal end of a dendrite of a sensory neuron responds to a stimulus in the internal or external environment and produces a nerve impulse.
2. The impulse is passed by the receptor to the CNS.
3. The incoming impulse is directed to a center usually within the CNS where it is blocked, transmitted, or rerouted. This is usually accomplished with an association neuron that lies between the sensory neuron and the motor neuron.
4. The motor neuron transmits the impulse to the tissue, organ, or gland that must respond to the stimulus.
5. The tissue, organ, or gland, called an effector, responds to the stimulus.

The axons of neurons in a reflex arc do not ever touch the dendrites of the adjacent neuron in the nerve conduction pathway. The impulse must travel across a minute gap called a synapse. In addition, impulses can travel in only one direction from axon to synapse to dendrite.

Axon/synapse/dendrite

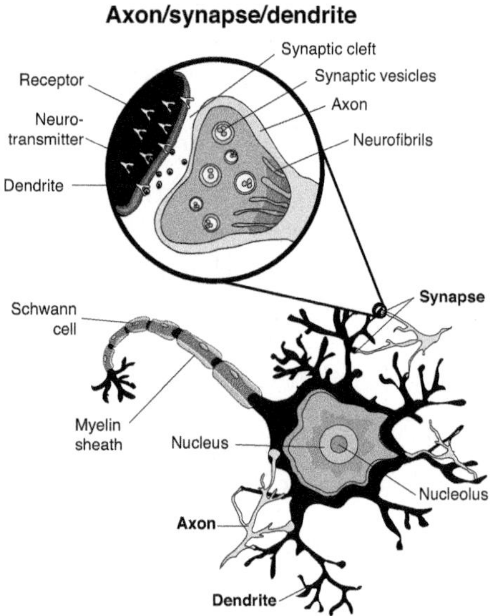

Nervous Tissue Injury

Unlike other tissues, nervous tissue has a very limited ability to regenerate. Specifically, if the cell body of a neuron is destroyed, the neuron cannot regenerate nor can other neurons reproduce and replace the damaged neuron. However, the human body is able to repair damaged nerve cells in which the cell body is intact and the axon has a neurilemma. Nerve cells in the peripheral nervous system generally have axons with a neurilemma while those in the brain and spinal cord do not. This means that a nerve injury of the hand has a good chance of healing while an injury of the brain or spinal cord is more often permanent.

ICD-10-CM Nervous System Coding Guidelines

See the table below for guidelines for Chapter 5, Mental, Behavioral and Neurodevelopmental Disorders and Chapter 6, Diseases of the Nervous System.

Chapter 5: Mental, Behavioral and Neurodevelopmental disorders (F01-F99)
1. Pain disorders related to psychological factors Assign code F45.41, for pain that is exclusively related to psychological disorders. As indicated by the Excludes 1 note under category G89, a code from category G89 should not be assigned with code F45.41. Code F45.42, Pain disorders with related psychological factors, should be used with a code from category G89, Pain, not elsewhere classified, if there is documentation of a psychological component for a patient with acute or chronic pain. *See Section I.C.6. Pain.*
2. Mental and behavioral disorders due to psychoactive substance use **a. In Remission** Selection of codes for "in remission" for categories F10-F19, Mental and behavioral disorders due to psychoactive substance use (categories F10-F19 with -.21) requires the provider's clinical judgment. The appropriate codes for "in remission" are assigned only on the basis of provider documentation (as defined in the Official Guidelines for Coding and Reporting). **b. Psychoactive Substance Use, Abuse And Dependence** When the provider documentation refers to use, abuse and dependence of the same substance (e.g. alcohol, opioid, cannabis, etc.), only one code should be assigned to identify the pattern of use based on the following hierarchy: i. If both use and abuse are documented, assign only the code for abuse ii. If both abuse and dependence are documented, assign only the code for dependence iii. If use, abuse and dependence are all documented, assign only the code for dependence iv. If both use and dependence are documented, assign only the code for dependence. **c. Psychoactive Substance Use** As with all other diagnoses, the codes for psychoactive substance use (F10.9-, F11.9-, F12.9-, F13.9-, F14.9-, F15.9-, F16.9-) should only be assigned based on provider documentation and when they meet the definition of a reportable diagnosis (see Section III, Reporting Additional Diagnoses). The codes are to be used only when the psychoactive substance use is associated with a mental or behavioral disorder, and such a relationship is documented by the provider.

Chapter 6: Diseases of the Nervous System (G00-G99)

1. **Dominant/nondominant side**

   Codes from category G81, Hemiplegia and hemiparesis, and subcategories, G83.1, Monoplegia of lower limb, G83.2, Monoplegia of upper limb, and G83.3, Monoplegia, unspecified, identify whether the dominant or nondominant side is affected. Should the affected side be documented, but not specified as dominant or nondominant, and the classification system does not indicate a default, code selection is as follows:

   - For ambidextrous patients, the default should be dominant.
   - If the left side is affected, the default is non-dominant.
   - If the right side is affected, the default is dominant.

2. **Pain – Category G89**

   a. **General coding information**

   Codes in category G89, Pain, not elsewhere classified, may be used in conjunction with codes from other categories and chapters to provide more detail about acute or chronic pain and neoplasm-related pain, unless otherwise indicated below.

   If the pain is not specified as acute or chronic, post-thoracotomy, postprocedural, or neoplasm-related, do not assign codes from category G89.

   A code from category G89 should not be assigned if the underlying (definitive) diagnosis is known, unless the reason for the encounter is pain control/ management and not management of the underlying condition.

   When an admission or encounter is for a procedure aimed at treating the underlying condition (e.g., spinal fusion, kyphoplasty), a code for the underlying condition (e.g., vertebral fracture, spinal stenosis) should be assigned as the principal diagnosis. No code from category G89 should be assigned.

3. **Category G89 codes as principal or first-listed diagnosis**

   Category G89 codes are acceptable as principal diagnosis or the first listed code:

   - When pain control or pain management is the reason for the admission/ encounter (e.g., a patient with displaced intervertebral disc, nerve impingement and severe back pain presents for injection of steroid into the spinal canal). The underlying cause of the pain should be reported as an additional diagnosis, if known.
   - When a patient is admitted for the insertion of a neurostimulator for pain control, assign the appropriate pain code as the principal or first listed diagnosis. When an admission or encounter is for a procedure aimed at treating the underlying condition and a neurostimulator is inserted for pain control during the same admission/ encounter, a code for the underlying condition should be assigned as the principal diagnosis and the appropriate pain code should be assigned as a secondary diagnosis.

Chapter 6: Diseases of the Nervous System (G00-G99)

4. **Use of Category G89 Codes in Conjunction with Site Specific Pain Codes**

   a. **Assigning Category G89 and Site-Specific Pain Codes**

   Codes from category G89 may be used in conjunction with codes that identify the site of pain (including codes from chapter 18) if the category G89 code provides additional information. For example, if the code describes the site of the pain, but does not fully describe whether the pain is acute or chronic, then both codes should be assigned.

   b. **Sequencing of Category G89 Codes with Site-Specific Pain Codes**

   The sequencing of category G89 codes with site-specific pain codes (including chapter 18 codes), is dependent on the circumstances of the encounter/ admission as follows:

   - If the encounter is for pain control or pain management, assign the code from category G89 followed by the code identifying the specific site of pain (e.g., encounter for pain management for acute neck pain from trauma is assigned code G89.11, Acute pain due to trauma, followed by code M54.2, Cervicalgia, to identify the site of pain).
   - If the encounter is for any other reason except pain control or pain management and a related definitive diagnosis has not been established (confirmed) by the provider, assign the code for the specific site of pain first, followed by the appropriate code from category G89.

5. **Pain due to devices, implants and grafts**

   See Section I.C.19. Pain due to medical devices

6. **Postoperative Pain**

   The provider's documentation should be used to guide the coding of postoperative pain, as well as Section III Reporting Additional Diagnoses and Section IV Diagnostic Coding and Reporting in the Outpatient Setting.

   The default for post-thoracotomy and other postoperative pain not specified as acute or chronic is the code for the acute form.

   Routine or expected postoperative pain immediately after surgery should not be coded.

   a. **Postoperative pain not associated with specific postoperative complication**

   Postoperative pain not associated with a specific postoperative complication is assigned to the appropriate postoperative pain code in category G89.

   b. **Postoperative pain associated with specific postoperative complication**

   Postoperative pain associated with a specific postoperative complication (such as painful wire sutures) is assigned to the appropriate code(s) found in Chapter 19, Injury, poisoning, and certain other consequences of external causes. If appropriate, use additional code(s) from category G89 to identify acute or chronic pain (G89.18 or G89.28).

7. **Chronic pain**

   Chronic pain is classified to subcategory G89.2. There is no time frame defining when pain becomes chronic pain. The provider's documentation should be used to guide use of these codes.

Chapter 6: Diseases of the Nervous System (G00-G99)
8. Neoplasm Related Pain Code G89.3 is assigned to pain documented as being related, associated or due to cancer, primary or secondary malignancy, or tumor. This code is assigned regardless of whether the pain is acute or chronic. This code may be assigned as the principal or first-listed code when the stated reason for the admission/encounter is documented as pain control/pain management. The underlying neoplasm should be reported as an additional diagnosis. When the reason for the admission/encounter is management of the neoplasm and the pain associated with the neoplasm is also documented, code G89.3 may be assigned as an additional diagnosis. It is not necessary to assign an additional code for the site of the pain. *See Section I.C.2 for instructions on the sequencing of neoplasms for all other stated reasons for the admission/ encounter (except for pain control/pain management).*
9. Chronic pain syndrome Central pain syndrome (G89.0) and chronic pain syndrome (G89.4) are different than the term "chronic pain," and therefore these codes should only be used when the provider has specifically documented this condition. *See Section I.C.5. Pain disorders related to psychological factors*

Documentation Elements of Nervous System

Key documentation elements for nervous system coding include the following:

- Dominant versus nondominant side
- Laterality
  - right
  - left
  - bilateral
- Episode of care for injuries and other external causes of mortality or morbidity
  - Initial encounter
  - Subsequent encounter
  - Sequela
- Loss of consciousness time duration

Diseases, Disorders, Injuries, and Other Conditions of the Nervous System

This section of the chapter looks at a variety of diseases, disorders, injuries, and other conditions involving the nervous system. The information presented in the anatomy and physiology section is expanded here to provide a better understanding regarding the part of the nervous system that is affected and how these conditions affect nervous system function. Specific information is provided for more commonly encountered conditions involving the nervous system.

Following the discussion of the various diseases, disease processes, disorders, injuries, and conditions, some diagnostic statements are provided with examples of coding in ICD-10-CM. The coding practice is followed by questions to help reinforce the student's knowledge of anatomy, physiology, and coding concepts. Answers to the coding questions can be found by reviewing the text or referring to the ICD-10-CM coding book.

Section 1 – Infectious/Parasitic Diseases

There are a number of infectious and parasitic diseases that affect the nervous system. Coding infectious and parasitic diseases can be problematic because some of these conditions are found in Chapter 6 – Diseases of the Nervous System while others are found in Chapter 1 – Infectious and Parasitic Diseases. In addition, some infections are captured by a single code while others have instructions to code the underlying disease first and still others have instructions to use a second code to identify the organism. Some of the more common infectious and parasitic diseases affecting the nervous system are described here.

Section 1a – Encephalitis and encephalomyelitis

Encephalitis is an inflammation of the encephalon. The encephalon is the portion of the nervous system enclosed within the cranium, which is more commonly referred to as the brain. The term encephalitis most commonly refers to an inflammation of the brain resulting from a viral infection. Encephalomyelitis refers to an inflammation of the brain and spinal cord.

West Nile encephalitis is a severe form of West Nile virus infection that becomes neuroinvasive and affects the brain. Although 4 out of 5 people infected with the West Nile virus do not develop any disease, about 20% will develop mild or moderate disease symptoms of fever, headache, body aches, fatigue, swollen glands, and a skin rash that can last a few days or several weeks. In less than 1 percent of infected persons, the disease affects the central nervous system, causing encephalitis, meningitis, or poliomyelitis. Symptoms manifest as headache, high fever, stiff neck, disorientation, stupor, muscle weakness, tremors or convulsions, even coma and paralysis.

Section 1a Coding Practice

Condition	ICD-10-CM
West Nile infection complicated by encephalitis	A92.31
Admission for treatment of acute disseminated encephalitis due to adverse effect of H. influenzae vaccine	G04.02, T50.B95A
Rasmussen encephalitis	G04.81
Idiopathic encephalitis	G04.90

ICD-10-CM Anatomy & Physiology

Section 1a Questions

Can the code for West Nile encephalitis be found under the term 'Infection' or 'Encephalitis'? If not, what term in the Alphabetic Index is used to locate the correct code for West Nile encephalitis?

Why is the vaccine coded in addition to the encephalitis when the vaccine is determined to be the cause of the encephalitis?

Which diagnosis listed above is reported with an unspecified or NOS code?

Which diagnosis listed above is reported using an NEC code?

What additional information is provided in the ICD-10-CM code when coding an adverse effect of vaccine?

See end of chapter for Coding Practice answers.

Section 1b – Herpes Zoster

Herpes zoster is caused by the varicella virus, more commonly referred to as chicken pox. Anyone who has had chicken pox can develop herpes zoster, also called shingles. After the initial varicella infection resolves, the varicella virus remains in a dormant state in some nerve cells. If the virus reactivates, it results in herpes zoster characterized initially by burning, itching, tingling or extreme sensitivity of the skin usually limited to one location on one side of the body. Next, a red rash develops followed by groups of blisters at the site of the rash. The outbreak lasts for 2-3 weeks. Following the outbreak, an individual can develop another condition called post-herpetic neuralgia.

Section 1b Coding Practice

Condition	ICD-10-CM
Herpes zoster encephalitis	B02.0
Herpes zoster meningitis	B02.1
Herpes zoster myelitis	B02.24
Herpes zoster trigeminal neuralgia	B02.22
Herpes zoster	B02.9

Section 1b Questions

What part of the nervous system is affected in herpes zoster encephalitis? In herpes zoster meningitis?

Which codes report an uncomplicated herpes zoster infection?

Which diagnoses report complications of herpes zoster?

Which codes report post-herpetic outbreak conditions?

How is post-herpetic radiculopathy reported?

See end of chapter for Coding Practice answers.

Section 1c – Meningitis

Meningitis is an inflammation of the meninges, which are the membranous coverings of the brain and spinal cord. They consist of three layers. The outer membrane is a tough fibrous tissue called the dura mater. The middle membrane is a delicate fibrous tissue called the arachnoid. The inner membrane, called the pia mater, is a transparent membrane that adheres to the brain and spinal cord. Meningitis usually involves the dura mater and/or the arachnoid. When the arachnoid is affected, the condition may be referred to as arachnoiditis. Meningitis may be the result of a bacterial or viral infection or due to another noninfectious cause. The condition may be acute or chronic.

Section 1c Coding Practice

Condition	ICD-10-CM
Meningitis due to Lyme disease	A69.21
Meningitis due to coccidioidomycosis	B38.4
Bacterial meningitis due to H. influenzae	G00.0
Spinal meningitis	G03.9
Meningitis due to Streptococcus pneumoniae infection	G00.2, B95.3
Viral meningitis	A87.9

Section 1c Questions

Why is only one code required for reporting meningitis due to Lyme disease?

Which conditions listed above are reported using ICD-10-CM unspecified or NOS codes?

Why are two codes reported for meningitis due to Streptococcus pneumoniae infection?

See end of chapter for Coding Practice answers.

Section 2 – Neoplasms

Neoplasms of the nervous system, like all neoplasms, are abnormal tissues in which the cells grow and divide more rapidly than that of normal tissue. Primary CNS neoplasms can occur in tissues of the brain or spinal cord but brain tumors are more common than spinal cord tumors. Brain tumors may be benign or malignant with statistics showing that almost half of all brain tumors are benign. However, even benign brain tumors can recur and can be fatal. The CNS, particularly the brain, is also a common site of secondary malignant or metastatic brain tumors. The PNS may also be the site of either benign or malignant neoplastic disease.

Gliomas

The most common types of nervous system tumors are connective tissue tumors called gliomas. Gliomas are differentiated by the type of connective tissue from which they arise and include:

Astrocytoma – A malignant neoplasm arising from astrocytes, the star-shaped glial cells that wrap around nerve cells to form a supporting network around the neurons in the brain and spinal cord. Astrocytomas may be subclassified by tumor grade as follows:

- Grade I, also called pilocytic astrocytomas
- Grade II, also called fibrillary astrocytomas
- Grade III, also called anaplastic astrocytomas
- Grade IV, also called glioblastoma multiforme

Brain stem glioma – A malignant tumor located in the lower part of the brain.

Ependymoma – A tumor that arises from the cells that line the ventricles and the subarachnoid space surrounding the brain and spinal cord through which cerebrospinal fluid flows. These tumors may be benign, malignant, or of uncertain behavior.

Oligodendroglioma – A tumor that arises from oligodendrocytes – cells that produce a thick, fatty sheath that covers and protects the nerve cells. These slow-growing malignant tumors are most common in the cerebrum.

Schwannoma – A tumor of the myelin sheath arising from Schwann cells. These tumors are peripheral nervous system tumors that can be benign or malignant. The most common type of benign schwannoma is an acoustic neuroma, which is a tumor of the vestibulocochlear cranial nerve (CN VIII). The most common sites for malignant schwannomas are the sciatic nerve, brachial plexus, and sacral plexus.

Other Nervous System Neoplasms

Medulloblastoma – A tumor of the cerebellum usually in the region of the fourth ventricle or central part of the cerebellum, or less frequently in the cerebellar hemispheres.

Meningioma – A tumor that develops in the membrane covering the brain and spinal cord. The majority of meningiomas are benign, although approximately 10 percent are classified as atypical or malignant.

Neuroma – A neuroma is a benign lesion of a nerve or a thickening of nervous tissue. Some specific types of neuromas, such as acoustic neuromas, are classified as neoplasms and reported with codes from the neoplasm chapter whereas other neuromas, such as Morton's neuromas, are classified as mononeuropathies and are coded in the nervous system chapter.

Neurofibromatosis – The term neurofibromatosis is most commonly associated with a genetic condition that causes benign tumors to grow on nervous tissue causing skin and bone abnormalities. This condition is known as neurofibromatosis type 1 (NF1) and is reported with a code from the chapter on congenital malformations, deformations, and chromosomal abnormalities. A less common type, neurofibromatosis type 2 (NF2), causes bilateral neurofibroma-like tumors of the acoustic nerve. NF2 is reported as a benign tumor of the acoustic nerve with a code from the neoplasm chapter. There is also a malignant form of neurofibromatosis, which is reported with a code from the neoplasm chapter.

Secondary Nervous System Neoplasms

Secondary neoplasms of the nervous system are neoplasms that have metastasized from another site to the nervous system. A common site of metastatic lesions is the brain. For example, primary malignant neoplasms of the breast or lung often metastasize to the brain.

Section 2 Coding Practice

Condition	ICD-10-CM
Low grade, pilocytic astrocytoma of the cerebellum	C71.6
Benign ependymoma at the base of the spinal cord	D33.4
Von Recklinghausen's disease	Q85.01
Malignant schwannoma, left sciatic nerve	C47.22
Meningothelial meningioma of the right frontal parasagittal region of the brain	D32.0
Subependymal glioma of the brain	D43.2
Spinal cord tumor, lumbosacral region	D49.7
Right upper outer quadrant breast cancer previously excised with admission for surgical treatment of metastasis to brain.	C79.31, Z85.3

Section 2 Questions

Why is neurofibromatosis type 1 reported with a code from Chapter 17, Congenital Malformations, Deformations, and Chromosomal Abnormalities?

What information is provided in the ICD-10-CM code for malignant schwannoma of the left sciatic nerve?

How are malignant neoplasms of peripheral nerves classified?

Even though meningothelial meningioma is not specifically described as a benign tumor, it is reported with a code for a benign neoplasm. Why?

See end of chapter for Coding Practice answers.

Section 3 – Systemic Atrophies Affecting the CNS

Systemic atrophies affecting the CNS are a group of motor neuron diseases that affect muscle control and strength. Many of these conditions have a hereditary component, meaning that they are caused by inherited genetic disorders. Terms used to describe these systemic atrophies include atrophy, ataxia, palsy, and sclerosis.

Huntington's disease is an autosomal dominant inherited disorder that manifests in adulthood and causes degeneration and death of certain nerve cells in the brain, accompanied by brain atrophy primarily in the basal ganglia and cerebral cortex. Symptoms of Huntington's disease include involuntary muscle movement, dementia, and behavioral changes.

Hereditary spastic paraplegia (HSP), also called familial spastic paraplegia (FSP), is a group of disorders, all of which are characterized by progressive weakness and spasticity or stiffness in the legs. Symptoms begin with mild stiffness of the legs and minor gait impairment. The condition usually progresses slowly with individuals eventually requiring the assistance of a cane, crutches, or wheelchair. Some forms of HSP are accompanied by other symptoms including optic nerve and retinal diseases, cataracts, generalized lack of muscle coordination (ataxia), epilepsy, cognitive impairment, peripheral neuropathy, and deafness. Several genetic disorders have been identified in individuals with HSP. Genetic testing can help identify the specific form of the disease.

Amyotrophic lateral sclerosis (ALS), also called Lou Gehrig's disease, is a progressive, fatal neurological disease. ALS belongs to a group of motor neuron diseases which are characterized by gradual degeneration and death of motor neurons. Motor neurons located in the brain, brain stem, and spinal cord are the control and communication pathways between the nervous system and voluntary muscles. Messages from upper motor neurons in the brain and brainstem are transmitted to lower motor neurons in the spinal cord and then along nerve fibers to specific voluntary muscles. In ALS, both upper and lower motor neurons degenerate and die. Because muscles no longer receive messages to move, the muscles weaken and atrophy. Eventually, the motor neurons in the brain lose the ability to control voluntary movement and all muscle control is lost. When control of the diaphragm and chest wall is lost, the individuals lose the ability to breathe on their own and ventilator support is necessary. Most people with ALS die from respiratory failure within 3-5 years of disease onset.

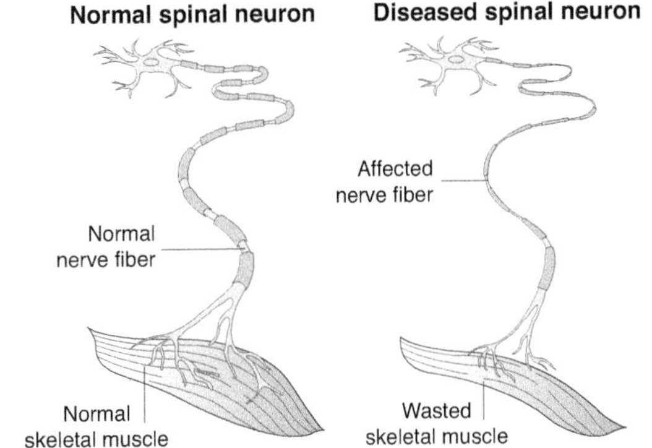

Section 3 Coding Practice

Condition	ICD-10-CM
Familial spastic paraplegia	G11.4
Late stage amyotrophic lateral sclerosis requiring ventilator support	G12.21, Z99.11
Huntington's dementia	G10
Spinal muscle atrophy, juvenile, type III	G12.1

Section 3 Questions

What terms in the ICD-10-CM Alphabetic Index are used to identify the code for continuous ventilator support?

What is another term for juvenile spinal muscle atrophy III?

See end of chapter for Coding Practice answers.

Section 4 – Parkinson's Disease

Parkinson's disease is a brain disorder in which nerve cells in an area of the brain known as the substantia negra become impaired or die. These nerve cells produce the chemical dopamine which is necessary for muscle coordination. Symptoms of Parkinson's disease include tremor, slow movement, rigidity, and problems with balance. Parkinson's disease can be primary or secondary. Primary Parkinson's disease is defined as disease that cannot be linked to another condition as the cause. Secondary Parkinson's disease is disease that can be linked to chemical or environmental toxins such as certain drugs, to a brain inflammation such as encephalitis, to cerebrovascular disease, or to another physiological condition.

Section 4 Coding Practice

Condition	ICD-10-CM
Parkinson's disease without dementia	G20
Parkinson's disease secondary to long-term haloperidol use, taken as prescribed	T43.4X5S, G21.11
Admission for malignant neuroleptic syndrome due to olanzapine (antipsychotic NEC), used as prescribed	T43.505A, G21.0
Atypical parkinsonism due to vascular compromise caused by cerebrovascular arteriosclerosis	I67.2, G21.4

Section 4 Questions

Why is the adverse effect code reported first?

How is Parkinson's disease with related dementia coded?

See end of chapter for Coding Practice answers.

Section 5 – Alzheimer's Disease and Other Degenerative Diseases of the Nervous System

Alzheimer's disease is a progressive fatal brain disease. The disease destroys brain cells, which leads to memory loss, confusion, disruption of thought processes, and behavioral disorders. In individuals with Alzheimer's disease, nerve impulses that form memory and influence thinking are disrupted both within the damaged nerve cells and at nerve synapses. This means that nerve impulses are not transmitted along nerve fibers or from one nerve cell to the next in the brain. Eventually, the nerve cells die and brain tissue atrophies. Damage occurs in the cortex which is responsible for thinking, planning, and remembering and is especially severe in the hippocampus which is responsible for the formation of new memories. As the brain atrophies, the fluid-filled ventricles enlarge.

Other degenerative diseases of the brain include frontotemporal dementia, senile degeneration of the brain not elsewhere classified, and degeneration due to alcohol abuse.

Section 5 Coding Practice

Condition	ICD-10-CM
Alzheimer's disease without behavioral disturbance	G30.9, F02.80
Alcoholic encephalopathy due to chronic alcoholism	G31.2, F10.20
Frontal lobe degeneration with dementia including agitated and aggressive behavior	G31.09, F02.81
Sub-acute necrotizing encephalopathy	G31.82

Section 5 Questions

What instruction for coding alcoholic encephalopathy is present in ICD-10-CM?

Under what term is the code for Alzheimer's disease found in the Alphabetic Index?

How is Alzheimer's disease classified in ICD-10-CM?

See end of chapter for Coding Practice answers.

Section 6 – Multiple Sclerosis and Other Demyelinating Diseases of the Nervous System

Multiple sclerosis is a chronic demyelinating disease of the central nervous system that may be disabling. While the cause is not known, it is believed to be an autoimmune disorder in which the body's defense system attacks myelin that surrounds and protects nerve fibers in the brain, spinal cord, and optic nerves. The nerve fibers may also be damaged. The damaged myelin then forms patches of scar tissue, also referred to as sclerosis or plaque. Symptoms include fatigue; weakness; numbness (paresthesia); dizziness (vertigo); disturbances in gait, balance, and coordination; bladder and bowel dysfunction; vision problems; and mood changes.

While multiple sclerosis is the most common type of demyelinating disease, there are a number of other types such as optic neuritis with demyelination, diffuse sclerosis of the central nervous system, and necrotizing myelitis of the central nervous system. Another common condition acute transverse myelitis is a spinal cord disorder which is an acute inflammation of the white and gray matter of one or more spinal cord segments, usually in the thoracic spine. Symptoms include bilateral motor, sensory and sphincter deficits below the level of the lesion that can progress over a short period to paraplegia, loss of sensation below the lesion, urinary retention and bowel incontinence.

Acute transverse myelitis is most commonly caused by multiple sclerosis however it has also been linked to neuromyelitis optica, infections, immunizations, autoimmune inflammation, vasculitis and certain drugs.

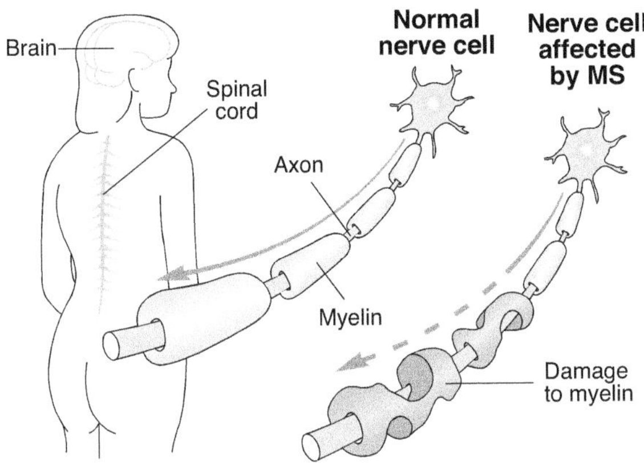

Section 6 Coding Practice

Condition	ICD-10-CM
Multiple sclerosis	G35
Demyelinating callosal encephalopathy	G37.1
Patient with multiple sclerosis is now diagnosed with neuromyelitis optica	G36.0, G35
Periaxial encephalitis	G37.0
Sub-acute necrotizing myelitis of the central nervous system (CNS)	G37.4

Section 6 Questions

In addition to Multiple Sclerosis, what other code categories are available for demyelinating diseases of the central nervous system?

How is Schilder's disease coded?

How is multiple sclerosis with acute transverse myelitis coded?

See end of chapter for Coding Practice answers.

Section 7 – Epilepsy, Seizure Disorders, and Seizures

Epilepsy, also referred to as a seizure disorder, is caused by a surge of electrical signals in all or a part of the brain. Seizure manifestations as well as the length of the seizure may vary considerably. A seizure may be exhibited by convulsions, loss of consciousness, blank staring, or jerky movements of the arms or legs. The seizure may last for a few seconds to several minutes. Only when an individual has two or more incidents of unprovoked seizure activity is a diagnosis of epilepsy made. There are many different types of epileptic seizures but these are generally divided into two broad categories, localization related seizures, also referred to as focal or partial seizures, and generalized seizures. These two broad categories are then further defined by whether the seizures are intractable or not and whether they present with status epilepticus or without status epilepticus. Intractable epilepsy is epilepsy that is not well controlled. Status epilepticus refers to recurrent or continuous seizure activity lasting more than 30 minutes.

A nonspecific diagnosis of seizure or convulsion disorder is reported with codes from the signs and symptoms chapter.

Section 7 Coding Practice

Condition	ICD-10-CM
Epilepsy with myoclonic seizures, intractable without status epilepticus	G40.319
Somatomotor epilepsy	G40.109
Petit mal seizures with status epilepticus	G40.A01
Seizure NOS	R56.9

Section 7 Questions

How is epilepsy with intractable seizures and status epilepticus coded?

Why is seizure NOS coded as a sign or symptom and not as epilepsy?

See end of chapter for Coding Practice answers.

Section 8 – Migraine

A migraine is a headache that can be extremely painful and can last for several hours or days. Some migraines are preceded by an aura or sensory warning that a migraine is imminent. The aura may consist of flashes of light, blind spots, and/or tingling in the arms or legs. The cause of migraines is not entirely understood, but they may be caused by changes in the trigeminal nerve and/or changes in serotonin levels in the brain. The trigeminal nerve is a major pain pathway. It is also known that serotonin levels drop during a migraine, which may cause the release of neuropeptides that then travel to the meninges causing the headache pain. It is also known that both internal and external environmental factors can trigger migraines. Known triggers include: hormone changes, some foods, stress, sensory stimuli, changes in wake-sleep patterns, physical exertion including sexual activity, changes in the weather or barometric pressure, and some medications.

Status migrainosus refers to a debilitating migraine lasting more than 72 hours. When coding status migrainosus, both the length of time and the debilitating nature of the attack must be documented.

Section 8 Coding Practice

Condition	ICD-10-CM
Migraine with aura, controlled with verapamil	G43.109
Persistent migraine aura, without cerebral infarction not intractable	G43.509
Migraine related to menstrual cycle, responsive to Imitrex	G43.829
Debilitating classic migraine for the past 4 days, unresponsive to medication	G43.111
Migraine with cyclical vomiting, not intractable, without status migrainosus	G43.A0

Section 8 Questions

When coding for migraine, what types of information need to be documented?

How are migraine variants coded in ICD-10-CM?

See end of chapter for Coding Practice answers.

Section 9 – Transient Ischemic Attacks

A transient ischemic attack (TIA) is a mini-stroke that typically lasts only a few minutes. A TIA is caused by an interruption of blood supply to a part of the brain. Symptoms may be similar to those of a stroke but typically resolve within 24 hours. Symptoms include: numbness or weakness in the face, arm, or leg usually only on one side; confusion; difficulty speaking or understanding speech; vision changes in one or both eyes; difficulty walking; dizziness; or loss of balance or coordination.

Section 9 Coding Practice

Condition	ICD-10-CM
TIA	G45.9
Recurrent focal cerebral ischemia	G45.8
Vertebrobasilar artery insufficiency	G45.0
Internal carotid artery syndrome	G45.1

Section 9 Questions

Why are transient ischemic attacks and related artery syndromes coded in the nervous system chapter instead of the circulatory system chapter?

How is cerebral artery spasm coded?

See end of chapter for Coding Practice answers.

Section 10 – Trigeminal Neuralgia and Other Nerve Disorders

Neuralgia refers to pain along the path of a nerve. Neuralgia may be caused by infection or inflammation, trauma, compression, or chemical irritation. The most common site of neuralgia is along the trigeminal nerve, also referred to as cranial nerve V (CN V). The trigeminal nerve is the main sensory nerve that innervates the side of the face and eye area. Symptoms include very painful, sharp spasms that typically last only a few seconds or minutes. Pain usually occurs on only one side of the face around the eye, cheek, and/or lower aspect of the face.

Other nerve disorders covered in this section include disorders of the facial nerve such as paralysis, twitching, and weakness. These types of disorders may be caused by an infection, injury, or tumor, but are more commonly idiopathic which means they are of unknown origin. If the nerve disorder is due to an infection, injury, or tumor, a code from one of those chapters would be used instead of a nervous system chapter code. Also many disorders of optic or acoustic nerves are covered in the chapters on the eye or ear.

Nonspecific diagnoses of neuralgia and neuritis are not reported with codes from the nervous system chapter. Instead, these nonspecific diagnoses are found in the musculoskeletal chapter.

Use caution when coding nerve disorders with the terminology of neuralgia, neuritis and neuropathy. Neuritis is an inflammation of the nerve and should not be coded in this section of ICD-10-CM.

Section 10 Coding Practice

Condition	ICD-10-CM
Trigeminal neuralgia	G50.0
Bell's palsy	G51.0
Glossopharyngeal neuralgia	G52.1
Neuralgia NOS	M79.2

Section 10 Questions

Neuralgia NOS is reported with a code from the musculoskeletal system chapter. Why is it listed in the musculoskeletal system chapter and not in the nervous system chapter?

How is clonic hemifacial spasm coded?

See end of chapter for Coding Practice answers.

Section 11 – Thoracic Outlet Syndrome and Other Nerve Root and Plexus Disorders

Nerve root and plexus disorders are typically caused by compression of these structures. Compression causes symptoms of pain and numbness. Compression caused by intervertebral disc disorders is considered to be a musculoskeletal condition and is reported with codes from the musculoskeletal system chapter.

The term 'thoracic outlet syndrome' refers to a condition in which the neurovascular structures just above the first rib and below the clavicle are compressed resulting in a number of symptoms. The brachial plexus is most commonly affected, although the subclavian artery or vein may also be compressed. The brachial plexus is formed by spinal nerves C5-T1. In thoracic outlet syndrome involving nervous system structures, usually the lower spinal nerve roots of C8-T1 are compressed causing pain and numbness along the ulnar nerve distribution. Sometimes the upper three spinal nerve roots C5-C7 are compressed causing pain and numbness in the neck, upper chest, upper back, and outer arm along the radial nerve distribution.

Section 11 Coding Practice

Condition	ICD-10-CM
Thoracic outlet syndrome	G54.0
Sacral plexus compression caused by metastatic lesions to the presacral soft tissues. Patient previously had a prostatectomy for prostate cancer	C79.89, G55, Z85.46
Supraclavicular lymphadenopathy due to non-Hodgkin's non-follicular lymphoma with compression of right brachial plexus	C83.91, G55
One year status post below-elbow amputation of right arm with painful phantom limb syndrome	G54.6, Z89.211

Section 11 Questions

What information is necessary to code amputation status accurately in ICD-10-CM?

What terminology is used in ICD-10-CM for diagnoses of brachial or lumbosacral plexus lesions and nerve root lesions?

How is compression of a nerve plexus coded when it is caused by another condition?

See end of chapter for Coding Practice answers.

Section 12 – Myasthenia Gravis, Muscular Dystrophy, and Other Diseases of the Myoneural Junction

Myoneural junction disorders, also called neuromuscular disorders, are caused by a defect in the transmission of nerve impulses from nerves to muscles. Transmission is interrupted at the (myoneural) junction where nerve cells connect to muscle tissue. Normally, when nerve impulses travel down a motor nerve, acetylcholine, a neurotransmitter, is released at the nerve ending. The acetylcholine travels across the neuromuscular junction and binds to receptors in the muscle, which activate causing the muscle to contract.

Myasthenia gravis is a chronic autoimmune neuromuscular disease caused by a defect in the transmission of nerve impulses from the nerve to the muscle it innervates. In myasthenia gravis, the body produces antibodies that block, alter, or destroy the acetylcholine receptors in the muscle tissue which prevents normal muscle contraction from occurring. Often the condition is more pronounced in muscles that control eye and eyelid movement, facial expression, chewing, talking, and swallowing; however, muscles that control breathing and movement in the neck and extremities may also be affected.

Muscular dystrophy is a group of more than 30 distinct genetic diseases that are characterized by progressive degeneration and weakness of the skeletal muscles that control movement. Some forms occur in infancy and childhood while others are not symptomatic until adolescence or adulthood. The different types also differ in respect to extent of muscle weakness, rate of progression, and pattern of inheritance. Duchenne's muscular dystrophy is the most common type and primarily affects boys. It is caused by the absence of dystrophin, a protein required to maintain the integrity of muscle tissue. Fascioscapulohumeral muscular dystrophy is the most common type manifesting in adolescence and affects muscles of the face, chest, shoulders, arms, and legs. Myotonic muscular dystrophy is the most common type manifesting in adulthood and is characterized by prolonged muscle spasms, cataracts, cardiac abnormalities, and endocrine disturbances.

Section 12 Coding Practice

Condition	ICD-10-CM
Myasthenia gravis	G70.00
Duchenne's muscular dystrophy	G71.0
Fascioscapulohumeral muscular dystrophy	G71.0
Myotonic muscular dystrophy	G71.11
Myasthenic syndrome due to uninodular goiter with thyrotoxicosis	E05.10, G73.3

Section 12 Questions

How is myasthenia gravis without documentation of exacerbation coded?

Is thyrotoxicosis the same thing as a thyrotoxic storm? If not, what is the difference?

How is initial encounter for accidental mercury induced myoneural disorder coded?

See end of chapter for Coding Practice answers.

Section 13 – Cerebral Palsy and Other Paralytic Syndromes

Cerebral palsy is a general term that can refer to a number of neurological disorders that manifest in infancy or early childhood. Cerebral palsy is caused by abnormalities in the brain in the areas that affect muscle control and movement. Most children are born with cerebral palsy but some develop it in infancy or early childhood following a brain infection or head injury. Cerebral palsy can cause a lack of muscle coordination when performing voluntary movements (ataxia); stiff or tight muscles and exaggerated reflexes (spasticity); muscle tone that is either too tight and stiff or too floppy; and gait abnormalities like dragging one foot or leg while walking, walking on toes, or moving with a crouched or scissored gait.

Also included in this section are hemiplegia, paraplegia, diplegia of upper limbs, and monoplegia, as well as other paralytic syndromes. These codes are used for a diagnosis of one of these conditions without further specification, when the condition is stated as old or longstanding, or in multiple coding scenarios.

Section 13 Coding Practice

Condition	ICD-10-CM
Congenital spastic diplegic cerebral palsy	G80.1
Long-term left-sided spastic hemiplegia (right side dominant)	G81.14
Long-standing locked-in state following brain stem stroke	I69.398, G83.5
Old cerebral infarction with right side dominant hemiplegia	I69.351

Section 13 Questions

Hereditary spastic paraplegia is not included in this code category. Where is it found and why is it listed in another category?

What does the term diplegic mean?

When hemiplegia is the result of a cerebral infarction, is a separate code required to describe the hemiplegia?

See end of chapter for Coding Practice answers.

Section 14 – Other Disorders of the Nervous System

The last section in the nervous system chapter includes pain and other disorders of the nervous system, including those of the autonomic nervous system, acquired hydrocephalus, complications of surgical procedures, and other conditions.

Pain

Pain codes in this section are for central pain syndrome, acute or chronic pain that is not classified elsewhere, neoplasm related pain, and chronic pain syndromes. More specific codes for pain are found in other chapters and in the chapter for signs, symptoms, and abnormal clinical and laboratory findings.

Disorders of the Autonomic Nervous System

The autonomic nervous system acts automatically and involuntarily to control smooth muscle, cardiac muscle, and glands. Disorders of the autonomic nervous system can affect heart rhythm, blood pressure, muscle tone, and facial sweating. Complex regional pain syndrome, a condition usually affecting a single extremity and characterized by burning or aching pain in the affected limb, swelling, skin discoloration, altered temperature, abnormal sweating, and hypersensitivity, is also found in this section.

Acquired Hydrocephalus

Acquired hydrocephalus occurs any time after birth and can occur at any age. It can be caused by injury or disease such as hemorrhage, neoplasm, cystic lesion, or infection. Hydrocephalus is broadly categorized as communicating or non-communicating. In communicating hydrocephalus, the flow of CSF is blocked after it exits the ventricles, but can still flow between ventricles. In non-communicating hydrocephalus, the flow of CSF is blocked along one of the narrow passageways connecting the ventricles which prevents flow between them. A common site of blockage is the aqueduct of Sylvius, which is a small passage between the third and fourth ventricles in the middle of the brain.

Complications of Procedures

Complications of surgical procedures and other procedural interventions covers a wide variety of conditions including cerebrospinal fluid leak or spinal headache following spinal puncture, intracranial hypotension following shunting procedure, intraoperative or post-procedural hemorrhage or hematoma of a nervous system structure, as well as other complications.

Section 14 Coding Practice

Condition	ICD-10-CM
Post-traumatic hydrocephalus	G91.3
Admission for pain management of acute tumor-related pain from primary malignancy of pancreas	G89.3, C25.9
Arnold-Chiari malformation type 1	G93.5
Carotid sinus syndrome	G90.01
Prolonged post-procedural encephalopathy following coronary artery bypass procedure	G97.82, G93.49, Z95.1

Section 14 Questions

What type of nervous system disorder is carotid sinus syndrome?

What term is used to find the correct code for Arnold-Chiari malformation type 1?

Why is a complication code from the nervous system chapter used to report encephalopathy following CABG?

Where are intraoperative and post-procedural complications affecting the nervous system found?

See end of chapter for Coding Practice answers.

Section 15 – Nervous System Conditions Originating in the Perinatal Period

These nervous system conditions originate in the perinatal period which is defined as the period before birth through the first 28 days after birth. Conditions that originate in the perinatal period and persist or cause morbidity later in life are also reported with codes from the chapter for certain conditions originating in the perinatal period. Examples of nervous system conditions listed in this chapter include newborn convulsions, disturbances of cerebral status, and disorders of muscle tone.

Cerebral or periventricular leukomalacia is an injury to the white matter of the cerebrum often associated with premature birth. It is considered to be a precursor for neurological impairment and cerebral palsy.

Transient neonatal myasthenia gravis is a neuromuscular postsynaptic transmission defect that sometimes occurs in infants born to mothers with myasthenia gravis. Sucking, swallowing, and respiratory difficulties are the most common symptoms. The condition generally resolves spontaneously, but supportive management and administration of medication prior to feedings is sometimes necessary until the condition resolves.

Section 15 Coding Practice

Condition	ICD-10-CM
Floppy baby syndrome	P94.2
Convulsions NOS in newborn	P90
Neonatal periventricular leukomalacia	P91.2
Transient neonatal myasthenia gravis	P94.0

Section 15 Questions

Myasthenia gravis in adults is classified as a myoneural disorder. How is transient neonatal myasthenia gravis classified?

See end of chapter for Coding Practice answers.

Section 16 – Congenital Malformations of the Nervous System

Many anomalies of the nervous system can be either congenital or acquired. Acquired anomalies are reported with codes from the nervous system chapter (G codes) while most congenital anomalies are reported with codes from the chapter on congenital malformations, deformation, and chromosomal abnormalities (Q codes). Types of conditions included in this section are congenital malformations of the brain, malformations of the spinal cord and meninges, and agenesis or displacement of a nerve or nerve plexus.

Anencephaly is a neural tube defect that results when the portion of neural tube that will form the brain fails to close during the third or fourth week of fetal development. This results in absence of a major portion of the brain including the forebrain and cerebrum. In many cases, the skull, soft tissues of the scalp and skin also fail to form leaving the brain stem and other brain tissue exposed. Anencephalic newborns are unable to see, hear, and feel pain. The absence of the cerebrum leaves the newborn in an unconscious state with only reflex actions such as breathing intact. Most live-born newborns with anencephaly die within hours or days of birth.

An **encephalocele** is also a neural tube defect that causes saclike protrusions of the brain and cerebral meninges through openings in the skull. This condition results from failure of the neural tube to close properly during fetal development and can result in deformities in the midline of the upper part of the skull, the area between the forehead and nose, or in the back of the skull. Newborns with encephaloceles usually have dramatic deformities evident at birth. Encephaloceles may present with craniofacial deformities or other brain malformations. Newborns with encephaloceles may have other medical conditions including hydrocephalus, spastic quadriplegia, microcephaly, ataxia, developmental delay, vision problems, mental and growth retardation, and seizures.

Spina bifida is another neural tube defect caused by failure of the spinal portion of the neural tube to close properly during the first month of fetal development. The extent of the defect can vary from an open defect with significant damage to the spinal cord and nerves to a closed defect with only failure of the vertebrae to form properly in that region. The three most common types are myelomeningocele, meningocele, and spina bifida occulta. Myelomeningocele is the most severe form and is characterized by protrusion of the spinal cord and meninges from a defect in the spine. Meningocele is characterized by normal development of the spinal cord but with protrusion of meninges through a defect in the spine. Spina bifida occulta is the least severe form characterized by failure of the vertebrae to form properly over the spinal cord and meninges which are covered only by a layer of skin. Spina bifida may occur with or without hydrocephalus.

Section 16 Coding Practice

Condition	ICD-10-CM
Spina bifida occulta	Q76.0
Myelomeningocele, thoracolumbar region, with hydrocephalus	Q05.1
Hemianencephaly	Q00.0
Meningoencephalocele frontal region	Q01.0
Congenital phrenic nerve agenesis with resulting pulmonary hypoplasia	Q07.8, Q33.6

Section 16 Questions

Why is spina bifida occulta listed under congenital malformation of the spine instead of under congenital malformations of the nervous system?

____

____

See end of chapter for Coding Practice answers.

Section 17 – Signs, Symptoms, and Abnormal Findings

There are a number of signs, symptoms, and abnormal clinical and laboratory findings that are indicators of nervous system diseases and disorders. Signs and symptoms specific to the nervous system include:

- Abnormal involuntary movement
- Abnormalities of gait and mobility
- Lack of coordination
- Abnormal reflexes
- Transient paralysis
- Repeated falls
- Facial droop

More general signs and symptoms that could be an indicator of nervous system disease include:

- Drowsiness
- Stupor
- Coma
- Disorientation
- Amnesia
- Other altered mental status
- Vertigo
- Speech disturbances
- Malaise
- Fatigue
- Convulsions

Abnormal laboratory findings include:

- Abnormal blood work
- Abnormal urine tests
- Abnormal cerebrospinal fluid findings
- Elevated tumor associated antigens (TAA) or tumor specific antigens (TSA)

Abnormal findings on diagnostic imaging include:

- Space occupying lesion of CNS
- Abnormal echoencephalogram
- Unspecified white matter disease

Abnormal results of function studies include those identified by:

- Electroencephalogram (EEG)
- Brain scan
- Nerve stimulation studies
- Electromyogram (EMG)

Section 17 Coding Practice

Condition	ICD-10-CM
Generalized weakness	R53.1
Lethargy	R53.83
Transient alteration of awareness	R40.4
Abnormal cell counts in CSF	R83.6
Abnormal PET scan, brain	R94.02

Section 17 Questions

What types of malaise and fatigue are identified in ICD-10-CM?

____

____

See end of chapter for Coding Practice answers.

Section 18 – Nervous System Injuries, Poisonings, and Other External Causes

Injuries to the nervous system are defined as those conditions that are due to some type of trauma. Some nervous system conditions, such as a subarachnoid hemorrhage, may be of traumatic or nontraumatic origin. Documentation is of paramount importance in determining whether to select a code from the chapter for nervous system diseases or from the chapter for injuries, poisoning, and certain other consequences of external causes.

Injuries, poisonings, and other external causes require a seventh character extender to define the episode of care. Episode of care for injuries to the nervous system must be specified as:

A Initial encounter

D Subsequent encounter

S Sequela

Poisonings from drugs, chemicals, or other substances include toxic and adverse effects of drugs as well as a new underdosing category. The correct poisoning code is initially identified in the Table of Drugs and Chemicals and then verified in the Tabular list. Poisonings, toxic and adverse effects, and underdosing usually require the use of multiple codes to identify the drug or chemical as well as the specific manifestations or other conditions associated with the poisoning.

Other consequences of external causes cover a wide variety of conditions. Examples of conditions related to the nervous system and to mental and behavioral disorders include:

- Abuse or neglect
- Traumatic shock
- Complications related to medical or surgical procedures
- Complications related to nervous system devices

Codes in this chapter may also require the use of external cause codes to provide data for how the injury occurred, the intent (unintentional/accidental versus intentional/suicide/assault), the place of occurrence, and the activity being performed.

Section 18 Coding Practice

Condition	ICD-10-CM
Admitted for subdural hemorrhage sustained in a fall when the patient slipped on ice while walking in the driveway of his home. Loss of consciousness less than 30 minutes	S06.5X1A, W00.0XXA, Y93.01, Y92.014
Initial visit for displacement of electrode used for deep brain stimulation in patient with essential tremor	T85.120A, G25.0
Follow-up visit for re-evaluation of injury of lumbosacral sympathetic nerve	S34.5XXD
Healed displaced fracture of the right anterior acetabular wall with concomitant femoral nerve injury. Two years status post injury, motor function has returned but the patient continues to have symptoms consistent with meralgia paresthetica.	G57.11, S32.411S, S74.11XS

Section 18 Questions

What are the time frames regarding the loss of consciousness related to head trauma?

____

____

Which codes listed in the coding practice examples above are external cause codes?

____

____

Which types of external cause codes require a 7th character extension to identify the episode of care?

____

____

What does the 7th character extension for the external cause codes specify?

____

____

See end of chapter for Coding Practice answers.

Section 19 – Mental and Behavioral Disorders

Mental and behavioral disorders have a dedicated chapter in ICD-10-CM. However, because mental and behavioral disorders are clearly related to, or are an integral part of nervous system function, mental and behavioral disorders are discussed here in the nervous system section of this course. There are several broad classifications of mental and behavioral disorders including:

Disorders Due to Physiological Condition – Mental disorders in this section are all caused by some type of physiological condition such as cerebral disease, brain injury, or some other type of cerebral dysfunction. Many codes in this section require that the underlying physiological condition be coded first.

Disorders Due to Psychoactive Substance Use and Dependence – Codes in this section include alcohol, drug, and inhalant use, abuse, and dependence; nicotine dependence; and other psychoactive substance related disorders. Note that nicotine use is not coded from this section but is instead reported with a code from Chapter 21 as a factor influencing health status.

Psychotic Disorders – Some of the more common types of psychotic disorders include schizophrenia, bipolar disorder, and major depressive disorders.

Non-Psychotic Disorders – Anxiety and dissociative and stress-related mental disorders are types of non-psychotic disorders.

Other Disorders – Other disorders and conditions reported with codes from Chapter 5 include: eating disorders, sleep disorders, sexual dysfunction not due to a substance or physiological condition, personality disorders, mental retardation, some developmental disorders, and behavioral and emotional disorders of childhood and adolescence.

Section 19 Coding Practice

Condition	ICD-10-CM
Late onset Alzheimer's disease with dementia and combative behavior	G30.1, F02.81
Parkinson's disease with dementia	G31.83, F02.80
Post-concussion syndrome following concussion three weeks ago with loss of consciousness less than 30 minutes.	S06.0X1S, F07.81
Acute alcohol intoxication with blood alcohol level 22 mg/100 ml	F10.920, Y90.1

Condition	ICD-10-CM
Recurrent major depression of moderate severity	F33.1
Chronic posttraumatic stress syndrome	F43.12
Developmental dyslexia	F81.0

Section 19 Questions

Is F02.80 ever reported as the primary (first listed) diagnosis code?

Why are two codes required to report post-concussion syndrome?

Why is code Y90.1 used in conjunction with F10.920 in the example above?

See end of chapter for Coding Practice answers.

Terminology

Arachnoid – One of the three membranes that protect the brain and spinal cord. The arachnoid is the middle membrane and is composed of delicate fibrous tissue.

Autonomic nervous system – The part of the nervous system that controls the smooth muscle, cardiac muscle, and glands. It functions automatically and involuntarily being regulated by several centers in the brain, including the cerebral cortex, hypothalamus, and the medulla oblongata. The autonomic system consists entirely of motor fibers that transmit impulses from the CNS to smooth muscle, cardiac muscle, and glandular epithelium and affects visceral functions.

Central nervous system (CNS) – One of two primary divisions of the nervous system, the CNS is composed of two organs, the brain and spinal cord.

Dura mater – One of three membranes that protect the brain and spinal cord. The dura mater is the outer membrane and is composed of a tough fibrous tissue.

Encephalon – The brain.

Extradural – Lying outside of the dura mater.

Extracranial – Lying outside the cranial cavity or skull.

Ganglion – A group of nerve cell bodies; a term usually used to refer to a group of nerve cell bodies located in the peripheral nervous system.

Intracranial – Lying within the cranial cavity or skull.

Intraspinal – Lying within the vertebral canal.

Meninges – The three membranes that cover the brain and spinal cord which include an outer membrane called the dura mater, a middle membrane called the arachnoid, and an inner membrane called the pia mater.

Nerve – A cordlike structure composed of one or more myelinated and/or unmyelinated nerve fibers that lie outside the central nervous system protected by connective tissue and nourished with blood vessels. Nerves transmit nerve impulses to and from the central nervous system.

Nerve reflex – An automatic response to a nerve stimulus.

Neuroglia – Connective tissue cells of the central nervous system.

Neuron – Nerve cell; the functional unit of the nervous system consisting of a cell body, dendrites, and an axon.

Peripheral nervous system – All neural tissue that lies outside the skull and vertebral column which includes nerve roots, nerves, nerve plexuses, and ganglions.

Pia mater – One of three membranes that protect the brain and spinal cord. The pia mater is the inner transparent layer containing blood vessels and is adherent to the surfaces of the brain and spinal cord.

Spinal nerve root – One of two bundles of nerve fibers, a sensory bundle and a motor bundle, that emerge from the spinal cord and then combine to form the mixed spinal nerve.

Subdural – Lying under the outermost membrane that covers the brain and spinal cord.

Quiz: Nervous System

1. Gliomas are:
   a. Malignant tumors of connective tissue cells in the CNS
   b. Malignant tumors of connective tissue cells in the PNS
   c. Malignant, benign, or uncertain behavior tumors of the connective tissue cells in the CNS
   d. Malignant, benign, or uncertain behavior tumors of the nerve cells (neurons) in the CNS
2. The white matter of the brain is composed of:
   a. Myelinated nerve fibers
   b. Unmyelinated axons
   c. Neurons
   d. Schwann cells
3. The cerebellum is the ______________________area of the brain.
   a. Sensory
   b. Motor
   c. Pain sensor
   d. Autonomic
4. Cauda equina refers to:
   a. A portion of the brain stem
   b. The mid-portion of the spinal cord
   c. The spinal nerve roots in the lumbosacral region
   d. The paired coccygeal nerves
5. Irritability is defined as:
   a. The ability of nerve cells to respond to stimuli and convert them into nerve impulses
   b. Any stimulus that is strong enough to initiate transmission of a nerve impulse
   c. A series of subthreshold stimuli
   d. The ability of the nerve cell to transmit an impulse to another nerve cell or another tissue
6. The code for a neuroma at an amputation site is reported with a code from:
   a. Chapter 2 Neoplasms
   b. Chapter 6 Diseases of the Nervous System
   c. Chapter 19 Injury, poisoning, and certain other consequences of external causes
   d. Multiple codes are required from different chapters
7. Infections of the nervous system:
   a. Are always reported with a code from Chapter 1 Infections
   b. Are always reported with a code from Chapter 6 Diseases of the Nervous System
   c. May be reported with a code from either chapter
   d. May require a single code from Chapter 1 Infections, a single code from Chapter 6 Diseases of the Nervous System, or one or more codes from both chapters
8. The human body is able to repair damaged nerve cells when the cell body is intact and the axon has a neurilemma. True or False?
   a. True
   b. False
9. Which disease listed below is NOT categorized as a demyelinating disease?
   a. Acute hemorrhagic leukoencephalitis
   b. Myasthenia gravis
   c. Multiple sclerosis
   d. Periaxial encephalitis
10. When reporting conditions such as hemiplegia and nerve injuries, documentation required to assign the most specific code includes information regarding which side(s) of the body that is (are) affected. This coding concept is known as:
    a. Dominant side identification
    b. Seventh character extension
    c. Sequencing
    d. Laterality

See next page for answers.

Quiz Answers—Nervous System

1. Gliomas are:

   c. Malignant, benign, or uncertain behavior tumors of the connective tissue cells in the CNS

2. The white matter of the brain is composed of:

   a. Myelinated nerve fibers

3. The cerebellum is the area of the brain.

   b. Motor

4. Cauda equina refers to:

   c. The spinal nerve roots in the lumbosacral region

5. Irritability is defined as:

   a. The ability of nerve cells to respond to stimuli and convert them into nerve impulse

6. The code for a neuroma at an amputation site is reported with an ICD-10-CM code from:

   c. Chapter 19, Injury, Poisoning, and Certain Other Consequences of External Causes

7. Infections of the nervous system:

   d. May require a single code from Chapter 1 Infections, a single code from Chapter 6 Diseases of the Nervous System, or one or more codes from both chapters

8. The human body is able to repair damaged nerve cells when the cell body is intact and the axon has a neurilemma: True or False?

   a. True

9. Which disease listed below is NOT categorized as a demyelinating disease:

   b. Myasthenia gravis

10. When reporting conditions such as hemiplegia and nerve injuries documentation required to assign the most specific code includes information on which side(s) of the body is affected. This coding concept is known as:

   d. Laterality

Coding Practice Answers

Section 1a Coding Practice

Question: Can the code for West Nile encephalitis be found under the term 'Infection' or 'Encephalitis'? If not, what term in the Alphabetic Index is used to locate the correct code for West Nile encephalitis?

Answer: The code for West Nile encephalitis can be found under 'Virus, West Nile, with, encephalitis'. The entry for 'Infection, West Nile' refers the coder to 'see Virus, West Nile'. The entry for 'Infection, brain' refers 'see also Encephalitis'; however West Nile is not listed under 'Encephalitis, viral, arthropod-borne, mosquito-borne'.

Question: Why is the vaccine coded in addition to the encephalitis when the vaccine is determined to be the cause of the encephalitis?

Answer: The vaccine is coded in addition to the postimmunization encephalitis because coding instructions state to identify the vaccine with an additional code.

Question: Which diagnosis listed above is reported with an unspecified or NOS code?

Answer: Idiopathic encephalitis is coded to an unspecified code.

Question: Which diagnosis listed above is reported using an NEC code?

Answer: Rasmussen encephalitis is coded to an 'other specified' or 'not elsewhere classified' code.

Question: What additional information is provided in the ICD-10-CM code when coding an adverse effect of vaccine?

Answer: Coding an adverse effect of vaccine also provides information about the intent (accidental, intentional, assault, undetermined as well as whether it is an initial or subsequent encounter or sequela

Section 1b Coding Practice

Question: What part of the nervous system is affected in herpes zoster encephalitis? In herpes zoster meningitis?

Answer: The brain is affected in herpes zoster encephalitis while the membranous coverings of the brain and/or spinal cord are affected in herpes zoster meningitis.

Question: Which codes report an uncomplicated herpes zoster infection?

Answer: B02.9 reports an uncomplicated herpes zoster infection.

Question: Which diagnoses report complications of herpes zoster?

Answer: The codes for herpes zoster encephalitis, meningitis, genticulate ganglionitis, myelitis, polyneuropathy, and trigeminal neuralgia all report nervous system complications of herpes zoster.

Question: Which codes report post-herpetic outbreak conditions?

Answer: Code B02.22 for trigeminal neuralgia and B02.29 other postherpetic nervous system involvement for neuralgia NEC report a post-herpetic outbreak condition. This is a condition that occurs as a second outbreak of the herpes zoster virus.

Question: How is post-herpetic radiculopathy reported?

Answer: B02.29 Other postherpetic nervous system involvement

Section 1c Coding Practice

Question: Why is only one code required for reporting meningitis due to Lyme disease?

Answer: Only one code is required to report meningitis due to Lyme disease because A69.21 is a combination code that clearly identifies the two conditions documented in the diagnosis.

Question: Which conditions listed above are reported using unspecified or NOS codes?

Answer: Spinal meningitis is reported with unspecified code G03.9, as the causative agent is not identified. Viral meningitis is also reported with an unspecified code, A87.9, since there is no further information specifying the virus.

Question: Why are two codes reported for meningitis due to Streptococcus pneumoniae infection?

Answer: Code G00.2 Streptococcal meningitis has a use additional code notation to further identify the organism. While Streptococcus is an organism it has multiple forms therefore the code is not specific to the organism. B95-B97.89 are codes for organisms as the cause of diseases listed elsewhere.

Section 2 Coding Practice

Question: Why is neurofibromatosis type 1 reported with a code from Chapter 17, Congenital Malformations, Deformations, and Chromosomal Abnormalities?

Answer: Neurofibromatosis type 1 is coded within the congenital malformations chapter because this is a genetic disease process that causes the growth of benign, tumor-like masses along nervous tissue as well as causing deformities of skin and bone. These tumor-like masses are not coded as individual morphologic neoplasms.

Question: What information is provided in the ICD-10-CM code for malignant schwannoma of the left sciatic nerve?

Answer: The ICD-10-CM code for a malignant schwannoma of the left sciatic nerve provides information regarding the type of connective and soft tissue affected being a peripheral nerve, and the lower limb on the left side.

Question: How are malignant neoplasms of peripheral nerves classified?

Answer: Malignant neoplasms of peripheral nerves are classified under a category provided specifically for peripheral nerves and autonomic nervous system and further identified by body area (head/neck/face, upper limb, lower limb, thorax, etc.) as well as laterality when appropriate.

Question: Even though meningothelial meningioma is not specifically described as a benign tumor, it is reported with a code for a benign neoplasm. Why?

Answer: Although most meningiomas are benign, do not assume the meningothelial meningioma is benign and reference the morphology in the index, which refers to 'see Neoplasm, meninges, benign'.

Section 3 Coding Practice

Question: What terms in the Alphabetic Index are used to identify the code for continuous ventilator support?

Answer: The code for continuous ventilator support, Z99.11, can be found under the index entry for 'Dependence, on, respirator' or Dependence, on, ventilator'.

Question: What is another term for juvenile spinal muscle atrophy III?

Answer: Kugelberg-Welander disease

Section 4 Coding Practice

Question: Why is the adverse effect code reported first?

Answer: Adverse effect codes from categories T36-T65 are combination codes that include the substance involved as well as the external cause and no additional external cause code is required. Because of this structure, the adverse effect code is sequenced first, followed by the code(s) that specify the exact nature or manifestation of the adverse effect, e.g. the neuroleptic-induced Parkinsonism

Question: How is Parkinson's disease with related dementia coded?

Answer: Assign G20 for the Parkinson's disease and F02.80 or F02.81 for dementia in other diseases classified elsewhere with/without behavioral disturbances. Do not code as G31.83 dementia with Parkinsonism. Parkinsonism is a disorder that is a combination of multiple disorders that result in Parkinson like traits but not all patients with Parkinsonism have Parkinson's disease.

Section 5 Coding Practice

Question: What instruction for coding alcoholic encephalopathy is present in ICD-10-CM?

Answer: Instructions for coding alcoholic encephalopathy include a note to 'code also the associated alcoholism' from category F10-.

Question: Under what term is the code for Alzheimer's disease found in the Alphabetic Index?

Answer: In the Alphabetic Index, the code for Alzheimer's disease is found under the entry 'Disease, Alzheimer's'.

Question: How is Alzheimer's disease classified in ICD-10-CM?

Answer: Alzheimer's disease is classified as being early onset G30.0), late onset (G30.1), other specified (G30.8), and unspecified (G30.9). Codes for delirium (F05), and dementia with (F02.81) or without (F02.80) behavioral disturbance are also coded.

Section 6 Coding Practice

Question: In addition to Multiple Sclerosis, what other code categories are available for demyelinating diseases of the central nervous system?

Answer: There are three code categories of diagnosis codes for demyelinating diseases of the central nervous system in ICD-10-CM:

G35 Multiple sclerosis

G36 Other acute disseminated demyelination

G37 Other demyelinating diseases of central nervous system

For other than multiple sclerosis these categories are further subdivided into the following subcategories:

G36.0 Neuromyelitis optica [Devic]

G36.1 Acute and subacute hemorrhagic leukoencephalitis (Hurst)

G36.8 Other specified acute disseminated Demyelination

G36.9 Acute disseminated demyelination, Unspecified

G37.0 Diffuse sclerosis of central nervous system

G37.1 Central demyelination of corpus callosum

G37.2 Central pontine myelinolysis

G37.3 cute transverse myelitis in demyelinating disease of central nervous system

G37.4 Subacute necrotizing myelitis of central nervous system

G37.5 Concentric sclerosis [Balo} of central nervous system

G37.8 Other specified demyelinating diseases of central nervous system

G37.9 Demyelinating disease of central nervous system, unspecified

Question: How is Schilder's disease coded?

Answer: Schilder's disease is coded as G37.0 Diffuse sclerosis of central nervous system. Schilder's disease is listed as an inclusion term under G37.0. When referencing the Alphabetic Index, the look-up is Schilder disease which directs to code G37.0.

Question: How is multiple sclerosis with acute transverse myelitis coded?

Answer: How this would be coded would be based upon the presenting reason for the encounter. There is an Excludes 1 note under G37.3 Acute transverse myelitis in demyelinating diseases of the central nervous system excluding reporting of G35.0 multiple sclerosis with G37.3. If a patient with MS is presenting for management of the acute transverse myelitis, only the acute transverse myelitis should be coded.

Section 7 Coding Practice

Question: How is epilepsy with intractable seizures and status epilepticus coded?

Answer: Combination codes are used in ICD-10-CM to identify the type of epilepsy, the level of seizure control, and whether or not seizures present with status epilepticus. Each type is coded as either 'intractable' or 'not intractable' and further specified as either 'with status epilepticus' or 'without status epilepticus' and all four possible combinations are an inclusive part of the code description.

Question: Why is seizure NOS coded as a sign or symptom and not as epilepsy?

Answer: Seizure is coded as a sign or symptom and not as epilepsy because a seizure or convulsion is a sign of another, causative condition. Having a seizure does not automatically mean a person actually has a diagnosis of epilepsy. A seizure may also occur with other medical conditions without having epilepsy.

Section 8 Coding Practice

Question: When coding for migraine what types of information needs to be documented?

Answer: The type of migraine, the presence/absence of aura, the level of control and whether or not it presents with status migrainosus. Each type is coded as either 'intractable' or 'not intractable' and further specified as either 'with status migrainosus' or 'without status migrainosus' and These are combination codes with each term being an inclusive part of the code description.

Question: How are migraine variants coded in ICD-10-CM?

Answer: Each type of migraine variant is coded within its own subcategory which is even further subdivided. Cyclical vomiting, ophthalmoplegic migraine, periodic headache syndromes in child or adolescent, and abdominal migraine each have their own subcategory and are coded as combination codes to state the level of control, and whether or not it presents with status migrainosus. Each type is coded as either 'intractable' or 'not intractable' and further specified as either 'with status migrainosus' or 'without status migrainosus' and these combinations are an inclusive part of the code description.

Section 9 Coding Practice

Question: Why are transient ischemic attacks and related artery syndromes coded in the nervous system chapter instead of the circulatory system chapter?

Answer: Transient ischemic attacks, basilar and carotid artery syndromes, and transient global amnesia are coded in the nervous system chapter because these conditions involve the brain or a temporary loss or obstruction of blood flow to areas of the brain, causing neurological pathology.

Question: How is cerebral artery spasm coded?

Answer: Cerebral artery spasm is an inclusion term listed under G45.9 Transient cerebral ischemic attack, unspecified. Alphabetic Index look-up of Spasm, cerebral (arterial) (venous) directs to G45.9.

Section 10 Coding Practice

Question: In ICD-10-CM, neuralgia NOS is reported with a code from the musculoskeletal system chapter. Why is it listed in the musculoskeletal system chapter and not in the nervous system chapter?

Answer: Neuralgia or neuritis NOS is coded in the musculoskeletal system chapter because unspecified pain is considered a general soft tissue disorder and not a disorder of a specific nerve, nerve root, or nerve plexus.

Question: How is clonic hemifacial spasm coded?

Answer: Clonic hemifacial spasm is coded using G51.3. Look-up in the Alphabetic Index is Spasm, hemifacial (clonic), G51.3.

Section 11 Coding Practice

Question: What information is necessary to code amputation status accurately in ICD-10-CM?

Answer: Level of amputation (upper arm, lower leg, above elbow, below knee, etc.) and laterality.

Question: What terminology is used for diagnoses of brachial or lumbosacral plexus lesions and nerve root lesions?

Answer: The diagnostic terminology of brachial or lumbosacral plexus disorders and nerve root disorders is used in the Tabular Index.

Question: How is compression of a nerve plexus coded when it is caused by another condition?

Answer: When a nerve plexus or root is compressed due to another underlying condition, it is coded to the specific plexus or root lesion in addition to the underlying condition. A separate, valid, three-digit category code is available for reporting all nerve root and plexus compressions in diseases classified elsewhere.

Section 12 Coding Practice

Question: How is myasthenia gravis without documentation of exacerbation coded?

Answer: When separate codes exist for with or without a specified manifestation/condition and it is not documented as with or without, the default is without.

Question: Is thyrotoxicosis the same thing as a thyrotoxic storm? If not, what is the difference?

Answer: Thyrotoxicosis is not the same thing as a thyrotoxic storm or crisis. Thyrotoxicosis is a clinically morbid condition caused by excessive amounts of thyroid hormones in the body, which may be caused from overactivity of the thyroid gland or ingestion of exogenous hormones. A thyrotoxic crisis or storm is a life-threatening condition that develops from an extremely exacerbated state of untreated or poorly treated hyperthyroidism. One can have thyrotoxicosis without thyrotoxic storm.

Question: How is initial encounter for accidental mercury induced Myoneural disorder coded?

Answer: Mercury induced myoneural disorder, accidental T56.1X1A and G70.1. ICD-10-CM coding instructions for G70.1 toxic myoneural disorders state to code first the T code (T51-T65) to identify the toxic agent. The T codes for toxic effects further require causation such as accidental, intentional(self-harm), assault and undetermined. Causation is defined in the 6th character. The Official ICD-10-CM guidelines direct to assign causation as undetermined when it is unknown. In addition to causation, these codes require a 7th character to define the stage of care.

Section 13 Coding Practice

Question: Hereditary spastic paraplegia is not included in this code category. Where is it found and why is it listed in another category?

Answer: Hereditary spastic paraplegia is coded to G11.4. This is an inherited systemic disease that causes atrophy. It is classified with hereditary ataxias and coded in the same grouping with Huntington's disease and other inherited muscular atrophies affecting the central nervous system.

Question: What does the term diplegic mean?

Answer: Diplegic means paralysis of the corresponding (symmetrical) parts on either side of the body.

Question: When hemiplegia is the result of a cerebral infarction, is a separate code required to describe the hemiplegia?

Answer: When hemiplegia is the result of a cerebral infarction, a separate code is not required in ICD-10-CM to describe the hemiplegia, because combination codes are available that classify the specific sequela as following a cerebral infarction.

Section 14 Coding Practice

Question: What type of nervous system disorder is carotid sinus syndrome?

Answer: Carotid sinus syndrome is an idiopathic neuropathy affecting the peripheral autonomic nervous system. It causes syncope or a brief loss of consciousness when pressure sensors in the carotid artery are stimulated.

Question: What term is used to find the correct code for Arnold-Chiari malformation type 1?

Answer: Arnold-Chiari malformation type I is found under the term 'Compression, brain (stem)' or 'Chiari's, malformation, type 1' Looking under 'Arnold-Chiari disease, obstruction, or syndrome' provides the codes for type II and type IV, with a 'see Encephalocele' reference for type III.

Question: Why is a complication code from the nervous system chapter used to report encephalopathy following CABG ?

Answer: A complication code from the nervous system chapter is used to report encephalopathy following CABG because it is a complication of a surgical procedure affecting the nervous system. Codes for intra- and postprocedural complications affecting a particular system are located within the specific chapter.

Question: Where are intraoperative and post-procedural complications affecting the nervous system found?

Answer: Intraoperative and post-procedural complications affecting the nervous system are found in Chapter 6, Diseases of the Nervous System under category G97.

Section 15 Coding Practice

Question: Myasthenia gravis in adults is classified as a myoneural disorder. How is transient neonatal myasthenia gravis classified?

Answer: Transient neonatal myasthenia gravis is classified as an endocrine and metabolic disturbance specific to the fetus or newborn. It is classified as a disorder of muscle tone of the newborn.

Section 16 Coding Practice

Question: Why is spina bifida occulta listed under congenital malformation of the spine instead of under congenital malformations of the nervous system?

Answer: Spina bifida occulta is listed under congenital malformation of the spine instead of congenital malformation of the nervous system because it is a condition involving the spinal column, or vertebrae, which protect the spinal cord. Normal vertebral bone anatomy is affected. Radiography shows abnormal spinous processes and neural arches, but it usually does not cause nervous system problems because the spinal cord and nerves are rarely affected.

Section 17 Coding Practice

Question: What types of malaise and fatigue are identified in ICD-10-CM?

Answer: Weakness or asthenia NOS (R53.1), neoplastic (malignant) related fatigue (R53.0), other malaise (R53.81), and other fatigue (R53.83).

Section 18 Coding Practice

Question: What are the time frames regarding the loss of consciousness related to head trauma?

Answer: Time frames for loss of consciousness are an inherent part of the code description:

- Without loss of consciousness
- With loss of consciousness of 30 min or less
- With loss of consciousness of 31 min to 59 min
- With loss of consciousness of 1 hour to 5 hours 59 min
- With loss of consciousness of 6 hours to 24 hours
- With loss of consciousness greater than 24 hours with return to pre-existing conscious level with patient surviving
- With loss of consciousness greater than 24 hours without return to pre-existing conscious level with patient surviving
- With loss of consciousness of any duration with death due to brain injury prior to regaining consciousness
- With loss of consciousness of any duration with death due to other cause prior to regaining consciousness
- With loss of consciousness of unspecified duration

Question: Which codes listed in the practice examples above are external cause codes?

Answer: Only the codes that begin with W and Y in the coding practice examples above are external causes of morbidity codes.

Question: Which types of external cause codes require a 7th character extension to identify the episode of care?

Answer: Almost all categories of external cause codes require the 7th character extension except complications of medical and surgical care (Y62-Y84), blood alcohol levels (Y90), and place of occurrence codes (Y92).

Question: What does the 7th character extension for the external cause codes specify?

Answer: The 7th character for the external cause codes specifies the initial or subsequent encounter, or sequela.

Section 19 Coding Practice

Question: Is F02.80 ever reported as the primary (first listed) diagnosis code?

Answer: Code F02.80 and F02.81 are manifestation codes and will never be reported as the first listed, primary diagnosis. Coding instructions require that the underlying physiological condition must be coded first.

Question: Why are two codes required to report postconcussion syndrome?

Answer: Two codes are required to report postconcussion syndrome per coding instructions for category F07 where postconcussion syndrome is classified. The underlying physiological condition must be coded first, so the appropriate concussion code with loss of consciousness is reported with a 7th digit denoting sequela, and the postconcussion syndrome code is listed next.

Question: Why is code Y90.1 used in conjunction with F10.920 in the example above?

Answer: Code Y90.1 in used in conjunction with F10.920 in the example above because an additional code is needed for the blood alcohol level, if applicable.

ICD-10-CM Documentation

Diseases and Disorders Affecting the Nervous System

Introduction

Diseases of the nervous system include disorders of the central nervous system that affect the brain and spinal cord, such as cerebral degeneration or Parkinson's disease, and diseases of the peripheral nervous system, such as polyneuropathy, myasthenia gravis, and muscular dystrophy. Some of the more commonly treated pain diagnoses are also classified as diseases of the nervous system, including: migraine and other headache syndromes, causalgia, complex regional pain syndrome I (CRPS I), neuralgia, and pain not elsewhere classified.

Physician documentation is the basis for code assignment and the importance of proper documentation is imperative. ICD-10-CM captures a greater level of specificity than in previous systems which will require more precise clinical information documented in the medical record. Updated and standardized clinical terminology is used in ICD-10-CM to be consistent with the current standards providers use when diagnosing and treating nervous system disorders. Clinical terms such as commonly used synonyms for "intractable" migraine and more current terminology for epilepsy are found in the code descriptions.

For example, the terms "epilepsy" and "seizure disorder" describe central nervous system disorders characterized by sudden-onset seizures and muscle contractions. Seizure disorders and recurrent seizures are classified with epilepsy; however, convulsions, seizures not otherwise specified, febrile seizures, and hysterical seizures are classified as non-epileptic. So, a detailed description of the seizure is needed in order to differentiate between epilepsy and other seizures and to distinguish between seizure types.

Many nervous system conditions are manifestations of other diseases and dual coding is often required to report both the underlying condition and the manifestation. Dual coding is frequently required for infectious diseases of the central nervous system and precise documentation is needed in order to determine whether the condition is coded to the nervous system or to an infectious disease combination code.

Combination codes for common etiologies and symptoms or manifestations (e.g., dementia with Parkinsonism) are common. The codes provide specific information and clinical detail. This places an even greater emphasis on the provider's documentation of the association between conditions, such as documenting the condition as "due to" a specified disease process.

Many diseases and conditions of the nervous system have additional elements which are captured in the code. For instance, providers routinely document the side of the body where disease or injury occurs (right, left, or bilateral), and laterality is included in many of the nervous system code description. Representative examples of documentation requirements are provided in this chapter to help identify documentation deficiencies so that physicians and coders are aware of the specificity needed for proper code assignment.

There are 11 code blocks for the central and peripheral nervous system. The table below shows the category blocks for nervous system disorders.

ICD-10-CM Blocks	
G00-G09	Inflammatory Diseases of the Central Nervous System
G10-G14	Systemic Atrophies Primarily Affecting the Central Nervous System
G20-G26	Extrapyramidal and Movement Disorders
G30-G32	Other Degenerative Diseases of the Nervous System
G35-G37	Demyelinating Diseases of the Central Nervous System
G40-G47	Episodic and Paroxysmal Disorders
G50-G59	Nerve, Nerve Root and Plexus Disorders
G60-G65	Polyneuropathies and other Disorders of the Peripheral Nervous System
G70-G73	Diseases of Myoneural Junction and Muscle
G80-G83	Cerebral Palsy and Other Paralytic Syndromes
G89-G99	Other Disorders of the Nervous System

The organization of nervous system diseases in ICD-10-CM includes:

- Hereditary and degenerative diseases of the central nervous system subdivided into four code blocks:
  - G10-G14 Systemic Atrophies Primarily Affecting the Central Nervous System
  - G20-G26 Extrapyramidal and Movement Disorders
  - G30-G32 Other Degenerative Diseases of the Nervous System
  - G35-G37 Demyelinating Diseases of the Central Nervous System
- Pain not elsewhere classified found in category G89 of code block G89-G99 Other Disorders of the Nervous System
- Other headache syndromes classified in category G44 in code block G40-G47 Episodic and Paroxysmal Disorders which also includes epilepsy (G40), migraine (G43), transient cerebral ischemic attacks and related syndromes (G45), vascular syndromes of brain in cerebrovascular diseases (G46), and sleep disorders (G47)

- Disorders of the peripheral nervous system subdivided into three code blocks:
  - G50-G59 Nerve, Nerve Root and Plexus Disorders
  - G60-G65 Polyneuropathies and other Disorders of the Peripheral Nervous System
  - G70-G73 Diseases of Myoneural Junction and Muscle
- Intraoperative and postprocedural complications specific to the nervous system classified in code block G89-G99 Other Disorders of the Nervous System

Because many underlying conditions can cause nervous system disorders, including infectious diseases, circulatory disorders, and external causes such as injury or drugs, careful review of the medical record documentation is needed in order to determine whether the condition is coded to the nervous system area.

Exclusions

There are no Excludes1 notes, but there are a number of Excludes2.

ICD-10-CM Excludes1	ICD-10-CM Excludes2
None	Certain conditions originating in the perinatal period (P04-P96) Certain infectious and parasitic diseases (A00-B99) Complications of pregnancy, childbirth and the puerperium (O00-O9A) Congenital malformations, deformations, and chromosomal abnormalities (Q00-Q99) Endocrine, nutritional and metabolic diseases (E00-E88) Injury, poisoning and certain other consequences of external causes (S00-T88) Neoplasms (C00-D49) Symptoms, signs and abnormal clinical and laboratory findings, not elsewhere classified (R00-R94)

Dominant/Nondominant Side

The side of the body affected (right, left) is a component of the code for conditions that affect one side of the body. Codes such as hemiplegia and hemiparesis (G81) and monoplegia of the upper limb (G83.2), and lower limb (G83.1) or unspecified monoplegia (G83.3) also identify whether the side affected is the dominant or nondominant side. When the documentation provides laterality but fails to identify the side affected as dominant or nondominant, and the classification system does not indicate a default, ICD-10-CM provides the following guidelines:

- For ambidextrous patients, the default should be dominant
- If the left side is affected, the default is non-dominant
- If the right side is affected, the default is dominant

Pain Not Elsewhere Classified (G89)

According to the guidelines, the pain codes in category G89 Pain, not elsewhere classified, are used in conjunction with codes from other categories and chapters to provide more detail about acute or chronic pain and neoplasm-related pain. However, if the pain is not specified in the provider documentation as acute or chronic, post-thoracotomy, postprocedural, or neoplasm-related, codes from category G89 are not assigned.

Codes from category G89 are not assigned when the underlying or definitive diagnosis is known, unless the reason for the encounter is pain management rather than management of the underlying condition. When an admission or encounter is for treatment of the underlying condition, a code for the underlying condition is assigned as the principal diagnosis and no code from category G89 is assigned. For example, when a patient is admitted for spinal fusion to treat a vertebral fracture, the code for the vertebral fracture would be assigned as the principal diagnosis but no pain code is assigned.

Category G89 Codes as Principal or First-Listed Diagnosis

Guidelines for assigning pain codes as the principal or first-listed diagnosis when pain control or pain management is the reason for the admission/encounter direct the user to assign a code for the underlying cause of the pain as an additional diagnosis, if known. A case example would be a patient with nerve impingement and severe back pain seen for a spinal canal steroid injection or a patient admitted for insertion of a neurostimulator for pain control; the appropriate pain code would be assigned as the principal or first-listed diagnosis. On the other hand, if the admission or encounter is for treatment of the underlying condition and a neurostimulator is also inserted for pain control during the same episode of care, the underlying condition is the principal diagnosis and the appropriate pain code should be assigned as a secondary diagnosis.

Category G89 Codes in Conjunction with Site-Specific Pain Codes

Pain codes from category G89 may be used in conjunction with site-specific pain codes that identify the site of pain if the category G89 code provides additional diagnostic information such as describing whether the pain is acute or chronic. The sequencing of codes is dependent on the circumstances of the admission/encounter, for example:

- The category G89 code is sequenced first followed by the code identifying the specific site of pain when the encounter is for pain control or pain management
- If the encounter is for any other reason and a related definitive diagnosis has not been confirmed in the provider's documentation, the specific site of the pain is coded first, followed by the category G89 code.

Postoperative Pain

Coding of postoperative pain is driven by the provider's documentation. For post-thoracotomy and other postoperative pain that is not specified as acute or chronic, the code for the acute form is the default.

Routine or expected postoperative pain immediately after surgery is not coded, but severe or an unexpected level of postoperative pain not associated with a specific postoperative complication is assigned to the appropriate postoperative pain code in category G89.

Chronic Pain

Codes in category G89 differentiate between acute and chronic pain. There is no time frame defining when pain becomes chronic pain so the provider's documentation directs the use of these codes. When chronic pain is documented, it is coded to subcategory G89.2. It is important to note that central pain syndrome (G89.0) and chronic pain syndrome (G89.4) are not the same as "chronic pain," so these codes should only be used when the provider has specifically documented these conditions.

Neoplasm Related Pain

Code G89.3 is assigned when the patient's pain is documented as being related to, associated with, or due to cancer, primary or secondary malignancy, or tumor. The code for neoplasm-related pain is assigned regardless of whether the pain is documented as acute or chronic. When the reason for the admission/ encounter is documented as pain control/pain management, G89.3 is assigned as the principal or first-listed code with the underlying neoplasm reported as an additional diagnosis. When the admission/encounter is for management of the neoplasm and the pain associated with the neoplasm is also documented, code G89.3 may be assigned as an additional diagnosis. It is not necessary to assign an additional code for the site of the pain.

General Documentation Requirements

General documentation requirements differ depending on the particular nervous system disease or disorder. In general, specificity of the type and cause of the nervous system disorder is required and must be documented in the medical record. Some of the general documentation requirements are discussed here, but greater detail for some of the more common diseases and conditions of the nervous system will be provided in the next section.

According to the *ICD-10-CM Official Guidelines for Coding and Reporting*, complete and accurate code assignment requires a joint effort between the provider and the coder. Without consistent, complete documentation in the medical record, accurate coding cannot be achieved. Much of the detail captured in the ICD-10-CM codes is routinely documented by providers, such as the severity or status of the disease in terms of acuity, the etiology (e.g., neoplasm-related pain), and the significance of related diagnostic findings (e.g., EEG confirms a seizure disorder). Beyond these basic medical record documentation requirements, specifically describing the site, such as the specific nerve (e.g., lesion of medial popliteal nerve, right lower limb) rather than a general anatomical site will ensure optimal code assignment for nervous system disorders.

Documentation in the patient's record should clearly specify the cause-and-effect relationship between a symptom, manifestation, or complication and a disease or a medical intervention. For example, documentation should specify whether a complication occurred intraoperatively, as in intraoperative hemorrhage, or postoperatively.

In addition to these general documentation requirements, there are specific diseases and disorders that require greater detail in documentation to ensure optimal code assignment.

Code-Specific Documentation Requirements

In this section, the ICD-10-CM code categories, subcategories, and subclassifications for some of the more commonly reported diseases and conditions affecting the nervous system are reviewed along with documentation requirements. Though not all of the codes with documentation requirements are discussed, this section will provide a representative sample of the type of additional documentation required for diseases affecting the nervous system. The section is organized alphabetically by the code category, subcategory, or subclassification, of the condition whether or not it is coded in the Nervous System Chapter or not.

Acoustic Nerve Disorders

Acoustic nerve disorders are caused by lesions or other dysfunction of the cochlea and acoustic nerve, rather than a problem of conduction. The eighth cranial nerve (the acoustic nerve) controls hearing, balance and head position. The acoustic nerve is known by several names including the auditory nerve, the vestibulocochlear nerve, the cochlear nerve and the vestibular nerve. The causes of acoustic neuritis are varied and include toxins, medications, injuries, tumors, infections, and other conditions that may damage the nerve.

In ICD-10-CM, codes for disorders of the acoustic nerve are found in category H93 Other disorders of ear, not elsewhere classified and in category H94 Other disorders of ear in diseases classified elsewhere. While the subcategory H93.3 Other disorders of the acoustic nerve does not provide codes for specific conditions, the subcategory H94.0 is specific to acoustic neuritis in infectious and parasitic diseases classified elsewhere.

Coding and Documentation Requirements

Identify type:

- Disorder of acoustic nerve
- Acoustic neuritis in infectious and parasitic diseases classified elsewhere

Identify laterality:

- Right acoustic nerve
- Left acoustic nerve
- Bilateral acoustic nerves
- Unspecified

For acoustic neuritis in infectious and parasitic diseases classified elsewhere, code first underlying disease, such as:

- Parasitic disease (B65-B89)

ICD-10-CM Code/Documentation	
Disorders of acoustic nerve	
H93.3X1	Right
H93.3X2	Left
H93.3X3	Bilateral
H93.3X9	Unspecified
Acoustic neuritis in infectious parasitic diseases classified elsewhere	
H94.00	Unspecified
H94.01	Right ear
H94.02	Left ear
H94.03	Bilateral

Documentation and Coding Example

Fifty-two-year-old Asian male returns for follow-up of dizziness and unsteady gait. Patient was in his usual state of good health 3 months ago when he developed a sudden onset of severe vertigo, nausea and vomiting. He thought it was a viral illness and self-treated with rest and fluids. The nausea and vomiting abated after 2 days but he continued to feel dizzy. He first presented to the clinic about 1 week after the onset of symptoms and was noted to have nystagmus in addition to an unsteady gait. His symptoms improved when lying down, intensified when sitting or standing. He was prescribed Meclizine initially and later used Scopolamine patches. He was seen 3 weeks later with continued symptoms and had an MRI to r/o tumor or stroke. MRI was negative and symptoms slowly began to improve. T 97.4, P 58, R 12, BP 136/80. On examination, this is a thin but muscular gentleman who looks younger that his stated age. Overall, he feels like he is almost back to normal. He states he still has some unsteadiness with balance when he gets fatigued but his gait is normal. He has had only 3-4 episodes of very mild vertigo in the past month that did not require medication.

Impression: **Acoustic neuritis bilaterally, resolving**.

Plan: RTC if symptoms worsen.

Diagnosis: **Bilateral acoustic neuritis.**

Diagnosis Code(s)

H93.3X3 Disorders of bilateral acoustic nerves

Coding Note(s)

The ICD-10-CM Index entries for Neuritis, acoustic (nerve) and Neuritis, auditory (nerve) direct the coder to subcategory H93.3. These codes also specify the affected ear(s).

Alteration of Consciousness

Category R40 Somnolence, stupor and coma has specific codes for somnolence (R40.0), stupor (R40.1), persistent vegetative state (R40.3), and transient alteration of awareness (R40.4). In addition to these codes, subcategory R40.2 Coma has a code for unspecified coma (R40.20), but more importantly, it contains coma scale codes and Glasgow coma scale total scores. The coma scale codes and coma scale total scores are used primarily by trauma registries but may also be reported by emergency medical services, acute care facilities, and other providers and facilities wanting to capture this information.

In order to complete the coma scale, information must be collected on the following:

- Eye opening response
- Best verbal response
- Best motor response

Eye opening response is scored as follows:

- No eye-opening response (1 point)
- Eye opening to pain only (not applied to face) (2 points)
- Eye opening to verbal stimuli, command, speech (3 points)
- Spontaneous – open with blinking at baseline (4 points)

Verbal response is scored as follows:

- No verbal response (1 point)
- Incomprehensible speech (2 points)
- Inappropriate words (3 points)
- Confused conversation, but able to answer questions (4 points)
- Oriented (5 points)

Motor response is scored as follows:

- No motor response (1 point)
- Extension response to pain (decerebrate posturing) (2 points)
- Flexion response to pain (decorticate posturing) (3 points)
- Withdraws in response to pain (flexion withdrawal) (4 points)
- Purposeful movement in response to painful stimulus (localizes pain) (5 points)
- Obeys commands for movement (6 points)

The scores for each of the three components are then added together to obtain the Glasgow Coma Scale (GCS) total score.

The total score is used to determine the severity of the head injury which is as follows:

- Severe head injury – GCS total score 3-8
- Moderate head injury – GCS total score 9-12
- Mild head injury – GCS total score 13-15

Coding and documentation requirements below are provided for the Glasgow Coma Scale components and total score.

Coding and Documentation Requirements

Coma Scale – Use individual scores, if known. All three elements—eye opening, best verbal response, and best motor response must be known to use individual scores. If all three elements are not documented, but the Glasgow Coma Scale total score is documented, use the code for the total score.

Identify individual scores:

- Eyes open:
  - Never
  - To pain

- To sound
- Spontaneous
- Best verbal response:
  - None
  - Incomprehensible words
  - Inappropriate words
  - Confused conversation
  - Oriented
- Best motor response:
  - None
  - Extension
  - Abnormal flexion
  - Flexion withdrawal
  - Localizes pain
  - Obeys commands

Identify time/place of coma score obtained:

- In the field (EMT/ambulance)
- At arrival to emergency department
- At hospital admission
- 24 hours or more after hospital admission
- Unspecified time -OR Identify

Glasgow coma scale total score:

- Glasgow score 13-15
- Glasgow score 9-12
- Glasgow score 3-8
- Other coma, without documented Glasgow coma scale score, or with partial score reported

Identify time/place of coma scale total score obtained:

- In the field (EMT/ambulance)
- At arrival to emergency department
- At hospital admission
- 24 hours or more after hospital admission
- Unspecified time

ICD-10-CM Code/Documentation	
R40.0	Somnolence
R40.1	Stupor
R40.3	Persistent vegetative state
R40.4	Transient alteration of awareness
R40.20	Unspecified coma
Coma Scale, Eyes Open	
R40.211-	Coma scale, eyes open, never
R40.212-	Coma scale, eyes open, to pain
R40.213-	Coma scale, eyes open, to sound
R40.214-	Coma scale, eyes open, spontaneous
Coma Scale, Best Verbal Response	
R40.221-	Coma scale, best verbal response, none
R40.222-	Coma scale, best verbal response, incomprehensible words

ICD-10-CM Code/Documentation	
R40.223-	Coma scale, best verbal response, inappropriate words
R40.224-	Coma scale, best verbal response, confused conversation
R40.225-	Coma scale, best verbal response, oriented
Coma Scale, Best Motor Response	
R40.231-	Coma scale, best motor response, none
R40.232-	Coma scale, best motor response, extension
R40.233-	Coma scale, best motor response, abnormal flexion
R40.234-	Coma scale, best motor response, flexion withdrawal
R40.235-	Coma scale, best motor response, localizes pain
R40.236-	Coma scale, best motor response, obeys commands
Glasgow Coma Scale, total score	
R40.241-	Glasgow coma scale score 13-15
R40.242-	Glasgow coma scale score 9-12
R40.243-	Glasgow coma scale score 3-8
R40.244-	Other coma, without documented Glasgow coma scale score, or with partial score reported

Note: A code from each coma scale subcategory is required to complete the coma scale and these codes should be used only when documentation is available for all three components (R40.21-, R40.22-, and R40.23-). Codes in subcategory R40.24 may be reported alone. Codes in all four of these subcategories require a 7th character to identify the site/time of the coma evaluation:

- 0 – Unspecified time
- 1 – In the field [EMT or ambulance]
- 2 – At arrival to emergency department
- 3 – At hospital admission
- 4 – 24 hours or more after hospital admission

Documentation and Coding Example

Sixteen-year-old Caucasian male transported to local ED via ambulance after he was found unresponsive at home by his mother. Patient has a fresh 4 cm x 5 cm hematoma on left temporal area. Mother states her son was surfing earlier in the day and was hit in the head by his board. He continued surfing for approximately 1 hour following the accident and drove himself home. He was alert and oriented all morning, only complaining of a headache, taking ibuprofen at 10 AM. He appeared to be sleeping at 1 PM when mother left to do errands and she was unable to arouse him when she returned 2 hours later. On examination, this is a well-developed, well-nourished, adolescent male. Temperature 97.4, HR 66, RR 12, BP 88/50. **Neurological examination reveals no spontaneous eye opening or response to verbal commands, there is withdrawal from painful stimuli. Score = 6 on Glasgow Coma Scale.** Call placed to Children's Hospital Trauma Center and life flight team dispatched. ETA 22 minutes. NSR on cardiac monitor. O2 saturation 92% by pulse oximetry, O2 started at 2 L/m via non-rebreather mask. HOB elevated 30%. IV line placed right forearm, LR infusing. Blood drawn for CBC, platelets, electrolytes, PT, PTT, type and hold and sent to lab. Bladder can be palpated above the pubic bone, Foley catheter placed without difficulty, 600 cc clear yellow urine returned.

Transport team note: Arrived in ED at 4:13 PM. Baseline lab tests all within normal limits. ABG drawn pH 7.32, pCO2 51, HCO3 25, pO2 88 %, SaO2 96 %. Patient intubated without difficulty, hand ventilated by RT. Transferred to life flight stretcher, on monitors, stable for transport. All consents obtained, parents following in private car. ETA Children's Hospital 17 minutes with neurosurgical team assembled and ready for patient. Uneventful helicopter transport. Patient taken directly from heliport to CT. Care assumed by neurosurgical team and radiology staff.

Code the Glasgow Coma Scale information only.

Diagnosis Code(s)

R40.2112 Coma scale, eyes open never, at arrival in emergency department

R40.2212 Coma scale, best verbal response, none, at arrival in emergency department

R40.2342 Coma scale, best motor response, flexion withdrawal, at arrival in emergency department

Reporting of the total score is not required since all three components are documented. If only the total score of 6 was reported it would be coded as follows:

R40.2432 Glasgow coma scale score 3-8, at arrival to emergency department

Coding Note(s)

Glasgow coma scale codes are reported additionally with fracture of skull (S02.-) and/or intracranial injury (S06.-) reported first.

Alzheimer's Disease

Alzheimer's disease is the most common form of dementia. The progressive degeneration of nerve cells in Alzheimer's disease manifests mental changes ranging from mild memory impairment to loss of cognitive function with dementia. Accurate code assignment of Alzheimer's disease, with or without associated dementia, requires comprehensive provider documentation that clearly distinguishes Alzheimer's dementia from senile dementia, senile degeneration, or senility.

Codes include more specificity so a diagnosis of Alzheimer's disease without further description of the onset (e.g., early onset, late onset) and the type of symptoms (e.g., depression, delusions) will not support optimal code assignment. It is essential that the provider documentation clarify dementia related to other conditions. Alzheimer's disease may also be associated with delirium or behavioral disturbances, so it is equally important to document these conditions when they are present.

Coding and Documentation Requirements

Identify type/onset of Alzheimer's disease:

- Early onset
- Late onset
- Other Alzheimer's disease
- Unspecified Alzheimer's disease

Use additional code when Alzheimer's disease is associated with:

- Delirium (F05)
- Dementia with behavioral disturbance (F02.81)
- Dementia without behavioral disturbance (F02.80)

ICD-10-CM Code/Documentation	
G30.0	Alzheimer's disease with early onset
G30.1	Alzheimer's disease with late onset
G30.8	Other Alzheimer's disease
G30.9	Alzheimer's disease, unspecified

Documentation and Coding Example

A 77-year-old woman was brought for neurological evaluation by her husband because of a 6-month history of increasing memory impairment. Her husband began noticing a gradual worsening in her memory and increased difficulty finding words. He also noted a decline in social activity which he describes as "extremely out of character" for his wife. She appeared to be in a chronic state of confusion and was unable to converse in a logical or coherent manner, and her responses to questions were frequently inappropriate. Her confusion and memory problems became even more pronounced and her husband reported she was not sleeping at night.

The patient is well-groomed, alert, and friendly with no specific complaints. She worked in a secretarial position until her retirement at age 65. Her past medical history is significant for hysterectomy and although elevated blood pressure was documented on several occasions, she was never diagnosed with or medicated for HTN. All of her recent evaluations, including a CT scan, were reported as normal.

General medical and neurological exams were normal. She scored 15 out of a possible 30 on the mini mental state examination MMSE. Her speech was highly paraphasic. She couldn't remember what she had for breakfast. She was able to provide her name, but when asked about her current age, she incorrectly stated her birth month, but then became aware of this and became very angry. She was unable to give the current year, or the name of the current president.

Formal testing was conducted and she scored well below average in all cognitive domains on the Wechsler Memory scale, the Wechsler Adult Intelligence Scale, the Visuospatial Construction, and the Graphomotor Alternation Test. The results of the evaluation indicate that she meets clinical criteria for **Alzheimer's disease.** Patient was started on an empirical trial of neurotransmitters therapy, discharged home with daily home health care assistance.

Diagnosis: **Dementia in late onset Alzheimer's disease**

Diagnosis Code(s)

G30.1 Alzheimer's disease with late onset

F02.80 Dementia in other diseases classified elsewhere without behavioral disturbance

Coding Note(s)

Alzheimer's disease with dementia requires dual with the underlying condition (Alzheimer's disease) coded first followed by a code for dementia with or without behavioral disturbance. Late onset Alzheimer's disease is coded to G30.1. When Alzheimer's associated dementia is present, code F02.8- is assigned as an additional code.

Causalgia

Causalgia, also referred to as complex regional pain syndrome type II (CRPS II), is a type of neuropathic pain that occurs following a distinct nerve injury, usually to a peripheral nerve in an extremity. Symptoms include continuous burning or throbbing pain along the peripheral nerve; sensitivity to cold and/or touch; changes in skin temperature, color, and/or texture; hair and nail changes; joint stiffness and muscle spasms; and weakness and/or atrophy.

Codes for causalgia are specified by upper and lower limb and laterality. Causalgia of the upper limb is reported with codes in subcategory G56.4. Causalgia of the lower limb is reported with codes from subcategory G57.7. Fifth characters for both the upper and lower limbs identify laterality as unspecified (0), right (1), or left (2).

Coding and Documentation Requirements

Identify site:

- Upper limb
  - Right
  - Left
  - Unspecified
- Lower limb
  - Right
  - Left
  - Unspecified

ICD-10-CM Code/Documentation	
G56.40	Causalgia of unspecified upper limb (complex regional pain syndrome II)
G56.41	Causalgia of right upper limb (complex regional pain syndrome II)
G56.42	Causalgia of left upper limb (complex regional pain syndrome II)
G57.70	Causalgia of unspecified lower limb (complex regional pain syndrome II)
G57.71	Causalgia of right lower limb (complex regional pain syndrome II)
G57.72	Causalgia of left lower limb (complex regional pain syndrome II)

Documentation and Coding Example

Patient is a 12-year-old Caucasian male referred to orthopedics by his pediatrician for evaluation of right foot pain and weakness. He is non-weight bearing on right lower extremity with use of crutches. The patient is accompanied to the appointment by his father. PMH includes seasonal allergies controlled with Cetirizine. Immunizations are up to date for age. Patient sustained a displaced fracture of the right fibula approximately two months ago complicated by right peroneal nerve injury while racing on a BMX course. He came over a jump, lost control of the bike and landed hard on his right leg. No other riders were involved. The accident occurred out of town and he was initially seen in an Urgent Care Center where X-rays showed a displaced fracture of the proximal fibular shaft with peroneal nerve compression. He underwent an ORIF with decompression of the peroneal nerve. He was placed in a hinged knee brace, given crutches to use, and told to follow up with PMD or orthopedist when he returned home. He was able to ambulate without pain initially but started noticing some weakness in his right foot two weeks after discontinuing the brace. As the weakness increased, he also began to have numbness and tingling on the top of the right foot. Walking and wearing shoes now cause unbearable pain. He denies any knee pain or loss of mobility. On examination, this is an anxious appearing, well nourished, thin, adolescent male. WT 84 lbs. (37th%) HT 62 in. (86th%). Cranial nerves grossly intact. Upper extremities are normal in strength, sensation, and movement. Cervical, thoracic, and lumbar spine all normal in appearance and movement. Hips and knees in good alignment with range of motion intact. Upper leg strength normal bilaterally. Left lower extremity has normal strength, sensation, and movement. Right lower extremity feels significantly warmer to touch than left and skin color is unusually red beginning 10 cm above ankle and extending though toes. He has hyperalgesia and marked allodynia on dorsal surface of right foot when skin is lightly stroked by examiners fingers. Hyperhidrosis is not appreciated. There is no muscle wasting noted but he has marked ankle weakness and right foot drop with attempted dorsiflexion. His is able to tolerate only a few steps weight bearing and he is noted to have a slapping gait with toe drag. Comprehensive x-rays obtained of right lower extremity including AP, lateral, and oblique views of knee; AP, lateral, and mortise views of the ankle; AP and lateral views of the tibia/fibula shafts which are negative for Maisonneuve injury but show **good calcification at the site of the transverse fracture of proximal fibula**.

Impression: **S/P right fibula fracture with secondary causalgia due to common peroneal nerve injury**.

Plan: MRI to include right knee, lower leg, and foot. Consider referral to neurology for EMG and pain management.

Diagnosis Code(s)

G57.71 Causalgia of right lower limb

S82.831S Other fracture of upper and lower end of right fibula, sequela

S84.11XS Injury of peroneal nerve at lower leg level, right leg, sequela

V18.0XXS Pedal cycle driver injured in noncollision transport accident in nontraffic accident, sequela

Coding Note(s)

The causalgia of the right leg is a sequela of a fracture resulting in a nerve injury of the upper end of the fibula. The causalgia is the first listed diagnosis code. Laterality is a component of the causalgia code. The code identifying the injury that resulted in the sequela is listed next. The patient had a transverse fracture of the upper end of the fibula with compression of the peroneal nerve. Both injuries are coded with 7th character S to indicate a sequela (late effect). While there are codes specific to transverse fracture of the shaft of the fibula, there is not a specific code for transverse fracture of the upper end so the code for other fracture of upper and lower end of the right fibula is reported. In this case, the use of "and" means "and/or" in the code descriptor for code S82.831S. The physician has also documented that there is good calcification at the fracture site which indicates that the fracture has healed normally. The code for the nerve injury is specific to the peroneal nerve. Laterality is also a component of both the fracture and nerve injury codes. The BMX rider was involved in a noncollision, nontraffic accident which is reported with the 7th character S to indicate that the patient is being treated for a sequela of the BMX accident.

Complex Regional Pain Syndrome I

Reflex sympathetic dystrophy (RSD) is now more commonly referred to as complex regional pain syndrome I (CRPS I). CRPS I is a type of severe, debilitating neuropathic pain that usually results from an injury, but in CRPS I there is no direct injury to the nerve itself. The precipitating injury may range from major to relatively minor trauma. It can also occur following an illness or it can occur without any known cause. Intense pain of the affected region can result even from light touch. Other symptoms related to abnormal function of the sympathetic nervous system may also be evident including abnormal circulation, temperature, and sweating. If not promptly diagnosed and treated there can be loss of function in the affected limb followed by muscle atrophy and even changes in hair and skin.

CRPS I is reported with codes from subcategory G90.5. Codes are specific to the upper or lower limbs and laterality is also a component of the codes.

Coding and Documentation Requirements

Identify the site:

- Upper limb
  - Right
  - Left
  - Bilateral
  - Unspecified side
- Lower limb
  - Right
  - Left
  - Bilateral
  - Unspecified side
- Other specified site
- Unspecified site

ICD-10-CM Code/Documentation	
G90.50	Complex regional pain syndrome I, unspecified
G90.511	Complex regional pain syndrome I of right upper limb
G90.512	Complex regional pain syndrome I of left upper limb
G90.513	Complex regional pain syndrome I of upper limb, bilateral
G90.519	Complex regional pain syndrome I of unspecified upper limb
G90.521	Complex regional pain syndrome I of right lower limb
G90.522	Complex regional pain syndrome I of left lower limb
G90.523	Complex regional pain syndrome I of lower limb, bilateral
G90.529	Complex regional pain syndrome I of unspecified lower limb
G90.59	Complex regional pain syndrome I of other specified site

Documentation and Coding Example

Seventy-one-year-old Asian female presents to PMD with **pain and swelling in both arms**. The patient was in her usual state of good health until one month ago when she was the **victim of an attempted purse snatching** outside a local restaurant. She held onto her purse which was looped over her left forearm, elbow bent, but she felt her **shoulder wrench and elbow twist** during the altercation. She declined medical attention at the time and treated her injury conservatively with heat and Aleve. She states the **left arm pain** has progressed from mild tingling to a continuous burning sensation extending from shoulder to fingertips. The initial **bruising on her left forearm** resolved within a week but swelling around the elbow has increased and now extends into the wrist and hand. She has difficulty with movement especially elbow extension. What is most concerning to her is that **in the past week her right arm, which was not injured at the time, has developed a tingling type pain and yesterday she noticed swelling in the wrist.** Temperature 94.2 HR 84 RR 16 BP 140/82. Current medications include Aleve, Os-Cal, and a multivitamin. On examination, this is a thin, athletic appearing woman who looks significantly younger than her stated age. Cranial nerves are grossly intact. PERRLA. Eyes are clear, nares patent, mucous membranes moist and pink. Neck supple without lymphadenopathy. HR regular, without bruits or rubs, Grade II, S1 ejection murmur is present. Breath sounds clear, equal bilaterally. Abdomen soft, non-distended with active bowel sounds. Lower extremities are completely benign with intact circulation, sensation, and movement. Right upper extremity has no bruising or discoloration noted. Shoulder is freely mobile without swelling or pain. Right elbow is not swollen but gentle manipulation elicits complaint of pain and obvious stiffness in the joint. Wrist is exquisitely tender and noticeably swollen over the carpal-metacarpal joint. Sensation is normal, skin warm, dry to touch. Examination of left upper extremity is difficult due to pain. Hyperalgesia is present from just below shoulder through fingertips. Swelling is most notable in the elbow and wrist with muscle wasting in the upper arm and forearm. Skin is pale in color, cool and moist to touch.

Impression: **Complex regional pain disorder, Type I, of both upper extremities. Sequela of direct injury to muscles/tendons left upper arm. No known injury or direct cause on the right**.

Plan: Comprehensive radiographs of bilateral upper extremities to r/o fracture and bone scan of same to assess for decreased bone density. Referral made to neurologist. Patient is offered a trial of physical therapy but she declines, stating she would prefer to wait until after she has been evaluated by neurology.

Diagnosis Code(s)

G90.513 Complex regional pain syndrome I of upper limb, bilateral

S46.902S Unspecified injury of unspecified muscle, fascia and tendon at shoulder and upper arm level, left arm, sequela

Y04.8XXS Assault by other bodily force, sequela

Coding Note(s)

The code descriptor has been changed from reflex sympathetic dystrophy (RSD) to complex regional pain syndrome I (CRPS

I) to reflect current terminology for the condition. Laterality is a component of the code which has been documented as bilateral. The CRPS I on the left is a sequela of the injury to the left arm so that should be coded additionally. There is no documented injury to the right arm, but CRPS I can also occur without a known cause. Sequela of injury is reported with an injury code with 7th character S. The site of the injury is documented as the muscles and tendons of the upper left arm, but the specific muscle(s)/tendon(s) are not identified and the specific type of injury is not documented so the code for unspecified injury of unspecified muscle/tendon is assigned. A code for the external cause is also assigned with 7th character S. The external cause is a pulling/wrenching injury in an attempt to snatch a purse which would be classified as an assault using bodily force. There is not a specific code for pulling/wrenching so the code for other bodily force is assigned.

Congenital Hydrocephalus

Congenital hydrocephalus is the excessive accumulation of cerebrospinal fluid (CSF) in the brain. Congenital hydrocephalus is a condition that is present at birth although it might not be diagnosed until later in infancy.

The ventricular system in the brain is made up of four ventricles connected by narrow passages. The ventricles are filled with CSF which is a clear fluid that surrounds the brain and spinal cord. Normally, CSF flows through the ventricles and then into cisterns which are closed spaces that serve as CSF reservoirs at the base of the brain. CSF bathes the surfaces of the brain and spinal cord and then is reabsorbed into the bloodstream. Any imbalance between production and absorption of CSF caused either by obstruction of CSF flow from one region of the brain to another, or by failure to reabsorb CSF, can cause an over-accumulation of CSF in the brain resulting in hydrocephalus.

Category Q03 Congenital hydrocephalus contains four codes:

- Code Q03.0 Malformations of the aqueduct of Sylvius identifies one of the most common causes of congenital hydrocephalus, which is stenosis or narrowing of this small passage between the third and fourth ventricles in the middle of the brain.
- Code Q03.1 Atresia of foramina of Magendie and Luschka, also called Dandy-Walker syndrome, is another common cause of obstructive internal hydrocephalus. An enlarged fourth ventricle and loss of the area between the two cerebellar hemispheres causes an increase in the fluid-filled spaces around the brain.
- There are also codes for other specified types of congenital hydrocephalus, Q03.8, and unspecified congenital hydrocephalus, Q03.9.

Careful attention must be paid to the documentation to ensure that the hydrocephalus is not associated with spina bifida or Arnold-Chiari syndrome Type II. Hydrocephalus with spina bifida is reported with codes Q05.0-Q05.4, and hydrocephalus associated with Arnold-Chiari syndrome Type II is reported with codes Q07.02 and Q07.03 (with both spina bifida and hydrocephalus).

Coding and Documentation Requirements

Identify the type of congenital hydrocephalus:

- Atresia of foramina of Magendie and Luschka (Dandy-Walker syndrome)
- Malformations of aqueduct of Sylvius
- Other specified type of congenital hydrocephalus
- Unspecified congenital hydrocephalus

ICD-10-CM Code/Documentation	
Q03.0	Malformations of aqueduct of Sylvius
Q03.1	Atresia of foramina of Magendie and Luschka
Q03.8	Other congenital hydrocephalus
Q03.9	Congenital hydrocephalus, unspecified

Documentation and Coding Example

Seven-month-old male infant is brought to ED by mother with irritability and vomiting. Mother states she has been concerned about her child for a few months due to increasing head size and decreased muscle tone. She expressed her concerns to the pediatrician one month ago at his 6-month check-up but the doctor just dismissed them and said he was fine. T 98.8, P 100, R 16, BP 100/40, Wt. 17 lbs. HC 48 cm. On examination, this is fussy infant with a large head and poor neck muscle control. Anterior fontanelle open and bulging. Sutures are widely separated and he has a large network of veins over the scalp. PERRL with papilledema, downward pupil gaze, and nystagmus noted on exam. Cranial nerves grossly intact. Heart rate regular, breath sounds clear. Abdomen soft, round with active bowel sounds. Mother states infant appears hungry and will breast feed but vomits soon after eating. He has refused solid foods today. Pediatric Neurology called to see infant and orders a CT scan under sedation, admit to pediatric floor following the scan.

Pediatric Neurology Admit Note: CT scan shows **atresia of the foramen Magendie and Luschka with hydrocephalus in the fourth ventricle**. Pediatric neurosurgery has been called to consult for shunt insertion. Pre-operative labs have been drawn including CBC, coagulation studies, comprehensive metabolic panel. Patient is NPO and receiving IV fluids for hydration.

Diagnosis Code(s)

Q03.1 Atresia of foramina of Magendie and Luschka

Coding Note(s)

The congenital hydrocephalus is due to congenital absence of the two foramina (openings) in the fourth ventricle of the brain preventing the normal flow of CSF and causing accumulation of fluid in this region of the brain. There is a specific code for this condition, Q03.1 Atresia of foramina of Magendie and Luschka.

Diabetes Mellitus

In ICD-10-CM, code categories include diabetes mellitus due to an underlying condition (E08); drug or chemical induced diabetes mellitus (E09); Type 1 diabetes mellitus (E10); Type 2 diabetes mellitus (E11); and other specified diabetes mellitus (E13). Other specified types of diabetes mellitus include diabetes due to identified genetic defects, such as defects of beta cell function or insulin action, as well as secondary diabetes due to surgery (postpancreatectomy, postprocedural). Diabetes not specified as due to an underlying cause and not specified as Type 1 or Type 2 is reported as Type 2 diabetes by default. Since these categories are available for identifying and reporting differing types of diabetes, it is important for the underlying cause of the diabetes to be documented.

Diabetes codes also capture the body system affected in the 4th character with the complication or manifestation typically identified by the 5th character. The 6th character allows for capture of multiple complications or manifestations often seen together such as diabetic retinopathy with macular degeneration. The 7th character denotes laterality, such as left eye or right eye. Each individual code does not, however, capture whether or not the diabetes is controlled or uncontrolled. Diabetes documented as uncontrolled or poorly controlled is captured by reporting an additional code for hyperglycemia. For example, Type II diabetes documented as poorly controlled as evidenced by elevated blood sugar (hyperglycemia) would be reported with code E11.65. As many diabetes codes as are necessary to report the complete clinical picture of all manifestations and complications of the diabetic patient should be reported.

The underlying condition, or drug or chemical poisoning identified as the cause of secondary diabetes is reported as the first-listed diagnosis with the secondary diabetes code listed next. Fourth character subcategories for secondary diabetes identify the body system affected by the complication, with the specific complication or manifestation identified by the fifth character. Some secondary diabetes codes capture multiple complications or manifestations with the sixth character, and some report laterality with a seventh character. This means that to capture the most specific code, providers will need to document not only the underlying cause but also clearly describe all complications and manifestations. Documenting any long-term insulin use is also required.

Capturing the correct code for diabetes mellitus requires clear and precise documentation of the underlying cause. Secondary diabetes is defined as a diabetic condition with an underlying cause other than genetics or environmental conditions and includes diabetes mellitus secondary to drugs and chemicals or due to an underlying disease, medical condition, surgical procedure, or trauma. Some of the drugs and chemical agents identified as causing secondary diabetes include:

- Anticonvulsants
- Antihypertensive drugs including diuretics and beta blockers
- Antipsychotics including lithium and some antidepressants
- Antiretroviral drugs
- Chemotherapy drugs
- Hormone supplements, including:
  - Anabolic steroids
  - Contraceptives
  - Estrogen
  - Growth hormones
  - Hormones prescribed for prostate cancer
- Immunosuppressive drugs including corticosteroids
- Some of the other causes of secondary diabetes include:
- Autoimmune diseases
- Carcinoid tumors of some sites, including:
  - Gastrointestinal tract
  - Lungs
- Endocrine disorders, including:
  - Cushing's syndrome
  - Excessive levels of growth hormones
  - Hyperthyroidism
- Hemochromatosis
- Liver diseases, including:
  - Hepatitis C
  - Fatty liver disease
- Pancreatic disease or injury, including:
  - Chronic pancreatitis
  - Pancreatic cancers
  - Pancreatic damage due to malnutrition
  - Other endocrine diseases that affect pancreatic function or damage the insulin-producing beta cells
- Trauma to the pancreas

Surgical procedures may also result in secondary diabetes mellitus. Procedures most often associated with secondary diabetes include total or partial removal of the pancreas for malignant neoplasm or severe pancreatic disease, or orchiectomy performed for testicular or prostate cancer.

Coding and Documentation Requirements

Identify the type of diabetes mellitus:

- Drug or chemical induced
- Due to underlying condition
- Type 1
- Type 2
- Other specified diabetes mellitus, which includes:
  - Due to genetic defects of beta-cell function
  - Due to genetic defects in insulin action
  - Postpancreatectomy
  - Postprocedural
  - Secondary diabetes not elsewhere classified

Identify the body system affected, the manifestations or complications, and laterality, when applicable:

- Arthropathy
  - Neuropathic
  - Other arthropathy
- Circulatory complications
  - Peripheral angiopathy
    - » With gangrene
    - » Without gangrene
  - Other specified circulatory complication

- Hyperglycemia
- Hyperosmolarity
  - with coma
  - without coma
- Hypoglycemia
  - With coma
  - Without coma
- Ketoacidosis
  - With coma
  - Without coma
- Kidney complications
  - Diabetic nephropathy
  - Chronic kidney disease
  - Other diabetic kidney complication
- Neurological complications
  - Amyotrophy
  - Autonomic (poly)neuropathy
  - Mononeuropathy
  - Polyneuropathy
  - Other specified neurological complication
  - Unspecified diabetic neuropathy
- Ophthalmic complications
  - Diabetic retinopathy
    - » Mild nonproliferative
      - With macular edema
      - Without macular edema
    - » Moderate nonproliferative
      - With macular edema
      - Without macular edema
    - » Severe nonproliferative

      With macular edema

      Without macular edema
    - » Proliferative
      - With macular edema
      - Without macular edema
      - With traction retinal detachment involving the macula
      - With traction retinal detachment not involving the macula
      - With combined traction retinal detachment and rhegmatogenous retinal detachment
    - » Stable proliferative
    - » Unspecified diabetic retinopathy
      - With macular edema
      - Without macular edema
  - Diabetic macular edema, resolved following treatment
  - Laterality
    - » Right eye
    - » Left eye
    - » Bilateral
    - » Unspecified eye
  - Diabetic cataract
  - Other diabetic ophthalmic complication
- Oral complications
  - Periodontal disease
  - Other oral complications
- Skin complication
  - Dermatitis
  - Foot ulcer
  - Other skin ulcer
  - Other skin complication
- Other specified complication
- Unspecified complication
- Without complications

ICD-10-CM Code/Documentation	
E08.41 Diabetes mellitus due to underlying condition with diabetic mononeuropathy	E08.40 Diabetes mellitus due to underlying condition with diabetic neuropathy, unspecified
E09.41 Drug or chemical induced diabetes mellitus with neurological complications with diabetic mononeuropathy	E09.40 Drug or chemical induced diabetes mellitus with neurological complications with diabetic neuropathy, unspecified
E13.41 Other specified diabetes mellitus with diabetic mononeuropathy	E13.40 Other specified diabetes mellitus with diabetic neuropathy, unspecified
E08.43 Diabetes mellitus due to underlying condition with diabetic autonomic (poly) neuropathy	E08.42 Diabetes mellitus due to underlying condition with diabetic polyneuropathy
E09.43 Drug or chemical induced diabetes mellitus with neurological complications with diabetic autonomic (poly) neuropathy	E09.42 Drug or chemical induced diabetes mellitus with neurological complications with diabetic polyneuropathy
E13.43 Other specified diabetes mellitus with diabetic autonomic (poly)neuropathy	E13.42 Other specified diabetes mellitus with diabetic polyneuropathy
E08.49 Diabetes mellitus due to underlying condition with other diabetic neurological complication	E08.44 Diabetes mellitus due to underlying condition with diabetic amyotrophy
E09.49 Drug or chemical induced diabetes mellitus with neurological complications with other diabetic neurological complication	E09.44 Drug or chemical induced diabetes mellitus with neurological complications with diabetic amyotrophy
E13.49 Other specified diabetes mellitus with other diabetic neurological complication	E13.44 Other specified diabetes mellitus with diabetic amyotrophy
E08.610 Diabetes mellitus due to underlying condition with diabetic neuropathic arthropathy	E09.610 Drug or chemical induced diabetes mellitus with diabetic neuropathic arthropathy
	E13.610 Other specified diabetes mellitus with diabetic neuropathic arthropathy

Documentation and Coding Example

Forty-four-year-old Caucasian female is seen by PMD for c/o fatigue, dizziness, and unusual sweating. Patient has a 20 + year history of excessive **alcohol use** and was diagnosed with **chronic calcifying pancreatitis 6 years ago** resulting from her excessive alcohol consumption. She developed diabetes 2 years ago as a result of the pancreatic disease. She has cut down on her consumption of alcohol but continues to drink **2-3 glasses of wine daily**. **Diabetes is fairly well controlled on Lantus and Novolog insulin**. She was experiencing low BG levels with Lantus at HS

but less since the dose was split and she is injecting BID. WT 126 lbs., T 97.8, P 62, R 12, BP 104/50, O2 Sat 98% on RA, BGL=206. On examination, this is a thin, athletic appearing woman who looks her stated age. Skin is very tan, mucous membranes moist and pink, eyes are clear. She states she normally is able to play tennis or work out at the gym daily for 60-90 minutes. For the past month she finds she is exhausted after exercising and in the past week has become fatigued during the workout and has to stop. She has also noticed excessive perspiration even when she is not active. The dizziness occurs upon rising from bed and sometimes from sitting to standing. She denies falls. PERRLA, neck supple. HR regular. Pulses full and intact in extremities. No evidence of edema. Reflexes 2 + and muscle tone is good. Breath sounds clear, equal bilaterally. Abdomen is soft and flat, bowel sounds present in all quadrants. Supine BP 110/52, Sitting 90/50,

Standing 90/52.

Impression: **Diabetes due to chronic calcifying pancreatitis with related new onset autonomic neuropathy, orthostatic hypotension, and excessive sweating**.

Plan: Increase salt in diet. Refer to cardiology for echocardiogram and treadmill to assess HR and BP during exercise. She is again counseled about her **use of alcohol including availability of inpatient treatment programs for her dependency**. She declines these services.

Note electronically sent to Cardiology and Endocrinologist. Follow up after Cardiology workup. Sooner if symptoms worsen.

Diagnosis Code(s)

K86.0 Alcohol-induced chronic pancreatitis

E08.43 Diabetes mellitus due to underlying condition with diabetic autonomic (poly)neuropathy

F10.20 Alcohol dependence, uncomplicated

R53.83 Other fatigue

I95.1 Orthostatic hypotension

R61 Generalized hyperhidrosis

Z79.4 Long term (current) use of insulin

Coding Note(s)

This patient has secondary diabetes which is due to chronic calcifying pancreatitis which has been more specifically documented as being caused by excessive alcohol use and dependence. She has developed a new manifestation of autonomic neuropathy which is due to her secondary diabetes. There is a code first note for category E08 indicating that the code for the underlying condition is listed first and the secondary diabetes code is listed as the second diagnosis.

Codes for secondary diabetes are combination codes that identify the body system affected and the type of complication, which has been identified as new onset diabetic autonomic neuropathy. The manner in which the diabetic autonomic neuropathy is manifesting could be any number of specified conditions, and since the actual neuropathic complication the patient is experiencing is not included in the code title, additional codes that further identify the specific autonomic complication(s) may also be reported.

Encephalocele

An encephalocele is a rare disorder in which the bones of the skull do not close completely. This results in a bone gap through which cerebral spinal fluid, brain tissue, and the meninges (membrane that covers the brain) can protrude. This results in a sac-like malformation outside the skull. An encephalocele is a type of neural tube defect. The neural tube is the embryonic tissue that forms the brain, spinal cord, and the surrounding bones of the skull. An encephalocele may also be referred to by the following terms:

- Cephalocele
- Cerebral meningocele
- Cranial hydromeningocele
- Encephalocystocele
- Encephalomyelocele
- Hydroencephalocele
- Meningoencephalocele

Another term used to refer to an encephalocele is Type III Arnold-Chiari syndrome. Careful review of documentation for Arnold-Chiari syndrome is required because only Type III is reported with a code from category Q01 Encephalocele. Arnold-Chiari syndrome Type II is reported with codes from subcategory Q07.0-, which are also the default codes for Arnold- Chiari syndrome not otherwise specified. There is also a Type IV Arnold Chiari syndrome which is reported with code Q04.8 Other specified congenital malformations of the brain.

Codes for encephalocele are found in category Q01. There are specific codes for the most common encephalocele locations which include midline of the upper anterior part of the skull (frontal), the area between the forehead and the nose (nasofrontal), and the back of the skull (occipital or basal).

Coding and Documentation Requirements

Identify site of encephalocele:

- Frontal
- Nasofrontal
- Occipital
- Other specified site
- Unspecified site

ICD-10-CM Code/Documentation	
Q01.0	Frontal encephalocele
Q01.1	Nasofrontal encephalocele
Q01.2	Occipital encephalocele
Q01.8	Encephalocele of other sites
Q01.9	Encephalocele, unspecified

Documentation and Coding Example

Patient is a two-month-old Caucasian female scheduled for elective cranial surgery to close an **occipital encephalocele**. The defect was found on prenatal ultrasound at 28 weeks gestation. Mother did not have an elevated AFP level and amniocentesis revealed normal 46 XX chromosome pattern. Infant was delivered via elective C-section at 39 weeks and she had an unremarkable neonatal period. MRI imaging at 2 days of age, revealed a 2 x 2 cm rhombic roof encephalocele, caudal to the torcula, containing cerebral spinal fluid but no brain tissue. Patient had a normal neurological workup and because she was somewhat small for gestational age, the team decided to postpone surgery until she had gained weight and was thriving. Patient is now 8 lbs. 4 oz., up from a BW of 5 lbs. 13 oz. She is exclusively breast fed. On examination, this is an active, alert infant. Fontanelles are open and soft, **encephalocele is noted at base of skull as a soft cystic mass**. Heart rate regular, breath sounds clear and equal bilaterally. Abdomen soft and round with active bowel sounds. No hip click, diaper area clean. Patient is healthy and cleared for surgery. Note electronically sent to hospital, neurosurgeon and anesthesia.

Diagnosis Code(s)

Q01.2 Occipital encephalocele

Coding Note(s)

Code Q01.2 is specific for an occipital encephalocele, which might also be documented as basal encephalocele.

Epilepsy and Recurrent Seizures

Epilepsy is a neurological condition characterized by recurrent seizures. The terms "epilepsy" and "seizure disorder" describe central nervous system disorders characterized by sudden onset seizures and muscle contractions. Epileptic seizures may be classified as idiopathic or symptomatic. Idiopathic seizures do not have a known cause but, in some cases, there is a family history of epilepsy. Symptomatic epilepsy is due to a specific cause, such as head trauma, stroke, brain tumors, alcohol or drug withdrawal, and other conditions. Epileptic seizures can also be a manifestation of neurologic or metabolic diseases. Different terminology may be used to describe epilepsy such as epileptic or epilepsia attack, convulsion, fit, and seizure; however, in the medical record documentation, epilepsy must be clearly differentiated from a diagnosis of seizure or convulsion which is reported with codes from the signs and symptoms chapter rather than a code for epilepsy from the nervous system chapter. This means that a clear distinction must be made between a patient who has one seizure and a patient with epilepsy. Due to legal consequences, a code of epilepsy cannot be assigned unless it is clearly diagnosed by the provider.

Accurate coding of epilepsy and recurrent seizures depends entirely on provider documentation. Current clinical terminology and codes that capture the required detail for the specific type of epilepsy and complications such as status epilepticus and intractability are found in the code options for epilepsy. In order to assign the most specific code, clinical terminology related to the different types of epilepsy must be understood. Below are definitions of the commonly used terms describing epilepsy and recurrent seizures.

Absence epileptic syndrome – A type of generalized epilepsy characterized by an alteration of consciousness of brief duration (usually less than 20 seconds) with sudden onset and termination. The alteration of consciousness may include impaired awareness and memory of ongoing events as evidenced by mental confusion, an inability to response to external stimuli, and amnesia. May also be referred to as absence petit mal seizure.

Cryptogenic epilepsy – Epilepsy that is likely due to a specific cause but the cause has not yet been identified.

Epilepsia partialis continua – Unique type of prolonged seizure consisting of prolonged simple partial (localized) motor seizures, now more commonly referred to as Kozhevnikov's (Kojevnikoff's, Kojewnikoff's, Kojevnikov's, Kojevnikov's) epilepsy.

Epileptic spasms – Epilepsy syndrome that is clinically similar to infantile spasms, but of a broader clinical classification that captures this syndrome when onset occurs in later childhood.

Note: Infantile spasms are classified to the more general code for epileptic spasms.

Focal epilepsy – Epilepsy that is localized or starts in one area of the brain (synonymous with partial epilepsy and localization related epilepsy).

Generalized epilepsy – Epilepsy that involves the entire brain at the same time.

Grand mal status – An obsolete term used to describe generalized tonic-clonic seizures.

Idiopathic epilepsy – Epilepsy with no known cause, and the person has no other signs of neurological disease.

Infantile spasms – Epilepsy syndrome of infancy and childhood also referred to as West Syndrome characterized by brief bobbing or bowing of the head followed by relaxation and a return of the head to a normal upright position. Infantile spasms are also associated with developmental regression and if not controlled can lead to mental retardation.

Juvenile myoclonic epilepsy – A type of generalized epilepsy with onset in childhood characterized by shock-like muscle contractions in a group of muscles usually in the arms or legs that result in a jerking motion and generalized tonic-clonic seizures. The patient may also experience absence seizures. May also be referred to as impulsive petit mal seizure.

Localization-related epilepsy – Epilepsy that is localized or starts in one area of the brain (synonymous with focal epilepsy and partial epilepsy).

Lennoux-Gastaut syndrome – Severe form of epilepsy usually beginning before age 4 and associated with impaired intellectual functioning, developmental delay, and behavioral disturbances. Seizure types vary but may include tonic, atonic, myoclonic, or absence seizures. The patient may experience periods of frequent seizures mixed with brief seizure-free periods. The cause is often identified with more common causes being brain malformations, perinatal asphyxia, severe head injury, central nervous system infection, and inherited degenerative or metabolic conditions. However, in about one-third of all cases no cause is identified.

Partial epilepsy – Epilepsy that is localized or starts in one area of the brain (synonymous with focal epilepsy and localization related epilepsy).

Petit mal status – An obsolete term used to describe a type of generalized epilepsy that does not involve tonic-clonic movements.

Status epilepticus – Repeated or prolonged seizures usually lasing more than 30 minutes. May be tonic-clonic (convulsive) type or nonconvulsive (absence) type.

Symptomatic epilepsy – Epilepsy due to a known cause.

Tonic-clonic seizures – Seizures characterized by an increase in muscle tone and rhythmic jerking of muscles in one part or all of the body.

In addition to the specific types of epilepsy and epileptic syndromes described above, epilepsy is also classified as intractable or not intractable. Intractable seizures are those that are not responding to treatment. Terms used to describe intractable seizures include: pharmacologically resistant, pharmacoresistant, poorly controlled, refractory, or treatment resistant. Seizures that are not intractable are responding to treatment. Documentation that supports classification as not intractable would be "under control", "well-controlled", and "seizure-free."

Seizure disorders and recurrent seizures are classified with epilepsy; however, convulsions, new-onset seizure, single seizure, febrile seizure, or hysterical seizure are classified as nonepileptic. Thorough documentation of the seizure is needed in order to differentiate between epilepsy and other seizures and to distinguish seizure types.

For some specific types of epilepsy, a distinction is made between idiopathic and symptomatic epilepsy. Localization related epilepsy must be documented as idiopathic (G40.0) or symptomatic (G40.1, G40.2). In addition, generalized epilepsy is specifically described as idiopathic (G40.3). There is also a specific subcategory for epileptic seizure related to external causes such as alcohol, drugs, hormonal changes, sleep deprivation, or stress. In addition, all types of epilepsy must be documented as intractable or not intractable and as with status epilepticus or without status epilepticus. Documentation should also clearly differentiate epilepsy and recurrent seizures from the following conditions which are reported elsewhere:

- Conversion disorder with seizures (F44.5)
- Convulsions NOS (R56.9)
- Hippocampal sclerosis (G93.81)
- Mesial temporal sclerosis (G93.81)
- Post traumatic seizures (R56.1)
- Seizure (convulsive) NOS (R56.9)
- Seizure of newborn (P90)
- Temporal sclerosis (G93.81)
- Todd's paralysis (G83.8)

Coding and Documentation Requirements

Identify type of epilepsy or recurrent seizures:

- Absence epileptic syndrome
- Due to external causes
- Generalized
  - Idiopathic
  - Other generalized type
- Juvenile myoclonic epilepsy (also known as impulsive petit mal)
- Localization-related (focal) (partial)
  - Idiopathic (with seizures of localized onset)
  - Symptomatic
    - With complex partial seizures
    - With simple partial seizures
- Other epilepsy and recurrent seizures
  - Epileptic spasms
  - Lennox-Gastaut syndrome
  - Other epilepsy
  - Other seizures
- Unspecified epilepsy

Identify response to treatment:

- With intractable epilepsy, which includes:
  - Pharmacoresistant or pharmacologically resistant
  - Poorly controlled
  - Treatment resistant
  - Refractory (medically)
- Without intractable epilepsy

Identify as with/without status epilepticus:

- With status epilepticus
- Without status epilepticus

ICD-10-CM Code/Documentation	
G40.001	Localization-related (focal) (partial) idiopathic epilepsy and epileptic syndromes with seizures of localized onset, not intractable, with status epilepticus
G40.009	Localization-related (focal) (partial) idiopathic epilepsy and epileptic syndromes with seizures of localized onset, not intractable, without status epilepticus
G40.011	Localization-related (focal) (partial) idiopathic epilepsy and epileptic syndromes with seizures of localized onset, intractable, with status epilepticus
G40.019	Localization-related (focal) (partial) idiopathic epilepsy and epileptic syndromes with seizures of localized onset, intractable, without status epilepticus

ICD-10-CM Code/Documentation	
G40.101	Localization-related (focal) (partial) symptomatic epilepsy and epileptic syndromes with simple partial seizures, not intractable, with status epilepticus
G40.109	Localization-related (focal) (partial) symptomatic epilepsy and epileptic syndromes with simple partial seizures, not intractable, without status epilepticus
G40.111	Localization-related (focal) (partial) symptomatic epilepsy and epileptic syndromes with simple partial seizures, intractable, with status epilepticus
G40.119	Localization-related (focal) (partial) symptomatic epilepsy and epileptic syndromes with simple partial seizures, intractable, without status epilepticus
G40.201	Localization-related (focal) (partial) symptomatic epilepsy and epileptic syndromes with complex partial seizures, not intractable, with status epilepticus
G40.209	Localization-related (focal) (partial) symptomatic epilepsy and epileptic syndromes with complex partial seizures, not intractable, without status epilepticus
G40.211	Localization-related (focal) (partial) symptomatic epilepsy and epileptic syndromes with complex partial seizures, intractable, with status epilepticus
G40.219	Localization-related (focal) (partial) symptomatic epilepsy and epileptic syndromes with complex partial seizures, intractable, without status epilepticus
G40.301	Generalized idiopathic epilepsy and epileptic syndromes, not intractable, with status epilepticus
G40.309	Generalized idiopathic epilepsy and epileptic syndromes, not intractable, without status epilepticus
G40.311	Generalized idiopathic epilepsy and epileptic syndromes, intractable, with status epilepticus
G40.319	Generalized idiopathic epilepsy and epileptic syndromes, intractable, without status epilepticus
G40.A01	Absence epileptic syndrome, not intractable, with status epilepticus
G40.A09	Absence epileptic syndrome, not intractable, without status epilepticus
G40.A11	Absence epileptic syndrome, intractable, with status epilepticus
G40.A19	Absence epileptic syndrome, intractable, without status epilepticus
G40.B01	Juvenile myoclonic epilepsy, not intractable, with status epilepticus
G40.B09	Juvenile myoclonic epilepsy, not intractable, without status epilepticus
G40.B11	Juvenile myoclonic epilepsy, intractable, with status epilepticus
G40.B19	Juvenile myoclonic epilepsy, intractable, without status epilepticus
G40.401	Other generalized epilepsy and epileptic syndromes, not intractable, with status epilepticus
G40.409	Other generalized epilepsy and epileptic syndromes, not intractable, without status epilepticus
G40.411	Other generalized epilepsy and epileptic syndromes, intractable, with status epilepticus

ICD-10-CM Code/Documentation	
G40.419	Other generalized epilepsy and epileptic syndromes, intractable, without status epilepticus
G40.501	Epileptic seizures related to external causes, not intractable, with status epilepticus
G40.509	Epileptic seizures related to external causes, not intractable, without status epilepticus
G40.801	Other epilepsy, not intractable, with status epilepticus
G40.802	Other epilepsy, not intractable, without status epilepticus
G40.803	Other epilepsy, intractable, with status epilepticus
G40.804	Other epilepsy, intractable, without status epilepticus
G40.811	Lennox-Gastaut syndrome, not intractable, with status epilepticus
G40.812	Lennox-Gastaut syndrome, not intractable, without status epilepticus
G40.813	Lennox-Gastaut syndrome, intractable, with status epilepticus
G40.814	Lennox-Gastaut syndrome, intractable, without status epilepticus
G40.821	Epileptic spasms, not intractable, with status epilepticus
G40.822	Epileptic spasms, not intractable, without status epilepticus
G40.823	Epileptic spasms, intractable, with status epilepticus
G40.824	Epileptic spasms, intractable, without status epilepticus
G40.89	Other seizures
G40.901	Epilepsy, unspecified, not intractable, with status epilepticus
G40.909	Epilepsy, unspecified, not intractable, without status epilepticus
G40.911	Epilepsy, unspecified, intractable, with status epilepticus
G40.919	Epilepsy, unspecified, intractable, without status epilepticus

Documentation and Coding Example

A previously healthy 9-year-old boy was admitted to the hospital from the Emergency Department following several episodes of vomiting over several days and then episodes of jerking movements of the left side of the body, predominantly the left leg, accompanied by an altered mental status. While in the ED, he had repeated episodes of generalized seizures and remained in status epilepticus despite treatment with intravenous pyridoxine (two doses, 100 mg each) and consequently was admitted.

He had been born at term and his developmental milestones were normal. There was no family history of seizures or mental retardation. The diagnostic workup done on admission was negative and included serum pyruvate, serum amino acids, blood lead, copper, and mercury levels, Epstein Barr virus IgG, herpes simplex virus, polymerase chain reaction and encephalitis panel, leptospira, mycoplasma, and rabies titers. The CSF protein and glucose were normal.

Initial scalp EEG recording showed frequent centrotemporal EEG spikes. Continuous scalp EEG monitoring showed multiple electroclinical seizures beginning in the right central region and spreading to both hemispheres. MRI demonstrated abnormally thickened cortex in the high right parietal lobe. Patient was treated with pentobarbital infusion and the clinical manifestations disappeared.

Diagnosis: **Refractory focal seizures, status epilepticus.**

Diagnosis Code(s)

G40.011 Localization-related (focal) (partial) idiopathic epilepsy and epileptic syndromes with seizures of localized onset, intractable, with status epilepticus

Coding Note(s)

Refractory is listed as a synonym for intractable. ICD-10-CM lists benign childhood epilepsy with centrotemporal EEG spikes under subcategory G40.0.

Extrapyramidal Disease and Movement Disorders

There are two systems of neural pathways that affect movement – the pyramidal system which is the direct activation pathway and the extrapyramidal system which is the indirect activation pathway. The pyramidal system is responsible for voluntary movement of the head, neck, and limbs. The extrapyramidal system is a second motor pathway that is responsible for control of movements. The extrapyramidal system modifies neural impulses that originate in the cerebral cortex and is responsible for selective activation and suppression of movements, initiation of movements, rate and force of movements, and coordination. Damage to the extrapyramidal system results in movement disorders.

Code block G20-G26 Extrapyramidal and Movement Disorders contains codes for reporting these conditions.

Many movement disorders present with similar extrapyramidal symptoms, such as akathisia, dyskinesias, and dystonias. These disorders often resemble Parkinson's disease, so it is important that the medical record documentation clearly describes extrapyramidal and movement disorders.

Specific and complete documentation is necessary to avoid confusion between disorders and ensure the most accurate code assignment. Tremors, for example, are commonly associated with Parkinson's disease, but essential tremor is the most common type of tremor and the two conditions differ. In addition, people with essential tremor sometimes develop other neurological signs and symptoms —such as an unsteady gait. Medical record documentation by the provider that clearly describes extrapyramidal and movement disorders is essential. Documentation should include characteristics of the specific disorder. The following list includes other types of extrapyramidal and movement disorders, such as tremor:

- Chorea
- Essential tremor
- Familial tremor
- Drug-induced movement disorder (identify drug):
  - Akathisia
  - Chorea
  - Tics
  - Tremor
  - Other
  - Unspecified
- Intention/other tremor
- Myoclonus, which includes:
  - Drug-induced myoclonus (identify drug)
  - Palatal myoclonus
- Other specified extrapyramidal and movement disorders
  - Benign shuddering attacks
  - Restless legs syndrome
  - Stiff man syndrome
- Tics of organic origin
- Unspecified movement disorder

The table below shows of the range of codes in the categories for extrapyramidal diseases and movement disorders. Four coding examples follow the table.

ICD-10-CM Category	ICD-10-CM Code/Documentation
G20 Parkinson's Disease	
G21 Secondary parkinsonism	G21.0 Malignant neurologic syndrome G21.11 Neuroleptic induced parkinsonism G21.19 Other drug induced secondary parkinsonism G21.2 Secondary parkinsonism due to other external agents G21.3 Postencephalitic parkinsonism G21.4 Vascular parkinsonism G21.8 Other secondary parkinsonism G21.9 Secondary parkinsonism, unspecified
G23 Other degenerative diseases of basal ganglia	G23.0 Hallervorden-Spatz disease G23.1 Progressive supranuclear ophthalmoplegia [Steele-Richardson-Olszewski] G23.2 Striatonigral degeneration G23.8 Other specified degenerative diseases of basal ganglia G23.9 Degenerative diseases of basal ganglia, unspecified
G24 Dystonia	G24.01 Drug-induced subacute dystonia G24.02 Drug induced acute dystonia G24.09 Other drug induced dystonia G24.1 Genetic torsion dystonia G24.2 Idiopathic nonfamilial dystonia G24.3 Spasmodic torticollis G24.4 Idiopathic orofacial dystonia G24.5 Blepharospasm G24.8 Other dystonia G24.9 Dystonia, unspecified

ICD-10-CM Category	ICD-10-CM Code/Documentation
G25 Other extrapyramidal and movement disorders	G25.0 Essential tremor G25.1 Drug-induced tremor G25.2 Other specified forms of tremor G25.3 Myoclonus G25.4 Drug-induced chorea G25.5 Other chorea G25.61 Drug induced tics G25.69 Other tics of organic origin G25.70 Drug induced movement disorder, unspecified G25.71 Drug induced akathisia G25.79 Other drug induced movement disorders G25.81 Restless legs syndrome G25.82 Stiff-man syndrome G25.83 Benign shuddering attacks G25.89 Other specified extrapyramidal and movement disorders G25.9 Extrapyramidal and movement disorder unspecified
G26 Extrapyramidal and movement disorders in diseases classified elsewhere	

Example 1

Secondary Parkinsonism

Parkinson's disease is a common debilitating disease affecting one out of every 100 people over the age of 60. The symptoms of Parkinson's disease include tremors, rigidity, and akinesia. The term "parkinsonism" refers to any condition that involves the types of movement changes seen in Parkinson's disease. Coding of secondary parkinsonism requires a clear understanding of the difference between Parkinson's disease and secondary parkinsonism. Parkinson's disease, also referred to as idiopathic parkinsonism, primary Parkinson's disease or primary parkinsonism, is not due to or caused by another underlying condition or external agent such as a drug. In contrast, secondary parkinsonism is always caused by an underlying condition or external agent, such as chemical or environmental toxins, drugs, encephalitis, cerebrovascular disease, or another physiological condition.

In the medical record documentation, secondary parkinsonism must be clearly differentiated from primary Parkinson's disease and the documentation must indicate the underlying cause of secondary parkinsonism. Parkinson's disease and secondary parkinsonism may also be associated with mental disorders such as dementia, depression, delirium, or behavioral disturbance. To ensure assignment of the most specific code, the documentation must specify the cause of secondary parkinsonism and indicate when the condition is associated with dementia, depression, delirium, or a behavioral disturbance.

Parkinson's disease and secondary parkinsonism codes are found under Extrapyramidal and movement disorders, categories G20-G21.

Coding and Documentation Requirements

Identify the cause of secondary parkinsonism:

- Drug-induced
  - Malignant neuroleptic syndrome
  - Neuroleptic induced parkinsonism
  - Other drug induced secondary parkinsonism
- Due to other external agents
- Postencephalitic
- Vascular
- Other specified cause
- Unspecified cause

For drug or external agent induced secondary parkinsonism, use an additional code to identify the substance.

ICD-10-CM Code/Documentation	
G21.0	Malignant neuroleptic syndrome
G21.11	Neuroleptic induced parkinsonism
G21.19	Other drug induced secondary Parkinsonism
G21.2	Secondary parkinsonism due to other external agents
G21.3	Postencephalitic parkinsonism
G21.4	Vascular parkinsonism
G21.8	Other secondary parkinsonism
G21.9	Secondary parkinsonism, unspecified

Documentation and Coding Example

Follow-up visit for evaluation of **parkinsonism due to adverse effect of metoclopramide**.

History and Physical: This otherwise healthy 55-year-old man was given **metoclopramide** to treat symptomatic gastroesophageal reflux. Six months later he developed severe parkinsonism exhibiting tremors, limited movements, rigidity, and postural instability. He was started on L-dopa because his primary care physician did not realize the parkinsonism was drug-induced, and the metoclopramide was continued. The patient was referred to me six months ago for evaluation of parkinsonism after one year of taking both drugs. At that time, it was recognized that **the parkinsonism was drug-induced**. The metoclopramide was stopped and the patient has been slowly withdrawn from the L-dopa over the past six-months. On exam today, the patient's parkinsonism has resolved completely.

Diagnosis: **Drug-induced secondary parkinsonism** has resolved completely

Plan: Patient is to return to the care of his primary care physician.

Diagnosis Code(s)

G21.19 Other drug induced secondary parkinsonism

T45.0X5D Adverse effect of antiallergic and antiemetic drugs, subsequent encounter

Coding Note(s)

An additional code is used to identify the drug responsible for the adverse effect. Metoclopramide is not classified as a neuroleptic drug, so the code for other drug induced secondary parkinsonism is assigned. An additional code is assigned for the adverse effect. The drug responsible for the adverse effect is identified with a code from categories T36-T50 with fifth or sixth character of 5. Adverse effect codes in ICD-10-CM include a seventh character to indicate the episode of care (e.g., initial encounter, subsequent encounter, or sequela). This is a follow-up encounter so 7th character D is assigned for subsequent encounter.

Example 2

Other Degenerative Diseases of Basal Ganglia

Included in the extrapyramidal and movement disorders category block are other degenerative diseases of the basal ganglia. Degenerative diseases are characterized by progressive neuron degeneration. The basal ganglia are nerve cells located within the brain involved in the initiation of voluntary movement. Damage to the basal ganglia causes muscle stiffness or spasticity and tremors. Because the deficits are primarily in motor function, the extrapyramidal system and basal ganglia have been associated with movement disorders.

Many different degenerative diseases affect the brain and produce similar symptoms, so specific documentation is necessary to avoid confusion between disorders. For example, progressive supranuclear palsy is sometimes mistaken for

Parkinson's disease, because both conditions are associated with stiffness, frequent falls, slurred speech, difficulty swallowing, and decreased spontaneous movement. Provider documentation in the medical record must clearly distinguish degenerative diseases of the basal ganglia from other degenerative diseases of the brain that are characterized by motor, cognitive, and psychiatric manifestations. To ensure assignment of the most specific code for degenerative diseases of the basal ganglia, provider documentation should describe:

- Etiology
- Location (e.g., the brainstem, basal ganglia, cerebellum)
- Clinical features
- Course of the disease

Coding and Documentation Requirements

Identify the type of basal ganglia degenerative disease:

- Hallervorden-Spatz disease
- Progressive supranuclear ophthalmoplegia
- [Steele-Richardson-Olszewski]
- Striatonigral degeneration
- Other specified basal ganglia degenerative disease, which includes:
    - Calcification of basal ganglia
- Unspecified basal ganglia degenerative disease

ICD-10-CM Code/Documentation	
G23.0	Hallervorden-Spatz disease
G23.1	Progressive supranuclear ophthalmoplegia [Steele-Richardson-Olszewski]
G23.2	Striatonigral degeneration
G23.8	Other specified degenerative diseases of basal ganglia
G23.9	Degenerative disease of basal ganglia, unspecified

Documentation and Coding Example

Follow-up Visit History: A 63-year-old male with a year-long history of headaches, dizziness, and progressive unsteadiness and stiffening of the left side of his body presented after experiencing several falls. There was no evidence of encephalitis or of previous ingestion of neuroleptic drugs, and no family history of Parkinson's. MRI scans of the brain ruled out stroke or hydrocephalus. On examination, there was akinesia and rigidity of all limbs, more pronounced on the left, and no tremor. Deep tendon reflexes were brisk, the plantar flexor sensation was intact. Command and pursuit eye movements were grossly impaired in all directions but Doll's eye movements were normal. Optokinetic nystagmus was markedly reduced in lateral gaze to either side and absent in the vertical plane, as was convergence, but the pupillary reactions were normal. There was no ptosis, nystagmus, oculomasticatory myorhythmia, or myoclonus. A diagnosis of **progressive supranuclear palsy** was considered based on the association of a supranuclear ophthalmoplegia and Parkinsonism, and the neuro-ophthalmic findings were consistent with a diagnosis of supranuclear ophthalmoplegia. He was started on trimethoprim 160 mg with sulfamethoxazole 800 mg twice daily and levodopa 100 mg with carbidopa 10 mg four times a day. There was rapid improvement in his eye movements with minimal residual restriction in upward gaze and gradual improvement in his other symptoms by day seven.

Diagnosis: **Progressive supranuclear ophthalmoplegia** responding well to current drug regimen.

Diagnosis Code(s)

G23.1 Progressive supranuclear ophthalmoplegia [Steele-Richardson-Olszewski]

Coding Note(s)

Progressive supranuclear ophthalmoplegia has a distinct code (G23.1).

Example 3

Tremor

There are three codes that describe specific types of tremors, G25.0 Essential tremor, G25.1 Drug-induced tremor, and G25.2 Other specified forms of tremor which includes intention tremor. It should be noted that a diagnosis of tremor that is not more specifically described in the documentation is reported with a symptom code, R25.1 Tremor unspecified. These codes are also found under the extrapyramidal and other movement disorders category.

Coding and Documentation Requirements

Identify the form of tremor:

- Drug-induced
- Essential/Familial
- Other specified form (includes intention tremor)

ICD-10-CM Code/Documentation	
G25.0	Essential tremor
G25.1	Drug-induced tremor
G25.2	Other specified forms of tremor

Documentation and Coding Example

Patient is a 64-year-old Caucasian female referred to Neurology by PMD for worsening tremor in her hands and head. PMH is significant for tremor that started in her hands at least twenty years ago and progressed slowly to arms and head/neck. Patient reports that most members of her family have the problem in varying degrees. She states that her symptoms have not interfered with ADLs or exercise. Her husband is a retired architect. She has not been employed outside the home in more than 40 years. The couple moved about 1 year ago from a relatively moist/cool coastal town to a warm/dry inland area to be closer to their children/grandchildren, and it was after the move that she noticed her tremor worsening. She states she spends 4-5 months of the year in England with family, and symptoms were less severe while she was there, but exacerbated upon her return home. This is a pleasant, impeccably groomed, thin but muscular woman who looks younger than her stated age. Her head nods continuously in yes/yes pattern, her voice quality is somewhat soft but she is easily understood, arm tremor is noted when she extends her right arm for a handshake, but not when her hands are resting in her lap. She states the tremor does seem to worsen when she is anxious or acutely ill. Her general health is good. She had laser surgery for acute glaucoma 10 years ago, uses Pilocarpine 2% eye gtts daily. Last eye exam was 6 weeks ago. She currently takes multivitamin and calcium supplements, but no other medications. On examination, WT 136 lbs., HT 67 inches, T 98.4, P 70, R 14, BP 130/78. PERRLA, eyes clear without redness or excessive tearing. TMs normal. Cranial nerves grossly intact. Upper extremities are negative for muscle atrophy, fasciculation, weakness, or tenderness. There is no drift, rigidity, or resistance. Reflexes are 2+, tone 4/5. Normal sensation to pin prick, temperature, and vibration. Lower extremities are the same with 3+ reflexes and 5/5 tone. Appendicular coordination normal, gait grossly normal. She has some stiffness in her left hip with a barely discernable limp which she states is residual injury from being struck by a car while walking across a street 13 years ago. Her tremor is limited to a gentle yes/yes nod of the head when upright and abates when she reclines and her head/neck is supported on a pillow. Her hand/arm tremor is characterized by a gentle, rhythmic shaking movement with all voluntary movement. It is quite pronounced when arms are extended out from the midline either forward or to the sides. She is able to hold a cup of water, bring it up to her mouth and drink using one hand but prefers to use both, especially with hot beverages to avoid spilling and possible burns. Pencil grip is normal and writing is legible but she performs the task slowly. She states she prefers to use a keyboard/computer. Using the small keyboard on her phone is laborious and she will voice activate most frequently called numbers and no longer does text messaging.

Impression: **Benign essential tremor** possibly exacerbated by move to warm climate. Discussed medication options including benefits and side effects and she agrees to a trial of propranolol. She is given samples of Inderal 40 mg to take BID and will return to clinic in 2 weeks for follow-up.

Diagnosis Code(s)

G25.0 Essential tremor

Coding Note(s)

There is a specific code for essential tremor, also referred to as benign essential tremor or familial tremor. Essential tremor is classified with other extrapyramidal and movement disorders in category G25.

Example 4

Restless Leg Syndrome (RLS)

Restless leg syndrome (RLS) is characterized by an irresistible need to move the legs due to uncomfortable sensations in them, such as creeping, crawling, tingling, or bubbling. However, movement does relieve the discomfort. Restless leg syndrome usually manifests at night or when sitting for long periods of time. The sensations are most often felt in the lower leg between the knee and ankle but can also be located in the upper leg or arms. RLS occurs most often in middle age or older adults and stress can exacerbate the condition.

Coding and Documentation Requirements

None.

ICD-10-CM Code/Documentation	
G25.81	Restless leg syndrome

Documentation and Coding Example

A 45-year-old woman presents to the office complaining of insomnia. She states she has had trouble falling asleep for many years, but the problem is worsening. In bed she feels an unbearable discomfort in the legs. She has also noticed this urge on long car rides. The problem is worse at night. She initially described the leg sensations as a "tingling" in her bones radiating from the ankles to the thighs, accompanied by the irresistible need to move her legs. Her symptoms improve when she gets up and walks around. The tingling sensation is now more like electrical shocks accompanied with involuntary, symmetrical limb jerks with restlessness occurring earlier (at 7 pm) and chronic insomnia.

Assessment/Plan: **Restless legs syndrome**. Start with small doses of pramipexole twice daily - 0.09 mg. at 6 pm and 0.18 mg at 10 pm.

Diagnosis Code(s)

G25.81 Restless legs syndrome

Coding Note(s)

There is a distinct code to report restless legs syndrome. The syndrome includes the characteristic symptoms which are not separately reported. There is no laterality requirement for this code.

Fracture of Skull

Fractures of the skull are captured with codes from subcategories S02.0- Fracture of vault of skull and S02.1- Fracture of base of skull (unspecified site of base of skull, fracture of the occiput or occipital condyle, other specified fractures of the base of the skull which includes anterior, middle, or posterior fossa, sphenoid bone, temporal bone, orbital roof, and ethmoid and frontal sinus). A 7th character extension identifies the fracture as open or closed and identifies the episode of care. A second code from category S06 is required to capture any intracranial injury with or without loss of consciousness. Intracranial injury codes are much more specific as to the type of injury. In addition, when there is a loss of consciousness, the codes are much more specific as to the period of time and to the outcome—including survival with or without return to previous conscious level for loss of consciousness greater than 24 hours, or death due to intracranial injury or other cause prior to regaining consciousness. In addition to the fracture and intracranial injury codes, one or more supplementary codes may be required to capture elements of any documented coma using the Glasgow coma scale classification.

Coding and Documentation Requirements

Identify skull fracture site:

- Vault of skull, which includes
  - Frontal bone
  - Parietal bone
- Base of skull, which includes
  - Anterior fossa
  - Ethmoid sinus
  - Frontal sinus
  - Middle fossa
  - Occipital bone
  - Orbital roof
  - Posterior fossa
  - Sphenoid bone
  - Temporal bone

Identify laterality:

- Right
- Left
- Unspecified side

Identify fracture as:

- Closed
- Open

Identify episode of care:

- Initial
- Subsequent
  - With routine fracture healing
  - With delayed fracture healing
  - With nonunion of fracture
- Sequela

Identify nature of any intracranial injury:

- Concussion
- Cerebral edema, which includes
  - Diffuse edema
  - Focal edema
- Contusion/laceration
  - Brainstem
  - Cerebellum
  - Cerebrum
    - » Right cerebrum
    - » Left cerebrum
    - » Unspecified site of cerebrum
- Diffuse traumatic brain injury
- Focal traumatic brain injury
- Hemorrhage
  - Intracranial
    - » Brainstem
    - » Cerebellum
    - » Cerebrum, left
    - » Cerebrum, right
    - » Cerebrum, unspecified
  - Epidural (extradural)
  - Subarachnoid
  - Subdural
- Other specified intracranial injury
  - Internal carotid artery, intracranial portion
    - » Left
    - » Right
  - Other specified intracranial injury
- Unspecified intracranial injury

Identify any loss of consciousness:

- No loss of consciousness
- 30 minutes or less
- 31 minutes to 59 minutes
- 1 hour to 5 hours 59 minutes
- 6 hours to 24 hours
- Greater than 24 hours
  - With return to pre-existing conscious level
  - Without return to pre-existing conscious level
- Any duration with death prior to regaining consciousness
  - Death due to brain injury
  - Death due to other cause
- Unspecified duration

Episode of care:

- Initial
- Subsequent
- Sequela

Coma Scale reporting requires the use of individual scores, if known. All three elements—eye opening, verbal response, and motor response must be known to use individual scores. If all three elements are not known, but Glasgow coma scale is documented, use the Glasgow coma scale total score.

Identify individual scores:

- Eyes open
  - Never
  - To pain
  - To sound
  - Spontaneous
- Best verbal response
  - None
  - Incomprehensible words
  - Inappropriate words
  - Confused conversation
  - Oriented
- Best motor response
  - None
  - Extension
  - Abnormal flexion
  - Flexion withdrawal
  - Localizes pain
  - Obeys commands

Identify Glasgow coma scale total score:

- Glasgow score 13-15
- Glasgow score 9-12
- Glasgow score 3-8

Identify time/place of coma score obtained:

- In the field (EMT/ambulance)
- At arrival in emergency department
- At hospital admission
- 24 hours or more after hospital admission
- Unspecified time

OR

- Other coma without documented Glasgow coma scale score or with partial score reported

Closed Fracture of Skull with Cerebral Edema

ICD-10-CM Code/Documentation	
Fracture Skull Vault	
S02.0XXA	Fracture of vault of skull, initial encounter for closed fracture
Traumatic Cerebral Edema/Loss of Consciousness	
S06.1X0A	Traumatic cerebral edema without loss of consciousness, initial encounter
Fracture Skull Vault	
S02.0XXA	Fracture of vault of skull, initial encounter for closed fracture
Traumatic Cerebral Edema/Loss of Consciousness	

ICD-10-CM Code/Documentation	
S06.1X1A	Traumatic cerebral edema with loss of consciousness ≤ 30 min, initial encounter
Fracture Skull Vault	
S02.0XXA	Fracture of vault of skull, initial encounter for closed fracture
S06.1X2A	Traumatic cerebral edema with loss of consciousness 31 min to 59 min, initial encounter
Fracture Skull Vault	
S02.0XXA	Fracture of vault of skull, initial encounter for closed fracture
Traumatic Cerebral Edema/Loss of Consciousness	
S06.1X3A	Traumatic cerebral edema with loss of consciousness 1 hr. to 5 hrs. 59 min, initial encounter
Fracture Skull Vault	
S02.0XXA	Fracture of vault of skull, initial encounter for closed fracture
S06.1X4A	Traumatic cerebral edema with loss of consciousness 6 hours to 24 hours, initial encounter
Fracture Skull Vault	
S02.0XXA	Fracture of vault of skull, initial encounter for closed fracture
Traumatic Cerebral Edema/Loss of Consciousness	
S06.1X5A	Traumatic cerebral edema with loss of consciousness greater than 24 hours with return to pre-existing conscious level, initial encounter
Fracture Skull Vault	
S02.0XXA	Fracture of vault of skull, initial encounter for closed fracture
Traumatic Cerebral Edema/Loss of Consciousness	
S06.1X6A	Traumatic cerebral edema with loss of consciousness greater than 24 hours without return to pre-existing conscious level with patient surviving, initial encounter
Fracture Skull Vault	
S02.0XXA	Fracture of vault of skull, initial encounter for closed fracture
Traumatic Cerebral Edema/Loss of Consciousness	
S06.1X7A	Traumatic cerebral edema with loss of consciousness of any duration with death due to brain injury prior to regaining consciousness
Fracture Skull Vault	
S02.0XXA	Fracture of vault of skull, initial encounter for closed fracture
Traumatic Cerebral Edema/Loss of Consciousness	
S06.1X8A	Traumatic cerebral edema with loss of consciousness of any duration with death due to other cause prior to regaining consciousness
Fracture Skull Vault	
S02.0XXA	Fracture of vault of skull, initial encounter for closed fracture
Traumatic Cerebral Edema/Loss of Consciousness	
S06.1X9A	Traumatic cerebral edema with loss of consciousness of unspecified duration, initial encounter

Note 1: An initial encounter for an open fracture of vault of skull without mention of intracranial injury is reported with the same codes listed above except that the 7th character extension 'A' is replaced with a 'B' for initial encounter for open fracture.

Note 2: The 7th character 'A' for codes in category S06 indicates only that this is the initial encounter, not whether or not the injury is open or closed.

Fracture of Skull with Cerebral Laceration/Contusion

ICD-10-CM Code/Documentation	
Fracture Skull Vault	
S02.0XXA	Fracture of vault of skull, initial encounter for closed fracture
Contusion/Laceration/Loss of Consciousness	
S06.319A	Contusion and laceration of right cerebrum with loss of consciousness of unspecified duration, initial encounter
S06.329A	Contusion and laceration of left cerebrum with loss of consciousness of unspecified duration, initial encounter
S06.339A	Contusion and laceration of unspecified cerebrum with loss of consciousness of unspecified duration, initial encounter
Fracture Skull Vault	
S02.0XXA	Fracture of vault of skull, initial encounter for closed fracture

ICD-10-CM Code/Documentation	
Contusion/Laceration/Loss of Consciousness	
S06.310A	Contusion and laceration of right cerebrum without loss of consciousness, initial encounter
S06.320A	Contusion and laceration of left cerebrum without loss of consciousness, initial encounter
S06.330A	Contusion and laceration of unspecified cerebrum without loss of consciousness, initial encounter
Fracture Skull Vault	
S02.0XXA	Fracture of vault of skull, initial encounter for closed fracture
Contusion/Laceration/Loss of Consciousness	
S06.311A	Contusion and laceration of right cerebrum with loss of consciousness ≤ 30 min, initial encounter
S06.312A	Contusion and laceration of right cerebrum with loss of consciousness 31 min to 59 min, initial encounter
S06.321A	Contusion and laceration of left cerebrum with loss of consciousness ≤ 30 min, initial encounter
S06.322A	Contusion and laceration of left cerebrum with loss of consciousness 31 min to 59 min, initial encounter
S06.331A	Contusion and laceration of unspecified cerebrum with loss of consciousness ≤ 30 min, initial encounter
S06.332A	Contusion and laceration of unspecified cerebrum with loss of consciousness 31 min to 59 min, initial encounter

ICD-10-CM Code/Documentation	
Fracture Skull Vault	
S02.0XXA	Fracture of vault of skull, initial encounter for closed fracture
Contusion/Laceration/Loss of Consciousness	
S06.313A	Contusion and laceration of right cerebrum with loss of consciousness 1 hr. to 5 hrs. 59 min, initial encounter
S06.314A	Contusion and laceration of right cerebrum with loss of consciousness 6 hrs. to 24 hrs., initial encounter
S06.323A	Contusion and laceration of left cerebrum with loss of consciousness 1 hr. to 5 hrs. 59 min, initial encounter
S06.324A	Contusion and laceration of left cerebrum with loss of consciousness 6 hrs. to 24 hrs., initial encounter
S06.333A	Contusion and laceration of unspecified cerebrum with loss of consciousness 1 hr. to 5 hrs. 59 min, initial encounter
S06.334A	Contusion and laceration of unspecified cerebrum with loss of consciousness 6 hrs. to 24 hrs., initial encounter
Fracture Skull Vault	
S02.0XXA	Fracture of vault of skull, initial encounter for closed fracture
Contusion/Laceration/Loss of Consciousness	
S06.315A	Contusion and laceration of right cerebrum with loss of consciousness greater than 24 hours with return to preexisting conscious level, initial encounter
S06.325A	Contusion and laceration of left cerebrum with loss of consciousness greater than 24 hours with return to preexisting conscious level, initial encounter
S06.335A	Contusion and laceration of unspecified cerebrum with loss of consciousness greater than 24 hours with return to preexisting conscious level, initial encounter
Fracture Skull Vault	
S02.0XXA	Fracture of vault of skull, initial encounter for closed fracture
Contusion/Laceration/Loss of Consciousness	
S06.316A	Contusion and laceration of right cerebrum with loss of consciousness greater than 24 hours without return to pre-existing conscious level with patient surviving, initial encounter
S06.326A	Contusion and laceration of left cerebrum with loss of consciousness greater than 24 hours without return to pre-existing conscious level with patient surviving, initial encounter
S06.336A	Contusion and laceration of unspecified cerebrum with loss of consciousness greater than 24 hours without return to pre-existing conscious level with patient surviving, initial encounter
Fracture Skull Vault	
S02.0XXA	Fracture of vault of skull, initial encounter for closed fracture

ICD-10-CM Code/Documentation	
Contusion/Laceration/Loss of Consciousness	
S06.319A	Contusion and laceration of right cerebrum with loss of consciousness of unspecified duration, initial encounter
S06.329A	Contusion and laceration of left cerebrum with loss of consciousness of unspecified duration, initial encounter
S06.339A	Contusion and laceration of unspecified cerebrum with loss of consciousness of unspecified duration, initial encounter
Fracture Skull Vault	
S02.0XXA	Fracture of vault of skull, initial encounter for closed fracture
Contusion/Laceration/Loss of Consciousness	
S06.319A	Contusion and laceration of right cerebrum with loss of consciousness of unspecified duration, initial encounter
S06.329A	Contusion and laceration of left cerebrum with loss of consciousness of unspecified duration, initial encounter
S06.339A	Contusion and laceration of unspecified cerebrum with loss of consciousness of unspecified duration, initial encounter

Note 1: An initial encounter for an open fracture of vault of skull with cerebral laceration and contusion is reported with the same codes listed above except that the 7th character extension 'A' is replaced with a 'B' for initial encounter for open fracture.

Note 2: The 7th character 'A' for codes in category S06 indicates only that this is the initial encounter, not whether or not the injury is open or closed.

Note 3: There are additional contusion and laceration codes that reflect death either due to the brain injury or other brain injury.

These codes are:

S06.017A Contusion and laceration of right cerebrum with loss of consciousness of any duration with death due to brain injury prior to regaining consciousness, initial encounter

S06.018A Contusion and laceration of right cerebrum with loss of consciousness of any duration with death due to other cause prior to regaining consciousness, initial encounter

S06.027A Contusion and laceration of left cerebrum with loss of consciousness of any duration with death due to brain injury prior to regaining consciousness, initial encounter

S06.028A Contusion and laceration of left cerebrum with loss of consciousness of any duration with death due to other cause prior to regaining consciousness, initial encounter

S06.037A Contusion and laceration of unspecified cerebrum with loss of consciousness of any duration with death due to brain injury prior to regaining consciousness, initial encounter

S06.038A Contusion and laceration of unspecified cerebrum with loss of consciousness of any duration with death due to other cause prior to regaining consciousness, initial encounter

Fracture of Skull with Subarachnoid, Subdural, and Extradural Hemorrhage

ICD-10-CM Code/Documentation	
Fracture Skull Vault	
S02.0XXA	Fracture of vault of skull, initial encounter for closed fracture
Hemorrhage/Loss of Consciousness	
S06.4X9A	Epidural hemorrhage with loss of consciousness of unspecified duration, initial encounter
S06.5X9A	Traumatic subdural hemorrhage with loss of consciousness of unspecified duration, initial encounter
S06.6X9A	Traumatic subarachnoid hemorrhage with loss of consciousness of unspecified duration, initial encounter
Fracture Skull Vault	
S02.0XXA	Fracture of vault of skull, initial encounter for closed fracture
Hemorrhage/Loss of Consciousness	
S06.4X0A	Epidural hemorrhage without loss of consciousness, initial encounter
S06.5X0A	Traumatic subdural hemorrhage without loss of consciousness, initial encounter
S06.6X0A	Traumatic subarachnoid hemorrhage without loss of consciousness, initial encounter
Fracture Skull Vault	
S02.0XXA	Fracture of vault of skull, initial encounter for closed fracture
Hemorrhage/Loss of Consciousness	
S06.4X1A	Epidural hemorrhage with loss of consciousness ≤ 30 min, initial encounter
S06.5X1A	Traumatic subdural hemorrhage with loss of consciousness ≤ 30 min, initial encounter
S06.6X1A	Traumatic subarachnoid hemorrhage with loss of consciousness ≤ 30 min, initial encounter
Fracture Skull Vault	
S02.0XXA	Fracture of vault of skull, initial encounter for closed fracture
Hemorrhage/Loss of Consciousness	
S06.4X2A	Epidural hemorrhage with loss of consciousness 31 min to 59 min, initial encounter
S06.5X2A	Traumatic subdural hemorrhage with loss of consciousness 31 min to 59 min, initial encounter
S06.6X2A	Traumatic subarachnoid hemorrhage with loss of consciousness 31 min to 59 min, initial encounter
Fracture Skull Vault	
S02.0XXA	Fracture of vault of skull, initial encounter for closed fracture
Hemorrhage/Loss of Consciousness	
S06.4X3A	Epidural hemorrhage with loss of consciousness 1 hr. to 5 hrs. 59 min, initial encounter
S06.5X3A	Traumatic subdural hemorrhage with loss of consciousness 1 hr. to 5 hrs. 59 min, initial encounter

ICD-10-CM Code/Documentation	
S06.6X3A	Traumatic subarachnoid hemorrhage with loss of consciousness 1 hr. to 5 hrs. 59 min, initial encounter
Fracture Skull Vault	
S02.0XXA	Fracture of vault of skull, initial encounter for closed fracture
Hemorrhage/Loss of Consciousness	
S06.4X4A	Epidural hemorrhage with loss of consciousness 6 hrs. to 24 hrs., initial enc1ounter
S06.5X4A	Traumatic subdural hemorrhage with loss of consciousness 6 hrs. to 24 hrs., initial encounter
S06.6X4A	Traumatic subarachnoid hemorrhage with loss of consciousness 6 hrs. to 24 hrs., initial encounter
Fracture Skull Vault	
S02.0XXA	Fracture of vault of skull, initial encounter for closed fracture
Hemorrhage/Loss of Consciousness	
S06.4X5A	Epidural hemorrhage with loss of consciousness greater than 24 hours with return to pre-existing conscious level, initial encounter
S06.5X5A	Traumatic subdural hemorrhage with loss of consciousness greater than 24 hours with return to pre-existing conscious level, initial encounter
S06.6X5A	Traumatic subarachnoid hemorrhage with loss of consciousness greater than 24 hours with return to preexisting conscious level, initial encounter
Fracture Skull Vault	
S02.0XXA	Fracture of vault of skull, initial encounter for closed fracture
Hemorrhage/Loss of Consciousness	
S06.4X6A	Epidural hemorrhage with loss of consciousness greater than 24 hours without return to pre-existing conscious level with patient surviving, initial encounter
S06.5X6A	Traumatic subdural hemorrhage with loss of consciousness greater than 24 hours without return to pre-existing conscious level with patient surviving, initial encounter
S06.6X6A	Traumatic subarachnoid hemorrhage with loss of consciousness greater than 24 hours without return to pre-existing conscious level with patient surviving, initial encounter
Fracture Skull Vault	
S02.0XXA	Fracture of vault of skull, initial encounter for closed fracture
Hemorrhage/Loss of Consciousness	
S06.4X9A	Epidural hemorrhage with loss of consciousness of unspecified duration, initial encounter
S06.5X9A	Traumatic subdural hemorrhage with loss of consciousness of unspecified duration, initial encounter
S06.6X9A	Traumatic subarachnoid hemorrhage with loss of consciousness of unspecified duration, initial encounter

Note 1: An initial encounter for an open fracture of vault of skull with subarachnoid, subdural, and extradural hemorrhage is reported with the same codes listed above except that the 7th character extension 'A' is replaced with a 'B' for initial encounter for open fracture.

Note 2: The 7th character 'A' for codes in category S06 indicates only that this is the initial encounter, not whether or not the injury is open or closed.

Note 3: There are ICD-10-CM epidural hemorrhage, traumatic subarachnoid hemorrhage, and traumatic subdural hemorrhage codes that reflect death either due to the brain injury or other brain injury. These codes are:

S06.4X7A Epidural hemorrhage with loss of consciousness of any duration with death due to brain injury prior to regaining consciousness, initial encounter

S06.4X8A Epidural hemorrhage with loss of consciousness of any duration with death due to other cause prior to regaining consciousness, initial encounter

S06.5X7A Traumatic subdural hemorrhage with loss of consciousness of any duration with death due to brain injury prior to regaining consciousness, initial encounter

S06.5X8A Traumatic subdural hemorrhage with loss of consciousness of any duration with death due to other cause prior to regaining consciousness, initial encounter

S06.6X7A Traumatic subarachnoid hemorrhage with loss of consciousness of any duration with death due to brain injury prior to regaining consciousness, initial encounter

S06.6X8A Traumatic subarachnoid hemorrhage with loss of consciousness of any duration with death due to other cause prior to regaining consciousness, initial encounter

Documentation and Coding Example

Sixteen-year-old Caucasian male transported to local ED via ambulance after he was found unresponsive at home by his mother. Patient has a fresh **4 cm x 5 cm hematoma on left temporal area.** Mother states her son was **surfing** earlier in the day and was hit in the head by his board. He continued surfing for approximately 1 hour following the accident and drove himself home. He was alert and oriented all morning, only complaining of a headache, taking ibuprofen at 10 AM. He **appeared to be sleeping at 1 PM when mother left to do errands and she was unable to arouse him when she returned 2 hours later.** On examination, this is a well-developed, well-nourished, adolescent male. Temperature 97.4, HR 66, RR 12, BP 88/50. **Neurological examination reveals no spontaneous eye opening or response to verbal commands, there is withdrawal from painful stimuli. Score = 6 on Glasgow Coma Scale.** Call placed to Children's Hospital Trauma Center and life flight team dispatched. ETA 22 minutes. NSR on cardiac monitor. O2 saturation 92% by pulse oximetry, O2 started at 2 L/m via non-rebreather mask. HOB elevated 30%. IV line placed right forearm, LR infusing. Blood drawn for CBC, platelets, electrolytes, PT, PTT, type and hold and sent to lab. Bladder can be palpated above the pubic bone, Foley catheter placed without difficulty, 600 cc clear yellow urine returned.

Transport Team Note: Arrived in ED at 4:13 PM. Baseline lab tests all within normal limits. ABG drawn pH 7.32, pCO2 51, HCO3 25, pO2 88 %, SaO2 96 %. Patient intubated without difficulty, hand ventilated by RT. Transferred to life flight stretcher, on monitors, stable for transport. All consents obtained, parents following in private car. ETA Children's Hospital 17 minutes with neurosurgical team assembled and ready for patient. Uneventful helicopter transport. Patient taken directly from heliport to CT. Care assumed by neurosurgical team and radiology staff.

Neurosurgical Note: CT scan reveals a linear fracture of the left parietal bone with large subdural hematoma. Patient taken to OR at 6:15 PM where a craniotomy was performed under general anesthesia. Hematoma evacuated and patient taken to Neurosurgical ICU with arterial line, CVP line, ICP catheter. Mannitol drip, prophylactic antibiotics, and anti-seizure medications.

Neurosurgical ICU Note: Patient arrived in unit at 9:50 PM. VSS stable on monitors. CVP, ICP pressures WNL. Patient comfortably sedated, taking spontaneous breaths on ventilator. Parents in to visit. **Opens eyes to parents' voices, localizes painful stimuli, unable to vocalize due to intubation, Glasgow coma scale=9**. Continued progress throughout night, extubated at 6 AM. Alert, recognizes parents, oriented to person only, last memory he has is surfing.

Discharge Note: Patient made an excellent physical recovery from surgery and is discharged on post-op day 5, wound staples removed prior to discharge. He has no residual weakness or visual deficits. He still has no memory of the time between surfing and waking up in the ICU. Patient weaned from antiseizure medications with normal EEG. He is discharged without medications and will be seen in Neurosurgical Clinic in 2 days.

Discharge diagnosis:

Linear skull fracture, left parietal bone

Large subdural hematoma

Total duration of loss of consciousness estimated at 6-7 hours

Diagnosis Code(s)

Note: Codes are for inpatient services at 2nd facility

S06.5X4A Traumatic subdural hemorrhage with loss of consciousness 6 hours to 24 hours, initial encounter

S02.0XXA Fracture of vault of skull, initial encounter for closed fracture

R40.2134 Coma scale, eyes open to sound, 24 hours or more after hospital admission

R40.2214 Coma scale, best verbal response, none, 24 hours or more after hospital admission

R40.2354 Coma scale, best motor response, localizes pain, 24 hours or more after hospital admission

W21.89XA Striking against or struck by other sports equipment, initial encounter

Y92.832 Beach as the place of occurrence of the external cause

Y93.18 Activity, surfing, windsurfing and boogie boarding

Y99.8 Other external cause status

Coding Note(s)

In ICD-10-CM, there is a sequencing note indicating that the intracranial injury is coded first. Glasgow coma scale codes are reported additionally with the fracture of skull (S02.-) and/or intracranial injury (S06.-) reported first. Both facilities and all physicians and ancillary service providers will report skull fracture codes with 7th character 'A' for initial episode of care because the services described above are related to the acute phase of the injury. The patient has a hematoma but no open wound of the head is documented, so the skull fracture is classified as a closed fracture which is also captured by the 7th character 'A'. The traumatic subdural hemorrhage is also reported with 7th character 'A'. There is documentation related to each element of the coma scale so each of the three components are coded rather than assigning the code for the Glasgow coma scale total score from subcategory R40.24. If only the total score had been reported, code R40.242 Glasgow coma scale score 9-12 would be assigned instead of the individual coma scores for eyes open, best verbal response, and best motor response.

Fracture of Cervical Vertebra with Spinal Cord Injury

Fractures of the cervical vertebra or other parts of the neck are reported with codes from category S12. If the fracture is associated with a cervical spinal cord injury, a code from category S14 is also required, and the code from category S14 is listed first. Fracture and spinal cord injury codes require the specific level of the fracture (C1, C2, C3, C4, C5, C6, C7). Associated spinal cord injuries require documentation of the type and extent of the injury to include incomplete lesion, Brown-Sequard syndrome, and a subcategory for other specified incomplete lesion.

Coding and Documentation Requirements

Fracture of cervical spine

Identify level/site of cervical spine fracture:

- C1
- C2
- C3
- C4
- C5
- C6
- C7

Identify type of fracture:

- For C1
  - Burst fracture
    - » Stable
    - » Unstable
  - » Posterior arch
  - » Lateral mass
  - » Other specified fracture
  - » Unspecified fracture

- For C2
  - Dens fracture
    - » Type II anterior displaced
    - » Type II posterior displaced
    - » Type II nondisplaced
    - » Other displaced
    - » Other nondisplaced
  - Traumatic spondylolisthesis
    - » Type III
    - » Other specified traumatic spondylolisthesis
    - » Unspecified traumatic spondylolisthesis
  - Other specified fracture
  - Unspecified fracture
- For C3-C7
  - Traumatic spondylolisthesis
    - » Type III
    - » Other specified traumatic spondylolisthesis
    - » Unspecified traumatic spondylolisthesis
  - Other specified fracture
  - Unspecified fracture

Identify fracture as nondisplaced or displaced as needed:

- Displaced
- Nondisplaced

Note: Some specific types of fractures are by definition either nondisplaced or displaced so this qualifier is not always required.

Identify fracture as:

- Closed
- Open

Identify episode of care:

- Initial
- Subsequent
  - With routine healing of fracture
  - With delayed healing of fracture
  - With nonunion of fracture
- Sequela

Spinal cord injury (if present)

Identify type of spinal cord injury:

- Anterior cord syndrome
- Brown-Sequard syndrome
- Central cord syndrome
- Complete lesion of cord
- Concussion/edema
- Other specified incomplete lesion of spinal cord
- Unspecified spinal cord injury

Identify highest level of cervical spinal cord injury:

- C1
- C2
- C3
- C4
- C5
- C6
- C7
- C8
- Unspecified level

Identify episode of care:

- Initial
- Subsequent
- Sequela

C5 Fracture with Spinal Cord Injury

ICD-10-CM Code/Documentation	
C5 Vertebral Fracture	
S12.400A	Unspecified displaced fracture of fifth cervical vertebrae, initial encounter for closed fracture
S12.401A	Unspecified nondisplaced fracture of fifth cervical vertebra, initial encounter for closed fracture
S12.430A	Unspecified traumatic displaced spondylolisthesis of fifth cervical vertebra, initial encounter for closed fracture
S12.431A	Unspecified traumatic nondisplaced spondylolisthesis of fifth cervical vertebra, initial encounter for closed fracture
S12.44XA	Type III traumatic spondylolisthesis of fifth cervical vertebra, initial encounter for closed fracture
S12.450A	Other traumatic displaced spondylolisthesis of fifth cervical vertebra, initial encounter for closed fracture
S12.451A	Other traumatic nondisplaced spondylolisthesis of fifth cervical vertebra, initial encounter for closed fracture
S12.490A	Other displaced fracture of fifth cervical vertebra, initial encounter for closed fracture
S12.491A	Other nondisplaced fracture of fifth cervical vertebra, initial encounter for closed fracture
C5 Spinal Cord Injury	
S14.105A	Unspecified injury at C5 level of cervical spinal cord, initial encounter
C5 Vertebral Fracture	
S12.400A	Unspecified displaced fracture of fifth cervical vertebrae, initial encounter for closed fracture
S12.401A	Unspecified nondisplaced fracture of fifth cervical vertebra, initial encounter for closed fracture
S12.430A	Unspecified traumatic displaced spondylolisthesis of fifth cervical vertebra, initial encounter for closed fracture
S12.431A	Unspecified traumatic nondisplaced spondylolisthesis of fifth cervical vertebra, initial encounter for closed fracture
S12.44XA	Type III traumatic spondylolisthesis of fifth cervical vertebra, initial encounter for closed fracture
S12.450A	Other traumatic displaced spondylolisthesis of fifth cervical vertebra, initial encounter for closed fracture
S12.451A	Other traumatic nondisplaced spondylolisthesis of fifth cervical vertebra, initial encounter for closed fracture
S12.490A	Other displaced fracture of fifth cervical vertebra, initial encounter for closed fracture

ICD-10-CM Code/Documentation	
S12.491A	Other nondisplaced fracture of fifth cervical vertebra, initial encounter for closed fracture
C5 Spinal Cord Injury	
S14.115A	Complete lesion at C5 level of cervical spinal cord, initial encounter
S12.451A	Other traumatic nondisplaced spondylolisthesis of fifth cervical vertebra, initial encounter for closed fracture
S12.490A	Other displaced fracture of fifth cervical vertebra, initial encounter for closed fracture
S12.491A	Other nondisplaced fracture of fifth cervical vertebra, initial encounter for closed fracture
C5 Spinal Cord Injury	
S14.135A	Anterior cord syndrome at C5 level of cervical spinal cord, initial encounter
C5 Vertebral Fracture	
S12.400A	Unspecified displaced fracture of fifth cervical vertebrae, initial encounter for closed fracture
S12.401A	Unspecified nondisplaced fracture of fifth cervical vertebra, initial encounter for closed fracture
S12.430A	Unspecified traumatic displaced spondylolisthesis of fifth cervical vertebra, initial encounter for closed fracture
S12.431A	Unspecified traumatic nondisplaced spondylolisthesis of fifth cervical vertebra, initial encounter for closed fracture
S12.44XA	Type III traumatic spondylolisthesis of fifth cervical vertebra, initial encounter for closed fracture
S12.450A	Other traumatic displaced spondylolisthesis of fifth cervical vertebra, initial encounter for closed fracture
S12.451A	Other traumatic nondisplaced spondylolisthesis of fifth cervical vertebra, initial encounter for closed fracture
S12.490A	Other displaced fracture of fifth cervical vertebra, initial encounter for closed fracture
S12.491A	Other nondisplaced fracture of fifth cervical vertebra, initial encounter for closed fracture
C5 Spinal Cord Injury	
S14.125A	Central cord syndrome at C5 level of cervical spinal cord, initial encounter
C5 Vertebral Fracture	
S12.400A	Unspecified displaced fracture of fifth cervical vertebrae, initial encounter for closed fracture
S12.401A	Unspecified nondisplaced fracture of fifth cervical vertebra, initial encounter for closed fracture
S12.430A	Unspecified traumatic displaced spondylolisthesis of fifth cervical vertebra, initial encounter for closed fracture
S12.431A	Unspecified traumatic nondisplaced spondylolisthesis of fifth cervical vertebra, initial encounter for closed fracture
S12.44XA	Type III traumatic spondylolisthesis of fifth cervical vertebra, initial encounter for closed fracture
S12.450A	Other traumatic displaced spondylolisthesis of fifth cervical vertebra, initial encounter for closed fracture
S12.451A	Other traumatic nondisplaced spondylolisthesis of fifth cervical vertebra, initial encounter for closed fracture
S12.490A	Other displaced fracture of fifth cervical vertebra, initial encounter for closed fracture

ICD-10-CM Code/Documentation	
S12.491A	Other nondisplaced fracture of fifth cervical vertebra, initial encounter for closed fracture
C5 Spinal Cord Injury	
S14.0XXA	Concussion and edema of cervical spinal cord, initial encounter
S14.145A	Brown-Sequard syndrome at C5 level of spinal cord, initial encounter
S14.155A	Other incomplete lesion at C5 level of spinal cord, initial encounter

Documentation and Coding Example

Patient is a thirty-eight-year-old Hispanic female brought to ED following **MVA**. Patient was an **unrestrained passenger** in the rear seat of a **car struck head on by another car at a high rate** of speed. She was completely ejected and found semi-conscious with no spontaneous movement on the pavement approximately 50 feet from the **crash site on I-15**. IV started in left antecubital, C-spine immobilized, placed on backboard and transported via ambulance to ED. On examination, this is a mildly obese, middle-aged female. She has **abrasions and contusions on face, upper right shoulder, and right thoracic region of back** consistent with sliding on asphalt. Patient **opens her eyes on command and can state her name**. She is able to recall being in a car accident, is not able to provide any medical history. Vocal quality is weak and breathless. PERRL. HR 50, RR 20, BP 84/50. O2 Sat. 93% on O2 4 L/m via mask. Color pale, skin diaphoretic. Breath sounds clear, shallow. Apical pulse irregular, peripheral pulses weak. SR on monitor with frequent PVCs. Abdomen soft, non-distended with poor tone. Bedside US reveals no free fluid in peritoneum. Foley catheter placed and returns clear yellow urine. Patient has no sensory awareness from shoulders down and no spontaneous muscle movement. She does complain of pain in her face, jaw, and neck. Findings are consistent with traumatic injury to the neck and spinal cord.

C-spine x-ray reveals a fracture of C5 with small fragment anteriorly and angulation of C5-C6 with displacement of C5 posteriorly. Neurosurgical team assembled and ready to assume care. CT reveals severe axial loading with propulsion of a teardrop bone fragment anteriorly and larger portion of the bone resting posterior against the spinal cord. MRI is consistent with soft tissue injury both anterior and posterior to the spinal cord. Patient is taken to surgery for decompression of spinal cord and stabilization of fracture.

Surgical ICU Note: Patient admitted from OR following decompression laminectomy, intubated, on ventilator, neck immobilized with hard cervical collar. Arterial line patent left wrist, peripheral IV lines in left antecubital and right hand. Abrasions cleaned in OR are covered with Xeroform gauze. There is no voluntary muscle movement and flaccid muscle tone from shoulders to toes. **Weaned from ventilator** on day four.

Step Down Unit Note: Transferred 5 days with one peripheral IV line. Patient has very flat affect, she reportedly lost all family members in the accident. Reflexes are consistent with a **complete spinal cord injury** at C5. She is able to perform a very weak shoulder shrug bilaterally but has no sensation or movement below that level. Patient receiving PT, OT, and ST.

Diagnosis Code(s)

S14.115A Complete lesion at C5 level of cervical spinal cord, initial encounter

S12.490A Other displaced fracture of fifth cervical vertebrae, initial encounter for closed fracture

S00.81XA Abrasion of other part of head, initial encounter

S00.83XA Contusion of other part of head, initial encounter

S20.221A Contusion of right back wall of thorax, initial encounter

S20.411A Abrasion of right back wall of thorax, initial encounter

S40.011A Contusion of right shoulder, initial encounter

S40.211A Abrasion of right shoulder, initial encounter

V43.62XA Car passenger injured in collision with other type car in traffic accident, initial encounter

Y92.411 Interstate highway as the place of occurrence of the external cause

Coding Note(s)

There is a note under category S14 to code also any transient paralysis (R29.5). Code R29.5 would not be reported as the patient has sustained an injury resulting in permanent paralysis.

Fracture of Dorsal (Thoracic) Vertebra

Similar to cervical spine fractures both the level of the fracture and the type of fracture must be specified. In addition, the fracture must be documented as open or closed and the episode of care must be known. For follow-up care, healing must be documented as routine, delayed, or with nonunion.

Coding and Documentation Requirements

Identify level of vertebral fracture:

- T1
- T2
- T3
- T4
- T5-T6
- T7-T8
- T9-T10
- T11-T12

Identify type of fracture:

- Burst
  - Stable
  - Unstable
- Wedge compression
- Other specified type of fracture
- Unspecified type of fracture

Identify fracture:

- Closed
- Open

Identify episode of care:

- Initial
- Subsequent
  - With routine healing of fracture
  - With delayed healing of fracture
  - With nonunion of fracture
- Sequela

Fracture of T11-T12 Vertebra

ICD-10-CM Code/Documentation	
Closed Fracture	
S22.080A	Wedge compression fracture of T11-T12 vertebra, initial encounter for closed fracture
S22.081A	Stable burst fracture of T11-T12 vertebra, initial encounter for closed fracture
S22.082A	Unstable burst fracture of T11-T12 vertebra, initial encounter for closed fracture
S22.088A	Other fracture of T11-T12 vertebra, initial encounter for closed fracture
S22.089A	Unspecified fracture of T11-T12 vertebra, initial encounter for closed fracture
Open Fracture	
S22.080B	Wedge compression fracture of T11-T12 vertebra, initial encounter for open fracture
S22.081B	Stable burst fracture of T11-T12 vertebra, initial encounter for open fracture
S22.082B	Unstable burst fracture of T11-T12 vertebra, initial encounter for open fracture
S22.088B	Other fracture of T11-T12 vertebra, initial encounter for open fracture
S22.089V	Unspecified fracture of T11-T12 vertebra, initial encounter for open fracture

Documentation and Coding Example

Thirty-nine-year-old male presents to ED with c/o moderate to severe pain in his back after falling approximately 15 feet from a boulder while **rock climbing**. Accident occurred approximately 2 hours ago. Patient is a well-developed, well-nourished male who looks younger than his stated age. He is muscular and very tan. He states he is a professional guide leading hiking tours and rock climbing expeditions. The accident today occurred in his **leisure time** on a familiar rock face and was witnessed by friends. As he descended from the top of the rock, his equipment malfunctioned and he dropped rapidly, landing with a hard jolt upright on both legs. He felt an immediate sharp pain in the mid back which is relieved somewhat by lying flat. He denies pain in his hips, knees, or ankles and was able to hike approximately 1/2 mile to a vehicle. On examination: Temperature 99 degrees, HR 72, RR 12, BP 114/60. Skin warm, slightly diaphoretic, outdoor temperature is in upper 80s. O2 saturation on RA 96%. PERRL, oriented x 3. No cervical spine tenderness and cranial nerves are grossly intact. Motor and sensory function is intact to upper extremities. Breath sounds clear and equal bilaterally, HR regular, no murmur or muffling of heart sounds appreciated. No visual deformities to spine but there is exquisite tenderness with muscle guarding at level of T10 to L4. There is no sign of crepitus. He has limited ROM when attempting flexion, extension, and rotation of spine due to pain. There are no neurological deficits in lower extremities. IV started in left forearm, D5 LR infusing. Medicated for pain with MS 2 mg IV push with good relief. AP and lateral spine x-rays reveal a possible **wedge compression fracture at T12**. CT confirms wedge compression fracture involving the anterior column at T12. Orthopedic consult obtained. Patient fitted with TLSO brace and discharged home with oral narcotic pain medication and instructions to schedule a follow-up in orthopedic clinic in 1 week.

Diagnosis Code(s)

S22.080A Wedge compression fracture of T11-T12 vertebra, initial encounter for closed fracture

W17.89XA Other fall from one level to another, initial encounter

Y93.31 Activity, mountain climbing, rock climbing, and wall climbing

Y92.838 Other recreation area as place of occurrence of the external cause

Y99.8 Other external cause status

Coding Note(s)

Y99.8 Other external cause status which includes leisure activity, is used instead of Y99.0 Civilian activity done for income or pay because even though the patient works as a guide on rock climbing expeditions, he incurred this injury during his leisure time not while he was working.

Hemiplegia and Hemiparesis

The terms hemiplegia and hemiparesis are often used interchangeably, but the two conditions are not the same. Hemiplegia is paralysis of one side of the body while hemiparesis is weakness on one side of the body. Hemiparesis is less severe than hemiplegia and both are a common side effect of stroke or cerebrovascular accident. Hemiplegia and hemiparesis must be clearly differentiated in the medical record documentation. Disability in these cases is determined by the underlying diagnosis, whether the paralysis is temporary or permanent, the extent of paralysis (monoplegia, hemiplegia, paraplegia, quadriplegia), and the body parts affected.

Hemiplegia and hemiparesis are frequently sequelae of cerebrovascular disease; however, cervical spinal cord diseases, peripheral nervous system diseases, and other conditions may manifest as hemiplegia. Precise, detailed provider documentation in the medical record is key to correct code assignment.

These conditions are reported with codes in category G81. There is a note indicating that codes in these categories are used only when hemiplegia or hemiparesis is documented without further specification, or is documented as old or longstanding of unspecified cause. The hemiplegia and hemiparesis codes may also be used in multiple coding scenarios to identify the specified types of hemiplegia resulting from any cause.

In hemiplegia and hemiparesis cases, the documentation needs to identify whether the dominant or nondominant side is affected.

If the affected side is documented but not specified as dominant or nondominant, Code selection for a specified side without documentation of which side is dominant is reported as follows:

- If the left side is affected, the default is non-dominant
- If the right side is affected, the default is dominant
- In ambidextrous patients, the default is dominant

It should be noted that hemiplegia documented as congenital or infantile, or due to sequela of a cerebrovascular accident or disease is not reported with codes from these categories. Congenital hemiplegia is used to describe hemiplegia demonstrated at birth while infantile hemiplegia refers to hemiplegia that develops in infancy or within the first few years of life. Congenital or infantile hemiplegia is reported with a code from category G80. Hemiplegia and hemiparesis due to sequelae of cerebrovascular disease is reported with codes from subcategories I69.05, I69.15, I69.25, I69.35, I69.85, and I69.95.

To assign the most specific code for hemiplegia or hemiparesis, the correct category must first be identified. Documentation should be reviewed for the following descriptors:

- Congenital or infantile
- Due to late effect of cerebrovascular accident
- Not otherwise specified

For hemiplegia or hemiparesis of long-standing duration, or not specified as to cause, or to report hemiplegia or hemiparesis in a multiple coding scenario, the type of hemiplegia or hemiparesis must be identified along with the side which should be specified as dominant or nondominant.

Coding and Documentation Requirements

Identify the type of hemiplegia or hemiparesis:

- Flaccid
- Spastic
- Unspecified

Identify the side affected:

- Right
  - Dominant side
  - Nondominant side
- Left
  - Dominant side
  - Nondominant side
- Unspecified side

ICD-10-CM Code/Documentation	
G81.00	Flaccid hemiplegia affecting unspecified side
G81.01	Flaccid hemiplegia affecting right dominant side
G81.02	Flaccid hemiplegia affecting left dominant side
G81.03	Flaccid hemiplegia affecting right nondominant side

ICD-10-CM Code/Documentation	
G81.04	Flaccid hemiplegia affecting left nondominant side
G81.10	Spastic hemiplegia affecting unspecified side
G81.11	Spastic hemiplegia affecting right dominant side
G81.12	Spastic hemiplegia affecting left dominant side
G81.13	Spastic hemiplegia affecting right nondominant side
G81.14	Spastic hemiplegia affecting left nondominant side
G81.90	Hemiplegia, unspecified affecting unspecified side
G81.91	Hemiplegia, unspecified affecting right dominant side
G81.92	Hemiplegia, unspecified affecting left dominant side
G81.93	Hemiplegia, unspecified affecting right nondominant side
G81.94	Hemiplegia, unspecified affecting left nondominant side

Documentation and Coding Example

Patient is a 78-year-old, **right-handed female with longstanding flaccid hemiplegia of unspecified cause affecting her left side.** On admission to the SNF, the patient is experiencing a largely flaccid hemiplegia with Chedoke-McMaster Staging scores on the left side of 1/7 in the hand and arm, 1/7 in the leg and 1/7 in the foot, and 1/7 for posture. There were no sensory problems noted. The patient uses a manual wheelchair with a lap tray for mobility. She was able to complete a 2-person pivot transfer despite problems with her balance. She requires set-up assistance with her meals and one person to assist her with dressing, grooming, and bathing. Due to her poor recovery prognosis, the plan of care will focus on minimizing contractures and palliation of pain. Ensure the flaccid arm is continuously supported when the patient is sitting or transferring—use lap tray or arm sling.

Very gentle range of motion exercises with physiotherapy.

Diagnosis: **Left-sided flaccid hemiplegia**

Diagnosis Code(s)

G81.04 Flaccid hemiplegia affecting left nondominant side

Coding Note(s)

This case is coded as flaccid hemiplegia of the nondominant side because the documentation describes the patient as righthanded, so the right side is the dominant side.

Malignant Neoplasm of Connective and Other Soft Tissue

Primary malignant neoplasms of connective and other soft tissues are classified as sarcomas and are extremely rare. There are many types of sarcomas and often the histological type is more specifically documented. Some histological types of connective tissue neoplasms are malignant fibrous histiocytoma, neurosarcoma, rhabdomyosarcoma, fibrosarcoma, hemangiopericytoma, and angiosarcoma. Gastrointestinal stromal tumors, or GIST, is another type of sarcoma that grows from the stromal cells of the digestive organs. Stromal cells are the connective tissue cells, such as fibroblasts, that support the function of the parenchymal cells of that organ.

When the histology of a neoplasm is documented, it is necessary to reference the histological type in the Alphabetic Index before proceeding to the Tabular List. Most of these histologic types refer the coder to Neoplasm, connective tissue, malignant. However, there are some exceptions. Neurosarcoma indicates that the correct code is found under Neoplasm, nerve, malignant. In the case of hemangiopericytoma, unless the documentation specifically identifies the neoplasm as malignant, the code for neoplasm, connective tissue, uncertain behavior is assigned.

Primary malignant neoplasms of connective and other soft tissue are separated into two categories. Category C47 reports primary malignant neoplasms of peripheral nerves and the autonomic nervous system. Category C49 reports primary malignant neoplasms of all other connective and soft tissues, including gastrointestinal stromal tumors. Both categories require laterality for reporting connective and soft tissue malignant neoplasms of the upper and lower limbs.

Coding and Documentation Requirements

Identify type of connective/soft tissue:

- Peripheral nerve/autonomic nervous system
- Other connective/soft tissue, which includes:
  - – Blood vessel
  - – Bursa
  - – Cartilage
  - – Fascia
  - – Fat
  - – Ligament, except uterine
  - – Lymphatic vessel
  - –Muscle
  - – Synovia
  - – Tendon (sheath)

Identify site:

- Abdomen
- Head/face/neck
- Lower limb, including hip
  - – Left
  - – Right
  - – Unspecified
- Overlapping sites
- Pelvis
- Thorax
- Trunk, unspecified
- Unspecified site

ICD-10-CM Code/Documentation	
C47.0	Malignant neoplasm of peripheral nerves of head, face and neck
C47.10	Malignant neoplasm of peripheral nerves of unspecified upper limb, including shoulder
C47.11	Malignant neoplasm of peripheral nerves of right upper limb, including shoulder

ICD-10-CM Code/Documentation	
C47.12	Malignant neoplasm of peripheral nerves of left upper limb, including shoulder
C47.20	Malignant neoplasm of peripheral nerves of unspecified lower limb, including hip
C47.21	Malignant neoplasm of peripheral nerves of right lower limb, including hip
C47.22	Malignant neoplasm of peripheral nerves of left lower limb, including hip
C47.3	Malignant neoplasm of peripheral nerves of thorax
C47.4	Malignant neoplasm of peripheral nerves of abdomen
C47.5	Malignant neoplasm of peripheral nerves of pelvis
C47.6	Malignant neoplasm of peripheral nerves of trunk, unspecified
C47.8	Malignant neoplasm of overlapping sites of peripheral nerves and autonomic nervous system
C47.9	Malignant neoplasm of peripheral nerves and autonomic system, unspecified
C49.0	Malignant neoplasm of connective and soft tissue of head, face and neck
C49.10	Malignant neoplasm of connective and soft tissue of unspecified upper limb, including shoulder
C49.11	Malignant neoplasm of connective and soft tissue of right upper limb, including shoulder
C49.12	Malignant neoplasm of connective and soft tissue of left upper limb, including shoulder
C49.20	Malignant neoplasm of connective and soft tissue of unspecified lower limb, including hip
C49.21	Malignant neoplasm of connective and soft tissue of right lower limb, including hip
C49.22	Malignant neoplasm of connective and soft tissue of left lower limb, including hip
C49.3	Malignant neoplasm of connective and soft tissue of thorax
C49.4	Malignant neoplasm of connective and soft tissue of abdomen
C49.5	Malignant neoplasm of connective and soft tissue of pelvis
C49.6	Malignant neoplasm of connective and soft tissue of trunk, unspecified
C49.8	Malignant neoplasm of overlapping sites of connective and soft tissue
C49.9	Malignant neoplasm of connective and soft tissue, unspecified
C49.A0	Gastrointestinal stromal tumor, unspecified site
C49.A1	Gastrointestinal stromal tumor of esophagus
C49.A2	Gastrointestinal stromal tumor of stomach
C49.A3	Gastrointestinal stromal tumor of small intestine
C49.A4	Gastrointestinal stromal tumor of large intestine
C49.A5	Gastrointestinal stromal tumor of rectum
C49.A9	Gastrointestinal stromal tumor of other sites

Documentation and Coding Example

Twenty-eight-year-old male presents with pain and swelling of the right upper arm, he can recall no injury or trauma to the area. Patient is right hand dominant and has a history of neurofibromatosis, type 1. Temperature 97.8, HR 62, RR 12, BP 104/66. On examination, this is a well-developed, well-nourished young man. He has at least 25 cafe-au-lait spots > 1cm in size on his upper body and freckling in the axilla bilaterally. Scattered pea size neurofibromas can be palpated beneath the skin on neck, torso, and both upper extremities. There are no observable skeletal deformities and his head appears to be of average size. PERRL, 4 Lisch nodules are present on right iris, 2 on left. Neck supple without lymphadenopathy. Mucous membranes are moist and pink. Weakness noted with flexion and supination of the right forearm, peripheral pulses intact. A 4 x 6 cm firm, tender mass is palpated in the right upper arm, 6 cm above the elbow along the mid-anterior area. The skin overlying the mass is of normal temperature and color. The skin on the lateral side of right forearm is cooler to touch and both sharp and dull sensation is decreased.

Impression: Neurofibroma of the right brachial plexus R/O peripheral nerve sheath tumor/soft tissue sarcoma. Labs/Tests: CBC, Sed Rate, CRP, RUE x-ray (including shoulder) and ultrasound. Radiologic and US studies confirm solid mass tumor. MRI indicates tumor with pseudocapsule and perilesional edema along musculocutaneous nerve. Ultrasound guided needle biopsy performed.

Diagnosis: **Malignant peripheral nerve sheath tumor.** Further testing ordered: CT scan of chest, PET scan, bone scan to identify any metastatic disease.

Diagnosis Code(s)

C47.11 Malignant neoplasm of peripheral nerves of right upper limb, including shoulder

Q85.01 Neurofibromatosis, type 1

Coding Note(s)

Under category C49 Malignant neoplasm of other connective and soft tissue there is an Excludes2 note for malignant neoplasm of peripheral nerves and autonomic nervous system (C47.-) indicating that it is possible to have both types of malignancies at the same time. In this case the malignancy is identified as being in the nerve sheath only, so only code C47.11 is reported. If the physician had indicated that surrounding soft tissue was also involved, it would be appropriate to report a code from both categories.

Malignant Neoplasm of Spinal Cord

In adults, the spinal cord extends from the foramen magnum at the base of the skull to the level of the first or second lumbar vertebrae. The terminal end of the spinal cord is referred to as the conus medullaris. Nerve roots that extend distal to the conus medullaris form the cauda equina which is a Latin term meaning horse's tail. The conus medullaris and cauda equina are the sites where the nervous system transitions from the central nervous system to the peripheral nervous system. The motor nerve roots of the cauda equina are considered part of the peripheral nervous system.

Primary malignant spinal cord and cauda equina tumors are those that originate in cells and tissue of the spinal cord and cauda equina respectively. Primary malignant neoplasms of both sites include ependymomas and astrocytomas. Ependymomas are the most common type. Most ependymomas are primary malignant neoplasms. However, some ependymomas, such as those described as myxopapillary or papillary, are classified under neoplasm, uncertain behavior. Astrocytomas are the second most common type and they are most often classified as primary malignant neoplasms, although for astrocytoma, subependymal, giant cell, the Alphabetic Index indicates that a code for neoplasm, uncertain behavior should be assigned. Schwannomas are another type of nervous system malignant neoplasm.

The site of the malignancy must be documented as the spinal cord or the cauda equina.

Coding and Documentation Requirements

Identify site:

- Spinal cord
- Cauda equina

ICD-10-CM Code/Documentation	
C72.0	Malignant neoplasm of spinal cord
C72.1	Malignant neoplasm of cauda equina

Documentation and Coding Example

Seventeen-year-old male presents to ED with severe low back pain not relieved with ice, rest, and ibuprofen. Student was in his usual state of good health until 1 day prior to admission when he had sudden onset of pain in his lower back radiating into his buttocks after a routine water polo practice at school. He was examined by the school's athletic trainer, told it was a muscle strain and advised to take 600 mg of ibuprofen q 8 hours RTC, ice for 20 minutes q 2 hours while awake and resume normal activities in 24 hours. Patient awoke this morning with a deep aching pain in lower back and sharp pain radiating through his buttocks and down both legs. He also noticed numbness in his groin and some urinary hesitancy and weakness of urine flow. Over the past 8 hours he has developed bilateral lower extremity weakness and sensory loss. Temperature 98.6, HR 100, RR 16, BP 106/66. On examination, this is an anxious appearing, well-developed, well-nourished teenager. He denies recent injury, illness, or drug use other than ibuprofen. PERRL, neck supple without lymphadenopathy. Upper extremity pulses and reflexes grossly intact. Heart rate regular, breath sounds clear and equal bilaterally. Abdomen soft with decreased bowel sounds. Bladder is distended. There is decreased anal sphincter tone on rectal exam. Patient states pain is constant, not relieved by any position change. There is decreased muscle tone and tendon reflexes in both lower extremities. Pulses are intact and there is no peripheral edema noted in lower extremities. Impression: Cauda equina syndrome, R/O tumor, infection, injury. Neurosurgical consult obtained. Labs/Tests: IV started and blood drawn for CBC, Sed Rate, CRP, PT, PTT, Metabolic Panel. Foley catheter placed and urine sent to lab for UA, culture. MRI of spine and pelvis with gadolinium contrast obtained and **reveals a 2 x 2.5 cm mass consistent with tumor, just below the dura in the posterior cauda equina.** IV dexamethasone and broad-spectrum antibiotics administered, emergency laminectomy performed, **biopsy reveals malignant neoplasm.** Tumor successfully removed.

Diagnosis: **Malignant neoplasm of cauda equina.**

Diagnosis Code(s)

C72.1 Malignant neoplasm of cauda equina

Migraine

Migraine is a common neurological disorder that often manifests as a headache. Usually unilateral and pulsating in nature, the headache results from abnormal brain activity along nerve pathways and brain chemical (neurotransmitter) changes. These affect blood flow in the brain and surrounding tissue and may trigger an "aura" or warning sign (visual, sensory, language, motor) before the onset of pain. Migraine headache is frequently accompanied by autonomic nervous system symptoms (nausea, vomiting, and sensitivity to light and/or sound). Triggers can include caffeine withdrawal, stress, lack of sleep. The various types of migraines are reported with codes in category G43. All migraines must be documented as intractable or not intractable. Terms that describe intractable migraine include: pharmacoresistant or pharmacologically resistant, treatment resistant, refractory, and poorly controlled. All migraines except cyclical vomiting (G43.A-), ophthalmoplegic (G43.B-), periodic headache syndromes child/adult (G43.C-) and abdominal migraines (G43.D-) must be documented as with status or without status migrainosus. Status migrainosus refers to a migraine that has lasted more than 72 hours.

Coding and Documentation Requirements

Identify migraine type:

- Abdominal
- Chronic without aura
- Cyclical vomiting
- Hemiplegic
- Menstrual
- Ophthalmoplegic
- Periodic headache syndromes child/adult
- Persistent aura
  - With cerebral infarction
  - Without cerebral infarction
- With aura
- Without aura
- Other migraine
- Unspecified

Identify presence/absence of intractability:

- Intractable
- Not intractable

Identify presence/absence of status migrainosus:

- With status migrainosus
- Without status migrainosus

Note – Status migrainosus is not required for migraines documented as abdominal, cyclical vomiting, ophthalmoplegic, or periodic head syndromes in child/adult.

Chronic Migraine without Aura

ICD-10-CM Code/Documentation	
G43.709	Chronic migraine without aura, not intractable, without status migrainosus
G43.719	Chronic migraine without aura, intractable, without status migrainosus
G43.701	Chronic migraine without aura, not intractable, with status migrainosus
G43.711	Chronic migraine without aura, intractable, with status migrainosus

Documentation and Coding Example

Presenting Complaint: Thirty-two-year-old Caucasian female is referred to Pain Management Clinic by her PMD for evaluation and treatment of **chronic migraine headache**.

History: PMH is significant for onset of migraines at age 13-14, typically associated with menstruation for 4-5 years and then becoming more frequent and unpredictable. Patient states her headaches are significantly worse in winter and summer since moving to the NE from Hawaii five years ago. She was initially treated with rizatriptan and ibuprofen for periodic pain management and when headaches became more frequent. she was started on daily propranolol. She experienced symptomatic hypotension on propranolol and was switched to amitriptyline which worked well for a few years with headache days numbering 4-5 per month. Gradually her headache days increased and she was switched to topiramate daily, with dose now at 50 mg BID and Treximet taken as needed on acute pain days. She reports **15-20 pain days per month** on these medications for the past 6 months. Headaches are negative for aura, usually bilateral in the supraorbital and/or temporal area with a pulsating quality. She typically experiences photophobia and nausea without vomiting. Patient is married with a 2-year-old son and works part time as a middle school guidance counselor.

Physical Examination: Temperature 97.9 HR 74 RR 14 BP 102/60 WT 122.5 lbs. On examination, this is a pleasant, well-nourished but tired appearing young woman who looks her stated age. At this time, she is experiencing a pulsating headache of moderate intensity, location bilateral with focal area temporal on the right and temporal-supraorbital on the left. She awoke with pain this morning and it has been ongoing for the past 3 days. She denies photophobia or nausea. She has taken topiramate as prescribed but has not taken Treximet in over a week because she ran out. Cranial nerves grossly intact. Both upper and lower extremities have normal strength, movement, and sensation. PERRLA, eyes negative for conjunctival injection and excess tearing. There is no evidence of ptosis or eyelid edema. No lymphadenopathy present. Oral mucosa normal, throat benign. Nares patent without rhinorrhea or congestion. HR regular without bruits, rubs, or murmur. Breath sounds clear, equal bilaterally. Abdomen soft and non-distended, bowel sounds present all quadrants. Liver is palpated at RCM, spleen is not palpated.

Impression: **Intractable chronic migraine headache syndrome not responsive to drug therapy**. Patient is a good candidate for OnabotulinumtoxinA (Botox) therapy. The procedure was explained to patient, questions answered and informed consent obtained.

Procedure Note: Skin over treatment area prepped with alcohol. Vacuum dried powdered Botox 200 units was reconstituted with 4 ml preservative free 0.9% sodium chloride per manufacturers specification. Using a 30-gauge 0.5 inch needle, a total of 155 units (0.1 ml=5 units) of Botox was injected at 31 points including corrugator muscle (10 units/2 sites), procerus muscle (5 units/1 site), frontalis muscle (20 units/4 sites), temporalis muscle (40 units/8 sites), occipitalis muscle (30 units/6 sites), cervical paraspinal muscle group (20 units/4 sites), and trapezius muscle (30 units/6 sites). Patient tolerated the procedure well. She has some mild ptosis noted in left eyelid but it does not obstruct vision.

Plan: Patient is advised to continue current medications as prescribed and that she may experience headache, tenderness at injection site, and mild muscle weakness in the next few days. She should call if she develops any other symptoms or problems. Return to clinic in 5 days for recheck.

Diagnosis Code(s)

G43.719 Chronic migraine without aura, intractable, without status migrainosus

Coding Note(s)

Use of the code for intractable migraine requires documentation that the migraine has not responded to treatment. In this case the patient has been referred to pain medicine because of intractable migraine and that is the stated diagnosis of the pain medicine specialist. The physician has also documented a diagnosis of chronic migraine. Chronic migraine is typically defined as 15 or more headache days per month. The documentation indicates that the patient experiences 15-20 headache days per month which further supports the diagnosis of chronic migraine. Status migrainosus refers to a migraine that has lasted for more than 72 hours. There is no documentation to support status migrainosus so, the code for without status migrainosus is assigned.

Migraine Variant

Migraine variant refers to a migraine that manifests in a form other than head pain. Migraine variants may be characterized by episodes of atypical sensory, motor, or visual aura, confusion, dysarthria, focal neurologic deficits, and other constitutional symptoms, with or without a headache. The provider documentation in the medical record must include enough detail to differentiate migraine variants from other migraines and other headache disorders. The diagnosis of migraine variant is determined by the provider's documentation. Typically, there is a history of paroxysmal signs and symptoms with or without cephalgia and without other disorders that may contribute to the symptoms. Many patients have a family history of migraine.

In the medical record documentation, migraine variants must be clearly differentiated from other headache disorders such as trigeminal autonomic cephalgias (cluster headaches), stabbing headache, thunderclap headaches, hypnic headaches and hemicrania continua, and headache syndromes associated with physical activity (e.g., exertional headaches). Chronic migraine and status migrainosus are not considered migraine variants.

Coding and Documentation Requirements

Identify migraine variant:

- Abdominal migraine
- Cyclical vomiting
- Ophthalmoplegic migraine
- Periodic headache syndromes in child/adult
- Other migraine

Identify response to treatment:

- Intractable
- Not intractable

For migraine variants classified under other migraine, identify any status migrainosus:

- With status migrainosus
- Without status migrainosus

ICD-10-CM Code/Documentation	
G43.A0	Cyclical vomiting, not intractable
G43.A1	Cyclical vomiting, intractable
G43.B0	Ophthalmoplegic migraine, not intractable
G43.B1	Ophthalmoplegic migraine, intractable
G43.C0	Periodic headache syndromes in child or adult, not intractable
G43.C1	Periodic headache syndromes in child or adult, intractable
G43.D0	Abdominal migraine, not intractable
G43.D1	Abdominal migraine, intractable
G43.801	Other migraine, not intractable, with status migrainosus
G43.809	Other migraine, not intractable, without status migrainosus
G43.811	Other migraine, intractable, with status migrainosus
G43.819	Other migraine, intractable, without status migrainosus

Documentation and Coding Example

A 7-year-old girl presented with complete right oculomotor palsy. She complained the previous day of a headache in the orbital region, severe and throbbing in nature. She was given children's Tylenol and went to bed early. She awakened the following morning with complete ptosis of the right upper lid, periorbital pain, and blurred vision. On examination, the right pupil was 6 mm and slightly reactive to light. The neurologic examination and skull x-rays were normal; diagnostic workup including the glucose tolerance test was all negative. MRI and magnetic resonance angiography ruled out aneurysm, tumor, and sphenoid sinus mucocele. Intermittent angle-closure glaucoma with mydriasis was also excluded on gonioscopy. She experienced near complete resolution of her symptoms following treatment with NSAIDs.

Diagnosis: **Ophthalmoplegic migraine**

Diagnosis Code(s)

G43.B0 Ophthalmoplegic migraine, not intractable

Coding Note(s)

Ophthalmoplegic migraine is specified as intractable (with refractory migraine) or not intractable (without refractory migraine). The documentation does not mention intractable migraine or refractory migraine. An intractable or refractory migraine is any migraine that is impossible to manage or resistant to usual therapies.

Other Headache Syndromes

A complaint of headache is a common reason for seeking medical care. Headaches have many causes and while most headaches are benign, a headache may also be a symptom of another underlying disease such as cerebral hemorrhage. A diagnosis of headache that is not further qualified as a specific type, such as tension or migraine, is reported with a symptom code. Other headache syndromes is a broad category that includes many specific headache types with the exception of migraine which has its own category. Below are characteristics of the various types of headaches classified under other headache syndromes.

Cluster headache – Headache characterized by a cyclical pattern of intense, usually unilateral pain with a rapid onset. They are vascular in origin, caused by the sudden dilatation of one or more blood vessels around the trigeminal nerve. The pain often centers behind or around the eye (retro-orbital, orbital, supraorbital) or in the temporal area and has a boring/drilling quality. The pain may be accompanied by one (or more) cranial autonomic nervous system symptoms. Cluster headaches are benign, but can be quite disabling. Individuals may have a genetic predisposition for this type of headache Disorders of the hypothalamus, smoking, and traumatic brain injury may also be causative factors. Cluster headaches are subclassified as episodic or chronic. Episodic cluster headaches typically occur at least once per day, often at the same time of day for several weeks. The headaches are followed by weeks, months, or years that are completely pain free. Chronic cluster headaches may have "high" or "low" cycles in the frequency or intensity of pain but no real remission.

Drug induced headache (medication overuse headache, analgesic rebound headache) – A serious and disabling condition that can occur when medication is taken daily for tension, migraine, or other acute or chronic headache or other pain. As the medication wears off, the pain returns and more medication is needed. This creates a cycle of pain, medicating to relieve the pain, and more intense pain. The condition is more common in women, typically between the ages of 30-40, but it can occur at any age. Pain is often described as a constant dull ache that is worse in the morning and after exercise. Medications associated with this rebound headache phenomena include: acetaminophen, ibuprofen, naproxen, aspirin, codeine, hydrocodone, tramadol, and ergotamine. Triptans (sumatriptan) used for vascular headaches can also induce these headaches. To stop the pain cycle, medication must be discontinued, preferably abruptly and entirely, but slow withdrawal may be necessary in certain situations. This often results in withdrawal symptoms including headache, anxiety, insomnia, and gastrointestinal upset (nausea, vomiting). Withdrawal symptoms can last as long as

12 weeks but typically subside in 7-10 days. Non-steroidal anti-inflammatory drugs (ibuprofen, naproxen) may be given to help relieve rebound headache phenomena when these drugs have not been used previously by the patient to treat the primary headache.

Hemicrania continua – A chronic, persistent, primary headache that often varies in severity as it cycles over a 24 period. It is most often unilateral in location and does not change sides. The incidence is somewhat higher in women with age of onset in early adulthood. There can be migrainous qualities including: pulsating/throbbing pain, nausea and vomiting, photophobia (light sensitivity), and phonophobia (noise sensitivity) along with autonomic nervous system symptoms. The most striking definitive characteristic of hemicrania continua is that it responds almost immediately to treatment with the drug indomethacin.

New daily persistent headache (NDPH) – A distinct, primary headache syndrome with symptoms that can mimic chronic migraine and tension-type headaches. The onset of NDPH is typically abrupt and reaches peak intensity within 3 days. Most individuals can recall the exact day/time of onset of the headache. In some instances, the pain will follow an infection or flu-like illness, surgery, or stressful life event. Autoimmune and/or inflammatory conditions and hypermobility of the cervical spine may also be contributing factors. The pain can be self-limiting (pain ends after a few months) or unrelenting (pain lasts for years) and is often unresponsive to standard therapy.

Paroxysmal hemicranias – Rare type of headache, more common in women, that usually begins during adulthood. The pain is similar to cluster headaches, but is distinguished by greater frequency and shorter duration of the individual episodes, presence of one or more cranial autonomic nervous system symptoms, and a favorable response to the drug indomethacin. Pain is unilateral (always on the same side) and severe, with a throbbing/boring quality behind or around the eye (retro-orbital, orbital, supraorbital) and/or in the temporal area. There can be localized dull pain or soreness in these areas between episodes of acute pain. Occasionally pain may radiate to the ipsilateral (same side) shoulder, arm, or neck. One or more cranial autonomic nervous system symptoms usually accompanies the pain, such as lacrimation (eye tearing), conjunctival injection (eye redness), nasal congestion, rhinorrhea (runny nose), miosis (constricted pupil), ptosis (eyelid drooping), or eyelid edema (swelling). Cause is not known and there is no familial tendency. Paroxysmal hemicranias are subclassified as episodic or chronic. Episodic paroxysmal hemicranias are less severe and less frequent. In some individuals, this non-chronic phase will be a "pass though" to chronic paroxysmal hemicranias. Chronic paroxysmal hemicranias, also referred to as Sjaastad syndrome, is more common than episodic paroxysmal hemicranias and is characterized by more severe and more frequent episodes.

Post-traumatic headache – Headache that occurs following a closed head injury or trauma to the neck area. It is a fairly common and self-limiting condition and may have characteristics of both tension and migrainous pain. The headache rarely occurs in isolation and accompanying symptoms can include: cervical (neck) pain, cognitive, behavioral, and/or somatic problems. Individuals with chronic pain disorders (other than headache), pre-existing headaches, and affective disorders are at greater risk for developing both acute and chronic post traumatic headache. The cycle of pain can be difficult to interrupt once it has been established and overuse of analgesics frequently results in rebound phenomena. This can lead to co-morbid psychiatric disorders, post-traumatic stress disorder, insomnia, substance abuse, and depression. Acute post-traumatic headache (APTH) can begin immediately or anytime in the 2 months following injury. Acute post-traumatic headache becomes chronic post- traumatic headache when the pain continues for longer than 2 months following injury.

Primary thunderclap headache – Relatively uncommon type of headache characterized by a dramatic, sudden, severe onset of pain anywhere in the head or neck area that peaks within 60 seconds and begins to fade in 1 hour. Residual pain/ discomfort may be present for up to 10 days. The sympathetic nervous system is believed to be involved and nausea and vomiting may occur with the pain; however, the headache usually cannot be attributed to any specific disorder. Thunderclap headache may signal a potentially life-threatening condition including: subarachnoid hemorrhage, cerebral venous sinus thrombosis, and cervical artery (carotid, vertebral artery) dissection.

Short-lasting unilateral neuralgiform headache with conjunctival injection and tearing (SUNCT) – A rare type of primary headache belonging to a group referred to as trigeminal autonomic cephalagia (TAC). This headache is triggered by the cranial autonomic nervous system at the trigeminal (5th cranial) nerve. Pain is usually described as moderate to severe with a burning, piercing, or stabbing quality. It is unilateral, centered in or around the eye (retro-orbital, orbital, supraorbital) and/or the temporal area. It is characterized by bursts of pain, lasting from a few seconds to 5-6 minutes and can occur up to 200 times per day (most commonly 5-6 times per hour). Cranial autonomic nervous system symptoms that accompany the pain include eye tearing (lacrimation) and conjunctival injection (eye redness). Nasal congestion, runny nose (rhinorrhea), constricted pupil (miosis), eyelid drooping (ptosis), or swelling (edema) may also occur. Men are affected more often than women with onset most commonly occurring after age 50. Pain may radiate to the teeth, neck, and around the ears. It is more common during daytime hours and can occur at regular or irregular intervals without a distinct refractory period.

Tension-type headache (muscle contraction headache, stress headache) – Characterized by pain that encircles the head without a throbbing or pulsating quality. Nausea/vomiting, disruption in normal activities, photophobia (light sensitivity) and phonophobia (sound sensitivity) are not normally associated with the condition. Onset is typically gradual, often in the middle of the day and pain can be exacerbated by fatigue, poor posture, emotions, and mental stress (including depression). This headache is more common in women and no familial tendency has been identified. Tension or stress headaches are the most common type of headaches among adults. The terms tension headache and tension-type headache are considered synonymous. Tension-type headache is subclassified as episodic or chronic. Episodic and chronic tension-type headaches are differentiated from each other by the frequency with which the headache occurs with episodic being defined as greater than 10 but less than 15 headache days per month and chronic being defined as more than 15 days per month. Episodic tension headaches occur randomly and are often the result of temporary stress, anxiety, or fatigue.

Vascular headache – A broad or generalized term that includes cluster headache, migraine headache, and toxic (fever, chemical) headache. For coding purposes, headaches described as vascular but without more specific information as to type are reported with the code for vascular headache not elsewhere classified. Vascular headaches all involve changes in blood flow or in the vascular (blood vessel) system of the brain which trigger head pain and other neurological symptoms. These symptoms can include nausea and vomiting, vertigo (dizziness), photophobia (light sensitivity), phonophobia (noise sensitivity), visual disturbances, numbness and tingling (in any area of the body), problems with speech, and muscle weakness.

Other headache syndromes are reported with codes from category G44 and include: cluster headaches, vascular headache not elsewhere classified, tension-type headaches, post-traumatic headaches, drug-induced headaches as well as others. Response to treatment is a component of many codes in category G44. Cluster headache, paroxysmal hemicranias, short lasting unilateral neuralgiform headache with conjunctival injection and tearing (SUNCT), other trigeminal autonomic cephalgias (TAC), tension-type headache, post-traumatic headache, and drug-induced headache must be specified as intractable or not intractable. Intractable refers to headache syndromes that are not responding to treatment. Terms that describe intractable migraine include: pharmacoresistant or pharmacologically resistant, treatment resistant, refractory, and poorly controlled. Not intractable describes a headache that is responsive to and well controlled with treatment. In addition, vascular headache not elsewhere classified is also classified in the nervous system chapter with other headache syndromes and is reported with code G44.1. Differentiation between the various types of headache can be difficult and patients often experience overlapping types of headache, so clearly documenting the type or types of headache the patient is experiencing is crucial to accurate diagnosis and appropriate treatment. This documentation is also needed for coding headache disorders.

Coding and Documentation Requirements

Identify the specific headache syndrome:

- Cluster headache syndrome
  - Chronic
  - Episodic
  - Unspecified
- Complicated headache syndromes
  - Hemicrania continua
  - New daily persistent headache (NDPH)
  - Primary thunderclap headache
  - Other complicated headache syndrome
- Drug induced headache, not elsewhere classified
- Other headache syndromes
  - Headache associated with sexual activity
  - Hypnic headache
  - Primary cough headache
  - Primary exertional headache
  - Primary stabbing headache
  - Other specified headache syndrome
- Other trigeminal autonomic cephalgias (TAC)
- Paroxysmal hemicranias
  - Chronic
  - Episodic
- Post-traumatic headache
  - Acute
  - Chronic
  - Unspecified
- Short lasting unilateral neuralgiform headache with conjunctival injection and tearing (SUNCT)
- Tension type headache
  - Chronic
  - Episodic
  - Unspecified
- Vascular headache, not elsewhere classified

Identify response to treatment for the following types: cluster, paroxysmal hemicranias, SUNCT, other TAC, tension-type, post-traumatic, and drug-induced:

- Intractable
- Not intractable

Cluster Headache Syndrome

ICD-10-CM Code/Documentation	
G44.001	Cluster headache syndrome, unspecified, intractable
G44.009	Cluster headache syndrome, unspecified, not intractable
G44.011	Episodic cluster headache, intractable
G44.009	Episodic cluster headache, not intractable
G44.021	Chronic cluster headache, intractable
G44.029	Chronic cluster headache, not intractable

Documentation and Coding Example

Thirty-seven-year-old Black male is referred to Pain Management Clinic by PCP for treatment of headaches. Patient is an attorney, working in a private, four-person firm focused on family law.

He is in a committed relationship with his partner of 6 years and they are expecting a baby girl with a surrogate in 2 months. PMH is significant for being struck in the left temple/eye area by a baseball ten months ago during a recreational game with friends. He had no loss of consciousness or visual changes, but significant pain and swelling of the face and eye. He was evaluated in the ED, where ophthalmology exam, x-rays, and a CT scan showed no eye damage, facial/skull fracture, or intracranial bleeding. The first headache occurred 2 months after this injury and woke him from sleep with intense stabbing pain in the left eye, accompanied by tearing and eye redness. The pain subsided in about 15 minutes only to reoccur twice in the next few hours. He was seen emergently by his ophthalmologist and the exam was entirely benign. The headaches continued, usually awakening him from sleep with a stabbing sensation in his left eye that lasted 30-

60 minutes. When the acute pain abated, he often had residual aching in the periorbital area and stabbing pain again within a few hours. His PCP advised taking ibuprofen which was not helpful, prescribed Toradol which was also not helpful and finally Percodan which patient states caused nausea and hallucinations. Patient has researched alternative treatment options and has tried acupuncture, melatonin, and removing foods containing tyramine and MSG from his diet. He estimates headache days were 1-3 per week at the beginning, gradually decreasing until he had a 6-week period that was pain free. The headaches began again one week ago and patient requested a referral to pain specialist. On examination, this is a soft spoken, slightly built young black male who looks his stated age. HT 69 inches, WT 150 lbs. T 96.8, P 58, R 14, BP 138/88. PERRLA, left eye has increased lacrimation, conjunctival injection and mild ptosis of the upper lid. Both nares are patent and the left naris has thin, clear mucus drainage. Oral mucosa moist and pink. Neck supple, without masses. Cranial nerves grossly intact. Upper extremities have brisk reflexes and good tone. Muscles are without atrophy, weakness, rigidity or tenderness. Heart rate regular, without bruit, murmur or rub. Breath sounds clear and equal bilaterally. Abdomen soft and non-tender with active bowel sounds in all quadrants. No evidence of hernia, normal male genitalia. Lower extremities have normal reflexes and good tone, no muscle atrophy, weakness, rigidity, or tenderness appreciated. Gait is normal. EKG is obtained and shows NSR.

Impression: **Episodic cluster headache, poorly controlled with current medications.** Consider a trial of verapamil for headache prophylaxis and sumatriptan nasal spray for acute headache.

Patient is commended for his diligence in seeking alternative treatment options and is assured that the pain management team will listen and work closely with him to ensure that his headaches are managed in a way that allows him to fully participate in and enjoy life. Treatment options discussed and patient agrees to try verapamil 40 mg PO BID for 2 weeks and RTC for re-evaluation. He declines sumatriptan nasal spray at this time. He is however interested in oxygen therapy and we will discuss that at his next visit.

Diagnosis Code(s)

G44.011 Episodic cluster headache, intractable

Coding Note(s)

Codes require identification of the headache syndrome as intractable or not intractable. These terms describe the response to treatment. Intractable indicates that the episodic cluster headache is not responding to current treatment. This is documented using the term 'poorly controlled' which, according to coding notes, is a term that is considered the equivalent of intractable.

Tension-Type Headaches

ICD-10-CM Code/Documentation	
G44.201	Tension-type headache, unspecified, intractable
G44.209	Tension-type headache, unspecified, not intractable
G44.211	Episodic tension-type headache, intractable
G44.219	Episodic tension-type headache, not intractable
G44.221	Chronic tension-type headache, intractable
G44.229	Chronic tension-type headache, not intractable

Documentation and Coding Example

HPI: This 36-year-old female complains of **headaches several times per week for several months, usually at the end of the day**. The headaches are reportedly worse after increased time at the computer. The pain starts at the base of the neck and moves up to her forehead. The patient has tried regulating eating and sleeping, drinking more water and decreasing caffeine intake, without relief. OTC headache medications have provided "little to no" relief. The only thing that helps is to lie down and close her eyes.

On examination, her neck muscles are very tight and tender. There are multiple trigger points in the sub-occipital muscles and in the sternocleidomastoid on the right. Pressure on the sub-occipital trigger points reproduces the headache. Range of motion is decreased in neck flexion and right rotation. Other testing for nerve, muscle, and joint involvement was negative and the temporomandibular joint (TMJ) is not contributory.

Assessment/Plan: **Classic tension headache**. Poor posture and fatigue cause excess tension in the posterior neck muscles, especially the sub- occipital muscle group. Treatment to include massage therapy to release the muscle tension and patient education on proper posture and ergonomics.

Diagnosis Code(s)

G44.209 Tension-type headache, unspecified, not intractable

Coding Note(s)

Under the main term Headache, the Alphabetical Index lists tension (-type) as a subterm. Tension headache NOS is listed as an inclusion term in the Tabular for tension-type headache. All types of tension headache are classified in Chapter 6 Diseases of the Nervous System, under other headache syndromes, in the subcategory G44.2. This subcategory includes: tension headache, tension-type headache, episodic tension-type headache, and chronic tension-type headache. Psychological factors affecting physical conditions (F54) has an Excludes2 note listing tension-type headache (G44.2). Headache frequency and the type and severity of symptoms should be described in the clinical documentation. Detailed documentation of the etiology and any associated mental or organic illness also is necessary. Documentation of tension headache should also describe the response to treatment.

Monoplegia of Lower/Upper Limb

Monoplegia is also known as paralysis of one limb or monoplegia disorder. Sensory loss is typically more prominent in the distal segments of the limbs. It is important that the provider clearly document the etiology or underlying cause as there are many possible causes and the underlying cause can affect code assignment. Examples of causes include:

- Cerebral palsy
- Stroke
- Brain tumor

- Multiple sclerosis
- Motor neuron disease
- Nerve trauma, impingement, or inflammation
- Mononeuritis multiplex

Like hemiplegia and hemiparesis, monoplegia of a limb is frequently due to sequela of cerebrovascular disease, cervical spinal cord diseases, or peripheral nervous system diseases. The specific type of monoplegia should be clearly described in the provider documentation. For example, congenital monoplegia (demonstrated at birth) and infantile monoplegia (develops within the first few years of life) are classified to other categories, as is monoplegia due to late effect (sequela) of cerebrovascular disease/accident. Clear, complete provider documentation in the medical record of the type and cause of the monoplegia is essential for correct code assignment.

Monoplegia is classified in the category for other paralytic syndromes. Monoplegia is also classified by whether the upper (G83.2) or limb lower (G83.1) is affected; the side of the body affected; and whether the side affected is dominant or nondominant.

There is a note indicating that codes in these categories are used only when the paralytic syndrome, in this case monoplegia, is documented without further specification, or is documented as old or longstanding of unspecified cause. The monoplegia codes may also be used in multiple coding scenarios to identify the specified types of monoplegia resulting from any cause.

For monoplegia cases, the documentation needs to identify whether the dominant or nondominant side is affected. If the affected side is documented but not specified as dominant or nondominant, Code selection for a specified side without documentation of which side is dominant is reported the same as hemiplegia:

- If the left side is affected, the default is non-dominant
- If the right side is affected, the default is dominant
- In ambidextrous patients, the default is dominant

Coding and Documentation Requirements

Identify the affected limb:

- Lower
- Upper
- Unspecified

Identify the side affected:

- Right
  - Dominant side
  - Nondominant side
- Left
  - Dominant side
  - Nondominant side
- Unspecified side

Monoplegia of Lower Limb

ICD-10-CM Code/Documentation	
G83.10	Monoplegia of lower limb affecting unspecified side
G83.11	Monoplegia of lower limb affecting right dominant side
G83.12	Monoplegia of lower limb affecting left dominant side
G83.13	Monoplegia of lower limb affecting right nondominant side
G83.14	Monoplegia of lower limb affecting left nondominant side

Documentation and Coding Example

A 46-year-old male patient presented with complaints of neck pain, numbing sensation, and right leg weakness. The physical examination showed monoplegia of right leg, with intact sensory function. The other extremities had no neurologic deficits. MR imaging showed spinal cord compression and high signal intensity of spinal cord at C6-7. Therefore, the cause of monoplegia of the leg was thought to be the spinal cord ischemia.

Diagnosis: **Monoplegia, right leg, due to spinal cord ischemia.**

Diagnosis Code(s)

G95.11 Acute infarction of spinal cord (embolic) (nonembolic)

G83.11 Monoplegia of lower limb affecting right dominant side

Coding Note(s)

In this case, the affected side is documented but not specified as dominant or nondominant. ICD-10-CM code selection hierarchy states that if the right side is affected, the default is dominant. It should also be noted that this is a multiple coding scenario, requiring a code for the spinal cord ischemia, which is listed first, and a second code identifying the monoplegia.

Monoplegia of Upper Limb

ICD-10-CM Code/Documentation	
G83.20	Monoplegia of upper limb affecting unspecified side
G83.21	Monoplegia of upper limb affecting right dominant side
G83.22	Monoplegia of upper limb affecting left dominant side
G83.23	Monoplegia of upper limb affecting right nondominant side
G83.24	Monoplegia of upper limb affecting left nondominant side

Documentation and Coding Example

A 75-year-old female presented to the emergency department with sudden onset right upper limb weakness and altered sensation. The patient was previously well with an unremarkable medical history. On examination, she was apyrexial, normotensive and normoglycemic with a GCS of 15/15. Neurological examination revealed right upper limb hypotonia and power of 0/5 in all hand and wrist muscle groups, 2/5 power in biceps and triceps, and 3/5 power in the shoulder girdle. Hypoesthesia was noted throughout the right upper limb. The remainder of the neurological examination did not reveal any other deficits.

Baseline labs were normal. On brain MRI, mild ischemic change was noted throughout the cerebral white matter in the absence of infarcts within the basal ganglia, brainstem or cerebellum and cerebral venography was not suggestive of a recent thrombosis.

Collectively the imaging studies were indicative of an acute parenchymal event with evidence of previous superficial bleeds. Following little improvement in right arm function after neurorehabilitation, the patient was discharged home.

Diagnosis: **Spontaneous right arm monoplegia secondary to probable cerebral amyloid angiopathy**.

Diagnosis Code(s)

G83.21 Monoplegia of upper limb affecting right dominant side

Coding Note(s)

Here again, the affected side is documented but not specified as dominant or nondominant. According to the code selection hierarchy in ICD-10-CM, the right side is affected so the default is dominant. ICD-10-CM Coding and Reporting Guidelines for Outpatient Services direct the user not to code diagnoses documented as "probable," "suspected," "questionable," "rule out," "working diagnosis," or other similar terms indicating uncertainty; therefore, no code is assigned for "probable cerebral amyloid angiopathy".

Viral Diseases of the Central Nervous System, Specified

Viruses can be spread through different mediums. Arthropods are invertebrates with an exoskeleton, jointed appendages, and a segmented body. Arthropod-borne infections are caused by viruses transmitted through invertebrates such as ticks and mosquitoes. Other invertebrates that are not arthropods, such as worms, may also transmit viruses. ICD-10-CM provides codes that distinguish arthropod-borne viral fevers and infections of the central nervous system by the vector of transmission, but there are no codes specifically designating non-arthropod borne viral illnesses. The codes for viral infections of the central nervous system are specific to site and must be specified as the brain (encephalon) (A85, A86) or meninges (A87). There are 3 codes available for reporting non-arthropod-borne viral encephalitis: enteroviral (A85.0), adenoviral (A85.1), and other specified viral encephalitis (A85.8). When the condition is not specified as encephalitis or meningitis, the code for other specified viral infections of the central nervous system not elsewhere classified (A88.8) is used. There is also a code for unspecified viral infection of central nervous system (A89).

Coding and Documentation Requirements

Specify viral type of encephalitis:

- Adenoviral
- Enteroviral
- Other viral, which may include the following descriptors:
  - Encephalitis lethargica
  - Von Economo disease
- Unspecified

Specify viral type of meningitis:

- Adenoviral
- Enteroviral, which may include:
  - coxsackievirus
  - echovirus
- Lymphocytic choriomeningitis
- Other viral
- Unspecified
- Other specified viral infection of the CNS

ICD-10-CM Code/Documentation	
A85.0	Enteroviral encephalitis
A85.1	Adenoviral encephalitis
A85.8	Other specified viral encephalitis
A70.0	Enteroviral meningitis
A87.1	Adenoviral meningitis
A87.2	Lymphocytic choriomeningitis
A87.8	Other viral meningitis
A88.8	Other specified viral infections of central nervous system

Documentation and Coding Example

Twenty-two-month-old male presents with a 4-day history of URI symptoms. Parent states he is usually very active and happy but has been irritable all day, crying inconsolably especially when touched or picked up. His URI symptoms have included fever to 102.6, nasal congestion, conjunctivitis, and cough. On examination, the patient has a maculopapular rash on the back of his head and neck. Child admitted to pediatric floor with **suspected acute viral meningitis** and placed in respiratory isolation. Neurological functioning continued to decline after admission. Symptoms included agitation, confusion, and seizures. Cross section and 3-D MRI imaging revealed **inclusion bodies** in the neurons and glial cells of the brain.

Diagnosis: **Acute inclusion body encephalitis**.

Diagnosis Code(s)

A85.8 Other specified viral encephalitis

Coding Note(s)

In the Alphabetic Index, the code is found under Encephalitis, acute, inclusion body.

Viral Diseases of Central Nervous System, Unspecified

There are two codes for unspecified viral diseases of the central nervous system, one for unspecified viral encephalitis (A86) and one for unspecified viral infection of the central nervous system when the condition is not specified as encephalitis or meningitis (A89).

Coding and Documentation Requirements

For viral infection of the CNS specify:

- Viral encephalitis/encephalomyelitis/
- meningoencephalitis NOS
- Viral infection of CNS, NOS

ICD-10-CM Code/Documentation	
A86	Unspecified viral encephalitis
A89	Unspecified viral infection of the central nervous system

Documentation and Coding Example

Thirty-year-old male presents with a 3-day history of flu-like symptoms, fever, headache, fatigue, muscle and joint pain, congestion and cough. Today he noticed neck stiffness and severe sensitivity to light. Patient denies exotic travel but recently spent a week skiing in Colorado. He denies falls or injuries but states he developed a large sore on this lip which he attributed to excessive sun exposure. On examination, this is an ill appearing, thin white male lying quietly with his eyes closed. Skin color is pale/pasty, skin is cool and clammy to touch. Temperature 98.2, HR 90, RR 20, BP 100/66. Unable to examine pupils due to extreme sensitivity to light. Limited anterior/ posterior neck flexion due to pain with movement. Mild lymph node swelling noted in cervical area. No other lymphadenopathy appreciated. Hyperactive reflexes noted in all extremities. HR regular without murmur. Fine scattered rales noted in lungs bilaterally, clear with coughing. Abdomen soft and non-tender. Liver palpated at RCM, spleen is not palpated. Denies flank pain or difficulty with urination. Lower extremities are without edema, pulses are intact. Blood samples obtained for CBC, culture, sed rate, herpes antibody testing. Neuroimaging obtained with MRI scan of head and neck. Lumbar puncture performed and CSF sent to lab for gram stain, cell count, culture, protein, glucose, lactic acid, IgG antibodies, CRP. Patient is admitted with a diagnosis of probable viral encephalomyelitis.

Final diagnosis: **Viral encephalomyelitis**.

Diagnosis Code(s)

A86 Unspecified viral encephalitis

Coding Note(s)

In the Alphabetic Index, under Encephalomyelitis, follow the instruction "see also Encephalitis". The code is found under Encephalitis, viral/virus. Since the specified type is not known, the code for unspecified viral encephalitis is reported.

Summary

ICD-10-CM classifies diseases affecting the nervous system by the type and cause of the disease or disorder, such as intraoperative and postprocedural complications, congenital conditions, infectious diseases, neoplasms, or traumatic injury. Documentation of the severity and/or status of the disease in terms of acute or chronic, as well as the site, etiology, and any secondary disease process are basic documentation requirements. Physician documentation of diagnostic test findings or confirmation of any diagnosis found in diagnostic test reports is also required documentation.

Nervous system coding requires a significant level of specificity, which makes the provider's medical 0record documentation particularly important. Precise clinical information will need to be documented in the medical record to accurately report the codes.

Resources

Documentation checklists are available in Appendix B for:

- Headache syndromes
- Migraine
- Seizures

Quiz

1. CRPS II is:
   a. severe neuropathic pain that may be a result of an illness or injury with intense pain to light touch, abnormal circulation, temperature and sweating
   b. usually occurs at night with an irresistible urge to move the legs due to unusual sensations such as tingling, creeping and crawling
   c. a type of neuropathic pain the occurs following a peripheral nerve injury resulting in burning or throbbing pain along the nerve, sensitivity to cold and touch, changes in skin color, temperature, texture, hair and nails
   d. Disease or damage to peripheral nerves resulting in impaired sensation, movement, gland or organ dysfunction.
2. How are seizure disorders and recurrent seizures classified?
   a. Seizure disorders and recurrent seizures are classified with epilepsy
   b. Seizure disorders and recurrent seizures are classified as non-epileptic
   c. Seizure disorders and recurrent seizures are classified as signs and symptoms
   d. None of the above
3. Which of the following is an alternate term for "intractable" migraine?
   a. Pharmacoresistant
   b. Refractory (medically)
   c. Poorly controlled
   d. All of the above
4. Where are coding and sequencing guidelines for diseases of the nervous system and complications due to the treatment of the diseases and conditions of the nervous system found?
   a. In the ICD-10-CM Official Guidelines for Coding and Reporting chapter specific guidelines for Chapter 6
   b. In the Alphabetic Index and the Tabular List and the chapter specific guidelines for Chapter 6
   c. In other chapter specific guidelines in the ICD-10-CM Official Guidelines for Coding and Reporting
   d. All of the above
5. What is the correct code assignment for an encounter for treatment of a condition causing pain?
   a. A code for the underlying condition is assigned as the principal diagnosis and a code from category G89 is assigned as an additional diagnosis.
   b. A code from category G89 is assigned as the principal diagnosis and no code is assigned for the underlying condition.
   c. A code for the underlying condition is assigned as the principal diagnosis and no code from category G89 is assigned.
   d. A code from category G89 is assigned as the principal diagnosis and a code for the underlying condition is assigned as an additional diagnosis.
6. Which of the following documentation is required for accurate coding of epilepsy?
   a. With or without intractable epilepsy
   b. Type of epilepsy
   c. With or without status epilepticus
   d. All of the above
7. When an admission is for treatment of an underlying condition and a neurostimulator is also inserted for pain control during the same episode of care, what is the correct code assignment?
   a. The underlying condition is the principal diagnosis and the appropriate pain code should be assigned as a secondary diagnosis.
   b. A code for the underlying condition is assigned as the principal diagnosis and no pain code is assigned as an additional diagnosis.
   c. A pain code is assigned as the principal diagnosis and a code for the underlying condition is assigned as an additional diagnosis.
   d. A code for insertion of a neurostimulator for pain control is assigned as the principal diagnosis and a pain code is assigned as an additional diagnosis.
8. Alzheimer's disease with dementia requires dual coding. What is the proper sequencing for Alzheimer's disease with dementia?
   a. The dementia is coded first with or without behavioral disturbance followed by a code for the underlying condition (Alzheimer's disease).
   b. Only the Alzheimer's disease is coded
   c. The Alzheimer's disease is coded first followed by a code for dementia with or without behavioral disturbance.
   d. The Alzheimer's disease is coded with an additional code for any behavioral disturbance.

9. In patients with hemiplegia, if the affected side is documented but not specified as dominant or nondominant, how is this coded?
   a. When the left side is affected, the default is nondominant
   b. When the right side is affected, the default is dominant
   c. When the patient is ambidextrous, the default is dominant
   d. All of the above
10. What is the correct coding of a diagnosis documented as post-thoracotomy pain without further specification as acute or chronic?
   a. A code from Chapter 19 Injury, poisoning, and certain other consequences of external causes, is assigned
   b. Post-thoracotomy pain is routine postoperative pain and is not coded
   c. The code for acute post-thoracotomy pain is the default
   d. The code for chronic post-thoracotomy pain is the default

See next page for answers and rationales.

Answers and Rationales

1. CRPS II is:

   c. a type of neuropathic pain the occurs following a peripheral nerve injury resulting in burning or throbbing pain along the nerve, sensitivity to cold and touch, changes in skin color, temperature, texture, hair and nails

   Rationale: CRPS II or chronic regional pain syndrome is pain as a result of a direct injury to a nerve vs RSD or CRPS I do not have to have a direct injury to a nerve. B is the definition for restless leg syndrome and d is the definition for neuropathy. For both CRPS I and CRPS II documentation of upper or lower extremity as well as laterality is required.

2. How are seizure disorders and recurrent seizures classified?

   a. Seizure disorders and recurrent seizures are classified with epilepsy

   Rationale: The Index entry for seizure disorder directs the user to see Epilepsy. Both Seizure disorder and recurrent seizures are indexed to G40.909 Epilepsy, unspecified.

3. Which of the following is an alternate term for "intractable" migraine?

   d. All of the above

   Rationale: According to the instructional note under category G40, the following terms are to be considered equivalent to intractable: pharmacoresistant (pharmacologically resistant), treatment resistant, refractory (medically), and poorly controlled.

4. Where are coding and sequencing guidelines for diseases of the nervous system and complications due to the treatment of the diseases and conditions of the nervous system found?

   b. In the Alphabetic Index and the Tabular List and the chapter specific guidelines for Chapter 6

   Rationale: the conventions and instructions of the classification along with the general and chapter-specific coding guidelines govern the selection and sequencing of ICD-10-CM codes. According to Section I.A of the ICD-10-CM coding guidelines, the conventions are the general rules for use of the classification independent of the guidelines. These conventions are incorporated within the Alphabetic Index and Tabular List of the ICD-10-CM as instructional notes.

5. What is the correct code assignment for an encounter for treatment of a condition causing pain?

   c. A code for the underlying condition is assigned as the principal diagnosis and no code from category G89 is assigned.

   Rationale: According to the chapter specific coding guidelines for Chapter 6 of ICD-10-CM, when an admission or encounter is for a procedure aimed at treating the underlying condition, a code for the underlying condition should be assigned as the principal diagnosis and no code from category G89 should be assigned.

6. Which of the following documentation is required for accurate coding of epilepsy?

   d. All of the above

   Rationale: Epilepsy is classified by the specific type and then as intractable or not intractable, and with or without status epilepticus. A note in lists the terms pharmacoresistant, pharmacologically resistant, poorly controlled, refractory, or treatment resistant as synonyms for intractable.

7. When an admission is for treatment of an underlying condition and a neurostimulator is also inserted for pain control during the same episode of care, what is the correct code assignment?

   a. The underlying condition is the principal diagnosis and the appropriate pain code should be assigned as a secondary diagnosis.

   Rationale: Section I.B.1.a of the ICD-10-CM coding guidelines provides specific direction on coding Category G89 codes as principal diagnosis or the first-listed code. According to these guidelines, when a patient is admitted for a procedure aimed at treating the underlying condition and a neurostimulator is inserted for pain control during the same admission/encounter, a code for the underlying condition should be assigned as the principal diagnosis and the appropriate pain code should be assigned as a secondary diagnosis.

8. What is the proper sequencing for Alzheimer's disease with dementia?

    c. The Alzheimer's disease is coded first followed by a code for dementia with or without behavioral disturbance.

    Rationale: An instructional note at category G30 directs the coder to use an additional code to identify delirium, dementia with or without behavioral disturbance.

9. In patients with hemiplegia, if the affected side is documented but not specified as dominant or nondominant?

    d. All of the above

    Rationale: Section I.C.6.a of the ICD-10-CM coding guidelines provides specific direction for cases where the affected side is documented, but not specified as dominant or nondominant. According to these guidelines, the default code is dominant for ambidextrous patients, nondominant when the left side is affected and dominant when the right side is affected.

10. What is the correct coding of a diagnosis documented as post-thoracotomy pain without further specification as acute or chronic?

    c. The code for acute post-thoracotomy pain is the default

    Rationale: According to Section I.C.6.b.3 of the ICD-10-CM coding guidelines, the default is the code for the acute form for post-thoracotomy pain when not specified as acute or chronic.

CPT® Procedural Coding

Introduction

Current Procedural Terminology (CPT) codes are published by the American Medical Association (AMA). The purpose of this coding system is to provide a uniform language for reporting services provided to patients.

A CPT Category I code is a five-digit numeric code used to describe medical, surgical, radiological, laboratory, anesthesiology, and evaluation management (E/M) services performed by physicians and other health care providers or entities. There are over 8,000 CPT codes ranging from 00100 through 99607. Beginning in 2002, the AMA added Category III (emerging technology) codes. In 2004, the AMA introduced Category II (supplemental tracking) codes. Both Category II and III codes are five-digit alphanumeric codes.

The entire family of procedure codes acceptable to Medicare is referred to as HCPCS, which is an acronym for:

H Healthcare

C Common

P Procedure

C Coding

S System

This family is comprised of two distinct parts or levels: Level I and Level II.

HCPCS Level I Codes (CPT)

HCPCS Level I codes consist of the five-digit codes listed in the *CPT®* codebook published by the American Medical Association. These are the most frequently used codes to report services and procedures, since the codebook mainly consists of physician procedures. The codes are updated annually, and the new codes for the upcoming year are available at the end of the preceding year for use on January 1.

HCPCS Level II Codes

HCPCS Level II codes consist of five-digit alphanumeric codes utilizing letters A-V, and were developed specifically by the Centers for Medicare & Medicaid Services (CMS) to report services and supplies not found in Level I. HCPCS Level II is a standardized coding system that is used primarily to identify products; supplies; drugs and biologicals; durable medical equipment, prosthetics, orthotics, and supplies (DMEPOS); quality reporting measures; some physician and non-physician provider services; and other services, such as ambulance services. HCPCS Level II codes are recognized by Medicare and many other third-party payers.

The CPT Codebook

This coding reference book, which is updated annually, is organized into nine sections, sixteen appendices, and an alphabetic index. There are specific guidelines listed in the CPT codebook at the beginning of each section. These guidelines indicate interpretations and appropriate reporting of codes contained in that particular section. The guidelines should be reviewed prior to using any code in that section. The sections include:

- **Introduction and Illustrated Anatomical and Procedural Review** — Contains basic instructions for using the CPT codebook and reviews basic medical terminology and anatomy with additional information, references, and illustrations.
- **Evaluation and Management** — Provides the codes and guidelines for reporting patient evaluation and management services, most of which are face-to-face with the provider and based on established or new patient status. The codes are broadly grouped into place of service, such as office, hospital, outpatient or ambulatory surgical center, emergency department, nursing home or other residential facility and/or type of service, such as observation, consultations, critical care, newborn care, and preventive care.
- **Anesthesia** — Provides guidelines, codes, and modifiers for reporting services involving the administration of anesthesia for different types of procedures and on various locations of the body.
- **Surgery** — Identifies surgical procedures performed across all specialties and body systems. The procedure normally includes the necessary, related services in the surgical package without being stated as part of the code description.
- **Radiology** — Lists codes for diagnostic imaging, ultrasound, radiological guidance, radiation oncology, and nuclear medicine. Procedures in this section include X-ray, fluoroscopy, computed tomography, magnetic resonance imaging, angiography, lymphangiography, mammography, radiological supervision and interpretation for therapeutic transcatheter procedures, bone studies, radiation treatment and planning for cancer, brachytherapy, and radiopharmaceutical procedures.
- **Pathology and Laboratory** — Contains codes for reporting procedures and services processed in a laboratory facility. Tests include organ or disease panels, drug assays, urinalysis, chemistry profiles, microorganism identification, immunoassays, pathological examination of surgical samples, and reproductive-related procedures.
- **Medicine** — Identifies procedures that usually do not require operating room services. The medicine codes provided in this section cover a wide spectrum of specialties and include both diagnostic and therapeutic procedures. This section includes procedures, such as neuromuscular testing, cardiac

catheterization, acupuncture, dialysis, chemotherapy, vaccine administration, and psychiatric services.

- **Category II Codes** — Lists supplemental, optional tracking codes composed of four digits and the letter F. These codes are intended to reduce the need for record abstraction and chart review and facilitate data collection by those seeking to measure quality of patient care.
- **Category III Codes** — Provide temporary codes composed of four digits and the letter T, established for reporting and tracking data for emerging technology, services, and procedures. When a Category III code is available, it must be used rather than reporting an unlisted code. These codes may or may not be assigned a Category I code at a future date.

The appendices include:

- **Appendix A – Modifiers** — Lists all the applicable modifiers for the CPT codes to identify when a service or procedure was altered by a specific circumstance or to provide additional information about the procedure performed. This includes anesthesia physical status modifiers, CPT Level I modifiers approved for ambulatory surgical centers and hospital outpatient departments, Category II modifiers, and HCPCS Level II National modifiers.
- **Appendix B – Summary of Additions, Deletions, and Revisions** — Shows the current year's changes that were made to the codes.
- **Appendix C – Clinical Examples** — Gives real-life clinical scenarios and examples of patient evaluation and management encounters to help medical offices in reporting services provided to the patient.
- **Appendix D – Summary of CPT Add-on Codes** — Lists in numerical sequence all the codes designated in CPT as add-on codes. The add-on codes are only to be assigned in addition to the principal procedure and never stand alone. Add-on codes are also not subject to modifier 51 rules. These codes are additionally identified with a ✚ symbol.
- **Appendix E – Summary of CPT Codes Exempt from Modifier 51** — Lists in numerical sequence all the CPT codes designated as exempt from the use of modifier 51 that have not been identified as add-on procedures or services. These codes are additionally identified with a ⦸ symbol.
- **Appendix F – Summary of CPT Codes Exempt from Modifier 63** — Lists in numerical sequence all the CPT codes designated as exempt from the use of modifier 63. These codes are additionally identified with a parenthetical instruction.
- **Appendix G – Summary of CPT Codes That Include Moderate (Conscious) Sedation** — Summary of CPT codes that include moderate (conscious) sedation (formerly Appendix G) has been removed from the CPT code set. The codes that were previously included were revised to remove the moderate (conscious) sedation symbol. For guidance on reporting codes formerly listed in Appendix G, refer to the guidelines for codes 99151-99153 and 99155-99157.
- **Appendix H – Alphabetical Clinical Topics Listing** — The Alphabetical Clinical Topics Listing (formerly Appendix H) has been removed from the CPT codebook. Since performance measures are subject to change each year, the alphabetic index to performance measures is now maintained on the AMA website at www.ama-assn.org/go/cpt. The online version will continue to provide measures in table format listed alphabetically by the disease or condition and crosswalked to the Category II codes used to report the quality measure.
- **Appendix I – Genetic Testing Code Modifiers** — The list of Genetic Testing Code Modifiers (formerly Appendix I) has been removed from the CPT code set. The addition of hundreds of molecular pathology codes resulted in the deletion of the stacking codes to which these modifiers applied. For the most current updates for molecular pathology coding in the CPT code set, see the AMA CPT website at www.ama-assn.org/go/cpt.
- **Appendix J – Electrodiagnostic Medicine Listing of Sensory, Motor, and Mixed Nerves** — Assigns each sensory, motor, and mixed nerve with its proper nerve conduction study code in order to improve accurate reporting of codes 95907-95913.
- **Appendix K – Product Pending FDA Approval** — Identifies vaccines that have already been assigned Category I codes that are still awaiting FDA approval. These are identified with the symbol ⚡.
- **Appendix L – Vascular Families** — Outlines the tree of vascular families and identifies first-, second-, and third-order branches, assuming the beginning point is the aorta, vena cava, pulmonary artery, or portal vein.
- **Appendix M – Renumbered CPT Codes – Citations Crosswalk** — This listing identifies codes that were deleted and renumbered from 2007 to 2009 and their crosswalk to current year code(s).
- **Appendix N – Summary of Resequenced CPT Codes** — This list identifies codes that do not appear in numeric sequence. Instead of deleting and renumbering existing codes that need to be moved, the existing codes are now being moved to the correct location without being renumbered. Resequenced codes are relocated to appear with codes for the appropriate code concept. The CPT codebook lists the code in numeric sequence without the code description. Instead, a parenthetical note is listed referencing the range of codes in which the resequenced code appears. The resequenced code is identified with a # symbol, and the full code description is listed for the resequenced code.
- **Appendix O – Multianalyte Assays with Algorithmic Analyses** — This list identifies codes for Multianalyte Assays with Algorithmic Analyses (MAAA) procedures that utilize multiple results derived from various types of assays (e.g., molecular pathology assays, non-nucleic acid based assays) that are typically unique to a single clinical laboratory or manufacturer.
- **Appendix P – CPT Codes That May Be Used For Synchronous Telemedicine Services** —This appendix first appeared in 2017 to list codes that may be used for reporting real-time telemedicine services when appended by modifier 95. These procedures include interactive electronic

communication using audio-visual telecommunications equipment. These are identified with the symbol ★.

Locating a CPT Code

Once familiar with the CPT codebook, identifying appropriate codes becomes less of a task. The numbers at the top of each page are for easy reference and give the range of codes located on that particular page.

Most sections list the sequence of codes in the following order:

- Top to bottom of body (head to toe)
- Central to peripheral in some subsections (i.e., cardiovascular and nervous system codes)
- Outside to inside of body (incision/excision)

There are two ways to locate a code in the CPT codebook:

- By anatomical site (numerically)
- The Index (alphabetically)

A code can be located simply by knowing the site or body system. For example, if a patient had an EKG performed in the emergency department, the user should try to locate a code through the Index. Alternatively, the coder could rationalize that a medicine service was performed to monitor the patient's heart, which is part of the cardiovascular system. Since those medicine codes are found in the 93000 series of codes, the coder could then look in this section of the CPT codebook to locate the appropriate code.

The Index is organized by main terms, shown in bold typeface. There are four primary classes of main entries:

- Procedure or service – e.g., Cardiac Catheterization, Angioplasty
- Organ or other anatomic site – e.g., Heart, Chest, Abdomen
- Condition – e.g., Angina, Myocardial Infarction
- Synonyms, eponyms, and abbreviations – e.g., EKG, EMG, DXA

The main term is divided into specific sub-terms that help in selecting the appropriate code.

Whenever more than one code applies to a given index entry, a code range is listed. If two or more nonsequential codes apply, they will be separated by a comma. For example:

Electrocardiography

Evaluation ... 0178T-0180T, 93000, 93010, 93660

If more than one sequential code applies, they will be separated by a hyphen. For example:

Office and/or Other Outpatient Services

Established patient ... 99211-99215

A cross-reference provides instructions to the user on where to look when entries are listed under another heading.

See directs the user to refer to the term listed. This is used primarily for synonyms, eponyms, and abbreviations, such as:

Ear Canal
See Auditory Canal

The alphabetic index is not a substitute for the main text of CPT. The user must always refer to the main text to ensure that the code selection is accurate and not assign any codes from the Index entry alone.

CPT Symbols

In addition to understanding the layout of CPT and knowing how to reference the book, the user must also understand symbols and their meanings.

● Indicates a new code has been added to the edition the coder is referencing. For example:

● 38573 Laparoscopy, surgical; with bilateral total pelvic lymphadenectomy and peri-aortic lymph node sampling, peritoneal washings, peritoneal biopsy(ies), omentectomy, and diaphragmatic washings, including diaphragmatic and other serosal biopsy(ies), when performed

▲ Indicates the code number is the same, but the definition or description has changed since the last edition

▲ 43112 Total or near total esophagectomy, with thoracotomy; with pharyngogastrostomy or cervical esophagogastrostomy, with or without pyloroplasty (ie, McKeown esophagectomy or tri-incisional esophagectomy)

; Indicates a selection of suffixes that append to the main portion (prefix) of the code. For example:

96372 Therapeutic, prophylactic, or diagnostic injection (specify substance or drug); **subcutaneous or intramuscular**

96373 Therapeutic, prophylactic, or diagnostic injection (specify substance or drug); **intra-arterial**

96374 Therapeutic, prophylactic, or diagnostic injection (specify substance or drug); intravenous push, single or initial substance/drug

⊘ Identifies codes that are exempt from the use of modifier 51 but have not been designated as add-on procedures/services.

⊘ 31500 Intubation, endotracheal, emergency procedure

Note: For more information on modifier 51, see the Modifier chapter.

★ Identifies telemedicine codes.

★ 90832 Psychotherapy, 30 minutes with patient

✗ Identifies codes that have been created for vaccines that are pending FDA approval (at the time of the publication of that year's CPT codebook).

✗ 90739 Hepatitis B vaccine, (HepB), adult dosage, 2 dose schedule, for intramuscular use

Add-on Codes

Add-on procedures or services are ones that are performed in addition to the primary procedure/service. In the CPT codebook, a ✚ indicates a CPT add-on code.

99291 Critical care, evaluation and management of the critically ill or critically injured patient; first 30-74 minutes

✚99292 each additional 30 minutes (List separately in addition to code for primary service)

The add-on procedure is performed on the same day by the same provider that performed the primary procedure/service. These codes should never be reported alone and should not be reported with modifier 51.

Modifiers

Modifiers consist of two numeric or alphanumeric digits appended to a code to indicate when a service or procedure that still fits the code description was altered by a specific circumstance or when additional information about the procedure performed needs to be provided.

Unlisted Procedure or Service

The procedure performed may not always be found with a designated code assignment in the CPT codebook. Unlisted procedure codes are provided in every section to be used in these cases. An accompanying operative report or other visit documentation is required when reporting unlisted codes in order for the payer to identify what the procedure entailed and determine its eligibility for reimbursement. An unlisted procedure code should not be used when a Category III code best describes the procedure performed.

Surgical Package

The concept of a global fee for surgical procedures is a long-established concept under which a single fee is billed that pays for all necessary services normally furnished by the surgeon before, during, and after the procedure. Since the fee schedule is based on uniform national relative values, it is necessary to have a uniform national definition of global surgery to assure that equivalent payment is made for the same amount of work and resources.

The following items are included in the global package reimbursement:

- Local anesthesia, digital block, or topical anesthesia
- After the decision for surgery is made, one E/M service one day before or the day of surgery
- Postoperative care that occurs directly after the procedure
- Examining the patient in the recovery area
- Any postoperative care occurring during the designated postoperative period

To assist in this uniform implementation, the CPT Editorial Panel created five modifiers (24, 25, 59, 78, and 79) to identify a service or procedure furnished during a global period that is not a part of the global surgery fee, such as a service unrelated to the condition requiring surgery or for treating the underlying condition and not for normal recovery from the surgery. Use of these modifiers allows such services to be reported in addition to the global fee.

Category II Codes

The Category II section of CPT contains a set of supplemental tracking codes that can be used for performance measurement. This section of codes was implemented in 2004 to facilitate data collection about the quality of care rendered for specific conditions. These codes report certain services and test results that support nationally established performance measures with evidence of contributing to increased quality patient care. It is not required for providers to report these codes; the use of these codes is optional.

Category II codes consist of five-digit alphanumeric codes that end in an F, and the following categories are included in this code set:

- Composite Codes
- Patient Management
- Patient History
- Physical Examination
- Diagnostic/Screening Processes or Results
- Therapeutic, Preventive, or Other Interventions
- Follow-up or Other Outcomes
- Patient Safety
- Structural Measures
- Nonmeasure Code Listing

Category III Codes

Category III codes are temporary codes that identify emerging technologies, services, and procedures, and allow for data collection to determine clinical efficacy, utilization, and outcomes. They are alphanumeric codes that consist of four numbers, followed by the letter T.

A Category III code should be reported instead of an unlisted code whenever it accurately describes the procedure that was performed. These temporary codes may or may not be assigned a Category I CPT code in the future.

2020 Neurology/Neurosurgery CPT Codes and Crosswalks

The 2020 Neurology and Neurosurgery CPT codes and crosswalks begin following the Surgery Guidelines section. Each code includes official CPT descriptions, official CPT Guidelines, Plain English Descriptions (PED), ICD-10-CM crosswalks, and Medicare-related information including: RVUs, Modifiers, and CCI edits (also known as NCCI).

Note: This Neurology and Neurosurgery coding book is not intended to replace the AMA's CPT codebook. Use this book in conjunction with the official AMA 2020 CPT codebook.

Surgery and Gastroenterology Guidelines

Guidelines to direct general reporting of services are presented in the **Introduction**. Some of the commonalities are repeated here for the convenience of those referring to this section on **Surgery**. Other definitions and items unique to Surgery and Gastroenterology are also listed.

Services

Services rendered in the office, home, or hospital, consultations, and other medical services are listed in the **Evaluation and Management Services** section (99201-99499) beginning on page 11.* "Special Services, Procedures, and Reports" (99000-99082) are listed in the **Medicine** section.

CPT Surgical Package Definition

By their very nature, the services to any patient are variable. The CPT codes that represent a readily identifiable surgical procedure thereby include, on a procedure-by-procedure basis, a variety of services. In defining the specific services "included" in a given CPT surgical code, the following services related to the surgery when furnished by the physician or other qualified health care professional who performs the surgery are included in addition to the operation per se:

- Evaluation and Management (E/M) service(s) subsequent to the decision for surgery on the day before and/or day of surgery (including history and physical)
- Local infiltration, metacarpal/metatarsal/digital block or topical anesthesia
- Immediate postoperative care, including dictating operative notes, talking with the family and other physicians or other qualified health care professionals
- Writing orders
- Evaluating the patient in the postanesthesia recovery area
- Typical postoperative follow-up care

Follow-Up Care for Diagnostic Procedures

Follow-up care for diagnostic procedures (e.g., endoscopy, arthroscopy, injection procedures for radiography) includes only that care related to recovery from the diagnostic procedure itself. Care of the condition for which the diagnostic procedure was performed or of other concomitant conditions is not included and may be listed separately.

Follow-Up Care for Therapeutic Surgical Procedures

Follow-up care for therapeutic surgical procedures includes only that care which is usually a part of the surgical service. Complications, exacerbations, recurrence, or the presence of other diseases or injuries requiring additional services should be separately reported.

Supplied Materials

Supplies and materials (e.g., sterile trays/drugs), over and above those usually included with the procedure(s) rendered are reported separately. List drugs, trays, supplies, and materials provided. Identify as 99070 or specific supply code.

Reporting More Than One Procedure/Service

When more than one procedure/service is performed on the same date, same session or during a post-operative period (subject to the "surgical package" concept), several CPT modifiers may apply (see Appendix A* for definition).

Separate Procedure

Some of the procedures or services listed in the CPT codebook that are commonly carried out as an integral component of a total service or procedure have been identified by the inclusion of the term "separate procedure." The codes designated as "separate procedure" should not be reported in addition to the code for the total procedure or service of which it is considered an integral component.

However, when a procedure or service that is designated as a "separate procedure" is carried out independently or considered to be unrelated or distinct from other procedures/services provided at that time, it may be reported by itself, or in addition to other procedures/services by appending modifier 59 to the specific "separate procedure" code to indicate that the procedure is not considered to be a component of another procedure, but is a distinct, independent procedure. This may represent a different session, different procedure or surgery, different site or organ system, separate incision/excision, separate lesion, or separate injury (or area of injury in extensive injuries).

 * Pages in this section refer to the AMA *CPT® 2020 Professional Edition.*

Unlisted Service or Procedure

A service or procedure may be provided that is not listed in this edition of the CPT codebook. When reporting such a service, the appropriate "Unlisted Procedure" code may be used to indicate the service, identifying it by "Special Report" as discussed in the section below. The "Unlisted Procedures" and accompanying codes for **Surgery** are as follows:

15999	Unlisted procedure, excision pressure ulcer
17999	Unlisted procedure, skin, mucous membrane and subcutaneous tissue
19499	Unlisted procedure, breast
20999	Unlisted procedure, musculoskeletal system, general
21089	Unlisted maxillofacial prosthetic procedure
21299	Unlisted craniofacial and maxillofacial procedure
21499	Unlisted musculoskeletal procedure, head
21899	Unlisted procedure, neck or thorax
22899	Unlisted procedure, spine
22999	Unlisted procedure, abdomen, musculoskeletal system
23929	Unlisted procedure, shoulder
24999	Unlisted procedure, humerus or elbow
25999	Unlisted procedure, forearm or wrist
26989	Unlisted procedure, hands or fingers
27299	Unlisted procedure, pelvis or hip joint
27599	Unlisted procedure, femur or knee
27899	Unlisted procedure, leg or ankle
28899	Unlisted procedure, foot or toes
29799	Unlisted procedure, casting or strapping
29999	Unlisted procedure, arthroscopy
30999	Unlisted procedure, nose
31299	Unlisted procedure, accessory sinuses
31599	Unlisted procedure, larynx
31899	Unlisted procedure, trachea, bronchi
32999	Unlisted procedure, lungs and pleura
33999	Unlisted procedure, cardiac surgery
36299	Unlisted procedure, vascular injection
37501	Unlisted vascular endoscopy procedure
37799	Unlisted procedure, vascular surgery
38129	Unlisted laparoscopy procedure, spleen
38589	Unlisted laparoscopy procedure, lymphatic system
38999	Unlisted procedure, hemic or lymphatic system
39499	Unlisted procedure, mediastinum
39599	Unlisted procedure, diaphragm
40799	Unlisted procedure, lips
40899	Unlisted procedure, vestibule of mouth
41599	Unlisted procedure, tongue, floor of mouth
41899	Unlisted procedure, dentoalveolar structures
42299	Unlisted procedure, palate, uvula
42699	Unlisted procedure, salivary glands or ducts
42999	Unlisted procedure, pharynx, adenoids, or tonsils
43289	Unlisted laparoscopy procedure, esophagus
43499	Unlisted procedure, esophagus
43659	Unlisted laparoscopy procedure, stomach
43999	Unlisted procedure, stomach
44238	Unlisted laparoscopy procedure, intestine (except rectum)
44799	Unlisted procedure, small intestine
44899	Unlisted procedure, Meckel's diverticulum and the mesentery
44979	Unlisted laparoscopy procedure, appendix
45399	Unlisted procedure, colon
45499	Unlisted laparoscopy procedure, rectum
45999	Unlisted procedure, rectum
46999	Unlisted procedure, anus
47379	Unlisted laparoscopic procedure, liver
47399	Unlisted procedure, liver
47579	Unlisted laparoscopy procedure, biliary tract
47999	Unlisted procedure, biliary tract
48999	Unlisted procedure, pancreas
49329	Unlisted laparoscopy procedure, abdomen, peritoneum and omentum
49659	Unlisted laparoscopy procedure, hernioplasty, herniorrhaphy, herniotomy
49999	Unlisted procedure, abdomen, peritoneum and omentum
50549	Unlisted laparoscopy procedure, renal
50949	Unlisted laparoscopy procedure, ureter
51999	Unlisted laparoscopy procedure, bladder
53899	Unlisted procedure, urinary system
54699	Unlisted laparoscopy procedure, testis
55559	Unlisted laparoscopy procedure, spermatic cord
55899	Unlisted procedure, male genital system
58578	Unlisted laparoscopy procedure, uterus
58579	Unlisted hysteroscopy procedure, uterus
58679	Unlisted laparoscopy procedure, oviduct, ovary

* Pages in this section refer to the AMA *CPT® 2020 Professional Edition.*

58999	Unlisted procedure, female genital system (nonobstetrical)
59897	Unlisted fetal invasive procedure, including ultrasound guidance, when performed
59898	Unlisted laparoscopy procedure, maternity care and delivery
59899	Unlisted procedure, maternity care and delivery
60659	Unlisted laparoscopy procedure, endocrine system
60699	Unlisted procedure, endocrine system
64999	Unlisted procedure, nervous system
66999	Unlisted procedure, anterior segment of eye
67299	Unlisted procedure, posterior segment
67399	Unlisted procedure, extraocular muscle
67599	Unlisted procedure, orbit
67999	Unlisted procedure, eyelids
68399	Unlisted procedure, conjunctiva
68899	Unlisted procedure, lacrimal system
69399	Unlisted procedure, external ear
69799	Unlisted procedure, middle ear
69949	Unlisted procedure, inner ear
69979	Unlisted procedure, temporal bone, middle fossa approach

Special Report

A service that is rarely provided, unusual, variable, or new may require a special report. Pertinent information should include an adequate definition or description of the nature, extent, and need for the procedure, and the time, effort, and

Imaging Guidance

When imaging guidance or imaging supervision and interpretation is included in a surgical procedure, guidelines for image documentation and report, included in the guidelines for Radiology (Including Nuclear Medicine and Diagnostic Ultrasound), will apply. Imaging guidance should not be reported for use of a nonimaging-guided tracking or localizing system (eg, radar signals, electromagnetic signals). Imaging guidance should only be reported when an imaging modality (eg, radiography, fluoroscopy, ultrasonography, magnetic resonance imaging, computed tomography, or nuclear medicine) is used and is appropriately documented.

Surgical Destruction

Surgical destruction is a part of a surgical procedure and different methods of destruction are not ordinarily listed separately unless the technique substantially alters the standard management of a problem or condition. Exceptions under special circumstances are provided for by separate code numbers.

Surgical Procedures on the Musculoskeletal System

Cast and strapping procedures appear at the end of this section.

The services listed below include the application and removal of the first cast or traction device only. Subsequent replacement of cast and/or traction device may require an additional listing.

Definitions

The terms "closed treatment," "open treatment," and "percutaneous skeletal fixation" have been carefully chosen to accurately reflect current orthopaedic procedural treatments.

Closed treatment specifically means that the fracture site is not surgically opened (exposed to the external environment and directly visualized). This terminology is used to describe procedures that treat fractures by three methods: (1) without manipulation; (2) with manipulation; or (3) with or without traction.

Open treatment is used when the fractured bone is either: (1) surgically opened (exposed to the external environment) and the fracture (bone ends) visualized and internal fixation may be used; or (2) the fractured bone is opened remote from the fracture site in order to insert an intramedullary nail across the fracture site (the fracture site is not opened and visualized).

Percutaneous skeletal fixation describes fracture treatment which is neither open nor closed. In this procedure, the fracture fragments are not visualized, but fixation (e.g., pins) is placed across the fracture site, usually under X-ray imaging.

The type of fracture (e.g., open, compound, closed) does not have any coding correlation with the type of treatment (e.g., closed, open, or percutaneous) provided.

The codes for treatment of fractures and joint injuries (dislocations) are categorized by the type of manipulation (reduction) and stabilization (fixation or immobilization). These codes can apply to either open (compound) or closed fractures or joint injuries.

Skeletal traction is the application of a force (distracting or traction force) to a limb segment through a wire, pin, screw, or clamp that is attached (e.g., penetrates) to bone.

Skin traction is the application of a force (longitudinal) to a limb using felt or strapping applied directly to skin only.

External fixation is the usage of skeletal pins plus an attaching mechanism/device used for temporary or definitive treatment of acute or chronic bony deformity.

Codes for obtaining autogenous bone grafts, cartilage, tendon, fascia lata grafts or other tissues through separate incisions are to be used only when the graft is not already listed as part of the basic procedure.

Re-reduction of a fracture and/or dislocation performed by the primary physician or other qualified health care professional may be identified by the addition of modifier 76 to the usual procedure number to indicate "Repeat Procedure or Service by Same Physician or Other Qualified Health Care Professional." (See Appendix A* guidelines.)

Codes for external fixation are to be used only when external fixation is not already listed as part of the basic procedure.

Manipulation is used throughout the musculoskeletal fracture and dislocation subsections to specifically mean the attempted reduction or restoration of a fracture or joint dislocation to its normal anatomic alignment by the application of manually applied forces.

Excision of subcutaneous soft connective tissue tumors (including simple or intermediate repair) involves the simple or marginal resection of tumors confined to subcutaneous tissue below the skin but above the deep fascia. These tumors are usually benign and are resected without removing a significant amount of surrounding normal tissue. Code selection is based on the location and size of the tumor. Code selection is determined by measuring the greatest diameter of the tumor plus that margin required for complete excision of the tumor. The margins refer to the most narrow margin required to adequately excise the tumor, based on the physician's judgment. The measurement of the tumor plus margin is made at the time of the excision. Appreciable vessel exploration and/or neuroplasty should be reported separately. Extensive undermining or other techniques to close a defect created by skin excision may require a complex repair which should be reported separately. Dissection or elevation of tissue planes to permit resection of the tumor is included in the excision. For excision of benign lesions of cutaneous origin (e.g., sebaceous cyst), see 11400-11446.

Excision of fascial or subfascial soft tissue tumors (including simple or intermediate repair) involves the resection of tumors confined to the tissue within or below the deep fascia, but not involving the bone. These tumors are usually benign, are often intramuscular, and are resected without removing a significant amount of surrounding normal tissue. Code selection is based on size and location of the tumor. Code selection is determined by measuring the greatest diameter of the tumor plus that margin required for complete excision of the tumor. The margins refer to the most narrow margin required to adequately excise the tumor, based on individual judgment. The measurement of the tumor plus margin is made at the time of the excision. Appreciable vessel exploration and/ or neuroplasty should be reported separately. Extensive undermining or other techniques to close a defect created by skin excision may require a complex repair which should be reported separately. Dissection or elevation of tissue planes to permit resection of the tumor is included in the excision.

Digital (i.e., fingers and toes) subfascial tumors are defined as those tumors involving the tendons, tendon sheaths, or joints of the digit. Tumors which simply abut but do not breach the tendon, tendon sheath, or joint capsule are considered subcutaneous soft tissue tumors.

Radical resection of soft connective tissue tumors (including simple or intermediate repair) involves the resection of the tumor with wide margins of normal tissue. Appreciable vessel exploration and/or neuroplasty repair or reconstruction (e.g., adjacent tissue transfer[s], flap[s]) should be reported separately. Extensive undermining or other techniques to close a defect created by skin excision may require a complex repair which should be reported separately. Dissection or elevation of tissue planes to permit resection of the tumor is included in the excision. Although these tumors may be confined to a specific layer (e.g., subcutaneous, subfascial), radical resection may involve removal of tissue from one or more layers. Radical resection of soft tissue tumors is most commonly used for malignant connective tissue tumors or very aggressive benign connective tissue tumors. Code selection is based on size and location of the tumor. Code selection is determined by measuring the greatest diameter of the tumor plus that margin required for complete excision of the tumor. The margins refer to the most narrow margin required to adequately excise the tumor, based on individual judgment. The measurement of the tumor plus margin is made at the time of the excision. For radical resection of tumor(s) of cutaneous origin (e.g., melanoma), see 11600-11646.

Radical resection of bone tumors (including simple or intermediate repair) involves the resection of the tumor with wide margins of normal tissue. Appreciable vessel exploration and/or neuroplasty and complex bone repair or reconstruction (e.g., adjacent tissue transfer[s], flap[s]) should be reported separately. Extensive undermining or other techniques to close a defect created by skin excision may require a complex repair which should be reported separately. Dissection or elevation of tissue planes to permit resection of the tumor is included in the excision. It may require removal of the entire bone if tumor growth is extensive (e.g., clavicle). Radical resection of bone tumors is usually performed for malignant tumors or very aggressive benign tumors. If surrounding soft tissue is removed during these procedures, the radical resection of soft tissue tumor codes should not be reported separately. Code selection is based solely on the location of the tumor, **not** on the size of the tumor or whether the tumor is benign or malignant, primary or metastatic.

Surgical Procedures on the Cardiovascular System

Selective vascular catheterizations should be coded to include introduction and all lesser order selective catheterizations used in the approach (e.g., the description for a selective right middle cerebral artery catheterization includes the introduction and placement catheterization of the right common and internal carotid arteries).

Additional second and/or third order arterial catheterizations within the same family of arteries supplied by a single first order artery should be expressed by 36218 or 36248. Additional first order or higher catheterizations in vascular families supplied by a first order vessel different from a previously selected and coded family should be separately coded using the conventions described above.

* Pages in this section refer to the AMA *CPT® 2020 Professional Edition.*

Operating Microscope Procedures

▶The surgical microscope is employed when the surgical services are performed using the techniques of microsurgery. Code 69990 should be reported (without modifier 51 appended) in addition to the code for the primary procedure performed. Do not use 69990 for visualization with magnifying loupes or corrected vision.

Do not report 69990 in addition to procedures where use of the operating microscope is an inclusive component (15756-15758, 15842, 19364, 19368, 20955-20962, 20969-20973, 22551, 22552, 22856-22861, 26551-26554, 26556, 31526, 31531, 31536, 31541, 31545, 31546, 31561, 31571, 43116, 43180, 43496, 46601, 46607, 49906, 61548, 63075-63078, 64727, 64820-64823, 64912, 65091-68850, 0184T, 0308T, 0402T, 0583T).◀

The Central Venous Access Procedures Table

	Non-tunneled	Tunneled Without Port or Pump	Central Tunneled	Tunneled With Port	Tunneled With Pump	Peripheral	<5 years	≥5 years	Any Age
Insertion									
Catheter (without imaging guidance)	36555						36555		
	36556							36556	
		36557	36557				36557		
		36558	36558					36558	
	36568 (w/o port or pump)					36568 (w/o port or pump)	36568 (w/o port or pump)		
	36569 (w/o port or pump)					36569 (w/o port or pump)		36569 (w/o port or pump)	
Catheter (with bundled imaging guidance)							36572 (w/o port or pump)	36572 (w/o port or pump)	
							36573 (w/o port or pump)		36573 (w/o port or pump)
Device			36560	36560			36560		
			36561	36561				36561	
			36563		36563				36563
		36565	36565						36565
			36566	36566					
	36570 (w/ port)			36570 (w/ port)		36570 (w/port)	36570 (w/ port)		
	36571 (w/ port)			36571 (w/ port)		36571 (w/port)		36571 (w/port)	
Repair									
Catheter	36575 (w/o port or pump)	36575 (w/o port or pump)	36575 (w/o port or pump)			36575 (w/o port or pump)			36575
Device	36576 (w/ port or pump)					36576 (w/port or pump)			36576
Partial Replacement - Central Venous Access Device (Catheter only)									
			36578	36578	36578	36578			36578
Complete Replacement - Central Venous Access Device (Through Same Venous Access Site)									
Catheter (without imaging guidance)	36580 (w/o port or pump)								36580
		36581	36581						36581
Catheter (with bundled imaging guidance)	36584 (w/o port or pump)					36584 (w/o port or pump)			36584 (w/o port or pump)
Device			36582	36582					36582
			36583		36583				36583
				36585 (w/ port)		36585 (w/port)			36585

* Pages in this section refer to the AMA *CPT® 2020 Professional Edition.*

Removal									
Catheter		36589							36589
Device			36590	36590	36590	36590			36590
Removal of Obstructive Material from Device									
	36595 (pericatheter)	36595 (pericatheter)	36595 (pericatheter)	36595 (pericatheter)	36595 (pericatheter)	36595 (pericatheter)			36595 (pericatheter)
	36596 (intraluminal)	36596 (intraluminal)	36596 (intraluminal)	36596 (intraluminal)	36596 (intraluminal)	36596 (intraluminal)			36596 (intraluminal)
Repositioning of Catheter									
	36597	36597	36597	36597	36597	36597	36597	36597	36597

10140-10160

10140 Incision and drainage of hematoma, seroma or fluid collection

10160 Puncture aspiration of abscess, hematoma, bulla, or cyst

(If imaging guidance is performed, see 76942, 77002, 77012, 77021)

AMA Coding Notes

Incision and Drainage Procedures on the Skin, Subcutaneous, and Accessory Structures

(For excision, see 11400, et seq)

AMA *CPT Assistant*

10140: Nov 14: 5

10160: Aug 17: 9

Plain English Description

In 10140, an incision is made with a scalpel and fluid is drained. Any blood clots are removed with a hemostat. Gauze packing or a cannula may be utilized to facilitate further drainage if fluids continue to enter the site. A pressure dressing usually is applied over the site. The incision may be closed or left open to heal secondarily. In 10160, the physician cleanses the skin above the subcutaneous fluid deposit. A large needle attached to a syringe is guided into the fluid deposit and aspirated with the syringe. A pressure dressing may be applied over the site of the procedure.

Hematoma/seroma/bulla/cyst drainage/aspiration

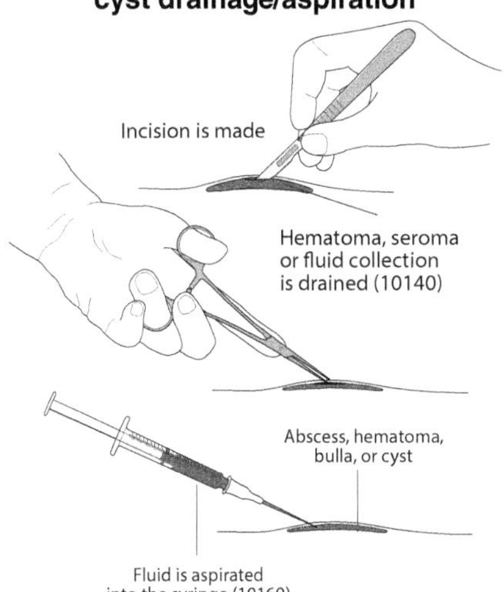

ICD-10-CM Diagnostic Codes

Code	Description
G97.61	Postprocedural hematoma of a nervous system organ or structure following a nervous system procedure
G97.62	Postprocedural hematoma of a nervous system organ or structure following other procedure
G97.63	Postprocedural seroma of a nervous system organ or structure following a nervous system procedure
G97.64	Postprocedural seroma of a nervous system organ or structure following other procedure
M79.81	Nontraumatic hematoma of soft tissue
➐ T79.2	Traumatic secondary and recurrent hemorrhage and seroma

ICD-10-CM Coding Notes

For codes requiring a 7th character extension, refer to your ICD-10-CM book. Review the character descriptions and coding guidelines for proper selection. For some procedures, only certain characters will apply.

CCI Edits

Refer to Appendix A for CCI edits.

Facility RVUs

Code	Work	PE Facility	MP	Total Facility
10140	1.58	1.61	0.22	3.41
10160	1.25	1.31	0.15	2.71

Non-facility RVUs

Code	Work	PE Non-Facility	MP	Total Non-Facility
10140	1.58	3.05	0.22	4.85
10160	1.25	2.31	0.15	3.71

Modifiers (PAR)

Code	Mod 50	Mod 51	Mod 62	Mod 66	Mod 80
10140	0	2	0	0	1
10160	0	2	0	0	1

Global Period

Code	Days
10140	010
10160	010

CPT® Procedural Coding

10180

10180 Incision and drainage, complex, postoperative wound infection
(For secondary closure of surgical wound, see 12020, 12021, 13160)

AMA Coding Notes

Incision and Drainage Procedures on the Skin, Subcutaneous, and Accessory Structures
(For excision, see 11400, et seq)

AMA *CPT Assistant*

10180: Nov 14: 5

Plain English Description

Incision and drainage are performed when infection occurs after an operation and the wound must be drained. The physician prepares the area by removing any sutures or staples or by creating additional incisions. Any necrotic (dead) tissue is removed after the wound has been drained. The wound is irrigated with saline and may be resutured or packed with gauze to allow additional drainage. Suction or latex drains may be used if the physician closes the wound. If the wound is left open, it may require future closure.

Incision and drainage, complex, postoperative wound infection

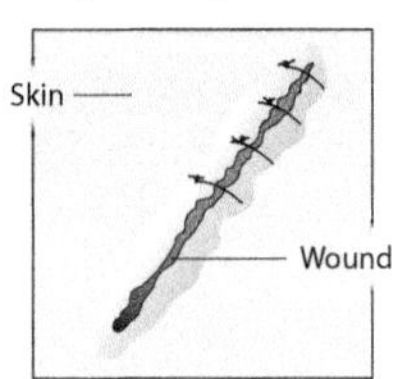

Sutures or staples are removed and wound is drained

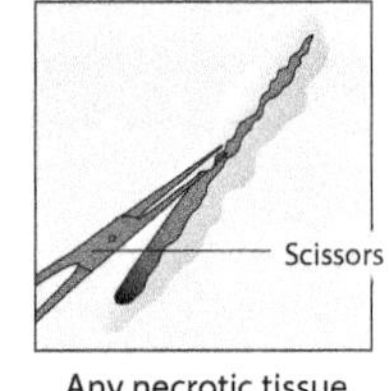

Any necrotic tissue is removed

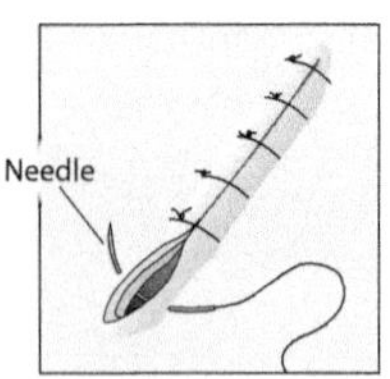

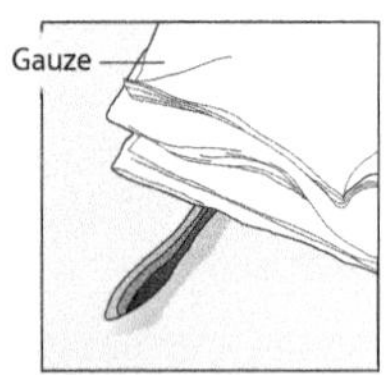

Wound is either resutured or packed with gauze

ICD-10-CM Diagnostic Codes

	Code	Description
	G97.82	Other postprocedural complications and disorders of nervous system
⑦	T81.41	Infection following a procedure, superficial incisional surgical site
⑦	T81.42	Infection following a procedure, deep incisional surgical site
⑦	T81.43	Infection following a procedure, organ and space surgical site
⑦	T84.63	Infection and inflammatory reaction due to internal fixation device of spine
⑦	T84.69	Infection and inflammatory reaction due to internal fixation device of other site
⑦	T85.732	Infection and inflammatory reaction due to implanted electronic neurostimulator of peripheral nerve, electrode (lead)
⑦	T85.733	Infection and inflammatory reaction due to implanted electronic neurostimulator of spinal cord, electrode (lead)
⑦	T85.734	Infection and inflammatory reaction due to implanted electronic neurostimulator, generator
⑦	T85.735	Infection and inflammatory reaction due to cranial or spinal infusion catheter
⑦	T85.738	Infection and inflammatory reaction due to other nervous system device, implant or graft

ICD-10-CM Coding Notes

For codes requiring a 7th character extension, refer to your ICD-10-CM book. Review the character descriptions and coding guidelines for proper selection. For some procedures, only certain characters will apply.

CCI Edits

Refer to Appendix A for CCI edits.

Facility RVUs

Code	Work	PE Facility	MP	Total Facility
10180	2.30	2.32	0.49	5.11

Non-facility RVUs

Code	Work	PE Non-Facility	MP	Total Non-Facility
10180	2.30	4.51	0.49	7.30

Modifiers (PAR)

Code	Mod 50	Mod 51	Mod 62	Mod 66	Mod 80
10180	0	2	0	0	1

Global Period

Code	Days
10180	010

11042-11047

11042 Debridement, subcutaneous tissue (includes epidermis and dermis, if performed); first 20 sq cm or less

(For debridement of skin [ie, epidermis and/or dermis only], see 97597, 97598)

11043 Debridement, muscle and/or fascia (includes epidermis, dermis, and subcutaneous tissue, if performed); first 20 sq cm or less

11044 Debridement, bone (includes epidermis, dermis, subcutaneous tissue, muscle and/or fascia, if performed); first 20 sq cm or less

+ **11045 Debridement, subcutaneous tissue (includes epidermis and dermis, if performed); each additional 20 sq cm, or part thereof (List separately in addition to code for primary procedure)**

(Use 11045 in conjunction with 11042)

+ **11047 Debridement, bone (includes epidermis, dermis, subcutaneous tissue, muscle and/or fascia, if performed); each additional 20 sq cm, or part thereof (List separately in addition to code for primary procedure)**

(Do not report 11042-11047 in conjunction with 97597-97602 for the same wound)

(Use 11047 in conjunction with 11044)

AMA Coding Guideline

Debridement Procedures on the Skin

Wound debridements (11042-11047) are reported by depth of tissue that is removed and by surface area of the wound. These services may be reported for injuries, infections, wounds and chronic ulcers. When performing debridement of a single wound, report depth using the deepest level of tissue removed. In multiple wounds, sum the surface area of those wounds that are at the same depth, but do not combine sums from different depths. For example: When bone is debrided from a 4 sq cm heel ulcer and from a 10 sq cm ischial ulcer, report the work with a single code, 11044. When subcutaneous tissue is debrided from a 16 sq cm dehisced abdominal wound and a 10 sq cm thigh wound, report the work with 11042 for the first 20 sq cm and 11045 for the second 6 sq cm. If all four wounds were debrided on the same day, use modifier 59 with either 11042, or 11044 as appropriate.

AMA Coding Notes

Debridement Procedures on the Skin

(For dermabrasions, see 15780-15783)

(For nail debridement, see 11720-11721)

(For burn(s), see 16000-16035)

(For pressure ulcers, see 15920-15999)

AMA *CPT Assistant* ☐

11042: Winter 92: 10, May 96: 6, Feb 97: 7, Aug 97: 6, Jun 05: 1, 10, Oct 07: 15, Nov 10: 9, May 11: 3, Sep 11: 11, Jan 12: 6, Mar 12: 3, Oct 12: 13, Feb 13: 16, Sep 13: 17, Oct 13: 15, Nov 14: 5, Feb 16: 14, Aug 16: 9, Oct 16: 3

11043: May 96: 6, Feb 97: 7, Apr 97: 11, Aug 97: 6, Dec 99: 10, Jun 05: 1, 10, Oct 07: 15, Nov 10: 9, May 11: 3, Sep 11: 11, Jan 12: 6, Mar 12: 3, Oct 12: 13, Feb 13: 16, Nov 14: 5, Aug 16: 9, Oct 16: 3

11044: Fall 93: 21, Mar 96: 10, May 96: 6, Feb 97: 7, Apr 97: 11, Aug 97: 6, Jun 05: 1, 10, Oct 07: 15, Nov 10: 9, May 11: 3, Sep 11: 11, Jan 12: 6, Mar 12: 3, Oct 12: 13, Feb 13: 16, Nov 14: 5, Aug 16: 9, Oct 16: 3

11045: May 11: 3, Sep 11: 11, Jan 12: 6, Mar 12: 3, Oct 12: 13, Nov 14: 5, Aug 16: 9, Oct 16: 3

11047: May 11: 3, Sep 11: 11, Jan 12: 6, Mar 12: 3, Oct 12: 13, Nov 14: 5, Aug 16: 9, Oct 16: 3

Plain English Description

Debridement of skin, subcutaneous tissue, muscle, and/or bone is performed and foreign material is removed. In 11042 and 11045, subcutaneous tissue, including epidermis and dermis, is debrided. Devascularized, necrotic skin is removed. Using sharp excision, nonviable epidermis, dermis, and subcutaneous tissue are removed until viable tissue is encountered as evidenced by bleeding. Foreign material is also removed. The physician may close the wound or cover the wound with gauze. Use 11042 for the first 20 sq cm debrided and 11045 for each additional 20 sq cm or part thereof. In 11043 and 11046, skin, subcutaneous tissue, and muscle are debrided. The wound is irrigated and skin and subcutaneous tissue are removed as described above. Muscle tissue is inspected for viability by checking color, consistency, contraction, and circulation. The fascia is incised parallel to the muscle fibers. Nonviable muscle tissue is identified and excised. Any foreign material is removed. When all nonviable tissue has been removed as indicated by bleeding in the exposed surfaces, the wound may be closed or packed with gauze, or a drain placed. Use 11043 for the first 20 sq cm debrided and 11046 for each additional 20 sq cm or part thereof. In 11044 and 11047, skin, subcutaneous tissue, muscle, and bone are debrided. Nonviable skin, subcutaneous tissue, muscle fascia, and muscle are removed as described above. All devascularized bone is removed until viable bone is encountered as evidenced by bleeding. The physician may close the wound, place a drain, or pack the wound with gauze. Use 11044 for the first 20 sq cm debrided and 11047 for each additional 20 sq cm or part thereof.

Debridement

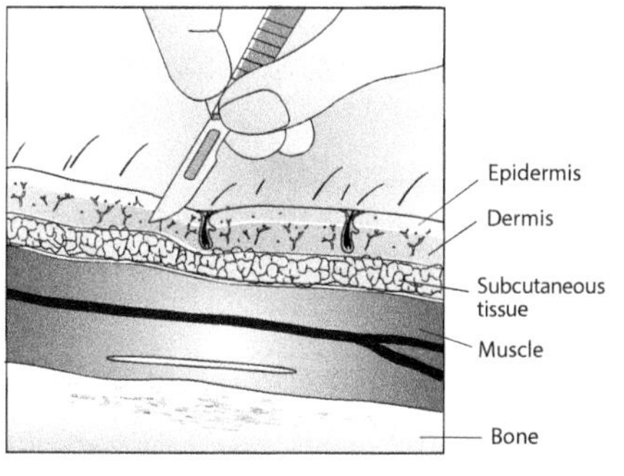

Subcutaneous tissue (11042, 11045); subcutaneous tissue, muscle and/or fascia (11043, 11046); subcutaneous tissue, muscle and/or fascia, bone (11044, 11047)

ICD-10-CM Diagnostic Codes

E08.621	Diabetes mellitus due to underlying condition with foot ulcer
E08.622	Diabetes mellitus due to underlying condition with other skin ulcer
E09.621	Drug or chemical induced diabetes mellitus with foot ulcer
E09.622	Drug or chemical induced diabetes mellitus with other skin ulcer
E10.621	Type 1 diabetes mellitus with foot ulcer
E10.622	Type 1 diabetes mellitus with other skin ulcer
E11.621	Type 2 diabetes mellitus with foot ulcer
E11.622	Type 2 diabetes mellitus with other skin ulcer
E13.621	Other specified diabetes mellitus with foot ulcer
E13.622	Other specified diabetes mellitus with other skin ulcer
I96	Gangrene, not elsewhere classified
L89.153	Pressure ulcer of sacral region, stage 3
L89.154	Pressure ulcer of sacral region, stage 4
L98.425	Non-pressure chronic ulcer of back with muscle involvement without evidence of necrosis
L98.426	Non-pressure chronic ulcer of back with bone involvement without evidence of necrosis
L98.428	Non-pressure chronic ulcer of back with other specified severity
L98.492	Non-pressure chronic ulcer of skin of other sites with fat layer exposed
L98.493	Non-pressure chronic ulcer of skin of other sites with necrosis of muscle
L98.494	Non-pressure chronic ulcer of skin of other sites with necrosis of bone
L98.495	Non-pressure chronic ulcer of skin of other sites with muscle involvement without evidence of necrosis
L98.496	Non-pressure chronic ulcer of skin of other sites with bone involvement without evidence of necrosis

	L98.498	Non-pressure chronic ulcer of skin of other sites with other specified severity
❼	T81.89	Other complications of procedures, not elsewhere classified

ICD-10-CM Coding Notes

For codes requiring a 7th character extension, refer to your ICD-10-CM book. Review the character descriptions and coding guidelines for proper selection. For some procedures, only certain characters will apply.

CCI Edits

Refer to Appendix A for CCI edits.

Facility RVUs ☐

Code	Work	PE Facility	MP	Total Facility
11042	1.01	0.62	0.12	1.75
11043	2.70	1.35	0.42	4.47
11044	4.10	1.82	0.64	6.56
11045	0.50	0.18	0.09	0.77
11047	1.80	0.71	0.35	2.86

Non-facility RVUs ☐

Code	Work	PE Non-Facility	MP	Total Non-Facility
11042	1.01	2.44	0.12	3.57
11043	2.70	3.52	0.42	6.64
11044	4.10	4.22	0.64	8.96
11045	0.50	0.60	0.09	1.19
11047	1.80	1.38	0.35	3.53

Modifiers (PAR) ☐

Code	Mod 50	Mod 51	Mod 62	Mod 66	Mod 80
11042	0	2	0	0	1
11043	0	2	0	0	1
11044	0	2	0	0	1
11045	0	0	0	0	0
11047	0	0	0	0	0

Global Period

Code	Days
11042	000
11043	000
11044	000
11045	ZZZ
11047	ZZZ

11104-11105

11104 Punch biopsy of skin (including simple closure, when performed); single lesion

+ **11105 Punch biopsy of skin (including simple closure, when performed); each separate/additional lesion (List separately in addition to code for primary procedure)**

(Report 11105 in conjunction with 11104, 11106, when different biopsy techniques are performed to sample separate/additional lesions for each type of biopsy technique used)

AMA Coding Guideline

Biopsy Procedures on the Skin

The use of a biopsy procedure code (eg, 11102, 11103, 11104, 11105, 11106, 11107) indicates that the procedure to obtain tissue solely for diagnostic histopathologic examination was performed independently, or was unrelated or distinct from other procedures/services provided at that time. Biopsies performed on different lesions or different sites on the same date of service may be reported separately, as they are not considered components of other procedures.

During certain surgical procedures in the integumentary system, such as excision, destruction, or shave removals, the removed tissue is often submitted for pathologic examination. The obtaining of tissue for pathology during the course of these procedures is a routine component of such procedures. This obtaining of tissue is not considered a separate biopsy procedure and is not separately reported.

Partial-thickness biopsies are those that sample a portion of the thickness of skin or mucous membrane and do not penetrate below the dermis or lamina propria. Full-thickness biopsies penetrate into tissue deep to the dermis or lamina propria, into the subcutaneous or submucosal space.

Sampling of stratum corneum only, by any modality (eg, skin scraping, tape stripping) does not constitute a skin biopsy procedure and is not separately reportable.

An appropriate biopsy technique is selected based on optimal tissue-sampling considerations for the type of neoplastic, inflammatory, or other lesion requiring a tissue diagnosis. Biopsy of the skin is reported under three distinct techniques:

Tangential biopsy (eg, shave, scoop, saucerize, curette) is performed with a sharp blade, such as a flexible biopsy blade, obliquely oriented scalpel or curette to remove a sample of epidermal tissue with or without portions of underlying dermis. The intent of a tangential biopsy (11102, 11103) is to obtain a tissue sample from a lesion for the purpose of diagnostic pathologic examination. Biopsy of lesions by tangential technique (11102, 11103) is not considered an excision. Tangential biopsy technique may be represented by a superficial sample and does not involve the full thickness of the dermis, which could result in portions of the lesion remaining in the deeper layers of the dermis.

For therapeutic removal of epidermal or dermal lesion(s) using shave technique, see 11300-11313. An indication for a shave removal (11300-11313) procedure may include a symptomatic lesion that rubs on waistband or bra, or any other reason why an elevated lesion is being completely removed with the shave technique, suggesting a therapeutic intent. It is the responsibility of the physician or qualified health care professional performing the procedure to clearly indicate the purpose of the procedure.

Punch biopsy requires a punch tool to remove a full-thickness cylindrical sample of skin. The intent of a punch biopsy (11104, 11105) is to obtain a cylindrical tissue sample of a cutaneous lesion for the purpose of diagnostic pathologic examination. Simple closure of the defect is included in the service. Manipulation of the biopsy defect to improve wound approximation is included in simple closure.

Incisional biopsy requires the use of a sharp blade (not a punch tool) to remove a full-thickness sample of tissue via a vertical incision or wedge, penetrating deep to the dermis, into the subcutaneous space. The intent of an incisional biopsy (11106, 11107) is to obtain a full-thickness tissue sample of a skin lesion for the purpose of diagnostic pathologic examination. This type of biopsy may sample subcutaneous fat, such as those performed for the evaluation of panniculitis. Although closure is usually performed on incisional biopsies, simple closure is not separately reported.

When multiple biopsy techniques are performed during the same encounter, only one primary lesion biopsy code (11102, 11104, 11106) is reported. Additional biopsy codes should be selected based on the following convention:

If multiple biopsies of the same type are performed, the primary code for that biopsy should be used along with the corresponding add-on code(s).

If an incisional biopsy is performed, report 11106 in combination with a tangential (11103), punch (11105), or incisional biopsy (11107) for the additional biopsy procedures.

If a punch biopsy is performed, report 11104 in combination with a tangential (11103), or punch (11105), for the additional biopsy procedures.

If multiple tangential biopsies are performed, report tangential biopsy (11102) in combination with 11103 for the additional tangential biopsy procedures.

When two or more biopsies of the same technique (ie, tangential, punch, or incisional) are performed on separate/additional lesions, use the appropriate add-on code (11103, 11105, 11107) to specify each additional biopsy. When two or three different biopsy techniques (ie, tangential, punch, or incisional) are performed to sample separate/additional lesions, select the appropriate biopsy code (11102, 11104, 11106) plus an additional add-on code (11103, 11105, 11107) for each additional biopsy performed.

The following table provides an illustration of the appropriate use of these codes for multiple biopsies:

Please see the Surgical Guidelines section for the following table: The Central Venous Access Procedures Table

AMA Coding Notes

Biopsy Procedures on the Skin

(For complete lesion excision with margins, see 11400-11646)

(For biopsy of nail unit, use 11755)

(For biopsy, intranasal, use 30100)

(For biopsy of lip, use 40490)

(For biopsy of vestibule of mouth, use 40808)

(For biopsy of tongue, anterior two-thirds, use 41100)

(For biopsy of floor of mouth, use 41108)

(For biopsy of penis, use 54100)

(For biopsy of vulva or perineum, see 56605, 56606)

(For biopsy of eyelid skin including lid margin, use 67810)

(For biopsy of conjunctiva, use 68100)

(For biopsy of ear, use 69100)

AMA *CPT Assistant* ▯

11104: Jan 19: 9
11105: Jan 19: 9

Plain English Description

A punch biopsy may be employed to remove or sample a variety of skin lesions including pigmented nevi, superficial inflammatory dermatoses, papulosquamous, granulomatous, bullous, or connective tissue disorders, and benign-appearing tumors. A punch biopsy removes a circular plug of skin, reticular dermis, and subcutaneous fat in a cylindrical sample. The skin is anesthetized and an appropriately sized punch tool is selected. The skin is stretched perpendicular to the tension lines and the punch tool is applied to the skin and rotated to penetrate to the desired depth. The tool is removed and the peripheral edge of the specimen is grasped with forceps, lifted, and cut at the base using a scissor. Bleeding can be controlled using electrocautery, aluminum chloride, or Monsel's solution. The deficit may be closed using simple suture, staple, gelfoam, or adhesive bandage including any simple manipulation to approximate the defect edges for better wound closure. Code 11104 reports a single lesion removed by punch biopsy including simple closure when performed. Code 11105 reports each additional lesion.

ICD-10-CM Diagnostic Codes

	Code	Description
	A69.20	Lyme disease, unspecified
	B20	Human immunodeficiency virus [HIV] disease
	D86.1	Sarcoidosis of lymph nodes
	D86.3	Sarcoidosis of skin
	D86.9	Sarcoidosis, unspecified
	E08.40	Diabetes mellitus due to underlying condition with diabetic neuropathy, unspecified
	E08.42	Diabetes mellitus due to underlying condition with diabetic polyneuropathy
	E09.40	Drug or chemical induced diabetes mellitus with neurological complications with diabetic neuropathy, unspecified
	E09.42	Drug or chemical induced diabetes mellitus with neurological complications with diabetic polyneuropathy
	E10.40	Type 1 diabetes mellitus with diabetic neuropathy, unspecified
	E10.42	Type 1 diabetes mellitus with diabetic polyneuropathy
	E11.40	Type 2 diabetes mellitus with diabetic neuropathy, unspecified
	E11.42	Type 2 diabetes mellitus with diabetic polyneuropathy
	E13.40	Other specified diabetes mellitus with diabetic neuropathy, unspecified
	E13.42	Other specified diabetes mellitus with diabetic polyneuropathy
	E75.21	Fabry (-Anderson) disease
	E78.2	Mixed hyperlipidemia
	E78.4	Other hyperlipidemia
	E78.49	Other hyperlipidemia
	E85.1	Neuropathic heredofamilial amyloidosis
	G60.9	Hereditary and idiopathic neuropathy, unspecified
	K90.0	Celiac disease
	M32.10	Systemic lupus erythematosus, organ or system involvement unspecified
	M35.00	Sicca syndrome, unspecified
	M35.09	Sicca syndrome with other organ involvement
⇄	M79.671	Pain in right foot
⇄	M79.672	Pain in left foot
❼	T45.1X1	Poisoning by antineoplastic and immunosuppressive drugs, accidental (unintentional)
❼	T45.1X2	Poisoning by antineoplastic and immunosuppressive drugs, intentional self-harm
❼	T45.1X3	Poisoning by antineoplastic and immunosuppressive drugs, assault
❼	T45.1X4	Poisoning by antineoplastic and immunosuppressive drugs, undetermined
❼	T45.1X5	Adverse effect of antineoplastic and immunosuppressive drugs

ICD-10-CM Coding Notes

For codes requiring a 7th character extension, refer to your ICD-10-CM book. Review the character descriptions and coding guidelines for proper selection. For some procedures, only certain characters will apply.

CCI Edits

Refer to Appendix A for CCI edits.

Facility RVUs ▯

Code	Work	PE Facility	MP	Total Facility
11104	0.83	0.48	0.09	1.40
11105	0.45	0.26	0.05	0.76

Non-facility RVUs ▯

Code	Work	PE Non-Facility	MP	Total Non-Facility
11104	0.83	2.65	0.09	3.57
11105	0.45	1.22	0.05	1.72

Modifiers (PAR) ▯

Code	Mod 50	Mod 51	Mod 62	Mod 66	Mod 80
11104	0	2	0	0	1
11105	0	0	0	0	1

Global Period

Code	Days
11104	000
11105	ZZZ

13160

13160 Secondary closure of surgical wound or dehiscence, extensive or complicated

(For packing or simple secondary wound closure, see 12020, 12021)

AMA Coding Guideline

Repair-Complex Procedures on the Integumentary System

Reconstructive procedures, complicated wound closure.

Sum of lengths of repairs for each group of anatomic sites.

Surgical Repair (Closure) Procedures on the Integumentary System

Use the codes in this section to designate wound closure utilizing sutures, staples, or tissue adhesives (eg, 2-cyanoacrylate), either singly or in combination with each other, or in combination with adhesive strips. Wound closure utilizing adhesive strips as the sole repair material should be coded using the appropriate E/M code.

Definitions

The repair of wounds may be classified as Simple, Intermediate, or Complex.

Simple repair is used when the wound is superficial; eg, involving primarily epidermis or dermis, or subcutaneous tissues without significant involvement of deeper structures, and requires simple one layer closure. This includes local anesthesia and chemical or electrocauterization of wounds not closed.

Intermediate repair includes the repair of wounds that, in addition to the above, require layered closure of one or more of the deeper layers of subcutaneous tissue and superficial (non-muscle) fascia, in addition to the skin (epidermal and dermal) closure. It includes limited undermining (defined as a distance less than the maximum width of the defect, measured perpendicular to the closure line, along at least one entire edge of the defect). Single-layer closure of heavily contaminated wounds that have required extensive cleaning or removal of particulate matter also constitutes intermediate repair.

Complex repair includes the repair of wounds that, in addition to the requirements for intermediate repair, require at least one of the following: exposure of bone, cartilage, tendon, or named neurovascular structure; debridement of wound edges (eg, traumatic lacerations or avulsions); extensive undermining (defined as a distance greater than or equal to the maximum width of the defect, measured perpendicular to the closure line along at least one entire edge of the defect); involvement of free margins of helical rim, vermilion border, or nostril rim; placement of retention sutures. Necessary preparation includes creation of a limited defect for repairs or the debridement of complicated lacerations or avulsions. Complex repair does not include excision of benign (11400-11446) or malignant (11600-11646) lesions, excisional preparation of a wound bed (15002-15005) or debridement of an open fracture or open dislocation.

Instructions for listing services at time of wound repair:

1. The repaired wound(s) should be measured and recorded in centimeters, whether curved, angular, or stellate.
2. When multiple wounds are repaired, add together the lengths of those in the same classification (see above) and from all anatomic sites that are grouped together into the same code descriptor. For example, add together the lengths of intermediate repairs to the trunk and extremities. Do not add lengths of repairs from different groupings of anatomic sites (eg, face and extremities). Also, do not add together lengths of different classifications (eg, intermediate and complex repairs).

When more than one classification of wounds is repaired, list the more complicated as the primary procedure and the less complicated as the secondary procedure, using modifier 59.

3. Decontamination and/or debridement: Debridement is considered a separate procedure only when gross contamination requires prolonged cleansing, when appreciable amounts of devitalized or contaminated tissue are removed, or when debridement is carried out separately without immediate primary closure.
4. Involvement of nerves, blood vessels and tendons: Report under appropriate system (Nervous, Cardiovascular, Musculoskeletal) for repair of these structures. The repair of these associated wounds is included in the primary procedure unless it qualifies as a complex repair, in which case modifier 59 applies.

Simple ligation of vessels in an open wound is considered as part of any wound closure.

Simple "exploration" of nerves, blood vessels or tendons exposed in an open wound is also considered part of the essential treatment of the wound and is not a separate procedure unless appreciable dissection is required. If the wound requires enlargement, extension of dissection (to determine penetration), debridement, removal of foreign body(s), ligation or coagulation of minor subcutaneous and/or muscular blood vessel(s) of the subcutaneous tissue, muscle fascia, and/or muscle, not requiring thoracotomy or laparotomy, use codes 20100-20103, as appropriate.

AMA Coding Notes

Repair-Complex Procedures on the Integumentary System

(For full thickness repair of lip or eyelid, see respective anatomical subsections)

Surgical Repair (Closure) Procedures on the Integumentary System

(For extensive debridement of soft tissue and/or bone, not associated with open fracture(s) and/or dislocation(s) resulting from penetrating and/or blunt trauma, see 11042-11047.)

(For extensive debridement of subcutaneous tissue, muscle fascia, muscle, and/or bone associated with open fracture(s) and/or dislocation(s), see 11010-11012.)

AMA *CPT Assistant* ▢

13160: Sep 97: 11, Dec 98: 5, Apr 00: 8, May 11: 4, Dec 12: 6

Plain English Description

Secondary closure of an extensive or complicated surgical wound or wound dehiscence is performed. This procedure covers two scenarios, one in which the surgical wound is not closed at the time of the original surgical procedure, and another in which a surgically closed wound opens along the previous suture line. Secondary surgical wound closure is performed on a date subsequent to the original surgical procedure during a separate surgical session or encounter. The edges of the open surgical wound are trimmed. The deepest layers may be closed with absorbable sutures, and the knot buried followed by closure of superficial layers with non-absorbable sutures. If retention sutures are used to hold the edges of the wound together without tension, they are placed through the entire thickness of the wound, a short length of plastic or rubber tubing is threaded over each suture, and each suture is then tied. Stents may also be used to hold tissue in place or maintain the opening of an orifice. Care is taken to carefully align wound edges to prevent scar depression. Secondary closure of a wound dehiscence is performed on a wound that has opened at the site of the earlier repair. The extent of the wound dehiscence is evaluated. The wound is irrigated with sterile saline or an antibiotic solution. The previously placed sutures are removed and the edges of the wound are trimmed. Any necrotic tissue is debrided. The wound is then repaired as described above.

Secondary closure of complicated surgical wound or dehiscence

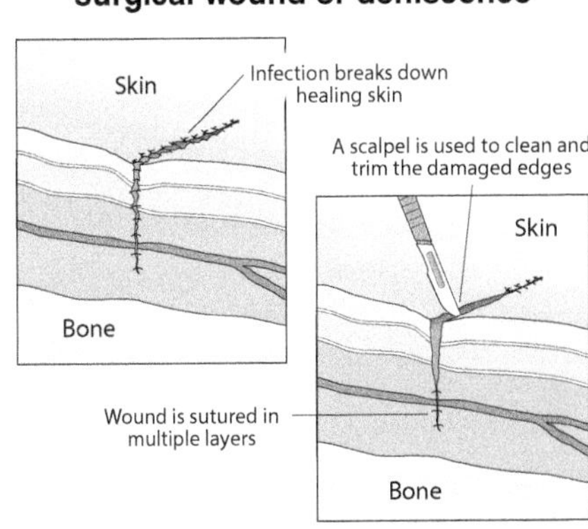

ICD-10-CM Diagnostic Codes

⑦	T81.30	Disruption of wound, unspecified
⑦	T81.31	Disruption of external operation (surgical) wound, not elsewhere classified

❼	T81.32	Disruption of internal operation (surgical) wound, not elsewhere classified
❼	T81.33	Disruption of traumatic injury wound repair
	Z48.1	Encounter for planned postprocedural wound closure

ICD-10-CM Coding Notes

For codes requiring a 7th character extension, refer to your ICD-10-CM book. Review the character descriptions and coding guidelines for proper selection. For some procedures, only certain characters will apply.

CCI Edits

Refer to Appendix A for CCI edits.

Facility RVUs

Code	Work	PE Facility	MP	Total Facility
13160	12.04	8.89	2.06	22.99

Non-facility RVUs

Code	Work	PE Non-Facility	MP	Total Non-Facility
13160	12.04	8.89	2.06	22.99

Modifiers (PAR)

Code	Mod 50	Mod 51	Mod 62	Mod 66	Mod 80
13160	0	2	0	0	1

Global Period

Code	Days
13160	090

20200-20205

20200 Biopsy, muscle; superficial
20205 Biopsy, muscle; deep

AMA Coding Guideline

Please see the Surgery Guidelines section for the following guidelines:

- *Surgical Procedures on the Musculoskeletal System*

Plain English Description

An incisional biopsy is performed on superficial (20200) or deep (20205) muscle tissue. This procedure is typically performed to diagnose diseases involving muscle tissue, such as muscular dystrophy, myasthenia gravis, polymyositis, dermatomyositis, amyotrophic lateral sclerosis (ALS), Friedreich's ataxia, and trichinosis or toxoplasmosis parasitic infections of the muscles. The planned biopsy site is cleansed. An incision is then made in the muscle and a tissue sample is obtained. The tissue sample is then sent for separately reportable pathology examination. Use 20200 for muscle biopsy involving a superficial incision or 20205 if a deeper incision with tissue dissection must be made to access the site.

Muscle biopsy

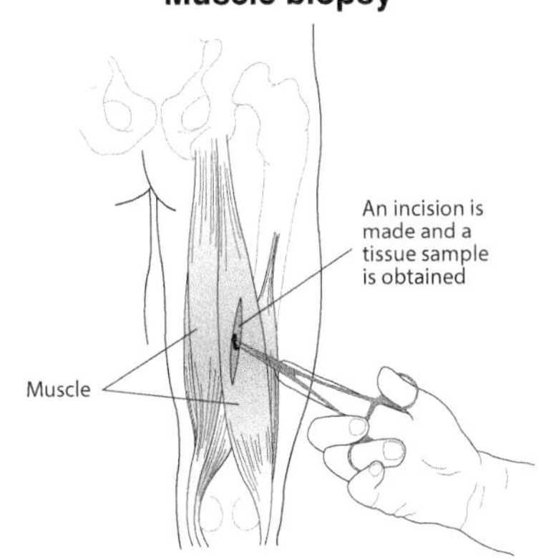

Tissue is obtained from a superficial muscle (20200), or a deep muscle (20205).

ICD-10-CM Diagnostic Codes

G12.23	Primary lateral sclerosis
G12.24	Familial motor neuron disease
G12.25	Progressive spinal muscle atrophy
G60.3	Idiopathic progressive neuropathy
G71.01	Duchenne or Becker muscular dystrophy
G71.02	Facioscapulohumeral muscular dystrophy
G71.09	Other specified muscular dystrophies
G71.2	Congenital myopathies
G71.3	Mitochondrial myopathy, not elsewhere classified
G71.8	Other primary disorders of muscles
G71.9	Primary disorder of muscle, unspecified
G72.2	Myopathy due to other toxic agents
G72.41	Inclusion body myositis [IBM]
G72.49	Other inflammatory and immune myopathies, not elsewhere classified
G72.89	Other specified myopathies
G73.7	Myopathy in diseases classified elsewhere
M33.00	Juvenile dermatomyositis, organ involvement unspecified
M33.01	Juvenile dermatomyositis with respiratory involvement
M33.03	Juvenile dermatomyositis without myopathy
M33.10	Other dermatomyositis, organ involvement unspecified
M33.11	Other dermatomyositis with respiratory involvement
M33.12	Other dermatomyositis with myopathy
M33.13	Other dermatomyositis without myopathy
M33.22	Polymyositis with myopathy
M33.91	Dermatopolymyositis, unspecified with respiratory involvement
M33.92	Dermatopolymyositis, unspecified with myopathy
M33.93	Dermatopolymyositis, unspecified without myopathy
M79.11	Myalgia of mastication muscle
M79.12	Myalgia of auxiliary muscles, head and neck
M79.18	Myalgia, other site

CCI Edits

Refer to Appendix A for CCI edits.

Facility RVUs

Code	Work	PE Facility	MP	Total Facility
20200	1.46	0.92	0.35	2.73
20205	2.35	1.49	0.60	4.44

Non-facility RVUs

Code	Work	PE Non-Facility	MP	Total Non-Facility
20200	1.46	4.26	0.35	6.07
20205	2.35	5.52	0.60	8.47

Modifiers (PAR)

Code	Mod 50	Mod 51	Mod 62	Mod 66	Mod 80
20200	0	2	0	0	1
20205	0	2	0	0	1

Global Period

Code	Days
20200	000
20205	000

20526

20526 Injection, therapeutic (eg, local anesthetic, corticosteroid), carpal tunnel

AMA Coding Guideline

Please see the Surgery Guidelines section for the following guidelines:

- *Surgical Procedures on the Musculoskeletal System*

AMA Coding Notes

General Introduction or Removal Procedures on the Musculoskeletal System

(For injection procedure for arthrography, see anatomical area)

(For injection of autologous adipose-derived regenerative cells, use 0490T)

AMA *CPT Assistant* □

20526: Mar 02: 7

Plain English Description

A therapeutic injection using a local anesthetic and/or corticosteroid is performed to treat symptoms of carpal tunnel syndrome. This procedure is referred to as a carpal tunnel or median nerve injection. The flexor carpi radialis (FCR) and palmaris longus (PL) muscles are located. The skin over the planned needle insertion site in the wrist on the palmar side is cleansed. The needle is inserted at a slight angle just distal to the wrist crease between the tendons of the FCR and PL muscles. The syringe is retracted to ensure the needle is clear of all blood vessels and a local anesthetic and/or steroid solution is injected, usually lidocaine with methylprednisolone. The needle is removed and the local anesthetic/steroid is allowed to disperse distally using gravity and finger motion. Carpal tunnel injection is generally more effective than other non-surgical treatments such as taking oral tablets or wearing a splint.

Carpal tunnel therapeutic injection

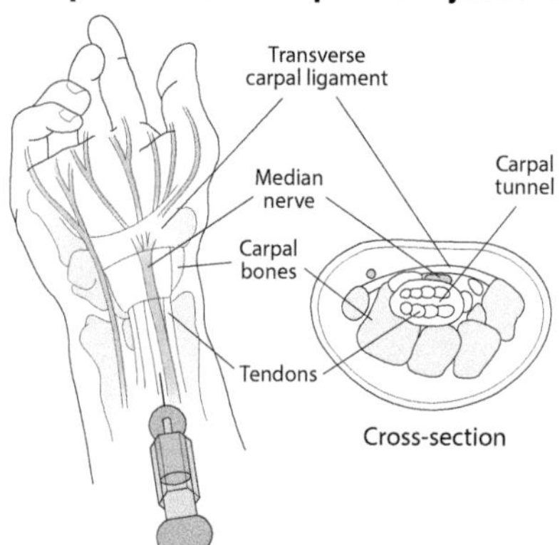

A therapeutic injection of corticosteroid or anesthetic is injected to help relieve the symptoms of carpal tunnel syndrome.

ICD-10-CM Diagnostic Codes

⇄	G56.01	Carpal tunnel syndrome, right upper limb
⇄	G56.02	Carpal tunnel syndrome, left upper limb
⇄	G56.03	Carpal tunnel syndrome, bilateral upper limbs
⇄	G56.11	Other lesions of median nerve, right upper limb
⇄	G56.12	Other lesions of median nerve, left upper limb
⇄	G56.13	Other lesions of median nerve, bilateral upper limbs
⇄	G56.41	Causalgia of right upper limb
⇄	G56.42	Causalgia of left upper limb
⇄	G56.43	Causalgia of bilateral upper limbs

CCI Edits

Refer to Appendix A for CCI edits.

Facility RVUs □

Code	Work	PE Facility	MP	Total Facility
20526	0.94	0.55	0.16	1.65

Non-facility RVUs □

Code	Work	PE Non-Facility	MP	Total Non-Facility
20526	0.94	1.15	0.16	2.25

Modifiers (PAR) □

Code	Mod 50	Mod 51	Mod 62	Mod 66	Mod 80
20526	1	2	0	0	1

Global Period

Code	Days
20526	000

20550-20551

20550 Injection(s); single tendon sheath, or ligament, aponeurosis (eg, plantar "fascia")

(For injection of Morton's neuroma, see 64455, 64632)

20551 Injection(s); single tendon origin/ insertion

(Do not report 20550, 20551 in conjunction with 0232T, 0481T)

(For harvesting, preparation, and injection[s] of platelet-rich plasma, use 0232T)

AMA Coding Guideline

Please see the Surgery Guidelines section for the following guidelines:

- *Surgical Procedures on the Musculoskeletal System*

AMA Coding Notes

General Introduction or Removal Procedures on the Musculoskeletal System

(For injection procedure for arthrography, see anatomical area)

(For injection of autologous adipose-derived regenerative cells, use 0490T)

AMA *CPT Assistant*

20550: Jan 96: 7, Jun 98: 10, Mar 02: 7, Aug 03: 14, Sep 03: 13, Dec 03: 11, Jan 09: 6, Jul 12: 14, Oct 14: 9

20551: Mar 02: 7, Sep 03: 13, Oct 14: 9, Dec 17: 16

Plain English Description

The physician injects a single tendon sheath, ligament, or aponeurosis (20550) or a single tendon origin or insertion (20551). In 20550, the site of maximum tenderness is identified by palpation. The needle is advanced into the tendon sheath, ligament, or aponeurosis and an anesthetic, steroid, or other therapeutic substance is injected. More than one injection to the same tendon sheath or ligament may be administered. In 20551, the tendon origin or insertion is located. A needle is advanced into the origin or insertion and an anesthetic, steroid, or other therapeutic substance is injected.

Injections

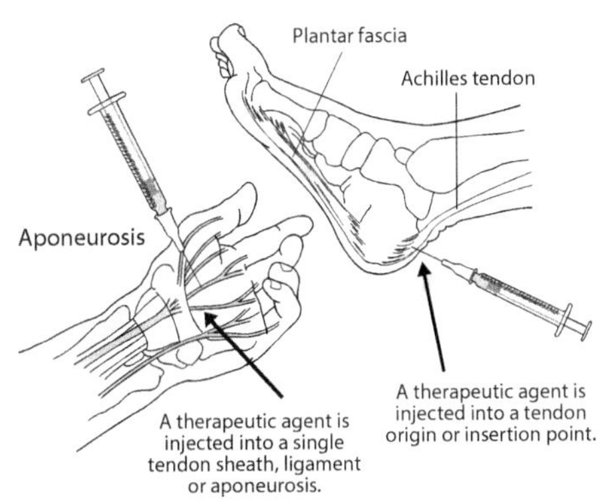

ICD-10-CM Diagnostic Codes

M46.01	Spinal enthesopathy, occipito-atlanto-axial region
M46.02	Spinal enthesopathy, cervical region
M46.03	Spinal enthesopathy, cervicothoracic region
M46.04	Spinal enthesopathy, thoracic region
M46.05	Spinal enthesopathy, thoracolumbar region
M46.06	Spinal enthesopathy, lumbar region
M46.07	Spinal enthesopathy, lumbosacral region
M46.08	Spinal enthesopathy, sacral and sacrococcygeal region
M46.09	Spinal enthesopathy, multiple sites in spine

CCI Edits

Refer to Appendix A for CCI edits.

Facility RVUs

Code	Work	PE Facility	MP	Total Facility
20550	0.75	0.29	0.09	1.13
20551	0.75	0.31	0.09	1.15

Non-facility RVUs

Code	Work	PE Non-Facility	MP	Total Non-Facility
20550	0.75	0.72	0.09	1.56
20551	0.75	0.76	0.09	1.60

Modifiers (PAR)

Code	Mod 50	Mod 51	Mod 62	Mod 66	Mod 80
20550	1	2	0	0	1
20551	0	2	0	0	1

Global Period

Code	Days
20550	000
20551	000

20552-20553

20552 Injection(s); single or multiple trigger point(s), 1 or 2 muscle(s)

20553 Injection(s); single or multiple trigger point(s), 3 or more muscles

(Do not report 20552, 20553 in conjunction with 20560, 20561 for the same muscle[s])

(If imaging guidance is performed, see 76942, 77002, 77021)

AMA Coding Guideline

Please see the Surgery Guidelines section for the following guidelines:

- *Surgical Procedures on the Musculoskeletal System*

AMA Coding Notes

General Introduction or Removal Procedures on the Musculoskeletal System

(For injection procedure for arthrography, see anatomical area)

(For injection of autologous adipose-derived regenerative cells, use 0490T)

AMA *CPT Assistant*

20552: Mar 02: 7, May 03: 19, Sep 03: 11, Feb 10: 9, Feb 11: 5, Jul 11: 16, Apr 12: 19, Oct 14: 9, Jun 17: 10, Dec 17: 16

20553: Mar 02: 7, May 03: 19, Sep 03: 11, Jun 08: 8, Feb 10: 9, Feb 11: 5, Jul 11: 16, Oct 14: 9, Jun 17: 10, Dec 18: 8

Plain English Description

The physician injects a single or multiple trigger points in one or two muscles (20552) or three or more muscles (20553). Trigger points are tiny contraction knots that develop in a muscle when it is injured or overworked. The physician identifies the trigger points by palpating the muscle. The needle is advanced into the muscle and an anesthetic, steroid, or other therapeutic substance is injected. This is repeated until all trigger points on all involved muscles have been treated.

Injection

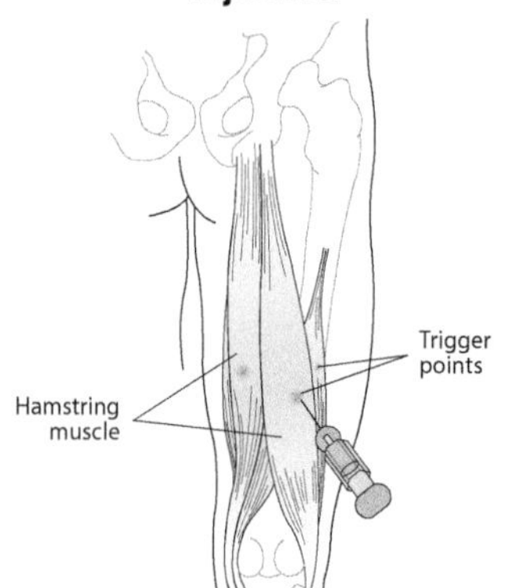

An anesthetic or therapeutic solution is injected into one or more trigger points in one or more muscles.

ICD-10-CM Diagnostic Codes

	Code	Description
	M53.3	Sacrococcygeal disorders, not elsewhere classified
	M54.2	Cervicalgia
	M54.5	Low back pain
	M54.6	Pain in thoracic spine
	M54.9	Dorsalgia, unspecified
⇄	M60.811	Other myositis, right shoulder
⇄	M60.812	Other myositis, left shoulder
⇄	M60.821	Other myositis, right upper arm
⇄	M60.822	Other myositis, left upper arm
⇄	M60.831	Other myositis, right forearm
⇄	M60.832	Other myositis, left forearm
⇄	M60.841	Other myositis, right hand
⇄	M60.842	Other myositis, left hand
⇄	M60.851	Other myositis, right thigh
⇄	M60.852	Other myositis, left thigh
⇄	M60.861	Other myositis, right lower leg
⇄	M60.862	Other myositis, left lower leg
⇄	M60.871	Other myositis, right ankle and foot
⇄	M60.872	Other myositis, left ankle and foot
	M60.89	Other myositis, multiple sites
	M79.11	Myalgia of mastication muscle
	M79.12	Myalgia of auxiliary muscles, head and neck
	M79.18	Myalgia, other site
⇄	M79.621	Pain in right upper arm
⇄	M79.622	Pain in left upper arm
⇄	M79.631	Pain in right forearm
⇄	M79.632	Pain in left forearm
⇄	M79.644	Pain in right finger(s)
⇄	M79.645	Pain in left finger(s)
⇄	M79.651	Pain in right thigh
⇄	M79.652	Pain in left thigh
⇄	M79.661	Pain in right lower leg
⇄	M79.662	Pain in left lower leg
⇄	M79.671	Pain in right foot
⇄	M79.672	Pain in left foot
⇄	M79.674	Pain in right toe(s)
⇄	M79.675	Pain in left toe(s)
	M79.7	Fibromyalgia
	R68.84	Jaw pain

CCI Edits

Refer to Appendix A for CCI edits.

Facility RVUs

Code	Work	PE Facility	MP	Total Facility
20552	0.66	0.36	0.09	1.11
20553	0.75	0.41	0.09	1.25

Non-facility RVUs

Code	Work	PE Non-Facility	MP	Total Non-Facility
20552	0.66	0.84	0.09	1.59
20553	0.75	0.98	0.09	1.82

Modifiers (PAR)

Code	Mod 50	Mod 51	Mod 62	Mod 66	Mod 80
20552	0	2	0	0	1
20553	0	2	0	0	1

Global Period

Code	Days
20552	000
20553	000

20660

20660 Application of cranial tongs, caliper, or stereotactic frame, including removal (separate procedure)

AMA Coding Guideline

Please see the Surgery Guidelines section for the following guidelines:

- *Surgical Procedures on the Musculoskeletal System*

AMA Coding Notes

General Introduction or Removal Procedures on the Musculoskeletal System

(For injection procedure for arthrography, see anatomical area)

(For injection of autologous adipose-derived regenerative cells, use 0490T)

AMA *CPT Assistant*

20660: Jun 96: 10, Nov 97: 14, Jan 06: 46, Dec 06: 10, Feb 08: 8, Jul 08: 10, Nov 09: 6, Apr 12: 11, Aug 12: 14

Plain English Description

The physician applies cranial tongs, a caliper, or a stereotactic frame for stabilization of the cervical spine. Local anesthesia is applied, after the pin placement locations have been shaved and Betadine has been applied. The pins from the device are simultaneously advanced into the cranial skin. The skull is not pierced. Lock nuts are tightened to maintain the appropriate depth and stability of the device. These nuts are checked every few hours for appropriate stability. The removal of this device is also included in this code.

Application of cranial tongs, caliper, or stereotactic frame, including removal (separate procedure)

Cranial stabilization device

Cervical spine

ICD-10-CM Diagnostic Codes

- M80.08 Age-related osteoporosis with current pathological fracture, vertebra(e)
- M80.88 Other osteoporosis with current pathological fracture, vertebra(e)
- M84.48 Pathological fracture, other site
- M84.58 Pathological fracture in neoplastic disease, other specified site
- M84.68 Pathological fracture in other disease, other site
- S12.000 Unspecified displaced fracture of first cervical vertebra
- S12.001 Unspecified nondisplaced fracture of first cervical vertebra
- S12.01 Stable burst fracture of first cervical vertebra
- S12.02 Unstable burst fracture of first cervical vertebra
- S12.030 Displaced posterior arch fracture of first cervical vertebra
- S12.031 Nondisplaced posterior arch fracture of first cervical vertebra
- S12.040 Displaced lateral mass fracture of first cervical vertebra
- S12.041 Nondisplaced lateral mass fracture of first cervical vertebra
- S12.090 Other displaced fracture of first cervical vertebra
- S12.091 Other nondisplaced fracture of first cervical vertebra
- S12.100 Unspecified displaced fracture of second cervical vertebra
- S12.101 Unspecified nondisplaced fracture of second cervical vertebra
- S12.110 Anterior displaced Type II dens fracture
- S12.111 Posterior displaced Type II dens fracture
- S12.112 Nondisplaced Type II dens fracture
- S12.120 Other displaced dens fracture
- S12.121 Other nondisplaced dens fracture
- S12.130 Unspecified traumatic displaced spondylolisthesis of second cervical vertebra
- S12.131 Unspecified traumatic nondisplaced spondylolisthesis of second cervical vertebra
- S12.14 Type III traumatic spondylolisthesis of second cervical vertebra
- S12.150 Other traumatic displaced spondylolisthesis of second cervical vertebra
- S12.151 Other traumatic nondisplaced spondylolisthesis of second cervical vertebra
- S12.190 Other displaced fracture of second cervical vertebra
- S12.191 Other nondisplaced fracture of second cervical vertebra
- S12.400 Unspecified displaced fracture of fifth cervical vertebra
- S12.401 Unspecified nondisplaced fracture of fifth cervical vertebra
- S12.500 Unspecified displaced fracture of sixth cervical vertebra
- S12.600 Unspecified displaced fracture of seventh cervical vertebra
- S12.601 Unspecified nondisplaced fracture of seventh cervical vertebra
- S13.100 Subluxation of unspecified cervical vertebrae
- S13.101 Dislocation of unspecified cervical vertebrae
- S13.110 Subluxation of C0/C1 cervical vertebrae
- S13.111 Dislocation of C0/C1 cervical vertebrae
- S13.120 Subluxation of C1/C2 cervical vertebrae
- S13.121 Dislocation of C1/C2 cervical vertebrae
- S13.130 Subluxation of C2/C3 cervical vertebrae
- S13.131 Dislocation of C2/C3 cervical vertebrae
- S13.140 Subluxation of C3/C4 cervical vertebrae
- S13.141 Dislocation of C3/C4 cervical vertebrae
- S13.150 Subluxation of C4/C5 cervical vertebrae
- S13.151 Dislocation of C4/C5 cervical vertebrae
- S13.160 Subluxation of C5/C6 cervical vertebrae
- S13.161 Dislocation of C5/C6 cervical vertebrae
- S13.170 Subluxation of C6/C7 cervical vertebrae
- S13.171 Dislocation of C6/C7 cervical vertebrae
- S13.180 Subluxation of C7/T1 cervical vertebrae
- S13.181 Dislocation of C7/T1 cervical vertebrae

ICD-10-CM Coding Notes

For codes requiring a 7th character extension, refer to your ICD-10-CM book. Review the character descriptions and coding guidelines for proper selection. For some procedures, only certain characters will apply.

CCI Edits

Refer to Appendix A for CCI edits.

Facility RVUs

Code	Work	PE Facility	MP	Total Facility
20660	4.00	1.85	1.15	7.00

Non-facility RVUs

Code	Work	PE Non-Facility	MP	Total Non-Facility
20660	4.00	1.85	1.15	7.00

Modifiers (PAR)

Code	Mod 50	Mod 51	Mod 62	Mod 66	Mod 80
20660	0	2	0	0	1

Global Period

Code	Days
20660	000

20930-20931

✚ **20930 Allograft, morselized, or placement of osteopromotive material, for spine surgery only (List separately in addition to code for primary procedure)**

(Use 20930 in conjunction with 22319, 22532, 22533, 22548-22558, 22590-22612, 22630, 22633, 22634, 22800-22812)

✚ **20931 Allograft, structural, for spine surgery only (List separately in addition to code for primary procedure)**

(Use 20931 in conjunction with 22319, 22532-22533, 22548-22558, 22590-22612, 22630, 22633, 22634, 22800-22812)

AMA Coding Guideline

General Grafts (or Implants) Procedures on the Musculoskeletal System

Codes for obtaining autogenous bone, cartilage, tendon, fascia lata grafts, bone marrow, or other tissues through separate skin/fascial incisions should be reported separately, unless the code descriptor references the harvesting of the graft or implant (eg, includes obtaining graft). Autologous grafts that are already defined in the CPT code set, including skin, bone, nerve, tendon, fascia lata, or vessels, should be reported with the more specific codes for each tissue type. Code 15769 may be used for other autologous soft tissue grafts harvested by direct excision. See 15771, 15772, 15773, 15774 for autologous fat grafting harvested by liposuction technique.

Do not append modifier 62 to bone graft codes 20900-20938.

Please see the Surgery Guidelines section for the following guidelines:

- *Surgical Procedures on the Musculoskeletal System*

AMA Coding Notes

General Grafts (or Implants) Procedures on the Musculoskeletal System

(For spinal surgery bone graft[s] see codes 20930-20938)

AMA *CPT Assistant*

20930: Feb 96: 6, Mar 96: 4, Sep 97: 8, Nov 99: 10, Feb 02: 6, Jan 04: 27, Dec 07: 1, Feb 08: 8, Nov 10: 8, Jul 11: 18, Dec 11: 15, Apr 12: 14, Jun 12: 11, Jul 13: 3, Jul 18: 14, May 19: 7

20931: Feb 96: 6, Feb 02: 6, Feb 05: 15, Feb 08: 8, Nov 10: 8, Jul 11: 18, Sep 11: 12, Dec 11: 15, Apr 12: 14, Jun 12: 11, Jul 13: 3, Jul 18: 14, May 19: 7

Plain English Description

A bone allograft or osteopromotive material is placed during a separately reportable surgical procedure on the spine. Bone allograft uses donor bone usually obtained from a cadaver. Bone allograft does not contain any osteoblasts (bone-growing cells) or bone morphogenic proteins (bone growing-proteins), so the graft provides only a calcium scaffolding for new bone to grow on (bone conduction). Osteopromotive materials induce bone growth and may be referred to as osteoinductive materials. These materials contain osteogenic proteins, which are natural growth factors that induce bone formation. One type called bone morphogenic proteins (BMP) causes mesenchymal cells to differentiate into chondroblasts and osteoblasts. BMP is combined with an absorbable collagen sponge and implanted into the bone defect to induce new bone growth. Other types include autogenous growth factor concentrate, bovine-derived osteoconductive protein, and recombinant human MP52. Use 20930 to report placement of a morcellized bone allograft consisting of donor bone that has been broken into small pieces (crushed), or the placement of osteopromotive material in the bone defect. Use 20931 to report the placement of a structural bone allograft, which is an intact piece of donor bone that has been configured or sculpted to fit into the bone defect.

Allograft for spinal surgery

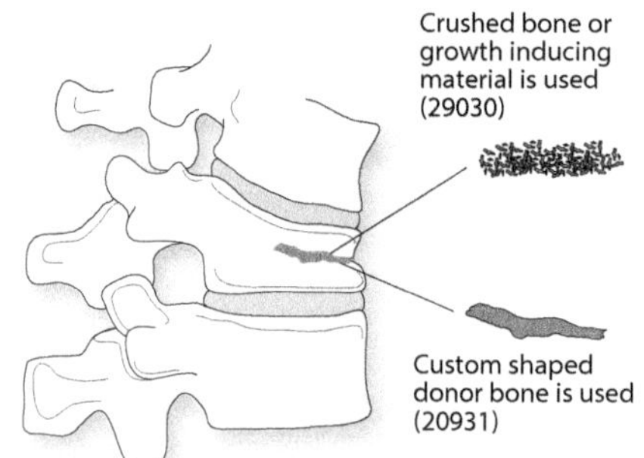

An allograft is used during a separately reportable surgery.

ICD-10-CM Diagnostic Codes

See Primary Procedure code for crosswalks.

CCI Edits

Refer to Appendix A for CCI edits.

Facility RVUs

Code	Work	PE Facility	MP	Total Facility
20930	0.00	0.00	0.00	0.00
20931	1.81	0.87	0.54	3.22

Non-facility RVUs

Code	Work	PE Non-Facility	MP	Total Non-Facility
20930	0.00	0.00	0.00	0.00
20931	1.81	0.87	0.54	3.22

Modifiers (PAR)

Code	Mod 50	Mod 51	Mod 62	Mod 66	Mod 80
20930	9	9	9	9	9
20931	0	0	1	0	1

Global Period

Code	Days
20930	XXX
20931	ZZZ

20936-20938

✚ **20936 Autograft for spine surgery only (includes harvesting the graft); local (eg, ribs, spinous process, or laminar fragments) obtained from same incision (List separately in addition to code for primary procedure)**

(Use 20936 in conjunction with 22319, 22532, 22533, 22548-22558, 22590-22612, 22630, 22633, 22634, 22800-22812)

✚ **20937 Autograft for spine surgery only (includes harvesting the graft); morselized (through separate skin or fascial incision) (List separately in addition to code for primary procedure)**

(Use 20937 in conjunction with 22319, 22532, 22533, 22548-22558, 22590-22612, 22630, 22633, 22634, 22800-22812)

✚ **20938 Autograft for spine surgery only (includes harvesting the graft); structural, bicortical or tricortical (through separate skin or fascial incision) (List separately in addition to code for primary procedure)**

(Use 20938 in conjunction with 22319, 22532, 22533, 22548-22558, 22590-22612, 22630, 22633, 22634, 22800-22812)

(For aspiration of bone marrow for bone grafting, spine surgery only, use 20939)

AMA Coding Guideline

General Grafts (or Implants) Procedures on the Musculoskeletal System

Codes for obtaining autogenous bone, cartilage, tendon, fascia lata grafts, bone marrow, or other tissues through separate skin/fascial incisions should be reported separately, unless the code descriptor references the harvesting of the graft or implant (eg, includes obtaining graft). Autologous grafts that are already defined in the CPT code set, including skin, bone, nerve, tendon, fascia lata, or vessels, should be reported with the more specific codes for each tissue type. Code 15769 may be used for other autologous soft tissue grafts harvested by direct excision. See 15771, 15772, 15773, 15774 for autologous fat grafting harvested by liposuction technique.

Do not append modifier 62 to bone graft codes 20900-20938.

Please see the Surgery Guidelines section for the following guidelines:

- *Surgical Procedures on the Musculoskeletal System*

AMA Coding Notes

General Grafts (or Implants) Procedures on the Musculoskeletal System

(For spinal surgery bone graft[s] see codes 20930-20938)

AMA *CPT Assistant* ▢

20936: Feb 96: 6, Sep 97: 8, Feb 02: 6, Feb 08: 8, Dec 11: 15, Apr 12: 14, Jun 12: 11, Jul 13: 3, Jul 18: 14

20937: Feb 96: 6, Sep 97: 8, Dec 99: 2, Feb 02: 6, Feb 08: 8, Dec 11: 15, Apr 12: 11, Jun 12: 11, Jul 13: 3, Jul 18: 14

20938: Feb 96: 6, Mar 96: 5, Sep 97: 8, Feb 02: 6, Feb 08: 8, Jul 11: 18, Dec 11: 15, Apr 12: 12, May 12: 11, Jun 12: 11, Jul 13: 3

Plain English Description

A bone autograft is placed during a separately reportable surgical procedure on the spine. An autologous bone graft is taken from the patient's own bone and can be harvested locally from the ribs, spinous process, or lamina through the same incision made for the spinal surgery (20936), or it can be harvested from a remote site, such as the iliac crest, through a separate incision. Autologous bone contains osteoblasts (bone-growing cells) and bone morphogenic proteins (bone-growing proteins) for new bone growth in addition to providing calcium scaffolding for new bone to grow on. In 20937, a morcellized bone graft is obtained through a separate incision, such as the iliac crest. An incision is made in the skin over the iliac crest and muscle is stripped to reveal the bone surface. The top portion of the iliac crest is excised and soft cancellous spongy bone is scooped out. The bone is crushed, or morcellized, and then packed into the bone defect in the spine and compressed to facilitate bone healing. Use 20938 for structural, bicortical, or tricortical bone graft obtained through a separate incision. Both cortical and cancellous bone is harvested, such as from the iliac crest, the bone is configured to fit into the bone defect, and then seated in the prepared space. The structural, bicortical, or tricortical bone graft may be secured using a screw or wire.

ICD-10-CM Diagnostic Codes

See Primary Procedure code for crosswalks.

CCI Edits

Refer to Appendix A for CCI edits.

Facility RVUs ▢

Code	Work	PE Facility	MP	Total Facility
20936	0.00	0.00	0.00	0.00
20937	2.79	1.36	0.70	4.85
20938	3.02	1.44	0.88	5.34

Non-facility RVUs ▢

Code	Work	PE Non-Facility	MP	Total Non-Facility
20936	0.00	0.00	0.00	0.00
20937	2.79	1.36	0.70	4.85
20938	3.02	1.44	0.88	5.34

Modifiers (PAR) ▢

Code	Mod 50	Mod 51	Mod 62	Mod 66	Mod 80
20936	9	9	9	9	9
20937	0	0	1	0	2
20938	0	0	1	0	2

Global Period

Code	Days
20936	XXX
20937	ZZZ
20938	ZZZ

20939

✚ **20939 Bone marrow aspiration for bone grafting, spine surgery only, through separate skin or fascial incision (List separately in addition to code for primary procedure)**

(Use 20939 in conjunction with 22319, 22532, 22533, 22534, 22548, 22551, 22552, 22554, 22556, 22558, 22590, 22595, 22600, 22610, 22612, 22630, 22633, 22634, 22800, 22802, 22804, 22808, 22810, 22812)

(For bilateral procedure, report 20939 twice. Do not report modifier 50 in conjunction with 20939)

(For aspiration of bone marrow for the purpose of bone grafting, other than spine surgery and other therapeutic musculoskeletal applications, use 20999)

(For bone marrow aspiration[s] for platelet-rich stem cell injection, use 0232T)

(For diagnostic bone marrow aspiration[s], see 38220, 38222)

AMA Coding Guideline

General Grafts (or Implants) Procedures on the Musculoskeletal System

Codes for obtaining autogenous bone, cartilage, tendon, fascia lata grafts, bone marrow, or other tissues through separate skin/fascial incisions should be reported separately, unless the code descriptor references the harvesting of the graft or implant (eg, includes obtaining graft). Autologous grafts that are already defined in the CPT code set, including skin, bone, nerve, tendon, fascia lata, or vessels, should be reported with the more specific codes for each tissue type. Code 15769 may be used for other autologous soft tissue grafts harvested by direct excision. See 15771, 15772, 15773, 15774 for autologous fat grafting harvested by liposuction technique.

Do not append modifier 62 to bone graft codes 20900-20938.

Please see the Surgery Guidelines section for the following guidelines:

- *Surgical Procedures on the Musculoskeletal System*

AMA Coding Notes

General Grafts (or Implants) Procedures on the Musculoskeletal System

(For spinal surgery bone graft[s] see codes 20930-20938)

AMA *CPT Assistant* ▢

20939: May 18: 3

Plain English Description

Bone marrow aspirate is used as a source of osteoprogenitor cells in spinal surgery to augment the site with autograft bone. Good technique ensures that the bone marrow is not diluted with peripheral blood. The anterior or posterior iliac crest is often used, although other sites such as the vertebral body are also used. This code is reported when bone marrow is aspirated through a separate skin or fascial incision in addition to the main procedure. Bone marrow cells are aspirated directly into syringes that are prepared with heparinized saline. For the anterior iliac crest, a small incision is made in the skin and the needle and cannula assembly are advanced about 4-5 cm behind the medial border, taking care to avoid the lateral femoral cutaneous nerve. For the posterior iliac crest, with the patient in the prone position, the needle and cannula is placed in the middle of the superficial cortex, carefully avoiding the cluneal nerves. Firm pressure is used to advance the needle up to 7 cm between the walls of the iliac crest, using an alternating clockwise/counterclockwise motion or taps with a mallet. With the cannula in place within cancellous bone, the needle is removed and the syringe is attached. The plunger is pulled back to aspirate the bone marrow. To remove additional bone marrow, the trocar needle is reattached and the assembly is pulled back and redirected, either through the same hole or by creating a new hole. The harvest site incision is closed.

Bone marrow aspiration for bone grafting, spine surgery only, through separate skin or fascial incision

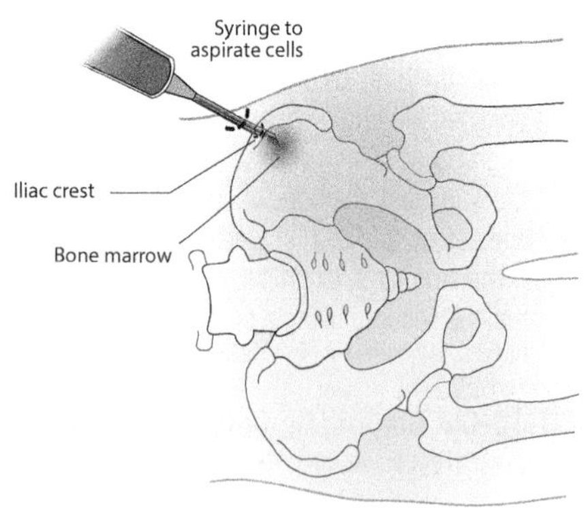

ICD-10-CM Diagnostic Codes

See Primary Procedure code for crosswalks.

CCI Edits

Refer to Appendix A for CCI edits.

Facility RVUs ▢

Code	Work	PE Facility	MP	Total Facility
20939	1.16	0.56	0.31	2.03

Non-facility RVUs ▢

Code	Work	PE Non-Facility	MP	Total Non-Facility
20939	1.16	0.56	0.31	2.03

Modifiers (PAR) ▢

Code	Mod 50	Mod 51	Mod 62	Mod 66	Mod 80
20939	1	0	0	0	0

Global Period

Code	Days
20939	ZZZ

22010-22015

22010 Incision and drainage, open, of deep abscess (subfascial), posterior spine; cervical, thoracic, or cervicothoracic

22015 Incision and drainage, open, of deep abscess (subfascial), posterior spine; lumbar, sacral, or lumbosacral

(Do not report 22015 in conjunction with 22010)

(Do not report 22015 in conjunction with instrumentation removal, 10180, 22850, 22852)

(For incision and drainage of abscess or hematoma, superficial, see 10060, 10140)

AMA Coding Guideline

Surgical Procedures on the Spine (Vertebral Column)

Cervical, thoracic, and lumbar spine.

Within the spine section, bone grafting procedures are reported separately and in addition to arthrodesis. For bone grafts in other Musculoskeletal sections, see specific code(s) descriptor(s) and/or accompanying guidelines.

To report bone grafts performed after arthrodesis, see 20930-20938. Do not append modifier 62 to bone graft codes 20900-20938.

Example:

Posterior arthrodesis of L5-S1 for degenerative disc disease utilizing morselized autogenous iliac bone graft harvested through a separate fascial incision.

Report as 22612 and 20937.

Within the spine section, instrumentation is reported separately and in addition to arthrodesis. To report instrumentation procedures performed with definitive vertebral procedure(s), see 22840-22855, 22859. Instrumentation procedure codes 22840-22848, 22853, 22854, 22859 are reported in addition to the definitive procedure(s). Modifier 62 may not be appended to the definitive or add-on spinal instrumentation procedure code(s) 22840-22848, 22850, 22852, 22853, 22854, 22859.

Example:

Posterior arthrodesis of L4-S1, utilizing morselized autogenous iliac bone graft harvested through separate fascial incision, and pedicle screw fixation.

Report as 22612, 22614, 22842, and 20937.

Vertebral procedures are sometimes followed by arthrodesis and in addition may include bone grafts and instrumentation.

When arthrodesis is performed in addition to another procedure, the arthrodesis should be reported in addition to the original procedure with modifier 51 (multiple procedures). Examples are after osteotomy, fracture care, vertebral corpectomy, and laminectomy. Bone grafts and instrumentation are never performed without arthrodesis.

Example:

Treatment of a burst fracture of L2 by corpectomy followed by arthrodesis of L1-L3, utilizing anterior instrumentation L1-L3 and structural allograft.

Report as 63090, 22558-51, 22585, 22845, and 20931.

When two surgeons work together as primary surgeons performing distinct part(s) of a single reportable procedure, each surgeon should report his/her distinct operative work by appending modifier 62 to the single definitive procedure code. If additional procedure(s) (including add-on procedure[s]) are performed during the same surgical session, separate code(s) may be reported by each co-surgeon, with modifier 62 appended (see Appendix A).

Example:

A 42-year-old male with a history of posttraumatic degenerative disc disease at L3-4 and L4-5 (internal disc disruption) underwent surgical repair. Surgeon A performed an anterior exposure of the spine with mobilization of the great vessels. Surgeon B performed anterior (minimal) discectomy and fusion at L3-4 and L4-5 using anterior interbody technique.

Report surgeon A: 22558 append modifier 62, 22585 append modifier 62

Report surgeon B: 22558 append modifier 62, 22585 append modifier 62, 20931

Please see the Surgery Guidelines section for the following guidelines:

- *Surgical Procedures on the Musculoskeletal System*

AMA Coding Notes

Surgical Procedures on the Spine (Vertebral Column)

(Do not append modifier 62 to bone graft code 20931)

(For injection procedure for myelography, use 62284)

(For injection procedure for discography, see 62290, 62291)

(For injection procedure, chemonucleolysis, single or multiple levels, use 62292)

(For injection procedure for facet joints, see 64490-64495, 64633-64636)

(For needle or trocar biopsy, see 20220-20225)

Plain English Description

An incision is made in the skin of the back over the abscess site. The incision is carried down through the soft tissue; the fascia is incised; and the abscess pocket is opened. Any loculations are broken up using blunt finger dissection. The abscess cavity is flushed with saline or antibiotic solution. Drains are placed as needed. The incision may be closed in layers or packed with gauze and left open. Use 22010 for incision and drainage of a deep, subfascial abscess in the cervical, thoracic, or cervicothoracic spine and 22015 for one located in the lumbar, sacral, or lumbosacral spine.

Incision and drainage of deep abscess of posterior spine

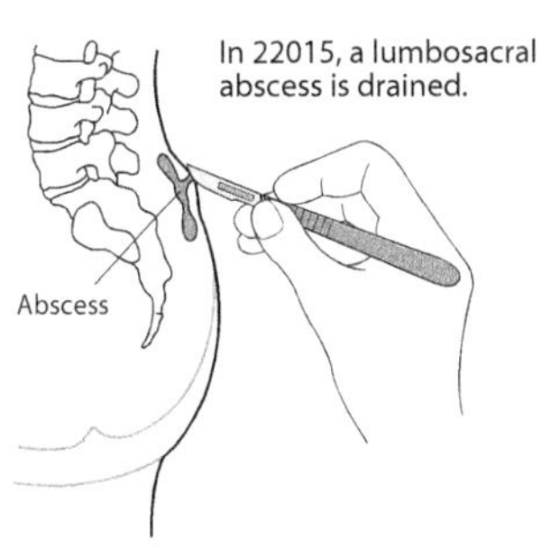

The physician makes an incision over the spine in the neck or the back to drain an abscess, or collection of pus, deep in the soft tissue. Report 22010 for drainage of a cervical, thoracic, or cervicothoracic abscess.

ICD-10-CM Diagnostic Codes

A18.01	Tuberculosis of spine
G06.1	Intraspinal abscess and granuloma
G07	Intracranial and intraspinal abscess and granuloma in diseases classified elsewhere
L02.212	Cutaneous abscess of back [any part, except buttock]
L03.221	Cellulitis of neck
L03.312	Cellulitis of back [any part except buttock]
M35.4	Diffuse (eosinophilic) fasciitis
M46.21	Osteomyelitis of vertebra, occipito-atlanto-axial region
M46.22	Osteomyelitis of vertebra, cervical region
M46.23	Osteomyelitis of vertebra, cervicothoracic region
M46.26	Osteomyelitis of vertebra, lumbar region
M46.27	Osteomyelitis of vertebra, lumbosacral region
M46.28	Osteomyelitis of vertebra, sacral and sacrococcygeal region
M46.31	Infection of intervertebral disc (pyogenic), occipito-atlanto-axial region
M46.32	Infection of intervertebral disc (pyogenic), cervical region
M46.33	Infection of intervertebral disc (pyogenic), cervicothoracic region
M46.34	Infection of intervertebral disc (pyogenic), thoracic region
M46.35	Infection of intervertebral disc (pyogenic), thoracolumbar region
M46.36	Infection of intervertebral disc (pyogenic), lumbar region
M46.37	Infection of intervertebral disc (pyogenic), lumbosacral region
M46.38	Infection of intervertebral disc (pyogenic), sacral and sacrococcygeal region
M46.39	Infection of intervertebral disc (pyogenic), multiple sites in spine
M72.6	Necrotizing fasciitis
M72.8	Other fibroblastic disorders

	M86.18	Other acute osteomyelitis, other site
	M86.28	Subacute osteomyelitis, other site
	M86.38	Chronic multifocal osteomyelitis, other site
	M86.48	Chronic osteomyelitis with draining sinus, other site
	M86.58	Other chronic hematogenous osteomyelitis, other site
❼	T81.42	Infection following a procedure, deep incisional surgical site
❼	T81.43	Infection following a procedure, organ and space surgical site

ICD-10-CM Coding Notes

For codes requiring a 7th character extension, refer to your ICD-10-CM book. Review the character descriptions and coding guidelines for proper selection. For some procedures, only certain characters will apply.

CCI Edits

Refer to Appendix A for CCI edits.

Facility RVUs ▯

Code	Work	PE Facility	MP	Total Facility
22010	12.75	11.39	3.58	27.72
22015	12.64	11.33	3.31	27.28

Non-facility RVUs ▯

Code	Work	PE Non-Facility	MP	Total Non-Facility
22010	12.75	11.39	3.58	27.72
22015	12.64	11.33	3.31	27.28

Modifiers (PAR) ▯

Code	Mod 50	Mod 51	Mod 62	Mod 66	Mod 80
22010	0	2	0	0	0
22015	0	2	0	0	1

Global Period

Code	Days
22010	090
22015	090

22206-22208

22206 Osteotomy of spine, posterior or posterolateral approach, 3 columns, 1 vertebral segment (eg, pedicle/vertebral body subtraction); thoracic

(Do not report 22206 in conjunction with 22207)

22207 Osteotomy of spine, posterior or posterolateral approach, 3 columns, 1 vertebral segment (eg, pedicle/vertebral body subtraction); lumbar

(Do not report 22207 in conjunction with 22206)

+ **22208 Osteotomy of spine, posterior or posterolateral approach, 3 columns, 1 vertebral segment (eg, pedicle/vertebral body subtraction); each additional vertebral segment (List separately in addition to code for primary procedure)**

(Use 22208 in conjunction with 22206, 22207)

(Do not report 22206, 22207, 22208 in conjunction with 22210-22226, 22830, 63001-63048, 63055-63066, 63075-63091, 63101-63103, when performed at the same level)

AMA Coding Guideline

Osteotomy Procedures on the Spine (Vertebral Column)

To report arthrodesis, see codes 22590-22632. (Report in addition to code[s] for the definitive procedure with modifier 51.)

To report instrumentation procedures, see 22840-22855, 22859. (Report in addition to code[s] for the definitive procedure[s].) Do not append modifier 62 to spinal instrumentation codes 22840-22848, 22850, 22852, 22853, 22854, 22859.

To report bone graft procedures, see 20930-20938. (Report in addition to code[s] for the definitive procedure[s].) Do not append modifier 62 to bone graft codes 20900-20938.

For the following codes, when two surgeons work together as primary surgeons performing distinct part(s) of an anterior spine osteotomy, each surgeon should report his/her distinct operative work by appending modifier 62 to the procedure code. In this situation, modifier 62 may be appended to the procedure code(s) 22210-22214, 22220-22224 and, as appropriate, to associated additional segment add-on code(s) 22216, 22226 as long as both surgeons continue to work together as primary surgeons.

Spinal osteotomy procedures are reported when a portion(s) of the vertebral segment(s) is cut and removed in preparation for re-aligning the spine as part of a spinal deformity correction. For excision of an intrinsic lesion of the vertebra without deformity correction, see 22100-22116. For decompression of the spinal cord and/or nerve roots, see 63001-63308.

The three columns are defined as anterior (anterior two-thirds of the vertebral body), middle (posterior third of the vertebral body and the pedicle), and posterior (articular facets, lamina, and spinous process).

Surgical Procedures on the Spine (Vertebral Column)

Cervical, thoracic, and lumbar spine.

Within the spine section, bone grafting procedures are reported separately and in addition to arthrodesis. For bone grafts in other Musculoskeletal sections, see specific code(s) descriptor(s) and/or accompanying guidelines.

To report bone grafts performed after arthrodesis, see 20930-20938. Do not append modifier 62 to bone graft codes 20900-20938.

Example:

Posterior arthrodesis of L5-S1 for degenerative disc disease utilizing morselized autogenous iliac bone graft harvested through a separate fascial incision.

Report as 22612 and 20937.

Within the spine section, instrumentation is reported separately and in addition to arthrodesis. To report instrumentation procedures performed with definitive vertebral procedure(s), see 22840-22855, 22859. Instrumentation procedure codes 22840-22848, 22853, 22854, 22859 are reported in addition to the definitive procedure(s). Modifier 62 may not be appended to the definitive or add-on spinal instrumentation procedure code(s) 22840-22848, 22850, 22852, 22853, 22854, 22859.

Example:

Posterior arthrodesis of L4-S1, utilizing morselized autogenous iliac bone graft harvested through separate fascial incision, and pedicle screw fixation.

Report as 22612, 22614, 22842, and 20937.

Vertebral procedures are sometimes followed by arthrodesis and in addition may include bone grafts and instrumentation.

When arthrodesis is performed in addition to another procedure, the arthrodesis should be reported in addition to the original procedure with modifier 51 (multiple procedures). Examples are after osteotomy, fracture care, vertebral corpectomy, and laminectomy. Bone grafts and instrumentation are never performed without arthrodesis.

Example:

Treatment of a burst fracture of L2 by corpectomy followed by arthrodesis of L1-L3, utilizing anterior instrumentation L1-L3 and structural allograft.

Report as 63090, 22558-51, 22585, 22845, and 20931.

When two surgeons work together as primary surgeons performing distinct part(s) of a single reportable procedure, each surgeon should report his/her distinct operative work by appending modifier 62 to the single definitive procedure code. If additional procedure(s) (including add-on procedure[s]) are performed during the same surgical session, separate code(s) may be reported by each co-surgeon, with modifier 62 appended (see Appendix A).

Example:

A 42-year-old male with a history of posttraumatic degenerative disc disease at L3-4 and L4-5 (internal disc disruption) underwent surgical repair. Surgeon A performed an anterior exposure of the spine with mobilization of the great vessels. Surgeon B performed anterior (minimal) discectomy and fusion at L3-4 and L4-5 using anterior interbody technique.

Report surgeon A: 22558 append modifier 62, 22585 append modifier 62

Report surgeon B: 22558 append modifier 62, 22585 append modifier 62, 20931

Please see the Surgery Guidelines section for the following guidelines:

- *Surgical Procedures on the Musculoskeletal System*

AMA Coding Notes

Surgical Procedures on the Spine (Vertebral Column)

(Do not append modifier 62 to bone graft code 20931)

(For injection procedure for myelography, use 62284)

(For injection procedure for discography, see 62290, 62291)

(For injection procedure, chemonucleolysis, single or multiple levels, use 62292)

(For injection procedure for facet joints, see 64490-64495, 64633-64636)

(For needle or trocar biopsy, see 20220-20225)

AMA *CPT Assistant* □

22206: Feb 08: 9, Jul 13: 3
22207: Feb 08: 9, Jul 13: 3
22208: Feb 08: 9

Plain English Description

A three-column osteotomy of the spine, also referred to as a pedicle subtraction osteotomy, is performed on a single thoracic segment using a posterior or posterolateral approach in 22206. The spine has three columns: anterior, middle, and posterior. The anterior column is composed of the vertebral body, the middle column is composed of two thick pedicles surrounding the vertebral foramen through which the spinal cord passes, and the posterior column is composed of the lamina, two transverse processes, and the spinous process. Thoracic and lumbar procedures for complex spinal deformities typically require osteotomy of all three columns. An incision is made in the skin of the back directly over the deformed vertebral segment or to the side of the vertebral segment requiring reconstruction. The fascia is incised. Subperiosteal dissection is performed along the spinal process, lamina, both transverse processes, and rib head of the vertebral segment. The posterior segment is resected, taking care to preserve the pedicles. This includes excision of the lamina (laminectomy), excision of the facets bilaterally (facetectomy), and resection of the ribs bilaterally. A cavity is created under the pedicles, which are resected. A wedge resection of the vertebral body is performed. A curette is used to thin the posterior vertebral wall until it is paper thin. The lateral portions of the vertebra are resected. A reverse angled curette is used to greenstick the posterior cortex of the vertebral body. The lateral vertebral body wall is resected at the level of the pedicles. The osteotomy is closed so that all columns are situated bone-on-bone. Correction of the deformity is evaluated by intraoperative imaging. Use 22207 for a three-column osteotomy of a lumbar segment and 22208 for three-column osteotomy of each additional vertebral segment.

ICD-10-CM Diagnostic Codes

M40.03	Postural kyphosis, cervicothoracic region
M40.04	Postural kyphosis, thoracic region
M40.05	Postural kyphosis, thoracolumbar region
M40.13	Other secondary kyphosis, cervicothoracic region
M40.14	Other secondary kyphosis, thoracic region
M40.15	Other secondary kyphosis, thoracolumbar region
M40.293	Other kyphosis, cervicothoracic region
M40.294	Other kyphosis, thoracic region
M40.295	Other kyphosis, thoracolumbar region
M40.35	Flatback syndrome, thoracolumbar region
M40.37	Flatback syndrome, lumbosacral region
M40.45	Postural lordosis, thoracolumbar region
M40.55	Lordosis, unspecified, thoracolumbar region
M41.03	Infantile idiopathic scoliosis, cervicothoracic region
M41.04	Infantile idiopathic scoliosis, thoracic region
M41.05	Infantile idiopathic scoliosis, thoracolumbar region
M41.113	Juvenile idiopathic scoliosis, cervicothoracic region
M41.114	Juvenile idiopathic scoliosis, thoracic region
M41.115	Juvenile idiopathic scoliosis, thoracolumbar region
M41.116	Juvenile idiopathic scoliosis, lumbar region
M41.117	Juvenile idiopathic scoliosis, lumbosacral region
M41.123	Adolescent idiopathic scoliosis, cervicothoracic region
M41.124	Adolescent idiopathic scoliosis, thoracic region
M41.125	Adolescent idiopathic scoliosis, thoracolumbar region
M41.23	Other idiopathic scoliosis, cervicothoracic region
M41.24	Other idiopathic scoliosis, thoracic region
M41.25	Other idiopathic scoliosis, thoracolumbar region
M41.34	Thoracogenic scoliosis, thoracic region
M41.35	Thoracogenic scoliosis, thoracolumbar region
M41.43	Neuromuscular scoliosis, cervicothoracic region
M41.44	Neuromuscular scoliosis, thoracic region
M41.45	Neuromuscular scoliosis, thoracolumbar region
M41.53	Other secondary scoliosis, cervicothoracic region
M41.54	Other secondary scoliosis, thoracic region
M41.55	Other secondary scoliosis, thoracolumbar region
M41.83	Other forms of scoliosis, cervicothoracic region
M41.84	Other forms of scoliosis, thoracic region
M41.85	Other forms of scoliosis, thoracolumbar region
M42.03	Juvenile osteochondrosis of spine, cervicothoracic region
M42.04	Juvenile osteochondrosis of spine, thoracic region
M42.05	Juvenile osteochondrosis of spine, thoracolumbar region
M45.3	Ankylosing spondylitis of cervicothoracic region
M45.4	Ankylosing spondylitis of thoracic region
M45.5	Ankylosing spondylitis of thoracolumbar region
M88.1	Osteitis deformans of vertebrae
M96.2	Postradiation kyphosis
M96.3	Postlaminectomy kyphosis
Q76.2	Congenital spondylolisthesis
Q76.413	Congenital kyphosis, cervicothoracic region
Q76.414	Congenital kyphosis, thoracic region
Q76.415	Congenital kyphosis, thoracolumbar region
Q76.425	Congenital lordosis, thoracolumbar region
Q76.49	Other congenital malformations of spine, not associated with scoliosis

CCI Edits

Refer to Appendix A for CCI edits.

Facility RVUs ▯

Code	Work	PE Facility	MP	Total Facility
22206	37.18	23.32	10.50	71.00
22207	36.68	23.08	9.70	69.46
22208	9.66	4.62	2.85	17.13

Non-facility RVUs ▯

Code	Work	PE Non-Facility	MP	Total Non-Facility
22206	37.18	23.32	10.50	71.00
22207	36.68	23.08	9.70	69.46
22208	9.66	4.62	2.85	17.13

Modifiers (PAR) ▯

Code	Mod 50	Mod 51	Mod 62	Mod 66	Mod 80
22206	0	2	1	0	2
22207	0	2	1	0	2
22208	0	0	1	0	2

Global Period

Code	Days
22206	090
22207	090
22208	ZZZ

22210-22216

22210 Osteotomy of spine, posterior or posterolateral approach, 1 vertebral segment; cervical

22212 Osteotomy of spine, posterior or posterolateral approach, 1 vertebral segment; thoracic

22214 Osteotomy of spine, posterior or posterolateral approach, 1 vertebral segment; lumbar

+ **22216 Osteotomy of spine, posterior or posterolateral approach, 1 vertebral segment; each additional vertebral segment (List separately in addition to primary procedure)**

(Use 22216 in conjunction with 22210, 22212, 22214)

AMA Coding Guideline

Osteotomy Procedures on the Spine (Vertebral Column)

To report arthrodesis, see codes 22590-22632. (Report in addition to code[s] for the definitive procedure with modifier 51.)

To report instrumentation procedures, see 22840-22855, 22859. (Report in addition to code[s] for the definitive procedure[s].) Do not append modifier 62 to spinal instrumentation codes 22840-22848, 22850, 22852, 22853, 22854, 22859.

To report bone graft procedures, see 20930-20938. (Report in addition to code[s] for the definitive procedure[s].) Do not append modifier 62 to bone graft codes 20900-20938.

For the following codes, when two surgeons work together as primary surgeons performing distinct part(s) of an anterior spine osteotomy, each surgeon should report his/her distinct operative work by appending modifier 62 to the procedure code. In this situation, modifier 62 may be appended to the procedure code(s) 22210-22214, 22220-22224 and, as appropriate, to associated additional segment add-on code(s) 22216, 22226 as long as both surgeons continue to work together as primary surgeons.

Spinal osteotomy procedures are reported when a portion(s) of the vertebral segment(s) is cut and removed in preparation for re-aligning the spine as part of a spinal deformity correction. For excision of an intrinsic lesion of the vertebra without deformity correction, see 22100-22116. For decompression of the spinal cord and/or nerve roots, see 63001-63308.

The three columns are defined as anterior (anterior two-thirds of the vertebral body), middle (posterior third of the vertebral body and the pedicle), and posterior (articular facets, lamina, and spinous process).

Surgical Procedures on the Spine (Vertebral Column)

Cervical, thoracic, and lumbar spine.

Within the spine section, bone grafting procedures are reported separately and in addition to arthrodesis. For bone grafts in other Musculoskeletal sections, see specific code(s) descriptor(s) and/or accompanying guidelines.

To report bone grafts performed after arthrodesis, see 20930-20938. Do not append modifier 62 to bone graft codes 20900-20938.

Example:

Posterior arthrodesis of L5-S1 for degenerative disc disease utilizing morselized autogenous iliac bone graft harvested through a separate fascial incision.

Report as 22612 and 20937.

Within the spine section, instrumentation is reported separately and in addition to arthrodesis. To report instrumentation procedures performed with definitive vertebral procedure(s), see 22840-22855, 22859. Instrumentation procedure codes 22840-22848, 22853, 22854, 22859 are reported in addition to the definitive procedure(s). Modifier 62 may not be appended to the definitive or add-on spinal instrumentation procedure code(s) 22840-22848, 22850, 22852, 22853, 22854, 22859.

Example:

Posterior arthrodesis of L4-S1, utilizing morselized autogenous iliac bone graft harvested through separate fascial incision, and pedicle screw fixation.

Report as 22612, 22614, 22842, and 20937.

Vertebral procedures are sometimes followed by arthrodesis and in addition may include bone grafts and instrumentation.

When arthrodesis is performed in addition to another procedure, the arthrodesis should be reported in addition to the original procedure with modifier 51 (multiple procedures). Examples are after osteotomy, fracture care, vertebral corpectomy, and laminectomy. Bone grafts and instrumentation are never performed without arthrodesis.

Example:

Treatment of a burst fracture of L2 by corpectomy followed by arthrodesis of L1-L3, utilizing anterior instrumentation L1-L3 and structural allograft.

Report as 63090, 22558-51, 22585, 22845, and 20931.

When two surgeons work together as primary surgeons performing distinct part(s) of a single reportable procedure, each surgeon should report his/her distinct operative work by appending modifier 62 to the single definitive procedure code. If additional procedure(s) (including add-on procedure[s]) are performed during the same surgical session, separate code(s) may be reported by each co-surgeon, with modifier 62 appended (see Appendix A).

Example:

A 42-year-old male with a history of posttraumatic degenerative disc disease at L3-4 and L4-5 (internal disc disruption) underwent surgical repair. Surgeon A performed an anterior exposure of the spine with mobilization of the great vessels. Surgeon B performed anterior (minimal) discectomy and fusion at L3-4 and L4-5 using anterior interbody technique.

Report surgeon A: 22558 append modifier 62, 22585 append modifier 62

Report surgeon B: 22558 append modifier 62, 22585 append modifier 62, 20931

Please see the Surgery Guidelines section for the following guidelines:

- *Surgical Procedures on the Musculoskeletal System*

AMA Coding Notes

Surgical Procedures on the Spine (Vertebral Column)

(Do not append modifier 62 to bone graft code 20931)

(For injection procedure for myelography, use 62284)

(For injection procedure for discography, see 62290, 62291)

(For injection procedure, chemonucleolysis, single or multiple levels, use 62292)

(For injection procedure for facet joints, see 64490-64495, 64633-64636)

(For needle or trocar biopsy, see 20220-20225)

AMA *CPT Assistant*

22210: Jul 13: 3

22212: Dec 07: 1, Jul 13: 3

22214: Dec 07: 1, Jul 13: 3, Dec 14: 16

22216: Dec 07: 1

Plain English Description

A spinal osteotomy involves removing part of the vertebra to correct a deformity, such as a flexion deformity. Excising a portion of the vertebra allows the vertebral segment to be realigned to improve function and stability of the spine and relieve pain. Using a posterior or posterolateral approach, an incision is made directly over the affected vertebral segment(s) or just lateral to the vertebra. The fascia is incised. Subperiosteal dissection is performed along the spinal process, lamina, both transverse processes, and rib head of the vertebral segment as needed. A wedge of bone is resected, which may include portions of the supraspinatus and infraspinatus ligaments and spinous processes. The patient is carefully repositioned as manual pressure is applied at the osteotomy site until the opposing ligaments tear. This is accomplished while keeping nerve roots and other vital structures under direct visualization to ensure that no impingement of these structures occurs as the vertebra is manipulated and the bony gap closed. Once the bony gap created by the wedge resection has been closed, separately reportable bone grafts and/or spinal instrumentation may be utilized to stabilize the spine. A body cast or jacket is applied as needed to immobilize the spine. Use 22210 for osteotomy of one cervical vertebral segment, 22212 for one thoracic segment, 22214 for one lumbar segment, and 22216 for each additional vertebral segment after the first.

ICD-10-CM Diagnostic Codes

G12.25	Progressive spinal muscle atrophy
M40.12	Other secondary kyphosis, cervical region
M40.13	Other secondary kyphosis, cervicothoracic region
M40.14	Other secondary kyphosis, thoracic region
M40.15	Other secondary kyphosis, thoracolumbar region
M40.292	Other kyphosis, cervical region
M40.293	Other kyphosis, cervicothoracic region
M40.294	Other kyphosis, thoracic region
M40.295	Other kyphosis, thoracolumbar region
M41.02	Infantile idiopathic scoliosis, cervical region
M41.03	Infantile idiopathic scoliosis, cervicothoracic region
M41.04	Infantile idiopathic scoliosis, thoracic region
M41.05	Infantile idiopathic scoliosis, thoracolumbar region
M41.112	Juvenile idiopathic scoliosis, cervical region
M41.113	Juvenile idiopathic scoliosis, cervicothoracic region
M41.114	Juvenile idiopathic scoliosis, thoracic region
M41.115	Juvenile idiopathic scoliosis, thoracolumbar region
M41.116	Juvenile idiopathic scoliosis, lumbar region
M41.117	Juvenile idiopathic scoliosis, lumbosacral region
M41.122	Adolescent idiopathic scoliosis, cervical region
M41.123	Adolescent idiopathic scoliosis, cervicothoracic region
M41.124	Adolescent idiopathic scoliosis, thoracic region
M41.125	Adolescent idiopathic scoliosis, thoracolumbar region
M41.126	Adolescent idiopathic scoliosis, lumbar region
M41.127	Adolescent idiopathic scoliosis, lumbosacral region
M41.22	Other idiopathic scoliosis, cervical region
M41.23	Other idiopathic scoliosis, cervicothoracic region
M41.24	Other idiopathic scoliosis, thoracic region
M41.25	Other idiopathic scoliosis, thoracolumbar region
M41.26	Other idiopathic scoliosis, lumbar region
M41.27	Other idiopathic scoliosis, lumbosacral region
M41.41	Neuromuscular scoliosis, occipito-atlanto-axial region
M41.42	Neuromuscular scoliosis, cervical region
M41.43	Neuromuscular scoliosis, cervicothoracic region
M41.44	Neuromuscular scoliosis, thoracic region
M41.45	Neuromuscular scoliosis, thoracolumbar region
M41.46	Neuromuscular scoliosis, lumbar region
M41.47	Neuromuscular scoliosis, lumbosacral region
M41.52	Other secondary scoliosis, cervical region
M41.53	Other secondary scoliosis, cervicothoracic region
M41.54	Other secondary scoliosis, thoracic region
M41.55	Other secondary scoliosis, thoracolumbar region
M41.56	Other secondary scoliosis, lumbar region
M41.57	Other secondary scoliosis, lumbosacral region
M41.82	Other forms of scoliosis, cervical region
M41.83	Other forms of scoliosis, cervicothoracic region
M41.84	Other forms of scoliosis, thoracic region
M41.85	Other forms of scoliosis, thoracolumbar region
M41.86	Other forms of scoliosis, lumbar region
M41.87	Other forms of scoliosis, lumbosacral region
M42.02	Juvenile osteochondrosis of spine, cervical region
M42.03	Juvenile osteochondrosis of spine, cervicothoracic region
M42.04	Juvenile osteochondrosis of spine, thoracic region
M42.05	Juvenile osteochondrosis of spine, thoracolumbar region
M42.06	Juvenile osteochondrosis of spine, lumbar region
M42.07	Juvenile osteochondrosis of spine, lumbosacral region
M45.2	Ankylosing spondylitis of cervical region
M45.3	Ankylosing spondylitis of cervicothoracic region
M45.4	Ankylosing spondylitis of thoracic region
M45.5	Ankylosing spondylitis of thoracolumbar region
M45.6	Ankylosing spondylitis lumbar region
M45.7	Ankylosing spondylitis of lumbosacral region
M48.02	Spinal stenosis, cervical region
M48.03	Spinal stenosis, cervicothoracic region
M48.04	Spinal stenosis, thoracic region
M48.05	Spinal stenosis, thoracolumbar region
M48.06	Spinal stenosis, lumbar region
M48.07	Spinal stenosis, lumbosacral region
M50.021	Cervical disc disorder at C4-C5 level with myelopathy
M50.022	Cervical disc disorder at C5-C6 level with myelopathy
M50.023	Cervical disc disorder at C6-C7 level with myelopathy
M50.03	Cervical disc disorder with myelopathy, cervicothoracic region
M53.2X2	Spinal instabilities, cervical region
M53.2X3	Spinal instabilities, cervicothoracic region
M53.2X4	Spinal instabilities, thoracic region
M53.2X5	Spinal instabilities, thoracolumbar region
M53.2X6	Spinal instabilities, lumbar region
M53.2X7	Spinal instabilities, lumbosacral region
M88.1	Osteitis deformans of vertebrae
M96.1	Postlaminectomy syndrome, not elsewhere classified
M96.2	Postradiation kyphosis
M96.3	Postlaminectomy kyphosis
Q76.2	Congenital spondylolisthesis
Q76.412	Congenital kyphosis, cervical region
Q76.413	Congenital kyphosis, cervicothoracic region
Q76.49	Other congenital malformations of spine, not associated with scoliosis

CCI Edits

Refer to Appendix A for CCI edits.

Facility RVUs

Code	Work	PE Facility	MP	Total Facility
22210	25.38	18.96	7.41	51.75
22212	20.99	16.72	5.54	43.25
22214	21.02	16.75	5.65	43.42
22216	6.03	2.92	1.61	10.56

Non-facility RVUs

Code	Work	PE Non-Facility	MP	Total Non-Facility
22210	25.38	18.96	7.41	51.75
22212	20.99	16.72	5.54	43.25
22214	21.02	16.75	5.65	43.42
22216	6.03	2.92	1.61	10.56

Modifiers (PAR)

Code	Mod 50	Mod 51	Mod 62	Mod 66	Mod 80
22210	0	2	1	0	2
22212	0	2	1	0	2
22214	0	2	1	0	2
22216	0	0	1	0	2

Global Period

Code	Days
22210	090
22212	090
22214	090
22216	ZZZ

22220-22226

22220 Osteotomy of spine, including discectomy, anterior approach, single vertebral segment; cervical

22222 Osteotomy of spine, including discectomy, anterior approach, single vertebral segment; thoracic

22224 Osteotomy of spine, including discectomy, anterior approach, single vertebral segment; lumbar

+ **22226 Osteotomy of spine, including discectomy, anterior approach, single vertebral segment; each additional vertebral segment (List separately in addition to code for primary procedure)**

(Use 22226 in conjunction with 22220, 22222, 22224)

(For vertebral corpectomy, see 63081-63091)

AMA Coding Guideline

Osteotomy Procedures on the Spine (Vertebral Column)

To report arthrodesis, see codes 22590-22632. (Report in addition to code[s] for the definitive procedure with modifier 51.)

To report instrumentation procedures, see 22840-22855, 22859. (Report in addition to code[s] for the definitive procedure[s].) Do not append modifier 62 to spinal instrumentation codes 22840-22848, 22850, 22852, 22853, 22854, 22859.

To report bone graft procedures, see 20930-20938. (Report in addition to code[s] for the definitive procedure[s].) Do not append modifier 62 to bone graft codes 20900-20938.

For the following codes, when two surgeons work together as primary surgeons performing distinct part(s) of an anterior spine osteotomy, each surgeon should report his/her distinct operative work by appending modifier 62 to the procedure code. In this situation, modifier 62 may be appended to the procedure code(s) 22210-22214, 22220-22224 and, as appropriate, to associated additional segment add-on code(s) 22216, 22226 as long as both surgeons continue to work together as primary surgeons.

Spinal osteotomy procedures are reported when a portion(s) of the vertebral segment(s) is cut and removed in preparation for re-aligning the spine as part of a spinal deformity correction. For excision of an intrinsic lesion of the vertebra without deformity correction, see 22100-22116. For decompression of the spinal cord and/or nerve roots, see 63001-63308.

The three columns are defined as anterior (anterior two-thirds of the vertebral body), middle (posterior third of the vertebral body and the pedicle), and posterior (articular facets, lamina, and spinous process).

Surgical Procedures on the Spine (Vertebral Column)

Cervical, thoracic, and lumbar spine.

Within the spine section, bone grafting procedures are reported separately and in addition to arthrodesis. For bone grafts in other Musculoskeletal sections, see specific code(s) descriptor(s) and/or accompanying guidelines.

To report bone grafts performed after arthrodesis, see 20930-20938. Do not append modifier 62 to bone graft codes 20900-20938.

Example:

Posterior arthrodesis of L5-S1 for degenerative disc disease utilizing morselized autogenous iliac bone graft harvested through a separate fascial incision.

Report as 22612 and 20937.

Within the spine section, instrumentation is reported separately and in addition to arthrodesis. To report instrumentation procedures performed with definitive vertebral procedure(s), see 22840-22855, 22859. Instrumentation procedure codes 22840-22848, 22853, 22854, 22859 are reported in addition to the definitive procedure(s). Modifier 62 may not be appended to the definitive or add-on spinal instrumentation procedure code(s) 22840-22848, 22850, 22852, 22853, 22854, 22859.

Example:

Posterior arthrodesis of L4-S1, utilizing morselized autogenous iliac bone graft harvested through separate fascial incision, and pedicle screw fixation.

Report as 22612, 22614, 22842, and 20937.

Vertebral procedures are sometimes followed by arthrodesis and in addition may include bone grafts and instrumentation.

When arthrodesis is performed in addition to another procedure, the arthrodesis should be reported in addition to the original procedure with modifier 51 (multiple procedures). Examples are after osteotomy, fracture care, vertebral corpectomy, and laminectomy. Bone grafts and instrumentation are never performed without arthrodesis.

Example:

Treatment of a burst fracture of L2 by corpectomy followed by arthrodesis of L1-L3, utilizing anterior instrumentation L1-L3 and structural allograft.

Report as 63090, 22558-51, 22585, 22845, and 20931.

When two surgeons work together as primary surgeons performing distinct part(s) of a single reportable procedure, each surgeon should report his/her distinct operative work by appending modifier 62 to the single definitive procedure code. If additional procedure(s) (including add-on procedure[s]) are performed during the same surgical session, separate code(s) may be reported by each co-surgeon, with modifier 62 appended (see Appendix A).

Example:

A 42-year-old male with a history of posttraumatic degenerative disc disease at L3-4 and L4-5 (internal disc disruption) underwent surgical repair. Surgeon A performed an anterior exposure of the spine with mobilization of the great vessels. Surgeon B performed anterior (minimal) discectomy and fusion at L3-4 and L4-5 using anterior interbody technique.

Report surgeon A: 22558 append modifier 62, 22585 append modifier 62

Report surgeon B: 22558 append modifier 62, 22585 append modifier 62, 20931

Please see the Surgery Guidelines section for the following guidelines:

- *Surgical Procedures on the Musculoskeletal System*

AMA Coding Notes

Surgical Procedures on the Spine (Vertebral Column)

(Do not append modifier 62 to bone graft code 20931)

(For injection procedure for myelography, use 62284)

(For injection procedure for discography, see 62290, 62291)

(For injection procedure, chemonucleolysis, single or multiple levels, use 62292)

(For injection procedure for facet joints, see 64490-64495, 64633-64636)

(For needle or trocar biopsy, see 20220-20225)

AMA *CPT Assistant*

22220: Feb 02: 4, Jul 13: 3
22222: Feb 02: 4
22224: Feb 02: 4, Jul 13: 3
22226: Feb 96: 6, Feb 02: 4

Plain English Description

A spinal osteotomy involves removing part of the vertebra to correct a deformity, such as a flexion deformity. Excising a portion of the vertebra allows the vertebral segment to be realigned to improve function and stability of the spine and relieve pain. Depending on the level and extent of the deformity, an anterior neck, thoracic, thoracoabdominal, abdominal, retropleural, or retroperitoneal incision is made. Soft tissues are dissected and the vertebrae are exposed. Subperiosteal dissection is performed along the vertebral segment as needed. Depending on the approach, a portion of the lamina may be removed to access the intervertebral disc. A curette is used to remove the intervertebral disc or disc fragments. A wedge of bone from the vertebral body is resected, which may include portions of the surrounding ligaments and spinous processes. The patient is carefully repositioned as manual pressure is applied at the osteotomy site until the opposing ligaments tear. This is accomplished while keeping nerve roots and other vital structures under direct visualization to ensure that no impingement of these structures occurs as the vertebra is manipulated and the bony gap closed. Once the bony gap created by the wedge resection has been closed, separately reportable bone grafts and/or spinal instrumentation may be utilized to stabilize the spine. A body cast or jacket is applied as needed to immobilize the spine. Use 22220 for osteotomy of one cervical vertebral segment, 22222 for one thoracic segment, 22224 for one lumbar segment, and 22226 for each additional vertebral segment after the first.

Osteotomy of spine

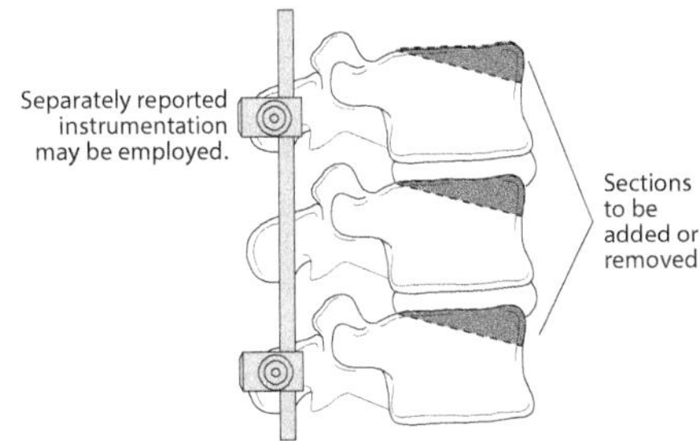

Code 22220 for a cervical osteotomy; 22222 for a thoracic osteotomy; 22224 for a lumbar osteotomy; and 22226 for each additional vertebra removed after the first. Any bone grafts should be reported separately.

ICD-10-CM Diagnostic Codes

E64.3	Sequelae of rickets
M40.03	Postural kyphosis, cervicothoracic region
M40.04	Postural kyphosis, thoracic region
M40.05	Postural kyphosis, thoracolumbar region
M40.12	Other secondary kyphosis, cervical region
M40.13	Other secondary kyphosis, cervicothoracic region
M40.14	Other secondary kyphosis, thoracic region
M40.15	Other secondary kyphosis, thoracolumbar region
M40.292	Other kyphosis, cervical region
M40.293	Other kyphosis, cervicothoracic region
M40.294	Other kyphosis, thoracic region
M40.295	Other kyphosis, thoracolumbar region
M40.35	Flatback syndrome, thoracolumbar region
M40.36	Flatback syndrome, lumbar region
M40.37	Flatback syndrome, lumbosacral region
M41.22	Other idiopathic scoliosis, cervical region
M41.23	Other idiopathic scoliosis, cervicothoracic region
M41.24	Other idiopathic scoliosis, thoracic region
M41.25	Other idiopathic scoliosis, thoracolumbar region
M41.26	Other idiopathic scoliosis, lumbar region
M41.82	Other forms of scoliosis, cervical region
M41.83	Other forms of scoliosis, cervicothoracic region
M41.84	Other forms of scoliosis, thoracic region
M41.85	Other forms of scoliosis, thoracolumbar region
M41.86	Other forms of scoliosis, lumbar region
M42.02	Juvenile osteochondrosis of spine, cervical region
M42.03	Juvenile osteochondrosis of spine, cervicothoracic region
M42.04	Juvenile osteochondrosis of spine, thoracic region
M42.05	Juvenile osteochondrosis of spine, thoracolumbar region
M42.06	Juvenile osteochondrosis of spine, lumbar region
M42.07	Juvenile osteochondrosis of spine, lumbosacral region
M45.2	Ankylosing spondylitis of cervical region
M45.3	Ankylosing spondylitis of cervicothoracic region
M45.4	Ankylosing spondylitis of thoracic region
M45.5	Ankylosing spondylitis of thoracolumbar region
M45.6	Ankylosing spondylitis lumbar region
M45.7	Ankylosing spondylitis of lumbosacral region
M47.14	Other spondylosis with myelopathy, thoracic region
M47.16	Other spondylosis with myelopathy, lumbar region
M48.04	Spinal stenosis, thoracic region
M48.33	Traumatic spondylopathy, cervicothoracic region
M48.34	Traumatic spondylopathy, thoracic region
M48.35	Traumatic spondylopathy, thoracolumbar region
M48.36	Traumatic spondylopathy, lumbar region
M48.37	Traumatic spondylopathy, lumbosacral region
M49.82	Spondylopathy in diseases classified elsewhere, cervical region
M49.83	Spondylopathy in diseases classified elsewhere, cervicothoracic region
M49.84	Spondylopathy in diseases classified elsewhere, thoracic region
M49.85	Spondylopathy in diseases classified elsewhere, thoracolumbar region
M49.86	Spondylopathy in diseases classified elsewhere, lumbar region
M49.87	Spondylopathy in diseases classified elsewhere, lumbosacral region
M51.04	Intervertebral disc disorders with myelopathy, thoracic region
M51.06	Intervertebral disc disorders with myelopathy, lumbar region
M51.34	Other intervertebral disc degeneration, thoracic region
M51.36	Other intervertebral disc degeneration, lumbar region
M51.44	Schmorl's nodes, thoracic region
M51.46	Schmorl's nodes, lumbar region
M88.1	Osteitis deformans of vertebrae
M96.1	Postlaminectomy syndrome, not elsewhere classified
M96.2	Postradiation kyphosis
M96.3	Postlaminectomy kyphosis
Q76.2	Congenital spondylolisthesis
Q76.412	Congenital kyphosis, cervical region
Q76.413	Congenital kyphosis, cervicothoracic region
Q76.414	Congenital kyphosis, thoracic region
Q76.415	Congenital kyphosis, thoracolumbar region

CCI Edits

Refer to Appendix A for CCI edits.

Facility RVUs ☐

Code	Work	PE Facility	MP	Total Facility
22220	22.94	17.54	6.87	47.35
22222	23.09	18.65	8.52	50.26
22224	23.09	17.38	5.63	46.10
22226	6.03	2.90	1.63	10.56

Non-facility RVUs ☐

Code	Work	PE Non-Facility	MP	Total Non-Facility
22220	22.94	17.54	6.87	47.35
22222	23.09	18.65	8.52	50.26
22224	23.09	17.38	5.63	46.10
22226	6.03	2.90	1.63	10.56

Modifiers (PAR) ☐

Code	Mod 50	Mod 51	Mod 62	Mod 66	Mod 80
22220	0	2	1	0	2
22222	0	2	1	0	2
22224	0	2	1	0	2
22226	0	0	1	0	2

Global Period

Code	Days
22220	090
22222	090
22224	090
22226	ZZZ

22310-22315

22310 Closed treatment of vertebral body fracture(s), without manipulation, requiring and including casting or bracing

(Do not report 22310 in conjunction with 22510, 22511, 22512, 22513, 22514, 22515, when performed at the same level)

22315 Closed treatment of vertebral fracture(s) and/or dislocation(s) requiring casting or bracing, with and including casting and/or bracing by manipulation or traction

(Do not report 22315 in conjunction with 22510, 22511, 22512, 22513, 22514, 22515, when performed at the same level)

(For spinal subluxation, use 97140)

AMA Coding Guideline

Fracture and/or Dislocation Procedures on the Spine (Vertebral Column)

To report arthrodesis, see codes 22590-22632. (Report in addition to code[s] for the definitive procedure with modifier 51.)

To report instrumentation procedures, see 22840-22855, 22859. (Report in addition to code[s] for the definitive procedure[s].) Do not append modifier 62 to spinal instrumentation codes 22840-22848, 22850, 22852, 22853, 22854, 22859.

To report bone graft procedures, see 20930-20938. (Report in addition to code[s] for the definitive procedure[s].) Do not append modifier 62 to bone graft codes 20900-20938.

For the following codes, when two surgeons work together as primary surgeons performing distinct part(s) of open fracture and/or dislocation procedure(s), each surgeon should report his/her distinct operative work by appending modifier 62 to the procedure code. In this situation, modifier 62 may be appended to the procedure code(s) 22318-22327 and, as appropriate, the associated additional fracture vertebrae or dislocated segment add-on code 22328 as long as both surgeons continue to work together as primary surgeons.

Surgical Procedures on the Spine (Vertebral Column)

Cervical, thoracic, and lumbar spine.

Within the spine section, bone grafting procedures are reported separately and in addition to arthrodesis. For bone grafts in other Musculoskeletal sections, see specific code(s) descriptor(s) and/or accompanying guidelines.

To report bone grafts performed after arthrodesis, see 20930-20938. Do not append modifier 62 to bone graft codes 20900-20938.

Example:

Posterior arthrodesis of L5-S1 for degenerative disc disease utilizing morselized autogenous iliac bone graft harvested through a separate fascial incision.

Report as 22612 and 20937.

Within the spine section, instrumentation is reported separately and in addition to arthrodesis. To report instrumentation procedures performed with definitive vertebral procedure(s), see 22840-22855, 22859. Instrumentation procedure codes 22840-22848, 22853, 22854, 22859 are reported in addition to the definitive procedure(s). Modifier 62 may not be appended to the definitive or add-on spinal instrumentation procedure code(s) 22840-22848, 22850, 22852, 22853, 22854, 22859.

Example:

Posterior arthrodesis of L4-S1, utilizing morselized autogenous iliac bone graft harvested through separate fascial incision, and pedicle screw fixation.

Report as 22612, 22614, 22842, and 20937.

Vertebral procedures are sometimes followed by arthrodesis and in addition may include bone grafts and instrumentation.

When arthrodesis is performed in addition to another procedure, the arthrodesis should be reported in addition to the original procedure with modifier 51 (multiple procedures). Examples are after osteotomy, fracture care, vertebral corpectomy, and laminectomy. Bone grafts and instrumentation are never performed without arthrodesis.

Example:

Treatment of a burst fracture of L2 by corpectomy followed by arthrodesis of L1-L3, utilizing anterior instrumentation L1-L3 and structural allograft.

Report as 63090, 22558-51, 22585, 22845, and 20931.

When two surgeons work together as primary surgeons performing distinct part(s) of a single reportable procedure, each surgeon should report his/her distinct operative work by appending modifier 62 to the single definitive procedure code. If additional procedure(s) (including add-on procedure[s]) are performed during the same surgical session, separate code(s) may be reported by each co-surgeon, with modifier 62 appended (see Appendix A).

Example:

A 42-year-old male with a history of posttraumatic degenerative disc disease at L3-4 and L4-5 (internal disc disruption) underwent surgical repair. Surgeon A performed an anterior exposure of the spine with mobilization of the great vessels. Surgeon B performed anterior (minimal) discectomy and fusion at L3-4 and L4-5 using anterior interbody technique.

Report surgeon A: 22558 append modifier 62, 22585 append modifier 62

Report surgeon B: 22558 append modifier 62, 22585 append modifier 62, 20931

Please see the Surgery Guidelines section for the following guidelines:

- *Surgical Procedures on the Musculoskeletal System*

AMA Coding Notes

Surgical Procedures on the Spine (Vertebral Column)

(Do not append modifier 62 to bone graft code 20931)

(For injection procedure for myelography, use 62284)

(For injection procedure for discography, see 62290, 62291)

(For injection procedure, chemonucleolysis, single or multiple levels, use 62292)

(For injection procedure for facet joints, see 64490-64495, 64633-64636)

(For needle or trocar biopsy, see 20220-20225)

AMA *CPT Assistant*

22310: Jun 12: 10, Jul 13: 3, Jul 14: 8
22315: Apr 12: 11, Jun 12: 10, Jul 13: 3

Plain English Description

Closed treatment of one or more vertebral body fractures is performed with casting or bracing. The vertebral body is the thick, disc-shaped anterior portion of the vertebra that is the weight-bearing part. Types of fractures typically treated with closed techniques include simple compression fractures and burst fractures. The superior and inferior surfaces attach to the intervertebral discs. A neurovascular exam is performed to ensure that nerves and blood vessels at the site of injury are intact. In 22310, no manipulation of fracture fragments is required. The patient is treated with pain medication and the spine is immobilized with a cervical collar, halo device, thoracic or lumbar corset, or a body cast or brace. In 22315, closed treatment of minimally displaced vertebral fractures and/or dislocations with no neurological deficit is performed using manipulation or traction and casting and/or bracing. The minimally displaced fracture and/or dislocated vertebrae are manually reduced (manipulated) into anatomic alignment. Alternatively, traction may be used to realign the spine. A longitudinal force is applied along the axis of the spine to decompress the fracture. Following reduction, separately reportable radiographs are again obtained to ensure anatomic alignment. The spine is then immobilized and hyperextended using a brace or cast.

Closed treatment of vertebral body fracture(s) requiring casting/bracing

Without (22310), or with (22315) manipulation/traction

ICD-10-CM Diagnostic Codes

M43.12 Spondylolisthesis, cervical region
M43.13 Spondylolisthesis, cervicothoracic region
M43.14 Spondylolisthesis, thoracic region
M43.15 Spondylolisthesis, thoracolumbar region
M43.16 Spondylolisthesis, lumbar region
M43.17 Spondylolisthesis, lumbosacral region
M48.42 Fatigue fracture of vertebra, cervical region
M48.43 Fatigue fracture of vertebra, cervicothoracic region
M48.44 Fatigue fracture of vertebra, thoracic region
M48.45 Fatigue fracture of vertebra, thoracolumbar region
M48.46 Fatigue fracture of vertebra, lumbar region
M48.47 Fatigue fracture of vertebra, lumbosacral region
M48.52 Collapsed vertebra, not elsewhere classified, cervical region
M48.53 Collapsed vertebra, not elsewhere classified, cervicothoracic region
M48.54 Collapsed vertebra, not elsewhere classified, thoracic region
M48.55 Collapsed vertebra, not elsewhere classified, thoracolumbar region
M48.56 Collapsed vertebra, not elsewhere classified, lumbar region
M80.08 Age-related osteoporosis with current pathological fracture, vertebra(e)
M84.48 Pathological fracture, other site
M84.58 Pathological fracture in neoplastic disease, other specified site
M84.68 Pathological fracture in other disease, other site
S12.01 Stable burst fracture of first cervical vertebra
S12.031 Nondisplaced posterior arch fracture of first cervical vertebra
S12.041 Nondisplaced lateral mass fracture of first cervical vertebra
S12.091 Other nondisplaced fracture of first cervical vertebra
S12.112 Nondisplaced Type II dens fracture
S12.121 Other nondisplaced dens fracture
S12.151 Other traumatic nondisplaced spondylolisthesis of second cervical vertebra
S12.191 Other nondisplaced fracture of second cervical vertebra
S12.24 Type III traumatic spondylolisthesis of third cervical vertebra
S12.251 Other traumatic nondisplaced spondylolisthesis of third cervical vertebra
S12.291 Other nondisplaced fracture of third cervical vertebra
S12.34 Type III traumatic spondylolisthesis of fourth cervical vertebra
S12.351 Other traumatic nondisplaced spondylolisthesis of fourth cervical vertebra
S12.391 Other nondisplaced fracture of fourth cervical vertebra
S12.44 Type III traumatic spondylolisthesis of fifth cervical vertebra
S12.451 Other traumatic nondisplaced spondylolisthesis of fifth cervical vertebra
S12.491 Other nondisplaced fracture of fifth cervical vertebra
S12.54 Type III traumatic spondylolisthesis of sixth cervical vertebra
S12.551 Other traumatic nondisplaced spondylolisthesis of sixth cervical vertebra
S12.591 Other nondisplaced fracture of sixth cervical vertebra
S12.64 Type III traumatic spondylolisthesis of seventh cervical vertebra
S12.651 Other traumatic nondisplaced spondylolisthesis of seventh cervical vertebra
S12.691 Other nondisplaced fracture of seventh cervical vertebra
S13.130 Subluxation of C2/C3 cervical vertebrae
S13.140 Subluxation of C3/C4 cervical vertebrae
S13.150 Subluxation of C4/C5 cervical vertebrae
S13.160 Subluxation of C5/C6 cervical vertebrae
S13.170 Subluxation of C6/C7 cervical vertebrae
S22.010 Wedge compression fracture of first thoracic vertebra
S22.011 Stable burst fracture of first thoracic vertebra
S22.018 Other fracture of first thoracic vertebra
S22.021 Stable burst fracture of second thoracic vertebra
S22.022 Unstable burst fracture of second thoracic vertebra
S22.028 Other fracture of second thoracic vertebra
S22.030 Wedge compression fracture of third thoracic vertebra
S22.031 Stable burst fracture of third thoracic vertebra
S22.038 Other fracture of third thoracic vertebra
S22.040 Wedge compression fracture of fourth thoracic vertebra
S22.041 Stable burst fracture of fourth thoracic vertebra
S22.048 Other fracture of fourth thoracic vertebra
S22.050 Wedge compression fracture of T5-T6 vertebra
S22.051 Stable burst fracture of T5-T6 vertebra
S22.058 Other fracture of T5-T6 vertebra
S22.060 Wedge compression fracture of T7-T8 vertebra
S22.061 Stable burst fracture of T7-T8 vertebra
S22.068 Other fracture of T7-T8 thoracic vertebra
S22.070 Wedge compression fracture of T9-T10 vertebra
S22.071 Stable burst fracture of T9-T10 vertebra
S22.078 Other fracture of T9-T10 vertebra
S22.080 Wedge compression fracture of T11-T12 vertebra
S22.081 Stable burst fracture of T11-T12 vertebra
S22.082 Unstable burst fracture of T11-T12 vertebra
S22.088 Other fracture of T11-T12 vertebra
S23.110 Subluxation of T1/T2 thoracic vertebra
S23.120 Subluxation of T2/T3 thoracic vertebra
S23.122 Subluxation of T3/T4 thoracic vertebra
S23.130 Subluxation of T4/T5 thoracic vertebra
S23.132 Subluxation of T5/T6 thoracic vertebra
S23.140 Subluxation of T6/T7 thoracic vertebra
S23.142 Subluxation of T7/T8 thoracic vertebra
S23.150 Subluxation of T8/T9 thoracic vertebra
S23.152 Subluxation of T9/T10 thoracic vertebra
S23.160 Subluxation of T10/T11 thoracic vertebra
S23.162 Subluxation of T11/T12 thoracic vertebra
S23.170 Subluxation of T12/L1 thoracic vertebra
S32.010 Wedge compression fracture of first lumbar vertebra
S32.011 Stable burst fracture of first lumbar vertebra
S32.018 Other fracture of first lumbar vertebra
S32.020 Wedge compression fracture of second lumbar vertebra
S32.021 Stable burst fracture of second lumbar vertebra
S32.028 Other fracture of second lumbar vertebra
S32.030 Wedge compression fracture of third lumbar vertebra
S32.031 Stable burst fracture of third lumbar vertebra
S32.038 Other fracture of third lumbar vertebra
S32.040 Wedge compression fracture of fourth lumbar vertebra

- S32.041 Stable burst fracture of fourth lumbar vertebra
- S32.048 Other fracture of fourth lumbar vertebra
- S32.050 Wedge compression fracture of fifth lumbar vertebra
- S32.051 Stable burst fracture of fifth lumbar vertebra
- S32.058 Other fracture of fifth lumbar vertebra
- S33.110 Subluxation of L1/L2 lumbar vertebra
- S33.120 Subluxation of L2/L3 lumbar vertebra
- S33.130 Subluxation of L3/L4 lumbar vertebra
- S33.140 Subluxation of L4/L5 lumbar vertebra

ICD-10-CM Coding Notes

For codes requiring a 7th character extension, refer to your ICD-10-CM book. Review the character descriptions and coding guidelines for proper selection. For some procedures, only certain characters will apply.

CCI Edits

Refer to Appendix A for CCI edits.

Facility RVUs

Code	Work	PE Facility	MP	Total Facility
22310	3.45	4.20	0.73	8.38
22315	10.11	9.75	2.35	22.21

Non-facility RVUs

Code	Work	PE Non-Facility	MP	Total Non-Facility
22310	3.45	4.52	0.73	8.70
22315	10.11	12.86	2.35	25.32

Modifiers (PAR)

Code	Mod 50	Mod 51	Mod 62	Mod 66	Mod 80
22310	0	2	0	0	1
22315	0	2	0	0	1

Global Period

Code	Days
22310	090
22315	090

22318-22319

22318 Open treatment and/or reduction of odontoid fracture(s) and or dislocation(s) (including os odontoideum), anterior approach, including placement of internal fixation; without grafting

22319 Open treatment and/or reduction of odontoid fracture(s) and or dislocation(s) (including os odontoideum), anterior approach, including placement of internal fixation; with grafting

AMA Coding Guideline

Fracture and/or Dislocation Procedures on the Spine (Vertebral Column)

To report arthrodesis, see codes 22590-22632. (Report in addition to code[s] for the definitive procedure with modifier 51.)

To report instrumentation procedures, see 22840-22855, 22859. (Report in addition to code[s] for the definitive procedure[s].) Do not append modifier 62 to spinal instrumentation codes 22840-22848, 22850, 22852, 22853, 22854, 22859.

To report bone graft procedures, see 20930-20938. (Report in addition to code[s] for the definitive procedure[s].) Do not append modifier 62 to bone graft codes 20900-20938.

For the following codes, when two surgeons work together as primary surgeons performing distinct part(s) of open fracture and/or dislocation procedure(s), each surgeon should report his/her distinct operative work by appending modifier 62 to the procedure code. In this situation, modifier 62 may be appended to the procedure code(s) 22318-22327 and, as appropriate, the associated additional fracture vertebrae or dislocated segment add-on code 22328 as long as both surgeons continue to work together as primary surgeons.

Surgical Procedures on the Spine (Vertebral Column)

Cervical, thoracic, and lumbar spine.

Within the spine section, bone grafting procedures are reported separately and in addition to arthrodesis. For bone grafts in other Musculoskeletal sections, see specific code(s) descriptor(s) and/or accompanying guidelines.

To report bone grafts performed after arthrodesis, see 20930-20938. Do not append modifier 62 to bone graft codes 20900-20938.

Example:

Posterior arthrodesis of L5-S1 for degenerative disc disease utilizing morselized autogenous iliac bone graft harvested through a separate fascial incision.

Report as 22612 and 20937.

Within the spine section, instrumentation is reported separately and in addition to arthrodesis. To report instrumentation procedures performed with definitive vertebral procedure(s), see 22840-22855, 22859. Instrumentation procedure codes 22840-22848, 22853, 22854, 22859 are reported in addition to the definitive procedure(s). Modifier 62 may not be appended to the definitive or add-on spinal instrumentation procedure code(s) 22840-22848, 22850, 22852, 22853, 22854, 22859.

Example:

Posterior arthrodesis of L4-S1, utilizing morselized autogenous iliac bone graft harvested through separate fascial incision, and pedicle screw fixation.

Report as 22612, 22614, 22842, and 20937.

Vertebral procedures are sometimes followed by arthrodesis and in addition may include bone grafts and instrumentation.

When arthrodesis is performed in addition to another procedure, the arthrodesis should be reported in addition to the original procedure with modifier 51 (multiple procedures). Examples are after osteotomy, fracture care, vertebral corpectomy, and laminectomy. Bone grafts and instrumentation are never performed without arthrodesis.

Example:

Treatment of a burst fracture of L2 by corpectomy followed by arthrodesis of L1-L3, utilizing anterior instrumentation L1-L3 and structural allograft.

Report as 63090, 22558-51, 22585, 22845, and 20931.

When two surgeons work together as primary surgeons performing distinct part(s) of a single reportable procedure, each surgeon should report his/her distinct operative work by appending modifier 62 to the single definitive procedure code. If additional procedure(s) (including add-on procedure[s]) are performed during the same surgical session, separate code(s) may be reported by each co-surgeon, with modifier 62 appended (see Appendix A).

Example:

A 42-year-old male with a history of posttraumatic degenerative disc disease at L3-4 and L4-5 (internal disc disruption) underwent surgical repair. Surgeon A performed an anterior exposure of the spine with mobilization of the great vessels. Surgeon B performed anterior (minimal) discectomy and fusion at L3-4 and L4-5 using anterior interbody technique.

Report surgeon A: 22558 append modifier 62, 22585 append modifier 62

Report surgeon B: 22558 append modifier 62, 22585 append modifier 62, 20931

Please see the Surgery Guidelines section for the following guidelines:

- *Surgical Procedures on the Musculoskeletal System*

AMA Coding Notes

Surgical Procedures on the Spine (Vertebral Column)

(Do not append modifier 62 to bone graft code 20931)

(For injection procedure for myelography, use 62284)

(For injection procedure for discography, see 62290, 62291)

(For injection procedure, chemonucleolysis, single or multiple levels, use 62292)

(For injection procedure for facet joints, see 64490-64495, 64633-64636)

(For needle or trocar biopsy, see 20220-20225)

AMA *CPT Assistant* ☐

22318: Nov 99: 11, Apr 12: 13, Jul 13: 3
22319: Nov 99: 11, Apr 12: 16, Jul 13: 3

Plain English Description

Internal fixation is used in open treatment of an odontoid fracture and/or dislocation through an anterior approach. The os odontoideum, or odontoid process, is the strong toothlike process that projects upward from the surface of the axis. The patient is placed in a supine position and the physician creates an incision through the muscle, carefully avoiding the carotid artery, trachea, and esophagus. The surrounding soft tissue is retracted and vessels may be ligated. Guide wires are used to stabilize the fracture or dislocation. Code 22318 if no bone grafting is necessary. Code 22319 if bone grafting is necessary. A drain may be inserted, and all incisions are closed.

ICD-10-CM Diagnostic Codes

	Code	Description
➐	M48.50	Collapsed vertebra, not elsewhere classified, site unspecified
➐	S12.110	Anterior displaced Type II dens fracture
➐	S12.111	Posterior displaced Type II dens fracture
➐	S12.112	Nondisplaced Type II dens fracture
➐	S12.120	Other displaced dens fracture
➐	S12.121	Other nondisplaced dens fracture
➐	S12.14	Type III traumatic spondylolisthesis of second cervical vertebra
➐	S12.150	Other traumatic displaced spondylolisthesis of second cervical vertebra
➐	S12.151	Other traumatic nondisplaced spondylolisthesis of second cervical vertebra

ICD-10-CM Coding Notes

For codes requiring a 7th character extension, refer to your ICD-10-CM book. Review the character descriptions and coding guidelines for proper selection. For some procedures, only certain characters will apply.

CCI Edits

Refer to Appendix A for CCI edits.

Facility RVUs

Code	Work	PE Facility	MP	Total Facility
22318	22.72	16.58	8.03	47.33
22319	25.33	17.97	9.35	52.65

Non-facility RVUs

Code	Work	PE Non-Facility	MP	Total Non-Facility
22318	22.72	16.58	8.03	47.33
22319	25.33	17.97	9.35	52.65

Modifiers (PAR)

Code	Mod 50	Mod 51	Mod 62	Mod 66	Mod 80
22318	0	2	2	0	2
22319	0	2	2	0	2

Global Period

Code	Days
22318	090
22319	090

22325-22328

22325 Open treatment and/or reduction of vertebral fracture(s) and/or dislocation(s), posterior approach, 1 fractured vertebra or dislocated segment; lumbar

(Do not report 22325 in conjunction with 22511, 22512, 22514, 22515 when performed at the same level)

22326 Open treatment and/or reduction of vertebral fracture(s) and/or dislocation(s), posterior approach, 1 fractured vertebra or dislocated segment; cervical

(Do not report 22326 in conjunction with 22510, 22512, when performed at the same level)

22327 Open treatment and/or reduction of vertebral fracture(s) and/or dislocation(s), posterior approach, 1 fractured vertebra or dislocated segment; thoracic

(Do not report 22327 in conjunction with 22510, 22512, 22513, 22515 when performed at the same level)

+ **22328 Open treatment and/or reduction of vertebral fracture(s) and/or dislocation(s), posterior approach, 1 fractured vertebra or dislocated segment; each additional fractured vertebra or dislocated segment (List separately in addition to code for primary procedure)**

(Use 22328 in conjunction with 22325-22327)

(For treatment of vertebral fracture by the anterior approach, see corpectomy 63081-63091, and appropriate arthrodesis, bone graft and instrument codes)

(For decompression of spine following fracture, see 63001-63091; for arthrodesis of spine following fracture, see 22548-22632)

AMA Coding Guideline

Fracture and/or Dislocation Procedures on the Spine (Vertebral Column)

To report arthrodesis, see codes 22590-22632. (Report in addition to code[s] for the definitive procedure with modifier 51.)

To report instrumentation procedures, see 22840-22855, 22859. (Report in addition to code[s] for the definitive procedure[s].) Do not append modifier 62 to spinal instrumentation codes 22840-22848, 22850, 22852, 22853, 22854, 22859.

To report bone graft procedures, see 20930-20938. (Report in addition to code[s] for the definitive procedure[s].) Do not append modifier 62 to bone graft codes 20900-20938.

For the following codes, when two surgeons work together as primary surgeons performing distinct part(s) of open fracture and/or dislocation procedure(s), each surgeon should report his/her distinct operative work by appending modifier 62 to the procedure code. In this situation, modifier 62 may be appended to the procedure code(s) 22318-22327 and, as appropriate, the associated additional fracture vertebrae or dislocated segment add-on code 22328 as long as both surgeons continue to work together as primary surgeons.

Surgical Procedures on the Spine (Vertebral Column)

Cervical, thoracic, and lumbar spine.

Within the spine section, bone grafting procedures are reported separately and in addition to arthrodesis. For bone grafts in other Musculoskeletal sections, see specific code(s) descriptor(s) and/or accompanying guidelines.

To report bone grafts performed after arthrodesis, see 20930-20938. Do not append modifier 62 to bone graft codes 20900-20938.

Example:

Posterior arthrodesis of L5-S1 for degenerative disc disease utilizing morselized autogenous iliac bone graft harvested through a separate fascial incision.

Report as 22612 and 20937.

Within the spine section, instrumentation is reported separately and in addition to arthrodesis. To report instrumentation procedures performed with definitive vertebral procedure(s), see 22840-22855, 22859. Instrumentation procedure codes 22840-22848, 22853, 22854, 22859 are reported in addition to the definitive procedure(s). Modifier 62 may not be appended to the definitive or add-on spinal instrumentation procedure code(s) 22840-22848, 22850, 22852, 22853, 22854, 22859.

Example:

Posterior arthrodesis of L4-S1, utilizing morselized autogenous iliac bone graft harvested through separate fascial incision, and pedicle screw fixation.

Report as 22612, 22614, 22842, and 20937.

Vertebral procedures are sometimes followed by arthrodesis and in addition may include bone grafts and instrumentation.

When arthrodesis is performed in addition to another procedure, the arthrodesis should be reported in addition to the original procedure with modifier 51 (multiple procedures). Examples are after osteotomy, fracture care, vertebral corpectomy, and laminectomy. Bone grafts and instrumentation are never performed without arthrodesis.

Example:

Treatment of a burst fracture of L2 by corpectomy followed by arthrodesis of L1-L3, utilizing anterior instrumentation L1-L3 and structural allograft.

Report as 63090, 22558-51, 22585, 22845, and 20931.

When two surgeons work together as primary surgeons performing distinct part(s) of a single reportable procedure, each surgeon should report his/her distinct operative work by appending modifier 62 to the single definitive procedure code. If additional procedure(s) (including add-on procedure[s]) are performed during the same surgical session, separate code(s) may be reported by each co-surgeon, with modifier 62 appended (see Appendix A).

Example:

A 42-year-old male with a history of posttraumatic degenerative disc disease at L3-4 and L4-5 (internal disc disruption) underwent surgical repair. Surgeon A performed an anterior exposure of the spine with mobilization of the great vessels. Surgeon B performed anterior (minimal) discectomy and fusion at L3-4 and L4-5 using anterior interbody technique.

Report surgeon A: 22558 append modifier 62, 22585 append modifier 62

Report surgeon B: 22558 append modifier 62, 22585 append modifier 62, 20931

Please see the Surgery Guidelines section for the following guidelines:

- *Surgical Procedures on the Musculoskeletal System*

AMA Coding Notes

Surgical Procedures on the Spine (Vertebral Column)

(Do not append modifier 62 to bone graft code 20931)

(For injection procedure for myelography, use 62284)

(For injection procedure for discography, see 62290, 62291)

(For injection procedure, chemonucleolysis, single or multiple levels, use 62292)

(For injection procedure for facet joints, see 64490-64495, 64633-64636)

(For needle or trocar biopsy, see 20220-20225)

AMA *CPT Assistant*

22325: Sep 97: 8, Jun 12: 10, Jul 13: 3, Aug 17: 9

22326: Sep 97: 8, Jul 13: 3

22327: Sep 97: 8, Jun 12: 10, Jul 13: 3

22328: Feb 96: 6

Plain English Description

The patient is placed in a prone position and the physician creates an incision over the fractured or dislocated vertebra or dislocated segment. The physician uses a rod to stabilize the area. Fusion may be necessary and is achieved via grafting (separately reportable) or internal fixation. The incision is closed. Code 22325 for a lumbar procedure; 22326 for cervical; 22327 for a thoracic site; and 22328 for each additional fractured or dislocated vertebra or segment in addition to the primary procedure.

Open treatment and/or reduction of vertebral fracture(s) and/or dislocation

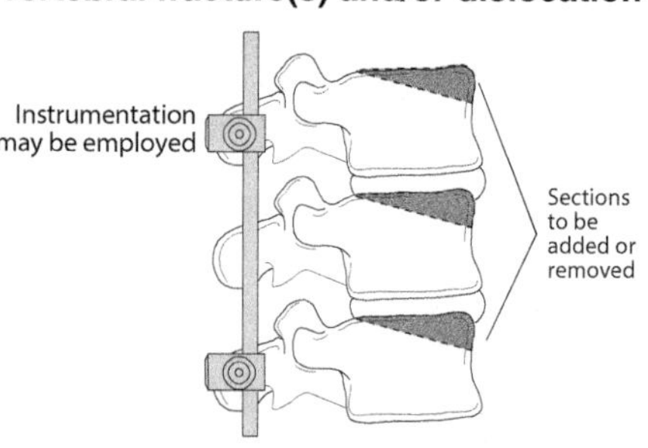

A rod is used to stabilize the area. Fusion may be necessary, and is achieved via grafting (separately reportable) or internal fixation. Code 22325 for a lumbar procedure; 22326 for cervical; 22327 for a thoracic site; and 22328 for each additional fractured or dislocated vertebra or segment in addition to the primary procedure.

ICD-10-CM Diagnostic Codes

- ❼ S12.030 Displaced posterior arch fracture of first cervical vertebra
- ❼ S12.190 Other displaced fracture of second cervical vertebra
- ❼ S12.290 Other displaced fracture of third cervical vertebra
- ❼ S12.390 Other displaced fracture of fourth cervical vertebra
- ❼ S12.490 Other displaced fracture of fifth cervical vertebra
- ❼ S12.590 Other displaced fracture of sixth cervical vertebra
- ❼ S12.690 Other displaced fracture of seventh cervical vertebra
- ❼ S22.010 Wedge compression fracture of first thoracic vertebra
- ❼ S22.011 Stable burst fracture of first thoracic vertebra
- ❼ S22.018 Other fracture of first thoracic vertebra
- ❼ S22.020 Wedge compression fracture of second thoracic vertebra
- ❼ S22.021 Stable burst fracture of second thoracic vertebra
- ❼ S22.022 Unstable burst fracture of second thoracic vertebra
- ❼ S22.028 Other fracture of second thoracic vertebra
- ❼ S22.030 Wedge compression fracture of third thoracic vertebra
- ❼ S22.031 Stable burst fracture of third thoracic vertebra
- ❼ S22.032 Unstable burst fracture of third thoracic vertebra
- ❼ S22.038 Other fracture of third thoracic vertebra
- ❼ S22.040 Wedge compression fracture of fourth thoracic vertebra
- ❼ S22.041 Stable burst fracture of fourth thoracic vertebra
- ❼ S22.042 Unstable burst fracture of fourth thoracic vertebra
- ❼ S22.048 Other fracture of fourth thoracic vertebra
- ❼ S22.050 Wedge compression fracture of T5-T6 vertebra
- ❼ S22.051 Stable burst fracture of T5-T6 vertebra
- ❼ S22.052 Unstable burst fracture of T5-T6 vertebra
- ❼ S22.058 Other fracture of T5-T6 vertebra
- ❼ S22.060 Wedge compression fracture of T7-T8 vertebra
- ❼ S22.061 Stable burst fracture of T7-T8 vertebra
- ❼ S22.062 Unstable burst fracture of T7-T8 vertebra
- ❼ S22.068 Other fracture of T7-T8 thoracic vertebra
- ❼ S22.070 Wedge compression fracture of T9-T10 vertebra
- ❼ S22.071 Stable burst fracture of T9-T10 vertebra
- ❼ S22.072 Unstable burst fracture of T9-T10 vertebra
- ❼ S22.078 Other fracture of T9-T10 vertebra
- ❼ S22.080 Wedge compression fracture of T11-T12 vertebra
- ❼ S22.081 Stable burst fracture of T11-T12 vertebra
- ❼ S22.082 Unstable burst fracture of T11-T12 vertebra
- ❼ S22.088 Other fracture of T11-T12 vertebra
- ❼ S32.010 Wedge compression fracture of first lumbar vertebra
- ❼ S32.011 Stable burst fracture of first lumbar vertebra
- ❼ S32.012 Unstable burst fracture of first lumbar vertebra
- ❼ S32.018 Other fracture of first lumbar vertebra
- ❼ S32.020 Wedge compression fracture of second lumbar vertebra
- ❼ S32.021 Stable burst fracture of second lumbar vertebra
- ❼ S32.022 Unstable burst fracture of second lumbar vertebra
- ❼ S32.028 Other fracture of second lumbar vertebra
- ❼ S32.031 Stable burst fracture of third lumbar vertebra
- ❼ S32.032 Unstable burst fracture of third lumbar vertebra
- ❼ S32.038 Other fracture of third lumbar vertebra
- ❼ S32.040 Wedge compression fracture of fourth lumbar vertebra
- ❼ S32.041 Stable burst fracture of fourth lumbar vertebra
- ❼ S32.042 Unstable burst fracture of fourth lumbar vertebra
- ❼ S32.048 Other fracture of fourth lumbar vertebra
- ❼ S32.050 Wedge compression fracture of fifth lumbar vertebra
- ❼ S32.051 Stable burst fracture of fifth lumbar vertebra
- ❼ S32.052 Unstable burst fracture of fifth lumbar vertebra
- ❼ S32.058 Other fracture of fifth lumbar vertebra

ICD-10-CM Coding Notes

For codes requiring a 7th character extension, refer to your ICD-10-CM book. Review the character descriptions and coding guidelines for proper selection. For some procedures, only certain characters will apply.

CCI Edits

Refer to Appendix A for CCI edits.

Facility RVUs ☐

Code	Work	PE Facility	MP	Total Facility
22325	19.87	16.21	5.91	41.99
22326	20.84	15.84	6.62	43.30
22327	20.77	16.66	6.30	43.73
22328	4.60	2.20	1.37	8.17

Non-facility RVUs ☐

Code	Work	PE Non-Facility	MP	Total Non-Facility
22325	19.87	16.21	5.91	41.99
22326	20.84	15.84	6.62	43.30
22327	20.77	16.66	6.30	43.73
22328	4.60	2.20	1.37	8.17

Modifiers (PAR) ☐

Code	Mod 50	Mod 51	Mod 62	Mod 66	Mod 80
22325	0	2	1	0	2
22326	0	2	1	0	2
22327	0	2	1	0	2
22328	0	0	1	0	2

Global Period

Code	Days
22325	090
22326	090
22327	090
22328	ZZZ

22513-22515

22513 Percutaneous vertebral augmentation, including cavity creation (fracture reduction and bone biopsy included when performed) using mechanical device (eg, kyphoplasty), 1 vertebral body, unilateral or bilateral cannulation, inclusive of all imaging guidance; thoracic

22514 Percutaneous vertebral augmentation, including cavity creation (fracture reduction and bone biopsy included when performed) using mechanical device (eg, kyphoplasty), 1 vertebral body, unilateral or bilateral cannulation, inclusive of all imaging guidance; lumbar

+ **22515 Percutaneous vertebral augmentation, including cavity creation (fracture reduction and bone biopsy included when performed) using mechanical device (eg, kyphoplasty), 1 vertebral body, unilateral or bilateral cannulation, inclusive of all imaging guidance; each additional thoracic or lumbar vertebral body (List separately in addition to code for primary procedure)**

(Use 22515 in conjunction with 22513, 22514)

(Do not report 22513, 22514, 22515 in conjunction with 20225, 22310, 22315, 22325, 22327, when performed at the same level as 22513, 22514, 22515)

AMA Coding Guideline

Percutaneous Vertebroplasty and Vertebral Augmentation Procedures

Codes 22510, 22511, 22512, 22513, 22514, 22515 describe procedures for percutaneous vertebral augmentation that include vertebroplasty of the cervical, thoracic, lumbar, and sacral spine and vertebral augmentation of the thoracic and lumbar spine.

For the purposes of reporting 22510, 22511, 22512, 22513, 22514, 22515, "vertebroplasty" is the process of injecting a material (cement) into the vertebral body to reinforce the structure of the body using image guidance. "Vertebral augmentation" is the process of cavity creation followed by the injection of the material (cement) under image guidance. For 0200T and 0201T, "sacral augmentation (sacroplasty)" refers to the creation of a cavity within a sacral vertebral body followed by injection of a material to fill that cavity.

The procedure codes are inclusive of bone biopsy, when performed, and imaging guidance necessary to perform the procedure. Use one primary procedure code and an add-on code for additional levels. When treating the sacrum, sacral procedures are reported only once per encounter.

Surgical Procedures on the Spine (Vertebral Column)

Cervical, thoracic, and lumbar spine.

Within the spine section, bone grafting procedures are reported separately and in addition to arthrodesis. For bone grafts in other Musculoskeletal sections, see specific code(s) descriptor(s) and/or accompanying guidelines.

To report bone grafts performed after arthrodesis, see 20930-20938. Do not append modifier 62 to bone graft codes 20900-20938.

Example:

Posterior arthrodesis of L5-S1 for degenerative disc disease utilizing morselized autogenous iliac bone graft harvested through a separate fascial incision.

Report as 22612 and 20937.

Within the spine section, instrumentation is reported separately and in addition to arthrodesis. To report instrumentation procedures performed with definitive vertebral procedure(s), see 22840-22855, 22859. Instrumentation procedure codes 22840-22848, 22853, 22854, 22859 are reported in addition to the definitive procedure(s). Modifier 62 may not be appended to the definitive or add-on spinal instrumentation procedure code(s) 22840-22848, 22850, 22852, 22853, 22854, 22859.

Example:

Posterior arthrodesis of L4-S1, utilizing morselized autogenous iliac bone graft harvested through separate fascial incision, and pedicle screw fixation.

Report as 22612, 22614, 22842, and 20937.

Vertebral procedures are sometimes followed by arthrodesis and in addition may include bone grafts and instrumentation.

When arthrodesis is performed in addition to another procedure, the arthrodesis should be reported in addition to the original procedure with modifier 51 (multiple procedures). Examples are after osteotomy, fracture care, vertebral corpectomy, and laminectomy. Bone grafts and instrumentation are never performed without arthrodesis.

Example:

Treatment of a burst fracture of L2 by corpectomy followed by arthrodesis of L1-L3, utilizing anterior instrumentation L1-L3 and structural allograft.

Report as 63090, 22558-51, 22585, 22845, and 20931.

When two surgeons work together as primary surgeons performing distinct part(s) of a single reportable procedure, each surgeon should report his/her distinct operative work by appending modifier 62 to the single definitive procedure code. If additional procedure(s) (including add-on procedure[s]) are performed during the same surgical session, separate code(s) may be reported by each co-surgeon, with modifier 62 appended (see Appendix A).

Example:

A 42-year-old male with a history of posttraumatic degenerative disc disease at L3-4 and L4-5 (internal disc disruption) underwent surgical repair. Surgeon A performed an anterior exposure of the spine with mobilization of the great vessels. Surgeon B performed anterior (minimal) discectomy and fusion at L3-4 and L4-5 using anterior interbody technique.

Report surgeon A: 22558 append modifier 62, 22585 append modifier 62

Report surgeon B: 22558 append modifier 62, 22585 append modifier 62, 20931

Please see the Surgery Guidelines section for the following guidelines:

- *Surgical Procedures on the Musculoskeletal System*

AMA Coding Notes

Surgical Procedures on the Spine (Vertebral Column)

(Do not append modifier 62 to bone graft code 20931)

(For injection procedure for myelography, use 62284)

(For injection procedure for discography, see 62290, 62291)

(For injection procedure, chemonucleolysis, single or multiple levels, use 62292)

(For injection procedure for facet joints, see 64490-64495, 64633-64636)

(For needle or trocar biopsy, see 20220-20225)

AMA *CPT Assistant*

22513: Jan 15: 8
22514: Jan 15: 8
22515: Jan 15: 8

Plain English Description

Percutaneous augmentation of the vertebra is performed to treat a compression fracture caused by osteoporosis, multiple myeloma, primary or metastatic malignant lesions, benign lesions, or traumatic injury of the spine. The patient is placed in a prone position. Using image guidance, a small skin incision is made over the affected vertebra. A working channel is created on one side of the vertebra by advancing a needle to the desired location in the vertebra. Needle biopsies are obtained as needed. A guidewire is then advanced through the needle. The needle is withdrawn and a cannula is advanced over the guidewire and the guidewire is removed. This is repeated on the opposite side for bilateral augmentation procedures. A mechanical device, such as a miniature expandable jack or expandable balloon tamp, is then placed through the cannula and expanded to create a cavity as contrast medium is simultaneously instilled. The fracture may also be reduced using the mechanical device. Once the cavity has been created, the mechanical device is removed. The cavity is then filled with morselized bone graft material, polymethylmethacrylate (PMMA) bone cement, or other bone graft substitute using a bone biopsy needle. The bone graft or cement is mixed with contrast medium so that the physician can observe filling of the cavity. Once the cavity is filled, the needle is withdrawn. A second injection may be performed on the opposite side of the vertebral body. For percutaneous augmentation of a single thoracic vertebral body, use 22513; for a single lumbar vertebral body, use 22514; and for each additional thoracic or lumbar vertebral body, use 22515.

Percutaneous vertebral augmentation, including cavity creation, using mechanical device; 1 vertebral body

Percutaneous injection in vertebrae

Patient in prone position

Cavity created by balloon insertion

Cavity filled with bone graft material

Thoracic (22513); lumbar (22514); each additional (22515)

ICD-10-CM Diagnostic Codes

	Code	Description
	C41.2	Malignant neoplasm of vertebral column
	C79.51	Secondary malignant neoplasm of bone
	C79.52	Secondary malignant neoplasm of bone marrow
	C7B.03	Secondary carcinoid tumors of bone
	C90.00	Multiple myeloma not having achieved remission
	C90.01	Multiple myeloma in remission
	C90.02	Multiple myeloma in relapse
	D16.6	Benign neoplasm of vertebral column
	D48.0	Neoplasm of uncertain behavior of bone and articular cartilage
	D49.2	Neoplasm of unspecified behavior of bone, soft tissue, and skin
	M48.34	Traumatic spondylopathy, thoracic region
	M48.35	Traumatic spondylopathy, thoracolumbar region
	M48.36	Traumatic spondylopathy, lumbar region
⑦	M48.54	Collapsed vertebra, not elsewhere classified, thoracic region
⑦	M48.55	Collapsed vertebra, not elsewhere classified, thoracolumbar region
⑦	M48.56	Collapsed vertebra, not elsewhere classified, lumbar region
	M54.5	Low back pain
	M54.6	Pain in thoracic spine
	M54.89	Other dorsalgia
	M54.9	Dorsalgia, unspecified
⑦	M80.08	Age-related osteoporosis with current pathological fracture, vertebra(e)
	M80.8	Other osteoporosis with current pathological fracture
⑦	M84.48	Pathological fracture, other site
⑦	M84.58	Pathological fracture in neoplastic disease, other specified site
⑦	M84.68	Pathological fracture in other disease, other site
	M85.88	Other specified disorders of bone density and structure, other site
	M85.89	Other specified disorders of bone density and structure, multiple sites
	M87.08	Idiopathic aseptic necrosis of bone, other site
	M87.38	Other secondary osteonecrosis, other site
	M87.88	Other osteonecrosis, other site
⑦	S22.010	Wedge compression fracture of first thoracic vertebra
⑦	S22.011	Stable burst fracture of first thoracic vertebra
⑦	S22.018	Other fracture of first thoracic vertebra
⑦	S22.020	Wedge compression fracture of second thoracic vertebra
⑦	S22.021	Stable burst fracture of second thoracic vertebra
⑦	S22.028	Other fracture of second thoracic vertebra
⑦	S22.030	Wedge compression fracture of third thoracic vertebra
⑦	S22.031	Stable burst fracture of third thoracic vertebra
⑦	S22.038	Other fracture of third thoracic vertebra
⑦	S22.040	Wedge compression fracture of fourth thoracic vertebra
⑦	S22.041	Stable burst fracture of fourth thoracic vertebra
⑦	S22.048	Other fracture of fourth thoracic vertebra
⑦	S22.050	Wedge compression fracture of T5-T6 vertebra
⑦	S22.051	Stable burst fracture of T5-T6 vertebra
⑦	S22.058	Other fracture of T5-T6 vertebra
⑦	S22.060	Wedge compression fracture of T7-T8 vertebra
⑦	S22.061	Stable burst fracture of T7-T8 vertebra
⑦	S22.068	Other fracture of T7-T8 thoracic vertebra
⑦	S22.070	Wedge compression fracture of T9-T10 vertebra
⑦	S22.071	Stable burst fracture of T9-T10 vertebra
⑦	S22.078	Other fracture of T9-T10 vertebra
⑦	S22.080	Wedge compression fracture of T11-T12 vertebra
⑦	S22.081	Stable burst fracture of T11-T12 vertebra
⑦	S22.088	Other fracture of T11-T12 vertebra
⑦	S32.010	Wedge compression fracture of first lumbar vertebra
⑦	S32.011	Stable burst fracture of first lumbar vertebra
⑦	S32.018	Other fracture of first lumbar vertebra
⑦	S32.020	Wedge compression fracture of second lumbar vertebra
⑦	S32.021	Stable burst fracture of second lumbar vertebra
⑦	S32.028	Other fracture of second lumbar vertebra
⑦	S32.030	Wedge compression fracture of third lumbar vertebra
⑦	S32.031	Stable burst fracture of third lumbar vertebra
⑦	S32.038	Other fracture of third lumbar vertebra
⑦	S32.040	Wedge compression fracture of fourth lumbar vertebra
⑦	S32.041	Stable burst fracture of fourth lumbar vertebra
⑦	S32.048	Other fracture of fourth lumbar vertebra
⑦	S32.050	Wedge compression fracture of fifth lumbar vertebra
⑦	S32.051	Stable burst fracture of fifth lumbar vertebra
⑦	S32.058	Other fracture of fifth lumbar vertebra

ICD-10-CM Coding Notes

For codes requiring a 7th character extension, refer to your ICD-10-CM book. Review the character descriptions and coding guidelines for proper selection. For some procedures, only certain characters will apply.

CCI Edits

Refer to Appendix A for CCI edits.

Facility RVUs

Code	Work	PE Facility	MP	Total Facility
22513	8.65	4.70	1.48	14.83
22514	7.99	4.46	1.38	13.83
22515	4.00	1.66	0.73	6.39

Non-facility RVUs

Code	Work	PE Non-Facility	MP	Total Non-Facility
22513	8.65	179.02	1.48	189.15
22514	7.99	178.97	1.38	188.34
22515	4.00	100.84	0.73	105.57

Modifiers (PAR)

Code	Mod 50	Mod 51	Mod 62	Mod 66	Mod 80
22513	0	2	0	0	1
22514	0	2	0	0	1
22515	0	0	0	0	1

Global Period

Code	Days
22513	010
22514	010
22515	ZZZ

22532-22534

22532 Arthrodesis, lateral extracavitary technique, including minimal discectomy to prepare interspace (other than for decompression); thoracic

22533 Arthrodesis, lateral extracavitary technique, including minimal discectomy to prepare interspace (other than for decompression); lumbar

✚ **22534 Arthrodesis, lateral extracavitary technique, including minimal discectomy to prepare interspace (other than for decompression); thoracic or lumbar, each additional vertebral segment (List separately in addition to code for primary procedure)**

(Use 22534 in conjunction with 22532 and 22533)

AMA Coding Guideline

Arthrodesis Procedures on the Spine (Vertebral Column)

Arthrodesis may be performed in the absence of other procedures and therefore when it is combined with another definitive procedure (eg, osteotomy, fracture care, vertebral corpectomy or laminectomy), modifier 51 is appropriate. However, arthrodesis codes 22585, 22614, and 22632 are considered add-on procedure codes and should not be used with modifier 51.

To report instrumentation procedures, see 22840-22855, 22859. (Codes 22840-22848, 22853, 22854, 22859 are reported in conjunction with code[s] for the definitive procedure[s]. When instrumentation reinsertion or removal is reported in conjunction with other definitive procedures, including arthrodesis, decompression, and exploration of fusion, append modifier 51 to 22849, 22850, 22852, and 22855.) To report exploration of fusion, use 22830. (When exploration is reported in conjunction with other definitive procedures, including arthrodesis and decompression, append modifier 51 to 22830.) Do not append modifier 62 to spinal instrumentation codes 22840-22848, 22850, 22852, 22853, 22854, 22859.

To report bone graft procedures, see 20930-20938. (Report in addition to code[s] for the definitive procedure[s].) Do not append modifier 62 to bone graft codes 20900-20938.

Surgical Procedures on the Spine (Vertebral Column)

Cervical, thoracic, and lumbar spine.

Within the spine section, bone grafting procedures are reported separately and in addition to arthrodesis. For bone grafts in other Musculoskeletal sections, see specific code(s) descriptor(s) and/or accompanying guidelines.

To report bone grafts performed after arthrodesis, see 20930-20938. Do not append modifier 62 to bone graft codes 20900-20938.

Example:

Posterior arthrodesis of L5-S1 for degenerative disc disease utilizing morselized autogenous iliac bone graft harvested through a separate fascial incision.

Report as 22612 and 20937.

Within the spine section, instrumentation is reported separately and in addition to arthrodesis. To report instrumentation procedures performed with definitive vertebral procedure(s), see 22840-22855, 22859. Instrumentation procedure codes 22840-22848, 22853, 22854, 22859 are reported in addition to the definitive procedure(s). Modifier 62 may not be appended to the definitive or add-on spinal instrumentation procedure code(s) 22840-22848, 22850, 22852, 22853, 22854, 22859.

Example:

Posterior arthrodesis of L4-S1, utilizing morselized autogenous iliac bone graft harvested through separate fascial incision, and pedicle screw fixation.

Report as 22612, 22614, 22842, and 20937.

Vertebral procedures are sometimes followed by arthrodesis and in addition may include bone grafts and instrumentation.

When arthrodesis is performed in addition to another procedure, the arthrodesis should be reported in addition to the original procedure with modifier 51 (multiple procedures). Examples are after osteotomy, fracture care, vertebral corpectomy, and laminectomy. Bone grafts and instrumentation are never performed without arthrodesis.

Example:

Treatment of a burst fracture of L2 by corpectomy followed by arthrodesis of L1-L3, utilizing anterior instrumentation L1-L3 and structural allograft.

Report as 63090, 22558-51, 22585, 22845, and 20931.

When two surgeons work together as primary surgeons performing distinct part(s) of a single reportable procedure, each surgeon should report his/her distinct operative work by appending modifier 62 to the single definitive procedure code. If additional procedure(s) (including add-on procedure[s]) are performed during the same surgical session, separate code(s) may be reported by each co-surgeon, with modifier 62 appended (see Appendix A).

Example:

A 42-year-old male with a history of posttraumatic degenerative disc disease at L3-4 and L4-5 (internal disc disruption) underwent surgical repair. Surgeon A performed an anterior exposure of the spine with mobilization of the great vessels. Surgeon B performed anterior (minimal) discectomy and fusion at L3-4 and L4-5 using anterior interbody technique.

Report surgeon A: 22558 append modifier 62, 22585 append modifier 62

Report surgeon B: 22558 append modifier 62, 22585 append modifier 62, 20931

Please see the Surgery Guidelines section for the following guidelines:

- *Surgical Procedures on the Musculoskeletal System*

AMA Coding Notes

Surgical Procedures on the Spine (Vertebral Column)

(Do not append modifier 62 to bone graft code 20931)

(For injection procedure for myelography, use 62284)

(For injection procedure for discography, see 62290, 62291)

(For injection procedure, chemonucleolysis, single or multiple levels, use 62292)

(For injection procedure for facet joints, see 64490-64495, 64633-64636)

(For needle or trocar biopsy, see 20220-20225)

AMA *CPT Assistant* ☐

22532: Apr 12: 16, Jul 13: 3

22533: Apr 12: 16, Jul 13: 3

Plain English Description

Arthrodesis by lateral extracavitary technique including minimal discectomy to prepare the interspace (other than for decompression) is performed. Lateral extracavitary approach requires resection of the ribs and exposure of the pleura, and/or peritoneum. A midline incision is made and extended laterally to expose the paraspinous muscle bundle over the thoracic or lumbar vertebral segment to be fused. The paraspinous muscles are elevated off the spinous processes and laminae. The paraspinous muscle bundle is then divided and elevated off the ribs. The rib is dissected from the intercostal muscles and pleura. The rib is resected and the intercostal nerve identified and protected. A high-speed drill is used to remove the associated transverse process and the lateral portion of the facet and pedicle. The dural sac and vertebral body are exposed. If the procedure involves the lumbar spine, the peritoneum is exposed and retracted. The nerve root is retracted to allow better visualization of the vertebral body. Degenerated disc material is removed to prepare the interspace for arthrodesis. Cartilage is removed from vertebral endplates and bone is decorticated. Separately reportable bone allograft or autograft is then placed between the vertebral endplates to facilitate the interbody arthrodesis. Drains are placed as needed and the incisions closed. Use code 22532 to report thoracic arthrodesis by lateral extracavitary technique, code 22533 for lumbar arthrodesis, and code 22534 for arthrodesis of each additional thoracic or lumbar vertebral segment.

Arthrodesis; thoracic

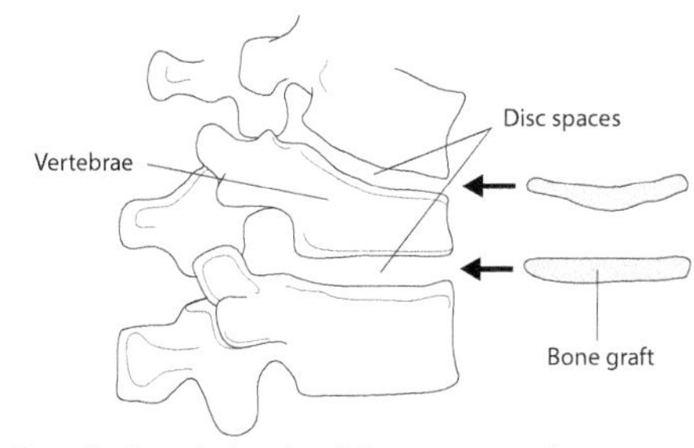

Part of a rib and a herniated disc are removed to access the space between two vertebrae in the upper back and a bone graft is then used to fuse the two vertebrae together. Code 22532 for thoracic vertebra; use 22533 for lumbar vertebra. Add 22534 for each additional vertebral segment that is fused.

ICD-10-CM Diagnostic Codes

C41.2	Malignant neoplasm of vertebral column
D16.6	Benign neoplasm of vertebral column
D48.0	Neoplasm of uncertain behavior of bone and articular cartilage
M47.14	Other spondylosis with myelopathy, thoracic region
M47.15	Other spondylosis with myelopathy, thoracolumbar region
M47.16	Other spondylosis with myelopathy, lumbar region
M47.814	Spondylosis without myelopathy or radiculopathy, thoracic region
M47.815	Spondylosis without myelopathy or radiculopathy, thoracolumbar region
M47.816	Spondylosis without myelopathy or radiculopathy, lumbar region
M51.04	Intervertebral disc disorders with myelopathy, thoracic region
M51.05	Intervertebral disc disorders with myelopathy, thoracolumbar region
M51.06	Intervertebral disc disorders with myelopathy, lumbar region
M51.14	Intervertebral disc disorders with radiculopathy, thoracic region
M51.15	Intervertebral disc disorders with radiculopathy, thoracolumbar region
M51.16	Intervertebral disc disorders with radiculopathy, lumbar region
M51.17	Intervertebral disc disorders with radiculopathy, lumbosacral region
M51.24	Other intervertebral disc displacement, thoracic region
M51.25	Other intervertebral disc displacement, thoracolumbar region
M51.26	Other intervertebral disc displacement, lumbar region
M51.27	Other intervertebral disc displacement, lumbosacral region
M51.34	Other intervertebral disc degeneration, thoracic region
M51.35	Other intervertebral disc degeneration, thoracolumbar region
M51.36	Other intervertebral disc degeneration, lumbar region
M51.37	Other intervertebral disc degeneration, lumbosacral region
M51.44	Schmorl's nodes, thoracic region
M51.45	Schmorl's nodes, thoracolumbar region
M53.2X3	Spinal instabilities, cervicothoracic region
M53.2X4	Spinal instabilities, thoracic region
M53.2X5	Spinal instabilities, thoracolumbar region
M53.2X6	Spinal instabilities, lumbar region
M96.1	Postlaminectomy syndrome, not elsewhere classified
M96.4	Postsurgical lordosis

CCI Edits

Refer to Appendix A for CCI edits.

Facility RVUs ▯

Code	Work	PE Facility	MP	Total Facility
22532	25.99	18.25	7.87	52.11
22533	24.79	17.34	5.91	48.04
22534	5.99	2.88	1.61	10.48

Non-facility RVUs ▯

Code	Work	PE Non-Facility	MP	Total Non-Facility
22532	25.99	18.25	7.87	52.11
22533	24.79	17.34	5.91	48.04
22534	5.99	2.88	1.61	10.48

Modifiers (PAR) ▯

Code	Mod 50	Mod 51	Mod 62	Mod 66	Mod 80
22532	0	2	2	0	2
22533	0	2	2	0	2
22534	0	0	2	0	2

Global Period

Code	Days
22532	090
22533	090
22534	ZZZ

22551-22552

22551 Arthrodesis, anterior interbody, including disc space preparation, discectomy, osteophytectomy and decompression of spinal cord and/or nerve roots; cervical below C2

+ **22552 Arthrodesis, anterior interbody, including disc space preparation, discectomy, osteophytectomy and decompression of spinal cord and/or nerve roots; cervical below C2, each additional interspace (List separately in addition to code for primary procedure)**

(Use 22552 in conjunction with 22551)

AMA Coding Guideline

Anterior or Anterolateral Approach Technique Arthrodesis Procedures on the Spine (Vertebral Column)

Procedure codes 22554-22558 are for SINGLE interspace; for additional interspaces, use 22585. A vertebral interspace is the non-bony compartment between two adjacent vertebral bodies, which contains the intervertebral disc, and includes the nucleus pulposus, annulus fibrosus, and two cartilaginous endplates.

For the following codes, when two surgeons work together as primary surgeons performing distinct part(s) of an anterior interbody arthrodesis, each surgeon should report his/her distinct operative work by appending modifier 62 to the procedure code. In this situation, modifier 62 may be appended to the procedure code(s) 22548-22558 and, as appropriate, to the associated additional interspace add-on code 22585 as long as both surgeons continue to work together as primary surgeons.

Arthrodesis Procedures on the Spine (Vertebral Column)

Arthrodesis may be performed in the absence of other procedures and therefore when it is combined with another definitive procedure (eg, osteotomy, fracture care, vertebral corpectomy or laminectomy), modifier 51 is appropriate. However, arthrodesis codes 22585, 22614, and 22632 are considered add-on procedure codes and should not be used with modifier 51.

To report instrumentation procedures, see 22840-22855, 22859. (Codes 22840-22848, 22853, 22854, 22859 are reported in conjunction with code[s] for the definitive procedure[s]. When instrumentation reinsertion or removal is reported in conjunction with other definitive procedures, including arthrodesis, decompression, and exploration of fusion, append modifier 51 to 22849, 22850, 22852, and 22855.) To report exploration of fusion, use 22830. (When exploration is reported in conjunction with other definitive procedures, including arthrodesis and decompression, append modifier 51 to 22830.) Do not append modifier 62 to spinal instrumentation codes 22840-22848, 22850, 22852, 22853, 22854, 22859.

To report bone graft procedures, see 20930-20938. (Report in addition to code[s] for the definitive procedure[s].) Do not append modifier 62 to bone graft codes 20900-20938.

Surgical Procedures on the Spine (Vertebral Column)

Cervical, thoracic, and lumbar spine.

Within the spine section, bone grafting procedures are reported separately and in addition to arthrodesis. For bone grafts in other Musculoskeletal sections, see specific code(s) descriptor(s) and/or accompanying guidelines.

To report bone grafts performed after arthrodesis, see 20930-20938. Do not append modifier 62 to bone graft codes 20900-20938.

Example:

Posterior arthrodesis of L5-S1 for degenerative disc disease utilizing morselized autogenous iliac bone graft harvested through a separate fascial incision.

Report as 22612 and 20937.

Within the spine section, instrumentation is reported separately and in addition to arthrodesis. To report instrumentation procedures performed with definitive vertebral procedure(s), see 22840-22855, 22859. Instrumentation procedure codes 22840-22848, 22853, 22854, 22859 are reported in addition to the definitive procedure(s). Modifier 62 may not be appended to the definitive or add-on spinal instrumentation procedure code(s) 22840-22848, 22850, 22852, 22853, 22854, 22859.

Example:

Posterior arthrodesis of L4-S1, utilizing morselized autogenous iliac bone graft harvested through separate fascial incision, and pedicle screw fixation.

Report as 22612, 22614, 22842, and 20937.

Vertebral procedures are sometimes followed by arthrodesis and in addition may include bone grafts and instrumentation.

When arthrodesis is performed in addition to another procedure, the arthrodesis should be reported in addition to the original procedure with modifier 51 (multiple procedures). Examples are after osteotomy, fracture care, vertebral corpectomy, and laminectomy. Bone grafts and instrumentation are never performed without arthrodesis.

Example:

Treatment of a burst fracture of L2 by corpectomy followed by arthrodesis of L1-L3, utilizing anterior instrumentation L1-L3 and structural allograft.

Report as 63090, 22558-51, 22585, 22845, and 20931.

When two surgeons work together as primary surgeons performing distinct part(s) of a single reportable procedure, each surgeon should report his/her distinct operative work by appending modifier 62 to the single definitive procedure code. If additional procedure(s) (including add-on procedure[s]) are performed during the same surgical session, separate code(s) may be reported by each co-surgeon, with modifier 62 appended (see Appendix A).

Example:

A 42-year-old male with a history of posttraumatic degenerative disc disease at L3-4 and L4-5 (internal disc disruption) underwent surgical repair. Surgeon A performed an anterior exposure of the spine with mobilization of the great vessels. Surgeon B performed anterior (minimal) discectomy and fusion at L3-4 and L4-5 using anterior interbody technique.

Report surgeon A: 22558 append modifier 62, 22585 append modifier 62

Report surgeon B: 22558 append modifier 62, 22585 append modifier 62, 20931

Please see the Surgery Guidelines section for the following guidelines:

- *Surgical Procedures on the Musculoskeletal System*

AMA Coding Notes

Surgical Procedures on the Spine (Vertebral Column)

(Do not append modifier 62 to bone graft code 20931)

(For injection procedure for myelography, use 62284)

(For injection procedure for discography, see 62290, 62291)

(For injection procedure, chemonucleolysis, single or multiple levels, use 62292)

(For injection procedure for facet joints, see 64490-64495, 64633-64636)

(For needle or trocar biopsy, see 20220-20225)

AMA *CPT Assistant*

22551: Apr 12: 16, Jul 13: 3, Jan 15: 13, May 16: 13, Aug 18: 10

22552: Apr 12: 16, Jul 13: 3, Aug 18: 10

Plain English Description

The damaged cervical vertebra below C2 is approached from the front (ventral) side of the body. The soft tissues and muscles overlying the cervical spine are dissected. The trachea and esophagus are retracted away from the surgical site. The affected portion of the cervical spine is exposed. A groove or channel is created in the vertebral body to expose the intervertebral disc and nerve roots. The intervertebral disc is exposed and carefully removed with the aid of the surgical microscope. Bone spurs and any bone impinging on the nerve roots is also removed along with the ligament that covers the spinal cord. Cartilage is removed from the vertebral endplates above and below the disc space and the bone is decorticated. Separately reportable bone allograft or autograft is then placed between the vertebral endplates to facilitate the interbody arthrodesis. Separately reportable internal fixation may also be used to stabilize the spine. Upon completion of the procedure, bleeding is controlled, drains are placed as needed, and soft tissues and skin are closed in layers. Use 22551 for a single cervical interspace and 22552 for each additional interspace.

Arthrodesis; anterior interbody, cervical below C-2

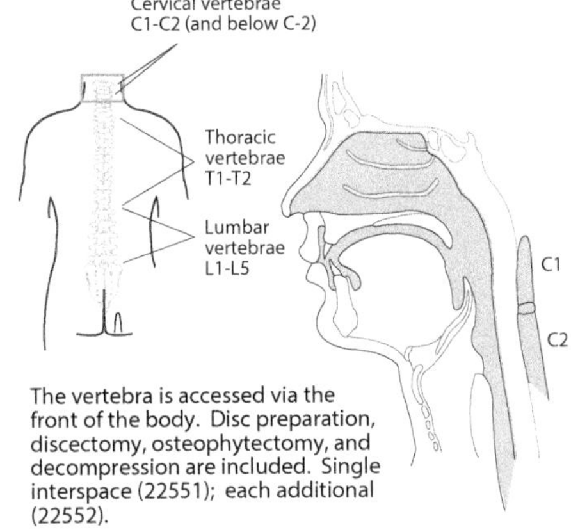

The vertebra is accessed via the front of the body. Disc preparation, discectomy, osteophytectomy, and decompression are included. Single interspace (22551); each additional (22552).

ICD-10-CM Diagnostic Codes

Code	Description
C41.2	Malignant neoplasm of vertebral column
D16.6	Benign neoplasm of vertebral column
M43.02	Spondylolysis, cervical region
M43.03	Spondylolysis, cervicothoracic region
M43.12	Spondylolisthesis, cervical region
M43.13	Spondylolisthesis, cervicothoracic region
M43.5X2	Other recurrent vertebral dislocation, cervical region
M43.8X2	Other specified deforming dorsopathies, cervical region
M43.8X3	Other specified deforming dorsopathies, cervicothoracic region
M46.02	Spinal enthesopathy, cervical region
M46.03	Spinal enthesopathy, cervicothoracic region
M47.12	Other spondylosis with myelopathy, cervical region
M47.13	Other spondylosis with myelopathy, cervicothoracic region
M47.22	Other spondylosis with radiculopathy, cervical region
M47.23	Other spondylosis with radiculopathy, cervicothoracic region
M47.812	Spondylosis without myelopathy or radiculopathy, cervical region
M47.813	Spondylosis without myelopathy or radiculopathy, cervicothoracic region
M47.892	Other spondylosis, cervical region
M47.893	Other spondylosis, cervicothoracic region
M48.02	Spinal stenosis, cervical region
M48.03	Spinal stenosis, cervicothoracic region
M48.42	Fatigue fracture of vertebra, cervical region
M48.43	Fatigue fracture of vertebra, cervicothoracic region
M49.82	Spondylopathy in diseases classified elsewhere, cervical region
M49.83	Spondylopathy in diseases classified elsewhere, cervicothoracic region
M50.03	Cervical disc disorder with myelopathy, cervicothoracic region
M50.11	Cervical disc disorder with radiculopathy, high cervical region
M50.121	Cervical disc disorder at C4-C5 level with radiculopathy
M50.122	Cervical disc disorder at C5-C6 level with radiculopathy
M50.123	Cervical disc disorder at C6-C7 level with radiculopathy
M50.13	Cervical disc disorder with radiculopathy, cervicothoracic region
M50.21	Other cervical disc displacement, high cervical region
M50.221	Other cervical disc displacement at C4-C5 level
M50.222	Other cervical disc displacement at C5-C6 level
M50.223	Other cervical disc displacement at C6-C7 level
M50.23	Other cervical disc displacement, cervicothoracic region
M50.31	Other cervical disc degeneration, high cervical region
M50.321	Other cervical disc degeneration at C4-C5 level
M50.322	Other cervical disc degeneration at C5-C6 level
M50.323	Other cervical disc degeneration at C6-C7 level
M50.33	Other cervical disc degeneration, cervicothoracic region
M50.81	Other cervical disc disorders, high cervical region
M50.821	Other cervical disc disorders at C4-C5 level
M50.822	Other cervical disc disorders at C5-C6 level
M50.823	Other cervical disc disorders at C6-C7 level
M50.83	Other cervical disc disorders, cervicothoracic region
M53.2X3	Spinal instabilities, cervicothoracic region
M80.08	Age-related osteoporosis with current pathological fracture, vertebra(e)
M80.88	Other osteoporosis with current pathological fracture, vertebra(e)
M96.1	Postlaminectomy syndrome, not elsewhere classified
S12.200	Unspecified displaced fracture of third cervical vertebra
S12.24	Type III traumatic spondylolisthesis of third cervical vertebra
S12.250	Other traumatic displaced spondylolisthesis of third cervical vertebra
S12.251	Other traumatic nondisplaced spondylolisthesis of third cervical vertebra
S12.290	Other displaced fracture of third cervical vertebra
S12.34	Type III traumatic spondylolisthesis of fourth cervical vertebra
S12.350	Other traumatic displaced spondylolisthesis of fourth cervical vertebra
S12.351	Other traumatic nondisplaced spondylolisthesis of fourth cervical vertebra
S12.390	Other displaced fracture of fourth cervical vertebra
S12.391	Other nondisplaced fracture of fourth cervical vertebra
S12.44	Type III traumatic spondylolisthesis of fifth cervical vertebra
S12.450	Other traumatic displaced spondylolisthesis of fifth cervical vertebra
S12.451	Other traumatic nondisplaced spondylolisthesis of fifth cervical vertebra
S12.490	Other displaced fracture of fifth cervical vertebra
S12.491	Other nondisplaced fracture of fifth cervical vertebra
S12.54	Type III traumatic spondylolisthesis of sixth cervical vertebra
S12.550	Other traumatic displaced spondylolisthesis of sixth cervical vertebra
S12.551	Other traumatic nondisplaced spondylolisthesis of sixth cervical vertebra
S12.590	Other displaced fracture of sixth cervical vertebra
S12.591	Other nondisplaced fracture of sixth cervical vertebra
S12.64	Type III traumatic spondylolisthesis of seventh cervical vertebra
S12.650	Other traumatic displaced spondylolisthesis of seventh cervical vertebra
S12.651	Other traumatic nondisplaced spondylolisthesis of seventh cervical vertebra
S12.690	Other displaced fracture of seventh cervical vertebra
S12.691	Other nondisplaced fracture of seventh cervical vertebra
S13.131	Dislocation of C2/C3 cervical vertebrae
S13.151	Dislocation of C4/C5 cervical vertebrae
S13.161	Dislocation of C5/C6 cervical vertebrae

ICD-10-CM Coding Notes

For codes requiring a 7th character extension, refer to your ICD-10-CM book. Review the character descriptions and coding guidelines for proper selection. For some procedures, only certain characters will apply.

CCI Edits

Refer to Appendix A for CCI edits.

Facility RVUs 🗋

Code	Work	PE Facility	MP	Total Facility
22551	25.00	16.72	7.66	49.38
22552	6.50	3.09	1.96	11.55

Non-facility RVUs 🗋

Code	Work	PE Non-Facility	MP	Total Non-Facility
22551	25.00	16.72	7.66	49.38
22552	6.50	3.09	1.96	11.55

Modifiers (PAR) 🗋

Code	Mod 50	Mod 51	Mod 62	Mod 66	Mod 80
22551	0	2	2	0	2
22552	0	0	2	0	2

Global Period

Code	Days
22551	090
22552	ZZZ

22554

22554 Arthrodesis, anterior interbody technique, including minimal discectomy to prepare interspace (other than for decompression); cervical below C2

(Do not report 22554 in conjunction with 63075, even if performed by a separate individual. To report anterior cervical discectomy and interbody fusion at the same level during the same session, use 22551)

AMA Coding Guideline

Anterior or Anterolateral Approach Technique Arthrodesis Procedures on the Spine (Vertebral Column)

Procedure codes 22554-22558 are for SINGLE interspace; for additional interspaces, use 22585. A vertebral interspace is the non-bony compartment between two adjacent vertebral bodies, which contains the intervertebral disc, and includes the nucleus pulposus, annulus fibrosus, and two cartilaginous endplates.

For the following codes, when two surgeons work together as primary surgeons performing distinct part(s) of an anterior interbody arthrodesis, each surgeon should report his/her distinct operative work by appending modifier 62 to the procedure code. In this situation, modifier 62 may be appended to the procedure code(s) 22548-22558 and, as appropriate, to the associated additional interspace add-on code 22585 as long as both surgeons continue to work together as primary surgeons.

Arthrodesis Procedures on the Spine (Vertebral Column)

Arthrodesis may be performed in the absence of other procedures and therefore when it is combined with another definitive procedure (eg, osteotomy, fracture care, vertebral corpectomy or laminectomy), modifier 51 is appropriate. However, arthrodesis codes 22585, 22614, and 22632 are considered add-on procedure codes and should not be used with modifier 51.

To report instrumentation procedures, see 22840-22855, 22859. (Codes 22840-22848, 22853, 22854, 22859 are reported in conjunction with code[s] for the definitive procedure[s]. When instrumentation reinsertion or removal is reported in conjunction with other definitive procedures, including arthrodesis, decompression, and exploration of fusion, append modifier 51 to 22849, 22850, 22852, and 22855.) To report exploration of fusion, use 22830. (When exploration is reported in conjunction with other definitive procedures, including arthrodesis and decompression, append modifier 51 to 22830.) Do not append modifier 62 to spinal instrumentation codes 22840-22848, 22850, 22852, 22853, 22854, 22859.

To report bone graft procedures, see 20930-20938. (Report in addition to code[s] for the definitive procedure[s].) Do not append modifier 62 to bone graft codes 20900-20938.

Surgical Procedures on the Spine (Vertebral Column)

Cervical, thoracic, and lumbar spine.

Within the spine section, bone grafting procedures are reported separately and in addition to arthrodesis. For bone grafts in other Musculoskeletal sections, see specific code(s) descriptor(s) and/or accompanying guidelines.

To report bone grafts performed after arthrodesis, see 20930-20938. Do not append modifier 62 to bone graft codes 20900-20938.

Example:

Posterior arthrodesis of L5-S1 for degenerative disc disease utilizing morselized autogenous iliac bone graft harvested through a separate fascial incision.

Report as 22612 and 20937.

Within the spine section, instrumentation is reported separately and in addition to arthrodesis. To report instrumentation procedures performed with definitive vertebral procedure(s), see 22840-22855, 22859. Instrumentation procedure codes 22840-22848, 22853, 22854, 22859 are reported in addition to the definitive procedure(s). Modifier 62 may not be appended to the definitive or add-on spinal instrumentation procedure code(s) 22840-22848, 22850, 22852, 22853, 22854, 22859.

Example:

Posterior arthrodesis of L4-S1, utilizing morselized autogenous iliac bone graft harvested through separate fascial incision, and pedicle screw fixation.

Report as 22612, 22614, 22842, and 20937.

Vertebral procedures are sometimes followed by arthrodesis and in addition may include bone grafts and instrumentation.

When arthrodesis is performed in addition to another procedure, the arthrodesis should be reported in addition to the original procedure with modifier 51 (multiple procedures). Examples are after osteotomy, fracture care, vertebral corpectomy, and laminectomy. Bone grafts and instrumentation are never performed without arthrodesis.

Example:

Treatment of a burst fracture of L2 by corpectomy followed by arthrodesis of L1-L3, utilizing anterior instrumentation L1-L3 and structural allograft.

Report as 63090, 22558-51, 22585, 22845, and 20931.

When two surgeons work together as primary surgeons performing distinct part(s) of a single reportable procedure, each surgeon should report his/her distinct operative work by appending modifier 62 to the single definitive procedure code. If additional procedure(s) (including add-on procedure[s]) are performed during the same surgical session, separate code(s) may be reported by each co-surgeon, with modifier 62 appended (see Appendix A).

Example:

A 42-year-old male with a history of posttraumatic degenerative disc disease at L3-4 and L4-5 (internal disc disruption) underwent surgical repair. Surgeon A performed an anterior exposure of the spine with mobilization of the great vessels. Surgeon B performed anterior (minimal) discectomy and fusion at L3-4 and L4-5 using anterior interbody technique.

Report surgeon A: 22558 append modifier 62, 22585 append modifier 62

Report surgeon B: 22558 append modifier 62, 22585 append modifier 62, 20931

Please see the Surgery Guidelines section for the following guidelines:

- *Surgical Procedures on the Musculoskeletal System*

AMA Coding Notes

Surgical Procedures on the Spine (Vertebral Column)

(Do not append modifier 62 to bone graft code 20931)

(For injection procedure for myelography, use 62284)

(For injection procedure for discography, see 62290, 62291)

(For injection procedure, chemonucleolysis, single or multiple levels, use 62292)

(For injection procedure for facet joints, see 64490-64495, 64633-64636)

(For needle or trocar biopsy, see 20220-20225)

AMA *CPT Assistant*

22554: Spring 93: 36, Sep 97: 8, Sep 00: 10, Jan 01: 12, Feb 02: 4, Apr 12: 16, Jul 13: 3, Apr 15: 7

Plain English Description

Spinal surgical immobilization of a joint, inducing the bones to grow solidly together, is performed for herniated disks, lesions, and stabilization of fractures and dislocations of the spine. Traction is applied to the head. The damaged vertebrae is approached from the front (ventral) side of the body. A cut is made through the neck, avoiding the esophagus, trachea, and thyroid. An instrument is used to hold the intervertebral muscles apart. A drill is inserted in the afflicted vertebrae and the positioning of the drill is confirmed via X-ray. The drill or saw is then used to cut a groove or channel in the front of the vertebrae. The area between the two adjacent vertebrae is cleaned out with spring-loaded forceps that are equipped with a sharp blade. The cartilage containing plates above and below the vertebrae to be fused is removed. The physician takes bone procured from a donor or the hip area of the individual undergoing the procedure. The bone graft is packed into the spaces, cleaned out, and trimmed to fit. The traction to the head is slowly lessened so the bone graft stays in place. The fibrous membranes covering the deep vertebral area are sutured, a drain is placed, and the incision is sutured.

ICD-10-CM Diagnostic Codes

C41.2 Malignant neoplasm of vertebral column
D16.6 Benign neoplasm of vertebral column
M43.02 Spondylolysis, cervical region
M43.03 Spondylolysis, cervicothoracic region
M43.12 Spondylolisthesis, cervical region
M43.13 Spondylolisthesis, cervicothoracic region
M43.5X2 Other recurrent vertebral dislocation, cervical region
M43.5X3 Other recurrent vertebral dislocation, cervicothoracic region
M43.8X2 Other specified deforming dorsopathies, cervical region
M43.8X3 Other specified deforming dorsopathies, cervicothoracic region
M46.02 Spinal enthesopathy, cervical region
M46.03 Spinal enthesopathy, cervicothoracic region
M47.12 Other spondylosis with myelopathy, cervical region
M47.13 Other spondylosis with myelopathy, cervicothoracic region
M47.22 Other spondylosis with radiculopathy, cervical region
M47.23 Other spondylosis with radiculopathy, cervicothoracic region
M47.812 Spondylosis without myelopathy or radiculopathy, cervical region
M47.813 Spondylosis without myelopathy or radiculopathy, cervicothoracic region
M47.892 Other spondylosis, cervical region
M47.893 Other spondylosis, cervicothoracic region
M48.02 Spinal stenosis, cervical region
M48.03 Spinal stenosis, cervicothoracic region
M50.10 Cervical disc disorder with radiculopathy, unspecified cervical region
M96.1 Postlaminectomy syndrome, not elsewhere classified
⑦ S12.24 Type III traumatic spondylolisthesis of third cervical vertebra
⑦ S12.250 Other traumatic displaced spondylolisthesis of third cervical vertebra
⑦ S12.251 Other traumatic nondisplaced spondylolisthesis of third cervical vertebra
⑦ S12.290 Other displaced fracture of third cervical vertebra
⑦ S12.291 Other nondisplaced fracture of third cervical vertebra
⑦ S12.34 Type III traumatic spondylolisthesis of fourth cervical vertebra
⑦ S12.350 Other traumatic displaced spondylolisthesis of fourth cervical vertebra
⑦ S12.351 Other traumatic nondisplaced spondylolisthesis of fourth cervical vertebra
⑦ S12.390 Other displaced fracture of fourth cervical vertebra
⑦ S12.391 Other nondisplaced fracture of fourth cervical vertebra
⑦ S12.44 Type III traumatic spondylolisthesis of fifth cervical vertebra
⑦ S12.450 Other traumatic displaced spondylolisthesis of fifth cervical vertebra
⑦ S12.451 Other traumatic nondisplaced spondylolisthesis of fifth cervical vertebra
⑦ S12.490 Other displaced fracture of fifth cervical vertebra
⑦ S12.491 Other nondisplaced fracture of fifth cervical vertebra
⑦ S12.54 Type III traumatic spondylolisthesis of sixth cervical vertebra
⑦ S12.550 Other traumatic displaced spondylolisthesis of sixth cervical vertebra
⑦ S12.551 Other traumatic nondisplaced spondylolisthesis of sixth cervical vertebra
⑦ S12.590 Other displaced fracture of sixth cervical vertebra
⑦ S12.591 Other nondisplaced fracture of sixth cervical vertebra
⑦ S12.64 Type III traumatic spondylolisthesis of seventh cervical vertebra
⑦ S12.650 Other traumatic displaced spondylolisthesis of seventh cervical vertebra
⑦ S12.651 Other traumatic nondisplaced spondylolisthesis of seventh cervical vertebra
⑦ S12.690 Other displaced fracture of seventh cervical vertebra
⑦ S12.691 Other nondisplaced fracture of seventh cervical vertebra
⑦ S13.100 Subluxation of unspecified cervical vertebrae
⑦ S13.161 Dislocation of C5/C6 cervical vertebrae
⑦ S13.181 Dislocation of C7/T1 cervical vertebrae

ICD-10-CM Coding Notes

For codes requiring a 7th character extension, refer to your ICD-10-CM book. Review the character descriptions and coding guidelines for proper selection. For some procedures, only certain characters will apply.

CCI Edits

Refer to Appendix A for CCI edits.

Facility RVUs ▯

Code	Work	PE Facility	MP	Total Facility
22554	17.69	13.39	5.25	36.33

Non-facility RVUs ▯

Code	Work	PE Non-Facility	MP	Total Non-Facility
22554	17.69	13.39	5.25	36.33

Modifiers (PAR) ▯

Code	Mod 50	Mod 51	Mod 62	Mod 66	Mod 80
22554	0	2	2	0	2

Global Period

Code	Days
22554	090

22558

22558 Arthrodesis, anterior interbody technique, including minimal discectomy to prepare interspace (other than for decompression); lumbar

(For arthrodesis using pre-sacral interbody technique, use 22586)

AMA Coding Guideline

Anterior or Anterolateral Approach Technique Arthrodesis Procedures on the Spine (Vertebral Column)

Procedure codes 22554-22558 are for SINGLE interspace; for additional interspaces, use 22585. A vertebral interspace is the non-bony compartment between two adjacent vertebral bodies, which contains the intervertebral disc, and includes the nucleus pulposus, annulus fibrosus, and two cartilaginous endplates.

For the following codes, when two surgeons work together as primary surgeons performing distinct part(s) of an anterior interbody arthrodesis, each surgeon should report his/her distinct operative work by appending modifier 62 to the procedure code. In this situation, modifier 62 may be appended to the procedure code(s) 22548-22558 and, as appropriate, to the associated additional interspace add-on code 22585 as long as both surgeons continue to work together as primary surgeons.

Arthrodesis Procedures on the Spine (Vertebral Column)

Arthrodesis may be performed in the absence of other procedures and therefore when it is combined with another definitive procedure (eg, osteotomy, fracture care, vertebral corpectomy or laminectomy), modifier 51 is appropriate. However, arthrodesis codes 22585, 22614, and 22632 are considered add-on procedure codes and should not be used with modifier 51.

To report instrumentation procedures, see 22840-22855, 22859. (Codes 22840-22848, 22853, 22854, 22859 are reported in conjunction with code[s] for the definitive procedure[s]. When instrumentation reinsertion or removal is reported in conjunction with other definitive procedures, including arthrodesis, decompression, and exploration of fusion, append modifier 51 to 22849, 22850, 22852, and 22855.) To report exploration of fusion, use 22830. (When exploration is reported in conjunction with other definitive procedures, including arthrodesis and decompression, append modifier 51 to 22830.) Do not append modifier 62 to spinal instrumentation codes 22840-22848, 22850, 22852, 22853, 22854, 22859.

To report bone graft procedures, see 20930-20938. (Report in addition to code[s] for the definitive procedure[s].) Do not append modifier 62 to bone graft codes 20900-20938.

Surgical Procedures on the Spine (Vertebral Column)

Cervical, thoracic, and lumbar spine.

Within the spine section, bone grafting procedures are reported separately and in addition to arthrodesis. For bone grafts in other Musculoskeletal sections, see specific code(s) descriptor(s) and/or accompanying guidelines.

To report bone grafts performed after arthrodesis, see 20930-20938. Do not append modifier 62 to bone graft codes 20900-20938.

Example:

Posterior arthrodesis of L5-S1 for degenerative disc disease utilizing morselized autogenous iliac bone graft harvested through a separate fascial incision.

Report as 22612 and 20937.

Within the spine section, instrumentation is reported separately and in addition to arthrodesis. To report instrumentation procedures performed with definitive vertebral procedure(s), see 22840-22855, 22859. Instrumentation procedure codes 22840-22848, 22853, 22854, 22859 are reported in addition to the definitive procedure(s). Modifier 62 may not be appended to the definitive or add-on spinal instrumentation procedure code(s) 22840-22848, 22850, 22852, 22853, 22854, 22859.

Example:

Posterior arthrodesis of L4-S1, utilizing morselized autogenous iliac bone graft harvested through separate fascial incision, and pedicle screw fixation.

Report as 22612, 22614, 22842, and 20937.

Vertebral procedures are sometimes followed by arthrodesis and in addition may include bone grafts and instrumentation.

When arthrodesis is performed in addition to another procedure, the arthrodesis should be reported in addition to the original procedure with modifier 51 (multiple procedures). Examples are after osteotomy, fracture care, vertebral corpectomy, and laminectomy. Bone grafts and instrumentation are never performed without arthrodesis.

Example:

Treatment of a burst fracture of L2 by corpectomy followed by arthrodesis of L1-L3, utilizing anterior instrumentation L1-L3 and structural allograft.

Report as 63090, 22558-51, 22585, 22845, and 20931.

When two surgeons work together as primary surgeons performing distinct part(s) of a single reportable procedure, each surgeon should report his/her distinct operative work by appending modifier 62 to the single definitive procedure code. If additional procedure(s) (including add-on procedure[s]) are performed during the same surgical session, separate code(s) may be reported by each co-surgeon, with modifier 62 appended (see Appendix A).

Example:

A 42-year-old male with a history of posttraumatic degenerative disc disease at L3-4 and L4-5 (internal disc disruption) underwent surgical repair. Surgeon A performed an anterior exposure of the spine with mobilization of the great vessels. Surgeon B performed anterior (minimal) discectomy and fusion at L3-4 and L4-5 using anterior interbody technique.

Report surgeon A: 22558 append modifier 62, 22585 append modifier 62

Report surgeon B: 22558 append modifier 62, 22585 append modifier 62, 20931

Please see the Surgery Guidelines section for the following guidelines:

- *Surgical Procedures on the Musculoskeletal System*

AMA Coding Notes

Surgical Procedures on the Spine (Vertebral Column)

(Do not append modifier 62 to bone graft code 20931)

(For injection procedure for myelography, use 62284)

(For injection procedure for discography, see 62290, 62291)

(For injection procedure, chemonucleolysis, single or multiple levels, use 62292)

(For injection procedure for facet joints, see 64490-64495, 64633-64636)

(For needle or trocar biopsy, see 20220-20225)

AMA *CPT Assistant* ▯

22558: Spring 93: 36, Mar 96: 6, Jul 96: 7, Sep 97: 8, Sep 00: 10, Feb 02: 4, Oct 09: 9, Apr 12: 16, Jul 13: 3, Mar 15: 9

Plain English Description

Spinal surgical immobilization of a joint, inducing bones to grow solidly together, is performed for herniated disks, lesions, and stabilization of fractures and dislocations of the spine. Traction is applied to the head. The damaged vertebrae is approached from the part of the lower back between the thorax and the pelvis (lumbar). A cut is made through the back. An instrument is used to hold the intervertebral muscles apart. A drill is inserted in the afflicted vertebrae and the positioning of the drill is confirmed via X-ray. The drill or saw is then used to cut a groove or channel in the front of the vertebrae. The area between the two adjacent vertebrae is cleaned out with spring-loaded forceps that are equipped with a sharp blade. The cartilage containing plates above and below the vertebrae to be fused is removed. The physician takes bone procured from a donor or the hip area of the individual undergoing the procedure. The bone graft is packed into the spaces, cleaned out, and trimmed to fit. The traction to the head is slowly lessened so the bone graft stays in place. The fibrous membranes covering the deep vertebral area are sutured, a drain is placed, and the incision is sutured.

ICD-10-CM Diagnostic Codes

	Code	Description
	C41.2	Malignant neoplasm of vertebral column
	C79.51	Secondary malignant neoplasm of bone
	D33.4	Benign neoplasm of spinal cord
	M40.36	Flatback syndrome, lumbar region
	M40.46	Postural lordosis, lumbar region
	M40.47	Postural lordosis, lumbosacral region
	M46.47	Discitis, unspecified, lumbosacral region
	M47.16	Other spondylosis with myelopathy, lumbar region
	M51.06	Intervertebral disc disorders with myelopathy, lumbar region
	M51.34	Other intervertebral disc degeneration, thoracic region
	M51.36	Other intervertebral disc degeneration, lumbar region
	M51.46	Schmorl's nodes, lumbar region
	M54.17	Radiculopathy, lumbosacral region
⇄	M54.31	Sciatica, right side
	M96.1	Postlaminectomy syndrome, not elsewhere classified
	Q76.2	Congenital spondylolisthesis

CCI Edits

Refer to Appendix A for CCI edits.

Facility RVUs ▯

Code	Work	PE Facility	MP	Total Facility
22558	23.53	14.91	5.95	44.39

Non-facility RVUs ▯

Code	Work	PE Non-Facility	MP	Total Non-Facility
22558	23.53	14.91	5.95	44.39

Modifiers (PAR) ▯

Code	Mod 50	Mod 51	Mod 62	Mod 66	Mod 80
22558	0	2	2	0	2

Global Period

Code	Days
22558	090

22585

✚ **22585 Arthrodesis, anterior interbody technique, including minimal discectomy to prepare interspace (other than for decompression); each additional interspace (List separately in addition to code for primary procedure)**

(Use 22585 in conjunction with 22554, 22556, 22558)

(Do not report 22585 in conjunction with 63075, even if performed by a separate individual. To report anterior cervical discectomy and interbody fusion at the same level during the same session, use 22552)

AMA Coding Guideline

Anterior or Anterolateral Approach Technique Arthrodesis Procedures on the Spine (Vertebral Column)

Procedure codes 22554-22558 are for SINGLE interspace; for additional interspaces, use 22585. A vertebral interspace is the non-bony compartment between two adjacent vertebral bodies, which contains the intervertebral disc, and includes the nucleus pulposus, annulus fibrosus, and two cartilaginous endplates.

For the following codes, when two surgeons work together as primary surgeons performing distinct part(s) of an anterior interbody arthrodesis, each surgeon should report his/her distinct operative work by appending modifier 62 to the procedure code. In this situation, modifier 62 may be appended to the procedure code(s) 22548-22558 and, as appropriate, to the associated additional interspace add-on code 22585 as long as both surgeons continue to work together as primary surgeons.

Arthrodesis Procedures on the Spine (Vertebral Column)

Arthrodesis may be performed in the absence of other procedures and therefore when it is combined with another definitive procedure (eg, osteotomy, fracture care, vertebral corpectomy or laminectomy), modifier 51 is appropriate. However, arthrodesis codes 22585, 22614, and 22632 are considered add-on procedure codes and should not be used with modifier 51.

To report instrumentation procedures, see 22840-22855, 22859. (Codes 22840-22848, 22853, 22854, 22859 are reported in conjunction with code[s] for the definitive procedure[s]. When instrumentation reinsertion or removal is reported in conjunction with other definitive procedures, including arthrodesis, decompression, and exploration of fusion, append modifier 51 to 22849, 22850, 22852, and 22855.) To report exploration of fusion, use 22830. (When exploration is reported in conjunction with other definitive procedures, including arthrodesis and decompression, append modifier 51 to 22830.) Do not append modifier 62 to spinal instrumentation codes 22840-22848, 22850, 22852, 22853, 22854, 22859.

To report bone graft procedures, see 20930-20938. (Report in addition to code[s] for the definitive procedure[s].) Do not append modifier 62 to bone graft codes 20900-20938.

Surgical Procedures on the Spine (Vertebral Column)

Cervical, thoracic, and lumbar spine.

Within the spine section, bone grafting procedures are reported separately and in addition to arthrodesis. For bone grafts in other Musculoskeletal sections, see specific code(s) descriptor(s) and/or accompanying guidelines.

To report bone grafts performed after arthrodesis, see 20930-20938. Do not append modifier 62 to bone graft codes 20900-20938.

Example:

Posterior arthrodesis of L5 S1 for degenerative disc disease utilizing morselized autogenous iliac bone graft harvested through a separate fascial incision.

Report as 22612 and 20937.

Within the spine section, instrumentation is reported separately and in addition to arthrodesis. To report instrumentation procedures performed with definitive vertebral procedure(s), see 22840-22855, 22859. Instrumentation procedure codes 22840-22848, 22853, 22854, 22859 are reported in addition to the definitive procedure(s). Modifier 62 may not be appended to the definitive or add-on spinal instrumentation procedure code(s) 22840-22848, 22850, 22852, 22853, 22854, 22859.

Example:

Posterior arthrodesis of L4-S1, utilizing morselized autogenous iliac bone graft harvested through separate fascial incision, and pedicle screw fixation.

Report as 22612, 22614, 22842, and 20937.

Vertebral procedures are sometimes followed by arthrodesis and in addition may include bone grafts and instrumentation.

When arthrodesis is performed in addition to another procedure, the arthrodesis should be reported in addition to the original procedure with modifier 51 (multiple procedures). Examples are after osteotomy, fracture care, vertebral corpectomy, and laminectomy. Bone grafts and instrumentation are never performed without arthrodesis.

Example:

Treatment of a burst fracture of L2 by corpectomy followed by arthrodesis of L1-L3, utilizing anterior instrumentation L1-L3 and structural allograft.

Report as 63090, 22558-51, 22585, 22845, and 20931.

When two surgeons work together as primary surgeons performing distinct part(s) of a single reportable procedure, each surgeon should report his/her distinct operative work by appending modifier 62 to the single definitive procedure code. If additional procedure(s) (including add-on procedure[s]) are performed during the same surgical session, separate code(s) may be reported by each co-surgeon, with modifier 62 appended (see Appendix A).

Example:

A 42-year-old male with a history of posttraumatic degenerative disc disease at L3-4 and L4-5 (internal disc disruption) underwent surgical repair. Surgeon A performed an anterior exposure of the spine with mobilization of the great vessels. Surgeon B performed anterior (minimal) discectomy and fusion at L3-4 and L4-5 using anterior interbody technique.

Report surgeon A: 22558 append modifier 62, 22585 append modifier 62

Report surgeon B: 22558 append modifier 62, 22585 append modifier 62, 20931

Please see the Surgery Guidelines section for the following guidelines:

- *Surgical Procedures on the Musculoskeletal System*

AMA Coding Notes

Surgical Procedures on the Spine (Vertebral Column)

(Do not append modifier 62 to bone graft code 20931)

(For injection procedure for myelography, use 62284)

(For injection procedure for discography, see 62290, 62291)

(For injection procedure, chemonucleolysis, single or multiple levels, use 62292)

(For injection procedure for facet joints, see 64490-64495, 64633-64636)

(For needle or trocar biopsy, see 20220-20225)

AMA *CPT Assistant* ☐

22585: Spring 93: 36, Feb 96: 6, Mar 96: 6, Sep 97: 8, Sep 00: 10, Feb 02: 4, Apr 08: 11

Plain English Description

Spinal surgical immobilization of a joint, inducing the bones to grow solidly together, is performed for herniated disks, lesions, and stabilization of fractures and dislocations of the spine. Traction is applied to the head. The damaged vertebrae is approached from the front (ventral) side of the body. A cut is made through the neck, avoiding the esophagus, trachea, and thyroid. An instrument is used to hold the intervertebral muscles apart. A drill is inserted in the afflicted vertebrae and the positioning of the drill is confirmed via X-ray. The drill or saw is then used to cut a groove or channel in the front of the vertebrae. The area between the two adjacent vertebrae is cleaned out with spring-loaded forceps that are equipped with a sharp blade. The cartilage containing plates above and below the vertebrae to be fused is removed. The physician takes bone procured from a donor or the hip area of the individual undergoing the procedure. The bone graft is packed into the spaces, cleaned out, and trimmed to fit. The traction to the head is slowly lessened so the bone graft stays in place. The fibrous membranes covering the deep vertebral area are sutured, a drain is placed, and the incision is sutured. This code is for each additional interspace. This code can be added to codes 22554, 22556, or 22558.

ICD-10-CM Diagnostic Codes

See Primary Procedure code for crosswalks.

CCI Edits

Refer to Appendix A for CCI edits.

Facility RVUs

Code	Work	PE Facility	MP	Total Facility
22585	5.52	2.52	1.47	9.51

Non-facility RVUs

Code	Work	PE Non-Facility	MP	Total Non-Facility
22585	5.52	2.52	1.47	9.51

Modifiers (PAR)

Code	Mod 50	Mod 51	Mod 62	Mod 66	Mod 80
22585	0	0	2	0	2

Global Period

Code	Days
22585	ZZZ

22600-22614

22600 Arthrodesis, posterior or posterolateral technique, single level; cervical below C2 segment

22610 Arthrodesis, posterior or posterolateral technique, single level; thoracic (with lateral transverse technique, when performed)

22612 Arthrodesis, posterior or posterolateral technique, single level; lumbar (with lateral transverse technique, when performed)

(Do not report 22612 in conjunction with 22630 for the same interspace and segment, use 22633)

+ **22614 Arthrodesis, posterior or posterolateral technique, single level; each additional vertebral segment (List separately in addition to code for primary procedure)**

(Use 22614 in conjunction with 22600, 22610, 22612, 22630 or 22633 when performed at a different level. When performing a posterior or posterolateral technique for fusion/arthrodesis at an additional level, use 22614. When performing a posterior interbody fusion arthrodesis at an additional level, use 22632. When performing a combined posterior or posterolateral technique with posterior interbody arthrodesis at an additional level, use 22634)

(For facet joint fusion, see 0219T-0222T)

(For placement of a posterior intrafacet implant, see 0219T-0222T)

AMA Coding Guideline

Posterior, Posterolateral or Lateral Transverse Process Technique Arthrodesis Procedures on the Spine (Vertebral Column)

To report instrumentation procedures, see 22840-22855, 22859. (Report in addition to code[s] for the definitive procedure[s].) Do not append modifier 62 to spinal instrumentation codes 22840-22848, 22850, 22852, 22853, 22854, 22859.

To report bone graft procedures, see 20930-20938. (Report in addition to code[s] for the definitive procedure[s].) Do not append modifier 62 to bone graft codes 20900-20938.

A vertebral segment describes the basic constituent part into which the spine may be divided. It represents a single complete vertebral bone with its associated articular processes and laminae. A vertebral interspace is the non-bony compartment between two adjacent vertebral bodies which contains the intervertebral disc, and includes the nucleus pulposus, annulus fibrosus, and two cartilaginous endplates.

Arthrodesis Procedures on the Spine (Vertebral Column)

Arthrodesis may be performed in the absence of other procedures and therefore when it is combined with another definitive procedure (eg, osteotomy, fracture care, vertebral corpectomy or laminectomy), modifier 51 is appropriate. However, arthrodesis codes 22585, 22614, and 22632 are considered add-on procedure codes and should not be used with modifier 51.

To report instrumentation procedures, see 22840-22855, 22859. (Codes 22840-22848, 22853, 22854, 22859 are reported in conjunction with code[s] for the definitive procedure[s]. When instrumentation reinsertion or removal is reported in conjunction with other definitive procedures, including arthrodesis, decompression, and exploration of fusion, append modifier 51 to 22849, 22850, 22852, and 22855.) To report exploration of fusion, use 22830. (When exploration is reported in conjunction with other definitive procedures, including arthrodesis and decompression, append modifier 51 to 22830.) Do not append modifier 62 to spinal instrumentation codes 22840-22848, 22850, 22852, 22853, 22854, 22859.

To report bone graft procedures, see 20930-20938. (Report in addition to code[s] for the definitive procedure[s].) Do not append modifier 62 to bone graft codes 20900-20938.

Surgical Procedures on the Spine (Vertebral Column)

Cervical, thoracic, and lumbar spine.

Within the spine section, bone grafting procedures are reported separately and in addition to arthrodesis. For bone grafts in other Musculoskeletal sections, see specific code(s) descriptor(s) and/or accompanying guidelines.

To report bone grafts performed after arthrodesis, see 20930-20938. Do not append modifier 62 to bone graft codes 20900-20938.

Example:

Posterior arthrodesis of L5-S1 for degenerative disc disease utilizing morselized autogenous iliac bone graft harvested through a separate fascial incision.

Report as 22612 and 20937.

Within the spine section, instrumentation is reported separately and in addition to arthrodesis. To report instrumentation procedures performed with definitive vertebral procedure(s), see 22840-22855, 22859. Instrumentation procedure codes 22840-22848, 22853, 22854, 22859 are reported in addition to the definitive procedure(s). Modifier 62 may not be appended to the definitive or add-on spinal instrumentation procedure code(s) 22840-22848, 22850, 22852, 22853, 22854, 22859.

Example:

Posterior arthrodesis of L4-S1, utilizing morselized autogenous iliac bone graft harvested through separate fascial incision, and pedicle screw fixation. Report as 22612, 22614, 22842, and 20937.

Vertebral procedures are sometimes followed by arthrodesis and in addition may include bone grafts and instrumentation.

When arthrodesis is performed in addition to another procedure, the arthrodesis should be reported in addition to the original procedure with modifier 51 (multiple procedures). Examples are after osteotomy, fracture care, vertebral corpectomy, and laminectomy. Bone grafts and instrumentation are never performed without arthrodesis.

Example:

Treatment of a burst fracture of L2 by corpectomy followed by arthrodesis of L1-L3, utilizing anterior instrumentation L1-L3 and structural allograft.

Report as 63090, 22558-51, 22585, 22845, and 20931.

When two surgeons work together as primary surgeons performing distinct part(s) of a single reportable procedure, each surgeon should report his/her distinct operative work by appending modifier 62 to the single definitive procedure code. If additional procedure(s) (including add-on procedure[s]) are performed during the same surgical session, separate code(s) may be reported by each co-surgeon, with modifier 62 appended (see Appendix A).

Example:

A 42-year-old male with a history of posttraumatic degenerative disc disease at L3-4 and L4-5 (internal disc disruption) underwent surgical repair. Surgeon A performed an anterior exposure of the spine with mobilization of the great vessels. Surgeon B performed anterior (minimal) discectomy and fusion at L3-4 and L4-5 using anterior interbody technique.

Report surgeon A: 22558 append modifier 62, 22585 append modifier 62

Report surgeon B: 22558 append modifier 62, 22585 append modifier 62, 20931

Please see the Surgery Guidelines section for the following guidelines:

- *Surgical Procedures on the Musculoskeletal System*

AMA Coding Notes

Surgical Procedures on the Spine (Vertebral Column)

(Do not append modifier 62 to bone graft code 20931)

(For injection procedure for myelography, use 62284)

(For injection procedure for discography, see 62290, 62291)

(For injection procedure, chemonucleolysis, single or multiple levels, use 62292)

(For injection procedure for facet joints, see 64490-64495, 64633-64636)

(For needle or trocar biopsy, see 20220-20225)

AMA *CPT Assistant* ☐

22600: Spring 93: 36, Sep 97: 8, Nov 10: 8, Apr 12: 16, Jun 12: 11, Jul 13: 3

22610: Spring 93: 36, Sep 97: 8, Nov 10: 8, Apr 12: 16, Jun 12: 10, Jul 13: 3

22612: Spring 93: 36, Mar 96: 7, Sep 97: 8, 11, Apr 08: 11, Jul 08: 7, Oct 09: 9, Nov 10: 8, Dec 11: 14, Jan 12: 3, Apr 12: 16, Jun 12: 10, Jul 13: 3, Dec 13: 14

22614: Feb 96: 6, Mar 96: 7, Nov 10: 8, Jun 12: 11, Jul 13: 3

Plain English Description

Posterior or posterolateral arthrodesis, also referred to as fusion, of one or more intervertebral joints is performed to treat a fracture or other instability. Fusion may be used alone or in conjunction with other procedures. If a posterior or posterolateral approach is used, an incision is made in the back of the neck or in the back over the affected vertebral joints. Soft tissues are dissected and the vertebrae are exposed. Separately reportable fracture treatment or decompression is performed as needed. The transverse processes, facet joints, and/or lamina are prepared for bone grafting. A separately reportable bone graft is obtained from the iliac crest or other site and prepared. Allograft bone obtained from a bone bank may also be used. The bone graft is placed. Drill holes are created in the facets or spinous processes of each vertebra and wires are threaded through the vertebrae to immobilize the joint. Alternatively, other reportable internal fixation devices may be placed through the pedicles or facets. A drain may be placed and the surgical wound is then closed in layers. Use 22600 for fusion of a single level of the cervical spine below the C2 segment; use 22610 for fusion of a single level of the thoracic spine; use 22612 for fusion of a single level of the lumbar spine. Use 22614 for fusion of each additional vertebral segment.

Arthrodesis, posterior or posterolateral technique

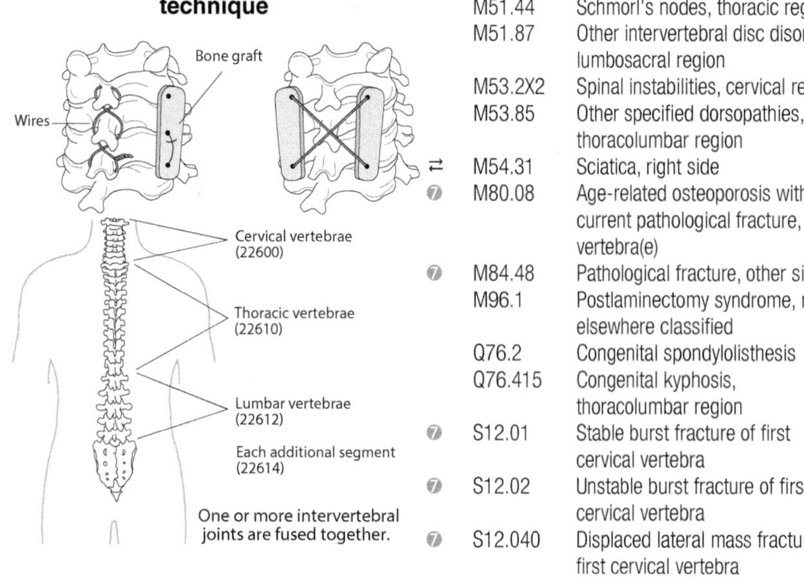

ICD-10-CM Diagnostic Codes

	Code	Description
	C41.2	Malignant neoplasm of vertebral column
	D16.6	Benign neoplasm of vertebral column
	M43.02	Spondylolysis, cervical region
	M43.03	Spondylolysis, cervicothoracic region
	M43.13	Spondylolisthesis, cervicothoracic region
	M46.45	Discitis, unspecified, thoracolumbar region
	M47.14	Other spondylosis with myelopathy, thoracic region
	M47.15	Other spondylosis with myelopathy, thoracolumbar region
	M47.16	Other spondylosis with myelopathy, lumbar region
	M47.26	Other spondylosis with radiculopathy, lumbar region
	M47.897	Other spondylosis, lumbosacral region
	M48.02	Spinal stenosis, cervical region
	M48.03	Spinal stenosis, cervicothoracic region
	M48.04	Spinal stenosis, thoracic region
	M48.05	Spinal stenosis, thoracolumbar region
	M48.061	Spinal stenosis, lumbar region without neurogenic claudication
	M48.062	Spinal stenosis, lumbar region with neurogenic claudication
	M48.07	Spinal stenosis, lumbosacral region
⑦	M48.46	Fatigue fracture of vertebra, lumbar region
	M50.23	Other cervical disc displacement, cervicothoracic region
	M51.24	Other intervertebral disc displacement, thoracic region
	M51.25	Other intervertebral disc displacement, thoracolumbar region
	M51.34	Other intervertebral disc degeneration, thoracic region
	M51.36	Other intervertebral disc degeneration, lumbar region
	M51.44	Schmorl's nodes, thoracic region
	M51.87	Other intervertebral disc disorders, lumbosacral region
	M53.2X2	Spinal instabilities, cervical region
	M53.85	Other specified dorsopathies, thoracolumbar region
⇄	M54.31	Sciatica, right side
⑦	M80.08	Age-related osteoporosis with current pathological fracture, vertebra(e)
⑦	M84.48	Pathological fracture, other site
	M96.1	Postlaminectomy syndrome, not elsewhere classified
	Q76.2	Congenital spondylolisthesis
	Q76.415	Congenital kyphosis, thoracolumbar region
⑦	S12.01	Stable burst fracture of first cervical vertebra
⑦	S12.02	Unstable burst fracture of first cervical vertebra
⑦	S12.040	Displaced lateral mass fracture of first cervical vertebra
⑦	S12.090	Other displaced fracture of first cervical vertebra
⑦	S12.110	Anterior displaced Type II dens fracture
⑦	S12.111	Posterior displaced Type II dens fracture
⑦	S12.112	Nondisplaced Type II dens fracture
⑦	S12.120	Other displaced dens fracture
⑦	S12.150	Other traumatic displaced spondylolisthesis of second cervical vertebra
⑦	S12.190	Other displaced fracture of second cervical vertebra
⑦	S13.100	Subluxation of unspecified cervical vertebrae
⑦	S13.161	Dislocation of C5/C6 cervical vertebrae
⑦	S13.181	Dislocation of C7/T1 cervical vertebrae
⑦	S22.018	Other fracture of first thoracic vertebra
⑦	S22.038	Other fracture of third thoracic vertebra
⑦	S22.058	Other fracture of T5-T6 vertebra
⑦	S22.068	Other fracture of T7-T8 thoracic vertebra
⑦	S22.088	Other fracture of T11-T12 vertebra
⑦	S23.111	Dislocation of T1/T2 thoracic vertebra
⑦	S23.122	Subluxation of T3/T4 thoracic vertebra
⑦	S23.123	Dislocation of T3/T4 thoracic vertebra
⑦	S23.132	Subluxation of T5/T6 thoracic vertebra
⑦	S23.171	Dislocation of T12/L1 thoracic vertebra
⑦	S32.018	Other fracture of first lumbar vertebra
⑦	S32.028	Other fracture of second lumbar vertebra
⑦	S32.038	Other fracture of third lumbar vertebra
⑦	S32.048	Other fracture of fourth lumbar vertebra
⑦	S32.058	Other fracture of fifth lumbar vertebra
⑦	S33.0	Traumatic rupture of lumbar intervertebral disc
⑦	S33.110	Subluxation of L1/L2 lumbar vertebra
⑦	S33.121	Dislocation of L2/L3 lumbar vertebra
⑦	S33.140	Subluxation of L4/L5 lumbar vertebra

ICD-10-CM Coding Notes

For codes requiring a 7th character extension, refer to your ICD-10-CM book. Review the character descriptions and coding guidelines for proper selection. For some procedures, only certain characters will apply.

CCI Edits

Refer to Appendix A for CCI edits.

Facility RVUs □

Code	Work	PE Facility	MP	Total Facility
22600	17.40	14.43	5.46	37.29
22610	17.28	14.25	5.13	36.66
22612	23.53	16.20	6.27	46.00
22614	6.43	3.09	1.86	11.38

Non-facility RVUs □

Code	Work	PE Non-Facility	MP	Total Non-Facility
22600	17.40	14.43	5.46	37.29
22610	17.28	14.25	5.13	36.66
22612	23.53	16.20	6.27	46.00
22614	6.43	3.09	1.86	11.38

Modifiers **(PAR)** □

Code	Mod 50	Mod 51	Mod 62	Mod 66	Mod 80
22600	0	2	2	0	2
22610	0	2	2	0	2
22612	0	2	2	0	2
22614	0	0	2	0	2

Global Period

Code	Days
22600	090
22610	090
22612	090
22614	ZZZ

22630-22632

22630 Arthrodesis, posterior interbody technique, including laminectomy and/or discectomy to prepare interspace (other than for decompression), single interspace; lumbar

(Do not report 22630 in conjunction with 22612 for the same interspace and segment, use 22633)

+ **22632 Arthrodesis, posterior interbody technique, including laminectomy and/or discectomy to prepare interspace (other than for decompression), single interspace; each additional interspace (List separately in addition to code for primary procedure)**

(Use 22632 in conjunction with 22612, 22630, or 22633 when performed at a different level. When performing a posterior interbody fusion arthrodesis at an additional level, use 22632. When performing a posterior or posterolateral technique for fusion/arthrodesis at an additional level, use 22614. When performing a combined posterior or posterolateral technique with posterior interbody arthrodesis at an additional level, use 22634)

AMA Coding Guideline

Posterior, Posterolateral or Lateral Transverse Process Technique Arthrodesis Procedures on the Spine (Vertebral Column)

To report instrumentation procedures, see 22840-22855, 22859. (Report in addition to code[s] for the definitive procedure[s].) Do not append modifier 62 to spinal instrumentation codes 22840-22848, 22850, 22852, 22853, 22854, 22859.

To report bone graft procedures, see 20930-20938. (Report in addition to code[s] for the definitive procedure[s].) Do not append modifier 62 to bone graft codes 20900-20938.

A vertebral segment describes the basic constituent part into which the spine may be divided. It represents a single complete vertebral bone with its associated articular processes and laminae. A vertebral interspace is the non-bony compartment between two adjacent vertebral bodies which contains the intervertebral disc, and includes the nucleus pulposus, annulus fibrosus, and two cartilaginous endplates.

Arthrodesis Procedures on the Spine (Vertebral Column)

Arthrodesis may be performed in the absence of other procedures and therefore when it is combined with another definitive procedure (eg, osteotomy, fracture care, vertebral corpectomy or laminectomy), modifier 51 is appropriate. However, arthrodesis codes 22585, 22614, and 22632 are considered add-on procedure codes and should not be used with modifier 51.

To report instrumentation procedures, see 22840-22855, 22859. (Codes 22840-22848, 22853, 22854, 22859 are reported in conjunction with code[s] for the definitive procedure[s]. When instrumentation reinsertion or removal is reported in conjunction with other definitive procedures, including arthrodesis, decompression, and exploration of fusion, append modifier 51 to 22849, 22850, 22852, and 22855.) To report exploration of fusion, use 22830. (When exploration is reported in conjunction with other definitive procedures, including arthrodesis and decompression, append modifier 51 to 22830.) Do not append modifier 62 to spinal instrumentation codes 22840-22848, 22850, 22852, 22853, 22854, 22859.

To report bone graft procedures, see 20930-20938. (Report in addition to code[s] for the definitive procedure[s].) Do not append modifier 62 to bone graft codes 20900-20938.

Surgical Procedures on the Spine (Vertebral Column)

Cervical, thoracic, and lumbar spine.

Within the spine section, bone grafting procedures are reported separately and in addition to arthrodesis. For bone grafts in other Musculoskeletal sections, see specific code(s) descriptor(s) and/or accompanying guidelines.

To report bone grafts performed after arthrodesis, see 20930-20938. Do not append modifier 62 to bone graft codes 20900-20938.

Example:

Posterior arthrodesis of L5-S1 for degenerative disc disease utilizing morselized autogenous iliac bone graft harvested through a separate fascial incision.

Report as 22612 and 20937.

Within the spine section, instrumentation is reported separately and in addition to arthrodesis. To report instrumentation procedures performed with definitive vertebral procedure(s), see 22840-22855, 22859. Instrumentation procedure codes 22840-22848, 22853, 22854, 22859 are reported in addition to the definitive procedure(s). Modifier 62 may not be appended to the definitive or add-on spinal instrumentation procedure code(s) 22840-22848, 22850, 22852, 22853, 22854, 22859.

Example:

Posterior arthrodesis of L4-S1, utilizing morselized autogenous iliac bone graft harvested through separate fascial incision, and pedicle screw fixation.

Report as 22612, 22614, 22842, and 20937.

Vertebral procedures are sometimes followed by arthrodesis and in addition may include bone grafts and instrumentation.

When arthrodesis is performed in addition to another procedure, the arthrodesis should be reported in addition to the original procedure with modifier 51 (multiple procedures). Examples are after osteotomy, fracture care, vertebral corpectomy, and laminectomy. Bone grafts and instrumentation are never performed without arthrodesis.

Example:

Treatment of a burst fracture of L2 by corpectomy followed by arthrodesis of L1-L3, utilizing anterior instrumentation L1-L3 and structural allograft.

Report as 63090, 22558-51, 22585, 22845, and 20931.

When two surgeons work together as primary surgeons performing distinct part(s) of a single reportable procedure, each surgeon should report his/her distinct operative work by appending modifier 62 to the single definitive procedure code. If additional procedure(s) (including add-on procedure[s]) are performed during the same surgical session, separate code(s) may be reported by each co-surgeon, with modifier 62 appended (see Appendix A).

Example:

A 42-year-old male with a history of posttraumatic degenerative disc disease at L3-4 and L4-5 (internal disc disruption) underwent surgical repair. Surgeon A performed an anterior exposure of the spine with mobilization of the great vessels. Surgeon B performed anterior (minimal) discectomy and fusion at L3-4 and L4-5 using anterior interbody technique.

Report surgeon A: 22558 append modifier 62, 22585 append modifier 62

Report surgeon B: 22558 append modifier 62, 22585 append modifier 62, 20931

Please see the Surgery Guidelines section for the following guidelines:

- *Surgical Procedures on the Musculoskeletal System*

AMA Coding Notes

Surgical Procedures on the Spine (Vertebral Column)

(Do not append modifier 62 to bone graft code 20931)

(For injection procedure for myelography, use 62284)

(For injection procedure for discography, see 62290, 62291)

(For injection procedure, chemonucleolysis, single or multiple levels, use 62292)

(For injection procedure for facet joints, see 64490-64495, 64633-64636)

(For needle or trocar biopsy, see 20220-20225)

AMA *CPT Assistant* □

22630: Spring 93: 36, Sep 97: 8, Nov 99: 11, Dec 99: 2, Jan 01: 12, Oct 09: 9, Nov 11: 10, Dec 11: 14, Jan 12: 3, Apr 12: 16, Jun 12: 11, Jul 13: 3

22632: Feb 96: 6, Sep 97: 8, Dec 99: 2, Jun 12: 11, Jul 13: 3

Plain English Description

Posterior interbody arthrodesis, also referred to as interbody fusion, of one or more intervertebral joints is performed to treat a vertebral fracture or instability. Fusion may be used alone or in conjunction with other procedures. An incision is made in the back over the affected lumbar vertebral joints. Soft tissues are dissected and the vertebrae are exposed. Muscle is retracted off the lamina. A bone drill is used to remove part of the lamina. The intervertebral disc is removed and the joint space is prepared for arthrodesis. Separately reportable fracture treatment or decompression may be performed as needed. A separately reportable bone graft is obtained from the iliac crest or other site and prepared. Allograft bone obtained from a bone bank may also be used. The bone graft is placed in the intervertebral joint space. Drill holes are created in the facets or spinous processes of each vertebra and wires are threaded through the vertebrae to immobilize the joint. Alternatively, other reportable internal fixation devices may be placed through the pedicles or facets. A drain may be placed and the surgical wound is then closed in layers. Use 22630 for fusion of a single lumbar intervertebral joint space. Use 22632 for fusion of each additional intervertebral space.

Spinal arthrodesis

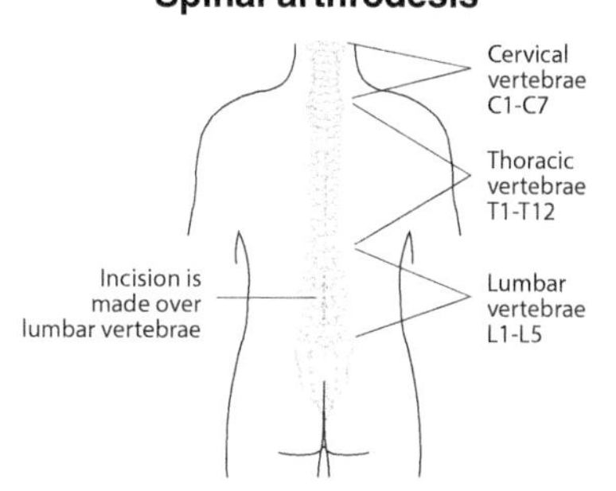

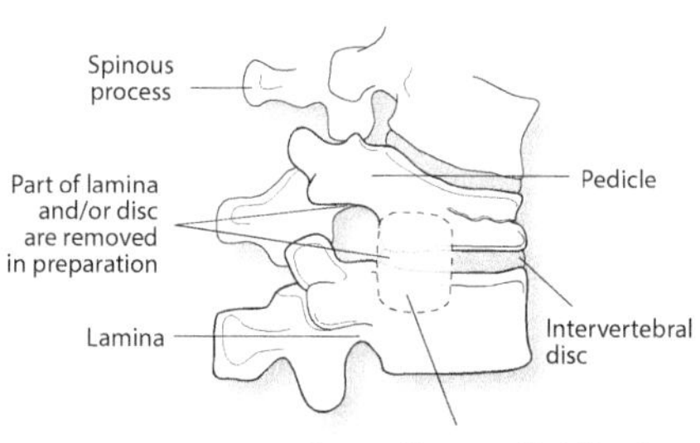

Bone grafts are used to bridge the laminae and fuse vertebrae together.

ICD-10-CM Diagnostic Codes

M24.80	Other specific joint derangements of unspecified joint, not elsewhere classified
M46.46	Discitis, unspecified, lumbar region
M47.16	Other spondylosis with myelopathy, lumbar region
M47.26	Other spondylosis with radiculopathy, lumbar region
M48.061	Spinal stenosis, lumbar region without neurogenic claudication
M48.062	Spinal stenosis, lumbar region with neurogenic claudication
M48.07	Spinal stenosis, lumbosacral region
➐ M48.56	Collapsed vertebra, not elsewhere classified, lumbar region
M51.06	Intervertebral disc disorders with myelopathy, lumbar region
M51.17	Intervertebral disc disorders with radiculopathy, lumbosacral region
M51.36	Other intervertebral disc degeneration, lumbar region
M53.85	Other specified dorsopathies, thoracolumbar region
➐ M80.88	Other osteoporosis with current pathological fracture, vertebra(e)
➐ M84.48	Pathological fracture, other site
M96.1	Postlaminectomy syndrome, not elsewhere classified
➐ S32.010	Wedge compression fracture of first lumbar vertebra
➐ S32.022	Unstable burst fracture of second lumbar vertebra
➐ S32.042	Unstable burst fracture of fourth lumbar vertebra

ICD-10-CM Coding Notes

For codes requiring a 7th character extension, refer to your ICD-10-CM book. Review the character descriptions and coding guidelines for proper selection. For some procedures, only certain characters will apply.

CCI Edits

Refer to Appendix A for CCI edits.

Facility RVUs ▯

Code	Work	PE Facility	MP	Total Facility
22630	22.09	16.38	7.12	45.59
22632	5.22	2.47	1.67	9.36

Non-facility RVUs ▯

Code	Work	PE Non-Facility	MP	Total Non-Facility
22630	22.09	16.38	7.12	45.59
22632	5.22	2.47	1.67	9.36

Modifiers (PAR) ▯

Code	Mod 50	Mod 51	Mod 62	Mod 66	Mod 80
22630	0	2	2	0	2
22632	0	0	2	0	2

Global Period

Code	Days
22630	090
22632	ZZZ

22633-22634

22633 Arthrodesis, combined posterior or posterolateral technique with posterior interbody technique including laminectomy and/ or discectomy sufficient to prepare interspace (other than for decompression), single interspace and segment; lumbar

(Do not report with 22612 or 22630 at the same level)

✚ **22634 Arthrodesis, combined posterior or posterolateral technique with posterior interbody technique including laminectomy and/ or discectomy sufficient to prepare interspace (other than for decompression), single interspace and segment; each additional interspace and segment (List separately in addition to code for primary procedure)**

(Use 22634 in conjunction with 22633)

AMA Coding Guideline

Posterior, Posterolateral or Lateral Transverse Process Technique Arthrodesis Procedures on the Spine (Vertebral Column)

To report instrumentation procedures, see 22840-22855, 22859. (Report in addition to code[s] for the definitive procedure[s].) Do not append modifier 62 to spinal instrumentation codes 22840-22848, 22850, 22852, 22853, 22854, 22859.

To report bone graft procedures, see 20930-20938. (Report in addition to code[s] for the definitive procedure[s].) Do not append modifier 62 to bone graft codes 20900-20938.

A vertebral segment describes the basic constituent part into which the spine may be divided. It represents a single complete vertebral bone with its associated articular processes and laminae. A vertebral interspace is the non-bony compartment between two adjacent vertebral bodies which contains the intervertebral disc, and includes the nucleus pulposus, annulus fibrosus, and two cartilaginous endplates.

Arthrodesis Procedures on the Spine (Vertebral Column)

Arthrodesis may be performed in the absence of other procedures and therefore when it is combined with another definitive procedure (eg, osteotomy, fracture care, vertebral corpectomy or laminectomy), modifier 51 is appropriate. However, arthrodesis codes 22585, 22614, and 22632 are considered add-on procedure codes and should not be used with modifier 51.

To report instrumentation procedures, see 22840-22855, 22859. (Codes 22840-22848, 22853, 22854, 22859 are reported in conjunction with code[s] for the definitive procedure[s]. When instrumentation reinsertion or removal is reported in conjunction with other definitive procedures, including arthrodesis, decompression, and exploration of fusion, append modifier 51 to 22849, 22850, 22852, and 22855.) To report exploration of fusion, use 22830. (When exploration is reported in conjunction with other definitive procedures, including arthrodesis and decompression, append modifier 51 to 22830.) Do not append modifier 62 to spinal instrumentation codes 22840-22848, 22850, 22852, 22853, 22854, 22859.

To report bone graft procedures, see 20930-20938. (Report in addition to code[s] for the definitive procedure[s].) Do not append modifier 62 to bone graft codes 20900-20938.

Surgical Procedures on the Spine (Vertebral Column)

Cervical, thoracic, and lumbar spine.

Within the spine section, bone grafting procedures are reported separately and in addition to arthrodesis. For bone grafts in other Musculoskeletal sections, see specific code(s) descriptor(s) and/or accompanying guidelines.

To report bone grafts performed after arthrodesis, see 20930-20938. Do not append modifier 62 to bone graft codes 20900-20938.

Example:

Posterior arthrodesis of L5-S1 for degenerative disc disease utilizing morselized autogenous iliac bone graft harvested through a separate fascial incision.

Report as 22612 and 20937.

Within the spine section, instrumentation is reported separately and in addition to arthrodesis. To report instrumentation procedures performed with definitive vertebral procedure(s), see 22840-22855, 22859. Instrumentation procedure codes 22840-22848, 22853, 22854, 22859 are reported in addition to the definitive procedure(s). Modifier 62 may not be appended to the definitive or add-on spinal instrumentation procedure code(s) 22840-22848, 22850, 22852, 22853, 22854, 22859.

Example:

Posterior arthrodesis of L4-S1, utilizing morselized autogenous iliac bone graft harvested through separate fascial incision, and pedicle screw fixation.

Report as 22612, 22614, 22842, and 20937.

Vertebral procedures are sometimes followed by arthrodesis and in addition may include bone grafts and instrumentation.

When arthrodesis is performed in addition to another procedure, the arthrodesis should be reported in addition to the original procedure with modifier 51 (multiple procedures). Examples are after osteotomy, fracture care, vertebral corpectomy, and laminectomy. Bone grafts and instrumentation are never performed without arthrodesis.

Example:

Treatment of a burst fracture of L2 by corpectomy followed by arthrodesis of L1-L3, utilizing anterior instrumentation L1-L3 and structural allograft.

Report as 63090, 22558-51, 22585, 22845, and 20931.

When two surgeons work together as primary surgeons performing distinct part(s) of a single reportable procedure, each surgeon should report his/her distinct operative work by appending modifier 62 to the single definitive procedure code. If additional procedure(s) (including add-on procedure[s]) are performed during the same surgical session, separate code(s) may be reported by each co-surgeon, with modifier 62 appended (see Appendix A).

Example:

A 42-year-old male with a history of posttraumatic degenerative disc disease at L3-4 and L4-5 (internal disc disruption) underwent surgical repair. Surgeon A performed an anterior exposure of the spine with mobilization of the great vessels. Surgeon B performed anterior (minimal) discectomy and fusion at L3-4 and L4-5 using anterior interbody technique.

Report surgeon A: 22558 append modifier 62, 22585 append modifier 62

Report surgeon B: 22558 append modifier 62, 22585 append modifier 62, 20931

Please see the Surgery Guidelines section for the following guidelines:

- *Surgical Procedures on the Musculoskeletal System*

AMA Coding Notes

Surgical Procedures on the Spine (Vertebral Column)

(Do not append modifier 62 to bone graft code 20931)

(For injection procedure for myelography, use 62284)

(For injection procedure for discography, see 62290, 62291)

(For injection procedure, chemonucleolysis, single or multiple levels, use 62292)

(For injection procedure for facet joints, see 64490-64495, 64633-64636)

(For needle or trocar biopsy, see 20220-20225)

AMA *CPT Assistant* ◻

22633: Dec 11: 14, Jan 12: 3, Jun 12: 10, Jul 13: 3, Oct 16: 11, May 18: 9, Jul 18: 14

22634: Dec 11: 14, Jan 12: 3, Jun 12: 10, Jul 13: 3, Jul 18: 14

Plain English Description

Fusion of one or more of the lumbar vertebral joints is performed to treat a fracture or other instability using a combined posterior or posterolateral technique with posterior interbody technique. Fusion may be used alone or in conjunction with other procedures. Using a posterior or posterolateral approach, an incision is made in the lower back over the affected lumbar vertebral joint(s). Soft tissues are dissected and the vertebrae are exposed. A bone drill is used to remove part of the lamina. The intervertebral disc is removed and the joint space is prepared for arthrodesis. Separately reportable fracture treatment or decompression may be performed as needed. The transverse processes, facet joints, and/or lamina are prepared for bone grafting. A separately reportable bone graft is obtained from the iliac crest or other site and prepared. Allograft bone obtained from a bone bank may also be used. The bone graft is placed in the intervertebral joint space to facilitate fusion of the vertebral bodies. Additional bone graft material is used as needed to fuse other sites in the vertebral joint such as the transverse processes, facet joints, or lamina. Drill holes are created in the facets or spinous processes of each vertebra and wires are threaded through the vertebrae to immobilize the joint. Alternatively, other separately reportable internal fixation devices may be placed through the pedicles or facets. A drain may be placed and the surgical wound is then closed in layers. Use 22633 for fusion of a single interspace and vertebral segment of the lumbar spine. Use 22634 for fusion of each additional interspace and vertebral segment.

Arthrodesis, combined posterior or posterolateral with posterior interbody technique

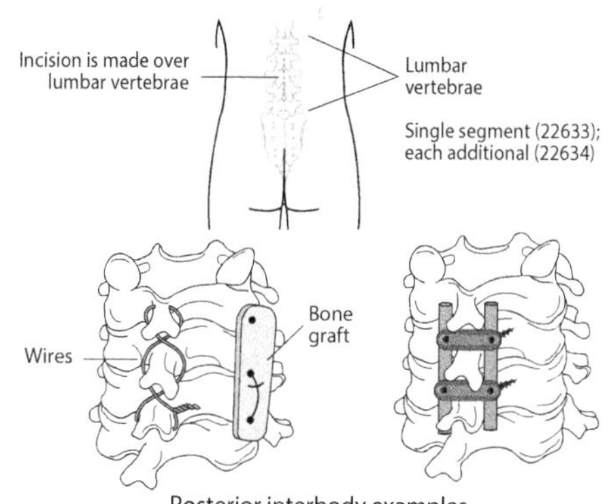

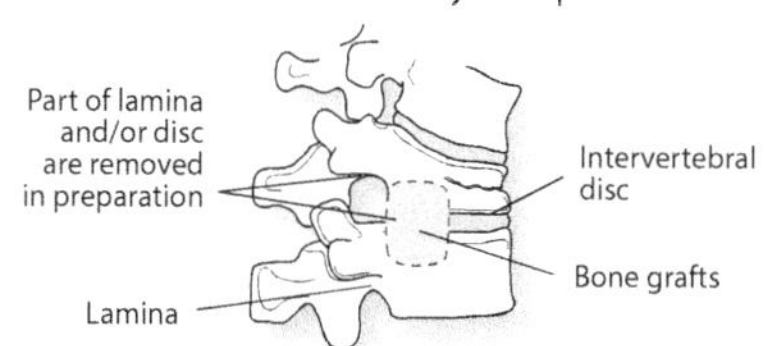

ICD-10-CM Diagnostic Codes

M46.46	Discitis, unspecified, lumbar region
M47.15	Other spondylosis with myelopathy, thoracolumbar region
M47.16	Other spondylosis with myelopathy, lumbar region
M47.26	Other spondylosis with radiculopathy, lumbar region
M47.817	Spondylosis without myelopathy or radiculopathy, lumbosacral region
M47.897	Other spondylosis, lumbosacral region
M48.061	Spinal stenosis, lumbar region without neurogenic claudication
M48.062	Spinal stenosis, lumbar region with neurogenic claudication
M48.07	Spinal stenosis, lumbosacral region
M48.16	Ankylosing hyperostosis [Forestier], lumbar region
M48.37	Traumatic spondylopathy, lumbosacral region
M49.86	Spondylopathy in diseases classified elsewhere, lumbar region
M51.06	Intervertebral disc disorders with myelopathy, lumbar region
M51.36	Other intervertebral disc degeneration, lumbar region
M53.2X6	Spinal instabilities, lumbar region
M96.1	Postlaminectomy syndrome, not elsewhere classified
Q76.2	Congenital spondylolisthesis

CCI Edits

Refer to Appendix A for CCI edits.

Facility RVUs □

Code	Work	PE Facility	MP	Total Facility
22633	27.75	18.02	7.90	53.67
22634	8.16	3.90	2.35	14.41

Non-facility RVUs □

Code	Work	PE Non-Facility	MP	Total Non-Facility
22633	27.75	18.02	7.90	53.67
22634	8.16	3.90	2.35	14.41

Modifiers (PAR) □

Code	Mod 50	Mod 51	Mod 62	Mod 66	Mod 80
22633	0	2	2	0	2
22634	0	0	2	0	2

Global Period

Code	Days
22633	090
22634	ZZZ

22830

22830 Exploration of spinal fusion

AMA Coding Guideline

Exploration Procedures on the Spine (Vertebral Column)

To report instrumentation procedures, see 22840-22855, 22859. (Codes 22840-22848, 22853, 22854, 22859 are reported in conjunction with code[s] for the definitive procedure[s]. When instrumentation reinsertion or removal is reported in conjunction with other definitive procedures, including arthrodesis, decompression, and exploration of fusion, append modifier 51 to 22849, 22850, 22852, and 22855.) Code 22849 should not be reported with 22850, 22852, and 22855 at the same spinal levels. To report exploration of fusion, see 22830. (When exploration is reported in conjunction with other definitive procedures, including arthrodesis and decompression, append modifier 51 to 22830.)

Surgical Procedures on the Spine (Vertebral Column)

Cervical, thoracic, and lumbar spine.

Within the spine section, bone grafting procedures are reported separately and in addition to arthrodesis. For bone grafts in other Musculoskeletal sections, see specific code(s) descriptor(s) and/or accompanying guidelines.

To report bone grafts performed after arthrodesis, see 20930-20938. Do not append modifier 62 to bone graft codes 20900-20938.

Example:

Posterior arthrodesis of L5-S1 for degenerative disc disease utilizing morselized autogenous iliac bone graft harvested through a separate fascial incision.

Report as 22612 and 20937.

Within the spine section, instrumentation is reported separately and in addition to arthrodesis. To report instrumentation procedures performed with definitive vertebral procedure(s), see 22840-22855, 22859. Instrumentation procedure codes 22840-22848, 22853, 22854, 22859 are reported in addition to the definitive procedure(s). Modifier 62 may not be appended to the definitive or add-on spinal instrumentation procedure code(s) 22840-22848, 22850, 22852, 22853, 22854, 22859.

Example:

Posterior arthrodesis of L4-S1, utilizing morselized autogenous iliac bone graft harvested through separate fascial incision, and pedicle screw fixation.

Report as 22612, 22614, 22842, and 20937.

Vertebral procedures are sometimes followed by arthrodesis and in addition may include bone grafts and instrumentation.

When arthrodesis is performed in addition to another procedure, the arthrodesis should be reported in addition to the original procedure with modifier 51 (multiple procedures). Examples are after osteotomy, fracture care, vertebral corpectomy, and laminectomy. Bone grafts and instrumentation are never performed without arthrodesis.

Example:

Treatment of a burst fracture of L2 by corpectomy followed by arthrodesis of L1-L3, utilizing anterior instrumentation L1-L3 and structural allograft.

Report as 63090, 22558-51, 22585, 22845, and 20931.

When two surgeons work together as primary surgeons performing distinct part(s) of a single reportable procedure, each surgeon should report his/her distinct operative work by appending modifier 62 to the single definitive procedure code. If additional procedure(s) (including add-on procedure[s]) are performed during the same surgical session, separate code(s) may be reported by each co-surgeon, with modifier 62 appended (see Appendix A).

Example:

A 42-year-old male with a history of posttraumatic degenerative disc disease at L3-4 and L4-5 (internal disc disruption) underwent surgical repair. Surgeon A performed an anterior exposure of the spine with mobilization of the great vessels. Surgeon B performed anterior (minimal) discectomy and fusion at L3-4 and L4-5 using anterior interbody technique.

Report surgeon A: 22558 append modifier 62, 22585 append modifier 62

Report surgeon B: 22558 append modifier 62, 22585 append modifier 62, 20931

Please see the Surgery Guidelines section for the following guidelines:

- *Surgical Procedures on the Musculoskeletal System*

AMA Coding Notes

Exploration Procedures on the Spine (Vertebral Column)

(To report bone graft procedures, see 20930-20938)

Surgical Procedures on the Spine (Vertebral Column)

(Do not append modifier 62 to bone graft code 20931)

(For injection procedure for myelography, use 62284)

(For injection procedure for discography, see 62290, 62291)

(For injection procedure, chemonucleolysis, single or multiple levels, use 62292)

(For injection procedure for facet joints, see 64490-64495, 64633-64636)

(For needle or trocar biopsy, see 20220-20225)

AMA *CPT Assistant* ☐

22830: Sep 97: 11, Mar 10: 9

Plain English Description

The patient is placed in position (e.g., posterior, posterolateral, anterior), depending on the site of the fusion. The physician examines the joint between two vertebrae that have been fused together for signs of damage or disease. The physician may also examine any instrumentation that had been placed during the fusion. The incision is closed with sutures.

Exploration of spinal fusion

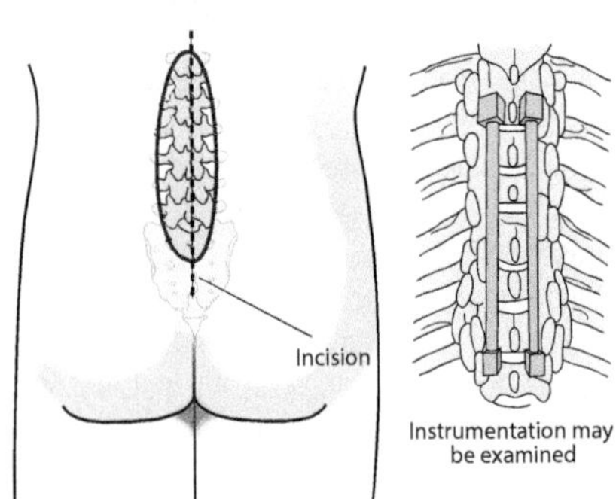

The joint is examined between two vertebrae that have been fused together for signs of damage or disease. The physician may also examine any instrumentation that had been placed during the fusion.

ICD-10-CM Diagnostic Codes

	Code	Description
	G89.28	Other chronic postprocedural pain
	M54.8	Other dorsalgia
	M96.0	Pseudarthrosis after fusion or arthrodesis
	M96.3	Postlaminectomy kyphosis
	M96.4	Postsurgical lordosis
❼	T84.318	Breakdown (mechanical) of other bone devices, implants and grafts
❼	T84.498	Other mechanical complication of other internal orthopedic devices, implants and grafts
	T86.831	Bone graft failure
	T86.838	Other complications of bone graft

ICD-10-CM Coding Notes

For codes requiring a 7th character extension, refer to your ICD-10-CM book. Review the character descriptions and coding guidelines for proper selection. For some procedures, only certain characters will apply.

CCI Edits

Refer to Appendix A for CCI edits.

Facility RVUs □

Code	Work	PE Facility	MP	Total Facility
22830	11.22	9.36	3.07	23.65

Non-facility RVUs □

Code	Work	PE Non-Facility	MP	Total Non-Facility
22830	11.22	9.36	3.07	23.65

Modifiers (PAR) □

Code	Mod 50	Mod 51	Mod 62	Mod 66	Mod 80
22830	0	2	1	0	2

Global Period

Code	Days
22830	090

22840

+ **22840 Posterior non-segmental instrumentation (eg, Harrington rod technique, pedicle fixation across 1 interspace, atlantoaxial transarticular screw fixation, sublaminar wiring at C1, facet screw fixation) (List separately in addition to code for primary procedure)**

(Use 22840 in conjunction with 22100-22102, 22110-22114, 22206, 22207, 22210-22214, 22220-22224, 22310-22327, 22532, 22533, 22548-22558, 22590-22612, 22630, 22633, 22634, 22800-22812, 63001-63030, 63040-63042, 63045-63047, 63050-63056, 63064, 63075, 63077, 63081, 63085, 63087, 63090, 63101, 63102, 63170-63290, 63300-63307)

AMA Coding Guideline

Spinal Instrumentation Procedures on the Spine (Vertebral Column)

Segmental instrumentation is defined as fixation at each end of the construct and at least one additional interposed bony attachment.

Non-segmental instrumentation is defined as fixation at each end of the construct and may span several vertebral segments without attachment to the intervening segments.

Insertion of spinal instrumentation is reported separately and in addition to arthrodesis. Instrumentation procedure codes 22840-22848, 22853, 22854, 22859 are reported in addition to the definitive procedure(s). Do not append modifier 62 to spinal instrumentation codes 22840-22848, 22850, 22852, 22853, 22854, 22859.

To report bone graft procedures, see 20930-20938. (Report in addition to code[s] for definitive procedure[s].) Do not append modifier 62 to bone graft codes 20900-20938.

A vertebral segment describes the basic constituent part into which the spine may be divided. It represents a single complete vertebral bone with its associated articular processes and laminae. A vertebral interspace is the non-bony compartment between two adjacent vertebral bodies, which contains the intervertebral disc, and includes the nucleus pulposus, annulus fibrosus, and two cartilaginous endplates.

Codes 22849, 22850, 22852, and 22855 are subject to modifier 51 if reported with other definitive procedure(s), including arthrodesis, decompression, and exploration of fusion. Code 22849 should not be reported in conjunction with 22850, 22852, and 22855 at the same spinal levels. Only the appropriate insertion code (22840-22848) should be reported when previously placed spinal instrumentation is being removed or revised during the same session where new instrumentation is inserted at levels including all or part of the previously instrumented segments. Do not report the reinsertion (22849) or removal (22850, 22852, 22855) procedures in addition to the insertion of the new instrumentation (22840-22848).

Surgical Procedures on the Spine (Vertebral Column)

Cervical, thoracic, and lumbar spine.

Within the spine section, bone grafting procedures are reported separately and in addition to arthrodesis. For bone grafts in other Musculoskeletal sections, see specific code(s) descriptor(s) and/or accompanying guidelines.

To report bone grafts performed after arthrodesis, see 20930-20938. Do not append modifier 62 to bone graft codes 20900-20938.

Example:

Posterior arthrodesis of L5-S1 for degenerative disc disease utilizing morselized autogenous iliac bone graft harvested through a separate fascial incision.

Report as 22612 and 20937.

Within the spine section, instrumentation is reported separately and in addition to arthrodesis. To report instrumentation procedures performed with definitive vertebral procedure(s), see 22840-22855, 22859. Instrumentation procedure codes 22840-22848, 22853, 22854, 22859 are reported in addition to the definitive procedure(s). Modifier 62 may not be appended to the definitive or add-on spinal instrumentation procedure code(s) 22840-22848, 22850, 22852, 22853, 22854, 22859.

Example:

Posterior arthrodesis of L4-S1, utilizing morselized autogenous iliac bone graft harvested through separate fascial incision, and pedicle screw fixation.

Report as 22612, 22614, 22842, and 20937.

Vertebral procedures are sometimes followed by arthrodesis and in addition may include bone grafts and instrumentation.

When arthrodesis is performed in addition to another procedure, the arthrodesis should be reported in addition to the original procedure with modifier 51 (multiple procedures). Examples are after osteotomy, fracture care, vertebral corpectomy, and laminectomy. Bone grafts and instrumentation are never performed without arthrodesis.

Example:

Treatment of a burst fracture of L2 by corpectomy followed by arthrodesis of L1-L3, utilizing anterior instrumentation L1-L3 and structural allograft.

Report as 63090, 22558-51, 22585, 22845, and 20931.

When two surgeons work together as primary surgeons performing distinct part(s) of a single reportable procedure, each surgeon should report his/her distinct operative work by appending modifier 62 to the single definitive procedure code. If additional procedure(s) (including add-on procedure[s]) are performed during the same surgical session, separate code(s) may be reported by each co-surgeon, with modifier 62 appended (see Appendix A).

Example:

A 42-year-old male with a history of posttraumatic degenerative disc disease at L3-4 and L4-5 (internal disc disruption) underwent surgical repair. Surgeon A performed an anterior exposure of the spine with mobilization of the great vessels. Surgeon B performed anterior (minimal) discectomy and fusion at L3-4 and L4-5 using anterior interbody technique.

Report surgeon A: 22558 append modifier 62, 22585 append modifier 62

Report surgeon B: 22558 append modifier 62, 22585 append modifier 62, 20931

Please see the Surgery Guidelines section for the following guidelines:

- *Surgical Procedures on the Musculoskeletal System*

AMA Coding Notes

Surgical Procedures on the Spine (Vertebral Column)

(Do not append modifier 62 to bone graft code 20931)

(For injection procedure for myelography, use 62284)

(For injection procedure for discography, see 62290, 62291)

(For injection procedure, chemonucleolysis, single or multiple levels, use 62292)

(For injection procedure for facet joints, see 64490-64495, 64633-64636)

(For needle or trocar biopsy, see 20220-20225)

AMA *CPT Assistant* ☐

22840: Feb 96: 6, Jul 96: 10, Sep 97: 8, Nov 99: 12, Feb 02: 6, Nov 10: 8, Jan 11: 9, Dec 11: 15, Apr 12: 12, Jun 12: 11, Jul 13: 3, Dec 13: 17, Oct 14: 15, Jun 17: 10

Plain English Description

Posterior non-segmental spine instrumentation is applied during a separately reportable arthrodesis (fusion) procedure on the spine. Spinal instrumentation is used to treat a deformity or instability of the spine. Posterior non-segmental fixation involves attaching the fixation device to the top and bottom vertebral segments without attaching it to any of the vertebral segments in between. Types of fixation include: Harrington rod technique, pedicle fixation across one interspace, atlantoaxial transarticular screw fixation, sublaminar wiring at C1, and facet screw fixation. Harrington rod technique involves placing a long rod spanning multiple vertebral segments fixed to the spine using hooks at the top and bottom vertebral segments only. Pedicle fixation across a single interspace, also referred to as transpedicular fixation, involves inserting a screw in a posteroanteromedial direction through the pedicle into the vertebral body on the vertebral segment above and below one single interspace. The screws are then secured to a plate or other fixator to provide stability. Atlantoaxial transarticular screw fixation involves placing a screw through the C1-2 vertebral bodies. Following preoperative 3D fluoroscopic assessment of anatomy and calculation of correct screw trajectory, a single (unilateral) pedicle screw or two (bilateral) pedicle screws are placed in the atlantoaxial complex through the pedicle of C2, traversing the C1-2 interspace, and penetrating the lateral mass of C1. C1 sublaminar wiring involves placing a wire through the C1-C2 lamina to provide stability. Facet screw fixation involves placing a short screw horizontally from the inferior articular process of the superior vertebra, traversing the interspace, and penetrating the articular process of the inferior vertebra. Alternatively, the facet screw can be angled and placed in the base of the pedicle or a translaminar facet screw can be placed through the spinous process and lamina of the contralateral side and penetrate the base of the pedicle.

Posterior non-segmental instrumentation

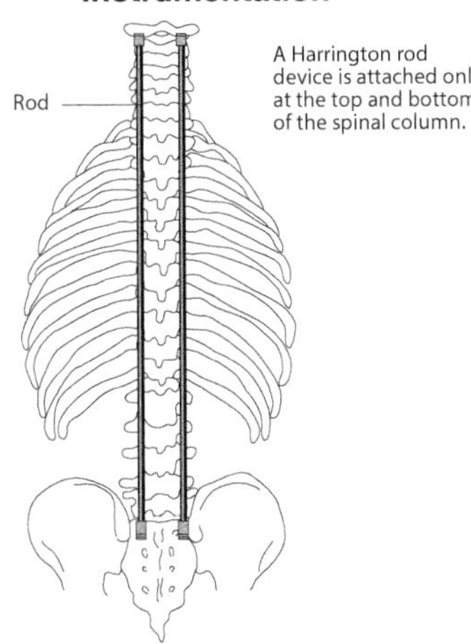

ICD-10-CM Diagnostic Codes

See Primary Procedure code for crosswalks.

CCI Edits

Refer to Appendix A for CCI edits.

Facility RVUs

Code	Work	PE Facility	MP	Total Facility
22840	12.52	6.01	3.55	22.08

Non-facility RVUs

Code	Work	PE Non-Facility	MP	Total Non-Facility
22840	12.52	6.01	3.55	22.08

Modifiers (PAR)

Code	Mod 50	Mod 51	Mod 62	Mod 66	Mod 80
22840	0	0	1	0	2

Global Period

Code	Days
22840	ZZZ

CPT® Procedural Coding

22842-22844

+ **22842 Posterior segmental instrumentation (eg, pedicle fixation, dual rods with multiple hooks and sublaminar wires); 3 to 6 vertebral segments (List separately in addition to code for primary procedure)**

(Use 22842 in conjunction with 22100-22102, 22110-22114, 22206, 22207, 22210-22214, 22220-22224, 22310-22327, 22532, 22533, 22548-22558, 22590-22612, 22630, 22633, 22634, 22800-22812, 63001-63030, 63040-63042, 63045-63047, 63050-63056, 63064, 63075, 63077, 63081, 63085, 63087, 63090, 63101, 63102, 63170-63290, 63300-63307)

+ **22843 Posterior segmental instrumentation (eg, pedicle fixation, dual rods with multiple hooks and sublaminar wires); 7 to 12 vertebral segments (List separately in addition to code for primary procedure)**

(Use 22843 in conjunction with 22100-22102, 22110-22114, 22206, 22207, 22210-22214, 22220-22224, 22310-22327, 22532, 22533, 22548-22558, 22590-22612, 22630, 22633, 22634, 22800-22812, 63001-63030, 63040-63042, 63045-63047, 63050-63056, 63064, 63075, 63077, 63081, 63085, 63087, 63090, 63101, 63102, 63170-63290, 63300-63307)

+ **22844 Posterior segmental instrumentation (eg, pedicle fixation, dual rods with multiple hooks and sublaminar wires); 13 or more vertebral segments (List separately in addition to code for primary procedure)**

(Use 22844 in conjunction with 22100-22102, 22110-22114, 22206, 22207, 22210-22214, 22220-22224, 22310-22327, 22532, 22533, 22548-22558, 22590-22612, 22630, 22633, 22634, 22800-22812, 63001-63030, 63040-63042, 63045-63047, 63050-63056, 63064, 63075, 63077, 63081, 63085, 63087, 63090, 63101, 63102, 63170-63290, 63300-63307)

AMA Coding Guideline

Spinal Instrumentation Procedures on the Spine (Vertebral Column)

Segmental instrumentation is defined as fixation at each end of the construct and at least one additional interposed bony attachment.

Non-segmental instrumentation is defined as fixation at each end of the construct and may span several vertebral segments without attachment to the intervening segments.

Insertion of spinal instrumentation is reported separately and in addition to arthrodesis. Instrumentation procedure codes 22840-22848, 22853, 22854, 22859 are reported in addition to the definitive procedure(s). Do not append modifier 62 to spinal instrumentation codes 22840-22848, 22850, 22852, 22853, 22854, 22859.

To report bone graft procedures, see 20930-20938. (Report in addition to code[s] for definitive procedure[s].) Do not append modifier 62 to bone graft codes 20900-20938.

A vertebral segment describes the basic constituent part into which the spine may be divided. It represents a single complete vertebral bone with its associated articular processes and laminae. A vertebral interspace is the non-bony compartment between two adjacent vertebral bodies, which contains the intervertebral disc, and includes the nucleus pulposus, annulus fibrosus, and two cartilaginous endplates.

Codes 22849, 22850, 22852, and 22855 are subject to modifier 51 if reported with other definitive procedure(s), including arthrodesis, decompression, and exploration of fusion. Code 22849 should not be reported in conjunction with 22850, 22852, and 22855 at the same spinal levels. Only the appropriate insertion code (22840-22848) should be reported when previously placed spinal instrumentation is being removed or revised during the same session where new instrumentation is inserted at levels including all or part of the previously instrumented segments. Do not report the reinsertion (22849) or removal (22850, 22852, 22855) procedures in addition to the insertion of the new instrumentation (22840-22848).

Surgical Procedures on the Spine (Vertebral Column)

Cervical, thoracic, and lumbar spine.

Within the spine section, bone grafting procedures are reported separately and in addition to arthrodesis. For bone grafts in other Musculoskeletal sections, see specific code(s) descriptor(s) and/or accompanying guidelines.

To report bone grafts performed after arthrodesis, see 20930-20938. Do not append modifier 62 to bone graft codes 20900-20938.

Example:

Posterior arthrodesis of L5-S1 for degenerative disc disease utilizing morselized autogenous iliac bone graft harvested through a separate fascial incision.

Report as 22612 and 20937.

Within the spine section, instrumentation is reported separately and in addition to arthrodesis. To report instrumentation procedures performed with definitive vertebral procedure(s), see 22840-22855, 22859. Instrumentation procedure codes 22840-22848, 22853, 22854, 22859 are reported in addition to the definitive procedure(s). Modifier 62 may not be appended to the definitive or add-on spinal instrumentation procedure code(s) 22840-22848, 22850, 22852, 22853, 22854, 22859.

Example:

Posterior arthrodesis of L4-S1, utilizing morselized autogenous iliac bone graft harvested through separate fascial incision, and pedicle screw fixation.

Report as 22612, 22614, 22842, and 20937.

Vertebral procedures are sometimes followed by arthrodesis and in addition may include bone grafts and instrumentation.

When arthrodesis is performed in addition to another procedure, the arthrodesis should be reported in addition to the original procedure with modifier 51 (multiple procedures). Examples are after osteotomy, fracture care, vertebral corpectomy, and laminectomy. Bone grafts and instrumentation are never performed without arthrodesis.

Example:

Treatment of a burst fracture of L2 by corpectomy followed by arthrodesis of L1-L3, utilizing anterior instrumentation L1-L3 and structural allograft.

Report as 63090, 22558-51, 22585, 22845, and 20931.

When two surgeons work together as primary surgeons performing distinct part(s) of a single reportable procedure, each surgeon should report his/her distinct operative work by appending modifier 62 to the single definitive procedure code. If additional procedure(s) (including add-on procedure[s]) are performed during the same surgical session, separate code(s) may be reported by each co-surgeon, with modifier 62 appended (see Appendix A).

Example:

A 42-year-old male with a history of posttraumatic degenerative disc disease at L3-4 and L4-5 (internal disc disruption) underwent surgical repair. Surgeon A performed an anterior exposure of the spine with mobilization of the great vessels. Surgeon B performed anterior (minimal) discectomy and fusion at L3-4 and L4-5 using anterior interbody technique.

Report surgeon A: 22558 append modifier 62, 22585 append modifier 62

Report surgeon B: 22558 append modifier 62, 22585 append modifier 62, 20931

Please see the Surgery Guidelines section for the following guidelines:

- *Surgical Procedures on the Musculoskeletal System*

AMA Coding Notes

Surgical Procedures on the Spine (Vertebral Column)

(Do not append modifier 62 to bone graft code 20931)

(For injection procedure for myelography, use 62284)

(For injection procedure for discography, see 62290, 62291)

(For injection procedure, chemonucleolysis, single or multiple levels, use 62292)

(For injection procedure for facet joints, see 64490-64495, 64633-64636)

(For needle or trocar biopsy, see 20220-20225)

AMA *CPT Assistant* ▯

22842: Feb 96: 6, Mar 96: 7, Sep 97: 8, Feb 02: 6, Dec 11: 15, Jun 12: 11, Jul 13: 3

22843: Feb 96: 6, Sep 97: 8, Feb 02: 6, Dec 11: 15, Jun 12: 11, Jul 13: 3, Jul 18: 14

22844: Feb 96: 6, Sep 97: 8, Feb 02: 6, Dec 11: 15, Jun 12: 11, Jul 13: 3

Plain English Description

Posterior segmental spinal instrumentation is applied during a separately reportable arthrodesis (fusion) procedure on the spine. Spinal instrumentation is used to treat a deformity or instability of the spine. Posterior segmental fixation involves attaching the fixation device to the top and bottom vertebral segments and at least one additional vertebral segment in between. Types of fixation include pedicle fixation across multiple interspaces and dual rods with multiple hooks and sublaminar wires. Pedicle fixation across multiple interspaces, also referred to as transpedicular fixation, involves inserting a screw in a posteroanteromedial direction through the pedicle into the vertebral body. This is performed across two or more interspaces (three or more vertebrae) and the screws are then secured to a plate or other fixator to provide stability. In dual rod fixation with multiple hooks and sublaminar wires, rods are placed on each side of the affected part of the spine and then fixed to each vertebral segment using hooks and/or sublaminar wires. Hooks may be fixed to the pedicle or lamina. If sublaminar wires are used, the wire loops are placed under the lamina of each vertebral segment and then around the rods and tightened. Use 22842 for posterior segmental instrumentation performed on 3 to 6 vertebral segments, 22843 for 7 to 12 vertebral segments, and 22844 for 13 or more vertebral segments.

Posterior segmental instrumentation

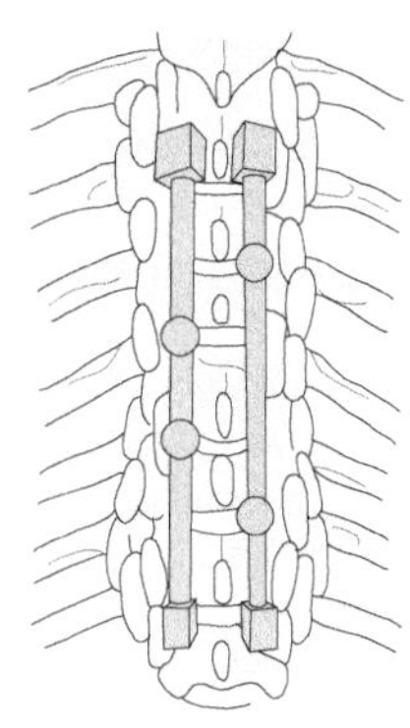

A device is attached to the vertebrae to treat a deformity or instability of the spine, 3-6 vertebrae (22842); 7-12 vertebrae (22843); 13 or more vertebrae (22844).

ICD-10-CM Diagnostic Codes

See Primary Procedure code for crosswalks.

CCI Edits

Refer to Appendix A for CCI edits.

Facility RVUs ▯

Code	Work	PE Facility	MP	Total Facility
22842	12.56	6.02	3.60	22.18
22843	13.44	6.46	3.80	23.70
22844	16.42	7.99	4.23	28.64

Non-facility RVUs ▯

Code	Work	PE Non-Facility	MP	Total Non-Facility
22842	12.56	6.02	3.60	22.18
22843	13.44	6.46	3.80	23.70
22844	16.42	7.99	4.23	28.64

Modifiers (PAR) ▯

Code	Mod 50	Mod 51	Mod 62	Mod 66	Mod 80
22842	0	0	2	0	2
22843	0	0	2	0	2
22844	0	0	2	0	2

Global Period

Code	Days
22842	ZZZ
22843	ZZZ
22844	ZZZ

22845-22847

✚ **22845 Anterior instrumentation; 2 to 3 vertebral segments (List separately in addition to code for primary procedure)**

(Use 22845 in conjunction with 22100-22102, 22110-22114, 22206, 22207, 22210-22214, 22220-22224, 22310-22327, 22532, 22533, 22548-22558, 22590-22612, 22630, 22633, 22634, 22800-22812, 63001-63030, 63040-63042, 63045-63047, 63050-63056, 63064, 63075, 63077, 63081, 63085, 63087, 63090, 63101, 63102, 63170-63290, 63300-63307)

✚ **22846 Anterior instrumentation; 4 to 7 vertebral segments (List separately in addition to code for primary procedure)**

(Use 22846 in conjunction with 22100-22102, 22110-22114, 22206, 22207, 22210-22214, 22220-22224, 22310-22327, 22532, 22533, 22548-22558, 22590-22612, 22630, 22633, 22634, 22800-22812, 63001-63030, 63040-63042, 63045-63047, 63050-63056, 63064, 63075, 63077, 63081, 63085, 63087, 63090, 63101, 63102, 63170-63290, 63300-63307)

✚ **22847 Anterior instrumentation; 8 or more vertebral segments (List separately in addition to code for primary procedure)**

(Use 22847 in conjunction with 22100-22102, 22110-22114, 22206, 22207, 22210-22214, 22220-22224, 22310-22327, 22532, 22533, 22548-22558, 22590-22612, 22630, 22633, 22634, 22800-22812, 63001-63030, 63040-63042, 63045-63047, 63050-63056, 63064, 63075, 63077, 63081, 63085, 63087, 63090, 63101, 63102, 63170-63290, 63300-63307)

AMA Coding Guideline

Spinal Instrumentation Procedures on the Spine (Vertebral Column)

Segmental instrumentation is defined as fixation at each end of the construct and at least one additional interposed bony attachment.

Non-segmental instrumentation is defined as fixation at each end of the construct and may span several vertebral segments without attachment to the intervening segments.

Insertion of spinal instrumentation is reported separately and in addition to arthrodesis. Instrumentation procedure codes 22840-22848, 22853, 22854, 22859 are reported in addition to the definitive procedure(s). Do not append modifier 62 to spinal instrumentation codes 22840-22848, 22850, 22852, 22853, 22854, 22859.

To report bone graft procedures, see 20930-20938. (Report in addition to code[s] for definitive procedure[s].) Do not append modifier 62 to bone graft codes 20900-20938.

A vertebral segment describes the basic constituent part into which the spine may be divided. It represents a single complete vertebral bone with its associated articular processes and laminae. A vertebral interspace is the non-bony compartment between two adjacent vertebral bodies, which contains the intervertebral disc, and includes the nucleus pulposus, annulus fibrosus, and two cartilaginous endplates.

Codes 22849, 22850, 22852, and 22855 are subject to modifier 51 if reported with other definitive procedure(s), including arthrodesis, decompression, and exploration of fusion. Code 22849 should not be reported in conjunction with 22850, 22852, and 22855 at the same spinal levels. Only the appropriate insertion code (22840-22848) should be reported when previously placed spinal instrumentation is being removed or revised during the same session where new instrumentation is inserted at levels including all or part of the previously instrumented segments. Do not report the reinsertion (22849) or removal (22850, 22852, 22855) procedures in addition to the insertion of the new instrumentation (22840-22848).

Surgical Procedures on the Spine (Vertebral Column)

Cervical, thoracic, and lumbar spine.

Within the spine section, bone grafting procedures are reported separately and in addition to arthrodesis. For bone grafts in other Musculoskeletal sections, see specific code(s) descriptor(s) and/or accompanying guidelines.

To report bone grafts performed after arthrodesis, see 20930-20938. Do not append modifier 62 to bone graft codes 20900-20938.

Example:

Posterior arthrodesis of L5-S1 for degenerative disc disease utilizing morselized autogenous iliac bone graft harvested through a separate fascial incision.

Report as 22612 and 20937.

Within the spine section, instrumentation is reported separately and in addition to arthrodesis. To report instrumentation procedures performed with definitive vertebral procedure(s), see 22840-22855, 22859. Instrumentation procedure codes 22840-22848, 22853, 22854, 22859 are reported in addition to the definitive procedure(s). Modifier 62 may not be appended to the definitive or add-on spinal instrumentation procedure code(s) 22840-22848, 22850, 22852, 22853, 22854, 22859.

Example:

Posterior arthrodesis of L4-S1, utilizing morselized autogenous iliac bone graft harvested through separate fascial incision, and pedicle screw fixation.

Report as 22612, 22614, 22842, and 20937.

Vertebral procedures are sometimes followed by arthrodesis and in addition may include bone grafts and instrumentation.

When arthrodesis is performed in addition to another procedure, the arthrodesis should be reported in addition to the original procedure with modifier 51 (multiple procedures). Examples are after osteotomy, fracture care, vertebral corpectomy, and laminectomy. Bone grafts and instrumentation are never performed without arthrodesis.

Example:

Treatment of a burst fracture of L2 by corpectomy followed by arthrodesis of L1-L3, utilizing anterior instrumentation L1-L3 and structural allograft.

Report as 63090, 22558-51, 22585, 22845, and 20931.

When two surgeons work together as primary surgeons performing distinct part(s) of a single reportable procedure, each surgeon should report his/her distinct operative work by appending modifier 62 to the single definitive procedure code. If additional procedure(s) (including add-on procedure[s]) are performed during the same surgical session, separate code(s) may be reported by each co-surgeon, with modifier 62 appended (see Appendix A).

Example:

A 42-year-old male with a history of posttraumatic degenerative disc disease at L3-4 and L4-5 (internal disc disruption) underwent surgical repair. Surgeon A performed an anterior exposure of the spine with mobilization of the great vessels. Surgeon B performed anterior (minimal) discectomy and fusion at L3-4 and L4-5 using anterior interbody technique.

Report surgeon A: 22558 append modifier 62, 22585 append modifier 62

Report surgeon B: 22558 append modifier 62, 22585 append modifier 62, 20931

Please see the Surgery Guidelines section for the following guidelines:

- *Surgical Procedures on the Musculoskeletal System*

AMA Coding Notes

Surgical Procedures on the Spine (Vertebral Column)

(Do not append modifier 62 to bone graft code 20931)

(For injection procedure for myelography, use 62284)

(For injection procedure for discography, see 62290, 62291)

(For injection procedure, chemonucleolysis, single or multiple levels, use 62292)

(For injection procedure for facet joints, see 64490-64495, 64633-64636)

(For needle or trocar biopsy, see 20220-20225)

AMA *CPT Assistant*

22845: Feb 96: 6, Mar 96: 10, Jul 96: 7, 10, Sep 97: 8, Feb 02: 6, Jun 12: 11, Jul 13: 3, Nov 14: 14, Jan 15: 13, Mar 15: 9, Apr 15: 7, May 16: 13, Mar 17: 7

22846: Feb 96: 6, Sep 97: 8, Feb 02: 6, Jun 12: 11, Jul 13: 3, May 16: 13

22847: Feb 96: 6, Sep 97: 8, Feb 02: 6, Jun 12: 11, Jul 13: 3, May 16: 13

Plain English Description

Anterior spinal instrumentation is applied during a separately reportable arthrodesis (fusion) procedure on the spine. Spinal instrumentation is used to treat a deformity or instability of the spine. Anterior spinal instrumentation is placed from the front of the body. Depending on the vertebral level, the access incision may be made in the front of the neck, the thorax, or the abdomen. Anterior instrumentation may also be placed from the side using an anterolateral approach. The appropriate approach is selected, overlying muscles are retracted, and blood vessels are retracted or ligated. The vertebrae are accessed and prepared, with muscles stripped. Separately reportable discectomy may be performed. A single or dual rod is placed and attached to the spine segments using hooks and/or screws and/or separately reportable intervertebral cage devices. Cages, hooks, and screws may be stabilized using separately reportable bone graft(s). Bone graft material is tightly packed and compressed around the cages, hooks, and/or screws. Use 22845 when anterior instrumentation is applied to 2 to 3 vertebral segments, 22846 for 4 to 7 vertebral segments, and 22847 for 8 or more vertebral segments.

Anterior instrumentation

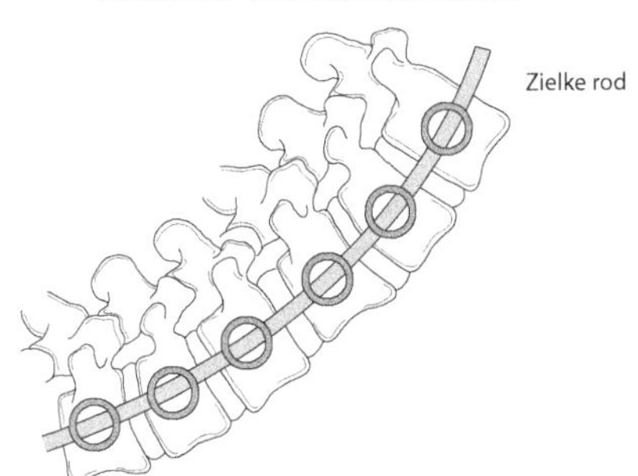

Anterior spinal instrumentation is applied during a separately reportable arthrodesis (fusion) procedure on the spine. Spinal instrumentation is used to treat a deformity or instability of the spine. Use 22845 for two to three segments; use 22846 for four to seven segments.; use 22847 for eight or more.

ICD-10-CM Diagnostic Codes

See Primary Procedure code for crosswalks.

CCI Edits

Refer to Appendix A for CCI edits.

Facility RVUs

Code	Work	PE Facility	MP	Total Facility
22845	11.94	5.67	3.56	21.17
22846	12.40	5.90	3.71	22.01
22847	13.78	6.91	2.74	23.43

Non-facility RVUs

Code	Work	PE Non-Facility	MP	Total Non-Facility
22845	11.94	5.67	3.56	21.17
22846	12.40	5.90	3.71	22.01
22847	13.78	6.91	2.74	23.43

Modifiers (PAR)

Code	Mod 50	Mod 51	Mod 62	Mod 66	Mod 80
22845	0	0	2	0	2
22846	0	0	2	0	2
22847	0	0	2	0	2

Global Period

Code	Days
22845	ZZZ
22846	ZZZ
22847	ZZZ

CPT® Procedural Coding

22849

22849 Reinsertion of spinal fixation device

AMA Coding Guideline

Spinal Instrumentation Procedures on the Spine (Vertebral Column)

Segmental instrumentation is defined as fixation at each end of the construct and at least one additional interposed bony attachment.

Non-segmental instrumentation is defined as fixation at each end of the construct and may span several vertebral segments without attachment to the intervening segments.

Insertion of spinal instrumentation is reported separately and in addition to arthrodesis. Instrumentation procedure codes 22840-22848, 22853, 22854, 22859 are reported in addition to the definitive procedure(s). Do not append modifier 62 to spinal instrumentation codes 22840-22848, 22850, 22852, 22853, 22854, 22859.

To report bone graft procedures, see 20930-20938. (Report in addition to code[s] for definitive procedure[s].) Do not append modifier 62 to bone graft codes 20900-20938.

A vertebral segment describes the basic constituent part into which the spine may be divided. It represents a single complete vertebral bone with its associated articular processes and laminae. A vertebral interspace is the non-bony compartment between two adjacent vertebral bodies, which contains the intervertebral disc, and includes the nucleus pulposus, annulus fibrosus, and two cartilaginous endplates.

Codes 22849, 22850, 22852, and 22855 are subject to modifier 51 if reported with other definitive procedure(s), including arthrodesis, decompression, and exploration of fusion. Code 22849 should not be reported in conjunction with 22850, 22852, and 22855 at the same spinal levels. Only the appropriate insertion code (22840-22848) should be reported when previously placed spinal instrumentation is being removed or revised during the same session where new instrumentation is inserted at levels including all or part of the previously instrumented segments. Do not report the reinsertion (22849) or removal (22850, 22852, 22855) procedures in addition to the insertion of the new instrumentation (22840-22848).

Surgical Procedures on the Spine (Vertebral Column)

Cervical, thoracic, and lumbar spine.

Within the spine section, bone grafting procedures are reported separately and in addition to arthrodesis. For bone grafts in other Musculoskeletal sections, see specific code(s) descriptor(s) and/or accompanying guidelines.

To report bone grafts performed after arthrodesis, see 20930-20938. Do not append modifier 62 to bone graft codes 20900-20938.

Example:

Posterior arthrodesis of L5-S1 for degenerative disc disease utilizing morselized autogenous iliac bone graft harvested through a separate fascial incision. Report as 22612 and 20937.

Within the spine section, instrumentation is reported separately and in addition to arthrodesis. To report instrumentation procedures performed with definitive vertebral procedure(s), see 22840-22855, 22859. Instrumentation procedure codes 22840-22848, 22853, 22854, 22859 are reported in addition to the definitive procedure(s). Modifier 62 may not be appended to the definitive or add-on spinal instrumentation procedure code(s) 22840-22848, 22850, 22852, 22853, 22854, 22859.

Example:

Posterior arthrodesis of L4-S1, utilizing morselized autogenous iliac bone graft harvested through separate fascial incision, and pedicle screw fixation. Report as 22612, 22614, 22842, and 20937.

Vertebral procedures are sometimes followed by arthrodesis and in addition may include bone grafts and instrumentation.

When arthrodesis is performed in addition to another procedure, the arthrodesis should be reported in addition to the original procedure with modifier 51 (multiple procedures). Examples are after osteotomy, fracture care, vertebral corpectomy, and laminectomy. Bone grafts and instrumentation are never performed without arthrodesis.

Example:

Treatment of a burst fracture of L2 by corpectomy followed by arthrodesis of L1-L3, utilizing anterior instrumentation L1-L3 and structural allograft. Report as 63090, 22558-51, 22585, 22845, and 20931.

When two surgeons work together as primary surgeons performing distinct part(s) of a single reportable procedure, each surgeon should report his/her distinct operative work by appending modifier 62 to the single definitive procedure code. If additional procedure(s) (including add-on procedure[s]) are performed during the same surgical session, separate code(s) may be reported by each co-surgeon, with modifier 62 appended (see Appendix A).

Example:

A 42-year-old male with a history of posttraumatic degenerative disc disease at L3-4 and L4-5 (internal disc disruption) underwent surgical repair. Surgeon A performed an anterior exposure of the spine with mobilization of the great vessels. Surgeon B performed anterior (minimal) discectomy and fusion at L3-4 and L4-5 using anterior interbody technique.

Report surgeon A: 22558 append modifier 62, 22585 append modifier 62

Report surgeon B: 22558 append modifier 62, 22585 append modifier 62, 20931

Please see the Surgery Guidelines section for the following guidelines:

- *Surgical Procedures on the Musculoskeletal System*

AMA Coding Notes

Surgical Procedures on the Spine (Vertebral Column)

(Do not append modifier 62 to bone graft code 20931)

(For injection procedure for myelography, use 62284)

(For injection procedure for discography, see 62290, 62291)

(For injection procedure, chemonucleolysis, single or multiple levels, use 62292)

(For injection procedure for facet joints, see 64490-64495, 64633-64636)

(For needle or trocar biopsy, see 20220-20225)

AMA *CPT Assistant*

22849: Feb 96: 6, Sep 97: 8, Feb 02: 6, Nov 02: 3, Oct 11: 10, Jun 12: 11, Jul 13: 3, May 16: 13, Jun 17: 10

Plain English Description

This procedure is performed to reattach a device to the spine that has become dislodged.

Reinsertion of spinal fixation device

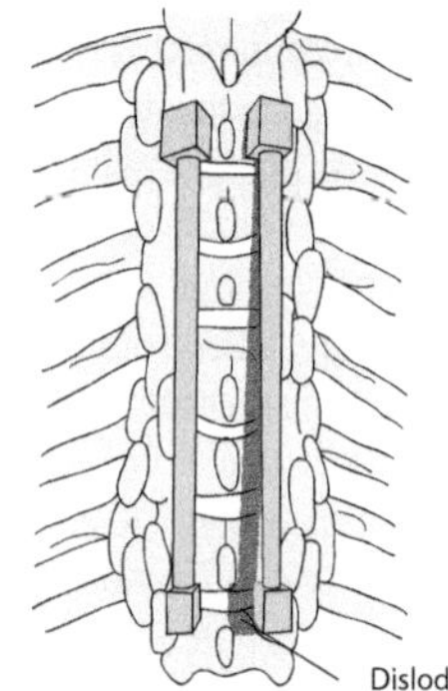

This procedure is performed to reattach a device to the spine that has become dislodged.

ICD-10-CM Diagnostic Codes

	Code	Description
	M96.0	Pseudarthrosis after fusion or arthrodesis
	M96.1	Postlaminectomy syndrome, not elsewhere classified
7	T84.216	Breakdown (mechanical) of internal fixation device of vertebrae
7	T84.226	Displacement of internal fixation device of vertebrae
7	T84.296	Other mechanical complication of internal fixation device of vertebrae
7	T84.428	Displacement of other internal orthopedic devices, implants and grafts
7	T84.498	Other mechanical complication of other internal orthopedic devices, implants and grafts
7	T84.82	Fibrosis due to internal orthopedic prosthetic devices, implants and grafts

- ➐ T84.84 Pain due to internal orthopedic prosthetic devices, implants and grafts
- ➐ T84.85 Stenosis due to internal orthopedic prosthetic devices, implants and grafts
- ➐ T84.89 Other specified complication of internal orthopedic prosthetic devices, implants and grafts

ICD-10-CM Coding Notes

For codes requiring a 7th character extension, refer to your ICD-10-CM book. Review the character descriptions and coding guidelines for proper selection. For some procedures, only certain characters will apply.

CCI Edits

Refer to Appendix A for CCI edits.

Facility RVUs ▯

Code	Work	PE Facility	MP	Total Facility
22849	19.17	13.33	5.25	37.75

Non-facility RVUs ▯

Code	Work	PE Non-Facility	MP	Total Non-Facility
22849	19.17	13.33	5.25	37.75

Modifiers **(PAR)** ▯

Code	Mod 50	Mod 51	Mod 62	Mod 66	Mod 80
22849	0	2	1	0	2

Global Period

Code	Days
22849	090

22850

22850 Removal of posterior nonsegmental instrumentation (eg, Harrington rod)

AMA Coding Guideline

Spinal Instrumentation Procedures on the Spine (Vertebral Column)

Segmental instrumentation is defined as fixation at each end of the construct and at least one additional interposed bony attachment.

Non-segmental instrumentation is defined as fixation at each end of the construct and may span several vertebral segments without attachment to the intervening segments.

Insertion of spinal instrumentation is reported separately and in addition to arthrodesis. Instrumentation procedure codes 22840-22848, 22853, 22854, 22859 are reported in addition to the definitive procedure(s). Do not append modifier 62 to spinal instrumentation codes 22840-22848, 22850, 22852, 22853, 22854, 22859.

To report bone graft procedures, see 20930-20938. (Report in addition to code[s] for definitive procedure[s].) Do not append modifier 62 to bone graft codes 20900-20938.

A vertebral segment describes the basic constituent part into which the spine may be divided. It represents a single complete vertebral bone with its associated articular processes and laminae. A vertebral interspace is the non-bony compartment between two adjacent vertebral bodies, which contains the intervertebral disc, and includes the nucleus pulposus, annulus fibrosus, and two cartilaginous endplates.

Codes 22849, 22850, 22852, and 22855 are subject to modifier 51 if reported with other definitive procedure(s), including arthrodesis, decompression, and exploration of fusion. Code 22849 should not be reported in conjunction with 22850, 22852, and 22855 at the same spinal levels. Only the appropriate insertion code (22840-22848) should be reported when previously placed spinal instrumentation is being removed or revised during the same session where new instrumentation is inserted at levels including all or part of the previously instrumented segments. Do not report the reinsertion (22849) or removal (22850, 22852, 22855) procedures in addition to the insertion of the new instrumentation (22840-22848).

Surgical Procedures on the Spine (Vertebral Column)

Cervical, thoracic, and lumbar spine.

Within the spine section, bone grafting procedures are reported separately and in addition to arthrodesis. For bone grafts in other Musculoskeletal sections, see specific code(s) descriptor(s) and/or accompanying guidelines.

To report bone grafts performed after arthrodesis, see 20930-20938. Do not append modifier 62 to bone graft codes 20900-20938.

Example:

Posterior arthrodesis of L5-S1 for degenerative disc disease utilizing morselized autogenous iliac bone graft harvested through a separate fascial incision.

Report as 22612 and 20937.

Within the spine section, instrumentation is reported separately and in addition to arthrodesis. To report instrumentation procedures performed with definitive vertebral procedure(s), see 22840-22855, 22859. Instrumentation procedure codes 22840-22848, 22853, 22854, 22859 are reported in addition to the definitive procedure(s). Modifier 62 may not be appended to the definitive or add-on spinal instrumentation procedure code(s) 22840-22848, 22850, 22852, 22853, 22854, 22859.

Example:

Posterior arthrodesis of L4-S1, utilizing morselized autogenous iliac bone graft harvested through separate fascial incision, and pedicle screw fixation.

Report as 22612, 22614, 22842, and 20937.

Vertebral procedures are sometimes followed by arthrodesis and in addition may include bone grafts and instrumentation.

When arthrodesis is performed in addition to another procedure, the arthrodesis should be reported in addition to the original procedure with modifier 51 (multiple procedures). Examples are after osteotomy, fracture care, vertebral corpectomy, and laminectomy. Bone grafts and instrumentation are never performed without arthrodesis.

Example:

Treatment of a burst fracture of L2 by corpectomy followed by arthrodesis of L1-L3, utilizing anterior instrumentation L1-L3 and structural allograft.

Report as 63090, 22558-51, 22585, 22845, and 20931.

When two surgeons work together as primary surgeons performing distinct part(s) of a single reportable procedure, each surgeon should report his/her distinct operative work by appending modifier 62 to the single definitive procedure code. If additional procedure(s) (including add-on procedure[s]) are performed during the same surgical session, separate code(s) may be reported by each co-surgeon, with modifier 62 appended (see Appendix A).

Example:

A 42-year-old male with a history of posttraumatic degenerative disc disease at L3-4 and L4-5 (internal disc disruption) underwent surgical repair. Surgeon A performed an anterior exposure of the spine with mobilization of the great vessels. Surgeon B performed anterior (minimal) discectomy and fusion at L3-4 and L4-5 using anterior interbody technique.

Report surgeon A: 22558 append modifier 62, 22585 append modifier 62

Report surgeon B: 22558 append modifier 62, 22585 append modifier 62, 20931

Please see the Surgery Guidelines section for the following guidelines:

- *Surgical Procedures on the Musculoskeletal System*

AMA Coding Notes

Surgical Procedures on the Spine (Vertebral Column)

(Do not append modifier 62 to bone graft code 20931)

(For injection procedure for myelography, use 62284)

(For injection procedure for discography, see 62290, 62291)

(For injection procedure, chemonucleolysis, single or multiple levels, use 62292)

(For injection procedure for facet joints, see 64490-64495, 64633-64636)

(For needle or trocar biopsy, see 20220-20225)

AMA *CPT Assistant*

22850: Feb 96: 6, Sep 97: 8, Feb 02: 6, Jun 12: 11, Jul 13: 3, May 16: 13, Jun 17: 10

Plain English Description

The physician removes a metal device, which is attached only at the top and bottom of the device from the spinal column.

Removal of posterior nonsegmental instrumentation

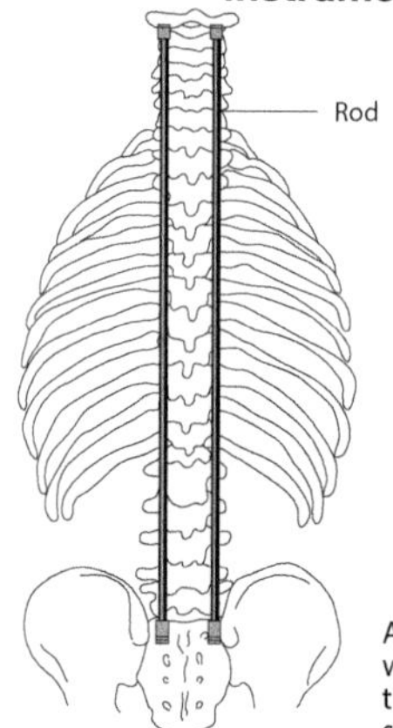

A metal device is removed, which is attached only at the top and bottom of the spinal column.

ICD-10-CM Diagnostic Codes

➐	T84.216	Breakdown (mechanical) of internal fixation device of vertebrae
➐	T84.226	Displacement of internal fixation device of vertebrae
➐	T84.296	Other mechanical complication of internal fixation device of vertebrae
➐	T84.428	Displacement of other internal orthopedic devices, implants and grafts
➐	T84.82	Fibrosis due to internal orthopedic prosthetic devices, implants and grafts
➐	T84.84	Pain due to internal orthopedic prosthetic devices, implants and grafts

⑦	T84.85	Stenosis due to internal orthopedic prosthetic devices, implants and grafts
⑦	T84.89	Other specified complication of internal orthopedic prosthetic devices, implants and grafts
	Z47.2	Encounter for removal of internal fixation device
	Z98.1	Arthrodesis status

ICD-10-CM Coding Notes

For codes requiring a 7th character extension, refer to your ICD-10-CM book. Review the character descriptions and coding guidelines for proper selection. For some procedures, only certain characters will apply.

CCI Edits

Refer to Appendix A for CCI edits.

Facility RVUs

Code	Work	PE Facility	MP	Total Facility
22850	9.82	8.55	2.72	21.09

Non-facility RVUs

Code	Work	PE Non-Facility	MP	Total Non-Facility
22850	9.82	8.55	2.72	21.09

Modifiers (PAR)

Code	Mod 50	Mod 51	Mod 62	Mod 66	Mod 80
22850	0	2	1	0	2

Global Period

Code	Days
22850	090

22852

22852 Removal of posterior segmental instrumentation

AMA Coding Guideline

Spinal Instrumentation Procedures on the Spine (Vertebral Column)

Segmental instrumentation is defined as fixation at each end of the construct and at least one additional interposed bony attachment.

Non-segmental instrumentation is defined as fixation at each end of the construct and may span several vertebral segments without attachment to the intervening segments.

Insertion of spinal instrumentation is reported separately and in addition to arthrodesis. Instrumentation procedure codes 22840-22848, 22853, 22854, 22859 are reported in addition to the definitive procedure(s). Do not append modifier 62 to spinal instrumentation codes 22840-22848, 22850, 22852, 22853, 22854, 22859.

To report bone graft procedures, see 20930-20938. (Report in addition to code[s] for definitive procedure[s].) Do not append modifier 62 to bone graft codes 20900-20938.

A vertebral segment describes the basic constituent part into which the spine may be divided. It represents a single complete vertebral bone with its associated articular processes and laminae. A vertebral interspace is the non-bony compartment between two adjacent vertebral bodies, which contains the intervertebral disc, and includes the nucleus pulposus, annulus fibrosus, and two cartilaginous endplates.

Codes 22849, 22850, 22852, and 22855 are subject to modifier 51 if reported with other definitive procedure(s), including arthrodesis, decompression, and exploration of fusion. Code 22849 should not be reported in conjunction with 22850, 22852, and 22855 at the same spinal levels. Only the appropriate insertion code (22840-22848) should be reported when previously placed spinal instrumentation is being removed or revised during the same session where new instrumentation is inserted at levels including all or part of the previously instrumented segments. Do not report the reinsertion (22849) or removal (22850, 22852, 22855) procedures in addition to the insertion of the new instrumentation (22840-22848).

Surgical Procedures on the Spine (Vertebral Column)

Cervical, thoracic, and lumbar spine.

Within the spine section, bone grafting procedures are reported separately and in addition to arthrodesis. For bone grafts in other Musculoskeletal sections, see specific code(s) descriptor(s) and/or accompanying guidelines.

To report bone grafts performed after arthrodesis, see 20930-20938. Do not append modifier 62 to bone graft codes 20900-20938.

Example:

Posterior arthrodesis of L5-S1 for degenerative disc disease utilizing morselized autogenous iliac bone graft harvested through a separate fascial incision. Report as 22612 and 20937.

Within the spine section, instrumentation is reported separately and in addition to arthrodesis. To report instrumentation procedures performed with definitive vertebral procedure(s), see 22840-22855, 22859. Instrumentation procedure codes 22840-22848, 22853, 22854, 22859 are reported in addition to the definitive procedure(s). Modifier 62 may not be appended to the definitive or add-on spinal instrumentation procedure code(s) 22840-22848, 22850, 22852, 22853, 22854, 22859.

Example:

Posterior arthrodesis of L4-S1, utilizing morselized autogenous iliac bone graft harvested through separate fascial incision, and pedicle screw fixation. Report as 22612, 22614, 22842, and 20937.

Vertebral procedures are sometimes followed by arthrodesis and in addition may include bone grafts and instrumentation.

When arthrodesis is performed in addition to another procedure, the arthrodesis should be reported in addition to the original procedure with modifier 51 (multiple procedures). Examples are after osteotomy, fracture care, vertebral corpectomy, and laminectomy. Bone grafts and instrumentation are never performed without arthrodesis.

Example:

Treatment of a burst fracture of L2 by corpectomy followed by arthrodesis of L1-L3, utilizing anterior instrumentation L1-L3 and structural allograft. Report as 63090, 22558-51, 22585, 22845, and 20931.

When two surgeons work together as primary surgeons performing distinct part(s) of a single reportable procedure, each surgeon should report his/her distinct operative work by appending modifier 62 to the single definitive procedure code. If additional procedure(s) (including add-on procedure[s]) are performed during the same surgical session, separate code(s) may be reported by each co-surgeon, with modifier 62 appended (see Appendix A).

Example:

A 42-year-old male with a history of posttraumatic degenerative disc disease at L3-4 and L4-5 (internal disc disruption) underwent surgical repair. Surgeon A performed an anterior exposure of the spine with mobilization of the great vessels. Surgeon B performed anterior (minimal) discectomy and fusion at L3-4 and L4-5 using anterior interbody technique.

Report surgeon A: 22558 append modifier 62, 22585 append modifier 62

Report surgeon B: 22558 append modifier 62, 22585 append modifier 62, 20931

Please see the Surgery Guidelines section for the following guidelines:

- *Surgical Procedures on the Musculoskeletal System*

AMA Coding Notes

Surgical Procedures on the Spine (Vertebral Column)

(Do not append modifier 62 to bone graft code 20931)

(For injection procedure for myelography, use 62284)

(For injection procedure for discography, see 62290, 62291)

(For injection procedure, chemonucleolysis, single or multiple levels, use 62292)

(For injection procedure for facet joints, see 64490-64495, 64633-64636)

(For needle or trocar biopsy, see 20220-20225)

AMA *CPT Assistant*

22852: Feb 96: 6, Sep 97: 8, Feb 02: 6, May 06: 16, Jun 12: 11, Jun 17: 10

Plain English Description

The physician removes a metal device, which is attached at the top, bottom, and various other places along the device from the spinal column.

Removal of posterior segmental instrumentation

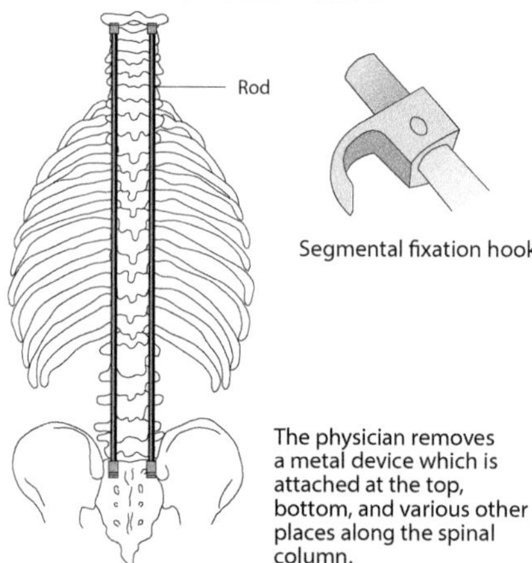

ICD-10-CM Diagnostic Codes

⑦	T84.216	Breakdown (mechanical) of internal fixation device of vertebrae
⑦	T84.226	Displacement of internal fixation device of vertebrae
⑦	T84.296	Other mechanical complication of internal fixation device of vertebrae
⑦	T84.428	Displacement of other internal orthopedic devices, implants and grafts
⑦	T84.82	Fibrosis due to internal orthopedic prosthetic devices, implants and grafts
⑦	T84.84	Pain due to internal orthopedic prosthetic devices, implants and grafts

⑦	T84.85	Stenosis due to internal orthopedic prosthetic devices, implants and grafts
⑦	T84.89	Other specified complication of internal orthopedic prosthetic devices, implants and grafts
	Z47.2	Encounter for removal of internal fixation device
	Z98.1	Arthrodesis status

ICD-10-CM Coding Notes

For codes requiring a 7th character extension, refer to your ICD-10-CM book. Review the character descriptions and coding guidelines for proper selection. For some procedures, only certain characters will apply.

CCI Edits

Refer to Appendix A for CCI edits.

Facility RVUs ▯

Code	Work	PE Facility	MP	Total Facility
22852	9.37	8.32	2.56	20.25

Non-facility RVUs ▯

Code	Work	PE Non-Facility	MP	Total Non-Facility
22852	9.37	8.32	2.56	20.25

Modifiers (PAR) ▯

Code	Mod 50	Mod 51	Mod 62	Mod 66	Mod 80
22852	0	2	1	0	2

Global Period

Code	Days
22852	090

22853-22854

+ **22853 Insertion of interbody biomechanical device(s) (eg, synthetic cage, mesh) with integral anterior instrumentation for device anchoring (eg, screws, flanges), when performed, to intervertebral disc space in conjunction with interbody arthrodesis, each interspace (List separately in addition to code for primary procedure)**

(Use 22853 in conjunction with 22100-22102, 22110-22114, 22206, 22207, 22210-22214, 22220-22224, 22310-22327, 22532, 22533, 22548-22558, 22590-22612, 22630, 22633, 22634, 22800-22812, 63001-63030, 63040-63042, 63045-63047, 63050-63056, 63064, 63075, 63077, 63081, 63085, 63087, 63090, 63101, 63102, 63170-63290, 63300-63307)

(Report 22853 for each treated intervertebral disc space)

+ **22854 Insertion of intervertebral biomechanical device(s) (eg, synthetic cage, mesh) with integral anterior instrumentation for device anchoring (eg, screws, flanges), when performed, to vertebral corpectomy(ies) (vertebral body resection, partial or complete) defect, in conjunction with interbody arthrodesis, each contiguous defect (List separately in addition to code for primary procedure)**

(Use 22854 in conjunction with 22100-22102, 22110-22114, 22206, 22207, 22210-22214, 22220-22224, 22310-22327, 22532, 22533, 22548-22558, 22590-22612, 22630, 22633, 22634, 22800-22812, 63001-63030, 63040-63042, 63045-63047, 63050-63056, 63064, 63075, 63077, 63081, 63085, 63087, 63090, 63101, 63102, 63170-63290, 63300-63307)

AMA Coding Guideline

Spinal Instrumentation Procedures on the Spine (Vertebral Column)

Segmental instrumentation is defined as fixation at each end of the construct and at least one additional interposed bony attachment.

Non-segmental instrumentation is defined as fixation at each end of the construct and may span several vertebral segments without attachment to the intervening segments.

Insertion of spinal instrumentation is reported separately and in addition to arthrodesis. Instrumentation procedure codes 22840-22848, 22853, 22854, 22859 are reported in addition to the definitive procedure(s). Do not append modifier 62 to spinal instrumentation codes 22840-22848, 22850, 22852, 22853, 22854, 22859.

To report bone graft procedures, see 20930-20938. (Report in addition to code[s] for definitive procedure[s].) Do not append modifier 62 to bone graft codes 20900-20938.

A vertebral segment describes the basic constituent part into which the spine may be divided. It represents a single complete vertebral bone with its associated articular processes and laminae. A vertebral interspace is the non-bony compartment between two adjacent vertebral bodies, which contains the intervertebral disc, and includes the nucleus pulposus, annulus fibrosus, and two cartilaginous endplates.

Codes 22849, 22850, 22852, and 22855 are subject to modifier 51 if reported with other definitive procedure(s), including arthrodesis, decompression, and exploration of fusion. Code 22849 should not be reported in conjunction with 22850, 22852, and 22855 at the same spinal levels. Only the appropriate insertion code (22840-22848) should be reported when previously placed spinal instrumentation is being removed or revised during the same session where new instrumentation is inserted at levels including all or part of the previously instrumented segments. Do not report the reinsertion (22849) or removal (22850, 22852, 22855) procedures in addition to the insertion of the new instrumentation (22840-22848).

Surgical Procedures on the Spine (Vertebral Column)

Cervical, thoracic, and lumbar spine.

Within the spine section, bone grafting procedures are reported separately and in addition to arthrodesis. For bone grafts in other Musculoskeletal sections, see specific code(s) descriptor(s) and/or accompanying guidelines.

To report bone grafts performed after arthrodesis, see 20930-20938. Do not append modifier 62 to bone graft codes 20900-20938.

Example:

Posterior arthrodesis of L5-S1 for degenerative disc disease utilizing morselized autogenous iliac bone graft harvested through a separate fascial incision.

Report as 22612 and 20937.

Within the spine section, instrumentation is reported separately and in addition to arthrodesis. To report instrumentation procedures performed with definitive vertebral procedure(s), see 22840-22855, 22859. Instrumentation procedure codes 22840-22848, 22853, 22854, 22859 are reported in addition to the definitive procedure(s). Modifier 62 may not be appended to the definitive or add-on spinal instrumentation procedure code(s) 22840-22848, 22850, 22852, 22853, 22854, 22859.

Example:

Posterior arthrodesis of L4-S1, utilizing morselized autogenous iliac bone graft harvested through separate fascial incision, and pedicle screw fixation.

Report as 22612, 22614, 22842, and 20937.

Vertebral procedures are sometimes followed by arthrodesis and in addition may include bone grafts and instrumentation.

When arthrodesis is performed in addition to another procedure, the arthrodesis should be reported in addition to the original procedure with modifier 51 (multiple procedures). Examples are after osteotomy, fracture care, vertebral corpectomy, and laminectomy. Bone grafts and instrumentation are never performed without arthrodesis.

Example:

Treatment of a burst fracture of L2 by corpectomy followed by arthrodesis of L1-L3, utilizing anterior instrumentation L1-L3 and structural allograft.

Report as 63090, 22558-51, 22585, 22845, and 20931.

When two surgeons work together as primary surgeons performing distinct part(s) of a single reportable procedure, each surgeon should report his/her distinct operative work by appending modifier 62 to the single definitive procedure code. If additional procedure(s) (including add-on procedure[s]) are performed during the same surgical session, separate code(s) may be reported by each co-surgeon, with modifier 62 appended (see Appendix A).

Example:

A 42-year-old male with a history of posttraumatic degenerative disc disease at L3-4 and L4-5 (internal disc disruption) underwent surgical repair. Surgeon A performed an anterior exposure of the spine with mobilization of the great vessels. Surgeon B performed anterior (minimal) discectomy and fusion at L3-4 and L4-5 using anterior interbody technique.

Report surgeon A: 22558 append modifier 62, 22585 append modifier 62

Report surgeon B: 22558 append modifier 62, 22585 append modifier 62, 20931

Please see the Surgery Guidelines section for the following guidelines:

- *Surgical Procedures on the Musculoskeletal System*

AMA Coding Notes

Surgical Procedures on the Spine (Vertebral Column)

(Do not append modifier 62 to bone graft code 20931)

(For injection procedure for myelography, use 62284)

(For injection procedure for discography, see 62290, 62291)

(For injection procedure, chemonucleolysis, single or multiple levels, use 62292)

(For injection procedure for facet joints, see 64490-64495, 64633-64636)

(For needle or trocar biopsy, see 20220-20225)

AMA *CPT Assistant*

22853: Mar 17: 7, Aug 17: 9, Jul 18: 14
22854: Mar 17: 7

Plain English Description

A procedure is performed to decompress the spinal cord and nerves and restore intervertebral disc space and anatomic alignment with insertion of an intervertebral biomechanical device. Surgical immobilization of the spine by fusing adjacent vertebrae (arthrodesis) and/or removing all or part of a vertebral body (corpectomy) may be done for degenerative disc disease, spinal stenosis, or bone spurs (osteophytes). The intervertebral biomechanical device is usually a cylindrical or square-shaped synthetic cage or that can be packed with autogenous bone material to promote arthrodesis. For cervical placement, a horizontal incision is made in the side of the neck. The platysma muscle is transected, the plane between the sternocleidomastoid muscle and strap muscles is entered, and the space between the trachea/esophagus and the carotid sheath is accessed. The fascia is dissected away from the disc space. For lumbar placement, an incision is made in the left side of the abdomen and the muscles retracted. The peritoneum is kept intact and retracted to the side as are vascular structures such as the aorta and vena cava. For both approaches, all or part of the intervertebral disc may be removed in a separately reported procedure. The biomechanical device is placed into the intervertebral disc space (22853) or vertebral body defect (22854) in conjunction with interbody arthrodesis. Bone graft material may be inserted into the device, with integral anterior fixation of the device, if performed, accomplished using screws/flanges. Report code 22859 when an intervertebral device, such as a synthetic cage, mesh, or methylmethacrylate, is inserted into the intervertebral disc space or vertebral body defect to maintain foraminal height or spinal cord/nerve decompression without arthrodesis, or fusing of adjacent vertebrae.

Insertion of interbody biomechanical device(s) (eg, synthetic cage, mesh) with integral anterior instrumentation for device anchoring (each interspace list separately)

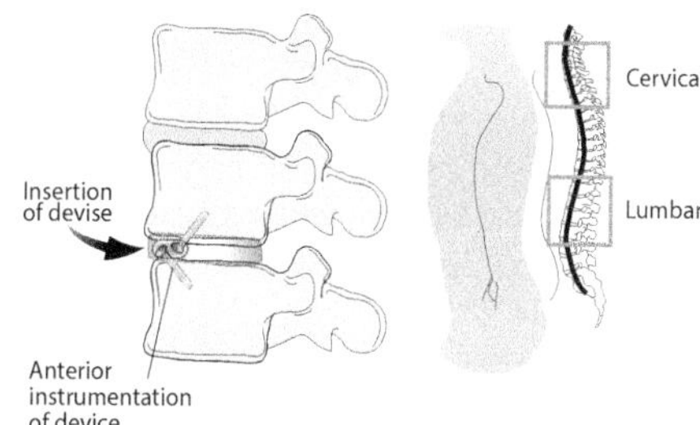

(22853) intervertebral disc space in conjunction with interbody arthrodesis; (22854) vertebral corpectomy(ies) vertebral body resection; (22859) without interbody arthrodesis

ICD-10-CM Diagnostic Codes

See Primary Procedure code for crosswalks.

CCI Edits

Refer to Appendix A for CCI edits.

Facility RVUs

Code	Work	PE Facility	MP	Total Facility
22853	4.25	2.03	1.24	7.52
22854	5.50	2.63	1.61	9.74

Non-facility RVUs

Code	Work	PE Non-Facility	MP	Total Non-Facility
22853	4.25	2.03	1.24	7.52
22854	5.50	2.63	1.61	9.74

Modifiers (PAR)

Code	Mod 50	Mod 51	Mod 62	Mod 66	Mod 80
22853	0	0	2	0	2
22854	0	0	2	0	2

Global Period

Code	Days
22853	ZZZ
22854	ZZZ

22855

22855 Removal of anterior instrumentation

AMA Coding Guideline

Spinal Instrumentation Procedures on the Spine (Vertebral Column)

Segmental instrumentation is defined as fixation at each end of the construct and at least one additional interposed bony attachment.

Non-segmental instrumentation is defined as fixation at each end of the construct and may span several vertebral segments without attachment to the intervening segments.

Insertion of spinal instrumentation is reported separately and in addition to arthrodesis. Instrumentation procedure codes 22840-22848, 22853, 22854, 22859 are reported in addition to the definitive procedure(s). Do not append modifier 62 to spinal instrumentation codes 22840-22848, 22850, 22852, 22853, 22854, 22859.

To report bone graft procedures, see 20930-20938. (Report in addition to code[s] for definitive procedure[s].) Do not append modifier 62 to bone graft codes 20900-20938.

A vertebral segment describes the basic constituent part into which the spine may be divided. It represents a single complete vertebral bone with its associated articular processes and laminae. A vertebral interspace is the non-bony compartment between two adjacent vertebral bodies, which contains the intervertebral disc, and includes the nucleus pulposus, annulus fibrosus, and two cartilaginous endplates.

Codes 22849, 22850, 22852, and 22855 are subject to modifier 51 if reported with other definitive procedure(s), including arthrodesis, decompression, and exploration of fusion. Code 22849 should not be reported in conjunction with 22850, 22852, and 22855 at the same spinal levels. Only the appropriate insertion code (22840-22848) should be reported when previously placed spinal instrumentation is being removed or revised during the same session where new instrumentation is inserted at levels including all or part of the previously instrumented segments. Do not report the reinsertion (22849) or removal (22850, 22852, 22855) procedures in addition to the insertion of the new instrumentation (22840-22848).

Surgical Procedures on the Spine (Vertebral Column)

Cervical, thoracic, and lumbar spine.

Within the spine section, bone grafting procedures are reported separately and in addition to arthrodesis. For bone grafts in other Musculoskeletal sections, see specific code(s) descriptor(s) and/or accompanying guidelines.

To report bone grafts performed after arthrodesis, see 20930-20938. Do not append modifier 62 to bone graft codes 20900-20938.

Example:

Posterior arthrodesis of L5-S1 for degenerative disc disease utilizing morselized autogenous iliac bone graft harvested through a separate fascial incision.

Report as 22612 and 20937.

Within the spine section, instrumentation is reported separately and in addition to arthrodesis. To report instrumentation procedures performed with definitive vertebral procedure(s), see 22840-22855, 22859. Instrumentation procedure codes 22840-22848, 22853, 22854, 22859 are reported in addition to the definitive procedure(s). Modifier 62 may not be appended to the definitive or add-on spinal instrumentation procedure code(s) 22840-22848, 22850, 22852, 22853, 22854, 22859.

Example:

Posterior arthrodesis of L4-S1, utilizing morselized autogenous iliac bone graft harvested through separate fascial incision, and pedicle screw fixation.

Report as 22612, 22614, 22842, and 20937.

Vertebral procedures are sometimes followed by arthrodesis and in addition may include bone grafts and instrumentation.

When arthrodesis is performed in addition to another procedure, the arthrodesis should be reported in addition to the original procedure with modifier 51 (multiple procedures). Examples are after osteotomy, fracture care, vertebral corpectomy, and laminectomy. Bone grafts and instrumentation are never performed without arthrodesis.

Example:

Treatment of a burst fracture of L2 by corpectomy followed by arthrodesis of L1-L3, utilizing anterior instrumentation L1-L3 and structural allograft.

Report as 63090, 22558-51, 22585, 22845, and 20931.

When two surgeons work together as primary surgeons performing distinct part(s) of a single reportable procedure, each surgeon should report his/her distinct operative work by appending modifier 62 to the single definitive procedure code. If additional procedure(s) (including add-on procedure[s]) are performed during the same surgical session, separate code(s) may be reported by each co-surgeon, with modifier 62 appended (see Appendix A).

Example:

A 42-year-old male with a history of posttraumatic degenerative disc disease at L3-4 and L4-5 (internal disc disruption) underwent surgical repair. Surgeon A performed an anterior exposure of the spine with mobilization of the great vessels. Surgeon B performed anterior (minimal) discectomy and fusion at L3-4 and L4-5 using anterior interbody technique.

Report surgeon A: 22558 append modifier 62, 22585 append modifier 62

Report surgeon B: 22558 append modifier 62, 22585 append modifier 62, 20931

Please see the Surgery Guidelines section for the following guidelines:

- *Surgical Procedures on the Musculoskeletal System*

AMA Coding Notes

Surgical Procedures on the Spine (Vertebral Column)

(Do not append modifier 62 to bone graft code 20931)

(For injection procedure for myelography, use 62284)

(For injection procedure for discography, see 62290, 62291)

(For injection procedure, chemonucleolysis, single or multiple levels, use 62292)

(For injection procedure for facet joints, see 64490-64495, 64633-64636)

(For needle or trocar biopsy, see 20220-20225)

AMA *CPT Assistant* ◻

22855: Feb 96: 6, Sep 97: 8, Feb 02: 6, Nov 02: 2, Jun 12: 11, Jun 17: 10

Plain English Description

The physician removes a metal instrument from the front of the spinal column.

Removal of anterior instrumentation

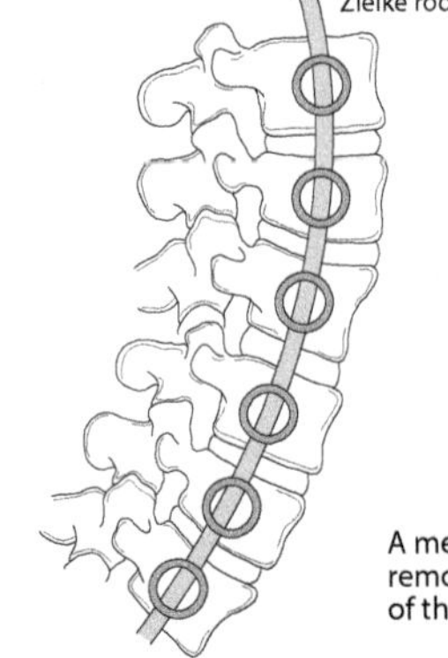

ICD-10-CM Diagnostic Codes

⑦	T84.216	Breakdown (mechanical) of internal fixation device of vertebrae
⑦	T84.226	Displacement of internal fixation device of vertebrae
⑦	T84.296	Other mechanical complication of internal fixation device of vertebrae
⑦	T84.428	Displacement of other internal orthopedic devices, implants and grafts
⑦	T84.63	Infection and inflammatory reaction due to internal fixation device of spine
⑦	T84.81	Embolism due to internal orthopedic prosthetic devices, implants and grafts
⑦	T84.82	Fibrosis due to internal orthopedic prosthetic devices, implants and grafts
⑦	T84.83	Hemorrhage due to internal orthopedic prosthetic devices, implants and grafts

➐	T84.84	Pain due to internal orthopedic prosthetic devices, implants and grafts
➐	T84.85	Stenosis due to internal orthopedic prosthetic devices, implants and grafts
➐	T84.86	Thrombosis due to internal orthopedic prosthetic devices, implants and grafts
➐	T84.89	Other specified complication of internal orthopedic prosthetic devices, implants and grafts
	Z47.2	Encounter for removal of internal fixation device
	Z98.1	Arthrodesis status

ICD-10-CM Coding Notes

For codes requiring a 7th character extension, refer to your ICD-10-CM book. Review the character descriptions and coding guidelines for proper selection. For some procedures, only certain characters will apply.

CCI Edits

Refer to Appendix A for CCI edits.

Facility RVUs

Code	Work	PE Facility	MP	Total Facility
22855	15.86	11.64	4.62	32.12

Non-facility RVUs

Code	Work	PE Non-Facility	MP	Total Non-Facility
22855	15.86	11.64	4.62	32.12

Modifiers (PAR)

Code	Mod 50	Mod 51	Mod 62	Mod 66	Mod 80
22855	0	2	1	0	2

Global Period

Code	Days
22855	090

22859

✚ **22859 Insertion of intervertebral biomechanical device(s) (eg, synthetic cage, mesh, methylmethacrylate) to intervertebral disc space or vertebral body defect without interbody arthrodesis, each contiguous defect (List separately in addition to code for primary procedure)**

(Use 22859 in conjunction with 22100-22102, 22110-22114, 22206, 22207, 22210-22214, 22220-22224, 22310-22327, 22532, 22533, 22548-22558, 22590-22612, 22630, 22633, 22634, 22800-22812, 63001-63030, 63040-63042, 63045-63047, 63050-63056, 63064, 63075, 63077, 63081, 63085, 63087, 63090, 63101, 63102, 63170-63290, 63300-63307)

(22853, 22854, 22859 may be reported more than once for noncontiguous defects)

(For application of an intervertebral bone device/graft, see 20930, 20931, 20936, 20937, 20938)

AMA Coding Guideline

Spinal Instrumentation Procedures on the Spine (Vertebral Column)

Segmental instrumentation is defined as fixation at each end of the construct and at least one additional interposed bony attachment.

Non-segmental instrumentation is defined as fixation at each end of the construct and may span several vertebral segments without attachment to the intervening segments.

Insertion of spinal instrumentation is reported separately and in addition to arthrodesis. Instrumentation procedure codes 22840-22848, 22853, 22854, 22859 are reported in addition to the definitive procedure(s). Do not append modifier 62 to spinal instrumentation codes 22840-22848, 22850, 22852, 22853, 22854, 22859.

To report bone graft procedures, see 20930-20938. (Report in addition to code[s] for definitive procedure[s].) Do not append modifier 62 to bone graft codes 20900-20938.

A vertebral segment describes the basic constituent part into which the spine may be divided. It represents a single complete vertebral bone with its associated articular processes and laminae. A vertebral interspace is the non-bony compartment between two adjacent vertebral bodies, which contains the intervertebral disc, and includes the nucleus pulposus, annulus fibrosus, and two cartilaginous endplates.

Codes 22849, 22850, 22852, and 22855 are subject to modifier 51 if reported with other definitive procedure(s), including arthrodesis, decompression, and exploration of fusion. Code 22849 should not be reported in conjunction with 22850, 22852, and 22855 at the same spinal levels. Only the appropriate insertion code (22840-22848) should be reported when previously placed spinal instrumentation is being removed or revised during the same session where new instrumentation is inserted at levels including all or part of the previously instrumented segments. Do not report the reinsertion (22849) or removal (22850, 22852, 22855) procedures in addition to the insertion of the new instrumentation (22840-22848).

Surgical Procedures on the Spine (Vertebral Column)

Cervical, thoracic, and lumbar spine.

Within the spine section, bone grafting procedures are reported separately and in addition to arthrodesis. For bone grafts in other Musculoskeletal sections, see specific code(s) descriptor(s) and/or accompanying guidelines.

To report bone grafts performed after arthrodesis, see 20930-20938. Do not append modifier 62 to bone graft codes 20900-20938.

Example:

Posterior arthrodesis of L5-S1 for degenerative disc disease utilizing morselized autogenous iliac bone graft harvested through a separate fascial incision.

Report as 22612 and 20937.

Within the spine section, instrumentation is reported separately and in addition to arthrodesis. To report instrumentation procedures performed with definitive vertebral procedure(s), see 22840-22855, 22859. Instrumentation procedure codes 22840-22848, 22853, 22854, 22859 are reported in addition to the definitive procedure(s). Modifier 62 may not be appended to the definitive or add-on spinal instrumentation procedure code(s) 22840-22848, 22850, 22852, 22853, 22854, 22859.

Example:

Posterior arthrodesis of L4-S1, utilizing morselized autogenous iliac bone graft harvested through separate fascial incision, and pedicle screw fixation.

Report as 22612, 22614, 22842, and 20937.

Vertebral procedures are sometimes followed by arthrodesis and in addition may include bone grafts and instrumentation.

When arthrodesis is performed in addition to another procedure, the arthrodesis should be reported in addition to the original procedure with modifier 51 (multiple procedures). Examples are after osteotomy, fracture care, vertebral corpectomy, and laminectomy. Bone grafts and instrumentation are never performed without arthrodesis.

Example:

Treatment of a burst fracture of L2 by corpectomy followed by arthrodesis of L1-L3, utilizing anterior instrumentation L1-L3 and structural allograft.

Report as 63090, 22558-51, 22585, 22845, and 20931.

When two surgeons work together as primary surgeons performing distinct part(s) of a single reportable procedure, each surgeon should report his/her distinct operative work by appending modifier 62 to the single definitive procedure code. If additional procedure(s) (including add-on procedure[s]) are performed during the same surgical session, separate code(s) may be reported by each co-surgeon, with modifier 62 appended (see Appendix A).

Example:

A 42-year-old male with a history of posttraumatic degenerative disc disease at L3-4 and L4-5 (internal disc disruption) underwent surgical repair. Surgeon A performed an anterior exposure of the spine with mobilization of the great vessels. Surgeon B performed anterior (minimal) discectomy and fusion at L3-4 and L4-5 using anterior interbody technique.

Report surgeon A: 22558 append modifier 62, 22585 append modifier 62

Report surgeon B: 22558 append modifier 62, 22585 append modifier 62, 20931

Please see the Surgery Guidelines section for the following guidelines:

- *Surgical Procedures on the Musculoskeletal System*

AMA Coding Notes

Surgical Procedures on the Spine (Vertebral Column)

(Do not append modifier 62 to bone graft code 20931)

(For injection procedure for myelography, use 62284)

(For injection procedure for discography, see 62290, 62291)

(For injection procedure, chemonucleolysis, single or multiple levels, use 62292)

(For injection procedure for facet joints, see 64490-64495, 64633-64636)

(For needle or trocar biopsy, see 20220-20225)

AMA *CPT Assistant* ☐

22859: Mar 17: 7

Plain English Description

A procedure is performed to decompress the spinal cord and nerves and restore intervertebral disc space and anatomic alignment with insertion of an intervertebral biomechanical device. Surgical immobilization of the spine by fusing adjacent vertebrae (arthrodesis) and/or removing all or part of a vertebral body (corpectomy) may be done for degenerative disc disease, spinal stenosis, or bone spurs (osteophytes). The intervertebral biomechanical device is usually a cylindrical or square-shaped synthetic cage that can be packed with autogenous bone material to promote arthrodesis. For cervical placement, a horizontal incision is made in the side of the neck. The platysma muscle is transected, the plane between the sternocleidomastoid muscle and strap muscles is entered, and the space between the trachea/esophagus and the carotid sheath is accessed. The fascia is dissected away from the disc space. For lumbar placement, an incision is made in the left side of the abdomen and the muscles retracted. The peritoneum is kept intact and retracted to the side as are vascular structures such as the aorta and vena cava. For both approaches, all or part of the intervertebral disc may be removed in a separately reported procedure. The biomechanical device is placed into the intervertebral disc space (22853) or vertebral body defect (22854) in conjunction with interbody arthrodesis. Bone graft material may be inserted into the device, with integral anterior fixation of the device, if performed, accomplished using screws/flanges. Report code 22859 when an intervertebral device, such as a synthetic cage, mesh, or methylmethacrylate, is inserted into the intervertebral disc space or vertebral body defect to maintain foraminal height or spinal cord/nerve decompression without arthrodesis, or fusing of adjacent vertebrae.

ICD-10-CM Diagnostic Codes

See Primary Procedure code for crosswalks.

CCI Edits

Refer to Appendix A for CCI edits.

Facility RVUs ▯

Code	Work	PE Facility	MP	Total Facility
22859	5.50	2.63	1.61	9.74

Non-facility RVUs ▯

Code	Work	PE Non-Facility	MP	Total Non-Facility
22859	5.50	2.63	1.61	9.74

Modifiers (PAR) ▯

Code	Mod 50	Mod 51	Mod 62	Mod 66	Mod 80
22859	0	0	2	0	2

Global Period

Code	Days
22859	ZZZ

22867-22868

22867 Insertion of interlaminar/interspinous process stabilization/distraction device, without fusion, including image guidance when performed, with open decompression, lumbar; single level

+ **22868 Insertion of interlaminar/interspinous process stabilization/distraction device, without fusion, including image guidance when performed, with open decompression, lumbar; second level (List separately in addition to code for primary procedure)**

(Use 22868 in conjunction with 22867)

(Do not report 22867, 22868 in conjunction with 22532, 22533, 22534, 22558, 22612, 22614, 22630, 22632, 22633, 22634, 22800, 22802, 22804, 22840, 22841, 22842, 22869, 22870, 63005, 63012, 63017, 63030, 63035, 63042, 63044, 63047, 63048, 77003 for the same level)

(For insertion of interlaminar/interspinous process stabilization/distraction device, without open decompression or fusion, see 22869, 22870)

AMA Coding Guideline

Spinal Instrumentation Procedures on the Spine (Vertebral Column)

Segmental instrumentation is defined as fixation at each end of the construct and at least one additional interposed bony attachment.

Non-segmental instrumentation is defined as fixation at each end of the construct and may span several vertebral segments without attachment to the intervening segments.

Insertion of spinal instrumentation is reported separately and in addition to arthrodesis. Instrumentation procedure codes 22840-22848, 22853, 22854, 22859 are reported in addition to the definitive procedure(s). Do not append modifier 62 to spinal instrumentation codes 22840-22848, 22850, 22852, 22853, 22854, 22859.

To report bone graft procedures, see 20930-20938. (Report in addition to code[s] for definitive procedure[s].) Do not append modifier 62 to bone graft codes 20900-20938.

A vertebral segment describes the basic constituent part into which the spine may be divided. It represents a single complete vertebral bone with its associated articular processes and laminae. A vertebral interspace is the non-bony compartment between two adjacent vertebral bodies, which contains the intervertebral disc, and includes the nucleus pulposus, annulus fibrosus, and two cartilaginous endplates.

Codes 22849, 22850, 22852, and 22855 are subject to modifier 51 if reported with other definitive procedure(s), including arthrodesis, decompression, and exploration of fusion. Code 22849 should not be reported in conjunction with 22850, 22852, and 22855 at the same spinal levels. Only the appropriate insertion code (22840-22848) should be reported when previously placed spinal instrumentation is being removed or revised during the same session where new instrumentation is inserted at levels including all or part of the previously instrumented segments. Do not report the reinsertion (22849) or removal (22850, 22852, 22855) procedures in addition to the insertion of the new instrumentation (22840-22848).

Surgical Procedures on the Spine (Vertebral Column)

Cervical, thoracic, and lumbar spine.

Within the spine section, bone grafting procedures are reported separately and in addition to arthrodesis. For bone grafts in other Musculoskeletal sections, see specific code(s) descriptor(s) and/or accompanying guidelines.

To report bone grafts performed after arthrodesis, see 20930-20938. Do not append modifier 62 to bone graft codes 20900-20938.

Example:

Posterior arthrodesis of L5-S1 for degenerative disc disease utilizing morselized autogenous iliac bone graft harvested through a separate fascial incision.

Report as 22612 and 20937.

Within the spine section, instrumentation is reported separately and in addition to arthrodesis. To report instrumentation procedures performed with definitive vertebral procedure(s), see 22840-22855, 22859. Instrumentation procedure codes 22840-22848, 22853, 22854, 22859 are reported in addition to the definitive procedure(s). Modifier 62 may not be appended to the definitive or add-on spinal instrumentation procedure code(s) 22840-22848, 22850, 22852, 22853, 22854, 22859.

Example:

Posterior arthrodesis of L4-S1, utilizing morselized autogenous iliac bone graft harvested through separate fascial incision, and pedicle screw fixation.

Report as 22612, 22614, 22842, and 20937.

Vertebral procedures are sometimes followed by arthrodesis and in addition may include bone grafts and instrumentation.

When arthrodesis is performed in addition to another procedure, the arthrodesis should be reported in addition to the original procedure with modifier 51 (multiple procedures). Examples are after osteotomy, fracture care, vertebral corpectomy, and laminectomy. Bone grafts and instrumentation are never performed without arthrodesis.

Example:

Treatment of a burst fracture of L2 by corpectomy followed by arthrodesis of L1-L3, utilizing anterior instrumentation L1-L3 and structural allograft.

Report as 63090, 22558-51, 22585, 22845, and 20931.

When two surgeons work together as primary surgeons performing distinct part(s) of a single reportable procedure, each surgeon should report his/her distinct operative work by appending modifier 62 to the single definitive procedure code. If additional procedure(s) (including add-on procedure[s]) are performed during the same surgical session, separate code(s) may be reported by each co-surgeon, with modifier 62 appended (see Appendix A).

Example:

A 42-year-old male with a history of posttraumatic degenerative disc disease at L3-4 and L4-5 (internal disc disruption) underwent surgical repair. Surgeon A performed an anterior exposure of the spine with mobilization of the great vessels. Surgeon B performed anterior (minimal) discectomy and fusion at L3-4 and L4-5 using anterior interbody technique.

Report surgeon A: 22558 append modifier 62, 22585 append modifier 62

Report surgeon B: 22558 append modifier 62, 22585 append modifier 62, 20931

Please see the Surgery Guidelines section for the following guidelines:

- *Surgical Procedures on the Musculoskeletal System*

AMA Coding Notes

Surgical Procedures on the Spine (Vertebral Column)

(Do not append modifier 62 to bone graft code 20931)

(For injection procedure for myelography, use 62284)

(For injection procedure for discography, see 62290, 62291)

(For injection procedure, chemonucleolysis, single or multiple levels, use 62292)

(For injection procedure for facet joints, see 64490-64495, 64633-64636)

(For needle or trocar biopsy, see 20220-20225)

AMA *CPT Assistant*

22867: Feb 17: 9

22868: Feb 17: 9

Plain English Description

A procedure is performed to insert one or more interlaminar/interspinous process implant(s) or spacer(s) to stabilize and/or open the neural foramen of the lumbar spine and decompress the spinal nerves. Interlaminar devices are implanted adjacent to the lamina and have 2 sets of wings that are placed around the inferior and superior spinous processes to restrict movement. Interspinous spacers are small devices implanted between the vertebral spinous processes and then expanded to relieve pressure on a nerve(s). These devices may be used in adults with spinal stenosis who have pain and/or neurogenic claudication. A small incision is made over the targeted lumbar disc(s) and carried down through the subcutaneous tissue. Dissection continues through the dorsolumbar fascia lateral to the midline and the multifidus is detached. The supraspinous ligaments attached to the fascia are preserved and the ligamentum flavum is elevated and resected. The superior and inferior laminae are partially resected. The exiting and transversing nerve roots are decompressed using a microscope if necessary. Partial facetectomies and foraminal decompression may be performed using a rongeur and/or drill. Incrementally sized dilators are inserted across the intraspinous space close to the posterior border of the facet joint. A sizing instrument is inserted and the appropriate device is inserted between the spinous processes as anterior to the intralaminar space as possible. The device is secured with screws. Drains may be placed before closure. Code 22867 reports the insertion of interlaminar/interspinous process stabilization/distraction device at a single level of the lumbar spine, with open decompression but without fusion, including image guidance when performed. Code 22868 reports additional device insertion at a second level of the lumbar spine.

Insertion of interlaminar/interspinous process stabilization/distraction device, without fusion, lumbar

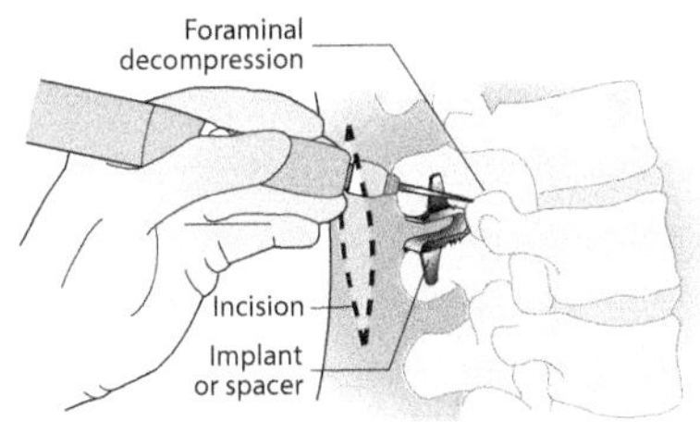

Single level (22867); second level (22868)

ICD-10-CM Diagnostic Codes

M48.061	Spinal stenosis, lumbar region without neurogenic claudication
M48.062	Spinal stenosis, lumbar region with neurogenic claudication
M48.07	Spinal stenosis, lumbosacral region

CCI Edits

Refer to Appendix A for CCI edits.

Facility RVUs

Code	Work	PE Facility	MP	Total Facility
22867	13.50	10.90	3.88	28.28
22868	4.00	1.90	1.18	7.08

Non-facility RVUs

Code	Work	PE Non-Facility	MP	Total Non-Facility
22867	13.50	10.90	3.88	28.28
22868	4.00	1.90	1.18	7.08

Modifiers (PAR)

Code	Mod 50	Mod 51	Mod 62	Mod 66	Mod 80
22867	0	2	0	0	2
22868	0	0	2	0	2

Global Period

Code	Days
22867	090
22868	ZZZ

27096

27096 Injection procedure for sacroiliac joint, anesthetic/steroid, with image guidance (fluoroscopy or CT) including arthrography when performed

(27096 is to be used only with CT or fluoroscopic imaging confirmation of intra-articular needle positioning)

(If CT or fluoroscopy imaging is not performed, use 20552)

(Code 27096 is a unilateral procedure. For bilateral procedure, use modifier 50)

AMA Coding Guideline

Surgical Procedures on the Pelvis and Hip Joint

Including head and neck of femur.

Please see the Surgery Guidelines section for the following guidelines:

- *Surgical Procedures on the Musculoskeletal System*

AMA *CPT Assistant* ☐

27096: Nov 99: 12, Apr 03: 8, Apr 04: 15, Jul 08: 9, Jan 12: 3, Aug 15: 6

Plain English Description

Injection of an anesthetic or steroid into the sacroiliac joint is performed with the use of fluoroscopic or CT guidance and joint arthrography as needed. The skin over the injection site is cleansed and a local anesthetic is injected. Using continuous fluoroscopic or CT guidance, a needle is inserted into the joint and fluid is aspirated as needed. If arthrography is performed, a radiopaque substance is injected into the sacroiliac joint. Once the radiopaque substance has been distributed throughout the joint, separately reportable radiographic images are obtained. An anesthetic or steroid injection is then administered.

Injection procedure for sacroiliac joint

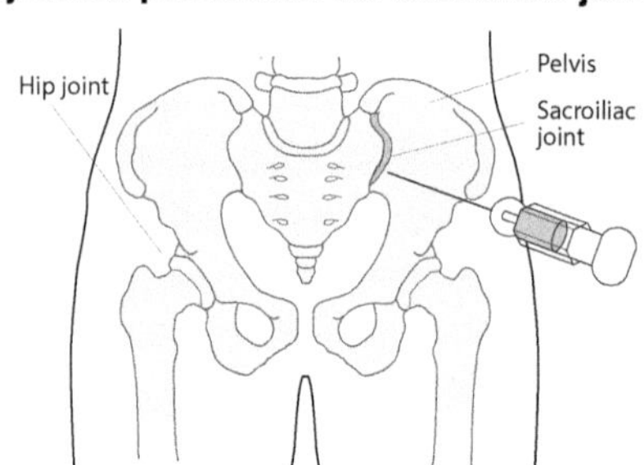

Using image guidance, anesthetic/steroid is injected into the sacroiliac joint. Includes arthrography.

ICD-10-CM Diagnostic Codes

	Code	Description
	G89.21	Chronic pain due to trauma
	G89.29	Other chronic pain
⇄	M05.051	Felty's syndrome, right hip
⇄	M05.052	Felty's syndrome, left hip
⇄	M05.451	Rheumatoid myopathy with rheumatoid arthritis of right hip
⇄	M05.452	Rheumatoid myopathy with rheumatoid arthritis of left hip
⇄	M05.851	Other rheumatoid arthritis with rheumatoid factor of right hip
⇄	M06.051	Rheumatoid arthritis without rheumatoid factor, right hip
⇄	M06.052	Rheumatoid arthritis without rheumatoid factor, left hip
⇄	M06.252	Rheumatoid bursitis, left hip
⇄	M08.251	Juvenile rheumatoid arthritis with systemic onset, right hip
⇄	M08.852	Other juvenile arthritis, left hip
	M12	Other and unspecified arthropathy
⇄	M12.551	Traumatic arthropathy, right hip
⇄	M12.552	Traumatic arthropathy, left hip
⇄	M13.851	Other specified arthritis, right hip
⇄	M13.852	Other specified arthritis, left hip
⇄	M16.11	Unilateral primary osteoarthritis, right hip
⇄	M16.12	Unilateral primary osteoarthritis, left hip
⇄	M16.31	Unilateral osteoarthritis resulting from hip dysplasia, right hip
⇄	M16.32	Unilateral osteoarthritis resulting from hip dysplasia, left hip
⇄	M16.51	Unilateral post-traumatic osteoarthritis, right hip
⇄	M16.52	Unilateral post-traumatic osteoarthritis, left hip
⇄	M25.851	Other specified joint disorders, right hip
⇄	M25.852	Other specified joint disorders, left hip
	M43.27	Fusion of spine, lumbosacral region
	M43.28	Fusion of spine, sacral and sacrococcygeal region
	M45.8	Ankylosing spondylitis sacral and sacrococcygeal region
	M46.08	Spinal enthesopathy, sacral and sacrococcygeal region
	M46.1	Sacroiliitis, not elsewhere classified
	M46.88	Other specified inflammatory spondylopathies, sacral and sacrococcygeal region
	M53.2X7	Spinal instabilities, lumbosacral region
	M53.2X8	Spinal instabilities, sacral and sacrococcygeal region
	M53.3	Sacrococcygeal disorders, not elsewhere classified
	M53.87	Other specified dorsopathies, lumbosacral region
	M53.88	Other specified dorsopathies, sacral and sacrococcygeal region
	M54.18	Radiculopathy, sacral and sacrococcygeal region
	M54.5	Low back pain
	M99.14	Subluxation complex (vertebral) of sacral region
❼⇄	S32.391	Other fracture of right ilium
❼⇄	S32.392	Other fracture of left ilium
❼	S33.2	Dislocation of sacroiliac and sacrococcygeal joint
❼	S33.6	Sprain of sacroiliac joint

ICD-10-CM Coding Notes

For codes requiring a 7th character extension, refer to your ICD-10-CM book. Review the character descriptions and coding guidelines for proper selection. For some procedures, only certain characters will apply.

CCI Edits

Refer to Appendix A for CCI edits.

Facility RVUs ☐

Code	Work	PE Facility	MP	Total Facility
27096	1.48	0.78	0.13	2.39

Non-facility RVUs ☐

Code	Work	PE Non-Facility	MP	Total Non-Facility
27096	1.48	3.00	0.13	4.61

Modifiers (PAR) ☐

Code	Mod 50	Mod 51	Mod 62	Mod 66	Mod 80
27096	1	2	0	0	1

Global Period

Code	Days
27096	000

● New ▲ Revised ✚ Add On ⊘Modifier 51 Exempt ★Telemedicine ☐ CPT QuickRef ✗FDA Pending ⇄ Laterality ❼ Seventh Character ♂Male ♀Female

27279

27279 Arthrodesis, sacroiliac joint, percutaneous or minimally invasive (indirect visualization), with image guidance, includes obtaining bone graft when performed, and placement of transfixing device

(For bilateral procedure, report 27279 with modifier 50)

AMA Coding Guideline

Surgical Procedures on the Pelvis and Hip Joint

Including head and neck of femur.

Please see the Surgery Guidelines section for the following guidelines:

- *Surgical Procedures on the Musculoskeletal System*

Plain English Description

Sacroiliac (SI) joint arthrodesis is a procedure used to artificially induce ossification between the spine (sacrum) and the pelvis (ilium) in patients with intractable joint pain often caused by fracture or arthritis. Fusion is accomplished by using a bone graft, synthetic bone substitute, or metal implant inserted across the SI joint. The percutaneous or minimally invasive technique uses fluoroscopic guidance to landmark the area and place the graft(s). If an autograft is used, the bone is first harvested from the iliac crest or rib of the patient. Allograft bone is obtained from a bone bank. A small incision is made in the skin and carried down to the fascia of the gluteal muscle. The muscle is penetrated and a Steinmann pin is inserted through the ilium, across the SI joint, and into the lateral sacrum. The uppermost implant is placed first followed by additional implants below. Holes for the implants are made first with a hollow pin. The bone grafting material is then inserted through the pin and the pin is removed. To avoid damage to nerves, additional implants are placed between the foramen openings at S1 and S2. The bone grafting material is packed into place to fuse the SI joint, and the fascia and skin are closed.

Arthrodesis, sacroiliac joint, percutaneous or minimally invasive, with image guidance, includes obtaining bone graft when performed, and placement of transfixing device

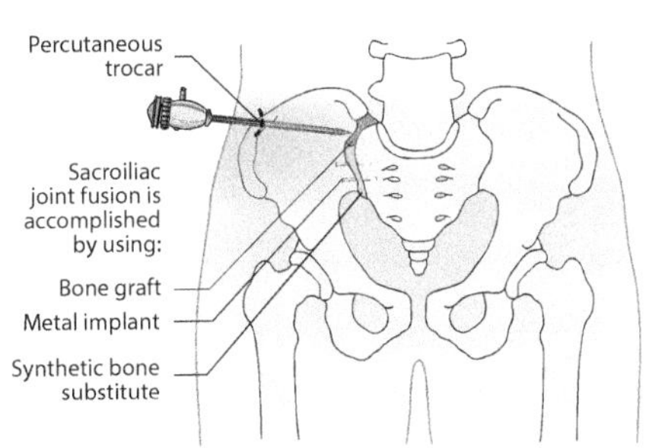

ICD-10-CM Diagnostic Codes

	Code	Description
⇄	M02.351	Reiter's disease, right hip
⇄	M02.352	Reiter's disease, left hip
⇄	M02.851	Other reactive arthropathies, right hip
⇄	M02.852	Other reactive arthropathies, left hip
	M02.88	Other reactive arthropathies, vertebrae
⇄	M05.051	Felty's syndrome, right hip
⇄	M05.052	Felty's syndrome, left hip
	M12.58	Traumatic arthropathy, other specified site
	M43.27	Fusion of spine, lumbosacral region
	M43.28	Fusion of spine, sacral and sacrococcygeal region
	M46.1	Sacroiliitis, not elsewhere classified
	M46.88	Other specified inflammatory spondylopathies, sacral and sacrococcygeal region
	M47.28	Other spondylosis with radiculopathy, sacral and sacrococcygeal region
	M47.818	Spondylosis without myelopathy or radiculopathy, sacral and sacrococcygeal region
	M48.38	Traumatic spondylopathy, sacral and sacrococcygeal region
	M53.2X7	Spinal instabilities, lumbosacral region
	M53.2X8	Spinal instabilities, sacral and sacrococcygeal region
	M53.3	Sacrococcygeal disorders, not elsewhere classified
	M53.87	Other specified dorsopathies, lumbosacral region
	M53.88	Other specified dorsopathies, sacral and sacrococcygeal region
➐	S33.2	Dislocation of sacroiliac and sacrococcygeal joint
➐	S33.6	Sprain of sacroiliac joint
➐	S33.8	Sprain of other parts of lumbar spine and pelvis

ICD-10-CM Coding Notes

For codes requiring a 7th character extension, refer to your ICD-10-CM book. Review the character descriptions and coding guidelines for proper selection. For some procedures, only certain characters will apply.

CCI Edits

Refer to Appendix A for CCI edits.

Facility RVUs ▯

Code	Work	PE Facility	MP	Total Facility
27279	12.13	9.96	3.25	25.34

Non-facility RVUs ▯

Code	Work	PE Non-Facility	MP	Total Non-Facility
27279	12.13	9.96	3.25	25.34

Modifiers (PAR) ▯

Code	Mod 50	Mod 51	Mod 62	Mod 66	Mod 80
27279	1	2	1	0	2

Global Period

Code	Days
27279	090

35301

35301 Thromboendarterectomy, including patch graft, if performed; carotid, vertebral, subclavian, by neck incision

AMA Coding Guideline

Surgical Procedures on Arteries and Veins

Primary vascular procedure listings include establishing both inflow and outflow by whatever procedures necessary. Also included is that portion of the operative arteriogram performed by the surgeon, as indicated. Sympathectomy, when done, is included in the listed aortic procedures. For unlisted vascular procedure, use 37799.

Please see the Surgery Guidelines section for the following guidelines:

- *Surgical Procedures on the Cardiovascular System*

AMA Coding Notes

Thromboendarterectomy Procedures on Arteries and Veins

(For coronary artery, see 33510-33536 and 33572)

(35301-35372 include harvest of saphenous or upper extremity vein when performed)

AMA *CPT Assistant*

35301: Jan 07: 7, Sep 10: 7

Plain English Description

Thromboendarterectomy is performed on the carotid, vertebral, or subclavian artery via a neck incision. This procedure removes a thrombus, such as a blood clot or atherosclerotic plaque that has adhered to vessels walls, along with the vessel intima from an occluded artery. An access incision is made in the neck over the affected artery. The thrombosed portion of the artery is isolated and dissected away from adjacent structures. Cerebral perfusion may be maintained by placement of a temporary shunt. Clamps are placed proximal and distal to the obstructed portion of the artery. The artery is incised and plaque and blood clot debris are removed. The artery lining (intima) is separated from the arterial walls and removed to increase the diameter of the artery. The edges of the remaining normal intima are sutured to the vessel walls. The artery is repaired primarily with sutures, or a venous or synthetic patch graft is applied to enlarge the diameter of the artery. If a shunt has been placed it, is removed. The vascular clamps are removed and blood flow through the affected artery reinitiated. The arterial suture line is checked for hemostasis. Overlying tissues are then closed in layers.

Thromboendarterectomy, including patch graft, if performed; carotid/vertebral/subclavian

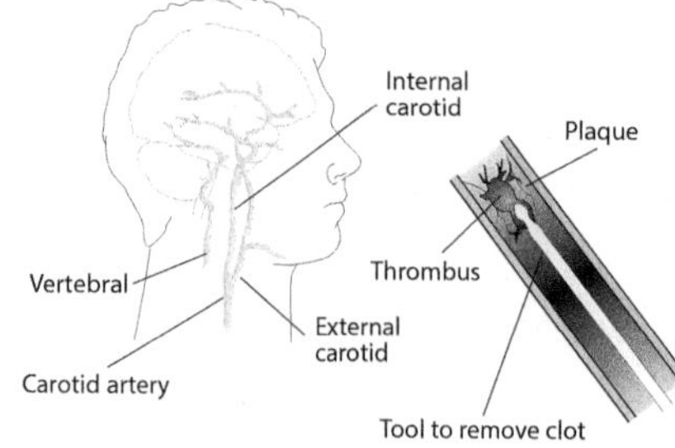

The neck vessel is opened and the blood clot or plaque and inner lining are removed. The vessel is closed. A graft may be used to enlarge its diameter.

ICD-10-CM Diagnostic Codes

	G45.0	Vertebro-basilar artery syndrome
	G45.1	Carotid artery syndrome (hemispheric)
	G45.2	Multiple and bilateral precerebral artery syndromes
	G45.3	Amaurosis fugax
	G45.9	Transient cerebral ischemic attack, unspecified
⇄	G81.91	Hemiplegia, unspecified affecting right dominant side
⇄	G81.92	Hemiplegia, unspecified affecting left dominant side
⇄	G81.93	Hemiplegia, unspecified affecting right nondominant side
⇄	G81.94	Hemiplegia, unspecified affecting left nondominant side
⇄	H53.131	Sudden visual loss, right eye
⇄	H53.132	Sudden visual loss, left eye
⇄	H53.133	Sudden visual loss, bilateral
	H53.8	Other visual disturbances
⇄	I65.21	Occlusion and stenosis of right carotid artery
⇄	I65.22	Occlusion and stenosis of left carotid artery
	I67.2	Cerebral atherosclerosis
	M62.81	Muscle weakness (generalized)
	R20.0	Anesthesia of skin
	R20.2	Paresthesia of skin
	R27.0	Ataxia, unspecified
	R27.8	Other lack of coordination
	R41.0	Disorientation, unspecified
	R42	Dizziness and giddiness
	R47.01	Aphasia
	R47.02	Dysphasia
	R47.81	Slurred speech
	R51	Headache
	R55	Syncope and collapse

CCI Edits

Refer to Appendix A for CCI edits.

Facility RVUs

Code	Work	PE Facility	MP	Total Facility
35301	21.16	6.67	5.07	32.90

Non-facility RVUs

Code	Work	PE Non-Facility	MP	Total Non-Facility
35301	21.16	6.67	5.07	32.90

Modifiers (PAR)

Code	Mod 50	Mod 51	Mod 62	Mod 66	Mod 80
35301	1	2	1	0	2

Global Period

Code	Days
35301	090

36000

36000 Introduction of needle or intracatheter, vein

AMA Coding Guideline

Intravenous Vascular Introduction and Injection Procedures

An intracatheter is a sheathed combination of needle and short catheter.

Vascular Introduction and Injection Procedures

Listed services for injection procedures include necessary local anesthesia, introduction of needles or catheter, injection of contrast media with or without automatic power injection, and/or necessary pre- and postinjection care specifically related to the injection procedure.

Selective vascular catheterization should be coded to include introduction and all lesser order selective catheterization used in the approach (eg, the description for a selective right middle cerebral artery catheterization includes the introduction and placement catheterization of the right common and internal carotid arteries).

Additional second and/or third order arterial catheterization within the same family of arteries or veins supplied by a single first order vessel should be expressed by 36012, 36218, or 36248.

Additional first order or higher catheterization in vascular families supplied by a first order vessel different from a previously selected and coded family should be separately coded using the conventions described above.

Surgical Procedures on Arteries and Veins

Primary vascular procedure listings include establishing both inflow and outflow by whatever procedures necessary. Also included is that portion of the operative arteriogram performed by the surgeon, as indicated. Sympathectomy, when done, is included in the listed aortic procedures. For unlisted vascular procedure, use 37799.

Please see the Surgery Guidelines section for the following guidelines:

- *Surgical Procedures on the Cardiovascular System*

AMA Coding Notes

Vascular Introduction and Injection Procedures

(For radiological supervision and interpretation, see Radiology)

(For injection procedures in conjunction with cardiac catheterization, see 93452-93461, 93563-93568)

(For chemotherapy of malignant disease, see 96401-96549)

AMA *CPT Assistant*

36000: Summer 95: 2, Apr 98: 1, 3, 7, Jul 98: 1, Apr 03: 26, Oct 03: 2, Jul 06: 4, Feb 07: 10, Jul 07: 1, Dec 08: 7, May 14: 4, Sep 14: 13, Oct 14: 6, Aug 19: 8

Plain English Description

The physician may place a metal needle, such as a butterfly or scalp needle; a plastic catheter mounted on a metal needle, also referred to as a plastic needle; or an intracatheter, which is a catheter inserted through a needle. The planned puncture site is selected and cleansed. The selected device is then introduced into the vein. A butterfly needle can be introduced into smaller veins in the hand. The butterfly shape stabilizes the hub on the skin surface. If a plastic needle is used, the metal tip is introduced into the vein and then removed. The plastic catheter is advanced into the vein. If an intracatheter is used, the metal needle is used to puncture the vein. The catheter is then introduced through the needle into the vein. The needle or intracatheter is secured to the skin with tape.

Introduction of needle or intracatheter, vein

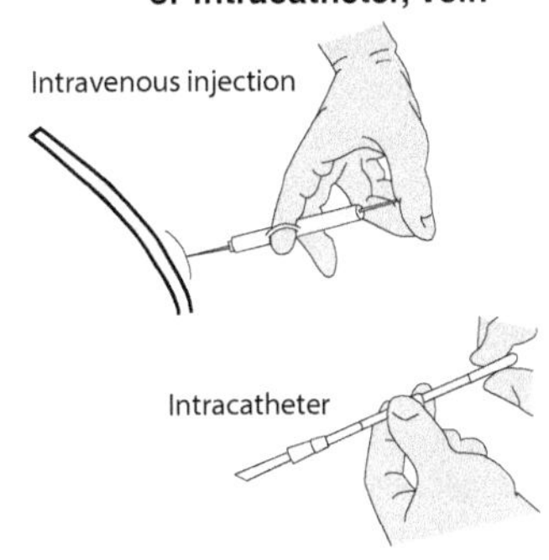

ICD-10-CM Diagnostic Codes

There are too many ICD-10-CM codes to list. Refer to ICD-10-CM code book for associated diagnostic codes.

CCI Edits

Refer to Appendix A for CCI edits.

Pub 100

36000: Pub 100-04, 12, 30.6.12

Facility RVUs

Code	Work	PE Facility	MP	Total Facility
36000	0.18	0.07	0.01	0.26

Non-facility RVUs

Code	Work	PE Non-Facility	MP	Total Non-Facility
36000	0.18	0.60	0.01	0.79

Modifiers (PAR)

Code	Mod 50	Mod 51	Mod 62	Mod 66	Mod 80
36000	9	9	9	9	9

Global Period

Code	Days
36000	XXX

36215-36218

36215 Selective catheter placement, arterial system; each first order thoracic or brachiocephalic branch, within a vascular family

(For catheter placement for coronary angiography, see 93454-93461)

36216 Selective catheter placement, arterial system; initial second order thoracic or brachiocephalic branch, within a vascular family

36217 Selective catheter placement, arterial system; initial third order or more selective thoracic or brachiocephalic branch, within a vascular family

+ **36218 Selective catheter placement, arterial system; additional second order, third order, and beyond, thoracic or brachiocephalic branch, within a vascular family (List in addition to code for initial second or third order vessel as appropriate)**

(Use 36218 in conjunction with 36216, 36217, 36225, 36226)

(For angiography, see 36222-36228, 75600-75774)

(For transluminal balloon angioplasty [except lower extremity artery[ies] for occlusive disease, intracranial, coronary, pulmonary, or dialysis circuit], see 37246, 37247)

(For transcatheter therapies, see 37200, 37211, 37213, 37214, 37236, 37237, 37238, 37239, 37241, 37242, 37243, 37244, 61624, 61626)

(When coronary artery, arterial conduit [eg, internal mammary, inferior epigastric or free radical artery] or venous bypass graft angiography is performed in conjunction with cardiac catheterization, see the appropriate cardiac catheterization, injection procedure, and imaging supervision code[s] [93455, 93457, 93459, 93461, 93530-93533, 93564] in the Medicine section. When internal mammary artery angiography only is performed without a concomitant cardiac catheterization, use 36216 or 36217 as appropriate)

Do not report 36218 or 75774 as part of diagnostic angiography of the extracranial and intracranial cervicocerebral vessels. It may be appropriate to report 36218 and 75774 for diagnostic angiography of upper extremities and other vascular beds of the neck and/or shoulder girdle performed in the same session as vertebral angiography (eg, workup of a neck tumor that requires catheterization and angiography of the vertebral artery as well as other brachiocephalic arteries).

AMA Coding Guideline

Diagnostic Studies of Cervicocerebral Arteries

Diagnostic Studies of Cervicocerebral Arteries: Codes 36221-36228 describe non-selective and selective arterial catheter placement and diagnostic imaging of the aortic arch, carotid, and vertebral arteries. Codes 36221-36226 include the work of accessing the vessel, placement of catheter(s), contrast injection(s), fluoroscopy, radiological supervision and interpretation, and closure of the arteriotomy by pressure, or application of an arterial closure device. Codes 36221-36228 describe arterial contrast injections with arterial, capillary, and venous phase imaging, when performed.

Code 36227 is an add-on code to report unilateral selective arterial catheter placement and diagnostic imaging of the ipsilateral external carotid circulation and includes all the work of accessing the additional vessel, placement of catheter(s), contrast injection(s), fluoroscopy, radiological supervision and interpretation. Code 36227 is reported in conjunction with 36222, 36223, or 36224.

Code 36228 is an add-on code to report unilateral selective arterial catheter placement and diagnostic imaging of the initial and each additional intracranial branch of the internal carotid or vertebral arteries. Code 36228 is reported in conjunction with 36223, 36224, 36225 or 36226. This includes any additional second or third order catheter selective placement in the same primary branch of the internal carotid, vertebral, or basilar artery and includes all the work of accessing the additional vessel, placement of catheter(s), contrast injection(s), fluoroscopy, radiological supervision and interpretation. It is not reported more than twice per side, regardless of the number of additional branches selectively catheterized.

Codes 36221-36226 are built on progressive hierarchies with more intensive services inclusive of less intensive services. The code inclusive of all of the services provided for that vessel should be reported (ie, use the code inclusive of the most intensive services provided). Only one code in the range 36222-36224 may be reported for each ipsilateral carotid territory. Only one code in the range 36225-36226 may be reported for each ipsilateral vertebral territory.

Code 36221 is reported for non-selective arterial catheter placement in the thoracic aorta and diagnostic imaging of the aortic arch and great vessel origins. Codes 36222-36228 are reported for unilateral artery catheterization. Do not report 36221 in conjunction with 36222-36226 as these selective codes include the work of 36221 when performed.

Do not report 36222, 36223, or 36224 together for ipsilateral angiography. Instead, select the code that represents the most comprehensive service using the following hierarchy of complexity (listed in descending order of complexity): 36224>36223>36222.

Do not report 36225 and 36226 together for ipsilateral angiography. Select the code that represents the more comprehensive service using the following hierarchy of complexity (listed in descending order of complexity): 36226>36225.

When bilateral carotid and/or vertebral arterial catheterization and imaging is performed, report 36222, 36223, 36224, 36225, 36226 with modifier 50, and report add-on codes 36227, 36228 twice (do not report modifier 50 in conjunction with 36227, 36228) if the same procedure is performed on both sides. For example, bilateral extracranial carotid angiography with selective catheterization of each common carotid artery would be reported with 36222 and modifier 50. However, when different territory(ies) is studied in the same session on both sides of the body, modifiers may be required to report the imaging performed. Use modifier 59 to denote that different carotid and/or vertebral arteries are being studied. For example, when selective right internal carotid artery catheterization accompanied by right extracranial and intracranial carotid angiography is followed by selective left common carotid artery catheterization with left extracranial carotid angiography, use 36224 to report the right side and 36222-59 to report the left side.

Diagnostic angiography of the cervicocerebral vessels may be followed by an interventional procedure at the same session. Interventional procedures may be separately reportable using standard coding conventions.

Do not report 36218 or 75774 as part of diagnostic angiography of the extracranial and intracranial cervicocerebral vessels. It may be appropriate to report 36218 and 75774 for diagnostic angiography of upper extremities and other vascular beds of the neck and/or shoulder girdle performed in the same session as vertebral angiography (eg, workup of a neck tumor that requires catheterization and angiography of the vertebral artery as well as other brachiocephalic arteries).

Report 76376 or 76377 for 3D rendering when performed in conjunction with 36221-36228.

Report 76937 for ultrasound guidance for vascular access, when performed in conjunction with 36221-36228.

Vascular Introduction and Injection Procedures

Listed services for injection procedures include necessary local anesthesia, introduction of needles or catheter, injection of contrast media with or without automatic power injection, and/or necessary pre- and postinjection care specifically related to the injection procedure.

Selective vascular catheterization should be coded to include introduction and all lesser order selective catheterization used in the approach (eg, the description for a selective right middle cerebral artery catheterization includes the introduction and placement catheterization of the right common and internal carotid arteries).

Additional second and/or third order arterial catheterization within the same family of arteries or veins supplied by a single first order vessel should be expressed by 36012, 36218, or 36248.

Additional first order or higher catheterization in vascular families supplied by a first order vessel different from a previously selected and coded family should be separately coded using the conventions described above.

Surgical Procedures on Arteries and Veins

Primary vascular procedure listings include establishing both inflow and outflow by whatever procedures necessary. Also included is that portion of the operative arteriogram performed by the surgeon, as indicated. Sympathectomy, when done, is included in the listed aortic procedures. For unlisted vascular procedure, use 37799.

Please see the Surgery Guidelines section for the following guidelines:

- *Surgical Procedures on the Cardiovascular System*

AMA Coding Notes

Intra-Arterial-Intra-Aortic Vascular Injection Procedures

(For radiological supervision and interpretation, see Radiology)

Vascular Introduction and Injection Procedures

(For radiological supervision and interpretation, see Radiology)

(For injection procedures in conjunction with cardiac catheterization, see 93452-93461, 93563-93568)

(For chemotherapy of malignant disease, see 96401-96549)

AMA *CPT Assistant* □

36215: Fall 93: 15, Aug 96: 3, Nov 97: 16, Apr 98: 9, Sep 00: 11, Oct 00: 4, Feb 03: 3, Apr 12: 4, Mar 17: 4, May 17: 8

36216: Fall 93: 15, Aug 96: 3, Oct 00: 4, Dec 07: 10, Dec 11: 12, Apr 12: 4, Nov 13: 14

36217: Fall 93: 15, Aug 96: 3, Oct 00: 4, Dec 07: 10, Dec 11: 12, Apr 12: 5

36218: Fall 93: 15, Aug 96: 3, Oct 00: 4, Jul 06: 7, Dec 07: 10, Apr 12: 5, May 13: 3, Oct 18: 3

Plain English Description

A selective catheter placement in a thoracic or brachiocephalic branch of a single vascular family of the arterial system is performed. A catheter is introduced into an extremity artery, with the preferred introduction site being a femoral artery, although an upper extremity artery may also be used. A small skin incision is made over the planned insertion site. An introducer sheath is placed in the artery and a guidewire inserted. If the right femoral artery is used, the guidewire is manipulated through the femoral and iliac arteries and into the aorta. A catheter is advanced over the guidewire into the aorta. The guidewire is advanced as needed and the physician then manipulates the catheter over the guidewire into a first-order thoracic or brachiocephalic branch off the aorta. The physician continues to selectively advance the guidewire and catheter through higher-order branches (second, third, and beyond) until the catheter is situated in the highest-order branch requiring evaluation. The guidewire is removed. Injection of medication and/or radiopaque contrast media is performed as needed. Use 36215 if a first-order branch is the highest-order branch catheterized within the vascular family, 36216 if a second-order branch if the highest-order branch catheterized, 36217 if a third- or higher-order branch is the highest-order branch catheterized. Use 36218 for catheterization of each additional second-, third-, or higher-order thoracic or brachiocephalic branch within the same vascular family.

Selective catheter placement, arterial system; thoracic/brachiocephalic

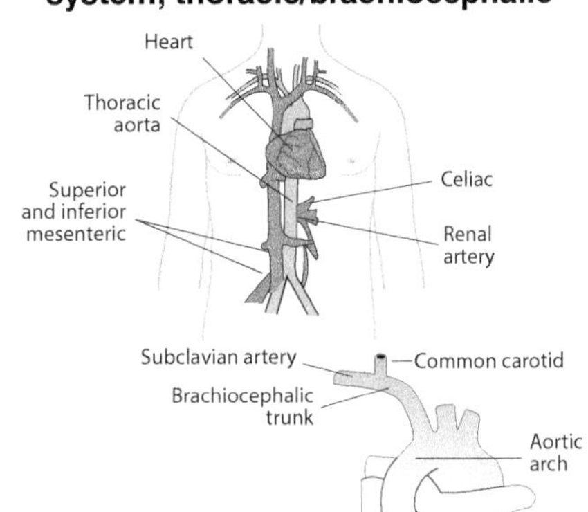

A catheter is placed via a needle/guidewire into the first order artery of the thoracic/brachiocephalic branch (36215); each additional branch of the same family (36216-36218).

ICD-10-CM Diagnostic Codes

There are too many ICD-10-CM codes to list. Refer to ICD-10-CM code book for associated diagnostic codes.

CCI Edits

Refer to Appendix A for CCI edits.

Facility RVUs □

Code	Work	PE Facility	MP	Total Facility
36215	4.17	1.42	0.54	6.13
36216	5.27	1.68	0.95	7.90
36217	6.29	2.02	1.21	9.52
36218	1.01	0.31	0.18	1.50

Non-facility RVUs □

Code	Work	PE Non-Facility	MP	Total Non-Facility
36215	4.17	26.01	0.54	30.72
36216	5.27	26.35	0.95	32.57
36217	6.29	46.44	1.21	53.94
36218	1.01	5.35	0.18	6.54

Modifiers (PAR) □

Code	Mod 50	Mod 51	Mod 62	Mod 66	Mod 80
36215	0	2	0	0	1
36216	0	2	0	0	1
36217	0	2	0	0	1
36218	0	0	0	0	1

Global Period

Code	Days
36215	000
36216	000
36217	000
36218	ZZZ

36222-36223

36222 Selective catheter placement, common carotid or innominate artery, unilateral, any approach, with angiography of the ipsilateral extracranial carotid circulation and all associated radiological supervision and interpretation, includes angiography of the cervicocerebral arch, when performed

(Do not report 36222 in conjunction with 37215, 37216, 37218 for the treated carotid artery)

36223 Selective catheter placement, common carotid or innominate artery, unilateral, any approach, with angiography of the ipsilateral intracranial carotid circulation and all associated radiological supervision and interpretation, includes angiography of the extracranial carotid and cervicocerebral arch, when performed

(Do not report 36223 in conjunction with 37215, 37216, 37218 for the treated carotid artery)

AMA Coding Guideline

Diagnostic Studies of Cervicocerebral Arteries

Diagnostic Studies of Cervicocerebral Arteries: Codes 36221-36228 describe non-selective and selective arterial catheter placement and diagnostic imaging of the aortic arch, carotid, and vertebral arteries. Codes 36221-36226 include the work of accessing the vessel, placement of catheter(s), contrast injection(s), fluoroscopy, radiological supervision and interpretation, and closure of the arteriotomy by pressure, or application of an arterial closure device. Codes 36221-36228 describe arterial contrast injections with arterial, capillary, and venous phase imaging, when performed.

Code 36227 is an add-on code to report unilateral selective arterial catheter placement and diagnostic imaging of the ipsilateral external carotid circulation and includes all the work of accessing the additional vessel, placement of catheter(s), contrast injection(s), fluoroscopy, radiological supervision and interpretation. Code 36227 is reported in conjunction with 36222, 36223, or 36224.

Code 36228 is an add-on code to report unilateral selective arterial catheter placement and diagnostic imaging of the initial and each additional intracranial branch of the internal carotid or vertebral arteries. Code 36228 is reported in conjunction with 36223, 36224, 36225 or 36226. This includes any additional second or third order catheter selective placement in the same primary branch of the internal carotid, vertebral, or basilar artery and includes all the work of accessing the additional vessel, placement of catheter(s), contrast injection(s), fluoroscopy, radiological supervision and interpretation. It is not reported more than twice per side, regardless of the number of additional branches selectively catheterized.

Codes 36221-36226 are built on progressive hierarchies with more intensive services inclusive of less intensive services. The code inclusive of all of the services provided for that vessel should be reported (ie, use the code inclusive of the most intensive services provided). Only one code in the range 36222-36224 may be reported for each ipsilateral carotid territory. Only one code in the range 36225-36226 may be reported for each ipsilateral vertebral territory.

Code 36221 is reported for non-selective arterial catheter placement in the thoracic aorta and diagnostic imaging of the aortic arch and great vessel origins. Codes 36222-36228 are reported for unilateral artery catheterization. Do not report 36221 in conjunction with 36222-36226 as these selective codes include the work of 36221 when performed.

Do not report 36222, 36223, or 36224 together for ipsilateral angiography. Instead, select the code that represents the most comprehensive service using the following hierarchy of complexity (listed in descending order of complexity): 36224>36223>36222.

Do not report 36225 and 36226 together for ipsilateral angiography. Select the code that represents the more comprehensive service using the following hierarchy of complexity (listed in descending order of complexity): 36226>36225.

When bilateral carotid and/or vertebral arterial catheterization and imaging is performed, report 36222, 36223, 36224, 36225, 36226 with modifier 50, and report add-on codes 36227, 36228 twice (do not report modifier 50 in conjunction with 36227, 36228) if the same procedure is performed on both sides. For example, bilateral extracranial carotid angiography with selective catheterization of each common carotid artery would be reported with 36222 and modifier 50. However, when different territory(ies) is studied in the same session on both sides of the body, modifiers may be required to report the imaging performed. Use modifier 59 to denote that different carotid and/or vertebral arteries are being studied. For example, when selective right internal carotid artery catheterization accompanied by right extracranial and intracranial carotid angiography is followed by selective left common carotid artery catheterization with left extracranial carotid angiography, use 36224 to report the right side and 36222-59 to report the left side.

Diagnostic angiography of the cervicocerebral vessels may be followed by an interventional procedure at the same session. Interventional procedures may be separately reportable using standard coding conventions.

Do not report 36218 or 75774 as part of diagnostic angiography of the extracranial and intracranial cervicocerebral vessels. It may be appropriate to report 36218 and 75774 for diagnostic angiography of upper extremities and other vascular beds of the neck and/or shoulder girdle performed in the same session as vertebral angiography (eg, workup of a neck tumor that requires catheterization and angiography of the vertebral artery as well as other brachiocephalic arteries).

Report 76376 or 76377 for 3D rendering when performed in conjunction with 36221-36228.

Report 76937 for ultrasound guidance for vascular access, when performed in conjunction with 36221-36228.

Vascular Introduction and Injection Procedures

Listed services for injection procedures include necessary local anesthesia, introduction of needles or catheter, injection of contrast media with or without automatic power injection, and/or necessary pre- and postinjection care specifically related to the injection procedure.

Selective vascular catheterization should be coded to include introduction and all lesser order selective catheterization used in the approach (eg, the description for a selective right middle cerebral artery catheterization includes the introduction and placement catheterization of the right common and internal carotid arteries).

Additional second and/or third order arterial catheterization within the same family of arteries or veins supplied by a single first order vessel should be expressed by 36012, 36218, or 36248.

Additional first order or higher catheterization in vascular families supplied by a first order vessel different from a previously selected and coded family should be separately coded using the conventions described above.

Surgical Procedures on Arteries and Veins

Primary vascular procedure listings include establishing both inflow and outflow by whatever procedures necessary. Also included is that portion of the operative arteriogram performed by the surgeon, as indicated. Sympathectomy, when done, is included in the listed aortic procedures. For unlisted vascular procedure, use 37799.

Please see the Surgery Guidelines section for the following guidelines:

- *Surgical Procedures on the Cardiovascular System*

AMA Coding Notes

Intra-Arterial-Intra-Aortic Vascular Injection Procedures

(For radiological supervision and interpretation, see Radiology)

Vascular Introduction and Injection Procedures

(For radiological supervision and interpretation, see Radiology)

(For injection procedures in conjunction with cardiac catheterization, see 93452-93461, 93563-93568)

(For chemotherapy of malignant disease, see 96401-96549)

AMA *CPT Assistant* ☐

36222: Feb 13: 17, May 13: 3, Jun 13: 12, Oct 13: 18, Nov 13: 14, Mar 14: 8, May 15: 7, Nov 15: 10

36223: Feb 13: 17, May 13: 3, Jun 13: 12, Oct 13: 18, Mar 14: 8

Plain English Description

Selective catheter placement in the right or left common carotid or right innominate (brachiocephalic) artery is performed by any approach including percutaneous placement via the femoral, axillary, brachial, or radial artery. A retrograde femoral artery approach is the most common. A small skin incision is made over the planned insertion site. An introducer sheath is placed in the artery and a guidewire is inserted. If the femoral artery is used, the guidewire is manipulated through the femoral and iliac arteries and into the aorta and along the aorta into the aortic arch to a point beyond the left common carotid artery or right innominate artery under continuous fluoroscopic guidance. A catheter is advanced over the guidewire into the aortic arch and positioned at the left common carotid or right innominate artery. The guidewire is retracted and manipulated into the left common carotid or right innominate artery/right common carotid artery. The catheter is again advanced over the guidewire and positioned 2-3 cm below the carotid bifurcation. The guidewire is removed. Radiopaque contrast media is injected. Angiography of the ipsilateral (same side) extracranial carotid circulation, including the cervicocerebral arch, is performed (36222). Arterial contrast injections with arterial, capillary, and venous phase imaging are also included when performed. Upon completion of the procedure, the catheter is removed and hemostasis is achieved by applying pressure to the arteriotomy site or using another closure technique. A written interpretation of findings is provided. Use 36223 when angiography of the ipsilateral intracranial carotid circulation, cervicocerebral arch, and the extracranial carotid circulation is performed.

ICD-10-CM Diagnostic Codes

	Code	Description
	G45.1	Carotid artery syndrome (hemispheric)
	G45.3	Amaurosis fugax
	G45.9	Transient cerebral ischemic attack, unspecified
⇄	G81.91	Hemiplegia, unspecified affecting right dominant side
⇄	G81.92	Hemiplegia, unspecified affecting left dominant side
⇄	G81.93	Hemiplegia, unspecified affecting right nondominant side
⇄	G81.94	Hemiplegia, unspecified affecting left nondominant side
⇄	H53.131	Sudden visual loss, right eye
⇄	H53.132	Sudden visual loss, left eye
⇄	H53.133	Sudden visual loss, bilateral
	H53.8	Other visual disturbances
⇄	I65.21	Occlusion and stenosis of right carotid artery
⇄	I65.22	Occlusion and stenosis of left carotid artery
	I67.2	Cerebral atherosclerosis
	I72.0	Aneurysm of carotid artery
	I77.71	Dissection of carotid artery
	M62.81	Muscle weakness (generalized)
	R20.0	Anesthesia of skin
	R20.2	Paresthesia of skin
	R27.0	Ataxia, unspecified
	R27.8	Other lack of coordination
	R41.0	Disorientation, unspecified
	R42	Dizziness and giddiness
	R47.01	Aphasia
	R47.02	Dysphasia
	R47.81	Slurred speech
	R51	Headache
	R55	Syncope and collapse

CCI Edits

Refer to Appendix A for CCI edits.

Facility RVUs ☐

Code	Work	PE Facility	MP	Total Facility
36222	5.28	1.75	1.16	8.19
36223	5.75	2.13	1.30	9.18

Non-facility RVUs ☐

Code	Work	PE Non-Facility	MP	Total Non-Facility
36222	5.28	29.11	1.16	35.55
36223	5.75	38.58	1.30	45.63

Modifiers (PAR) ☐

Code	Mod 50	Mod 51	Mod 62	Mod 66	Mod 80
36222	1	2	0	0	1
36223	1	2	0	0	1

Global Period

Code	Days
36222	000
36223	000

36224

36224 Selective catheter placement, internal carotid artery, unilateral, with angiography of the ipsilateral intracranial carotid circulation and all associated radiological supervision and interpretation, includes angiography of the extracranial carotid and cervicocerebral arch, when performed

(Do not report 36224 in conjunction with 37215, 37216, 37218 for the treated carotid artery)

AMA Coding Guideline

Diagnostic Studies of Cervicocerebral Arteries

Diagnostic Studies of Cervicocerebral Arteries: Codes 36221-36228 describe non-selective and selective arterial catheter placement and diagnostic imaging of the aortic arch, carotid, and vertebral arteries. Codes 36221-36226 include the work of accessing the vessel, placement of catheter(s), contrast injection(s), fluoroscopy, radiological supervision and interpretation, and closure of the arteriotomy by pressure, or application of an arterial closure device. Codes 36221-36228 describe arterial contrast injections with arterial, capillary, and venous phase imaging, when performed.

Code 36227 is an add-on code to report unilateral selective arterial catheter placement and diagnostic imaging of the ipsilateral external carotid circulation and includes all the work of accessing the additional vessel, placement of catheter(s), contrast injection(s), fluoroscopy, radiological supervision and interpretation. Code 36227 is reported in conjunction with 36222, 36223, or 36224.

Code 36228 is an add-on code to report unilateral selective arterial catheter placement and diagnostic imaging of the initial and each additional intracranial branch of the internal carotid or vertebral arteries. Code 36228 is reported in conjunction with 36223, 36224, 36225 or 36226. This includes any additional second or third order catheter selective placement in the same primary branch of the internal carotid, vertebral, or basilar artery and includes all the work of accessing the additional vessel, placement of catheter(s), contrast injection(s), fluoroscopy, radiological supervision and interpretation. It is not reported more than twice per side, regardless of the number of additional branches selectively catheterized.

Codes 36221-36226 are built on progressive hierarchies with more intensive services inclusive of less intensive services. The code inclusive of all of the services provided for that vessel should be reported (ie, use the code inclusive of the most intensive services provided). Only one code in the range 36222-36224 may be reported for each ipsilateral carotid territory. Only one code in the range 36225-36226 may be reported for each ipsilateral vertebral territory.

Code 36221 is reported for non-selective arterial catheter placement in the thoracic aorta and diagnostic imaging of the aortic arch and great vessel origins. Codes 36222-36228 are reported for unilateral artery catheterization. Do not report 36221 in conjunction with 36222-36226 as these selective codes include the work of 36221 when performed.

Do not report 36222, 36223, or 36224 together for ipsilateral angiography. Instead, select the code that represents the most comprehensive service using the following hierarchy of complexity (listed in descending order of complexity): 36224>36223>36222.

Do not report 36225 and 36226 together for ipsilateral angiography. Select the code that represents the more comprehensive service using the following hierarchy of complexity (listed in descending order of complexity): 36226>36225.

When bilateral carotid and/or vertebral arterial catheterization and imaging is performed, report 36222, 36223, 36224, 36225, 36226 with modifier 50, and report add-on codes 36227, 36228 twice (do not report modifier 50 in conjunction with 36227, 36228) if the same procedure is performed on both sides. For example, bilateral extracranial carotid angiography with selective catheterization of each common carotid artery would be reported with 36222 and modifier 50. However, when different territory(ies) is studied in the same session on both sides of the body, modifiers may be required to report the imaging performed. Use modifier 59 to denote that different carotid and/or vertebral arteries are being studied. For example, when selective right internal carotid artery catheterization accompanied by right extracranial and intracranial carotid angiography is followed by selective left common carotid artery catheterization with left extracranial carotid angiography, use 36224 to report the right side and 36222-59 to report the left side.

Diagnostic angiography of the cervicocerebral vessels may be followed by an interventional procedure at the same session. Interventional procedures may be separately reportable using standard coding conventions.

Do not report 36218 or 75774 as part of diagnostic angiography of the extracranial and intracranial cervicocerebral vessels. It may be appropriate to report 36218 and 75774 for diagnostic angiography of upper extremities and other vascular beds of the neck and/or shoulder girdle performed in the same session as vertebral angiography (eg, workup of a neck tumor that requires catheterization and angiography of the vertebral artery as well as other brachiocephalic arteries).

Report 76376 or 76377 for 3D rendering when performed in conjunction with 36221-36228.

Report 76937 for ultrasound guidance for vascular access, when performed in conjunction with 36221-36228.

Vascular Introduction and Injection Procedures

Listed services for injection procedures include necessary local anesthesia, introduction of needles or catheter, injection of contrast media with or without automatic power injection, and/or necessary pre- and postinjection care specifically related to the injection procedure.

Selective vascular catheterization should be coded to include introduction and all lesser order selective catheterization used in the approach (eg, the description for a selective right middle cerebral artery catheterization includes the introduction and placement catheterization of the right common and internal carotid arteries).

Additional second and/or third order arterial catheterization within the same family of arteries or veins supplied by a single first order vessel should be expressed by 36012, 36218, or 36248.

Additional first order or higher catheterization in vascular families supplied by a first order vessel different from a previously selected and coded family should be separately coded using the conventions described above.

Surgical Procedures on Arteries and Veins

Primary vascular procedure listings include establishing both inflow and outflow by whatever procedures necessary. Also included is that portion of the operative arteriogram performed by the surgeon, as indicated. Sympathectomy, when done, is included in the listed aortic procedures. For unlisted vascular procedure, use 37799.

Please see the Surgery Guidelines section for the following guidelines:

- *Surgical Procedures on the Cardiovascular System*

AMA Coding Notes

Intra-Arterial-Intra-Aortic Vascular Injection Procedures

(For radiological supervision and interpretation, see Radiology)

Vascular Introduction and Injection Procedures

(For radiological supervision and interpretation, see Radiology)

(For injection procedures in conjunction with cardiac catheterization, see 93452-93461, 93563-93568)

(For chemotherapy of malignant disease, see 96401-96549)

AMA *CPT Assistant*

36224: Feb 13: 17, May 13: 3, Jun 13: 12, Oct 13: 18, Mar 14: 8

Plain English Description

Selective catheter placement in the right or left internal carotid artery is performed by percutaneous catheter placement via the femoral, axillary, brachial, or radial artery. A retrograde femoral artery approach is the most common. A small skin incision is made over the planned insertion site. An introducer sheath is placed in the artery and a guidewire is inserted. If the femoral artery is used, the guidewire is manipulated through the femoral and iliac arteries and into the aorta. The guidewire is advanced along the aorta into the aortic arch to a point beyond the left common carotid artery or right innominate artery under continuous fluoroscopic guidance. A catheter is advanced over the guidewire into the aortic arch and positioned at the left common carotid or right innominate artery. The guidewire is retracted and manipulated into the left common carotid or right innominate artery/right common carotid artery. The catheter is again advanced over the guidewire and positioned below the carotid bifurcation. The guidewire is then manipulated into the right or left internal carotid artery, followed by the catheter, which is positioned within the internal carotid artery. The guidewire is removed. Radiopaque contrast media is injected. Angiography of the ipsilateral (same side) intracranial carotid circulation including the cervicocerebral arch is performed. Angiography of the external carotid artery may also be performed. Arterial contrast injections with arterial, capillary, and venous phase imaging are also included when performed. Upon completion of the procedure, the catheter is removed and hemostasis is achieved by applying pressure to the arteriotomy site or using another closure technique. A written interpretation of findings is provided.

ICD-10-CM Diagnostic Codes

	G45.1	Carotid artery syndrome (hemispheric)
	G45.3	Amaurosis fugax
	G45.9	Transient cerebral ischemic attack, unspecified
⇄	G81.91	Hemiplegia, unspecified affecting right dominant side
⇄	G81.92	Hemiplegia, unspecified affecting left dominant side
⇄	G81.93	Hemiplegia, unspecified affecting right nondominant side
⇄	G81.94	Hemiplegia, unspecified affecting left nondominant side
⇄	H53.131	Sudden visual loss, right eye
⇄	H53.132	Sudden visual loss, left eye
⇄	H53.133	Sudden visual loss, bilateral
	H53.8	Other visual disturbances
⇄	I65.21	Occlusion and stenosis of right carotid artery
⇄	I65.22	Occlusion and stenosis of left carotid artery
	I67.2	Cerebral atherosclerosis
	I72.0	Aneurysm of carotid artery
	I77.71	Dissection of carotid artery
	M62.81	Muscle weakness (generalized)
	R20.0	Anesthesia of skin
	R20.2	Paresthesia of skin
	R27.0	Ataxia, unspecified
	R27.8	Other lack of coordination
	R41.0	Disorientation, unspecified
	R42	Dizziness and giddiness
	R47.01	Aphasia
	R47.02	Dysphasia
	R47.81	Slurred speech
	R51	Headache
	R55	Syncope and collapse

CCI Edits

Refer to Appendix A for CCI edits.

Facility RVUs ☐

Code	Work	PE Facility	MP	Total Facility
36224	6.25	2.61	1.57	10.43

Non-facility RVUs ☐

Code	Work	PE Non-Facility	MP	Total Non-Facility
36224	6.25	51.11	1.57	58.93

Modifiers (PAR) ☐

Code	Mod 50	Mod 51	Mod 62	Mod 66	Mod 80
36224	1	2	0	0	1

Global Period

Code	Days
36224	000

36225-36226

36225 Selective catheter placement, subclavian or innominate artery, unilateral, with angiography of the ipsilateral vertebral circulation and all associated radiological supervision and interpretation, includes angiography of the cervicocerebral arch, when performed

36226 Selective catheter placement, vertebral artery, unilateral, with angiography of the ipsilateral vertebral circulation and all associated radiological supervision and interpretation, includes angiography of the cervicocerebral arch, when performed

AMA Coding Guideline

Diagnostic Studies of Cervicocerebral Arteries

Diagnostic Studies of Cervicocerebral Arteries: Codes 36221-36228 describe non-selective and selective arterial catheter placement and diagnostic imaging of the aortic arch, carotid, and vertebral arteries. Codes 36221-36226 include the work of accessing the vessel, placement of catheter(s), contrast injection(s), fluoroscopy, radiological supervision and interpretation, and closure of the arteriotomy by pressure, or application of an arterial closure device. Codes 36221-36228 describe arterial contrast injections with arterial, capillary, and venous phase imaging, when performed.

Code 36227 is an add-on code to report unilateral selective arterial catheter placement and diagnostic imaging of the ipsilateral external carotid circulation and includes all the work of accessing the additional vessel, placement of catheter(s), contrast injection(s), fluoroscopy, radiological supervision and interpretation. Code 36227 is reported in conjunction with 36222, 36223, or 36224.

Code 36228 is an add-on code to report unilateral selective arterial catheter placement and diagnostic imaging of the initial and each additional intracranial branch of the internal carotid or vertebral arteries. Code 36228 is reported in conjunction with 36223, 36224, 36225 or 36226. This includes any additional second or third order catheter selective placement in the same primary branch of the internal carotid, vertebral, or basilar artery and includes all the work of accessing the additional vessel, placement of catheter(s), contrast injection(s), fluoroscopy, radiological supervision and interpretation. It is not reported more than twice per side, regardless of the number of additional branches selectively catheterized.

Codes 36221-36226 are built on progressive hierarchies with more intensive services inclusive of less intensive services. The code inclusive of all of the services provided for that vessel should be reported (ie, use the code inclusive of the most intensive services provided). Only one code in the range 36222-36224 may be reported for each ipsilateral carotid territory. Only one code in the range 36225-36226 may be reported for each ipsilateral vertebral territory.

Code 36221 is reported for non-selective arterial catheter placement in the thoracic aorta and diagnostic imaging of the aortic arch and great vessel origins. Codes 36222-36228 are reported for unilateral artery catheterization. Do not report 36221 in conjunction with 36222-36226 as these selective codes include the work of 36221 when performed.

Do not report 36222, 36223, or 36224 together for ipsilateral angiography. Instead, select the code that represents the most comprehensive service using the following hierarchy of complexity (listed in descending order of complexity): 36224>36223>36222.

Do not report 36225 and 36226 together for ipsilateral angiography. Select the code that represents the more comprehensive service using the following hierarchy of complexity (listed in descending order of complexity): 36226>36225.

When bilateral carotid and/or vertebral arterial catheterization and imaging is performed, report 36222, 36223, 36224, 36225, 36226 with modifier 50, and report add-on codes 36227, 36228 twice (do not report modifier 50 in conjunction with 36227, 36228) if the same procedure is performed on both sides. For example, bilateral extracranial carotid angiography with selective catheterization of each common carotid artery would be reported with 36222 and modifier 50. However, when different territory(ies) is studied in the same session on both sides of the body, modifiers may be required to report the imaging performed. Use modifier 59 to denote that different carotid and/or vertebral arteries are being studied. For example, when selective right internal carotid artery catheterization accompanied by right extracranial and intracranial carotid angiography is followed by selective left common carotid artery catheterization with left extracranial carotid angiography, use 36224 to report the right side and 36222-59 to report the left side.

Diagnostic angiography of the cervicocerebral vessels may be followed by an interventional procedure at the same session. Interventional procedures may be separately reportable using standard coding conventions.

Do not report 36218 or 75774 as part of diagnostic angiography of the extracranial and intracranial cervicocerebral vessels. It may be appropriate to report 36218 and 75774 for diagnostic angiography of upper extremities and other vascular beds of the neck and/or shoulder girdle performed in the same session as vertebral angiography (eg, workup of a neck tumor that requires catheterization and angiography of the vertebral artery as well as other brachiocephalic arteries).

Report 76376 or 76377 for 3D rendering when performed in conjunction with 36221-36228.

Report 76937 for ultrasound guidance for vascular access, when performed in conjunction with 36221-36228.

Vascular Introduction and Injection Procedures

Listed services for injection procedures include necessary local anesthesia, introduction of needles or catheter, injection of contrast media with or without automatic power injection, and/or necessary pre- and postinjection care specifically related to the injection procedure.

Selective vascular catheterization should be coded to include introduction and all lesser order selective catheterization used in the approach (eg, the description for a selective right middle cerebral artery catheterization includes the introduction and placement catheterization of the right common and internal carotid arteries).

Additional second and/or third order arterial catheterization within the same family of arteries or veins supplied by a single first order vessel should be expressed by 36012, 36218, or 36248.

Additional first order or higher catheterization in vascular families supplied by a first order vessel different from a previously selected and coded family should be separately coded using the conventions described above.

Surgical Procedures on Arteries and Veins

Primary vascular procedure listings include establishing both inflow and outflow by whatever procedures necessary. Also included is that portion of the operative arteriogram performed by the surgeon, as indicated. Sympathectomy, when done, is included in the listed aortic procedures. For unlisted vascular procedure, use 37799.

Please see the Surgery Guidelines section for the following guidelines:

- *Surgical Procedures on the Cardiovascular System*

AMA Coding Notes

Intra-Arterial-Intra-Aortic Vascular Injection Procedures

(For radiological supervision and interpretation, see Radiology)

Vascular Introduction and Injection Procedures

(For radiological supervision and interpretation, see Radiology)

(For injection procedures in conjunction with cardiac catheterization, see 93452-93461, 93563-93568)

(For chemotherapy of malignant disease, see 96401-96549)

AMA *CPT Assistant* ☐

36225: May 13: 3, Jun 13: 12, Oct 13: 18, Nov 13: 14, Mar 14: 8

36226: May 13: 3, Jun 13: 12, Oct 13: 18, Mar 14: 8

Plain English Description

Selective catheter placement in the right innominate (brachiocephalic)/subclavian artery or left subclavian artery is performed by percutaneous catheter placement via the femoral, axillary, brachial, or radial artery. A retrograde femoral artery approach is the most common. A small skin incision is made over the planned insertion site. An introducer sheath is placed in the artery and a guidewire is inserted. If the femoral artery is used, the guidewire is manipulated through the femoral and iliac arteries into the aorta. The guidewire is advanced along the aorta into the aortic arch to a point beyond the left subclavian artery or right innominate artery under continuous fluoroscopic guidance. A catheter is advanced over the guidewire into the aortic arch and positioned at the left subclavian or right subclavian/innominate artery. The guidewire is retracted and manipulated into the left subclavian or right innominate/right subclavian artery. The catheter is again advanced over the guidewire and positioned below the vertebral artery branch. Use code 36225 when the catheter is not advanced beyond the right innominate/right subclavian artery or left subclavian artery. Use 36226 when the catheter is advanced into the vertebral artery. The guidewire is removed. Radiopaque contrast media is injected. Angiography of the ipsilateral (same side) vertebral circulation is performed. Angiography of the cervicocerebral arch may also be performed. Arterial contrast injections with arterial, capillary, and venous phase imaging are also included when performed. Upon completion of the procedure, the catheter is removed and hemostasis is achieved by applying pressure to the arteriotomy site or using another closure technique. A written interpretation of findings is provided.

ICD-10-CM Diagnostic Codes

	G45.0	Vertebro-basilar artery syndrome
	G45.3	Amaurosis fugax
	G45.9	Transient cerebral ischemic attack, unspecified
⇄	G81.91	Hemiplegia, unspecified affecting right dominant side
⇄	G81.92	Hemiplegia, unspecified affecting left dominant side
⇄	G81.93	Hemiplegia, unspecified affecting right nondominant side
⇄	G81.94	Hemiplegia, unspecified affecting left nondominant side
⇄	H53.131	Sudden visual loss, right eye
⇄	H53.132	Sudden visual loss, left eye
⇄	H53.133	Sudden visual loss, bilateral
	H53.8	Other visual disturbances
⇄	I65.01	Occlusion and stenosis of right vertebral artery
⇄	I65.02	Occlusion and stenosis of left vertebral artery
	I72.6	Aneurysm of vertebral artery
	I77.74	Dissection of vertebral artery
	M62.81	Muscle weakness (generalized)
	R20.0	Anesthesia of skin
	R20.2	Paresthesia of skin
	R27.0	Ataxia, unspecified
	R27.8	Other lack of coordination
	R41.0	Disorientation, unspecified
	R42	Dizziness and giddiness
	R47.01	Aphasia
	R47.02	Dysphasia
	R47.81	Slurred speech
	R51	Headache
	R55	Syncope and collapse

CCI Edits

Refer to Appendix A for CCI edits.

Facility RVUs ☐

Code	Work	PE Facility	MP	Total Facility
36225	5.75	2.07	1.33	9.15
36226	6.25	2.53	1.50	10.28

Non-facility RVUs ☐

Code	Work	PE Non-Facility	MP	Total Non-Facility
36225	5.75	36.67	1.33	43.75
36226	6.25	47.96	1.50	55.71

Modifiers **(PAR)** ☐

Code	Mod 50	Mod 51	Mod 62	Mod 66	Mod 80
36225	1	2	0	0	1
36226	1	2	0	0	1

Global Period

Code	Days
36225	000
36226	000

36227

+ 36227 Selective catheter placement, external carotid artery, unilateral, with angiography of the ipsilateral external carotid circulation and all associated radiological supervision and interpretation (List separately in addition to code for primary procedure)

(Use 36227 in conjunction with 36222, 36223, or 36224)

(Do not report 36221-36227 in conjunction with 37217 for ipsilateral services)

AMA Coding Guideline

Diagnostic Studies of Cervicocerebral Arteries

Diagnostic Studies of Cervicocerebral Arteries: Codes 36221-36228 describe non-selective and selective arterial catheter placement and diagnostic imaging of the aortic arch, carotid, and vertebral arteries. Codes 36221-36226 include the work of accessing the vessel, placement of catheter(s), contrast injection(s), fluoroscopy, radiological supervision and interpretation, and closure of the arteriotomy by pressure, or application of an arterial closure device. Codes 36221-36228 describe arterial contrast injections with arterial, capillary, and venous phase imaging, when performed.

Code 36227 is an add-on code to report unilateral selective arterial catheter placement and diagnostic imaging of the ipsilateral external carotid circulation and includes all the work of accessing the additional vessel, placement of catheter(s), contrast injection(s), fluoroscopy, radiological supervision and interpretation. Code 36227 is reported in conjunction with 36222, 36223, or 36224.

Code 36228 is an add-on code to report unilateral selective arterial catheter placement and diagnostic imaging of the initial and each additional intracranial branch of the internal carotid or vertebral arteries. Code 36228 is reported in conjunction with 36223, 36224, 36225 or 36226. This includes any additional second or third order catheter selective placement in the same primary branch of the internal carotid, vertebral, or basilar artery and includes all the work of accessing the additional vessel, placement of catheter(s), contrast injection(s), fluoroscopy, radiological supervision and interpretation. It is not reported more than twice per side, regardless of the number of additional branches selectively catheterized.

Codes 36221-36226 are built on progressive hierarchies with more intensive services inclusive of less intensive services. The code inclusive of all of the services provided for that vessel should be reported (ie, use the code inclusive of the most intensive services provided). Only one code in the range 36222-36224 may be reported for each ipsilateral carotid territory. Only one code in the range 36225-36226 may be reported for each ipsilateral vertebral territory.

Code 36221 is reported for non-selective arterial catheter placement in the thoracic aorta and diagnostic imaging of the aortic arch and great vessel origins. Codes 36222-36228 are reported for unilateral artery catheterization. Do not report 36221 in conjunction with 36222-36226 as these selective codes include the work of 36221 when performed.

Do not report 36222, 36223, or 36224 together for ipsilateral angiography. Instead, select the code that represents the most comprehensive service using the following hierarchy of complexity (listed in descending order of complexity): 36224>36223>36222.

Do not report 36225 and 36226 together for ipsilateral angiography. Select the code that represents the more comprehensive service using the following hierarchy of complexity (listed in descending order of complexity): 36226>36225.

When bilateral carotid and/or vertebral arterial catheterization and imaging is performed, report 36222, 36223, 36224, 36225, 36226 with modifier 50, and report add-on codes 36227, 36228 twice (do not report modifier 50 in conjunction with 36227, 36228) if the same procedure is performed on both sides. For example, bilateral extracranial carotid angiography with selective catheterization of each common carotid artery would be reported with 36222 and modifier 50. However, when different territory(ies) is studied in the same session on both sides of the body, modifiers may be required to report the imaging performed. Use modifier 59 to denote that different carotid and/or vertebral arteries are being studied. For example, when selective right internal carotid artery catheterization accompanied by right extracranial and intracranial carotid angiography is followed by selective left common carotid artery catheterization with left extracranial carotid angiography, use 36224 to report the right side and 36222-59 to report the left side.

Diagnostic angiography of the cervicocerebral vessels may be followed by an interventional procedure at the same session. Interventional procedures may be separately reportable using standard coding conventions.

Do not report 36218 or 75774 as part of diagnostic angiography of the extracranial and intracranial cervicocerebral vessels. It may be appropriate to report 36218 and 75774 for diagnostic angiography of upper extremities and other vascular beds of the neck and/or shoulder girdle performed in the same session as vertebral angiography (eg, workup of a neck tumor that requires catheterization and angiography of the vertebral artery as well as other brachiocephalic arteries).

Report 76376 or 76377 for 3D rendering when performed in conjunction with 36221-36228.

Report 76937 for ultrasound guidance for vascular access, when performed in conjunction with 36221-36228.

Vascular Introduction and Injection Procedures

Listed services for injection procedures include necessary local anesthesia, introduction of needles or catheter, injection of contrast media with or without automatic power injection, and/or necessary pre- and postinjection care specifically related to the injection procedure.

Selective vascular catheterization should be coded to include introduction and all lesser order selective catheterization used in the approach (eg, the description for a selective right middle cerebral artery catheterization includes the introduction and placement catheterization of the right common and internal carotid arteries).

Additional second and/or third order arterial catheterization within the same family of arteries or veins supplied by a single first order vessel should be expressed by 36012, 36218, or 36248.

Additional first order or higher catheterization in vascular families supplied by a first order vessel different from a previously selected and coded family should be separately coded using the conventions described above.

Surgical Procedures on Arteries and Veins

Primary vascular procedure listings include establishing both inflow and outflow by whatever procedures necessary. Also included is that portion of the operative arteriogram performed by the surgeon, as indicated. Sympathectomy, when done, is included in the listed aortic procedures. For unlisted vascular procedure, use 37799.

Please see the Surgery Guidelines section for the following guidelines:

- *Surgical Procedures on the Cardiovascular System*

AMA Coding Notes

Intra-Arterial-Intra-Aortic Vascular Injection Procedures

(For radiological supervision and interpretation, see Radiology)

Vascular Introduction and Injection Procedures

(For radiological supervision and interpretation, see Radiology)

(For injection procedures in conjunction with cardiac catheterization, see 93452-93461, 93563-93568)

(For chemotherapy of malignant disease, see 96401-96549)

AMA *CPT Assistant* ▫

36227: Feb 13: 17, May 13: 3, Jun 13: 12, Oct 13: 18, Mar 14: 8, Nov 15: 10

Plain English Description

Selective catheter placement in the right or left external carotid artery is performed by percutaneous catheter placement via the femoral, axillary, brachial, or radial artery. A retrograde femoral artery approach is the most common. A small skin incision is made over the planned insertion site. An introducer sheath is placed in the artery and a guidewire is inserted. If the femoral artery is used, the guidewire is manipulated through the femoral and iliac arteries into the aorta. The guidewire is advanced along the aorta into the aortic arch to a point beyond the left common carotid artery or right innominate artery under continuous fluoroscopic guidance. A catheter is advanced over the guidewire into the aortic arch and positioned at the left common carotid or right innominate artery. The guidewire is retracted and manipulated into the left common carotid or right innominate/common carotid artery. The catheter is again advanced over the guidewire and positioned below the carotid bifurcation. The guidewire is then manipulated into the right or left external carotid artery, followed by the catheter, which is positioned within the external carotid artery. The guidewire is removed. Radiopaque contrast media is injected. Angiography of the ipsilateral (same side) external carotid circulation is performed. Arterial contrast injections with arterial, capillary, and venous phase imaging are also included when performed. Upon completion of the procedure, the catheter is removed and hemostasis is achieved by applying pressure to the arteriotomy site or using another closure technique. A written interpretation of findings is provided.

ICD-10-CM Diagnostic Codes

See Primary Procedure code for crosswalks.

CCI Edits

Refer to Appendix A for CCI edits.

Facility RVUs

Code	Work	PE Facility	MP	Total Facility
36227	2.09	0.81	0.51	3.41

Non-facility RVUs

Code	Work	PE Non-Facility	MP	Total Non-Facility
36227	2.09	4.51	0.51	7.11

Modifiers (PAR)

Code	Mod 50	Mod 51	Mod 62	Mod 66	Mod 80
36227	1	0	0	0	1

Global Period

Code	Days
36227	ZZZ

36228

✚ **36228 Selective catheter placement, each intracranial branch of the internal carotid or vertebral arteries, unilateral, with angiography of the selected vessel circulation and all associated radiological supervision and interpretation (eg, middle cerebral artery, posterior inferior cerebellar artery) (List separately in addition to code for primary procedure)**

(Use 36228 in conjunction with 36223, 36224, 36225 or 36226)

(Do not report 36228 more than twice per side)

AMA Coding Guideline

Diagnostic Studies of Cervicocerebral Arteries

Diagnostic Studies of Cervicocerebral Arteries: Codes 36221-36228 describe non-selective and selective arterial catheter placement and diagnostic imaging of the aortic arch, carotid, and vertebral arteries. Codes 36221-36226 include the work of accessing the vessel, placement of catheter(s), contrast injection(s), fluoroscopy, radiological supervision and interpretation, and closure of the arteriotomy by pressure, or application of an arterial closure device. Codes 36221-36228 describe arterial contrast injections with arterial, capillary, and venous phase imaging, when performed.

Code 36227 is an add-on code to report unilateral selective arterial catheter placement and diagnostic imaging of the ipsilateral external carotid circulation and includes all the work of accessing the additional vessel, placement of catheter(s), contrast injection(s), fluoroscopy, radiological supervision and interpretation. Code 36227 is reported in conjunction with 36222, 36223, or 36224.

Code 36228 is an add-on code to report unilateral selective arterial catheter placement and diagnostic imaging of the initial and each additional intracranial branch of the internal carotid or vertebral arteries. Code 36228 is reported in conjunction with 36223, 36224, 36225 or 36226. This includes any additional second or third order catheter selective placement in the same primary branch of the internal carotid, vertebral, or basilar artery and includes all the work of accessing the additional vessel, placement of catheter(s), contrast injection(s), fluoroscopy, radiological supervision and interpretation. It is not reported more than twice per side, regardless of the number of additional branches selectively catheterized.

Codes 36221-36226 are built on progressive hierarchies with more intensive services inclusive of less intensive services. The code inclusive of all of the services provided for that vessel should be reported (ie, use the code inclusive of the most intensive services provided). Only one code in the range 36222-36224 may be reported for each ipsilateral carotid territory. Only one code in the range 36225-36226 may be reported for each ipsilateral vertebral territory.

Code 36221 is reported for non-selective arterial catheter placement in the thoracic aorta and diagnostic imaging of the aortic arch and great vessel origins. Codes 36222-36228 are reported for unilateral artery catheterization. Do not report 36221 in conjunction with 36222-36226 as these selective codes include the work of 36221 when performed.

Do not report 36222, 36223, or 36224 together for ipsilateral angiography. Instead, select the code that represents the most comprehensive service using the following hierarchy of complexity (listed in descending order of complexity): 36224>36223>36222.

Do not report 36225 and 36226 together for ipsilateral angiography. Select the code that represents the more comprehensive service using the following hierarchy of complexity (listed in descending order of complexity): 36226>36225.

When bilateral carotid and/or vertebral arterial catheterization and imaging is performed, report 36222, 36223, 36224, 36225, 36226 with modifier 50, and report add-on codes 36227, 36228 twice (do not report modifier 50 in conjunction with 36227, 36228) if the same procedure is performed on both sides. For example, bilateral extracranial carotid angiography with selective catheterization of each common carotid artery would be reported with 36222 and modifier 50. However, when different territory(ies) is studied in the same session on both sides of the body, modifiers may be required to report the imaging performed. Use modifier 59 to denote that different carotid and/or vertebral arteries are being studied. For example, when selective right internal carotid artery catheterization accompanied by right extracranial and intracranial carotid angiography is followed by selective left common carotid artery catheterization with left extracranial carotid angiography, use 36224 to report the right side and 36222-59 to report the left side.

Diagnostic angiography of the cervicocerebral vessels may be followed by an interventional procedure at the same session. Interventional procedures may be separately reportable using standard coding conventions.

Do not report 36218 or 75774 as part of diagnostic angiography of the extracranial and intracranial cervicocerebral vessels. It may be appropriate to report 36218 and 75774 for diagnostic angiography of upper extremities and other vascular beds of the neck and/or shoulder girdle performed in the same session as vertebral angiography (eg, workup of a neck tumor that requires catheterization and angiography of the vertebral artery as well as other brachiocephalic arteries).

Report 76376 or 76377 for 3D rendering when performed in conjunction with 36221-36228.

Report 76937 for ultrasound guidance for vascular access, when performed in conjunction with 36221-36228.

Vascular Introduction and Injection Procedures

Listed services for injection procedures include necessary local anesthesia, introduction of needles or catheter, injection of contrast media with or without automatic power injection, and/or necessary pre- and postinjection care specifically related to the injection procedure.

Selective vascular catheterization should be coded to include introduction and all lesser order selective catheterization used in the approach (eg, the description for a selective right middle cerebral artery catheterization includes the introduction and placement catheterization of the right common and internal carotid arteries).

Additional second and/or third order arterial catheterization within the same family of arteries or veins supplied by a single first order vessel should be expressed by 36012, 36218, or 36248. Additional first order or higher catheterization in vascular families supplied by a first order vessel different from a previously selected and coded family should be separately coded using the conventions described above.

Surgical Procedures on Arteries and Veins

Primary vascular procedure listings include establishing both inflow and outflow by whatever procedures necessary. Also included is that portion of the operative arteriogram performed by the surgeon, as indicated. Sympathectomy, when done, is included in the listed aortic procedures. For unlisted vascular procedure, use 37799.

Please see the Surgery Guidelines section for the following guidelines:

- *Surgical Procedures on the Cardiovascular System*

AMA Coding Notes

Intra-Arterial-Intra-Aortic Vascular Injection Procedures

(For radiological supervision and interpretation, see Radiology)

Vascular Introduction and Injection Procedures

(For radiological supervision and interpretation, see Radiology)

(For injection procedures in conjunction with cardiac catheterization, see 93452-93461, 93563-93568)

(For chemotherapy of malignant disease, see 96401-96549)

AMA *CPT Assistant* ☐

36228: Feb 13: 17, May 13: 3, Jun 13: 12, Oct 13: 18

Plain English Description

Selective catheter placement in intracranial branches beyond the internal carotid arteries or vertebral arteries is performed, which may include the middle cerebral artery, posterior inferior cerebellar artery, or other higher-level branches. Selective catheter placement to the level of the internal carotid or vertebral arteries is reported separately. If catheterization and angiography for evaluation of circulation of a higher-level artery is needed, the guidewire and catheter are advanced into the selected higher-level artery or arteries. The guidewire is removed. Radiopaque contrast media is injected. Angiography of the selected higher-level vessel circulation is performed. Arterial contrast injections with arterial, capillary, and venous phase imaging are also included when performed. Upon completion of the procedure, the catheter is removed and a written report of findings is provided. Report 36228 for each additional higher-level artery on which selective catheterization and angiography are performed.

ICD-10-CM Diagnostic Codes

See Primary Procedure code for crosswalks.

CCI Edits

Refer to Appendix A for CCI edits.

Facility RVUs ▯

Code	Work	PE Facility	MP	Total Facility
36228	4.25	1.66	1.07	6.98

Non-facility RVUs ▯

Code	Work	PE Non-Facility	MP	Total Non-Facility
36228	4.25	32.35	1.07	37.67

Modifiers (PAR) ▯

Code	Mod 50	Mod 51	Mod 62	Mod 66	Mod 80
36228	1	0	0	0	1

Global Period

Code	Days
36228	ZZZ

36415-36416

36415 Collection of venous blood by venipuncture

(Do not report modifier 63 in conjunction with 36415)

36416 Collection of capillary blood specimen (eg, finger, heel, ear stick)

AMA Coding Guideline

Venous Procedures

Venipuncture, needle or catheter for diagnostic study or intravenous therapy, percutaneous. These codes are also used to report the therapy as specified. For collection of a specimen from an established catheter, use 36592. For collection of a specimen from a completely implantable venous access device, use 36591.

Vascular Introduction and Injection Procedures

Listed services for injection procedures include necessary local anesthesia, introduction of needles or catheter, injection of contrast media with or without automatic power injection, and/or necessary pre- and postinjection care specifically related to the injection procedure.

Selective vascular catheterization should be coded to include introduction and all lesser order selective catheterization used in the approach (eg, the description for a selective right middle cerebral artery catheterization includes the introduction and placement catheterization of the right common and internal carotid arteries).

Additional second and/or third order arterial catheterization within the same family of arteries or veins supplied by a single first order vessel should be expressed by 36012, 36218, or 36248.

Additional first order or higher catheterization in vascular families supplied by a first order vessel different from a previously selected and coded family should be separately coded using the conventions described above.

Surgical Procedures on Arteries and Veins

Primary vascular procedure listings include establishing both inflow and outflow by whatever procedures necessary. Also included is that portion of the operative arteriogram performed by the surgeon, as indicated. Sympathectomy, when done, is included in the listed aortic procedures. For unlisted vascular procedure, use 37799.

Please see the Surgery Guidelines section for the following guidelines:

- *Surgical Procedures on the Cardiovascular System*

AMA Coding Notes

Vascular Introduction and Injection Procedures

(For radiological supervision and interpretation, see Radiology)

(For injection procedures in conjunction with cardiac catheterization, see 93452-93461, 93563-93568)

(For chemotherapy of malignant disease, see 96401-96549)

AMA *CPT Assistant*

36415: Jun 96: 10, Mar 98: 10, Oct 99: 11, Aug 00: 2, Feb 07: 10, Jul 07: 1, Dec 08: 7, May 14: 4

Plain English Description

In 36415, an appropriate vein is selected, usually one of the larger antecubital veins such as the median cubital, basilic, or cephalic vein. A tourniquet is placed above the planned puncture site. The site is disinfected with an alcohol pad. A needle is attached to a hub and the vein is punctured. A Vacutainer tube is attached to the hub and the blood specimen is collected. The Vacutainer tube is removed. Depending on the specific blood tests required, multiple Vacutainers may be filled from the same puncture site. In 36416, a blood sample is obtained by capillary puncture usually performed on the fingertip, ear lobe, heel, or toe. Heel and toe sites are typically used only on neonates and infants. The planned puncture site is cleaned with an alcohol pad. A lancet is used to puncture the skin. A drop of blood is allowed to form at the puncture site and is then touched with a capillary tube to collect the specimen.

Collection of blood specimen

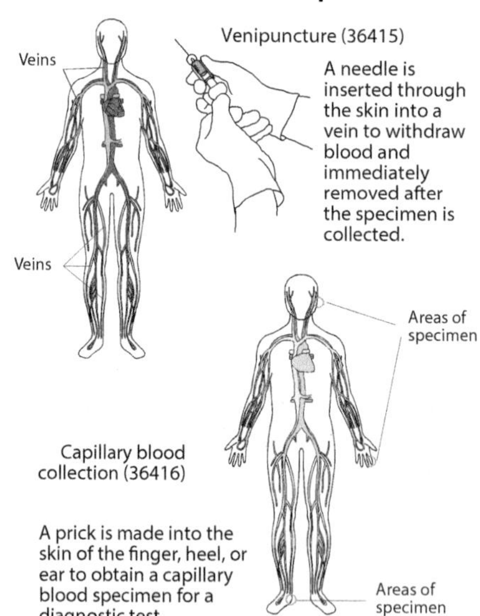

ICD-10-CM Diagnostic Codes

There are too many ICD-10-CM codes to list. Refer to ICD-10-CM code book for associated diagnostic codes.

CCI Edits

Refer to Appendix A for CCI edits.

Pub 100

36415: Pub 100-04, 12, 30.6.12, Pub 100-04, 16, 60.1.4

Facility RVUs

Code	Work	PE Facility	MP	Total Facility
36415	0.00	0.00	0.00	0.00
36416	0.00	0.00	0.00	0.00

Non-facility RVUs

Code	Work	PE Non-Facility	MP	Total Non-Facility
36415	0.00	0.00	0.00	0.00
36416	0.00	0.00	0.00	0.00

Modifiers (PAR)

Code	Mod 50	Mod 51	Mod 62	Mod 66	Mod 80
36415	9	9	9	9	9
36416	9	9	9	9	9

Global Period

Code	Days
36415	XXX
36416	XXX

37215-37216

37215 Transcatheter placement of intravascular stent(s), cervical carotid artery, open or percutaneous, including angioplasty, when performed, and radiological supervision and interpretation; with distal embolic protection

37216 Transcatheter placement of intravascular stent(s), cervical carotid artery, open or percutaneous, including angioplasty, when performed, and radiological supervision and interpretation; without distal embolic protection

(37215 and 37216 include all ipsilateral selective carotid catheterization, all diagnostic imaging for ipsilateral, cervical and cerebral carotid arteriography, and all related radiological supervision and interpretation. When ipsilateral carotid arteriogram (including imaging and selective catheterization) confirms the need for carotid stenting, 37215 and 37216 are inclusive of these services. If carotid stenting is not indicated, then the appropriate codes for carotid catheterization and imaging should be reported in lieu of 37215 and 37216)

(Do not report 37215, 37216 in conjunction with 36222-36224 for the treated carotid artery)

(For open or percutaneous transcatheter placement of extracranial vertebral artery stent[s], see Category III codes 0075T, 0076T)

AMA Coding Guideline

Surgical Procedures on Arteries and Veins

Primary vascular procedure listings include establishing both inflow and outflow by whatever procedures necessary. Also included is that portion of the operative arteriogram performed by the surgeon, as indicated. Sympathectomy, when done, is included in the listed aortic procedures. For unlisted vascular procedure, use 37799.

Please see the Surgery Guidelines section for the following guidelines:

- *Surgical Procedures on the Cardiovascular System*
- *Transcatheter Procedures on Arteries and Veins*

AMA *CPT Assistant*

37215: May 05: 7, Feb 13: 3, Mar 14: 8

37216: May 05: 7, Feb 13: 3, Mar 14: 8

Plain English Description

Transcatheter placement of intravascular stent(s) in a stenosed cervical carotid artery is performed. For a percutaneous approach, the femoral or other artery is punctured and the introducer sheath is inserted. A guidewire is introduced and advanced into the aortic arch. A carotid configuration catheter is advanced over the guidewire into the aortic arch. Roadmapping angiograms are obtained of the common carotid artery. The guidewire is removed and a hydrophilic wire is introduced. The carotid configuration catheter is inserted over the hydrophilic wire and configured at the aortic arch to conform to the patient's anatomy. The catheter is advanced into the common carotid artery. For the open approach, the introducer sheath is inserted through a surgically exposed common carotid artery via a small skin incision. The open approach is best employed in cases of severe arteriosclerotic disease of the femoral or iliac arteries, or the aorta. Roadmapping angiography is performed on the cervical carotid artery and measurements are made of the artery and area of stenosis. The hydrophilic wire is advanced into the external carotid artery and the carotid catheter is advanced over the wire. The hydrophilic wire is removed and a stiff wire is advanced to the site of the stenosis. A long guiding sheath is advanced over the carotid catheter and stiff wire. The carotid catheter and stiff wire are removed, leaving the long guiding sheath in place. In 37215, a distal embolic protection device is used. The deployment device is advanced across the lesion and positioned in the extracranial aspect of the internal carotid artery. The umbrella filter is opened and the embolic protection deployment device is removed. Angioplasty may then be performed before placing the stent. A balloon catheter is advanced to the site of the lesion and inflated. The area of stenosis is dilated, and the balloon catheter is removed. The stent delivery catheter is then advanced to the site of the lesion and carefully positioned. The stent is deployed and the delivery catheter is removed. A balloon catheter may again be advanced and inflated to seat the stent. All catheters are removed and pressure is applied to the venous access site. Use 37215 when cervical carotid artery stent(s) are placed with a distal embolic protection device and 37216 when the procedure is performed without a distal embolic protection device.

Transcatheter placement of intravascular stent(s), cervical carotid artery

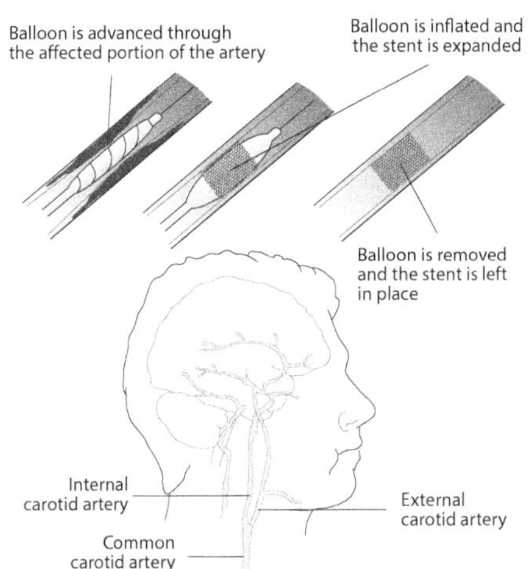

A needle is inserted through the skin to introduce a catheter into the cervical carotid artery.

ICD-10-CM Diagnostic Codes

	Code	Description
	G45.1	Carotid artery syndrome (hemispheric)
	G45.3	Amaurosis fugax
	G45.9	Transient cerebral ischemic attack, unspecified
⇄	G81.91	Hemiplegia, unspecified affecting right dominant side
⇄	G81.92	Hemiplegia, unspecified affecting left dominant side
⇄	G81.93	Hemiplegia, unspecified affecting right nondominant side
⇄	G81.94	Hemiplegia, unspecified affecting left nondominant side
⇄	H53.131	Sudden visual loss, right eye
⇄	H53.132	Sudden visual loss, left eye
⇄	H53.133	Sudden visual loss, bilateral
	H53.8	Other visual disturbances
⇄	I65.21	Occlusion and stenosis of right carotid artery
⇄	I65.22	Occlusion and stenosis of left carotid artery
⇄	I65.23	Occlusion and stenosis of bilateral carotid arteries
	I67.2	Cerebral atherosclerosis
	I72.0	Aneurysm of carotid artery
	I77.71	Dissection of carotid artery
	M62.81	Muscle weakness (generalized)
	R20.0	Anesthesia of skin
	R20.2	Paresthesia of skin
	R27.0	Ataxia, unspecified
	R27.8	Other lack of coordination
	R41.0	Disorientation, unspecified
	R42	Dizziness and giddiness
	R47.01	Aphasia
	R47.02	Dysphasia
	R47.81	Slurred speech
	R51	Headache
	R55	Syncope and collapse

CCI Edits

Refer to Appendix A for CCI edits.

Facility RVUs

Code	Work	PE Facility	MP	Total Facility
37215	17.75	7.13	4.16	29.04
37216	17.98	8.87	1.42	28.27

Non-facility RVUs

Code	Work	PE Non-Facility	MP	Total Non-Facility
37215	17.75	7.13	4.16	29.04
37216	17.98	8.87	1.42	28.27

Modifiers (PAR)

Code	Mod 50	Mod 51	Mod 62	Mod 66	Mod 80
37215	1	2	0	0	0
37216	9	9	9	9	9

Global Period

Code	Days
37215	090
37216	090

51784-51785

51784 Electromyography studies (EMG) of anal or urethral sphincter, other than needle, any technique

(Do not report 51784 in conjunction with 51792)

51785 Needle electromyography studies (EMG) of anal or urethral sphincter, any technique

AMA Coding Guideline

Urodynamic Procedures on the Bladder

The following section (51725-51798) lists procedures that may be used separately or in many and varied combinations.

When multiple procedures are performed in the same investigative session, modifier 51 should be employed.

All procedures in this section imply that these services are performed by, or are under the direct supervision of, a physician or other qualified health care professional and that all instruments, equipment, fluids, gases, probes, catheters, technician's fees, medications, gloves, trays, tubing, and other sterile supplies be provided by that individual. When the individual only interprets the results and/or operates the equipment, a professional component, modifier 26, should be used to identify these services.

AMA Coding Notes

Surgical Procedures on the Urinary System

(For provision of chemotherapeutic agents, report both the specific service in addition to code(s) for the specific substance(s) or drug(s) provided)

AMA *CPT Assistant*

51784: Sep 02: 6, Feb 10: 7, Feb 14: 11, Sep 14: 14

51785: Apr 02: 6, Sep 02: 6, Jul 04: 13, Feb 10: 7

Plain English Description

Electromyography (EMG) measures the electrical activity in the anal or urethral sphincter muscles. Muscles and nerves generate electrical impulses that facilitate sphincter contraction and relaxation. If electrical impulses are impaired, the sphincter will not open and close properly. In 51784, an EMG electrode patch is placed around the urethral sphincter or anal sphincter and muscle impulses recorded. EMG of the anal or urethral sphincter using an electrode patch is performed at the time of separately reportable complex cystometrogram (CMG) or voiding pressure (VP) studies. Electrical activity is recorded during filling and emptying of the bladder. In 51785, needles are placed in the urethral or anal sphincter to obtain information on pelvic floor muscle activity. This test is performed during separately reportable complex CMG in patients with neurological disease to record electrical impulses during filling and emptying of the bladder.

Electromyography studies (EMG) of anal or urethral sphincter

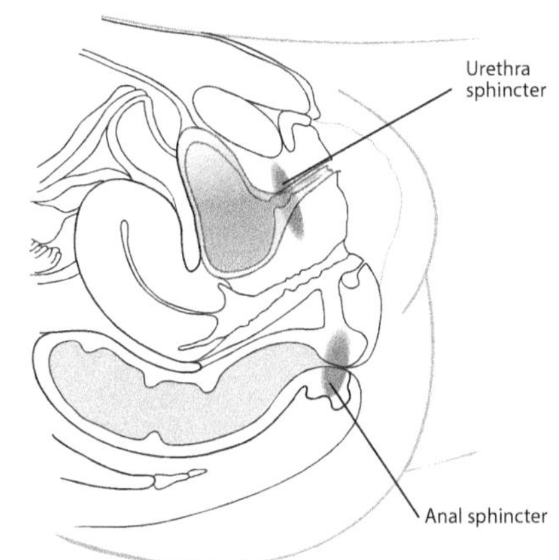

Other than needle, any technique (51784); needle, any technique (51785)

ICD-10-CM Diagnostic Codes

G54.1	Lumbosacral plexus disorders
G63	Polyneuropathy in diseases classified elsewhere
G83.4	Cauda equina syndrome
G95.89	Other specified diseases of spinal cord
M62.58	Muscle wasting and atrophy, not elsewhere classified, other site
N31.0	Uninhibited neuropathic bladder, not elsewhere classified
N31.1	Reflex neuropathic bladder, not elsewhere classified
N31.2	Flaccid neuropathic bladder, not elsewhere classified
N31.8	Other neuromuscular dysfunction of bladder
N31.9	Neuromuscular dysfunction of bladder, unspecified
N32.81	Overactive bladder
N36.41	Hypermobility of urethra
N36.42	Intrinsic sphincter deficiency (ISD)
N36.43	Combined hypermobility of urethra and intrinsic sphincter deficiency
N36.44	Muscular disorders of urethra
N39.3	Stress incontinence (female) (male)
N39.41	Urge incontinence
N39.42	Incontinence without sensory awareness
N39.44	Nocturnal enuresis
N39.45	Continuous leakage
N39.46	Mixed incontinence
N39.490	Overflow incontinence
N39.491	Coital incontinence
N39.492	Postural (urinary) incontinence
N39.498	Other specified urinary incontinence
N81.82	Incompetence or weakening of pubocervical tissue ♀
N81.83	Incompetence or weakening of rectovaginal tissue ♀
N81.84	Pelvic muscle wasting ♀
N99.89	Other postprocedural complications and disorders of genitourinary system
R15.0	Incomplete defecation
R15.1	Fecal smearing
R15.2	Fecal urgency
R15.9	Full incontinence of feces
R30.0	Dysuria
R30.1	Vesical tenesmus
R33.8	Other retention of urine
R33.9	Retention of urine, unspecified
R35.0	Frequency of micturition
R35.1	Nocturia
R39.11	Hesitancy of micturition
R39.14	Feeling of incomplete bladder emptying
R39.15	Urgency of urination
R39.81	Functional urinary incontinence

CCI Edits

Refer to Appendix A for CCI edits.

Facility RVUs

Code	Work	PE Facility	MP	Total Facility
51784	0.75	1.08	0.09	1.92
51785	1.53	8.65	0.46	10.64

Non-facility RVUs

Code	Work	PE Non-Facility	MP	Total Non-Facility
51784	0.75	1.08	0.09	1.92
51785	1.53	8.65	0.46	10.64

Modifiers (PAR)

Code	Mod 50	Mod 51	Mod 62	Mod 66	Mod 80
51784	0	2	0	0	1
51785	0	2	0	0	0

Global Period

Code	Days
51784	XXX
51785	XXX

CPT® Procedural Coding

61020-61026

61020 Ventricular puncture through previous burr hole, fontanelle, suture, or implanted ventricular catheter/reservoir; without injection

61026 Ventricular puncture through previous burr hole, fontanelle, suture, or implanted ventricular catheter/reservoir; with injection of medication or other substance for diagnosis or treatment

AMA Coding Notes

Surgical Procedures on the Skull, Meninges, and Brain

(For injection procedure for cerebral angiography, see 36100-36218)

(For injection procedure for ventriculography, see 61026, 61120)

(For injection procedure for pneumoencephalography, use 61055)

Plain English Description

A ventricular puncture through a previous burr hole, fontanelle, suture, or an implanted ventricular catheter/reservoir is performed without injection. The hair is cut or the scalp is shaved over the planned puncture site. If the procedure is performed through a previous burr hole, fontanelle, or suture, a spinal needle is advanced through the skin and into the ventricle. The stylet is removed and cerebrospinal fluid and blood are drained. The stylet is then replaced, the needle removed, and a dressing applied. If the procedure is performed through an implanted ventricular catheter/reservoir, the needle is inserted at a 30 to 45 degree angle through the skin into the reservoir bladder. Cerebrospinal fluid and blood are drained. As the intracranial pressure reduces, the flow rate will slow. When the pressure has been reduced sufficiently, the needle is removed and firm pressure is applied to the puncture site until drainage has stopped. Use code 61026 when ventricular puncture is performed through a previous burr hole, fontanelle, suture, or an implanted ventricular catheter/reservoir with injection of medication or other substance for diagnosis or treatment. The puncture procedure is performed as described above. As cerebrospinal fluid is withdrawn from the ventricle, an equal amount of medication or other substance, such as gas, contrast media, dye, or radioactive material, is instilled. The head is then rotated to disperse the medication or other substance. If the injection is performed for ventriculography, separately reportable radiographs are obtained.

Ventricular puncture through previous burr hole, fontanelle, suture, or implanted ventricular catheter/reservoir

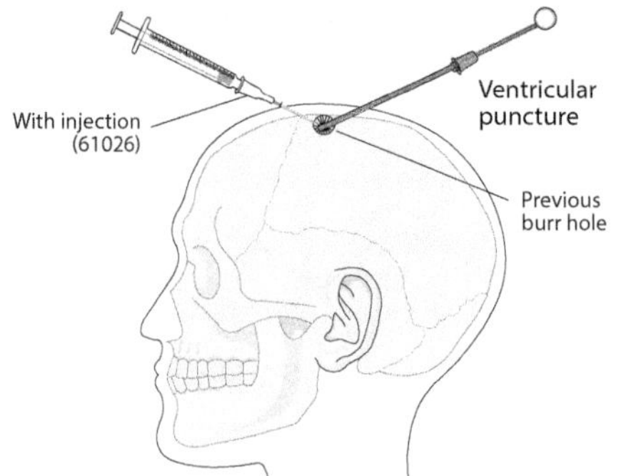

Without injection (61020); with injection of medication or other substance for diagnosis or treatment (61026)

ICD-10-CM Diagnostic Codes

	Code	Description
	C71.0	Malignant neoplasm of cerebrum, except lobes and ventricles
	C71.1	Malignant neoplasm of frontal lobe
	C71.2	Malignant neoplasm of temporal lobe
	C71.3	Malignant neoplasm of parietal lobe
	C71.4	Malignant neoplasm of occipital lobe
	C71.5	Malignant neoplasm of cerebral ventricle
	C71.6	Malignant neoplasm of cerebellum
	C71.8	Malignant neoplasm of overlapping sites of brain
	C79.31	Secondary malignant neoplasm of brain
	D33.0	Benign neoplasm of brain, supratentorial
	G91.0	Communicating hydrocephalus
	G91.1	Obstructive hydrocephalus
	G91.2	(Idiopathic) normal pressure hydrocephalus
	G91.3	Post-traumatic hydrocephalus, unspecified
	G91.4	Hydrocephalus in diseases classified elsewhere
	G91.8	Other hydrocephalus
	G91.9	Hydrocephalus, unspecified
	G92	Toxic encephalopathy
	G93.0	Cerebral cysts
	G93.40	Encephalopathy, unspecified
	G93.41	Metabolic encephalopathy
	G93.49	Other encephalopathy
	G93.6	Cerebral edema
	G93.7	Reye's syndrome
	G97.31	Intraoperative hemorrhage and hematoma of a nervous system organ or structure complicating a nervous system procedure
	G97.32	Intraoperative hemorrhage and hematoma of a nervous system organ or structure complicating other procedure
	G97.51	Postprocedural hemorrhage of a nervous system organ or structure following a nervous system procedure
	G97.52	Postprocedural hemorrhage of a nervous system organ or structure following other procedure
	G97.61	Postprocedural hematoma of a nervous system organ or structure following a nervous system procedure
	G97.62	Postprocedural hematoma of a nervous system organ or structure following other procedure
	G97.63	Postprocedural seroma of a nervous system organ or structure following a nervous system procedure
	G97.64	Postprocedural seroma of a nervous system organ or structure following other procedure
	H47.11	Papilledema associated with increased intracranial pressure
	I67.4	Hypertensive encephalopathy
	Q04.6	Congenital cerebral cysts
	R83.2	Abnormal level of other drugs, medicaments and biological substances in cerebrospinal fluid
	R83.3	Abnormal level of substances chiefly nonmedicinal as to source in cerebrospinal fluid
	R83.4	Abnormal immunological findings in cerebrospinal fluid
	R83.5	Abnormal microbiological findings in cerebrospinal fluid
	R83.6	Abnormal cytological findings in cerebrospinal fluid
	R83.8	Other abnormal findings in cerebrospinal fluid
⑦	S06.1X0	Traumatic cerebral edema without loss of consciousness
⑦	S06.1X9	Traumatic cerebral edema with loss of consciousness of unspecified duration
⑦	S06.2X0	Diffuse traumatic brain injury without loss of consciousness
⑦	S06.2X9	Diffuse traumatic brain injury with loss of consciousness of unspecified duration
⑦ ⇄	S06.310	Contusion and laceration of right cerebrum without loss of consciousness
⑦ ⇄	S06.319	Contusion and laceration of right cerebrum with loss of consciousness of unspecified duration
⑦ ⇄	S06.320	Contusion and laceration of left cerebrum without loss of consciousness
⑦ ⇄	S06.329	Contusion and laceration of left cerebrum with loss of consciousness of unspecified duration
⑦ ⇄	S06.340	Traumatic hemorrhage of right cerebrum without loss of consciousness
⑦ ⇄	S06.349	Traumatic hemorrhage of right cerebrum with loss of consciousness of unspecified duration
⑦ ⇄	S06.350	Traumatic hemorrhage of left cerebrum without loss of consciousness

● New ▲ Revised ✚ Add On ⊘Modifier 51 Exempt ★Telemedicine ▯ CPT QuickRef ⁄FDA Pending ⇄ Laterality ⑦ Seventh Character ♂Male ♀Female

⑦⇄	S06.359	Traumatic hemorrhage of left cerebrum with loss of consciousness of unspecified duration
⑦	S06.6X0	Traumatic subarachnoid hemorrhage without loss of consciousness
⑦	S06.6X9	Traumatic subarachnoid hemorrhage with loss of consciousness of unspecified duration
⑦	T85.730	Infection and inflammatory reaction due to ventricular intracranial (communicating) shunt
⑦	T85.731	Infection and inflammatory reaction due to implanted electronic neurostimulator of brain, electrode (lead)
⑦	T85.735	Infection and inflammatory reaction due to cranial or spinal infusion catheter

ICD-10-CM Coding Notes

For codes requiring a 7th character extension, refer to your ICD-10-CM book. Review the character descriptions and coding guidelines for proper selection. For some procedures, only certain characters will apply.

CCI Edits

Refer to Appendix A for CCI edits.

Facility RVUs

Code	Work	PE Facility	MP	Total Facility
61020	1.51	1.03	0.49	3.03
61026	1.69	1.04	0.35	3.08

Non-facility RVUs

Code	Work	PE Non-Facility	MP	Total Non-Facility
61020	1.51	1.03	0.49	3.03
61026	1.69	1.04	0.35	3.08

Modifiers (PAR)

Code	Mod 50	Mod 51	Mod 62	Mod 66	Mod 80
61020	0	2	0	0	1
61026	0	2	0	0	1

Global Period

Code	Days
61020	000
61026	000

61070

61070 Puncture of shunt tubing or reservoir for aspiration or injection procedure

(For radiological supervision and interpretation, use 75809)

AMA Coding Notes

Surgical Procedures on the Skull, Meninges, and Brain

(For injection procedure for cerebral angiography, see 36100-36218)

(For injection procedure for ventriculography, see 61026, 61120)

(For injection procedure for pneumoencephalography, use 61055)

Plain English Description

The physician punctures shunt tubing or a reservoir in the skull, meninges, or brain and aspirates fluid or injects medication or another substance. The puncture site is disinfected. A needle with a syringe is advanced into the shunt tubing or reservoir. Cerebrospinal fluid and blood are aspirated, or a medication or other substance is injected through the shunt tubing or into the reservoir.

Puncture of shunt tubing or reservoir for aspiration or injection procedure

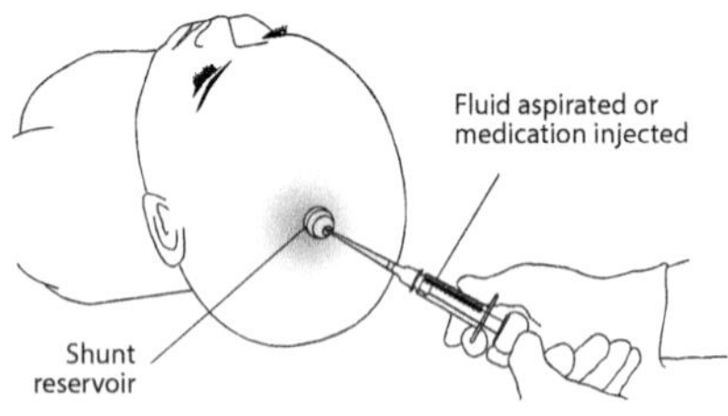

ICD-10-CM Diagnostic Codes

There are too many ICD-10-CM codes to list. Refer to ICD-10-CM code book for associated diagnostic codes.

CCI Edits

Refer to Appendix A for CCI edits.

Facility RVUs

Code	Work	PE Facility	MP	Total Facility
61070	0.89	0.59	0.15	1.63

Non-facility RVUs

Code	Work	PE Non-Facility	MP	Total Non-Facility
61070	0.89	0.59	0.15	1.63

Modifiers (PAR)

Code	Mod 50	Mod 51	Mod 62	Mod 66	Mod 80
61070	0	2	0	0	1

Global Period

Code	Days
61070	000

61105-61107

61105 Twist drill hole for subdural or ventricular puncture

⊘ **61107 Twist drill hole(s) for subdural, intracerebral, or ventricular puncture; for implanting ventricular catheter, pressure recording device, or other intracerebral monitoring device**

(For intracranial neuroendoscopic ventricular catheter placement, use 62160)

AMA Coding Notes

Surgical Procedures on the Skull, Meninges, and Brain

(For injection procedure for cerebral angiography, see 36100-36218)

(For injection procedure for ventriculography, see 61026, 61120)

(For injection procedure for pneumoencephalography, use 61055)

Plain English Description

A twist drill hole is created in the skull for subdural or ventricular puncture. A twist drill hole is created using a hand twist drill with the safety stop set to the expected thickness of the skull at the drill hole site. The drill is advanced through the outer and inner table of the skull until a change in resistance indicates that the inner table of the skull has been penetrated and the dura punctured. A needle is then inserted through the drill hole into the subdural space or one of the brain ventricles and cerebrospinal fluid is aspirated. Use code 61107 when a twist drill hole is created in the skull for subdural, intracerebral, or ventricular puncture with implantation of intraventricular catheter, pressure recording device, or other intracerebral monitoring device. Intracerebral monitoring devices measure diverse physiological parameters including intracerebral oxygenation, blood flow, and temperature. The twist drill hole is created as described above. A catheter is advanced into the space between the dural and arachnoid membranes (subdural space), cerebrum, or one of the ventricles. The catheter is attached to drainage tubing, a pressure transducer, or other intracerebral monitoring device. Catheter patency is tested and/or the monitoring system is tested and calibrated.

Twist drill hole for subdural or ventricular puncture

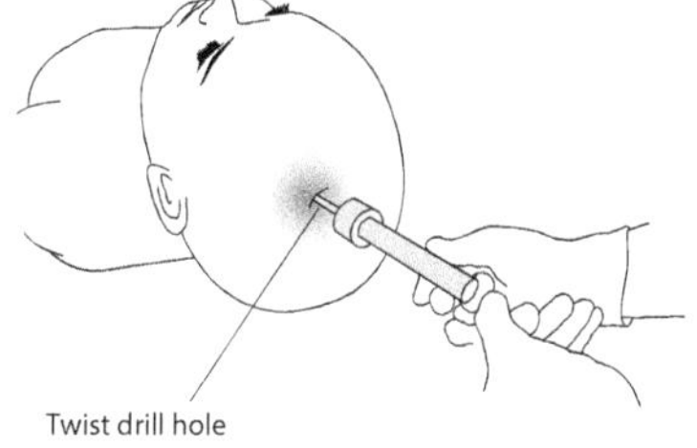

Twist drill hole for subdural or ventricular puncture (61105); twist drill hole(s) for subdural, intracerebral, or ventricular puncture; for implanting ventricular catheter, pressure recording device, or other intracerebral monitoring device

ICD-10-CM Diagnostic Codes

Code	Description
C71.0	Malignant neoplasm of cerebrum, except lobes and ventricles
C71.1	Malignant neoplasm of frontal lobe
C71.2	Malignant neoplasm of temporal lobe
C71.3	Malignant neoplasm of parietal lobe
C71.4	Malignant neoplasm of occipital lobe
C71.5	Malignant neoplasm of cerebral ventricle
C71.6	Malignant neoplasm of cerebellum
C71.8	Malignant neoplasm of overlapping sites of brain
C79.31	Secondary malignant neoplasm of brain
D33.0	Benign neoplasm of brain, supratentorial
G91.0	Communicating hydrocephalus
G91.1	Obstructive hydrocephalus
G91.2	(Idiopathic) normal pressure hydrocephalus
G91.3	Post-traumatic hydrocephalus, unspecified
G91.4	Hydrocephalus in diseases classified elsewhere
G91.8	Other hydrocephalus
G91.9	Hydrocephalus, unspecified
G92	Toxic encephalopathy
G93.0	Cerebral cysts
G93.40	Encephalopathy, unspecified
G93.41	Metabolic encephalopathy
G93.49	Other encephalopathy
G93.6	Cerebral edema
G93.7	Reye's syndrome
G97.31	Intraoperative hemorrhage and hematoma of a nervous system organ or structure complicating a nervous system procedure
G97.32	Intraoperative hemorrhage and hematoma of a nervous system organ or structure complicating other procedure
G97.51	Postprocedural hemorrhage of a nervous system organ or structure following a nervous system procedure
G97.52	Postprocedural hemorrhage of a nervous system organ or structure following other procedure
G97.61	Postprocedural hematoma of a nervous system organ or structure following a nervous system procedure
G97.63	Postprocedural seroma of a nervous system organ or structure following a nervous system procedure
H47.11	Papilledema associated with increased intracranial pressure
I67.4	Hypertensive encephalopathy
Q04.6	Congenital cerebral cysts
R83.2	Abnormal level of other drugs, medicaments and biological substances in cerebrospinal fluid
R83.3	Abnormal level of substances chiefly nonmedicinal as to source in cerebrospinal fluid
R83.4	Abnormal immunological findings in cerebrospinal fluid
R83.5	Abnormal microbiological findings in cerebrospinal fluid
R83.6	Abnormal cytological findings in cerebrospinal fluid
R83.8	Other abnormal findings in cerebrospinal fluid
⓻ S06.1X0	Traumatic cerebral edema without loss of consciousness
⓻ S06.1X9	Traumatic cerebral edema with loss of consciousness of unspecified duration
⓻ S06.2X0	Diffuse traumatic brain injury without loss of consciousness
⓻ S06.2X9	Diffuse traumatic brain injury with loss of consciousness of unspecified duration
⓻⇄ S06.310	Contusion and laceration of right cerebrum without loss of consciousness
⓻⇄ S06.319	Contusion and laceration of right cerebrum with loss of consciousness of unspecified duration
⓻⇄ S06.320	Contusion and laceration of left cerebrum without loss of consciousness
⓻⇄ S06.329	Contusion and laceration of left cerebrum with loss of consciousness of unspecified duration
⓻⇄ S06.340	Traumatic hemorrhage of right cerebrum without loss of consciousness
⓻⇄ S06.349	Traumatic hemorrhage of right cerebrum with loss of consciousness of unspecified duration
⓻⇄ S06.350	Traumatic hemorrhage of left cerebrum without loss of consciousness
⓻⇄ S06.359	Traumatic hemorrhage of left cerebrum with loss of consciousness of unspecified duration
⓻ S06.5X0	Traumatic subdural hemorrhage without loss of consciousness
⓻ S06.5X9	Traumatic subdural hemorrhage with loss of consciousness of unspecified duration

❼	S06.6X0	Traumatic subarachnoid hemorrhage without loss of consciousness
❼	S06.6X9	Traumatic subarachnoid hemorrhage with loss of consciousness of unspecified duration
❼	T85.730	Infection and inflammatory reaction due to ventricular intracranial (communicating) shunt
❼	T85.731	Infection and inflammatory reaction due to implanted electronic neurostimulator of brain, electrode (lead)
❼	T85.735	Infection and inflammatory reaction due to cranial or spinal infusion catheter
	Z45.41	Encounter for adjustment and management of cerebrospinal fluid drainage device

ICD-10-CM Coding Notes

For codes requiring a 7th character extension, refer to your ICD-10-CM book. Review the character descriptions and coding guidelines for proper selection. For some procedures, only certain characters will apply.

CCI Edits

Refer to Appendix A for CCI edits.

Facility RVUs ▢

Code	Work	PE Facility	MP	Total Facility
61105	5.45	5.81	1.99	13.25
61107	4.99	2.29	1.80	9.08

Non-facility RVUs ▢

Code	Work	PE Non-Facility	MP	Total Non-Facility
61105	5.45	5.81	1.99	13.25
61107	4.99	2.29	1.80	9.08

Modifiers (PAR) ▢

Code	Mod 50	Mod 51	Mod 62	Mod 66	Mod 80
61105	0	2	0	0	0
61107	0	0	0	0	1

Global Period

Code	Days
61105	090
61107	000

61108

61108 Twist drill hole(s) for subdural, intracerebral, or ventricular puncture; for evacuation and/or drainage of subdural hematoma

AMA Coding Notes

Surgical Procedures on the Skull, Meninges, and Brain

(For injection procedure for cerebral angiography, see 36100-36218)

(For injection procedure for ventriculography, see 61026, 61120)

(For injection procedure for pneumoencephalography, use 61055)

Plain English Description

A twist drill hole is created in the skull for evacuation of a subdural hematoma. A twist drill hole is created using a hand twist drill with the safety stop set to the expected thickness of the skull at the drill site. The drill is advanced through the outer and inner table of the skull until a change in resistance indicates that the inner table of the skull has been penetrated and the dura punctured. A syringe is then inserted through the drill hole into the subdural space and the subdural hematoma is flushed out.

Drainage of a hematoma

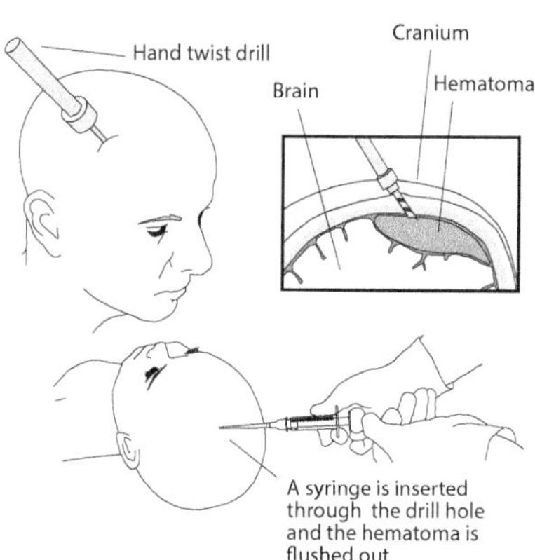

A twist drill is used to create a hole in the cranium.

ICD-10-CM Diagnostic Codes

	Code	Description
	G97.31	Intraoperative hemorrhage and hematoma of a nervous system organ or structure complicating a nervous system procedure
	G97.32	Intraoperative hemorrhage and hematoma of a nervous system organ or structure complicating other procedure
	G97.41	Accidental puncture or laceration of dura during a procedure
	G97.48	Accidental puncture and laceration of other nervous system organ or structure during a nervous system procedure
	G97.49	Accidental puncture and laceration of other nervous system organ or structure during other procedure
	G97.61	Postprocedural hematoma of a nervous system organ or structure following a nervous system procedure
	G97.62	Postprocedural hematoma of a nervous system organ or structure following other procedure
➐	S06.5X0	Traumatic subdural hemorrhage without loss of consciousness
➐	S06.5X1	Traumatic subdural hemorrhage with loss of consciousness of 30 minutes or less
➐	S06.5X2	Traumatic subdural hemorrhage with loss of consciousness of 31 minutes to 59 minutes
➐	S06.5X3	Traumatic subdural hemorrhage with loss of consciousness of 1 hour to 5 hours 59 minutes
➐	S06.5X4	Traumatic subdural hemorrhage with loss of consciousness of 6 hours to 24 hours
➐	S06.5X9	Traumatic subdural hemorrhage with loss of consciousness of unspecified duration

ICD-10-CM Coding Notes

For codes requiring a 7th character extension, refer to your ICD-10-CM book. Review the character descriptions and coding guidelines for proper selection. For some procedures, only certain characters will apply.

CCI Edits

Refer to Appendix A for CCI edits.

Facility RVUs ☐

Code	Work	PE Facility	MP	Total Facility
61108	11.64	10.14	4.05	25.83

Non-facility RVUs ☐

Code	Work	PE Non-Facility	MP	Total Non-Facility
61108	11.64	10.14	4.05	25.83

Modifiers (PAR) ☐

Code	Mod 50	Mod 51	Mod 62	Mod 66	Mod 80
61108	0	2	0	0	1

Global Period

Code	Days
61108	090

61140

61140 Burr hole(s) or trephine; with biopsy of brain or intracranial lesion

AMA Coding Notes

Surgical Procedures on the Skull, Meninges, and Brain

(For injection procedure for cerebral angiography, see 36100-36218)

(For injection procedure for ventriculography, see 61026, 61120)

(For injection procedure for pneumoencephalography, use 61055)

Plain English Description

A burr or trephine is used to make a small opening in the skull and obtain a biopsy of the brain or an intracranial lesion. The scalp is incised and flapped forward. A burr hole is created with a surgical drill or perforator. Alternatively, a small disc of bone may be removed using a trephine. The dura is incised. Bleeding is controlled by electrocautery. A biopsy needle is inserted and a tissue sample is obtained from the brain or intracranial lesion. The needle is withdrawn; the dura is closed; and the skull defect is repaired by replacing the bone disc or applying bone wax.

Burr hole(s) or trephine; with biopsy of brain or intracranial lesion

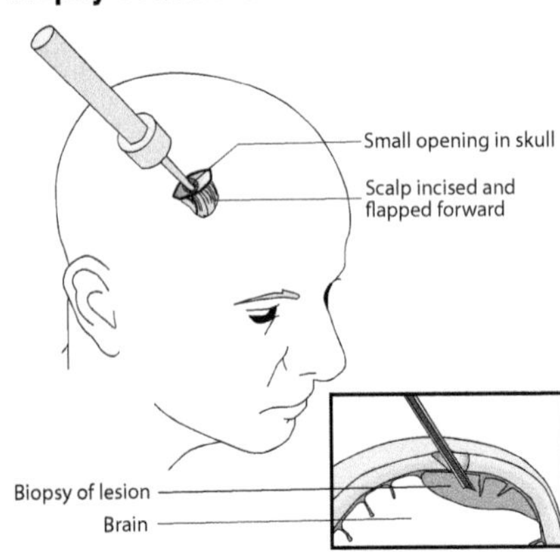

ICD-10-CM Diagnostic Codes

C70.0	Malignant neoplasm of cerebral meninges
C71.0	Malignant neoplasm of cerebrum, except lobes and ventricles
C71.1	Malignant neoplasm of frontal lobe
C71.2	Malignant neoplasm of temporal lobe
C71.3	Malignant neoplasm of parietal lobe
C71.4	Malignant neoplasm of occipital lobe
C71.5	Malignant neoplasm of cerebral ventricle
C71.6	Malignant neoplasm of cerebellum
C71.7	Malignant neoplasm of brain stem
C71.8	Malignant neoplasm of overlapping sites of brain
C79.31	Secondary malignant neoplasm of brain
C79.32	Secondary malignant neoplasm of cerebral meninges
D32.0	Benign neoplasm of cerebral meninges
D33.0	Benign neoplasm of brain, supratentorial
D33.1	Benign neoplasm of brain, infratentorial
D42.0	Neoplasm of uncertain behavior of cerebral meninges
D43.0	Neoplasm of uncertain behavior of brain, supratentorial
D43.1	Neoplasm of uncertain behavior of brain, infratentorial
D49.6	Neoplasm of unspecified behavior of brain
G06.0	Intracranial abscess and granuloma
G93.0	Cerebral cysts
Q04.6	Congenital cerebral cysts

CCI Edits

Refer to Appendix A for CCI edits.

Facility RVUs ☐

Code	Work	PE Facility	MP	Total Facility
61140	17.23	12.98	6.33	36.54

Non-facility RVUs ☐

Code	Work	PE Non-Facility	MP	Total Non-Facility
61140	17.23	12.98	6.33	36.54

Modifiers (PAR) ☐

Code	Mod 50	Mod 51	Mod 62	Mod 66	Mod 80
61140	0	2	0	0	2

Global Period

Code	Days
61140	090

61150-61151

61150 Burr hole(s) or trephine; with drainage of brain abscess or cyst

61151 Burr hole(s) or trephine; with subsequent tapping (aspiration) of intracranial abscess or cyst

AMA Coding Notes

Surgical Procedures on the Skull, Meninges, and Brain

(For injection procedure for cerebral angiography, see 36100-36218)

(For injection procedure for ventriculography, see 61026, 61120)

(For injection procedure for pneumoencephalography, use 61055)

Plain English Description

A burr or trephine is used to make a small opening in the skull followed by drainage of a brain abscess or cyst. The scalp is incised and flapped forward. A burr hole is created with a surgical drill or perforator. Alternatively, a small disc of bone may be removed using a trephine. The dura is incised. Bleeding is controlled by electrocautery. A needle is inserted and advanced to the abscess or cyst site. The abscess or cyst capsule is perforated. The obturator in the needle is removed and a syringe attached to the needle. The cyst or abscess is drained. The needle is withdrawn, the dura closed, and the skull defect repaired by replacing the bone disc or applying bone wax. Use code 61150 for the initial drainage of the brain abscess or cyst and 61151 when a subsequent tapping with aspiration of the intracranial abscess or cyst is performed.

Burr hole(s) or trephine

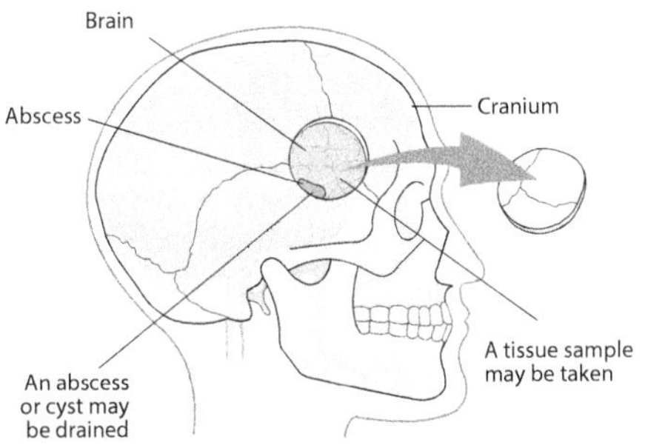

A burr drill or trephine is used to create a hole in the cranium. With drainage of brain abscess or cyst (61150); with subsequent tapping of intracranial abscess or cyst (61151)

ICD-10-CM Diagnostic Codes

A06.6	Amebic brain abscess
A17.81	Tuberculoma of brain and spinal cord
A54.82	Gonococcal brain abscess
B43.1	Pheomycotic brain abscess
G06.0	Intracranial abscess and granuloma
G93.0	Cerebral cysts
Q04.6	Congenital cerebral cysts

CCI Edits

Refer to Appendix A for CCI edits.

Facility RVUs ▯

Code	Work	PE Facility	MP	Total Facility
61150	18.90	13.14	6.97	39.01
61151	13.49	10.18	4.96	28.63

Non-facility RVUs ▯

Code	Work	PE Non-Facility	MP	Total Non-Facility
61150	18.90	13.14	6.97	39.01
61151	13.49	10.18	4.96	28.63

Modifiers (PAR) ▯

Code	Mod 50	Mod 51	Mod 62	Mod 66	Mod 80
61150	0	2	1	0	1
61151	0	2	0	0	1

Global Period

Code	Days
61150	090
61151	090

61154-61156

61154 Burr hole(s) with evacuation and/or drainage of hematoma, extradural or subdural

(For bilateral procedure, report 61154 with modifier 50)

61156 Burr hole(s); with aspiration of hematoma or cyst, intracerebral

AMA Coding Notes

Surgical Procedures on the Skull, Meninges, and Brain

(For injection procedure for cerebral angiography, see 36100-36218)

(For injection procedure for ventriculography, see 61026, 61120)

(For injection procedure for pneumoencephalography, use 61055)

Plain English Description

A burr hole craniotomy is performed for drainage of a subdural or extradural hematoma. The scalp is incised and flapped forward. A burr hole is created with a surgical drill or perforator through the outer and inner table of the skull. For an extradural hematoma, the collection of blood is located between the inner table of the skull and the dural membrane. A cannula with a stylet is inserted through a guide. A syringe is inserted and the collection of blood flushed from the hematoma site. For a subdural hematoma, the dura is incised and the collection of blood between the dura and arachnoid membranes located. A cannula with stylet is inserted. A syringe is inserted and the collection of blood flushed from the hematoma site. The syringe is withdrawn, the dura closed, and the skull defect repaired using bone wax. Use 61156 for aspiration of an intracerebral hematoma or cyst. An intracerebral hematoma or cyst, also referred to as a cerebral hematoma or cyst, is a collection of blood or fluid within the brain in the substance of the cerebrum. The cannula is advanced into the intracerebral hematoma or cyst and blood or fluid removed using gentle suction.

Burr hole(s)

With evacuation and/or drainage of hematoma, extradural or subdural (61154); with aspiration of hematoma or cyst, intracerebral (61156)

ICD-10-CM Diagnostic Codes

	Code	Description
	G93.0	Cerebral cysts
	G97.31	Intraoperative hemorrhage and hematoma of a nervous system organ or structure complicating a nervous system procedure
	G97.32	Intraoperative hemorrhage and hematoma of a nervous system organ or structure complicating other procedure
	G97.41	Accidental puncture or laceration of dura during a procedure
	G97.48	Accidental puncture and laceration of other nervous system organ or structure during a nervous system procedure
	G97.49	Accidental puncture and laceration of other nervous system organ or structure during other procedure
	G97.61	Postprocedural hematoma of a nervous system organ or structure following a nervous system procedure
	G97.62	Postprocedural hematoma of a nervous system organ or structure following other procedure
	Q04.6	Congenital cerebral cysts
➐⇄	S06.340	Traumatic hemorrhage of right cerebrum without loss of consciousness
➐⇄	S06.341	Traumatic hemorrhage of right cerebrum with loss of consciousness of 30 minutes or less
➐⇄	S06.342	Traumatic hemorrhage of right cerebrum with loss of consciousness of 31 minutes to 59 minutes
➐⇄	S06.343	Traumatic hemorrhage of right cerebrum with loss of consciousness of 1 hours to 5 hours 59 minutes
➐⇄	S06.344	Traumatic hemorrhage of right cerebrum with loss of consciousness of 6 hours to 24 hours
➐⇄	S06.345	Traumatic hemorrhage of right cerebrum with loss of consciousness greater than 24 hours with return to pre-existing conscious level
➐⇄	S06.349	Traumatic hemorrhage of right cerebrum with loss of consciousness of unspecified duration
➐⇄	S06.350	Traumatic hemorrhage of left cerebrum without loss of consciousness
➐⇄	S06.351	Traumatic hemorrhage of left cerebrum with loss of consciousness of 30 minutes or less
➐⇄	S06.352	Traumatic hemorrhage of left cerebrum with loss of consciousness of 31 minutes to 59 minutes
➐⇄	S06.353	Traumatic hemorrhage of left cerebrum with loss of consciousness of 1 hours to 5 hours 59 minutes
➐⇄	S06.354	Traumatic hemorrhage of left cerebrum with loss of consciousness of 6 hours to 24 hours
➐⇄	S06.355	Traumatic hemorrhage of left cerebrum with loss of consciousness greater than 24 hours with return to pre-existing conscious level
➐⇄	S06.359	Traumatic hemorrhage of left cerebrum with loss of consciousness of unspecified duration
➐	S06.4X0	Epidural hemorrhage without loss of consciousness
➐	S06.4X1	Epidural hemorrhage with loss of consciousness of 30 minutes or less
➐	S06.4X2	Epidural hemorrhage with loss of consciousness of 31 minutes to 59 minutes
➐	S06.4X3	Epidural hemorrhage with loss of consciousness of 1 hour to 5 hours 59 minutes
➐	S06.4X4	Epidural hemorrhage with loss of consciousness of 6 hours to 24 hours
➐	S06.4X5	Epidural hemorrhage with loss of consciousness greater than 24 hours with return to pre-existing conscious level
➐	S06.4X9	Epidural hemorrhage with loss of consciousness of unspecified duration
➐	S06.5X0	Traumatic subdural hemorrhage without loss of consciousness
➐	S06.5X1	Traumatic subdural hemorrhage with loss of consciousness of 30 minutes or less
➐	S06.5X2	Traumatic subdural hemorrhage with loss of consciousness of 31 minutes to 59 minutes
➐	S06.5X3	Traumatic subdural hemorrhage with loss of consciousness of 1 hour to 5 hours 59 minutes
➐	S06.5X4	Traumatic subdural hemorrhage with loss of consciousness of 6 hours to 24 hours
➐	S06.5X9	Traumatic subdural hemorrhage with loss of consciousness of unspecified duration

ICD-10-CM Coding Notes

For codes requiring a 7th character extension, refer to your ICD-10-CM book. Review the character descriptions and coding guidelines for proper selection. For some procedures, only certain characters will apply.

CCI Edits

Refer to Appendix A for CCI edits.

Facility RVUs

Code	Work	PE Facility	MP	Total Facility
61154	17.07	13.37	6.24	36.68
61156	17.45	11.98	6.41	35.84

Non-facility RVUs

Code	Work	PE Non-Facility	MP	Total Non-Facility
61154	17.07	13.37	6.24	36.68
61156	17.45	11.98	6.41	35.84

Modifiers (PAR)

Code	Mod 50	Mod 51	Mod 62	Mod 66	Mod 80
61154	1	2	1	0	2
61156	0	2	1	0	2

Global Period

Code	Days
61154	090
61156	090

61210

61210 Burr hole(s); for implanting ventricular catheter, reservoir, EEG electrode(s), pressure recording device, or other cerebral monitoring device (separate procedure)

(For intracranial neuroendoscopic ventricular catheter placement, use 62160)

AMA Coding Notes

Surgical Procedures on the Skull, Meninges, and Brain

(For injection procedure for cerebral angiography, see 36100-36218)

(For injection procedure for ventriculography, see 61026, 61120)

(For injection procedure for pneumoencephalography, use 61055)

Plain English Description

One or more cranial burr holes are created to allow for implantation of a ventricular catheter, reservoir, EEG electrode(s), pressure recording device, or other cerebral monitoring device. The area over the burr hole site(s) is shaved. A small incision is made through the skin and fascia. Overlying muscle is separated and the periosteum is incised. A drill cutter is used to create a small hole through the entire thickness of the skull. The opening is enlarged using a conical or cylindrical burr. If a larger opening is required, a rongeur may be used.

Burr hole(s) for implanting ventricular catheter/reservoir/EEG electrode(s)/ pressure recording device/ other cerebral monitoring devise

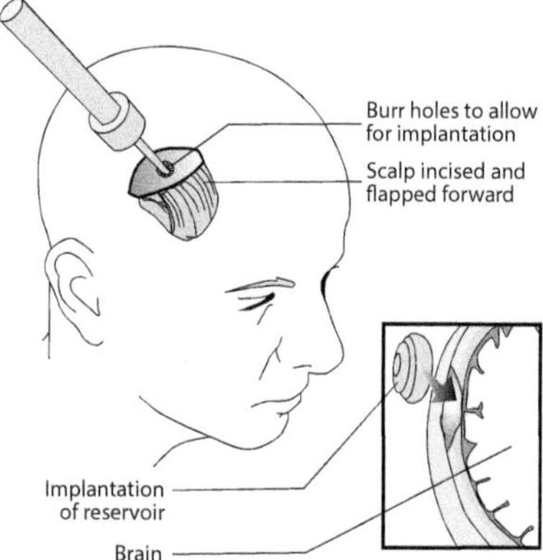

ICD-10-CM Diagnostic Codes

C71.0 Malignant neoplasm of cerebrum, except lobes and ventricles
C71.1 Malignant neoplasm of frontal lobe
C71.2 Malignant neoplasm of temporal lobe
C71.3 Malignant neoplasm of parietal lobe
C71.4 Malignant neoplasm of occipital lobe
C71.5 Malignant neoplasm of cerebral ventricle
C71.6 Malignant neoplasm of cerebellum
C71.8 Malignant neoplasm of overlapping sites of brain
C79.31 Secondary malignant neoplasm of brain
D33.0 Benign neoplasm of brain, supratentorial
G40.211 Localization-related (focal) (partial) symptomatic epilepsy and epileptic syndromes with complex partial seizures, intractable, with status epilepticus
G40.219 Localization-related (focal) (partial) symptomatic epilepsy and epileptic syndromes with complex partial seizures, intractable, without status epilepticus
G40.311 Generalized idiopathic epilepsy and epileptic syndromes, intractable, with status epilepticus
G40.319 Generalized idiopathic epilepsy and epileptic syndromes, intractable, without status epilepticus
G40.803 Other epilepsy, intractable, with status epilepticus
G40.804 Other epilepsy, intractable, without status epilepticus
G40.B11 Juvenile myoclonic epilepsy, intractable, with status epilepticus
G40.B19 Juvenile myoclonic epilepsy, intractable, without status epilepticus
G91.0 Communicating hydrocephalus
G91.1 Obstructive hydrocephalus
G91.2 (Idiopathic) normal pressure hydrocephalus
G91.3 Post-traumatic hydrocephalus, unspecified
G91.4 Hydrocephalus in diseases classified elsewhere
G91.8 Other hydrocephalus
G91.9 Hydrocephalus, unspecified
G92 Toxic encephalopathy
G93.0 Cerebral cysts
G93.40 Encephalopathy, unspecified
G93.41 Metabolic encephalopathy
G93.49 Other encephalopathy
G93.6 Cerebral edema
G93.7 Reye's syndrome
G97.31 Intraoperative hemorrhage and hematoma of a nervous system organ or structure complicating a nervous system procedure
G97.32 Intraoperative hemorrhage and hematoma of a nervous system organ or structure complicating other procedure
G97.51 Postprocedural hemorrhage of a nervous system organ or structure following a nervous system procedure
G97.52 Postprocedural hemorrhage of a nervous system organ or structure following other procedure
G97.61 Postprocedural hematoma of a nervous system organ or structure following a nervous system procedure
G97.63 Postprocedural seroma of a nervous system organ or structure following a nervous system procedure
H47.11 Papilledema associated with increased intracranial pressure
I67.4 Hypertensive encephalopathy
Q04.6 Congenital cerebral cysts
R83.2 Abnormal level of other drugs, medicaments and biological substances in cerebrospinal fluid
R83.3 Abnormal level of substances chiefly nonmedicinal as to source in cerebrospinal fluid
R83.4 Abnormal immunological findings in cerebrospinal fluid
R83.5 Abnormal microbiological findings in cerebrospinal fluid
R83.6 Abnormal cytological findings in cerebrospinal fluid
R83.8 Other abnormal findings in cerebrospinal fluid
⑦ S06.1X0 Traumatic cerebral edema without loss of consciousness
⑦ S06.1X9 Traumatic cerebral edema with loss of consciousness of unspecified duration
⑦ S06.2X0 Diffuse traumatic brain injury without loss of consciousness
⑦ S06.2X9 Diffuse traumatic brain injury with loss of consciousness of unspecified duration
⑦⇄ S06.310 Contusion and laceration of right cerebrum without loss of consciousness
⑦⇄ S06.319 Contusion and laceration of right cerebrum with loss of consciousness of unspecified duration
⑦⇄ S06.320 Contusion and laceration of left cerebrum without loss of consciousness
⑦⇄ S06.329 Contusion and laceration of left cerebrum with loss of consciousness of unspecified duration
⑦⇄ S06.340 Traumatic hemorrhage of right cerebrum without loss of consciousness
⑦⇄ S06.349 Traumatic hemorrhage of right cerebrum with loss of consciousness of unspecified duration
⑦⇄ S06.350 Traumatic hemorrhage of left cerebrum without loss of consciousness
⑦⇄ S06.359 Traumatic hemorrhage of left cerebrum with loss of consciousness of unspecified duration
⑦ S06.5X0 Traumatic subdural hemorrhage without loss of consciousness
⑦ S06.5X9 Traumatic subdural hemorrhage with loss of consciousness of unspecified duration

⑦	S06.6X0	Traumatic subarachnoid hemorrhage without loss of consciousness
⑦	S06.6X9	Traumatic subarachnoid hemorrhage with loss of consciousness of unspecified duration
⑦	T85.730	Infection and inflammatory reaction due to ventricular intracranial (communicating) shunt
⑦	T85.731	Infection and inflammatory reaction due to implanted electronic neurostimulator of brain, electrode (lead)
⑦	T85.735	Infection and inflammatory reaction due to cranial or spinal infusion catheter
	Z45.41	Encounter for adjustment and management of cerebrospinal fluid drainage device

ICD-10-CM Coding Notes

For codes requiring a 7th character extension, refer to your ICD-10-CM book. Review the character descriptions and coding guidelines for proper selection. For some procedures, only certain characters will apply.

CCI Edits

Refer to Appendix A for CCI edits.

Facility RVUs ☐

Code	Work	PE Facility	MP	Total Facility
61210	5.83	2.69	2.13	10.65

Non-facility RVUs ☐

Code	Work	PE Non-Facility	MP	Total Non-Facility
61210	5.83	2.69	2.13	10.65

Modifiers (PAR) ☐

Code	Mod 50	Mod 51	Mod 62	Mod 66	Mod 80
61210	0	2	0	0	1

Global Period

Code	Days
61210	000

61215

61215 Insertion of subcutaneous reservoir, pump or continuous infusion system for connection to ventricular catheter

(For refilling and maintenance of an implantable infusion pump for spinal or brain drug therapy, use 95990)

(For chemotherapy, use 96450)

AMA Coding Notes

Surgical Procedures on the Skull, Meninges, and Brain

(For injection procedure for cerebral angiography, see 36100-36218)

(For injection procedure for ventriculography, see 61026, 61120)

(For injection procedure for pneumoencephalography, use 61055)

AMA *CPT Assistant*

61215: Spring 93: 13

Plain English Description

The physician inserts a subcutaneous reservoir, pump, or continuous infusion system for connection to a ventricular catheter. An implantable reservoir, pump, or continuous infusion system may be used to deliver medication directly into the brain or to drain excess cerebrospinal fluid from the ventricles. An incision is made in the skin under the infraclavicular fossa and a subcutaneous pocket is created. The reservoir, pump, or continuous infusion system is placed within the subcutaneous pocket and connected to a previously placed ventricular catheter. The skin is closed over the reservoir, pump, or continuous infusion system.

Insertion of subcutaneous reservoir, pump or continuous infusion system for connection to ventricular catheter

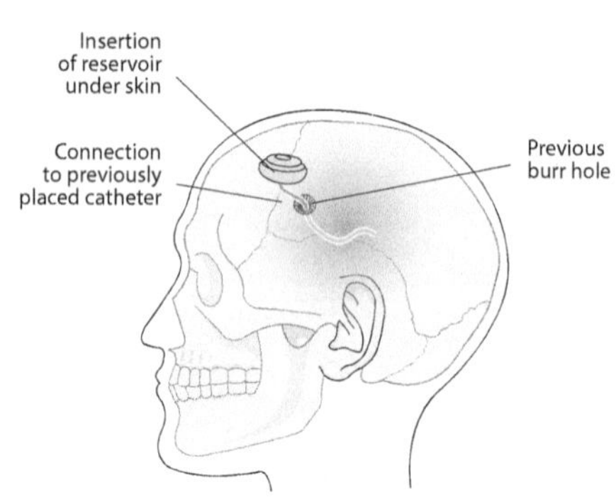

ICD-10-CM Diagnostic Codes

C71.0	Malignant neoplasm of cerebrum, except lobes and ventricles
C71.1	Malignant neoplasm of frontal lobe
C71.2	Malignant neoplasm of temporal lobe
C71.3	Malignant neoplasm of parietal lobe
C71.4	Malignant neoplasm of occipital lobe
C71.5	Malignant neoplasm of cerebral ventricle
C71.6	Malignant neoplasm of cerebellum
C71.7	Malignant neoplasm of brain stem
C71.8	Malignant neoplasm of overlapping sites of brain
C79.31	Secondary malignant neoplasm of brain
D43.0	Neoplasm of uncertain behavior of brain, supratentorial
D43.1	Neoplasm of uncertain behavior of brain, infratentorial

CCI Edits

Refer to Appendix A for CCI edits.

Facility RVUs

Code	Work	PE Facility	MP	Total Facility
61215	5.85	6.60	2.13	14.58

Non-facility RVUs

Code	Work	PE Non-Facility	MP	Total Non-Facility
61215	5.85	6.60	2.13	14.58

Modifiers (PAR)

Code	Mod 50	Mod 51	Mod 62	Mod 66	Mod 80
61215	0	2	1	0	1

Global Period

Code	Days
61215	090

61304-61305

61304 Craniectomy or craniotomy, exploratory; supratentorial

61305 Craniectomy or craniotomy, exploratory; infratentorial (posterior fossa)

AMA Coding Notes

Surgical Procedures on the Skull, Meninges, and Brain

(For injection procedure for cerebral angiography, see 36100-36218)

(For injection procedure for ventriculography, see 61026, 61120)

(For injection procedure for pneumoencephalography, use 61055)

Plain English Description

An exploratory supratentorial craniectomy or craniotomy is performed. The supratentorial region is the part of the brain that lies above the tentorium cerebelli, a fold of dura mater that separates the frontal and occipital lobes of the cerebrum from the cerebellum. A craniectomy is performed by creating scalp flaps, followed by several burr holes. The bone between the burr holes is then cut with a saw or craniotome and a large bone flap raised for temporary or permanent removal. A craniotomy is performed by incising the scalp and then raising scalp, bone, and dural flaps to expose the cerebrum. A suspected defect or injury to the supratentorial region of the brain is explored and any abnormalities noted. No definitive surgery is performed. When the exploratory procedure is complete, the dural flap is placed over the exposed brain and approximated with sutures, taking care to tightly close the dura to prevent leakage of cerebrospinal fluid. The bone flap is then placed over the dura and anchored with steel sutures. Alternatively, a craniectomy defect may be plugged with bone wax or silicone. The fascia and muscle are closed followed by the scalp in a layered fashion. Use code 61305 for an exploratory infratentorial craniectomy or craniotomy of the cerebellar region. The infratentorial region is the part of the brain that lies below the tentorium cerebelli.

Craniectomy or craniotomy, exploratory

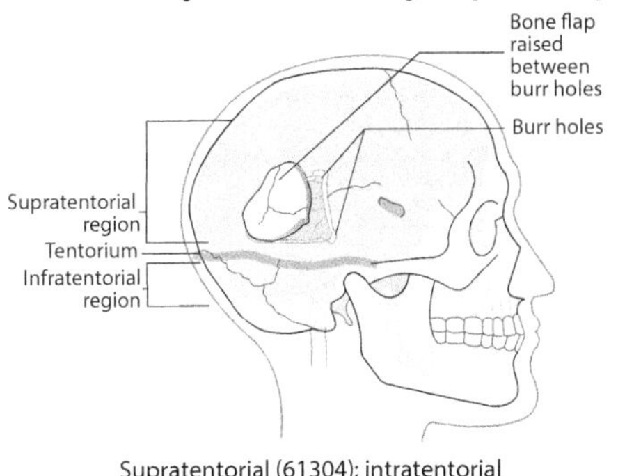

Supratentorial (61304); intratentorial (posterior fossa) (61305)

ICD-10-CM Diagnostic Codes

Code	Description
A06.6	Amebic brain abscess
A17.81	Tuberculoma of brain and spinal cord
A54.82	Gonococcal brain abscess
B43.1	Pheomycotic brain abscess
B94.8	Sequelae of other specified infectious and parasitic diseases
B95.0	Streptococcus, group A, as the cause of diseases classified elsewhere
B95.1	Streptococcus, group B, as the cause of diseases classified elsewhere
B95.2	Enterococcus as the cause of diseases classified elsewhere
B95.3	Streptococcus pneumoniae as the cause of diseases classified elsewhere
B95.4	Other streptococcus as the cause of diseases classified elsewhere
B95.5	Unspecified streptococcus as the cause of diseases classified elsewhere
B95.61	Methicillin susceptible Staphylococcus aureus infection as the cause of diseases classified elsewhere
B95.62	Methicillin resistant Staphylococcus aureus infection as the cause of diseases classified elsewhere
B95.7	Other staphylococcus as the cause of diseases classified elsewhere
B95.8	Unspecified staphylococcus as the cause of diseases classified elsewhere
B96.3	Hemophilus influenzae [H. influenzae] as the cause of diseases classified elsewhere
C70.0	Malignant neoplasm of cerebral meninges
C71.0	Malignant neoplasm of cerebrum, except lobes and ventricles
C71.1	Malignant neoplasm of frontal lobe
C71.2	Malignant neoplasm of temporal lobe
C71.3	Malignant neoplasm of parietal lobe
C71.4	Malignant neoplasm of occipital lobe
C71.5	Malignant neoplasm of cerebral ventricle
C71.6	Malignant neoplasm of cerebellum
C71.7	Malignant neoplasm of brain stem
C71.8	Malignant neoplasm of overlapping sites of brain
C79.31	Secondary malignant neoplasm of brain
C79.32	Secondary malignant neoplasm of cerebral meninges
D32.0	Benign neoplasm of cerebral meninges
D33.0	Benign neoplasm of brain, supratentorial
D33.1	Benign neoplasm of brain, infratentorial
D42.0	Neoplasm of uncertain behavior of cerebral meninges
D43.0	Neoplasm of uncertain behavior of brain, supratentorial
D43.1	Neoplasm of uncertain behavior of brain, infratentorial
D49.6	Neoplasm of unspecified behavior of brain
D49.7	Neoplasm of unspecified behavior of endocrine glands and other parts of nervous system
G06.0	Intracranial abscess and granuloma
G07	Intracranial and intraspinal abscess and granuloma in diseases classified elsewhere
G09	Sequelae of inflammatory diseases of central nervous system
G93.0	Cerebral cysts
Q04.6	Congenital cerebral cysts
S01.84XS	Puncture wound with foreign body of other part of head, sequela
S02.0XXS	Fracture of vault of skull, sequela
⇄ S02.11AS	Type I occipital condyle fracture, right side, sequela
⇄ S02.11BS	Type I occipital condyle fracture, left side, sequela
⇄ S02.11CS	Type II occipital condyle fracture, right side, sequela
⇄ S02.11DS	Type II occipital condyle fracture, left side, sequela
⇄ S02.11ES	Type III occipital condyle fracture, right side, sequela
⇄ S02.11FS	Type III occipital condyle fracture, left side, sequela
⇄ S02.11GS	Other fracture of occiput, right side, sequela
S02.2XXS	Fracture of nasal bones, sequela
⇄ S02.31XS	Fracture of orbital floor, right side, sequela
⇄ S02.32XS	Fracture of orbital floor, left side, sequela

CCI Edits

Refer to Appendix A for CCI edits.

Pub 100

61304: Pub 100-04, 12, 20.4.5

61305: Pub 100-04, 12, 20.4.5

Facility RVUs

Code	Work	PE Facility	MP	Total Facility
61304	23.41	15.54	8.47	47.42
61305	28.64	18.73	10.58	57.95

Non-facility RVUs

Code	Work	PE Non-Facility	MP	Total Non-Facility
61304	23.41	15.54	8.47	47.42
61305	28.64	18.73	10.58	57.95

Modifiers (PAR)

Code	Mod 50	Mod 51	Mod 62	Mod 66	Mod 80
61304	0	2	1	0	2
61305	0	2	1	0	2

Global Period

Code	Days
61304	090
61305	090

61312-61313

61312 Craniectomy or craniotomy for evacuation of hematoma, supratentorial; extradural or subdural

61313 Craniectomy or craniotomy for evacuation of hematoma, supratentorial; intracerebral

AMA Coding Notes

Surgical Procedures on the Skull, Meninges, and Brain

(For injection procedure for cerebral angiography, see 36100-36218)

(For injection procedure for ventriculography, see 61026, 61120)

(For injection procedure for pneumoencephalography, use 61055)

Plain English Description

A supratentorial craniectomy or craniotomy is performed for evacuation of an extradural or subdural hematoma (61312). The supratentorial region is the part of the brain that lies above the tentorium cerebelli, a fold of dura mater that separates the frontal and occipital lobes of the cerebrum from the cerebellum. An extradural hematoma is a collection of blood between the inner table of the skull and the dural membrane. A subdural hematoma is a collection of blood between the dural and arachnoid membranes. A craniectomy is performed by creating scalp flaps, followed by several burr holes. The bone between the burr holes is then cut with a saw or craniotome and a bone flap raised for temporary or permanent removal. A craniotomy is performed by incising the scalp and then raising scalp and bone flaps to expose an extradural hematoma. If a subdural hematoma is present, dural flaps are raised. The collection of blood is removed using biopsy forceps, gentle suction, and irrigation. When the procedure is complete, the dural flap is placed over the exposed brain and approximated with sutures, taking care to tightly close the dura to prevent leakage of cerebrospinal fluid. Alternatively, a temporary drain may be placed in the subdural space to drain residual fluid. The bone flap is then placed over the dura and anchored with steel sutures. Alternatively, a craniectomy defect may be plugged with bone wax or silicone. The fascia and muscle are closed and then the scalp in a layered fashion. Use code 61313 for a supratentorial craniectomy or craniotomy for evacuation of an intracerebral hematoma. An intracerebral hematoma, also referred to as a cerebral hematoma, is a collection of blood within the brain in the substance of the cerebrum usually caused by rupture of an artery.

Craniectomy or craniotomy for evacuation of hematoma, supratentorial

Extradural or subdural (61312); intracerebral (61313)

ICD-10-CM Diagnostic Codes

	Code	Description
	G97.61	Postprocedural hematoma of a nervous system organ or structure following a nervous system procedure
	G97.62	Postprocedural hematoma of a nervous system organ or structure following other procedure
⑦⇄	S06.340	Traumatic hemorrhage of right cerebrum without loss of consciousness
⑦⇄	S06.341	Traumatic hemorrhage of right cerebrum with loss of consciousness of 30 minutes or less
⑦⇄	S06.342	Traumatic hemorrhage of right cerebrum with loss of consciousness of 31 minutes to 59 minutes
⑦⇄	S06.343	Traumatic hemorrhage of right cerebrum with loss of consciousness of 1 hours to 5 hours 59 minutes
⑦⇄	S06.344	Traumatic hemorrhage of right cerebrum with loss of consciousness of 6 hours to 24 hours
⑦⇄	S06.345	Traumatic hemorrhage of right cerebrum with loss of consciousness greater than 24 hours with return to pre-existing conscious level
⑦⇄	S06.349	Traumatic hemorrhage of right cerebrum with loss of consciousness of unspecified duration
⑦⇄	S06.350	Traumatic hemorrhage of left cerebrum without loss of consciousness
⑦⇄	S06.351	Traumatic hemorrhage of left cerebrum with loss of consciousness of 30 minutes or less
⑦⇄	S06.352	Traumatic hemorrhage of left cerebrum with loss of consciousness of 31 minutes to 59 minutes
⑦⇄	S06.353	Traumatic hemorrhage of left cerebrum with loss of consciousness of 1 hours to 5 hours 59 minutes
⑦⇄	S06.354	Traumatic hemorrhage of left cerebrum with loss of consciousness of 6 hours to 24 hours
⑦⇄	S06.355	Traumatic hemorrhage of left cerebrum with loss of consciousness greater than 24 hours with return to pre-existing conscious level
⑦⇄	S06.359	Traumatic hemorrhage of left cerebrum with loss of consciousness of unspecified duration
⑦	S06.4X0	Epidural hemorrhage without loss of consciousness
⑦	S06.4X1	Epidural hemorrhage with loss of consciousness of 30 minutes or less
⑦	S06.4X2	Epidural hemorrhage with loss of consciousness of 31 minutes to 59 minutes
⑦	S06.4X3	Epidural hemorrhage with loss of consciousness of 1 hour to 5 hours 59 minutes
⑦	S06.4X4	Epidural hemorrhage with loss of consciousness of 6 hours to 24 hours
⑦	S06.4X5	Epidural hemorrhage with loss of consciousness greater than 24 hours with return to pre-existing conscious level
⑦	S06.4X9	Epidural hemorrhage with loss of consciousness of unspecified duration
⑦	S06.5X0	Traumatic subdural hemorrhage without loss of consciousness
⑦	S06.5X1	Traumatic subdural hemorrhage with loss of consciousness of 30 minutes or less
⑦	S06.5X2	Traumatic subdural hemorrhage with loss of consciousness of 31 minutes to 59 minutes
⑦	S06.5X3	Traumatic subdural hemorrhage with loss of consciousness of 1 hour to 5 hours 59 minutes
⑦	S06.5X4	Traumatic subdural hemorrhage with loss of consciousness of 6 hours to 24 hours
⑦	S06.5X9	Traumatic subdural hemorrhage with loss of consciousness of unspecified duration

ICD-10-CM Coding Notes

For codes requiring a 7th character extension, refer to your ICD-10-CM book. Review the character descriptions and coding guidelines for proper selection. For some procedures, only certain characters will apply.

CCI Edits

Refer to Appendix A for CCI edits.

Pub 100

61312: Pub 100-04, 12, 20.4.5
61313: Pub 100-04, 12, 20.4.5

Facility RVUs

Code	Work	PE Facility	MP	Total Facility
61312	30.17	18.71	11.09	59.97
61313	28.09	18.85	10.31	57.25

Non-facility RVUs

Code	Work	PE Non-Facility	MP	Total Non-Facility
61312	30.17	18.71	11.09	59.97
61313	28.09	18.85	10.31	57.25

Modifiers (PAR)

Code	Mod 50	Mod 51	Mod 62	Mod 66	Mod 80
61312	0	2	1	0	2
61313	0	2	1	0	2

Global Period

Code	Days
61312	090
61313	090

61314-61315

61314 Craniectomy or craniotomy for evacuation of hematoma, infratentorial; extradural or subdural

61315 Craniectomy or craniotomy for evacuation of hematoma, infratentorial; intracerebellar

AMA Coding Notes

Surgical Procedures on the Skull, Meninges, and Brain

(For injection procedure for cerebral angiography, see 36100-36218)

(For injection procedure for ventriculography, see 61026, 61120)

(For injection procedure for pneumoencephalography, use 61055)

Plain English Description

An infratentorial craniectomy or craniotomy is performed for evacuation of an extradural or subdural hematoma (61314). The infratentorial region is the part of the brain that lies below the tentorium cerebelli, a fold of dura mater that separates the frontal and occipital lobes of the cerebrum from the cerebellum. An extradural hematoma is a collection of blood between the inner table of the skull and the dural membrane. A subdural hematoma is a collection of blood between the dural and arachnoid membranes. A craniectomy is performed by creating scalp flaps, followed by several burr holes. The bone between the burr holes is then cut with a saw or craniotome and a bone flap raised for temporary or permanent removal. A craniotomy is performed by incising the scalp and then raising scalp and bone flaps to expose an extradural hematoma. If a subdural hematoma is present, dural flaps are raised. The collection of blood is removed using biopsy forceps, gentle suction, and irrigation. When the procedure is complete, the dural flap is placed over the exposed brain and approximated with sutures, taking care to tightly close the dura to prevent leakage of cerebrospinal fluid. Alternatively, a temporary drain may be placed in subdural space to drain residual fluid. The bone flap is then placed over the dura and anchored with steel sutures. Alternatively, a craniectomy defect may be plugged with bone wax or silicone. The fascia and muscle are closed and then the scalp in a layered fashion. Use code 61315 for an infratentorial craniectomy or craniotomy for evacuation of an intracerebellar hematoma. An intracerebellar hematoma, also referred to as a cerebellar hematoma, is a collection of blood within the brain in the substance of the cerebellum usually caused by rupture of an artery.

Craniectomy or craniotomy for evacuation of hematoma, infratentorial

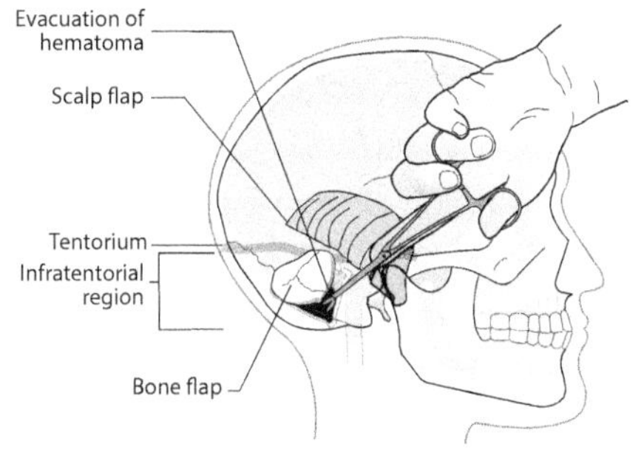

Extradural or subdural (61314); intracerebral (61315)

ICD-10-CM Diagnostic Codes

	Code	Description
	G97.61	Postprocedural hematoma of a nervous system organ or structure following a nervous system procedure
	G97.62	Postprocedural hematoma of a nervous system organ or structure following other procedure
⑦	S06.370	Contusion, laceration, and hemorrhage of cerebellum without loss of consciousness
⑦	S06.371	Contusion, laceration, and hemorrhage of cerebellum with loss of consciousness of 30 minutes or less
⑦	S06.372	Contusion, laceration, and hemorrhage of cerebellum with loss of consciousness of 31 minutes to 59 minutes
⑦	S06.373	Contusion, laceration, and hemorrhage of cerebellum with loss of consciousness of 1 hour to 5 hours 59 minutes
⑦	S06.374	Contusion, laceration, and hemorrhage of cerebellum with loss of consciousness of 6 hours to 24 hours
⑦	S06.375	Contusion, laceration, and hemorrhage of cerebellum with loss of consciousness greater than 24 hours with return to pre-existing conscious level
⑦	S06.379	Contusion, laceration, and hemorrhage of cerebellum with loss of consciousness of unspecified duration
⑦	S06.4X0	Epidural hemorrhage without loss of consciousness
⑦	S06.4X1	Epidural hemorrhage with loss of consciousness of 30 minutes or less
⑦	S06.4X2	Epidural hemorrhage with loss of consciousness of 31 minutes to 59 minutes
⑦	S06.4X3	Epidural hemorrhage with loss of consciousness of 1 hour to 5 hours 59 minutes
⑦	S06.4X4	Epidural hemorrhage with loss of consciousness of 6 hours to 24 hours
⑦	S06.4X5	Epidural hemorrhage with loss of consciousness greater than 24 hours with return to pre-existing conscious level
⑦	S06.4X9	Epidural hemorrhage with loss of consciousness of unspecified duration
⑦	S06.5X0	Traumatic subdural hemorrhage without loss of consciousness
⑦	S06.5X1	Traumatic subdural hemorrhage with loss of consciousness of 30 minutes or less
⑦	S06.5X2	Traumatic subdural hemorrhage with loss of consciousness of 31 minutes to 59 minutes
⑦	S06.5X3	Traumatic subdural hemorrhage with loss of consciousness of 1 hour to 5 hours 59 minutes
⑦	S06.5X4	Traumatic subdural hemorrhage with loss of consciousness of 6 hours to 24 hours
⑦	S06.5X9	Traumatic subdural hemorrhage with loss of consciousness of unspecified duration

ICD-10-CM Coding Notes

For codes requiring a 7th character extension, refer to your ICD-10-CM book. Review the character descriptions and coding guidelines for proper selection. For some procedures, only certain characters will apply.

CCI Edits

Refer to Appendix A for CCI edits.

Pub 100

61314: Pub 100-04, 12, 20.4.5
61315: Pub 100-04, 12, 20.4.5

Facility RVUs ☐

Code	Work	PE Facility	MP	Total Facility
61314	25.90	17.39	9.47	52.76
61315	29.65	19.13	10.90	59.68

Non-facility RVUs ☐

Code	Work	PE Non-Facility	MP	Total Non-Facility
61314	25.90	17.39	9.47	52.76
61315	29.65	19.13	10.90	59.68

Modifiers (PAR) ☐

Code	Mod 50	Mod 51	Mod 62	Mod 66	Mod 80
61314	0	2	1	0	2
61315	0	2	1	0	2

Global Period

Code	Days
61314	090
61315	090

61316

✚ **61316 Incision and subcutaneous placement of cranial bone graft (List separately in addition to code for primary procedure)**

(Use 61316 in conjunction with 61304, 61312, 61313, 61322, 61323, 61340, 61570, 61571, 61680-61705)

AMA Coding Notes

Surgical Procedures on the Skull, Meninges, and Brain

(For injection procedure for cerebral angiography, see 36100-36218)

(For injection procedure for ventriculography, see 61026, 61120)

(For injection procedure for pneumoencephalography, use 61055)

Plain English Description

A cranial bone graft removed at the time of a separately reportable craniectomy procedure is placed in a subcutaneous pocket to be used for future reconstruction of the skull defect. Subcutaneous storage, also referred to as subcutaneous banking, of the removed cranial bone flap preserves the viability of the bone for future use as an autogenous bone graft. An incision is made in the skin of the abdomen and a subcutaneous pocket is fashioned. The cranial bone flap removed during the craniectomy procedure is placed in the subcutaneous pocket and the skin and subcutaneous tissue are closed over the bone flap.

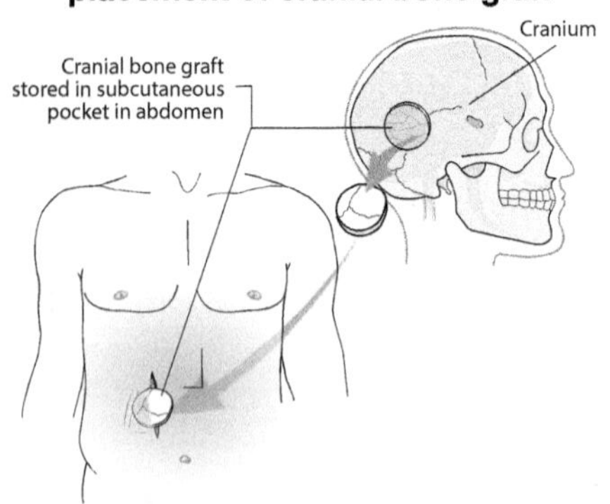

ICD-10-CM Diagnostic Codes

See Primary Procedure code for crosswalks.

CCI Edits

Refer to Appendix A for CCI edits.

Pub 100

61316: Pub 100-04, 12, 20.4.5

Facility RVUs ☐

Code	Work	PE Facility	MP	Total Facility
61316	1.39	0.64	0.51	2.54

Non-facility RVUs ☐

Code	Work	PE Non-Facility	MP	Total Non-Facility
61316	1.39	0.64	0.51	2.54

Modifiers (PAR) ☐

Code	Mod 50	Mod 51	Mod 62	Mod 66	Mod 80
61316	0	0	0	0	1

Global Period

Code	Days
61316	ZZZ

61320-61321

61320 Craniectomy or craniotomy, drainage of intracranial abscess; supratentorial

61321 Craniectomy or craniotomy, drainage of intracranial abscess; infratentorial

AMA Coding Notes

Surgical Procedures on the Skull, Meninges, and Brain

(For injection procedure for cerebral angiography, see 36100-36218)

(For injection procedure for ventriculography, see 61026, 61120)

(For injection procedure for pneumoencephalography, use 61055)

Plain English Description

A supratentorial craniectomy or craniotomy is performed for drainage of intracranial abscess. The supratentorial region is the part of the brain that lies above the tentorium cerebelli, a fold of dura mater that separates the frontal and occipital lobes of the cerebrum from the cerebellum. An intracranial abscess in the supratentorial region is a collection of pus in the cerebrum, the subdural space, or the extradural space. A craniectomy is performed by creating scalp flaps, followed by several burr holes. The bone between the burr holes is then cut with a saw or craniotome and a bone flap raised for temporary or permanent removal. A craniotomy is performed by incising the scalp and then raising scalp and bone flaps to expose an extradural abscess. If a subdural abscess is present, dural flaps are raised. Several approaches and techniques are employed depending on the location of the abscess and whether or not abscess resides in an eloquent or non-eloquent region of the brain. The eloquent brain includes the sensorimotor, language, and visual cortex; the hypothalamus and thalamus; the internal capsule, brainstem; and deep cerebellar nuclei and peduncles. If the abscess is in a non-eloquent region, the abscess wall is dissected from the surrounding brain to allow enucleation of the lesion. If the abscess is in an eloquent region, an operative microscope is used to visualize and preserve cortical vessels within the sulcus. The abscess wall is located and opened widely to create a pouch (marsupialization) and pus is aspirated. The cavity is then irrigated with saline solution. When the procedure is complete, the dural flap is placed over the exposed brain and approximated with sutures, taking care to tightly close the dura to prevent leakage of cerebrospinal fluid. The bone flap is then placed over the dura and anchored with steel sutures. Alternatively, a craniectomy defect may be plugged with bone wax or silicone. The fascia and muscle are closed and then the scalp in a layered fashion. Use code 61321 for drainage of an intracranial abscess in the infratentorial region of the brain, the region below the tentorium cerebelli that includes the cerebellum and brainstem.

Craniectomy or craniotomy, drainage of intercranial abscess

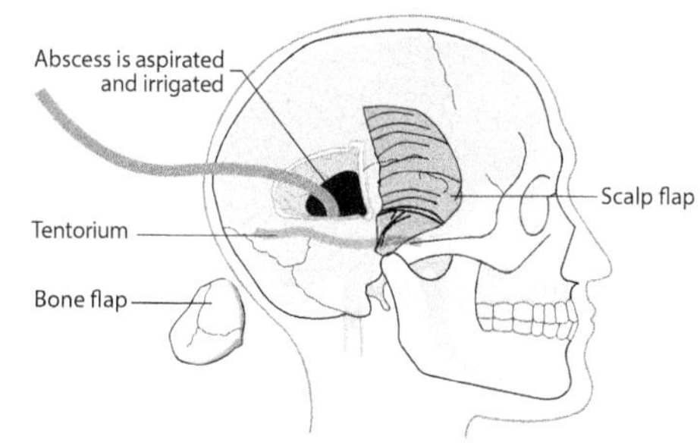

Supratentorial (61320); infratentorial (61321)

ICD-10-CM Diagnostic Codes

	Code	Description
	A06.6	Amebic brain abscess
	A17.81	Tuberculoma of brain and spinal cord
	A54.82	Gonococcal brain abscess
	B43.1	Pheomycotic brain abscess
	B95.0	Streptococcus, group A, as the cause of diseases classified elsewhere
	B95.1	Streptococcus, group B, as the cause of diseases classified elsewhere
	B95.3	Streptococcus pneumoniae as the cause of diseases classified elsewhere
	B95.4	Other streptococcus as the cause of diseases classified elsewhere
	B95.5	Unspecified streptococcus as the cause of diseases classified elsewhere
	B95.61	Methicillin susceptible Staphylococcus aureus infection as the cause of diseases classified elsewhere
	B95.62	Methicillin resistant Staphylococcus aureus infection as the cause of diseases classified elsewhere
	B95.7	Other staphylococcus as the cause of diseases classified elsewhere
	B95.8	Unspecified staphylococcus as the cause of diseases classified elsewhere
	B96.3	Hemophilus influenzae [H. influenzae] as the cause of diseases classified elsewhere
	G06.0	Intracranial abscess and granuloma
	G07	Intracranial and intraspinal abscess and granuloma in diseases classified elsewhere
	G09	Sequelae of inflammatory diseases of central nervous system
	S01.84XS	Puncture wound with foreign body of other part of head, sequela
	S02.0XXS	Fracture of vault of skull, sequela
⇄	S02.101S	Fracture of base of skull, right side, sequela
⇄	S02.102S	Fracture of base of skull, left side, sequela
⇄	S02.11AS	Type I occipital condyle fracture, right side, sequela
⇄	S02.11BS	Type I occipital condyle fracture, left side, sequela
⇄	S02.11CS	Type II occipital condyle fracture, right side, sequela
⇄	S02.11DS	Type II occipital condyle fracture, left side, sequela
⇄	S02.11ES	Type III occipital condyle fracture, right side, sequela
⇄	S02.11FS	Type III occipital condyle fracture, left side, sequela
⇄	S02.11GS	Other fracture of occiput, right side, sequela
	S02.19XS	Other fracture of base of skull, sequela
	S02.2XXS	Fracture of nasal bones, sequela
⇄	S02.31XS	Fracture of orbital floor, right side, sequela
⇄	S02.32XS	Fracture of orbital floor, left side, sequela

CCI Edits

Refer to Appendix A for CCI edits.

Pub 100

61320: Pub 100-04, 12, 20.4.5

61321: Pub 100-04, 12, 20.4.5

Facility RVUs ▢

Code	Work	PE Facility	MP	Total Facility
61320	27.42	17.43	10.00	54.85
61321	30.53	19.60	11.31	61.44

Non-facility RVUs ▢

Code	Work	PE Non-Facility	MP	Total Non-Facility
61320	27.42	17.43	10.00	54.85
61321	30.53	19.60	11.31	61.44

Modifiers (PAR) ▢

Code	Mod 50	Mod 51	Mod 62	Mod 66	Mod 80
61320	0	2	1	0	2
61321	0	2	1	0	2

Global Period

Code	Days
61320	090
61321	090

61322-61323

61322 Craniectomy or craniotomy, decompressive, with or without duraplasty, for treatment of intracranial hypertension, without evacuation of associated intraparenchymal hematoma; without lobectomy

(Do not report 61313 in addition to 61322)

(For subtemporal decompression, use 61340)

61323 Craniectomy or craniotomy, decompressive, with or without duraplasty, for treatment of intracranial hypertension, without evacuation of associated intraparenchymal hematoma; with lobectomy

(Do not report 61313 in addition to 61323)

(For subtemporal decompression, use 61340)

AMA Coding Notes

Surgical Procedures on the Skull, Meninges, and Brain

(For injection procedure for cerebral angiography, see 36100-36218)

(For injection procedure for ventriculography, see 61026, 61120)

(For injection procedure for pneumoencephalography, use 61055)

AMA *CPT Assistant* ◻

61322: Aug 18: 11

Plain English Description

A decompressive craniectomy or craniotomy is performed with or without duraplasty to treat intracranial hypertension without evacuation of intraparenchymal hematoma and without lobectomy. A craniectomy is performed by creating scalp flaps, followed by several burr holes. The bone between the burr holes is then cut with a saw or craniotome and a bone flap raised for temporary or permanent removal. A craniotomy is performed by incising the scalp and then raising scalp and bone flaps. The dura is opened. A duraplasty may be performed using an autologous galeal flap graft, a cultured dermal graft, or a synthetic patch graft to enlarge the dura allowing decompression of the brain. The dura and/or dural graft is tightly sutured to prevent leakage of cerebrospinal fluid. A drain is placed. The bone flap is then placed over the dura and anchored with steel sutures. Alternatively, the bone flap may be excised and stored in an abdominal pocket or bone bank until cerebral swelling has resolved. In 61323, the procedure is performed with a lobectomy. The procedure is performed as described above, and then swollen brain tissue is removed to control intracranial pressure.

Craniectomy or craniotomy, decompressive, for treatment of intracranial hypertension

Cultured dermal graft for duraplasty

Brain

Cranium

Bone flap

Without lobectomy (61322); with lobectomy (61323)

ICD-10-CM Diagnostic Codes

	Code	Description
	C71.0	Malignant neoplasm of cerebrum, except lobes and ventricles
	C71.1	Malignant neoplasm of frontal lobe
	C71.2	Malignant neoplasm of temporal lobe
	C71.3	Malignant neoplasm of parietal lobe
	C71.4	Malignant neoplasm of occipital lobe
	C71.5	Malignant neoplasm of cerebral ventricle
	C71.6	Malignant neoplasm of cerebellum
	C71.8	Malignant neoplasm of overlapping sites of brain
	C79.31	Secondary malignant neoplasm of brain
	G91.1	Obstructive hydrocephalus
	G91.3	Post-traumatic hydrocephalus, unspecified
	G91.4	Hydrocephalus in diseases classified elsewhere
	G91.8	Other hydrocephalus
	G92	Toxic encephalopathy
	G93.41	Metabolic encephalopathy
	G93.49	Other encephalopathy
	G93.6	Cerebral edema
	G93.7	Reye's syndrome
	G97.51	Postprocedural hemorrhage of a nervous system organ or structure following a nervous system procedure
	G97.52	Postprocedural hemorrhage of a nervous system organ or structure following other procedure
	H47.11	Papilledema associated with increased intracranial pressure
	I61.0	Nontraumatic intracerebral hemorrhage in hemisphere, subcortical
	I61.1	Nontraumatic intracerebral hemorrhage in hemisphere, cortical
	I61.2	Nontraumatic intracerebral hemorrhage in hemisphere, unspecified
	I61.3	Nontraumatic intracerebral hemorrhage in brain stem
	I61.4	Nontraumatic intracerebral hemorrhage in cerebellum
	I61.5	Nontraumatic intracerebral hemorrhage, intraventricular
	I61.6	Nontraumatic intracerebral hemorrhage, multiple localized
	I61.8	Other nontraumatic intracerebral hemorrhage
	I61.9	Nontraumatic intracerebral hemorrhage, unspecified
	I67.4	Hypertensive encephalopathy
⑦	S06.1X0	Traumatic cerebral edema without loss of consciousness
⑦	S06.1X1	Traumatic cerebral edema with loss of consciousness of 30 minutes or less
⑦	S06.1X2	Traumatic cerebral edema with loss of consciousness of 31 minutes to 59 minutes
⑦	S06.1X3	Traumatic cerebral edema with loss of consciousness of 1 hour to 5 hours 59 minutes
⑦	S06.1X4	Traumatic cerebral edema with loss of consciousness of 6 hours to 24 hours
⑦	S06.1X5	Traumatic cerebral edema with loss of consciousness greater than 24 hours with return to pre-existing conscious level
⑦	S06.1X6	Traumatic cerebral edema with loss of consciousness greater than 24 hours without return to pre-existing conscious level with patient surviving
⑦	S06.1X9	Traumatic cerebral edema with loss of consciousness of unspecified duration
⑦	S06.2X0	Diffuse traumatic brain injury without loss of consciousness
⑦	S06.2X1	Diffuse traumatic brain injury with loss of consciousness of 30 minutes or less
⑦	S06.2X2	Diffuse traumatic brain injury with loss of consciousness of 31 minutes to 59 minutes
⑦	S06.2X3	Diffuse traumatic brain injury with loss of consciousness of 1 hour to 5 hours 59 minutes
⑦	S06.2X4	Diffuse traumatic brain injury with loss of consciousness of 6 hours to 24 hours
⑦	S06.2X5	Diffuse traumatic brain injury with loss of consciousness greater than 24 hours with return to pre-existing conscious levels
⑦	S06.2X9	Diffuse traumatic brain injury with loss of consciousness of unspecified duration
⑦⇄	S06.310	Contusion and laceration of right cerebrum without loss of consciousness
⑦⇄	S06.311	Contusion and laceration of right cerebrum with loss of consciousness of 30 minutes or less
⑦⇄	S06.312	Contusion and laceration of right cerebrum with loss of consciousness of 31 minutes to 59 minutes

⑦⇄ S06.313 Contusion and laceration of right cerebrum with loss of consciousness of 1 hour to 5 hours 59 minutes
⑦⇄ S06.314 Contusion and laceration of right cerebrum with loss of consciousness of 6 hours to 24 hours
⑦⇄ S06.315 Contusion and laceration of right cerebrum with loss of consciousness greater than 24 hours with return to pre-existing conscious level
⑦⇄ S06.319 Contusion and laceration of right cerebrum with loss of consciousness of unspecified duration
⑦⇄ S06.320 Contusion and laceration of left cerebrum without loss of consciousness
⑦⇄ S06.321 Contusion and laceration of left cerebrum with loss of consciousness of 30 minutes or less
⑦⇄ S06.322 Contusion and laceration of left cerebrum with loss of consciousness of 31 minutes to 59 minutes
⑦⇄ S06.323 Contusion and laceration of left cerebrum with loss of consciousness of 1 hour to 5 hours 59 minutes
⑦⇄ S06.324 Contusion and laceration of left cerebrum with loss of consciousness of 6 hours to 24 hours
⑦⇄ S06.325 Contusion and laceration of left cerebrum with loss of consciousness greater than 24 hours with return to pre-existing conscious level
⑦⇄ S06.329 Contusion and laceration of left cerebrum with loss of consciousness of unspecified duration
⑦⇄ S06.340 Traumatic hemorrhage of right cerebrum without loss of consciousness
⑦⇄ S06.342 Traumatic hemorrhage of right cerebrum with loss of consciousness of 31 minutes to 59 minutes
⑦⇄ S06.343 Traumatic hemorrhage of right cerebrum with loss of consciousness of 1 hours to 5 hours 59 minutes
⑦⇄ S06.344 Traumatic hemorrhage of right cerebrum with loss of consciousness of 6 hours to 24 hours
⑦⇄ S06.345 Traumatic hemorrhage of right cerebrum with loss of consciousness greater than 24 hours with return to pre-existing conscious level
⑦⇄ S06.349 Traumatic hemorrhage of right cerebrum with loss of consciousness of unspecified duration
⑦⇄ S06.350 Traumatic hemorrhage of left cerebrum without loss of consciousness
⑦⇄ S06.351 Traumatic hemorrhage of left cerebrum with loss of consciousness of 30 minutes or less
⑦⇄ S06.352 Traumatic hemorrhage of left cerebrum with loss of consciousness of 31 minutes to 59 minutes
⑦⇄ S06.353 Traumatic hemorrhage of left cerebrum with loss of consciousness of 1 hours to 5 hours 59 minutes
⑦⇄ S06.354 Traumatic hemorrhage of left cerebrum with loss of consciousness of 6 hours to 24 hours
⑦⇄ S06.355 Traumatic hemorrhage of left cerebrum with loss of consciousness greater than 24 hours with return to pre-existing conscious level
⑦⇄ S06.359 Traumatic hemorrhage of left cerebrum with loss of consciousness of unspecified duration

ICD-10-CM Coding Notes

For codes requiring a 7th character extension, refer to your ICD-10-CM book. Review the character descriptions and coding guidelines for proper selection. For some procedures, only certain characters will apply.

CCI Edits

Refer to Appendix A for CCI edits.

Pub 100

61322: Pub 100-04, 12, 20.4.5
61323: Pub 100-04, 12, 20.4.5

Facility RVUs

Code	Work	PE Facility	MP	Total Facility
61322	34.26	21.83	12.63	68.72
61323	35.06	21.15	13.04	69.25

Non-facility RVUs

Code	Work	PE Non-Facility	MP	Total Non-Facility
61322	34.26	21.83	12.63	68.72
61323	35.06	21.15	13.04	69.25

Modifiers (PAR)

Code	Mod 50	Mod 51	Mod 62	Mod 66	Mod 80
61322	0	2	1	0	2
61323	0	2	1	0	2

Global Period

Code	Days
61322	090
61323	090

61343

61343 Craniectomy, suboccipital with cervical laminectomy for decompression of medulla and spinal cord, with or without dural graft (eg, Arnold-Chiari malformation)

AMA Coding Notes

Surgical Procedures on the Skull, Meninges, and Brain

(For injection procedure for cerebral angiography, see 36100-36218)

(For injection procedure for ventriculography, see 61026, 61120)

(For injection procedure for pneumoencephalography, use 61055)

Plain English Description

This procedure is performed to decompress the medulla and spinal cord when compression is caused by bony defects in the suboccipital region of the skull and the C1-C2 region of the spine. This condition is referred to as an Arnold-Chiari malformation. The bony defects put pressure on the medulla oblongata, which is the most inferior aspect of the brain stem and also forms the upper portion of the spinal cord. Pressure on the medulla can cause dizziness, muscle weakness, numbness, vision problems, headache, and problems with balance and coordination. The head is fixed in a neutral position using tongs or a Mayfield head holder. A midline incision is made over the lower aspect of the skull, and the occiput and C1 and C2 vertebrae are exposed. A pericranial graft is harvested as needed. Laminectomy retractors are placed at the superior and inferior wound margins. At C1 and C2, the spinous processes are removed with a cutting rongeur and the laminae with a punch rongeur. The ligamentum flavum is incised as needed. Burr holes are created in the suboccipital region and a saw is then used to connect the burr holes and create a bone flap that extends to the posterior margin of the foramen magnum. The posterior margin of the foramen magnum is removed using a high-speed drill. The bone flap is elevated. Decompression of the medulla and spinal cord may require opening the dura. The dura is then enlarged using the previously harvested pericranial graft. Alternatively, a cultured dermal graft or synthetic patch graft may be used to enlarge the dura. The dura and dural graft are tightly sutured to prevent cerebrospinal fluid leakage. A drain may be placed. The bone flap is then replaced and anchored with steel sutures.

Craniectomy, suboccipital with cervical laminectomy; decompression of medulla and spinal cord

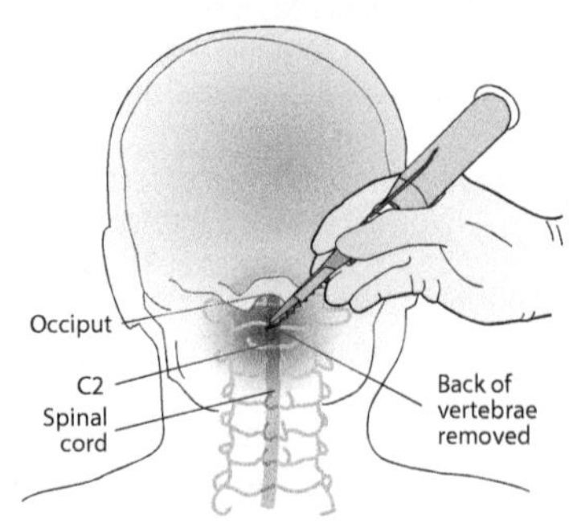

ICD-10-CM Diagnostic Codes

G93.5	Compression of brain
G95.0	Syringomyelia and syringobulbia
Q01.2	Occipital encephalocele
Q01.8	Encephalocele of other sites
Q04.8	Other specified congenital malformations of brain
Q07.00	Arnold-Chiari syndrome without spina bifida or hydrocephalus
Q07.01	Arnold-Chiari syndrome with spina bifida
Q07.02	Arnold-Chiari syndrome with hydrocephalus
Q07.03	Arnold-Chiari syndrome with spina bifida and hydrocephalus

CCI Edits

Refer to Appendix A for CCI edits.

Pub 100

61343: Pub 100-04, 12, 20.4.5

Facility RVUs ▯

Code	Work	PE Facility	MP	Total Facility
61343	31.86	19.99	11.58	63.43

Non-facility RVUs ▯

Code	Work	PE Non-Facility	MP	Total Non-Facility
61343	31.86	19.99	11.58	63.43

Modifiers (PAR) ▯

Code	Mod 50	Mod 51	Mod 62	Mod 66	Mod 80
61343	0	2	1	0	2

Global Period

Code	Days
61343	090

61345

61345 Other cranial decompression, posterior fossa

(For orbital decompression by lateral wall approach, Kroenlein type, use 67445)

AMA Coding Notes

Surgical Procedures on the Skull, Meninges, and Brain

(For injection procedure for cerebral angiography, see 36100-36218)

(For injection procedure for ventriculography, see 61026, 61120)

(For injection procedure for pneumoencephalography, use 61055)

Plain English Description

A posterior fossa cranial decompression is often done in symptomatic cases of Arnold-Chiari malformation with tonsillar herniation causing headache, hydrocephalus, or syringomyelia. The cerebellum is located low down in the back of the head near the brainstem and has two small areas at the bottom called the cerebellar tonsils. Normally, these structures sit entirely within the skull. In Arnold-Chiari malformation, the cerebellar tonsils, sometimes with the brainstem, herniate through the foramen magnum, down into the spinal canal. Posterior fossa decompression removes the bone at the back of the skull to relieve pressure on the brain and spinal cord, make more room for the herniated cerebellum, and restore normal CSF flow. After the patient is prepped with the head in a skull-fixation device, an incision is made approximately 3 inches down the midline at the base of the head to the upper neck. The muscles attached to the back of the skull and upper vertebrae are elevated and lifted back. A small section of skull at the back of the head is removed to relieve compression of the cerebellar tonsils and expose the dura. Sometimes, bony removal alone restores normal CSF flow and relieves compression. The surgeon may open the dura to observe the tonsils. Electrocautery may be used to shrink the herniated tonsils and unblock CSF flow. If duraplasty is required to expand the opening and space around the tonsils, a patch of synthetic material or a piece of the patient's own pericranium is used and sutured into place in a watertight fashion. Dural sealant is used around the suture line to prevent leakage of CSF. The neck muscles and skin are replaced and sutured together.

Other cranial decompression, posterior fossa

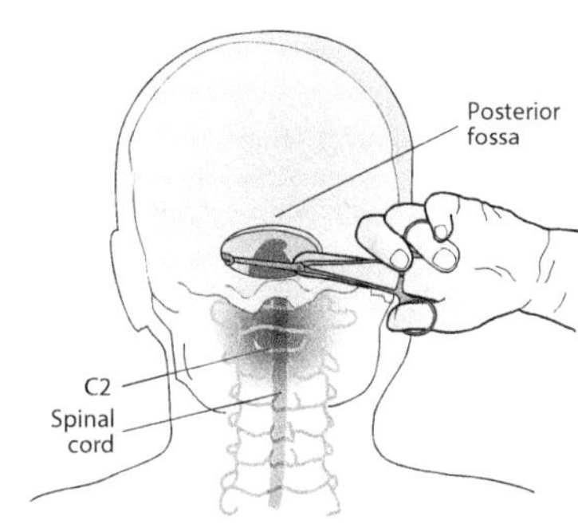

ICD-10-CM Diagnostic Codes

G93.5	Compression of brain
G95.0	Syringomyelia and syringobulbia
Q01.2	Occipital encephalocele
Q01.8	Encephalocele of other sites
Q04.8	Other specified congenital malformations of brain
Q07.00	Arnold-Chiari syndrome without spina bifida or hydrocephalus
Q07.01	Arnold-Chiari syndrome with spina bifida
Q07.02	Arnold-Chiari syndrome with hydrocephalus
Q07.03	Arnold-Chiari syndrome with spina bifida and hydrocephalus

CCI Edits

Refer to Appendix A for CCI edits.

Pub 100

61345: Pub 100-04, 12, 20.4.5

Facility RVUs

Code	Work	PE Facility	MP	Total Facility
61345	29.23	18.91	10.81	58.95

Non-facility RVUs

Code	Work	PE Non-Facility	MP	Total Non-Facility
61345	29.23	18.91	10.81	58.95

Modifiers (PAR)

Code	Mod 50	Mod 51	Mod 62	Mod 66	Mod 80
61345	0	2	1	0	2

Global Period

Code	Days
61345	090

CPT® Procedural Coding

61450

61450 Craniectomy, subtemporal, for section, compression, or decompression of sensory root of gasserian ganglion

AMA Coding Notes

Surgical Procedures on the Skull, Meninges, and Brain

(For injection procedure for cerebral angiography, see 36100-36218)

(For injection procedure for ventriculography, see 61026, 61120)

(For injection procedure for pneumoencephalography, use 61055)

Plain English Description

The Gasserian ganglion is a sensory ganglion of the trigeminal nerve (cranial nerve V) (CN V), and is more commonly referred to as the trigeminal ganglion. It is located in a cavity in the dura mater called Meckel's cave near the apex of the petrous portion of the temporal bone. Section, compression, or decompression is performed to treat pain symptoms caused by compression of the Gasserian ganglion. A small curvilinear incision is made behind the ear. The temporal muscle is divided and muscle fibers are separated from the bone to expose the temporal fossa. A small piece of the temporal bone is excised to allow access to the sensory root of the Gasserian ganglion. Nerve fibers may be divided, a balloon used to temporarily compress the nerve root freeing it from surrounding structures, or the vascular structures compressing the trigeminal nerve may be dissected away from the nerve. That latter procedure, also referred to as microvascular decompression, is the most common procedure. Blood vessels are dissected away from the nerve and a Teflon pad placed between the nerve and blood vessels. The excised portion of temporal bone is replaced and secured with wire sutures. Overlying tissues are closed in layers.

ICD-10-CM Diagnostic Codes

B02.22	Postherpetic trigeminal neuralgia
G44.001	Cluster headache syndrome, unspecified, intractable
G44.021	Chronic cluster headache, intractable
G44.041	Chronic paroxysmal hemicrania, intractable
G44.091	Other trigeminal autonomic cephalgias (TAC), intractable
G44.51	Hemicrania continua
G50.0	Trigeminal neuralgia
G50.8	Other disorders of trigeminal nerve

CCI Edits

Refer to Appendix A for CCI edits.

Pub 100

61450: Pub 100-04, 12, 20.4.5

Facility RVUs

Code	Work	PE Facility	MP	Total Facility
61450	27.69	17.55	10.24	55.48

Non-facility RVUs

Code	Work	PE Non-Facility	MP	Total Non-Facility
61450	27.69	17.55	10.24	55.48

Modifiers (PAR)

Code	Mod 50	Mod 51	Mod 62	Mod 66	Mod 80
61450	0	2	1	0	2

Global Period

Code	Days
61450	090

61458-61460

61458 Craniectomy, suboccipital; for exploration or decompression of cranial nerves

61460 Craniectomy, suboccipital; for section of 1 or more cranial nerves

AMA Coding Notes

Surgical Procedures on the Skull, Meninges, and Brain

(For injection procedure for cerebral angiography, see 36100-36218)

(For injection procedure for ventriculography, see 61026, 61120)

(For injection procedure for pneumoencephalography, use 61055)

Plain English Description

Cranial nerves become compressed when blood vessels cross the nerves, putting pressure on them. This compression can cause a variety of symptoms depending on which nerves are affected, including vertigo (dizziness) when the vestibular nerve is compressed or tinnitus (ringing or other noise in the ears) when the cochlear nerve is compressed. The patient is placed supine and the head fixed in a Mayfield clamp. The head is rotated to the side and flexed to allow access to the surgical site. A curvilinear skin incision is made behind the ear, taking care to avoid the greater and lesser occipital nerves. A small section of bone is removed using a cutting bur. The dura is incised, the posterior fossa decompressed, and the cerebellopontine angle exposed. In 61458, cranial nerves are explored and/or decompressed with the aid of an operating microscope. Microvascular decompression is accomplished by placing small synthetic sponges between the compressing blood vessels and the affected cranial nerves. In 61460, one or more cranial nerves are sectioned (cut). Cranial nerve section is performed to treat conditions such as severe vertigo caused by Meniere's disease or vestibular neuritis. Following completion of the cranial nerve decompression or cranial nerve section, the dura is reapproximated and exposed mastoid air cells sealed with bone wax. Gelfoam is placed over the dura followed by Gelfilm and muscle, fascia, and skin are closed in layers.

ICD-10-CM Diagnostic Codes

There are too many ICD-10-CM codes to list. Refer to ICD-10-CM code book for associated diagnostic codes.

CCI Edits

Refer to Appendix A for CCI edits.

Pub 100

61458: Pub 100-04, 12, 20.4.5

61460: Pub 100-04, 12, 20.4.5

Facility RVUs ▯

Code	Work	PE Facility	MP	Total Facility
61458	28.84	18.66	10.58	58.08
61460	30.24	19.38	11.21	60.83

Non-facility RVUs ▯

Code	Work	PE Non-Facility	MP	Total Non-Facility
61458	28.84	18.66	10.58	58.08
61460	30.24	19.38	11.21	60.83

Modifiers (PAR) ▯

Code	Mod 50	Mod 51	Mod 62	Mod 66	Mod 80
61458	0	2	1	0	2
61460	0	2	2	0	2

Global Period

Code	Days
61458	090
61460	090

61500

61500 Craniectomy; with excision of tumor or other bone lesion of skull

AMA Coding Notes

Surgical Procedures on the Skull, Meninges, and Brain

(For injection procedure for cerebral angiography, see 36100-36218)

(For injection procedure for ventriculography, see 61026, 61120)

(For injection procedure for pneumoencephalography, use 61055)

AMA *CPT Assistant*

61500: Jan 14: 9

Plain English Description

Skull tumors or lesions may originate in the bone, cartilage, blood or blood vessels, or other connective tissue, neuroepithelial cells, squamous cells, or they may be metastatic in nature. Incision is made in the skin and carried down through the soft tissue overlying the site of the tumor or bone lesion in the skull. The periosteum is incised and elevated. The tumor or lesion and a margin of healthy tissue is excised. If the periosteum is healthy, it is closed over the defect. If the periosteum is not healthy and must be excised, the defect may be plugged with bone wax or silicone. The fascia and muscle are closed over the defect and the scalp is closed in a layered fashion.

ICD-10-CM Diagnostic Codes

	Code	Description
	B90.2	Sequelae of tuberculosis of bones and joints
	B94.8	Sequelae of other specified infectious and parasitic diseases
	C41.0	Malignant neoplasm of bones of skull and face
	C79.51	Secondary malignant neoplasm of bone
	D16.4	Benign neoplasm of bones of skull and face
	D48.0	Neoplasm of uncertain behavior of bone and articular cartilage
	M89.78	Major osseous defect, other site
	S02.0XXS	Fracture of vault of skull, sequela
⇄	S02.11AS	Type I occipital condyle fracture, right side, sequela
⇄	S02.11BS	Type I occipital condyle fracture, left side, sequela
⇄	S02.11CS	Type II occipital condyle fracture, right side, sequela
⇄	S02.11DS	Type II occipital condyle fracture, left side, sequela
⇄	S02.11ES	Type III occipital condyle fracture, right side, sequela
⇄	S02.11FS	Type III occipital condyle fracture, left side, sequela
⇄	S02.11GS	Other fracture of occiput, right side, sequela
⇄	S02.11HS	Other fracture of occiput, left side, sequela
	S02.19XS	Other fracture of base of skull, sequela

CCI Edits

Refer to Appendix A for CCI edits.

Pub 100

61500: Pub 100-04, 12, 20.4.5

Facility RVUs

Code	Work	PE Facility	MP	Total Facility
61500	19.18	13.22	5.49	37.89

Non-facility RVUs

Code	Work	PE Non-Facility	MP	Total Non-Facility
61500	19.18	13.22	5.49	37.89

Modifiers (PAR)

Code	Mod 50	Mod 51	Mod 62	Mod 66	Mod 80
61500	0	2	1	0	2

Global Period

Code	Days
61500	090

61501

61501 Craniectomy; for osteomyelitis

AMA Coding Notes

Surgical Procedures on the Skull, Meninges, and Brain

(For injection procedure for cerebral angiography, see 36100-36218)

(For injection procedure for ventriculography, see 61026, 61120)

(For injection procedure for pneumoencephalography, use 61055)

AMA *CPT Assistant*

61501: Jan 14: 9

Plain English Description

A craniectomy is performed for osteomyelitis of the skull. This procedure may also be referred to as a sequestrectomy of the skull. A sequestrum is a piece of necrotic bone that has become separated from healthy surrounding bone. An incision is made in the skin and carried down through the soft tissue overlying the site of the osteomyelitis. If the periosteum is soft and viable, it is elevated off the necrotic sequestrum. The necrotic bone is excised and the ribbon of elevated periosteum is then approximated over the cortical bone defect. If the periosteum is not viable and an involucrum has formed around the sequestrum, the necrotic bone is removed leaving the involucrum, which will form new bone in the cortical bone defect. The incisions in the soft tissue and skin are closed and a dressing is applied.

ICD-10-CM Diagnostic Codes

A02.24	Salmonella osteomyelitis
A54.43	Gonococcal osteomyelitis
B67.2	Echinococcus granulosus infection of bone
M85.38	Osteitis condensans, other site
M86.08	Acute hematogenous osteomyelitis, other sites
M86.18	Other acute osteomyelitis, other site
M86.28	Subacute osteomyelitis, other site
M86.38	Chronic multifocal osteomyelitis, other site
M86.48	Chronic osteomyelitis with draining sinus, other site
M86.58	Other chronic hematogenous osteomyelitis, other site
M86.68	Other chronic osteomyelitis, other site
M86.8X8	Other osteomyelitis, other site
M87.08	Idiopathic aseptic necrosis of bone, other site
M87.28	Osteonecrosis due to previous trauma, other site
M87.38	Other secondary osteonecrosis, other site
M87.88	Other osteonecrosis, other site
M89.78	Major osseous defect, other site

CCI Edits

Refer to Appendix A for CCI edits.

Pub 100

61501: Pub 100-04, 12, 20.4.5

Facility RVUs

Code	Work	PE Facility	MP	Total Facility
61501	16.35	12.08	4.46	32.89

Non-facility RVUs

Code	Work	PE Non-Facility	MP	Total Non-Facility
61501	16.35	12.08	4.46	32.89

Modifiers (PAR)

Code	Mod 50	Mod 51	Mod 62	Mod 66	Mod 80
61501	0	2	1	0	2

Global Period

Code	Days
61501	090

61510-61512

61510 Craniectomy, trephination, bone flap craniotomy; for excision of brain tumor, supratentorial, except meningioma

61512 Craniectomy, trephination, bone flap craniotomy; for excision of meningioma, supratentorial

AMA Coding Notes

Surgical Procedures on the Skull, Meninges, and Brain

(For injection procedure for cerebral angiography, see 36100-36218)

(For injection procedure for ventriculography, see 61026, 61120)

(For injection procedure for pneumoencephalography, use 61055)

Plain English Description

The supratentorial region is the part of the brain that lies above the tentorium cerebelli, a fold in the dura mater that separates the frontal and occipital lobes of the cerebrum from the cerebellum. A craniectomy is performed by creating scalp flaps, followed by burr holes. The bone between the burr holes is then cut with a saw or craniotome and a bone flap elevated and removed either temporarily or permanently. Trephination involves removing a circular button of the skull. Craniotomy involves creating scalp and bone flaps, which are then elevated to expose the region of the brain with the tumor. In 61510, a brain tumor or lesion other than a meningioma is excised. The dura is incised and a dural flap is created. An operative microscope is used to visualize and preserve cortical blood vessels and other critical structures. The brain tumor is located and carefully dissected from the surrounding brain tissue. The physician attempts to resect the tumor in its entirety. If critical structures are involved, as much of the tumor as can safely be removed is excised. The dura is repaired. Bone flaps are placed over the dura and secured with steel sutures. Alternatively, the skull defect may be plugged with bone wax or silicone. The scalp flap is reapproximated and the skin incision closed. In 61512, a meningioma is excised. A meningioma is a tumor of the meninges, which are the membranes that cover the brain and spinal cord. Meningiomas are usually slow-growing benign tumors. Malignant meningiomas do occur although they are quite rare. The meningioma is exposed. The arterial feeders to the meningioma are identified and coagulated. The meningioma is completely resected including any involved dura and any involved or hyperostotic bone. The dura is then repaired using an autograft of pericranium or fascia lata. Alternatively, a synthetic dural substitute may be used. The skull defect, scalp flap, and skin are repaired as described above.

ICD-10-CM Diagnostic Codes

C70.0	Malignant neoplasm of cerebral meninges
C71.0	Malignant neoplasm of cerebrum, except lobes and ventricles
C71.1	Malignant neoplasm of frontal lobe
C71.2	Malignant neoplasm of temporal lobe
C71.3	Malignant neoplasm of parietal lobe
C71.4	Malignant neoplasm of occipital lobe
C71.5	Malignant neoplasm of cerebral ventricle
C71.8	Malignant neoplasm of overlapping sites of brain
C79.31	Secondary malignant neoplasm of brain
C79.32	Secondary malignant neoplasm of cerebral meninges
D32.0	Benign neoplasm of cerebral meninges
D33.0	Benign neoplasm of brain, supratentorial
D42.0	Neoplasm of uncertain behavior of cerebral meninges
D43.0	Neoplasm of uncertain behavior of brain, supratentorial
D49.6	Neoplasm of unspecified behavior of brain
D49.7	Neoplasm of unspecified behavior of endocrine glands and other parts of nervous system

CCI Edits

Refer to Appendix A for CCI edits.

Pub 100

61510: Pub 100-04, 12, 20.4.5

61512: Pub 100-04, 12, 20.4.5

Facility RVUs ▯

Code	Work	PE Facility	MP	Total Facility
61510	30.83	21.15	11.38	63.36
61512	37.14	22.95	13.73	73.82

Non-facility RVUs ▯

Code	Work	PE Non-Facility	MP	Total Non-Facility
61510	30.83	21.15	11.38	63.36
61512	37.14	22.95	13.73	73.82

Modifiers (PAR) ▯

Code	Mod 50	Mod 51	Mod 62	Mod 66	Mod 80
61510	0	2	1	0	2
61512	0	2	1	0	2

Global Period

Code	Days
61510	090
61512	090

61514-61516

61514 Craniectomy, trephination, bone flap craniotomy; for excision of brain abscess, supratentorial

61516 Craniectomy, trephination, bone flap craniotomy; for excision or fenestration of cyst, supratentorial

(For excision of pituitary tumor or craniopharyngioma, see 61545, 61546, 61548)

AMA Coding Notes

Surgical Procedures on the Skull, Meninges, and Brain

(For injection procedure for cerebral angiography, see 36100-36218)

(For injection procedure for ventriculography, see 61026, 61120)

(For injection procedure for pneumoencephalography, use 61055)

Plain English Description

The supratentorial region is the part of the brain that lies above the tentorium cerebelli, a fold in the dura mater that separates the frontal and occipital lobes of the cerebrum from the cerebellum. A craniectomy is performed by creating scalp flaps, followed by burr holes. The bone between the burr holes is then cut with a saw or craniotome and a bone flap elevated and removed either temporarily or permanently. Trephination involves removing a circular button of the skull. Craniotomy involves creating scalp and bone flaps, which are then elevated to expose the region of the brain with the brain abscess or cyst. In 61514, a brain abscess is excised. The abscess wall is dissected from surrounding brain tissue and the entire abscess pocket removed without rupturing the abscess wall. In 61516, a cyst is excised or fenestrated. If the cyst is excised, it is carefully dissected from surrounding brain tissue and removed in its entirety without rupturing the cyst wall. If it is fenestrated, the cyst is incised and an opening created so that the cyst can drain into the cerebrospinal fluid pathway. The dura is repaired. Bone flaps are placed over the dura and secured with steel sutures. Alternatively. the skull defect may be plugged with bone wax or silicone. The scalp flap is reapproximated and the skin incision closed.

ICD-10-CM Diagnostic Codes

	Code	Description
	A06.6	Amebic brain abscess
	A17.81	Tuberculoma of brain and spinal cord
	A54.82	Gonococcal brain abscess
	B43.1	Pheomycotic brain abscess
	B94.8	Sequelae of other specified infectious and parasitic diseases
	B95.0	Streptococcus, group A, as the cause of diseases classified elsewhere
	B95.1	Streptococcus, group B, as the cause of diseases classified elsewhere
	B95.2	Enterococcus as the cause of diseases classified elsewhere
	B95.3	Streptococcus pneumoniae as the cause of diseases classified elsewhere
	B95.4	Other streptococcus as the cause of diseases classified elsewhere
	B95.5	Unspecified streptococcus as the cause of diseases classified elsewhere
	B95.61	Methicillin susceptible Staphylococcus aureus infection as the cause of diseases classified elsewhere
	B95.62	Methicillin resistant Staphylococcus aureus infection as the cause of diseases classified elsewhere
	B95.7	Other staphylococcus as the cause of diseases classified elsewhere
	B95.8	Unspecified staphylococcus as the cause of diseases classified elsewhere
	B96.3	Hemophilus influenzae [H. influenzae] as the cause of diseases classified elsewhere
	G06.0	Intracranial abscess and granuloma
	G07	Intracranial and intraspinal abscess and granuloma in diseases classified elsewhere
	G09	Sequelae of inflammatory diseases of central nervous system
	G93.0	Cerebral cysts
	Q04.6	Congenital cerebral cysts
	S01.84XS	Puncture wound with foreign body of other part of head, sequela
	S02.0XXS	Fracture of vault of skull, sequela
⇄	S02.11AS	Type I occipital condyle fracture, right side, sequela
⇄	S02.11BS	Type I occipital condyle fracture, left side, sequela
⇄	S02.11CS	Type II occipital condyle fracture, right side, sequela
⇄	S02.11DS	Type II occipital condyle fracture, left side, sequela
⇄	S02.11ES	Type III occipital condyle fracture, right side, sequela
⇄	S02.11FS	Type III occipital condyle fracture, left side, sequela
⇄	S02.11GS	Other fracture of occiput, right side, sequela
	S02.2XXS	Fracture of nasal bones, sequela
⇄	S02.31XS	Fracture of orbital floor, right side, sequela
⇄	S02.32XS	Fracture of orbital floor, left side, sequela

CCI Edits

Refer to Appendix A for CCI edits.

Pub 100

61514: Pub 100-04, 12, 20.4.5
61516: Pub 100-04, 12, 20.4.5

Facility RVUs

Code	Work	PE Facility	MP	Total Facility
61514	27.23	17.95	9.96	55.14
61516	26.58	17.68	9.78	54.04

Non-facility RVUs

Code	Work	PE Non-Facility	MP	Total Non-Facility
61514	27.23	17.95	9.96	55.14
61516	26.58	17.68	9.78	54.04

Modifiers (PAR)

Code	Mod 50	Mod 51	Mod 62	Mod 66	Mod 80
61514	0	2	1	0	2
61516	0	2	1	0	2

Global Period

Code	Days
61514	090
61516	090

61517

✚ **61517 Implantation of brain intracavitary chemotherapy agent (List separately in addition to code for primary procedure)**

(Use 61517 only in conjunction with 61510 or 61518)

(Do not report 61517 for brachytherapy insertion. For intracavitary insertion of radioelement sources or ribbons, see 77770, 77771, 77772)

AMA Coding Notes

Surgical Procedures on the Skull, Meninges, and Brain

(For injection procedure for cerebral angiography, see 36100-36218)

(For injection procedure for ventriculography, see 61026, 61120)

(For injection procedure for pneumoencephalography, use 61055)

Plain English Description

Following resection of a malignant neoplasm of the brain, an intracavity chemotherapy agent is implanted. The chemotherapy agent is removed from the packaging and handled as instructed in the manufacturer's guidelines. The chemotherapy agent is then placed in the resection cavity and secured per the manufacturer's guidelines, taking care to avoid covering the ventricles and large vascular structures. Following placement of the chemotherapy agent, the cavity may be irrigated. The dura is then tightly closed to prevent cerebrospinal fluid leakage.

ICD-10-CM Diagnostic Codes

See Primary Procedure code for crosswalks.

CCI Edits

Refer to Appendix A for CCI edits.

Pub 100

61517: Pub 100-04, 12, 20.4.5

Facility RVUs ☐

Code	Work	PE Facility	MP	Total Facility
61517	1.38	0.64	0.51	2.53

Non-facility RVUs ☐

Code	Work	PE Non-Facility	MP	Total Non-Facility
61517	1.38	0.64	0.51	2.53

Modifiers (PAR) ☐

Code	Mod 50	Mod 51	Mod 62	Mod 66	Mod 80
61517	0	0	0	0	1

Global Period

Code	Days
61517	ZZZ

61518-61519

61518 Craniectomy for excision of brain tumor, infratentorial or posterior fossa; except meningioma, cerebellopontine angle tumor, or midline tumor at base of skull

61519 Craniectomy for excision of brain tumor, infratentorial or posterior fossa; meningioma

AMA Coding Notes

Surgical Procedures on the Skull, Meninges, and Brain

(For injection procedure for cerebral angiography, see 36100-36218)

(For injection procedure for ventriculography, see 61026, 61120)

(For injection procedure for pneumoencephalography, use 61055)

Plain English Description

The infratentorial region of the brain is the region below the tentorium cerebelli and includes the cerebellum and brainstem. A craniectomy is performed by creating scalp flaps, followed by burr holes. The bone between the burr holes is then cut with a saw or craniotome and a bone flap elevated and removed either temporarily or permanently. Trephination involves removing a circular button of the skull. Craniotomy involves creating scalp and bone flaps, which are then elevated to expose the region of the brain with the brain tumor. In 61518, a brain tumor or lesion other than a meningioma, cerebellopontine angle tumor, or midline tumor at the base of the skull is excised. The dura is incised and a dural flap is created. An operative microscope is used to visualize and preserve cortical blood vessels and other critical structures. The brain tumor is located and carefully dissected from the surrounding brain tissue. The physician attempts to resect the tumor in its entirety. If critical structures are involved, as much of the tumor as can safely be removed is excised. In 61519, a meningioma is excised. A meningioma is a tumor of the meninges, the membranes that cover and protect the brain and spinal cord. Meningiomas are usually slow-growing benign tumors. Malignant meningiomas do occur although they are quite rare. The meningioma is located and exposed. The arterial feeders to the meningioma are identified and coagulated. The meningioma is completely resected, including any involved dura and any involved or hyperostotic bone. After lesion removal, the dura is repaired using an autograft of pericranium or fascia lata or a synthetic dural substitute. Care is taken to seal the dura from cerebrospinal fluid leakage. Bone flaps are placed over the dura and secured with steel sutures. Alternatively, the skull defect may be plugged with bone wax or silicone. The scalp flap is reapproximated and the skin incision is closed.

ICD-10-CM Diagnostic Codes

C70.0	Malignant neoplasm of cerebral meninges
C71.6	Malignant neoplasm of cerebellum
C71.7	Malignant neoplasm of brain stem
C71.9	Malignant neoplasm of brain, unspecified
C79.31	Secondary malignant neoplasm of brain
C79.32	Secondary malignant neoplasm of cerebral meninges
D32.0	Benign neoplasm of cerebral meninges
D33.1	Benign neoplasm of brain, infratentorial
D33.2	Benign neoplasm of brain, unspecified
D42.0	Neoplasm of uncertain behavior of cerebral meninges
D43.1	Neoplasm of uncertain behavior of brain, infratentorial
D43.2	Neoplasm of uncertain behavior of brain, unspecified
D49.6	Neoplasm of unspecified behavior of brain
D49.7	Neoplasm of unspecified behavior of endocrine glands and other parts of nervous system

CCI Edits

Refer to Appendix A for CCI edits.

Pub 100

61518: Pub 100-04, 12, 20.4.5
61519: Pub 100-04, 12, 20.4.5

Facility RVUs

Code	Work	PE Facility	MP	Total Facility
61518	39.89	25.29	14.77	79.95
61519	43.43	25.85	16.17	85.45

Non-facility RVUs

Code	Work	PE Non-Facility	MP	Total Non-Facility
61518	39.89	25.29	14.77	79.95
61519	43.43	25.85	16.17	85.45

Modifiers (PAR)

Code	Mod 50	Mod 51	Mod 62	Mod 66	Mod 80
61518	0	2	1	0	2
61519	0	2	1	0	2

Global Period

Code	Days
61518	090
61519	090

61520

61520 Craniectomy for excision of brain tumor, infratentorial or posterior fossa; cerebellopontine angle tumor

AMA Coding Notes

Surgical Procedures on the Skull, Meninges, and Brain

(For injection procedure for cerebral angiography, see 36100-36218)

(For injection procedure for ventriculography, see 61026, 61120)

(For injection procedure for pneumoencephalography, use 61055)

Plain English Description

Cerebellopontine angle tumors are the most common site of intracranial posterior fossa tumors. The cerebellopontine angle is a bilateral space that is filled with cerebrospinal fluid. The medial boundary is the brain stem, the cerebellum lies just above the space, and the temporal bone forms the lateral boundary. The floor of the cerebellopontine angle is formed by the lower cranial nerves (IX, X, XI). The most common type of cerebellopontine angel tumor is an acoustic neuroma, which may also be referred to as a vestibular schwannoma. Acoustic neuromas are slow-growing tumors of the acoustic nerve, which is located behind the ear and below the cerebellum. Other less common types of tumors in this region include other types of benign tumors and primary or metastatic malignant tumors. Using a retrosigmoid approach, an occipital craniotomy is performed. The dura is opened and the arachnoid is incised. The tumor is exposed and carefully debulked. The posterior wall of the internal auditory canal is removed so that tumor within the auditory canal can be excised. The dura is opened and the tumor debulking in the auditory canal continues until only the tumor capsule remains. Adherent portions of the tumor capsule are carefully dissected from the brain stem and from the facial nerve (cranial nerve VII). The skull defect, scalp flap, and skin are repaired as described above. Following complete removal of the tumor, the dura is closed and the craniotomy repaired.

ICD-10-CM Diagnostic Codes

C71.6	Malignant neoplasm of cerebellum
C79.31	Secondary malignant neoplasm of brain
D33.1	Benign neoplasm of brain, infratentorial
D43.1	Neoplasm of uncertain behavior of brain, infratentorial
D49.6	Neoplasm of unspecified behavior of brain

CCI Edits

Refer to Appendix A for CCI edits.

Pub 100

61520: Pub 100-04, 12, 20.4.5

Facility RVUs

Code	Work	PE Facility	MP	Total Facility
61520	57.09	32.08	19.31	108.48

Non-facility RVUs

Code	Work	PE Non-Facility	MP	Total Non-Facility
61520	57.09	32.08	19.31	108.48

Modifiers (PAR)

Code	Mod 50	Mod 51	Mod 62	Mod 66	Mod 80
61520	0	2	2	0	2

Global Period

Code	Days
61520	090

61521

61521 Craniectomy for excision of brain tumor, infratentorial or posterior fossa; midline tumor at base of skull

AMA Coding Notes

Surgical Procedures on the Skull, Meninges, and Brain

(For injection procedure for cerebral angiography, see 36100-36218)

(For injection procedure for ventriculography, see 61026, 61120)

(For injection procedure for pneumoencephalography, use 61055)

Plain English Description

The infratentorial region lies below the tentorium cerebelli and includes the cerebellum and the brainstem. The tentorium cerebelli is the second largest fold in the dura mater that provides a strong, arched, membranous covering over the cerebellum, supports the occipital lobes, and separates the two structures. A craniectomy for the infratentorial or posterior fossa region is performed by making a midline incision at the base of the skull down to the upper vertebrae, creating scalp flaps, and elevating the muscles, followed by burr holes. The bone between the burr holes is then cut with a saw or craniotome and the piece of bone is elevated and removed, either temporarily or permanently. The dura is incised and a dural flap is created. An operative microscope is used to visualize and preserve cortical blood vessels and other critical structures. The midline brain tumor at the base of the skull is located and carefully dissected from the surrounding brain tissue. The physician attempts to resect the tumor in its entirety. If critical structures are involved, as much of the tumor as can safely be removed is excised. The dura is repaired using an autograft of pericranium or fascia lata, or a synthetic dural substitute. Care is taken to seal the dura from cerebrospinal fluid leakage. Bone flaps are replaced over the dura and secured with steel sutures. Alternatively, the skull defect may be plugged with bone wax or silicone. The muscles and scalp flap are re-approximated and the skin incision is closed.

ICD-10-CM Diagnostic Codes

C71.7	Malignant neoplasm of brain stem
C71.9	Malignant neoplasm of brain, unspecified
C79.31	Secondary malignant neoplasm of brain
D33.1	Benign neoplasm of brain, infratentorial
D33.2	Benign neoplasm of brain, unspecified
D43.1	Neoplasm of uncertain behavior of brain, infratentorial
D43.2	Neoplasm of uncertain behavior of brain, unspecified
D49.6	Neoplasm of unspecified behavior of brain

CCI Edits

Refer to Appendix A for CCI edits.

Pub 100

61521: Pub 100-04, 12, 20.4.5

Facility RVUs ▯

Code	Work	PE Facility	MP	Total Facility
61521	46.99	27.54	17.72	92.25

Non-facility RVUs ▯

Code	Work	PE Non-Facility	MP	Total Non-Facility
61521	46.99	27.54	17.72	92.25

Modifiers (PAR) ▯

Code	Mod 50	Mod 51	Mod 62	Mod 66	Mod 80
61521	0	2	1	0	2

Global Period

Code	Days
61521	090

61522-61524

61522 Craniectomy, infratentorial or posterior fossa; for excision of brain abscess

61524 Craniectomy, infratentorial or posterior fossa; for excision or fenestration of cyst

AMA Coding Notes

Surgical Procedures on the Skull, Meninges, and Brain

(For injection procedure for cerebral angiography, see 36100-36218)

(For injection procedure for ventriculography, see 61026, 61120)

(For injection procedure for pneumoencephalography, use 61055)

Plain English Description

The infratentorial region of the brain is the region below the tentorium cerebelli and includes the cerebellum and brainstem. A craniectomy is performed by creating scalp flaps, followed by burr holes. The bone between the burr holes is then cut with a saw or craniotome and a bone flap elevated and removed either temporarily or permanently. Trephination involves removing a circular button of the skull. Craniotomy involves creating scalp and bone flaps, which are then elevated to expose the region of the brain with the brain abscess or cyst. In 61522, a brain abscess is excised. The abscess wall is dissected from surrounding brain tissue and the entire abscess pocket removed without rupturing the abscess wall. In 61524, a cyst is excised or fenestrated. If the cyst is excised, it is carefully dissected from surrounding brain tissue and removed in its entirety without rupturing the cyst wall. If it is fenestrated, the cyst is incised and an opening created so that the cyst can drain into the cerebrospinal fluid pathway. The dura is repaired. Bone flaps are placed over the dura and secured with steel sutures. Alternatively, the skull defect may be plugged with bone wax or silicone. The scalp flap is reapproximated and the skin incision closed.

ICD-10-CM Diagnostic Codes

	Code	Description
	A06.6	Amebic brain abscess
	A17.81	Tuberculoma of brain and spinal cord
	A54.82	Gonococcal brain abscess
	B43.1	Pheomycotic brain abscess
	B94.8	Sequelae of other specified infectious and parasitic diseases
	B95.0	Streptococcus, group A, as the cause of diseases classified elsewhere
	B95.1	Streptococcus, group B, as the cause of diseases classified elsewhere
	B95.3	Streptococcus pneumoniae as the cause of diseases classified elsewhere
	B95.4	Other streptococcus as the cause of diseases classified elsewhere
	B95.5	Unspecified streptococcus as the cause of diseases classified elsewhere
	B95.61	Methicillin susceptible Staphylococcus aureus infection as the cause of diseases classified elsewhere
	B95.62	Methicillin resistant Staphylococcus aureus infection as the cause of diseases classified elsewhere
	B95.7	Other staphylococcus as the cause of diseases classified elsewhere
	B95.8	Unspecified staphylococcus as the cause of diseases classified elsewhere
	B96.3	Hemophilus influenzae [H. influenzae] as the cause of diseases classified elsewhere
	G06.0	Intracranial abscess and granuloma
	G07	Intracranial and intraspinal abscess and granuloma in diseases classified elsewhere
	G09	Sequelae of inflammatory diseases of central nervous system
	G93.0	Cerebral cysts
	Q04.6	Congenital cerebral cysts
	S01.84XS	Puncture wound with foreign body of other part of head, sequela
⇄	S02.101S	Fracture of base of skull, right side, sequela
⇄	S02.102S	Fracture of base of skull, left side, sequela
⇄	S02.11AS	Type I occipital condyle fracture, right side, sequela
⇄	S02.11BS	Type I occipital condyle fracture, left side, sequela
⇄	S02.11CS	Type II occipital condyle fracture, right side, sequela
⇄	S02.11DS	Type II occipital condyle fracture, left side, sequela
⇄	S02.11ES	Type III occipital condyle fracture, right side, sequela
⇄	S02.11FS	Type III occipital condyle fracture, left side, sequela
⇄	S02.11GS	Other fracture of occiput, right side, sequela
	S02.19XS	Other fracture of base of skull, sequela

CCI Edits

Refer to Appendix A for CCI edits.

Pub 100

61522: Pub 100-04, 12, 20.4.5

61524: Pub 100-04, 12, 20.4.5

Facility RVUs ▯

Code	Work	PE Facility	MP	Total Facility
61522	31.54	19.98	11.69	63.21
61524	29.89	19.22	11.06	60.17

Non-facility RVUs ▯

Code	Work	PE Non-Facility	MP	Total Non-Facility
61522	31.54	19.98	11.69	63.21
61524	29.89	19.22	11.06	60.17

Modifiers (PAR) ▯

Code	Mod 50	Mod 51	Mod 62	Mod 66	Mod 80
61522	0	2	1	0	2
61524	0	2	1	0	2

Global Period

Code	Days
61522	090
61524	090

61526-61530

61526 Craniectomy, bone flap craniotomy, transtemporal (mastoid) for excision of cerebellopontine angle tumor

61530 Craniectomy, bone flap craniotomy, transtemporal (mastoid) for excision of cerebellopontine angle tumor; combined with middle/posterior fossa craniotomy/craniectomy

AMA Coding Notes

Surgical Procedures on the Skull, Meninges, and Brain

(For injection procedure for cerebral angiography, see 36100-36218)

(For injection procedure for ventriculography, see 61026, 61120)

(For injection procedure for pneumoencephalography, use 61055)

AMA *CPT Assistant* ◻

61526: Summer 91: 8, Mar 18: 11

Plain English Description

Cerebellopontine angle tumors are the most common site of intracranial posterior fossa tumors. The cerebellopontine angle is a bilateral space that is filled with cerebrospinal fluid. The medial boundary is the brain stem, the cerebellum lies just above the space, and the temporal bone forms the lateral boundary. The floor of the cerebellopontine angle is formed by the lower cranial nerves (IX, X, XI). The most common type of cerebellopontine angel tumor is an acoustic neuroma, which may also be referred to as a vestibular schwannoma. Acoustic neuromas are slow-growing tumors of the acoustic nerve, which is located behind the ear and below the cerebellum. Other less common types of tumors in this region include other types of benign tumors and primary or metastatic malignant tumors. In 61526, a transtemporal approach is used. A postauricular skin flap is developed and the temporalis muscle and mastoid periosteum exposed. The mastoid periosteum is incised and elevated off the mastoid bone. A mastoidectomy is performed. The middle and posterior fossa dura are exposed. Bone is removed and the temporal lobe dura and the sigmoid sinus exposed and retracted. The antrum, lateral semicircular canal, and vertical facial nerve are identified. The incus, is removed, the tensor tympani tendon sectioned, and the Eustachian tube packed with oxidized cellulose packing. The middle ear space is packed with temporalis muscle. A labyrinthectomy is performed. The jugular bulb is identified. The internal auditory canal is exposed and inferior and superior troughs developed so that the bone of the internal auditory canal can be removed. The facial nerve is identified. The superior vestibular nerve is followed to the ampullated end of the superior semicircular canal. The superior vestibular nerve is reflected inferiorly from the ampullated end of the superior semicircular canal. The facial nerve is located and integrity confirmed using a facial nerve stimulator. The tumor is debulked and dissected free of the facial nerve. The tumor is completely removed. The posterior fossa dura is reapproximated. Fat is packed into the surgical defect. The periosteum is closed followed by layered closure of overlying soft tissue and skin. In 61530, the transtemporal approach is combined with a middle/posterior fossa craniectomy to provide better exposure of the tumor. A skin incision is made either anterior or posterior to the external auditory meatus. The temporalis muscle is incised or reflected inferiorly. A temporal craniotomy is performed. The dura is elevated from the floor of the middle cranial fossa. The temporal lobe dura is elevated off the surface of the temporal bone. The petrosal sinus is identified and protected. Dissection continues until the lateral posterior end of the internal auditory canal is exposed. The greater superficial petrosal nerve is identified and followed retrograde to the geniculate ganglion. The geniculate ganglion is completely exposed. The labyrinthine portion of the nerve is identified and followed medially and inferiorly into the internal auditory canal. Once the medial end of the internal auditory canal is identified, overlying bone is removed until adequate exposure has been attained, including exposure of the superior vestibular nerve where it penetrates the labyrinthine bone to innervate the ampulla. The tumor is then completely removed as described above. Bone is used to fill air cells to prevent leakage of cerebrospinal fluid. Fat is packed into the internal auditory canal. The dura is repaired. The skull is replaced and secured with miniplates. The soft tissues are closed in layers.

ICD-10-CM Diagnostic Codes

C71.6	Malignant neoplasm of cerebellum
C79.31	Secondary malignant neoplasm of brain
D33.1	Benign neoplasm of brain, infratentorial
D43.1	Neoplasm of uncertain behavior of brain, infratentorial
D49.6	Neoplasm of unspecified behavior of brain

CCI Edits

Refer to Appendix A for CCI edits.

Pub 100

61526: Pub 100-04, 12, 20.4.5

61530: Pub 100-04, 12, 20.4.5

Facility RVUs ◻

Code	Work	PE Facility	MP	Total Facility
61526	54.08	28.60	14.26	96.94
61530	45.56	26.44	17.16	89.16

Non-facility RVUs ◻

Code	Work	PE Non-Facility	MP	Total Non-Facility
61526	54.08	28.60	14.26	96.94
61530	45.56	26.44	17.16	89.16

Modifiers (PAR) ◻

Code	Mod 50	Mod 51	Mod 62	Mod 66	Mod 80
61526	0	2	2	0	1
61530	0	2	2	0	1

Global Period

Code	Days
61526	090
61530	090

61531-61533

61531 Subdural implantation of strip electrodes through 1 or more burr or trephine hole(s) for long-term seizure monitoring

(For stereotactic implantation of electrodes, use 61760)

(For craniotomy for excision of intracranial arteriovenous malformation, see 61680-61692)

61533 Craniotomy with elevation of bone flap; for subdural implantation of an electrode array, for long-term seizure monitoring

(For continuous EEG monitoring, see 95700-95726)

AMA Coding Notes

Surgical Procedures on the Skull, Meninges, and Brain

(For injection procedure for cerebral angiography, see 36100-36218)

(For injection procedure for ventriculography, see 61026, 61120)

(For injection procedure for pneumoencephalography, use 61055)

AMA *CPT Assistant*

61531: Jul 19: 11

Plain English Description

Different types of electrodes are implanted subdurally for long-term seizure monitoring. In 61531, strip electrodes that consist of a single row of electrodes are placed into the subdural region through burr or trephine holes. The scalp is incised and flapped forward. A burr hole is created with a surgical drill or perforator. Alternatively, a small disc of bone may be removed using a trephine. The dura is incised. Bleeding is controlled by electrocautery. A strip electrode is inserted into the subdural region. The strip electrode is tested to ensure that it is functioning properly. The dura is closed and the skull defect is repaired by replacing the bone disc or applying bone wax. The procedure is repeated at each strip electrode implantation site. In 61533, an electrode array that contains multiple rows of electrodes on a square grid is implanted subdurally through a craniotomy. The skin is incised and scalp flaps are created followed by burr holes. The bone between the burr holes is cut with a saw or craniotome and the bone flap is elevated. The dura is opened and retracted. The electrode array is placed at the desired site in the subdural region and tested to ensure that it is functioning properly. The electrode array is secured with sutures and the dura is closed over the array. The bone flap is replaced and secured with sutures, wires, or a miniplate and screws. The overlying muscle is repaired and the galea and skin are closed in layers.

ICD-10-CM Diagnostic Codes

G40.011 Localization-related (focal) (partial) idiopathic epilepsy and epileptic syndromes with seizures of localized onset, intractable, with status epilepticus

G40.019 Localization-related (focal) (partial) idiopathic epilepsy and epileptic syndromes with seizures of localized onset, intractable, without status epilepticus

G40.111 Localization-related (focal) (partial) symptomatic epilepsy and epileptic syndromes with simple partial seizures, intractable, with status epilepticus

G40.119 Localization-related (focal) (partial) symptomatic epilepsy and epileptic syndromes with simple partial seizures, intractable, without status epilepticus

G40.211 Localization-related (focal) (partial) symptomatic epilepsy and epileptic syndromes with complex partial seizures, intractable, with status epilepticus

G40.219 Localization-related (focal) (partial) symptomatic epilepsy and epileptic syndromes with complex partial seizures, intractable, without status epilepticus

CCI Edits

Refer to Appendix A for CCI edits.

Pub 100

61531: Pub 100-04, 12, 20.4.5

61533: Pub 100-04, 12, 20.4.5, Pub 100-04, 12, 40.1

Facility RVUs

Code	Work	PE Facility	MP	Total Facility
61531	16.41	12.77	6.04	35.22
61533	21.46	14.68	7.92	44.06

Non-facility RVUs

Code	Work	PE Non-Facility	MP	Total Non-Facility
61531	16.41	12.77	6.04	35.22
61533	21.46	14.68	7.92	44.06

Modifiers (PAR)

Code	Mod 50	Mod 51	Mod 62	Mod 66	Mod 80
61531	0	2	2	0	2
61533	0	2	1	0	2

Global Period

Code	Days
61531	090
61533	090

61534

61534 Craniotomy with elevation of bone flap; for excision of epileptogenic focus without electrocorticography during surgery

AMA Coding Notes

Surgical Procedures on the Skull, Meninges, and Brain

(For injection procedure for cerebral angiography, see 36100-36218)

(For injection procedure for ventriculography, see 61026, 61120)

(For injection procedure for pneumoencephalography, use 61055)

Plain English Description

In some patients with epilepsy, a lesional or localized epileptogenic focus can be identified. The site of the lesion is located and confirmed using separately reportable electroencephalography studies and MRI as needed. If the lesion is not in an eloquent region of the brain, the lesion may be excised without the use of intraoperative electrocorticography. The skin is incised and scalp flaps created followed by burr holes. The bone between the burr holes is cut with a saw or craniotome and a bone flap elevated. The dura is opened and retracted. The region of the lesional or localized epileptogenic focus is identified and the abnormal brain tissue is excised. Following removal of all abnormal brain tissue, the dura is closed. The bone flap is replaced and secured with sutures, wires, or miniplate and screws. The overlying muscle is repaired and the galea and skin closed in layers.

ICD-10-CM Diagnostic Codes

G40.011 Localization-related (focal) (partial) idiopathic epilepsy and epileptic syndromes with seizures of localized onset, intractable, with status epilepticus

G40.019 Localization-related (focal) (partial) idiopathic epilepsy and epileptic syndromes with seizures of localized onset, intractable, without status epilepticus

G40.111 Localization-related (focal) (partial) symptomatic epilepsy and epileptic syndromes with simple partial seizures, intractable, with status epilepticus

G40.119 Localization-related (focal) (partial) symptomatic epilepsy and epileptic syndromes with simple partial seizures, intractable, without status epilepticus

G40.211 Localization-related (focal) (partial) symptomatic epilepsy and epileptic syndromes with complex partial seizures, intractable, with status epilepticus

G40.219 Localization-related (focal) (partial) symptomatic epilepsy and epileptic syndromes with complex partial seizures, intractable, without status epilepticus

CCI Edits

Refer to Appendix A for CCI edits.

Pub 100

61534: Pub 100-04, 12, 20.4.5, Pub 100-04, 12, 40.1

Facility RVUs ☐

Code	Work	PE Facility	MP	Total Facility
61534	23.01	16.05	8.47	47.53

Non-facility RVUs ☐

Code	Work	PE Non-Facility	MP	Total Non-Facility
61534	23.01	16.05	8.47	47.53

Modifiers (PAR) ☐

Code	Mod 50	Mod 51	Mod 62	Mod 66	Mod 80
61534	0	2	1	0	2

Global Period

Code	Days
61534	090

61535-61536

61535 Craniotomy with elevation of bone flap; for removal of epidural or subdural electrode array, without excision of cerebral tissue (separate procedure)

61536 Craniotomy with elevation of bone flap; for excision of cerebral epileptogenic focus, with electrocorticography during surgery (includes removal of electrode array)

AMA Coding Notes

Surgical Procedures on the Skull, Meninges, and Brain

(For injection procedure for cerebral angiography, see 36100-36218)

(For injection procedure for ventriculography, see 61026, 61120)

(For injection procedure for pneumoencephalography, use 61055)

AMA *CPT Assistant*

61535: Jul 19: 11

Plain English Description

Following a previous surgery in which an epidural or subdural electrode array was placed to allow identification of an epileptogenic focus, the craniotomy site is reopened and the array is removed and/or the epileptogenic focus is excised. In 61535, the electrode array is removed without excision of any brain tissue. A skin incision is made along the previous incision lines. Scalp flaps are raised and a bone flap elevated. If an epidural electrode array is present, it is removed from the surface of the dura. If a subdural electrode array is present, the dura is opened and the subdural array removed. In 61536, the electrode array is removed as described above and then the epileptogenic focus is also excised with the help of intraoperative electrocorticography. To perform electrocorticography electrodes are placed on the surface of the cerebral cortex and additional electrodes are inserted into deeper regions of the brain as needed. Brain waves are recorded with and without stimuli. The boundaries of the epileptogenic focus are identified. The region of the lesional or localized epileptogenic focus is identified and the abnormal brain tissue is excised. Following removal of all abnormal brain tissue, the electrocorticography electrodes are removed and the dura is closed. The bone flap is replaced and secured with sutures, wires, or miniplate and screws. The overlying muscle is repaired and the galea and skin are closed in layers.

ICD-10-CM Diagnostic Codes

G40.011 Localization-related (focal) (partial) idiopathic epilepsy and epileptic syndromes with seizures of localized onset, intractable, with status epilepticus

G40.019 Localization-related (focal) (partial) idiopathic epilepsy and epileptic syndromes with seizures of localized onset, intractable, without status epilepticus

G40.111 Localization-related (focal) (partial) symptomatic epilepsy and epileptic syndromes with simple partial seizures, intractable, with status epilepticus

G40.119 Localization-related (focal) (partial) symptomatic epilepsy and epileptic syndromes with simple partial seizures, intractable, without status epilepticus

G40.211 Localization-related (focal) (partial) symptomatic epilepsy and epileptic syndromes with complex partial seizures, intractable, with status epilepticus

G40.219 Localization-related (focal) (partial) symptomatic epilepsy and epileptic syndromes with complex partial seizures, intractable, without status epilepticus

CCI Edits

Refer to Appendix A for CCI edits.

Pub 100

61535: Pub 100-04, 12, 20.4.5, Pub 100-04, 12, 40.1

61536: Pub 100-04, 12, 20.4.5, Pub 100-04, 12, 40.1

Facility RVUs

Code	Work	PE Facility	MP	Total Facility
61535	13.15	10.85	4.83	28.83
61536	37.72	22.83	14.05	74.60

Non-facility RVUs

Code	Work	PE Non-Facility	MP	Total Non-Facility
61535	13.15	10.85	4.83	28.83
61536	37.72	22.83	14.05	74.60

Modifiers (PAR)

Code	Mod 50	Mod 51	Mod 62	Mod 66	Mod 80
61535	0	2	1	0	2
61536	0	2	1	0	2

Global Period

Code	Days
61535	090
61536	090

61537-61540

61537 Craniotomy with elevation of bone flap; for lobectomy, temporal lobe, without electrocorticography during surgery

61538 Craniotomy with elevation of bone flap; for lobectomy, temporal lobe, with electrocorticography during surgery

61539 Craniotomy with elevation of bone flap; for lobectomy, other than temporal lobe, partial or total, with electrocorticography during surgery

61540 Craniotomy with elevation of bone flap; for lobectomy, other than temporal lobe, partial or total, without electrocorticography during surgery

AMA Coding Notes

Surgical Procedures on the Skull, Meninges, and Brain

(For injection procedure for cerebral angiography, see 36100-36218)

(For injection procedure for ventriculography, see 61026, 61120)

(For injection procedure for pneumoencephalography, use 61055)

Plain English Description

One of the temporal lobes is excised usually for control of epileptic seizures. Temporal lobectomy may be performed with or without intraoperative electrocorticography, also referred to as brain mapping. This involves recording electrical potentials directly from the cerebral cortex and/or adjacent structures to help identify the boundaries of the epileptogenic zone and to help identify the extent of the required resection of the temporal lobe. The skin is incised and scalp flaps are created followed by burr holes. The bone between the burr holes is cut with a saw or craniotome and the bone flap elevated. The dura is opened and retracted. The anterior aspect of the temporal lobe is measured and the location of cortical incisions is determined. If electrocorticography is used, electrodes are placed on the surface of the cerebral cortex and additional electrodes are inserted into deeper regions of the brain. Brain waves are recorded with and without stimuli. The boundaries of the epileptogenic zone are identified. The cortex is incised and dissection carried deep to the cortex using an ultrasonic aspirator. Dissection continues along the coronal plane to the temporal horn of the lateral ventricle and hippocampus. Attention then turns to the pia mater of the medial cortex. A subpial dissection is performed and the pia is opened. The anterior and lateral portion of the temporal lobe is removed. Attention is then directed to the hippocampus, amygdala, and uncus, which are carefully dissected while taking care to coagulate and divide perforating arteries from the posterior cerebral artery without damaging it. As dissection continues, care is taken to preserve the anterior choroidal artery and the pia arachnoid overlying the ambient cistern, which contains the internal carotid artery, posterior cerebral artery, CN III, CN IV, CN V, and CN VI, the basilar vein of Rosenthal, the optic tract, the lateral geniculate and the brainstem. The hippocampus, amygdala, and uncus are excised, which completes the excision of the temporal lobe. The dura is repaired and the bone flap replaced and secured with sutures, wires, or miniplate and screws. The temporalis muscle is repaired and the galea and skin are closed in layers. Use 61537 if the procedure is performed without electrocorticography and 61538 if electrocorticography is used. Report code 61539 when a lobe, other than the temporal lobe, is removed in a similar manner either partially or totally using electrocorticography and 61540 without electrocorticography.

ICD-10-CM Diagnostic Codes

G40.011	Localization-related (focal) (partial) idiopathic epilepsy and epileptic syndromes with seizures of localized onset, intractable, with status epilepticus
G40.019	Localization-related (focal) (partial) idiopathic epilepsy and epileptic syndromes with seizures of localized onset, intractable, without status epilepticus
G40.111	Localization-related (focal) (partial) symptomatic epilepsy and epileptic syndromes with simple partial seizures, intractable, with status epilepticus
G40.119	Localization-related (focal) (partial) symptomatic epilepsy and epileptic syndromes with simple partial seizures, intractable, without status epilepticus
G40.211	Localization-related (focal) (partial) symptomatic epilepsy and epileptic syndromes with complex partial seizures, intractable, with status epilepticus
G40.219	Localization-related (focal) (partial) symptomatic epilepsy and epileptic syndromes with complex partial seizures, intractable, without status epilepticus

CCI Edits

Refer to Appendix A for CCI edits.

Pub 100

61537: Pub 100-04, 12, 20.4.5

61538: Pub 100-04, 12, 20.4.5

61539: Pub 100-04, 12, 20.4.5, Pub 100-04, 12, 40.1

61540: Pub 100-04, 12, 20.4.5

Facility RVUs

Code	Work	PE Facility	MP	Total Facility
61537	36.45	21.32	13.56	71.33
61538	39.45	22.96	14.72	77.13
61539	34.28	21.24	12.73	68.25
61540	31.43	19.91	11.63	62.97

Non-facility RVUs

Code	Work	PE Non-Facility	MP	Total Non-Facility
61537	36.45	21.32	13.56	71.33
61538	39.45	22.96	14.72	77.13
61539	34.28	21.24	12.73	68.25
61540	31.43	19.91	11.63	62.97

Modifiers (PAR)

Code	Mod 50	Mod 51	Mod 62	Mod 66	Mod 80
61537	0	2	1	0	2
61538	0	2	1	0	2
61539	0	2	1	0	2
61540	0	2	1	0	2

Global Period

Code	Days
61537	090
61538	090
61539	090
61540	090

61541

61541 Craniotomy with elevation of bone flap; for transection of corpus callosum

AMA Coding Notes

Surgical Procedures on the Skull, Meninges, and Brain

(For injection procedure for cerebral angiography, see 36100-36218)

(For injection procedure for ventriculography, see 61026, 61120)

(For injection procedure for pneumoencephalography, use 61055)

Plain English Description

The brain is divided into right and left cerebral hemispheres. Each hemisphere has an outer layer of gray matter called the cerebral cortex and an inner layer of white matter. The two hemispheres are separated by the corpus callosum. Transection of the corpus callosum is performed to treat generalized seizure disorders. These types of seizures begin in the cerebral cortex and then spread through the commissural pathways. Transection of the corpus callosum interrupts the generalized or bilateral pathway and can reduce or eliminate certain types of seizures. A long skin incision is made beginning anterior to the coronal suture on the left side of the skull and carried across the midline to the right side. A scalp flap is created. Burr holes are drilled slightly to the left of midline, the bone between the burr holes is cut with a saw or craniotome, and a bone flap elevated. The dura is opened in a curvilinear fashion beginning at the sagittal sinus and retracted. Using a surgical microscope, dissection is carried down the interhemispheric fissure. A self-retaining retractor is used to retract the right frontal lobe and a second retractor is used on the falx or contralateral cingulate gyrus to allow adequate exposure of the corpus callosum. The callosal margin and pericallosal arteries are identified passing over the callosum. Callosal fibers are initially divided using suction aspiration and bipolar coagulation through the genu and anterior callosum while taking care to protect the pericallosal arteries. The midline raphe, which is the septum between the lateral ventricles, is identified and a ball dissector is then used to divide the perpendicular fibers in the posterior aspect of the corpus callosum. Once the transection is complete, the dura is closed. The bone flap is replaced and secured with sutures, wires, or miniplate and screws. The overlying muscle is repaired and the galea and skin closed in layers.

ICD-10-CM Diagnostic Codes

G40.311	Generalized idiopathic epilepsy and epileptic syndromes, intractable, with status epilepticus
G40.319	Generalized idiopathic epilepsy and epileptic syndromes, intractable, without status epilepticus
G40.411	Other generalized epilepsy and epileptic syndromes, intractable, with status epilepticus
G40.419	Other generalized epilepsy and epileptic syndromes, intractable, without status epilepticus

CCI Edits

Refer to Appendix A for CCI edits.

Pub 100

61541: Pub 100-04, 12, 20.4.5, Pub 100-04, 12, 40

Facility RVUs ▯

Code	Work	PE Facility	MP	Total Facility
61541	30.94	19.70	11.46	62.10

Non-facility RVUs ▯

Code	Work	PE Non-Facility	MP	Total Non-Facility
61541	30.94	19.70	11.46	62.10

Modifiers (PAR) ▯

Code	Mod 50	Mod 51	Mod 62	Mod 66	Mod 80
61541	0	2	1	0	2

Global Period

Code	Days
61541	090

61545

61545 Craniotomy with elevation of bone flap; for excision of craniopharyngioma

(For craniotomy for selective amygdalohippocampectomy, use 61566)

(For craniotomy for multiple subpial transections during surgery, use 61567)

AMA Coding Notes

Surgical Procedures on the Skull, Meninges, and Brain

(For injection procedure for cerebral angiography, see 36100-36218)

(For injection procedure for ventriculography, see 61026, 61120)

(For injection procedure for pneumoencephalography, use 61055)

Plain English Description

A craniopharyngioma is a benign tumor with both cystic and solid components that arises from the remnants of the craniopharyngeal duct near the base of the pituitary gland. The skin is incised above the eyebrows and the tumor approached via a supraorbital craniotomy. Scalp flaps are created followed by burr holes in the supraorbital region. The bone between the burr holes is cut with a saw or craniotome and a bone flap elevated. The dura is opened and retracted. Brain tissue is dissected, taking care to preserve critical structures, and the tumor is exposed. The tumor is carefully dissected from surrounding tissue and excised. Separately reportable intraoperative evaluation by a pathologist is performed to assess the margins. If the margins are not free of abnormal tissue, additional tissue is excised if critical structures can be spared. Excision of tissue continues until the margins are clear or until the neurosurgeon determines that he/she has removed as much of the tumor as can be safely removed. The dura is closed. The bone flap is replaced and secured with sutures, wires, or miniplate and screws. The overlying muscle is repaired and the skin closed in layers.

Craniotomy with elevation of bone flap; for excision of craniopharyngioma

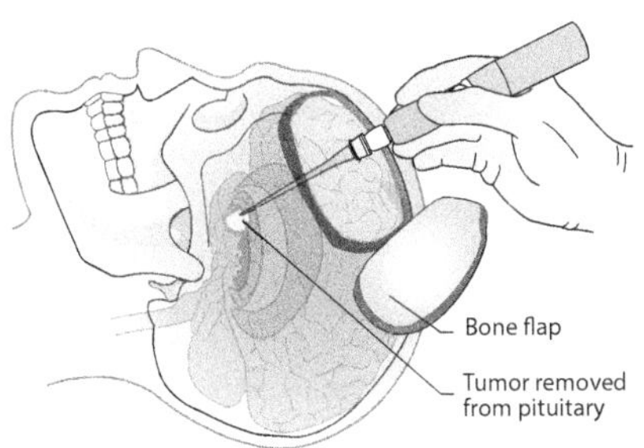

ICD-10-CM Diagnostic Codes

D35.3	Benign neoplasm of craniopharyngeal duct
D44.4	Neoplasm of uncertain behavior of craniopharyngeal duct

CCI Edits

Refer to Appendix A for CCI edits.

Pub 100

61545: Pub 100-04, 12, 20.4.5

Facility RVUs

Code	Work	PE Facility	MP	Total Facility
61545	46.43	28.39	17.49	92.31

Non-facility RVUs

Code	Work	PE Non-Facility	MP	Total Non-Facility
61545	46.43	28.39	17.49	92.31

Modifiers (PAR)

Code	Mod 50	Mod 51	Mod 62	Mod 66	Mod 80
61545	0	2	1	0	2

Global Period

Code	Days
61545	090

CPT® Procedural Coding

61546-61548

61546 Craniotomy for hypophysectomy or excision of pituitary tumor, intracranial approach

61548 Hypophysectomy or excision of pituitary tumor, transnasal or transseptal approach, nonstereotactic

(Do not report code 69990 in addition to code 61548)

AMA Coding Notes

Surgical Procedures on the Skull, Meninges, and Brain

(For injection procedure for cerebral angiography, see 36100-36218)

(For injection procedure for ventriculography, see 61026, 61120)

(For injection procedure for pneumoencephalography, use 61055)

AMA *CPT Assistant* ▯

61548: Nov 98: 17, Jul 11: 13

Plain English Description

The pituitary gland or a pituitary tumor is surgically removed. The pituitary gland is a small pea-sized endocrine gland that is located at the center and base of the skull immediately behind the bridge of the nose in a small depression in the skull called the sella turcica. The pituitary gland can be accessed via an intracranial, transnasal, or transseptal approach. In 61546, an intracranial approach is used usually to access a tumor that extends beyond the sella turcica. The skin is incised above the eyebrows and the tumor approached via a supraorbital craniotomy. Scalp flaps are created followed by burr holes in the supraorbital region. The bone between the burr holes is cut with a saw or craniotome and a bone flap elevated. The dura is opened and retracted. The frontal lobe is elevated and the pituitary gland or tumor exposed. The pituitary gland or tumor is carefully dissected from surrounding tissue and excised. Separately reportable intraoperative evaluation by a pathologist is performed to assess the margins. If the margins are not free of abnormal tissue, additional tissue is excised if critical structures can be spared. Excision of tissue continues until the margins are clear or until the neurosurgeon determines that he/she has removed as much of the tumor as can be safely removed. The dura is closed. The bone flap is replaced and secured with sutures, wires, or miniplate and screws. The overlying muscle is repaired and the skin closed in layers. In 61548, a transnasal or transseptal approach is used. Stents are placed in the nose, secured with sutures to the nasal septum, and the nose is packed with gauze or sponges to absorb drainage from the operative site. An incision is made in the mouth just below the upper lip at the junction with the upper gum. Soft tissue is dissected and the nasal cavity is entered. A speculum is inserted and the pituitary gland or tumor located. The dura is incised. The pituitary gland may be grasped with forceps and removed or the gland or tumor may be carefully dissected from surrounding tissue and excised. Once the gland or tumor has been completely excised, the dura is closed. This may require a fat graft, which is usually harvested from the inner thigh. The speculum is removed and the surgical wound closed in layers.

Hypophysectomy or excision of pituitary tumor

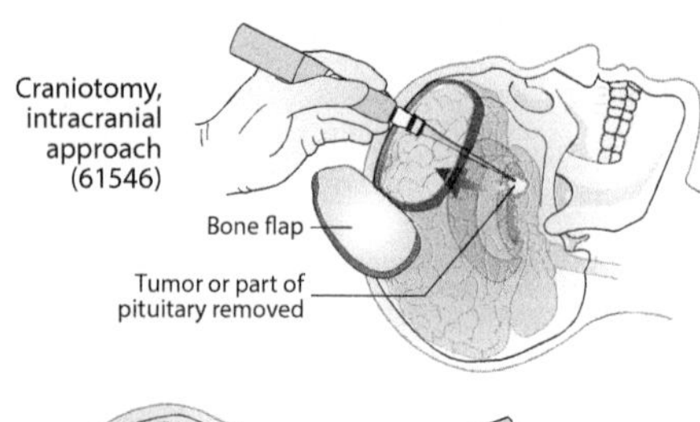

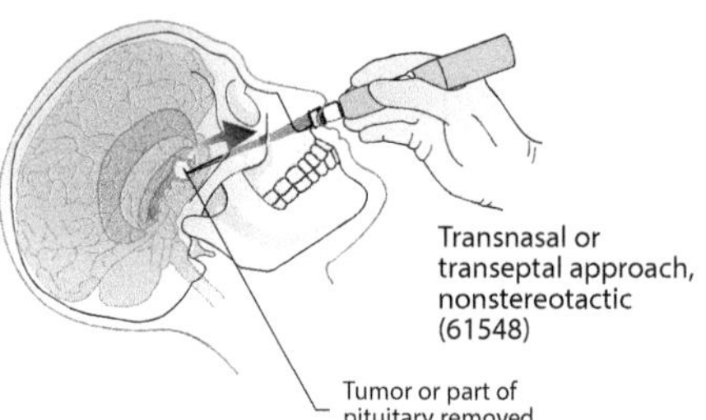

ICD-10-CM Diagnostic Codes

C75.1	Malignant neoplasm of pituitary gland
C79.89	Secondary malignant neoplasm of other specified sites
D09.3	Carcinoma in situ of thyroid and other endocrine glands
D35.2	Benign neoplasm of pituitary gland
D44.3	Neoplasm of uncertain behavior of pituitary gland
D44.4	Neoplasm of uncertain behavior of craniopharyngeal duct
D49.7	Neoplasm of unspecified behavior of endocrine glands and other parts of nervous system
E24.0	Pituitary-dependent Cushing's disease
Q89.2	Congenital malformations of other endocrine glands

CCI Edits

Refer to Appendix A for CCI edits.

Pub 100

61546: Pub 100-04, 12, 20.4.5

Facility RVUs ▯

Code	Work	PE Facility	MP	Total Facility
61546	33.44	20.85	12.40	66.69
61548	23.37	14.52	7.31	45.20

Non-facility RVUs ▯

Code	Work	PE Non-Facility	MP	Total Non-Facility
61546	33.44	20.85	12.40	66.69
61548	23.37	14.52	7.31	45.20

Modifiers (PAR) ▯

Code	Mod 50	Mod 51	Mod 62	Mod 66	Mod 80
61546	0	2	1	0	2
61548	0	2	2	0	2

Global Period

Code	Days
61546	090
61548	090

61566-61567

61566 Craniotomy with elevation of bone flap; for selective amygdalohippocampectomy

61567 Craniotomy with elevation of bone flap; for multiple subpial transections, with electrocorticography during surgery

AMA Coding Notes

Surgical Procedures on the Skull, Meninges, and Brain

(For injection procedure for cerebral angiography, see 36100-36218)

(For injection procedure for ventriculography, see 61026, 61120)

(For injection procedure for pneumoencephalography, use 61055)

Plain English Description

Craniotomy with elevation of bone flap for selective amygdalohippocampectomy (SAH) or multiple subpial transections (MST) with intraoperative electrocorticography (ECoG) may be performed through a subtemporal approach (below the temporal lobe), transcortical approach (through the cortex and gray matter), or transsylvian approach (via wide dissection of the sylvian fissure). SAH and/or MST may be used to treat mesial temporal lobe epilepsy that is unresponsive to medical therapy. With the patient's head secured using three-pin fixation, the temporal area is incised to expose the temporalis fascia, which is then opened and separated from the periosteum. The skin and muscle flap are retracted laterally and a bone flap is elevated using burr hole(s) and craniotome. The dura is opened and flapped anteriorly to expose the brain cortex for SAH (61566) or MST with ECoG (61567) using the selected approach. For SAH (61566), the intraventricular anatomy is identified including the dural floor of the middle fossa, pial boundary overlying the suprasellar cistern containing the carotid artery and third cranial nerve, uncus of the temporal lobe, medial prominence of the hippocampus, and choriod plexus fissure. The parahippocampal gyrus is then resected medially and posteriorly, preserving the mesial pial border, and the hippocampus is mobilized laterally into the cavity. The resection continues anteriorly and posteriorly to the level of the tectal plate and the tissue is removed. For MST with ECoG (61567), following exposure of the brain cortex, electrodes are placed directly on the surface to identify and delineate the interface between the epileptogenic zones and functional cortex substance of the brain. The electrophysiological activity of the brain is then mapped and small, shallow, parallel incisions are made in the nerve fibers of the gray matter just below the pia mater (subpial). At the conclusion of either procedure, bleeding is controlled using electrocautery and/or gelfoam, the dura is closed, and the bone flap is plated. The temporalis muscle is reapproximated and the scalp is closed in layers.

Craniotomy with elevation of bone flap

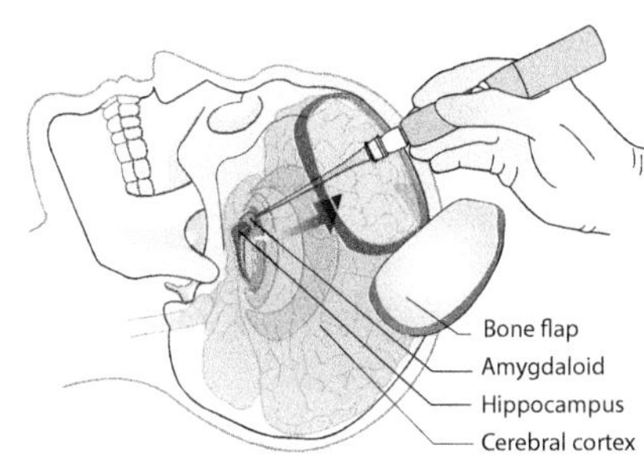

For selective amygdalohippocampectomy (61566); for multiple subpial transections, with electocorticography during surgery (61567)

ICD-10-CM Diagnostic Codes

G40.011	Localization-related (focal) (partial) idiopathic epilepsy and epileptic syndromes with seizures of localized onset, intractable, with status epilepticus
G40.019	Localization-related (focal) (partial) idiopathic epilepsy and epileptic syndromes with seizures of localized onset, intractable, without status epilepticus
G40.111	Localization-related (focal) (partial) symptomatic epilepsy and epileptic syndromes with simple partial seizures, intractable, with status epilepticus
G40.119	Localization-related (focal) (partial) symptomatic epilepsy and epileptic syndromes with simple partial seizures, intractable, without status epilepticus
G40.211	Localization-related (focal) (partial) symptomatic epilepsy and epileptic syndromes with complex partial seizures, intractable, with status epilepticus
G40.219	Localization-related (focal) (partial) symptomatic epilepsy and epileptic syndromes with complex partial seizures, intractable, without status epilepticus

CCI Edits

Refer to Appendix A for CCI edits.

Pub 100

61566: Pub 100-04, 12, 20.4.5

61567: Pub 100-04, 12, 20.4.5

Facility RVUs

Code	Work	PE Facility	MP	Total Facility
61566	32.45	20.38	12.03	64.86
61567	37.00	23.16	13.78	73.94

Non-facility RVUs

Code	Work	PE Non-Facility	MP	Total Non-Facility
61566	32.45	20.38	12.03	64.86
61567	37.00	23.16	13.78	73.94

Modifiers (PAR)

Code	Mod 50	Mod 51	Mod 62	Mod 66	Mod 80
61566	0	2	1	0	2
61567	0	2	1	0	2

Global Period

Code	Days
61566	090
61567	090

61580-61581

61580 Craniofacial approach to anterior cranial fossa; extradural, including lateral rhinotomy, ethmoidectomy, sphenoidectomy, without maxillectomy or orbital exenteration

61581 Craniofacial approach to anterior cranial fossa; extradural, including lateral rhinotomy, orbital exenteration, ethmoidectomy, sphenoidectomy and/or maxillectomy

AMA Coding Guideline

Skull Base Surgical Procedures

The surgical management of lesions involving the skull base (base of anterior, middle, and posterior cranial fossae) often requires the skills of several surgeons of different surgical specialties working together or in tandem during the operative session. These operations are usually not staged because of the need for definitive closure of dura, subcutaneous tissues, and skin to avoid serious infections such as osteomyelitis and/or meningitis.

The procedures are categorized according to:

The approach procedure is described according to anatomical area involved, ie, anterior cranial fossa, middle cranial fossa, posterior cranial fossa, and brain stem or upper spinal cord.

The definitive procedure(s) describes the repair, biopsy, resection, or excision of various lesions of the skull base and, when appropriate, primary closure of the dura, mucous membranes, and skin.

The repair/reconstruction procedure(s) is reported separately if extensive dural grafting, cranioplasty, local or regional myocutaneous pedicle flaps, or extensive skin grafts are required.

For primary closure, see the appropriate codes (ie, 15730, 15733, 15756, 15757, 15758).

When one surgeon performs the approach procedure, another surgeon performs the definitive procedure, and another surgeon performs the repair/reconstruction procedure, each surgeon reports only the code for the specific procedure performed.

If one surgeon performs more than one procedure (ie, approach procedure and definitive procedure), then both codes are reported, adding modifier 51 to the secondary, additional procedure(s).

AMA Coding Notes

Skull Base Surgical Procedures

(1) approach procedure necessary to obtain adequate exposure to the lesion (pathologic entity), (2) definitive procedure(s) necessary to biopsy, excise or otherwise treat the lesion, and (3) repair/reconstruction of the defect present following the definitive procedure(s).

Surgical Procedures on the Skull, Meninges, and Brain

(For injection procedure for cerebral angiography, see 36100-36218)

(For injection procedure for ventriculography, see 61026, 61120)

(For injection procedure for pneumoencephalography, use 61055)

AMA *CPT Assistant* ☐

61580: Winter 93: 17, Spring 94: 11

61581: Winter 93: 17, Spring 94: 11

Plain English Description

An extradural lesion is exposed using a craniofacial approach to the anterior cranial fossa. In 61580, an incision is made beginning at the medial edge of the eyebrow and extends down the side of the nose (lateral rhinotomy) around the nasal ala and down the center of the lip. A second incision line is made from the upper aspect of the side of the nose to the inner canthus and carried below the eye to the outer canthus and along the maxilla into the temporal region. The facial nerve is mobilized and transected using a technique that will allow reanastomosis of the nerve at the end of the procedure. Subperiosteal dissection is then carried down to the intraorbital nerve, which is transected and tagged. A flap is created composed of the upper lip, cheek, lower eyelid, and parotid gland. Mucosa and bone of the ethmoid and sphenoid sinuses are completely resected (ethmoidectomy, sphenoidectomy) to provide access to the extradural lesion. In 61581, the exposure is performed as described above, but an orbital exenteration is performed, which typically requires a maxillectomy. This type of approach is typically performed for malignant tumors that have invaded the maxillary sinus. Orbital structures are removed when the tumor has invaded the periorbital region. The maxillary sinus is exposed. Mucosa and bone of the maxillary sinus are completely resected. Traction sutures are placed posterior to the margins of the closed lids. An incision is made in the superior aspect through the skin of the eyelid behind the eye lashes. The full-thickness skin incision is carried around the entire circumference of the eye and includes the skin around the outer and inner canthi. The incision is carried through the subcutaneous tissues and into the periosteum around the orbital rim. Periorbital elevators are used to free the periosteum from underlying bone. The eyeball and the entire contents of the orbit are removed en bloc. The lesion is now exposed. Once all neurovascular structures are identified and preserved, lesion dissection begins and is reported separately.

Craniofacial approach to anterior cranial fossa

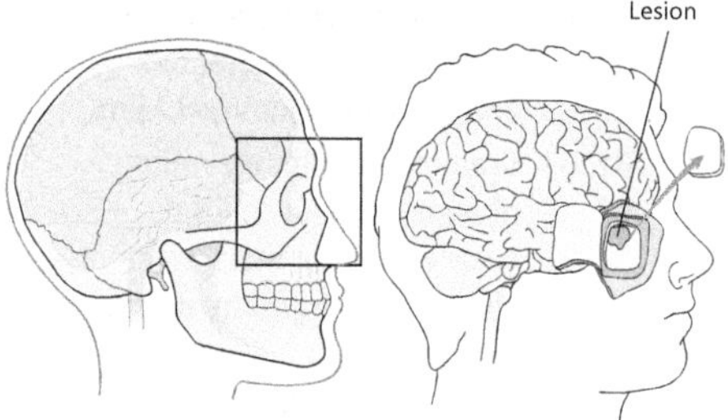

A lesion lying outside of the membrane that lines the skull is accessed through the face (61580), or through the lower sinus/eye socket (60581).

ICD-10-CM Diagnostic Codes

	Code	Description
	A17.1	Meningeal tuberculoma
	A17.81	Tuberculoma of brain and spinal cord
	B95.0	Streptococcus, group A, as the cause of diseases classified elsewhere
	B95.1	Streptococcus, group B, as the cause of diseases classified elsewhere
	B95.3	Streptococcus pneumoniae as the cause of diseases classified elsewhere
	B95.4	Other streptococcus as the cause of diseases classified elsewhere
	B95.61	Methicillin susceptible Staphylococcus aureus infection as the cause of diseases classified elsewhere
	B95.62	Methicillin resistant Staphylococcus aureus infection as the cause of diseases classified elsewhere
	B95.7	Other staphylococcus as the cause of diseases classified elsewhere
	B96.3	Hemophilus influenzae [H. influenzae] as the cause of diseases classified elsewhere
	B96.89	Other specified bacterial agents as the cause of diseases classified elsewhere
	C31.0	Malignant neoplasm of maxillary sinus
	C31.1	Malignant neoplasm of ethmoidal sinus
	C31.3	Malignant neoplasm of sphenoid sinus
	C31.8	Malignant neoplasm of overlapping sites of accessory sinuses
	C41.0	Malignant neoplasm of bones of skull and face
	C49.0	Malignant neoplasm of connective and soft tissue of head, face and neck
⇄	C69.61	Malignant neoplasm of right orbit
⇄	C69.62	Malignant neoplasm of left orbit
	C78.39	Secondary malignant neoplasm of other respiratory organs
	C79.49	Secondary malignant neoplasm of other parts of nervous system
	C79.51	Secondary malignant neoplasm of bone

C79.89	Secondary malignant neoplasm of other specified sites
D16.4	Benign neoplasm of bones of skull and face
D48.0	Neoplasm of uncertain behavior of bone and articular cartilage
G06.0	Intracranial abscess and granuloma
J32.0	Chronic maxillary sinusitis
J32.1	Chronic frontal sinusitis
J32.2	Chronic ethmoidal sinusitis
J32.3	Chronic sphenoidal sinusitis
J32.4	Chronic pansinusitis
J32.8	Other chronic sinusitis

CCI Edits

Refer to Appendix A for CCI edits.

Pub 100

61580: Pub 100-04, 12, 20.4.5
61581: Pub 100-04, 12, 20.4.5

Facility RVUs

Code	Work	PE Facility	MP	Total Facility
61580	34.51	29.44	6.59	70.54
61581	39.13	32.14	5.34	76.61

Non-facility RVUs

Code	Work	PE Non-Facility	MP	Total Non-Facility
61580	34.51	29.44	6.59	70.54
61581	39.13	32.14	5.34	76.61

Modifiers (PAR)

Code	Mod 50	Mod 51	Mod 62	Mod 66	Mod 80
61580	1	2	1	2	1
61581	1	2	2	2	1

Global Period

Code	Days
61580	090
61581	090

61582-61583

61582 Craniofacial approach to anterior cranial fossa; extradural, including unilateral or bifrontal craniotomy, elevation of frontal lobe(s), osteotomy of base of anterior cranial fossa

61583 Craniofacial approach to anterior cranial fossa; intradural, including unilateral or bifrontal craniotomy, elevation or resection of frontal lobe, osteotomy of base of anterior cranial fossa

AMA Coding Guideline

Skull Base Surgical Procedures

The surgical management of lesions involving the skull base (base of anterior, middle, and posterior cranial fossae) often requires the skills of several surgeons of different surgical specialties working together or in tandem during the operative session. These operations are usually not staged because of the need for definitive closure of dura, subcutaneous tissues, and skin to avoid serious infections such as osteomyelitis and/or meningitis.

The procedures are categorized according to:

The approach procedure is described according to anatomical area involved, ie, anterior cranial fossa, middle cranial fossa, posterior cranial fossa, and brain stem or upper spinal cord.

The definitive procedure(s) describes the repair, biopsy, resection, or excision of various lesions of the skull base and, when appropriate, primary closure of the dura, mucous membranes, and skin.

The repair/reconstruction procedure(s) is reported separately if extensive dural grafting, cranioplasty, local or regional myocutaneous pedicle flaps, or extensive skin grafts are required.

For primary closure, see the appropriate codes (ie, 15730, 15733, 15756, 15757, 15758).

When one surgeon performs the approach procedure, another surgeon performs the definitive procedure, and another surgeon performs the repair/reconstruction procedure, each surgeon reports only the code for the specific procedure performed.

If one surgeon performs more than one procedure (ie, approach procedure and definitive procedure), then both codes are reported, adding modifier 51 to the secondary, additional procedure(s).

AMA Coding Notes

Skull Base Surgical Procedures

(1) approach procedure necessary to obtain adequate exposure to the lesion (pathologic entity), (2) definitive procedure(s) necessary to biopsy, excise or otherwise treat the lesion, and (3) repair/reconstruction of the defect present following the definitive procedure(s).

Surgical Procedures on the Skull, Meninges, and Brain

(For injection procedure for cerebral angiography, see 36100-36218)

(For injection procedure for ventriculography, see 61026, 61120)

(For injection procedure for pneumoencephalography, use 61055)

AMA *CPT Assistant* ▯

61582: Winter 93: 17, Spring 94: 11

61583: Winter 93: 17, Spring 94: 11, Dec 17: 13

Plain English Description

The craniofacial approach to the anterior cranial fossa (ACF) may be used to resect neoplastic tumors and vascular lesions of the sinus and orbit. The ACF is formed by the frontal, ethmoid, and sphenoid bones laterally with the floor of the ACF corresponding to the roof of the orbits and centrally to the vault of the nasal cavity and the fovea ethmoidalis. A unilateral craniotomy incision starts <1 cm anteriorly to the tragus, just above the zygomatic arch and continues superiorly ending at the frontal midline. A bifrontal (bicoronal) craniotomy extends ear to ear, also starting <1 cm anterior to the tragus and ending on each side just above the zygomatic arch behind the hairline. After opening the skin, dissection continues down through the subcutaneous tissue, galea, and superficial temporalis fascia laterally and the pericranium centrally. A flap may be harvested from the pericranium or temporalis fascia for later use in closing the dura. A scalp flap is retracted to expose the bone. For unilateral craniotomy, 2-4 burr holes are made. Two holes are drilled medial to the sagittal sinus, one as far anteriorly as possible, the other as far posteriorly as possible. The additional 2 holes can be placed at the junction of the superior temporal line and the orbital rim, posterior to the sphenoid wing depression. For bilateral craniotomy, 2holes are placed on either side of the sagittal sinus and 2 are placed laterally. A curette or rongeur is used to widen the holes and the craniotomy is completed using a craniotome. The bone flap is elevated; the dura is separated from the bone; and the flap is removed. The extradural procedure (61582) continues with dissection in a lateral to medial direction to identify the cribriform plate and remove the cristal galli. For an intradural procedure (61583), the dura is incised and the frontal lobe is retracted superiorly to expose the anterior skull base from above. The cutting or removal of bone at the base of the ACF may be necessary to widen the surgical field. Cuts are typically made at the paired anterior ethmoidal foramen connecting the ACF with each orbit and/or the cribriform foramina, an opening in the ethmoid bone cribriform plate connecting the ACF to the nasal cavity.

Craniofacial approach to anterior cranial fossa
(includes unilateral/bifrontal craniotomy, elevation of frontal lobe(s), osteotomy of base)

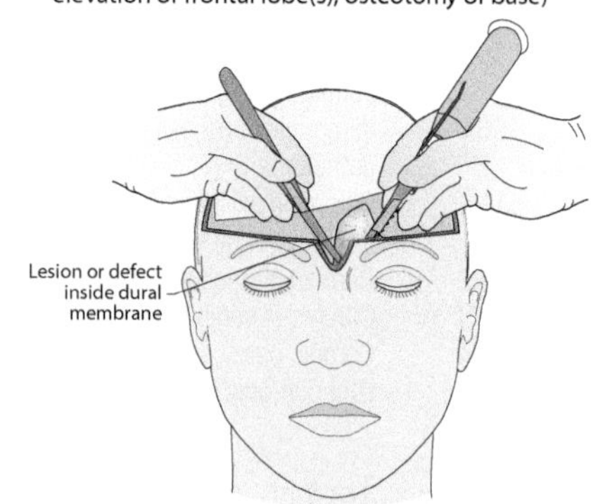

Extradural (61582); intradural (61583)

ICD-10-CM Diagnostic Codes

	Code	Description
	C49.0	Malignant neoplasm of connective and soft tissue of head, face and neck
	C70.0	Malignant neoplasm of cerebral meninges
	C79.32	Secondary malignant neoplasm of cerebral meninges
	C79.49	Secondary malignant neoplasm of other parts of nervous system
	C79.51	Secondary malignant neoplasm of bone
	C79.89	Secondary malignant neoplasm of other specified sites
	D32.0	Benign neoplasm of cerebral meninges
	D42.0	Neoplasm of uncertain behavior of cerebral meninges
⇄	H47.091	Other disorders of optic nerve, not elsewhere classified, right eye
⇄	H47.092	Other disorders of optic nerve, not elsewhere classified, left eye
⇄	H47.093	Other disorders of optic nerve, not elsewhere classified, bilateral
	H47.11	Papilledema associated with increased intracranial pressure
⇄	H47.141	Foster-Kennedy syndrome, right eye
⇄	H47.142	Foster-Kennedy syndrome, left eye
⇄	H47.143	Foster-Kennedy syndrome, bilateral
	H53.8	Other visual disturbances
	R41.3	Other amnesia
	R43.0	Anosmia

CCI Edits

Refer to Appendix A for CCI edits.

Pub 100

61582: Pub 100-04, 12, 20.4.5

61583: Pub 100-04, 12, 20.4.5

Facility RVUs ▯

Code	Work	PE Facility	MP	Total Facility
61582	35.14	40.54	13.05	88.73
61583	38.50	31.60	13.24	83.34

Non-facility RVUs ▯

Code	Work	PE Non-Facility	MP	Total Non-Facility
61582	35.14	40.54	13.05	88.73
61583	38.50	31.60	13.24	83.34

Modifiers (PAR) ▯

Code	Mod 50	Mod 51	Mod 62	Mod 66	Mod 80
61582	0	2	1	2	2
61583	0	2	1	2	2

Global Period

Code	Days
61582	090
61583	090

61584-61585

61584 Orbitocranial approach to anterior cranial fossa, extradural, including supraorbital ridge osteotomy and elevation of frontal and/or temporal lobe(s); without orbital exenteration

61585 Orbitocranial approach to anterior cranial fossa, extradural, including supraorbital ridge osteotomy and elevation of frontal and/or temporal lobe(s); with orbital exenteration

AMA Coding Guideline

Skull Base Surgical Procedures

The surgical management of lesions involving the skull base (base of anterior, middle, and posterior cranial fossae) often requires the skills of several surgeons of different surgical specialties working together or in tandem during the operative session. These operations are usually not staged because of the need for definitive closure of dura, subcutaneous tissues, and skin to avoid serious infections such as osteomyelitis and/or meningitis.

The procedures are categorized according to:

The approach procedure is described according to anatomical area involved, ie, anterior cranial fossa, middle cranial fossa, posterior cranial fossa, and brain stem or upper spinal cord.

The definitive procedure(s) describes the repair, biopsy, resection, or excision of various lesions of the skull base and, when appropriate, primary closure of the dura, mucous membranes, and skin.

The repair/reconstruction procedure(s) is reported separately if extensive dural grafting, cranioplasty, local or regional myocutaneous pedicle flaps, or extensive skin grafts are required.

For primary closure, see the appropriate codes (ie, 15730, 15733, 15756, 15757, 15758).

When one surgeon performs the approach procedure, another surgeon performs the definitive procedure, and another surgeon performs the repair/reconstruction procedure, each surgeon reports only the code for the specific procedure performed.

If one surgeon performs more than one procedure (ie, approach procedure and definitive procedure), then both codes are reported, adding modifier 51 to the secondary, additional procedure(s).

AMA Coding Notes

Skull Base Surgical Procedures

(1) approach procedure necessary to obtain adequate exposure to the lesion (pathologic entity), (2) definitive procedure(s) necessary to biopsy, excise or otherwise treat the lesion, and (3) repair/reconstruction of the defect present following the definitive procedure(s).

Surgical Procedures on the Skull, Meninges, and Brain

(For injection procedure for cerebral angiography, see 36100-36218)

(For injection procedure for ventriculography, see 61026, 61120)

(For injection procedure for pneumoencephalography, use 61055)

AMA *CPT Assistant* □

61584: Winter 93: 18
61585: Winter 93: 18

Plain English Description

The extradural orbitocranial approach to the anterior fossa may be used to resect malignant tumors or infectious diseases and to treat traumatic injuries of the orbit and paranasal sinuses, with or without orbital exenteration (removal of the periorbita, eyeball, appendages, eyelids, and surrounding skin). The scalp is incised along the inferior border of the zygomatic arch and extended upward and forward in a curve to intersect at the contralateral midpupillary line behind the hairline. The frontal periosteum is elevated in a separate layer and left attached along the bone. With the subgaleal fat pad exposed, the temporalis fascia, muscle, and periosteal flap are elevated together with the scalp, extending from the inferior aspect of the scalp incision up to the superior temporal bone. A fascial cuff may be created for later facilitation of temporalis muscle layer reapproximation. The temporalis muscle is elevated from the periosteum of the underlying bone. A flap may be harvested from the pericranium or temporalis fascia for later use in closing the dura. The muscle is mobilized over the lateral orbit to expose the frontozygomatic suture. The mobilized myofascial flap is retracted inferiorly. The periorbita is then freed along the supralateral orbit, including the supraorbital notch medially and the frontozygomatic suture laterally. The periorbital dissection is initiated near the lacrimal gland, medial to the frontozygomatic suture, detached from the bone suture, and continued from the inferior orbital fissure laterally to the supraorbital notch medially. After exposure of the supraorbital ridge, an osteotome or rongeur may be used to thin or contour the bone for better exposure of the orbit. The approach necessary for completing the separately reported definitive procedure also includes elevation of the frontal and/or temporal lobe(s) without orbital exenteration (61584). Code 61585 reports the procedure with orbital exenteration, which may include palpebral skin and conjunctiva sparing (Type I), palpebral skin-sparing, eyeball and appendages removed with the conjunctiva (Type II), both eyelids removed along with the orbital contents (Type III), or removal of eyeball, eyelids, and appendages with involved bone structures (Type IV).

ICD-10-CM Diagnostic Codes

	Code	Description
	C31.0	Malignant neoplasm of maxillary sinus
	C31.1	Malignant neoplasm of ethmoidal sinus
	C31.2	Malignant neoplasm of frontal sinus
	C31.3	Malignant neoplasm of sphenoid sinus
	C31.8	Malignant neoplasm of overlapping sites of accessory sinuses
	C41.0	Malignant neoplasm of bones of skull and face
	C41.9	Malignant neoplasm of bone and articular cartilage, unspecified
⇄	C69.61	Malignant neoplasm of right orbit
⇄	C69.62	Malignant neoplasm of left orbit
⇄	C69.81	Malignant neoplasm of overlapping sites of right eye and adnexa
⇄	C69.82	Malignant neoplasm of overlapping sites of left eye and adnexa
	C78.39	Secondary malignant neoplasm of other respiratory organs
	C79.49	Secondary malignant neoplasm of other parts of nervous system
	C79.51	Secondary malignant neoplasm of bone
	D02.3	Carcinoma in situ of other parts of respiratory system
	D14.0	Benign neoplasm of middle ear, nasal cavity and accessory sinuses
	D16.4	Benign neoplasm of bones of skull and face
⇄	D31.6	Benign neoplasm of unspecified site of orbit
	D38.5	Neoplasm of uncertain behavior of other respiratory organs
	D48.0	Neoplasm of uncertain behavior of bone and articular cartilage
	D48.7	Neoplasm of uncertain behavior of other specified sites

CCI Edits

Refer to Appendix A for CCI edits.

Pub 100

61584: Pub 100-04, 12, 20.4.5
61585: Pub 100-04, 12, 20.4.5

Facility RVUs ▯

Code	Work	PE Facility	MP	Total Facility
61584	37.70	31.98	13.20	82.88
61585	42.57	35.53	15.96	94.06

Non-facility RVUs ▯

Code	Work	PE Non-Facility	MP	Total Non-Facility
61584	37.70	31.98	13.20	82.88
61585	42.57	35.53	15.96	94.06

Modifiers **(PAR)** ▯

Code	Mod 50	Mod 51	Mod 62	Mod 66	Mod 80
61584	1	2	1	2	2
61585	1	2	1	2	2

Global Period

Code	Days
61584	090
61585	090

61590

61590 Infratemporal pre-auricular approach to middle cranial fossa (parapharyngeal space, infratemporal and midline skull base, nasopharynx), with or without disarticulation of the mandible, including parotidectomy, craniotomy, decompression and/or mobilization of the facial nerve and/or petrous carotid artery

AMA Coding Guideline

Skull Base Surgical Procedures

The surgical management of lesions involving the skull base (base of anterior, middle, and posterior cranial fossae) often requires the skills of several surgeons of different surgical specialties working together or in tandem during the operative session. These operations are usually not staged because of the need for definitive closure of dura, subcutaneous tissues, and skin to avoid serious infections such as osteomyelitis and/or meningitis.

The procedures are categorized according to:

The approach procedure is described according to anatomical area involved, ie, anterior cranial fossa, middle cranial fossa, posterior cranial fossa, and brain stem or upper spinal cord.

The definitive procedure(s) describes the repair, biopsy, resection, or excision of various lesions of the skull base and, when appropriate, primary closure of the dura, mucous membranes, and skin.

The repair/reconstruction procedure(s) is reported separately if extensive dural grafting, cranioplasty, local or regional myocutaneous pedicle flaps, or extensive skin grafts are required.

For primary closure, see the appropriate codes (ie, 15730, 15733, 15756, 15757, 15758).

When one surgeon performs the approach procedure, another surgeon performs the definitive procedure, and another surgeon performs the repair/reconstruction procedure, each surgeon reports only the code for the specific procedure performed.

If one surgeon performs more than one procedure (ie, approach procedure and definitive procedure), then both codes are reported, adding modifier 51 to the secondary, additional procedure(s).

AMA Coding Notes

Skull Base Surgical Procedures

(1) approach procedure necessary to obtain adequate exposure to the lesion (pathologic entity), (2) definitive procedure(s) necessary to biopsy, excise or otherwise treat the lesion, and (3) repair/reconstruction of the defect present following the definitive procedure(s).

Surgical Procedures on the Skull, Meninges, and Brain

(For injection procedure for cerebral angiography, see 36100-36218)

(For injection procedure for ventriculography, see 61026, 61120)

(For injection procedure for pneumoencephalography, use 61055)

AMA *CPT Assistant* ▢

61590: Winter 93: 18

Plain English Description

An extradural or intradural lesion is exposed using an infratemporal pre-auricular approach to the middle cranial fossa. This approach provides access to lesions in the parapharyngeal space, infratemporal and midline skull base, and the nasopharynx. The incision begins near the midline at the top of the skull, extends laterally over the temporal region, and is then carried down in front of the ear along the pre-auricular crease to the level of the tragus. The incision is then extended down into the neck to provide access to and control of the internal carotid artery. The scalp flap is elevated. The temporalis muscle is elevated off the temporal fossa. The fascia of the masseter muscle is dissected and the parotid gland is exposed and removed (parotidectomy). For wider exposure, the mandible may be exposed and severed from its attachments to the temporal bone (mandibular disarticulation). A temporal craniotomy is performed with the exact placement of the osteotomies determined by the location of the lesion. Once the cranium is opened, the orbital soft tissues are protected. The frontal lobe is retracted. Soft tissues are then dissected off the infratemporal skull base. The facial nerve is identified and decompressed or mobilized as needed. The petrous carotid artery is also identified and decompressed or mobilized. Once all neurovascular structures are identified and preserved, lesion dissection begins and is reported separately

Infratemporal pre-auricular approach to middle cranial fossa

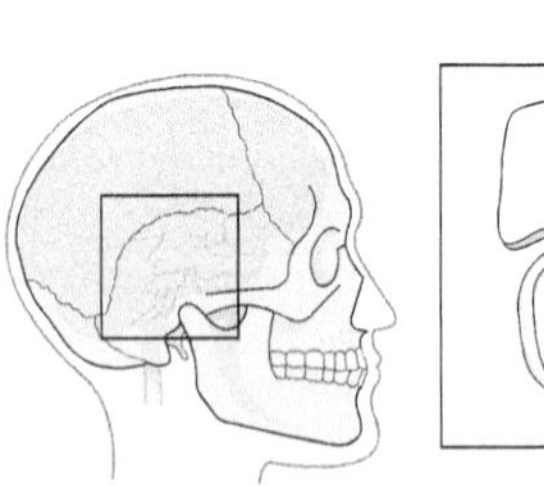

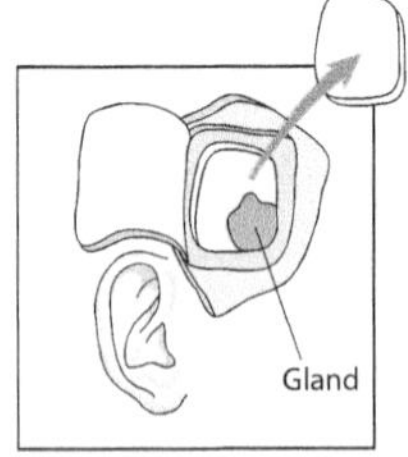

The middle of the head is accessed by removing the section of bone in front of and above the ear.

ICD-10-CM Diagnostic Codes

C07	Malignant neoplasm of parotid gland
C11.0	Malignant neoplasm of superior wall of nasopharynx
C11.1	Malignant neoplasm of posterior wall of nasopharynx
C11.2	Malignant neoplasm of lateral wall of nasopharynx
C11.3	Malignant neoplasm of anterior wall of nasopharynx
C11.8	Malignant neoplasm of overlapping sites of nasopharynx
C41.0	Malignant neoplasm of bones of skull and face
C49.0	Malignant neoplasm of connective and soft tissue of head, face and neck
C70.0	Malignant neoplasm of cerebral meninges
C79.49	Secondary malignant neoplasm of other parts of nervous system
C79.51	Secondary malignant neoplasm of bone
C79.89	Secondary malignant neoplasm of other specified sites
D10.6	Benign neoplasm of nasopharynx
D11.0	Benign neoplasm of parotid gland
D16.4	Benign neoplasm of bones of skull and face
D21.0	Benign neoplasm of connective and other soft tissue of head, face and neck
D32.0	Benign neoplasm of cerebral meninges
D37.030	Neoplasm of uncertain behavior of the parotid salivary glands
D37.05	Neoplasm of uncertain behavior of pharynx
D42.0	Neoplasm of uncertain behavior of cerebral meninges
D48.0	Neoplasm of uncertain behavior of bone and articular cartilage
D48.1	Neoplasm of uncertain behavior of connective and other soft tissue
G53	Cranial nerve disorders in diseases classified elsewhere
J38.01	Paralysis of vocal cords and larynx, unilateral
J38.02	Paralysis of vocal cords and larynx, bilateral
R13.19	Other dysphagia
R47.81	Slurred speech
R49.0	Dysphonia

CCI Edits

Refer to Appendix A for CCI edits.

Pub 100

61590: Pub 100-04, 12, 20.4.5

Facility RVUs

Code	Work	PE Facility	MP	Total Facility
61590	47.04	31.92	8.72	87.68

Non-facility RVUs

Code	Work	PE Non-Facility	MP	Total Non-Facility
61590	47.04	31.92	8.72	87.68

Modifiers (PAR)

Code	Mod 50	Mod 51	Mod 62	Mod 66	Mod 80
61590	1	2	1	2	2

Global Period

Code	Days
61590	090

61591

61591 Infratemporal post-auricular approach to middle cranial fossa (internal auditory meatus, petrous apex, tentorium, cavernous sinus, parasellar area, infratemporal fossa) including mastoidectomy, resection of sigmoid sinus, with or without decompression and/or mobilization of contents of auditory canal or petrous carotid artery

AMA Coding Guideline

Skull Base Surgical Procedures

The surgical management of lesions involving the skull base (base of anterior, middle, and posterior cranial fossae) often requires the skills of several surgeons of different surgical specialties working together or in tandem during the operative session. These operations are usually not staged because of the need for definitive closure of dura, subcutaneous tissues, and skin to avoid serious infections such as osteomyelitis and/or meningitis.

The procedures are categorized according to:

The approach procedure is described according to anatomical area involved, ie, anterior cranial fossa, middle cranial fossa, posterior cranial fossa, and brain stem or upper spinal cord.

The definitive procedure(s) describes the repair, biopsy, resection, or excision of various lesions of the skull base and, when appropriate, primary closure of the dura, mucous membranes, and skin.

The repair/reconstruction procedure(s) is reported separately if extensive dural grafting, cranioplasty, local or regional myocutaneous pedicle flaps, or extensive skin grafts are required.

For primary closure, see the appropriate codes (ie, 15730, 15733, 15756, 15757, 15758).

When one surgeon performs the approach procedure, another surgeon performs the definitive procedure, and another surgeon performs the repair/reconstruction procedure, each surgeon reports only the code for the specific procedure performed.

If one surgeon performs more than one procedure (ie, approach procedure and definitive procedure), then both codes are reported, adding modifier 51 to the secondary, additional procedure(s).

AMA Coding Notes

Skull Base Surgical Procedures

(1) approach procedure necessary to obtain adequate exposure to the lesion (pathologic entity), (2) definitive procedure(s) necessary to biopsy, excise or otherwise treat the lesion, and (3) repair/ reconstruction of the defect present following the definitive procedure(s).

Surgical Procedures on the Skull, Meninges, and Brain

(For injection procedure for cerebral angiography, see 36100-36218)

(For injection procedure for ventriculography, see 61026, 61120)

(For injection procedure for pneumoencephalography, use 61055)

AMA *CPT Assistant*

61591: Winter 93: 18

Plain English Description

An extradural or intradural lesion is exposed using an infratemporal post-auricular approach to the middle cranial fossa. This approach allows access to lesions in the internal auditory meatus, petrous apex, tentorium, cavernous sinus, parasellar area, and infratemporal fossa. The incision begins in the temporal area and extends behind the ear over the mastoid bone and down into the neck to provide access to and control of the internal carotid artery. The scalp flap is elevated. The temporalis muscle is elevated off the temporal fossa. A mastoidectomy is performed along with resection of the sigmoid sinus to allow exposure of the middle cranial fossa. The middle ear may be sacrificed during the approach. The facial nerve is skeletonized and protected if possible but it may be resected if the tumor has invaded the facial nerve. A temporal craniotomy is performed with the exact placement of the osteotomies determined by the location of the lesion. The frontal lobe is retracted. Soft tissues are then dissected off the infratemporal skull base. If the middle ear has not been sacrificed, the auditory canal is decompressed and mobilized. The petrous carotid artery is also decompressed or mobilized. Once all neurovascular structures are identified and preserved, lesion dissection begins.

ICD-10-CM Diagnostic Codes

	Code	Description
	C41.0	Malignant neoplasm of bones of skull and face
	C49.0	Malignant neoplasm of connective and soft tissue of head, face and neck
	C70.0	Malignant neoplasm of cerebral meninges
⇄	C72.41	Malignant neoplasm of right acoustic nerve
⇄	C72.42	Malignant neoplasm of left acoustic nerve
	C72.9	Malignant neoplasm of central nervous system, unspecified
	C76.0	Malignant neoplasm of head, face and neck
	C79.49	Secondary malignant neoplasm of other parts of nervous system
	C79.51	Secondary malignant neoplasm of bone
	C79.89	Secondary malignant neoplasm of other specified sites
	D16.4	Benign neoplasm of bones of skull and face
	D21.0	Benign neoplasm of connective and other soft tissue of head, face and neck
	D32.0	Benign neoplasm of cerebral meninges
	D33.3	Benign neoplasm of cranial nerves
	D33.9	Benign neoplasm of central nervous system, unspecified
	D42.0	Neoplasm of uncertain behavior of cerebral meninges
	D43.3	Neoplasm of uncertain behavior of cranial nerves
	D43.8	Neoplasm of uncertain behavior of other specified parts of central nervous system
	D48.0	Neoplasm of uncertain behavior of bone and articular cartilage
	D48.1	Neoplasm of uncertain behavior of connective and other soft tissue
	G06.0	Intracranial abscess and granuloma
	G06.2	Extradural and subdural abscess, unspecified
	G08	Intracranial and intraspinal phlebitis and thrombophlebitis
	G46.0	Middle cerebral artery syndrome
	G53	Cranial nerve disorders in diseases classified elsewhere
	I67.6	Nonpyogenic thrombosis of intracranial venous system
	Q28.2	Arteriovenous malformation of cerebral vessels
	Q28.3	Other malformations of cerebral vessels

CCI Edits

Refer to Appendix A for CCI edits.

Pub 100

61591: Pub 100-04, 12, 20.4.5

Facility RVUs

Code	Work	PE Facility	MP	Total Facility
61591	47.02	31.98	9.65	88.65

Non-facility RVUs

Code	Work	PE Non-Facility	MP	Total Non-Facility
61591	47.02	31.98	9.65	88.65

Modifiers (PAR)

Code	Mod 50	Mod 51	Mod 62	Mod 66	Mod 80
61591	1	2	1	2	2

Global Period

Code	Days
61591	090

61592

61592 Orbitocranial zygomatic approach to middle cranial fossa (cavernous sinus and carotid artery, clivus, basilar artery or petrous apex) including osteotomy of zygoma, craniotomy, extra- or intradural elevation of temporal lobe

AMA Coding Guideline

Skull Base Surgical Procedures

The surgical management of lesions involving the skull base (base of anterior, middle, and posterior cranial fossae) often requires the skills of several surgeons of different surgical specialties working together or in tandem during the operative session. These operations are usually not staged because of the need for definitive closure of dura, subcutaneous tissues, and skin to avoid serious infections such as osteomyelitis and/or meningitis.

The procedures are categorized according to:

The approach procedure is described according to anatomical area involved, ie, anterior cranial fossa, middle cranial fossa, posterior cranial fossa, and brain stem or upper spinal cord.

The definitive procedure(s) describes the repair, biopsy, resection, or excision of various lesions of the skull base and, when appropriate, primary closure of the dura, mucous membranes, and skin.

The repair/reconstruction procedure(s) is reported separately if extensive dural grafting, cranioplasty, local or regional myocutaneous pedicle flaps, or extensive skin grafts are required.

For primary closure, see the appropriate codes (ie, 15730, 15733, 15756, 15757, 15758).

When one surgeon performs the approach procedure, another surgeon performs the definitive procedure, and another surgeon performs the repair/reconstruction procedure, each surgeon reports only the code for the specific procedure performed.

If one surgeon performs more than one procedure (ie, approach procedure and definitive procedure), then both codes are reported, adding modifier 51 to the secondary, additional procedure(s).

AMA Coding Notes

Skull Base Surgical Procedures

(1) approach procedure necessary to obtain adequate exposure to the lesion (pathologic entity), (2) definitive procedure(s) necessary to biopsy, excise or otherwise treat the lesion, and (3) repair/ reconstruction of the defect present following the definitive procedure(s).

Surgical Procedures on the Skull, Meninges, and Brain

(For injection procedure for cerebral angiography, see 36100-36218)

(For injection procedure for ventriculography, see 61026, 61120)

(For injection procedure for pneumoencephalography, use 61055)

AMA *CPT Assistant* ▢

61592: Winter 93: 18

Plain English Description

The orbitocranial zygomatic approach to the middle cranial fossa (MCF) may be used to resect neoplastic tumors and vascular lesions of the orbit, sinus, and auditory structures. The MCF lies between the anterior and posterior fossas, with the floor of the MCF formed by the body and greater wings of the sphenoid bone, the squamous part of the temporal bone, and the anterior surface of the temporal petrous bone. The scalp is incised along the inferior border of the zygomatic arch and extended upward and forward in a curve to intersect at the contralateral midpupillary line behind the hairline. The scalp flap is elevated to expose the temporal fascia, which is incised, taking care to preserve the frontal branch of the facial nerve. The fascia is elevated to expose the zygoma and superior orbital rim. The deep fascia is then dissected off the zygomatic arch periosteum to expose the bone. A flap may be harvested from the pericranium or muscle fascia for later use in closing the dura. Next, the temporal muscle is sharply incised along the edges of the fascia and elevated. Subperiosteal dissection continues along the orbital rim. The skin flaps are retracted and the periosteum is freed from the lateral and superior aspects of the orbital walls medial to the supraorbital nerve. A drill is used to create burr holes in the temporal bone and the holes are connected using a craniotome or saw to create the temporal bone flap. The bone flap is elevated and the dura is tacked to the edges. A saw is then used to complete the orbital and zygomatic osteotomies and free the orbitozygomatic bone flap in a single piece. First the root of the zygomatic process is divided obliquely and then cut to divide it from the lateral orbital rim. Beginning intraorbitally with the tip of the saw in the inferior fissure, the osteotomy is extended posteriorly and laterally completing the division of the zygomatic bone. The dura is then elevated to expose the superior and lateral walls of the orbits. The superior orbital rim and roof are then divided, and the lateral orbital wall is freed by connecting cuts along the inferior and superior orbital fissures. Once the orbitozygomatic bone flap is freed and the middle cranial fossa is exposed, the cavernous sinus, carotid artery, clivus, basilar artery, and petrous apex can be examined, and the temporal lobe elevated for removal of neoplastic tumors or vascular disorders.

Orbitocranial zygomatic approach to middle cranial fossa

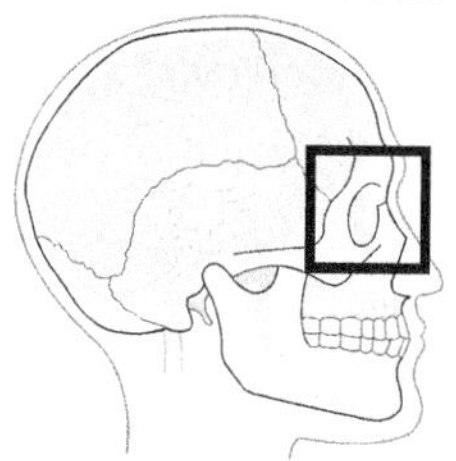

The physician removes the small skull bone behind the eye socket, giving the physician access to the middle of the skull. The physician will make incisions in this area and will elevate the part of the brain in the temple.

ICD-10-CM Diagnostic Codes

C41.0	Malignant neoplasm of bones of skull and face
C70.0	Malignant neoplasm of cerebral meninges
C72.50	Malignant neoplasm of unspecified cranial nerve
C72.9	Malignant neoplasm of central nervous system, unspecified
C79.32	Secondary malignant neoplasm of cerebral meninges
C79.49	Secondary malignant neoplasm of other parts of nervous system
C79.51	Secondary malignant neoplasm of bone
D16.4	Benign neoplasm of bones of skull and face
D32.0	Benign neoplasm of cerebral meninges
D33.3	Benign neoplasm of cranial nerves
D33.9	Benign neoplasm of central nervous system, unspecified
D42.0	Neoplasm of uncertain behavior of cerebral meninges
D43.3	Neoplasm of uncertain behavior of cranial nerves
D43.8	Neoplasm of uncertain behavior of other specified parts of central nervous system
D48.0	Neoplasm of uncertain behavior of bone and articular cartilage
G06.0	Intracranial abscess and granuloma
G06.2	Extradural and subdural abscess, unspecified
G08	Intracranial and intraspinal phlebitis and thrombophlebitis
Q28.2	Arteriovenous malformation of cerebral vessels
Q28.3	Other malformations of cerebral vessels

CCI Edits

Refer to Appendix A for CCI edits.

Pub 100

61592: Pub 100-04, 12, 20.4.5

Facility RVUs ☐

Code	Work	PE Facility	MP	Total Facility
61592	43.08	33.83	14.85	91.76

Non-facility RVUs ☐

Code	Work	PE Non-Facility	MP	Total Non-Facility
61592	43.08	33.83	14.85	91.76

Modifiers (PAR) ☐

Code	Mod 50	Mod 51	Mod 62	Mod 66	Mod 80
61592	1	2	1	2	2

Global Period

Code	Days
61592	090

61595

61595 Transtemporal approach to posterior cranial fossa, jugular foramen or midline skull base, including mastoidectomy, decompression of sigmoid sinus and/or facial nerve, with or without mobilization

AMA Coding Guideline

Skull Base Surgical Procedures

The surgical management of lesions involving the skull base (base of anterior, middle, and posterior cranial fossae) often requires the skills of several surgeons of different surgical specialties working together or in tandem during the operative session. These operations are usually not staged because of the need for definitive closure of dura, subcutaneous tissues, and skin to avoid serious infections such as osteomyelitis and/or meningitis.

The procedures are categorized according to:

The approach procedure is described according to anatomical area involved, ie, anterior cranial fossa, middle cranial fossa, posterior cranial fossa, and brain stem or upper spinal cord.

The definitive procedure(s) describes the repair, biopsy, resection, or excision of various lesions of the skull base and, when appropriate, primary closure of the dura, mucous membranes, and skin.

The repair/reconstruction procedure(s) is reported separately if extensive dural grafting, cranioplasty, local or regional myocutaneous pedicle flaps, or extensive skin grafts are required.

For primary closure, see the appropriate codes (ie, 15730, 15733, 15756, 15757, 15758).

When one surgeon performs the approach procedure, another surgeon performs the definitive procedure, and another surgeon performs the repair/reconstruction procedure, each surgeon reports only the code for the specific procedure performed.

If one surgeon performs more than one procedure (ie, approach procedure and definitive procedure), then both codes are reported, adding modifier 51 to the secondary, additional procedure(s).

AMA Coding Notes

Skull Base Surgical Procedures

(1) approach procedure necessary to obtain adequate exposure to the lesion (pathologic entity), (2) definitive procedure(s) necessary to biopsy, excise or otherwise treat the lesion, and (3) repair/ reconstruction of the defect present following the definitive procedure(s).

Surgical Procedures on the Skull, Meninges, and Brain

(For injection procedure for cerebral angiography, see 36100-36218)

(For injection procedure for ventriculography, see 61026, 61120)

(For injection procedure for pneumoencephalography, use 61055)

AMA *CPT Assistant* □

61595: Winter 93: 18, Mar 18: 11

Plain English Description

A C-shaped incision is made beginning above the ear over the temporal bone, extending in a wide arc around the ear and down the neck. A flap is elevated to expose the temporal muscle, mastoid, and neck structures. A complete mastoidectomy along with removal of the mastoid tip is performed. The sigmoid sinus, a small S-shaped cavity behind the mastoid bone, is denuded of bone except for a small rectangle of bone called Bill's island. The internal carotid artery is exposed and protected. The internal jugular vein is exposed and ligated. The facial nerve is identified and protected. A transtemporal craniotomy is performed with the exact placement of the osteotomies determined by the location of the lesion. Once all neurovascular structures are identified and preserved, lesion dissection begins and is reported separately.

Transtemporal approach to posterior cranial fossa, jugular foramen or midline skull base

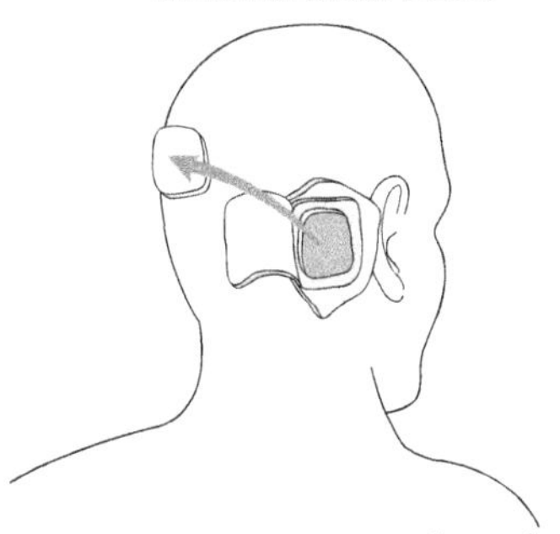

The physician removes a piece of bone above and behind the ear. The physician will decompress the sinus by the ear and/or the facial nerve. The facial nerve may be moved.

ICD-10-CM Diagnostic Codes

C71.6	Malignant neoplasm of cerebellum
C71.7	Malignant neoplasm of brain stem
C79.31	Secondary malignant neoplasm of brain
D33.1	Benign neoplasm of brain, infratentorial
D43.1	Neoplasm of uncertain behavior of brain, infratentorial
D43.3	Neoplasm of uncertain behavior of cranial nerves
G91.4	Hydrocephalus in diseases classified elsewhere

CCI Edits

Refer to Appendix A for CCI edits.

Pub 100

61595: Pub 100-04, 12, 20.4.5

Facility RVUs □

Code	Work	PE Facility	MP	Total Facility
61595	33.74	26.90	7.62	68.26

Non-facility RVUs □

Code	Work	PE Non-Facility	MP	Total Non-Facility
61595	33.74	26.90	7.62	68.26

Modifiers (PAR) □

Code	Mod 50	Mod 51	Mod 62	Mod 66	Mod 80
61595	1	2	1	2	1

Global Period

Code	Days
61595	090

● New ▲ Revised ✚ Add On ⊘Modifier 51 Exempt ★Telemedicine □ CPT QuickRef ⁄FDA Pending ⇄ Laterality Seventh Character ♂Male ♀Female

61597

61597 Transcondylar (far lateral) approach to posterior cranial fossa, jugular foramen or midline skull base, including occipital condylectomy, mastoidectomy, resection of C1-C3 vertebral body(s), decompression of vertebral artery, with or without mobilization

AMA Coding Guideline

Skull Base Surgical Procedures

The surgical management of lesions involving the skull base (base of anterior, middle, and posterior cranial fossae) often requires the skills of several surgeons of different surgical specialties working together or in tandem during the operative session. These operations are usually not staged because of the need for definitive closure of dura, subcutaneous tissues, and skin to avoid serious infections such as osteomyelitis and/or meningitis.

The procedures are categorized according to:

The approach procedure is described according to anatomical area involved, ie, anterior cranial fossa, middle cranial fossa, posterior cranial fossa, and brain stem or upper spinal cord.

The definitive procedure(s) describes the repair, biopsy, resection, or excision of various lesions of the skull base and, when appropriate, primary closure of the dura, mucous membranes, and skin.

The repair/reconstruction procedure(s) is reported separately if extensive dural grafting, cranioplasty, local or regional myocutaneous pedicle flaps, or extensive skin grafts are required.

For primary closure, see the appropriate codes (ie, 15730, 15733, 15756, 15757, 15758).

When one surgeon performs the approach procedure, another surgeon performs the definitive procedure, and another surgeon performs the repair/reconstruction procedure, each surgeon reports only the code for the specific procedure performed.

If one surgeon performs more than one procedure (ie, approach procedure and definitive procedure), then both codes are reported, adding modifier 51 to the secondary, additional procedure(s).

AMA Coding Notes

Skull Base Surgical Procedures

(1) approach procedure necessary to obtain adequate exposure to the lesion (pathologic entity), (2) definitive procedure(s) necessary to biopsy, excise or otherwise treat the lesion, and (3) repair/reconstruction of the defect present following the definitive procedure(s).

Surgical Procedures on the Skull, Meninges, and Brain

(For injection procedure for cerebral angiography, see 36100-36218)

(For injection procedure for ventriculography, see 61026, 61120)

(For injection procedure for pneumoencephalography, use 61055)

AMA *CPT Assistant*

61597: Winter 93: 18

Plain English Description

The transcondylar (far lateral) approach to the posterior cranial fossa, jugular foramen, or midline skull base may be used for resection of neoplastic tumors and vascular lesions, and decompression of the vertebral artery and cranial nerves. The posterior fossa lies at the lowest part of the internal cranial base and contains the cerebellum and brainstem. The jugular foramen is a canal between the petrous temporal bone and the occipital bone that transmits cranial nerves IX, X, and XI, and also contains the sigmoid sinus, which becomes the jugular vein and branches of the occipital artery. With the head immobilized, the scalp is opened using a curved incision starting 2-3 cm behind the ear and extending into the neck along the posterior border of the sternocleidomastoid muscle to C3-C4. The skin and galea are elevated to expose the pericranium above the superficial neck fascia, which may be harvested for later use as a tissue graft for closing the dura. The pericranium and superficial neck fascia are elevated exposing the muscle layers. The trapezius and sternocleidomastoid are encountered first, followed by the splenius capitis, longissimus capitis, and semispinalis capitis. All muscle layers are incised and reflected together to expose the suboccipital triangle, which is bound by a third deeper layer of muscle: the rectus capitis posterior major (medially), the inferior oblique (inferiorly), and superior oblique (supralaterally). The suboccipital triangle is incised to expose the C1 lamina and vertebral artery (VA) and may be extended to expose C2-C3 as necessary. The nerve roots between the cervical vertebrae are identified along with the extradural VA, which is explored from the foramen transversarium of C2 to the occiput, and any decompression completed. Next a suboccipital craniotomy is performed using a drill and/or rongeur and extending to the foramen magnum inferiorly and the occipital condyle laterally. The occipital condyles are a paired part of the occipital bone flanking the foramen magnum that connect the skull to the vertebral column to form the craniovertebral joint (CVJ). The condyle(s) may be reduced for maximum exposure of the CVJ. The craniotomy can be extended up to the transverse sigmoid junction as necessary. The sigmoid sinus and jugular bulb are then exposed, taking care to preserve major blood vessels. By alternating elevating the sigmoid sinus and the presigmoid dura off the mastoid bone, a mastoidectomy may be performed. A hemilaminectomy of C1 (extending to C2-C3 as necessary) is performed and the atlantooccipital membrane is sharply divided to expose the dura. The dura opening may be extended anteriorly to the junction of the transverse and sigmoid sinuses to increase exposure. The dura mater is reflected laterally and tacked with sutures before the definitive procedure.

ICD-10-CM Diagnostic Codes

C41.0	Malignant neoplasm of bones of skull and face
C41.2	Malignant neoplasm of vertebral column
C70.0	Malignant neoplasm of cerebral meninges
C71.6	Malignant neoplasm of cerebellum
C71.7	Malignant neoplasm of brain stem
C72.59	Malignant neoplasm of other cranial nerves
C79.32	Secondary malignant neoplasm of cerebral meninges
C79.49	Secondary malignant neoplasm of other parts of nervous system
C79.51	Secondary malignant neoplasm of bone
D16.6	Benign neoplasm of vertebral column
D32.0	Benign neoplasm of cerebral meninges
D33.1	Benign neoplasm of brain, infratentorial
D43.1	Neoplasm of uncertain behavior of brain, infratentorial
D43.3	Neoplasm of uncertain behavior of cranial nerves
G06.0	Intracranial abscess and granuloma
G06.2	Extradural and subdural abscess, unspecified
G08	Intracranial and intraspinal phlebitis and thrombophlebitis
G91.4	Hydrocephalus in diseases classified elsewhere
Q28.2	Arteriovenous malformation of cerebral vessels
Q28.3	Other malformations of cerebral vessels

CCI Edits

Refer to Appendix A for CCI edits.

Pub 100

61597: Pub 100-04, 12, 20.4.5

Facility RVUs

Code	Work	PE Facility	MP	Total Facility
61597	40.82	29.96	14.21	84.99

Non-facility RVUs

Code	Work	PE Non-Facility	MP	Total Non-Facility
61597	40.82	29.96	14.21	84.99

Modifiers (PAR)

Code	Mod 50	Mod 51	Mod 62	Mod 66	Mod 80
61597	1	2	1	2	2

Global Period

Code	Days
61597	090

61598

61598 Transpetrosal approach to posterior cranial fossa, clivus or foramen magnum, including ligation of superior petrosal sinus and/or sigmoid sinus

AMA Coding Guideline

Skull Base Surgical Procedures

The surgical management of lesions involving the skull base (base of anterior, middle, and posterior cranial fossae) often requires the skills of several surgeons of different surgical specialties working together or in tandem during the operative session. These operations are usually not staged because of the need for definitive closure of dura, subcutaneous tissues, and skin to avoid serious infections such as osteomyelitis and/or meningitis.

The procedures are categorized according to:

The approach procedure is described according to anatomical area involved, ie, anterior cranial fossa, middle cranial fossa, posterior cranial fossa, and brain stem or upper spinal cord.

The definitive procedure(s) describes the repair, biopsy, resection, or excision of various lesions of the skull base and, when appropriate, primary closure of the dura, mucous membranes, and skin.

The repair/reconstruction procedure(s) is reported separately if extensive dural grafting, cranioplasty, local or regional myocutaneous pedicle flaps, or extensive skin grafts are required.

For primary closure, see the appropriate codes (ie, 15730, 15733, 15756, 15757, 15758).

When one surgeon performs the approach procedure, another surgeon performs the definitive procedure, and another surgeon performs the repair/reconstruction procedure, each surgeon reports only the code for the specific procedure performed.

If one surgeon performs more than one procedure (ie, approach procedure and definitive procedure), then both codes are reported, adding modifier 51 to the secondary, additional procedure(s).

AMA Coding Notes

Skull Base Surgical Procedures

(1) approach procedure necessary to obtain adequate exposure to the lesion (pathologic entity), (2) definitive procedure(s) necessary to biopsy, excise or otherwise treat the lesion, and (3) repair/reconstruction of the defect present following the definitive procedure(s).

Surgical Procedures on the Skull, Meninges, and Brain

(For injection procedure for cerebral angiography, see 36100-36218)

(For injection procedure for ventriculography, see 61026, 61120)

(For injection procedure for pneumoencephalography, use 61055)

AMA *CPT Assistant* ▢

61598: Winter 93: 18

Plain English Description

The transpetrosal approach to the posterior cranial fossa, clivus, or foramen magnum may be used to resect neoplastic tumors and vascular lesions. With the head immobilized, the skin is incised starting about 1 cm anterior to the tragus and continuing to the superior temporal line, turned posterior and then caudal to about 6 cm posterior to the external auditory canal and terminating at the mastoid tip. The skin flap is elevated off the temporalis muscle, pericranium, and suboccipital muscles. A flap may be harvested from the pericranium or temporalis fascia for later use in closing the dura. The muscles are then elevated and retracted to expose the bone. A temporo-suboccipital craniotomy is performed by placing multiple burr holes. Using a drill or craniotome to connect the burr holes, the bone flap is then lifted to expose the posterior fossa dura and the transverse sinus. To improve visualization, the squamous temporal bone may be flattened with the drill to the middle fossa floor. The middle fossa dura is elevated toward the petrous ridge, taking care to preserve blood vessels and nerves. Once the ridge has been reached, elevation continues posteriorly toward the arcuate eminence. The sigmoid sinus and presigmoid dura are alternatingly elevated off the mastoid bone facing the sigmoid sinus, and the bone may be resected using cutting burrs and rongeurs. The posterior semicircular canal is identified. The cortical bone is skeletonized, preserving the facial nerve, followed by identification and skeletonization of the superior semicircular canal (SSC). The petrous ridge is then resected at the petrous apex from the SSC to the trigeminal nerve. The posterior fossa is opened along the anterior border of the sigmoid sinus, and the opening is extended caudal to the superior petrosal sinus. The dura is opened through the trigeminal dural ring, retracted, and tacked with stay sutures to allow a clear view of the petroclival region of the brain.

ICD-10-CM Diagnostic Codes

C71.6	Malignant neoplasm of cerebellum
C71.7	Malignant neoplasm of brain stem
C79.31	Secondary malignant neoplasm of brain
D33.1	Benign neoplasm of brain, infratentorial
D43.1	Neoplasm of uncertain behavior of brain, infratentorial
D43.3	Neoplasm of uncertain behavior of cranial nerves
G91.4	Hydrocephalus in diseases classified elsewhere
Q28.2	Arteriovenous malformation of cerebral vessels
Q28.3	Other malformations of cerebral vessels

CCI Edits

Refer to Appendix A for CCI edits.

Pub 100

61598: Pub 100-04, 12, 20.4.5

Facility RVUs ▢

Code	Work	PE Facility	MP	Total Facility
61598	36.53	32.32	13.59	82.44

Non-facility RVUs ▢

Code	Work	PE Non-Facility	MP	Total Non-Facility
61598	36.53	32.32	13.59	82.44

Modifiers (PAR) ▢

Code	Mod 50	Mod 51	Mod 62	Mod 66	Mod 80
61598	0	2	1	2	2

Global Period

Code	Days
61598	090

61600-61601

61600 Resection or excision of neoplastic, vascular or infectious lesion of base of anterior cranial fossa; extradural

61601 Resection or excision of neoplastic, vascular or infectious lesion of base of anterior cranial fossa; intradural, including dural repair, with or without graft

AMA Coding Guideline

Skull Base Surgical Procedures

The surgical management of lesions involving the skull base (base of anterior, middle, and posterior cranial fossae) often requires the skills of several surgeons of different surgical specialties working together or in tandem during the operative session. These operations are usually not staged because of the need for definitive closure of dura, subcutaneous tissues, and skin to avoid serious infections such as osteomyelitis and/or meningitis.

The procedures are categorized according to:

The approach procedure is described according to anatomical area involved, ie, anterior cranial fossa, middle cranial fossa, posterior cranial fossa, and brain stem or upper spinal cord.

The definitive procedure(s) describes the repair, biopsy, resection, or excision of various lesions of the skull base and, when appropriate, primary closure of the dura, mucous membranes, and skin.

The repair/reconstruction procedure(s) is reported separately if extensive dural grafting, cranioplasty, local or regional myocutaneous pedicle flaps, or extensive skin grafts are required.

For primary closure, see the appropriate codes (ie, 15730, 15733, 15756, 15757, 15758).

When one surgeon performs the approach procedure, another surgeon performs the definitive procedure, and another surgeon performs the repair/reconstruction procedure, each surgeon reports only the code for the specific procedure performed.

If one surgeon performs more than one procedure (ie, approach procedure and definitive procedure), then both codes are reported, adding modifier 51 to the secondary, additional procedure(s).

AMA Coding Notes

Skull Base Surgical Procedures

(1) approach procedure necessary to obtain adequate exposure to the lesion (pathologic entity), (2) definitive procedure(s) necessary to biopsy, excise or otherwise treat the lesion, and (3) repair/reconstruction of the defect present following the definitive procedure(s).

Surgical Procedures on the Skull, Meninges, and Brain

(For injection procedure for cerebral angiography, see 36100-36218)

(For injection procedure for ventriculography, see 61026, 61120)

(For injection procedure for pneumoencephalography, use 61055)

AMA *CPT Assistant* ☐

61600: Winter 93: 19, Spring 94: 12, Nov 96: 12

61601: Winter 93: 19, Spring 94: 12

Plain English Description

The anterior fossa is accessed using a separately reported approach. The extradural resection or excision proceeds in a lateral to medial direction and the cribriform plate is examined. If it is determined that the cribriform plate has lesion involvement, osteotomies are performed and the cribriform plate is removed en bloc with the surrounding neoplastic, vascular, or infectious lesion, taking care to preserve the olfactory bulb, cranial nerves, and blood vessels, if possible. The sinus may be explored and a rhinotomy, ethmoidectomy, maxillectomy, or maxillotomy performed as necessary. If the dura can be left intact, it is retracted back to the planum sphenoidale and a drill or chisel is employed to cut bone as necessary to complete the resection or excision of the lesion (61600). If the lesion extends intradurally, the dural sleeves extending along the olfactory nerves are divided; the dura is opened; and resection or excision of the remaining lesion is carried out (61601). The dural defect is then repaired using suture only or interposing a graft material such as autologous pericranium or synthetic adherent such as acellular human dermis or collagen matrix to secure a watertight seal and prevent cerebrospinal fluid leakage. The extradural defect may be filled with autologous graft material such as fascia or fat. The skull deficit is closed using the patient's excised bone, cadaver bone graft, or metal plate, and the incision is sutured in layers. The skin may be closed using staples.

Resection or excision of neoplastic, vascular or infectious lesion of anterior cranial fossa

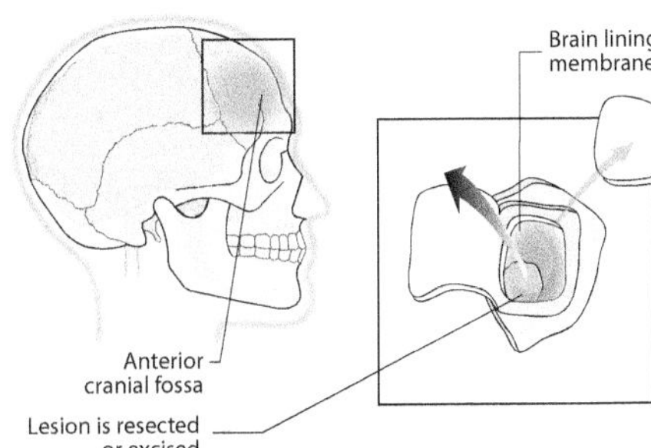

Extradural (61600); intradural, including dural repair, with or without graft (61601)

ICD-10-CM Diagnostic Codes

	Code	Description
	A17.1	Meningeal tuberculoma
	A17.81	Tuberculoma of brain and spinal cord
	B95.0	Streptococcus, group A, as the cause of diseases classified elsewhere
	B95.1	Streptococcus, group B, as the cause of diseases classified elsewhere
	B95.3	Streptococcus pneumoniae as the cause of diseases classified elsewhere
	B95.4	Other streptococcus as the cause of diseases classified elsewhere
	B95.61	Methicillin susceptible Staphylococcus aureus infection as the cause of diseases classified elsewhere
	B95.62	Methicillin resistant Staphylococcus aureus infection as the cause of diseases classified elsewhere
	B95.7	Other staphylococcus as the cause of diseases classified elsewhere
	B96.3	Hemophilus influenzae [H. influenzae] as the cause of diseases classified elsewhere
	B96.89	Other specified bacterial agents as the cause of diseases classified elsewhere
	C31.0	Malignant neoplasm of maxillary sinus
	C31.1	Malignant neoplasm of ethmoidal sinus
	C31.3	Malignant neoplasm of sphenoid sinus
	C31.8	Malignant neoplasm of overlapping sites of accessory sinuses
	C41.0	Malignant neoplasm of bones of skull and face
	C41.9	Malignant neoplasm of bone and articular cartilage, unspecified
	C49.0	Malignant neoplasm of connective and soft tissue of head, face and neck
⇄	C69.61	Malignant neoplasm of right orbit
⇄	C69.62	Malignant neoplasm of left orbit
⇄	C69.81	Malignant neoplasm of overlapping sites of right eye and adnexa
⇄	C69.82	Malignant neoplasm of overlapping sites of left eye and adnexa
	C70.0	Malignant neoplasm of cerebral meninges
	C72.50	Malignant neoplasm of unspecified cranial nerve
	C72.59	Malignant neoplasm of other cranial nerves
	C78.39	Secondary malignant neoplasm of other respiratory organs
	C79.32	Secondary malignant neoplasm of cerebral meninges
	C79.49	Secondary malignant neoplasm of other parts of nervous system
	C79.51	Secondary malignant neoplasm of bone
	C79.89	Secondary malignant neoplasm of other specified sites
	D16.4	Benign neoplasm of bones of skull and face
⇄	D31.6	Benign neoplasm of unspecified site of orbit

	D32.0	Benign neoplasm of cerebral meninges
	D33.3	Benign neoplasm of cranial nerves
	D42.0	Neoplasm of uncertain behavior of cerebral meninges
	D43.3	Neoplasm of uncertain behavior of cranial nerves
	D48.0	Neoplasm of uncertain behavior of bone and articular cartilage
	D48.7	Neoplasm of uncertain behavior of other specified sites
	F07.0	Personality change due to known physiological condition
	G06.0	Intracranial abscess and granuloma
	G06.2	Extradural and subdural abscess, unspecified
	G08	Intracranial and intraspinal phlebitis and thrombophlebitis
	G46.0	Middle cerebral artery syndrome
⇄	H47.091	Other disorders of optic nerve, not elsewhere classified, right eye
⇄	H47.092	Other disorders of optic nerve, not elsewhere classified, left eye
⇄	H47.093	Other disorders of optic nerve, not elsewhere classified, bilateral
	H47.11	Papilledema associated with increased intracranial pressure
⇄	H47.141	Foster-Kennedy syndrome, right eye
⇄	H47.142	Foster-Kennedy syndrome, left eye
⇄	H47.143	Foster-Kennedy syndrome, bilateral
	H53.8	Other visual disturbances
⇄	I60.11	Nontraumatic subarachnoid hemorrhage from right middle cerebral artery
⇄	I60.12	Nontraumatic subarachnoid hemorrhage from left middle cerebral artery
	I60.7	Nontraumatic subarachnoid hemorrhage from unspecified intracranial artery
	I60.8	Other nontraumatic subarachnoid hemorrhage
	I61.1	Nontraumatic intracerebral hemorrhage in hemisphere, cortical
	I61.8	Other nontraumatic intracerebral hemorrhage
	J32.0	Chronic maxillary sinusitis
	J32.1	Chronic frontal sinusitis
	J32.2	Chronic ethmoidal sinusitis
	J32.3	Chronic sphenoidal sinusitis
	J32.4	Chronic pansinusitis
	J32.8	Other chronic sinusitis
	Q28.2	Arteriovenous malformation of cerebral vessels
	Q28.3	Other malformations of cerebral vessels
	R41.3	Other amnesia
	R43.0	Anosmia

CCI Edits

Refer to Appendix A for CCI edits.

Pub 100

61600: Pub 100-04, 12, 20.4.5
61601: Pub 100-04, 12, 20.4.5

Facility RVUs ▯

Code	Work	PE Facility	MP	Total Facility
61600	30.01	25.23	6.12	61.36
61601	31.14	27.89	10.58	69.61

Non-facility RVUs ▯

Code	Work	PE Non-Facility	MP	Total Non-Facility
61600	30.01	25.23	6.12	61.36
61601	31.14	27.89	10.58	69.61

Modifiers (PAR) ▯

Code	Mod 50	Mod 51	Mod 62	Mod 66	Mod 80
61600	0	2	1	2	2
61601	0	2	1	2	2

Global Period

Code	Days
61600	090
61601	090

61605-61606

61605 Resection or excision of neoplastic, vascular or infectious lesion of infratemporal fossa, parapharyngeal space, petrous apex; extradural

61606 Resection or excision of neoplastic, vascular or infectious lesion of infratemporal fossa, parapharyngeal space, petrous apex; intradural, including dural repair, with or without graft

AMA Coding Guideline

Skull Base Surgical Procedures

The surgical management of lesions involving the skull base (base of anterior, middle, and posterior cranial fossae) often requires the skills of several surgeons of different surgical specialties working together or in tandem during the operative session. These operations are usually not staged because of the need for definitive closure of dura, subcutaneous tissues, and skin to avoid serious infections such as osteomyelitis and/or meningitis.

The procedures are categorized according to:

The approach procedure is described according to anatomical area involved, ie, anterior cranial fossa, middle cranial fossa, posterior cranial fossa, and brain stem or upper spinal cord.

The definitive procedure(s) describes the repair, biopsy, resection, or excision of various lesions of the skull base and, when appropriate, primary closure of the dura, mucous membranes, and skin.

The repair/reconstruction procedure(s) is reported separately if extensive dural grafting, cranioplasty, local or regional myocutaneous pedicle flaps, or extensive skin grafts are required.

For primary closure, see the appropriate codes (ie, 15730, 15733, 15756, 15757, 15758).

When one surgeon performs the approach procedure, another surgeon performs the definitive procedure, and another surgeon performs the repair/ reconstruction procedure, each surgeon reports only the code for the specific procedure performed.

If one surgeon performs more than one procedure (ie, approach procedure and definitive procedure), then both codes are reported, adding modifier 51 to the secondary, additional procedure(s).

AMA Coding Notes

Skull Base Surgical Procedures

(1) approach procedure necessary to obtain adequate exposure to the lesion (pathologic entity), (2) definitive procedure(s) necessary to biopsy, excise or otherwise treat the lesion, and (3) repair/ reconstruction of the defect present following the definitive procedure(s).

Surgical Procedures on the Skull, Meninges, and Brain

(For injection procedure for cerebral angiography, see 36100-36218)

(For injection procedure for ventriculography, see 61026, 61120)

(For injection procedure for pneumoencephalography, use 61055)

AMA *CPT Assistant*

61605: Winter 93: 19
61606: Winter 93: 20

Plain English Description

The infratemporal fossa, parapharyngeal space, and petrous apex are accessed using a separately reportable approach. The extradural space between the periosteal dura layer attached to the cranium and the endosteal dura layer protecting the brain is explored and lesion(s) are resected as necessary (61605). For an intradural procedure (61606), the endosteal dura is entered and resection or excision proceeds with skeletonization of the infratemporal fossa to the base of the middle cranial fossa in a posteroanterior direction. The cartilaginous Eustachian tube is examined for lesions and resected as necessary. Care is taken to preserve the maxillary artery and trigeminal nerve and their branches. The parapharyngeal space is explored and any lesion is resected/excised as necessary. The pterygoid muscles are examined and resected, preserving or ligating the pterygoid venous plexus as necessary. The lateral and medial pterygoid plates and the petrous apex may be drilled or chiseled to remove lesions. The dural defect is repaired using suture only or interposing a graft material such as autologous pericranium or a synthetic adherent, such as acellular human dermis or collagen matrix, to secure a watertight seal and prevent cerebrospinal fluid leakage. The extradural deficit may be filled with autologous graft material such as fascia or fat. The zygomatic arch is wired; the incision is sutured in layers; and the skin may be closed using staples.

Resection or excision of neoplastic, vascular or infectious lesion of infratemporal fossa, parapharyngeal space, petrous apex

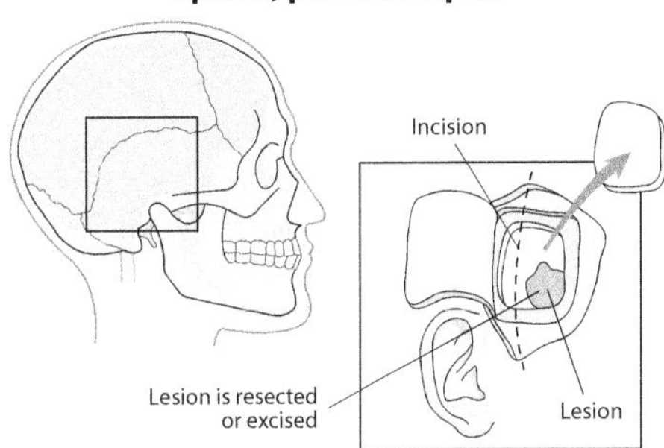

ICD-10-CM Diagnostic Codes

C11.0	Malignant neoplasm of superior wall of nasopharynx
C11.1	Malignant neoplasm of posterior wall of nasopharynx
C11.2	Malignant neoplasm of lateral wall of nasopharynx
C11.3	Malignant neoplasm of anterior wall of nasopharynx
C11.8	Malignant neoplasm of overlapping sites of nasopharynx
C41.0	Malignant neoplasm of bones of skull and face
C49.0	Malignant neoplasm of connective and soft tissue of head, face and neck
C70.0	Malignant neoplasm of cerebral meninges
C72.59	Malignant neoplasm of other cranial nerves
C79.49	Secondary malignant neoplasm of other parts of nervous system
C79.51	Secondary malignant neoplasm of bone
C79.89	Secondary malignant neoplasm of other specified sites
D10.6	Benign neoplasm of nasopharynx
D16.4	Benign neoplasm of bones of skull and face
D21.0	Benign neoplasm of connective and other soft tissue of head, face and neck
D32.0	Benign neoplasm of cerebral meninges
D33.3	Benign neoplasm of cranial nerves
D37.05	Neoplasm of uncertain behavior of pharynx
D42.0	Neoplasm of uncertain behavior of cerebral meninges
D48.0	Neoplasm of uncertain behavior of bone and articular cartilage
D48.1	Neoplasm of uncertain behavior of connective and other soft tissue
G06.0	Intracranial abscess and granuloma
G53	Cranial nerve disorders in diseases classified elsewhere
J38.01	Paralysis of vocal cords and larynx, unilateral
J38.02	Paralysis of vocal cords and larynx, bilateral
R13.19	Other dysphagia
R47.81	Slurred speech
R49.0	Dysphonia

CCI Edits

Refer to Appendix A for CCI edits.

Pub 100

61605: Pub 100-04, 12, 20.4.5
61606: Pub 100-04, 12, 20.4.5

Facility RVUs ▯

Code	Work	PE Facility	MP	Total Facility
61605	32.57	24.71	4.96	62.24
61606	42.05	29.61	13.14	84.80

Non-facility RVUs ▯

Code	Work	PE Non-Facility	MP	Total Non-Facility
61605	32.57	24.71	4.96	62.24
61606	42.05	29.61	13.14	84.80

Modifiers (PAR) ▯

Code	Mod 50	Mod 51	Mod 62	Mod 66	Mod 80
61605	0	2	1	2	2
61606	0	2	1	2	2

Global Period

Code	Days
61605	090
61606	090

61607-61608

61607 Resection or excision of neoplastic, vascular or infectious lesion of parasellar area, cavernous sinus, clivus or midline skull base; extradural

61608 Resection or excision of neoplastic, vascular or infectious lesion of parasellar area, cavernous sinus, clivus or midline skull base; intradural, including dural repair, with or without graft

AMA Coding Guideline

Skull Base Surgical Procedures

The surgical management of lesions involving the skull base (base of anterior, middle, and posterior cranial fossae) often requires the skills of several surgeons of different surgical specialties working together or in tandem during the operative session. These operations are usually not staged because of the need for definitive closure of dura, subcutaneous tissues, and skin to avoid serious infections such as osteomyelitis and/or meningitis.

The procedures are categorized according to:

The approach procedure is described according to anatomical area involved, ie, anterior cranial fossa, middle cranial fossa, posterior cranial fossa, and brain stem or upper spinal cord.

The definitive procedure(s) describes the repair, biopsy, resection, or excision of various lesions of the skull base and, when appropriate, primary closure of the dura, mucous membranes, and skin.

The repair/reconstruction procedure(s) is reported separately if extensive dural grafting, cranioplasty, local or regional myocutaneous pedicle flaps, or extensive skin grafts are required.

For primary closure, see the appropriate codes (ie, 15730, 15733, 15756, 15757, 15758).

When one surgeon performs the approach procedure, another surgeon performs the definitive procedure, and another surgeon performs the repair/reconstruction procedure, each surgeon reports only the code for the specific procedure performed.

If one surgeon performs more than one procedure (ie, approach procedure and definitive procedure), then both codes are reported, adding modifier 51 to the secondary, additional procedure(s).

AMA Coding Notes

Skull Base Surgical Procedures

(1) approach procedure necessary to obtain adequate exposure to the lesion (pathologic entity), (2) definitive procedure(s) necessary to biopsy, excise or otherwise treat the lesion, and (3) repair/reconstruction of the defect present following the definitive procedure(s).

Surgical Procedures on the Skull, Meninges, and Brain

(For injection procedure for cerebral angiography, see 36100-36218)

(For injection procedure for ventriculography, see 61026, 61120)

(For injection procedure for pneumoencephalography, use 61055)

AMA *CPT Assistant*

61607: Winter 93: 20
61608: Winter 93: 20

Plain English Description

The parasellar area, cavernous sinus, clivus, or midline skull base is accessed using a separately reportable approach. Resection or excision of the neoplastic, vascular, or infectious lesion proceeds through the sella turcica, the central area of the sphenoid bone covered by dura housing the hypothalamus, optic chiasm, and pituitary gland. It then extends laterally into the cavernous sinus containing a network of blood vessels and nerves. Care is taken to preserve the carotid arteries, cranial nerves III, IV, and VI inside the cavernous sinus, and cranial nerve V outside its walls. Dura forms the inside walls of the cavernous sinus, which maintains separation of the pituitary gland from the brain. The dural tent is opened (61608) using blunt or sharp dissection toward the clivus, the shallow depression behind the dorsum sellae, which slopes sharply backwards to the anterior portion of the basilar occipital bone or midline skull base where it joins the sphenoid bone. The lesion is removed en bloc whenever possible or debulked to the greatest extent and the surgical area is checked for bleeding. The dural defect is then repaired using suture only (primary closure) or interposing a graft material such as autologous pericranium or synthetic adherent such as acellular human dermis or collagen matrix to secure a watertight seal and prevent cerebrospinal fluid (CSF) leakage. The extradural deficit may be filled with autologous graft material (fascia, fat, the bone). The skull deficit is closed using the patient's excised bone, cadaver bone graft, or metal plate; the incision is sutured in layers; and the skin may be closed using staples. If the dura is not opened for the lesion to be excised or resected, report 61607.

Resection or excision of neoplastic, vascular or infectious lesion of parasellar area, cavernous sinus, clivus or midline skull base; Intradural

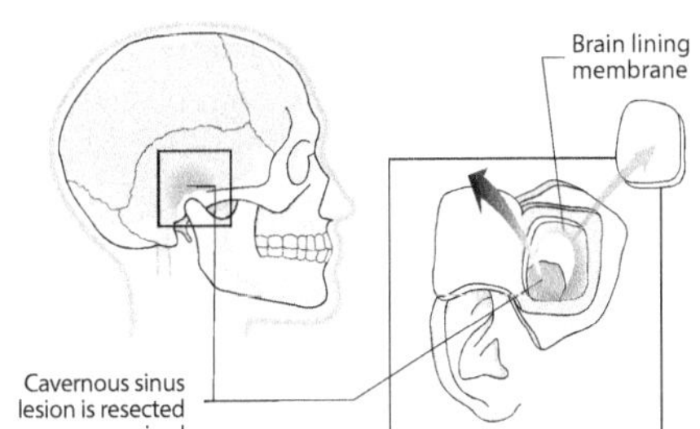

Extradural (61607; intradural (61608)

ICD-10-CM Diagnostic Codes

C41.0	Malignant neoplasm of bones of skull and face
C70.0	Malignant neoplasm of cerebral meninges
C72.50	Malignant neoplasm of unspecified cranial nerve
C72.9	Malignant neoplasm of central nervous system, unspecified
C79.32	Secondary malignant neoplasm of cerebral meninges
C79.49	Secondary malignant neoplasm of other parts of nervous system
C79.51	Secondary malignant neoplasm of bone
D16.4	Benign neoplasm of bones of skull and face
D32.0	Benign neoplasm of cerebral meninges
D33.3	Benign neoplasm of cranial nerves
D33.9	Benign neoplasm of central nervous system, unspecified
D42.0	Neoplasm of uncertain behavior of cerebral meninges
D43.3	Neoplasm of uncertain behavior of cranial nerves
D43.8	Neoplasm of uncertain behavior of other specified parts of central nervous system
D48.0	Neoplasm of uncertain behavior of bone and articular cartilage
G06.0	Intracranial abscess and granuloma
G06.2	Extradural and subdural abscess, unspecified
G08	Intracranial and intraspinal phlebitis and thrombophlebitis

CCI Edits

Refer to Appendix A for CCI edits.

Pub 100

61607: Pub 100-04, 12, 20.4.5
61608: Pub 100-04, 12, 20.4.5

Facility RVUs

Code	Work	PE Facility	MP	Total Facility
61607	40.93	26.69	9.69	77.31
61608	45.54	32.61	16.05	94.20

Non-facility RVUs

Code	Work	PE Non-Facility	MP	Total Non-Facility
61607	40.93	26.69	9.69	77.31
61608	45.54	32.61	16.05	94.20

Modifiers (PAR)

Code	Mod 50	Mod 51	Mod 62	Mod 66	Mod 80
61607	0	2	1	2	2
61608	0	2	1	2	2

Global Period

Code	Days
61607	090
61608	090

61615-61616

61615 Resection or excision of neoplastic, vascular or infectious lesion of base of posterior cranial fossa, jugular foramen, foramen magnum, or C1-C3 vertebral bodies; extradural

61616 Resection or excision of neoplastic, vascular or infectious lesion of base of posterior cranial fossa, jugular foramen, foramen magnum, or C1-C3 vertebral bodies; intradural, including dural repair, with or without graft

AMA Coding Guideline

Skull Base Surgical Procedures

The surgical management of lesions involving the skull base (basc of anterior, middle, and posterior cranial fossae) often requires the skills of several surgeons of different surgical specialties working together or in tandem during the operative session. These operations are usually not staged because of the need for definitive closure of dura, subcutaneous tissues, and skin to avoid serious infections such as osteomyelitis and/or meningitis.

The procedures are categorized according to:

The approach procedure is described according to anatomical area involved, ie, anterior cranial fossa, middle cranial fossa, posterior cranial fossa, and brain stem or upper spinal cord.

The definitive procedure(s) describes the repair, biopsy, resection, or excision of various lesions of the skull base and, when appropriate, primary closure of the dura, mucous membranes, and skin.

The repair/reconstruction procedure(s) is reported separately if extensive dural grafting, cranioplasty, local or regional myocutaneous pedicle flaps, or extensive skin grafts are required.

For primary closure, see the appropriate codes (ie, 15730, 15733, 15756, 15757, 15758).

When one surgeon performs the approach procedure, another surgeon performs the definitive procedure, and another surgeon performs the repair/reconstruction procedure, each surgeon reports only the code for the specific procedure performed.

If one surgeon performs more than one procedure (ie, approach procedure and definitive procedure), then both codes are reported, adding modifier 51 to the secondary, additional procedure(s).

AMA Coding Notes

Skull Base Surgical Procedures

(1) approach procedure necessary to obtain adequate exposure to the lesion (pathologic entity), (2) definitive procedure(s) necessary to biopsy, excise or otherwise treat the lesion, and (3) repair/reconstruction of the defect present following the definitive procedure(s).

Surgical Procedures on the Skull, Meninges, and Brain

(For injection procedure for cerebral angiography, see 36100-36218)

(For injection procedure for ventriculography, see 61026, 61120)

(For injection procedure for pneumoencephalography, use 61055)

AMA *CPT Assistant*

61615: Winter 93: 20

61616: Mar 18: 11

Plain English Description

The physician removes a lesion from the base of the skull. The lesion may be behind one of the top three vertebrae directly under the back of the head, and is located outside of the membrane that covers the brain.

Resection or excision of neoplastic, vascular or infectious lesion of base of posterior cranial fossa, jugular foramen, foramen magnum, or C1-C3 vertebral bodies

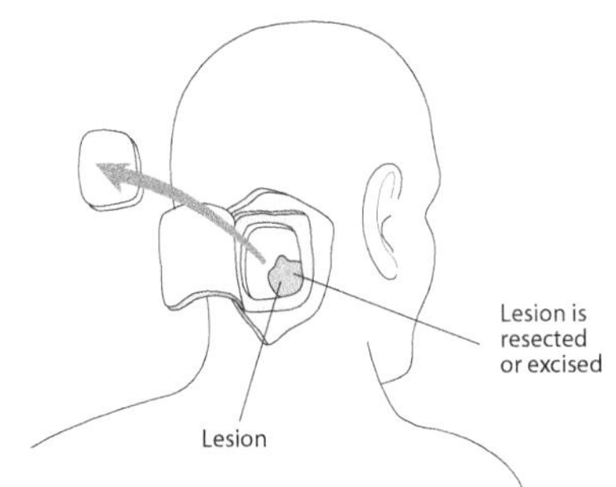

ICD-10-CM Diagnostic Codes

C41.0	Malignant neoplasm of bones of skull and face
C41.2	Malignant neoplasm of vertebral column
C70.0	Malignant neoplasm of cerebral meninges
C71.6	Malignant neoplasm of cerebellum
C71.7	Malignant neoplasm of brain stem
C72.59	Malignant neoplasm of other cranial nerves
C79.32	Secondary malignant neoplasm of cerebral meninges
C79.49	Secondary malignant neoplasm of other parts of nervous system
C79.51	Secondary malignant neoplasm of bone
D16.6	Benign neoplasm of vertebral column
D32.0	Benign neoplasm of cerebral meninges
D33.1	Benign neoplasm of brain, infratentorial
D43.1	Neoplasm of uncertain behavior of brain, infratentorial
D43.3	Neoplasm of uncertain behavior of cranial nerves
G06.0	Intracranial abscess and granuloma
G06.2	Extradural and subdural abscess, unspecified
G08	Intracranial and intraspinal phlebitis and thrombophlebitis
G91.4	Hydrocephalus in diseases classified elsewhere
Q28.2	Arteriovenous malformation of cerebral vessels
Q28.3	Other malformations of cerebral vessels

CCI Edits

Refer to Appendix A for CCI edits.

Pub 100

61615: Pub 100-04, 12, 20.4.5

61616: Pub 100-04, 12, 20.4.5

Facility RVUs

Code	Work	PE Facility	MP	Total Facility
61615	35.77	32.23	13.30	81.30
61616	46.74	34.29	15.02	96.05

Non-facility RVUs

Code	Work	PE Non-Facility	MP	Total Non-Facility
61615	35.77	32.23	13.30	81.30
61616	46.74	34.29	15.02	96.05

Modifiers (PAR)

Code	Mod 50	Mod 51	Mod 62	Mod 66	Mod 80
61615	0	2	1	2	2
61616	0	2	1	2	2

Global Period

Code	Days
61615	090
61616	090

61618-61619

61618 Secondary repair of dura for cerebrospinal fluid leak, anterior, middle or posterior cranial fossa following surgery of the skull base; by free tissue graft (eg, pericranium, fascia, tensor fascia lata, adipose tissue, homologous or synthetic grafts)

61619 Secondary repair of dura for cerebrospinal fluid leak, anterior, middle or posterior cranial fossa following surgery of the skull base; by local or regionalized vascularized pedicle flap or myocutaneous flap (including galea, temporalis, frontalis or occipitalis muscle)

AMA Coding Guideline

Skull Base Surgical Procedures

The surgical management of lesions involving the skull base (base of anterior, middle, and posterior cranial fossae) often requires the skills of several surgeons of different surgical specialties working together or in tandem during the operative session. These operations are usually not staged because of the need for definitive closure of dura, subcutaneous tissues, and skin to avoid serious infections such as osteomyelitis and/or meningitis.

The procedures are categorized according to:

The approach procedure is described according to anatomical area involved, ie, anterior cranial fossa, middle cranial fossa, posterior cranial fossa, and brain stem or upper spinal cord.

The definitive procedure(s) describes the repair, biopsy, resection, or excision of various lesions of the skull base and, when appropriate, primary closure of the dura, mucous membranes, and skin.

The repair/reconstruction procedure(s) is reported separately if extensive dural grafting, cranioplasty, local or regional myocutaneous pedicle flaps, or extensive skin grafts are required.

For primary closure, see the appropriate codes (ie, 15730, 15733, 15756, 15757, 15758).

When one surgeon performs the approach procedure, another surgeon performs the definitive procedure, and another surgeon performs the repair/reconstruction procedure, each surgeon reports only the code for the specific procedure performed.

If one surgeon performs more than one procedure (ie, approach procedure and definitive procedure), then both codes are reported, adding modifier 51 to the secondary, additional procedure(s).

AMA Coding Notes

Skull Base Surgical Procedures

(1) approach procedure necessary to obtain adequate exposure to the lesion (pathologic entity), (2) definitive procedure(s) necessary to biopsy, excise or otherwise treat the lesion, and (3) repair/reconstruction of the defect present following the definitive procedure(s).

Surgical Procedures on the Skull, Meninges, and Brain

(For injection procedure for cerebral angiography, see 36100-36218)

(For injection procedure for ventriculography, see 61026, 61120)

(For injection procedure for pneumoencephalography, use 61055)

AMA *CPT Assistant*

61618: Winter 93: 20, Spring 94: 19, Mar 00: 11
61619: Winter 93: 20, Spring 94: 19, Mar 00: 11

Plain English Description

Secondary repair of the dura may be required to manage leakage of cerebrospinal fluid (CSF) from the anterior, middle, or posterior cranial fossa(s) when primary closure fails following surgery of the skull base and resection of tumors or repair of vascular lesions. A free tissue graft (61618), harvested during the surgical approach (pericranium, fascia, tensor fascia lata) or with a separately reported procedure (adipose tissue, homologous graft) or synthetic graft (titanium mesh, high-viscosity polymethylmethacrylate, porcine dermis), are trimmed to the desired size and shape and placed over the dural deficit. Beginning at the inferior midline and continuing bilaterally around the dural deficit, the graft is sutured into place creating a watertight closure. The graft may be checked for leakage by irrigating inside the graft with saline before placing the final closing sutures and reinforcing where necessary. For closure using local or regionalized vascularized pedical flap or myocutaneous flap (61619) including the galea, temporalis, frontalis, or occipital muscle, the flap is unrolled and evaluated for viability. The graft is then rotated, trimmed to fit the deficit, tacked to the dura, and closed in layers using sutures ensuring a watertight seal as described for code 61618.

Secondary repair of dura for cerebrospinal fluid leak/anterior/middle/posterior cranial fossa; local/regionalized vascularized pedicle/myocutaneous flap

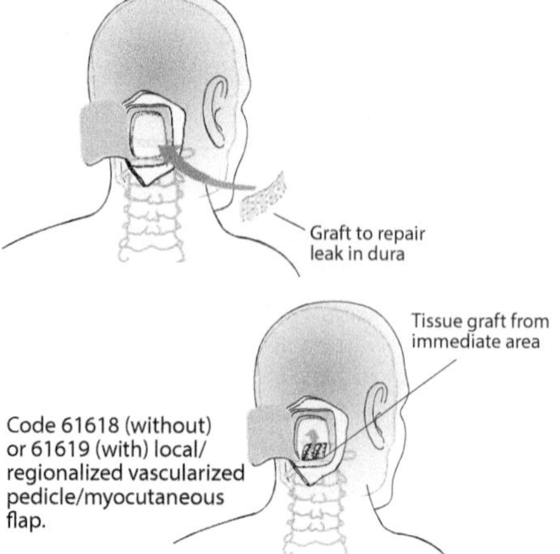

ICD-10-CM Diagnostic Codes

G96.0	Cerebrospinal fluid leak
G97.82	Other postprocedural complications and disorders of nervous system

CCI Edits

Refer to Appendix A for CCI edits.

Pub 100

61618: Pub 100-04, 12, 20.4.5
61619: Pub 100-04, 12, 20.4.5

Facility RVUs

Code	Work	PE Facility	MP	Total Facility
61618	18.69	12.68	5.49	36.86
61619	22.10	13.46	5.07	40.63

Non-facility RVUs

Code	Work	PE Non-Facility	MP	Total Non-Facility
61618	18.69	12.68	5.49	36.86
61619	22.10	13.46	5.07	40.63

Modifiers (PAR)

Code	Mod 50	Mod 51	Mod 62	Mod 66	Mod 80
61618	0	2	1	2	2
61619	0	2	1	2	2

Global Period

Code	Days
61618	090
61619	090

61623

61623 Endovascular temporary balloon arterial occlusion, head or neck (extracranial/intracranial) including selective catheterization of vessel to be occluded, positioning and inflation of occlusion balloon, concomitant neurological monitoring, and radiologic supervision and interpretation of all angiography required for balloon occlusion and to exclude vascular injury post occlusion

(If selective catheterization and angiography of arteries other than artery to be occluded is performed, use appropriate catheterization and radiologic supervision and interpretation codes)

(If complete diagnostic angiography of the artery to be occluded is performed immediately prior to temporary occlusion, use appropriate radiologic supervision and interpretation codes only)

AMA Coding Notes

Surgical Procedures on the Skull, Meninges, and Brain

(For injection procedure for cerebral angiography, see 36100-36218)

(For injection procedure for ventriculography, see 61026, 61120)

(For injection procedure for pneumoencephalography, use 61055)

Plain English Description

Temporary balloon occlusion is performed prior to permanent occlusion to determine whether permanent occlusion of the artery can be performed without causing neurovascular compromise or injury such as a stroke. An access artery is selected and punctured. An introducer sheath is placed over the needle and the needle withdrawn. A guidewire is inserted and advanced to the target vessel in the head or neck under fluoroscopic guidance. A neuroangiography catheter is advanced over the guidewire and the guidewire removed. Diagnostic angiography is performed to confirm the vascular anomaly and to evaluate the vasculature prior to balloon occlusion. Following completion of the diagnostic angiography, the angiography catheter is positioned in the artery to be occluded. A guidewire is reintroduced through the catheter and advanced to the target vessel. The angiography catheter is removed and the temporary balloon occlusion catheter advanced over the guidewire. A neurological examination is performed prior to deployment of the balloon. Intra-arterial pressure measurements are obtained within the target vessel. The balloon is inflated and the artery occluded. Contrast is injected to confirm vessel occlusion. Arterial pressures are again obtained and a neurological examination performed to confirm neurological stability. Timed neurological evaluation and arterial pressure measurements are performed over the next 30 minutes to ensure that there is no change in neurological status. The temporary occlusion balloon is then deflated and removed. A completion angiogram is performed to exclude any vascular injury following the temporary occlusion procedure.

Endovascular temporary balloon arterial occlusion, head or neck

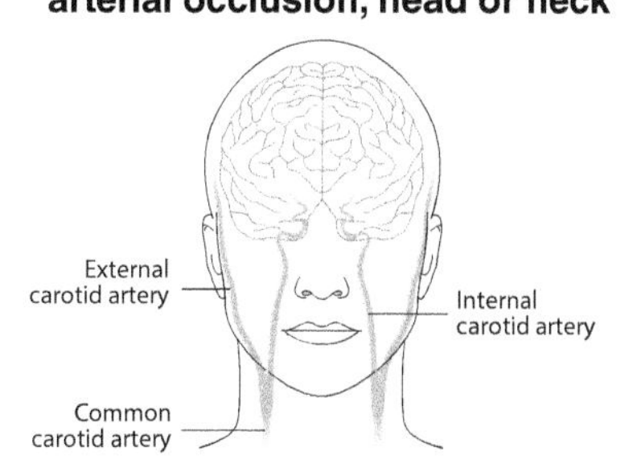

Balloon is delivered by catheter

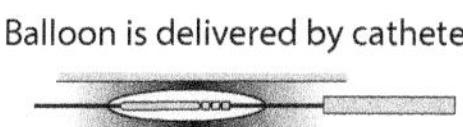

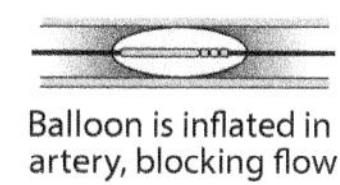

Balloon is inflated in artery, blocking flow

A balloon is inserted into an artery in the head or neck and inflated to cause temporary blockage.

ICD-10-CM Diagnostic Codes

C49.0	Malignant neoplasm of connective and soft tissue of head, face and neck
C70.0	Malignant neoplasm of cerebral meninges
C71.0	Malignant neoplasm of cerebrum, except lobes and ventricles
C71.1	Malignant neoplasm of frontal lobe
C71.2	Malignant neoplasm of temporal lobe
C71.3	Malignant neoplasm of parietal lobe
C71.4	Malignant neoplasm of occipital lobe
C71.5	Malignant neoplasm of cerebral ventricle
C71.6	Malignant neoplasm of cerebellum
C71.7	Malignant neoplasm of brain stem
C71.8	Malignant neoplasm of overlapping sites of brain
C72.59	Malignant neoplasm of other cranial nerves
C79.31	Secondary malignant neoplasm of brain
C79.32	Secondary malignant neoplasm of cerebral meninges
C79.49	Secondary malignant neoplasm of other parts of nervous system
C79.89	Secondary malignant neoplasm of other specified sites
I67.0	Dissection of cerebral arteries, nonruptured
I67.1	Cerebral aneurysm, nonruptured
I72.0	Aneurysm of carotid artery
I72.5	Aneurysm of other precerebral arteries
I72.6	Aneurysm of vertebral artery
I72.8	Aneurysm of other specified arteries
I77.71	Dissection of carotid artery
I77.74	Dissection of vertebral artery
I77.75	Dissection of other precerebral arteries
Q28.0	Arteriovenous malformation of precerebral vessels
Q28.1	Other malformations of precerebral vessels
Q28.2	Arteriovenous malformation of cerebral vessels
Q28.3	Other malformations of cerebral vessels

CCI Edits

Refer to Appendix A for CCI edits.

Pub 100

61623: Pub 100-04, 12, 20.4.5

Facility RVUs

Code	Work	PE Facility	MP	Total Facility
61623	9.95	4.02	2.59	16.56

Non-facility RVUs

Code	Work	PE Non-Facility	MP	Total Non-Facility
61623	9.95	4.02	2.59	16.56

Modifiers (PAR)

Code	Mod 50	Mod 51	Mod 62	Mod 66	Mod 80
61623	0	2	0	0	1

Global Period

Code	Days
61623	000

61624-61626

61624 Transcatheter permanent occlusion or embolization (eg, for tumor destruction, to achieve hemostasis, to occlude a vascular malformation), percutaneous, any method; central nervous system (intracranial, spinal cord)

(For non-central nervous system and non-head or neck embolization, see 37241-37244)

(For radiological supervision and interpretation, use 75894)

61626 Transcatheter permanent occlusion or embolization (eg, for tumor destruction, to achieve hemostasis, to occlude a vascular malformation), percutaneous, any method; non-central nervous system, head or neck (extracranial, brachiocephalic branch)

(For non-central nervous system and non-head or neck embolization, see 37241-37244)

(For radiological supervision and interpretation, use 75894)

AMA Coding Notes

Surgical Procedures on the Skull, Meninges, and Brain

(For injection procedure for cerebral angiography, see 36100-36218)

(For injection procedure for ventriculography, see 61026, 61120)

(For injection procedure for pneumoencephalography, use 61055)

AMA *CPT Assistant*

61624: Jun 99: 10, Nov 06: 8, Nov 13: 6

61626: Nov 13: 6

Plain English Description

The physician performs a permanent percutaneous transcatheter occlusion or embolization procedure on a central nervous system (CNS) artery (61624) or non-CNS head or neck artery (61626). Occlusion or embolization procedures are performed for tumor destruction, to achieve hemostasis, or to occlude a vascular malformation. CNS arteries include intracranial and spinal cord arteries. Non-CNS arteries include extracranial arteries and arterial branches off the brachiocephalic arteries. An access artery is selected and punctured. An introducer sheath is placed over the needle and the needle withdrawn. A guidewire is inserted and advanced to the target vessel using separately reportable imaging guidance. An angiography catheter is advanced over the guidewire and the guidewire removed. Diagnostic angiography is performed to confirm the vascular anomaly and to evaluate the vasculature prior to the permanent occlusion or embolization procedure. Following completion of the diagnostic angiography, the angiography catheter is positioned in the artery to be occluded. A guidewire is reintroduced through the catheter and advanced to the target vessel. The angiography catheter is removed and the embolization or occlusion catheter advanced over the guidewire. A neurological examination is performed prior to placing the occlusion device or injecting the embolizing agent. The occlusion device is then inserted through the catheter and deployed or the embolizing agent is injected. Contrast is injected to confirm vessel occlusion. A post-procedure neurological examination is performed to confirm neurological stability.

Transcatheter permanent occlusion or embolization, percutaneous, any method

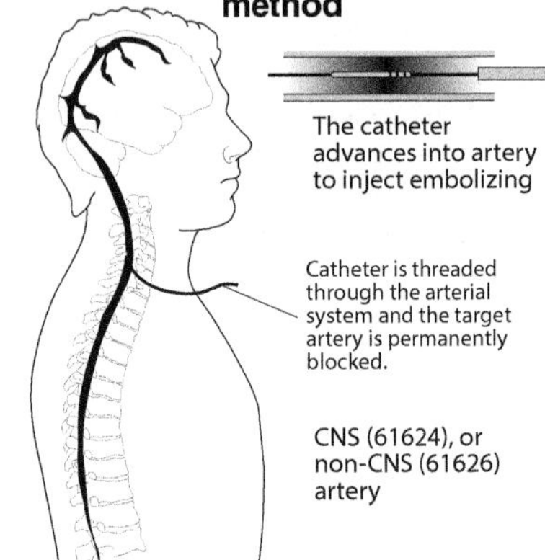

ICD-10-CM Diagnostic Codes

C49.0	Malignant neoplasm of connective and soft tissue of head, face and neck
C70.0	Malignant neoplasm of cerebral meninges
C71.0	Malignant neoplasm of cerebrum, except lobes and ventricles
C71.1	Malignant neoplasm of frontal lobe
C71.2	Malignant neoplasm of temporal lobe
C71.3	Malignant neoplasm of parietal lobe
C71.4	Malignant neoplasm of occipital lobe
C71.5	Malignant neoplasm of cerebral ventricle
C71.6	Malignant neoplasm of cerebellum
C71.7	Malignant neoplasm of brain stem
C71.8	Malignant neoplasm of overlapping sites of brain
C72.59	Malignant neoplasm of other cranial nerves
C79.31	Secondary malignant neoplasm of brain
C79.32	Secondary malignant neoplasm of cerebral meninges
C79.49	Secondary malignant neoplasm of other parts of nervous system
C79.89	Secondary malignant neoplasm of other specified sites
I60.7	Nontraumatic subarachnoid hemorrhage from unspecified intracranial artery
I60.8	Other nontraumatic subarachnoid hemorrhage
I67.0	Dissection of cerebral arteries, nonruptured
I67.1	Cerebral aneurysm, nonruptured
I72.0	Aneurysm of carotid artery
I72.5	Aneurysm of other precerebral arteries
I72.6	Aneurysm of vertebral artery
I72.8	Aneurysm of other specified arteries
I77.2	Rupture of artery
I77.71	Dissection of carotid artery
I77.74	Dissection of vertebral artery
I77.75	Dissection of other precerebral arteries
Q28.0	Arteriovenous malformation of precerebral vessels
Q28.1	Other malformations of precerebral vessels
Q28.2	Arteriovenous malformation of cerebral vessels
Q28.3	Other malformations of cerebral vessels
Q28.8	Other specified congenital malformations of circulatory system

CCI Edits

Refer to Appendix A for CCI edits.

Pub 100

61624: Pub 100-04, 12, 20.4.5

61626: Pub 100-04, 12, 20.4.5

Facility RVUs

Code	Work	PE Facility	MP	Total Facility
61624	20.12	8.06	5.16	33.34
61626	16.60	6.03	2.98	25.61

Non-facility RVUs

Code	Work	PE Non-Facility	MP	Total Non-Facility
61624	20.12	8.06	5.16	33.34
61626	16.60	6.03	2.98	25.61

Modifiers (PAR)

Code	Mod 50	Mod 51	Mod 62	Mod 66	Mod 80
61624	0	2	0	0	1
61626	0	2	0	0	1

Global Period

Code	Days
61624	000
61626	000

● New ▲ Revised ✚ Add On ⊘Modifier 51 Exempt ★Telemedicine ▯CPT QuickRef ⁄⁄FDA Pending ⇄ Laterality ❼Seventh Character ♂Male ♀Female

61630-61635

61630 Balloon angioplasty, intracranial (eg, atherosclerotic stenosis), percutaneous

61635 Transcatheter placement of intravascular stent(s), intracranial (eg, atherosclerotic stenosis), including balloon angioplasty, if performed

(61630 and 61635 include all selective vascular catheterization of the target vascular territory, all diagnostic imaging for arteriography of the target vascular territory, and all related radiological supervision and interpretation. When diagnostic arteriogram (including imaging and selective catheterization) confirms the need for angioplasty or stent placement, 61630 and 61635 are inclusive of these services. If angioplasty or stenting are not indicated, then the appropriate codes for selective catheterization and imaging should be reported in lieu of 61630 and 61635)

(Do not report 61630 or 61635 in conjunction with 61645 for the same vascular territory)

(For definition of vascular territory, see the Nervous System Endovascular Therapy guidelines)

AMA Coding Notes

Surgical Procedures on the Skull, Meninges, and Brain

(For injection procedure for cerebral angiography, see 36100-36218)

(For injection procedure for ventriculography, see 61026, 61120)

(For injection procedure for pneumoencephalography, use 61055)

AMA *CPT Assistant*

61630: Apr 17: 10
61635: Mar 14: 8

Plain English Description

An intracranial arterial stenosis is treated by percutaneous balloon angioplasty and/or stent placement. The skin is cleansed over the catheter access site. A local anesthetic is injected. A small stab incision is made in the skin and a needle is inserted into the blood vessel followed by a sheath. A microcatheter or neurointerventional guidewire is threaded from the access artery to the carotid circulation. The intracranial artery to be treated is then selectively catheterized by advancing an arteriography catheter over the guide catheter wire. A diagnostic arteriography is performed to evaluate the anatomy and determine whether balloon angioplasty is indicated. In 61630, a balloon angioplasty is performed. Additional angiograms are obtained to evaluate the stenotic artery and determine the proper placement and diameter of the angioplasty balloon. The angioplasty balloon catheter is then prepared. A steerable micro-guidewire and microcatheter are advanced through the guide catheter into the intracranial arteries and across the stenosed artery. The micro-guidewire is removed and replaced with an exchange wire. The microcatheter is removed and the angioplasty balloon catheter is advanced over the exchange wire and situated across the stenotic region. The balloon is inflated and the stenotic region dilated under fluoroscopic control. Once adequate dilation has been achieved, the balloon catheter is withdrawn into the access artery but not removed. The guidewire is left in place while post-procedure angiograms are obtained to evaluate for hyperacute thrombosis or rebound stenosis. Additional interventional measures are initiated if these conditions occur. Once the stenotic lesion has been successfully dilated and any complications addressed, the catheters and guidewires are removed. In 61635, an intracranial intravascular stent is placed. If indicated, a balloon angioplasty is performed as described above. Following completion of arteriography studies and balloon angioplasty, the exchange wire or catheter is left in place. The stent delivery system is then advanced over the wire or catheter until it is positioned across the area of stenosis. The stent is deployed and the delivery system withdrawn into the access artery leaving the exchange catheter or wire in place. Angiograms are obtained and the position of the stent evaluated. After a 15-minute interval additional angiograms are obtained to rule out complications. All catheters and wires are removed.

Angioplasty or transcatheter placement of intravascular stent(s), intracranial

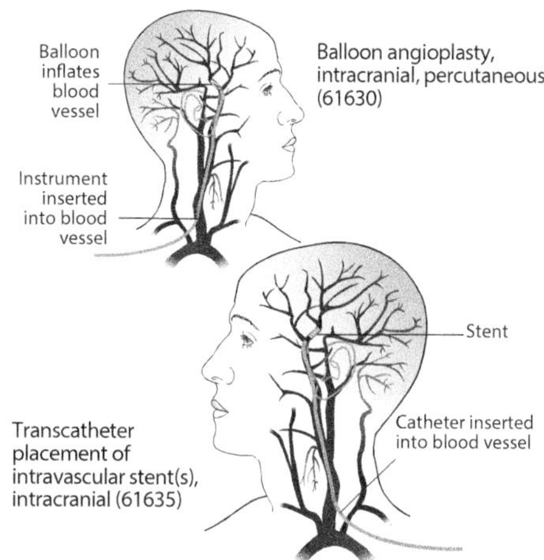

ICD-10-CM Diagnostic Codes

⇄	I66.01	Occlusion and stenosis of right middle cerebral artery
⇄	I66.02	Occlusion and stenosis of left middle cerebral artery
⇄	I66.03	Occlusion and stenosis of bilateral middle cerebral arteries
⇄	I66.11	Occlusion and stenosis of right anterior cerebral artery
⇄	I66.12	Occlusion and stenosis of left anterior cerebral artery
⇄	I66.13	Occlusion and stenosis of bilateral anterior cerebral arteries
⇄	I66.21	Occlusion and stenosis of right posterior cerebral artery
⇄	I66.22	Occlusion and stenosis of left posterior cerebral artery
⇄	I66.23	Occlusion and stenosis of bilateral posterior cerebral arteries
	I66.3	Occlusion and stenosis of cerebellar arteries
	I66.8	Occlusion and stenosis of other cerebral arteries
	I66.9	Occlusion and stenosis of unspecified cerebral artery
	I67.2	Cerebral atherosclerosis
	I70.9	Other and unspecified atherosclerosis
	I77.1	Stricture of artery

CCI Edits

Refer to Appendix A for CCI edits.

Pub 100

61630: Pub 100-04, 12, 20.4.5
61635: Pub 100-04, 12, 20.4.5

Facility RVUs

Code	Work	PE Facility	MP	Total Facility
61630	22.07	11.52	5.93	39.52
61635	24.28	11.96	5.77	42.01

Non-facility RVUs

Code	Work	PE Non-Facility	MP	Total Non-Facility
61630	22.07	11.52	5.93	39.52
61635	24.28	11.96	5.77	42.01

Modifiers (PAR)

Code	Mod 50	Mod 51	Mod 62	Mod 66	Mod 80
61630	0	2	1	0	2
61635	0	2	1	0	2

Global Period

Code	Days
61630	XXX
61635	XXX

61640-61642

61640 Balloon dilatation of intracranial vasospasm, percutaneous; initial vessel

✚ **61641 Balloon dilatation of intracranial vasospasm, percutaneous; each additional vessel in same vascular territory (List separately in addition to code for primary procedure)**

✚ **61642 Balloon dilatation of intracranial vasospasm, percutaneous; each additional vessel in different vascular territory (List separately in addition to code for primary procedure)**

(Use 61641 and 61642 in conjunction with 61640)

(61640, 61641, 61642 include all selective vascular catheterization of the target vessel, contrast injection[s], vessel measurement, roadmapping, postdilatation angiography, and fluoroscopic guidance for the balloon dilatation)

(Do not report 61640, 61642 in conjunction with 61650 or 61651 for the same vascular territory)

(For definition of vascular territory, see the Nervous System Endovascular Therapy guidelines)

AMA Coding Notes

Surgical Procedures on the Skull, Meninges, and Brain

(For injection procedure for cerebral angiography, see 36100-36218)

(For injection procedure for ventriculography, see 61026, 61120)

(For injection procedure for pneumoencephalography, use 61055)

AMA *CPT Assistant* ☐

61640: May 14: 10
61641: May 14: 10
61642: May 14: 10

Plain English Description

Intracranial endovascular balloon dilatation is performed to treat vasospasm of the smooth muscle lining. Vasospasm may occur following subarachnoid hemorrhage, which causes changes in the intima that can result in luminal narrowing and rigidity of the vessel wall. The skin is cleansed over the catheter access site. A local anesthetic is injected. A small stab incision is made in the skin and a needle is inserted into the blood vessel followed by a sheath. A microcatheter or neurointerventional guidewire is threaded from the access artery to the carotid circulation. The intracranial artery to be treated is then selectively catheterized by advancing an arteriography catheter over the guidewire. A diagnostic arteriography is performed to evaluate the anatomy and determine whether balloon dilatation is indicated. In 61640, a balloon dilatation of the initial vessel is performed. Additional angiograms are obtained to evaluate the arterial lesion and determine the proper placement and diameter of the balloon. The balloon catheter is then prepared. A steerable micro-guidewire and microcatheter are advanced through the guide catheter into the intracranial arteries and across the arterial lesion. The micro-guidewire is removed and replaced with an exchange wire. The microcatheter is removed and the angioplasty balloon catheter is advanced over the exchange wire and situated across the lesion. The balloon is inflated and the arterial lesion is dilated under fluoroscopic control. Once adequate dilatation has been achieved, the balloon catheter is withdrawn into the access artery but not removed. The guidewire is left in place while post-procedure angiograms are obtained to evaluate for hyperacute thrombosis or rebound stenosis. Additional interventional measures are initiated if these conditions occur. Once the arterial lesion has been successfully dilated and any complications addressed, the catheters and guidewires are removed. Use 61641 for each additional vessel in the same vascular territory treated with balloon dilatation. Use 61642 for each additional vessel in a different vascular territory treated with balloon dilatation.

Balloon dilatation of intracranial vasospasm, percutaneous

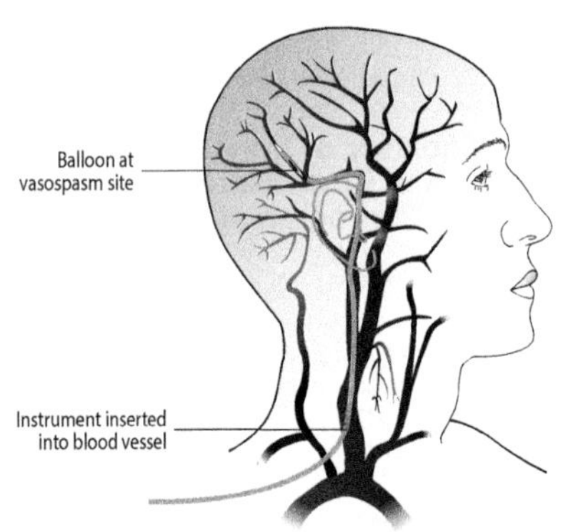

Initial vessel (61640); each additional vessel in same vascular family (61641); each additional vessel in different vascular family (61642)

ICD-10-CM Diagnostic Codes

I67.841	Reversible cerebrovascular vasoconstriction syndrome
I67.848	Other cerebrovascular vasospasm and vasoconstriction

CCI Edits

Refer to Appendix A for CCI edits.

Pub 100

61640: Pub 100-04, 12, 20.4.5
61641: Pub 100-04, 12, 20.4.5
61642: Pub 100-04, 12, 20.4.5

Facility RVUs ☐

Code	Work	PE Facility	MP	Total Facility
61640	12.32	0.00	1.69	14.01
61641	4.33	0.00	0.59	4.92
61642	8.66	0.00	1.18	9.84

Non-facility RVUs ☐

Code	Work	PE Non-Facility	MP	Total Non-Facility
61640	12.32	0.00	1.69	14.01
61641	4.33	0.00	0.59	4.92
61642	8.66	0.00	1.18	9.84

Modifiers (PAR) ☐

Code	Mod 50	Mod 51	Mod 62	Mod 66	Mod 80
61640	9	9	9	9	9
61641	9	9	9	9	9
61642	9	9	9	9	9

Global Period

Code	Days
61640	000
61641	ZZZ
61642	ZZZ

61645

61645 Percutaneous arterial transluminal mechanical thrombectomy and/or infusion for thrombolysis, intracranial, any method, including diagnostic angiography, fluoroscopic guidance, catheter placement, and intraprocedural pharmacological thrombolytic injection(s)

(Do not report 61645 in conjunction with 36221, 36222, 36223, 36224, 36225, 36226, 37184, 61630, 61635, 61650, 61651 for the same vascular territory)

(To report venous mechanical thrombectomy and/or thrombolysis, see 37187, 37188, 37212, 37214)

AMA Coding Guideline

Cerebral Endovascular Therapeutic Interventions

Codes 61645, 61650, 61651 describe cerebral endovascular therapeutic interventions in any intracranial artery. They include selective catheterization, diagnostic angiography, and all subsequent angiography including associated radiological supervision and interpretation within the treated vascular territory, fluoroscopic guidance, neurologic and hemodynamic monitoring of the patient, and closure of the arteriotomy by manual pressure, an arterial closure device, or suture.

For purposes of reporting services described by 61645, 61650, 61651, the intracranial arteries are divided into three vascular territories: 1) right carotid circulation; 2) left carotid circulation; 3) vertebro-basilar circulation. Code 61645 may be reported once for each intracranial vascular territory treated. Code 61650 is reported once for the first intracranial vascular territory treated with intra-arterial prolonged administration of pharmacologic agent(s). If additional intracranial vascular territory(ies) is also treated with intra-arterial prolonged administration of pharmacologic agent(s) during the same session, the treatment of each additional vascular territory(ies) is reported using 61651 (may be reported maximally two times per day).

Code 61645 describes endovascular revascularization of thrombotic/embolic occlusion of intracranial arterial vessel(s) via any method, including mechanical thrombectomy (eg, mechanical retrieval device, aspiration catheter) and/or the administration of any agent(s) for the purpose of revascularization, such as thrombolytics or IIB/IIIA inhibitors.

Codes 61650, 61651 describe the cerebral endovascular continuous or intermittent therapeutic prolonged administration of any non-thrombolytic agent(s) (eg, spasmolytics or chemotherapy) into an artery to treat non-iatrogenic central nervous system diseases or sequelae thereof. These codes should not be used to report administration of agents (eg, heparin, nitroglycerin, saline) usually administered during endovascular interventions. These codes are used for prolonged administrations, ie, of at least 10 minutes continuous or intermittent duration.

Do not report 61645, 61650, or 61651 in conjunction with 36221, 36226, 36228, 37184, or 37186 for the treated vascular territory. Do not report 61645 in conjunction with 61650 or 61651 for the same vascular distribution. Diagnostic angiography of a non-treated vascular territory may be reported separately. For example, angiography of the left carotid and/or the vertebral circulations may be reported if the intervention is performed in the right carotid circulation.

AMA Coding Notes

Surgical Procedures on the Skull, Meninges, and Brain

(For injection procedure for cerebral angiography, see 36100-36218)

(For injection procedure for ventriculography, see 61026, 61120)

(For injection procedure for pneumoencephalography, use 61055)

AMA *CPT Assistant* □

61645: Nov 15: 3, Dec 15: 17, Mar 16: 3

Plain English Description

A procedure is performed to remove mechanically and/or dissolve with thrombolytic drugs an intracranial blood clot. Percutaneous access to the intracranial blood vessel(s) is established through a peripheral artery. A needle is introduced into the artery under fluoroscopic guidance and a thin wire is threaded through the needle and advanced to the occluded area. If diagnostic angiography is performed, a catheter is introduced over the guidewire and advanced to the occlusion. The guidewire is removed and dye is injected to obtain detailed images of the intracranial blood vessels. The guidewire is then reinserted and advanced as far as possible through the clot. A mechanical device such as an aspiration catheter, micro-guidewire, micro-snare, or retriever is advanced over the guidewire and the clot is evacuated. An infusion of a thrombolytic agent such as tissue plasminogen activator, urokinase, streptokinase, alteplase, reteplase, and tenacteplase may be used to assists with clot degradation. An infusion catheter is introduced over the guidewire to the clot area and medication is delivered as bolus injection(s) or continuous infusion while clot lysis is monitored with periodic angiograms. The catheter is removed at the end of the treatment period. Code 61645 includes diagnostic angiography and fluoroscopic guidance, catheter placement, and intraprocedural pharmacological thrombolytic injection(s).

ICD-10-CM Diagnostic Codes

⇄	I66.01	Occlusion and stenosis of right middle cerebral artery
⇄	I66.02	Occlusion and stenosis of left middle cerebral artery
⇄	I66.03	Occlusion and stenosis of bilateral middle cerebral arteries
⇄	I66.11	Occlusion and stenosis of right anterior cerebral artery
⇄	I66.12	Occlusion and stenosis of left anterior cerebral artery
⇄	I66.13	Occlusion and stenosis of bilateral anterior cerebral arteries
⇄	I66.21	Occlusion and stenosis of right posterior cerebral artery
⇄	I66.22	Occlusion and stenosis of left posterior cerebral artery
⇄	I66.23	Occlusion and stenosis of bilateral posterior cerebral arteries
	I66.3	Occlusion and stenosis of cerebellar arteries
	I66.8	Occlusion and stenosis of other cerebral arteries
	I66.9	Occlusion and stenosis of unspecified cerebral artery
	I67.2	Cerebral atherosclerosis

CCI Edits

Refer to Appendix A for CCI edits.

Pub 100

61645: Pub 100-04, 12, 20.4.5

Facility RVUs □

Code	Work	PE Facility	MP	Total Facility
61645	15.00	5.82	3.37	24.19

Non-facility RVUs □

Code	Work	PE Non-Facility	MP	Total Non-Facility
61645	15.00	5.82	3.37	24.19

Modifiers (PAR) □

Code	Mod 50	Mod 51	Mod 62	Mod 66	Mod 80
61645	1	0	0	0	0

Global Period

Code	Days
61645	000

61650-61651

61650 Endovascular intracranial prolonged administration of pharmacologic agent(s) other than for thrombolysis, arterial, including catheter placement, diagnostic angiography, and imaging guidance; initial vascular territory

+ **61651 Endovascular intracranial prolonged administration of pharmacologic agent(s) other than for thrombolysis, arterial, including catheter placement, diagnostic angiography, and imaging guidance; each additional vascular territory (List separately in addition to code for primary procedure)**

(Use 61651 in conjunction with 61650)

(Do not report 61650 or 61651 in conjunction with 36221, 36222, 36223, 36224, 36225, 36226, 61640, 61641, 61642, 61645 for the same vascular territory)

(Do not report 61650 or 61651 in conjunction with 96420, 96422, 96423, 96425 for the same vascular territory)

AMA Coding Guideline

Cerebral Endovascular Therapeutic Interventions

Codes 61645, 61650, 61651 describe cerebral endovascular therapeutic interventions in any intracranial artery. They include selective catheterization, diagnostic angiography, and all subsequent angiography including associated radiological supervision and interpretation within the treated vascular territory, fluoroscopic guidance, neurologic and hemodynamic monitoring of the patient, and closure of the arteriotomy by manual pressure, an arterial closure device, or suture.

For purposes of reporting services described by 61645, 61650, 61651, the intracranial arteries are divided into three vascular territories: 1) right carotid circulation; 2) left carotid circulation; 3) vertebro-basilar circulation. Code 61645 may be reported once for each intracranial vascular territory treated. Code 61650 is reported once for the first intracranial vascular territory treated with intra-arterial prolonged administration of pharmacologic agent(s). If additional intracranial vascular territory(ies) is also treated with intra-arterial prolonged administration of pharmacologic agent(s) during the same session, the treatment of each additional vascular territory(ies) is reported using 61651 (may be reported maximally two times per day).

Code 61645 describes endovascular revascularization of thrombotic/embolic occlusion of intracranial arterial vessel(s) via any method, including mechanical thrombectomy (eg, mechanical retrieval device, aspiration catheter) and/or the administration of any agent(s) for the purpose of revascularization, such as thrombolytics or IIB/IIIA inhibitors.

Codes 61650, 61651 describe the cerebral endovascular continuous or intermittent therapeutic prolonged administration of any non-thrombolytic agent(s) (eg, spasmolytics or chemotherapy) into an artery to treat non-iatrogenic central nervous system diseases or sequelae thereof. These codes should not be used to report administration of agents (eg, heparin, nitroglycerin, saline) usually administered during endovascular interventions. These codes are used for prolonged administrations, ie, of at least 10 minutes continuous or intermittent duration.

Do not report 61645, 61650, or 61651 in conjunction with 36221, 36226, 36228, 37184, or 37186 for the treated vascular territory. Do not report 61645 in conjunction with 61650 or 61651 for the same vascular distribution. Diagnostic angiography of a non-treated vascular territory may be reported separately. For example, angiography of the left carotid and/or the vertebral circulations may be reported if the intervention is performed in the right carotid circulation.

AMA Coding Notes

Surgical Procedures on the Skull, Meninges, and Brain

(For injection procedure for cerebral angiography, see 36100-36218)

(For injection procedure for ventriculography, see 61026, 61120)

(For injection procedure for pneumoencephalography, use 61055)

AMA *CPT Assistant*

61650: Nov 15: 3, Mar 16: 3

61651: Nov 15: 3, Mar 16: 3

Plain English Description

A procedure is performed to administer endovascular intracranial pharmacologic agent(s) other than for thrombolysis. These agents may include papaverine, nicardipine, and verapamil used to treat arterial vasospasm following stroke. Access to intracranial blood vessels is established through a peripheral artery. A needle is introduced into the artery under fluoroscopic guidance; a thin wire is threaded through the needle and advanced to the targeted vascular area. If diagnostic angiography is performed, a catheter is introduced over the guidewire and the guidewire is removed. Dye is injected to obtain detailed images of the intracranial blood vessels. The guidewire is then reinserted and the angiography catheter is removed. An infusion catheter is introduced over the guidewire to the targeted vascular territory and the pharmacologic agent is delivered as prolonged continuous infusion. The catheter may be moved to access additional vascular territories (61651) with subsequent delivery of pharmacologic agents before being removed at the end of the treatment period. These codes include diagnostic angiography and imaging guidance.

ICD-10-CM Diagnostic Codes

A52.04	Syphilitic cerebral arteritis
B95.0	Streptococcus, group A, as the cause of diseases classified elsewhere
B95.1	Streptococcus, group B, as the cause of diseases classified elsewhere
B95.3	Streptococcus pneumoniae as the cause of diseases classified elsewhere
B95.4	Other streptococcus as the cause of diseases classified elsewhere
B95.61	Methicillin susceptible Staphylococcus aureus infection as the cause of diseases classified elsewhere
B95.62	Methicillin resistant Staphylococcus aureus infection as the cause of diseases classified elsewhere
B95.7	Other staphylococcus as the cause of diseases classified elsewhere
C70.0	Malignant neoplasm of cerebral meninges
C71.0	Malignant neoplasm of cerebrum, except lobes and ventricles
C71.1	Malignant neoplasm of frontal lobe
C71.2	Malignant neoplasm of temporal lobe
C71.3	Malignant neoplasm of parietal lobe
C71.4	Malignant neoplasm of occipital lobe
C71.5	Malignant neoplasm of cerebral ventricle
C71.6	Malignant neoplasm of cerebellum
C71.7	Malignant neoplasm of brain stem
C79.31	Secondary malignant neoplasm of brain
C79.32	Secondary malignant neoplasm of cerebral meninges
G45.9	Transient cerebral ischemic attack, unspecified
I33.0	Acute and subacute infective endocarditis
I60.7	Nontraumatic subarachnoid hemorrhage from unspecified intracranial artery
I63.81	Other cerebral infarction due to occlusion or stenosis of small artery
I67.848	Other cerebrovascular vasospasm and vasoconstriction
I68.2	Cerebral arteritis in other diseases classified elsewhere
I69.098	Other sequelae following nontraumatic subarachnoid hemorrhage
I69.898	Other sequelae of other cerebrovascular disease

CCI Edits

Refer to Appendix A for CCI edits.

Pub 100

61650: Pub 100-04, 12, 20.4.5
61651: Pub 100-04, 12, 20.4.5

Facility RVUs

Code	Work	PE Facility	MP	Total Facility
61650	10.00	3.92	2.59	16.51
61651	4.25	1.71	1.11	7.07

Non-facility RVUs

Code	Work	PE Non-Facility	MP	Total Non-Facility
61650	10.00	3.92	2.59	16.51
61651	4.25	1.71	1.11	7.07

Modifiers (PAR)

Code	Mod 50	Mod 51	Mod 62	Mod 66	Mod 80
61650	0	2	0	0	1
61651	0	0	0	0	1

Global Period

Code	Days
61650	000
61651	ZZZ

61680-61686

61680 Surgery of intracranial arteriovenous malformation; supratentorial, simple
61682 Surgery of intracranial arteriovenous malformation; supratentorial, complex
61684 Surgery of intracranial arteriovenous malformation; infratentorial, simple
61686 Surgery of intracranial arteriovenous malformation; infratentorial, complex

AMA Coding Guideline

Surgery for Aneurysm, Arteriovenous Malformation or Vascular Disease Procedures on the Skull, Meninges, and Brain

Includes craniotomy when appropriate for procedure.

AMA Coding Notes

Surgical Procedures on the Skull, Meninges, and Brain

(For injection procedure for cerebral angiography, see 36100-36218)

(For injection procedure for ventriculography, see 61026, 61120)

(For injection procedure for pneumoencephalography, use 61055)

AMA *CPT Assistant*

61682: Jun 13: 14
61686: Jun 13: 14

Plain English Description

An arteriovenous malformation (AVM) is an abnormal connection between the arterial and venous systems in which one or more arteries and veins connect directly with each other without blood first passing through the capillary system. Intracranial AVMs are congenital malformations. The direct connection between the arterial and venous systems results in shunting of blood into the venous system at high pressure. This can result in rupture of the blood vessels and hemorrhage as well as other complications. An AVM in the supratentorial region lies above the tentorium cerebelli, a fold in the dura mater that separates the frontal and occipital lobes of the cerebrum from the cerebellum and contains the cerebral hemispheres, lateral and third ventricles, choroid plexus, hypothalamus, and pineal and pituitary glands. An AVM in the infratentorial region lies below the tentorium cerebelli and contains the cerebellum, cerebellopontine angle, the fourth ventricle, and the brain stem. A craniotomy is performed by creating scalp flaps, followed by burr holes. The bone between the burr holes is then cut with a saw or craniotome and a bone flap is elevated. The dura is opened and the AVM is exposed. Separately reportable angiography may be performed intraoperatively to identify which blood vessels are involved. Using microsurgical technique, the arterial feeders are located, suture ligated, and divided. The mass of involved blood vessels is then dissected from surrounding tissue and the draining vein(s) isolated, suture ligated, and divided. The AVM is completely excised. Additional angiograms are obtained to ensure that the entire AVM has been removed. Once the AVM has been completely excised, the dura is closed; the bone flap is replaced and secured with sutures, wire, or miniplate and screws; and the overlying skin flap is closed with sutures. Use 61680 for a simple supratentorial AVM. A simple AVM is a smaller mass of vessels that typically does not have normal vessels incorporated in the mass and is not located in a critical region of the brain. Use 61682 for a complex supratentorial AVM. A complex AVM is a larger mass of vessels that may have normal vessels incorporated in the mass or is located in a critical region of the brain. Use 61684 for a simple infratentorial AVM and 61686 for a complex infratentorial AVM.

Surgery of intracranial arteriovenous malformations

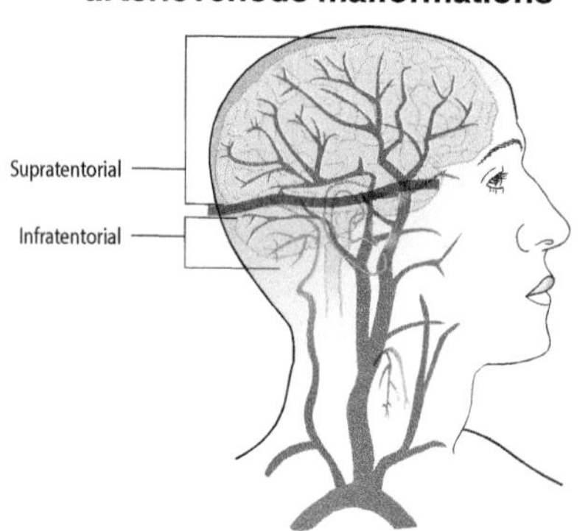

Supratentorial, simple (61680); supratentorial, complex (61682); infratentorial, simple (61684); infratentorial, complex (61686)

ICD-10-CM Diagnostic Codes

Q28.2	Arteriovenous malformation of cerebral vessels
Q28.3	Other malformations of cerebral vessels

CCI Edits

Refer to Appendix A for CCI edits.

Pub 100

61680: Pub 100-04, 12, 20.4.5
61682: Pub 100-04, 12, 20.4.5
61684: Pub 100-04, 12, 20.4.5
61686: Pub 100-04, 12, 20.4.5

Facility RVUs

Code	Work	PE Facility	MP	Total Facility
61680	32.55	20.70	11.88	65.13
61682	63.41	34.00	26.32	123.73
61684	41.64	25.08	15.60	82.32
61686	67.50	37.43	29.24	134.17

Non-facility RVUs

Code	Work	PE Non-Facility	MP	Total Non-Facility
61680	32.55	20.70	11.88	65.13
61682	63.41	34.00	26.32	123.73
61684	41.64	25.08	15.60	82.32
61686	67.50	37.43	29.24	134.17

Modifiers (PAR)

Code	Mod 50	Mod 51	Mod 62	Mod 66	Mod 80
61680	0	2	1	0	2
61682	0	2	1	0	2
61684	0	2	1	0	2
61686	0	2	1	0	2

Global Period

Code	Days
61680	090
61682	090
61684	090
61686	090

61690-61692

61690 Surgery of intracranial arteriovenous malformation; dural, simple

61692 Surgery of intracranial arteriovenous malformation; dural, complex

AMA Coding Guideline

Surgery for Aneurysm, Arteriovenous Malformation or Vascular Disease Procedures on the Skull, Meninges, and Brain

Includes craniotomy when appropriate for procedure.

AMA Coding Notes

Surgical Procedures on the Skull, Meninges, and Brain

(For injection procedure for cerebral angiography, see 36100-36218)

(For injection procedure for ventriculography, see 61026, 61120)

(For injection procedure for pneumoencephalography, use 61055)

AMA *CPT Assistant*

61692: Jun 13: 14

Plain English Description

An arteriovenous malformation (AVM) is an abnormal connection between the arterial and venous systems in which one or more arteries and veins connect directly with each other without blood first passing through capillary system. Intracranial AVMs are congenital malformations. The direct connection between the arterial and venous systems results in shunting of blood into the venous system at high pressure. This can result in rupture of the blood vessels and hemorrhage as well as other complications. These surgeries are performed on an AVM in the dura, which is the tough fibrous outer membrane that covers the central nervous system. A craniotomy is performed by creating scalp flaps, followed by burr holes. The bone between the burr holes is then cut with a saw or craniotome and a bone flap elevated, taking care to carefully dissect the periosteal layer of the dura from the overlying bone. The AVM is exposed. Separately reportable angiography may be performed intraoperatively to identify which blood vessels are involved. Using microsurgical technique, the arterial feeders are located, suture ligated and divided. The mass of involved blood vessels is then dissected from surrounding tissue and the draining vein or veins isolated, suture ligated and divided. The AVM is completely excised. Additional angiograms are obtained to ensure that the entire AVM has been removed. Once the AVM has been completely excised, the dura is repaired, the bone flap replaced and secured with sutures, wire, or miniplate and screws, and the overlying skin flap closed with sutures. Use 61690 for a simple dural AVM. A simple AVM is a smaller mass of vessels that typically does not have normal vessels incorporated in the mass and is typically not located in a critical region of the brain. Use 61692 for a complex dural AVM. A complex AVM is a larger mass of vessels that may have normal vessels incorporated in the mass or be located in a critical region of the brain.

Surgery of intracranial arteriovenous malformations; dural

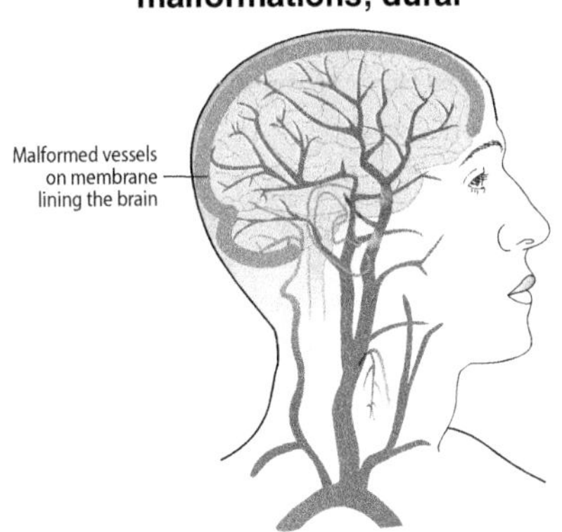

Simple (61690); complex (61692)

ICD-10-CM Diagnostic Codes

Q28.2	Arteriovenous malformation of cerebral vessels
Q28.3	Other malformations of cerebral vessels

CCI Edits

Refer to Appendix A for CCI edits.

Pub 100

61690: Pub 100-04, 12, 20.4.5

61692: Pub 100-04, 12, 20.4.5

Facility RVUs

Code	Work	PE Facility	MP	Total Facility
61690	31.34	20.08	11.62	63.04
61692	54.59	30.80	20.72	106.11

Non-facility RVUs

Code	Work	PE Non-Facility	MP	Total Non-Facility
61690	31.34	20.08	11.62	63.04
61692	54.59	30.80	20.72	106.11

Modifiers (PAR)

Code	Mod 50	Mod 51	Mod 62	Mod 66	Mod 80
61690	0	2	1	0	2
61692	0	2	1	0	2

Global Period

Code	Days
61690	090
61692	090

61697-61698

61697 Surgery of complex intracranial aneurysm, intracranial approach; carotid circulation

61698 Surgery of complex intracranial aneurysm, intracranial approach; vertebrobasilar circulation

(61697, 61698 involve aneurysms that are larger than 15 mm or with calcification of the aneurysm neck, or with incorporation of normal vessels into the aneurysm neck, or a procedure requiring temporary vessel occlusion, trapping, or cardiopulmonary bypass to successfully treat the aneurysm)

AMA Coding Guideline

Surgery for Aneurysm, Arteriovenous Malformation or Vascular Disease Procedures on the Skull, Meninges, and Brain

Includes craniotomy when appropriate for procedure.

AMA Coding Notes

Surgical Procedures on the Skull, Meninges, and Brain

(For injection procedure for cerebral angiography, see 36100-36218)

(For injection procedure for ventriculography, see 61026, 61120)

(For injection procedure for pneumoencephalography, use 61055)

AMA *CPT Assistant*

61697: Dec 17: 13

Plain English Description

Surgery is performed on a complex intracranial aneurysm of the carotid (61697) or vertebrobasilar (61698) circulation via an intracranial approach. Complex intracranial aneurysms are those that are larger than 15 mm, have calcification of the aneurysm neck, and/or have normal vessels incorporated into the aneurysm neck. If the surgery requires temporary vessel occlusion, trapping, or cardiopulmonary bypass for successful treatment, the aneurysm is also classified as complex. The approach depends on the exact location of the aneurysm. An approach through the interhemispheric fissure or pterion may be used. After the skin and subcutaneous tissue have been incised and overlying bone removed (craniectomy), the dura mater is opened. The arachnoid is nicked and cerebrospinal fluid is drained as needed to allow maximal exposure of the internal carotid or vertebrobasilar artery. The artery is located and separated from the arachnoid membrane and the aneurysm is exposed. The aneurysm may be treated by clipping and resecting the mass lesion. Vessel reconstruction is then performed using direct repair with bypass graft. Alternatively, if collateral circulation is adequate, the aneurysm may be trapped and clips applied above and below the lesion to become completely occluded.

Surgery of complex intracranial aneurysm, intracranial approach

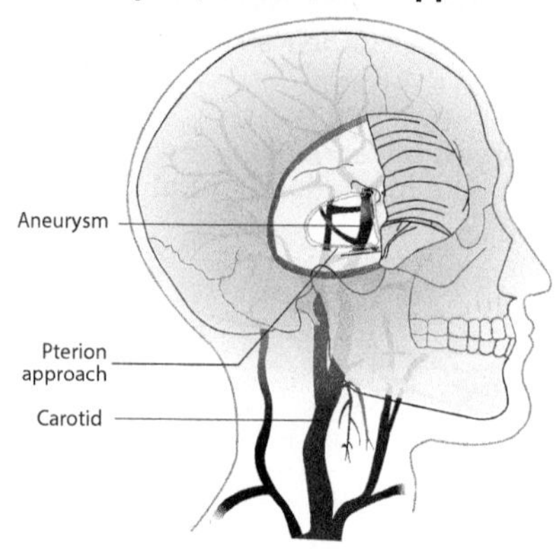

Carotid circulation (61697); vertebrobasilar circulation (616987)

ICD-10-CM Diagnostic Codes

I67.0	Dissection of cerebral arteries, nonruptured
I67.1	Cerebral aneurysm, nonruptured
I72.0	Aneurysm of carotid artery
I72.5	Aneurysm of other precerebral arteries
I72.6	Aneurysm of vertebral artery
I72.8	Aneurysm of other specified arteries
I77.71	Dissection of carotid artery
I77.74	Dissection of vertebral artery
I77.75	Dissection of other precerebral arteries
Q28.1	Other malformations of precerebral vessels
Q28.3	Other malformations of cerebral vessels

CCI Edits

Refer to Appendix A for CCI edits.

Pub 100

61697: Pub 100-04, 12, 20.4.5

61698: Pub 100-04, 12, 20.4.5

Facility RVUs

Code	Work	PE Facility	MP	Total Facility
61697	63.40	35.11	24.16	122.67
61698	69.63	38.40	30.01	138.04

Non-facility RVUs

Code	Work	PE Non-Facility	MP	Total Non-Facility
61697	63.40	35.11	24.16	122.67
61698	69.63	38.40	30.01	138.04

Modifiers (PAR)

Code	Mod 50	Mod 51	Mod 62	Mod 66	Mod 80
61697	0	2	1	0	2
61698	0	2	1	0	2

Global Period

Code	Days
61697	090
61698	090

61700-61702

61700 Surgery of simple intracranial aneurysm, intracranial approach; carotid circulation

61702 Surgery of simple intracranial aneurysm, intracranial approach; vertebrobasilar circulation

AMA Coding Guideline

Surgery for Aneurysm, Arteriovenous Malformation or Vascular Disease Procedures on the Skull, Meninges, and Brain

Includes craniotomy when appropriate for procedure.

AMA Coding Notes

Surgical Procedures on the Skull, Meninges, and Brain

(For injection procedure for cerebral angiography, see 36100-36218)

(For injection procedure for ventriculography, see 61026, 61120)

(For injection procedure for pneumoencephalography, use 61055)

AMA *CPT Assistant* ▯

61700: Jun 99: 11, Jul 99: 10, Dec 17: 13

Plain English Description

Surgery is performed on a simple intracranial aneurysm of the carotid (61700) or vertebrobasilar (61702) artery via an intracranial approach. Simple intracranial aneurysms are those that are 15 mm or less, do not have calcification of the aneurysm neck, and do not have normal vessels incorporated into the aneurysm neck. Simple aneurysm repair does not require temporary vessel occlusion, trapping, or cardiopulmonary bypass for successful treatment. The approach depends on the exact location of the aneurysm. An approach through the interhemispheric fissure or pterion may be used. After the skin and subcutaneous tissue have been incised and overlying bone removed (craniectomy), the dura mater is opened. The arachnoid is nicked and cerebrospinal fluid is drained as needed to allow maximal exposure of the internal carotid or vertebrobasilar artery. The artery is located and separated from the arachnoid membrane and the aneurysm is exposed. Simple aneurysms are typically treated by applying a clip to permanently exclude the aneurysm from the intracranial circulation.

Surgery of an intracranial aneurysm

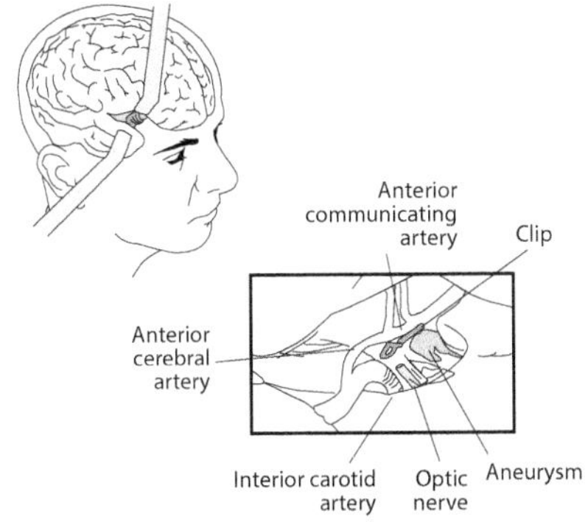

Use 61700 for carotid circulation; use 61702 for vertebrobasilar circulation.

ICD-10-CM Diagnostic Codes

I67.0	Dissection of cerebral arteries, nonruptured
I67.1	Cerebral aneurysm, nonruptured
I72.0	Aneurysm of carotid artery
I72.5	Aneurysm of other precerebral arteries
I72.6	Aneurysm of vertebral artery
I72.8	Aneurysm of other specified arteries
I77.71	Dissection of carotid artery
I77.74	Dissection of vertebral artery
I77.75	Dissection of other precerebral arteries
Q28.1	Other malformations of precerebral vessels
Q28.3	Other malformations of cerebral vessels

CCI Edits

Refer to Appendix A for CCI edits.

Pub 100

61700: Pub 100-04, 12, 20.4.5

61702: Pub 100-04, 12, 20.4.5

Facility RVUs ▯

Code	Work	PE Facility	MP	Total Facility
61700	50.62	29.34	18.81	98.77
61702	60.04	33.98	23.08	117.10

Non-facility RVUs ▯

Code	Work	PE Non-Facility	MP	Total Non-Facility
61700	50.62	29.34	18.81	98.77
61702	60.04	33.98	23.08	117.10

Modifiers (PAR) ▯

Code	Mod 50	Mod 51	Mod 62	Mod 66	Mod 80
61700	0	2	1	0	2
61702	0	2	1	0	2

Global Period

Code	Days
61700	090
61702	090

61703

61703 Surgery of intracranial aneurysm, cervical approach by application of occluding clamp to cervical carotid artery (Selverstone-Crutchfield type)

(For cervical approach for direct ligation of carotid artery, see 37600-37606)

AMA Coding Guideline

Surgery for Aneurysm, Arteriovenous Malformation or Vascular Disease Procedures on the Skull, Meninges, and Brain

Includes craniotomy when appropriate for procedure.

AMA Coding Notes

Surgical Procedures on the Skull, Meninges, and Brain

(For injection procedure for cerebral angiography, see 36100-36218)

(For injection procedure for ventriculography, see 61026, 61120)

(For injection procedure for pneumoencephalography, use 61055)

Plain English Description

An intracranial aneurysm, also called a cerebral or intracerebral aneurysm, is a weakened area in a blood vessel wall that expands and fills with blood. Depending on the size and location, it can put pressure on surrounding brain tissue, causing pain and neurological deficits. It can also rupture, causing an intracranial hemorrhage. Intracranial aneurysms may be congenital or acquired. An intracranial aneurysm that is fed by the cervical carotid artery is occluded by application of a Selverstone-Crutchfield type clamp via a cervical approach. An incision is made on the side of the neck over the proximal aspect of the internal carotid artery that feeds the aneurysm. The artery is dissected from surrounding tissue and an adjustable clamp is placed around the artery to partially occlude it. Partial occlusion of the artery allows the arterial walls to thicken and clotting to occur within the aneurysmal sac, thereby reducing the risk of enlargement or rupture of the aneurysm. This type of clamp can be adjusted postoperatively because a tightening device that is part of the clamp extends to the skin surface. Once the desired amount of occlusion has been achieved, overlying tissues are closed in layers around the tightening device.

Surgery of intracranial aneurysm, cervical approach by application of occluding clamp to cervical carotid artery

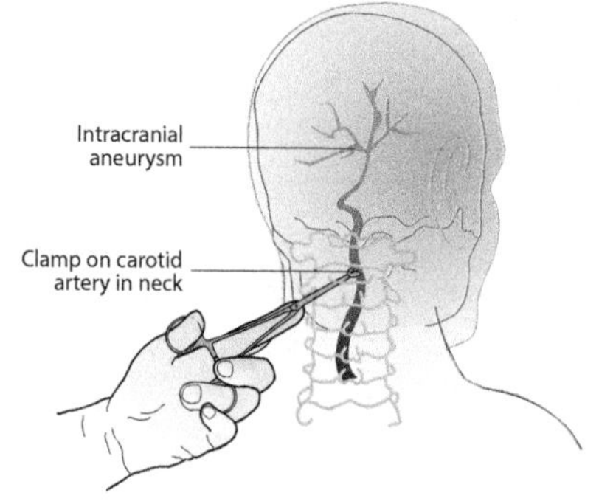

ICD-10-CM Diagnostic Codes

I67.0	Dissection of cerebral arteries, nonruptured
I67.1	Cerebral aneurysm, nonruptured
Q28.1	Other malformations of precerebral vessels
Q28.3	Other malformations of cerebral vessels

CCI Edits

Refer to Appendix A for CCI edits.

Pub 100

61703: Pub 100-04, 12, 20.4.5

Facility RVUs

Code	Work	PE Facility	MP	Total Facility
61703	18.80	13.45	6.94	39.19

Non-facility RVUs

Code	Work	PE Non-Facility	MP	Total Non-Facility
61703	18.80	13.45	6.94	39.19

Modifiers (PAR)

Code	Mod 50	Mod 51	Mod 62	Mod 66	Mod 80
61703	0	2	1	0	2

Global Period

Code	Days
61703	090

61705

61705 Surgery of aneurysm, vascular malformation or carotid-cavernous fistula; by intracranial and cervical occlusion of carotid artery

AMA Coding Guideline

Surgery for Aneurysm, Arteriovenous Malformation or Vascular Disease Procedures on the Skull, Meninges, and Brain

Includes craniotomy when appropriate for procedure.

AMA Coding Notes

Surgical Procedures on the Skull, Meninges, and Brain

(For injection procedure for cerebral angiography, see 36100-36218)

(For injection procedure for ventriculography, see 61026, 61120)

(For injection procedure for pneumoencephalography, use 61055)

Plain English Description

Blood flow to an intracranial aneurysm, vascular malformation, or carotid-cavernous fistula is interrupted using a combined intracranial and cervical approach to clamp the internal or external artery. An intracranial aneurysm, also called a cerebral or intracerebral aneurysm, is a weakened area in a blood vessel wall that expands and fills with blood. Depending on the size and location, it can put pressure on surrounding brain tissue, causing pain and neurological deficits. It can also rupture, causing an intracranial hemorrhage. Intracranial aneurysms may be congenital or acquired. A vascular malformation refers to any type of abnormality of the blood vessels. A carotid-cavernous fistula is an abnormal communication between the external or internal carotid artery and the venous cavernous sinus located behind the eyes. An incision is made on the side of the neck over the proximal aspect of the internal carotid artery that feeds the aneurysm. The artery is dissected from surrounding tissue and an adjustable clamp is placed around the artery to partially occlude it. Next, a craniotomy is performed by creating scalp flaps, followed by burr holes. The bone between the burr holes is then cut with a saw or craniotome and a bone flap is elevated. The dura is opened. The portion of the internal or external carotid artery that supplies the aneurysm, vascular malformation, or carotid-cavernous fistula is exposed and dissected free of surrounding tissue using microsurgical technique. A clamp is then placed around the carotid artery and slowly closed. Once the artery has been partially or completely occluded, the dura is closed; the bone flap is replaced and secured with sutures, wire, or miniplate and screws; and the overlying skin flap is closed with sutures.

Surgery of aneurysm, vascular malformation or carotid-cavernous fistula; by intracranial and cervical occlusion of carotid artery

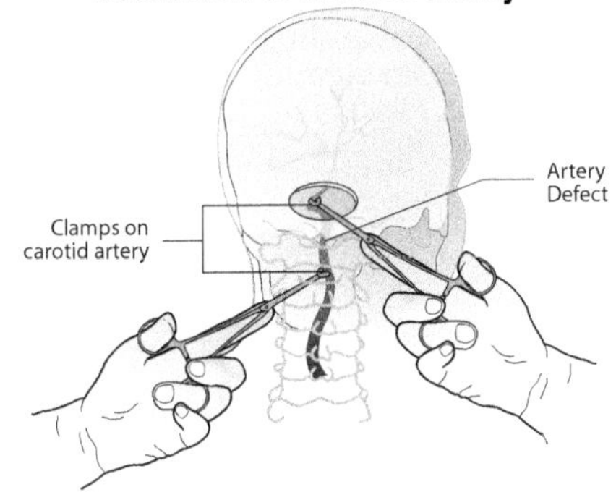

ICD-10-CM Diagnostic Codes

I67.0	Dissection of cerebral arteries, nonruptured
I67.1	Cerebral aneurysm, nonruptured
Q28.0	Arteriovenous malformation of precerebral vessels
Q28.1	Other malformations of precerebral vessels
Q28.2	Arteriovenous malformation of cerebral vessels
Q28.3	Other malformations of cerebral vessels

CCI Edits

Refer to Appendix A for CCI edits.

Pub 100

61705: Pub 100-04, 12, 20.4.5

Facility RVUs ☐

Code	Work	PE Facility	MP	Total Facility
61705	38.10	23.00	14.19	75.29

Non-facility RVUs ☐

Code	Work	PE Non-Facility	MP	Total Non-Facility
61705	38.10	23.00	14.19	75.29

Modifiers (PAR) ☐

Code	Mod 50	Mod 51	Mod 62	Mod 66	Mod 80
61705	0	2	1	0	2

Global Period

Code	Days
61705	090

61708

61708 Surgery of aneurysm, vascular malformation or carotid-cavernous fistula; by intracranial electrothrombosis

(For ligation or gradual occlusion of internal/common carotid artery, see 37605, 37606)

AMA Coding Guideline

Surgery for Aneurysm, Arteriovenous Malformation or Vascular Disease Procedures on the Skull, Meninges, and Brain

Includes craniotomy when appropriate for procedure.

AMA Coding Notes

Surgical Procedures on the Skull, Meninges, and Brain

(For injection procedure for cerebral angiography, see 36100-36218)

(For injection procedure for ventriculography, see 61026, 61120)

(For injection procedure for pneumoencephalography, use 61055)

Plain English Description

Blood flow to an intracranial aneurysm, vascular malformation, or carotid-cavernous fistula is interrupted using intracranial electrothrombosis. An intracranial aneurysm, also called a cerebral or intracerebral aneurysm, is a weakened area in the blood vessel wall that expands and fills with blood. Depending on the size and location, it can put pressure on surrounding brain tissue, causing pain and neurological deficits. It can also rupture, causing an intracranial hemorrhage. Intracranial aneurysms may be congenital or acquired. A vascular malformation refers to any type of abnormality of the blood vessels. A carotid-cavernous fistula is an abnormal communication between the external or internal carotid artery and the venous cavernous sinus located behind the eyes. A craniotomy is performed by creating scalp flaps, followed by burr holes. The bone between the burr holes is then cut with a saw or craniotome and a bone flap is elevated. The dura is opened. A catheter is inserted into the carotid artery that supplies the aneurysm, vascular malformation, or carotid-cavernous fistula. A microcatheter is advanced and positioned in the vascular target area. A coil is introduced via a delivery wire. A positive electrical current is applied to the proximal end of the delivery wire. This attracts negatively charged red and white blood cells, platelets, and fibrinogen to the positively charged coil. A thrombus develops in the aneurysmal sac, vascular malformation, or fistula. The positive current is applied for several minutes until the coils have dissolved in the thrombus. Once the aneurysm, malformation, or fistula has been completely occluded, the microcatheter is removed; the dura is closed; the bone flap is replaced and secured with sutures, wire, or miniplate and screws; and the overlying skin flap is closed with sutures.

Surgery of aneurysm, vascular malformation or carotid-cavernous fistula; by intracranial electrothrombosis

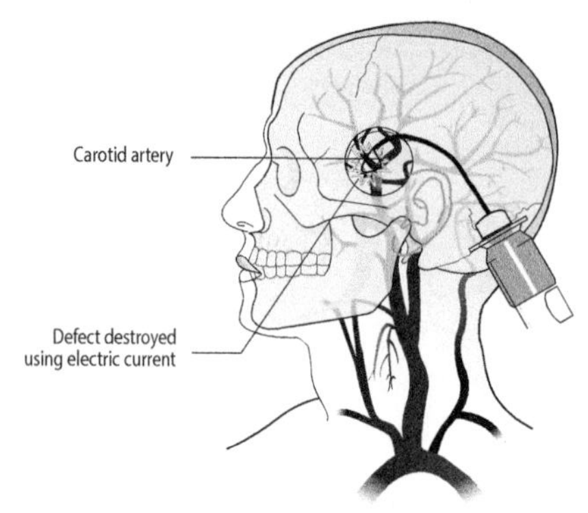

ICD-10-CM Diagnostic Codes

I67.0	Dissection of cerebral arteries, nonruptured
I67.1	Cerebral aneurysm, nonruptured
Q28.0	Arteriovenous malformation of precerebral vessels
Q28.1	Other malformations of precerebral vessels
Q28.2	Arteriovenous malformation of cerebral vessels
Q28.3	Other malformations of cerebral vessels

CCI Edits

Refer to Appendix A for CCI edits.

Pub 100

61708: Pub 100-04, 12, 20.4.5

Facility RVUs

Code	Work	PE Facility	MP	Total Facility
61708	37.20	22.59	13.84	73.63

Non-facility RVUs

Code	Work	PE Non-Facility	MP	Total Non-Facility
61708	37.20	22.59	13.84	73.63

Modifiers (PAR)

Code	Mod 50	Mod 51	Mod 62	Mod 66	Mod 80
61708	0	2	0	0	2

Global Period

Code	Days
61708	090

61710

61710 Surgery of aneurysm, vascular malformation or carotid-cavernous fistula; by intra-arterial embolization, injection procedure, or balloon catheter

AMA Coding Guideline

Surgery for Aneurysm, Arteriovenous Malformation or Vascular Disease Procedures on the Skull, Meninges, and Brain

Includes craniotomy when appropriate for procedure.

AMA Coding Notes

Surgical Procedures on the Skull, Meninges, and Brain

(For injection procedure for cerebral angiography, see 36100-36218)

(For injection procedure for ventriculography, see 61026, 61120)

(For injection procedure for pneumoencephalography, use 61055)

AMA *CPT Assistant*

61710: Nov 13: 6

Plain English Description

Blood flow to an intracranial aneurysm, vascular malformation, or carotid-cavernous fistula is interrupted using intra-arterial embolization, injection, or balloon catheter placement. An intracranial aneurysm, also called a cerebral or intracerebral aneurysm, is a weakened area in a blood vessel that expands and fills with blood. Depending on the size and location, it can put pressure on surrounding brain tissue, causing pain and neurological deficits. It can also rupture, causing an intracranial hemorrhage. Intracranial aneurysms may be congenital or acquired.
A vascular malformation refers to any type of abnormality of the blood vessels. A carotid-cavernous fistula is an abnormal communication between the external or internal carotid artery and the venous cavernous sinus located behind the eyes. A catheter is inserted through the skin into the access artery and maneuvered into the carotid artery that supplies the aneurysm, vascular malformation, or carotid-cavernous fistula. A microcatheter is advanced and positioned in the sac of the aneurysm, vascular malformation, or in the carotid cavernous fistula. One or more coils or a balloon catheter with detachable balloons is introduced via the microcatheter. The coil or balloon is deployed and secured at the site of the aneurysm, malformation, or fistula. The balloon immediately occludes the aneurysm, malformation, or fistula. In the case of the coils, blood clots will form around the coils and block the flow of blood. Alternatively, an injection procedure may be performed. Angiograms are obtained to ensure that the devices are properly placed. Once the aneurysmal sac, vascular malformation or fistula has been completely occluded or the coils are in place, the catheter is removed.

Surgery of aneurysm, vascular malformation, or carotid-cavernous fistula; by intra-arterial embolization, injection procedure, or balloon catheter

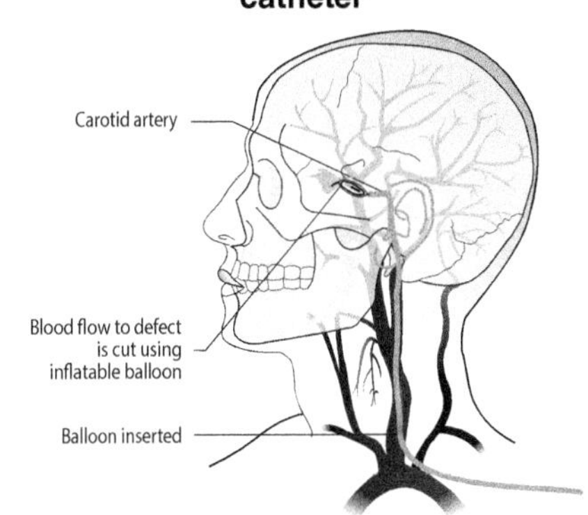

ICD-10-CM Diagnostic Codes

I67.0	Dissection of cerebral arteries, nonruptured
I67.1	Cerebral aneurysm, nonruptured
Q28.0	Arteriovenous malformation of precerebral vessels
Q28.1	Other malformations of precerebral vessels
Q28.2	Arteriovenous malformation of cerebral vessels
Q28.3	Other malformations of cerebral vessels

CCI Edits

Refer to Appendix A for CCI edits.

Pub 100

61710: Pub 100-04, 12, 20.4.5

Facility RVUs

Code	Work	PE Facility	MP	Total Facility
61710	31.29	19.21	11.59	62.09

Non-facility RVUs

Code	Work	PE Non-Facility	MP	Total Non-Facility
61710	31.29	19.21	11.59	62.09

Modifiers (PAR)

Code	Mod 50	Mod 51	Mod 62	Mod 66	Mod 80
61710	0	2	0	0	0

Global Period

Code	Days
61710	090

61711

61711 Anastomosis, arterial, extracranial-intracranial (eg, middle cerebral/cortical) arteries

(For carotid or vertebral thromboendarterectomy, use 35301)

(Use 69990 when the surgical microscope is employed for the microsurgical procedure. Do not use 69990 for visualization with magnifying loupes or corrected vision)

AMA Coding Guideline

Surgery for Aneurysm, Arteriovenous Malformation or Vascular Disease Procedures on the Skull, Meninges, and Brain

Includes craniotomy when appropriate for procedure.

AMA Coding Notes

Surgical Procedures on the Skull, Meninges, and Brain

(For injection procedure for cerebral angiography, see 36100-36218)

(For injection procedure for ventriculography, see 61026, 61120)

(For injection procedure for pneumoencephalography, use 61055)

Plain English Description

An extracranial to intracranial anastomosis is a bypass procedure performed to augment cerebral blood flow. It typically involves connection of the superficial temporal artery to a branch of the middle cerebral or cortical arteries, although it can be performed on other arteries as well. A craniotomy is performed by creating scalp flaps, followed by burr holes. The bone between the burr holes is then cut with a saw or craniotome and a bone flap elevated. The dura is opened and the affected intracranial artery exposed. The donor artery is also exposed. If needed, a vein bypass graft may be harvested, usually the saphenous vein in the leg. Using microscopic technique, the obstructed portion of the middle cerebral branch or cortical artery is bypassed either by direct bypass or using a bypass graft. If direct bypass is used, the donor artery is mobilized and transected. The obstructed artery is incised at a point beyond the obstruction and the donor artery is sutured to the obstructed artery. If a vein graft is used, the donor and obstructed arteries are incised and the vein graft sutured to these arteries to provide a conduit that bypasses the obstructed region. Intraoperative angiograms are obtained to verify patency at the anastomosis site and to evaluate blood flow in the brain. The dura is closed, the bone flap replaced and secured with sutures, wire, or miniplate and screws, and the overlying skin flap closed with sutures

Anastomosis, arterial, extracranial-intracranial

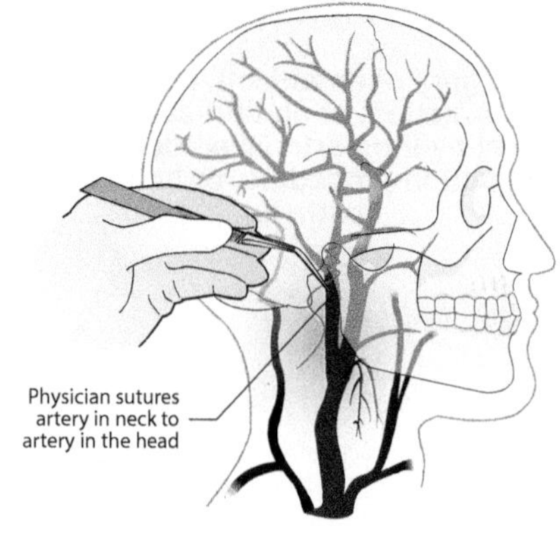

ICD-10-CM Diagnostic Codes

	Code	Description
	G46.0	Middle cerebral artery syndrome
	G46.1	Anterior cerebral artery syndrome
	I63.81	Other cerebral infarction due to occlusion or stenosis of small artery
⇄	I65.21	Occlusion and stenosis of right carotid artery
⇄	I65.22	Occlusion and stenosis of left carotid artery
⇄	I65.23	Occlusion and stenosis of bilateral carotid arteries
⇄	I66.01	Occlusion and stenosis of right middle cerebral artery
⇄	I66.02	Occlusion and stenosis of left middle cerebral artery
⇄	I66.03	Occlusion and stenosis of bilateral middle cerebral arteries
⇄	I66.11	Occlusion and stenosis of right anterior cerebral artery
⇄	I66.12	Occlusion and stenosis of left anterior cerebral artery
⇄	I66.13	Occlusion and stenosis of bilateral anterior cerebral arteries
	I67.1	Cerebral aneurysm, nonruptured
	I67.5	Moyamoya disease
	I67.82	Cerebral ischemia

CCI Edits

Refer to Appendix A for CCI edits.

Pub 100

61711: Pub 100-04, 12, 20.4.5

Facility RVUs ▯

Code	Work	PE Facility	MP	Total Facility
61711	38.23	22.92	13.79	74.94

Non-facility RVUs ▯

Code	Work	PE Non-Facility	MP	Total Non-Facility
61711	38.23	22.92	13.79	74.94

Modifiers (PAR) ▯

Code	Mod 50	Mod 51	Mod 62	Mod 66	Mod 80
61711	0	2	1	0	2

Global Period

Code	Days
61711	090

● New ▲ Revised ✚ Add On ⊘Modifier 51 Exempt ★Telemedicine ▯ CPT QuickRef ✗FDA Pending ⇄ Laterality ⓻ Seventh Character ♂Male ♀Female

61720-61735

61720 Creation of lesion by stereotactic method, including burr hole(s) and localizing and recording techniques, single or multiple stages; globus pallidus or thalamus

61735 Creation of lesion by stereotactic method, including burr hole(s) and localizing and recording techniques, single or multiple stages; subcortical structure(s) other than globus pallidus or thalamus

AMA Coding Notes

Surgical Procedures on the Skull, Meninges, and Brain

(For injection procedure for cerebral angiography, see 36100-36218)

(For injection procedure for ventriculography, see 61026, 61120)

(For injection procedure for pneumoencephalography, use 61055)

AMA *CPT Assistant*

61720: Jul 11: 12, Jul 14: 9

61735: Jul 11: 12

Plain English Description

The globus pallidus and thalamus are subcortical structures in the brain, which means that they lie below the cerebral cortex. These two structures are located in the forebrain. The globus pallidus is a pale-appearing spherical area that is part of the lentiform nucleus, which is a component of the basal ganglia. The basal ganglia are the large masses of gray matter at the base of the cerebral hemisphere of the brain. The thalamus is a large oval structure immediately above the midbrain. Other subcortical structures of the forebrain include the limbic system, which contains the hippocampus, amygdala, cingulate gyrus and others, and the hypothalamus. The midbrain and hindbrain are also subcortical structures. The midbrain contains the tectum and tegmentum, and the hindbrain contains the cerebellum, reticular formation, pons, and medulla. Stereotactic lesion creation of the subcortical structures is a type of psychosurgical procedure and is considered investigational or experimental by many payers. A special frame is attached to the skull. MRI or CT scans are used to map out the procedure and determine where the lesions will be created. Surgical apparatus attached to the head frame are adjusted to the MRI or CT coordinates of the target region. Alternatively, frameless stereotactic surgery may be performed using fiduciary markers. One or more small incisions are made over the lateral aspect of the skull and the skull is exposed. Burr holes are created to access the subcortical region of the brain. Electrocautery probes are inserted through the burr holes, and using the stereotactic coordinates, the probes are advanced to the region where the lesion is to be created. A radiofrequency current is then generated and the desired tissue is ablated. If the desired result is not attained during the first surgical session, the procedure is repeated during a subsequent surgery on another day. Use 61720 for creation of a lesion in the globus pallidus or thalamus. Use 61735 for creation of a lesion in other subcortical structures.

Creation of lesion by stereotactic method, Including burr hole(s) and recording techniques

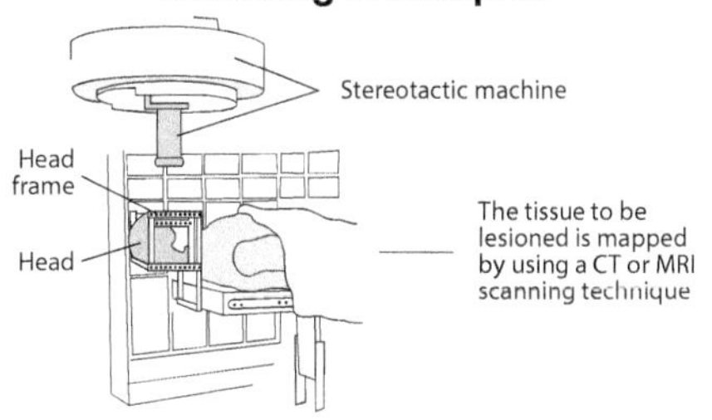

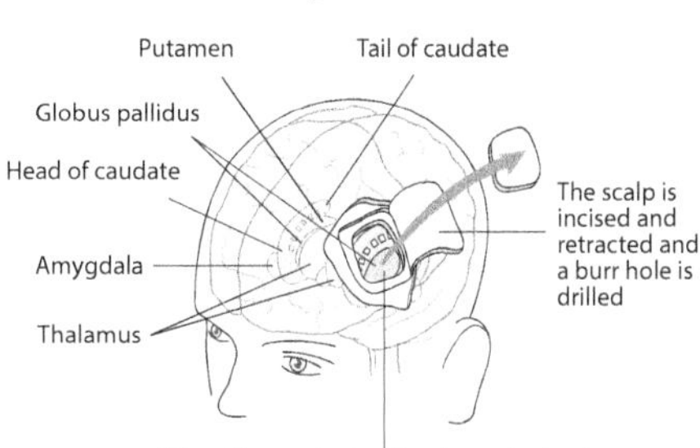

ICD-10-CM Diagnostic Codes

G20	Parkinson's disease
G21.3	Postencephalitic parkinsonism
G21.4	Vascular parkinsonism
G21.8	Other secondary parkinsonism
G21.9	Secondary parkinsonism, unspecified
G24.1	Genetic torsion dystonia
G24.3	Spasmodic torticollis
G24.8	Other dystonia
G25.0	Essential tremor
G25.5	Other chorea

CCI Edits

Refer to Appendix A for CCI edits.

Facility RVUs

Code	Work	PE Facility	MP	Total Facility
61720	17.62	12.54	6.49	36.65
61735	22.35	15.37	8.23	45.95

Non-facility RVUs

Code	Work	PE Non-Facility	MP	Total Non-Facility
61720	17.62	12.54	6.49	36.65
61735	22.35	15.37	8.23	45.95

Modifiers (PAR)

Code	Mod 50	Mod 51	Mod 62	Mod 66	Mod 80
61720	0	2	0	0	1
61735	0	2	1	0	1

Global Period

Code	Days
61720	090
61735	090

61750-61751

61750 Stereotactic biopsy, aspiration, or excision, including burr hole(s), for intracranial lesion

61751 Stereotactic biopsy, aspiration, or excision, including burr hole(s), for intracranial lesion; with computed tomography and/or magnetic resonance guidance

(For radiological supervision and interpretation of computerized tomography, see 70450, 70460, or 70470 as appropriate)

(For radiological supervision and interpretation of magnetic resonance imaging, see 70551, 70552, or 70553 as appropriate)

AMA Coding Notes

Surgical Procedures on the Skull, Meninges, and Brain

(For injection procedure for cerebral angiography, see 36100-36218)

(For injection procedure for ventriculography, see 61026, 61120)

(For injection procedure for pneumoencephalography, use 61055)

AMA *CPT Assistant* □

61750: Nov 99: 30

61751: Jun 96: 10, Nov 99: 30, Dec 04: 20, Jul 11: 12

Plain English Description

Stereotactic biopsy, aspiration, or excision is performed on a deep mass, tumor, or lesion that cannot be approached using an open technique. A special frame is attached to the skull. MRI or CT scans are used to map out the location of the mass, tumor, or lesion and determine where the lesions will be created. Alternatively, angiography may be used. To obtain a biopsy, a stereotactic biopsy apparatus is attached to the head frame and adjusted to the MRI, CT, or angiogram coordinates of the target region. Alternatively, frameless stereotactic surgery may be performed using fiduciary markers. An incision is made in the skin overlying the site where the burr hole will be created. The burr hole is drilled and the biopsy probe is inserted through the burr hole. Using the stereotactic coordinates, the biopsy probe is advanced to the site of the mass, tumor, or lesion. Tissue samples are obtained. The same technique is used for an aspiration procedure except that a stereotactic aspiration device is used. To excise a mass, tumor, or lesion, stereotactic surgical instruments are passed through one or more burr holes and the tumor is removed in a piecemeal fashion. Once the procedure is complete, the burr hole is filled with bone wax and the skin incision is closed. The stereotactic frame is removed. Use 61750 when the procedure is performed without CT or MRI guidance. Use 61751 when CT or MRI guidance is used.

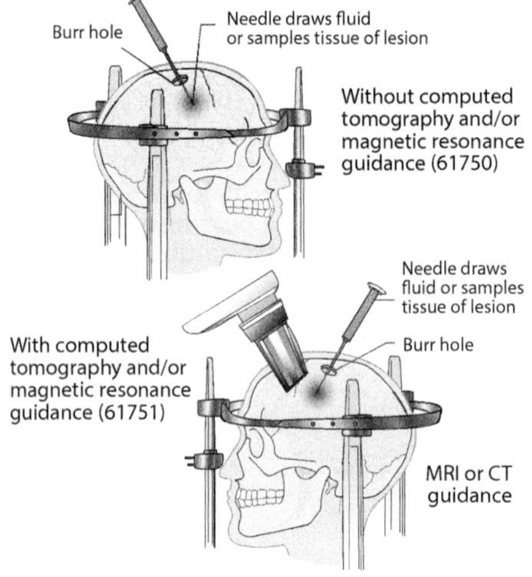

ICD-10-CM Diagnostic Codes

	Code	Description
	A06.6	Amebic brain abscess
	A17.81	Tuberculoma of brain and spinal cord
	A54.82	Gonococcal brain abscess
	B43.1	Pheomycotic brain abscess
	B94.8	Sequelae of other specified infectious and parasitic diseases
	B95.0	Streptococcus, group A, as the cause of diseases classified elsewhere
	B95.1	Streptococcus, group B, as the cause of diseases classified elsewhere
	B95.3	Streptococcus pneumoniae as the cause of diseases classified elsewhere
	B95.4	Other streptococcus as the cause of diseases classified elsewhere
	B95.5	Unspecified streptococcus as the cause of diseases classified elsewhere
	B95.61	Methicillin susceptible Staphylococcus aureus infection as the cause of diseases classified elsewhere
	B95.62	Methicillin resistant Staphylococcus aureus infection as the cause of diseases classified elsewhere
	B95.7	Other staphylococcus as the cause of diseases classified elsewhere
	B95.8	Unspecified staphylococcus as the cause of diseases classified elsewhere
	B96.3	Hemophilus influenzae [H. influenzae] as the cause of diseases classified elsewhere
	C70.0	Malignant neoplasm of cerebral meninges
	C71.0	Malignant neoplasm of cerebrum, except lobes and ventricles
	C71.1	Malignant neoplasm of frontal lobe
	C71.2	Malignant neoplasm of temporal lobe
	C71.3	Malignant neoplasm of parietal lobe
	C71.4	Malignant neoplasm of occipital lobe
	C71.5	Malignant neoplasm of cerebral ventricle
	C71.8	Malignant neoplasm of overlapping sites of brain
	C79.31	Secondary malignant neoplasm of brain
	C79.32	Secondary malignant neoplasm of cerebral meninges
	D32.0	Benign neoplasm of cerebral meninges
	D33.0	Benign neoplasm of brain, supratentorial
	D33.3	Benign neoplasm of cranial nerves
	D42.0	Neoplasm of uncertain behavior of cerebral meninges
	D43.0	Neoplasm of uncertain behavior of brain, supratentorial
	D49.6	Neoplasm of unspecified behavior of brain
	D49.7	Neoplasm of unspecified behavior of endocrine glands and other parts of nervous system
	G06.0	Intracranial abscess and granuloma
	G07	Intracranial and intraspinal abscess and granuloma in diseases classified elsewhere
	G09	Sequelae of inflammatory diseases of central nervous system
	G93.0	Cerebral cysts
	Q04.6	Congenital cerebral cysts
	S01.84XS	Puncture wound with foreign body of other part of head, sequela
	S02.0XXS	Fracture of vault of skull, sequela
⇄	S02.101S	Fracture of base of skull, right side, sequela
⇄	S02.102S	Fracture of base of skull, left side, sequela
⇄	S02.11AS	Type I occipital condyle fracture, right side, sequela
⇄	S02.11BS	Type I occipital condyle fracture, left side, sequela
⇄	S02.11CS	Type II occipital condyle fracture, right side, sequela
⇄	S02.11DS	Type II occipital condyle fracture, left side, sequela
⇄	S02.11ES	Type III occipital condyle fracture, right side, sequela
⇄	S02.11FS	Type III occipital condyle fracture, left side, sequela
⇄	S02.11GS	Other fracture of occiput, right side, sequela
	S02.19XS	Other fracture of base of skull, sequela
	S02.2XXS	Fracture of nasal bones, sequela
⇄	S02.31XS	Fracture of orbital floor, right side, sequela
⇄	S02.32XS	Fracture of orbital floor, left side, sequela

CCI Edits

Refer to Appendix A for CCI edits.

Facility RVUs

Code	Work	PE Facility	MP	Total Facility
61750	19.83	13.53	7.28	40.64
61751	18.79	14.11	6.87	39.77

Non-facility RVUs

Code	Work	PE Non-Facility	MP	Total Non-Facility
61750	19.83	13.53	7.28	40.64
61751	18.79	14.11	6.87	39.77

Modifiers (PAR)

Code	Mod 50	Mod 51	Mod 62	Mod 66	Mod 80
61750	0	2	1	0	1
61751	0	2	1	0	1

Global Period

Code	Days
61750	090
61751	090

61760

61760 Stereotactic implantation of depth electrodes into the cerebrum for long-term seizure monitoring

AMA Coding Notes

Surgical Procedures on the Skull, Meninges, and Brain

(For injection procedure for cerebral angiography, see 36100-36218)

(For injection procedure for ventriculography, see 61026, 61120)

(For injection procedure for pneumoencephalography, use 61055)

AMA *CPT Assistant* ▢

61760: Jul 11: 12

Plain English Description

Stereotactic implantation of depth electrodes in the deep tissues of the cerebrum for long-term seizure monitoring is performed. A special frame is attached to the skull. MRI or CT scans are used to map out the site where the depth electrodes will be placed. An insertion apparatus containing the depth electrodes is attached to the head frame and adjusted to the MRI or CT coordinates. Alternatively, frameless stereotactic surgery may be performed using fiduciary markers. An incision is made in the skin overlying the site where the burr hole will be created. The burr hole is drilled and the depth electrodes are inserted through the burr hole. Using the stereotactic coordinates, the depth electrodes are advanced to the desired site in the deep tissues of the cerebrum. The electrodes are tested to ensure they are functioning properly. The burr hole is filled with bone wax and the skin incision is closed. The stereotactic frame is removed.

Stereotactic implantation of depth electrodes into the cerebrum for long term seizure monitoring

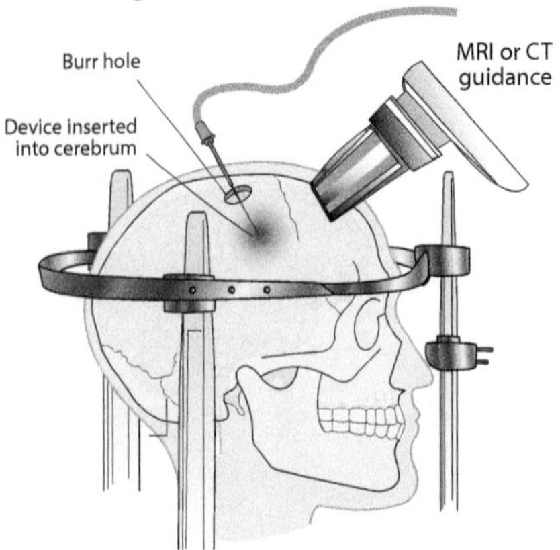

ICD-10-CM Diagnostic Codes

G40.011	Localization-related (focal) (partial) idiopathic epilepsy and epileptic syndromes with seizures of localized onset, intractable, with status epilepticus
G40.019	Localization-related (focal) (partial) idiopathic epilepsy and epileptic syndromes with seizures of localized onset, intractable, without status epilepticus
G40.111	Localization-related (focal) (partial) symptomatic epilepsy and epileptic syndromes with simple partial seizures, intractable, with status epilepticus
G40.119	Localization-related (focal) (partial) symptomatic epilepsy and epileptic syndromes with simple partial seizures, intractable, without status epilepticus
G40.211	Localization-related (focal) (partial) symptomatic epilepsy and epileptic syndromes with complex partial seizures, intractable, with status epilepticus
G40.219	Localization-related (focal) (partial) symptomatic epilepsy and epileptic syndromes with complex partial seizures, intractable, without status epilepticus

CCI Edits

Refer to Appendix A for CCI edits.

Facility RVUs ▢

Code	Work	PE Facility	MP	Total Facility
61760	22.39	15.01	8.21	45.61

Non-facility RVUs ▢

Code	Work	PE Non-Facility	MP	Total Non-Facility
61760	22.39	15.01	8.21	45.61

Modifiers (PAR) ▢

Code	Mod 50	Mod 51	Mod 62	Mod 66	Mod 80
61760	0	2	2	0	1

Global Period

Code	Days
61760	090

61781-61782

+ **61781 Stereotactic computer-assisted (navigational) procedure; cranial, intradural (List separately in addition to code for primary procedure)**

(Do not report 61781 in conjunction with 61720-61791, 61796-61799, 61863-61868, 62201, 77371-77373, 77432)

+ **61782 Stereotactic computer-assisted (navigational) procedure; cranial, extradural (List separately in addition to code for primary procedure)**

(Do not report 61781, 61782 by the same individual during the same surgical session)

AMA Coding Notes

Surgical Procedures on the Skull, Meninges, and Brain

(For injection procedure for cerebral angiography, see 36100-36218)

(For injection procedure for ventriculography, see 61026, 61120)

(For injection procedure for pneumoencephalography, use 61055)

AMA *CPT Assistant* ☐

61781: Jul 11: 12, Jul 14: 9, Sep 14: 14

61782: Jul 11: 12

Plain English Description

Stereotactic procedures are those that are done in a defined three-dimensional space using a computer system. The use of computer-assisted stereotaxis in conjunction with a definitive procedure on the brain allows the physician to perform the procedure without general anesthesia, through much smaller skin incisions and bone openings, and to locate the surgical site more precisely. A local anesthetic is injected into the planned pin sites on the skull. The stereotactic ring is positioned over the skull and pins are placed through the skin and into the skull to immobilize the head. A second localizing ring is then temporarily placed on the stereotactic ring and a CT scan is performed. The information obtained from the CT scan is then analyzed using navigational computer software that provides a set of coordinates to identify the precise optimal location for the skin incision and bone cuts and to locate the lesion or region of the brain precisely on which the definitive procedure will be performed. The physician then uses the stereotactic equipment and the coordinates obtained from the CT scan to perform the separately reportable definitive procedure. Use 61781 for a procedure within or beneath the dura mater (intradural); use 61782 for a procedure outside the dura mater (extradural).

Stereotactic computer-assisted procedure, cranial

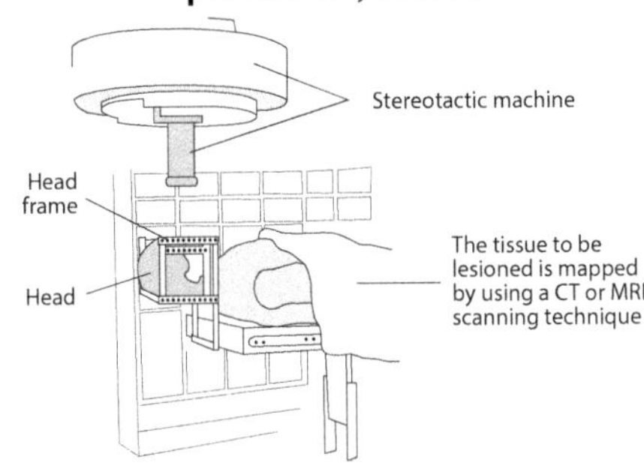

Intradural (61781), extradural (61782)

ICD-10-CM Diagnostic Codes

See Primary Procedure code for crosswalks.

CCI Edits

Refer to Appendix A for CCI edits.

Facility RVUs ☐

Code	Work	PE Facility	MP	Total Facility
61781	3.75	1.72	1.34	6.81
61782	3.18	1.37	0.46	5.01

Non-facility RVUs ☐

Code	Work	PE Non-Facility	MP	Total Non-Facility
61781	3.75	1.72	1.34	6.81
61782	3.18	1.37	0.46	5.01

Modifiers (PAR) ☐

Code	Mod 50	Mod 51	Mod 62	Mod 66	Mod 80
61781	0	0	0	0	0
61782	0	0	0	0	0

Global Period

Code	Days
61781	ZZZ
61782	ZZZ

61783

+ **61783 Stereotactic computer-assisted (navigational) procedure; spinal (List separately in addition to code for primary procedure)**

(Do not report 61783 in conjunction with 63620, 63621)

AMA Coding Notes

Surgical Procedures on the Skull, Meninges, and Brain

(For injection procedure for cerebral angiography, see 36100-36218)

(For injection procedure for ventriculography, see 61026, 61120)

(For injection procedure for pneumoencephalography, use 61055)

AMA *CPT Assistant*

61783: Jul 11: 12

Plain English Description

Stereotactic procedures are those that are done in a defined three-dimensional space using a computer system. The use of computer-assisted stereotaxis in conjunction with a definitive procedure on the spine allows the physician to perform the procedure without general anesthesia, through much smaller incisions, and to locate the surgical site more precisely. The patient is immobilized and a CT scan is performed on the region of the spine where the definitive procedure will be performed. The information obtained from the CT scan is then analyzed using navigational computer software that provides a set of coordinates to identify the precise optimal location for the skin incision and bone cuts and to locate precisely the lesion or region of the spine on which the definitive procedure will be performed. The physician then uses the stereotactic equipment and the coordinates obtained from the CT scan to perform the separately reportable definitive procedure.

Stereotactic computer-assisted procedure, spinal

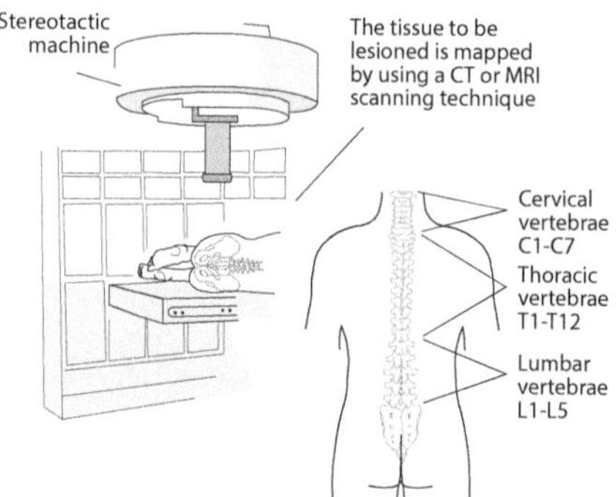

ICD-10-CM Diagnostic Codes

See Primary Procedure code for crosswalks.

CCI Edits

Refer to Appendix A for CCI edits.

Facility RVUs

Code	Work	PE Facility	MP	Total Facility
61783	3.75	1.76	1.25	6.76

Non-facility RVUs

Code	Work	PE Non-Facility	MP	Total Non-Facility
61783	3.75	1.76	1.25	6.76

Modifiers (PAR)

Code	Mod 50	Mod 51	Mod 62	Mod 66	Mod 80
61783	0	0	0	0	0

Global Period

Code	Days
61783	ZZZ

61790-61791

61790 Creation of lesion by stereotactic method, percutaneous, by neurolytic agent (eg, alcohol, thermal, electrical, radiofrequency); gasserian ganglion

61791 Creation of lesion by stereotactic method, percutaneous, by neurolytic agent (eg, alcohol, thermal, electrical, radiofrequency); trigeminal medullary tract

AMA Coding Notes

Surgical Procedures on the Skull, Meninges, and Brain

(For injection procedure for cerebral angiography, see 36100-36218)

(For injection procedure for ventriculography, see 61026, 61120)

(For injection procedure for pneumoencephalography, use 61055)

AMA *CPT Assistant*

61790: Jul 11: 12

61791: Jul 11: 12, Jul 14: 9

Plain English Description

A special frame is attached to the skull. MRI or CT scans are used to map out the procedure and determine where the lesions in the gasserian ganglion or trigeminal medullary tract will be created. Depending on the type of destruction procedure performed, a needle or probe apparatus is attached to the head frame and adjusted to the MRI or CT coordinates of the target region. Alternatively, frameless stereotactic surgery may be performed using fiduciary markers. The needle or probe is then advanced through the skin to the region where the lesion will be created using the stereotactic coordinates. If an injection procedure is performed, a neurolytic agent such as alcohol is injected. If an electric or radiofrequency probe is used, the probe is activated and the desired tissue is ablated. Use 61790 for creation of a lesion in the gasserian ganglion. Use 61791 for creation of a lesion in the trigeminal medullary tract.

Creation of lesion by stereotactic method, percutaneous, by neurolytic agent

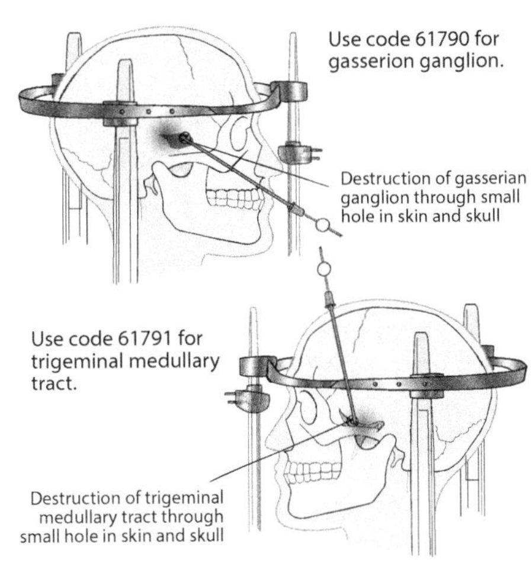

ICD-10-CM Diagnostic Codes

B02.22	Postherpetic trigeminal neuralgia
G44.001	Cluster headache syndrome, unspecified, intractable
G44.021	Chronic cluster headache, intractable
G44.041	Chronic paroxysmal hemicrania, intractable
G44.091	Other trigeminal autonomic cephalgias (TAC), intractable
G44.51	Hemicrania continua
G50.0	Trigeminal neuralgia
G50.8	Other disorders of trigeminal nerve

CCI Edits

Refer to Appendix A for CCI edits.

Facility RVUs

Code	Work	PE Facility	MP	Total Facility
61790	11.60	9.52	4.19	25.31
61791	15.41	11.38	5.66	32.45

Non-facility RVUs

Code	Work	PE Non-Facility	MP	Total Non-Facility
61790	11.60	9.52	4.19	25.31
61791	15.41	11.38	5.66	32.45

Modifiers (PAR)

Code	Mod 50	Mod 51	Mod 62	Mod 66	Mod 80
61790	1	2	0	0	1
61791	1	2	0	0	0

Global Period

Code	Days
61790	090
61791	090

61796-61797

61796 Stereotactic radiosurgery (particle beam, gamma ray, or linear accelerator); 1 simple cranial lesion

(Do not report 61796 more than once per course of treatment)

(Do not report 61796 in conjunction with 61798)

✚ **61797 Stereotactic radiosurgery (particle beam, gamma ray, or linear accelerator); each additional cranial lesion, simple (List separately in addition to code for primary procedure)**

(Use 61797 in conjunction with 61796, 61798)

(For each course of treatment, 61797 and 61799 may be reported no more than once per lesion. Do not report any combination of 61797 and 61799 more than 4 times for entire course of treatment regardless of number of lesions treated)

AMA Coding Guideline

Stereotactic Radiosurgery (Cranial) Procedures on the Skull, Meninges, and Brain

Cranial stereotactic radiosurgery is a distinct procedure that utilizes externally generated ionizing radiation to inactivate or eradicate defined target(s) in the head without the need to make an incision. The target is defined by and the treatment is delivered using high-resolution stereotactic imaging. Stereotactic radiosurgery codes and headframe application procedures are reported by the neurosurgeon. The radiation oncologist reports the appropriate code(s) for clinical treatment planning, physics and dosimetry, treatment delivery, and management from the Radiation Oncology section (77261-77790). Any necessary planning, dosimetry, targeting, positioning, or blocking by the neurosurgeon is included in the stereotactic radiation surgery services. The same individual should not report stereotactic radiosurgery services with radiation treatment management codes (77427-77435).

Cranial stereotactic radiosurgery is typically performed in a single planning and treatment session, using a rigidly attached stereotactic guiding device, other immobilization technology and/or a stereotactic image-guidance system, but can be performed with more than one planning session and in a limited number of treatment sessions, up to a maximum of five sessions. Do not report stereotactic radiosurgery more than once per lesion per course of treatment when the treatment requires more than one session.

Codes 61796 and 61797 involve stereotactic radiosurgery for simple cranial lesions. Simple cranial lesions are lesions less than 3.5 cm in maximum dimension that do not meet the definition of a complex lesion provided below. Report code 61796 when all lesions are simple.

Codes 61798 and 61799 involve stereotactic radiosurgery for complex cranial lesions and procedures that create therapeutic lesions (eg, thalamotomy or pallidotomy). All lesions 3.5 cm in maximum dimension or greater are complex. When performing therapeutic lesion creation procedures, report code 61798 only once regardless of the number of lesions created. Schwannomas, arterio-venous malformations, pituitary tumors, glomus tumors, pineal region tumors and cavernous sinus/parasellar/petroclival tumors are complex. Any lesion that is adjacent (5mm or less) to the optic nerve/optic chasm/optic tract or within the brainstem is complex. If treating multiple lesions, and any single lesion treated is complex, use 61798.

Do not report codes 61796-61800 in conjunction with code 20660.

Codes 61796-61799 include computer-assisted planning. Do not report codes 61796-61799 in conjunction with 61781-61783.

AMA Coding Notes

Stereotactic Radiosurgery (Cranial) Procedures on the Skull, Meninges, and Brain

(For intensity modulated beam delivery plan and treatment, see 77301, 77385, 77386. For stereotactic body radiation therapy, see 77373, 77435)

Surgical Procedures on the Skull, Meninges, and Brain

(For injection procedure for cerebral angiography, see 36100-36218)

(For injection procedure for ventriculography, see 61026, 61120)

(For injection procedure for pneumoencephalography, use 61055)

AMA *CPT Assistant*

61796: Jul 11: 12, Apr 12: 11, Jul 14: 9, Jun 15: 6

61797: Jul 11: 12, Apr 12: 11, Jun 15: 6

Plain English Description

Stereotactic radiosurgery using a particle beam, gamma ray, or linear accelerator is performed on a single, simple cranial lesion in 61796. Stereotactic radiosurgery delivers a very high radiation dose to a precise location using multiple intersecting beams of radiation. Particle beam or cyclotron technology has limited use in the United States. Gamma ray technology uses a gamma knife composed of 201 beams of highly focused gamma rays to treat small to medium-sized cranial lesions. Linear accelerator (LINAC) technology uses high-energy X-ray photons or electrons in curving paths around the head and can be used to treat larger cranial lesions. A rigid stereotactic frame is attached to the head in a separately reportable procedure to secure the head in a fixed position and ensure that the radiation beams are directed at the lesion with the necessary precision. During a separately reportable planning procedure, the lesion is visualized using three-dimensional MRI or CT scans. The required treatment is defined and includes determination of lesion location and volume, identification of surrounding structures and assessment of risk of damage to these structures, and dose computation. If a gamma knife is used, the patient is placed on the gamma bed. A helmet with several hundred holes is attached to the head frame. The gamma bed moves backward into the treatment area. The helmet locks into the radiation source and the radiation dose is delivered. If a linear accelerator is used, a computer is used in conjunction with a micro-multileaf collimator attached to the linear accelerator, which arranges and shapes high-energy radiation beams in the exact configuration of the lesion. The gantry rotates around the patient and delivers the planned radiation dose to the lesion. Use code 61796 for a single, simple cranial lesion and code 61797 for each additional simple cranial lesion.

Stereotactic radiosurgery (particle beam, gamma ray, or linear accelerator)

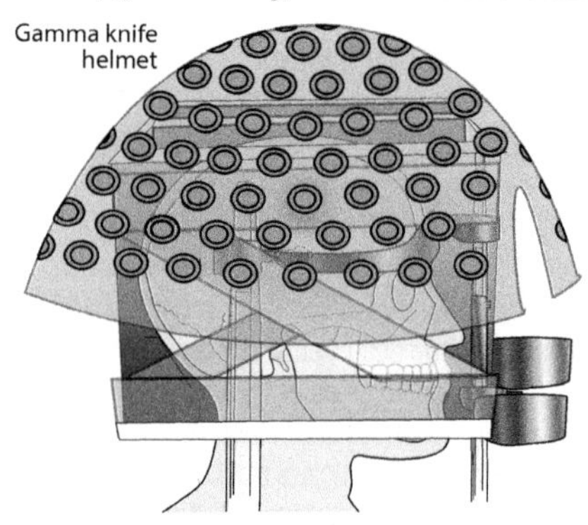

1 simple cranial lesion (61796); each additional cranial lesion, simple (61797)

ICD-10-CM Diagnostic Codes

C41.0	Malignant neoplasm of bones of skull and face
C71.0	Malignant neoplasm of cerebrum, except lobes and ventricles
C71.1	Malignant neoplasm of frontal lobe
C71.2	Malignant neoplasm of temporal lobe
C71.3	Malignant neoplasm of parietal lobe
C71.4	Malignant neoplasm of occipital lobe
C71.5	Malignant neoplasm of cerebral ventricle
C79.31	Secondary malignant neoplasm of brain
C79.51	Secondary malignant neoplasm of bone

D16.4	Benign neoplasm of bones of skull and face
D33.0	Benign neoplasm of brain, supratentorial
D43.0	Neoplasm of uncertain behavior of brain, supratentorial

CCI Edits

Refer to Appendix A for CCI edits.

Facility RVUs

Code	Work	PE Facility	MP	Total Facility
61796	13.93	10.23	5.08	29.24
61797	3.48	1.60	1.27	6.35

Non-facility RVUs

Code	Work	PE Non-Facility	MP	Total Non-Facility
61796	13.93	10.23	5.08	29.24
61797	3.48	1.60	1.27	6.35

Modifiers (PAR)

Code	Mod 50	Mod 51	Mod 62	Mod 66	Mod 80
61796	0	0	0	0	2
61797	0	0	0	0	2

Global Period

Code	Days
61796	090
61797	ZZZ

61798-61799

61798 Stereotactic radiosurgery (particle beam, gamma ray, or linear accelerator); 1 complex cranial lesion

(Do not report 61798 more than once per course of treatment)

(Do not report 61798 in conjunction with 61796)

+ **61799 Stereotactic radiosurgery (particle beam, gamma ray, or linear accelerator); each additional cranial lesion, complex (List separately in addition to code for primary procedure)**

(Use 61799 in conjunction with 61798)

(For each course of treatment, 61797 and 61799 may be reported no more than once per lesion. Do not report any combination of 61797 and 61799 more than 4 times for entire course of treatment regardless of number of lesions treated)

AMA Coding Guideline

Stereotactic Radiosurgery (Cranial) Procedures on the Skull, Meninges, and Brain

Cranial stereotactic radiosurgery is a distinct procedure that utilizes externally generated ionizing radiation to inactivate or eradicate defined target(s) in the head without the need to make an incision. The target is defined by and the treatment is delivered using high-resolution stereotactic imaging. Stereotactic radiosurgery codes and headframe application procedures are reported by the neurosurgeon. The radiation oncologist reports the appropriate code(s) for clinical treatment planning, physics and dosimetry, treatment delivery, and management from the Radiation Oncology section (77261-77790). Any necessary planning, dosimetry, targeting, positioning, or blocking by the neurosurgeon is included in the stereotactic radiation surgery services. The same individual should not report stereotactic radiosurgery services with radiation treatment management codes (77427-77435).

Cranial stereotactic radiosurgery is typically performed in a single planning and treatment session, using a rigidly attached stereotactic guiding device, other immobilization technology and/or a stereotactic image-guidance system, but can be performed with more than one planning session and in a limited number of treatment sessions, up to a maximum of five sessions. Do not report stereotactic radiosurgery more than once per lesion per course of treatment when the treatment requires more than one session.

Codes 61796 and 61797 involve stereotactic radiosurgery for simple cranial lesions. Simple cranial lesions are lesions less than 3.5 cm in maximum dimension that do not meet the definition of a complex lesion provided below. Report code 61796 when all lesions are simple.

Codes 61798 and 61799 involve stereotactic radiosurgery for complex cranial lesions and procedures that create therapeutic lesions (eg, thalamotomy or pallidotomy). All lesions 3.5 cm in maximum dimension or greater are complex. When performing therapeutic lesion creation procedures, report code 61798 only once regardless of the number of lesions created. Schwannomas, arterio-venous malformations, pituitary tumors, glomus tumors, pineal region tumors and cavernous sinus/parasellar/petroclival tumors are complex. Any lesion that is adjacent (5mm or less) to the optic nerve/optic chasm/optic tract or within the brainstem is complex. If treating multiple lesions, and any single lesion treated is complex, use 61798.

Do not report codes 61796-61800 in conjunction with code 20660.

Codes 61796-61799 include computer-assisted planning. Do not report codes 61796-61799 in conjunction with 61781-61783.

AMA Coding Notes

Stereotactic Radiosurgery (Cranial) Procedures on the Skull, Meninges, and Brain

(For intensity modulated beam delivery plan and treatment, see 77301, 77385, 77386. For stereotactic body radiation therapy, see 77373, 77435)

Surgical Procedures on the Skull, Meninges, and Brain

(For injection procedure for cerebral angiography, see 36100-36218)

(For injection procedure for ventriculography, see 61026, 61120)

(For injection procedure for pneumoencephalography, use 61055)

AMA *CPT Assistant* ☐

61798: Jul 11: 12, Apr 12: 11, Jun 15: 6

61799: Jul 11: 12, Apr 12: 11, Jul 14: 9, Jun 15: 6

Plain English Description

Stereotactic radiosurgery using a particle beam, gamma ray, or linear accelerator is performed on a single, complex cranial lesion in 61798. Stereotactic radiosurgery delivers a very high radiation dose to a precise location using multiple intersecting beams of radiation. Particle beam or cyclotron technology has limited use in the United States. Gamma ray technology uses a gamma knife composed of 201 beams of highly focused gamma rays to treat small to medium-sized cranial lesions. Linear accelerator (LINAC) technology uses high-energy X-ray photons or electrons in curving paths around the head and can be used to treat larger cranial lesions. A rigid stereotactic frame is attached to the head in a separately reportable procedure to secure the head in a fixed position and ensure that the radiation beams are directed at the lesion with the necessary precision. During a separately reportable planning procedure, the lesion is visualized using three-dimensional MRI or CT scans. The required treatment is defined and includes determination of lesion location and volume, identification of surrounding structures and assessment of risk of damage to these structures, and dose computation. If a gamma knife is used, the patient is placed on the gamma bed. A helmet with several hundred holes is attached to the head frame. The gamma bed moves backward into the treatment area. The helmet locks into the radiation source and the radiation dose is delivered. If a linear accelerator is used, a computer is used in conjunction with a micro-multileaf collimator attached to the linear accelerator, which arranges and shapes high-energy radiation beams in the exact configuration of the lesion. The gantry rotates around the patient and delivers the planned radiation dose to the lesion. Use code 61798 for a single, complex cranial lesion and code 61799 for each additional complex cranial lesion.

Stereotactic radiosurgery (particle beam, gamma ray, or linear accelerator) complex

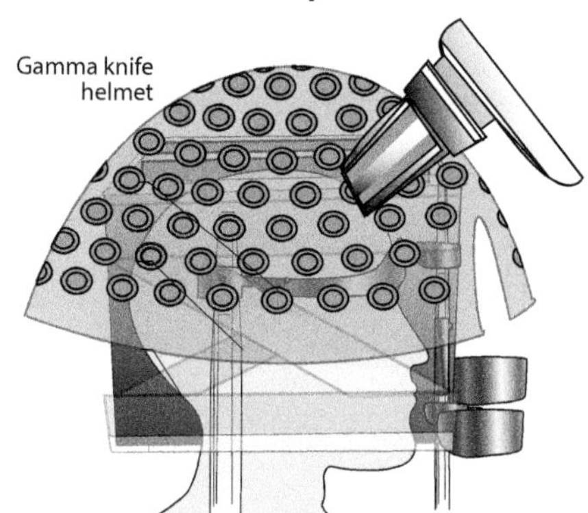

1 complex cranial lesion (61798);
each additional cranial lesion, complex (61799)

ICD-10-CM Diagnostic Codes

	Code	Description
	C41.0	Malignant neoplasm of bones of skull and face
	C70.0	Malignant neoplasm of cerebral meninges
	C71.0	Malignant neoplasm of cerebrum, except lobes and ventricles
	C71.7	Malignant neoplasm of brain stem
	C71.9	Malignant neoplasm of brain, unspecified
⇄	C72.21	Malignant neoplasm of right olfactory nerve
⇄	C72.22	Malignant neoplasm of left olfactory nerve
⇄	C72.31	Malignant neoplasm of right optic nerve
⇄	C72.32	Malignant neoplasm of left optic nerve
⇄	C72.41	Malignant neoplasm of right acoustic nerve
⇄	C72.42	Malignant neoplasm of left acoustic nerve

C72.59	Malignant neoplasm of other cranial nerves
C75.1	Malignant neoplasm of pituitary gland
C75.2	Malignant neoplasm of craniopharyngeal duct
C75.3	Malignant neoplasm of pineal gland
C79.31	Secondary malignant neoplasm of brain
C79.32	Secondary malignant neoplasm of cerebral meninges
C79.49	Secondary malignant neoplasm of other parts of nervous system
C79.51	Secondary malignant neoplasm of bone
C79.89	Secondary malignant neoplasm of other specified sites
D09.3	Carcinoma in situ of thyroid and other endocrine glands
D16.4	Benign neoplasm of bones of skull and face
D18.02	Hemangioma of intracranial structures
D32.0	Benign neoplasm of cerebral meninges
D33.0	Benign neoplasm of brain, supratentorial
D33.1	Benign neoplasm of brain, infratentorial
D33.2	Benign neoplasm of brain, unspecified
D33.3	Benign neoplasm of cranial nerves
D35.2	Benign neoplasm of pituitary gland
D35.3	Benign neoplasm of craniopharyngeal duct
D35.4	Benign neoplasm of pineal gland
D42.0	Neoplasm of uncertain behavior of cerebral meninges
D43.1	Neoplasm of uncertain behavior of brain, infratentorial
D43.3	Neoplasm of uncertain behavior of cranial nerves
D44.3	Neoplasm of uncertain behavior of pituitary gland
D44.4	Neoplasm of uncertain behavior of craniopharyngeal duct
D44.5	Neoplasm of uncertain behavior of pineal gland
Q28.2	Arteriovenous malformation of cerebral vessels

CCI Edits

Refer to Appendix A for CCI edits.

Facility RVUs ▯

Code	Work	PE Facility	MP	Total Facility
61798	19.85	12.84	7.11	39.80
61799	4.81	2.21	1.76	8.78

Non-facility RVUs ▯

Code	Work	PE Non-Facility	MP	Total Non-Facility
61798	19.85	12.84	7.11	39.80
61799	4.81	2.21	1.76	8.78

Modifiers (PAR) ▯

Code	Mod 50	Mod 51	Mod 62	Mod 66	Mod 80
61798	0	0	0	0	2
61799	0	0	0	0	2

Global Period

Code	Days
61798	090
61799	ZZZ

61800

+ **61800 Application of stereotactic headframe for stereotactic radiosurgery (List separately in addition to code for primary procedure)**

(Use 61800 in conjunction with 61796, 61798)

AMA Coding Guideline

Stereotactic Radiosurgery (Cranial) Procedures on the Skull, Meninges, and Brain

Cranial stereotactic radiosurgery is a distinct procedure that utilizes externally generated ionizing radiation to inactivate or eradicate defined target(s) in the head without the need to make an incision. The target is defined by and the treatment is delivered using high-resolution stereotactic imaging. Stereotactic radiosurgery codes and headframe application procedures are reported by the neurosurgeon. The radiation oncologist reports the appropriate code(s) for clinical treatment planning, physics and dosimetry, treatment delivery, and management from the Radiation Oncology section (77261-77790). Any necessary planning, dosimetry, targeting, positioning, or blocking by the neurosurgeon is included in the stereotactic radiation surgery services. The same individual should not report stereotactic radiosurgery services with radiation treatment management codes (77427-77435).

Cranial stereotactic radiosurgery is typically performed in a single planning and treatment session, using a rigidly attached stereotactic guiding device, other immobilization technology and/or a stereotactic image-guidance system, but can be performed with more than one planning session and in a limited number of treatment sessions, up to a maximum of five sessions. Do not report stereotactic radiosurgery more than once per lesion per course of treatment when the treatment requires more than one session.

Codes 61796 and 61797 involve stereotactic radiosurgery for simple cranial lesions. Simple cranial lesions are lesions less than 3.5 cm in maximum dimension that do not meet the definition of a complex lesion provided below. Report code 61796 when all lesions are simple.

Codes 61798 and 61799 involve stereotactic radiosurgery for complex cranial lesions and procedures that create therapeutic lesions (eg, thalamotomy or pallidotomy). All lesions 3.5 cm in maximum dimension or greater are complex. When performing therapeutic lesion creation procedures, report code 61798 only once regardless of the number of lesions created. Schwannomas, arterio-venous malformations, pituitary tumors, glomus tumors, pineal region tumors and cavernous sinus/parasellar/petroclival tumors are complex. Any lesion that is adjacent (5mm or less) to the optic nerve/optic chasm/optic tract or within the brainstem is complex. If treating multiple lesions, and any single lesion treated is complex, use 61798.

Do not report codes 61796-61800 in conjunction with code 20660.

Codes 61796-61799 include computer-assisted planning. Do not report codes 61796-61799 in conjunction with 61781-61783.

AMA Coding Notes

Stereotactic Radiosurgery (Cranial) Procedures on the Skull, Meninges, and Brain

(For intensity modulated beam delivery plan and treatment, see 77301, 77385, 77386. For stereotactic body radiation therapy, see 77373, 77435)

Surgical Procedures on the Skull, Meninges, and Brain

(For injection procedure for cerebral angiography, see 36100-36218)

(For injection procedure for ventriculography, see 61026, 61120)

(For injection procedure for pneumoencephalography, use 61055)

AMA *CPT Assistant*

61800: Apr 12: 11, Jun 15: 6

Plain English Description

A stereotactic head frame is applied for a separately reportable stereotactic radiosurgery procedure. A local anesthetic is injected at each of the stabilization sites in the skull. The frame is then fitted to the patient's head and attached to the skull using metal screws.

Application of stereotactic headframe for stereotactic radiosurgery

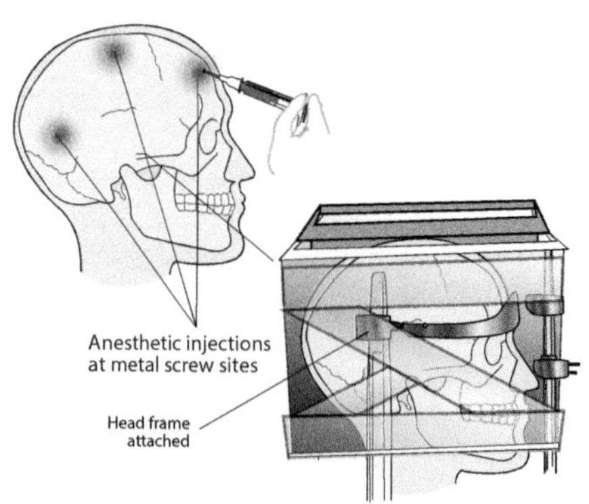

ICD-10-CM Diagnostic Codes

See Primary Procedure code for crosswalks.

CCI Edits

Refer to Appendix A for CCI edits.

Facility RVUs

Code	Work	PE Facility	MP	Total Facility
61800	2.25	1.34	0.81	4.40

Non-facility RVUs

Code	Work	PE Non-Facility	MP	Total Non-Facility
61800	2.25	1.34	0.81	4.40

Modifiers (PAR)

Code	Mod 50	Mod 51	Mod 62	Mod 66	Mod 80
61800	0	0	0	0	2

Global Period

Code	Days
61800	ZZZ

61863-61864

61863 Twist drill, burr hole, craniotomy, or craniectomy with stereotactic implantation of neurostimulator electrode array in subcortical site (eg, thalamus, globus pallidus, subthalamic nucleus, periventricular, periaqueductal gray), without use of intraoperative microelectrode recording; first array

+ **61864 Twist drill, burr hole, craniotomy, or craniectomy with stereotactic implantation of neurostimulator electrode array in subcortical site (eg, thalamus, globus pallidus, subthalamic nucleus, periventricular, periaqueductal gray), without use of intraoperative microelectrode recording; each additional array (List separately in addition to primary procedure)**

(Use 61864 in conjunction with 61863)

AMA Coding Guideline

Neurostimulators (Intracranial) Procedures on the Skull, Meninges, and Brain

For electronic analysis with programming, when performed, of cranial nerve and brain neurostimulator pulse generator/transmitters, see codes 95970, 95976, 95977, 95983, 95984. Test stimulation to confirm correct target site placement of the electrode array(s) and/or to confirm the functional status of the system is inherent to placement and is not separately reported as electronic analysis or programming of the neurostimulator system. Electronic analysis (95970) at the time of implantation is not separately reported.

Microelectrode recording, when performed by the operating surgeon in association with implantation of neurostimulator electrode arrays, is an inclusive service and should not be reported separately. If another individual participates in neurophysiological mapping during a deep brain stimulator implantation procedure, this service may be reported by the second individual with codes 95961-95962.

AMA Coding Notes

Surgical Procedures on the Skull, Meninges, and Brain

(For injection procedure for cerebral angiography, see 36100-36218)

(For injection procedure for ventriculography, see 61026, 61120)

(For injection procedure for pneumoencephalography, use 61055)

AMA *CPT Assistant* □

61863: Sep 99: 5, Oct 10: 10, Jul 11: 12, Jul 14: 9

61864: Sep 99: 5, Jul 11: 12

Plain English Description

Implantation of a neurostimulator array in the subcortical region of the brain is performed to treat functional disorders due to Parkinson's disease, various types of tremors, multiple sclerosis, medically intractable primary dystonias, and those due to psychotropic medications, bradykinesia, dyskinesia, rigidity, and severe pain from cancer or other causes. A stereotactic frame is attached to the skull. MRI or CT scans are used to map out the procedure and determine how many electrode arrays will be placed and where they will be placed. The trajectories for the array placements in the target regions are also determined. The components required to implant the arrays are attached to the stereotactic head frame. If twist holes or burr holes are used to access the implantation sites, the entry points are localized, marked on the skin and the skin is incised. The twist holes or burr holes are then created. The dura is coagulated and punctured. Alternatively, a craniotomy or craniectomy is performed. Scalp flaps are developed. Burr holes are drilled and the bone between the burr holes is then cut with a saw or craniotome. A bone flap is elevated or a portion of the skull is removed. The dura is opened and the surface of the brain exposed. The entry site for the guide cannula is inspected to ensure there are no large vessels and the brain surface is coagulated. The guide cannula is inserted into the brain. The deep brain stimulation array is introduced and positioned in the target area. Test stimulation is performed and the adjustment made in the position of the array until the desired functional results are achieved. The guide cannula is then removed, leaving the electrode array in place. An anchoring device is used to maintain the array in the desired position. The lead is coiled in a subgaleal pocket. The procedure is repeated if more than one array is implanted. The galea is closed with sutures followed by the skin. The stereotactic frame is removed. Use 61863 for implantation of the first array without the use of intraoperative microelectrode recording (MER) and 61864 for each additional array placed without MER.

Twist drill, burr hole, craniotomy, or craniectomy

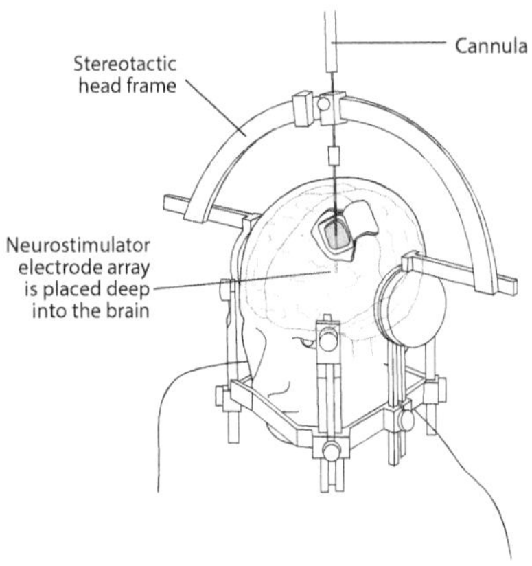

ICD-10-CM Diagnostic Codes

G40.011	Localization-related (focal) (partial) idiopathic epilepsy and epileptic syndromes with seizures of localized onset, intractable, with status epilepticus
G40.019	Localization-related (focal) (partial) idiopathic epilepsy and epileptic syndromes with seizures of localized onset, intractable, without status epilepticus
G40.111	Localization-related (focal) (partial) symptomatic epilepsy and epileptic syndromes with simple partial seizures, intractable, with status epilepticus
G40.119	Localization-related (focal) (partial) symptomatic epilepsy and epileptic syndromes with simple partial seizures, intractable, without status epilepticus
G40.211	Localization-related (focal) (partial) symptomatic epilepsy and epileptic syndromes with complex partial seizures, intractable, with status epilepticus
G40.219	Localization-related (focal) (partial) symptomatic epilepsy and epileptic syndromes with complex partial seizures, intractable, without status epilepticus

CCI Edits

Refer to Appendix A for CCI edits.

Facility RVUs

Code	Work	PE Facility	MP	Total Facility
61863	20.71	15.01	7.63	43.35
61864	4.49	2.06	1.65	8.20

Non-facility RVUs

Code	Work	PE Non-Facility	MP	Total Non-Facility
61863	20.71	15.01	7.63	43.35
61864	4.49	2.06	1.65	8.20

Modifiers (PAR)

Code	Mod 50	Mod 51	Mod 62	Mod 66	Mod 80
61863	1	2	1	0	2
61864	0	0	1	0	2

Global Period

Code	Days
61863	090
61864	ZZZ

61867-61868

61867 Twist drill, burr hole, craniotomy, or craniectomy with stereotactic implantation of neurostimulator electrode array in subcortical site (eg, thalamus, globus pallidus, subthalamic nucleus, periventricular, periaqueductal gray), with use of intraoperative microelectrode recording; first array

✚ **61868 Twist drill, burr hole, craniotomy, or craniectomy with stereotactic implantation of neurostimulator electrode array in subcortical site (eg, thalamus, globus pallidus, subthalamic nucleus, periventricular, periaqueductal gray), with use of intraoperative microelectrode recording; each additional array (List separately in addition to primary procedure)**

(Use 61868 in conjunction with 61867)

AMA Coding Guideline

Neurostimulators (Intracranial) Procedures on the Skull, Meninges, and Brain

For electronic analysis with programming, when performed, of cranial nerve and brain neurostimulator pulse generator/transmitters, see codes 95970, 95976, 95977, 95983, 95984. Test stimulation to confirm correct target site placement of the electrode array(s) and/or to confirm the functional status of the system is inherent to placement and is not separately reported as electronic analysis or programming of the neurostimulator system. Electronic analysis (95970) at the time of implantation is not separately reported.

Microelectrode recording, when performed by the operating surgeon in association with implantation of neurostimulator electrode arrays, is an inclusive service and should not be reported separately. If another individual participates in neurophysiological mapping during a deep brain stimulator implantation procedure, this service may be reported by the second individual with codes 95961-95962.

AMA Coding Notes

Surgical Procedures on the Skull, Meninges, and Brain

(For injection procedure for cerebral angiography, see 36100-36218)

(For injection procedure for ventriculography, see 61026, 61120)

(For injection procedure for pneumoencephalography, use 61055)

AMA *CPT Assistant* ▯

61867: Jul 11: 12

61868: Jul 11: 12, Jul 14: 9

Plain English Description

Implantation of a neurostimulator array in the subcortical region of the brain is performed to treat functional disorders due to Parkinson's disease, various types of tremors, multiple sclerosis, medically intractable primary dystonias, and those due to psychotropic medications, bradykinesia, dyskinesia, rigidity and severe pain from cancer or other causes. A stereotactic frame is attached to the skull. MRI or CT scans are used to map out the procedure and determine how many electrode arrays will be placed and where they will be placed. The trajectories for the array placements in the target regions are also determined. The components required to implant the arrays are attached to a stereotactic head frame. If twist holes or burr holes are used to access the implantation sites, the entry points are localized, marked on the skin and the skin is incised. The twist holes or burr holes are then created. The dura is coagulated and punctured. Alternatively, a craniotomy or craniectomy is performed. Scalp flaps are developed. Burr holes are drilled and the bone between the burr holes is then cut with a saw or craniotome. A bone flap is elevated or a portion of the skull is removed. The dura is opened and the surface of the brain exposed. The entry site for the guide cannula is inspected to ensure there are no large vessels, and the brain surface is coagulated. The guide cannula is inserted into the brain. A microdrive/electrode assembly component is attached to the stereotactic frame and a microelectrode inserted into the guide cannula. As the microelectrode is advanced into the brain tissue, recordings from individual neurons are obtained and response of these neurons to light touch, passive joint movement, and other stimuli is evaluated. Multiple microelectrode tracks may be required to identify the optimal target region for electrode array placement. Once optimal placement of the electrode array is determined, the microelectrode is removed. The deep brain stimulation array is introduced and positioned in the target area. Test stimulation is performed and the adjustment made in the position of the array until the desired functional results are achieved. The guide cannula is then removed, leaving the electrode array in place. An anchoring device is used to maintain the array in the desired position. The lead is coiled in a subgaleal pocket. The procedure is repeated if more than one array is implanted. The galea is closed with sutures followed by the skin. The stereotactic frame is removed. Use 61867 for implantation of the first array with the use of intraoperative microelectrode recording (MER) and 61868 for each additional array placed with MER.

Stereotactic implantation

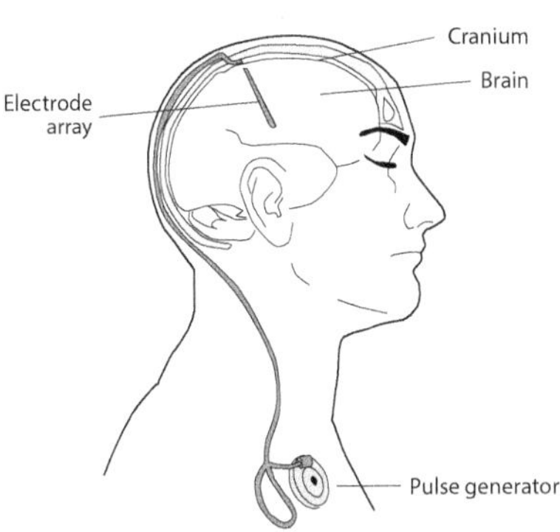

Use 61867 for initial implantation and electrode; use 61868 for each additional electrode

ICD-10-CM Diagnostic Codes

G40.011	Localization-related (focal) (partial) idiopathic epilepsy and epileptic syndromes with seizures of localized onset, intractable, with status epilepticus
G40.019	Localization-related (focal) (partial) idiopathic epilepsy and epileptic syndromes with seizures of localized onset, intractable, without status epilepticus
G40.111	Localization-related (focal) (partial) symptomatic epilepsy and epileptic syndromes with simple partial seizures, intractable, with status epilepticus
G40.119	Localization-related (focal) (partial) symptomatic epilepsy and epileptic syndromes with simple partial seizures, intractable, without status epilepticus
G40.211	Localization-related (focal) (partial) symptomatic epilepsy and epileptic syndromes with complex partial seizures, intractable, with status epilepticus
G40.219	Localization-related (focal) (partial) symptomatic epilepsy and epileptic syndromes with complex partial seizures, intractable, without status epilepticus

CCI Edits

Refer to Appendix A for CCI edits.

Facility RVUs

Code	Work	PE Facility	MP	Total Facility
61867	33.03	20.67	12.21	65.91
61868	7.91	3.63	2.91	14.45

Non-facility RVUs

Code	Work	PE Non-Facility	MP	Total Non-Facility
61867	33.03	20.67	12.21	65.91
61868	7.91	3.63	2.91	14.45

Modifiers (PAR)

Code	Mod 50	Mod 51	Mod 62	Mod 66	Mod 80
61867	1	2	1	0	2
61868	0	0	1	0	2

Global Period

Code	Days
61867	090
61868	ZZZ

61880

61880 Revision or removal of intracranial neurostimulator electrodes

AMA Coding Guideline

Neurostimulators (Intracranial) Procedures on the Skull, Meninges, and Brain

For electronic analysis with programming, when performed, of cranial nerve and brain neurostimulator pulse generator/transmitters, see codes 95970, 95976, 95977, 95983, 95984. Test stimulation to confirm correct target site placement of the electrode array(s) and/or to confirm the functional status of the system is inherent to placement and is not separately reported as electronic analysis or programming of the neurostimulator system. Electronic analysis (95970) at the time of implantation is not separately reported.

Microelectrode recording, when performed by the operating surgeon in association with implantation of neurostimulator electrode arrays, is an inclusive service and should not be reported separately. If another individual participates in neurophysiological mapping during a deep brain stimulator implantation procedure, this service may be reported by the second individual with codes 95961-95962.

AMA Coding Notes

Surgical Procedures on the Skull, Meninges, and Brain

(For injection procedure for cerebral angiography, see 36100-36218)

(For injection procedure for ventriculography, see 61026, 61120)

(For injection procedure for pneumoencephalography, use 61055)

Plain English Description

To revise or remove an intracranial neurostimulator electrode(s), an incision is made through the scalp to expose the skull, burr hole(s), wire electrode(s), and plastic cap(s) covering the burr hole(s) that keep the thin electrode wire in place. The plastic caps are removed, and the electrode(s) are repositioned in the brain as necessary or pulled through the burr hole(s) and removed from contact with the brain. For revision, the plastic cap(s) are replaced over the burr hole(s) to hold the electrode wire(s) in the new brain location and the scalp incision is closed with sutures or staples. For partial removal, the electrode wire is coiled beneath the skin, next to the skull, and the skin is then closed with sutures or staples. For complete removal, a small incision is made in the skin over the stimulator, usually located in the anterior chest below the clavicle, the electrode wire is disconnected from that device, pulled out through one end of the skin tunnel between the cranium and chest, and both incisions are then closed with sutures or staples.

Revision or removal of intracranial neurostimulator electrodes

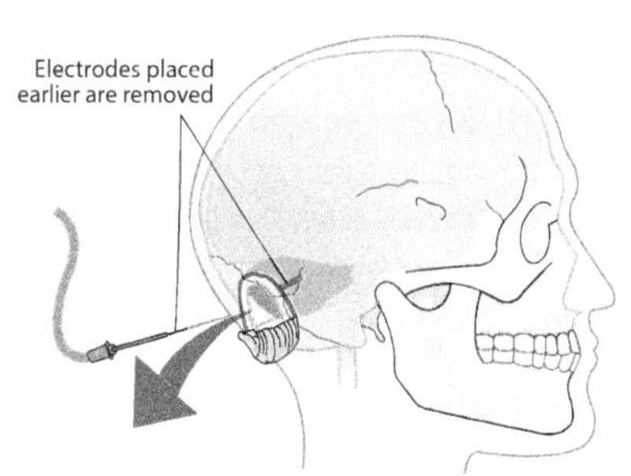

ICD-10-CM Diagnostic Codes

	Code	Description
	G40.011	Localization-related (focal) (partial) idiopathic epilepsy and epileptic syndromes with seizures of localized onset, intractable, with status epilepticus
	G40.019	Localization-related (focal) (partial) idiopathic epilepsy and epileptic syndromes with seizures of localized onset, intractable, without status epilepticus
	G40.111	Localization-related (focal) (partial) symptomatic epilepsy and epileptic syndromes with simple partial seizures, intractable, with status epilepticus
	G40.119	Localization-related (focal) (partial) symptomatic epilepsy and epileptic syndromes with simple partial seizures, intractable, without status epilepticus
	G40.211	Localization-related (focal) (partial) symptomatic epilepsy and epileptic syndromes with complex partial seizures, intractable, with status epilepticus
	G40.219	Localization-related (focal) (partial) symptomatic epilepsy and epileptic syndromes with complex partial seizures, intractable, without status epilepticus
➐	T85.110	Breakdown (mechanical) of implanted electronic neurostimulator of brain electrode (lead)
➐	T85.120	Displacement of implanted electronic neurostimulator of brain electrode (lead)
➐	T85.190	Other mechanical complication of implanted electronic neurostimulator of brain electrode (lead)
➐	T85.731	Infection and inflammatory reaction due to implanted electronic neurostimulator of brain, electrode (lead)

ICD-10-CM Coding Notes

For codes requiring a 7th character extension, refer to your ICD-10-CM book. Review the character descriptions and coding guidelines for proper selection. For some procedures, only certain characters will apply.

CCI Edits

Refer to Appendix A for CCI edits.

Pub 100

61880: Pub 100-04, 32, 50.4.3

Facility RVUs ▯

Code	Work	PE Facility	MP	Total Facility
61880	6.95	7.12	2.55	16.62

Non-facility RVUs ▯

Code	Work	PE Non-Facility	MP	Total Non-Facility
61880	6.95	7.12	2.55	16.62

Modifiers (PAR) ▯

Code	Mod 50	Mod 51	Mod 62	Mod 66	Mod 80
61880	1	2	1	0	2

Global Period

Code	Days
61880	090

61885-61888

61885 Insertion or replacement of cranial neurostimulator pulse generator or receiver, direct or inductive coupling; with connection to a single electrode array

61886 Insertion or replacement of cranial neurostimulator pulse generator or receiver, direct or inductive coupling; with connection to 2 or more electrode arrays

(For percutaneous placement of cranial nerve (eg, vagus, trigeminal) neurostimulator electrode(s), use 64553)

(For revision or removal of cranial nerve (eg, vagus, trigeminal) neurostimulator electrode array, use 64569)

61888 Revision or removal of cranial neurostimulator pulse generator or receiver

(Do not report 61888 in conjunction with 61885 or 61886 for the same pulse generator)

AMA Coding Guideline

Neurostimulators (Intracranial) Procedures on the Skull, Meninges, and Brain

For electronic analysis with programming, when performed, of cranial nerve and brain neurostimulator pulse generator/transmitters, see codes 95970, 95976, 95977, 95983, 95984. Test stimulation to confirm correct target site placement of the electrode array(s) and/or to confirm the functional status of the system is inherent to placement and is not separately reported as electronic analysis or programming of the neurostimulator system. Electronic analysis (95970) at the time of implantation is not separately reported.

Microelectrode recording, when performed by the operating surgeon in association with implantation of neurostimulator electrode arrays, is an inclusive service and should not be reported separately. If another individual participates in neurophysiological mapping during a deep brain stimulator implantation procedure, this service may be reported by the second individual with codes 95961-95962.

AMA Coding Notes

Surgical Procedures on the Skull, Meninges, and Brain

(For injection procedure for cerebral angiography, see 36100-36218)

(For injection procedure for ventriculography, see 61026, 61120)

(For injection procedure for pneumoencephalography, use 61055)

AMA *CPT Assistant* □

61885: Sep 99: 5, Nov 99: 30, Jun 00: 3, Apr 01: 8, Sep 03: 3, Dec 10: 14, Feb 11: 5, Sep 11: 8

61886: Nov 99: 30, Jun 00: 3, Apr 01: 8, Feb 11: 5, Sep 11: 8

61888: Sep 11: 8

Plain English Description

To insert a cranial neurostimulator pulse generator or receiver, an incision is made in the anterior chest, just below the clavicle, carried down to the subcutaneous tissue and a small pocket is fashioned. To replace a cranial neurostimulator pulse generator or receiver, an incision is made over the existing device and carried down to the subcutaneous pocket to expose the device. The electrode(s) are then disconnected and the device is dissected free of surrounding tissue and removed. The new neurostimulator pulse generator or receiver is then placed into the existing or newly fashioned subcutaneous pocket and connected to the cranial electrode wire(s). The pulse generator or receiver is programmed and the incision is closed in layers with sutures. The skin may be closed with staples. Report code 61885 for connection to a single electrode array and code 61886 for insertion or replacement of a cranial neurostimulator pulse generator or receiver with connection to 2 or more electrode arrays. To revise or remove a cranial neurostimulator pulse generator or receiver (61888), an incision is made over the existing device and carried down to the subcutaneous pocket to expose the device and electrode wire(s). Revisions to the device are made and the electrode wire(s) is reconnected, or the device is dissected free of surrounding tissue and removed from the body.

Cranial neurostimulator pulse generator or receiver

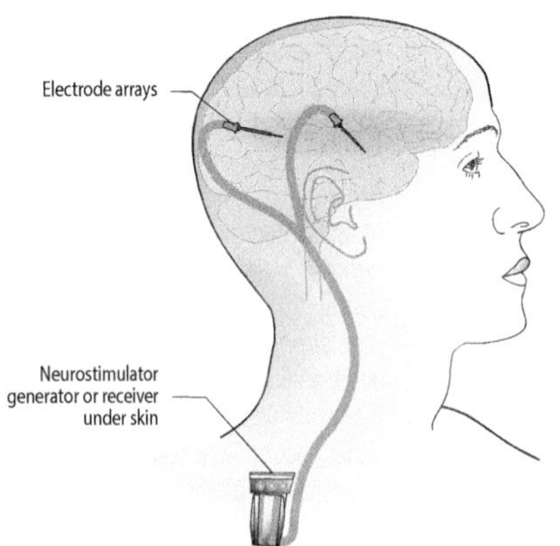

For insertion or replacement use code 61885 for single electrode array; use code 61886 for 2 or more. For revision or removal use code 61888.

ICD-10-CM Diagnostic Codes

	Code	Description
	G40.011	Localization-related (focal) (partial) idiopathic epilepsy and epileptic syndromes with seizures of localized onset, intractable, with status epilepticus
	G40.019	Localization-related (focal) (partial) idiopathic epilepsy and epileptic syndromes with seizures of localized onset, intractable, without status epilepticus
	G40.111	Localization-related (focal) (partial) symptomatic epilepsy and epileptic syndromes with simple partial seizures, intractable, with status epilepticus
	G40.119	Localization-related (focal) (partial) symptomatic epilepsy and epileptic syndromes with simple partial seizures, intractable, without status epilepticus
	G40.211	Localization-related (focal) (partial) symptomatic epilepsy and epileptic syndromes with complex partial seizures, intractable, with status epilepticus
	G40.219	Localization-related (focal) (partial) symptomatic epilepsy and epileptic syndromes with complex partial seizures, intractable, without status epilepticus
⑦	T85.113	Breakdown (mechanical) of implanted electronic neurostimulator, generator
⑦	T85.123	Displacement of implanted electronic neurostimulator, generator
⑦	T85.193	Other mechanical complication of implanted electronic neurostimulator, generator
⑦	T85.734	Infection and inflammatory reaction due to implanted electronic neurostimulator, generator

ICD-10-CM Coding Notes

For codes requiring a 7th character extension, refer to your ICD-10-CM book. Review the character descriptions and coding guidelines for proper selection. For some procedures, only certain characters will apply.

CCI Edits

Refer to Appendix A for CCI edits.

Pub 100

61885: Pub 100-04, 32, 50.4.3, 50.5

61886: Pub 100-04, 32, 50.4.3

61888: Pub 100-04, 32, 50.4.3, 50.5

Facility RVUs

Code	Work	PE Facility	MP	Total Facility
61885	6.05	6.76	2.12	14.93
61886	9.93	11.12	3.64	24.69
61888	5.23	4.34	1.82	11.39

Non-facility RVUs

Code	Work	PE Non-Facility	MP	Total Non-Facility
61885	6.05	6.76	2.12	14.93
61886	9.93	11.12	3.64	24.69
61888	5.23	4.34	1.82	11.39

Modifiers (PAR)

Code	Mod 50	Mod 51	Mod 62	Mod 66	Mod 80
61885	1	2	0	0	0
61886	0	2	0	0	0
61888	1	2	0	0	1

Global Period

Code	Days
61885	090
61886	090
61888	010

62000-62010

62000 Elevation of depressed skull fracture; simple, extradural

62005 Elevation of depressed skull fracture; compound or comminuted, extradural

62010 Elevation of depressed skull fracture; with repair of dura and/or debridement of brain

AMA Coding Notes

Surgical Procedures on the Skull, Meninges, and Brain

(For injection procedure for cerebral angiography, see 36100-36218)

(For injection procedure for ventriculography, see 61026, 61120)

(For injection procedure for pneumoencephalography, use 61055)

Plain English Description

A depressed skull fracture results from a high-energy, direct blow to a small surface area of the skull from a blunt object. Depressed skull fractures may be open or closed and may result in loss of consciousness. A depressed skull fracture may also be associated with intracranial injuries such epidural or subdural hematoma and dural tearing. In 62000, elevation of a closed fracture without a dural tear is performed. A closed skull fracture is one in which the skin is intact at the site of the fracture. A lazy-S or horseshoe incision is made over the depressed region and the bone exposed. The bone is elevated. The depressed area is inspected to ensure that the dura is intact. In 62005, elevation of an open fracture or a fracture in which there is fragmentation of the bone is performed. The skin is inspected and debrided as needed. The skin laceration may be extended to allow inspection of the skull. Fracture fragments are detached using a pneumatic drill. The dura is inspected and found to be intact. The bone fragments are washed in antiseptic solution. The skull is reconstructed and the fracture fragments secured with sutures, wire, or miniplates and screws. In 62010, a depressed skull fracture complicated by a dural tear and/or contamination or damage to brain tissue is performed. Fracture fragments are detached and cleansed as described above. Debris including fracture fragments is removed from the brain. Any damaged or contaminated tissue is carefully debrided. The dura is then repaired with sutures, fibrin glue, or a patch graft. The skull is reconstructed as described above. Overlying soft tissues and skin are closed in layers.

Elevation of depressed skull fracture

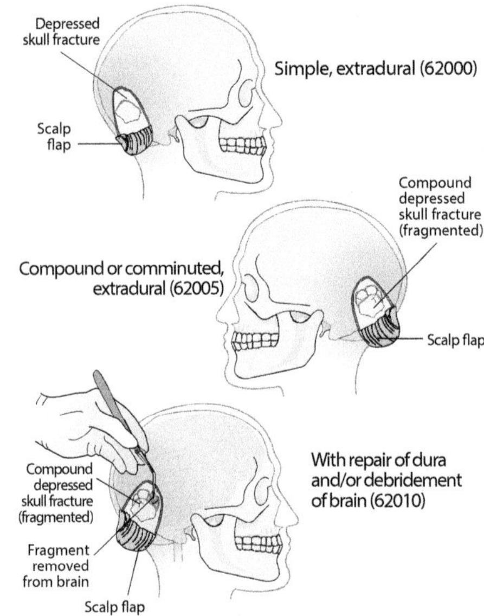

ICD-10-CM Diagnostic Codes

⑦⇄	S02.101	Fracture of base of skull, right side
⑦⇄	S02.102	Fracture of base of skull, left side
⑦⇄	S02.11A	Type I occipital condyle fracture, right side
⑦⇄	S02.11B	Type I occipital condyle fracture, left side
⑦⇄	S02.11C	Type II occipital condyle fracture, right side
⑦⇄	S02.11D	Type II occipital condyle fracture, left side
⑦⇄	S02.11E	Type III occipital condyle fracture, right side
⑦⇄	S02.11F	Type III occipital condyle fracture, left side
⑦⇄	S02.11G	Other fracture of occiput, right side
⑦⇄	S02.11H	Other fracture of occiput, left side
⑦⇄	S02.121	Fracture of orbital roof, right side
⑦⇄	S02.122	Fracture of orbital roof, left side
⑦	S02.19	Other fracture of base of skull
⑦⇄	S02.841	Fracture of lateral orbital wall, right side
⑦⇄	S02.842	Fracture of lateral orbital wall, left side

ICD-10-CM Coding Notes

For codes requiring a 7th character extension, refer to your ICD-10-CM book. Review the character descriptions and coding guidelines for proper selection. For some procedures, only certain characters will apply.

CCI Edits

Refer to Appendix A for CCI edits.

Pub 100

62010: Pub 100-04, 12, 20.4.5

Facility RVUs ☐

Code	Work	PE Facility	MP	Total Facility
62000	13.93	10.69	5.13	29.75
62005	17.63	12.54	6.49	36.66
62010	21.43	14.95	7.90	44.28

Non-facility RVUs ☐

Code	Work	PE Non-Facility	MP	Total Non-Facility
62000	13.93	10.69	5.13	29.75
62005	17.63	12.54	6.49	36.66
62010	21.43	14.95	7.90	44.28

Modifiers (PAR) ☐

Code	Mod 50	Mod 51	Mod 62	Mod 66	Mod 80
62000	0	2	0	0	1
62005	0	2	1	0	2
62010	0	2	1	0	2

Global Period

Code	Days
62000	090
62005	090
62010	090

62100

62100 Craniotomy for repair of dural/cerebrospinal fluid leak, including surgery for rhinorrhea/otorrhea

(For repair of spinal dural/CSF leak, see 63707, 63709)

AMA Coding Notes

Surgical Procedures on the Skull, Meninges, and Brain

(For injection procedure for cerebral angiography, see 36100-36218)

(For injection procedure for ventriculography, see 61026, 61120)

(For injection procedure for pneumoencephalography, use 61055)

Plain English Description

A cerebrospinal fluid (CSF) leak may occur from the nose (rhinorrhea), external auditory canal (otorrhea), or other tear in the dura as a result of trauma or a complication of surgery. Separately reportable radiological studies are performed to identify the site of the cerebrospinal fluid leak. An incision is made over the skull at the site of the CSF leak and the skull is exposed. Burr holes are created in the skull and a saw is then used to connect the burr holes and create a bone flap. The bone flap is elevated and the dura exposed. The dural tear is located and repaired with sutures, fibrin glue, or a dural patch. The bone flap is replaced and secured with sutures, wire, or miniplates and screws. Overlying soft tissue and skin are closed in layers.

Craniotomy for repair of dural/cerebrospinal fluid leak, including surgery for rhinorrhea/otorrhea

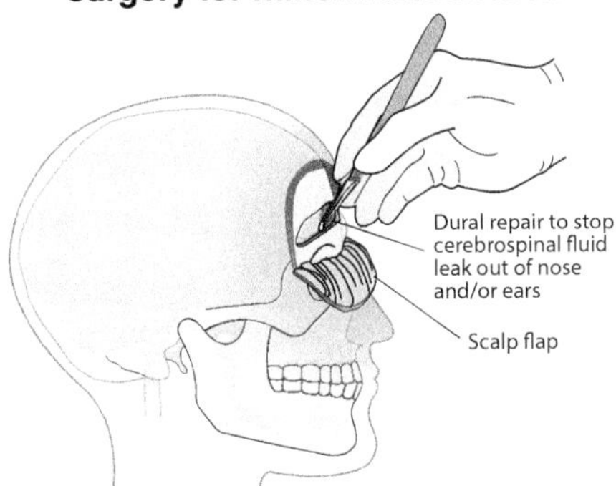

ICD-10-CM Diagnostic Codes

G96.0 Cerebrospinal fluid leak

CCI Edits

Refer to Appendix A for CCI edits.

Pub 100

62100: Pub 100-04, 12, 20.4.5

Facility RVUs

Code	Work	PE Facility	MP	Total Facility
62100	23.53	14.80	7.30	45.63

Non-facility RVUs

Code	Work	PE Non-Facility	MP	Total Non-Facility
62100	23.53	14.80	7.30	45.63

Modifiers (PAR)

Code	Mod 50	Mod 51	Mod 62	Mod 66	Mod 80
62100	0	2	1	0	2

Global Period

Code	Days
62100	090

62120-62121

62120 Repair of encephalocele, skull vault, including cranioplasty

62121 Craniotomy for repair of encephalocele, skull base

AMA Coding Notes

Surgical Procedures on the Skull, Meninges, and Brain

(For injection procedure for cerebral angiography, see 36100-36218)

(For injection procedure for ventriculography, see 61026, 61120)

(For injection procedure for pneumoencephalography, use 61055)

Plain English Description

An encephalocele is a congenital anomaly in which intracranial contents protrude through a skull defect. An encephalocele may contain only cerebral spinal fluid or it may contain brain tissue as well. Encephaloceles are divided into two broad categories, those that protrude from the skull vault and those that protrude at the skull base. Cranial vault encephaloceles occur in the outer aspect of the skull, usually along the suture lines in the frontal, parietal, or occipital regions or, less commonly, at the pterion and result in a visible external bulge. Skull base encephaloceles are subclassified into two types based on site. Skull base frontoethmoidal encephaloceles project forward causing a mass in the face while basal encephaloceles project downward producing a mass in the nasopharynx. The exact procedure depends on the site and the contents of the encephalocele. A skin flap is created to allow exposure of the encephalocele. Burr holes are created in the skull and a saw is then used to connect the burr holes to create a bone flap around the skull defect. The bone flap is elevated around the encephalocele and the stalk identified. If there is no brain or other tissue in the encephalocele, the stalk is suture ligated and the encephalocele excised. If brain or other tissue is present in the encephalocele, it is reduced back into the skull vault and the encephalocele is then excised. The dura is repaired with a sutures or a patch graft. Bone flaps are replaced and the defect in the skull is then repaired using a bone graft, bone wax, or other techniques. Bone flaps are secured with sutures, wire, or miniplates and screws. Use 62120 for repair of an encephalocele of the skull vault and 62121 for repair of an encephalocele located in the skull base.

ICD-10-CM Diagnostic Codes

Q01.0	Frontal encephalocele
Q01.1	Nasofrontal encephalocele
Q01.2	Occipital encephalocele
Q01.8	Encephalocele of other sites
Q01.9	Encephalocele, unspecified

CCI Edits

Refer to Appendix A for CCI edits.

Facility RVUs

Code	Work	PE Facility	MP	Total Facility
62120	24.59	26.96	9.08	60.63
62121	23.03	16.81	5.20	45.04

Non-facility RVUs

Code	Work	PE Non-Facility	MP	Total Non-Facility
62120	24.59	26.96	9.08	60.63
62121	23.03	16.81	5.20	45.04

Modifiers (PAR)

Code	Mod 50	Mod 51	Mod 62	Mod 66	Mod 80
62120	0	2	1	0	2
62121	0	2	1	0	2

Global Period

Code	Days
62120	090
62121	090

62140-62141

62140 Cranioplasty for skull defect; up to 5 cm diameter

62141 Cranioplasty for skull defect; larger than 5 cm diameter

AMA Coding Notes

Surgical Procedures on the Skull, Meninges, and Brain

(For injection procedure for cerebral angiography, see 36100-36218)

(For injection procedure for ventriculography, see 61026, 61120)

(For injection procedure for pneumoencephalography, use 61055)

AMA *CPT Assistant*

62140: Jan 14: 9

62141: Jan 14: 9

Plain English Description

A cranioplasty to repair a skull defect may be performed using a cranial bone graft or other materials. The site of the skull defect is exposed. If a previously removed cranial bone is used, it is retrieved from the subcutaneous pocket in a separately reportable procedure. The cranial bone graft is returned to the site of the skull defect and secured with sutures, wires, or miniplate and screws. Alternatively, a prosthetic plate may be used to repair the defect. Use 62140 for repair of a skull defect up to 5 cm in diameter. Use 62141 for repair of a skull defect larger than 5 cm.

ICD-10-CM Diagnostic Codes

M95.2	Other acquired deformity of head
Q67.0	Congenital facial asymmetry
Q75.0	Craniosynostosis
Q75.1	Craniofacial dysostosis
Q75.8	Other specified congenital malformations of skull and face bones
Z62.810	Personal history of physical and sexual abuse in childhood
Z85.841	Personal history of malignant neoplasm of brain
Z86.011	Personal history of benign neoplasm of the brain
Z86.69	Personal history of other diseases of the nervous system and sense organs
Z86.73	Personal history of transient ischemic attack (TIA), and cerebral infarction without residual deficits
Z87.39	Personal history of other diseases of the musculoskeletal system and connective tissue
Z87.728	Personal history of other specified (corrected) congenital malformations of nervous system and sense organs
Z87.76	Personal history of (corrected) congenital malformations of integument, limbs and musculoskeletal system
Z87.81	Personal history of (healed) traumatic fracture
Z87.820	Personal history of traumatic brain injury
Z87.828	Personal history of other (healed) physical injury and trauma
Z91.410	Personal history of adult physical and sexual abuse

CCI Edits

Refer to Appendix A for CCI edits.

Facility RVUs

Code	Work	PE Facility	MP	Total Facility
62140	14.55	10.40	4.63	29.58
62141	16.07	11.53	5.33	32.93

Non-facility RVUs

Code	Work	PE Non-Facility	MP	Total Non-Facility
62140	14.55	10.40	4.63	29.58
62141	16.07	11.53	5.33	32.93

Modifiers (PAR)

Code	Mod 50	Mod 51	Mod 62	Mod 66	Mod 80
62140	0	2	1	0	2
62141	0	2	1	0	2

Global Period

Code	Days
62140	090
62141	090

62142

62142 Removal of bone flap or prosthetic plate of skull

AMA Coding Notes

Surgical Procedures on the Skull, Meninges, and Brain

(For injection procedure for cerebral angiography, see 36100-36218)

(For injection procedure for ventriculography, see 61026, 61120)

(For injection procedure for pneumoencephalography, use 61055)

AMA *CPT Assistant*

62142: Jan 14: 9

Plain English Description

The physician removes a flap of bone or a prosthetic plate that was implanted in a previous procedure to cover a defect. A U-incision is made over the site of the bone flap or prosthetic plate. A skin flap is elevated and the bone flap or prosthetic plate exposed. Any external fixation such as wire or miniplates and screws is removed. The bone flap or prosthetic plate is separated from skull using a drill, saw, or other device. The bone flap or prosthetic plate is then removed. The dura is inspected to ensure that it is intact. A separately reportable procedure may then be used to repair the skull defect.

Removal of bone flap or prosthetic plate of skull

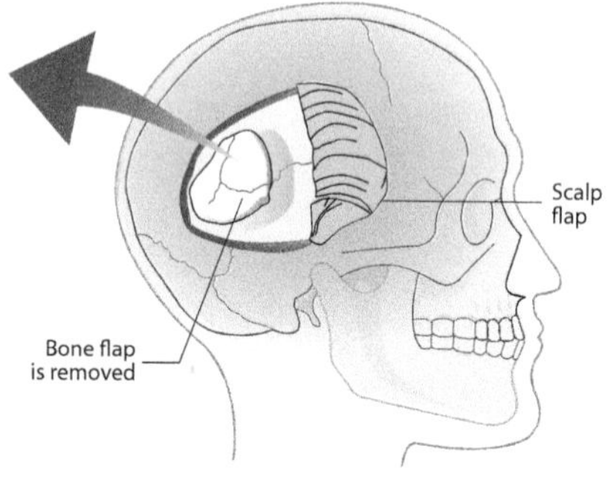

ICD-10-CM Diagnostic Codes

There are too many ICD-10-CM codes to list. Refer to ICD-10-CM code book for associated diagnostic codes.

CCI Edits

Refer to Appendix A for CCI edits.

Facility RVUs

Code	Work	PE Facility	MP	Total Facility
62142	11.83	9.60	4.10	25.53

Non-facility RVUs

Code	Work	PE Non-Facility	MP	Total Non-Facility
62142	11.83	9.60	4.10	25.53

Modifiers (PAR)

Code	Mod 50	Mod 51	Mod 62	Mod 66	Mod 80
62142	0	2	0	0	2

Global Period

Code	Days
62142	090

62143

62143 Replacement of bone flap or prosthetic plate of skull

AMA Coding Notes

Surgical Procedures on the Skull, Meninges, and Brain

(For injection procedure for cerebral angiography, see 36100-36218)

(For injection procedure for ventriculography, see 61026, 61120)

(For injection procedure for pneumoencephalography, use 61055)

AMA *CPT Assistant*

62143: Jan 14: 9

Plain English Description

The site of the skull injury or defect is exposed. If a previously removed cranial bone is used, it is retrieved from the subcutaneous pocket in a separately reportable procedure. The cranial bone graft is returned to the site of the skull defect and secured with sutures, wires, or miniplate and screws. Alternatively, a prosthetic plate may be used to repair the defect. An appropriately sized plate is selected and secured with wires or a miniplate and screws. Overlying soft tissue and skin are repaired in layers.

Removal of bone flap or prosthetic plate of skull

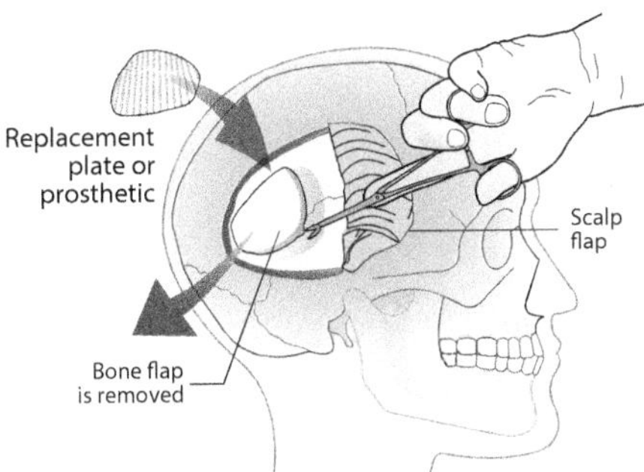

ICD-10-CM Diagnostic Codes

Code	Description
M95.2	Other acquired deformity of head
M96.6	Fracture of bone following insertion of orthopedic implant, joint prosthesis, or bone plate
Q67.0	Congenital facial asymmetry
Q75.0	Craniosynostosis
Q75.1	Craniofacial dysostosis
Q75.8	Other specified congenital malformations of skull and face bones
T84.328	Displacement of other bone devices, implants and grafts
T84.398	Other mechanical complication of other bone devices, implants and grafts
Z62.810	Personal history of physical and sexual abuse in childhood
Z85.841	Personal history of malignant neoplasm of brain
Z86.011	Personal history of benign neoplasm of the brain
Z86.69	Personal history of other diseases of the nervous system and sense organs
Z86.73	Personal history of transient ischemic attack (TIA), and cerebral infarction without residual deficits
Z87.39	Personal history of other diseases of the musculoskeletal system and connective tissue
Z87.728	Personal history of other specified (corrected) congenital malformations of nervous system and sense organs
Z87.76	Personal history of (corrected) congenital malformations of integument, limbs and musculoskeletal system
Z87.81	Personal history of (healed) traumatic fracture
Z87.820	Personal history of traumatic brain injury
Z87.828	Personal history of other (healed) physical injury and trauma
Z91.410	Personal history of adult physical and sexual abuse

ICD-10-CM Coding Notes

For codes requiring a 7th character extension, refer to your ICD-10-CM book. Review the character descriptions and coding guidelines for proper selection. For some procedures, only certain characters will apply.

CCI Edits

Refer to Appendix A for CCI edits.

Facility RVUs

Code	Work	PE Facility	MP	Total Facility
62143	14.15	10.82	5.06	30.03

Non-facility RVUs

Code	Work	PE Non-Facility	MP	Total Non-Facility
62143	14.15	10.82	5.06	30.03

Modifiers (PAR)

Code	Mod 50	Mod 51	Mod 62	Mod 66	Mod 80
62143	0	2	1	0	2

Global Period

Code	Days
62143	090

62145

62145 Cranioplasty for skull defect with reparative brain surgery

AMA Coding Notes

Surgical Procedures on the Skull, Meninges, and Brain

(For injection procedure for cerebral angiography, see 36100-36218)

(For injection procedure for ventriculography, see 61026, 61120)

(For injection procedure for pneumoencephalography, use 61055)

AMA *CPT Assistant*

62145: Jan 14: 9

Plain English Description

A cranioplasty to repair a skull injury or defect is performed at the time of reparative brain surgery. The site of the skull injury or defect is exposed. If a temporary prosthetic plate has been placed over the defect, it is removed. The reparative procedure performed is dependent on the type of brain injury. Following the reparative procedure, the skull is repaired. If a previously removed cranial bone is used, it is retrieved from the subcutaneous pocket in a separately reportable procedure. The cranial bone graft is returned to the site of the skull defect and secured with sutures, wires, or miniplate and screws. Use of a local bone graft is accomplished by taking a large bone graft from another site in the skull, splitting the bone with a chisel, replacing the cortical bone at the donor site, and then repairing the skull defect with the inner plate of the donor bone. Both sites are repaired with sutures or wires. Alternatively, the bone graft may be harvested from tibia, scapula, ribs, or iliac crest. The bone graft is configured to the size and shape of the defect. The bone graft is then secured as described above. Another option is the use of a prosthetic plate that is secured with wires or miniplate and screws. The overlying soft tissue and skin is then closed in layers.

Cranioplasty for skull defect with reparative brain surgery

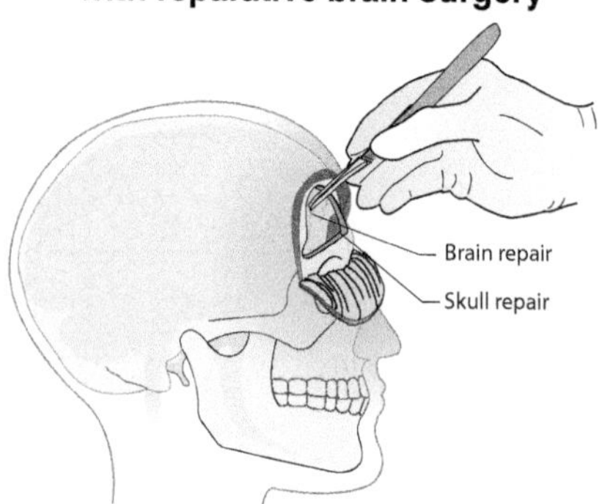

ICD-10-CM Diagnostic Codes

M95.2	Other acquired deformity of head
Q01.0	Frontal encephalocele
Q01.1	Nasofrontal encephalocele
Q01.2	Occipital encephalocele
Q01.8	Encephalocele of other sites
Q01.9	Encephalocele, unspecified
Q02	Microcephaly
Q03.8	Other congenital hydrocephalus
Q75.8	Other specified congenital malformations of skull and face bones
Z62.810	Personal history of physical and sexual abuse in childhood
Z85.841	Personal history of malignant neoplasm of brain
Z86.011	Personal history of benign neoplasm of the brain
Z86.69	Personal history of other diseases of the nervous system and sense organs
Z86.73	Personal history of transient ischemic attack (TIA), and cerebral infarction without residual deficits
Z87.39	Personal history of other diseases of the musculoskeletal system and connective tissue
Z87.728	Personal history of other specified (corrected) congenital malformations of nervous system and sense organs
Z87.76	Personal history of (corrected) congenital malformations of integument, limbs and musculoskeletal system
Z87.81	Personal history of (healed) traumatic fracture
Z87.820	Personal history of traumatic brain injury
Z87.828	Personal history of other (healed) physical injury and trauma
Z91.410	Personal history of adult physical and sexual abuse

CCI Edits

Refer to Appendix A for CCI edits.

Facility RVUs

Code	Work	PE Facility	MP	Total Facility
62145	20.09	13.68	7.31	41.08

Non-facility RVUs

Code	Work	PE Non-Facility	MP	Total Non-Facility
62145	20.09	13.68	7.31	41.08

Modifiers (PAR)

Code	Mod 50	Mod 51	Mod 62	Mod 66	Mod 80
62145	0	2	1	0	2

Global Period

Code	Days
62145	090

62146-62147

62146 Cranioplasty with autograft (includes obtaining bone grafts); up to 5 cm diameter

62147 Cranioplasty with autograft (includes obtaining bone grafts); larger than 5 cm diameter

AMA Coding Notes

Surgical Procedures on the Skull, Meninges, and Brain

(For injection procedure for cerebral angiography, see 36100-36218)

(For injection procedure for ventriculography, see 61026, 61120)

(For injection procedure for pneumoencephalography, use 61055)

AMA *CPT Assistant*

62146: Jan 14: 9

62147: Jan 14: 9

Plain English Description

A cranioplasty to repair a skull defect may be performed using a bone graft. The site of the skull injury or defect is exposed. If a previously removed cranial bone is used, it is retrieved from the subcutaneous pocket in a separately reportable procedure. The cranial bone graft is returned to the site of the skull defect and secured with sutures, wires, or miniplate and screws. Use of a local bone graft is accomplished by taking a large bone graft from another site in the skull, splitting the bone with a chisel, replacing the cortical bone at the donor site, and then repairing the skull defect with the inner plate of the donor bone. Both sites are repaired with sutures or wires. Alternatively, the bone graft may be harvested from tibia, scapula, ribs, or iliac crest. The bone graft is configured to the size and shape of the defect. The bone graft is then secured as described above. Use 62146 for repair of a skull defect up to 5 cm in diameter. Use 62147 for repair of a skull defect larger than 5 cm.

Cranioplasty with autograft

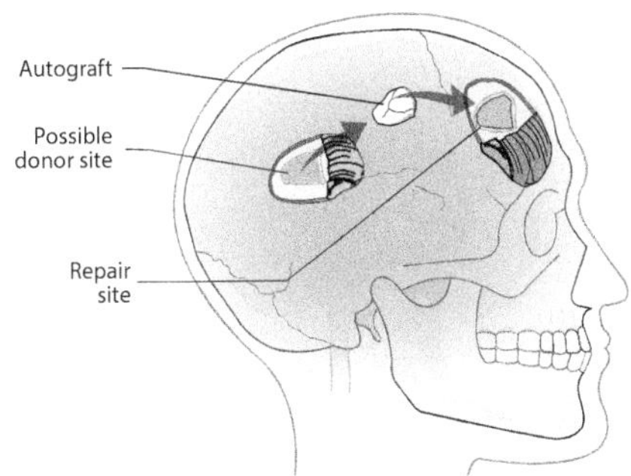

ICD-10-CM Diagnostic Codes

M95.2	Other acquired deformity of head
Q75.8	Other specified congenital malformations of skull and face bones
Z62.810	Personal history of physical and sexual abuse in childhood
Z85.841	Personal history of malignant neoplasm of brain
Z86.011	Personal history of benign neoplasm of the brain
Z86.69	Personal history of other diseases of the nervous system and sense organs
Z86.73	Personal history of transient ischemic attack (TIA), and cerebral infarction without residual deficits
Z87.39	Personal history of other diseases of the musculoskeletal system and connective tissue
Z87.728	Personal history of other specified (corrected) congenital malformations of nervous system and sense organs
Z87.76	Personal history of (corrected) congenital malformations of integument, limbs and musculoskeletal system
Z87.81	Personal history of (healed) traumatic fracture
Z87.820	Personal history of traumatic brain injury
Z87.828	Personal history of other (healed) physical injury and trauma
Z91.410	Personal history of adult physical and sexual abuse

CCI Edits

Refer to Appendix A for CCI edits.

Facility RVUs

Code	Work	PE Facility	MP	Total Facility
62146	17.28	11.05	4.29	32.62
62147	20.67	13.67	6.69	41.03

Non-facility RVUs

Code	Work	PE Non-Facility	MP	Total Non-Facility
62146	17.28	11.05	4.29	32.62
62147	20.67	13.67	6.69	41.03

Modifiers (PAR)

Code	Mod 50	Mod 51	Mod 62	Mod 66	Mod 80
62146	0	2	1	0	2
62147	0	2	1	0	2

Global Period

Code	Days
62146	090
62147	090

62148

✚ **62148 Incision and retrieval of subcutaneous cranial bone graft for cranioplasty (List separately in addition to code for primary procedure)**

(Use 62148 in conjunction with 62140-62147)

AMA Coding Notes

Surgical Procedures on the Skull, Meninges, and Brain

(For injection procedure for cerebral angiography, see 36100-36218)

(For injection procedure for ventriculography, see 61026, 61120)

(For injection procedure for pneumoencephalography, use 61055)

Plain English Description

A previously placed cranial bone graft is removed from the subcutaneous pocket and used to repair the skull defect. The subcutaneous pocket is opened along the previous incision. The bone graft is located, freed from surrounding tissue, and placed in an antibiotic solution until it is needed for the separately reportable cranioplasty. The subcutaneous pocket is irrigated, hemostasis obtained by electrocautery, and the skin pocket is closed.

ICD-10-CM Diagnostic Codes

See Primary Procedure code for crosswalks.

CCI Edits

Refer to Appendix A for CCI edits.

Facility RVUs ▯

Code	Work	PE Facility	MP	Total Facility
62148	2.00	0.93	0.74	3.67

Non-facility RVUs ▯

Code	Work	PE Non-Facility	MP	Total Non-Facility
62148	2.00	0.93	0.74	3.67

Modifiers (PAR) ▯

Code	Mod 50	Mod 51	Mod 62	Mod 66	Mod 80
62148	0	0	0	0	1

Global Period

Code	Days
62148	ZZZ

62160

+ **62160 Neuroendoscopy, intracranial, for placement or replacement of ventricular catheter and attachment to shunt system or external drainage (List separately in addition to code for primary procedure)**

(Use 62160 only in conjunction with 61107, 61210, 62220-62230, 62258)

AMA Coding Guideline

Neuroendoscopy Procedures on the Skull, Meninges, and Brain

Surgical endoscopy always includes diagnostic endoscopy.

AMA Coding Notes

Surgical Procedures on the Skull, Meninges, and Brain

(For injection procedure for cerebral angiography, see 36100-36218)

(For injection procedure for ventriculography, see 61026, 61120)

(For injection procedure for pneumoencephalography, use 61055)

AMA *CPT Assistant*

62160: Jun 07: 11, Dec 12: 14

Plain English Description

An intracranial neuroendoscopy is performed during a separately reportable ventricular catheter placement or replacement. A small incision is made in the scalp and the skull exposed. The periosteum is incised and a burr hole strategically created to allow visualization of the ventricular catheter. A neuroendoscope is inserted through the burr hole and advanced into the ventricle and surrounding intracranial structures identified and inspected. If the ventricular catheter is being replaced, the existing catheter is located using the neuroendoscope and removed under direct visualization. In a placement or replacement procedure, a ventricular catheter is then advanced into the ventricle using the neuroendoscope to ensure the catheter is properly positioned. The neuroendoscope is removed and the burr hole filled with bone graft or bone wax. The periosteum is closed followed by soft tissues and skin.

Neuroendoscopy, intracranial, ventricular catheter and attachment to shunt system

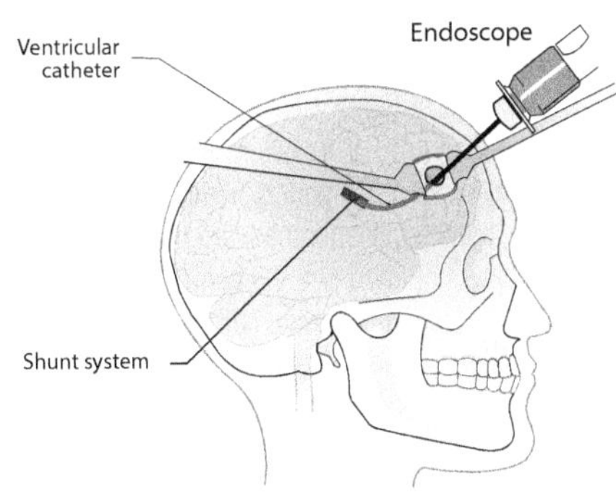

ICD-10-CM Diagnostic Codes

See Primary Procedure code for crosswalks.

CCI Edits

Refer to Appendix A for CCI edits.

Facility RVUs

Code	Work	PE Facility	MP	Total Facility
62160	3.00	1.38	1.09	5.47

Non-facility RVUs

Code	Work	PE Non-Facility	MP	Total Non-Facility
62160	3.00	1.38	1.09	5.47

Modifiers (PAR)

Code	Mod 50	Mod 51	Mod 62	Mod 66	Mod 80
62160	0	0	0	0	1

Global Period

Code	Days
62160	ZZZ

62161-62162

62161 Neuroendoscopy, intracranial; with dissection of adhesions, fenestration of septum pellucidum or intraventricular cysts (including placement, replacement, or removal of ventricular catheter)

62162 Neuroendoscopy, intracranial; with fenestration or excision of colloid cyst, including placement of external ventricular catheter for drainage

AMA Coding Guideline

Neuroendoscopy Procedures on the Skull, Meninges, and Brain

Surgical endoscopy always includes diagnostic endoscopy.

AMA Coding Notes

Surgical Procedures on the Skull, Meninges, and Brain

(For injection procedure for cerebral angiography, see 36100-36218)

(For injection procedure for ventriculography, see 61026, 61120)

(For injection procedure for pneumoencephalography, use 61055)

Plain English Description

A small incision is made in the scalp and the skull exposed. A burr hole is strategically created to allow visualization of the site where the adhesions or cyst is located or to allow visualization of the septum pellucidum. The dura is incised and a neuroendoscope is inserted through the burr hole. The brain cortex is inspected to ensure that large blood vessels are not in the path of the planned trocar insertion site. A trocar is then introduced into the ventricle. The inner stylet is removed from the trocar and the neuroendoscope inserted and advanced to the site of the adhesions, cyst, or septum pellucidum. In 62161, any adhesions obstructing the flow of cerebrospinal fluid are dissected. If an intraventricular cyst is present, the cyst wall is opened. The neuroendoscope is advanced into the cyst and a second opening created in the opposite side (back) of the cyst wall. The openings are enlarged. The neuroendoscope is advanced within the ventricular system, which is inspected to ensure that there is good communication of cerebrospinal fluid throughout the system. The septum pellucidum may be opened to allow better circulation of cerebrospinal fluid. The septum pellucidum is a thin plate of brain tissue dividing the column and body of the fornix below and the corpus callosum above and anteriorly. It is usually fused in the middle, forming a partition between the left and right frontal horn of the lateral ventricles. The neuroendoscope is removed. If a ventricular catheter is needed, it is advanced into the ventricle through the trocar and positioned in the ventricle. The trocar is removed. The catheter is cut to the desired length, attached to a one-way, flow-controlled valve proximally. Shunt tubing distal to the valve is then tunneled through the scalp to the neck and into the jugular vein or other shunt termination site in a separately reportable procedure. All incisions are closed. In 62162, a colloid cyst is opened or excised. The neuroendoscope is advanced toward the colloid cyst. The cyst is opened and the contents of the cyst evacuated using a suction catheter. The suction catheter is removed and a cautery device advanced through the working channel of the neuroendoscope. The site of attachment of the cyst wall is located and coagulated. The cautery device is removed and a cutting device inserted. The attachment is cut. The cutting device is removed and a grasping device inserted. The cyst is then removed, the area inspected for bleeding, and the neuroendoscope removed. A ventricular catheter is inserted as described above but instead of being tunneled to the internal shunt system, it is attached to an external drainage system.

Neuroendoscopy, intracranial; dissection of adhesions, fenestration of septum pellucidum/intraventricular cysts

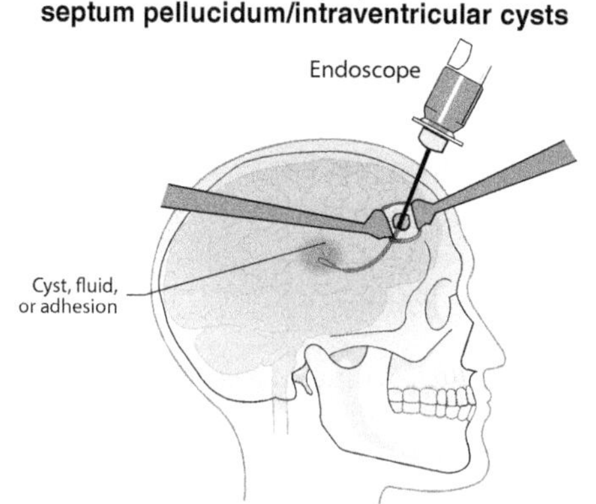

With dissection of adhesions, fenestration of septum pellucidum or intraventricular cyst, including placement, replacement, or removal of ventricular catheter (62161); with fenestration or excision of colloid cyst, including placement of external ventricular catheter for drainage (62162)

ICD-10-CM Diagnostic Codes

G91.4	Hydrocephalus in diseases classified elsewhere
G91.8	Other hydrocephalus
G93.0	Cerebral cysts
G96.12	Meningeal adhesions (cerebral) (spinal)
I67.4	Hypertensive encephalopathy
Q04.6	Congenital cerebral cysts
Q07.8	Other specified congenital malformations of nervous system

CCI Edits

Refer to Appendix A for CCI edits.

Facility RVUs

Code	Work	PE Facility	MP	Total Facility
62161	21.23	14.73	7.69	43.65
62162	26.80	17.83	9.90	54.53

Non-facility RVUs

Code	Work	PE Non-Facility	MP	Total Non-Facility
62161	21.23	14.73	7.69	43.65
62162	26.80	17.83	9.90	54.53

Modifiers (PAR)

Code	Mod 50	Mod 51	Mod 62	Mod 66	Mod 80
62161	0	2	1	0	2
62162	0	2	1	0	2

Global Period

Code	Days
62161	090
62162	090

62164

62164 Neuroendoscopy, intracranial; with excision of brain tumor, including placement of external ventricular catheter for drainage

AMA Coding Guideline

Neuroendoscopy Procedures on the Skull, Meninges, and Brain

Surgical endoscopy always includes diagnostic endoscopy.

AMA Coding Notes

Surgical Procedures on the Skull, Meninges, and Brain

(For injection procedure for cerebral angiography, see 36100-36218)

(For injection procedure for ventriculography, see 61026, 61120)

(For injection procedure for pneumoencephalography, use 61055)

Plain English Description

A brain tumor is excised using neuroendoscopy. A small incision is made in the scalp and the skull exposed. A burr hole is strategically placed to allow insertion of the neuroendoscope into the ventricular system. The dura is incised and a neuroendoscope is inserted through the burr hole. The brain cortex is inspected to ensure that large blood vessels are not in the path of the planned trocar insertion site. A trocar is then introduced into the ventricle. The ventricular system is inspected as the neuroendoscope is advanced to the tumor site. A tissue sample may be obtained and sent for separately reportable pathological examination. The tumor is then excised. A large tumor may require multiple passes and the use of a variety of instruments such as forceps, curettes, and suction devices. Following removal of the tumor, a cautery device is advanced through the working channel of the neuroendoscope to control bleeding. The neuroendoscope is removed. If a ventricular catheter is needed, it is advanced into the ventricle through the trocar and positioned in the ventricle. The trocar is removed. The catheter is cut to the desired length and attached to an external drainage system.

Neuroendoscopy, intracranial; with retrieval of foreign body

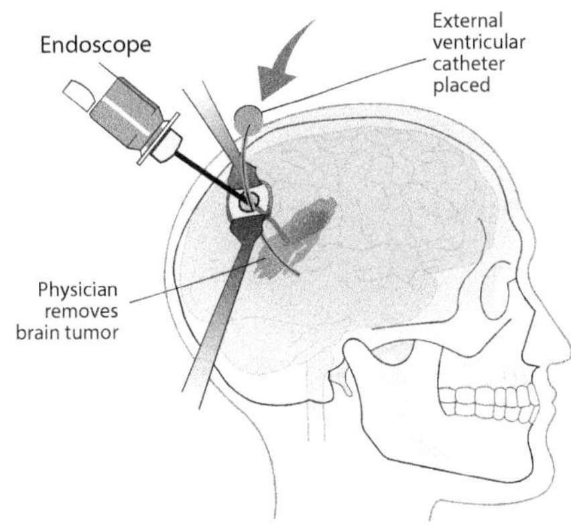

ICD-10-CM Diagnostic Codes

C70.0	Malignant neoplasm of cerebral meninges
C71.0	Malignant neoplasm of cerebrum, except lobes and ventricles
C71.1	Malignant neoplasm of frontal lobe
C71.2	Malignant neoplasm of temporal lobe
C71.3	Malignant neoplasm of parietal lobe
C71.4	Malignant neoplasm of occipital lobe
C71.5	Malignant neoplasm of cerebral ventricle
C71.6	Malignant neoplasm of cerebellum
C71.7	Malignant neoplasm of brain stem
C71.8	Malignant neoplasm of overlapping sites of brain
C79.31	Secondary malignant neoplasm of brain
C79.32	Secondary malignant neoplasm of cerebral meninges
D32.0	Benign neoplasm of cerebral meninges
D33.0	Benign neoplasm of brain, supratentorial
D33.1	Benign neoplasm of brain, infratentorial
D33.2	Benign neoplasm of brain, unspecified
D42.0	Neoplasm of uncertain behavior of cerebral meninges
D43.0	Neoplasm of uncertain behavior of brain, supratentorial
D43.1	Neoplasm of uncertain behavior of brain, infratentorial
D43.2	Neoplasm of uncertain behavior of brain, unspecified
D49.6	Neoplasm of unspecified behavior of brain
D49.7	Neoplasm of unspecified behavior of endocrine glands and other parts of nervous system

CCI Edits

Refer to Appendix A for CCI edits.

Facility RVUs ▢

Code	Work	PE Facility	MP	Total Facility
62164	29.43	20.05	10.90	60.38

Non-facility RVUs ▢

Code	Work	PE Non-Facility	MP	Total Non-Facility
62164	29.43	20.05	10.90	60.38

Modifiers (PAR) ▢

Code	Mod 50	Mod 51	Mod 62	Mod 66	Mod 80
62164	0	2	1	0	2

Global Period

Code	Days
62164	090

CPT® Procedural Coding

62165

62165 Neuroendoscopy, intracranial; with excision of pituitary tumor, transnasal or trans-sphenoidal approach

AMA Coding Guideline

Neuroendoscopy Procedures on the Skull, Meninges, and Brain

Surgical endoscopy always includes diagnostic endoscopy.

AMA Coding Notes

Surgical Procedures on the Skull, Meninges, and Brain

(For injection procedure for cerebral angiography, see 36100-36218)

(For injection procedure for ventriculography, see 61026, 61120)

(For injection procedure for pneumoencephalography, use 61055)

AMA *CPT Assistant* ▯

62165: Dec 17: 14

Plain English Description

A pituitary tumor is excised using neuroendoscopy via a transnasal or transsphenoidal approach. The neuroendoscope is inserted into one of the nostrils to the sphenoid ostium. The sphenoid ostium is opened using a rongeur. The sphenoid mucosa is stripped and bleeding controlled with electrocautery. The sinus is irrigated with antibiotic solution. Using endoscopic guidance, a small osteotome is used to remove the floor of the sella and expose the dura. The dura is incised. The pituitary tumor is visualized through the endoscope. A tissue sample may be obtained and sent for separately reportable pathological examination. The tumor is then excised. A large tumor may require multiple passes and the use of a variety of instruments such as forceps, curettes, and suction devices. Following removal of the tumor, a cautery device is advanced through the working channel of the endoscope to control bleeding. The endoscope is retracted into the nasal sinus so that the dural repair and sella reconstruction can be performed under direct visualization. The dural defect is packed with Gelfoam and the sella floor repaired. The sphenoid sinus is packed with Vaseline-impregnated gauze. The endoscope is withdrawn.

Neuroendoscopy, intracranial; with excision of pituitary tumor

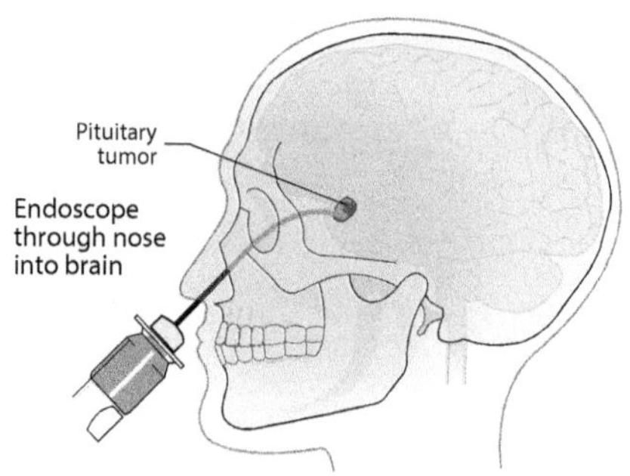

ICD-10-CM Diagnostic Codes

C75.1	Malignant neoplasm of pituitary gland
C79.89	Secondary malignant neoplasm of other specified sites
D09.3	Carcinoma in situ of thyroid and other endocrine glands
D35.2	Benign neoplasm of pituitary gland
D44.3	Neoplasm of uncertain behavior of pituitary gland

CCI Edits

Refer to Appendix A for CCI edits.

Facility RVUs ▯

Code	Work	PE Facility	MP	Total Facility
62165	23.23	14.44	6.23	43.90

Non-facility RVUs ▯

Code	Work	PE Non-Facility	MP	Total Non-Facility
62165	23.23	14.44	6.23	43.90

Modifiers (PAR) ▯

Code	Mod 50	Mod 51	Mod 62	Mod 66	Mod 80
62165	0	2	1	0	0

Global Period

Code	Days
62165	090

62190-62192

62190 Creation of shunt; subarachnoid/subdural-atrial, -jugular, -auricular

62192 Creation of shunt; subarachnoid/subdural-peritoneal, -pleural, other terminus

AMA Coding Notes

Surgical Procedures on the Skull, Meninges, and Brain

(For injection procedure for cerebral angiography, see 36100-36218)

(For injection procedure for ventriculography, see 61026, 61120)

(For injection procedure for pneumoencephalography, use 61055)

Plain English Description

A shunt is placed in the subarachnoid or subdural space in the brain to drain excess cerebrospinal fluid. In 62190, the shunt terminates in the right atrium of the heart, the atrial appendage (auricle), or the jugular vein. A curved skin incision is made in the scalp to create a skin flap. The scalp is flapped forward and a single burr hole created with a perforator. A second incision is then made in the skin of the neck for access to the jugular vein or common facial vein. A needle is inserted into the selected vein and a guidewire and vessel dilator are inserted through the needle into the jugular or facial vein. The dura is opened using pinhole cautery and the shunt (catheter) is then placed into the subarachnoid or subdural space. The proximal catheter and distal catheter are then connected to the shunt valve and the shunt valve is tested to ensure that cerebrospinal fluid (CSF) is flowing through the valve. If the shunt system is functioning properly, the distal catheter is then tunneled from the head into the neck. A cannula is placed under the scalp at the site of the coronal flap and advanced through the subgaleal space of the head and then between the subcuticular layer of the skin and the fascia of the superficial muscles of the neck. The distal catheter is advanced over the previously placed guidewire into the jugular vein. The catheter may terminate in the jugular vein or be advanced through the wall of the jugular and terminate in the right atrium or atrial appendage (auricle). In 62192, the shunt terminates in the peritoneum, pleural cavity, or other site in the body. The procedure is performed as described above except that the second incision is made in the skin of the chest or abdomen and the pleural space or peritoneum is exposed. The cannula is advanced between the subcuticular layer of the skin and the fascia of the superficial muscles of the neck and chest for a subarachnoid/subdural-pleural shunt. If the shunt terminates in the peritoneum, the cannula is advanced to abdomen. The terminal (distal) end of the catheter is then passed through the tunnel and positioned in the pleural space, peritoneum, or other prepared site.

Ventriculocisternostomy

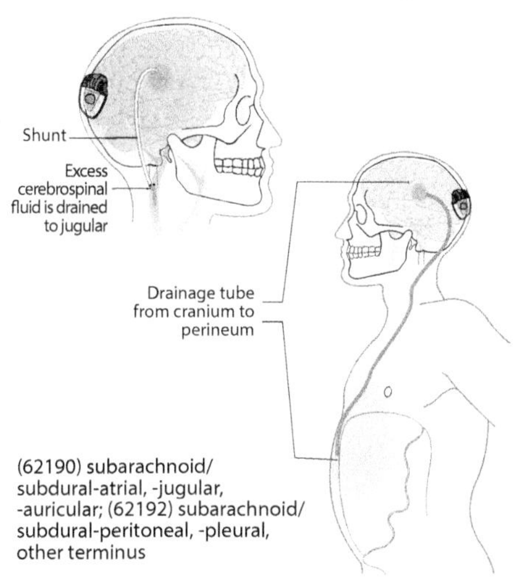

ICD-10-CM Diagnostic Codes

Code	Description
A17.0	Tuberculous meningitis
A39.0	Meningococcal meningitis
A42.81	Actinomycotic meningitis
A87.0	Enteroviral meningitis
A87.1	Adenoviral meningitis
A87.8	Other viral meningitis
B37.5	Candidal meningitis
C70.0	Malignant neoplasm of cerebral meninges
C71.5	Malignant neoplasm of cerebral ventricle
C71.6	Malignant neoplasm of cerebellum
C71.7	Malignant neoplasm of brain stem
C79.31	Secondary malignant neoplasm of brain
C79.32	Secondary malignant neoplasm of cerebral meninges
D32.9	Benign neoplasm of meninges, unspecified
D33.0	Benign neoplasm of brain, supratentorial
D33.1	Benign neoplasm of brain, infratentorial
D43.0	Neoplasm of uncertain behavior of brain, supratentorial
D43.1	Neoplasm of uncertain behavior of brain, infratentorial
G00.0	Hemophilus meningitis
G00.1	Pneumococcal meningitis
G00.2	Streptococcal meningitis
G00.3	Staphylococcal meningitis
G00.8	Other bacterial meningitis
G00.9	Bacterial meningitis, unspecified
G03.0	Nonpyogenic meningitis
G03.1	Chronic meningitis
G03.2	Benign recurrent meningitis [Mollaret]
G03.8	Meningitis due to other specified causes
G03.9	Meningitis, unspecified
G91.0	Communicating hydrocephalus
G91.1	Obstructive hydrocephalus
G91.2	(Idiopathic) normal pressure hydrocephalus
G91.3	Post-traumatic hydrocephalus, unspecified
G91.4	Hydrocephalus in diseases classified elsewhere
G91.8	Other hydrocephalus
G91.9	Hydrocephalus, unspecified
G93.0	Cerebral cysts
I61.5	Nontraumatic intracerebral hemorrhage, intraventricular
P37.1	Congenital toxoplasmosis
Q03.0	Malformations of aqueduct of Sylvius
Q03.1	Atresia of foramina of Magendie and Luschka
Q03.8	Other congenital hydrocephalus
Q03.9	Congenital hydrocephalus, unspecified
Q05.0	Cervical spina bifida with hydrocephalus
Q05.1	Thoracic spina bifida with hydrocephalus
Q05.2	Lumbar spina bifida with hydrocephalus
Q05.3	Sacral spina bifida with hydrocephalus
Q05.4	Unspecified spina bifida with hydrocephalus
Q07.0	Arnold-Chiari syndrome
Q07.02	Arnold-Chiari syndrome with hydrocephalus
Q07.03	Arnold-Chiari syndrome with spina bifida and hydrocephalus

CCI Edits

Refer to Appendix A for CCI edits.

Facility RVUs ▯

Code	Work	PE Facility	MP	Total Facility
62190	12.17	10.02	4.49	26.68
62192	13.35	10.23	4.74	28.32

Non-facility RVUs ▯

Code	Work	PE Non-Facility	MP	Total Non-Facility
62190	12.17	10.02	4.49	26.68
62192	13.35	10.23	4.74	28.32

Modifiers (PAR) ▯

Code	Mod 50	Mod 51	Mod 62	Mod 66	Mod 80
62190	0	2	1	0	1
62192	0	2	1	0	2

Global Period

Code	Days
62190	090
62192	090

CPT® Procedural Coding

62194

62194 Replacement or irrigation, subarachnoid/subdural catheter

AMA Coding Notes

Surgical Procedures on the Skull, Meninges, and Brain

(For injection procedure for cerebral angiography, see 36100-36218)

(For injection procedure for ventriculography, see 61026, 61120)

(For injection procedure for pneumoencephalography, use 61055)

AMA *CPT Assistant*

62194: Dec 11: 6

Plain English Description

An obstructed or malfunctioning subarachnoid or subdural catheter is irrigated or replaced. To irrigate the catheter, a needle is inserted into the catheter tubing. Aspiration may first be attempted to dislodge small obstructing particles. If this fails, a second needle is inserted and the catheter is irrigated and aspirated simultaneously. If the obstruction cannot be eliminated by irrigation and aspiration, the catheter is removed and replaced. A skin incision is made over the malfunctioning catheter. The proximal catheter is disconnected from the shunt valve. A guidewire is inserted into the proximal catheter and advanced to the subarachnoid or subdural space. The catheter is removed over the guidewire and a new catheter advanced into the subarachnoid or subdural space. The guidewire is removed and the new catheter secured and connected to the valve component.

Replacement or irrigation; subarachnoid/subdural catheter

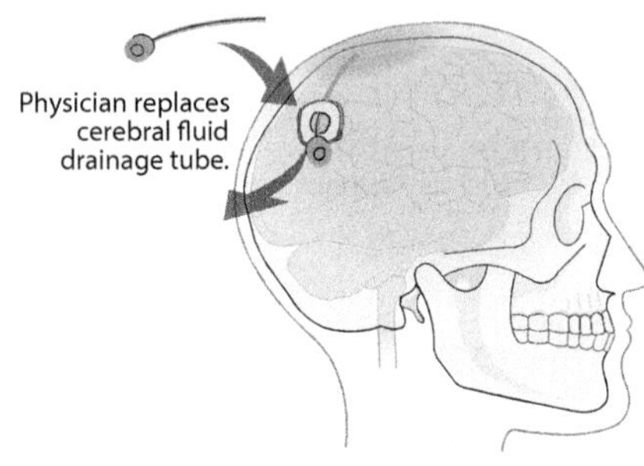

ICD-10-CM Diagnostic Codes

	Code	Description
	A17.0	Tuberculous meningitis
	A39.0	Meningococcal meningitis
	A42.81	Actinomycotic meningitis
	A87.0	Enteroviral meningitis
	A87.1	Adenoviral meningitis
	A87.8	Other viral meningitis
	B37.5	Candidal meningitis
	C70.0	Malignant neoplasm of cerebral meninges
	C71.5	Malignant neoplasm of cerebral ventricle
	C71.6	Malignant neoplasm of cerebellum
	C71.7	Malignant neoplasm of brain stem
	C79.31	Secondary malignant neoplasm of brain
	C79.32	Secondary malignant neoplasm of cerebral meninges
	D32.9	Benign neoplasm of meninges, unspecified
	D33.0	Benign neoplasm of brain, supratentorial
	D33.1	Benign neoplasm of brain, infratentorial
	D43.0	Neoplasm of uncertain behavior of brain, supratentorial
	D43.1	Neoplasm of uncertain behavior of brain, infratentorial
	G00.0	Hemophilus meningitis
	G00.1	Pneumococcal meningitis
	G00.2	Streptococcal meningitis
	G00.3	Staphylococcal meningitis
	G00.8	Other bacterial meningitis
	G00.9	Bacterial meningitis, unspecified
	G03.0	Nonpyogenic meningitis
	G03.1	Chronic meningitis
	G03.2	Benign recurrent meningitis [Mollaret]
	G03.8	Meningitis due to other specified causes
	G03.9	Meningitis, unspecified
	G91.0	Communicating hydrocephalus
	G91.1	Obstructive hydrocephalus
	G91.2	(Idiopathic) normal pressure hydrocephalus
	G91.3	Post-traumatic hydrocephalus, unspecified
	G91.4	Hydrocephalus in diseases classified elsewhere
	G91.8	Other hydrocephalus
	G91.9	Hydrocephalus, unspecified
	G93.0	Cerebral cysts
	I61.5	Nontraumatic intracerebral hemorrhage, intraventricular
	P37.1	Congenital toxoplasmosis
	Q03.0	Malformations of aqueduct of Sylvius
	Q03.1	Atresia of foramina of Magendie and Luschka
	Q03.8	Other congenital hydrocephalus
	Q03.9	Congenital hydrocephalus, unspecified
	Q05.0	Cervical spina bifida with hydrocephalus
	Q05.1	Thoracic spina bifida with hydrocephalus
	Q05.2	Lumbar spina bifida with hydrocephalus
	Q05.3	Sacral spina bifida with hydrocephalus
	Q05.4	Unspecified spina bifida with hydrocephalus
	Q07.0	Arnold-Chiari syndrome
	Q07.02	Arnold-Chiari syndrome with hydrocephalus
	Q07.03	Arnold-Chiari syndrome with spina bifida and hydrocephalus
❼	T85.01	Breakdown (mechanical) of ventricular intracranial (communicating) shunt
❼	T85.02	Displacement of ventricular intracranial (communicating) shunt
❼	T85.03	Leakage of ventricular intracranial (communicating) shunt
❼	T85.09	Other mechanical complication of ventricular intracranial (communicating) shunt
❼	T85.730	Infection and inflammatory reaction due to ventricular intracranial (communicating) shunt
❼	T85.810	Embolism due to nervous system prosthetic devices, implants and grafts
❼	T85.820	Fibrosis due to nervous system prosthetic devices, implants and grafts
❼	T85.830	Hemorrhage due to nervous system prosthetic devices, implants and grafts
❼	T85.840	Pain due to nervous system prosthetic devices, implants and grafts
❼	T85.850	Stenosis due to nervous system prosthetic devices, implants and grafts
❼	T85.860	Thrombosis due to nervous system prosthetic devices, implants and grafts
❼	T85.890	Other specified complication of nervous system prosthetic devices, implants and grafts
❼	T85.9	Unspecified complication of internal prosthetic device, implant and graft
	Z45.41	Encounter for adjustment and management of cerebrospinal fluid drainage device

ICD-10-CM Coding Notes

For codes requiring a 7th character extension, refer to your ICD-10-CM book. Review the character descriptions and coding guidelines for proper selection. For some procedures, only certain characters will apply.

CCI Edits

Refer to Appendix A for CCI edits.

Facility RVUs

Code	Work	PE Facility	MP	Total Facility
62194	5.78	6.15	2.13	14.06

Non-facility RVUs

Code	Work	PE Non-Facility	MP	Total Non-Facility
62194	5.78	6.15	2.13	14.06

Modifiers (PAR)

Code	Mod 50	Mod 51	Mod 62	Mod 66	Mod 80
62194	0	2	0	0	0

Global Period

Code	Days
62194	010

62200

62200 Ventriculocisternostomy, third ventricle

AMA Coding Notes

Surgical Procedures on the Skull, Meninges, and Brain

(For injection procedure for cerebral angiography, see 36100-36218)

(For injection procedure for ventriculography, see 61026, 61120)

(For injection procedure for pneumoencephalography, use 61055)

Plain English Description

An open ventriculocisternostomy is performed to create a communication (opening) between the third ventricle and the subarachnoid space (cistern). A circular incision is made in the scalp in the right frontal area and a skin flap is moved forward. A craniotomy is then created, the dura is opened, and the frontal horn of the lateral ventricle is identified. The lateral ventricle is catheterized and intracranial pressures are taken. The catheter is then advanced into the third ventricle and the floor is punctured to create an opening between the third ventricle and the subarachnoid cistern. The opening is enlarged until good flow of cerebrospinal fluid (CSF) is evidenced. If good CSF flow is not seen, the prepontine cistern is explored and any arachnoid bands obstructing flow are lysed. If an imperforate membrane of Liliequist is identified, it is disrupted. A second communication may be created if good flow of CSF is not seen following disruption of the obstruction. After good communication is verified, closing intracranial pressures are obtained. If pressures are elevated, an external ventricular drain is placed.

Ventriculocisternostomy, third ventricle

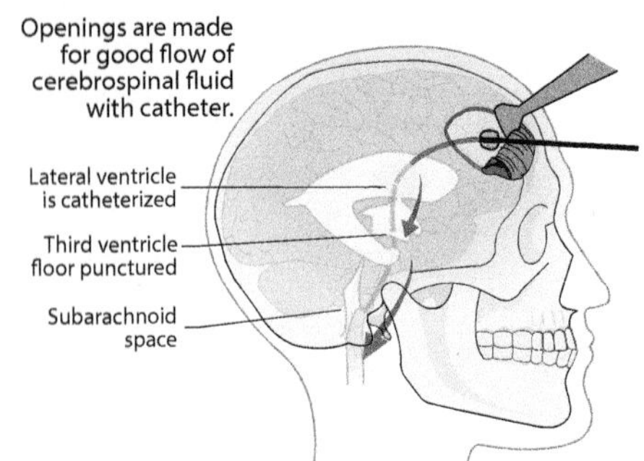

ICD-10-CM Diagnostic Codes

C70.0	Malignant neoplasm of cerebral meninges
C79.31	Secondary malignant neoplasm of brain
C79.32	Secondary malignant neoplasm of cerebral meninges
D32.9	Benign neoplasm of meninges, unspecified
D33.0	Benign neoplasm of brain, supratentorial
D33.1	Benign neoplasm of brain, infratentorial
G91.0	Communicating hydrocephalus
G91.1	Obstructive hydrocephalus
G91.2	(Idiopathic) normal pressure hydrocephalus
G91.3	Post-traumatic hydrocephalus, unspecified
G91.4	Hydrocephalus in diseases classified elsewhere
G91.8	Other hydrocephalus
G91.9	Hydrocephalus, unspecified
G93.0	Cerebral cysts
I61.5	Nontraumatic intracerebral hemorrhage, intraventricular
P37.1	Congenital toxoplasmosis
Q03.0	Malformations of aqueduct of Sylvius
Q03.1	Atresia of foramina of Magendie and Luschka
Q03.8	Other congenital hydrocephalus
Q03.9	Congenital hydrocephalus, unspecified
Q05.0	Cervical spina bifida with hydrocephalus
Q05.1	Thoracic spina bifida with hydrocephalus
Q05.2	Lumbar spina bifida with hydrocephalus
Q05.3	Sacral spina bifida with hydrocephalus
Q05.4	Unspecified spina bifida with hydrocephalus
Q07.0	Arnold-Chiari syndrome
Q07.02	Arnold-Chiari syndrome with hydrocephalus
Q07.03	Arnold-Chiari syndrome with spina bifida and hydrocephalus

CCI Edits

Refer to Appendix A for CCI edits.

Facility RVUs

Code	Work	PE Facility	MP	Total Facility
62200	19.29	13.31	7.12	39.72

Non-facility RVUs

Code	Work	PE Non-Facility	MP	Total Non-Facility
62200	19.29	13.31	7.12	39.72

Modifiers (PAR)

Code	Mod 50	Mod 51	Mod 62	Mod 66	Mod 80
62200	0	2	1	0	2

Global Period

Code	Days
62200	090

62201

62201 Ventriculocisternostomy, third ventricle; stereotactic, neuroendoscopic method

(For intracranial neuroendoscopic procedures, see 62161-62165)

AMA Coding Notes

Surgical Procedures on the Skull, Meninges, and Brain

(For injection procedure for cerebral angiography, see 36100-36218)

(For injection procedure for ventriculography, see 61026, 61120)

(For injection procedure for pneumoencephalography, use 61055)

AMA *CPT Assistant*

62201: Aug 07: 15, Jul 11: 12, Jul 14: 9

Plain English Description

A stereotactic neuroendoscopic third ventricle ventriculocisternostomy, also referred to as endoscopic third ventriculostomy (ETV), is performed. The scalp is incised; a skin flap is created and retracted; and a single burr hole is created in the skull with a perforator. The dura is then perforated using pinhole cautery. A neuroendoscope and ventricular catheter system are introduced into the frontal horn of the lateral ventricle. The neuroendoscope is removed, leaving the ventricular catheter in place and intracranial pressures are measured. The neuroendoscope is reinserted, the foramen of Monro is visualized, and the ventricular catheter is then advanced into the third ventricle. The basilar artery is identified. Care is taken to avoid puncturing the basilar artery as the floor of the third ventricle is opened (fenestrated) using the neuroendoscope, which is then passed into the subarachnoid space (cistern). The opening in the floor of the third ventricle is enlarged using the ventricular catheter. The catheter and neuroendoscope are then withdrawn to the third ventricle and flow of CSF is verified as evidenced by CSF pulsation. If good CSF flow is not evidenced, a second opening may be created or the prepontine cistern may be explored and any obstructing arachnoid bands or an imperforate Liliequist's membrane disrupted using the ventricular catheter to perform gentle dissection. After good communication is verified, closing intracranial pressures are obtained. If the pressures are elevated, an external ventricular drain is placed.

Ventriculocisternostomy, third ventricle; stereotactic, neuroendoscopic method

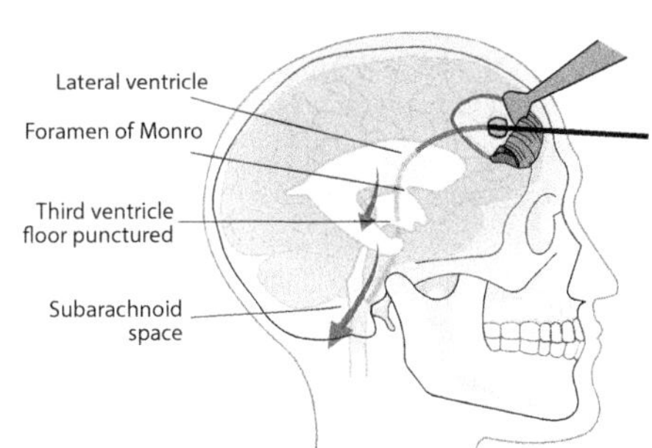

Neuroendoscope and ventricular catheter is introduced to increase flow of CSF.

ICD-10-CM Diagnostic Codes

Code	Description
C70.0	Malignant neoplasm of cerebral meninges
C79.31	Secondary malignant neoplasm of brain
C79.32	Secondary malignant neoplasm of cerebral meninges
D32.9	Benign neoplasm of meninges, unspecified
D33.0	Benign neoplasm of brain, supratentorial
D33.1	Benign neoplasm of brain, infratentorial
G91.0	Communicating hydrocephalus
G91.1	Obstructive hydrocephalus
G91.2	(Idiopathic) normal pressure hydrocephalus
G91.3	Post-traumatic hydrocephalus, unspecified
G91.4	Hydrocephalus in diseases classified elsewhere
G91.8	Other hydrocephalus
G91.9	Hydrocephalus, unspecified
G93.0	Cerebral cysts
I61.5	Nontraumatic intracerebral hemorrhage, intraventricular
P37.1	Congenital toxoplasmosis
Q03.0	Malformations of aqueduct of Sylvius
Q03.1	Atresia of foramina of Magendie and Luschka
Q03.8	Other congenital hydrocephalus
Q03.9	Congenital hydrocephalus, unspecified
Q05.0	Cervical spina bifida with hydrocephalus
Q05.1	Thoracic spina bifida with hydrocephalus
Q05.2	Lumbar spina bifida with hydrocephalus
Q05.3	Sacral spina bifida with hydrocephalus
Q05.4	Unspecified spina bifida with hydrocephalus
Q07.0	Arnold-Chiari syndrome
Q07.02	Arnold-Chiari syndrome with hydrocephalus
Q07.03	Arnold-Chiari syndrome with spina bifida and hydrocephalus

CCI Edits

Refer to Appendix A for CCI edits.

Facility RVUs

Code	Work	PE Facility	MP	Total Facility
62201	16.04	12.89	5.87	34.80

Non-facility RVUs

Code	Work	PE Non-Facility	MP	Total Non-Facility
62201	16.04	12.89	5.87	34.80

Modifiers (PAR)

Code	Mod 50	Mod 51	Mod 62	Mod 66	Mod 80
62201	0	2	0	0	1

Global Period

Code	Days
62201	090

62220-62223

62220 Creation of shunt; ventriculo-atrial, -jugular, -auricular

(For intracranial neuroendoscopic ventricular catheter placement, use 62160)

62223 Creation of shunt; ventriculo-peritoneal, -pleural, other terminus

(For intracranial neuroendoscopic ventricular catheter placement, use 62160)

AMA Coding Notes

Surgical Procedures on the Skull, Meninges, and Brain

(For injection procedure for cerebral angiography, see 36100-36218)

(For injection procedure for ventriculography, see 61026, 61120)

(For injection procedure for pneumoencephalography, use 61055)

Plain English Description

A shunt is placed in a ventricle in the brain, usually the lateral ventricle, to drain excess cerebrospinal fluid from the brain into the right atrium of the heart, the atrial appendage (auricle), or the jugular vein. A curved skin incision is made in the scalp to create a skin flap. The scalp is flapped forward and a single burr hole created with a perforator. The dura is perforated using pinhole cautery. A second incision is then made in the skin of the neck for access to the jugular vein or common facial vein. A needle is inserted into the selected vein and a guidewire and vessel dilator are inserted through the needle into the jugular or facial vein. Using a stylet, the ventricular shunt (catheter) is then placed through the previously created opening in the dura, advanced through the pia, into the gray and white matter, through the ependymal lining, and positioned in the lateral ventricle. The stylet is then removed. The ventricular (proximal) catheter and distal catheter are then connected to the shunt valve and the shunt valve is tested to ensure that cerebrospinal fluid (CSF) is flowing through the valve. If the shunt system is functioning properly, the distal catheter is then tunneled from the head into the neck. A cannula is placed under the scalp at the site of the coronal flap and advanced through the subgaleal space of the head and then between the subcuticular layer of the skin and the fascia of the superficial muscles of the neck. The distal catheter is then advanced over the previously placed guidewire into the jugular vein. The catheter may terminate in the jugular vein or be advanced through the wall of the jugular and terminate in the right atrium or atrial appendage (auricle). Use code 62223 when a shunt is placed in a ventricle in the brain to drain excess cerebrospinal fluid from the brain into the peritoneum, pleural cavity, or other site in the body. The procedure is performed as described above except that the second incision is made in the skin of the chest or abdomen and the pleural space or peritoneum is exposed. The cannula is advanced between the subcuticular layer of the skin and the fascia of the superficial muscles of the neck and chest for a ventriculo-pleural shunt. If the shunt terminates in the peritoneum, the cannula is advanced to the abdomen. The terminal (distal) end of the catheter is then passed through the tunnel and positioned in the pleural space, peritoneum, or other prepared site.

Creation of shunt

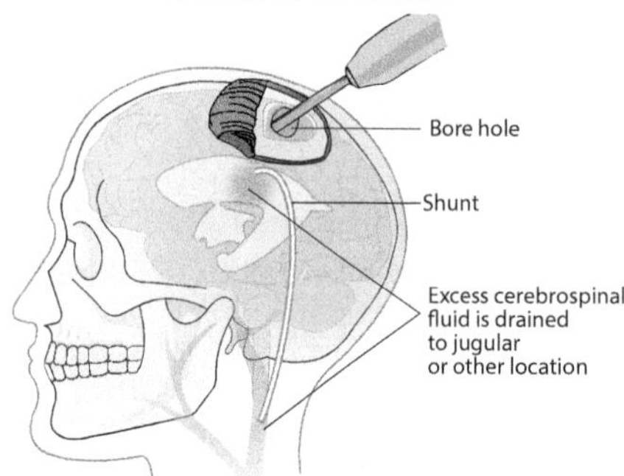

Ventriculo-atrial, -jugular, -auricular (62220);
Ventriculo-peritoneal, -pleural, other terminus (62223)

ICD-10-CM Diagnostic Codes

Code	Description
A17.0	Tuberculous meningitis
A39.0	Meningococcal meningitis
A42.81	Actinomycotic meningitis
A87.0	Enteroviral meningitis
A87.1	Adenoviral meningitis
A87.8	Other viral meningitis
B37.5	Candidal meningitis
C70.0	Malignant neoplasm of cerebral meninges
C71.5	Malignant neoplasm of cerebral ventricle
C71.6	Malignant neoplasm of cerebellum
C71.7	Malignant neoplasm of brain stem
C79.31	Secondary malignant neoplasm of brain
C79.32	Secondary malignant neoplasm of cerebral meninges
D32.9	Benign neoplasm of meninges, unspecified
D33.0	Benign neoplasm of brain, supratentorial
D33.1	Benign neoplasm of brain, infratentorial
D43.0	Neoplasm of uncertain behavior of brain, supratentorial
D43.1	Neoplasm of uncertain behavior of brain, infratentorial
G00.0	Hemophilus meningitis
G00.1	Pneumococcal meningitis
G00.2	Streptococcal meningitis
G00.3	Staphylococcal meningitis
G00.8	Other bacterial meningitis
G00.9	Bacterial meningitis, unspecified
G03.0	Nonpyogenic meningitis
G03.1	Chronic meningitis
G03.2	Benign recurrent meningitis [Mollaret]
G03.8	Meningitis due to other specified causes
G03.9	Meningitis, unspecified
G91.0	Communicating hydrocephalus
G91.1	Obstructive hydrocephalus
G91.2	(Idiopathic) normal pressure hydrocephalus
G91.3	Post-traumatic hydrocephalus, unspecified
G91.4	Hydrocephalus in diseases classified elsewhere
G91.8	Other hydrocephalus
G91.9	Hydrocephalus, unspecified
G93.0	Cerebral cysts
I61.5	Nontraumatic intracerebral hemorrhage, intraventricular
P37.1	Congenital toxoplasmosis
Q03.0	Malformations of aqueduct of Sylvius
Q03.1	Atresia of foramina of Magendie and Luschka
Q03.8	Other congenital hydrocephalus
Q03.9	Congenital hydrocephalus, unspecified
Q05.0	Cervical spina bifida with hydrocephalus
Q05.1	Thoracic spina bifida with hydrocephalus
Q05.2	Lumbar spina bifida with hydrocephalus
Q05.3	Sacral spina bifida with hydrocephalus
Q05.4	Unspecified spina bifida with hydrocephalus
Q07.0	Arnold-Chiari syndrome
Q07.02	Arnold-Chiari syndrome with hydrocephalus
Q07.03	Arnold-Chiari syndrome with spina bifida and hydrocephalus

CCI Edits

Refer to Appendix A for CCI edits.

Facility RVUs ☐

Code	Work	PE Facility	MP	Total Facility
62220	14.10	9.69	4.69	28.48
62223	14.05	11.17	4.80	30.02

Non-facility RVUs ☐

Code	Work	PE Non-Facility	MP	Total Non-Facility
62220	14.10	9.69	4.69	28.48
62223	14.05	11.17	4.80	30.02

Modifiers (PAR) ☐

Code	Mod 50	Mod 51	Mod 62	Mod 66	Mod 80
62220	0	2	1	0	2
62223	0	2	1	0	2

Global Period

Code	Days
62220	090
62223	090

62225

62225 Replacement or irrigation, ventricular catheter

(For intracranial neuroendoscopic ventricular catheter placement, use 62160)

AMA Coding Notes

Surgical Procedures on the Skull, Meninges, and Brain

(For injection procedure for cerebral angiography, see 36100-36218)

(For injection procedure for ventriculography, see 61026, 61120)

(For injection procedure for pneumoencephalography, use 61055)

AMA *CPT Assistant*

62225: Dec 11: 6

Plain English Description

An obstructed or malfunctioning ventricular catheter is irrigated or replaced. To irrigate the catheter, a needle is inserted into the catheter tubing. Aspiration may first be attempted to dislodge small obstructing particles. If this fails, a second needle is inserted and the catheter is irrigated and aspirated simultaneously. If the obstruction cannot be eliminated by irrigation and aspiration, the catheter is removed and replaced. A skin incision is made over the malfunctioning catheter. The proximal catheter is disconnected from the shunt valve. A guidewire is inserted into the proximal catheter and advanced into the ventricle. The catheter is removed over the guidewire and a new catheter advanced into the ventricle. The guidewire is removed and the new catheter secured and connected to the valve component.

Replacement or irrigation, ventricular catheter

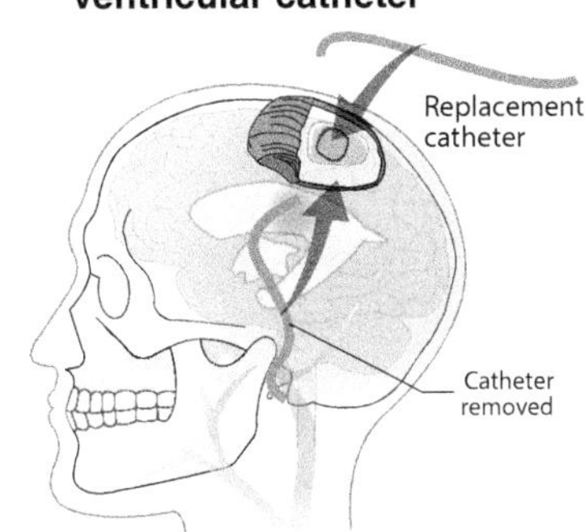

ICD-10-CM Diagnostic Codes

Code	Description
A17.0	Tuberculous meningitis
A39.0	Meningococcal meningitis
A42.81	Actinomycotic meningitis
A87.0	Enteroviral meningitis
A87.1	Adenoviral meningitis
A87.8	Other viral meningitis
B37.5	Candidal meningitis
C70.0	Malignant neoplasm of cerebral meninges
C71.5	Malignant neoplasm of cerebral ventricle
C71.6	Malignant neoplasm of cerebellum
C71.7	Malignant neoplasm of brain stem
C79.31	Secondary malignant neoplasm of brain
C79.32	Secondary malignant neoplasm of cerebral meninges
D32.9	Benign neoplasm of meninges, unspecified
D33.0	Benign neoplasm of brain, supratentorial
D33.1	Benign neoplasm of brain, infratentorial
D43.0	Neoplasm of uncertain behavior of brain, supratentorial
D43.1	Neoplasm of uncertain behavior of brain, infratentorial
G00.0	Hemophilus meningitis
G00.1	Pneumococcal meningitis
G00.2	Streptococcal meningitis
G00.3	Staphylococcal meningitis
G00.8	Other bacterial meningitis
G00.9	Bacterial meningitis, unspecified
G03.0	Nonpyogenic meningitis
G03.1	Chronic meningitis
G03.2	Benign recurrent meningitis [Mollaret]
G03.8	Meningitis due to other specified causes
G03.9	Meningitis, unspecified
G91.0	Communicating hydrocephalus
G91.1	Obstructive hydrocephalus
G91.2	(Idiopathic) normal pressure hydrocephalus
G91.3	Post-traumatic hydrocephalus, unspecified
G91.4	Hydrocephalus in diseases classified elsewhere
G91.8	Other hydrocephalus
G91.9	Hydrocephalus, unspecified
G93.0	Cerebral cysts
I61.5	Nontraumatic intracerebral hemorrhage, intraventricular
P37.1	Congenital toxoplasmosis
Q03.0	Malformations of aqueduct of Sylvius
Q03.1	Atresia of foramina of Magendie and Luschka
Q03.8	Other congenital hydrocephalus
Q03.9	Congenital hydrocephalus, unspecified
Q05.0	Cervical spina bifida with hydrocephalus
Q05.1	Thoracic spina bifida with hydrocephalus
Q05.2	Lumbar spina bifida with hydrocephalus
Q05.3	Sacral spina bifida with hydrocephalus
Q05.4	Unspecified spina bifida with hydrocephalus
Q07.0	Arnold-Chiari syndrome
Q07.02	Arnold-Chiari syndrome with hydrocephalus
Q07.03	Arnold-Chiari syndrome with spina bifida and hydrocephalus
⑦ T85.01	Breakdown (mechanical) of ventricular intracranial (communicating) shunt
⑦ T85.02	Displacement of ventricular intracranial (communicating) shunt
⑦ T85.03	Leakage of ventricular intracranial (communicating) shunt
⑦ T85.09	Other mechanical complication of ventricular intracranial (communicating) shunt
⑦ T85.730	Infection and inflammatory reaction due to ventricular intracranial (communicating) shunt
⑦ T85.810	Embolism due to nervous system prosthetic devices, implants and grafts
⑦ T85.820	Fibrosis due to nervous system prosthetic devices, implants and grafts
⑦ T85.830	Hemorrhage due to nervous system prosthetic devices, implants and grafts
⑦ T85.840	Pain due to nervous system prosthetic devices, implants and grafts
⑦ T85.850	Stenosis due to nervous system prosthetic devices, implants and grafts
⑦ T85.860	Thrombosis due to nervous system prosthetic devices, implants and grafts
⑦ T85.890	Other specified complication of nervous system prosthetic devices, implants and grafts
⑦ T85.9	Unspecified complication of internal prosthetic device, implant and graft
Z45.41	Encounter for adjustment and management of cerebrospinal fluid drainage device

ICD-10-CM Coding Notes

For codes requiring a 7th character extension, refer to your ICD-10-CM book. Review the character descriptions and coding guidelines for proper selection. For some procedures, only certain characters will apply.

CCI Edits

Refer to Appendix A for CCI edits.

Facility RVUs

Code	Work	PE Facility	MP	Total Facility
62225	6.19	6.73	2.25	15.17

Non-facility RVUs

Code	Work	PE Non-Facility	MP	Total Non-Facility
62225	6.19	6.73	2.25	15.17

Modifiers (PAR)

Code	Mod 50	Mod 51	Mod 62	Mod 66	Mod 80
62225	0	2	0	0	1

Global Period

Code	Days
62225	090

62230

62230 Replacement or revision of cerebrospinal fluid shunt, obstructed valve, or distal catheter in shunt system

(For intracranial neuroendoscopic ventricular catheter placement, use 62160)

(For replacement of only the valve and proximal catheter, use 62230 in conjunction with 62225)

AMA Coding Notes

Surgical Procedures on the Skull, Meninges, and Brain

(For injection procedure for cerebral angiography, see 36100-36218)

(For injection procedure for ventriculography, see 61026, 61120)

(For injection procedure for pneumoencephalography, use 61055)

AMA *CPT Assistant* □

62230: Dec 11: 6, Dec 12: 14

Plain English Description

A malfunctioning or obstructed cerebrospinal fluid (CSF) shunt, valve, or distal catheter is replaced or revised. The shunt, valve, or distal catheter can become obstructed with protein deposits when there is excess protein in the CSF. Another cause of malfunction of the distal catheter is if it becomes dislodged. This is particularly common when the shunt terminates in the peritoneum. The shunt system is evaluated to determine which component is obstructed or malfunctioning. If the ventricular shunt is malfunctioning, it may be repositioned or replaced. A skin incision is made over the malfunctioning shunt. A guidewire is advanced through the catheter to the proximal end. The catheter may be advanced or retracted. Flow of CSF is evaluated. If repositioning the catheter does not correct the malfunction, the proximal catheter is disconnected from the shunt valve. A guidewire is inserted into the proximal catheter and advanced into the ventricle. The catheter is removed over the guidewire and a new catheter advanced into the ventricle. The guidewire is removed and the new catheter secured and connected to the valve component. If the valve is malfunctioning or obstructed, the shunt may be flushed to help dislodge any protein deposits that are obstructing the valve. If this is not effective, the valve is disconnected from the proximal and distal catheters, and they are connected to a replacement valve. If the distal catheter is malfunctioning, it may be irrigated to relieve the obstruction. Alternatively, a guidewire may be inserted and the end of the distal catheter repositioned in an attempt to relieve the obstruction. If this does not work, the distal catheter is removed over the guidewire and a new catheter advanced over the guidewire. Contrast is injected as needed and the position of the catheter checked. The revised or replaced components are then secured to surrounding skin and subcutaneous tissues.

Replacement or revision of cerebrospinal fluid shunt, obstructed valve, or distal catheter in shunt system

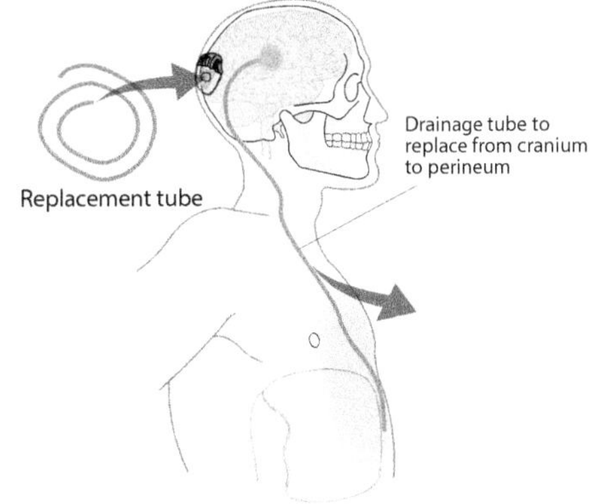

ICD-10-CM Diagnostic Codes

Code	Description
A17.0	Tuberculous meningitis
A39.0	Meningococcal meningitis
A42.81	Actinomycotic meningitis
A87.0	Enteroviral meningitis
A87.1	Adenoviral meningitis
A87.8	Other viral meningitis
B37.5	Candidal meningitis
C70.0	Malignant neoplasm of cerebral meninges
C71.5	Malignant neoplasm of cerebral ventricle
C71.6	Malignant neoplasm of cerebellum
C71.7	Malignant neoplasm of brain stem
C79.31	Secondary malignant neoplasm of brain
C79.32	Secondary malignant neoplasm of cerebral meninges
D32.9	Benign neoplasm of meninges, unspecified
D33.0	Benign neoplasm of brain, supratentorial
D33.1	Benign neoplasm of brain, infratentorial
D43.0	Neoplasm of uncertain behavior of brain, supratentorial
D43.1	Neoplasm of uncertain behavior of brain, infratentorial
G00.0	Hemophilus meningitis
G00.1	Pneumococcal meningitis
G00.2	Streptococcal meningitis
G00.3	Staphylococcal meningitis
G00.8	Other bacterial meningitis
G00.9	Bacterial meningitis, unspecified
G03.0	Nonpyogenic meningitis
G03.1	Chronic meningitis
G03.2	Benign recurrent meningitis [Mollaret]
G03.8	Meningitis due to other specified causes
G03.9	Meningitis, unspecified
G91.0	Communicating hydrocephalus
G91.1	Obstructive hydrocephalus
G91.2	(Idiopathic) normal pressure hydrocephalus
G91.3	Post-traumatic hydrocephalus, unspecified
G91.4	Hydrocephalus in diseases classified elsewhere
G91.8	Other hydrocephalus
G91.9	Hydrocephalus, unspecified
G93.0	Cerebral cysts
I61.5	Nontraumatic intracerebral hemorrhage, intraventricular
P37.1	Congenital toxoplasmosis
Q03.0	Malformations of aqueduct of Sylvius
Q03.1	Atresia of foramina of Magendie and Luschka
Q03.8	Other congenital hydrocephalus
Q03.9	Congenital hydrocephalus, unspecified
Q05.0	Cervical spina bifida with hydrocephalus
Q05.1	Thoracic spina bifida with hydrocephalus
Q05.2	Lumbar spina bifida with hydrocephalus
Q05.3	Sacral spina bifida with hydrocephalus
Q05.4	Unspecified spina bifida with hydrocephalus
Q07.0	Arnold-Chiari syndrome
Q07.02	Arnold-Chiari syndrome with hydrocephalus
Q07.03	Arnold-Chiari syndrome with spina bifida and hydrocephalus
⑦ T85.01	Breakdown (mechanical) of ventricular intracranial (communicating) shunt
⑦ T85.02	Displacement of ventricular intracranial (communicating) shunt
⑦ T85.03	Leakage of ventricular intracranial (communicating) shunt
⑦ T85.09	Other mechanical complication of ventricular intracranial (communicating) shunt
⑦ T85.730	Infection and inflammatory reaction due to ventricular intracranial (communicating) shunt
⑦ T85.810	Embolism due to nervous system prosthetic devices, implants and grafts
⑦ T85.820	Fibrosis due to nervous system prosthetic devices, implants and grafts
⑦ T85.830	Hemorrhage due to nervous system prosthetic devices, implants and grafts
⑦ T85.840	Pain due to nervous system prosthetic devices, implants and grafts
⑦ T85.850	Stenosis due to nervous system prosthetic devices, implants and grafts
⑦ T85.860	Thrombosis due to nervous system prosthetic devices, implants and grafts
⑦ T85.890	Other specified complication of nervous system prosthetic devices, implants and grafts
⑦ T85.9	Unspecified complication of internal prosthetic device, implant and graft

Z45.41	Encounter for adjustment and management of cerebrospinal fluid drainage device

ICD-10-CM Coding Notes

For codes requiring a 7th character extension, refer to your ICD-10-CM book. Review the character descriptions and coding guidelines for proper selection. For some procedures, only certain characters will apply.

CCI Edits

Refer to Appendix A for CCI edits.

Facility RVUs

Code	Work	PE Facility	MP	Total Facility
62230	11.43	8.84	4.00	24.27

Non-facility RVUs

Code	Work	PE Non-Facility	MP	Total Non-Facility
62230	11.43	8.84	4.00	24.27

Modifiers (PAR)

Code	Mod 50	Mod 51	Mod 62	Mod 66	Mod 80
62230	0	2	1	0	2

Global Period

Code	Days
62230	090

62252

62252 Reprogramming of programmable cerebrospinal shunt

AMA Coding Notes

Surgical Procedures on the Skull, Meninges, and Brain

(For injection procedure for cerebral angiography, see 36100-36218)

(For injection procedure for ventriculography, see 61026, 61120)

(For injection procedure for pneumoencephalography, use 61055)

Plain English Description

A programmable cerebrospinal fluid (CSF) shunt is reprogrammed. This non-invasive procedure is used to adjust pressure settings in a previously placed intracranial CSF shunt and can correct over- or under-drainage of CSF in a patient with hydrocephalus. These types of shunts are also used in patients with fluid-filled cysts or other fluid accumulations in the brain, and reprogramming may be used to treat under-drainage in these patients. Reprogramming is also required following MRI. The previously implanted valve on the CSF shunt is palpated through the skin. The valve is typically located behind the ear. The transmitter head of the programmer is placed over the valve. The programming console is set to the desired pressure and an electromagnetic transmitter device is used to send a coded magnetic signal through the skin to the valve to reset the pressure setting. Following reprogramming, a separately reportable radiograph is obtained to verify that the pressure setting has been reset. The physician may repeat the procedure if the radiograph reveals that the desired setting has not been achieved.

Reprogramming of programmable cerebrospinal shunt

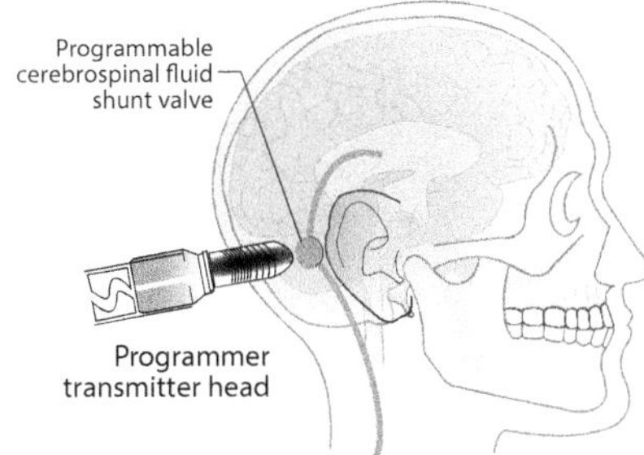

ICD-10-CM Diagnostic Codes

A17.0	Tuberculous meningitis
A39.0	Meningococcal meningitis
A42.81	Actinomycotic meningitis
A87.0	Enteroviral meningitis
A87.1	Adenoviral meningitis
A87.8	Other viral meningitis
B37.5	Candidal meningitis
C70.0	Malignant neoplasm of cerebral meninges
C71.5	Malignant neoplasm of cerebral ventricle
C71.6	Malignant neoplasm of cerebellum
C71.7	Malignant neoplasm of brain stem
C79.31	Secondary malignant neoplasm of brain
C79.32	Secondary malignant neoplasm of cerebral meninges
D32.9	Benign neoplasm of meninges, unspecified
D33.0	Benign neoplasm of brain, supratentorial
D33.1	Benign neoplasm of brain, infratentorial
D43.0	Neoplasm of uncertain behavior of brain, supratentorial
D43.1	Neoplasm of uncertain behavior of brain, infratentorial
G00.0	Hemophilus meningitis
G00.1	Pneumococcal meningitis
G00.2	Streptococcal meningitis
G00.3	Staphylococcal meningitis
G00.8	Other bacterial meningitis
G00.9	Bacterial meningitis, unspecified
G03.0	Nonpyogenic meningitis
G03.1	Chronic meningitis
G03.2	Benign recurrent meningitis [Mollaret]
G03.8	Meningitis due to other specified causes
G03.9	Meningitis, unspecified
G91.0	Communicating hydrocephalus
G91.1	Obstructive hydrocephalus
G91.2	(Idiopathic) normal pressure hydrocephalus
G91.3	Post-traumatic hydrocephalus, unspecified
G91.4	Hydrocephalus in diseases classified elsewhere
G91.8	Other hydrocephalus
G91.9	Hydrocephalus, unspecified
G93.0	Cerebral cysts
I61.5	Nontraumatic intracerebral hemorrhage, intraventricular
P37.1	Congenital toxoplasmosis
Q03.0	Malformations of aqueduct of Sylvius
Q03.1	Atresia of foramina of Magendie and Luschka
Q03.8	Other congenital hydrocephalus
Q03.9	Congenital hydrocephalus, unspecified
Q05.0	Cervical spina bifida with hydrocephalus
Q05.1	Thoracic spina bifida with hydrocephalus
Q05.2	Lumbar spina bifida with hydrocephalus
Q05.3	Sacral spina bifida with hydrocephalus
Q05.4	Unspecified spina bifida with hydrocephalus
Q07.0	Arnold-Chiari syndrome
Q07.02	Arnold-Chiari syndrome with hydrocephalus
Q07.03	Arnold-Chiari syndrome with spina bifida and hydrocephalus
Z45.41	Encounter for adjustment and management of cerebrospinal fluid drainage device

CCI Edits

Refer to Appendix A for CCI edits.

Facility RVUs

Code	Work	PE Facility	MP	Total Facility
62252	0.74	1.31	0.26	2.31

Non-facility RVUs

Code	Work	PE Non-Facility	MP	Total Non-Facility
62252	0.74	1.31	0.26	2.31

Modifiers (PAR)

Code	Mod 50	Mod 51	Mod 62	Mod 66	Mod 80
62252	0	0	0	0	0

Global Period

Code	Days
62252	XXX

62256-62258

62256 Removal of complete cerebrospinal fluid shunt system; without replacement

62258 Removal of complete cerebrospinal fluid shunt system; with replacement by similar or other shunt at same operation

(For percutaneous irrigation or aspiration of shunt reservoir, use 61070)

(For reprogramming of programmable CSF shunt, use 62252)

(For intracranial neuroendoscopic ventricular catheter placement, use 62160)

AMA Coding Notes

Surgical Procedures on the Skull, Meninges, and Brain

(For injection procedure for cerebral angiography, see 36100-36218)

(For injection procedure for ventriculography, see 61026, 61120)

(For injection procedure for pneumoencephalography, use 61055)

AMA *CPT Assistant*

62258: Dec 11: 6

Plain English Description

A cerebrospinal fluid shunt system may be removed if it was placed temporarily or for a complication such as obstruction or infection. In 62256, the shunt system is removed without replacement. The shunt valve is exposed. The proximal and distal catheters are detached from the shunt valve and the shunt valve is removed. The proximal and distal catheters are then removed. To remove the proximal catheter, a skin incision is made over the shunt. Overlying soft tissues are dissected and any anchoring sutures are cut. A guidewire is advanced through the catheter to the proximal end. The catheter is removed over the guidewire. A temporary drain may be placed over the guidewire or the guidewire may be removed and the dura closed. To remove the distal catheter, a guidewire is placed. The subcutaneous tunnel is opened and the shunt is dissected free of the tunnel and the terminal end removed. In 62258, the shunt system is removed as described above and replaced with a new shunt system during the same surgical session. After removing the shunt valve and the existing proximal catheter over the guidewire, a new catheter is inserted into the ventricle, subarachnoid, or subdural space. The new proximal catheter and new distal catheter are then connected to the new shunt valve and the shunt valve is tested to ensure that cerebrospinal fluid (CSF) is flowing through the valve. If the shunt system is functioning properly, the distal catheter is then advanced into the termination site over the guidewire that was placed when the existing distal catheter was removed. Alternatively, if the distal catheter is rerouted to a new termination site, a cannula is placed under the scalp. If the new termination site is the jugular, right atrium, or atrial appendage, the cannula is advanced through the subgaleal space of the head and then between the subcuticular layer of the skin and the fascia of the superficial muscles of the neck. The distal catheter is then advanced over a previously placed guidewire into the jugular vein. The catheter may remain in the jugular vein or be advanced through the wall of the jugular and terminate in the right atrium or atrial appendage (auricle). If the shunt terminates in the peritoneum, pleural cavity, or other site in the body, the procedure is performed as described above except that the second incision is made in the skin of the chest or abdomen and the pleural space or peritoneum is exposed. The cannula is advanced between the subcuticular layer of the skin and the fascia of the superficial muscles of the neck and chest for a subarachnoid/subdural-pleural shunt. If the shunt terminates in the peritoneum, the cannula is advanced to the abdomen. The terminal (distal) end of the catheter is then passed through the tunnel and positioned in the pleural space, peritoneum, or other prepared site.

Removal of complete cerebrospinal fluid shunt system

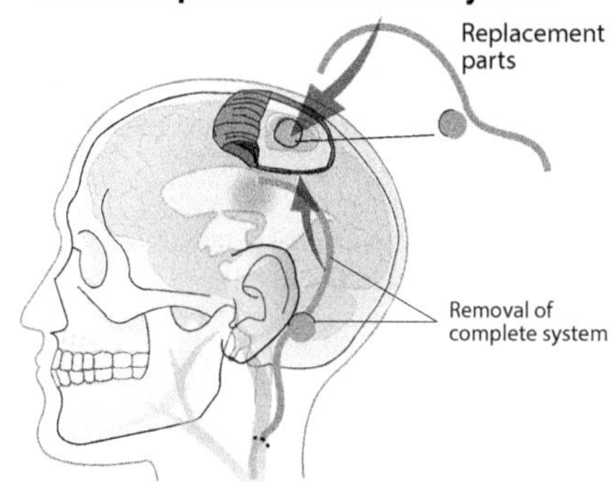

Without replacement (62256); with replacement by similar or other shunt at same operation (62258)

ICD-10-CM Diagnostic Codes

A17.0	Tuberculous meningitis
A39.0	Meningococcal meningitis
A42.81	Actinomycotic meningitis
A87.0	Enteroviral meningitis
A87.1	Adenoviral meningitis
A87.8	Other viral meningitis
B37.5	Candidal meningitis
C70.0	Malignant neoplasm of cerebral meninges
C71.5	Malignant neoplasm of cerebral ventricle
C71.6	Malignant neoplasm of cerebellum
C71.7	Malignant neoplasm of brain stem
C79.31	Secondary malignant neoplasm of brain
C79.32	Secondary malignant neoplasm of cerebral meninges
D32.9	Benign neoplasm of meninges, unspecified
D33.0	Benign neoplasm of brain, supratentorial
D33.1	Benign neoplasm of brain, infratentorial
D43.0	Neoplasm of uncertain behavior of brain, supratentorial
D43.1	Neoplasm of uncertain behavior of brain, infratentorial
G00.0	Hemophilus meningitis
G00.1	Pneumococcal meningitis
G00.2	Streptococcal meningitis
G00.3	Staphylococcal meningitis
G00.8	Other bacterial meningitis
G00.9	Bacterial meningitis, unspecified
G03.0	Nonpyogenic meningitis
G03.1	Chronic meningitis
G03.2	Benign recurrent meningitis [Mollaret]
G03.8	Meningitis due to other specified causes
G03.9	Meningitis, unspecified
G91.0	Communicating hydrocephalus
G91.1	Obstructive hydrocephalus
G91.2	(Idiopathic) normal pressure hydrocephalus
G91.3	Post-traumatic hydrocephalus, unspecified
G91.4	Hydrocephalus in diseases classified elsewhere
G91.8	Other hydrocephalus
G91.9	Hydrocephalus, unspecified
G93.0	Cerebral cysts
I61.5	Nontraumatic intracerebral hemorrhage, intraventricular
P37.1	Congenital toxoplasmosis
Q03.0	Malformations of aqueduct of Sylvius
Q03.1	Atresia of foramina of Magendie and Luschka
Q03.8	Other congenital hydrocephalus
Q03.9	Congenital hydrocephalus, unspecified
Q05.0	Cervical spina bifida with hydrocephalus
Q05.1	Thoracic spina bifida with hydrocephalus
Q05.2	Lumbar spina bifida with hydrocephalus
Q05.3	Sacral spina bifida with hydrocephalus
Q05.4	Unspecified spina bifida with hydrocephalus
Q07.0	Arnold-Chiari syndrome
Q07.02	Arnold-Chiari syndrome with hydrocephalus
Q07.03	Arnold-Chiari syndrome with spina bifida and hydrocephalus
⑦ T85.01	Breakdown (mechanical) of ventricular intracranial (communicating) shunt
⑦ T85.02	Displacement of ventricular intracranial (communicating) shunt
⑦ T85.03	Leakage of ventricular intracranial (communicating) shunt
⑦ T85.09	Other mechanical complication of ventricular intracranial (communicating) shunt

❼	T85.730	Infection and inflammatory reaction due to ventricular intracranial (communicating) shunt
❼	T85.810	Embolism due to nervous system prosthetic devices, implants and grafts
❼	T85.820	Fibrosis due to nervous system prosthetic devices, implants and grafts
❼	T85.830	Hemorrhage due to nervous system prosthetic devices, implants and grafts
❼	T85.840	Pain due to nervous system prosthetic devices, implants and grafts
❼	T85.850	Stenosis due to nervous system prosthetic devices, implants and grafts
❼	T85.860	Thrombosis due to nervous system prosthetic devices, implants and grafts
❼	T85.890	Other specified complication of nervous system prosthetic devices, implants and grafts
❼	T85.9	Unspecified complication of internal prosthetic device, implant and graft
	Z45.41	Encounter for adjustment and management of cerebrospinal fluid drainage device

ICD-10-CM Coding Notes

For codes requiring a 7th character extension, refer to your ICD-10-CM book. Review the character descriptions and coding guidelines for proper selection. For some procedures, only certain characters will apply.

CCI Edits

Refer to Appendix A for CCI edits.

Facility RVUs ▯

Code	Work	PE Facility	MP	Total Facility
62256	7.38	7.29	2.70	17.37
62258	15.64	11.01	5.39	32.04

Non-facility RVUs ▯

Code	Work	PE Non-Facility	MP	Total Non-Facility
62256	7.38	7.29	2.70	17.37
62258	15.64	11.01	5.39	32.04

Modifiers (PAR) ▯

Code	Mod 50	Mod 51	Mod 62	Mod 66	Mod 80
62256	0	2	0	0	2
62258	0	2	1	0	2

Global Period

Code	Days
62256	090
62258	090

62263-62264

62263 Percutaneous lysis of epidural adhesions using solution injection (eg, hypertonic saline, enzyme) or mechanical means (eg, catheter) including radiologic localization (includes contrast when administered), multiple adhesiolysis sessions; 2 or more days

(62263 includes codes 72275 and 77003)

62264 Percutaneous lysis of epidural adhesions using solution injection (eg, hypertonic saline, enzyme) or mechanical means (eg, catheter) including radiologic localization (includes contrast when administered), multiple adhesiolysis sessions; 1 day

(Do not report 62264 with 62263)

(62264 includes codes 72275 and 77003)

AMA Coding Guideline

Injection, Drainage, or Aspiration Procedures on the Spine and Spinal Cord

Injection of contrast during fluoroscopic guidance and localization is an inclusive component of 62263, 62264, 62267, 62273, 62280, 62281, 62282, 62302, 62303, 62304, 62305, 62321, 62323, 62325, 62327, 62328, 62329. Fluoroscopic guidance and localization is reported with 77003, unless a formal contrast study (myelography, epidurography, or arthrography) is performed, in which case the use of fluoroscopy is included in the supervision and interpretation codes or the myelography via lumbar injection code. Image guidance and the injection of contrast are inclusive components and are required for the performance of myelography, as described by codes 62302, 62303, 62304, 62305.

For radiologic supervision and interpretation of epidurography, use 72275. Code 72275 is only to be used when an epidurogram is performed, images documented, and a formal radiologic report is issued.

Code 62263 describes a catheter-based treatment involving targeted injection of various substances (eg, hypertonic saline, steroid, anesthetic) via an indwelling epidural catheter. Code 62263 includes percutaneous insertion and removal of an epidural catheter (remaining in place over a several-day period), for the administration of multiple injections of a neurolytic agent(s) performed during serial treatment sessions (ie, spanning two or more treatment days). If required, adhesions or scarring may also be lysed by mechanical means. Code 62263 is not reported for each adhesiolysis treatment, but should be reported once to describe the entire series of injections/infusions spanning two or more treatment days.

Code 62264 describes multiple adhesiolysis treatment sessions performed on the same day. Adhesions or scarring may be lysed by injections of neurolytic agent(s). If required, adhesions or scarring may also be lysed mechanically using a percutaneously-deployed catheter.

Codes 62263 and 62264 include the procedure of injections of contrast for epidurography (72275) and fluoroscopic guidance and localization (77003) during initial or subsequent sessions.

Fluoroscopy or CT and any injection of contrast are inclusive components of 62321, 62323, 62325, 62327. For epidurography, use 72275.

The placement and use of a catheter to administer one or more epidural or subarachnoid injections on a single calendar day should be reported in the same manner as if a needle had been used, ie, as a single injection using either 62320, 62321, 62322, or 62323. Such injections should not be reported with 62324, 62325, 62326, or 62327.

Threading a catheter into the epidural space, injecting substances at one or more levels and then removing the catheter should be treated as a single injection (62320, 62321, 62322, 62323). If the catheter is left in place to deliver substance(s) over a prolonged period (ie, more than a single calendar day) either continuously or via intermittent bolus, use 62324, 62325, 62326, 62327 as appropriate.

When reporting 62320, 62321, 62322, 62323, 62324, 62325, 62326, 62327 code choice is based on the region at which the needle or catheter entered the body (eg, lumbar). Codes 62320, 62321, 62322, 62323, 62324, 62325, 62326, 62327 should be reported only once, when the substance injected spreads or catheter tip insertion moves into another spinal region (eg, 62322 is reported only once for injection or catheter insertion at L3-4 with spread of the substance or placement of the catheter tip to the thoracic region).

Percutaneous spinal procedures are done with indirect visualization (eg, image guidance) (eg, 62287). Endoscopic assistance during an open procedure with continuous and direct visualization (light-based) is reported using excision codes (eg, 63020-63035).

Definitions

For purposes of CPT coding, the following definitions of approach and visualization apply. The primary approach and visualization define the service, whether another method is incidentally applied. Surgical services are presumed open, unless otherwise specified.

Percutaneous: Image-guided procedures (eg, computer tomography [CT] or fluoroscopy) performed with indirect visualization of the spine without the use of any device that allows visualization through a surgical incision.

Endoscopic: Spinal procedures performed with continuous direct visualization of the spine through an endoscope.

Open: Spinal procedures performed with continuous direct visualization of the spine through a surgical opening.

Indirect visualization: Image-guided (eg, CT or fluoroscopy), not light-based visualization.

Direct visualization: Light-based visualization; can be performed by eye, or with surgical loupes, microscope, or endoscope.

AMA Coding Notes

Injection, Drainage, or Aspiration Procedures on the Spine and Spinal Cord

(For transforaminal epidural injection, see 64479-64484)

(Report 01996 for daily hospital management of continuous epidural or subarachnoid drug administration performed in conjunction with 62324, 62325, 62326, 62327)

(For the techniques of microsurgery and/or use of microscope, use 69990)

Surgical Procedures on the Spine and Spinal Cord

(For application of caliper or tongs, use 20660)

(For treatment of fracture or dislocation of spine, see 22310-22327)

AMA *CPT Assistant* ▢

62263: Nov 99: 33, Dec 99: 11, Mar 02: 11, Dec 02: 10, Nov 05: 14, Jul 08: 9, Oct 09: 12, Nov 10: 3, Jan 11: 8, Jun 12: 12

62264: Nov 05: 14, Jul 08: 9, Oct 09: 12, Nov 10: 3, Jan 11: 8, Jun 12: 12

Plain English Description

One or more substances used to lyse adhesions are injected via an indwelling epidural catheter. The skin is cleansed over the planned injection site and a local anesthetic is administered. Using fluoroscopic or other radiological guidance as needed, a spinal needle is advanced into the epidural space or caudal vertebral space at the desired vertebral level. A catheter is advanced over the needle into the epidural space and the needle is withdrawn. The catheter is manipulated through the bands of scar tissue to the target spinal nerve or nerve root. Contrast is injected to confirm proper placement of the catheter and to evaluate nerve roots and spinal nerves in the area. Free flow of contrast within the epidural space is confirmed. The number of injections and the substances that will be used to lyse the adhesions are determined. Typically, hyaluronidase, a local anesthetic, and a steroid are injected followed by an injection of hypertonic saline 30 minutes later. The catheter is secured. The first injection or series of injections is administered. Before each injection or series of injections, contrast is again injected and the catheter position checked. The epidural space at the injection site is evaluated and the destruction of scar tissue and amount of opening of the epidural space around the target nerves or nerve roots are also noted prior to each injection. Use 62263 when a series of injections are administered over two or more days. Use 62264 when injections are administered over a single day.

Percutaneous lysis of epidural adhesions using solution injection

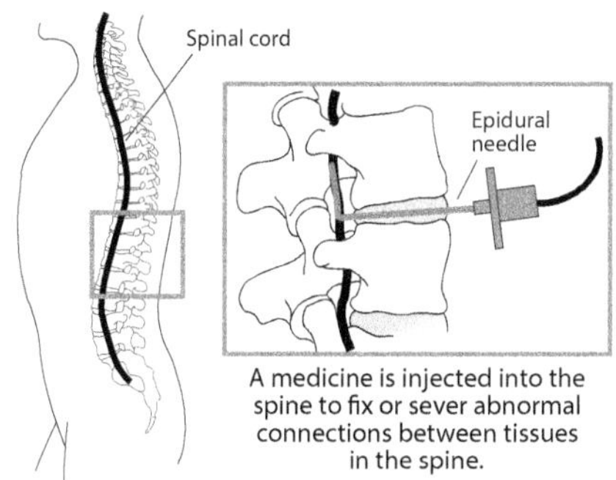

Multiple adhesiolysis sessions, (62263) 2 or more days; (62264) 1 day

ICD-10-CM Diagnostic Codes

G96.12	Meningeal adhesions (cerebral) (spinal)
Q07.8	Other specified congenital malformations of nervous system

CCI Edits

Refer to Appendix A for CCI edits.

Facility RVUs

Code	Work	PE Facility	MP	Total Facility
62263	5.00	3.43	0.47	8.90
62264	4.42	2.15	0.44	7.01

Non-facility RVUs

Code	Work	PE Non-Facility	MP	Total Non-Facility
62263	5.00	12.03	0.47	17.50
62264	4.42	7.67	0.44	12.53

Modifiers (PAR)

Code	Mod 50	Mod 51	Mod 62	Mod 66	Mod 80
62263	0	2	0	0	1
62264	0	2	0	0	1

Global Period

Code	Days
62263	010
62264	010

62267

62267 Percutaneous aspiration within the nucleus pulposus, intervertebral disc, or paravertebral tissue for diagnostic purposes

(For imaging, use 77003)

(Do not report 62267 in conjunction with 10005, 10006, 10007, 10008, 10009, 10010, 10011, 10012, 20225, 62287, 62290, 62291)

AMA Coding Guideline

Injection, Drainage, or Aspiration Procedures on the Spine and Spinal Cord

Injection of contrast during fluoroscopic guidance and localization is an inclusive component of 62263, 62264, 62267, 62273, 62280, 62281, 62282, 62302, 62303, 62304, 62305, 62321, 62323, 62325, 62327, 62328, 62329. Fluoroscopic guidance and localization is reported with 77003, unless a formal contrast study (myelography, epidurography, or arthrography) is performed, in which case the use of fluoroscopy is included in the supervision and interpretation codes or the myelography via lumbar injection code. Image guidance and the injection of contrast are inclusive components and are required for the performance of myelography, as described by codes 62302, 62303, 62304, 62305.

For radiologic supervision and interpretation of epidurography, use 72275. Code 72275 is only to be used when an epidurogram is performed, images documented, and a formal radiologic report is issued.

Code 62263 describes a catheter-based treatment involving targeted injection of various substances (eg, hypertonic saline, steroid, anesthetic) via an indwelling epidural catheter. Code 62263 includes percutaneous insertion and removal of an epidural catheter (remaining in place over a several-day period), for the administration of multiple injections of a neurolytic agent(s) performed during serial treatment sessions (ie, spanning two or more treatment days). If required, adhesions or scarring may also be lysed by mechanical means. Code 62263 is not reported for each adhesiolysis treatment, but should be reported once to describe the entire series of injections/infusions spanning two or more treatment days.

Code 62264 describes multiple adhesiolysis treatment sessions performed on the same day. Adhesions or scarring may be lysed by injections of neurolytic agent(s). If required, adhesions or scarring may also be lysed mechanically using a percutaneously-deployed catheter.

Codes 62263 and 62264 include the procedure of injections of contrast for epidurography (72275) and fluoroscopic guidance and localization (77003) during initial or subsequent sessions.

Fluoroscopy or CT and any injection of contrast are inclusive components of 62321, 62323, 62325, 62327. For epidurography, use 72275.

The placement and use of a catheter to administer one or more epidural or subarachnoid injections on a single calendar day should be reported in the same manner as if a needle had been used, ie, as a single injection using either 62320, 62321, 62322, or 62323. Such injections should not be reported with 62324, 62325, 62326, or 62327.

Threading a catheter into the epidural space, injecting substances at one or more levels and then removing the catheter should be treated as a single injection (62320, 62321, 62322, 62323). If the catheter is left in place to deliver substance(s) over a prolonged period (ie, more than a single calendar day) either continuously or via intermittent bolus, use 62324, 62325, 62326, 62327 as appropriate.

When reporting 62320, 62321, 62322, 62323, 62324, 62325, 62326, 62327 code choice is based on the region at which the needle or catheter entered the body (eg, lumbar). Codes 62320, 62321, 62322, 62323, 62324, 62325, 62326, 62327 should be reported only once, when the substance injected spreads or catheter tip insertion moves into another spinal region (eg, 62322 is reported only once for injection or catheter insertion at L3-4 with spread of the substance or placement of the catheter tip to the thoracic region).

Percutaneous spinal procedures are done with indirect visualization (eg, image guidance) (eg, 62287). Endoscopic assistance during an open procedure with continuous and direct visualization (light-based) is reported using excision codes (eg, 63020-63035).

Definitions

For purposes of CPT coding, the following definitions of approach and visualization apply. The primary approach and visualization define the service, whether another method is incidentally applied. Surgical services are presumed open, unless otherwise specified.

Percutaneous: Image-guided procedures (eg, computer tomography [CT] or fluoroscopy) performed with indirect visualization of the spine without the use of any device that allows visualization through a surgical incision.

Endoscopic: Spinal procedures performed with continuous direct visualization of the spine through an endoscope.

Open: Spinal procedures performed with continuous direct visualization of the spine through a surgical opening.

Indirect visualization: Image-guided (eg, CT or fluoroscopy), not light-based visualization.

Direct visualization: Light-based visualization; can be performed by eye, or with surgical loupes, microscope, or endoscope.

AMA Coding Notes

Injection, Drainage, or Aspiration Procedures on the Spine and Spinal Cord

(For transforaminal epidural injection, see 64479-64484)

(Report 01996 for daily hospital management of continuous epidural or subarachnoid drug administration performed in conjunction with 62324, 62325, 62326, 62327)

(For the techniques of microsurgery and/or use of microscope, use 69990)

Surgical Procedures on the Spine and Spinal Cord

(For application of caliper or tongs, use 20660)

(For treatment of fracture or dislocation of spine, see 22310-22327)

AMA *CPT Assistant*

62267: Nov 10: 3, Jan 11: 8, Jul 12: 3

Plain English Description

The physician performs a diagnostic percutaneous aspiration within the nucleus pulposus, intervertebral disc, or paravertebral tissue. Fluid is aspirated or cells are harvested to evaluate infectious discitis, spinal or paraverteral fluid accumulations, or other conditions. The skin is cleansed and a local anesthetic is administered at the planned puncture site. The needle is then inserted into the disc or paraspinal tissue using separately reportable image guidance. Fluid and/or tissue are aspirated. The needle is moved as needed and additional fluid or tissue samples are aspirated. The needle is removed and the fluid or tissue is sent for laboratory analysis.

Percutaneous aspiration within the nucleus pulposus, intervertebral disc, or paravertebral tissue for diagnostic purposes

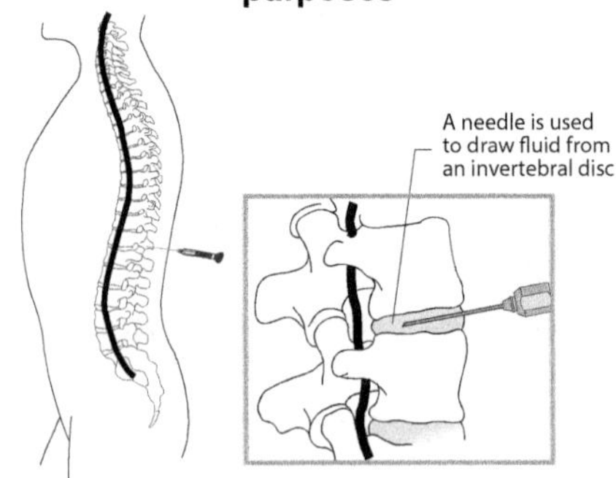

ICD-10-CM Diagnostic Codes

C41.2	Malignant neoplasm of vertebral column
C79.51	Secondary malignant neoplasm of bone
D16.6	Benign neoplasm of vertebral column
D48.0	Neoplasm of uncertain behavior of bone and articular cartilage
M46.20	Osteomyelitis of vertebra, site unspecified

M46.22	Osteomyelitis of vertebra, cervical region
M46.23	Osteomyelitis of vertebra, cervicothoracic region
M46.24	Osteomyelitis of vertebra, thoracic region
M46.25	Osteomyelitis of vertebra, thoracolumbar region
M46.26	Osteomyelitis of vertebra, lumbar region
M46.27	Osteomyelitis of vertebra, lumbosacral region
M46.28	Osteomyelitis of vertebra, sacral and sacrococcygeal region
M46.30	Infection of intervertebral disc (pyogenic), site unspecified
M46.31	Infection of intervertebral disc (pyogenic), occipito-atlanto-axial region
M46.32	Infection of intervertebral disc (pyogenic), cervical region
M46.33	Infection of intervertebral disc (pyogenic), cervicothoracic region
M46.34	Infection of intervertebral disc (pyogenic), thoracic region
M46.35	Infection of intervertebral disc (pyogenic), thoracolumbar region
M46.36	Infection of intervertebral disc (pyogenic), lumbar region
M46.37	Infection of intervertebral disc (pyogenic), lumbosacral region
M46.38	Infection of intervertebral disc (pyogenic), sacral and sacrococcygeal region
M46.41	Discitis, unspecified, occipito-atlanto-axial region
M46.42	Discitis, unspecified, cervical region
M46.43	Discitis, unspecified, cervicothoracic region
M46.44	Discitis, unspecified, thoracic region
M46.45	Discitis, unspecified, thoracolumbar region
M46.46	Discitis, unspecified, lumbar region
M46.47	Discitis, unspecified, lumbosacral region
M46.48	Discitis, unspecified, sacral and sacrococcygeal region
M50.31	Other cervical disc degeneration, high cervical region
M50.321	Other cervical disc degeneration at C4-C5 level
M50.322	Other cervical disc degeneration at C5-C6 level
M50.323	Other cervical disc degeneration at C6-C7 level
M50.33	Other cervical disc degeneration, cervicothoracic region
M51.34	Other intervertebral disc degeneration, thoracic region
M51.35	Other intervertebral disc degeneration, thoracolumbar region
M51.36	Other intervertebral disc degeneration, lumbar region
M51.37	Other intervertebral disc degeneration, lumbosacral region
M88.1	Osteitis deformans of vertebrae
M90.6	Osteitis deformans in neoplastic diseases

CCI Edits

Refer to Appendix A for CCI edits.

Facility RVUs ▯

Code	Work	PE Facility	MP	Total Facility
62267	3.00	1.27	0.27	4.54

Non-facility RVUs ▯

Code	Work	PE Non-Facility	MP	Total Non-Facility
62267	3.00	4.33	0.27	7.60

Modifiers (PAR) ▯

Code	Mod 50	Mod 51	Mod 62	Mod 66	Mod 80
62267	0	2	0	0	0

Global Period

Code	Days
62267	000

CPT® Procedural Coding

62270-62272

▲ **62270 Spinal puncture, lumbar, diagnostic**

▲ **62272 Spinal puncture, therapeutic, for drainage of cerebrospinal fluid (by needle or catheter)**

AMA Coding Guideline

Injection, Drainage, or Aspiration Procedures on the Spine and Spinal Cord

Injection of contrast during fluoroscopic guidance and localization is an inclusive component of 62263, 62264, 62267, 62273, 62280, 62281, 62282, 62302, 62303, 62304, 62305, 62321, 62323, 62325, 62327, 62328, 62329. Fluoroscopic guidance and localization is reported with 77003, unless a formal contrast study (myelography, epidurography, or arthrography) is performed, in which case the use of fluoroscopy is included in the supervision and interpretation codes or the myelography via lumbar injection code. Image guidance and the injection of contrast are inclusive components and are required for the performance of myelography, as described by codes 62302, 62303, 62304, 62305.

For radiologic supervision and interpretation of epidurography, use 72275. Code 72275 is only to be used when an epidurogram is performed, images documented, and a formal radiologic report is issued.

Code 62263 describes a catheter-based treatment involving targeted injection of various substances (eg, hypertonic saline, steroid, anesthetic) via an indwelling epidural catheter. Code 62263 includes percutaneous insertion and removal of an epidural catheter (remaining in place over a several-day period), for the administration of multiple injections of a neurolytic agent(s) performed during serial treatment sessions (ie, spanning two or more treatment days). If required, adhesions or scarring may also be lysed by mechanical means. Code 62263 is not reported for each adhesiolysis treatment, but should be reported once to describe the entire series of injections/infusions spanning two or more treatment days.

Code 62264 describes multiple adhesiolysis treatment sessions performed on the same day. Adhesions or scarring may be lysed by injections of neurolytic agent(s). If required, adhesions or scarring may also be lysed mechanically using a percutaneously-deployed catheter.

Codes 62263 and 62264 include the procedure of injections of contrast for epidurography (72275) and fluoroscopic guidance and localization (77003) during initial or subsequent sessions.

Fluoroscopy or CT and any injection of contrast are inclusive components of 62321, 62323, 62325, 62327. For epidurography, use 72275.

The placement and use of a catheter to administer one or more epidural or subarachnoid injections on a single calendar day should be reported in the same manner as if a needle had been used, ie, as a single injection using either 62320, 62321, 62322, or 62323. Such injections should not be reported with 62324, 62325, 62326, or 62327.

Threading a catheter into the epidural space, injecting substances at one or more levels and then removing the catheter should be treated as a single injection (62320, 62321, 62322, 62323). If the catheter is left in place to deliver substance(s) over a prolonged period (ie, more than a single calendar day) either continuously or via intermittent bolus, use 62324, 62325, 62326, 62327 as appropriate.

When reporting 62320, 62321, 62322, 62323, 62324, 62325, 62326, 62327 code choice is based on the region at which the needle or catheter entered the body (eg, lumbar). Codes 62320, 62321, 62322, 62323, 62324, 62325, 62326, 62327 should be reported only once, when the substance injected spreads or catheter tip insertion moves into another spinal region (eg, 62322 is reported only once for injection or catheter insertion at L3-4 with spread of the substance or placement of the catheter tip to the thoracic region).

Percutaneous spinal procedures are done with indirect visualization (eg, image guidance) (eg, 62287). Endoscopic assistance during an open procedure with continuous and direct visualization (light-based) is reported using excision codes (eg, 63020-63035).

Definitions

For purposes of CPT coding, the following definitions of approach and visualization apply. The primary approach and visualization define the service, whether another method is incidentally applied. Surgical services are presumed open, unless otherwise specified.

Percutaneous: Image-guided procedures (eg, computer tomography [CT] or fluoroscopy) performed with indirect visualization of the spine without the use of any device that allows visualization through a surgical incision.

Endoscopic: Spinal procedures performed with continuous direct visualization of the spine through an endoscope.

Open: Spinal procedures performed with continuous direct visualization of the spine through a surgical opening.

Indirect visualization: Image-guided (eg, CT or fluoroscopy), not light-based visualization.

Direct visualization: Light-based visualization; can be performed by eye, or with surgical loupes, microscope, or endoscope.

AMA Coding Notes

Injection, Drainage, or Aspiration Procedures on the Spine and Spinal Cord

(For transforaminal epidural injection, see 64479-64484)

(Report 01996 for daily hospital management of continuous epidural or subarachnoid drug administration performed in conjunction with 62324, 62325, 62326, 62327)

(For the techniques of microsurgery and/or use of microscope, use 69990)

Surgical Procedures on the Spine and Spinal Cord

(For application of caliper or tongs, use 20660)

(For treatment of fracture or dislocation of spine, see 22310-22327)

AMA *CPT Assistant* ▢

62270: Nov 99: 32, 33, Oct 03: 2, Jul 06: 4, Jul 07: 1, Oct 09: 12, Nov 10: 3, Jan 11: 8, Mar 12: 3

62272: Nov 99: 32, 33, Nov 10: 3, Dec 13: 14

Plain English Description

A lumbar spinal puncture is performed for diagnostic or therapeutic purposes. In 62270, a diagnostic lumbar puncture is performed for symptoms that may be indicative of an infection, such as meningitis; a malignant neoplasm; bleeding, such as subarachnoid hemorrhage; multiple sclerosis; or Guillain-Barre syndrome. Diagnostic lumbar puncture may also be performed to measure cerebrospinal fluid (CSF) pressure. The skin over the lumbar spine is disinfected and a local anesthetic is administered. A lumbar puncture needle is then inserted into the spinal canal and CSF specimens are collected. The CSF specimens are sent to the laboratory for separately reportable evaluation. In 62272, a therapeutic spinal puncture is performed for elevated CSF pressure and CSF is drained using a needle or catheter placed as described above. CSF pressure is monitored during the drainage procedure, and when the desired pressure is reached, the needle or catheter is removed.

Spinal puncture

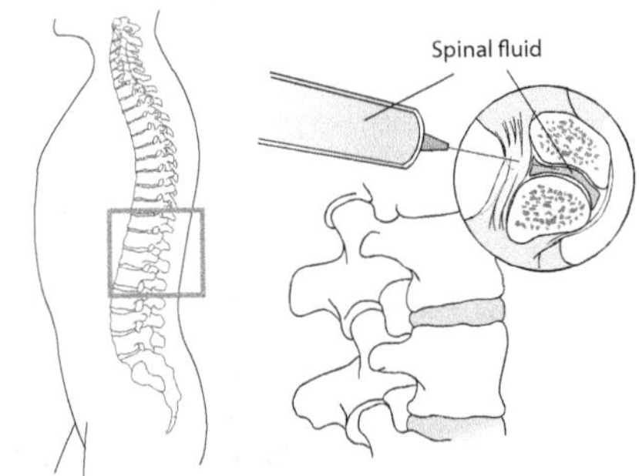

Cerebrospinal fluid is removed for diagnostic (62270) or therapeutic (62272) purposes.

ICD-10-CM Diagnostic Codes

A17.0	Tuberculous meningitis
A17.82	Tuberculous meningoencephalitis
A32.11	Listerial meningitis
A32.12	Listerial meningoencephalitis
A39.0	Meningococcal meningitis
A39.81	Meningococcal encephalitis
A42.81	Actinomycotic meningitis
A42.82	Actinomycotic encephalitis
A50.41	Late congenital syphilitic meningitis
A50.42	Late congenital syphilitic encephalitis
A52.13	Late syphilitic meningitis

A52.14	Late syphilitic encephalitis
A69.21	Meningitis due to Lyme disease
A69.22	Other neurologic disorders in Lyme disease
A83.3	St Louis encephalitis
A83.5	California encephalitis
A85.0	Enteroviral encephalitis
A85.1	Adenoviral encephalitis
A85.8	Other specified viral encephalitis
A87.0	Enteroviral meningitis
A87.1	Adenoviral meningitis
A87.2	Lymphocytic choriomeningitis
A87.8	Other viral meningitis
A87.9	Viral meningitis, unspecified
A92.31	West Nile virus infection with encephalitis
B00.3	Herpesviral meningitis
B00.4	Herpesviral encephalitis
B01.0	Varicella meningitis
B01.11	Varicella encephalitis and encephalomyelitis
B02.0	Zoster encephalitis
B02.1	Zoster meningitis
B10.01	Human herpesvirus 6 encephalitis
B10.09	Other human herpesvirus encephalitis
B38.4	Coccidioidomycosis meningitis
B40.81	Blastomycotic meningoencephalitis
C70.0	Malignant neoplasm of cerebral meninges
C70.1	Malignant neoplasm of spinal meninges
G00.0	Hemophilus meningitis
G00.1	Pneumococcal meningitis
G00.2	Streptococcal meningitis
G00.3	Staphylococcal meningitis
G00.8	Other bacterial meningitis
G00.9	Bacterial meningitis, unspecified
G01	Meningitis in bacterial diseases classified elsewhere
G02	Meningitis in other infectious and parasitic diseases classified elsewhere
G37.8	Other specified demyelinating diseases of central nervous system
G44.52	New daily persistent headache (NDPH)
G61.0	Guillain-Barre syndrome
G61.81	Chronic inflammatory demyelinating polyneuritis
G93.2	Benign intracranial hypertension
I60.8	Other nontraumatic subarachnoid hemorrhage
I60.9	Nontraumatic subarachnoid hemorrhage, unspecified
P10.3	Subarachnoid hemorrhage due to birth injury
P52.5	Subarachnoid (nontraumatic) hemorrhage of newborn
R51	Headache

CCI Edits

Refer to Appendix A for CCI edits.

Facility RVUs

Code	Work	PE Facility	MP	Total Facility
62270	1.22	0.41	0.16	1.79
62272	1.58	0.64	0.32	2.54

Non-facility RVUs

Code	Work	PE Non-Facility	MP	Total Non-Facility
62270	1.22	2.59	0.16	3.97
62272	1.58	3.32	0.32	5.22

Modifiers (PAR)

Code	Mod 50	Mod 51	Mod 62	Mod 66	Mod 80
62270	0	2	0	0	1
62272	0	2	0	0	1

Global Period

Code	Days
62270	000
62272	000

62273

62273 Injection, epidural, of blood or clot patch

(For injection of diagnostic or therapeutic substance[s], see 62320, 62321, 62322, 62323, 62324, 62325, 62326, 62327)

AMA Coding Guideline

Injection, Drainage, or Aspiration Procedures on the Spine and Spinal Cord

Injection of contrast during fluoroscopic guidance and localization is an inclusive component of 62263, 62264, 62267, 62273, 62280, 62281, 62282, 62302, 62303, 62304, 62305, 62321, 62323, 62325, 62327, 62328, 62329. Fluoroscopic guidance and localization is reported with 77003, unless a formal contrast study (myelography, epidurography, or arthrography) is performed, in which case the use of fluoroscopy is included in the supervision and interpretation codes or the myelography via lumbar injection code. Image guidance and the injection of contrast are inclusive components and are required for the performance of myelography, as described by codes 62302, 62303, 62304, 62305.

For radiologic supervision and interpretation of epidurography, use 72275. Code 72275 is only to be used when an epidurogram is performed, images documented, and a formal radiologic report is issued.

Code 62263 describes a catheter-based treatment involving targeted injection of various substances (eg, hypertonic saline, steroid, anesthetic) via an indwelling epidural catheter. Code 62263 includes percutaneous insertion and removal of an epidural catheter (remaining in place over a several-day period), for the administration of multiple injections of a neurolytic agent(s) performed during serial treatment sessions (ie, spanning two or more treatment days). If required, adhesions or scarring may also be lysed by mechanical means. Code 62263 is not reported for each adhesiolysis treatment, but should be reported once to describe the entire series of injections/infusions spanning two or more treatment days.

Code 62264 describes multiple adhesiolysis treatment sessions performed on the same day. Adhesions or scarring may be lysed by injections of neurolytic agent(s). If required, adhesions or scarring may also be lysed mechanically using a percutaneously-deployed catheter.

Codes 62263 and 62264 include the procedure of injections of contrast for epidurography (72275) and fluoroscopic guidance and localization (77003) during initial or subsequent sessions.

Fluoroscopy or CT and any injection of contrast are inclusive components of 62321, 62323, 62325, 62327. For epidurography, use 72275.

The placement and use of a catheter to administer one or more epidural or subarachnoid injections on a single calendar day should be reported in the same manner as if a needle had been used, ie, as a single injection using either 62320, 62321, 62322, or 62323. Such injections should not be reported with 62324, 62325, 62326, or 62327.

Threading a catheter into the epidural space, injecting substances at one or more levels and then removing the catheter should be treated as a single injection (62320, 62321, 62322, 62323). If the catheter is left in place to deliver substance(s) over a prolonged period (ie, more than a single calendar day) either continuously or via intermittent bolus, use 62324, 62325, 62326, 62327 as appropriate.

When reporting 62320, 62321, 62322, 62323, 62324, 62325, 62326, 62327 code choice is based on the region at which the needle or catheter entered the body (eg, lumbar). Codes 62320, 62321, 62322, 62323, 62324, 62325, 62326, 62327 should be reported only once, when the substance injected spreads or catheter tip insertion moves into another spinal region (eg, 62322 is reported only once for injection or catheter insertion at L3-4 with spread of the substance or placement of the catheter tip to the thoracic region).

Percutaneous spinal procedures are done with indirect visualization (eg, image guidance) (eg, 62287). Endoscopic assistance during an open procedure with continuous and direct visualization (light-based) is reported using excision codes (eg, 63020-63035).

Definitions

For purposes of CPT coding, the following definitions of approach and visualization apply. The primary approach and visualization define the service, whether another method is incidentally applied. Surgical services are presumed open, unless otherwise specified.

Percutaneous: Image-guided procedures (eg, computer tomography [CT] or fluoroscopy) performed with indirect visualization of the spine without the use of any device that allows visualization through a surgical incision.

Endoscopic: Spinal procedures performed with continuous direct visualization of the spine through an endoscope.

Open: Spinal procedures performed with continuous direct visualization of the spine through a surgical opening.

Indirect visualization: Image-guided (eg, CT or fluoroscopy), not light-based visualization.

Direct visualization: Light-based visualization; can be performed by eye, or with surgical loupes, microscope, or endoscope.

AMA Coding Notes

Injection, Drainage, or Aspiration Procedures on the Spine and Spinal Cord

(For transforaminal epidural injection, see 64479-64484)

(Report 01996 for daily hospital management of continuous epidural or subarachnoid drug administration performed in conjunction with 62324, 62325, 62326, 62327)

(For the techniques of microsurgery and/or use of microscope, use 69990)

Surgical Procedures on the Spine and Spinal Cord

(For application of caliper or tongs, use 20660)

(For treatment of fracture or dislocation of spine, see 22310-22327)

AMA *CPT Assistant*

62273: Nov 99: 32, 34, Oct 09: 12, Nov 10: 3

Plain English Description

The physician injects a blood or clot patch into the epidural space. Epidural blood patches are used to treat the complication of severe headache caused by a leak of spinal fluid into the epidural space following epidural anesthesia or diagnostic or therapeutic spinal punctures. The skin over the lower back is disinfected and local anesthetic injected. A separate site is prepared for a venipuncture and an intravenous catheter is placed in the vein. The epidural needle is placed in the epidural space near the site of the previous puncture site. Blood is withdrawn from the venous catheter and the blood is then injected into the epidural space. The patient rests for approximately 30 minutes while the blood forms a patch over the cerebrospinal (CSF) leak.

Blood or clot patch injection

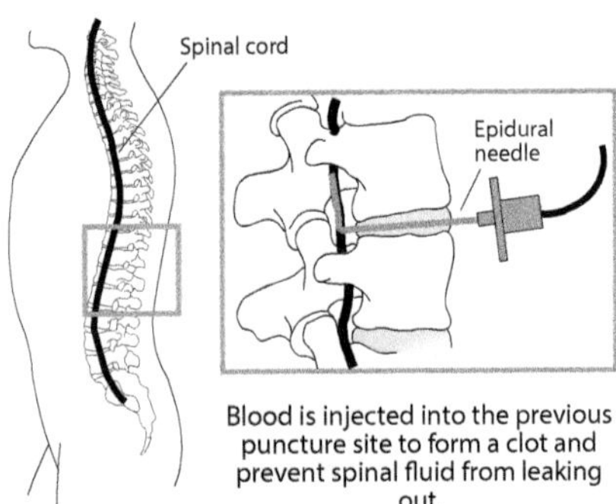

ICD-10-CM Diagnostic Codes

G97.0	Cerebrospinal fluid leak from spinal puncture
G97.1	Other reaction to spinal and lumbar puncture

CCI Edits

Refer to Appendix A for CCI edits.

Facility RVUs □

Code	Work	PE Facility	MP	Total Facility
62273	2.15	0.92	0.19	3.26

Non-facility RVUs □

Code	Work	PE Non-Facility	MP	Total Non-Facility
62273	2.15	2.56	0.19	4.90

Modifiers (PAR) □

Code	Mod 50	Mod 51	Mod 62	Mod 66	Mod 80
62273	0	2	0	0	1

Global Period

Code	Days
62273	000

62280-62282

62280 Injection/infusion of neurolytic substance (eg, alcohol, phenol, iced saline solutions), with or without other therapeutic substance; subarachnoid

62281 Injection/infusion of neurolytic substance (eg, alcohol, phenol, iced saline solutions), with or without other therapeutic substance; epidural, cervical or thoracic

62282 Injection/infusion of neurolytic substance (eg, alcohol, phenol, iced saline solutions), with or without other therapeutic substance; epidural, lumbar, sacral (caudal)

AMA Coding Guideline

Injection, Drainage, or Aspiration Procedures on the Spine and Spinal Cord

Injection of contrast during fluoroscopic guidance and localization is an inclusive component of 62263, 62264, 62267, 62273, 62280, 62281, 62282, 62302, 62303, 62304, 62305, 62321, 62323, 62325, 62327, 62328, 62329. Fluoroscopic guidance and localization is reported with 77003, unless a formal contrast study (myelography, epidurography, or arthrography) is performed, in which case the use of fluoroscopy is included in the supervision and interpretation codes or the myelography via lumbar injection code. Image guidance and the injection of contrast are inclusive components and are required for the performance of myelography, as described by codes 62302, 62303, 62304, 62305.

For radiologic supervision and interpretation of epidurography, use 72275. Code 72275 is only to be used when an epidurogram is performed, images documented, and a formal radiologic report is issued.

Code 62263 describes a catheter-based treatment involving targeted injection of various substances (eg, hypertonic saline, steroid, anesthetic) via an indwelling epidural catheter. Code 62263 includes percutaneous insertion and removal of an epidural catheter (remaining in place over a several-day period), for the administration of multiple injections of a neurolytic agent(s) performed during serial treatment sessions (ie, spanning two or more treatment days). If required, adhesions or scarring may also be lysed by mechanical means. Code 62263 is not reported for each adhesiolysis treatment, but should be reported once to describe the entire series of injections/infusions spanning two or more treatment days.

Code 62264 describes multiple adhesiolysis treatment sessions performed on the same day. Adhesions or scarring may be lysed by injections of neurolytic agent(s). If required, adhesions or scarring may also be lysed mechanically using a percutaneously-deployed catheter.

Codes 62263 and 62264 include the procedure of injections of contrast for epidurography (72275) and fluoroscopic guidance and localization (77003) during initial or subsequent sessions.

Fluoroscopy or CT and any injection of contrast are inclusive components of 62321, 62323, 62325, 62327. For epidurography, use 72275.

The placement and use of a catheter to administer one or more epidural or subarachnoid injections on a single calendar day should be reported in the same manner as if a needle had been used, ie, as a single injection using either 62320, 62321, 62322, or 62323. Such injections should not be reported with 62324, 62325, 62326, or 62327.

Threading a catheter into the epidural space, injecting substances at one or more levels and then removing the catheter should be treated as a single injection (62320, 62321, 62322, 62323). If the catheter is left in place to deliver substance(s) over a prolonged period (ie, more than a single calendar day) either continuously or via intermittent bolus, use 62324, 62325, 62326, 62327 as appropriate.

When reporting 62320, 62321, 62322, 62323, 62324, 62325, 62326, 62327 code choice is based on the region at which the needle or catheter entered the body (eg, lumbar). Codes 62320, 62321, 62322, 62323, 62324, 62325, 62326, 62327 should be reported only once, when the substance injected spreads or catheter tip insertion moves into another spinal region (eg, 62322 is reported only once for injection or catheter insertion at L3-4 with spread of the substance or placement of the catheter tip to the thoracic region).

Percutaneous spinal procedures are done with indirect visualization (eg, image guidance) (eg, 62287). Endoscopic assistance during an open procedure with continuous and direct visualization (light-based) is reported using excision codes (eg, 63020-63035).

Definitions

For purposes of CPT coding, the following definitions of approach and visualization apply. The primary approach and visualization define the service, whether another method is incidentally applied. Surgical services are presumed open, unless otherwise specified.

Percutaneous: Image-guided procedures (eg, computer tomography [CT] or fluoroscopy) performed with indirect visualization of the spine without the use of any device that allows visualization through a surgical incision.

Endoscopic: Spinal procedures performed with continuous direct visualization of the spine through an endoscope.

Open: Spinal procedures performed with continuous direct visualization of the spine through a surgical opening.

Indirect visualization: Image-guided (eg, CT or fluoroscopy), not light-based visualization.

Direct visualization: Light-based visualization; can be performed by eye, or with surgical loupes, microscope, or endoscope.

AMA Coding Notes

Injection, Drainage, or Aspiration Procedures on the Spine and Spinal Cord

(For transforaminal epidural injection, see 64479-64484)

(Report 01996 for daily hospital management of continuous epidural or subarachnoid drug administration performed in conjunction with 62324, 62325, 62326, 62327)

(For the techniques of microsurgery and/or use of microscope, use 69990)

Surgical Procedures on the Spine and Spinal Cord

(For application of caliper or tongs, use 20660)

(For treatment of fracture or dislocation of spine, see 22310-22327)

AMA *CPT Assistant* ☐

62280: Nov 99: 32, 34, Jan 00: 2, Jul 08: 9, Oct 09: 12, Feb 10: 11, Nov 10: 3, Jan 11: 8, Jun 12: 12

62281: Apr 96: 11, Nov 99: 32, 34, Jan 00: 2, Jul 08: 9, Oct 09: 12, Feb 10: 11, May 10: 10, Nov 10: 3, Jan 11: 8, Jun 12: 12

62282: Apr 96: 11, Nov 99: 32, 34, Jan 00: 2, Jul 08: 9, Oct 09: 12, Feb 10: 11, Nov 10: 3, Jan 11: 8, Jun 12: 12

Plain English Description

This procedure may also be referred to as a neurolytic block. Neurolytic substances such as alcohol, phenol, or iced saline destroy neural structures involved in pain perception and provide long-lasting pain relief. Types of conditions treated include chronic, intractable, non-terminal pain that is not responsive to other pain management modalities or cancer pain. Neurolytic blocks can be performed by injection or infusion of a neurolytic substance into the subarachnoid space, which lies between the arachnoid mater and pia mater, or into the epidural space, which lies between the bone and the outermost membrane covering the spinal cord or dura mater. The patient is positioned on an X-ray table with the back exposed. The site where the injection is to be performed is cleansed and a local anesthetic administered. Using separately reportable fluoroscopic guidance, a spinal needle or cannula is inserted into the subarachnoid or epidural space. A small amount of contrast is injected to ensure that the needle or cannula is properly positioned. The neurolytic substance is then injected or infused. Use 62280 for a subarachnoid injection or infusion at any level of the spine; use 62281 for an epidural injection or infusion in the cervical or thoracic region; and use 62282 for an epidural injection or infusion in the lumbar or sacral (caudal) region.

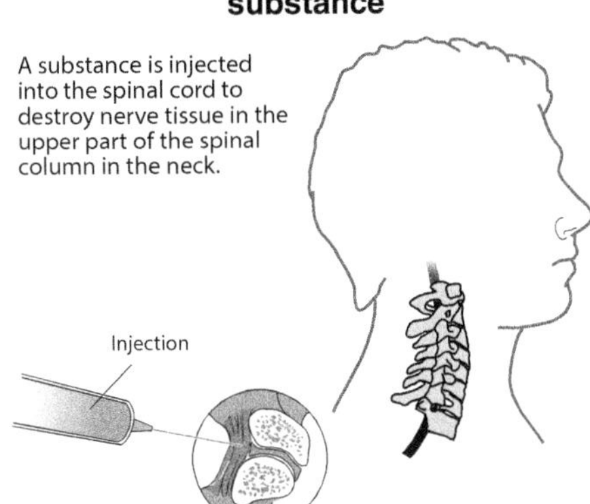

ICD-10-CM Diagnostic Codes

C76.0	Malignant neoplasm of head, face and neck
C76.1	Malignant neoplasm of thorax
C76.2	Malignant neoplasm of abdomen
C76.3	Malignant neoplasm of pelvis
C79.51	Secondary malignant neoplasm of bone
C79.89	Secondary malignant neoplasm of other specified sites
G89.11	Acute pain due to trauma
G89.12	Acute post-thoracotomy pain
G89.18	Other acute postprocedural pain
G89.21	Chronic pain due to trauma
G89.22	Chronic post-thoracotomy pain
G89.28	Other chronic postprocedural pain
G89.29	Other chronic pain
G89.3	Neoplasm related pain (acute) (chronic)
G89.4	Chronic pain syndrome
M54.11	Radiculopathy, occipito-atlanto-axial region
M54.12	Radiculopathy, cervical region
M54.13	Radiculopathy, cervicothoracic region
M54.14	Radiculopathy, thoracic region
M54.15	Radiculopathy, thoracolumbar region
M54.16	Radiculopathy, lumbar region
M54.17	Radiculopathy, lumbosacral region
M54.18	Radiculopathy, sacral and sacrococcygeal region
M54.2	Cervicalgia
⇄ M54.31	Sciatica, right side
⇄ M54.32	Sciatica, left side
⇄ M54.41	Lumbago with sciatica, right side
⇄ M54.42	Lumbago with sciatica, left side
M54.5	Low back pain
M54.6	Pain in thoracic spine
M54.81	Occipital neuralgia
M54.89	Other dorsalgia
M54.9	Dorsalgia, unspecified

CCI Edits

Refer to Appendix A for CCI edits.

Facility RVUs

Code	Work	PE Facility	MP	Total Facility
62280	2.63	1.75	0.52	4.90
62281	2.66	1.66	0.26	4.58
62282	2.33	1.58	0.22	4.13

Non-facility RVUs

Code	Work	PE Non-Facility	MP	Total Non-Facility
62280	2.63	6.97	0.52	10.12
62281	2.66	3.91	0.26	6.83
62282	2.33	6.21	0.22	8.76

Modifiers (PAR)

Code	Mod 50	Mod 51	Mod 62	Mod 66	Mod 80
62280	0	2	0	0	1
62281	0	2	0	0	1
62282	0	2	0	0	1

Global Period

Code	Days
62280	010
62281	010
62282	010

62284

62284 Injection procedure for myelography and/or computed tomography, lumbar

(Do not report 62284 in conjunction with 62302, 62303, 62304, 62305, 72240, 72255, 72265, 72270)

(When both 62284 and 72240, 72255, 72265, 72270 are performed by the same physician or other qualified health care professional for myelography, see 62302, 62303, 62304, 62305)

(For injection procedure at C1-C2, use 61055)

(For radiological supervision and interpretation, see Radiology)

AMA Coding Guideline

Injection, Drainage, or Aspiration Procedures on the Spine and Spinal Cord

Injection of contrast during fluoroscopic guidance and localization is an inclusive component of 62263, 62264, 62267, 62273, 62280, 62281, 62282, 62302, 62303, 62304, 62305, 62321, 62323, 62325, 62327, 62328, 62329. Fluoroscopic guidance and localization is reported with 77003, unless a formal contrast study (myelography, epidurography, or arthrography) is performed, in which case the use of fluoroscopy is included in the supervision and interpretation codes or the myelography via lumbar injection code. Image guidance and the injection of contrast are inclusive components and are required for the performance of myelography, as described by codes 62302, 62303, 62304, 62305.

For radiologic supervision and interpretation of epidurography, use 72275. Code 72275 is only to be used when an epidurogram is performed, images documented, and a formal radiologic report is issued.

Code 62263 describes a catheter-based treatment involving targeted injection of various substances (eg, hypertonic saline, steroid, anesthetic) via an indwelling epidural catheter. Code 62263 includes percutaneous insertion and removal of an epidural catheter (remaining in place over a several-day period), for the administration of multiple injections of a neurolytic agent(s) performed during serial treatment sessions (ie, spanning two or more treatment days). If required, adhesions or scarring may also be lysed by mechanical means. Code 62263 is not reported for each adhesiolysis treatment, but should be reported once to describe the entire series of injections/infusions spanning two or more treatment days.

Code 62264 describes multiple adhesiolysis treatment sessions performed on the same day. Adhesions or scarring may be lysed by injections of neurolytic agent(s). If required, adhesions or scarring may also be lysed mechanically using a percutaneously-deployed catheter.

Codes 62263 and 62264 include the procedure of injections of contrast for epidurography (72275) and fluoroscopic guidance and localization (77003) during initial or subsequent sessions.

Fluoroscopy or CT and any injection of contrast are inclusive components of 62321, 62323, 62325, 62327. For epidurography, use 72275.

The placement and use of a catheter to administer one or more epidural or subarachnoid injections on a single calendar day should be reported in the same manner as if a needle had been used, ie, as a single injection using either 62320, 62321, 62322, or 62323. Such injections should not be reported with 62324, 62325, 62326, or 62327.

Threading a catheter into the epidural space, injecting substances at one or more levels and then removing the catheter should be treated as a single injection (62320, 62321, 62322, 62323). If the catheter is left in place to deliver substance(s) over a prolonged period (ie, more than a single calendar day) either continuously or via intermittent bolus, use 62324, 62325, 62326, 62327 as appropriate.

When reporting 62320, 62321, 62322, 62323, 62324, 62325, 62326, 62327 code choice is based on the region at which the needle or catheter entered the body (eg, lumbar). Codes 62320, 62321, 62322, 62323, 62324, 62325, 62326, 62327 should be reported only once, when the substance injected spreads or catheter tip insertion moves into another spinal region (eg, 62322 is reported only once for injection or catheter insertion at L3-4 with spread of the substance or placement of the catheter tip to the thoracic region).

Percutaneous spinal procedures are done with indirect visualization (eg, image guidance) (eg, 62287). Endoscopic assistance during an open procedure with continuous and direct visualization (light-based) is reported using excision codes (eg, 63020-63035).

Definitions

For purposes of CPT coding, the following definitions of approach and visualization apply. The primary approach and visualization define the service, whether another method is incidentally applied. Surgical services are presumed open, unless otherwise specified.

Percutaneous: Image-guided procedures (eg, computer tomography [CT] or fluoroscopy) performed with indirect visualization of the spine without the use of any device that allows visualization through a surgical incision.

Endoscopic: Spinal procedures performed with continuous direct visualization of the spine through an endoscope.

Open: Spinal procedures performed with continuous direct visualization of the spine through a surgical opening.

Indirect visualization: Image-guided (eg, CT or fluoroscopy), not light-based visualization.

Direct visualization: Light-based visualization; can be performed by eye, or with surgical loupes, microscope, or endoscope.

AMA Coding Notes

Injection, Drainage, or Aspiration Procedures on the Spine and Spinal Cord

(For transforaminal epidural injection, see 64479-64484)

(Report 01996 for daily hospital management of continuous epidural or subarachnoid drug administration performed in conjunction with 62324, 62325, 62326, 62327)

(For the techniques of microsurgery and/or use of microscope, use 69990)

Surgical Procedures on the Spine and Spinal Cord

(For application of caliper or tongs, use 20660)

(For treatment of fracture or dislocation of spine, see 22310-22327)

AMA *CPT Assistant*

62284: Fall 93: 13, Sep 04: 13

Plain English Description

The spinal canal (subarachnoid space) is injected with contrast material to visualize structures including the spinal cord and spinal nerve roots for separately reportable myelography and/or computed tomography (CT). This code is used to report injection procedures of the lumbar region of the spine. The patient is placed face-down on the examination table. The spine is visualized using separately reportable fluoroscopy. The skin over the planned injection site, usually the lower lumbar spine, is cleansed and a local anesthetic is injected. The patient may be repositioned if needed on the side or in a sitting position. A needle is then inserted into the subarachnoid space and contrast material is then injected and observed as it moves through the subarachnoid space enhancing visualization of the spinal cord, nerve roots, and surrounding soft tissues.

Injection procedure for myelography/CT

The spinal canal (subarachnoid space) is injected with contrast material to visualize the spinal cord and nerve roots.

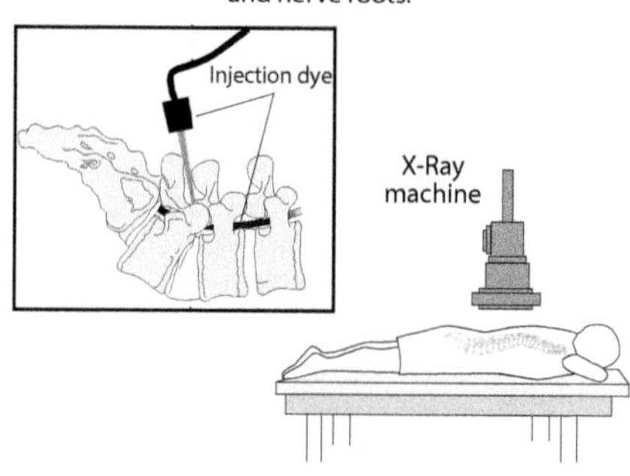

ICD-10-CM Diagnostic Codes

A17.82	Tuberculous meningoencephalitis
A39.81	Meningococcal encephalitis

A69.22 Other neurologic disorders in Lyme disease
A87.0 Enteroviral meningitis
A87.2 Lymphocytic choriomeningitis
B37.5 Candidal meningitis
B40.81 Blastomycotic meningoencephalitis
B45.1 Cerebral cryptococcosis
B57.41 Meningitis in Chagas' disease
B57.42 Meningoencephalitis in Chagas' disease
C70.9 Malignant neoplasm of meninges, unspecified
C79.49 Secondary malignant neoplasm of other parts of nervous system
D32.9 Benign neoplasm of meninges, unspecified
D42.9 Neoplasm of uncertain behavior of meninges, unspecified
G00.0 Hemophilus meningitis
G00.1 Pneumococcal meningitis
G00.2 Streptococcal meningitis
G00.3 Staphylococcal meningitis
G00.8 Other bacterial meningitis
G03.8 Meningitis due to other specified causes
G04.2 Bacterial meningoencephalitis and meningomyelitis, not elsewhere classified
G05.3 Encephalitis and encephalomyelitis in diseases classified elsewhere
G05.4 Myelitis in diseases classified elsewhere
G92 Toxic encephalopathy
G96.12 Meningeal adhesions (cerebral) (spinal)
G96.9 Disorder of central nervous system, unspecified
M43.05 Spondylolysis, thoracolumbar region
M43.06 Spondylolysis, lumbar region
M43.07 Spondylolysis, lumbosacral region
M43.15 Spondylolisthesis, thoracolumbar region
M43.16 Spondylolisthesis, lumbar region
M43.17 Spondylolisthesis, lumbosacral region
M45.5 Ankylosing spondylitis of thoracolumbar region
M45.6 Ankylosing spondylitis lumbar region
M46.25 Osteomyelitis of vertebra, thoracolumbar region
M46.26 Osteomyelitis of vertebra, lumbar region
M46.27 Osteomyelitis of vertebra, lumbosacral region
M46.35 Infection of intervertebral disc (pyogenic), thoracolumbar region
M46.36 Infection of intervertebral disc (pyogenic), lumbar region
M46.37 Infection of intervertebral disc (pyogenic), lumbosacral region
M46.45 Discitis, unspecified, thoracolumbar region
M46.46 Discitis, unspecified, lumbar region
M46.47 Discitis, unspecified, lumbosacral region
M46.55 Other infective spondylopathies, thoracolumbar region
M46.56 Other infective spondylopathies, lumbar region
M46.57 Other infective spondylopathies, lumbosacral region
M46.85 Other specified inflammatory spondylopathies, thoracolumbar region
M46.86 Other specified inflammatory spondylopathies, lumbar region
M46.87 Other specified inflammatory spondylopathies, lumbosacral region
M47.15 Other spondylosis with myelopathy, thoracolumbar region
M47.16 Other spondylosis with myelopathy, lumbar region
M47.25 Other spondylosis with radiculopathy, thoracolumbar region
M47.26 Other spondylosis with radiculopathy, lumbar region
M47.27 Other spondylosis with radiculopathy, lumbosacral region
M47.815 Spondylosis without myelopathy or radiculopathy, thoracolumbar region
M47.816 Spondylosis without myelopathy or radiculopathy, lumbar region
M47.817 Spondylosis without myelopathy or radiculopathy, lumbosacral region
M48.06 Spinal stenosis, lumbar region
M48.15 Ankylosing hyperostosis [Forestier], thoracolumbar region
M48.16 Ankylosing hyperostosis [Forestier], lumbar region
M48.17 Ankylosing hyperostosis [Forestier], lumbosacral region
M51.05 Intervertebral disc disorders with myelopathy, thoracolumbar region
M51.06 Intervertebral disc disorders with myelopathy, lumbar region
M51.15 Intervertebral disc disorders with radiculopathy, thoracolumbar region
M51.16 Intervertebral disc disorders with radiculopathy, lumbar region
M51.17 Intervertebral disc disorders with radiculopathy, lumbosacral region
M51.25 Other intervertebral disc displacement, thoracolumbar region
M51.26 Other intervertebral disc displacement, lumbar region
M51.27 Other intervertebral disc displacement, lumbosacral region
M51.35 Other intervertebral disc degeneration, thoracolumbar region
M51.36 Other intervertebral disc degeneration, lumbar region
M51.37 Other intervertebral disc degeneration, lumbosacral region
M51.45 Schmorl's nodes, thoracolumbar region
M51.46 Schmorl's nodes, lumbar region
M51.47 Schmorl's nodes, lumbosacral region
M51.85 Other intervertebral disc disorders, thoracolumbar region
M51.86 Other intervertebral disc disorders, lumbar region
M51.87 Other intervertebral disc disorders, lumbosacral region
M54.15 Radiculopathy, thoracolumbar region
M54.16 Radiculopathy, lumbar region
M54.17 Radiculopathy, lumbosacral region
⇄ M54.31 Sciatica, right side
⇄ M54.32 Sciatica, left side
⇄ M54.41 Lumbago with sciatica, right side
⇄ M54.42 Lumbago with sciatica, left side
M54.5 Low back pain
M54.89 Other dorsalgia
M96.1 Postlaminectomy syndrome, not elsewhere classified

CCI Edits

Refer to Appendix A for CCI edits.

Facility RVUs

Code	Work	PE Facility	MP	Total Facility
62284	1.54	0.78	0.18	2.50

Non-facility RVUs

Code	Work	PE Non-Facility	MP	Total Non-Facility
62284	1.54	3.94	0.18	5.66

Modifiers (PAR)

Code	Mod 50	Mod 51	Mod 62	Mod 66	Mod 80
62284	0	2	0	0	1

Global Period

Code	Days
62284	000

62287

62287 Decompression procedure, percutaneous, of nucleus pulposus of intervertebral disc, any method utilizing needle based technique to remove disc material under fluoroscopic imaging or other form of indirect visualization, with discography and/or epidural injection(s) at the treated level(s), when performed, single or multiple levels, lumbar

(Do not report 62287 in conjunction with 62267, 62290, 62322, 77003, 77012, 72295, when performed at same level)

(For non-needle based technique for percutaneous decompression of nucleus pulposus of intervertebral disc, see 0274T, 0275T)

AMA Coding Guideline

Injection, Drainage, or Aspiration Procedures on the Spine and Spinal Cord

Injection of contrast during fluoroscopic guidance and localization is an inclusive component of 62263, 62264, 62267, 62273, 62280, 62281, 62282, 62302, 62303, 62304, 62305, 62321, 62323, 62325, 62327, 62328, 62329. Fluoroscopic guidance and localization is reported with 77003, unless a formal contrast study (myelography, epidurography, or arthrography) is performed, in which case the use of fluoroscopy is included in the supervision and interpretation codes or the myelography via lumbar injection code. Image guidance and the injection of contrast are inclusive components and are required for the performance of myelography, as described by codes 62302, 62303, 62304, 62305.

For radiologic supervision and interpretation of epidurography, use 72275. Code 72275 is only to be used when an epidurogram is performed, images documented, and a formal radiologic report is issued.

Code 62263 describes a catheter-based treatment involving targeted injection of various substances (eg, hypertonic saline, steroid, anesthetic) via an indwelling epidural catheter. Code 62263 includes percutaneous insertion and removal of an epidural catheter (remaining in place over a several-day period), for the administration of multiple injections of a neurolytic agent(s) performed during serial treatment sessions (ie, spanning two or more treatment days). If required, adhesions or scarring may also be lysed by mechanical means. Code 62263 is not reported for each adhesiolysis treatment, but should be reported once to describe the entire series of injections/infusions spanning two or more treatment days.

Code 62264 describes multiple adhesiolysis treatment sessions performed on the same day. Adhesions or scarring may be lysed by injections of neurolytic agent(s). If required, adhesions or scarring may also be lysed mechanically using a percutaneously-deployed catheter.

Codes 62263 and 62264 include the procedure of injections of contrast for epidurography (72275) and fluoroscopic guidance and localization (77003) during initial or subsequent sessions.

Fluoroscopy or CT and any injection of contrast are inclusive components of 62321, 62323, 62325, 62327. For epidurography, use 72275.

The placement and use of a catheter to administer one or more epidural or subarachnoid injections on a single calendar day should be reported in the same manner as if a needle had been used, ie, as a single injection using either 62320, 62321, 62322, or 62323. Such injections should not be reported with 62324, 62325, 62326, or 62327.

Threading a catheter into the epidural space, injecting substances at one or more levels and then removing the catheter should be treated as a single injection (62320, 62321, 62322, 62323). If the catheter is left in place to deliver substance(s) over a prolonged period (ie, more than a single calendar day) either continuously or via intermittent bolus, use 62324, 62325, 62326, 62327 as appropriate.

When reporting 62320, 62321, 62322, 62323, 62324, 62325, 62326, 62327 code choice is based on the region at which the needle or catheter entered the body (eg, lumbar). Codes 62320, 62321, 62322, 62323, 62324, 62325, 62326, 62327 should be reported only once, when the substance injected spreads or catheter tip insertion moves into another spinal region (eg, 62322 is reported only once for injection or catheter insertion at L3-4 with spread of the substance or placement of the catheter tip to the thoracic region).

Percutaneous spinal procedures are done with indirect visualization (eg, image guidance) (eg, 62287). Endoscopic assistance during an open procedure with continuous and direct visualization (light-based) is reported using excision codes (eg, 63020-63035).

Definitions

For purposes of CPT coding, the following definitions of approach and visualization apply. The primary approach and visualization define the service, whether another method is incidentally applied. Surgical services are presumed open, unless otherwise specified.

Percutaneous: Image-guided procedures (eg, computer tomography [CT] or fluoroscopy) performed with indirect visualization of the spine without the use of any device that allows visualization through a surgical incision.

Endoscopic: Spinal procedures performed with continuous direct visualization of the spine through an endoscope.

Open: Spinal procedures performed with continuous direct visualization of the spine through a surgical opening.

Indirect visualization: Image-guided (eg, CT or fluoroscopy), not light-based visualization.

Direct visualization: Light-based visualization; can be performed by eye, or with surgical loupes, microscope, or endoscope.

AMA Coding Notes

Injection, Drainage, or Aspiration Procedures on the Spine and Spinal Cord

(For transforaminal epidural injection, see 64479-64484)

(Report 01996 for daily hospital management of continuous epidural or subarachnoid drug administration performed in conjunction with 62324, 62325, 62326, 62327)

(For the techniques of microsurgery and/or use of microscope, use 69990)

Surgical Procedures on the Spine and Spinal Cord

(For application of caliper or tongs, use 20660)

(For treatment of fracture or dislocation of spine, see 22310-22327)

AMA *CPT Assistant* ▯

62287: Nov 99: 34, Mar 02: 11, Oct 10: 9, Jul 12: 3, Oct 12: 14, Apr 14: 11, Mar 15: 10, Feb 17: 12

Plain English Description

Percutaneous decompression of the nucleus pulposus of a herniated lumbar intervertebral disc is done by needle-based technique to remove disc material using fluoroscopic imaging or other form of indirect visualization. Percutaneous disc decompression is done for patients with a contained herniated disc that is bulging without rupture. Different percutaneous procedures include manual, automated, and radiofrequency or laser methods. All types of procedures involve inserting small instruments through a needle placed between the vertebrae into the middle of the disc. Radiographic monitoring, such as fluoroscopy, is used to guide the instruments as herniated tissue is removed. Laser instruments burn or evaporate the disc. One method called coblation nucleoplasty uses low-frequency radio waves to carve tunnels in the disc by causing tissue to disintegrate into gases at the molecular level. Using fluoroscopic guidance, the needle is advanced through the skin and into the disc using a trajectory that avoids the spinal canal. Small amounts of contrast may be injected to ensure that the needle is properly positioned in the disc. A nucleoplasty cannula is then advanced through the needle and into the disc. The nucleoplasty catheter is activated and the nucleus pulposus is vaporized. As the catheter is withdrawn, coagulation is used to shrink the channel created by the coblation process, which further decompresses the disc. Usually 6-12 channels are created using this technique. Another method, called DISC nucleoplasty, uses special plasma technology, instead of heat energy, to remove the tissue from the center of the disc. A SpineWand is inserted through a needle into the center of the disc. A series of channels are made to remove tissue precisely and without trauma. As tissue is removed from the nucleus, the disc is decompressed and the pressure exerted on the nearby nerve root is relieved. Use this code for percutaneous decompression of single or multiple lumbar levels.

Decompression procedure, percutaneous, of nucleus pulposus of intervertebral disc any method

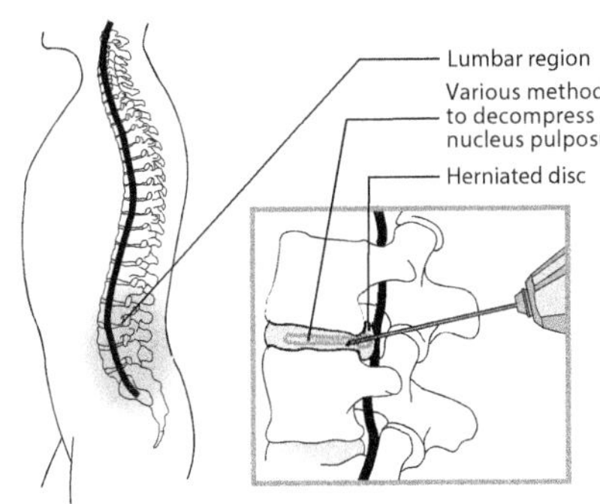

ICD-10-CM Diagnostic Codes

M46.45	Discitis, unspecified, thoracolumbar region
M46.46	Discitis, unspecified, lumbar region
M46.47	Discitis, unspecified, lumbosacral region
M51.05	Intervertebral disc disorders with myelopathy, thoracolumbar region
M51.06	Intervertebral disc disorders with myelopathy, lumbar region
M51.15	Intervertebral disc disorders with radiculopathy, thoracolumbar region
M51.16	Intervertebral disc disorders with radiculopathy, lumbar region
M51.17	Intervertebral disc disorders with radiculopathy, lumbosacral region
M51.25	Other intervertebral disc displacement, thoracolumbar region
M51.26	Other intervertebral disc displacement, lumbar region
M51.27	Other intervertebral disc displacement, lumbosacral region
M51.35	Other intervertebral disc degeneration, thoracolumbar region
M51.36	Other intervertebral disc degeneration, lumbar region
M51.37	Other intervertebral disc degeneration, lumbosacral region
M51.45	Schmorl's nodes, thoracolumbar region
M51.46	Schmorl's nodes, lumbar region
M51.47	Schmorl's nodes, lumbosacral region
M51.85	Other intervertebral disc disorders, thoracolumbar region
M51.86	Other intervertebral disc disorders, lumbar region
M51.87	Other intervertebral disc disorders, lumbosacral region
M54.15	Radiculopathy, thoracolumbar region
M54.16	Radiculopathy, lumbar region
M54.17	Radiculopathy, lumbosacral region
⇄ M54.31	Sciatica, right side
⇄ M54.32	Sciatica, left side
⇄ M54.41	Lumbago with sciatica, right side
⇄ M54.42	Lumbago with sciatica, left side
M54.5	Low back pain
M54.89	Other dorsalgia
M96.1	Postlaminectomy syndrome, not elsewhere classified

CCI Edits

Refer to Appendix A for CCI edits.

Facility RVUs ▯

Code	Work	PE Facility	MP	Total Facility
62287	9.03	6.58	1.15	16.76

Non-facility RVUs ▯

Code	Work	PE Non-Facility	MP	Total Non-Facility
62287	9.03	6.58	1.15	16.76

Modifiers (PAR) ▯

Code	Mod 50	Mod 51	Mod 62	Mod 66	Mod 80
62287	0	2	0	0	1

Global Period

Code	Days
62287	090

62290-62291

62290 Injection procedure for discography, each level; lumbar

62291 Injection procedure for discography, each level; cervical or thoracic

(For radiological supervision and interpretation, see 72285, 72295)

AMA Coding Guideline

Injection, Drainage, or Aspiration Procedures on the Spine and Spinal Cord

Injection of contrast during fluoroscopic guidance and localization is an inclusive component of 62263, 62264, 62267, 62273, 62280, 62281, 62282, 62302, 62303, 62304, 62305, 62321, 62323, 62325, 62327, 62328, 62329. Fluoroscopic guidance and localization is reported with 77003, unless a formal contrast study (myelography, epidurography, or arthrography) is performed, in which case the use of fluoroscopy is included in the supervision and interpretation codes or the myelography via lumbar injection code. Image guidance and the injection of contrast are inclusive components and are required for the performance of myelography, as described by codes 62302, 62303, 62304, 62305.

For radiologic supervision and interpretation of epidurography, use 72275. Code 72275 is only to be used when an epidurogram is performed, images documented, and a formal radiologic report is issued.

Code 62263 describes a catheter-based treatment involving targeted injection of various substances (eg, hypertonic saline, steroid, anesthetic) via an indwelling epidural catheter. Code 62263 includes percutaneous insertion and removal of an epidural catheter (remaining in place over a several-day period), for the administration of multiple injections of a neurolytic agent(s) performed during serial treatment sessions (ie, spanning two or more treatment days). If required, adhesions or scarring may also be lysed by mechanical means. Code 62263 is not reported for each adhesiolysis treatment, but should be reported once to describe the entire series of injections/infusions spanning two or more treatment days.

Code 62264 describes multiple adhesiolysis treatment sessions performed on the same day. Adhesions or scarring may be lysed by injections of neurolytic agent(s). If required, adhesions or scarring may also be lysed mechanically using a percutaneously-deployed catheter.

Codes 62263 and 62264 include the procedure of injections of contrast for epidurography (72275) and fluoroscopic guidance and localization (77003) during initial or subsequent sessions.

Fluoroscopy or CT and any injection of contrast are inclusive components of 62321, 62323, 62325, 62327. For epidurography, use 72275.

The placement and use of a catheter to administer one or more epidural or subarachnoid injections on a single calendar day should be reported in the same manner as if a needle had been used, ie, as a single injection using either 62320, 62321, 62322, or 62323. Such injections should not be reported with 62324, 62325, 62326, or 62327.

Threading a catheter into the epidural space, injecting substances at one or more levels and then removing the catheter should be treated as a single injection (62320, 62321, 62322, 62323). If the catheter is left in place to deliver substance(s) over a prolonged period (ie, more than a single calendar day) either continuously or via intermittent bolus, use 62324, 62325, 62326, 62327 as appropriate.

When reporting 62320, 62321, 62322, 62323, 62324, 62325, 62326, 62327 code choice is based on the region at which the needle or catheter entered the body (eg, lumbar). Codes 62320, 62321, 62322, 62323, 62324, 62325, 62326, 62327 should be reported only once, when the substance injected spreads or catheter tip insertion moves into another spinal region (eg, 62322 is reported only once for injection or catheter insertion at L3-4 with spread of the substance or placement of the catheter tip to the thoracic region).

Percutaneous spinal procedures are done with indirect visualization (eg, image guidance) (eg, 62287). Endoscopic assistance during an open procedure with continuous and direct visualization (light-based) is reported using excision codes (eg, 63020-63035).

Definitions

For purposes of CPT coding, the following definitions of approach and visualization apply. The primary approach and visualization define the service, whether another method is incidentally applied. Surgical services are presumed open, unless otherwise specified.

Percutaneous: Image-guided procedures (eg, computer tomography [CT] or fluoroscopy) performed with indirect visualization of the spine without the use of any device that allows visualization through a surgical incision.

Endoscopic: Spinal procedures performed with continuous direct visualization of the spine through an endoscope.

Open: Spinal procedures performed with continuous direct visualization of the spine through a surgical opening.

Indirect visualization: Image-guided (eg, CT or fluoroscopy), not light-based visualization.

Direct visualization: Light-based visualization; can be performed by eye, or with surgical loupes, microscope, or endoscope.

AMA Coding Notes

Injection, Drainage, or Aspiration Procedures on the Spine and Spinal Cord

(For transforaminal epidural injection, see 64479-64484)

(Report 01996 for daily hospital management of continuous epidural or subarachnoid drug administration performed in conjunction with 62324, 62325, 62326, 62327)

(For the techniques of microsurgery and/or use of microscope, use 69990)

Surgical Procedures on the Spine and Spinal Cord

(For application of caliper or tongs, use 20660)

(For treatment of fracture or dislocation of spine, see 22310-22327)

AMA *CPT Assistant*

62290: Nov 99: 35, Apr 03: 27, Mar 11: 7, Jul 12: 3

62291: Nov 99: 35, Mar 11: 7

Plain English Description

Discography is performed to determine if an intervertebral disc abnormality is the cause of back pain. The patient is positioned on the side and the site of the injection is cleansed with an antiseptic solution. A local anesthetic is injected. Using separately reportable fluoroscopic supervision, a large- bore needle is advanced through the skin to the disc. A discography needle is advanced through the first needle and into the center of the disc. Contrast is injected and separately reportable radiographs obtained. The procedure may be repeated on multiple discs and is reported for each level injected. Use 62290 for each lumbar disc injected; use 62291 for each cervical or thoracic disc injected.

Injection procedure for discography, each level

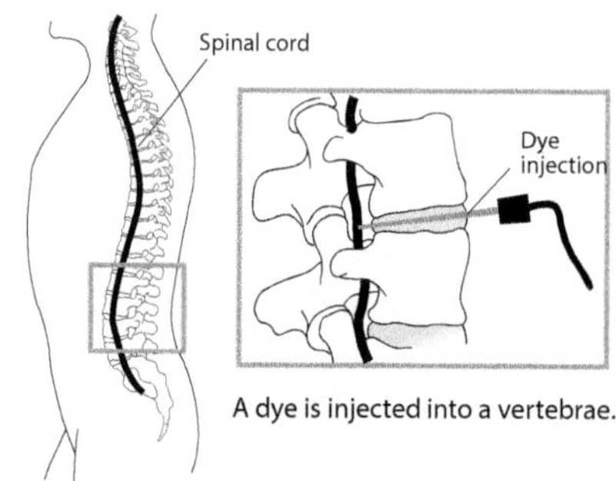

Lumbar (62290), cervical or thoracic (62291)

ICD-10-CM Diagnostic Codes

M46.31	Infection of intervertebral disc (pyogenic), occipito-atlanto-axial region
M46.32	Infection of intervertebral disc (pyogenic), cervical region
M46.33	Infection of intervertebral disc (pyogenic), cervicothoracic region
M46.34	Infection of intervertebral disc (pyogenic), thoracic region
M46.35	Infection of intervertebral disc (pyogenic), thoracolumbar region
M46.36	Infection of intervertebral disc (pyogenic), lumbar region
M46.41	Discitis, unspecified, occipito-atlanto-axial region

M46.42	Discitis, unspecified, cervical region
M46.43	Discitis, unspecified, cervicothoracic region
M46.44	Discitis, unspecified, thoracic region
M46.45	Discitis, unspecified, thoracolumbar region
M46.46	Discitis, unspecified, lumbar region
M46.47	Discitis, unspecified, lumbosacral region
M50.01	Cervical disc disorder with myelopathy, high cervical region
M50.021	Cervical disc disorder at C4-C5 level with myelopathy
M50.022	Cervical disc disorder at C5-C6 level with myelopathy
M50.023	Cervical disc disorder at C6-C7 level with myelopathy
M50.03	Cervical disc disorder with myelopathy, cervicothoracic region
M50.11	Cervical disc disorder with radiculopathy, high cervical region
M50.121	Cervical disc disorder at C4-C5 level with radiculopathy
M50.122	Cervical disc disorder at C5-C6 level with radiculopathy
M50.123	Cervical disc disorder at C6-C7 level with radiculopathy
M50.13	Cervical disc disorder with radiculopathy, cervicothoracic region
M50.21	Other cervical disc displacement, high cervical region
M50.221	Other cervical disc displacement at C4-C5 level
M50.222	Other cervical disc displacement at C5-C6 level
M50.223	Other cervical disc displacement at C6-C7 level
M50.23	Other cervical disc displacement, cervicothoracic region
M50.31	Other cervical disc degeneration, high cervical region
M50.321	Other cervical disc degeneration at C4-C5 level
M50.322	Other cervical disc degeneration at C5-C6 level
M50.323	Other cervical disc degeneration at C6-C7 level
M50.33	Other cervical disc degeneration, cervicothoracic region
M50.81	Other cervical disc disorders, high cervical region
M50.821	Other cervical disc disorders at C4-C5 level
M50.822	Other cervical disc disorders at C5-C6 level
M50.823	Other cervical disc disorders at C6-C7 level
M50.83	Other cervical disc disorders, cervicothoracic region
M51.04	Intervertebral disc disorders with myelopathy, thoracic region
M51.05	Intervertebral disc disorders with myelopathy, thoracolumbar region
M51.06	Intervertebral disc disorders with myelopathy, lumbar region
M51.14	Intervertebral disc disorders with radiculopathy, thoracic region
M51.15	Intervertebral disc disorders with radiculopathy, thoracolumbar region
M51.16	Intervertebral disc disorders with radiculopathy, lumbar region
M51.17	Intervertebral disc disorders with radiculopathy, lumbosacral region
M51.24	Other intervertebral disc displacement, thoracic region
M51.25	Other intervertebral disc displacement, thoracolumbar region
M51.26	Other intervertebral disc displacement, lumbar region
M51.27	Other intervertebral disc displacement, lumbosacral region
M51.34	Other intervertebral disc degeneration, thoracic region
M51.35	Other intervertebral disc degeneration, thoracolumbar region
M51.36	Other intervertebral disc degeneration, lumbar region
M51.37	Other intervertebral disc degeneration, lumbosacral region
M51.44	Schmorl's nodes, thoracic region
M51.45	Schmorl's nodes, thoracolumbar region
M51.46	Schmorl's nodes, lumbar region
M51.47	Schmorl's nodes, lumbosacral region
M51.84	Other intervertebral disc disorders, thoracic region
M51.85	Other intervertebral disc disorders, thoracolumbar region
M51.86	Other intervertebral disc disorders, lumbar region
M51.87	Other intervertebral disc disorders, lumbosacral region
M54.12	Radiculopathy, cervical region
M54.13	Radiculopathy, cervicothoracic region
M54.14	Radiculopathy, thoracic region
M54.15	Radiculopathy, thoracolumbar region
M54.16	Radiculopathy, lumbar region
M54.17	Radiculopathy, lumbosacral region
M54.2	Cervicalgia
⇄ M54.31	Sciatica, right side
⇄ M54.32	Sciatica, left side
⇄ M54.41	Lumbago with sciatica, right side
⇄ M54.42	Lumbago with sciatica, left side
M54.5	Low back pain
M54.6	Pain in thoracic spine
M96.1	Postlaminectomy syndrome, not elsewhere classified

CCI Edits

Refer to Appendix A for CCI edits.

Facility RVUs

Code	Work	PE Facility	MP	Total Facility
62290	3.00	1.51	0.28	4.79
62291	2.91	1.39	0.27	4.57

Non-facility RVUs

Code	Work	PE Non-Facility	MP	Total Non-Facility
62290	3.00	6.80	0.28	10.08
62291	2.91	6.37	0.27	9.55

Modifiers (PAR)

Code	Mod 50	Mod 51	Mod 62	Mod 66	Mod 80
62290	0	2	0	0	1
62291	0	2	0	0	1

Global Period

Code	Days
62290	000
62291	000

62292

62292 Injection procedure for chemonucleolysis, including discography, intervertebral disc, single or multiple levels, lumbar

AMA Coding Guideline

Injection, Drainage, or Aspiration Procedures on the Spine and Spinal Cord

Injection of contrast during fluoroscopic guidance and localization is an inclusive component of 62263, 62264, 62267, 62273, 62280, 62281, 62282, 62302, 62303, 62304, 62305, 62321, 62323, 62325, 62327, 62328, 62329. Fluoroscopic guidance and localization is reported with 77003, unless a formal contrast study (myelography, epidurography, or arthrography) is performed, in which case the use of fluoroscopy is included in the supervision and interpretation codes or the myelography via lumbar injection code. Image guidance and the injection of contrast are inclusive components and are required for the performance of myelography, as described by codes 62302, 62303, 62304, 62305.

For radiologic supervision and interpretation of epidurography, use 72275. Code 72275 is only to be used when an epidurogram is performed, images documented, and a formal radiologic report is issued.

Code 62263 describes a catheter-based treatment involving targeted injection of various substances (eg, hypertonic saline, steroid, anesthetic) via an indwelling epidural catheter. Code 62263 includes percutaneous insertion and removal of an epidural catheter (remaining in place over a several-day period), for the administration of multiple injections of a neurolytic agent(s) performed during serial treatment sessions (ie, spanning two or more treatment days). If required, adhesions or scarring may also be lysed by mechanical means. Code 62263 is not reported for each adhesiolysis treatment, but should be reported once to describe the entire series of injections/infusions spanning two or more treatment days.

Code 62264 describes multiple adhesiolysis treatment sessions performed on the same day. Adhesions or scarring may be lysed by injections of neurolytic agent(s). If required, adhesions or scarring may also be lysed mechanically using a percutaneously-deployed catheter.

Codes 62263 and 62264 include the procedure of injections of contrast for epidurography (72275) and fluoroscopic guidance and localization (77003) during initial or subsequent sessions.

Fluoroscopy or CT and any injection of contrast are inclusive components of 62321, 62323, 62325, 62327. For epidurography, use 72275.

The placement and use of a catheter to administer one or more epidural or subarachnoid injections on a single calendar day should be reported in the same manner as if a needle had been used, ie, as a single injection using either 62320, 62321, 62322, or 62323. Such injections should not be reported with 62324, 62325, 62326, or 62327. Threading a catheter into the epidural space, injecting substances at one or more levels and then removing the catheter should be treated as a single injection (62320, 62321, 62322, 62323). If the catheter is left in place to deliver substance(s) over a prolonged period (ie, more than a single calendar day) either continuously or via intermittent bolus, use 62324, 62325, 62326, 62327 as appropriate.

When reporting 62320, 62321, 62322, 62323, 62324, 62325, 62326, 62327 code choice is based on the region at which the needle or catheter entered the body (eg, lumbar). Codes 62320, 62321, 62322, 62323, 62324, 62325, 62326, 62327 should be reported only once, when the substance injected spreads or catheter tip insertion moves into another spinal region (eg, 62322 is reported only once for injection or catheter insertion at L3-4 with spread of the substance or placement of the catheter tip to the thoracic region).

Percutaneous spinal procedures are done with indirect visualization (eg, image guidance) (eg, 62287). Endoscopic assistance during an open procedure with continuous and direct visualization (light-based) is reported using excision codes (eg, 63020-63035).

Definitions

For purposes of CPT coding, the following definitions of approach and visualization apply. The primary approach and visualization define the service, whether another method is incidentally applied. Surgical services are presumed open, unless otherwise specified.

Percutaneous: Image-guided procedures (eg, computer tomography [CT] or fluoroscopy) performed with indirect visualization of the spine without the use of any device that allows visualization through a surgical incision.

Endoscopic: Spinal procedures performed with continuous direct visualization of the spine through an endoscope.

Open: Spinal procedures performed with continuous direct visualization of the spine through a surgical opening.

Indirect visualization: Image-guided (eg, CT or fluoroscopy), not light-based visualization.

Direct visualization: Light-based visualization; can be performed by eye, or with surgical loupes, microscope, or endoscope.

AMA Coding Notes

Injection, Drainage, or Aspiration Procedures on the Spine and Spinal Cord

(For transforaminal epidural injection, see 64479-64484)

(Report 01996 for daily hospital management of continuous epidural or subarachnoid drug administration performed in conjunction with 62324, 62325, 62326, 62327)

(For the techniques of microsurgery and/or use of microscope, use 69990)

Surgical Procedures on the Spine and Spinal Cord

(For application of caliper or tongs, use 20660)

(For treatment of fracture or dislocation of spine, see 22310-22327)

AMA *CPT Assistant* ▢

62292: Oct 99: 10

Plain English Description

Chemonucleolysis involves the injection of the enzyme chymopapain into the gelatinous center of the intervertebral disc to treat herniated nucleus pulposus. This enzyme dissolves the gelatinous nucleus pulposus. The patient is positioned on the side and the site of the injection is cleansed with an antiseptic solution. A local anesthetic is injected. Using separately reportable fluoroscopic supervision, a large bore needle is advanced through the skin to the disc. A discography needle is advanced through the first needle and into the center of the disc. Saline or water may be injected to ensure that the correct disc has been penetrated. The saline or water injection will reproduce the patient's pain. Alternatively, contrast may be injected and separately reportable radiographs obtained. Once placement in the correct disc has been verified, a small test dose of chymopapain is injected to determine whether the patient is hypersensitive to the enzyme. The patient is observed for 10-15 minutes, and if no adverse effects are noted, a full dose of chymopapain is injected. The procedure may be repeated on multiple lumbar discs.

Injection procedure for chemonucleolysis, including discography, intervertebral disc

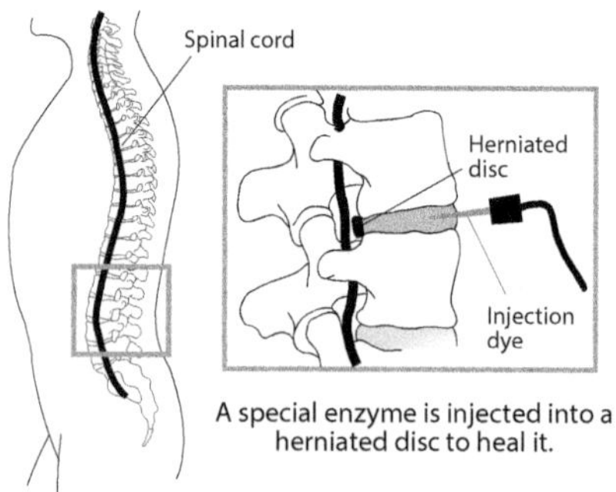

A special enzyme is injected into a herniated disc to heal it.

ICD-10-CM Diagnostic Codes

M51.06	Intervertebral disc disorders with myelopathy, lumbar region
M51.16	Intervertebral disc disorders with radiculopathy, lumbar region
M51.26	Other intervertebral disc displacement, lumbar region
M51.36	Other intervertebral disc degeneration, lumbar region
M51.86	Other intervertebral disc disorders, lumbar region

CCI Edits

Refer to Appendix A for CCI edits.

Facility RVUs

Code	Work	PE Facility	MP	Total Facility
62292	9.24	6.48	0.97	16.69

Non-facility RVUs

Code	Work	PE Non-Facility	MP	Total Non-Facility
62292	9.24	6.48	0.97	16.69

Modifiers (PAR)

Code	Mod 50	Mod 51	Mod 62	Mod 66	Mod 80
62292	0	2	0	0	0

Global Period

Code	Days
62292	090

62302-62305

62302 Myelography via lumbar injection, including radiological supervision and interpretation; cervical

(Do not report 62302 in conjunction with 62284, 62303, 62304, 62305, 72240, 72255, 72265, 72270)

62303 Myelography via lumbar injection, including radiological supervision and interpretation; thoracic

(Do not report 62303 in conjunction with 62284, 62302, 62304, 62305, 72240, 72255, 72265, 72270)

62304 Myelography via lumbar injection, including radiological supervision and interpretation; lumbosacral

(Do not report 62304 in conjunction with 62284, 62302, 62303, 62305, 72240, 72255, 72265, 72270)

62305 Myelography via lumbar injection, including radiological supervision and interpretation; 2 or more regions (eg, lumbar/thoracic, cervical/thoracic, lumbar/cervical, lumbar/thoracic/cervical)

(Do not report 62305 in conjunction with 62284, 62302, 62303, 62304, 72240, 72255, 72265, 72270)

(For myelography lumbar injection and imaging performed by different physicians or other qualified health care professionals, see 62284 or 72240, 72255, 72265, 72270)

(For injection procedure at C1-C2, use 61055)

AMA Coding Guideline

Injection, Drainage, or Aspiration Procedures on the Spine and Spinal Cord

Injection of contrast during fluoroscopic guidance and localization is an inclusive component of 62263, 62264, 62267, 62273, 62280, 62281, 62282, 62302, 62303, 62304, 62305, 62321, 62323, 62325, 62327, 62328, 62329. Fluoroscopic guidance and localization is reported with 77003, unless a formal contrast study (myelography, epidurography, or arthrography) is performed, in which case the use of fluoroscopy is included in the supervision and interpretation codes or the myelography via lumbar injection code. Image guidance and the injection of contrast are inclusive components and are required for the performance of myelography, as described by codes 62302, 62303, 62304, 62305.

For radiologic supervision and interpretation of epidurography, use 72275. Code 72275 is only to be used when an epidurogram is performed, images documented, and a formal radiologic report is issued.

Code 62263 describes a catheter-based treatment involving targeted injection of various substances (eg, hypertonic saline, steroid, anesthetic) via an indwelling epidural catheter. Code 62263 includes percutaneous insertion and removal of an epidural catheter (remaining in place over a several-day period), for the administration of multiple injections of a neurolytic agent(s) performed during serial treatment sessions (ie, spanning two or more treatment days). If required, adhesions or scarring may also be lysed by mechanical means. Code 62263 is not reported for each adhesiolysis treatment, but should be reported once to describe the entire series of injections/infusions spanning two or more treatment days.

Code 62264 describes multiple adhesiolysis treatment sessions performed on the same day. Adhesions or scarring may be lysed by injections of neurolytic agent(s). If required, adhesions or scarring may also be lysed mechanically using a percutaneously-deployed catheter.

Codes 62263 and 62264 include the procedure of injections of contrast for epidurography (72275) and fluoroscopic guidance and localization (77003) during initial or subsequent sessions.

Fluoroscopy or CT and any injection of contrast are inclusive components of 62321, 62323, 62325, 62327. For epidurography, use 72275.

The placement and use of a catheter to administer one or more epidural or subarachnoid injections on a single calendar day should be reported in the same manner as if a needle had been used, ie, as a single injection using either 62320, 62321, 62322, or 62323. Such injections should not be reported with 62324, 62325, 62326, or 62327.

Threading a catheter into the epidural space, injecting substances at one or more levels and then removing the catheter should be treated as a single injection (62320, 62321, 62322, 62323). If the catheter is left in place to deliver substance(s) over a prolonged period (ie, more than a single calendar day) either continuously or via intermittent bolus, use 62324, 62325, 62326, 62327 as appropriate.

When reporting 62320, 62321, 62322, 62323, 62324, 62325, 62326, 62327 code choice is based on the region at which the needle or catheter entered the body (eg, lumbar). Codes 62320, 62321, 62322, 62323, 62324, 62325, 62326, 62327 should be reported only once, when the substance injected spreads or catheter tip insertion moves into another spinal region (eg, 62322 is reported only once for injection or catheter insertion at L3-4 with spread of the substance or placement of the catheter tip to the thoracic region).

Percutaneous spinal procedures are done with indirect visualization (eg, image guidance) (eg, 62287). Endoscopic assistance during an open procedure with continuous and direct visualization (light-based) is reported using excision codes (eg, 63020-63035).

Definitions

For purposes of CPT coding, the following definitions of approach and visualization apply. The primary approach and visualization define the service, whether another method is incidentally applied. Surgical services are presumed open, unless otherwise specified.

Percutaneous: Image-guided procedures (eg, computer tomography [CT] or fluoroscopy) performed with indirect visualization of the spine without the use of any device that allows visualization through a surgical incision.

Endoscopic: Spinal procedures performed with continuous direct visualization of the spine through an endoscope.

Open: Spinal procedures performed with continuous direct visualization of the spine through a surgical opening.

Indirect visualization: Image-guided (eg, CT or fluoroscopy), not light-based visualization.

Direct visualization: Light-based visualization; can be performed by eye, or with surgical loupes, microscope, or endoscope.

AMA Coding Notes

Injection, Drainage, or Aspiration Procedures on the Spine and Spinal Cord

(For transforaminal epidural injection, see 64479-64484)

(Report 01996 for daily hospital management of continuous epidural or subarachnoid drug administration performed in conjunction with 62324, 62325, 62326, 62327)

(For the techniques of microsurgery and/or use of microscope, use 69990)

Surgical Procedures on the Spine and Spinal Cord

(For application of caliper or tongs, use 20660)

(For treatment of fracture or dislocation of spine, see 22310-22327)

Plain English Description

Myelography is an imaging technique that provides a detailed picture of the spinal canal, spinal cord, and spinal nerve roots using real-time fluoroscopy, and X-rays. The procedure is done under the direct supervision of a radiologist and may be used to diagnose intervertebral disc herniation, spinal stenosis, tumors, infection, inflammation, and other lesions caused by disease or trauma. The patient is positioned lying on the abdomen or side. Under fluoroscopy, a spinal needle is advanced into the spinal canal at the lumbar region until a free flow of cerebrospinal fluid (CSF) is observed. A contrast material (non-ionic dye) is injected through the needle into the subarachnoid space and the needle is withdrawn. The procedure table is slowly tilted up or down to allow the contrast dye to flow within the subarachnoid space. The flow of dye is monitored using fluoroscopy and X-rays may then be obtained to document abnormalities. When the procedure is complete, the table is returned to a horizontal position and the patient is allowed to assume a comfortable position. Code 62302 is used for examination of the cervical region of the spine; code 62303 for the thoracic region; code

62304 for the lumbosacral area; and code 62305 is reported when 2 or more areas of the spine are examined.

ICD-10-CM Diagnostic Codes

A17.82	Tuberculous meningoencephalitis
A39.81	Meningococcal encephalitis
A69.22	Other neurologic disorders in Lyme disease
A87.0	Enteroviral meningitis
A87.2	Lymphocytic choriomeningitis
B37.5	Candidal meningitis
B40.81	Blastomycotic meningoencephalitis
B45.1	Cerebral cryptococcosis
B57.41	Meningitis in Chagas' disease
B57.42	Meningoencephalitis in Chagas' disease
C70.9	Malignant neoplasm of meninges, unspecified
C79.49	Secondary malignant neoplasm of other parts of nervous system
D32.9	Benign neoplasm of meninges, unspecified
D42.9	Neoplasm of uncertain behavior of meninges, unspecified
G00.0	Hemophilus meningitis
G00.1	Pneumococcal meningitis
G00.2	Streptococcal meningitis
G00.3	Staphylococcal meningitis
G00.8	Other bacterial meningitis
G03.8	Meningitis due to other specified causes
G04.2	Bacterial meningoencephalitis and meningomyelitis, not elsewhere classified
G05.3	Encephalitis and encephalomyelitis in diseases classified elsewhere
G05.4	Myelitis in diseases classified elsewhere
G92	Toxic encephalopathy
G96.12	Meningeal adhesions (cerebral) (spinal)
G96.9	Disorder of central nervous system, unspecified
M43.01	Spondylolysis, occipito-atlanto-axial region
M43.02	Spondylolysis, cervical region
M43.03	Spondylolysis, cervicothoracic region
M43.04	Spondylolysis, thoracic region
M43.15	Spondylolisthesis, thoracolumbar region
M43.16	Spondylolisthesis, lumbar region
M43.17	Spondylolisthesis, lumbosacral region
M43.19	Spondylolisthesis, multiple sites in spine
M45.0	Ankylosing spondylitis of multiple sites in spine
M45.1	Ankylosing spondylitis of occipito-atlanto-axial region
M45.2	Ankylosing spondylitis of cervical region
M45.3	Ankylosing spondylitis of cervicothoracic region
M45.4	Ankylosing spondylitis of thoracic region
M45.5	Ankylosing spondylitis of thoracolumbar region
M45.6	Ankylosing spondylitis lumbar region
M46.22	Osteomyelitis of vertebra, cervical region
M46.23	Osteomyelitis of vertebra, cervicothoracic region
M46.24	Osteomyelitis of vertebra, thoracic region
M46.25	Osteomyelitis of vertebra, thoracolumbar region
M46.26	Osteomyelitis of vertebra, lumbar region
M46.27	Osteomyelitis of vertebra, lumbosacral region
M46.31	Infection of intervertebral disc (pyogenic), occipito-atlanto-axial region
M46.32	Infection of intervertebral disc (pyogenic), cervical region
M46.33	Infection of intervertebral disc (pyogenic), cervicothoracic region
M46.34	Infection of intervertebral disc (pyogenic), thoracic region
M46.35	Infection of intervertebral disc (pyogenic), thoracolumbar region
M46.36	Infection of intervertebral disc (pyogenic), lumbar region
M46.37	Infection of intervertebral disc (pyogenic), lumbosacral region
M46.41	Discitis, unspecified, occipito-atlanto-axial region
M46.42	Discitis, unspecified, cervical region
M46.43	Discitis, unspecified, cervicothoracic region
M46.44	Discitis, unspecified, thoracic region
M46.45	Discitis, unspecified, thoracolumbar region
M46.46	Discitis, unspecified, lumbar region
M46.47	Discitis, unspecified, lumbosacral region
M46.51	Other infective spondylopathies, occipito-atlanto-axial region
M46.52	Other infective spondylopathies, cervical region
M46.53	Other infective spondylopathies, cervicothoracic region
M46.54	Other infective spondylopathies, thoracic region
M46.55	Other infective spondylopathies, thoracolumbar region
M46.56	Other infective spondylopathies, lumbar region
M46.57	Other infective spondylopathies, lumbosacral region
M46.81	Other specified inflammatory spondylopathies, occipito-atlanto-axial region
M46.82	Other specified inflammatory spondylopathies, cervical region
M46.83	Other specified inflammatory spondylopathies, cervicothoracic region
M46.84	Other specified inflammatory spondylopathies, thoracic region
M46.85	Other specified inflammatory spondylopathies, thoracolumbar region
M46.86	Other specified inflammatory spondylopathies, lumbar region
M46.87	Other specified inflammatory spondylopathies, lumbosacral region
M47.11	Other spondylosis with myelopathy, occipito-atlanto-axial region
M47.12	Other spondylosis with myelopathy, cervical region
M47.13	Other spondylosis with myelopathy, cervicothoracic region
M47.14	Other spondylosis with myelopathy, thoracic region
M47.15	Other spondylosis with myelopathy, thoracolumbar region
M47.16	Other spondylosis with myelopathy, lumbar region
M47.21	Other spondylosis with radiculopathy, occipito-atlanto-axial region
M47.22	Other spondylosis with radiculopathy, cervical region
M47.23	Other spondylosis with radiculopathy, cervicothoracic region
M47.24	Other spondylosis with radiculopathy, thoracic region
M47.25	Other spondylosis with radiculopathy, thoracolumbar region
M47.26	Other spondylosis with radiculopathy, lumbar region
M47.27	Other spondylosis with radiculopathy, lumbosacral region
M48.02	Spinal stenosis, cervical region
M48.04	Spinal stenosis, thoracic region
M48.06	Spinal stenosis, lumbar region
M50.01	Cervical disc disorder with myelopathy, high cervical region
M50.021	Cervical disc disorder at C4-C5 level with myelopathy
M50.022	Cervical disc disorder at C5-C6 level with myelopathy
M50.023	Cervical disc disorder at C6-C7 level with myelopathy
M50.03	Cervical disc disorder with myelopathy, cervicothoracic region
M51.04	Intervertebral disc disorders with myelopathy, thoracic region
M51.05	Intervertebral disc disorders with myelopathy, thoracolumbar region
M51.06	Intervertebral disc disorders with myelopathy, lumbar region
M51.14	Intervertebral disc disorders with radiculopathy, thoracic region
M51.15	Intervertebral disc disorders with radiculopathy, thoracolumbar region
M51.16	Intervertebral disc disorders with radiculopathy, lumbar region
M53.0	Cervicocranial syndrome
M53.1	Cervicobrachial syndrome
M54.12	Radiculopathy, cervical region
M54.14	Radiculopathy, thoracic region
M54.16	Radiculopathy, lumbar region
M54.2	Cervicalgia

⇄ M54.41 Lumbago with sciatica, right side
⇄ M54.42 Lumbago with sciatica, left side

CCI Edits

Refer to Appendix A for CCI edits.

Facility RVUs ▯

Code	Work	PE Facility	MP	Total Facility
62302	2.29	1.02	0.19	3.50
62303	2.29	1.02	0.19	3.50
62304	2.25	1.01	0.19	3.45
62305	2.35	1.05	0.19	3.59

Non-facility RVUs ▯

Code	Work	PE Non-Facility	MP	Total Non-Facility
62302	2.29	4.89	0.19	7.37
62303	2.29	5.03	0.19	7.51
62304	2.25	4.83	0.19	7.27
62305	2.35	5.37	0.19	7.91

Modifiers (PAR) ▯

Code	Mod 50	Mod 51	Mod 62	Mod 66	Mod 80
62302	0	2	0	0	1
62303	0	2	0	0	1
62304	0	2	0	0	1
62305	0	2	0	0	1

Global Period

Code	Days
62302	000
62303	000
62304	000
62305	000

62320-62323

62320 Injection(s), of diagnostic or therapeutic substance(s) (eg, anesthetic, antispasmodic, opioid, steroid, other solution), not including neurolytic substances, including needle or catheter placement, interlaminar epidural or subarachnoid, cervical or thoracic; without imaging guidance

62321 Injection(s), of diagnostic or therapeutic substance(s) (eg, anesthetic, antispasmodic, opioid, steroid, other solution), not including neurolytic substances, including needle or catheter placement, interlaminar epidural or subarachnoid, cervical or thoracic; with imaging guidance (ie, fluoroscopy or CT)

(Do not report 62321 in conjunction with 77003, 77012, 76942)

62322 Injection(s), of diagnostic or therapeutic substance(s) (eg, anesthetic, antispasmodic, opioid, steroid, other solution), not including neurolytic substances, including needle or catheter placement, interlaminar epidural or subarachnoid, lumbar or sacral (caudal); without imaging guidance

62323 Injection(s), of diagnostic or therapeutic substance(s) (eg, anesthetic, antispasmodic, opioid, steroid, other solution), not including neurolytic substances, including needle or catheter placement, interlaminar epidural or subarachnoid, lumbar or sacral (caudal); with imaging guidance (ie, fluoroscopy or CT)

(Do not report 62323 in conjunction with 77003, 77012, 76942)

AMA Coding Guideline

Injection, Drainage, or Aspiration Procedures on the Spine and Spinal Cord

Injection of contrast during fluoroscopic guidance and localization is an inclusive component of 62263, 62264, 62267, 62273, 62280, 62281, 62282, 62302, 62303, 62304, 62305, 62321, 62323, 62325, 62327, 62328, 62329. Fluoroscopic guidance and localization is reported with 77003, unless a formal contrast study (myelography, epidurography, or arthrography) is performed, in which case the use of fluoroscopy is included in the supervision and interpretation codes or the myelography via lumbar injection code. Image guidance and the injection of contrast are inclusive components and are required for the performance of myelography, as described by codes 62302, 62303, 62304, 62305.

For radiologic supervision and interpretation of epidurography, use 72275. Code 72275 is only to be used when an epidurogram is performed, images documented, and a formal radiologic report is issued.

Code 62263 describes a catheter-based treatment involving targeted injection of various substances (eg, hypertonic saline, steroid, anesthetic) via an indwelling epidural catheter. Code 62263 includes percutaneous insertion and removal of an epidural catheter (remaining in place over a several-day period), for the administration of multiple injections of a neurolytic agent(s) performed during serial treatment sessions (ie, spanning two or more treatment days). If required, adhesions or scarring may also be lysed by mechanical means. Code 62263 is not reported for each adhesiolysis treatment, but should be reported once to describe the entire series of injections/infusions spanning two or more treatment days.

Code 62264 describes multiple adhesiolysis treatment sessions performed on the same day. Adhesions or scarring may be lysed by injections of neurolytic agent(s). If required, adhesions or scarring may also be lysed mechanically using a percutaneously-deployed catheter.

Codes 62263 and 62264 include the procedure of injections of contrast for epidurography (72275) and fluoroscopic guidance and localization (77003) during initial or subsequent sessions.

Fluoroscopy or CT and any injection of contrast are inclusive components of 62321, 62323, 62325, 62327. For epidurography, use 72275.

The placement and use of a catheter to administer one or more epidural or subarachnoid injections on a single calendar day should be reported in the same manner as if a needle had been used, ie, as a single injection using either 62320, 62321, 62322, or 62323. Such injections should not be reported with 62324, 62325, 62326, or 62327.

Threading a catheter into the epidural space, injecting substances at one or more levels and then removing the catheter should be treated as a single injection (62320, 62321, 62322, 62323). If the catheter is left in place to deliver substance(s) over a prolonged period (ie, more than a single calendar day) either continuously or via intermittent bolus, use 62324, 62325, 62326, 62327 as appropriate.

When reporting 62320, 62321, 62322, 62323, 62324, 62325, 62326, 62327 code choice is based on the region at which the needle or catheter entered the body (eg, lumbar). Codes 62320, 62321, 62322, 62323, 62324, 62325, 62326, 62327 should be reported only once, when the substance injected spreads or catheter tip insertion moves into another spinal region (eg, 62322 is reported only once for injection or catheter insertion at L3-4 with spread of the substance or placement of the catheter tip to the thoracic region).

Percutaneous spinal procedures are done with indirect visualization (eg, image guidance) (eg, 62287). Endoscopic assistance during an open procedure with continuous and direct visualization (light-based) is reported using excision codes (eg, 63020-63035).

Definitions

For purposes of CPT coding, the following definitions of approach and visualization apply. The primary approach and visualization define the service, whether another method is incidentally applied. Surgical services are presumed open, unless otherwise specified.

Percutaneous: Image-guided procedures (eg, computer tomography [CT] or fluoroscopy) performed with indirect visualization of the spine without the use of any device that allows visualization through a surgical incision.

Endoscopic: Spinal procedures performed with continuous direct visualization of the spine through an endoscope.

Open: Spinal procedures performed with continuous direct visualization of the spine through a surgical opening.

Indirect visualization: Image-guided (eg, CT or fluoroscopy), not light-based visualization.

Direct visualization: Light-based visualization; can be performed by eye, or with surgical loupes, microscope, or endoscope.

AMA Coding Notes

Injection, Drainage, or Aspiration Procedures on the Spine and Spinal Cord

(For transforaminal epidural injection, see 64479-64484)

(Report 01996 for daily hospital management of continuous epidural or subarachnoid drug administration performed in conjunction with 62324, 62325, 62326, 62327)

(For the techniques of microsurgery and/or use of microscope, use 69990)

Surgical Procedures on the Spine and Spinal Cord

(For application of caliper or tongs, use 20660)

(For treatment of fracture or dislocation of spine, see 22310-22327)

AMA *CPT Assistant*

62320: Sep 17: 6
62321: Sep 17: 6
62322: Sep 17: 6
62323: Sep 17: 6

Plain English Description

The skin over the spinal region to be injected is cleansed with an antiseptic solution and a local anesthetic is injected. A thin spinal needle or catheter is inserted into the back of the epidural or subarachnoid space through a paramedian or midline interlaminar approach, usually under fluoroscopic guidance. The epidural space is the outermost area of the spinal canal filled with cerebrospinal fluid that lies between the outermost protective membrane (dura mater) surrounding the nerve roots and the vertebral wall. The subarachnoid space lies closer to the spinal cord and is located between the middle protective membrane, the arachnoid, and the innermost delicate membrane surrounding the spinal cord, the pia mater. Contrast dye may be injected first to confirm proper needle placement, to perform an epidurography, and to see that the medication is traveling into the desired area. A diagnostic or therapeutic substance, such as an anesthetic, antispasmodic, opioid, steroid, or other solution, such as a steroid and local anesthetic mix, excluding a neurolytic substance, is injected into the epidural or subarachnoid space. Following injection, the patient is monitored for any adverse effects. Use 62320 for interlaminar epidural or subarachnoid injection(s) in the cervical or thoracic region without imaging guidance and 62322 for the lumbar or sacral (caudal) region. Use 62321 for similar injection(s) done with imaging guidance, such as fluoroscopy or computed tomography (CT), in the cervical or thoracic region and 62323 for the lumbar or sacral (caudal) region.

ICD-10-CM Diagnostic Codes

G89.11 Acute pain due to trauma
G89.12 Acute post-thoracotomy pain
G89.18 Other acute postprocedural pain
G89.21 Chronic pain due to trauma
G89.22 Chronic post-thoracotomy pain
G89.28 Other chronic postprocedural pain
G89.29 Other chronic pain
G89.3 Neoplasm related pain (acute) (chronic)
M43.02 Spondylolysis, cervical region
M43.03 Spondylolysis, cervicothoracic region
M43.04 Spondylolysis, thoracic region
M43.05 Spondylolysis, thoracolumbar region
M43.06 Spondylolysis, lumbar region
M43.07 Spondylolysis, lumbosacral region
M43.08 Spondylolysis, sacral and sacrococcygeal region
M43.12 Spondylolisthesis, cervical region
M43.13 Spondylolisthesis, cervicothoracic region
M43.14 Spondylolisthesis, thoracic region
M43.15 Spondylolisthesis, thoracolumbar region
M43.16 Spondylolisthesis, lumbar region
M43.17 Spondylolisthesis, lumbosacral region
M43.18 Spondylolisthesis, sacral and sacrococcygeal region
M47.12 Other spondylosis with myelopathy, cervical region
M47.13 Other spondylosis with myelopathy, cervicothoracic region
M47.14 Other spondylosis with myelopathy, thoracic region
M47.15 Other spondylosis with myelopathy, thoracolumbar region
M47.16 Other spondylosis with myelopathy, lumbar region
M47.17 Other spondylosis with myelopathy, lumbosacral region
M47.18 Other spondylosis with myelopathy, sacral and sacrococcygeal region
M47.22 Other spondylosis with radiculopathy, cervical region
M47.23 Other spondylosis with radiculopathy, cervicothoracic region
M47.24 Other spondylosis with radiculopathy, thoracic region
M47.25 Other spondylosis with radiculopathy, thoracolumbar region
M47.26 Other spondylosis with radiculopathy, lumbar region
M47.27 Other spondylosis with radiculopathy, lumbosacral region
M47.28 Other spondylosis with radiculopathy, sacral and sacrococcygeal region
M47.812 Spondylosis without myelopathy or radiculopathy, cervical region
M47.813 Spondylosis without myelopathy or radiculopathy, cervicothoracic region
M47.814 Spondylosis without myelopathy or radiculopathy, thoracic region
M47.815 Spondylosis without myelopathy or radiculopathy, thoracolumbar region
M47.816 Spondylosis without myelopathy or radiculopathy, lumbar region
M47.817 Spondylosis without myelopathy or radiculopathy, lumbosacral region
M47.818 Spondylosis without myelopathy or radiculopathy, sacral and sacrococcygeal region
M47.892 Other spondylosis, cervical region
M47.893 Other spondylosis, cervicothoracic region
M47.894 Other spondylosis, thoracic region
M47.895 Other spondylosis, thoracolumbar region
M47.896 Other spondylosis, lumbar region
M47.897 Other spondylosis, lumbosacral region
M47.898 Other spondylosis, sacral and sacrococcygeal region
M48.02 Spinal stenosis, cervical region
M48.03 Spinal stenosis, cervicothoracic region
M48.04 Spinal stenosis, thoracic region
M48.05 Spinal stenosis, thoracolumbar region
M48.061 Spinal stenosis, lumbar region without neurogenic claudication
M48.062 Spinal stenosis, lumbar region with neurogenic claudication
M48.07 Spinal stenosis, lumbosacral region
M48.08 Spinal stenosis, sacral and sacrococcygeal region
M50.01 Cervical disc disorder with myelopathy, high cervical region
M50.021 Cervical disc disorder at C4-C5 level with myelopathy
M50.022 Cervical disc disorder at C5-C6 level with myelopathy
M50.023 Cervical disc disorder at C6-C7 level with myelopathy
M50.03 Cervical disc disorder with myelopathy, cervicothoracic region
M50.11 Cervical disc disorder with radiculopathy, high cervical region
M50.121 Cervical disc disorder at C4-C5 level with radiculopathy
M50.122 Cervical disc disorder at C5-C6 level with radiculopathy
M50.123 Cervical disc disorder at C6-C7 level with radiculopathy
M50.13 Cervical disc disorder with radiculopathy, cervicothoracic region
M50.21 Other cervical disc displacement, high cervical region
M50.221 Other cervical disc displacement at C4-C5 level
M50.222 Other cervical disc displacement at C5-C6 level
M50.223 Other cervical disc displacement at C6-C7 level
M50.23 Other cervical disc displacement, cervicothoracic region
M50.31 Other cervical disc degeneration, high cervical region
M50.321 Other cervical disc degeneration at C4-C5 level
M50.322 Other cervical disc degeneration at C5-C6 level
M50.323 Other cervical disc degeneration at C6-C7 level
M50.33 Other cervical disc degeneration, cervicothoracic region
M50.81 Other cervical disc disorders, high cervical region
M50.821 Other cervical disc disorders at C4-C5 level
M50.822 Other cervical disc disorders at C5-C6 level
M50.823 Other cervical disc disorders at C6-C7 level
M50.83 Other cervical disc disorders, cervicothoracic region
M51.04 Intervertebral disc disorders with myelopathy, thoracic region
M51.05 Intervertebral disc disorders with myelopathy, thoracolumbar region
M51.06 Intervertebral disc disorders with myelopathy, lumbar region
M51.14 Intervertebral disc disorders with radiculopathy, thoracic region
M51.15 Intervertebral disc disorders with radiculopathy, thoracolumbar region
M51.16 Intervertebral disc disorders with radiculopathy, lumbar region
M51.17 Intervertebral disc disorders with radiculopathy, lumbosacral region
M51.24 Other intervertebral disc displacement, thoracic region
M51.25 Other intervertebral disc displacement, thoracolumbar region
M51.26 Other intervertebral disc displacement, lumbar region

	M51.27	Other intervertebral disc displacement, lumbosacral region
	M51.34	Other intervertebral disc degeneration, thoracic region
	M51.35	Other intervertebral disc degeneration, thoracolumbar region
	M51.36	Other intervertebral disc degeneration, lumbar region
	M51.37	Other intervertebral disc degeneration, lumbosacral region
	M51.44	Schmorl's nodes, thoracic region
	M51.45	Schmorl's nodes, thoracolumbar region
	M51.46	Schmorl's nodes, lumbar region
	M51.47	Schmorl's nodes, lumbosacral region
	M51.84	Other intervertebral disc disorders, thoracic region
	M51.85	Other intervertebral disc disorders, thoracolumbar region
	M51.86	Other intervertebral disc disorders, lumbar region
	M51.87	Other intervertebral disc disorders, lumbosacral region
	M54.11	Radiculopathy, occipito-atlanto-axial region
	M54.12	Radiculopathy, cervical region
	M54.13	Radiculopathy, cervicothoracic region
	M54.14	Radiculopathy, thoracic region
	M54.15	Radiculopathy, thoracolumbar region
	M54.16	Radiculopathy, lumbar region
	M54.17	Radiculopathy, lumbosacral region
	M54.18	Radiculopathy, sacral and sacrococcygeal region
	M54.2	Cervicalgia
⇄	M54.31	Sciatica, right side
⇄	M54.32	Sciatica, left side
⇄	M54.41	Lumbago with sciatica, right side
⇄	M54.42	Lumbago with sciatica, left side
	M54.6	Pain in thoracic spine

CCI Edits

Refer to Appendix A for CCI edits.

Facility RVUs ▯

Code	Work	PE Facility	MP	Total Facility
62320	1.80	0.88	0.18	2.86
62321	1.95	0.96	0.18	3.09
62322	1.55	0.73	0.15	2.43
62323	1.80	0.88	0.18	2.86

Non-facility RVUs ▯

Code	Work	PE Non-Facility	MP	Total Non-Facility
62320	1.80	2.69	0.18	4.67
62321	1.95	5.24	0.18	7.37
62322	1.55	2.57	0.15	4.27
62323	1.80	5.31	0.18	7.29

Modifiers (PAR) ▯

Code	Mod 50	Mod 51	Mod 62	Mod 66	Mod 80
62320	9	2	0	0	1
62321	9	2	0	0	1
62322	9	2	0	0	1
62323	9	2	0	0	1

Global Period

Code	Days
62320	000
62321	000
62322	000
62323	000

62324-62327

62324 Injection(s), including indwelling catheter placement, continuous infusion or intermittent bolus, of diagnostic or therapeutic substance(s) (eg, anesthetic, antispasmodic, opioid, steroid, other solution), not including neurolytic substances, interlaminar epidural or subarachnoid, cervical or thoracic; without imaging guidance

62325 Injection(s), including indwelling catheter placement, continuous infusion or intermittent bolus, of diagnostic or therapeutic substance(s) (eg, anesthetic, antispasmodic, opioid, steroid, other solution), not including neurolytic substances, interlaminar epidural or subarachnoid, cervical or thoracic; with imaging guidance (ie, fluoroscopy or CT)

(Do not report 62325 in conjunction with 77003, 77012, 76942)

62326 Injection(s), including indwelling catheter placement, continuous infusion or intermittent bolus, of diagnostic or therapeutic substance(s) (eg, anesthetic, antispasmodic, opioid, steroid, other solution), not including neurolytic substances, interlaminar epidural or subarachnoid, lumbar or sacral (caudal); without imaging guidance

62327 Injection(s), including indwelling catheter placement, continuous infusion or intermittent bolus, of diagnostic or therapeutic substance(s) (eg, anesthetic, antispasmodic, opioid, steroid, other solution), not including neurolytic substances, interlaminar epidural or subarachnoid, lumbar or sacral (caudal); with imaging guidance (ie, fluoroscopy or CT)

(Do not report 62327 in conjunction with 77003, 77012, 76942)

(Report 01996 for daily hospital management of continuous epidural or subarachnoid drug administration performed in conjunction with 62324, 62325, 62326, 62327)

AMA Coding Guideline

Injection, Drainage, or Aspiration Procedures on the Spine and Spinal Cord

Injection of contrast during fluoroscopic guidance and localization is an inclusive component of 62263, 62264, 62267, 62273, 62280, 62281, 62282, 62302, 62303, 62304, 62305, 62321, 62323, 62325, 62327, 62328, 62329. Fluoroscopic guidance and localization is reported with 77003, unless a formal contrast study (myelography, epidurography, or arthrography) is performed, in which case the use of fluoroscopy is included in the supervision and interpretation codes or the myelography via lumbar injection code. Image guidance and the injection of contrast are inclusive components and are required for the performance of myelography, as described by codes 62302, 62303, 62304, 62305.

For radiologic supervision and interpretation of epidurography, use 72275. Code 72275 is only to be used when an epidurogram is performed, images documented, and a formal radiologic report is issued.

Code 62263 describes a catheter-based treatment involving targeted injection of various substances (eg, hypertonic saline, steroid, anesthetic) via an indwelling epidural catheter. Code 62263 includes percutaneous insertion and removal of an epidural catheter (remaining in place over a several-day period), for the administration of multiple injections of a neurolytic agent(s) performed during serial treatment sessions (ie, spanning two or more treatment days). If required, adhesions or scarring may also be lysed by mechanical means. Code 62263 is not reported for each adhesiolysis treatment, but should be reported once to describe the entire series of injections/infusions spanning two or more treatment days.

Code 62264 describes multiple adhesiolysis treatment sessions performed on the same day. Adhesions or scarring may be lysed by injections of neurolytic agent(s). If required, adhesions or scarring may also be lysed mechanically using a percutaneously-deployed catheter.

Codes 62263 and 62264 include the procedure of injections of contrast for epidurography (72275) and fluoroscopic guidance and localization (77003) during initial or subsequent sessions.

Fluoroscopy or CT and any injection of contrast are inclusive components of 62321, 62323, 62325, 62327. For epidurography, use 72275.

The placement and use of a catheter to administer one or more epidural or subarachnoid injections on a single calendar day should be reported in the same manner as if a needle had been used, ie, as a single injection using either 62320, 62321, 62322, or 62323. Such injections should not be reported with 62324, 62325, 62326, or 62327. Threading a catheter into the epidural space, injecting substances at one or more levels and then removing the catheter should be treated as a single injection (62320, 62321, 62322, 62323). If the catheter is left in place to deliver substance(s) over a prolonged period (ie, more than a single calendar day) either continuously or via intermittent bolus, use 62324, 62325, 62326, 62327 as appropriate.

When reporting 62320, 62321, 62322, 62323, 62324, 62325, 62326, 62327 code choice is based on the region at which the needle or catheter entered the body (eg, lumbar). Codes 62320, 62321, 62322, 62323, 62324, 62325, 62326, 62327 should be reported only once, when the substance injected spreads or catheter tip insertion moves into another spinal region (eg, 62322 is reported only once for injection or catheter insertion at L3-4 with spread of the substance or placement of the catheter tip to the thoracic region).

Percutaneous spinal procedures are done with indirect visualization (eg, image guidance) (eg, 62287). Endoscopic assistance during an open procedure with continuous and direct visualization (light-based) is reported using excision codes (eg, 63020-63035).

Definitions

For purposes of CPT coding, the following definitions of approach and visualization apply. The primary approach and visualization define the service, whether another method is incidentally applied. Surgical services are presumed open, unless otherwise specified.

Percutaneous: Image-guided procedures (eg, computer tomography [CT] or fluoroscopy) performed with indirect visualization of the spine without the use of any device that allows visualization through a surgical incision.

Endoscopic: Spinal procedures performed with continuous direct visualization of the spine through an endoscope.

Open: Spinal procedures performed with continuous direct visualization of the spine through a surgical opening.

Indirect visualization: Image-guided (eg, CT or fluoroscopy), not light-based visualization.

Direct visualization: Light-based visualization; can be performed by eye, or with surgical loupes, microscope, or endoscope.

AMA Coding Notes

Injection, Drainage, or Aspiration Procedures on the Spine and Spinal Cord

(For transforaminal epidural injection, see 64479-64484)

(Report 01996 for daily hospital management of continuous epidural or subarachnoid drug administration performed in conjunction with 62324, 62325, 62326, 62327)

(For the techniques of microsurgery and/or use of microscope, use 69990)

Surgical Procedures on the Spine and Spinal Cord

(For application of caliper or tongs, use 20660)

(For treatment of fracture or dislocation of spine, see 22310-22327)

AMA *CPT Assistant*

62324: May 17: 10, Sep 17: 6
62325: May 17: 10, Sep 17: 6
62326: May 17: 10, Sep 17: 7
62327: May 17: 10, Sep 17: 7

Plain English Description

The skin over the spinal region to be catheterized is cleansed with an antiseptic solution and a local anesthetic is injected. A spinal needle is inserted into the back of the epidural or subarachnoid space through a paramedian or midline interlaminar approach, usually under fluoroscopic guidance. The epidural space is the outermost area of the spinal canal filled with cerebrospinal fluid that lies between the outermost protective membrane (dura mater) surrounding the nerve roots and the vertebral wall. The subarachnoid space lies closer to the spinal cord and is located between the middle protective membrane, the arachnoid, and the innermost delicate membrane surrounding the spinal cord, the pia mater. Contrast dye may be injected first to confirm proper needle placement or perform an epidurography. A catheter is then threaded through the needle and advanced within the target space to ensure secure placement. A diagnostic or therapeutic substance, such as an anesthetic, antispasmodic, opioid, steroid, or other solution, such as a steroid and local anesthetic mix, excluding a neurolytic substance, is then continuously infused or injected as an intermittent bolus into the epidural or subarachnoid space. Following infusion, the patient is monitored for any adverse effects. Use 62324 for interlaminar epidural or subarachnoid continuous infusion or intermittent bolus injection(s) in the cervical or thoracic region without imaging guidance and 62325 with imaging guidance. Use 62326 for interlaminar epidural or subarachnoid infusion or bolus injection(s) in the lumbar or sacral (caudal) region without imaging guidance and 62327 with imaging guidance.

ICD-10-CM Diagnostic Codes

G89.11 Acute pain due to trauma
G89.12 Acute post-thoracotomy pain
G89.18 Other acute postprocedural pain
G89.21 Chronic pain due to trauma
G89.22 Chronic post-thoracotomy pain
G89.28 Other chronic postprocedural pain
G89.29 Other chronic pain
G89.3 Neoplasm related pain (acute) (chronic)
G89.4 Chronic pain syndrome
M43.02 Spondylolysis, cervical region
M43.03 Spondylolysis, cervicothoracic region
M43.04 Spondylolysis, thoracic region
M43.05 Spondylolysis, thoracolumbar region
M43.06 Spondylolysis, lumbar region
M43.07 Spondylolysis, lumbosacral region
M43.08 Spondylolysis, sacral and sacrococcygeal region
M43.12 Spondylolisthesis, cervical region
M43.13 Spondylolisthesis, cervicothoracic region
M43.14 Spondylolisthesis, thoracic region
M43.15 Spondylolisthesis, thoracolumbar region
M43.16 Spondylolisthesis, lumbar region
M43.17 Spondylolisthesis, lumbosacral region
M43.18 Spondylolisthesis, sacral and sacrococcygeal region
M47.12 Other spondylosis with myelopathy, cervical region
M47.13 Other spondylosis with myelopathy, cervicothoracic region
M47.14 Other spondylosis with myelopathy, thoracic region
M47.15 Other spondylosis with myelopathy, thoracolumbar region
M47.16 Other spondylosis with myelopathy, lumbar region
M47.17 Other spondylosis with myelopathy, lumbosacral region
M47.18 Other spondylosis with myelopathy, sacral and sacrococcygeal region
M47.21 Other spondylosis with radiculopathy, occipito-atlanto-axial region
M47.22 Other spondylosis with radiculopathy, cervical region
M47.23 Other spondylosis with radiculopathy, cervicothoracic region
M47.24 Other spondylosis with radiculopathy, thoracic region
M47.25 Other spondylosis with radiculopathy, thoracolumbar region
M47.26 Other spondylosis with radiculopathy, lumbar region
M47.27 Other spondylosis with radiculopathy, lumbosacral region
M47.28 Other spondylosis with radiculopathy, sacral and sacrococcygeal region
M47.812 Spondylosis without myelopathy or radiculopathy, cervical region
M47.813 Spondylosis without myelopathy or radiculopathy, cervicothoracic region
M47.814 Spondylosis without myelopathy or radiculopathy, thoracic region
M47.815 Spondylosis without myelopathy or radiculopathy, thoracolumbar region
M47.816 Spondylosis without myelopathy or radiculopathy, lumbar region
M47.817 Spondylosis without myelopathy or radiculopathy, lumbosacral region
M47.818 Spondylosis without myelopathy or radiculopathy, sacral and sacrococcygeal region
M47.892 Other spondylosis, cervical region
M47.893 Other spondylosis, cervicothoracic region
M47.894 Other spondylosis, thoracic region
M47.895 Other spondylosis, thoracolumbar region
M47.896 Other spondylosis, lumbar region
M47.897 Other spondylosis, lumbosacral region
M47.898 Other spondylosis, sacral and sacrococcygeal region
M48.01 Spinal stenosis, occipito-atlanto-axial region
M48.02 Spinal stenosis, cervical region
M48.03 Spinal stenosis, cervicothoracic region
M48.04 Spinal stenosis, thoracic region
M48.05 Spinal stenosis, thoracolumbar region
M48.061 Spinal stenosis, lumbar region without neurogenic claudication
M48.062 Spinal stenosis, lumbar region with neurogenic claudication
M48.07 Spinal stenosis, lumbosacral region
M48.08 Spinal stenosis, sacral and sacrococcygeal region
M50.01 Cervical disc disorder with myelopathy, high cervical region
M50.021 Cervical disc disorder at C4-C5 level with myelopathy
M50.022 Cervical disc disorder at C5-C6 level with myelopathy
M50.023 Cervical disc disorder at C6-C7 level with myelopathy
M50.03 Cervical disc disorder with myelopathy, cervicothoracic region
M50.11 Cervical disc disorder with radiculopathy, high cervical region
M50.121 Cervical disc disorder at C4-C5 level with radiculopathy
M50.122 Cervical disc disorder at C5-C6 level with radiculopathy
M50.123 Cervical disc disorder at C6-C7 level with radiculopathy
M50.13 Cervical disc disorder with radiculopathy, cervicothoracic region
M50.21 Other cervical disc displacement, high cervical region
M50.221 Other cervical disc displacement at C4-C5 level
M50.222 Other cervical disc displacement at C5-C6 level
M50.223 Other cervical disc displacement at C6-C7 level
M50.23 Other cervical disc displacement, cervicothoracic region
M50.31 Other cervical disc degeneration, high cervical region
M50.321 Other cervical disc degeneration at C4-C5 level
M50.322 Other cervical disc degeneration at C5-C6 level
M50.323 Other cervical disc degeneration at C6-C7 level
M50.33 Other cervical disc degeneration, cervicothoracic region
M50.81 Other cervical disc disorders, high cervical region
M50.821 Other cervical disc disorders at C4-C5 level
M50.822 Other cervical disc disorders at C5-C6 level
M50.823 Other cervical disc disorders at C6-C7 level

M50.83	Other cervical disc disorders, cervicothoracic region
M51.04	Intervertebral disc disorders with myelopathy, thoracic region
M51.05	Intervertebral disc disorders with myelopathy, thoracolumbar region
M51.06	Intervertebral disc disorders with myelopathy, lumbar region
M51.14	Intervertebral disc disorders with radiculopathy, thoracic region
M51.15	Intervertebral disc disorders with radiculopathy, thoracolumbar region
M51.16	Intervertebral disc disorders with radiculopathy, lumbar region
M51.17	Intervertebral disc disorders with radiculopathy, lumbosacral region
M51.24	Other intervertebral disc displacement, thoracic region
M51.25	Other intervertebral disc displacement, thoracolumbar region
M51.26	Other intervertebral disc displacement, lumbar region
M51.27	Other intervertebral disc displacement, lumbosacral region
M51.34	Other intervertebral disc degeneration, thoracic region
M51.35	Other intervertebral disc degeneration, thoracolumbar region
M51.36	Other intervertebral disc degeneration, lumbar region
M51.37	Other intervertebral disc degeneration, lumbosacral region
M51.44	Schmorl's nodes, thoracic region
M51.45	Schmorl's nodes, thoracolumbar region
M51.46	Schmorl's nodes, lumbar region
M51.47	Schmorl's nodes, lumbosacral region
M51.84	Other intervertebral disc disorders, thoracic region
M51.85	Other intervertebral disc disorders, thoracolumbar region
M51.86	Other intervertebral disc disorders, lumbar region
M51.87	Other intervertebral disc disorders, lumbosacral region
M54.11	Radiculopathy, occipito-atlanto-axial region
M54.12	Radiculopathy, cervical region
M54.13	Radiculopathy, cervicothoracic region
M54.14	Radiculopathy, thoracic region
M54.15	Radiculopathy, thoracolumbar region
M54.16	Radiculopathy, lumbar region
M54.17	Radiculopathy, lumbosacral region
M54.18	Radiculopathy, sacral and sacrococcygeal region
M54.2	Cervicalgia
⇄ M54.31	Sciatica, right side
⇄ M54.32	Sciatica, left side
⇄ M54.41	Lumbago with sciatica, right side
⇄ M54.42	Lumbago with sciatica, left side
M54.6	Pain in thoracic spine

CCI Edits

Refer to Appendix A for CCI edits.

Facility RVUs ▯

Code	Work	PE Facility	MP	Total Facility
62324	1.89	0.54	0.15	2.58
62325	2.20	0.74	0.19	3.13
62326	1.78	0.59	0.15	2.52
62327	1.90	0.81	0.18	2.89

Non-facility RVUs ▯

Code	Work	PE Non-Facility	MP	Total Non-Facility
62324	1.89	2.02	0.15	4.06
62325	2.20	4.55	0.19	6.94
62326	1.78	2.25	0.15	4.18
62327	1.90	4.99	0.18	7.07

Modifiers (PAR) ▯

Code	Mod 50	Mod 51	Mod 62	Mod 66	Mod 80
62324	9	2	0	0	1
62325	9	2	0	0	1
62326	9	2	0	0	1
62327	9	2	0	0	1

Global Period

Code	Days
62324	000
62325	000
62326	000
62327	000

62328-62329

- ● **62328 Spinal puncture, lumbar, diagnostic; with fluoroscopic or CT guidance**

  (Do not report 62270, 62328 in conjunction with 77003, 77012)

  (If ultrasound or MRI guidance is performed, see 76942, 77021)

- ● **62329 Spinal puncture, therapeutic, for drainage of cerebrospinal fluid (by needle or catheter); with fluoroscopic or CT guidance**

  (Do not report 62272, 62329 in conjunction with 77003, 77012)

  (If ultrasound or MRI guidance is performed, see 76942, 77021)

AMA Coding Guideline

Injection, Drainage, or Aspiration Procedures on the Spine and Spinal Cord

Injection of contrast during fluoroscopic guidance and localization is an inclusive component of 62263, 62264, 62267, 62273, 62280, 62281, 62282, 62302, 62303, 62304, 62305, 62321, 62323, 62325, 62327, 62328, 62329. Fluoroscopic guidance and localization is reported with 77003, unless a formal contrast study (myelography, epidurography, or arthrography) is performed, in which case the use of fluoroscopy is included in the supervision and interpretation codes or the myelography via lumbar injection code. Image guidance and the injection of contrast are inclusive components and are required for the performance of myelography, as described by codes 62302, 62303, 62304, 62305.

For radiologic supervision and interpretation of epidurography, use 72275. Code 72275 is only to be used when an epidurogram is performed, images documented, and a formal radiologic report is issued.

Code 62263 describes a catheter-based treatment involving targeted injection of various substances (eg, hypertonic saline, steroid, anesthetic) via an indwelling epidural catheter. Code 62263 includes percutaneous insertion and removal of an epidural catheter (remaining in place over a several-day period), for the administration of multiple injections of a neurolytic agent(s) performed during serial treatment sessions (ie, spanning two or more treatment days). If required, adhesions or scarring may also be lysed by mechanical means. Code 62263 is not reported for each adhesiolysis treatment, but should be reported once to describe the entire series of injections/infusions spanning two or more treatment days.

Code 62264 describes multiple adhesiolysis treatment sessions performed on the same day. Adhesions or scarring may be lysed by injections of neurolytic agent(s). If required, adhesions or scarring may also be lysed mechanically using a percutaneously-deployed catheter.

Codes 62263 and 62264 include the procedure of injections of contrast for epidurography (72275) and fluoroscopic guidance and localization (77003) during initial or subsequent sessions.

Fluoroscopy or CT and any injection of contrast are inclusive components of 62321, 62323, 62325, 62327. For epidurography, use 72275.

The placement and use of a catheter to administer one or more epidural or subarachnoid injections on a single calendar day should be reported in the same manner as if a needle had been used, ie, as a single injection using either 62320, 62321, 62322, or 62323. Such injections should not be reported with 62324, 62325, 62326, or 62327.

Threading a catheter into the epidural space, injecting substances at one or more levels and then removing the catheter should be treated as a single injection (62320, 62321, 62322, 62323). If the catheter is left in place to deliver substance(s) over a prolonged period (ie, more than a single calendar day) either continuously or via intermittent bolus, use 62324, 62325, 62326, 62327 as appropriate.

When reporting 62320, 62321, 62322, 62323, 62324, 62325, 62326, 62327 code choice is based on the region at which the needle or catheter entered the body (eg, lumbar). Codes 62320, 62321, 62322, 62323, 62324, 62325, 62326, 62327 should be reported only once, when the substance injected spreads or catheter tip insertion moves into another spinal region (eg, 62322 is reported only once for injection or catheter insertion at L3-4 with spread of the substance or placement of the catheter tip to the thoracic region).

Percutaneous spinal procedures are done with indirect visualization (eg, image guidance) (eg, 62287). Endoscopic assistance during an open procedure with continuous and direct visualization (light-based) is reported using excision codes (eg, 63020-63035).

Definitions

For purposes of CPT coding, the following definitions of approach and visualization apply. The primary approach and visualization define the service, whether another method is incidentally applied. Surgical services are presumed open, unless otherwise specified.

Percutaneous: Image-guided procedures (eg, computer tomography [CT] or fluoroscopy) performed with indirect visualization of the spine without the use of any device that allows visualization through a surgical incision.

Endoscopic: Spinal procedures performed with continuous direct visualization of the spine through an endoscope.

Open: Spinal procedures performed with continuous direct visualization of the spine through a surgical opening.

Indirect visualization: Image-guided (eg, CT or fluoroscopy), not light-based visualization.

Direct visualization: Light-based visualization; can be performed by eye, or with surgical loupes, microscope, or endoscope.

AMA Coding Notes

Injection, Drainage, or Aspiration Procedures on the Spine and Spinal Cord

(For transforaminal epidural injection, see 64479-64484)

(Report 01996 for daily hospital management of continuous epidural or subarachnoid drug administration performed in conjunction with 62324, 62325, 62326, 62327)

(For the techniques of microsurgery and/or use of microscope, use 69990)

Surgical Procedures on the Spine and Spinal Cord

(For application of caliper or tongs, use 20660)

(For treatment of fracture or dislocation of spine, see 22310-22327)

Plain English Description

A lumbar spinal puncture is performed under fluoroscopic or CT guidance for diagnostic or therapeutic purposes. In 62328, a diagnostic lumbar puncture is performed for symptoms that may be indicative of an infection, such as meningitis; a malignant neoplasm; bleeding, such as subarachnoid hemorrhage; multiple sclerosis; or Guillain-Barre syndrome. Diagnostic lumbar puncture may also be performed to measure cerebrospinal fluid (CSF) pressure. The skin over the lumbar spine is disinfected and a local anesthetic is administered. A lumbar puncture needle is then inserted under imaging guidance into the spinal canal and CSF specimens are collected. The CSF specimens are sent to the laboratory for separately reportable evaluation. In 62329, a therapeutic spinal puncture is performed for elevated CSF pressure and CSF is drained using a needle or catheter placed as described above. CSF pressure is monitored during the drainage procedure and when the desired pressure is reached, the needle or catheter is removed.

Spinal puncture

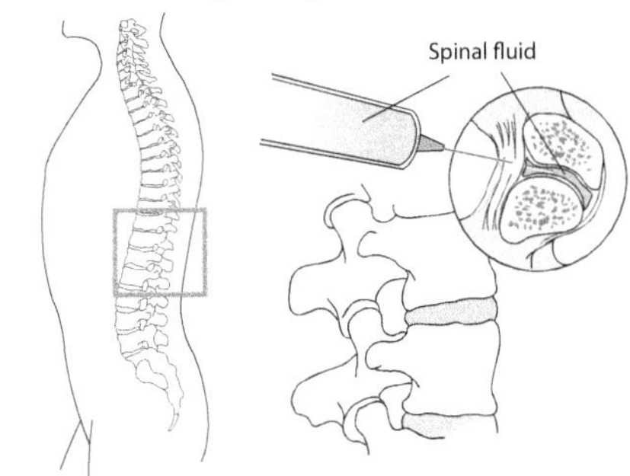

Cerebrospinal fluid is removed for diagnostic (62328) or therapeutic (62329) purposes using imaging guidance.

ICD-10-CM Diagnostic Codes

A17.0	Tuberculous meningitis
A17.82	Tuberculous meningoencephalitis

A32.11	Listerial meningitis
A32.12	Listerial meningoencephalitis
A39.0	Meningococcal meningitis
A39.81	Meningococcal encephalitis
A42.81	Actinomycotic meningitis
A42.82	Actinomycotic encephalitis
A50.41	Late congenital syphilitic meningitis
A50.42	Late congenital syphilitic encephalitis
A52.13	Late syphilitic meningitis
A52.14	Late syphilitic encephalitis
A69.21	Meningitis due to Lyme disease
A69.22	Other neurologic disorders in Lyme disease
A83.3	St Louis encephalitis
A83.5	California encephalitis
A85.0	Enteroviral encephalitis
A85.1	Adenoviral encephalitis
A85.8	Other specified viral encephalitis
A87.0	Enteroviral meningitis
A87.1	Adenoviral meningitis
A87.2	Lymphocytic choriomeningitis
A87.8	Other viral meningitis
A87.9	Viral meningitis, unspecified
A92.31	West Nile virus infection with encephalitis
B00.3	Herpesviral meningitis
B00.4	Herpesviral encephalitis
B01.0	Varicella meningitis
B01.11	Varicella encephalitis and encephalomyelitis
B02.0	Zoster encephalitis
B02.1	Zoster meningitis
B10.01	Human herpesvirus 6 encephalitis
B10.09	Other human herpesvirus encephalitis
B38.4	Coccidioidomycosis meningitis
B40.81	Blastomycotic meningoencephalitis
C70.0	Malignant neoplasm of cerebral meninges
C70.1	Malignant neoplasm of spinal meninges
G00.0	Hemophilus meningitis
G00.1	Pneumococcal meningitis
G00.2	Streptococcal meningitis
G00.3	Staphylococcal meningitis
G00.8	Other bacterial meningitis
G00.9	Bacterial meningitis, unspecified
G01	Meningitis in bacterial diseases classified elsewhere
G02	Meningitis in other infectious and parasitic diseases classified elsewhere
G37.8	Other specified demyelinating diseases of central nervous system
G44.52	New daily persistent headache (NDPH)
G61.0	Guillain-Barre syndrome
G61.81	Chronic inflammatory demyelinating polyneuritis
G93.2	Benign intracranial hypertension
I60.8	Other nontraumatic subarachnoid hemorrhage
I60.9	Nontraumatic subarachnoid hemorrhage, unspecified
P10.3	Subarachnoid hemorrhage due to birth injury
P52.5	Subarachnoid (nontraumatic) hemorrhage of newborn
R51	Headache

CCI Edits

Refer to Appendix A for CCI edits.

Facility RVUs ▯

Code	Work	PE Facility	MP	Total Facility
62328	1.73	0.62	0.24	2.59
62329	2.03	0.80	0.43	3.26

Non-facility RVUs ▯

Code	Work	PE Non-Facility	MP	Total Non-Facility
62328	1.73	5.43	0.24	7.40
62329	2.03	6.73	0.43	9.19

Modifiers (PAR) ▯

Code	Mod 50	Mod 51	Mod 62	Mod 66	Mod 80
62328	0	2	0	0	1
62329	0	2	0	0	1

Global Period

Code	Days
62328	000
62329	000

62350-62351

62350 Implantation, revision or repositioning of tunneled intrathecal or epidural catheter, for long-term medication administration via an external pump or implantable reservoir/infusion pump; without laminectomy

62351 Implantation, revision or repositioning of tunneled intrathecal or epidural catheter, for long-term medication administration via an external pump or implantable reservoir/infusion pump; with laminectomy

(For refilling and maintenance of an implantable infusion pump for spinal or brain drug therapy, see 95990, 95991)

AMA Coding Notes

Catheter Implantation Procedures on the Spine and Spinal Cord

(For percutaneous placement of intrathecal or epidural catheter, see 62270, 62272, 62273, 62280, 62281, 62282, 62284, 62320, 62321, 62322, 62323, 62324, 62325, 62326, 62327, 62328, 62329)

Surgical Procedures on the Spine and Spinal Cord

(For application of caliper or tongs, use 20660)

(For treatment of fracture or dislocation of spine, see 22310-22327)

AMA *CPT Assistant* □

62350: Nov 99: 36

62351: Nov 99: 36

Plain English Description

Implantation, revision, or repositioning of an intrathecal or epidural catheter may be performed with or without a laminectomy. In 62350, the procedure is performed without a laminectomy. For initial implantation, the overlying skin is cleansed with an antiseptic solution and a local anesthetic injected. A spinal needle is inserted into the skin and advanced into the intrathecal or epidural space. A catheter is then threaded through the needle and the catheter tip advanced cephalad to the selected level for pain control or other medication administration. The catheter is then tunneled subcutaneously approximately 5-10 cm away from the insertion site. The catheter is secured with sutures. The catheter is then connected to an external pump or an implantable reservoir or infusion pump. If revision of the catheter is performed, the catheter is exposed and the connection site at the reservoir or pump is inspected. The catheter may be disconnected and trimmed and reconnected or other revisions made. If repositioning is performed, the catheter is disconnected from the internal or external pump or reservoir. The catheter is manipulated into a different site within the intrathecal or epidural space. The revised or repositioned catheter is secured with sutures and reconnected to the pump or reservoir. In 62351, the procedure is performed with a laminectomy. The skin is incised over the catheter placement site and extended down to the spinous processes. Muscle is retracted off the lamina and facet joint. A bone drill is used to remove part or all of the lamina. The intrathecal or epidural catheter is implanted, revised, or repositioned as described above. The catheter is tunneled through the subcutaneous tissue and connected to the pump or reservoir. The surgical wound is closed.

Implantation, revision or repositioning of tunneled intrathecal or epidural catheter

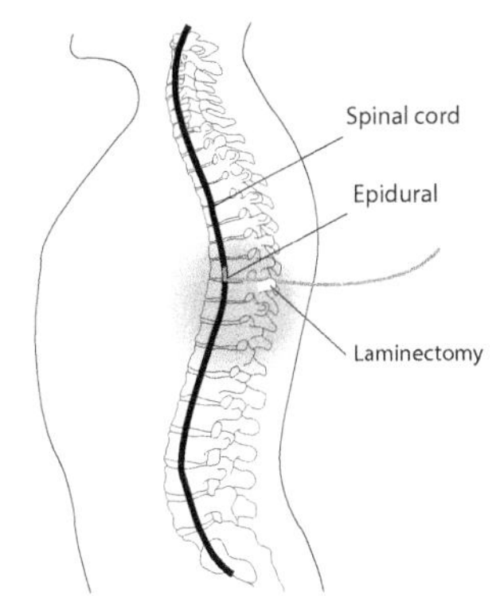

Without laminectomy (62350); with laminectomy (62351)

ICD-10-CM Diagnostic Codes

	Code	Description
	C16.0	Malignant neoplasm of cardia
	C16.1	Malignant neoplasm of fundus of stomach
	C16.2	Malignant neoplasm of body of stomach
	C16.3	Malignant neoplasm of pyloric antrum
	C16.4	Malignant neoplasm of pylorus
	C16.5	Malignant neoplasm of lesser curvature of stomach, unspecified
	C16.6	Malignant neoplasm of greater curvature of stomach, unspecified
	C16.8	Malignant neoplasm of overlapping sites of stomach
	C16.9	Malignant neoplasm of stomach, unspecified
	C17.0	Malignant neoplasm of duodenum
	C17.1	Malignant neoplasm of jejunum
	C17.2	Malignant neoplasm of ileum
	C17.3	Meckel's diverticulum, malignant
	C17.8	Malignant neoplasm of overlapping sites of small intestine
	C18.0	Malignant neoplasm of cecum
	C18.2	Malignant neoplasm of ascending colon
	C18.3	Malignant neoplasm of hepatic flexure
	C18.4	Malignant neoplasm of transverse colon
	C18.5	Malignant neoplasm of splenic flexure
	C18.6	Malignant neoplasm of descending colon
	C18.7	Malignant neoplasm of sigmoid colon
	C18.8	Malignant neoplasm of overlapping sites of colon
	C22.0	Liver cell carcinoma
	C22.1	Intrahepatic bile duct carcinoma
	C22.2	Hepatoblastoma
	C22.3	Angiosarcoma of liver
	C22.4	Other sarcomas of liver
	C22.7	Other specified carcinomas of liver
	C22.8	Malignant neoplasm of liver, primary, unspecified as to type
	C22.9	Malignant neoplasm of liver, not specified as primary or secondary
	C25.0	Malignant neoplasm of head of pancreas
	C25.1	Malignant neoplasm of body of pancreas
	C25.2	Malignant neoplasm of tail of pancreas
	C25.3	Malignant neoplasm of pancreatic duct
	C25.4	Malignant neoplasm of endocrine pancreas
	C25.7	Malignant neoplasm of other parts of pancreas
	C25.8	Malignant neoplasm of overlapping sites of pancreas
	C25.9	Malignant neoplasm of pancreas, unspecified
	C26.0	Malignant neoplasm of intestinal tract, part unspecified
	C26.9	Malignant neoplasm of ill-defined sites within the digestive system
⇄	C34.81	Malignant neoplasm of overlapping sites of right bronchus and lung
⇄	C34.82	Malignant neoplasm of overlapping sites of left bronchus and lung
	C39.9	Malignant neoplasm of lower respiratory tract, part unspecified
⇄	C40.21	Malignant neoplasm of long bones of right lower limb
⇄	C40.22	Malignant neoplasm of long bones of left lower limb
	C41.0	Malignant neoplasm of bones of skull and face
	C41.2	Malignant neoplasm of vertebral column
	C41.3	Malignant neoplasm of ribs, sternum and clavicle
	C41.4	Malignant neoplasm of pelvic bones, sacrum and coccyx
	C41.9	Malignant neoplasm of bone and articular cartilage, unspecified
	C48.0	Malignant neoplasm of retroperitoneum
	C48.1	Malignant neoplasm of specified parts of peritoneum
	C48.8	Malignant neoplasm of overlapping sites of retroperitoneum and peritoneum
	C76.0	Malignant neoplasm of head, face and neck
	C76.1	Malignant neoplasm of thorax
	C76.2	Malignant neoplasm of abdomen
	C76.3	Malignant neoplasm of pelvis

C78.7	Secondary malignant neoplasm of liver and intrahepatic bile duct
C79.51	Secondary malignant neoplasm of bone
C79.89	Secondary malignant neoplasm of other specified sites
G89.11	Acute pain due to trauma
G89.12	Acute post-thoracotomy pain
G89.18	Other acute postprocedural pain
G89.21	Chronic pain due to trauma
G89.22	Chronic post-thoracotomy pain
G89.28	Other chronic postprocedural pain
G89.29	Other chronic pain
G89.3	Neoplasm related pain (acute) (chronic)
M96.1	Postlaminectomy syndrome, not elsewhere classified

CCI Edits

Refer to Appendix A for CCI edits.

Facility RVUs ▯

Code	Work	PE Facility	MP	Total Facility
62350	6.05	4.28	1.12	11.45
62351	11.66	10.07	3.39	25.12

Non-facility RVUs ▯

Code	Work	PE Non-Facility	MP	Total Non-Facility
62350	6.05	4.28	1.12	11.45
62351	11.66	10.07	3.39	25.12

Modifiers **(PAR)** ▯

Code	Mod 50	Mod 51	Mod 62	Mod 66	Mod 80
62350	0	2	1	0	1
62351	0	2	2	0	2

Global Period

Code	Days
62350	010
62351	090

62355

62355 Removal of previously implanted intrathecal or epidural catheter

AMA Coding Notes

Catheter Implantation Procedures on the Spine and Spinal Cord

(For percutaneous placement of intrathecal or epidural catheter, see 62270, 62272, 62273, 62280, 62281, 62282, 62284, 62320, 62321, 62322, 62323, 62324, 62325, 62326, 62327, 62328, 62329)

Surgical Procedures on the Spine and Spinal Cord

(For application of caliper or tongs, use 20660)

(For treatment of fracture or dislocation of spine, see 22310-22327)

Plain English Description

The previously placed intrathecal or epidural catheter is exposed at the distal aspect of the tunnel and disconnected from the pump or reservoir. Distal sutures are removed. The tunneled portion of the catheter is then palpated from the pump or reservoir site to the site where it enters the spinal canal. A small incision is made over the site where the catheter enters the spinal canal. The subcutaneous tunneled portion of the catheter is removed. Proximal sutures are removed. The catheter is then removed from the intrathecal or epidural space. The skin is closed with a suture or steristrips.

Removal of previously implanted intrathecal or epidural catheter

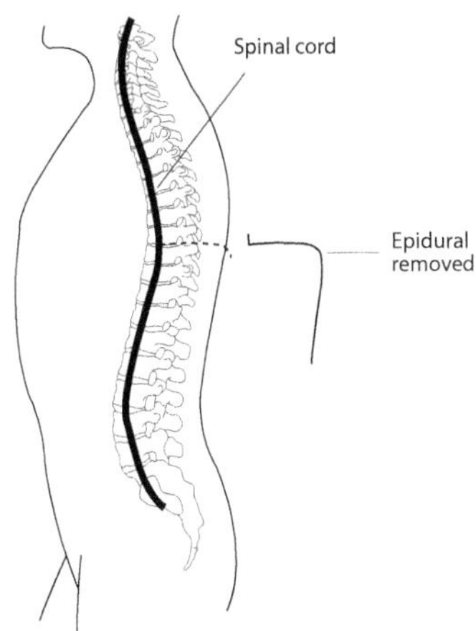

ICD-10-CM Diagnostic Codes

	Code	Description
⑦	T85.610	Breakdown (mechanical) of cranial or spinal infusion catheter
⑦	T85.620	Displacement of cranial or spinal infusion catheter
⑦	T85.630	Leakage of cranial or spinal infusion catheter
⑦	T85.690	Other mechanical complication of cranial or spinal infusion catheter
⑦	T85.735	Infection and inflammatory reaction due to cranial or spinal infusion catheter
⑦	T85.810	Embolism due to nervous system prosthetic devices, implants and grafts
⑦	T85.820	Fibrosis due to nervous system prosthetic devices, implants and grafts
⑦	T85.830	Hemorrhage due to nervous system prosthetic devices, implants and grafts
⑦	T85.840	Pain due to nervous system prosthetic devices, implants and grafts
⑦	T85.850	Stenosis due to nervous system prosthetic devices, implants and grafts
⑦	T85.860	Thrombosis due to nervous system prosthetic devices, implants and grafts
⑦	T85.890	Other specified complication of nervous system prosthetic devices, implants and grafts
	Z45.1	Encounter for adjustment and management of infusion pump
	Z45.49	Encounter for adjustment and management of other implanted nervous system device

ICD-10-CM Coding Notes

For codes requiring a 7th character extension, refer to your ICD-10-CM book. Review the character descriptions and coding guidelines for proper selection. For some procedures, only certain characters will apply.

CCI Edits

Refer to Appendix A for CCI edits.

Facility RVUs ▢

Code	Work	PE Facility	MP	Total Facility
62355	3.55	3.46	0.78	7.79

Non-facility RVUs ▢

Code	Work	PE Non-Facility	MP	Total Non-Facility
62355	3.55	3.46	0.78	7.79

Modifiers (PAR) ▢

Code	Mod 50	Mod 51	Mod 62	Mod 66	Mod 80
62355	0	2	0	0	0

Global Period

Code	Days
62355	010

62360-62362

62360 Implantation or replacement of device for intrathecal or epidural drug infusion; subcutaneous reservoir

62361 Implantation or replacement of device for intrathecal or epidural drug infusion; nonprogrammable pump

62362 Implantation or replacement of device for intrathecal or epidural drug infusion; programmable pump, including preparation of pump, with or without programming

AMA Coding Notes

Surgical Procedures on the Spine and Spinal Cord

(For application of caliper or tongs, use 20660)

(For treatment of fracture or dislocation of spine, see 22310-22327)

AMA *CPT Assistant* ☐

62362: Mar 97: 11

Plain English Description

For initial implantation of a subcutaneous reservoir or pump, the skin is incised, typically in the lateral aspect of the lower abdomen. A subcutaneous pocket is fashioned. The subcutaneous reservoir or pump is connected to the catheter and placed in the pocket. The skin is closed over the device. For replacement of a subcutaneous reservoir or pump, the old device is first removed in a separately reportable procedure. The new device is then inserted. Use 62360 for placement of a subcutaneous reservoir. Use 62361 for placement of a nonprogrammable pump. Use 62362 for placement of a programmable pump. Placement of a programmable pump requires preparation of the pump. The reservoir and alarm status are checked to ensure that the pump will function properly once implanted. Dosing, continuous infusion rate, and/or time intervals for bolus infusion may be programmed at this time.

Implantation or replacement of device for intrathecal or epidural drug infusion; programmable pump

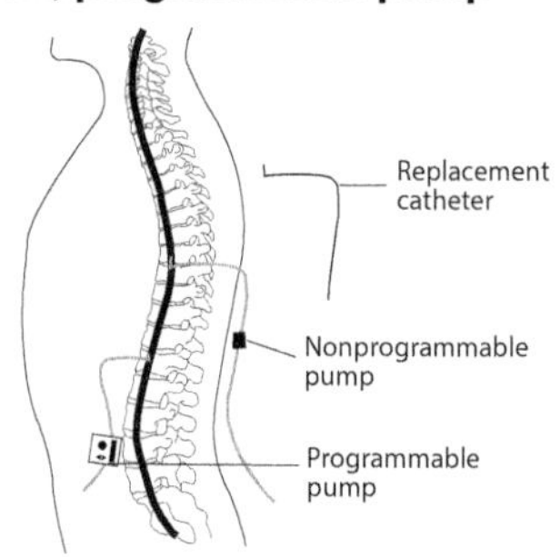

Subcutaneous reservoir (62360); nonprogrammable pump (62361); programmable pump (62362)

ICD-10-CM Diagnostic Codes

	Code	Description
	C16.0	Malignant neoplasm of cardia
	C16.1	Malignant neoplasm of fundus of stomach
	C16.2	Malignant neoplasm of body of stomach
	C16.3	Malignant neoplasm of pyloric antrum
	C16.4	Malignant neoplasm of pylorus
	C16.5	Malignant neoplasm of lesser curvature of stomach, unspecified
	C16.6	Malignant neoplasm of greater curvature of stomach, unspecified
	C16.8	Malignant neoplasm of overlapping sites of stomach
	C16.9	Malignant neoplasm of stomach, unspecified
	C17.0	Malignant neoplasm of duodenum
	C17.1	Malignant neoplasm of jejunum
	C17.2	Malignant neoplasm of ileum
	C17.3	Meckel's diverticulum, malignant
	C17.8	Malignant neoplasm of overlapping sites of small intestine
	C18.0	Malignant neoplasm of cecum
	C18.2	Malignant neoplasm of ascending colon
	C18.3	Malignant neoplasm of hepatic flexure
	C18.4	Malignant neoplasm of transverse colon
	C18.5	Malignant neoplasm of splenic flexure
	C18.6	Malignant neoplasm of descending colon
	C18.7	Malignant neoplasm of sigmoid colon
	C18.8	Malignant neoplasm of overlapping sites of colon
	C22.0	Liver cell carcinoma
	C22.1	Intrahepatic bile duct carcinoma
	C22.2	Hepatoblastoma
	C22.3	Angiosarcoma of liver
	C22.4	Other sarcomas of liver
	C22.7	Other specified carcinomas of liver
	C22.8	Malignant neoplasm of liver, primary, unspecified as to type
	C22.9	Malignant neoplasm of liver, not specified as primary or secondary
	C25.0	Malignant neoplasm of head of pancreas
	C25.1	Malignant neoplasm of body of pancreas
	C25.2	Malignant neoplasm of tail of pancreas
	C25.3	Malignant neoplasm of pancreatic duct
	C25.4	Malignant neoplasm of endocrine pancreas
	C25.7	Malignant neoplasm of other parts of pancreas
	C25.8	Malignant neoplasm of overlapping sites of pancreas
	C25.9	Malignant neoplasm of pancreas, unspecified
	C26.0	Malignant neoplasm of intestinal tract, part unspecified
	C26.9	Malignant neoplasm of ill-defined sites within the digestive system
⇄	C34.81	Malignant neoplasm of overlapping sites of right bronchus and lung
⇄	C34.82	Malignant neoplasm of overlapping sites of left bronchus and lung
	C39.9	Malignant neoplasm of lower respiratory tract, part unspecified
⇄	C40.21	Malignant neoplasm of long bones of right lower limb
⇄	C40.22	Malignant neoplasm of long bones of left lower limb
	C41.0	Malignant neoplasm of bones of skull and face
	C41.2	Malignant neoplasm of vertebral column
	C41.3	Malignant neoplasm of ribs, sternum and clavicle
	C41.4	Malignant neoplasm of pelvic bones, sacrum and coccyx
	C41.9	Malignant neoplasm of bone and articular cartilage, unspecified
	C48.0	Malignant neoplasm of retroperitoneum
	C48.1	Malignant neoplasm of specified parts of peritoneum
	C48.8	Malignant neoplasm of overlapping sites of retroperitoneum and peritoneum
	C76.0	Malignant neoplasm of head, face and neck
	C76.1	Malignant neoplasm of thorax
	C76.2	Malignant neoplasm of abdomen
	C76.3	Malignant neoplasm of pelvis
	C78.7	Secondary malignant neoplasm of liver and intrahepatic bile duct
	C79.51	Secondary malignant neoplasm of bone
	C79.89	Secondary malignant neoplasm of other specified sites
	G89.11	Acute pain due to trauma
	G89.12	Acute post-thoracotomy pain
	G89.18	Other acute postprocedural pain
	G89.21	Chronic pain due to trauma
	G89.22	Chronic post-thoracotomy pain
	G89.28	Other chronic postprocedural pain
	G89.29	Other chronic pain
	G89.3	Neoplasm related pain (acute) (chronic)
	M96.1	Postlaminectomy syndrome, not elsewhere classified
❼	T85.610	Breakdown (mechanical) of cranial or spinal infusion catheter
❼	T85.620	Displacement of cranial or spinal infusion catheter
❼	T85.630	Leakage of cranial or spinal infusion catheter
❼	T85.690	Other mechanical complication of cranial or spinal infusion catheter
❼	T85.735	Infection and inflammatory reaction due to cranial or spinal infusion catheter
❼	T85.810	Embolism due to nervous system prosthetic devices, implants and grafts
❼	T85.820	Fibrosis due to nervous system prosthetic devices, implants and grafts
❼	T85.830	Hemorrhage due to nervous system prosthetic devices, implants and grafts

⑦	T85.840	Pain due to nervous system prosthetic devices, implants and grafts
⑦	T85.850	Stenosis due to nervous system prosthetic devices, implants and grafts
⑦	T85.860	Thrombosis due to nervous system prosthetic devices, implants and grafts
⑦	T85.890	Other specified complication of nervous system prosthetic devices, implants and grafts
	Z45.1	Encounter for adjustment and management of infusion pump
	Z45.49	Encounter for adjustment and management of other implanted nervous system device

ICD-10-CM Coding Notes

For codes requiring a 7th character extension, refer to your ICD-10-CM book. Review the character descriptions and coding guidelines for proper selection. For some procedures, only certain characters will apply.

CCI Edits

Refer to Appendix A for CCI edits.

Facility RVUs ▯

Code	Work	PE Facility	MP	Total Facility
62360	4.33	3.80	0.91	9.04
62361	5.00	5.47	1.85	12.32
62362	5.60	4.26	1.17	11.03

Non-facility RVUs ▯

Code	Work	PE Non-Facility	MP	Total Non-Facility
62360	4.33	3.80	0.91	9.04
62361	5.00	5.47	1.85	12.32
62362	5.60	4.26	1.17	11.03

Modifiers (PAR) ▯

Code	Mod 50	Mod 51	Mod 62	Mod 66	Mod 80
62360	0	2	1	0	0
62361	0	2	1	0	0
62362	0	2	1	0	0

Global Period

Code	Days
62360	010
62361	010
62362	010

62365

62365 Removal of subcutaneous reservoir or pump, previously implanted for intrathecal or epidural infusion

AMA Coding Notes

Surgical Procedures on the Spine and Spinal Cord

(For application of caliper or tongs, use 20660)

(For treatment of fracture or dislocation of spine, see 22310-22327)

Plain English Description

An incision is made in the skin over the implanted reservoir or pump. The device is exposed and dissected free of subcutaneous tissue. The device is disconnected from the intrathecal or epidural catheter and removed. Separately reportable procedures are then performed either to remove the catheter or to replace the reservoir or pump.

Removal of subcutaneous reservoir or pump, previously implanted for intrathecal

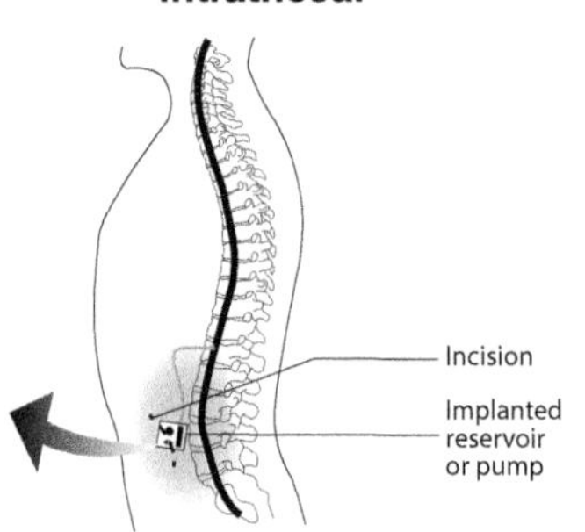

ICD-10-CM Diagnostic Codes

- ➐ T85.610 Breakdown (mechanical) of cranial or spinal infusion catheter
- ➐ T85.620 Displacement of cranial or spinal infusion catheter
- ➐ T85.630 Leakage of cranial or spinal infusion catheter
- ➐ T85.690 Other mechanical complication of cranial or spinal infusion catheter
- ➐ T85.735 Infection and inflammatory reaction due to cranial or spinal infusion catheter
- ➐ T85.810 Embolism due to nervous system prosthetic devices, implants and grafts
- ➐ T85.820 Fibrosis due to nervous system prosthetic devices, implants and grafts
- ➐ T85.830 Hemorrhage due to nervous system prosthetic devices, implants and grafts
- ➐ T85.840 Pain due to nervous system prosthetic devices, implants and grafts
- ➐ T85.850 Stenosis due to nervous system prosthetic devices, implants and grafts
- ➐ T85.860 Thrombosis due to nervous system prosthetic devices, implants and grafts
- ➐ T85.890 Other specified complication of nervous system prosthetic devices, implants and grafts
- Z45.1 Encounter for adjustment and management of infusion pump
- Z45.49 Encounter for adjustment and management of other implanted nervous system device

ICD-10-CM Coding Notes

For codes requiring a 7th character extension, refer to your ICD-10-CM book. Review the character descriptions and coding guidelines for proper selection. For some procedures, only certain characters will apply.

CCI Edits

Refer to Appendix A for CCI edits.

Facility RVUs

Code	Work	PE Facility	MP	Total Facility
62365	3.93	3.65	0.90	8.48

Non-facility RVUs

Code	Work	PE Non-Facility	MP	Total Non-Facility
62365	3.93	3.65	0.90	8.48

Modifiers (PAR)

Code	Mod 50	Mod 51	Mod 62	Mod 66	Mod 80
62365	0	2	0	0	0

Global Period

Code	Days
62365	010

62367-62370

62367 Electronic analysis of programmable, implanted pump for intrathecal or epidural drug infusion (includes evaluation of reservoir status, alarm status, drug prescription status); without reprogramming or refill

62368 Electronic analysis of programmable, implanted pump for intrathecal or epidural drug infusion (includes evaluation of reservoir status, alarm status, drug prescription status); with reprogramming

(For refilling and maintenance of an implantable infusion pump for spinal or brain drug therapy, see 95990-95991)

62369 Electronic analysis of programmable, implanted pump for intrathecal or epidural drug infusion (includes evaluation of reservoir status, alarm status, drug prescription status); with reprogramming and refill

62370 Electronic analysis of programmable, implanted pump for intrathecal or epidural drug infusion (includes evaluation of reservoir status, alarm status, drug prescription status); with reprogramming and refill (requiring skill of a physician or other qualified health care professional)

(Do not report 62367-62370 in conjunction with 95990, 95991. For refilling and maintenance of a reservoir or an implantable infusion pump for spinal or brain drug delivery without reprogramming, see 95990, 95991)

AMA Coding Notes

Surgical Procedures on the Spine and Spinal Cord

(For application of caliper or tongs, use 20660)

(For treatment of fracture or dislocation of spine, see 22310-22327)

AMA *CPT Assistant*

62367: Jul 12: 5, 6, Aug 12: 10, 11, 12, 15

62368: Nov 02: 10, Jul 06: 1, Jul 12: 5, 6, Aug 12: 10, 11, 12, 15

62369: Jul 12: 5, 6, Aug 12: 10, 11, 12, 15

62370: Jul 12: 5, 6, Aug 12: 10, 11, 12, 15

Plain English Description

A previously placed programmable, implanted intrathecal or epidural drug infusion pump is evaluated using electronic analysis. A connection is established between the programmable pump and the interrogation device. The interrogation device provides information on reservoir status, alarm status, and drug flow rates, which are evaluated to ensure that these are within normal parameters. The technician or physician reviews the data obtained by the interrogation device and determines if any reprogramming is needed. If so, reprogramming is performed using a telemetry device and may include adjusting alarm parameters and drug flow rates. The new settings are verified with the interrogation device. The pump may also be refilled. A written report of findings is provided. Report 62367 for electronic analysis and evaluation when the pump is not reprogrammed or refilled. Report 62368 when the pump is reprogrammed but not refilled. Use 62369 when evaluation, reprogramming, and refilling of the pump is performed by a technician and 62370 when the same service requires the skill of a physician or other qualified health care professional.

Electronic analysis of programmable, implanted pump for intrathecal or epidural drug infusion

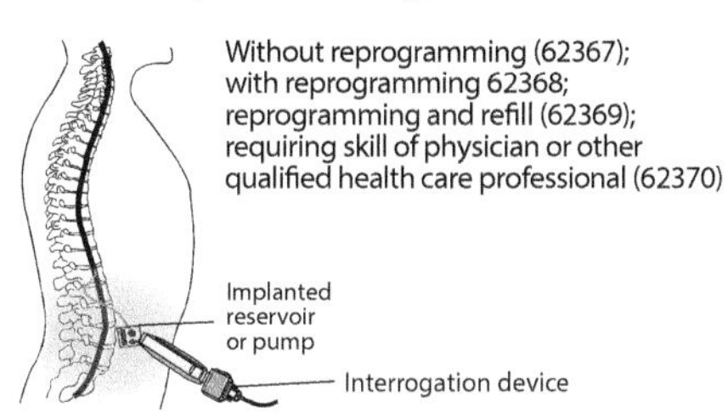

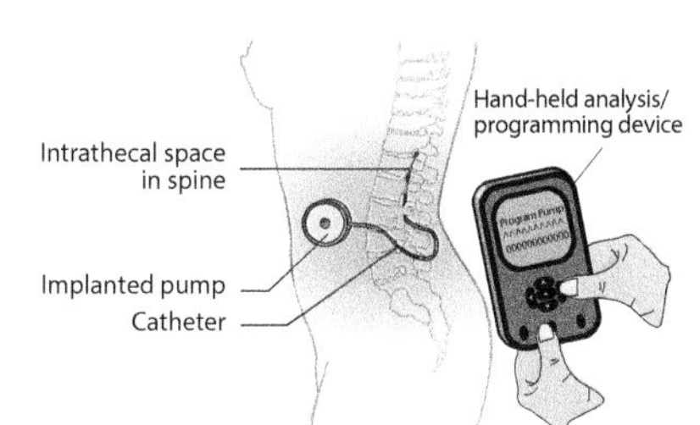

ICD-10-CM Diagnostic Codes

Z45.1	Encounter for adjustment and management of infusion pump
Z45.49	Encounter for adjustment and management of other implanted nervous system device

CCI Edits

Refer to Appendix A for CCI edits.

Facility RVUs

Code	Work	PE Facility	MP	Total Facility
62367	0.48	0.19	0.06	0.73
62368	0.67	0.27	0.09	1.03
62369	0.67	0.27	0.09	1.03
62370	0.90	0.35	0.09	1.34

Non-facility RVUs

Code	Work	PE Non-Facility	MP	Total Non-Facility
62367	0.48	0.38	0.06	0.92
62368	0.67	0.53	0.09	1.29
62369	0.67	1.97	0.09	2.73
62370	0.90	1.84	0.09	2.83

Modifiers (PAR)

Code	Mod 50	Mod 51	Mod 62	Mod 66	Mod 80
62367	0	0	0	0	1
62368	0	0	0	0	1
62369	0	0	0	0	1
62370	0	0	0	0	1

Global Period

Code	Days
62367	XXX
62368	XXX
62369	XXX
62370	XXX

62380

62380 Endoscopic decompression of spinal cord, nerve root(s), including laminotomy, partial facetectomy, foraminotomy, discectomy and/or excision of herniated intervertebral disc, 1 interspace, lumbar

(For open procedures, see 63030, 63056)

(For bilateral procedure, report 62380 with modifier 50)

AMA Coding Guideline

Endoscopic Decompression of Neural Elements and/or Excision of Herniated Intervertebral Discs

Definitions

For purposes of CPT coding, the following definitions of approach and visualization apply. The primary approach and visualization define the service, whether another method is incidentally applied. Surgical services are presumed open, unless otherwise specified.

Percutaneous: Image-guided procedures (eg, computer tomography [CT] or fluoroscopy) performed with indirect visualization of the spine without the use of any device that allows visualization through a surgical incision.

Endoscopic: Spinal procedures performed with continuous direct visualization of the spine through an endoscope.

Open: Spinal procedures performed with continuous direct visualization of the spine through a surgical opening.

Indirect visualization: Image-guided (eg, CT or fluoroscopy), not light-based visualization.

Direct visualization: Light-based visualization; can be performed by eye, or with surgical loupes, microscope, or endoscope.

AMA Coding Notes

Endoscopic Decompression of Neural Elements and/or Excision of Herniated Intervertebral Discs

(For the techniques of microsurgery and/or use of microscope, use 69990)

(For percutaneous decompression, see 62287, 0274T, 0275T)

Surgical Procedures on the Spine and Spinal Cord

(For application of caliper or tongs, use 20660)

(For treatment of fracture or dislocation of spine, see 22310-22327)

AMA *CPT Assistant* ☐

62380: Feb 17: 12

Plain English Description

Spinal cord and/or nerve root(s) decompression is done endoscopically. Compression symptoms include local or radiating pain, reduced mobility, and neurologic compromise. A needle/guidewire is inserted through the skin on one side of the midline and advanced to the involved level using fluoroscopic guidance. Small incisions are made around the needle/guidewire. Metal dilating tubes in graduating sizes are passed over the guidewire, gently spreading soft tissue and muscles away from the vertebrae. The needle/guidewire is removed. A hollow metal cylinder is passed over the metal dilator and the dilator is removed. The endoscope is inserted through the metal cylinder and the surgeon visualizes the targeted area on a projection screen. A nerve retractor is passed down a working channel of the endoscope and the spinal nerve is gently moved aside. Surgical instruments are then passed down another working channel of the endoscope and bony lamina is removed (laminotomy), as well as facet joints (partial facetectomy) and bone from around the neural foramen (foraminotomy). Herniated intervertebral disc may be partially or totally removed (discectomy). The retracted nerve is allowed to move back into place. The endoscope is removed. The metal cylinder is removed, allowing soft tissue to close the incision. Skin may be closed with suture or staple or covered with a dressing.

ICD-10-CM Diagnostic Codes

	M51.05	Intervertebral disc disorders with myelopathy, thoracolumbar region
	M51.06	Intervertebral disc disorders with myelopathy, lumbar region
	M51.15	Intervertebral disc disorders with radiculopathy, thoracolumbar region
	M51.16	Intervertebral disc disorders with radiculopathy, lumbar region
	M51.17	Intervertebral disc disorders with radiculopathy, lumbosacral region
	M51.25	Other intervertebral disc displacement, thoracolumbar region
	M51.26	Other intervertebral disc displacement, lumbar region
	M51.27	Other intervertebral disc displacement, lumbosacral region
	M51.35	Other intervertebral disc degeneration, thoracolumbar region
	M51.36	Other intervertebral disc degeneration, lumbar region
	M51.37	Other intervertebral disc degeneration, lumbosacral region
	M51.46	Schmorl's nodes, lumbar region
	M51.47	Schmorl's nodes, lumbosacral region
	M51.85	Other intervertebral disc disorders, thoracolumbar region
	M51.86	Other intervertebral disc disorders, lumbar region
	M51.87	Other intervertebral disc disorders, lumbosacral region
	M53.85	Other specified dorsopathies, thoracolumbar region
	M53.86	Other specified dorsopathies, lumbar region
	M53.87	Other specified dorsopathies, lumbosacral region
	M54.15	Radiculopathy, thoracolumbar region
	M54.16	Radiculopathy, lumbar region
	M54.17	Radiculopathy, lumbosacral region
⇄	M54.31	Sciatica, right side
⇄	M54.32	Sciatica, left side
	M54.89	Other dorsalgia
	M99.53	Intervertebral disc stenosis of neural canal of lumbar region
	M99.73	Connective tissue and disc stenosis of intervertebral foramina of lumbar region

CCI Edits

Refer to Appendix A for CCI edits.

Facility RVUs ☐

Code	Work	PE Facility	MP	Total Facility
62380	0.00	0.00	0.00	0.00

Non-facility RVUs ☐

Code	Work	PE Non-Facility	MP	Total Non-Facility
62380	0.00	0.00	0.00	0.00

Modifiers (PAR) ☐

Code	Mod 50	Mod 51	Mod 62	Mod 66	Mod 80
62380	1	2	2	0	2

Global Period

Code	Days
62380	090

63001-63011

63001 Laminectomy with exploration and/or decompression of spinal cord and/or cauda equina, without facetectomy, foraminotomy or discectomy (eg, spinal stenosis), 1 or 2 vertebral segments; cervical

63003 Laminectomy with exploration and/or decompression of spinal cord and/or cauda equina, without facetectomy, foraminotomy or discectomy (eg, spinal stenosis), 1 or 2 vertebral segments; thoracic

63005 Laminectomy with exploration and/or decompression of spinal cord and/or cauda equina, without facetectomy, foraminotomy or discectomy (eg, spinal stenosis), 1 or 2 vertebral segments; lumbar, except for spondylolisthesis

63011 Laminectomy with exploration and/or decompression of spinal cord and/or cauda equina, without facetectomy, foraminotomy or discectomy (eg, spinal stenosis), 1 or 2 vertebral segments; sacral

AMA Coding Guideline

Posterior Extradural Laminotomy or Laminectomy for Exploration/ Decompression of Neural Elements or Excision of Herniated Intervertebral Disks Procedures

Definitions

For purposes of CPT coding, the following definitions of approach and visualization apply. The primary approach and visualization define the service, whether another method is incidentally applied. Surgical services are presumed open, unless otherwise specified.

Percutaneous: Image-guided procedures (eg, computer tomography [CT] or fluoroscopy) performed with indirect visualization of the spine without the use of any device that allows visualization through a surgical incision.

Endoscopic: Spinal procedures performed with continuous direct visualization of the spine through an endoscope.

Open: Spinal procedures performed with continuous direct visualization of the spine through a surgical opening.

Indirect visualization: Image-guided (eg, CT or fluoroscopy), not light-based visualization.

Direct visualization: Light-based visualization; can be performed by eye, or with surgical loupes, microscope, or endoscope.

AMA Coding Notes

Posterior Extradural Laminotomy or Laminectomy for Exploration/ Decompression of Neural Elements or Excision of Herniated Intervertebral Disks Procedures

(When 63001-63048 are followed by arthrodesis, see 22590-22614)

(For the techniques of microsurgery and/or use of microscope, use 69990)

(For percutaneous decompression, see 62287, 0274T, 0275T)

Surgical Procedures on the Spine and Spinal Cord

(For application of caliper or tongs, use 20660)

(For treatment of fracture or dislocation of spine, see 22310-22327)

AMA *CPT Assistant* □

63001: Jan 01: 12, Jun 07: 1, Jul 11: 13, Jul 12: 3, Jul 13: 3

63003: Jan 01: 12, Jul 12: 3, Jul 13: 3

63005: Jan 01: 12, Jul 12: 3, Jul 13: 3, Dec 13: 17

63011: Jan 01: 12, Jul 13: 3

Plain English Description

Laminectomy (lamina excision) is performed to determine the cause of back pain and to relieve pressure on the spinal cord, spinal nerve roots, and/or cauda equina. The lamina is the portion of the vertebra that forms the posterior aspect of the vertebral arch. A posterior skin incision is made over the affected portion of the spine. Overlying fat and muscle are retracted off the lamina. The lamina is excised. The underlying paired ligaments (ligamentum flavum) that bind the lamina of contiguous vertebrae together are also excised. The spinal canal is exposed and explored. Adhesions between the dura and ligamentum flavum are lysed. The spinal nerve roots and/or cauda equina are carefully dissected and freed within the intervertebral foramen. The procedure may be performed on a single vertebra or two contiguous vertebrae. Separately reportable arthrodesis is performed as needed to stabilize the spine. Laminectomy of 1 or 2 vertebral segments of the cervical spine is reported with 63001, thoracic spine with 63003, lumbar spine with 63005, and sacral spine with 63011.

Laminectomy with exploration and/or decompression of spinal cord, 1 or 2 vertebral segments

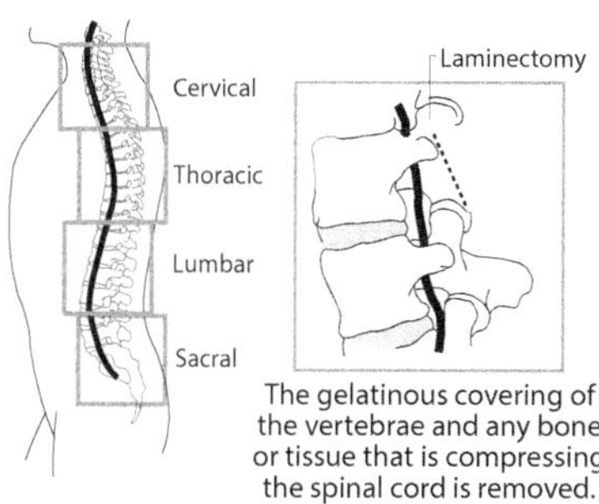

The gelatinous covering of the vertebrae and any bone or tissue that is compressing the spinal cord is removed.

ICD-10-CM Diagnostic Codes

G12.25	Progressive spinal muscle atrophy
G54.1	Lumbosacral plexus disorders
G83.4	Cauda equina syndrome
G95.29	Other cord compression
M46.02	Spinal enthesopathy, cervical region
M46.03	Spinal enthesopathy, cervicothoracic region
M46.04	Spinal enthesopathy, thoracic region
M46.05	Spinal enthesopathy, thoracolumbar region
M46.06	Spinal enthesopathy, lumbar region
M46.07	Spinal enthesopathy, lumbosacral region
M46.08	Spinal enthesopathy, sacral and sacrococcygeal region
M46.42	Discitis, unspecified, cervical region
M46.43	Discitis, unspecified, cervicothoracic region
M46.45	Discitis, unspecified, thoracolumbar region
M46.46	Discitis, unspecified, lumbar region
M46.47	Discitis, unspecified, lumbosacral region
M47.011	Anterior spinal artery compression syndromes, occipito-atlanto-axial region
M47.012	Anterior spinal artery compression syndromes, cervical region
M47.013	Anterior spinal artery compression syndromes, cervicothoracic region
M47.014	Anterior spinal artery compression syndromes, thoracic region
M47.015	Anterior spinal artery compression syndromes, thoracolumbar region
M47.016	Anterior spinal artery compression syndromes, lumbar region
M47.12	Other spondylosis with myelopathy, cervical region
M47.13	Other spondylosis with myelopathy, cervicothoracic region
M47.14	Other spondylosis with myelopathy, thoracic region
M47.15	Other spondylosis with myelopathy, thoracolumbar region
M47.16	Other spondylosis with myelopathy, lumbar region
M48.02	Spinal stenosis, cervical region
M48.03	Spinal stenosis, cervicothoracic region

M48.04 Spinal stenosis, thoracic region
M48.05 Spinal stenosis, thoracolumbar region
M48.061 Spinal stenosis, lumbar region without neurogenic claudication
M48.062 Spinal stenosis, lumbar region with neurogenic claudication
M48.07 Spinal stenosis, lumbosacral region
M48.08 Spinal stenosis, sacral and sacrococcygeal region
⑦ M48.52 Collapsed vertebra, not elsewhere classified, cervical region
⑦ M48.53 Collapsed vertebra, not elsewhere classified, cervicothoracic region
⑦ M48.54 Collapsed vertebra, not elsewhere classified, thoracic region
⑦ M48.55 Collapsed vertebra, not elsewhere classified, thoracolumbar region
⑦ M48.56 Collapsed vertebra, not elsewhere classified, lumbar region
⑦ M48.57 Collapsed vertebra, not elsewhere classified, lumbosacral region
M48.8X2 Other specified spondylopathies, cervical region
M48.8X3 Other specified spondylopathies, cervicothoracic region
M48.8X4 Other specified spondylopathies, thoracic region
M48.8X5 Other specified spondylopathies, thoracolumbar region
M48.8X6 Other specified spondylopathies, lumbar region
M48.8X7 Other specified spondylopathies, lumbosacral region
M50.01 Cervical disc disorder with myelopathy, high cervical region
M50.021 Cervical disc disorder at C4-C5 level with myelopathy
M50.022 Cervical disc disorder at C5-C6 level with myelopathy
M50.023 Cervical disc disorder at C6-C7 level with myelopathy
M50.121 Cervical disc disorder at C4-C5 level with radiculopathy
M50.122 Cervical disc disorder at C5-C6 level with radiculopathy
M50.123 Cervical disc disorder at C6-C7 level with radiculopathy
M50.821 Other cervical disc disorders at C4-C5 level
M50.822 Other cervical disc disorders at C5-C6 level
M50.823 Other cervical disc disorders at C6-C7 level
M50.83 Other cervical disc disorders, cervicothoracic region
M51.04 Intervertebral disc disorders with myelopathy, thoracic region
M51.05 Intervertebral disc disorders with myelopathy, thoracolumbar region
M51.06 Intervertebral disc disorders with myelopathy, lumbar region
M51.07 Intervertebral disc disorders with myelopathy, lumbosacral region
M51.15 Intervertebral disc disorders with radiculopathy, thoracolumbar region
M51.17 Intervertebral disc disorders with radiculopathy, lumbosacral region
M51.24 Other intervertebral disc displacement, thoracic region
M51.25 Other intervertebral disc displacement, thoracolumbar region
M51.26 Other intervertebral disc displacement, lumbar region
M51.27 Other intervertebral disc displacement, lumbosacral region
M51.34 Other intervertebral disc degeneration, thoracic region
M51.35 Other intervertebral disc degeneration, thoracolumbar region
M51.36 Other intervertebral disc degeneration, lumbar region
M51.37 Other intervertebral disc degeneration, lumbosacral region
M54.12 Radiculopathy, cervical region
M54.13 Radiculopathy, cervicothoracic region
M54.14 Radiculopathy, thoracic region
M54.15 Radiculopathy, thoracolumbar region
M54.16 Radiculopathy, lumbar region
M54.17 Radiculopathy, lumbosacral region
M96.1 Postlaminectomy syndrome, not elsewhere classified
⑦ S14.153 Other incomplete lesion at C3 level of cervical spinal cord
⑦ S14.154 Other incomplete lesion at C4 level of cervical spinal cord
⑦ S14.155 Other incomplete lesion at C5 level of cervical spinal cord
⑦ S14.156 Other incomplete lesion at C6 level of cervical spinal cord
⑦ S14.157 Other incomplete lesion at C7 level of cervical spinal cord
⑦ S14.158 Other incomplete lesion at C8 level of cervical spinal cord
⑦ S24.151 Other incomplete lesion at T1 level of thoracic spinal cord
⑦ S24.152 Other incomplete lesion at T2-T6 level of thoracic spinal cord
⑦ S24.153 Other incomplete lesion at T7-T10 level of thoracic spinal cord
⑦ S24.154 Other incomplete lesion at T11-T12 level of thoracic spinal cord

ICD-10-CM Coding Notes

For codes requiring a 7th character extension, refer to your ICD-10-CM book. Review the character descriptions and coding guidelines for proper selection. For some procedures, only certain characters will apply.

CCI Edits

Refer to Appendix A for CCI edits.

Facility RVUs ▯

Code	Work	PE Facility	MP	Total Facility
63001	17.61	12.27	5.84	35.72
63003	17.74	12.31	5.70	35.75
63005	16.43	12.70	5.31	34.44
63011	15.91	11.59	3.92	31.42

Non-facility RVUs ▯

Code	Work	PE Non-Facility	MP	Total Non-Facility
63001	17.61	12.27	5.84	35.72
63003	17.74	12.31	5.70	35.75
63005	16.43	12.70	5.31	34.44
63011	15.91	11.59	3.92	31.42

Modifiers (PAR) ▯

Code	Mod 50	Mod 51	Mod 62	Mod 66	Mod 80
63001	0	2	2	0	2
63003	0	2	2	0	2
63005	0	2	2	0	2
63011	0	2	2	0	2

Global Period

Code	Days
63001	090
63003	090
63005	090
63011	090

63012

63012 Laminectomy with removal of abnormal facets and/or pars inter-articularis with decompression of cauda equina and nerve roots for spondylolisthesis, lumbar (Gill type procedure)

AMA Coding Guideline

Posterior Extradural Laminotomy or Laminectomy for Exploration/ Decompression of Neural Elements or Excision of Herniated Intervertebral Disks Procedures

Definitions

For purposes of CPT coding, the following definitions of approach and visualization apply. The primary approach and visualization define the service, whether another method is incidentally applied. Surgical services are presumed open, unless otherwise specified.

Percutaneous: Image-guided procedures (eg, computer tomography [CT] or fluoroscopy) performed with indirect visualization of the spine without the use of any device that allows visualization through a surgical incision.

Endoscopic: Spinal procedures performed with continuous direct visualization of the spine through an endoscope.

Open: Spinal procedures performed with continuous direct visualization of the spine through a surgical opening.

Indirect visualization: Image-guided (eg, CT or fluoroscopy), not light-based visualization.

Direct visualization: Light-based visualization; can be performed by eye, or with surgical loupes, microscope, or endoscope.

AMA Coding Notes

Posterior Extradural Laminotomy or Laminectomy for Exploration/ Decompression of Neural Elements or Excision of Herniated Intervertebral Disks Procedures

(When 63001-63048 are followed by arthrodesis, see 22590-22614)

(For the techniques of microsurgery and/or use of microscope, use 69990)

(For percutaneous decompression, see 62287, 0274T, 0275T)

Surgical Procedures on the Spine and Spinal Cord

(For application of caliper or tongs, use 20660)

(For treatment of fracture or dislocation of spine, see 22310-22327)

AMA *CPT Assistant* ▯

63012: Jan 01: 12, Jul 13: 3

Plain English Description

Spondylolisthesis is a condition in which one of the lower lumbar vertebral bodies, usually the fifth vertebral body, slips forward on the vertebral body below it. The condition begins with spondylolysis, which refers to degeneration or deficient development of the pars interarticularis of the slipped vertebra. The pars interarticularis is the segment of bone between the superior and inferior articular facets. A posterior skin incision is made over the affected vertebrae of the lumbar spine. Overlying fat and muscle are retracted off the lamina. The lamina is excised. The underlying paired ligaments (ligamentum flavum) that bind the lamina of contiguous vertebrae together are also excised. The superior and inferior articular facets and the pars interarticularis are inspected and smoothed or excised as needed. The spinal canal is exposed and explored. Adhesions between the dura and ligamentum flavum are lysed. The spinal nerve roots and/or cauda equina are carefully dissected and freed within the intervertebral foramen. The surgical wound is closed in layers.

Laminectomy with removal of abnormal facets and/or pars inter-articularis with decompression of cauda equina and nerve roots for spondylolisthesis

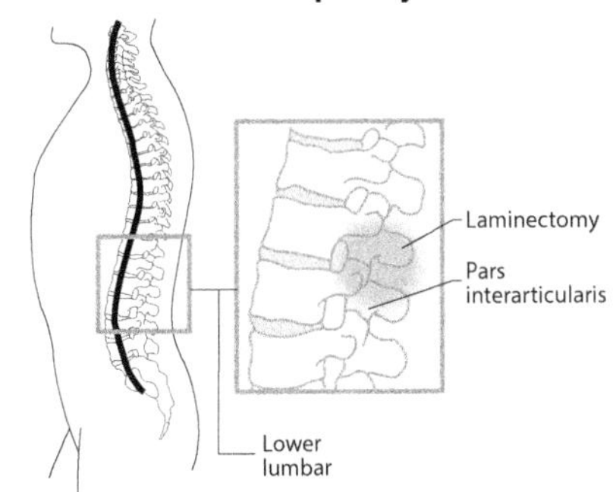

ICD-10-CM Diagnostic Codes

G83.4	Cauda equina syndrome
M43.15	Spondylolisthesis, thoracolumbar region
M43.16	Spondylolisthesis, lumbar region
M43.17	Spondylolisthesis, lumbosacral region
M43.18	Spondylolisthesis, sacral and sacrococcygeal region
M51.06	Intervertebral disc disorders with myelopathy, lumbar region
M51.16	Intervertebral disc disorders with radiculopathy, lumbar region
Q06.3	Other congenital cauda equina malformations
Q76.2	Congenital spondylolisthesis

CCI Edits

Refer to Appendix A for CCI edits.

Facility RVUs ▯

Code	Work	PE Facility	MP	Total Facility
63012	16.85	12.43	5.26	34.54

Non-facility RVUs ▯

Code	Work	PE Non-Facility	MP	Total Non-Facility
63012	16.85	12.43	5.26	34.54

Modifiers (PAR) ▯

Code	Mod 50	Mod 51	Mod 62	Mod 66	Mod 80
63012	0	2	2	0	2

Global Period

Code	Days
63012	090

63015-63017

63015 Laminectomy with exploration and/or decompression of spinal cord and/or cauda equina, without facetectomy, foraminotomy or discectomy (eg, spinal stenosis), more than 2 vertebral segments; cervical

63016 Laminectomy with exploration and/or decompression of spinal cord and/or cauda equina, without facetectomy, foraminotomy or discectomy (eg, spinal stenosis), more than 2 vertebral segments; thoracic

63017 Laminectomy with exploration and/or decompression of spinal cord and/or cauda equina, without facetectomy, foraminotomy or discectomy (eg, spinal stenosis), more than 2 vertebral segments; lumbar

AMA Coding Guideline

Posterior Extradural Laminotomy or Laminectomy for Exploration/ Decompression of Neural Elements or Excision of Herniated Intervertebral Disks Procedures

Definitions

For purposes of CPT coding, the following definitions of approach and visualization apply. The primary approach and visualization define the service, whether another method is incidentally applied. Surgical services are presumed open, unless otherwise specified.

Percutaneous: Image-guided procedures (eg, computer tomography [CT] or fluoroscopy) performed with indirect visualization of the spine without the use of any device that allows visualization through a surgical incision.

Endoscopic: Spinal procedures performed with continuous direct visualization of the spine through an endoscope.

Open: Spinal procedures performed with continuous direct visualization of the spine through a surgical opening.

Indirect visualization: Image-guided (eg, CT or fluoroscopy), not light-based visualization.

Direct visualization: Light-based visualization; can be performed by eye, or with surgical loupes, microscope, or endoscope.

AMA Coding Notes

Posterior Extradural Laminotomy or Laminectomy for Exploration/ Decompression of Neural Elements or Excision of Herniated Intervertebral Disks Procedures

(When 63001-63048 are followed by arthrodesis, see 22590-22614)

(For the techniques of microsurgery and/or use of microscope, use 69990)

(For percutaneous decompression, see 62287, 0274T, 0275T)

Surgical Procedures on the Spine and Spinal Cord

(For application of caliper or tongs, use 20660)

(For treatment of fracture or dislocation of spine, see 22310-22327)

AMA *CPT Assistant* ▯

63015: Jan 01: 12, Jul 13: 3
63016: Jan 01: 12, Jul 13: 3
63017: Jan 01: 12, Jul 13: 3

Plain English Description

Laminectomy (lamina excision) is performed to determine the cause of back pain and to relieve pressure on the spinal cord, spinal nerve roots, and/or cauda equina. The lamina is the portion of the vertebra that forms the posterior aspect of the vertebral arch. A posterior skin incision is made over the affected portion of the spine. Overlying fat and muscle are retracted off the lamina. The lamina is excised. The underlying paired ligaments (ligamentum flavum) that bind the lamina of contiguous vertebrae together are also excised. The spinal canal is exposed and explored. Adhesions between the dura and ligamentum flavum are lysed. The spinal nerve roots and/or cauda equina are carefully dissected and freed within the intervertebral foramen. The procedure is performed on more than two contiguous vertebrae. Separately reportable arthrodesis is performed as needed to stabilize the spine. Laminectomy of more than 2 vertebral segments of the cervical spine is reported with 63015, more than 2 vertebral segments of the thoracic spine with 63016, and more than 2 vertebral segments of the lumbar spine with 63017.

Laminectomy with exploration and/or decompression of spinal cord, more than two vertebral segments

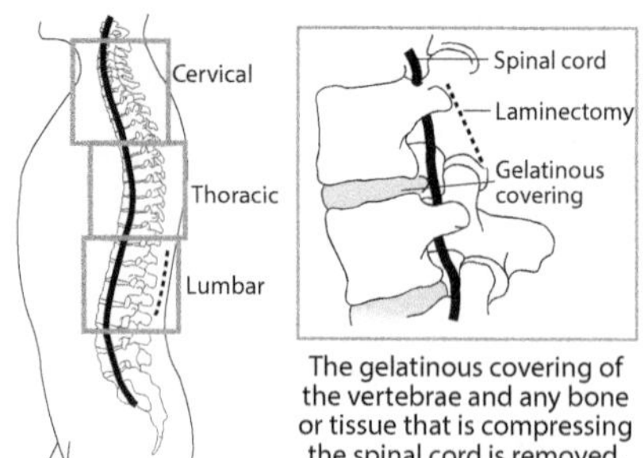

Cervical (63015); thoracic (63016); lumbar (63017)

ICD-10-CM Diagnostic Codes

	Code	Description
	G12.25	Progressive spinal muscle atrophy
	G54.1	Lumbosacral plexus disorders
	G83.4	Cauda equina syndrome
	G95.29	Other cord compression
	M46.02	Spinal enthesopathy, cervical region
	M46.03	Spinal enthesopathy, cervicothoracic region
	M46.04	Spinal enthesopathy, thoracic region
	M46.05	Spinal enthesopathy, thoracolumbar region
	M46.06	Spinal enthesopathy, lumbar region
	M46.07	Spinal enthesopathy, lumbosacral region
	M46.08	Spinal enthesopathy, sacral and sacrococcygeal region
	M46.42	Discitis, unspecified, cervical region
	M46.43	Discitis, unspecified, cervicothoracic region
	M46.45	Discitis, unspecified, thoracolumbar region
	M46.46	Discitis, unspecified, lumbar region
	M46.47	Discitis, unspecified, lumbosacral region
	M47.011	Anterior spinal artery compression syndromes, occipito-atlanto-axial region
	M47.012	Anterior spinal artery compression syndromes, cervical region
	M47.013	Anterior spinal artery compression syndromes, cervicothoracic region
	M47.014	Anterior spinal artery compression syndromes, thoracic region
	M47.015	Anterior spinal artery compression syndromes, thoracolumbar region
	M47.016	Anterior spinal artery compression syndromes, lumbar region
	M47.12	Other spondylosis with myelopathy, cervical region
	M47.13	Other spondylosis with myelopathy, cervicothoracic region
	M47.14	Other spondylosis with myelopathy, thoracic region
	M47.15	Other spondylosis with myelopathy, thoracolumbar region
	M47.16	Other spondylosis with myelopathy, lumbar region
	M48.02	Spinal stenosis, cervical region
	M48.03	Spinal stenosis, cervicothoracic region
	M48.04	Spinal stenosis, thoracic region
	M48.05	Spinal stenosis, thoracolumbar region
	M48.061	Spinal stenosis, lumbar region without neurogenic claudication
	M48.062	Spinal stenosis, lumbar region with neurogenic claudication
	M48.07	Spinal stenosis, lumbosacral region
	M48.08	Spinal stenosis, sacral and sacrococcygeal region
❼	M48.52	Collapsed vertebra, not elsewhere classified, cervical region
❼	M48.53	Collapsed vertebra, not elsewhere classified, cervicothoracic region
❼	M48.54	Collapsed vertebra, not elsewhere classified, thoracic region
❼	M48.55	Collapsed vertebra, not elsewhere classified, thoracolumbar region
❼	M48.56	Collapsed vertebra, not elsewhere classified, lumbar region

⑦	M48.57	Collapsed vertebra, not elsewhere classified, lumbosacral region
	M48.8X2	Other specified spondylopathies, cervical region
	M48.8X3	Other specified spondylopathies, cervicothoracic region
	M48.8X4	Other specified spondylopathies, thoracic region
	M48.8X5	Other specified spondylopathies, thoracolumbar region
	M48.8X6	Other specified spondylopathies, lumbar region
	M48.8X7	Other specified spondylopathies, lumbosacral region
	M50.021	Cervical disc disorder at C4-C5 level with myelopathy
	M50.022	Cervical disc disorder at C5-C6 level with myelopathy
	M50.023	Cervical disc disorder at C6-C7 level with myelopathy
	M50.121	Cervical disc disorder at C4-C5 level with radiculopathy
	M50.122	Cervical disc disorder at C5-C6 level with radiculopathy
	M50.123	Cervical disc disorder at C6-C7 level with radiculopathy
	M50.821	Other cervical disc disorders at C4-C5 level
	M50.822	Other cervical disc disorders at C5-C6 level
	M50.823	Other cervical disc disorders at C6-C7 level
	M50.83	Other cervical disc disorders, cervicothoracic region
	M51.04	Intervertebral disc disorders with myelopathy, thoracic region
	M51.05	Intervertebral disc disorders with myelopathy, thoracolumbar region
	M51.06	Intervertebral disc disorders with myelopathy, lumbar region
	M51.07	Intervertebral disc disorders with myelopathy, lumbosacral region
	M51.15	Intervertebral disc disorders with radiculopathy, thoracolumbar region
	M51.17	Intervertebral disc disorders with radiculopathy, lumbosacral region
	M51.24	Other intervertebral disc displacement, thoracic region
	M51.25	Other intervertebral disc displacement, thoracolumbar region
	M51.26	Other intervertebral disc displacement, lumbar region
	M51.27	Other intervertebral disc displacement, lumbosacral region
	M51.34	Other intervertebral disc degeneration, thoracic region
	M51.35	Other intervertebral disc degeneration, thoracolumbar region
	M51.36	Other intervertebral disc degeneration, lumbar region
	M51.37	Other intervertebral disc degeneration, lumbosacral region
	M54.12	Radiculopathy, cervical region
	M54.13	Radiculopathy, cervicothoracic region
	M54.14	Radiculopathy, thoracic region
	M54.15	Radiculopathy, thoracolumbar region
	M54.16	Radiculopathy, lumbar region
	M54.17	Radiculopathy, lumbosacral region
	M96.1	Postlaminectomy syndrome, not elsewhere classified
⑦	S14.153	Other incomplete lesion at C3 level of cervical spinal cord
⑦	S14.154	Other incomplete lesion at C4 level of cervical spinal cord
⑦	S14.155	Other incomplete lesion at C5 level of cervical spinal cord
⑦	S14.156	Other incomplete lesion at C6 level of cervical spinal cord
⑦	S14.157	Other incomplete lesion at C7 level of cervical spinal cord
⑦	S14.158	Other incomplete lesion at C8 level of cervical spinal cord
⑦	S24.151	Other incomplete lesion at T1 level of thoracic spinal cord
⑦	S24.152	Other incomplete lesion at T2-T6 level of thoracic spinal cord
⑦	S24.153	Other incomplete lesion at T7-T10 level of thoracic spinal cord
⑦	S24.154	Other incomplete lesion at T11-T12 level of thoracic spinal cord

ICD-10-CM Coding Notes

For codes requiring a 7th character extension, refer to your ICD-10-CM book. Review the character descriptions and coding guidelines for proper selection. For some procedures, only certain characters will apply.

CCI Edits

Refer to Appendix A for CCI edits.

Facility RVUs ▯

Code	Work	PE Facility	MP	Total Facility
63015	20.85	14.87	7.05	42.77
63016	22.03	14.86	7.12	44.01
63017	17.33	13.22	5.84	36.39

Non-facility RVUs ▯

Code	Work	PE Non-Facility	MP	Total Non-Facility
63015	20.85	14.87	7.05	42.77
63016	22.03	14.86	7.12	44.01
63017	17.33	13.22	5.84	36.39

Modifiers (PAR) ▯

Code	Mod 50	Mod 51	Mod 62	Mod 66	Mod 80
63015	0	2	2	0	2
63016	0	2	2	0	2
63017	0	2	2	0	2

Global Period

Code	Days
63015	090
63016	090
63017	090

63020-63035

63020 Laminotomy (hemilaminectomy), with decompression of nerve root(s), including partial facetectomy, foraminotomy and/or excision of herniated intervertebral disc; 1 interspace, cervical

(For bilateral procedure, report 63020 with modifier 50)

63030 Laminotomy (hemilaminectomy), with decompression of nerve root(s), including partial facetectomy, foraminotomy and/or excision of herniated intervertebral disc; 1 interspace, lumbar

(For bilateral procedure, report 63030 with modifier 50)

✚ **63035 Laminotomy (hemilaminectomy), with decompression of nerve root(s), including partial facetectomy, foraminotomy and/or excision of herniated intervertebral disc; each additional interspace, cervical or lumbar (List separately in addition to code for primary procedure)**

(Use 63035 in conjunction with 63020-63030)

(For bilateral procedure, report 63035 twice. Do not report modifier 50 in conjunction with 63035)

(For percutaneous endoscopic approach, see 0274T, 0275T)

AMA Coding Guideline

Posterior Extradural Laminotomy or Laminectomy for Exploration/ Decompression of Neural Elements or Excision of Herniated Intervertebral Disks Procedures

Definitions

For purposes of CPT coding, the following definitions of approach and visualization apply. The primary approach and visualization define the service, whether another method is incidentally applied. Surgical services are presumed open, unless otherwise specified.

Percutaneous: Image-guided procedures (eg, computer tomography [CT] or fluoroscopy) performed with indirect visualization of the spine without the use of any device that allows visualization through a surgical incision.

Endoscopic: Spinal procedures performed with continuous direct visualization of the spine through an endoscope.

Open: Spinal procedures performed with continuous direct visualization of the spine through a surgical opening.

Indirect visualization: Image-guided (eg, CT or fluoroscopy), not light-based visualization.

Direct visualization: Light-based visualization; can be performed by eye, or with surgical loupes, microscope, or endoscope.

AMA Coding Notes

Posterior Extradural Laminotomy or Laminectomy for Exploration/ Decompression of Neural Elements or Excision of Herniated Intervertebral Disks Procedures

(When 63001-63048 are followed by arthrodesis, see 22590-22614)

(For the techniques of microsurgery and/or use of microscope, use 69990)

(For percutaneous decompression, see 62287, 0274T, 0275T)

Surgical Procedures on the Spine and Spinal Cord

(For application of caliper or tongs, use 20660)

(For treatment of fracture or dislocation of spine, see 22310-22327)

AMA *CPT Assistant*

63020: Nov 99: 36, Jan 01: 12, Jul 12: 4, Dec 12: 13, Jul 13: 3

63030: Mar 96: 7, Nov 99: 36, Jan 01: 12, Feb 01: 10, Sep 02: 10, Oct 04: 12, Oct 08: 10, Oct 09: 9, Nov 10: 4, Mar 11: 7, Jul 11: 13, Jul 12: 3, 4, Dec 12: 13, Jul 13: 3, Dec 13: 17, May 16: 13, Feb 17: 13

63035: Fall 91: 8, Mar 96: 7, Nov 99: 36, Jan 01: 12, Feb 01: 10, Jul 12: 4

Plain English Description

A posterior approach laminotomy or hemilaminectomy with nerve root decompression is carried out on one interspace, including partial facetectomy, foraminotomy, and/or excision of a herniated intervertebral disc. A laminotomy is an incision into the lamina of the vertebral arch to open the space and decompress the spinal cord or nerve roots. It is sometimes performed as a hemilaminectomy, removing a portion of the lamina from the left or right side, usually with a portion of the facet joint also. The skin incision is marked out and carried down to the spinous processes. Muscle is retracted off the lamina and facet joint. The level is verified radiographically, and an operating microscope is brought in. A bone drill is used to remove part of the lamina and the facet joint (partial facetectomy) to allow more room for the compressed nerve(s). The ligamentum flavum attaching the vertebral lamina may be removed to expose the dura and compressed nerves. The openings under the facet joints where the nerve runs through are checked, and a portion of the bone around the opening may be removed for additional pressure relief, if necessary (foraminotomy). Ruptured disc fragments or bulging nucleus pulposus are also removed to decompress the nerve(s). The surgical wound is closed in layers.

Code 63020 reports one cervical interspace; code 63030 reports one lumbar interspace; and code 63035 is used for each additional interspace, either cervical or lumbar.

Laminotomy (hemilaminectomy) with decompression of nerve root(s)

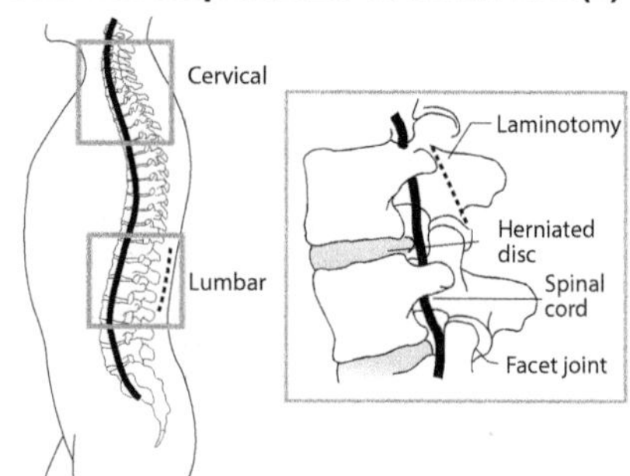

1 interspace, cervical (63020); 1 interspace lumbar (63030); each additional interspace, cervical or lumbar (63035)

ICD-10-CM Diagnostic Codes

G54.1	Lumbosacral plexus disorders
G54.2	Cervical root disorders, not elsewhere classified
G54.4	Lumbosacral root disorders, not elsewhere classified
G54.8	Other nerve root and plexus disorders
G55	Nerve root and plexus compressions in diseases classified elsewhere
G95.29	Other cord compression
M43.12	Spondylolisthesis, cervical region
M43.13	Spondylolisthesis, cervicothoracic region
M45.2	Ankylosing spondylitis of cervical region
M45.6	Ankylosing spondylitis lumbar region
M46.02	Spinal enthesopathy, cervical region
M46.06	Spinal enthesopathy, lumbar region
M46.42	Discitis, unspecified, cervical region
M46.46	Discitis, unspecified, lumbar region
M46.82	Other specified inflammatory spondylopathies, cervical region
M46.86	Other specified inflammatory spondylopathies, lumbar region
M47.012	Anterior spinal artery compression syndromes, cervical region
M47.016	Anterior spinal artery compression syndromes, lumbar region
M47.022	Vertebral artery compression syndromes, cervical region
M47.16	Other spondylosis with myelopathy, lumbar region
M47.22	Other spondylosis with radiculopathy, cervical region
M47.26	Other spondylosis with radiculopathy, lumbar region
M48.02	Spinal stenosis, cervical region
M48.062	Spinal stenosis, lumbar region with neurogenic claudication
M48.07	Spinal stenosis, lumbosacral region
M48.32	Traumatic spondylopathy, cervical region

	M48.36	Traumatic spondylopathy, lumbar region
⑦	M48.52	Collapsed vertebra, not elsewhere classified, cervical region
⑦	M48.56	Collapsed vertebra, not elsewhere classified, lumbar region
	M48.8X2	Other specified spondylopathies, cervical region
	M48.8X6	Other specified spondylopathies, lumbar region
	M50.11	Cervical disc disorder with radiculopathy, high cervical region
	M50.121	Cervical disc disorder at C4-C5 level with radiculopathy
	M50.122	Cervical disc disorder at C5-C6 level with radiculopathy
	M50.123	Cervical disc disorder at C6-C7 level with radiculopathy
	M50.21	Other cervical disc displacement, high cervical region
	M50.221	Other cervical disc displacement at C4-C5 level
	M50.222	Other cervical disc displacement at C5-C6 level
	M50.223	Other cervical disc displacement at C6-C7 level
	M50.81	Other cervical disc disorders, high cervical region
	M50.821	Other cervical disc disorders at C4-C5 level
	M50.822	Other cervical disc disorders at C5-C6 level
	M50.823	Other cervical disc disorders at C6-C7 level
	M51.16	Intervertebral disc disorders with radiculopathy, lumbar region
	M51.26	Other intervertebral disc displacement, lumbar region
	M51.36	Other intervertebral disc degeneration, lumbar region
	M54.12	Radiculopathy, cervical region
	M54.16	Radiculopathy, lumbar region

ICD-10-CM Coding Notes

For codes requiring a 7th character extension, refer to your ICD-10-CM book. Review the character descriptions and coding guidelines for proper selection. For some procedures, only certain characters will apply.

CCI Edits

Refer to Appendix A for CCI edits.

Facility RVUs ▯

Code	Work	PE Facility	MP	Total Facility
63020	16.20	12.41	4.87	33.48
63030	13.18	11.01	3.92	28.11
63035	3.15	1.50	0.90	5.55

Non-facility RVUs ▯

Code	Work	PE Non-Facility	MP	Total Non-Facility
63020	16.20	12.41	4.87	33.48
63030	13.18	11.01	3.92	28.11
63035	3.15	1.50	0.90	5.55

Modifiers (PAR) ▯

Code	Mod 50	Mod 51	Mod 62	Mod 66	Mod 80
63020	1	2	2	0	2
63030	1	2	2	0	2
63035	1	0	2	0	2

Global Period

Code	Days
63020	090
63030	090
63035	ZZZ

63040-63044

63040 Laminotomy (hemilaminectomy), with decompression of nerve root(s), including partial facetectomy, foraminotomy and/or excision of herniated intervertebral disc, reexploration, single interspace; cervical

(For bilateral procedure, report 63040 with modifier 50)

63042 Laminotomy (hemilaminectomy), with decompression of nerve root(s), including partial facetectomy, foraminotomy and/or excision of herniated intervertebral disc, reexploration, single interspace; lumbar

(For bilateral procedure, report 63042 with modifier 50)

+ **63043 Laminotomy (hemilaminectomy), with decompression of nerve root(s), including partial facetectomy, foraminotomy and/or excision of herniated intervertebral disc, reexploration, single interspace; each additional cervical interspace (List separately in addition to code for primary procedure)**

(Use 63043 in conjunction with 63040)

(For bilateral procedure, report 63043 twice. Do not report modifier 50 in conjunction with 63043)

+ **63044 Laminotomy (hemilaminectomy), with decompression of nerve root(s), including partial facetectomy, foraminotomy and/or excision of herniated intervertebral disc, reexploration, single interspace; each additional lumbar interspace (List separately in addition to code for primary procedure)**

(Use 63044 in conjunction with 63042)

(For bilateral procedure, report 63044 twice. Do not report modifier 50 in conjunction with 63044)

AMA Coding Guideline

Posterior Extradural Laminotomy or Laminectomy for Exploration/ Decompression of Neural Elements or Excision of Herniated Intervertebral Disks Procedures

Definitions

For purposes of CPT coding, the following definitions of approach and visualization apply. The primary approach and visualization define the service, whether another method is incidentally applied. Surgical services are presumed open, unless otherwise specified.

Percutaneous: Image-guided procedures (eg, computer tomography [CT] or fluoroscopy) performed with indirect visualization of the spine without the use of any device that allows visualization through a surgical incision.

Endoscopic: Spinal procedures performed with continuous direct visualization of the spine through an endoscope.

Open: Spinal procedures performed with continuous direct visualization of the spine through a surgical opening.

Indirect visualization: Image-guided (eg, CT or fluoroscopy), not light-based visualization.

Direct visualization: Light-based visualization; can be performed by eye, or with surgical loupes, microscope, or endoscope.

AMA Coding Notes

Posterior Extradural Laminotomy or Laminectomy for Exploration/ Decompression of Neural Elements or Excision of Herniated Intervertebral Disks Procedures

(When 63001-63048 are followed by arthrodesis, see 22590-22614)

(For the techniques of microsurgery and/or use of microscope, use 69990)

(For percutaneous decompression, see 62287, 0274T, 0275T)

Surgical Procedures on the Spine and Spinal Cord

(For application of caliper or tongs, use 20660)

(For treatment of fracture or dislocation of spine, see 22310-22327)

AMA *CPT Assistant*

63040: Jan 99: 11, Jan 01: 12, Jul 13: 3
63042: Jan 99: 11, Jan 01: 12, Oct 08: 10, Oct 09: 9, Jul 11: 13, Jul 13: 3

Plain English Description

Laminotomy (hemilaminectomy) for re-exploration of a previously explored cervical (63040, 63043) or lumbar (63042, 63044) disc space is performed with decompression of nerve roots. This procedure may include partial facetectomy, foraminotomy, and/or excision of herniated intervertebral disc. The previous skin incision is reopened and the disc space is exposed. Scar tissue over the laminae is removed and the laminotomy is enlarged. Scar tissue within the disc space is dissected. The nerve root is identified and explored. Scar tissue and bony spurs are removed. A portion of the flat articular surface (facet) of the vertebra may be excised (facetectomy). The foramen is enlarged as needed (foraminotomy). If a herniated disc is found, disc material is curetted from the disc space to decompress the nerve root. Upon completion of the procedure, bleeding is controlled by coagulation; the wound is irrigated; and incisions are closed. Use 63040 for laminotomy and re-exploration of a single cervical interspace and 63043 for each additional cervical interspace. Use 63042 for laminotomy and re-exploration of a single lumbar interspace and 63044 for each additional lumbar interspace.

Laminotomy (hemilaminectomy) with decompression of nerve root(s)

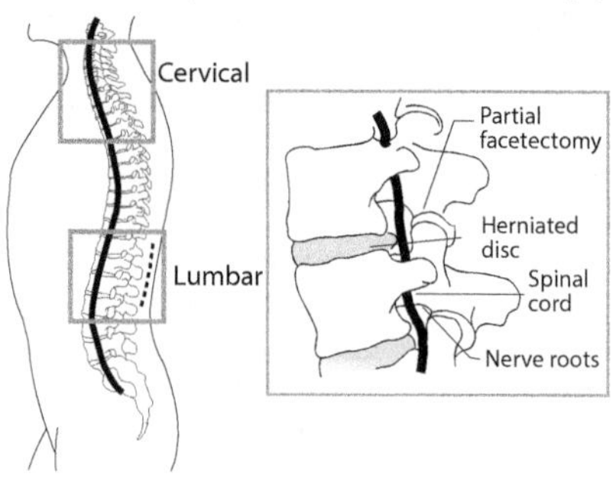

Cervical (63040); lumbar (63042); each additional cervical interspace (63043); each additional lumbar interspace (63044)

ICD-10-CM Diagnostic Codes

G12.25	Progressive spinal muscle atrophy
G54.1	Lumbosacral plexus disorders
G54.2	Cervical root disorders, not elsewhere classified
G54.4	Lumbosacral root disorders, not elsewhere classified
G54.8	Other nerve root and plexus disorders
G55	Nerve root and plexus compressions in diseases classified elsewhere
G95.29	Other cord compression
M43.12	Spondylolisthesis, cervical region
M43.13	Spondylolisthesis, cervicothoracic region
M45.2	Ankylosing spondylitis of cervical region
M45.6	Ankylosing spondylitis lumbar region
M46.02	Spinal enthesopathy, cervical region
M46.06	Spinal enthesopathy, lumbar region
M46.42	Discitis, unspecified, cervical region
M46.46	Discitis, unspecified, lumbar region
M46.82	Other specified inflammatory spondylopathies, cervical region
M46.86	Other specified inflammatory spondylopathies, lumbar region
M47.012	Anterior spinal artery compression syndromes, cervical region
M47.016	Anterior spinal artery compression syndromes, lumbar region
M47.022	Vertebral artery compression syndromes, cervical region
M47.22	Other spondylosis with radiculopathy, cervical region
M47.26	Other spondylosis with radiculopathy, lumbar region
M48.02	Spinal stenosis, cervical region
M48.062	Spinal stenosis, lumbar region with neurogenic claudication
M48.07	Spinal stenosis, lumbosacral region
M48.32	Traumatic spondylopathy, cervical region

	M48.36	Traumatic spondylopathy, lumbar region
➐	M48.52	Collapsed vertebra, not elsewhere classified, cervical region
➐	M48.56	Collapsed vertebra, not elsewhere classified, lumbar region
	M48.8X2	Other specified spondylopathies, cervical region
	M48.8X6	Other specified spondylopathies, lumbar region
	M50.021	Cervical disc disorder at C4-C5 level with myelopathy
	M50.022	Cervical disc disorder at C5-C6 level with myelopathy
	M50.023	Cervical disc disorder at C6-C7 level with myelopathy
	M50.11	Cervical disc disorder with radiculopathy, high cervical region
	M50.121	Cervical disc disorder at C4-C5 level with radiculopathy
	M50.122	Cervical disc disorder at C5-C6 level with radiculopathy
	M50.123	Cervical disc disorder at C6-C7 level with radiculopathy
	M50.21	Other cervical disc displacement, high cervical region
	M50.221	Other cervical disc displacement at C4-C5 level
	M50.222	Other cervical disc displacement at C5-C6 level
	M50.223	Other cervical disc displacement at C6-C7 level
	M50.81	Other cervical disc disorders, high cervical region
	M50.821	Other cervical disc disorders at C4-C5 level
	M50.822	Other cervical disc disorders at C5-C6 level
	M50.823	Other cervical disc disorders at C6-C7 level
	M51.16	Intervertebral disc disorders with radiculopathy, lumbar region
	M51.26	Other intervertebral disc displacement, lumbar region
	M51.27	Other intervertebral disc displacement, lumbosacral region
	M51.36	Other intervertebral disc degeneration, lumbar region
	M54.12	Radiculopathy, cervical region
	M54.16	Radiculopathy, lumbar region

ICD-10-CM Coding Notes

For codes requiring a 7th character extension, refer to your ICD-10-CM book. Review the character descriptions and coding guidelines for proper selection. For some procedures, only certain characters will apply.

CCI Edits

Refer to Appendix A for CCI edits.

Facility RVUs 🗋

Code	Work	PE Facility	MP	Total Facility
63040	20.31	14.01	5.97	40.29
63042	18.76	13.57	5.21	37.54
63043	0.00	0.00	0.00	0.00
63044	0.00	0.00	0.00	0.00

Non-facility RVUs 🗋

Code	Work	PE Non-Facility	MP	Total Non-Facility
63040	20.31	14.01	5.97	40.29
63042	18.76	13.57	5.21	37.54
63043	0.00	0.00	0.00	0.00
63044	0.00	0.00	0.00	0.00

Modifiers (PAR) 🗋

Code	Mod 50	Mod 51	Mod 62	Mod 66	Mod 80
63040	1	2	2	0	2
63042	1	2	2	0	2
63043	1	0	2	0	2
63044	1	0	2	0	2

Global Period

Code	Days
63040	090
63042	090
63043	ZZZ
63044	ZZZ

63045-63048

63045 Laminectomy, facetectomy and foraminotomy (unilateral or bilateral with decompression of spinal cord, cauda equina and/or nerve root[s], [eg, spinal or lateral recess stenosis]), single vertebral segment; cervical

63046 Laminectomy, facetectomy and foraminotomy (unilateral or bilateral with decompression of spinal cord, cauda equina and/or nerve root[s], [eg, spinal or lateral recess stenosis]), single vertebral segment; thoracic

63047 Laminectomy, facetectomy and foraminotomy (unilateral or bilateral with decompression of spinal cord, cauda equina and/or nerve root[s], [eg, spinal or lateral recess stenosis]), single vertebral segment; lumbar

+ **63048 Laminectomy, facetectomy and foraminotomy (unilateral or bilateral with decompression of spinal cord, cauda equina and/or nerve root[s], [eg, spinal or lateral recess stenosis]), single vertebral segment; each additional segment, cervical, thoracic, or lumbar (List separately in addition to code for primary procedure)**

(Use 63048 in conjunction with 63045-63047)

AMA Coding Guideline

Posterior Extradural Laminotomy or Laminectomy for Exploration/ Decompression of Neural Elements or Excision of Herniated Intervertebral Disks Procedures

Definitions

For purposes of CPT coding, the following definitions of approach and visualization apply. The primary approach and visualization define the service, whether another method is incidentally applied. Surgical services are presumed open, unless otherwise specified.

Percutaneous: Image-guided procedures (eg, computer tomography [CT] or fluoroscopy) performed with indirect visualization of the spine without the use of any device that allows visualization through a surgical incision.

Endoscopic: Spinal procedures performed with continuous direct visualization of the spine through an endoscope.

Open: Spinal procedures performed with continuous direct visualization of the spine through a surgical opening.

Indirect visualization: Image-guided (eg, CT or fluoroscopy), not light-based visualization.

Direct visualization: Light-based visualization; can be performed by eye, or with surgical loupes, microscope, or endoscope.

AMA Coding Notes

Posterior Extradural Laminotomy or Laminectomy for Exploration/ Decompression of Neural Elements or Excision of Herniated Intervertebral Disks Procedures

(When 63001-63048 are followed by arthrodesis, see 22590-22614)

(For the techniques of microsurgery and/or use of microscope, use 69990)

(For percutaneous decompression, see 62287, 0274T, 0275T)

Surgical Procedures on the Spine and Spinal Cord

(For application of caliper or tongs, use 20660)

(For treatment of fracture or dislocation of spine, see 22310-22327)

AMA *CPT Assistant*

63045: Jan 01: 12, Dec 12: 13, Jul 13: 3

63046: Jan 99: 11, Jan 01: 12, Dec 12: 13, Jul 13: 3

63047: Jan 99: 11, Jan 01: 12, Feb 01: 10, Nov 02: 11, Apr 08: 11, Jul 08: 7, Oct 08: 10, Oct 09: 9, Nov 10: 4, Jul 11: 13, Dec 12: 13, Jul 13: 3, Dec 13: 17, Dec 14: 16, Oct 16: 11, Feb 17: 13, May 18: 9

63048: Fall 91: 8, Jan 99: 11, Jan 01: 12, Dec 12: 13

Plain English Description

Laminectomy (lamina excision) is performed to determine the cause of back pain and to relieve pressure on the spinal cord, spinal nerve roots, and/or cauda equina. The lamina is the portion of the vertebra that forms posterior aspect of the vertebral arch. A posterior skin incision is made over the affected portion of the spine down to the spinous process. Overlying fat and muscle are retracted off the lamina. The lamina is excised. The underlying paired ligaments (ligamentum flavum) that bind the lamina of contiguous vertebrae together are also excised. The superior and inferior articular facets and the pars interarticularis are inspected. The openings under the facet joints where the spinal nerves emerge are explored and bone is removed as needed to decompress the nerve roots. The spinal canal is exposed and explored. The intervertebral foramen is enlarged to decompress the spinal cord. Adhesions between the dura and ligamentum flavum are lysed. The spinal nerve roots and/or cauda equina are carefully dissected and freed within the intervertebral foramen. The surgical wound is closed in layers. Separately reportable arthrodesis is performed as needed to stabilize the spine. Laminectomy, facetectomy, and foraminotomy of a single vertebral segment of the cervical spine are reported with 63045, thoracic spine with 63046, and lumbar spine with 63047, and each additional cervical, thoracic, or lumbar segment is reported with 63048.

Laminectomy, facetectomy and foraminotomy (unilateral or bilateral), single vertebral segment

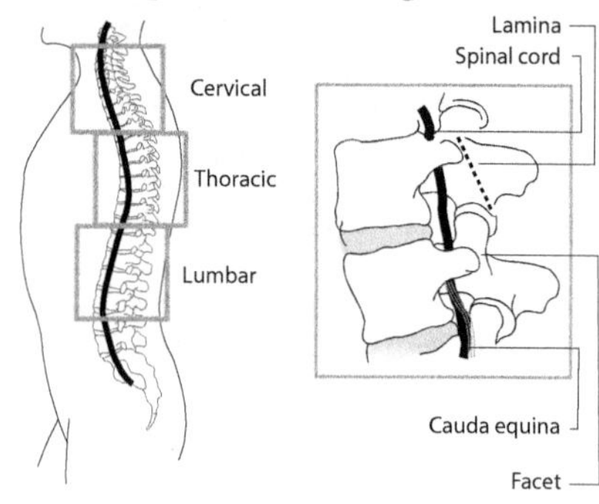

Cervical (63045); thoracic (63046); lumbar (63047); each additional segment, cervical, thoracic, or lumbar (63048)

ICD-10-CM Diagnostic Codes

Code	Description
C41.2	Malignant neoplasm of vertebral column
C72.0	Malignant neoplasm of spinal cord
D16.6	Benign neoplasm of vertebral column
D33.4	Benign neoplasm of spinal cord
G12.25	Progressive spinal muscle atrophy
G54.1	Lumbosacral plexus disorders
G54.2	Cervical root disorders, not elsewhere classified
G54.4	Lumbosacral root disorders, not elsewhere classified
G54.8	Other nerve root and plexus disorders
G55	Nerve root and plexus compressions in diseases classified elsewhere
G83.4	Cauda equina syndrome
G95.29	Other cord compression
M43.12	Spondylolisthesis, cervical region
M43.13	Spondylolisthesis, cervicothoracic region
M43.14	Spondylolisthesis, thoracic region
M43.15	Spondylolisthesis, thoracolumbar region
M43.16	Spondylolisthesis, lumbar region
M43.17	Spondylolisthesis, lumbosacral region
M45.2	Ankylosing spondylitis of cervical region
M45.3	Ankylosing spondylitis of cervicothoracic region
M45.4	Ankylosing spondylitis of thoracic region
M45.5	Ankylosing spondylitis of thoracolumbar region
M45.6	Ankylosing spondylitis lumbar region
M45.7	Ankylosing spondylitis of lumbosacral region
M46.02	Spinal enthesopathy, cervical region
M46.03	Spinal enthesopathy, cervicothoracic region

M46.04 Spinal enthesopathy, thoracic region
M46.05 Spinal enthesopathy, thoracolumbar region
M46.06 Spinal enthesopathy, lumbar region
M46.07 Spinal enthesopathy, lumbosacral region
M46.42 Discitis, unspecified, cervical region
M46.43 Discitis, unspecified, cervicothoracic region
M46.45 Discitis, unspecified, thoracolumbar region
M46.46 Discitis, unspecified, lumbar region
M46.47 Discitis, unspecified, lumbosacral region
M46.82 Other specified inflammatory spondylopathies, cervical region
M46.83 Other specified inflammatory spondylopathies, cervicothoracic region
M46.84 Other specified inflammatory spondylopathies, thoracic region
M46.85 Other specified inflammatory spondylopathies, thoracolumbar region
M46.86 Other specified inflammatory spondylopathies, lumbar region
M46.87 Other specified inflammatory spondylopathies, lumbosacral region
M47.012 Anterior spinal artery compression syndromes, cervical region
M47.013 Anterior spinal artery compression syndromes, cervicothoracic region
M47.014 Anterior spinal artery compression syndromes, thoracic region
M47.015 Anterior spinal artery compression syndromes, thoracolumbar region
M47.016 Anterior spinal artery compression syndromes, lumbar region
M47.022 Vertebral artery compression syndromes, cervical region
M47.12 Other spondylosis with myelopathy, cervical region
M47.13 Other spondylosis with myelopathy, cervicothoracic region
M47.14 Other spondylosis with myelopathy, thoracic region
M47.15 Other spondylosis with myelopathy, thoracolumbar region
M47.16 Other spondylosis with myelopathy, lumbar region
M47.17 Other spondylosis with myelopathy, lumbosacral region
M47.22 Other spondylosis with radiculopathy, cervical region
M47.23 Other spondylosis with radiculopathy, cervicothoracic region
M47.24 Other spondylosis with radiculopathy, thoracic region
M47.25 Other spondylosis with radiculopathy, thoracolumbar region
M47.26 Other spondylosis with radiculopathy, lumbar region
M47.27 Other spondylosis with radiculopathy, lumbosacral region
M48.02 Spinal stenosis, cervical region
M48.03 Spinal stenosis, cervicothoracic region
M48.04 Spinal stenosis, thoracic region
M48.05 Spinal stenosis, thoracolumbar region
M48.061 Spinal stenosis, lumbar region without neurogenic claudication
M48.062 Spinal stenosis, lumbar region with neurogenic claudication
M48.07 Spinal stenosis, lumbosacral region
M48.32 Traumatic spondylopathy, cervical region
M48.33 Traumatic spondylopathy, cervicothoracic region
M48.34 Traumatic spondylopathy, thoracic region
M48.35 Traumatic spondylopathy, thoracolumbar region
M48.36 Traumatic spondylopathy, lumbar region
M48.37 Traumatic spondylopathy, lumbosacral region
⑦ M48.52 Collapsed vertebra, not elsewhere classified, cervical region
⑦ M48.53 Collapsed vertebra, not elsewhere classified, cervicothoracic region
⑦ M48.54 Collapsed vertebra, not elsewhere classified, thoracic region
⑦ M48.55 Collapsed vertebra, not elsewhere classified, thoracolumbar region
⑦ M48.56 Collapsed vertebra, not elsewhere classified, lumbar region
⑦ M48.57 Collapsed vertebra, not elsewhere classified, lumbosacral region
M48.8X2 Other specified spondylopathies, cervical region
M48.8X3 Other specified spondylopathies, cervicothoracic region
M48.8X4 Other specified spondylopathies, thoracic region
M48.8X5 Other specified spondylopathies, thoracolumbar region
M48.8X6 Other specified spondylopathies, lumbar region
M48.8X7 Other specified spondylopathies, lumbosacral region
M50.021 Cervical disc disorder at C4-C5 level with myelopathy
M50.022 Cervical disc disorder at C5-C6 level with myelopathy
M50.023 Cervical disc disorder at C6-C7 level with myelopathy
M50.03 Cervical disc disorder with myelopathy, cervicothoracic region
M50.11 Cervical disc disorder with radiculopathy, high cervical region
M50.121 Cervical disc disorder at C4-C5 level with radiculopathy
M50.122 Cervical disc disorder at C5-C6 level with radiculopathy
M50.123 Cervical disc disorder at C6-C7 level with radiculopathy
M50.13 Cervical disc disorder with radiculopathy, cervicothoracic region
M50.21 Other cervical disc displacement, high cervical region
M50.221 Other cervical disc displacement at C4-C5 level
M50.222 Other cervical disc displacement at C5-C6 level
M50.223 Other cervical disc displacement at C6-C7 level
M50.23 Other cervical disc displacement, cervicothoracic region
M50.81 Other cervical disc disorders, high cervical region
M50.821 Other cervical disc disorders at C4-C5 level
M50.822 Other cervical disc disorders at C5-C6 level
M50.823 Other cervical disc disorders at C6-C7 level
M50.83 Other cervical disc disorders, cervicothoracic region
M51.04 Intervertebral disc disorders with myelopathy, thoracic region
M51.05 Intervertebral disc disorders with myelopathy, thoracolumbar region
M51.06 Intervertebral disc disorders with myelopathy, lumbar region
M51.07 Intervertebral disc disorders with myelopathy, lumbosacral region
M51.15 Intervertebral disc disorders with radiculopathy, thoracolumbar region
M51.16 Intervertebral disc disorders with radiculopathy, lumbar region
M51.17 Intervertebral disc disorders with radiculopathy, lumbosacral region
M51.24 Other intervertebral disc displacement, thoracic region
M51.25 Other intervertebral disc displacement, thoracolumbar region
M51.26 Other intervertebral disc displacement, lumbar region
M51.27 Other intervertebral disc displacement, lumbosacral region
M51.34 Other intervertebral disc degeneration, thoracic region
M51.35 Other intervertebral disc degeneration, thoracolumbar region
M51.36 Other intervertebral disc degeneration, lumbar region
M51.37 Other intervertebral disc degeneration, lumbosacral region
M54.12 Radiculopathy, cervical region
M54.13 Radiculopathy, cervicothoracic region
M54.14 Radiculopathy, thoracic region
M54.15 Radiculopathy, thoracolumbar region
M54.16 Radiculopathy, lumbar region
M54.17 Radiculopathy, lumbosacral region
M96.1 Postlaminectomy syndrome, not elsewhere classified
Q76.2 Congenital spondylolisthesis
⑦ S14.153 Other incomplete lesion at C3 level of cervical spinal cord
⑦ S14.154 Other incomplete lesion at C4 level of cervical spinal cord
⑦ S14.155 Other incomplete lesion at C5 level of cervical spinal cord

➐	S14.156	Other incomplete lesion at C6 level of cervical spinal cord
➐	S14.157	Other incomplete lesion at C7 level of cervical spinal cord
➐	S14.158	Other incomplete lesion at C8 level of cervical spinal cord
➐	S24.151	Other incomplete lesion at T1 level of thoracic spinal cord
➐	S24.152	Other incomplete lesion at T2-T6 level of thoracic spinal cord
➐	S24.153	Other incomplete lesion at T7-T10 level of thoracic spinal cord
➐	S24.154	Other incomplete lesion at T11-T12 level of thoracic spinal cord

ICD-10-CM Coding Notes

For codes requiring a 7th character extension, refer to your ICD-10-CM book. Review the character descriptions and coding guidelines for proper selection. For some procedures, only certain characters will apply.

CCI Edits

Refer to Appendix A for CCI edits.

Facility RVUs ▯

Code	Work	PE Facility	MP	Total Facility
63045	17.95	13.41	5.83	37.19
63046	17.25	12.98	5.26	35.49
63047	15.37	12.02	4.51	31.90
63048	3.47	1.66	1.00	6.13

Non-facility RVUs ▯

Code	Work	PE Non-Facility	MP	Total Non-Facility
63045	17.95	13.41	5.83	37.19
63046	17.25	12.98	5.26	35.49
63047	15.37	12.02	4.51	31.90
63048	3.47	1.66	1.00	6.13

Modifiers (PAR) ▯

Code	Mod 50	Mod 51	Mod 62	Mod 66	Mod 80
63045	2	2	2	0	2
63046	2	2	2	0	2
63047	2	2	2	0	2
63048	0	0	2	0	2

Global Period

Code	Days
63045	090
63046	090
63047	090
63048	ZZZ

63050-63051

63050 Laminoplasty, cervical, with decompression of the spinal cord, 2 or more vertebral segments

63051 Laminoplasty, cervical, with decompression of the spinal cord, 2 or more vertebral segments; with reconstruction of the posterior bony elements (including the application of bridging bone graft and non-segmental fixation devices [eg, wire, suture, mini-plates], when performed)

(Do not report 63050 or 63051 in conjunction with 22600, 22614, 22840-22842, 63001, 63015, 63045, 63048, 63295 for the same vertebral segment(s))

AMA Coding Guideline

Posterior Extradural Laminotomy or Laminectomy for Exploration/ Decompression of Neural Elements or Excision of Herniated Intervertebral Disks Procedures

Definitions

For purposes of CPT coding, the following definitions of approach and visualization apply. The primary approach and visualization define the service, whether another method is incidentally applied. Surgical services are presumed open, unless otherwise specified.

Percutaneous: Image-guided procedures (eg, computer tomography [CT] or fluoroscopy) performed with indirect visualization of the spine without the use of any device that allows visualization through a surgical incision.

Endoscopic: Spinal procedures performed with continuous direct visualization of the spine through an endoscope.

Open: Spinal procedures performed with continuous direct visualization of the spine through a surgical opening.

Indirect visualization: Image-guided (eg, CT or fluoroscopy), not light-based visualization.

Direct visualization: Light-based visualization; can be performed by eye, or with surgical loupes, microscope, or endoscope.

AMA Coding Notes

Posterior Extradural Laminotomy or Laminectomy for Exploration/ Decompression of Neural Elements or Excision of Herniated Intervertebral Disks Procedures

(When 63001-63048 are followed by arthrodesis, see 22590-22614)

(For the techniques of microsurgery and/or use of microscope, use 69990)

(For percutaneous decompression, see 62287, 0274T, 0275T)

Surgical Procedures on the Spine and Spinal Cord

(For application of caliper or tongs, use 20660)

(For treatment of fracture or dislocation of spine, see 22310-22327)

AMA *CPT Assistant*

63050: Jul 13: 3

63051: Jul 11: 13, Jul 13: 3

Plain English Description

Cervical laminoplasty is performed to treat spinal stenosis. The aim of the procedure is to put pressure on the spinal cord while maintaining posterior stability of the spine. This is accomplished by partially cutting the bony posterior elements on one side to create a hinge and completely cutting posterior bone on the opposite side to form a partially opened door. A posterior incision is made over the cervical spine. Paraspinous muscles are retracted and the laminae, spinous processes, and facet joints over the affected vertebral bodies are exposed. Complete osteotomy of 2 or more vertebral segments is performed on the side that will form the open door component. The ligamentum flavum is divided. On the opposite side, a hinge is created by scoring each vertebra with a drill at the junction of the facet and lamina. An elevator is used to open the side on which the complete osteotomy has been performed, relieving pressure on the spinal cord. In 63050, reconstruction of the bony elements is not performed. In 63051, reconstruction using bone grafts and/or a nonsegmental fixation device is performed following the laminoplasty. If bone grafts are used, the separately reportable bone allografts or autografts are configured to fit the bony defects. The bone grafts are then placed into the defects in each vertebra on the side of the complete osteotomy to maintain the opening. Fixation devices, such as wire, suture, or mini-plates, are then applied as needed across the osteotomy to secure the bone grafts. The surgical wound is closed in layers.

Laminoplasty, cervical, with decompression of the spinal cord, 2 or more vertebral segments

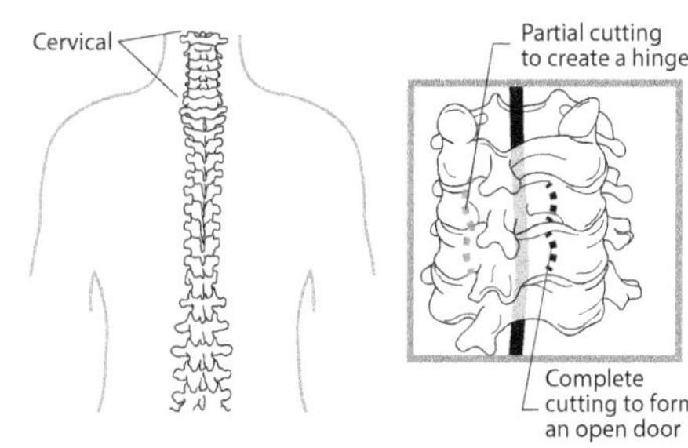

Laminoplasty (63050); laminoplasty with reconstruction of the posterior bony elements (63051)

ICD-10-CM Diagnostic Codes

G95.29	Other cord compression
G95.9	Disease of spinal cord, unspecified
M47.012	Anterior spinal artery compression syndromes, cervical region
M47.12	Other spondylosis with myelopathy, cervical region
M47.13	Other spondylosis with myelopathy, cervicothoracic region
M48.02	Spinal stenosis, cervical region
M48.03	Spinal stenosis, cervicothoracic region
M50.01	Cervical disc disorder with myelopathy, high cervical region
M50.021	Cervical disc disorder at C4-C5 level with myelopathy
M50.022	Cervical disc disorder at C5-C6 level with myelopathy
M50.023	Cervical disc disorder at C6-C7 level with myelopathy
M50.03	Cervical disc disorder with myelopathy, cervicothoracic region
M50.11	Cervical disc disorder with radiculopathy, high cervical region
M50.121	Cervical disc disorder at C4-C5 level with radiculopathy
M50.122	Cervical disc disorder at C5-C6 level with radiculopathy
M50.123	Cervical disc disorder at C6-C7 level with radiculopathy
M50.13	Cervical disc disorder with radiculopathy, cervicothoracic region

CCI Edits

Refer to Appendix A for CCI edits.

Facility RVUs

Code	Work	PE Facility	MP	Total Facility
63050	22.01	15.07	6.44	43.52
63051	25.51	16.72	7.14	49.37

Non-facility RVUs

Code	Work	PE Non-Facility	MP	Total Non-Facility
63050	22.01	15.07	6.44	43.52
63051	25.51	16.72	7.14	49.37

Modifiers (PAR)

Code	Mod 50	Mod 51	Mod 62	Mod 66	Mod 80
63050	0	2	2	0	2
63051	0	2	2	0	2

Global Period

Code	Days
63050	090
63051	090

63055-63057

63055 Transpedicular approach with decompression of spinal cord, equina and/or nerve root(s) (eg, herniated intervertebral disc), single segment; thoracic

63056 Transpedicular approach with decompression of spinal cord, equina and/or nerve root(s) (eg, herniated intervertebral disc), single segment; lumbar (including transfacet, or lateral extraforaminal approach) (eg, far lateral herniated intervertebral disc)

+ **63057 Transpedicular approach with decompression of spinal cord, equina and/or nerve root(s) (eg, herniated intervertebral disc), single segment; each additional segment, thoracic or lumbar (List separately in addition to code for primary procedure)**

(Use 63057 in conjunction with 63055, 63056)

AMA Coding Notes

Surgical Procedures on the Spine and Spinal Cord

(For application of caliper or tongs, use 20660)

(For treatment of fracture or dislocation of spine, see 22310-22327)

AMA *CPT Assistant*

63055: Nov 99: 36, Jul 13: 3

63056: Nov 99: 36, Oct 09: 9, Nov 11: 10, Jul 12: 3, Jul 13: 3, Jan 14: 9

63057: Nov 99: 36

Plain English Description

A transpedicular approach requires removal of part of one of the two pedicles. The pedicles are short, thick bony processes that project posteriorly from the body of the vertebra and unite with the lamina to form the vertebral arch, which contains the spinal cord. A skin incision is made at the lateral margin of the spinous process of the affected cervical disc. The paraspinal muscles are elevated off the spinous process, lamina, and transverse process. The lamina and facet joint are exposed. The medial portion of the facet and the lateral portion of the lamina are removed using a high-speed drill. The pedicle is partially removed and the lateral margin of the spinal cord is exposed. The spinal nerve root and herniated portion of the intervertebral disc are identified. Any bone spurs at the site of the herniation are excised and a cavity is created. The cavity is enlarged and ruptured disc fragments or bulging nucleus pulposus impinging on the spinal cord, nerve root, and/or cauda equina are removed. Additional bone is removed as needed to relieve pressure on the nerve. Bleeding is controlled and the surgical wound is closed in layers. Use code 63055 for transpedicular decompression of a single segment of the thoracic spine; use 63056 for a single segment of the lumbar spine; and 63057 for each additional thoracic or lumbar segment.

Transpedicular approach with decompression of spinal cord, equina, and/or nerve root(s), single segment

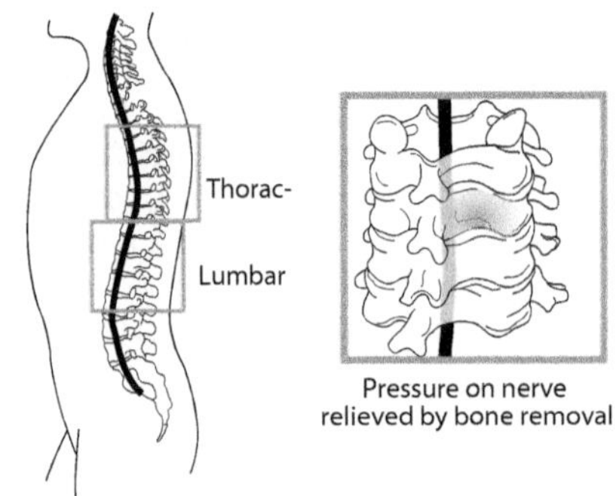

Thoracic (63055); lumbar (63056); each additional segment, thoracic or lumbar (63057)

ICD-10-CM Diagnostic Codes

M47.14	Other spondylosis with myelopathy, thoracic region
M47.15	Other spondylosis with myelopathy, thoracolumbar region
M47.16	Other spondylosis with myelopathy, lumbar region
M47.24	Other spondylosis with radiculopathy, thoracic region
M47.25	Other spondylosis with radiculopathy, thoracolumbar region
M47.26	Other spondylosis with radiculopathy, lumbar region
M48.04	Spinal stenosis, thoracic region
M48.05	Spinal stenosis, thoracolumbar region
M48.062	Spinal stenosis, lumbar region with neurogenic claudication
M51.04	Intervertebral disc disorders with myelopathy, thoracic region
M51.05	Intervertebral disc disorders with myelopathy, thoracolumbar region
M51.06	Intervertebral disc disorders with myelopathy, lumbar region
M51.14	Intervertebral disc disorders with radiculopathy, thoracic region
M51.15	Intervertebral disc disorders with radiculopathy, thoracolumbar region
M51.16	Intervertebral disc disorders with radiculopathy, lumbar region
M51.17	Intervertebral disc disorders with radiculopathy, lumbosacral region
M51.24	Other intervertebral disc displacement, thoracic region
M51.25	Other intervertebral disc displacement, thoracolumbar region
M51.26	Other intervertebral disc displacement, lumbar region
M51.27	Other intervertebral disc displacement, lumbosacral region
M51.34	Other intervertebral disc degeneration, thoracic region
M51.35	Other intervertebral disc degeneration, thoracolumbar region
M51.36	Other intervertebral disc degeneration, lumbar region
M96.1	Postlaminectomy syndrome, not elsewhere classified

CCI Edits

Refer to Appendix A for CCI edits.

Facility RVUs

Code	Work	PE Facility	MP	Total Facility
63055	23.55	15.68	7.80	47.03
63056	21.86	14.71	6.51	43.08
63057	5.25	2.51	1.52	9.28

Non-facility RVUs

Code	Work	PE Non-Facility	MP	Total Non-Facility
63055	23.55	15.68	7.80	47.03
63056	21.86	14.71	6.51	43.08
63057	5.25	2.51	1.52	9.28

Modifiers (PAR)

Code	Mod 50	Mod 51	Mod 62	Mod 66	Mod 80
63055	0	2	1	0	2
63056	0	2	1	0	2
63057	0	0	1	0	2

Global Period

Code	Days
63055	090
63056	090
63057	ZZZ

63064-63066

63064 Costovertebral approach with decompression of spinal cord or nerve root(s) (eg, herniated intervertebral disc), thoracic; single segment

+ 63066 Costovertebral approach with decompression of spinal cord or nerve root(s) (eg, herniated intervertebral disc), thoracic; each additional segment (List separately in addition to code for primary procedure)

(Use 63066 in conjunction with 63064)

(For excision of thoracic intraspinal lesions by laminectomy, see 63266, 63271, 63276, 63281, 63286)

Costovertebral approach with decompression of spinal cord or nerve roots

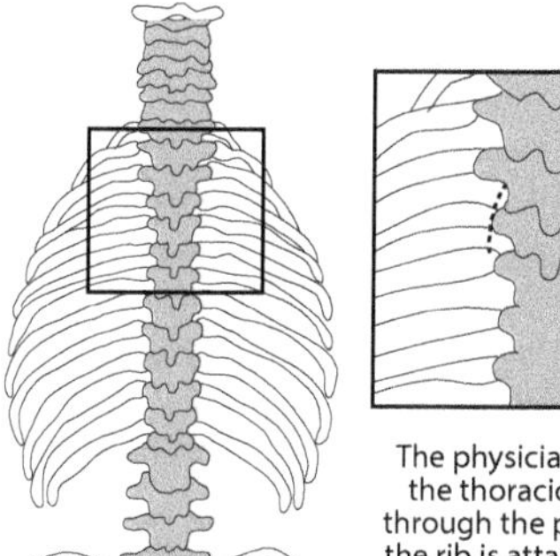

Single segment (63064); each additional segment

AMA Coding Notes

Surgical Procedures on the Spine and Spinal Cord

(For application of caliper or tongs, use 20660)

(For treatment of fracture or dislocation of spine, see 22310-22327)

AMA *CPT Assistant*

63064: Fall 92: 19, Jul 13: 3

Plain English Description

A costovertebral approach involves partial rib excision and removal of the transverse process on the affected side of the vertebra so that a ventral window can be created for visualization of the spinal cord and nerve roots. The transverse processes extend laterally from the neural arch at the point where the pedicles and lamina join on each side of the vertebra. The transverse processes of the thoracic spine are longer and heavier than those in other regions and have facets that articulate with the tubercles (heads) of the ribs. A semilunar skin incision is made at the appropriate level over the thoracic spine and extended over the posterior aspect of the rib. Overlying soft tissue and muscle are dissected and the posterior aspect of the rib exposed. The paraspinal muscles are elevated off the spinous process, lamina, and transverse process. The lamina and facet joint are exposed. A portion of the rib and transverse process are removed using a high-speed drill to create a window. The spinal cord and nerve roots are exposed. The intervertebral disc is exposed and any herniation noted. Bone spurs are excised and a cavity is created. The cavity is enlarged and any ruptured disc fragments or bulging nucleus pulposus impinging on the spinal cord and/or nerve root are removed. Additional bone is removed as needed to relieve pressure on the nerve. Bleeding is controlled and the surgical wound is closed in layers. Use 63064 for a single thoracic vertebral segment and 63066 for each additional thoracic vertebral segment.

ICD-10-CM Diagnostic Codes

C41.2	Malignant neoplasm of vertebral column
C79.49	Secondary malignant neoplasm of other parts of nervous system
M46.24	Osteomyelitis of vertebra, thoracic region
M46.44	Discitis, unspecified, thoracic region
M46.45	Discitis, unspecified, thoracolumbar region
M48.04	Spinal stenosis, thoracic region
M48.05	Spinal stenosis, thoracolumbar region
M51.04	Intervertebral disc disorders with myelopathy, thoracic region
M51.05	Intervertebral disc disorders with myelopathy, thoracolumbar region
M51.14	Intervertebral disc disorders with radiculopathy, thoracic region
M51.15	Intervertebral disc disorders with radiculopathy, thoracolumbar region
M51.24	Other intervertebral disc displacement, thoracic region
M51.25	Other intervertebral disc displacement, thoracolumbar region
M51.34	Other intervertebral disc degeneration, thoracic region
M51.35	Other intervertebral disc degeneration, thoracolumbar region

CCI Edits

Refer to Appendix A for CCI edits.

Facility RVUs

Code	Work	PE Facility	MP	Total Facility
63064	26.22	16.87	8.44	51.53
63066	3.26	1.50	1.21	5.97

Non-facility RVUs

Code	Work	PE Non-Facility	MP	Total Non-Facility
63064	26.22	16.87	8.44	51.53
63066	3.26	1.50	1.21	5.97

Modifiers (PAR)

Code	Mod 50	Mod 51	Mod 62	Mod 66	Mod 80
63064	0	2	1	0	2
63066	0	0	1	0	2

Global Period

Code	Days
63064	090
63066	ZZZ

63075-63076

63075 Discectomy, anterior, with decompression of spinal cord and/or nerve root(s), including osteophytectomy; cervical, single interspace

(Do not report 63075 in conjunction with 22554, even if performed by separate individuals. To report anterior cervical discectomy and interbody fusion at the same level during the same session, use 22551)

✚ **63076 Discectomy, anterior, with decompression of spinal cord and/or nerve root(s), including osteophytectomy; cervical, each additional interspace (List separately in addition to code for primary procedure)**

(Do not report 63076 in conjunction with 22554, even if performed by separate individuals. To report anterior cervical discectomy and interbody fusion at the same level during the same session, use 22552)

(Use 63076 in conjunction with 63075)

AMA Coding Guideline

Anterior or Anterolateral Approach for Extradural Exploration/Decompression Procedures on the Spine and Spinal Cord

For the following codes, when two surgeons work together as primary surgeons performing distinct part(s) of spinal cord exploration/decompression operation, each surgeon should report his/her distinct operative work by appending modifier 62 to the procedure code (and any associated add-on codes for that procedure code as long as both surgeons continue to work together as primary surgeons). In this situation, modifier 62 may be appended to the definitive procedure code(s) 63075, 63077, 63081, 63085, 63087, 63090 and, as appropriate, to associated additional interspace add-on code(s) 63076, 63078 or additional segment add-on code(s) 63082, 63086, 63088, 63091 as long as both surgeons continue to work together as primary surgeons.

For vertebral corpectomy, the term partial is used to describe removal of a substantial portion of the body of the vertebra. In the cervical spine, the amount of bone removed is defined as at least one-half of the vertebral body. In the thoracic and lumbar spine, the amount of bone removed is defined as at least one-third of the vertebral body.

AMA Coding Notes

Surgical Procedures on the Spine and Spinal Cord

(For application of caliper or tongs, use 20660)

(For treatment of fracture or dislocation of spine, see 22310-22327)

AMA *CPT Assistant* ▢

63075: Nov 98: 18, Jan 01: 12, Feb 02: 4, Jul 13: 3, Apr 15: 7

63076: Nov 98: 18, Jan 01: 12, Feb 02: 4

Plain English Description

Anterior discectomy of the cervical spine is performed through a skin incision in the anterior aspect of the neck. The soft tissues and muscles overlying the cervical spine are dissected. The trachea and esophagus are retracted away from the surgical site. The affected portion of the cervical spine is exposed. The intervertebral disc is exposed and carefully removed with the aid of the surgical microscope. Bone spurs and any bone impinging on the nerve roots are also removed, along with the ligament that covers the spinal cord. If a separately reportable bone graft is needed, the bone is contoured for placement of the graft. Separately reportable internal fixation may also be used to stabilize the spine. Upon completion of the procedure, bleeding is controlled and soft tissues and skin are closed in layers. Use 63075 for a single cervical interspace and 63076 for each additional interspace.

Discectomy, anterior, with decompression of spinal cord and/or nerve root, including osteophytectomy; cervical

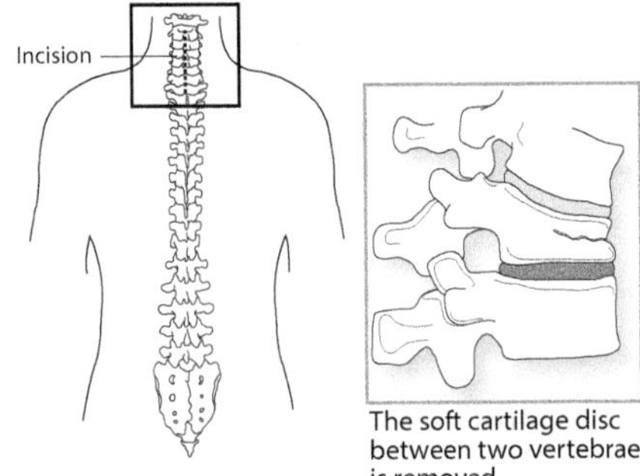

Single interspace (63075), each additional interspace (63076)

ICD-10-CM Diagnostic Codes

Code	Description
G06.1	Intraspinal abscess and granuloma
G95.20	Unspecified cord compression
M25.78	Osteophyte, vertebrae
M46.32	Infection of intervertebral disc (pyogenic), cervical region
M46.33	Infection of intervertebral disc (pyogenic), cervicothoracic region
M46.42	Discitis, unspecified, cervical region
M46.43	Discitis, unspecified, cervicothoracic region
M46.52	Other infective spondylopathies, cervical region
M46.53	Other infective spondylopathies, cervicothoracic region
M46.82	Other specified inflammatory spondylopathies, cervical region
M46.83	Other specified inflammatory spondylopathies, cervicothoracic region
M47.012	Anterior spinal artery compression syndromes, cervical region
M47.013	Anterior spinal artery compression syndromes, cervicothoracic region
M47.12	Other spondylosis with myelopathy, cervical region
M47.13	Other spondylosis with myelopathy, cervicothoracic region
M47.22	Other spondylosis with radiculopathy, cervical region
M47.23	Other spondylosis with radiculopathy, cervicothoracic region
M48.02	Spinal stenosis, cervical region
M48.03	Spinal stenosis, cervicothoracic region
M48.8X2	Other specified spondylopathies, cervical region
M48.8X3	Other specified spondylopathies, cervicothoracic region
M50.01	Cervical disc disorder with myelopathy, high cervical region
M50.021	Cervical disc disorder at C4-C5 level with myelopathy
M50.022	Cervical disc disorder at C5-C6 level with myelopathy
M50.023	Cervical disc disorder at C6-C7 level with myelopathy
M50.03	Cervical disc disorder with myelopathy, cervicothoracic region
M50.11	Cervical disc disorder with radiculopathy, high cervical region
M50.121	Cervical disc disorder at C4-C5 level with radiculopathy
M50.122	Cervical disc disorder at C5-C6 level with radiculopathy
M50.123	Cervical disc disorder at C6-C7 level with radiculopathy
M50.13	Cervical disc disorder with radiculopathy, cervicothoracic region
M50.21	Other cervical disc displacement, high cervical region
M50.221	Other cervical disc displacement at C4-C5 level
M50.222	Other cervical disc displacement at C5-C6 level
M50.223	Other cervical disc displacement at C6-C7 level
M50.23	Other cervical disc displacement, cervicothoracic region
M50.31	Other cervical disc degeneration, high cervical region
M50.321	Other cervical disc degeneration at C4-C5 level
M50.322	Other cervical disc degeneration at C5-C6 level
M50.323	Other cervical disc degeneration at C6-C7 level
M50.33	Other cervical disc degeneration, cervicothoracic region
M50.81	Other cervical disc disorders, high cervical region
M50.821	Other cervical disc disorders at C4-C5 level
M50.822	Other cervical disc disorders at C5-C6 level
M50.823	Other cervical disc disorders at C6-C7 level

M96.1	Postlaminectomy syndrome, not elsewhere classified

CCI Edits

Refer to Appendix A for CCI edits.

Facility RVUs □

Code	Work	PE Facility	MP	Total Facility
63075	19.60	13.77	5.73	39.10
63076	4.04	1.93	1.17	7.14

Non-facility RVUs □

Code	Work	PE Non-Facility	MP	Total Non-Facility
63075	19.60	13.77	5.73	39.10
63076	4.04	1.93	1.17	7.14

Modifiers (PAR) □

Code	Mod 50	Mod 51	Mod 62	Mod 66	Mod 80
63075	0	2	2	0	2
63076	0	0	2	0	2

Global Period

Code	Days
63075	090
63076	ZZZ

CPT® Procedural Coding

63077-63078

63077 Discectomy, anterior, with decompression of spinal cord and/or nerve root(s), including osteophytectomy; thoracic, single interspace

+ **63078 Discectomy, anterior, with decompression of spinal cord and/or nerve root(s), including osteophytectomy; thoracic, each additional interspace (List separately in addition to code for primary procedure)**

(Use 63078 in conjunction with 63077)

(Do not report code 69990 in addition to codes 63075-63078)

AMA Coding Guideline

Anterior or Anterolateral Approach for Extradural Exploration/Decompression Procedures on the Spine and Spinal Cord

For the following codes, when two surgeons work together as primary surgeons performing distinct part(s) of spinal cord exploration/decompression operation, each surgeon should report his/her distinct operative work by appending modifier 62 to the procedure code (and any associated add-on codes for that procedure code as long as both surgeons continue to work together as primary surgeons). In this situation, modifier 62 may be appended to the definitive procedure code(s) 63075, 63077, 63081, 63085, 63087, 63090 and, as appropriate, to associated additional interspace add-on code(s) 63076, 63078 or additional segment add-on code(s) 63082, 63086, 63088, 63091 as long as both surgeons continue to work together as primary surgeons.

For vertebral corpectomy, the term partial is used to describe removal of a substantial portion of the body of the vertebra. In the cervical spine, the amount of bone removed is defined as at least one-half of the vertebral body. In the thoracic and lumbar spine, the amount of bone removed is defined as at least one-third of the vertebral body.

AMA Coding Notes

Surgical Procedures on the Spine and Spinal Cord

(For application of caliper or tongs, use 20660)

(For treatment of fracture or dislocation of spine, see 22310-22327)

AMA *CPT Assistant*

63077: Nov 98: 18, Jan 01: 12, Feb 02: 4, Jul 13: 3

63078: Nov 98: 18, Jan 01: 12, Feb 02: 4

Plain English Description

Anterior discectomy of the thoracic spine is performed using a thoracic approach, which requires a thoracotomy. Typically, a team approach is used with the exposure being performed by a thoracic surgeon and the discectomy performed by a spine surgeon. The skin over the thorax is incised to allow access to the appropriate level of the thoracic spine. Overlying muscles are dissected and a rib is resected. Rib spreaders are used to allow adequate exposure of the spine. The affected portion of the thoracic spine is exposed. The intervertebral disc is exposed and carefully removed with the aid of the surgical microscope. Bone spurs and any bone impinging on the nerve roots are also removed along with the ligament that covers the spinal cord. If a separately reportable bone graft is needed, the bone is contoured for placement of the graft. Separately reportable internal fixation may also be used to stabilize the spine. Upon completion of the procedure, bleeding is controlled, a chest tube is placed, and the thorax is closed in layers. Use 63077 for a single thoracic interspace and 63078 for each additional interspace.

Discectomy, anterior, with decompression of spinal cord and/or nerve root, including osteophytectomy; thoracic

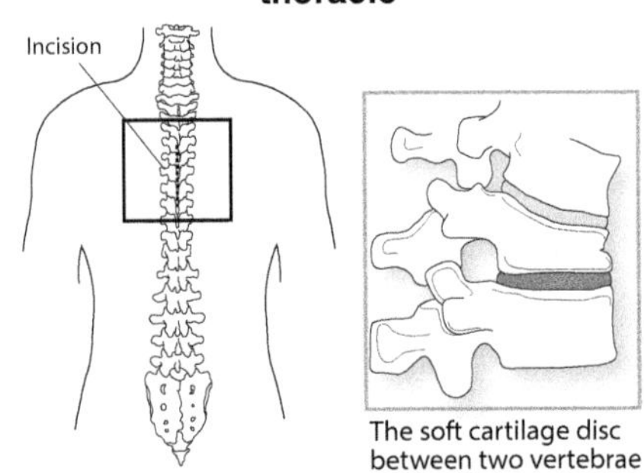

Single interspace (63077); each additional interspace (63078)

ICD-10-CM Diagnostic Codes

G06.1	Intraspinal abscess and granuloma
G54.3	Thoracic root disorders, not elsewhere classified
G95.20	Unspecified cord compression
M25.78	Osteophyte, vertebrae
M46.34	Infection of intervertebral disc (pyogenic), thoracic region
M46.35	Infection of intervertebral disc (pyogenic), thoracolumbar region
M46.44	Discitis, unspecified, thoracic region
M46.45	Discitis, unspecified, thoracolumbar region
M46.54	Other infective spondylopathies, thoracic region
M46.55	Other infective spondylopathies, thoracolumbar region
M46.82	Other specified inflammatory spondylopathies, cervical region
M46.83	Other specified inflammatory spondylopathies, cervicothoracic region
M46.84	Other specified inflammatory spondylopathies, thoracic region
M46.85	Other specified inflammatory spondylopathies, thoracolumbar region
M47.014	Anterior spinal artery compression syndromes, thoracic region
M47.015	Anterior spinal artery compression syndromes, thoracolumbar region
M47.14	Other spondylosis with myelopathy, thoracic region
M47.15	Other spondylosis with myelopathy, thoracolumbar region
M47.24	Other spondylosis with radiculopathy, thoracic region
M47.25	Other spondylosis with radiculopathy, thoracolumbar region
M48.04	Spinal stenosis, thoracic region
M48.05	Spinal stenosis, thoracolumbar region
M48.8X4	Other specified spondylopathies, thoracic region
M48.8X5	Other specified spondylopathies, thoracolumbar region
M51.04	Intervertebral disc disorders with myelopathy, thoracic region
M51.05	Intervertebral disc disorders with myelopathy, thoracolumbar region
M51.14	Intervertebral disc disorders with radiculopathy, thoracic region
M51.15	Intervertebral disc disorders with radiculopathy, thoracolumbar region
M51.24	Other intervertebral disc displacement, thoracic region
M51.25	Other intervertebral disc displacement, thoracolumbar region
M51.34	Other intervertebral disc degeneration, thoracic region
M51.35	Other intervertebral disc degeneration, thoracolumbar region
M51.84	Other intervertebral disc disorders, thoracic region
M51.85	Other intervertebral disc disorders, thoracolumbar region
M96.1	Postlaminectomy syndrome, not elsewhere classified

CCI Edits

Refer to Appendix A for CCI edits.

Facility RVUs

Code	Work	PE Facility	MP	Total Facility
63077	22.88	14.51	6.23	43.62
63078	3.28	1.51	1.22	6.01

Non-facility RVUs

Code	Work	PE Non-Facility	MP	Total Non-Facility
63077	22.88	14.51	6.23	43.62
63078	3.28	1.51	1.22	6.01

Modifiers (PAR)

Code	Mod 50	Mod 51	Mod 62	Mod 66	Mod 80
63077	0	2	2	0	2
63078	0	0	2	0	2

Global Period

Code	Days
63077	090
63078	ZZZ

63081-63082

63081 Vertebral corpectomy (vertebral body resection), partial or complete, anterior approach with decompression of spinal cord and/or nerve root(s); cervical, single segment

+ **63082 Vertebral corpectomy (vertebral body resection), partial or complete, anterior approach with decompression of spinal cord and/or nerve root(s); cervical, each additional segment (List separately in addition to code for primary procedure)**

(Use 63082 in conjunction with 63081)

(For transoral approach, see 61575, 61576)

AMA Coding Guideline

Anterior or Anterolateral Approach for Extradural Exploration/Decompression Procedures on the Spine and Spinal Cord

For the following codes, when two surgeons work together as primary surgeons performing distinct part(s) of spinal cord exploration/decompression operation, each surgeon should report his/her distinct operative work by appending modifier 62 to the procedure code (and any associated add-on codes for that procedure code as long as both surgeons continue to work together as primary surgeons). In this situation, modifier 62 may be appended to the definitive procedure code(s) 63075, 63077, 63081, 63085, 63087, 63090 and, as appropriate, to associated additional interspace add-on code(s) 63076, 63078 or additional segment add-on code(s) 63082, 63086, 63088, 63091 as long as both surgeons continue to work together as primary surgeons.

For vertebral corpectomy, the term partial is used to describe removal of a substantial portion of the body of the vertebra. In the cervical spine, the amount of bone removed is defined as at least one-half of the vertebral body. In the thoracic and lumbar spine, the amount of bone removed is defined as at least one-third of the vertebral body.

AMA Coding Notes

Surgical Procedures on the Spine and Spinal Cord

(For application of caliper or tongs, use 20660)

(For treatment of fracture or dislocation of spine, see 22310-22327)

AMA *CPT Assistant* □

63081: Spring 93: 37, Feb 02: 4, Jul 13: 3, Jun 15: 10, Apr 16: 8

63082: Spring 93: 37, Feb 02: 4, Apr 16: 8

Plain English Description

Vertebral corpectomy involves removal of the vertebral body as well as the vertebral discs above and below the vertebra. The procedure is typically performed to treat severe spinal stenosis with bone spurs arising from the vertebral body as well as the vertebral arch. The procedure may also be performed to treat fracture, tumor, or infection of the spine. Often multiple vertebral segments are involved. The cervical spine is exposed via an anterior approach, beginning with a skin incision in the anterior aspect of the neck. The soft tissues and muscles overlying the cervical spine are dissected. The trachea and esophagus are retracted. The affected segment of the cervical spine is exposed. The intervertebral discs above and below the vertebral body are removed first with the aid of the surgical microscope. The discs are carefully dissected from surrounding tissue and removed. Bone spurs and any bone impinging on the nerve roots are also removed along with the ligament that covers the spinal cord. The vertebral body is then excised. Separately reportable bone grafting and fusion procedures are performed. The bone graft is placed in the surgical defect to support the anterior aspect of the spine where the discs and vertebral body have been removed. Surrounding bone is contoured for placement of the graft and to ensure fusion of the graft and adjacent bone. Separately reportable internal fixation may also be used to stabilize the spine. Upon completion of the procedure, bleeding is controlled and soft tissues and skin are closed in layers. Use 63081 for a single cervical segment and 63082 for each additional cervical segment.

Vertebral corpectomy, partial or complete, anterior approach with decompression of spinal cord and/or nerve roots

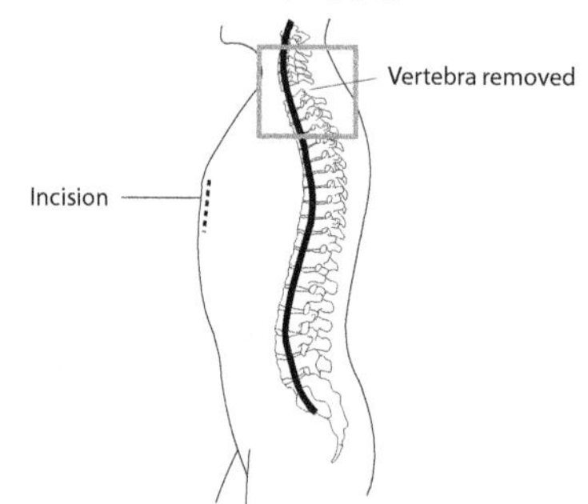

Cervical, single segment (63081); cervical, each additional segment (63082)

ICD-10-CM Diagnostic Codes

	Code	Description
	C41.2	Malignant neoplasm of vertebral column
	C79.51	Secondary malignant neoplasm of bone
	D16.6	Benign neoplasm of vertebral column
	G06.1	Intraspinal abscess and granuloma
	G95.20	Unspecified cord compression
	G95.89	Other specified diseases of spinal cord
	M25.78	Osteophyte, vertebrae
	M45.2	Ankylosing spondylitis of cervical region
	M45.3	Ankylosing spondylitis of cervicothoracic region
	M46.22	Osteomyelitis of vertebra, cervical region
	M46.23	Osteomyelitis of vertebra, cervicothoracic region
	M47.012	Anterior spinal artery compression syndromes, cervical region
	M47.013	Anterior spinal artery compression syndromes, cervicothoracic region
	M47.12	Other spondylosis with myelopathy, cervical region
	M47.13	Other spondylosis with myelopathy, cervicothoracic region
	M47.22	Other spondylosis with radiculopathy, cervical region
	M47.23	Other spondylosis with radiculopathy, cervicothoracic region
❼	M48.42	Fatigue fracture of vertebra, cervical region
❼	M48.43	Fatigue fracture of vertebra, cervicothoracic region
❼	M48.52	Collapsed vertebra, not elsewhere classified, cervical region
❼	M48.53	Collapsed vertebra, not elsewhere classified, cervicothoracic region
❼	M84.58	Pathological fracture in neoplastic disease, other specified site
❼	M84.68	Pathological fracture in other disease, other site
	M86.68	Other chronic osteomyelitis, other site

ICD-10-CM Coding Notes

For codes requiring a 7th character extension, refer to your ICD-10-CM book. Review the character descriptions and coding guidelines for proper selection. For some procedures, only certain characters will apply.

CCI Edits

Refer to Appendix A for CCI edits.

Pub 100

63081: Pub 100-04, 12, 20.4.5

63082: Pub 100-04, 12, 20.4.5

Facility RVUs □

Code	Work	PE Facility	MP	Total Facility
63081	26.10	17.06	7.79	50.95
63082	4.36	2.08	1.28	7.72

Non-facility RVUs □

Code	Work	PE Non-Facility	MP	Total Non-Facility
63081	26.10	17.06	7.79	50.95
63082	4.36	2.08	1.28	7.72

Modifiers (PAR) □

Code	Mod 50	Mod 51	Mod 62	Mod 66	Mod 80
63081	0	2	1	2	2
63082	0	0	1	2	2

Global Period

Code	Days
63081	090
63082	ZZZ

63085-63086

63085 Vertebral corpectomy (vertebral body resection), partial or complete, transthoracic approach with decompression of spinal cord and/or nerve root(s); thoracic, single segment

+ **63086 Vertebral corpectomy (vertebral body resection), partial or complete, transthoracic approach with decompression of spinal cord and/or nerve root(s); thoracic, each additional segment (List separately in addition to code for primary procedure)**

(Use 63086 in conjunction with 63085)

AMA Coding Guideline

Anterior or Anterolateral Approach for Extradural Exploration/Decompression Procedures on the Spine and Spinal Cord

For the following codes, when two surgeons work together as primary surgeons performing distinct part(s) of spinal cord exploration/decompression operation, each surgeon should report his/her distinct operative work by appending modifier 62 to the procedure code (and any associated add-on codes for that procedure code as long as both surgeons continue to work together as primary surgeons). In this situation, modifier 62 may be appended to the definitive procedure code(s) 63075, 63077, 63081, 63085, 63087, 63090 and, as appropriate, to associated additional interspace add-on code(s) 63076, 63078 or additional segment add-on code(s) 63082, 63086, 63088, 63091 as long as both surgeons continue to work together as primary surgeons.

For vertebral corpectomy, the term partial is used to describe removal of a substantial portion of the body of the vertebra. In the cervical spine, the amount of bone removed is defined as at least one-half of the vertebral body. In the thoracic and lumbar spine, the amount of bone removed is defined as at least one-third of the vertebral body.

AMA Coding Notes

Surgical Procedures on the Spine and Spinal Cord

(For application of caliper or tongs, use 20660)

(For treatment of fracture or dislocation of spine, see 22310-22327)

AMA *CPT Assistant* ▯

63085: Spring 93: 37, Feb 02: 4, Jul 13: 3, Apr 16: 8

63086: Spring 93: 37, Feb 02: 4, Apr 16: 8

Plain English Description

Vertebral corpectomy involves removal of the vertebral body as well as the vertebral discs above and below the vertebra. The procedure is typically performed to treat severe spinal stenosis with bone spurs arising from the vertebral body as well as the vertebral arch. The procedure may also be performed to treat fracture, tumor, or infection of the spine. Often multiple vertebral segments are involved. Vertebral corpectomy of the thoracic spine is performed using a transthoracic approach, which requires a thoracotomy. Typically a co-surgeon or team approach is used, with the exposure being performed by a thoracic surgeon and the corpectomy performed by a spine surgeon. The skin over the thorax is incised to allow access to the appropriate levels of the thoracic spine. Overlying muscles are dissected and one or more ribs are resected. Rib spreaders are used to allow adequate exposure of the spine. The affected portion of the thoracic spine is exposed. The intervertebral discs above and below the vertebral body are removed first with the aid of the surgical microscope. The discs are carefully dissected from surrounding tissue and removed. Bone spurs and any bone impinging on the nerve roots are also removed along with the ligament that covers the spinal cord. The vertebral body is then excised. Separately reportable bone grafting and fusion procedures are performed. The bone graft is placed in the surgical defect to support the anterior aspect of the spine where the discs and vertebral body have been removed. Surrounding bone is contoured for placement of the graft and to ensure fusion of the graft and adjacent bone. Separately reportable internal fixation may also be used to stabilize the spine. Upon completion of the procedure, bleeding is controlled, a chest tube is placed, and the thorax is closed in layers. Use 63085 for a single thoracic segment and 63086 for each additional thoracic segment.

Vertebral corpectomy, partial or complete, transthoracic approach with decompression of spinal cord and/or

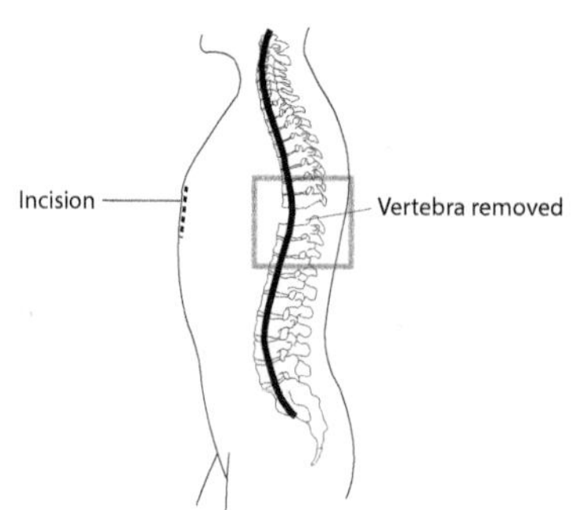

Thoracic, single segment (63085); thoracic, each additional segment (63086)

ICD-10-CM Diagnostic Codes

C41.2	Malignant neoplasm of vertebral column
C72.0	Malignant neoplasm of spinal cord
C79.49	Secondary malignant neoplasm of other parts of nervous system
C79.51	Secondary malignant neoplasm of bone
D16.6	Benign neoplasm of vertebral column
G06.1	Intraspinal abscess and granuloma
G95.20	Unspecified cord compression
G95.89	Other specified diseases of spinal cord
M25.78	Osteophyte, vertebrae
M45.4	Ankylosing spondylitis of thoracic region
M46.24	Osteomyelitis of vertebra, thoracic region
M47.014	Anterior spinal artery compression syndromes, thoracic region
M47.14	Other spondylosis with myelopathy, thoracic region
M47.24	Other spondylosis with radiculopathy, thoracic region
M48.04	Spinal stenosis, thoracic region
⑦ M48.44	Fatigue fracture of vertebra, thoracic region
⑦ M48.54	Collapsed vertebra, not elsewhere classified, thoracic region
⑦ M84.58	Pathological fracture in neoplastic disease, other specified site
⑦ M84.68	Pathological fracture in other disease, other site
M86.68	Other chronic osteomyelitis, other site

ICD-10-CM Coding Notes

For codes requiring a 7th character extension, refer to your ICD-10-CM book. Review the character descriptions and coding guidelines for proper selection. For some procedures, only certain characters will apply.

CCI Edits

Refer to Appendix A for CCI edits.

Pub 100

63085: Pub 100-04, 12, 20.4.5

63086: Pub 100-04, 12, 20.4.5

Facility RVUs ▯

Code	Work	PE Facility	MP	Total Facility
63085	29.47	17.80	8.46	55.73
63086	3.19	1.46	0.88	5.53

Non-facility RVUs ▯

Code	Work	PE Non-Facility	MP	Total Non-Facility
63085	29.47	17.80	8.46	55.73
63086	3.19	1.46	0.88	5.53

Modifiers (PAR) ▯

Code	Mod 50	Mod 51	Mod 62	Mod 66	Mod 80
63085	0	2	2	2	2
63086	0	0	2	2	2

Global Period

Code	Days
63085	090
63086	ZZZ

63087-63088

63087 Vertebral corpectomy (vertebral body resection), partial or complete, combined thoracolumbar approach with decompression of spinal cord, cauda equina or nerve root(s), lower thoracic or lumbar; single segment

+ **63088 Vertebral corpectomy (vertebral body resection), partial or complete, combined thoracolumbar approach with decompression of spinal cord, cauda equina or nerve root(s), lower thoracic or lumbar; each additional segment (List separately in addition to code for primary procedure)**

(Use 63088 in conjunction with 63087)

AMA Coding Guideline

Anterior or Anterolateral Approach for Extradural Exploration/Decompression Procedures on the Spine and Spinal Cord

For the following codes, when two surgeons work together as primary surgeons performing distinct part(s) of spinal cord exploration/decompression operation, each surgeon should report his/her distinct operative work by appending modifier 62 to the procedure code (and any associated add-on codes for that procedure code as long as both surgeons continue to work together as primary surgeons). In this situation, modifier 62 may be appended to the definitive procedure code(s) 63075, 63077, 63081, 63085, 63087, 63090 and, as appropriate, to associated additional interspace add-on code(s) 63076, 63078 or additional segment add-on code(s) 63082, 63086, 63088, 63091 as long as both surgeons continue to work together as primary surgeons.

For vertebral corpectomy, the term partial is used to describe removal of a substantial portion of the body of the vertebra. In the cervical spine, the amount of bone removed is defined as at least one-half of the vertebral body. In the thoracic and lumbar spine, the amount of bone removed is defined as at least one-third of the vertebral body.

AMA Coding Notes

Surgical Procedures on the Spine and Spinal Cord

(For application of caliper or tongs, use 20660)

(For treatment of fracture or dislocation of spine, see 22310-22327)

AMA *CPT Assistant*

63087: Spring 93: 37, Feb 02: 4, Jul 13: 3, Apr 16: 8

63088: Spring 93: 37, Feb 02: 4, Apr 16: 8

Plain English Description

Vertebral corpectomy involves removal of the vertebral body as well as the vertebral discs above and below the vertebra. The procedure is typically performed to treat severe spinal stenosis with bone spurs arising from the vertebral body as well as the vertebral arch. The procedure may also be performed to treat fracture, tumor, or infection of the spine. Often multiple vertebral segments are involved. Vertebral corpectomy of the lower thoracic or lumbar spine is performed using a combined thoracolumbar approach. Typically, a co-surgeon team approach is used, with the exposure being performed by a thoracic surgeon and the corpectomy performed by a spine surgeon. The skin over the thorax is incised to allow access to the appropriate levels of the thoracic spine. Overlying muscles are dissected and one or more ribs are resected. Rib spreaders are used to allow adequate exposure of the thoracic spine. The thoracic incision is extended over the abdomen to allow adequate exposure of all diseased or damaged lower thoracic and lumbar segments. Once the spine is adequately exposed, intervertebral discs above and below the vertebral body are removed with the aid of the surgical microscope. The discs are carefully dissected from surrounding tissue and removed. Bone spurs and any bone impinging on the nerve roots are also removed, along with the ligament that covers the spinal cord. The vertebral body is then excised. Separately reportable bone grafting and fusion procedures are performed. The bone graft is placed in the surgical defect to support the anterior aspect of the spine where the discs and vertebral body have been removed. Surrounding bone is contoured for placement of the graft and to ensure fusion of the graft and adjacent bone. Separately reportable internal fixation may also be used to stabilize the spine. Upon completion of the procedure, bleeding is controlled, a chest tube is placed, and the thorax and abdomen are closed in layers. Use 63087 for a single lower thoracic or lumbar segment and 63088 for each additional segment.

Vertebral corpectomy, combined thoracolumbar approach with decompression

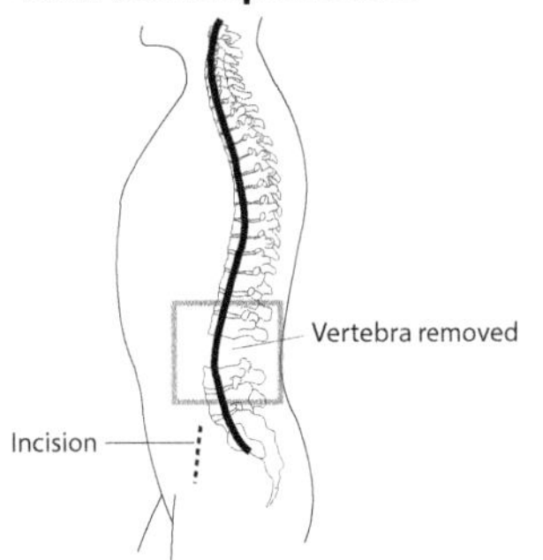

Lower thoracic or lumbar, single segment (63087); lower thoracic or lumbar, each additional segment (63088)

ICD-10-CM Diagnostic Codes

	Code	Description
	C41.2	Malignant neoplasm of vertebral column
	C72.0	Malignant neoplasm of spinal cord
	C79.49	Secondary malignant neoplasm of other parts of nervous system
	C79.51	Secondary malignant neoplasm of bone
	D16.6	Benign neoplasm of vertebral column
	G06.1	Intraspinal abscess and granuloma
	G12.25	Progressive spinal muscle atrophy
	G95.20	Unspecified cord compression
	G95.81	Conus medullaris syndrome
	G95.89	Other specified diseases of spinal cord
	M25.78	Osteophyte, vertebrae
	M40.35	Flatback syndrome, thoracolumbar region
	M40.36	Flatback syndrome, lumbar region
	M45.5	Ankylosing spondylitis of thoracolumbar region
	M45.6	Ankylosing spondylitis lumbar region
	M46.25	Osteomyelitis of vertebra, thoracolumbar region
	M46.26	Osteomyelitis of vertebra, lumbar region
	M47.015	Anterior spinal artery compression syndromes, thoracolumbar region
	M47.016	Anterior spinal artery compression syndromes, lumbar region
	M47.15	Other spondylosis with myelopathy, thoracolumbar region
	M47.16	Other spondylosis with myelopathy, lumbar region
	M47.25	Other spondylosis with radiculopathy, thoracolumbar region
	M47.26	Other spondylosis with radiculopathy, lumbar region
	M48.05	Spinal stenosis, thoracolumbar region
	M48.061	Spinal stenosis, lumbar region without neurogenic claudication
	M48.062	Spinal stenosis, lumbar region with neurogenic claudication
⓻	M48.45	Fatigue fracture of vertebra, thoracolumbar region
⓻	M48.46	Fatigue fracture of vertebra, lumbar region
⓻	M48.55	Collapsed vertebra, not elsewhere classified, thoracolumbar region
⓻	M48.56	Collapsed vertebra, not elsewhere classified, lumbar region
⓻	M84.58	Pathological fracture in neoplastic disease, other specified site
⓻	M84.68	Pathological fracture in other disease, other site
	M86.68	Other chronic osteomyelitis, other site

ICD-10-CM Coding Notes

For codes requiring a 7th character extension, refer to your ICD-10-CM book. Review the character descriptions and coding guidelines for proper selection. For some procedures, only certain characters will apply.

CCI Edits

Refer to Appendix A for CCI edits.

Pub 100

63087: Pub 100-04, 12, 20.4.5
63088: Pub 100-04, 12, 20.4.5

Facility RVUs

Code	Work	PE Facility	MP	Total Facility
63087	37.53	21.51	10.76	69.80
63088	4.32	1.95	1.16	7.43

Non-facility RVUs

Code	Work	PE Non-Facility	MP	Total Non-Facility
63087	37.53	21.51	10.76	69.80
63088	4.32	1.95	1.16	7.43

Modifiers (PAR)

Code	Mod 50	Mod 51	Mod 62	Mod 66	Mod 80
63087	0	2	2	2	2
63088	0	0	2	2	2

Global Period

Code	Days
63087	090
63088	ZZZ

63090-63091

63090 Vertebral corpectomy (vertebral body resection), partial or complete, transperitoneal or retroperitoneal approach with decompression of spinal cord, cauda equina or nerve root(s), lower thoracic, lumbar, or sacral; single segment

✚ **63091 Vertebral corpectomy (vertebral body resection), partial or complete, transperitoneal or retroperitoneal approach with decompression of spinal cord, cauda equina or nerve root(s), lower thoracic, lumbar, or sacral; each additional segment (List separately in addition to code for primary procedure)**

(Use 63091 in conjunction with 63090)

(Procedures 63081-63091 include discectomy above and/or below vertebral segment)

(If followed by arthrodesis, see 22548-22812)

(For reconstruction of spine, use appropriate vertebral corpectomy codes 63081-63091, bone graft codes 20930-20938, arthrodesis codes 22548-22812, and spinal instrumentation codes 22840-22855, 22859)

AMA Coding Guideline

Anterior or Anterolateral Approach for Extradural Exploration/Decompression Procedures on the Spine and Spinal Cord

For the following codes, when two surgeons work together as primary surgeons performing distinct part(s) of spinal cord exploration/decompression operation, each surgeon should report his/her distinct operative work by appending modifier 62 to the procedure code (and any associated add-on codes for that procedure code as long as both surgeons continue to work together as primary surgeons). In this situation, modifier 62 may be appended to the definitive procedure code(s) 63075, 63077, 63081, 63085, 63087, 63090 and, as appropriate, to associated additional interspace add-on code(s) 63076, 63078 or additional segment add-on code(s) 63082, 63086, 63088, 63091 as long as both surgeons continue to work together as primary surgeons.

For vertebral corpectomy, the term partial is used to describe removal of a substantial portion of the body of the vertebra. In the cervical spine, the amount of bone removed is defined as at least one-half of the vertebral body. In the thoracic and lumbar spine, the amount of bone removed is defined as at least one-third of the vertebral body.

AMA Coding Notes

Surgical Procedures on the Spine and Spinal Cord

(For application of caliper or tongs, use 20660)

(For treatment of fracture or dislocation of spine, see 22310-22327)

AMA *CPT Assistant* ▯

63090: Spring 93: 37, Mar 96: 6, Feb 02: 4, Jul 13: 3, Apr 16: 8

63091: Spring 93: 37, Mar 96: 6, Feb 02: 4, Apr 16: 8

Plain English Description

Vertebral corpectomy involves removal of the vertebral body as well as the vertebral discs above and below the vertebra. The procedure is typically performed to treat severe spinal stenosis with bone spurs arising from the vertebral body as well as the vertebral arch. The procedure may also be performed to treat fracture, tumor, or infection of the spine. Often multiple vertebral segments are involved. Vertebral corpectomy of the lower thoracic, lumbar, or sacral spine is performed using an anterior or anterolateral approach. A co-surgeon or team approach may be used, with the exposure being performed by a general surgeon and the corpectomy performed by a spine surgeon. If a transperitoneal (anterior) approach is used, the abdomen is incised and the peritoneum entered. The bowel is moved out of the way. If a retroperitoneal (anterolateral) approach is used, a flank incision is made. Surrounding tissues are dissected, taking care to protect vital structures. All diseased or damaged lower thoracic, lumbar, and/or sacral segments are exposed. Intervertebral discs above and below the vertebral body are removed with the aid of the surgical microscope. The discs are carefully dissected from surrounding tissue and removed. Bone spurs and any bone impinging on the nerve roots and/or cauda equina are also removed, along with the ligament that covers the spinal cord. The vertebral body is then excised. Separately reportable bone grafting and fusion procedures are performed. The bone graft is placed in the surgical defect to support the anterior aspect of the spine where the discs and vertebral body have been removed. Surrounding bone is contoured for placement of the graft and to ensure fusion of the graft and adjacent bone. Separately reportable internal fixation may also be used to stabilize the spine. Upon completion of the procedure, bleeding is controlled, drains placed as needed, and the surgical wound is closed in layers. Use 63090 for a single lower thoracic, lumbar, or sacral segment and 63091 for each additional segment.

Vertebral corpectomy, transperitoneal or retroperitoneal approach

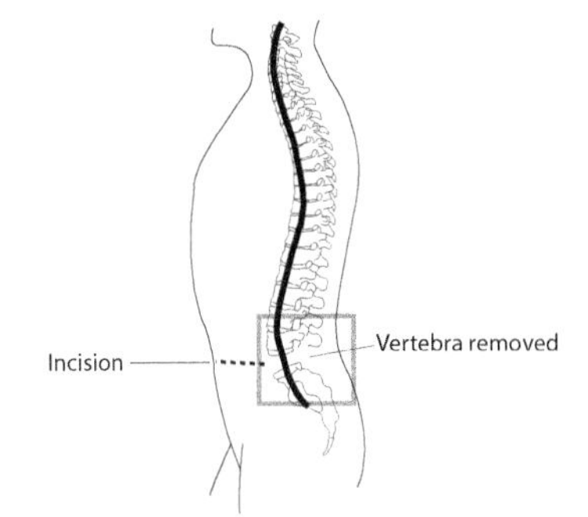

Lower thoracic, lumbar, or sacral, single segment (63090); lower thoracic, lumbar, or sacral, each additional segment (63091)

ICD-10-CM Diagnostic Codes

C41.2	Malignant neoplasm of vertebral column
C72.0	Malignant neoplasm of spinal cord
C79.49	Secondary malignant neoplasm of other parts of nervous system
C79.51	Secondary malignant neoplasm of bone
D16.6	Benign neoplasm of vertebral column
G06.1	Intraspinal abscess and granuloma
G12.25	Progressive spinal muscle atrophy
G83.4	Cauda equina syndrome
G95.20	Unspecified cord compression
G95.81	Conus medullaris syndrome
G95.89	Other specified diseases of spinal cord
M25.78	Osteophyte, vertebrae
M40.35	Flatback syndrome, thoracolumbar region
M40.36	Flatback syndrome, lumbar region
M45.5	Ankylosing spondylitis of thoracolumbar region
M45.6	Ankylosing spondylitis lumbar region
M45.7	Ankylosing spondylitis of lumbosacral region
M45.8	Ankylosing spondylitis sacral and sacrococcygeal region
M46.25	Osteomyelitis of vertebra, thoracolumbar region
M46.26	Osteomyelitis of vertebra, lumbar region
M46.27	Osteomyelitis of vertebra, lumbosacral region
M46.28	Osteomyelitis of vertebra, sacral and sacrococcygeal region
M47.015	Anterior spinal artery compression syndromes, thoracolumbar region
M47.016	Anterior spinal artery compression syndromes, lumbar region
M47.15	Other spondylosis with myelopathy, thoracolumbar region
M47.16	Other spondylosis with myelopathy, lumbar region
M47.17	Other spondylosis with myelopathy, lumbosacral region
M47.25	Other spondylosis with radiculopathy, thoracolumbar region

	Code	Description
	M47.26	Other spondylosis with radiculopathy, lumbar region
	M47.27	Other spondylosis with radiculopathy, lumbosacral region
	M47.28	Other spondylosis with radiculopathy, sacral and sacrococcygeal region
	M48.05	Spinal stenosis, thoracolumbar region
	M48.061	Spinal stenosis, lumbar region without neurogenic claudication
	M48.062	Spinal stenosis, lumbar region with neurogenic claudication
	M48.07	Spinal stenosis, lumbosacral region
❼	M48.45	Fatigue fracture of vertebra, thoracolumbar region
❼	M48.46	Fatigue fracture of vertebra, lumbar region
❼	M48.47	Fatigue fracture of vertebra, lumbosacral region
❼	M48.55	Collapsed vertebra, not elsewhere classified, thoracolumbar region
❼	M48.56	Collapsed vertebra, not elsewhere classified, lumbar region
❼	M48.57	Collapsed vertebra, not elsewhere classified, lumbosacral region
	M51.06	Intervertebral disc disorders with myelopathy, lumbar region
	M51.07	Intervertebral disc disorders with myelopathy, lumbosacral region
	M51.36	Other intervertebral disc degeneration, lumbar region
	M51.37	Other intervertebral disc degeneration, lumbosacral region
❼	M84.58	Pathological fracture in neoplastic disease, other specified site
❼	M84.68	Pathological fracture in other disease, other site
	M86.68	Other chronic osteomyelitis, other site
	M96.0	Pseudarthrosis after fusion or arthrodesis
	M96.1	Postlaminectomy syndrome, not elsewhere classified

ICD-10-CM Coding Notes

For codes requiring a 7th character extension, refer to your ICD-10-CM book. Review the character descriptions and coding guidelines for proper selection. For some procedures, only certain characters will apply.

CCI Edits

Refer to Appendix A for CCI edits.

Pub 100

63090: Pub 100-04, 12, 20.4.5
63091: Pub 100-04, 12, 20.4.5

Facility RVUs ▯

Code	Work	PE Facility	MP	Total Facility
63090	30.93	18.33	7.62	56.88
63091	3.03	1.41	0.74	5.18

Non-facility RVUs ▯

Code	Work	PE Non-Facility	MP	Total Non-Facility
63090	30.93	18.33	7.62	56.88
63091	3.03	1.41	0.74	5.18

Modifiers (PAR) ▯

Code	Mod 50	Mod 51	Mod 62	Mod 66	Mod 80
63090	0	2	2	2	2
63091	0	0	2	2	2

Global Period

Code	Days
63090	090
63091	ZZZ

63101-63103

63101 Vertebral corpectomy (vertebral body resection), partial or complete, lateral extracavitary approach with decompression of spinal cord and/or nerve root(s) (eg, for tumor or retropulsed bone fragments); thoracic, single segment

63102 Vertebral corpectomy (vertebral body resection), partial or complete, lateral extracavitary approach with decompression of spinal cord and/or nerve root(s) (eg, for tumor or retropulsed bone fragments); lumbar, single segment

✚ **63103 Vertebral corpectomy (vertebral body resection), partial or complete, lateral extracavitary approach with decompression of spinal cord and/or nerve root(s) (eg, for tumor or retropulsed bone fragments); thoracic or lumbar, each additional segment (List separately in addition to code for primary procedure)**

(Use 63103 in conjunction with 63101 and 63102)

AMA Coding Guideline

Lateral Extracavitary Approach for Extradural Exploration/Decompression Procedures on the Spine and Spinal Cord

For vertebral corpectomy, the term partial is used to describe removal of a substantial portion of the body of the vertebra. In the cervical spine, the amount of bone removed is defined as at least one-half of the vertebral body. In the thoracic and lumbar spine, the amount of bone removed is defined as at least one-third of the vertebral body.

AMA Coding Notes

Surgical Procedures on the Spine and Spinal Cord

(For application of caliper or tongs, use 20660)

(For treatment of fracture or dislocation of spine, see 22310-22327)

AMA *CPT Assistant*

63101: Jul 13: 3

63102: Jul 13: 3

Plain English Description

Vertebral corpectomy involves removal of the vertebral body as well as the vertebral discs above and below the vertebra. In this procedure a lateral extracavity approach is used. This approach is more commonly used to treat tumor or fractures with retropulsed bone fragments, although it may also be used for severe spinal stenosis and infection. A co-surgeon or team approach may be used with the exposure being performed by a general or thoracic surgeon and the corpectomy performed by a spine surgeon. The skin of the back is incised in the midline over the involved vertebral segments and then carried laterally to allow exposure of the paraspinal muscles. Overlying muscles are elevated and the spinous processes and laminae exposed. The paraspinal muscle bundle is divided lateral to the spine and elevated off the ribs. The tumor, fracture, or other condition is identified using intraoperative imaging as needed. The ribs may be resected. The intercostal nerves are identified and protected. The spinous processes, facets, and pedicles are removed using a high-speed drill. The dural sac is exposed, along with the lateral aspect of the vertebral body. For a thoracic corpectomy, the parietal pleura are retracted as needed to allow more complete exposure of the vertebral body. The nerve root may be divided or retracted superiorly to allow better visualization of the vertebra. The vertebral body is partially or completely excised. The discs inferior and superior to the vertebral body are also removed. Any remaining tumor tissue, bone fragments, bone spurs, or other lesions are removed. The site is then prepared for separately reportable bone grafts, fusion, and internal fixation devices. Use 63101 for vertebral corpectomy of a single thoracic segment, 63102 for a single lumbar segment, and 63103 for each additional thoracic or lumbar segment.

Vertebral corpectomy, lateral extracavitary approach

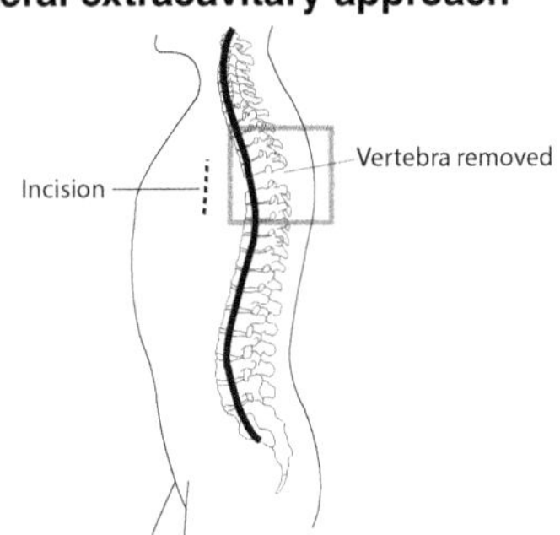

Thoracic, single segment (63101); thoracic, each additional segment (63103)

ICD-10-CM Diagnostic Codes

	Code	Description
	C41.2	Malignant neoplasm of vertebral column
	C72.0	Malignant neoplasm of spinal cord
	C79.49	Secondary malignant neoplasm of other parts of nervous system
	C79.51	Secondary malignant neoplasm of bone
	D16.6	Benign neoplasm of vertebral column
	D33.4	Benign neoplasm of spinal cord
	D43.4	Neoplasm of uncertain behavior of spinal cord
	D48.0	Neoplasm of uncertain behavior of bone and articular cartilage
⑦	M48.44	Fatigue fracture of vertebra, thoracic region
⑦	M48.45	Fatigue fracture of vertebra, thoracolumbar region
⑦	M48.46	Fatigue fracture of vertebra, lumbar region
⑦	M48.54	Collapsed vertebra, not elsewhere classified, thoracic region
⑦	M48.55	Collapsed vertebra, not elsewhere classified, thoracolumbar region
⑦	M48.56	Collapsed vertebra, not elsewhere classified, lumbar region
⑦	M80.88	Other osteoporosis with current pathological fracture, vertebra(e)
⑦	M84.58	Pathological fracture in neoplastic disease, other specified site
⑦	M84.68	Pathological fracture in other disease, other site
⑦	S22.012	Unstable burst fracture of first thoracic vertebra
⑦	S22.022	Unstable burst fracture of second thoracic vertebra
⑦	S22.032	Unstable burst fracture of third thoracic vertebra
⑦	S22.042	Unstable burst fracture of fourth thoracic vertebra
⑦	S22.052	Unstable burst fracture of T5-T6 vertebra
⑦	S22.062	Unstable burst fracture of T7-T8 vertebra
⑦	S22.072	Unstable burst fracture of T9-T10 vertebra
⑦	S22.082	Unstable burst fracture of T11-T12 vertebra
⑦	S32.012	Unstable burst fracture of first lumbar vertebra
⑦	S32.022	Unstable burst fracture of second lumbar vertebra
⑦	S32.032	Unstable burst fracture of third lumbar vertebra
⑦	S32.042	Unstable burst fracture of fourth lumbar vertebra
⑦	S32.052	Unstable burst fracture of fifth lumbar vertebra

ICD-10-CM Coding Notes

For codes requiring a 7th character extension, refer to your ICD-10-CM book. Review the character descriptions and coding guidelines for proper selection. For some procedures, only certain characters will apply.

CCI Edits

Refer to Appendix A for CCI edits.

Pub 100

63101: Pub 100-04, 12, 20.4.5

63102: Pub 100-04, 12, 20.4.5

63103: Pub 100-04, 12, 20.4.5

Facility RVUs

Code	Work	PE Facility	MP	Total Facility
63101	34.10	22.19	10.98	67.27
63102	34.10	21.82	9.61	65.53
63103	4.82	2.29	1.42	8.53

Non-facility RVUs

Code	Work	PE Non-Facility	MP	Total Non-Facility
63101	34.10	22.19	10.98	67.27
63102	34.10	21.82	9.61	65.53
63103	4.82	2.29	1.42	8.53

Modifiers (PAR)

Code	Mod 50	Mod 51	Mod 62	Mod 66	Mod 80
63101	0	2	1	0	2
63102	0	2	1	0	2
63103	0	0	1	0	2

Global Period

Code	Days
63101	090
63102	090
63103	ZZZ

63172-63173

63172 Laminectomy with drainage of intramedullary cyst/syrinx; to subarachnoid space

63173 Laminectomy with drainage of intramedullary cyst/syrinx; to peritoneal or pleural space

AMA Coding Notes

Surgical Procedures on the Spine and Spinal Cord

(For application of caliper or tongs, use 20660)

(For treatment of fracture or dislocation of spine, see 22310-22327)

AMA *CPT Assistant* □

63172: Jul 13: 3

63173: Jul 13: 3

Plain English Description

An intramedullary cyst or syrinx is a rare lesion consisting of a fluid-filled cavity within the spinal cord. The skin is incised over the cervical, thoracic, or thoracolumbar region where the intramedullary cyst or syrinx is located and extended down to the spinous processes. Muscle is retracted off the lamina and facet joint. A bone drill is used to remove part or all of the lamina, the spinal cord is exposed, and the cyst or syrinx evaluated. The lesion is incised and drained. A drain is placed in the lesion. The drain is tunneled and secured. In 63172, a short drain is placed that terminates in the subarachnoid space, which is the space between the arachnoid, the middle membrane covering the spinal cord, and the pia mater, the innermost membrane that is adherent to the spinal cord. In 63173, the drain is tunneled to the planned exit site in the peritoneal or pleural cavity. The peritoneum or pleura is incised and the drain is placed into the peritoneal or pleural cavity. The drain is secured and the surgical incisions are closed.

Laminectomy with drainage of intramedullary cyst/syrinx

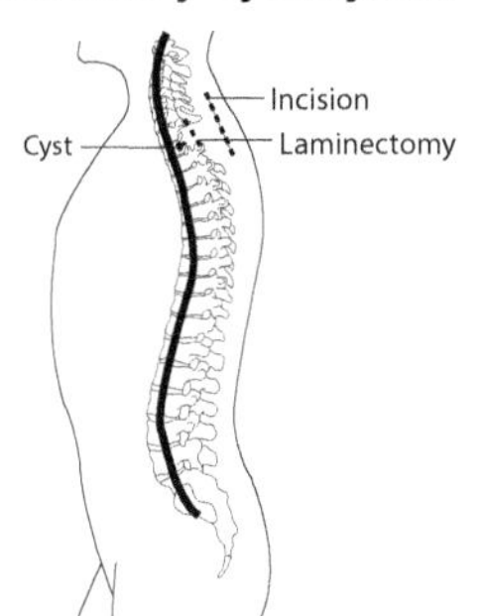

The lamina is removed from around a vertebra and a cyst is drained; into spinal cord (63172); into abdominal/chest cavity (63173).

ICD-10-CM Diagnostic Codes

D33.4	Benign neoplasm of spinal cord
G95.0	Syringomyelia and syringobulbia
G95.89	Other specified diseases of spinal cord
Q06.4	Hydromyelia

CCI Edits

Refer to Appendix A for CCI edits.

Pub 100

63172: Pub 100-04, 12, 20.4.5

63173: Pub 100-04, 12, 20.4.5

Facility RVUs □

Code	Work	PE Facility	MP	Total Facility
63172	19.76	13.61	6.64	40.01
63173	24.31	16.51	8.97	49.79

Non-facility RVUs □

Code	Work	PE Non-Facility	MP	Total Non-Facility
63172	19.76	13.61	6.64	40.01
63173	24.31	16.51	8.97	49.79

Modifiers (PAR) □

Code	Mod 50	Mod 51	Mod 62	Mod 66	Mod 80
63172	0	2	1	0	2
63173	0	2	1	0	2

Global Period

Code	Days
63172	090
63173	090

63185-63190

63185 Laminectomy with rhizotomy; 1 or 2 segments

63190 Laminectomy with rhizotomy; more than 2 segments

AMA Coding Notes

Surgical Procedures on the Spine and Spinal Cord

(For application of caliper or tongs, use 20660)

(For treatment of fracture or dislocation of spine, see 22310-22327)

AMA *CPT Assistant*

63185: Jul 13: 3

63190: Jul 13: 3

Plain English Description

Rhizotomy is performed to treat spasticity that has not responded to oral medications or less invasive treatment modalities, such as facet joint or nerve root injections of botulinum toxin, phenol, or alcohol. The procedure is most commonly used to treat severe lower extremity spasticity caused by cerebral palsy. The skin is incised over the spine in the region where the rhizotomy will be performed. The incision is extended down to the spinous processes. Muscle is retracted off the lamina and facet joint. A bone drill is used to remove part or all of the lamina, and the spinal cord and nerve roots are exposed. Electrical stimulation is applied selectively to individual nerve rootlets to identify the motor nerve rootlets that are causing the spasticity and the nerve rootlets are cut. Use 63185 when the procedure is performed on one or two vertebral segments. Use 63190 when rhizotomy is performed on more than two vertebral segments.

Laminectomy with rhizotomy

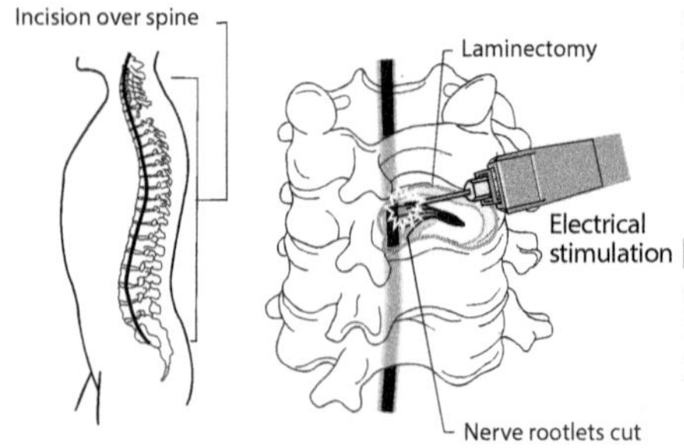

1 or 2 segments (63185); more than 2 segments (63190)

ICD-10-CM Diagnostic Codes

G80.1	Spastic diplegic cerebral palsy
G80.2	Spastic hemiplegic cerebral palsy
G83.4	Cauda equina syndrome
M47.23	Other spondylosis with radiculopathy, cervicothoracic region
M47.24	Other spondylosis with radiculopathy, thoracic region
M47.25	Other spondylosis with radiculopathy, thoracolumbar region
M47.26	Other spondylosis with radiculopathy, lumbar region
M47.27	Other spondylosis with radiculopathy, lumbosacral region
M50.121	Cervical disc disorder at C4-C5 level with radiculopathy
M50.122	Cervical disc disorder at C5-C6 level with radiculopathy
M50.123	Cervical disc disorder at C6-C7 level with radiculopathy
M50.13	Cervical disc disorder with radiculopathy, cervicothoracic region
M50.80	Other cervical disc disorders, unspecified cervical region
M51.14	Intervertebral disc disorders with radiculopathy, thoracic region
M51.15	Intervertebral disc disorders with radiculopathy, thoracolumbar region
M51.16	Intervertebral disc disorders with radiculopathy, lumbar region
M51.17	Intervertebral disc disorders with radiculopathy, lumbosacral region
M54.5	Low back pain
M54.6	Pain in thoracic spine
M54.8	Other dorsalgia
M62.830	Muscle spasm of back
M96.1	Postlaminectomy syndrome, not elsewhere classified

CCI Edits

Refer to Appendix A for CCI edits.

Pub 100

63185: Pub 100-04, 12, 20.4.5

63190: Pub 100-04, 12, 20.4.5

Facility RVUs

Code	Work	PE Facility	MP	Total Facility
63185	16.49	12.18	4.48	33.15
63190	18.89	13.39	3.75	36.03

Non-facility RVUs

Code	Work	PE Non-Facility	MP	Total Non-Facility
63185	16.49	12.18	4.48	33.15
63190	18.89	13.39	3.75	36.03

Modifiers (PAR)

Code	Mod 50	Mod 51	Mod 62	Mod 66	Mod 80
63185	0	2	1	0	2
63190	0	2	1	0	2

Global Period

Code	Days
63185	090
63190	090

63198-63199

63198 Laminectomy with cordotomy with section of both spinothalamic tracts, 2 stages within 14 days; cervical

63199 Laminectomy with cordotomy with section of both spinothalamic tracts, 2 stages within 14 days; thoracic

AMA Coding Notes

Surgical Procedures on the Spine and Spinal Cord

(For application of caliper or tongs, use 20660)

(For treatment of fracture or dislocation of spine, see 22310-22327)

AMA *CPT Assistant* ▯

63198: Jul 13: 3

63199: Jul 13: 3

Plain English Description

Cordotomy is performed to selectively destroy the anterior spinothalamic tract, which is the primary pain-transmitting pathway of the spinal cord. The procedure may be performed in a single operation or a two-stage procedure, unilaterally or bilaterally. The spinothalamic tract is located on both sides of the spine in the anterolateral aspect of the spinal cord. The spinothalamic tract on one side of the spinal cord carries sensory stimuli from the opposite side of the body to the brain. With the advent of new pain treatment modalities, a cordotomy is rarely performed today except for severe unilateral pain due to malignancy in terminally ill patients. The skin is incised over vertebra in the cervical or thoracic spine where the spinothalamic tract is to be destroyed. The incision is extended down to the spinous processes. Muscle is retracted off the lamina and facet joint. A bone drill is used to remove part or all of the lamina, and the spinal cord is exposed. The spinothalamic tract is identified and cut. Use 63198 for a bilateral two-stage cordotomy of the cervical spine with the second stage being performed within 14 days of the first stage or 63199 if a two-stage procedure is performed on the thoracic spine.

Laminectomy with cordotomy, with section of both spinothalamic tracts, 2 stages within 14 days

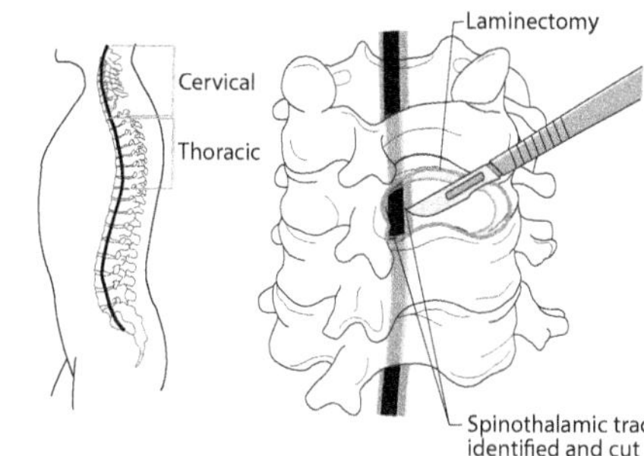

Cervical (63198); thoracic (63199)

ICD-10-CM Diagnostic Codes

C45.0	Mesothelioma of pleura
C45.1	Mesothelioma of peritoneum
C45.2	Mesothelioma of pericardium
C45.7	Mesothelioma of other sites
C45.9	Mesothelioma, unspecified
C72.0	Malignant neoplasm of spinal cord
C79.49	Secondary malignant neoplasm of other parts of nervous system
G89.0	Central pain syndrome
G89.21	Chronic pain due to trauma
G89.22	Chronic post-thoracotomy pain
G89.28	Other chronic postprocedural pain
G89.29	Other chronic pain
G89.3	Neoplasm related pain (acute) (chronic)
G89.4	Chronic pain syndrome

CCI Edits

Refer to Appendix A for CCI edits.

Pub 100

63198: Pub 100-04, 12, 20.4.5

63199: Pub 100-04, 12, 20.4.5

Facility RVUs ▯

Code	Work	PE Facility	MP	Total Facility
63198	29.90	19.39	11.07	60.36
63199	31.47	20.12	11.66	63.25

Non-facility RVUs ▯

Code	Work	PE Non-Facility	MP	Total Non-Facility
63198	29.90	19.39	11.07	60.36
63199	31.47	20.12	11.66	63.25

Modifiers (PAR) ▯

Code	Mod 50	Mod 51	Mod 62	Mod 66	Mod 80
63198	0	2	1	0	2
63199	0	2	1	0	2

Global Period

Code	Days
63198	090
63199	090

63200

63200 Laminectomy, with release of tethered spinal cord, lumbar

AMA Coding Notes

Surgical Procedures on the Spine and Spinal Cord

(For application of caliper or tongs, use 20660)

(For treatment of fracture or dislocation of spine, see 22310-22327)

AMA *CPT Assistant*

63200: Jul 13: 3

Plain English Description

Normally the distal aspect of the spinal cord, called the conus medullaris, floats freely in the spinal fluid that surrounds it. A tethered spinal cord is a condition where the end of the spinal cord is immobile due to attachment to the tissues that form the spinal canal. The condition is typically a congenital anomaly that is often associated with spina bifida and myelomeningocele; however, it can occur alone or it can result from trauma to the spinal cord. Tethering causes the spinal cord to stretch during movement and as a child grows. This stretching causes neurologic symptoms such as muscle weakness, sensory disturbances, loss of bladder and bowel control, and orthopedic deformities. The skin is incised over vertebra in the lumbar spine where the spinal cord is tethered. The incision is extended down to the spinous processes. Muscle is retracted off the lamina and facet joint. A bone drill is used to remove part or all of the lamina and the tethered end of the spinal cord is exposed. The dura mater is incised. The spinal cord is gently teased away from surrounding tissue, scar tissue, and/or fat with the aid of an operating microscope. When the spinal cord has been completely mobilized, the overlying meninges are closed with sutures or a dural patch graft.

Laminectomy, with release of tethered spinal cord, lumbar

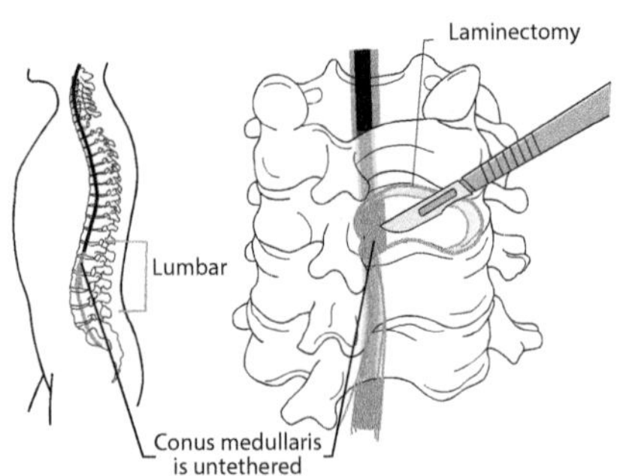

ICD-10-CM Diagnostic Codes

D33.4	Benign neoplasm of spinal cord
G95.81	Conus medullaris syndrome
G95.89	Other specified diseases of spinal cord
Q05.2	Lumbar spina bifida with hydrocephalus
Q05.6	Thoracic spina bifida without hydrocephalus
Q05.7	Lumbar spina bifida without hydrocephalus
Q05.9	Spina bifida, unspecified
Q06.1	Hypoplasia and dysplasia of spinal cord
Q06.2	Diastematomyelia
Q06.3	Other congenital cauda equina malformations
Q06.9	Congenital malformation of spinal cord, unspecified
Q07.8	Other specified congenital malformations of nervous system
Q67.5	Congenital deformity of spine
Q76.0	Spina bifida occulta
Q76.49	Other congenital malformations of spine, not associated with scoliosis

CCI Edits

Refer to Appendix A for CCI edits.

Pub 100

63200: Pub 100-04, 12, 20.4.5

Facility RVUs

Code	Work	PE Facility	MP	Total Facility
63200	21.44	15.15	7.60	44.19

Non-facility RVUs

Code	Work	PE Non-Facility	MP	Total Non-Facility
63200	21.44	15.15	7.60	44.19

Modifiers (PAR)

Code	Mod 50	Mod 51	Mod 62	Mod 66	Mod 80
63200	0	2	0	0	2

Global Period

Code	Days
63200	090

63250-63252

63250 Laminectomy for excision or occlusion of arteriovenous malformation of spinal cord; cervical

63251 Laminectomy for excision or occlusion of arteriovenous malformation of spinal cord; thoracic

63252 Laminectomy for excision or occlusion of arteriovenous malformation of spinal cord; thoracolumbar

Laminectomy for excision or occlusion of arteriovenous malformation of spinal cord

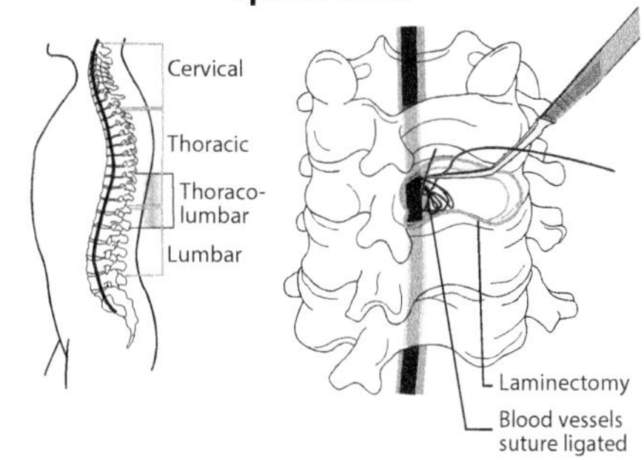

Cervical (63250); thoracic (63251); thoracolumbar (63252)

AMA Coding Notes

Surgical Procedures on the Spine and Spinal Cord

(For application of caliper or tongs, use 20660)

(For treatment of fracture or dislocation of spine, see 22310-22327)

AMA *CPT Assistant*

63250: Jul 13: 3
63251: Jul 13: 3
63252: Jul 13: 3

Plain English Description

Spinal cord arteriovenous malformation (AVM) is an extremely rare congenital anomaly that is characterized by abnormally tangled arteries and veins on, in, or near the spinal cord. An AVM may prevent oxygenated blood from reaching all the cells and tissues in and around the spinal cord, causing the tissue to die. Other complications of AVM include rupture of weakened blood vessels or compression of the spinal cord. The skin is incised over the cervical, thoracic, or thoracolumbar region where the AVM is located and extended down to the spinous processes. Muscle is retracted off the lamina and facet joint. A bone drill is used to remove part or all of the lamina, and the spinal cord is exposed. The AVM is located. Blood vessels supplying the AVM are located and suture ligated The AVM may be excised or permanently occluded using sutures or clamps. Use 63250 for an AVM in the cervical region, 63251 for an AVM in the thoracic region, or 63252 for one in the thoracolumbar region.

ICD-10-CM Diagnostic Codes

Q28.8	Other specified congenital malformations of circulatory system

CCI Edits

Refer to Appendix A for CCI edits.

Pub 100

63250: Pub 100-04, 12, 20.4.5
63251: Pub 100-04, 12, 20.4.5
63252: Pub 100-04, 12, 20.4.5

Facility RVUs

Code	Work	PE Facility	MP	Total Facility
63250	43.86	25.65	16.48	85.99
63251	44.64	26.47	16.78	87.89
63252	44.63	26.46	16.78	87.87

Non-facility RVUs

Code	Work	PE Non-Facility	MP	Total Non-Facility
63250	43.86	25.65	16.48	85.99
63251	44.64	26.47	16.78	87.89
63252	44.63	26.46	16.78	87.87

Modifiers (PAR)

Code	Mod 50	Mod 51	Mod 62	Mod 66	Mod 80
63250	0	2	1	0	2
63251	0	2	1	0	2
63252	0	2	1	0	2

Global Period

Code	Days
63250	090
63251	090
63252	090

63265-63268

63265 Laminectomy for excision or evacuation of intraspinal lesion other than neoplasm, extradural; cervical

63266 Laminectomy for excision or evacuation of intraspinal lesion other than neoplasm, extradural; thoracic

63267 Laminectomy for excision or evacuation of intraspinal lesion other than neoplasm, extradural; lumbar

63268 Laminectomy for excision or evacuation of intraspinal lesion other than neoplasm, extradural; sacral

AMA Coding Notes

Surgical Procedures on the Spine and Spinal Cord

(For application of caliper or tongs, use 20660)

(For treatment of fracture or dislocation of spine, see 22310-22327)

AMA *CPT Assistant* □

63265: Jul 13: 3

63267: Jul 13: 3

63268: Jul 13: 3

Plain English Description

Non-neoplastic intraspinal lesions include infectious lesions such as those caused by tuberculosis, syphilis, cytomegalovirus, herpes simplex virus, bacteria, or parasites; non-infectious lesions include those caused by sarcoid, multiple sclerosis, or systemic lupus erythematosus; and inflammatory lesions, which may be caused by idiopathic necrotizing or radiation myelopathy. In this procedure, a non-neoplastic intraspinal lesion located outside the dura mater (extradural) is excised or evacuated. The skin is incised over the cervical, thoracic, lumbar, or sacral region where the intraspinal lesion is located and extended down to the spinous processes. Muscle is retracted off the lamina and facet joint. A bone drill is used to remove part or all of the lamina, and the spinal cord is exposed. The lesion is identified. The extent of the lesion is explored and determined to be limited to tissue outside the dura mater. A tissue sample may be obtained and sent for a separate pathology examination. Once the nature of the lesion has been determined, it is carefully dissected away from surrounding tissue. Dissection may be performed with the help of an operating microscope, which is reported separately. When it is completely free of all surrounding tissue, it is removed. Alternatively, the lesion may be evacuated using a suction device. Use 63265 for a non-neoplastic intraspinal lesion in the cervical region, 63266 for one in the thoracic region, 63267 for one in the lumbar region, or 63268 for one in the sacral region.

Laminectomy for excision or evacuation of intraspinal lesion other than neoplasm, extradural

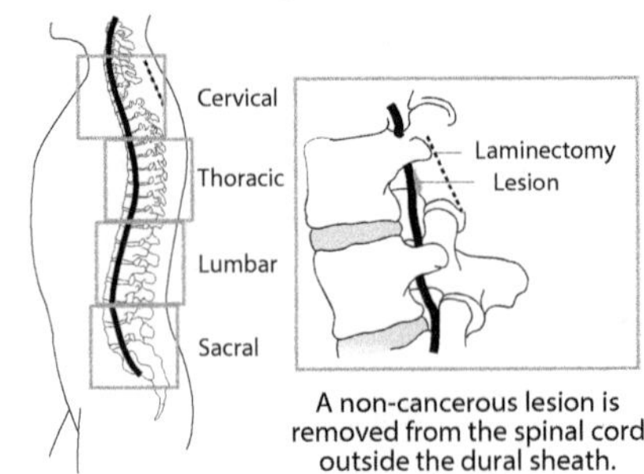

Cervical (63265); thoracic (63266); lumbar (63267); sacral (63268)

ICD-10-CM Diagnostic Codes

A17.81	Tuberculoma of brain and spinal cord
G06.1	Intraspinal abscess and granuloma
G06.2	Extradural and subdural abscess, unspecified
G07	Intracranial and intraspinal abscess and granuloma in diseases classified elsewhere
M71.38	Other bursal cyst, other site

CCI Edits

Refer to Appendix A for CCI edits.

Pub 100

63265: Pub 100-04, 12, 20.4.5

63266: Pub 100-04, 12, 20.4.5

63267: Pub 100-04, 12, 20.4.5

63268: Pub 100-04, 12, 20.4.5

Facility RVUs □

Code	Work	PE Facility	MP	Total Facility
63265	23.82	16.26	8.20	48.28
63266	24.68	16.63	8.44	49.75
63267	19.45	14.07	6.16	39.68
63268	20.02	14.33	6.58	40.93

Non-facility RVUs □

Code	Work	PE Non-Facility	MP	Total Non-Facility
63265	23.82	16.26	8.20	48.28
63266	24.68	16.63	8.44	49.75
63267	19.45	14.07	6.16	39.68
63268	20.02	14.33	6.58	40.93

Modifiers (PAR) □

Code	Mod 50	Mod 51	Mod 62	Mod 66	Mod 80
63265	0	2	1	0	2
63266	0	2	1	0	2
63267	0	2	1	0	2
63268	0	2	1	0	2

Global Period

Code	Days
63265	090
63266	090
63267	090
63268	090

63270-63273

63270 Laminectomy for excision of intraspinal lesion other than neoplasm, intradural; cervical

63271 Laminectomy for excision of intraspinal lesion other than neoplasm, intradural; thoracic

63272 Laminectomy for excision of intraspinal lesion other than neoplasm, intradural; lumbar

63273 Laminectomy for excision of intraspinal lesion other than neoplasm, intradural; sacral

AMA Coding Notes

Surgical Procedures on the Spine and Spinal Cord

(For application of caliper or tongs, use 20660)

(For treatment of fracture or dislocation of spine, see 22310-22327)

AMA *CPT Assistant*

63270: Jul 13: 3
63271: Jul 13: 3
63272: Jul 13: 3
63273: Jul 13: 3

Plain English Description

Non-neoplastic intraspinal lesions include infectious lesions such as those caused by tuberculosis, syphilis, cytomegalovirus, herpes simplex virus, bacteria, or parasites; non-infectious lesions include those caused by sarcoid, multiple sclerosis, or systemic lupus erythematosus; and inflammatory lesions, which may be caused by idiopathic necrotizing or radiation myelopathy.

In this procedure, a non-neoplastic intraspinal lesion located within the dura mater (intradural) is excised. The skin is incised over the cervical, thoracic, lumbar, or sacral region where the intraspinal lesion is located and extended down to the spinous processes. Muscle is retracted off the lamina and facet joint. A bone drill is used to remove part or all of the lamina, and the spinal cord is exposed. The lesion is identified within the dura mater. The dura is incised over the site of the lesion. The extent of the lesion is explored. A tissue sample may be obtained and sent for separate pathology examination. Once the nature of the lesion has been determined, it is carefully dissected away from surrounding tissue with the help of an operating microscope. When it is completely free of all surrounding tissue, it is removed. Use 63270 for a non-neoplastic intraspinal intradural lesion in the cervical region; 63271 for one in the thoracic region; 63272 for one in the lumbar region; or 63273 for one in the sacral region.

Laminectomy for excision of intraspinal lesion other than neoplasm, intradural

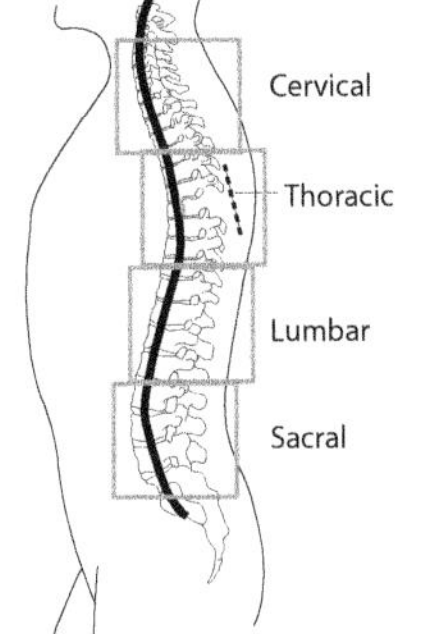

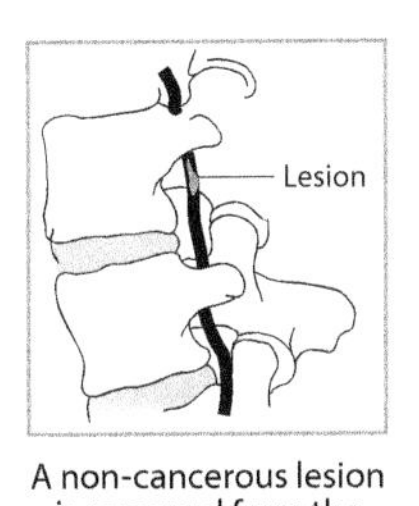

A non-cancerous lesion is removed from the spinal cord inside the dural sheath.

Cervical (63270); thoracic (63271); lumbar (63272); sacral (63273)

ICD-10-CM Diagnostic Codes

G06.1	Intraspinal abscess and granuloma
G95.0	Syringomyelia and syringobulbia
G95.89	Other specified diseases of spinal cord
G96.12	Meningeal adhesions (cerebral) (spinal)
G96.19	Other disorders of meninges, not elsewhere classified
G96.8	Other specified disorders of central nervous system
Q06.4	Hydromyelia

CCI Edits

Refer to Appendix A for CCI edits.

Pub 100

63270: Pub 100-04, 12, 20.4.5
63271: Pub 100-04, 12, 20.4.5
63272: Pub 100-04, 12, 20.4.5
63273: Pub 100-04, 12, 20.4.5

Facility RVUs

Code	Work	PE Facility	MP	Total Facility
63270	29.80	19.17	11.04	60.01
63271	29.92	19.16	10.76	59.84
63272	27.50	17.95	9.14	54.59
63273	26.47	17.64	9.77	53.88

Non-facility RVUs

Code	Work	PE Non-Facility	MP	Total Non-Facility
63270	29.80	19.17	11.04	60.01
63271	29.92	19.16	10.76	59.84
63272	27.50	17.95	9.14	54.59
63273	26.47	17.64	9.77	53.88

Modifiers (PAR)

Code	Mod 50	Mod 51	Mod 62	Mod 66	Mod 80
63270	0	2	1	0	2
63271	0	2	1	0	2
63272	0	2	1	0	2
63273	0	2	0	0	2

Global Period

Code	Days
63270	090
63271	090
63272	090
63273	090

63275-63278

63275 Laminectomy for biopsy/ excision of intraspinal neoplasm; extradural, cervical
63276 Laminectomy for biopsy/ excision of intraspinal neoplasm; extradural, thoracic
63277 Laminectomy for biopsy/ excision of intraspinal neoplasm; extradural, lumbar
63278 Laminectomy for biopsy/ excision of intraspinal neoplasm; extradural, sacral

AMA Coding Notes

Surgical Procedures on the Spine and Spinal Cord

(For application of caliper or tongs, use 20660)

(For treatment of fracture or dislocation of spine, see 22310-22327)

AMA *CPT Assistant*

63275: Jul 13: 3
63276: Jul 13: 3
63277: Jul 13: 3
63278: Jul 13: 3

Plain English Description

An intraspinal neoplasm may be benign, malignant, or of uncertain behavior. In this procedure, a neoplastic intraspinal tumor located outside the dura mater (extradural) is biopsied or excised. The skin is incised over the cervical, thoracic, lumbar, or sacral region where the tumor is located. The incision is extended down to the spinous processes. Muscle is retracted off the lamina and facet joint. A bone drill is used to remove part or all of the lamina, and the spinal cord is exposed. The tumor is identified. The extent of the tumor is explored and determined to be limited to tissue outside the dura mater. A tissue sample may be obtained and sent for separate pathology examination. Following the tissue biopsy, the physician may close the surgical site or excise the tumor. If the tumor can be excised, it is carefully dissected away from surrounding tissue with the help of an operating microscope. When it is completely free of all surrounding tissue, it is removed. Use 63275 for a neoplastic intraspinal tumor in the cervical region; 63276 for one in the thoracic region; 63277 for one in the lumbar region; or 63278 for one in the sacral region.

Laminectomy for biopsy/excision of intraspinal neoplasm; extradural

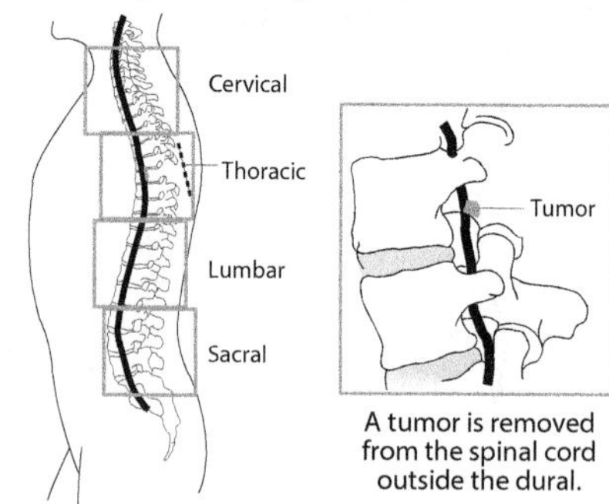

Cervical (63275); thoracic (63276); lumbar (63277); sacral (63278)

ICD-10-CM Diagnostic Codes

C41.2	Malignant neoplasm of vertebral column
C41.4	Malignant neoplasm of pelvic bones, sacrum and coccyx
C70.1	Malignant neoplasm of spinal meninges
C79.49	Secondary malignant neoplasm of other parts of nervous system
C79.51	Secondary malignant neoplasm of bone
D16.6	Benign neoplasm of vertebral column
D32.1	Benign neoplasm of spinal meninges
D42.1	Neoplasm of uncertain behavior of spinal meninges
D48.0	Neoplasm of uncertain behavior of bone and articular cartilage

CCI Edits

Refer to Appendix A for CCI edits.

Pub 100

63275: Pub 100-04, 12, 20.4.5
63276: Pub 100-04, 12, 20.4.5
63277: Pub 100-04, 12, 20.4.5
63278: Pub 100-04, 12, 20.4.5

Facility RVUs

Code	Work	PE Facility	MP	Total Facility
63275	25.86	17.25	9.03	52.14
63276	25.69	17.13	8.91	51.73
63277	22.39	15.49	7.21	45.09
63278	22.12	15.64	8.15	45.91

Non-facility RVUs

Code	Work	PE Non-Facility	MP	Total Non-Facility
63275	25.86	17.25	9.03	52.14
63276	25.69	17.13	8.91	51.73
63277	22.39	15.49	7.21	45.09
63278	22.12	15.64	8.15	45.91

Modifiers (PAR)

Code	Mod 50	Mod 51	Mod 62	Mod 66	Mod 80
63275	0	2	1	0	2
63276	0	2	1	0	2
63277	0	2	1	0	2
63278	0	2	1	0	2

Global Period

Code	Days
63275	090
63276	090
63277	090
63278	090

63280-63283

63280 Laminectomy for biopsy/excision of intraspinal neoplasm; intradural, extramedullary, cervical

63281 Laminectomy for biopsy/excision of intraspinal neoplasm; intradural, extramedullary, thoracic

63282 Laminectomy for biopsy/excision of intraspinal neoplasm; intradural, extramedullary, lumbar

63283 Laminectomy for biopsy/excision of intraspinal neoplasm; intradural, sacral

AMA Coding Notes

Surgical Procedures on the Spine and Spinal Cord

(For application of caliper or tongs, use 20660)

(For treatment of fracture or dislocation of spine, see 22310-22327)

AMA *CPT Assistant*

63280: Jul 13: 3
63281: Jul 13: 3
63282: Jul 13: 3
63283: Jul 13: 3

Plain English Description

An intraspinal neoplasm may be benign, malignant, or of uncertain behavior. In this procedure, a neoplastic intraspinal tumor located within the dura mater (intradural) but outside of the spinal cord (extramedullary) is biopsied or excised. The tumor does not extend outside the dura into the extradural tissues. The skin is incised over the cervical, thoracic, lumbar, or sacral region where the tumor is located. The incision is extended down to the spinous processes. Muscle is retracted off the lamina and facet joint. A bone drill is used to remove part or all of the lamina, and the spinal cord is exposed. The tumor is identified within the dura mater. The dura is incised over the site of the tumor. The tumor is determined to lie outside of the spinal cord. A tissue sample may be obtained and sent for separate pathology examination. Following the tissue biopsy, the physician may close the surgical site or excise the tumor. If the tumor can be excised, it is carefully dissected away from surrounding tissue with the help of an operating microscope. When it is completely free of all surrounding tissue, it is removed. The dura is then closed with sutures or a dural patch graft. Use 63280 for a neoplastic intraspinal tumor in the cervical region; 63281 for one in the thoracic region; 63282 for one in the lumbar region; or 63283 for one in the sacral region.

Laminectomy for biopsy/excision of intraspinal neoplasm; intradural, extramedullary

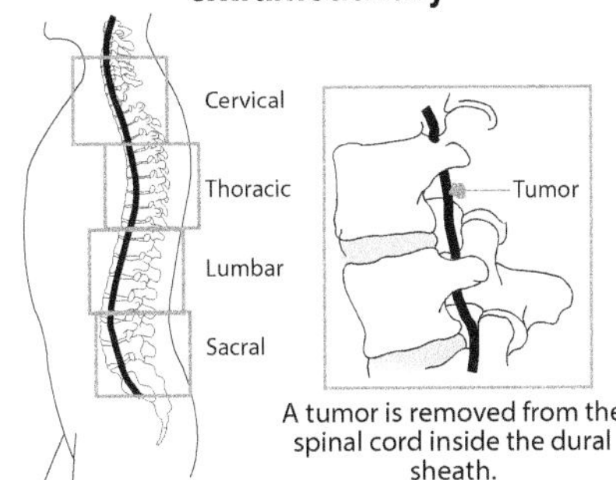

Cervical (63280); thoracic (63281); lumbar (63282); sacral (63283)

ICD-10-CM Diagnostic Codes

C70.1	Malignant neoplasm of spinal meninges
C72.0	Malignant neoplasm of spinal cord
C72.1	Malignant neoplasm of cauda equina
C79.49	Secondary malignant neoplasm of other parts of nervous system
D32.1	Benign neoplasm of spinal meninges
D33.4	Benign neoplasm of spinal cord
D42.1	Neoplasm of uncertain behavior of spinal meninges
D43.4	Neoplasm of uncertain behavior of spinal cord

CCI Edits

Refer to Appendix A for CCI edits.

Pub 100

63280: Pub 100-04, 12, 20.4.5
63281: Pub 100-04, 12, 20.4.5
63282: Pub 100-04, 12, 20.4.5
63283: Pub 100-04, 12, 20.4.5

Facility RVUs

Code	Work	PE Facility	MP	Total Facility
63280	30.29	19.84	11.10	61.23
63281	29.99	19.61	10.92	60.52
63282	28.15	18.76	10.17	57.08
63283	26.76	18.23	9.88	54.87

Non-facility RVUs

Code	Work	PE Non-Facility	MP	Total Non-Facility
63280	30.29	19.84	11.10	61.23
63281	29.99	19.61	10.92	60.52
63282	28.15	18.76	10.17	57.08
63283	26.76	18.23	9.88	54.87

Modifiers (PAR)

Code	Mod 50	Mod 51	Mod 62	Mod 66	Mod 80
63280	0	2	1	0	2
63281	0	2	1	0	2
63282	0	2	1	0	2
63283	0	2	1	0	2

Global Period

Code	Days
63280	090
63281	090
63282	090
63283	090

63285-63287

63285 Laminectomy for biopsy/excision of intraspinal neoplasm; intradural, intramedullary, cervical

63286 Laminectomy for biopsy/excision of intraspinal neoplasm; intradural, intramedullary, thoracic

63287 Laminectomy for biopsy/excision of intraspinal neoplasm; intradural, intramedullary, thoracolumbar

AMA Coding Notes

Surgical Procedures on the Spine and Spinal Cord

(For application of caliper or tongs, use 20660)

(For treatment of fracture or dislocation of spine, see 22310-22327)

AMA *CPT Assistant*

63285: Jul 13: 3
63286: Jul 13: 3
63287: Jul 13: 3

Plain English Description

An intraspinal neoplasm may be benign, malignant, or of uncertain behavior. In this procedure, a neoplastic intraspinal tumor located within the dura mater (intradural) and extending into the tissues of the spinal cord (intramedullary) is biopsied or excised. The tumor does not extend outside the dura into the extradural tissues. The skin is incised over the cervical, thoracic, or lumbar region where the tumor is located. The incision is extended down to the spinous processes. Muscle is retracted off the lamina and facet joint. A bone drill is used to remove part or all of the lamina, and the spinal cord is exposed. The tumor is identified within the dura mater. The dura is incised over the site of the tumor. The tumor is determined to extend into tissues of the spinal cord. A tissue sample may be obtained and sent for separate pathology examination. Following the tissue biopsy, the physician may close the surgical site or excise the tumor. If the tumor can be excised, it is carefully dissected away from surrounding tissue with the help of an operating microscope. When it is completely free of all surrounding tissue, it is removed. The dura is then closed with sutures or a dural patch graft. Use 63285 for a neoplastic intraspinal tumor in the cervical region; 63286 for one in the thoracic region; or 63287 for one in the thoracolumbar region.

Laminectomy for biopsy/excision of intraspinal neoplasm; intradural, intramedullary

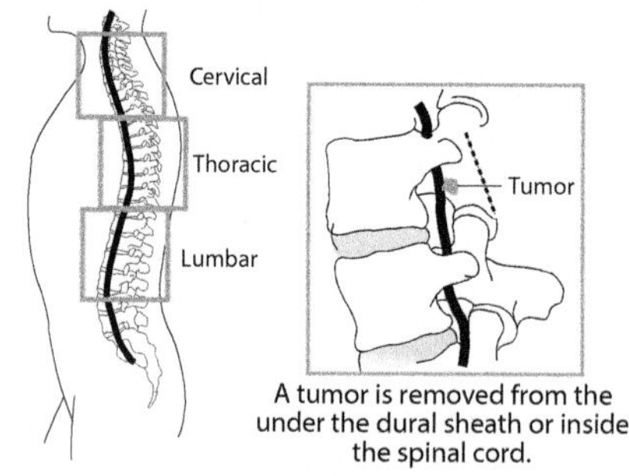

A tumor is removed from the under the dural sheath or inside the spinal cord.

ICD-10-CM Diagnostic Codes

C72.0	Malignant neoplasm of spinal cord
C79.49	Secondary malignant neoplasm of other parts of nervous system
D33.4	Benign neoplasm of spinal cord
D43.4	Neoplasm of uncertain behavior of spinal cord

CCI Edits

Refer to Appendix A for CCI edits.

Pub 100

63285: Pub 100-04, 12, 20.4.5
63286: Pub 100-04, 12, 20.4.5
63287: Pub 100-04, 12, 20.4.5

Facility RVUs

Code	Work	PE Facility	MP	Total Facility
63285	38.05	23.42	14.18	75.65
63286	37.62	23.22	13.91	74.75
63287	40.08	24.36	14.97	79.41

Non-facility RVUs

Code	Work	PE Non-Facility	MP	Total Non-Facility
63285	38.05	23.42	14.18	75.65
63286	37.62	23.22	13.91	74.75
63287	40.08	24.36	14.97	79.41

Modifiers (PAR)

Code	Mod 50	Mod 51	Mod 62	Mod 66	Mod 80
63285	0	2	1	0	2
63286	0	2	1	0	2
63287	0	2	1	0	2

Global Period

Code	Days
63285	090
63286	090
63287	090

63290

63290 Laminectomy for biopsy/excision of intraspinal neoplasm; combined extradural-intradural lesion, any level

(For drainage of intramedullary cyst/syrinx, use 63172, 63173)

AMA Coding Notes

Surgical Procedures on the Spine and Spinal Cord

(For application of caliper or tongs, use 20660)

(For treatment of fracture or dislocation of spine, see 22310-22327)

AMA *CPT Assistant*

63290: Jul 13: 3

Plain English Description

An intraspinal neoplasm may be benign, malignant, or of uncertain behavior. In this procedure, the tumor is located outside the dura mater with extension of the tumor into the dura. The tumor is biopsied or excised. The skin is incised over the cervical, thoracic, lumbar, or sacral region where the tumor is located. The incision is extended down to the spinous processes. Muscle is retracted off the lamina and facet joint. A bone drill is used to remove part or all of the lamina, and the spinal cord is exposed. The tumor outside the dura mater is located, evaluated, and determined to extend beyond the dura mater. The dura is incised over the site of the lesion. A tissue sample may be obtained and sent for separate pathology examination. Following the tissue biopsy, the physician may close the surgical site or excise the tumor. If the tumor can be excised, it is carefully dissected away from surrounding tissue with the help of an operating microscope. When it is completely free of all surrounding tissue, it is removed. The dura is then closed with sutures or a dural patch graft. Use 63290 for an extradural-intradural intraspinal neoplasm at any level of the spine.

Laminectomy for biopsy/excision of intraspinal neoplasm; combined extradural-intradural lesion

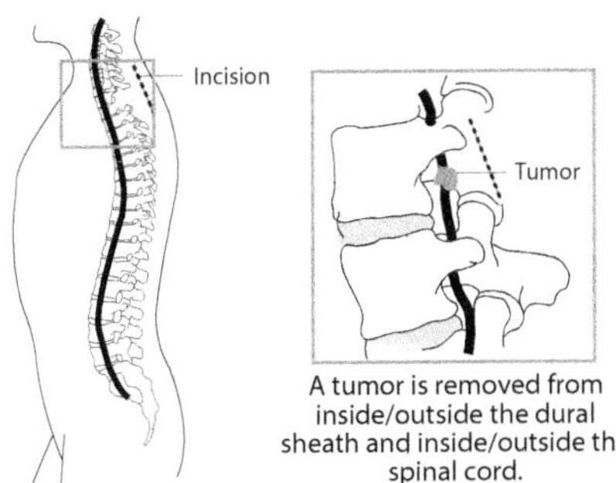

A tumor is removed from inside/outside the dural sheath and inside/outside the spinal cord.

ICD-10-CM Diagnostic Codes

C41.2	Malignant neoplasm of vertebral column
C41.4	Malignant neoplasm of pelvic bones, sacrum and coccyx
C70.1	Malignant neoplasm of spinal meninges
C72.0	Malignant neoplasm of spinal cord
C79.49	Secondary malignant neoplasm of other parts of nervous system
C79.51	Secondary malignant neoplasm of bone
D16.6	Benign neoplasm of vertebral column
D32.1	Benign neoplasm of spinal meninges
D33.4	Benign neoplasm of spinal cord
D42.1	Neoplasm of uncertain behavior of spinal meninges
D43.4	Neoplasm of uncertain behavior of spinal cord
D48.0	Neoplasm of uncertain behavior of bone and articular cartilage

CCI Edits

Refer to Appendix A for CCI edits.

Pub 100

63290: Pub 100-04, 12, 20.4.5

Facility RVUs

Code	Work	PE Facility	MP	Total Facility
63290	40.82	24.71	15.25	80.78

Non-facility RVUs

Code	Work	PE Non-Facility	MP	Total Non-Facility
63290	40.82	24.71	15.25	80.78

Modifiers (PAR)

Code	Mod 50	Mod 51	Mod 62	Mod 66	Mod 80
63290	0	2	1	0	2

Global Period

Code	Days
63290	090

63300

63300 Vertebral corpectomy (vertebral body resection), partial or complete, for excision of intraspinal lesion, single segment; extradural, cervical

AMA Coding Guideline

Excision, Anterior or Anterolateral Approach, Intraspinal Lesion Procedures on the Spine and Spinal Cord

For the following codes, when two surgeons work together as primary surgeons performing distinct part(s) of an anterior approach for an intraspinal excision, each surgeon should report his/her distinct operative work by appending modifier 62 to the single definitive procedure code. In this situation, modifier 62 may be appended to the definitive procedure code(s) 63300-63307 and, as appropriate, to the associated additional segment add-on code 63308 as long as both surgeons continue to work together as primary surgeons.

For vertebral corpectomy, the term partial is used to describe removal of a substantial portion of the body of the vertebra. In the cervical spine, the amount of bone removed is defined as at least one-half of the vertebral body. In the thoracic and lumbar spine, the amount of bone removed is defined as at least one-third of the vertebral body.

AMA Coding Notes

Excision, Anterior or Anterolateral Approach, Intraspinal Lesion Procedures on the Spine and Spinal Cord

(For arthrodesis, see 22548-22585)

(For reconstruction of spine, see 20930-20938)

Surgical Procedures on the Spine and Spinal Cord

(For application of caliper or tongs, use 20660)

(For treatment of fracture or dislocation of spine, see 22310-22327)

AMA *CPT Assistant* ▯

63300: Feb 02: 4, Jul 13: 3

Plain English Description

Vertebral corpectomy involves removal of the vertebral body as well as the vertebral discs above and below the vertebra. In this procedure, vertebral corpectomy is performed to excise a lesion or tumor that is located within the spinal canal (intraspinal) but outside the dura mater (extradural). Resection is performed on only one vertebral segment in the cervical spine. The cervical spine is exposed via an anterior approach beginning with a skin incision in the anterior aspect of the neck. The soft tissues and muscles overlying the cervical spine are dissected. The trachea and esophagus are retracted. The affected segment of the cervical spine is exposed. The intervertebral discs above and below the vertebral body are removed first with the aid of the surgical microscope. The discs are carefully dissected from surrounding tissue and removed. The vertebral body is excised and the lesion or tumor in the spinal canal identified and explored. It is determined that the lesion or tumor lies outside the dura. The lesion or tumor is carefully dissected free of surrounding tissues with the aid of an operating microscope. Once the lesion or tumor has been completely excised, separately reportable bone grafting and fusion procedures are performed. The bone graft is placed in the surgical defect to support the anterior aspect of the spine where the discs and vertebral body have been removed. Surrounding bone is contoured for placement of the graft and to ensure fusion of the graft and adjacent bone. Separately reportable spine instrumentation may also be used to stabilize the spine. Upon completion of the procedure, bleeding is controlled and soft tissues and skin are closed in layers.

Vertebral corpectomy, partial or complete, for excision of intraspinal

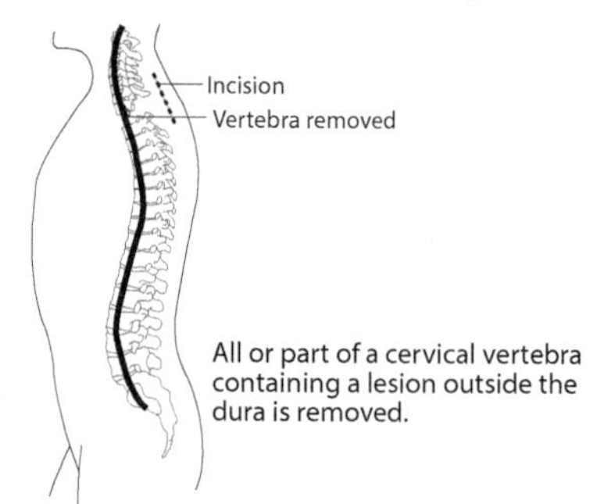

ICD-10-CM Diagnostic Codes

C41.2	Malignant neoplasm of vertebral column
C70.1	Malignant neoplasm of spinal meninges
C79.49	Secondary malignant neoplasm of other parts of nervous system
C79.51	Secondary malignant neoplasm of bone
D16.6	Benign neoplasm of vertebral column
D32.1	Benign neoplasm of spinal meninges
D42.1	Neoplasm of uncertain behavior of spinal meninges
D48.0	Neoplasm of uncertain behavior of bone and articular cartilage
G06.1	Intraspinal abscess and granuloma
G06.2	Extradural and subdural abscess, unspecified
G07	Intracranial and intraspinal abscess and granuloma in diseases classified elsewhere

CCI Edits

Refer to Appendix A for CCI edits.

Pub 100

63300: Pub 100-04, 12, 20.4.5

Facility RVUs ▯

Code	Work	PE Facility	MP	Total Facility
63300	26.80	17.48	8.87	53.15

Non-facility RVUs ▯

Code	Work	PE Non-Facility	MP	Total Non-Facility
63300	26.80	17.48	8.87	53.15

Modifiers (PAR) ▯

Code	Mod 50	Mod 51	Mod 62	Mod 66	Mod 80
63300	0	2	1	0	2

Global Period

Code	Days
63300	090

63301-63302

63301 Vertebral corpectomy (vertebral body resection), partial or complete, for excision of intraspinal lesion, single segment; extradural, thoracic by transthoracic approach

63302 Vertebral corpectomy (vertebral body resection), partial or complete, for excision of intraspinal lesion, single segment; extradural, thoracic by thoracolumbar approach

AMA Coding Guideline

Excision, Anterior or Anterolateral Approach, Intraspinal Lesion Procedures on the Spine and Spinal Cord

For the following codes, when two surgeons work together as primary surgeons performing distinct part(s) of an anterior approach for an intraspinal excision, each surgeon should report his/her distinct operative work by appending modifier 62 to the single definitive procedure code. In this situation, modifier 62 may be appended to the definitive procedure code(s) 63300-63307 and, as appropriate, to the associated additional segment add-on code 63308 as long as both surgeons continue to work together as primary surgeons.

For vertebral corpectomy, the term partial is used to describe removal of a substantial portion of the body of the vertebra. In the cervical spine, the amount of bone removed is defined as at least one-half of the vertebral body. In the thoracic and lumbar spine, the amount of bone removed is defined as at least one-third of the vertebral body.

AMA Coding Notes

Excision, Anterior or Anterolateral Approach, Intraspinal Lesion Procedures on the Spine and Spinal Cord

(For arthrodesis, see 22548-22585)

(For reconstruction of spine, see 20930-20938)

Surgical Procedures on the Spine and Spinal Cord

(For application of caliper or tongs, use 20660)

(For treatment of fracture or dislocation of spine, see 22310-22327)

AMA *CPT Assistant* ▢

63301: Feb 02: 4, Jul 13: 3

63302: Feb 02: 4, Jul 13: 3

Plain English Description

Vertebral corpectomy involves removal of the vertebral body as well as the vertebral discs above and below the vertebra. In this procedure, vertebral corpectomy is performed to excise a lesion or tumor that is located within the spinal canal (intraspinal) but outside the dura mater (extradural). Resection is performed on only one vertebral segment in the thoracic spine. The thoracic spine is exposed using either a transthoracic approach (63301) or a thoracolumbar approach (63302), both of which require a thoracotomy. Typically, a co-surgeon or team approach is used, with the exposure being performed by a thoracic surgeon and the corpectomy performed by a spine surgeon. The skin over the thorax is incised to allow access to the appropriate levels of the thoracic spine. Overlying muscles are dissected. In 63301, one or more of the upper ribs are resected. Rib spreaders are used to allow adequate exposure of the spine. The pleura are incised and the affected portion of the thoracic spine is exposed. In 63302, the incision is made at the 10th rib and extended across the abdomen. The rib is cut at the costochondral junction and resected. The pleural cavity is opened along the bed of the 10th rib and the appropriate level of the thoracic spine exposed. The intervertebral discs above and below the vertebral body are removed first with the aid of the surgical microscope. The discs are carefully dissected from surrounding tissue and removed. The vertebral body is excised and the lesion or tumor in the spinal canal identified and explored. It is determined that the lesion or tumor lies outside the dura. The lesion or tumor is carefully dissected free of surrounding tissues with the aid of an operating microscope. Once the lesion or tumor has been completely excised, separately reportable bone grafting and fusion procedures are performed. The bone graft is placed in the surgical defect to support the anterior aspect of the spine where the discs and vertebral body have been removed. Surrounding bone is contoured for placement of the graft and to ensure fusion of the graft and adjacent bone. Separately reportable spine instrumentation may also be used to stabilize the spine. Upon completion of the procedure, bleeding is controlled and soft tissues and skin are closed in layers.

Vertebral corpectomy for excision of intraspinal lesion, extradural

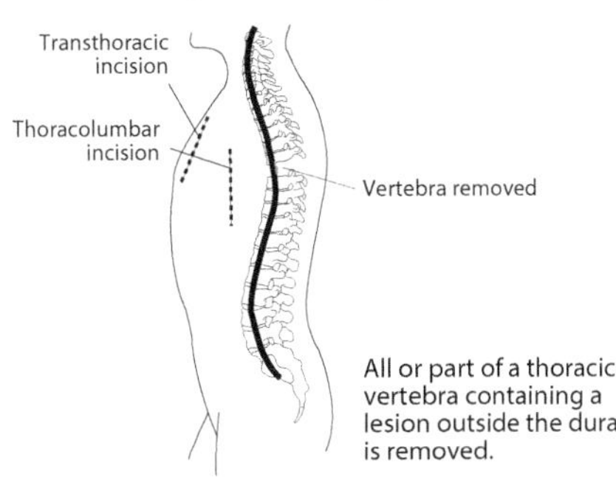

ICD-10-CM Diagnostic Codes

C41.2	Malignant neoplasm of vertebral column
C70.1	Malignant neoplasm of spinal meninges
C79.49	Secondary malignant neoplasm of other parts of nervous system
C79.51	Secondary malignant neoplasm of bone
D16.6	Benign neoplasm of vertebral column
D32.1	Benign neoplasm of spinal meninges
D42.1	Neoplasm of uncertain behavior of spinal meninges
D48.0	Neoplasm of uncertain behavior of bone and articular cartilage
G06.1	Intraspinal abscess and granuloma
G06.2	Extradural and subdural abscess, unspecified
G07	Intracranial and intraspinal abscess and granuloma in diseases classified elsewhere

CCI Edits

Refer to Appendix A for CCI edits.

Pub 100

63301: Pub 100-04, 12, 20.4.5

63302: Pub 100-04, 12, 20.4.5

Facility RVUs ▢

Code	Work	PE Facility	MP	Total Facility
63301	31.57	20.44	11.70	63.71
63302	31.15	20.25	11.54	62.94

Non-facility RVUs ▢

Code	Work	PE Non-Facility	MP	Total Non-Facility
63301	31.57	20.44	11.70	63.71
63302	31.15	20.25	11.54	62.94

Modifiers (PAR) ▢

Code	Mod 50	Mod 51	Mod 62	Mod 66	Mod 80
63301	0	2	1	0	2
63302	0	2	1	0	2

Global Period

Code	Days
63301	090
63302	090

CPT® Procedural Coding

63303

63303 Vertebral corpectomy (vertebral body resection), partial or complete, for excision of intraspinal lesion, single segment; extradural, lumbar or sacral by transperitoneal or retroperitoneal approach

AMA Coding Guideline

Excision, Anterior or Anterolateral Approach, Intraspinal Lesion Procedures on the Spine and Spinal Cord

For the following codes, when two surgeons work together as primary surgeons performing distinct part(s) of an anterior approach for an intraspinal excision, each surgeon should report his/her distinct operative work by appending modifier 62 to the single definitive procedure code. In this situation, modifier 62 may be appended to the definitive procedure code(s) 63300-63307 and, as appropriate, to the associated additional segment add-on code 63308 as long as both surgeons continue to work together as primary surgeons.

For vertebral corpectomy, the term partial is used to describe removal of a substantial portion of the body of the vertebra. In the cervical spine, the amount of bone removed is defined as at least one-half of the vertebral body. In the thoracic and lumbar spine, the amount of bone removed is defined as at least one-third of the vertebral body.

AMA Coding Notes

Excision, Anterior or Anterolateral Approach, Intraspinal Lesion Procedures on the Spine and Spinal Cord

(For arthrodesis, see 22548-22585)

(For reconstruction of spine, see 20930-20938)

Surgical Procedures on the Spine and Spinal Cord

(For application of caliper or tongs, use 20660)

(For treatment of fracture or dislocation of spine, see 22310-22327)

AMA *CPT Assistant* ▢

63303: Feb 02: 4, Jul 13: 3

Plain English Description

Vertebral corpectomy involves removal of the vertebral body as well as the vertebral discs above and below the vertebra. In this procedure, vertebral corpectomy is performed to excise a lesion or tumor that is located within the spinal canal (intraspinal) but outside the dura mater (extradural). Resection is performed on only one vertebral segment in the lumbar or sacral spine. If a transperitoneal (anterior) approach is used, the abdomen is incised and the peritoneum entered. The bowel is moved out of the way. If a retroperitoneal (anterolateral) approach is used, a flank incision is made. Surrounding tissues are dissected, taking care to protect vital structures. The affected lumbar or sacral segment is exposed. The intervertebral discs above and below the vertebral body are removed first with the aid of the surgical microscope. The discs are carefully dissected from surrounding tissue and removed. The vertebral body is excised and the lesion or tumor in the spinal canal identified and explored. It is determined that the lesion or tumor lies outside the dura. The lesion or tumor is carefully dissected free of surrounding tissues with the aid of an operating microscope. Once the lesion or tumor has been completely excised, separately reportable bone grafting and fusion procedures are performed. The bone graft is placed in the surgical defect to support the anterior aspect of the spine where the discs and vertebral body have been removed. Surrounding bone is contoured for placement of the graft and to ensure fusion of the graft and adjacent bone. Separately reportable spinal instrumentation may also be used to stabilize the spine. Upon completion of the procedure, bleeding is controlled and soft tissues and skin are closed in layers.

Vertebral corpectomy for excision of intraspinal lesion, extradural

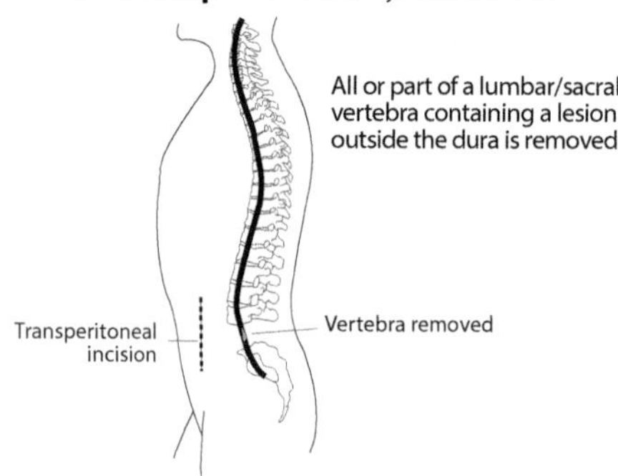

ICD-10-CM Diagnostic Codes

A17.81	Tuberculoma of brain and spinal cord
C41.2	Malignant neoplasm of vertebral column
C41.4	Malignant neoplasm of pelvic bones, sacrum and coccyx
C70.1	Malignant neoplasm of spinal meninges
C79.49	Secondary malignant neoplasm of other parts of nervous system
C79.51	Secondary malignant neoplasm of bone
D16.6	Benign neoplasm of vertebral column
D32.1	Benign neoplasm of spinal meninges
D42.1	Neoplasm of uncertain behavior of spinal meninges
D48.0	Neoplasm of uncertain behavior of bone and articular cartilage
G07	Intracranial and intraspinal abscess and granuloma in diseases classified elsewhere

CCI Edits

Refer to Appendix A for CCI edits.

Pub 100

63303: Pub 100-04, 12, 20.4.5

Facility RVUs ▢

Code	Work	PE Facility	MP	Total Facility
63303	33.55	20.90	12.46	66.91

Non-facility RVUs ▢

Code	Work	PE Non-Facility	MP	Total Non-Facility
63303	33.55	20.90	12.46	66.91

Modifiers (PAR) ▢

Code	Mod 50	Mod 51	Mod 62	Mod 66	Mod 80
63303	0	2	1	0	2

Global Period

Code	Days
63303	090

63304

63304 Vertebral corpectomy (vertebral body resection), partial or complete, for excision of intraspinal lesion, single segment; intradural, cervical

AMA Coding Guideline

Excision, Anterior or Anterolateral Approach, Intraspinal Lesion Procedures on the Spine and Spinal Cord

For the following codes, when two surgeons work together as primary surgeons performing distinct part(s) of an anterior approach for an intraspinal excision, each surgeon should report his/her distinct operative work by appending modifier 62 to the single definitive procedure code. In this situation, modifier 62 may be appended to the definitive procedure code(s) 63300-63307 and, as appropriate, to the associated additional segment add-on code 63308 as long as both surgeons continue to work together as primary surgeons.

For vertebral corpectomy, the term partial is used to describe removal of a substantial portion of the body of the vertebra. In the cervical spine, the amount of bone removed is defined as at least one-half of the vertebral body. In the thoracic and lumbar spine, the amount of bone removed is defined as at least one-third of the vertebral body.

AMA Coding Notes

Excision, Anterior or Anterolateral Approach, Intraspinal Lesion Procedures on the Spine and Spinal Cord

(For arthrodesis, see 22548-22585)

(For reconstruction of spine, see 20930-20938)

Surgical Procedures on the Spine and Spinal Cord

(For application of caliper or tongs, use 20660)

(For treatment of fracture or dislocation of spine, see 22310-22327)

AMA *CPT Assistant*

63304: Feb 02: 4, Jul 13: 3

Plain English Description

Vertebral corpectomy involves removal of the vertebral body as well as the vertebral discs above and below the vertebra. In this procedure, vertebral corpectomy is performed to excise a lesion or tumor that is located within the spinal canal (intraspinal) and extends into or lies within the dura mater (intradural). Resection is performed on only one vertebral segment in the cervical spine. The cervical spine is exposed via an anterior approach beginning with a skin incision in the anterior aspect of the neck. The soft tissues and muscles overlying the cervical spine are dissected. The trachea and esophagus are retracted. The affected segment of the cervical spine is exposed. The intervertebral discs above and below the vertebral body are removed first with the aid of the surgical microscope. The discs are carefully dissected from surrounding tissue and removed. The vertebral body is excised and the lesion or tumor in the spinal canal identified and explored. If it is determined that the lesion or tumor lies within or extends into the dura, the dura is incised. The lesion or tumor is carefully dissected free of surrounding tissues with the aid of an operating microscope and removed. The dura is then repaired with sutures or a dural graft. Separately reportable bone grafting and fusion procedures are performed. The bone graft is placed in the surgical defect to support the anterior aspect of the spine where the discs and vertebral body have been removed. Surrounding bone is contoured for placement of the graft and to ensure fusion of the graft and adjacent bone. Separately reportable spine instrumentation may also be used to stabilize the spine. Upon completion of the procedure, bleeding is controlled and soft tissues and skin are closed in layers.

Vertebral corpectomy for excision of intraspinal lesion, intradural

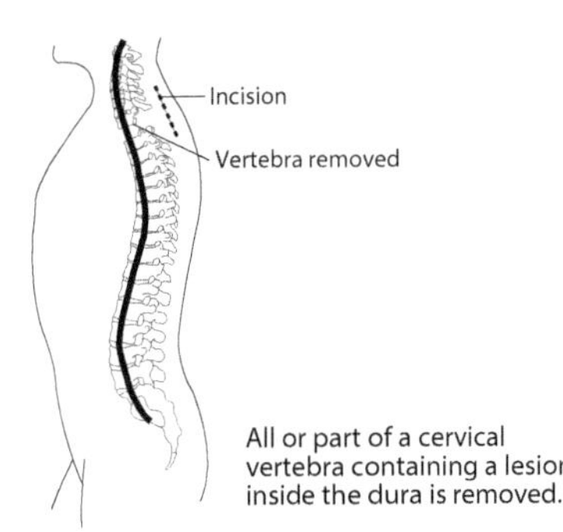

ICD-10-CM Diagnostic Codes

Code	Description
A17.81	Tuberculoma of brain and spinal cord
C70.1	Malignant neoplasm of spinal meninges
C79.49	Secondary malignant neoplasm of other parts of nervous system
C79.51	Secondary malignant neoplasm of bone
D16.6	Benign neoplasm of vertebral column
D32.1	Benign neoplasm of spinal meninges
D42.1	Neoplasm of uncertain behavior of spinal meninges
D48.0	Neoplasm of uncertain behavior of bone and articular cartilage
G06.1	Intraspinal abscess and granuloma
G06.2	Extradural and subdural abscess, unspecified
G07	Intracranial and intraspinal abscess and granuloma in diseases classified elsewhere
G95.0	Syringomyelia and syringobulbia
G95.19	Other vascular myelopathies

CCI Edits

Refer to Appendix A for CCI edits.

Pub 100

63304: Pub 100-04, 12, 20.4.5

Facility RVUs

Code	Work	PE Facility	MP	Total Facility
63304	33.85	21.49	12.55	67.89

Non-facility RVUs

Code	Work	PE Non-Facility	MP	Total Non-Facility
63304	33.85	21.49	12.55	67.89

Modifiers (PAR)

Code	Mod 50	Mod 51	Mod 62	Mod 66	Mod 80
63304	0	2	1	0	2

Global Period

Code	Days
63304	090

63305-63306

63305 Vertebral corpectomy (vertebral body resection), partial or complete, for excision of intraspinal lesion, single segment; intradural, thoracic by transthoracic approach

63306 Vertebral corpectomy (vertebral body resection), partial or complete, for excision of intraspinal lesion, single segment; intradural, thoracic by thoracolumbar approach

AMA Coding Guideline

Excision, Anterior or Anterolateral Approach, Intraspinal Lesion Procedures on the Spine and Spinal Cord

For the following codes, when two surgeons work together as primary surgeons performing distinct part(s) of an anterior approach for an intraspinal excision, each surgeon should report his/her distinct operative work by appending modifier 62 to the single definitive procedure code. In this situation, modifier 62 may be appended to the definitive procedure code(s) 63300-63307 and, as appropriate, to the associated additional segment add-on code 63308 as long as both surgeons continue to work together as primary surgeons.

For vertebral corpectomy, the term partial is used to describe removal of a substantial portion of the body of the vertebra. In the cervical spine, the amount of bone removed is defined as at least one-half of the vertebral body. In the thoracic and lumbar spine, the amount of bone removed is defined as at least one-third of the vertebral body.

AMA Coding Notes

Excision, Anterior or Anterolateral Approach, Intraspinal Lesion Procedures on the Spine and Spinal Cord

(For arthrodesis, see 22548-22585)

(For reconstruction of spine, see 20930-20938)

Surgical Procedures on the Spine and Spinal Cord

(For application of caliper or tongs, use 20660)

(For treatment of fracture or dislocation of spine, see 22310-22327)

AMA *CPT Assistant* ▯

63305: Feb 02: 4, Jul 13: 3

63306: Feb 02: 4, Jul 13: 3

Plain English Description

Vertebral corpectomy involves removal of the vertebral body as well as the vertebral discs above and below the vertebra. In this procedure, vertebral corpectomy is performed to excise a lesion or tumor that is located within the spinal canal (intraspinal) and within or extending into the dura mater (intradural). Resection is performed on only one vertebral segment in the thoracic spine. The thoracic spine is exposed using either a transthoracic approach (63305) or a thoracolumbar approach (63306) both of which require a thoracotomy. Typically, a co-surgeon or team approach is used, with the exposure being performed by a thoracic surgeon and the corpectomy performed by a spine surgeon. The skin over the thorax is incised to allow access to the appropriate levels of the thoracic spine. Overlying muscles are dissected. In 63305, one or more of the upper ribs are resected. Rib spreaders are used to allow adequate exposure of the spine. The pleura are incised and the affected portion of the thoracic spine is exposed. In 63306, the incision is made at the 10th rib and extended across the abdomen. The rib is cut at the costochondral junction and resected. The pleural cavity is opened along the bed of the 10th rib and the appropriate level of the thoracic spine exposed. The intervertebral discs above and below the vertebral body are removed first with the aid of the surgical microscope. The discs are carefully dissected from surrounding tissue and removed. The vertebral body is excised and the lesion or tumor in the spinal canal identified and explored. If it is determined that the lesion or tumor lies within or extends into the dura, the dura is incised. The lesion or tumor is carefully dissected free of surrounding tissues with the aid of an operating microscope and removed. The dura is then repaired with sutures or a dural graft. Separately reportable bone grafting and fusion procedures are performed. The bone graft is placed in the surgical defect to support the anterior aspect of the spine where the discs and vertebral body have been removed. Surrounding bone is contoured for placement of the graft and to ensure fusion of the graft and adjacent bone. Separately reportable spine instrumentation may also be used to stabilize the spine.

Vertebral corpectomy for excision of intraspinal lesion, intradural

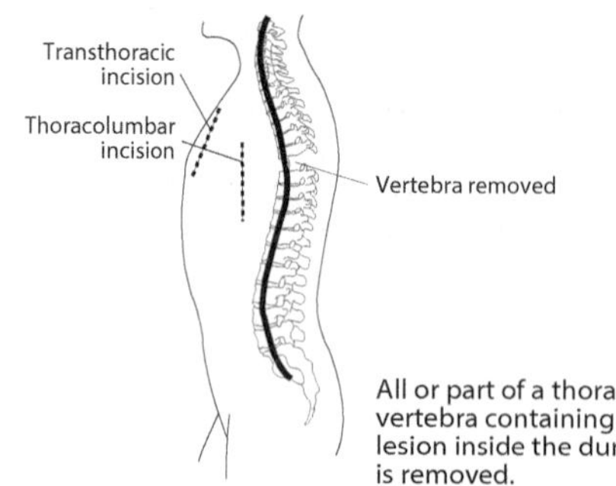

ICD-10-CM Diagnostic Codes

A17.81	Tuberculoma of brain and spinal cord
C41.2	Malignant neoplasm of vertebral column
C70.1	Malignant neoplasm of spinal meninges
C79.49	Secondary malignant neoplasm of other parts of nervous system
C79.51	Secondary malignant neoplasm of bone
D16.6	Benign neoplasm of vertebral column
D32.1	Benign neoplasm of spinal meninges
D42.1	Neoplasm of uncertain behavior of spinal meninges
D48.0	Neoplasm of uncertain behavior of bone and articular cartilage
G06.1	Intraspinal abscess and granuloma
G06.2	Extradural and subdural abscess, unspecified
G07	Intracranial and intraspinal abscess and granuloma in diseases classified elsewhere
G95.0	Syringomyelia and syringobulbia
G95.19	Other vascular myelopathies

CCI Edits

Refer to Appendix A for CCI edits.

Pub 100

63305: Pub 100-04, 12, 20.4.5

63306: Pub 100-04, 12, 20.4.5

Facility RVUs ▯

Code	Work	PE Facility	MP	Total Facility
63305	36.24	22.60	13.46	72.30
63306	35.55	22.28	13.22	71.05

Non-facility RVUs ▯

Code	Work	PE Non-Facility	MP	Total Non-Facility
63305	36.24	22.60	13.46	72.30
63306	35.55	22.28	13.22	71.05

Modifiers (PAR) ▯

Code	Mod 50	Mod 51	Mod 62	Mod 66	Mod 80
63305	0	2	1	0	2
63306	0	2	1	0	2

Global Period

Code	Days
63305	090
63306	090

63307

63307 Vertebral corpectomy (vertebral body resection), partial or complete, for excision of intraspinal lesion, single segment; intradural, lumbar or sacral by transperitoneal or retroperitoneal approach

AMA Coding Guideline

Excision, Anterior or Anterolateral Approach, Intraspinal Lesion Procedures on the Spine and Spinal Cord

For the following codes, when two surgeons work together as primary surgeons performing distinct part(s) of an anterior approach for an intraspinal excision, each surgeon should report his/her distinct operative work by appending modifier 62 to the single definitive procedure code. In this situation, modifier 62 may be appended to the definitive procedure code(s) 63300-63307 and, as appropriate, to the associated additional segment add-on code 63308 as long as both surgeons continue to work together as primary surgeons.

For vertebral corpectomy, the term partial is used to describe removal of a substantial portion of the body of the vertebra. In the cervical spine, the amount of bone removed is defined as at least one-half of the vertebral body. In the thoracic and lumbar spine, the amount of bone removed is defined as at least one-third of the vertebral body.

AMA Coding Notes

Excision, Anterior or Anterolateral Approach, Intraspinal Lesion Procedures on the Spine and Spinal Cord

(For arthrodesis, see 22548-22585)

(For reconstruction of spine, see 20930-20938)

Surgical Procedures on the Spine and Spinal Cord

(For application of caliper or tongs, use 20660)

(For treatment of fracture or dislocation of spine, see 22310-22327)

AMA *CPT Assistant* ☐

63307: Feb 02: 4, Jul 13: 3

Plain English Description

Vertebral corpectomy involves removal of the vertebral body as well as the vertebral discs above and below the vertebra. In this procedure, vertebral corpectomy is performed to excise a lesion or tumor that is located within the spinal canal (intraspinal) and within or extending into the dura mater (intradural). Resection is performed on only one vertebral segment in the lumbar or sacral spine. If a transperitoneal (anterior) approach is used, the abdomen is incised and the peritoneum entered. The bowel is moved out of the way. If a retroperitoneal (anterolateral) approach is used, a flank incision is made. Surrounding tissues are dissected taking care to protect vital structures. The affected lumbar or sacral segment is exposed. The intervertebral discs above and below the vertebral body are removed first with the aid of the surgical microscope. The discs are dissected from surrounding tissue and removed. The vertebral body is excised and the lesion or tumor in the spinal canal identified and explored. If it is determined that the lesion or tumor lies within or extends into the dura, the dura is incised. The lesion or tumor is carefully dissected free of surrounding tissues with the aid of an operating microscope and removed. The dura is then repaired with sutures or a dural graft. Separately reportable bone grafting and fusion procedures are performed. The bone graft is placed in the surgical defect to support the anterior aspect of the spine where the discs and vertebral body have been removed. Surrounding bone is contoured for placement of the graft and to ensure fusion of the graft and adjacent bone. Separately reportable spine instrumentation may also be used to stabilize the spine.

Vertebral corpectomy, for excision of intraspinal lesion, intradural

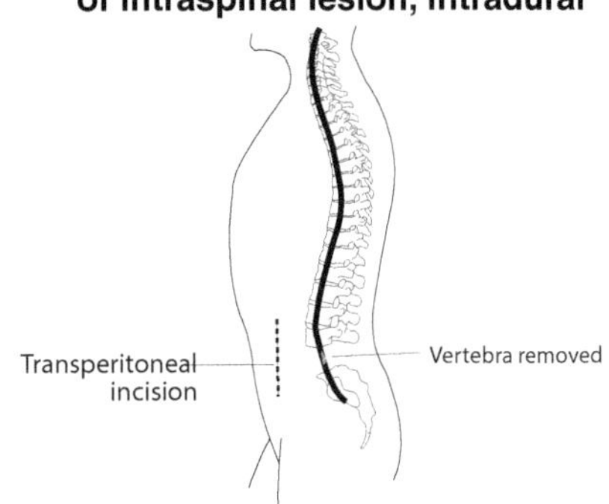

All or part of a lumbar/sacral vertebra in the back containing a lesion inside the dura is removed.

ICD-10-CM Diagnostic Codes

A17.81	Tuberculoma of brain and spinal cord
C41.2	Malignant neoplasm of vertebral column
C70.1	Malignant neoplasm of spinal meninges
C72.0	Malignant neoplasm of spinal cord
C79.49	Secondary malignant neoplasm of other parts of nervous system
C79.51	Secondary malignant neoplasm of bone
D16.6	Benign neoplasm of vertebral column
D32.1	Benign neoplasm of spinal meninges
D33.4	Benign neoplasm of spinal cord
D42.1	Neoplasm of uncertain behavior of spinal meninges
D43.4	Neoplasm of uncertain behavior of spinal cord
D48.0	Neoplasm of uncertain behavior of bone and articular cartilage
G06.1	Intraspinal abscess and granuloma
G06.2	Extradural and subdural abscess, unspecified
G07	Intracranial and intraspinal abscess and granuloma in diseases classified elsewhere
G95.0	Syringomyelia and syringobulbia
G95.19	Other vascular myelopathies

CCI Edits

Refer to Appendix A for CCI edits.

Pub 100

63307: Pub 100-04, 12, 20.4.5

Facility RVUs ☐

Code	Work	PE Facility	MP	Total Facility
63307	34.96	21.63	12.99	69.58

Non-facility RVUs ☐

Code	Work	PE Non-Facility	MP	Total Non-Facility
63307	34.96	21.63	12.99	69.58

Modifiers (PAR) ☐

Code	Mod 50	Mod 51	Mod 62	Mod 66	Mod 80
63307	0	2	1	0	2

Global Period

Code	Days
63307	090

63308

✚ **63308 Vertebral corpectomy (vertebral body resection), partial or complete, for excision of intraspinal lesion, single segment; each additional segment (List separately in addition to codes for single segment)**

(Use 63308 in conjunction with 63300-63307)

AMA Coding Guideline

Excision, Anterior or Anterolateral Approach, Intraspinal Lesion Procedures on the Spine and Spinal Cord

For the following codes, when two surgeons work together as primary surgeons performing distinct part(s) of an anterior approach for an intraspinal excision, each surgeon should report his/her distinct operative work by appending modifier 62 to the single definitive procedure code. In this situation, modifier 62 may be appended to the definitive procedure code(s) 63300-63307 and, as appropriate, to the associated additional segment add-on code 63308 as long as both surgeons continue to work together as primary surgeons.

For vertebral corpectomy, the term partial is used to describe removal of a substantial portion of the body of the vertebra. In the cervical spine, the amount of bone removed is defined as at least one-half of the vertebral body. In the thoracic and lumbar spine, the amount of bone removed is defined as at least one-third of the vertebral body.

AMA Coding Notes

Excision, Anterior or Anterolateral Approach, Intraspinal Lesion Procedures on the Spine and Spinal Cord

(For arthrodesis, see 22548-22585)

(For reconstruction of spine, see 20930-20938)

Surgical Procedures on the Spine and Spinal Cord

(For application of caliper or tongs, use 20660)

(For treatment of fracture or dislocation of spine, see 22310-22327)

AMA *CPT Assistant* ▯

63308: Feb 02: 4

Plain English Description

Following exposure of the spine as described in the primary procedure, it is determined that vertebral body resection on more than one vertebral segment is required. The first vertebral segment and superior and inferior intervertebral discs are excised as described in the primary procedure. One or more additional contiguous vertebral segments are resected in the same manner. The intervertebral discs above and below the vertebral body are removed first followed by removal of vertebral body. Use 63308 for each additional vertebral body resection.

Vertebral corpectomy for excision of intraspinal lesion

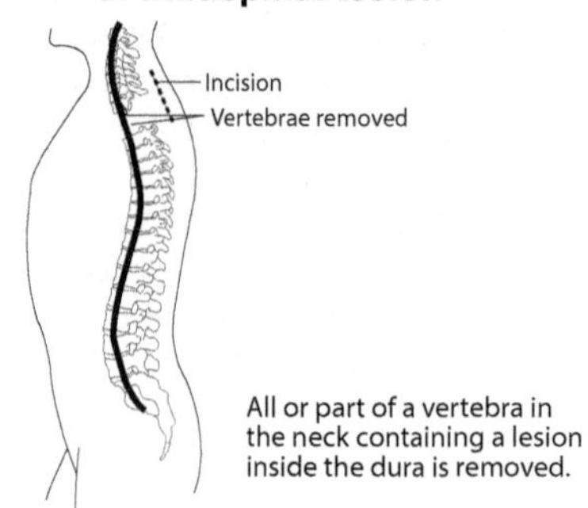

All or part of a vertebra in the neck containing a lesion inside the dura is removed.

ICD-10-CM Diagnostic Codes

See Primary Procedure code for crosswalks.

CCI Edits

Refer to Appendix A for CCI edits.

Pub 100

63308: Pub 100-04, 12, 20.4.5

Facility RVUs ▯

Code	Work	PE Facility	MP	Total Facility
63308	5.24	2.44	1.69	9.37

Non-facility RVUs ▯

Code	Work	PE Non-Facility	MP	Total Non-Facility
63308	5.24	2.44	1.69	9.37

Modifiers (PAR) ▯

Code	Mod 50	Mod 51	Mod 62	Mod 66	Mod 80
63308	0	0	1	0	2

Global Period

Code	Days
63308	ZZZ

63620-63621

63620 Stereotactic radiosurgery (particle beam, gamma ray, or linear accelerator); 1 spinal lesion

(Do not report 63620 more than once per course of treatment)

+ **63621 Stereotactic radiosurgery (particle beam, gamma ray, or linear accelerator); each additional spinal lesion (List separately in addition to code for primary procedure)**

(Report 63621 in conjunction with 63620)

(For each course of treatment, 63621 may be reported no more than once per lesion. Do not report 63621 more than 2 times for entire course of treatment regardless of number of lesions treated)

AMA Coding Guideline

Stereotactic Radiosurgery (Spinal) Procedures on the Spine and Spinal Cord

Spinal stereotactic radiosurgery is a distinct procedure that utilizes externally generated ionizing radiation to inactivate or eradicate defined target(s) in the spine without the need to make an incision. The target is defined by and the treatment is delivered using high-resolution stereotactic imaging. These codes are reported by the surgeon. The radiation oncologist reports the appropriate code(s) for clinical treatment planning, physics and dosimetry, treatment delivery and management from the Radiation Oncology section (77261-77790). Any necessary planning, dosimetry, targeting, positioning, or blocking by the neurosurgeon is included in the stereotactic radiation surgery services. The same individual should not report stereotactic radiosurgery services with radiation treatment management codes (77427-77432).

Spinal stereotactic radiosurgery is typically performed in a single planning and treatment session using a stereotactic image-guidance system, but can be performed with a planning session and in a limited number of treatment sessions, up to a maximum of five sessions. Do not report stereotactic radiosurgery more than once per lesion per course of treatment when the treatment requires greater than one session.

Stereotactic spinal surgery is only used when the tumor being treated affects spinal neural tissue or abuts the dura mater. Arteriovenous malformations must be subdural. For other radiation services of the spine, see Radiation Oncology services.

Codes 63620, 63621 include computer-assisted planning. Do not report 63620, 63621 in conjunction with 61781-61783.

AMA Coding Notes

Stereotactic Radiosurgery (Spinal) Procedures on the Spine and Spinal Cord

(For intensity modulated beam delivery plan and treatment, see 77301, 77385, 77386. For stereotactic body radiation therapy, see 77373, 77435)

Surgical Procedures on the Spine and Spinal Cord

(For application of caliper or tongs, use 20660)

(For treatment of fracture or dislocation of spine, see 22310-22327)

AMA *CPT Assistant* □

63620: Oct 10: 3, Jul 11: 12, Jun 15: 6

63621: Oct 10: 3, Jul 11: 12, Jun 15: 6

Plain English Description

Stereotactic radiosurgery using a particle beam, gamma ray, or linear accelerator is performed on a single spinal lesion. Stereotactic radiosurgery delivers a very high radiation dose to a precise location using multiple intersecting beams of radiation. Particle beam or cyclotron technology has limited use in the United States. Gamma ray technology uses a gamma knife composed of 201 beams of highly focused gamma rays to treat small to medium-sized lesions. Linear accelerator (LINAC) technology uses high-energy X-ray photons or electrons in curving paths and can be used to treat larger lesions. During a separately reportable planning procedure, the lesion is visualized using three-dimensional MRI or CT scans. Spinal lesions are treated using a frameless technique. If the lesion is in the cervical spine, a molded face mask may be used to stabilize the head and neck. If the lesion is in the thoracic or lumbar spine, gold fiducial markers are placed into the pedicles adjacent to the lesion. The implanted fiducials are used to direct the radiation beams. An immobilization device such as an alpha cradle may also be used. The required treatment is defined and includes determination of lesion location and volume, identification of surrounding structures and assessment of risk of damage to these structures, and dose computation. If a gamma knife is used, the patient is placed on the gamma bed. The gamma bed moves backward into the treatment area and is locked into the radiation source. The radiation dose is delivered. If a linear accelerator is used, a computer is used in conjunction with a micro-multileaf collimator attached to the linear accelerator, which arranges and shapes high-energy radiation beams in the exact configuration of the lesion. The gantry rotates around the patient and delivers the planned radiation dose to the lesion. Use code 63620 for a single spinal lesion and code 63621 for each additional spinal lesion.

Stereotactic radiosurgery

(particle beam, gamma ray, or linear accelerator)

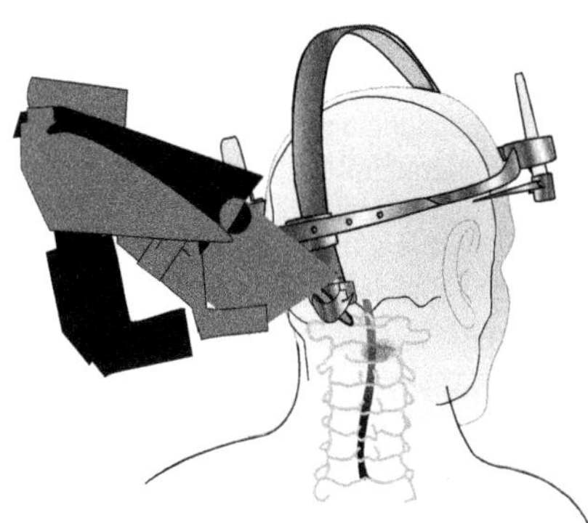

1 spinal lesion (63620); each additional spinal lesion (63621)

ICD-10-CM Diagnostic Codes

C41.2	Malignant neoplasm of vertebral column
C41.4	Malignant neoplasm of pelvic bones, sacrum and coccyx
C70.1	Malignant neoplasm of spinal meninges
C72.0	Malignant neoplasm of spinal cord
C79.49	Secondary malignant neoplasm of other parts of nervous system
C79.51	Secondary malignant neoplasm of bone

CCI Edits

Refer to Appendix A for CCI edits.

Facility RVUs □

Code	Work	PE Facility	MP	Total Facility
63620	15.60	11.01	5.68	32.29
63621	4.00	1.84	1.46	7.30

Non-facility RVUs □

Code	Work	PE Non-Facility	MP	Total Non-Facility
63620	15.60	11.01	5.68	32.29
63621	4.00	1.84	1.46	7.30

Modifiers (PAR) □

Code	Mod 50	Mod 51	Mod 62	Mod 66	Mod 80
63620	0	0	0	0	2
63621	0	0	0	0	2

Global Period

Code	Days
63620	090
63621	ZZZ

63650-63655

63650 Percutaneous implantation of neurostimulator electrode array, epidural

63655 Laminectomy for implantation of neurostimulator electrodes, plate/ paddle, epidural

AMA Coding Guideline

Neurostimulators (Spinal) Procedures

For electronic analysis with programming, when performed, of spinal cord neurostimulator pulse generator/transmitters, see codes 95970, 95971, 95972. Test stimulation to confirm correct target site placement of the electrode array(s) and/ or to confirm the functional status of the system is inherent to placement, and is not separately reported as electronic analysis or programming of the neurostimulator system. Electronic analysis (95970) at the time of implantation is not separately reported.

Codes 63650, 63655, and 63661-63664 describe the operative placement, revision, replacement, or removal of the spinal neurostimulator system components to provide spinal electrical stimulation. A neurostimulator system includes an implanted neurostimulator, external controller, extension, and collection of contacts. Multiple contacts or electrodes (4 or more) provide the actual electrical stimulation in the epidural space.

For percutaneously placed neurostimulator systems (63650, 63661, 63663), the contacts are on a catheter-like lead. An array defines the collection of contacts that are on one catheter.

For systems placed via an open surgical exposure (63655, 63662, 63664), the contacts are on a plate or paddle-shaped surface.

Do not report 63661 or 63663 when removing or replacing a temporary percutaneously placed array for an external generator.

AMA Coding Notes

Surgical Procedures on the Spine and Spinal Cord

(For application of caliper or tongs, use 20660)

(For treatment of fracture or dislocation of spine, see 22310-22327)

AMA *CPT Assistant* □

63650: Jun 98: 3, 4, Nov 98: 18, Mar 99: 11, Apr 99: 10, Sep 99: 3, Dec 08: 8, Feb 10: 9, Aug 10: 8, Dec 10: 14, Apr 11: 10, Oct 13: 19, Dec 15: 17, Jan 16: 12, Dec 17: 16, Oct 18: 11

63655: Jun 98: 3, 4, Nov 98: 18, Sep 99: 3, 4, Dec 08: 8, Aug 10: 8, Dec 10: 14, Apr 11: 10

Plain English Description

Placement of an implantable spinal cord stimulation system is performed to treat chronic back and/ or leg pain. Electrical stimulation of the spinal cord alleviates pain by activating pain-inhibiting neurons and inducing a tingling sensation that masks pain sensations. In 63650, percutaneous placement of an electrode array in the epidural space is performed. Using separately reportable fluoroscopic guidance, a small incision is made in the skin over the planned insertion site. The vertebra is exposed and a small portion of the lamina removed (laminotomy). The electrode array, also referred to as leads, is advanced into the epidural space and secured with sutures. The patient is then awakened and the array tested to ensure that the neurostimulator is properly placed and that there is no pain from the electrode array implant itself. The neurostimulator will be tested at various settings, and once the optimal settings are determined, they will be used to program the pulse generator or receiver that will be implanted in a separately reportable procedure. The lead wires are then tunneled to the pulse generator/ receiver pocket where they are attached to the generator/receiver. In 63655, an electrode plate or paddle is placed in the epidural space using an open technique requiring a laminectomy. An incision between 2-5 inches in length is made over the spine. Overlying soft tissue is dissected and the lamina exposed. Part or all of the lamina is excised to allow access to the epidural space. The plate or paddle is positioned in the epidural space and secured to the spine. Once the plate or paddle is in place, the patient is awakened and the device is tested. Tunneling of the leads to the pulse generator/receiver pocket and connection of the leads is performed as described above.

Implantation of neurostimulator electrode array, epidural

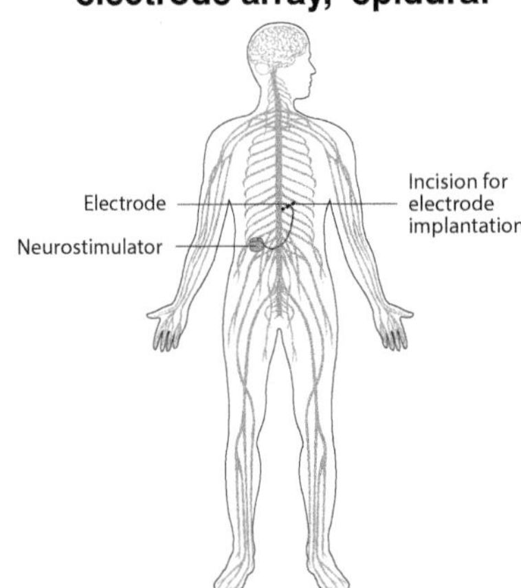

Percutaneous array (63650); plate/paddle laminectomy (63655)

ICD-10-CM Diagnostic Codes

	Code	Description
	G03.1	Chronic meningitis
⇄	G56.41	Causalgia of right upper limb
⇄	G56.42	Causalgia of left upper limb
⇄	G56.43	Causalgia of bilateral upper limbs
⇄	G57.71	Causalgia of right lower limb
⇄	G57.72	Causalgia of left lower limb
⇄	G57.73	Causalgia of bilateral lower limbs
	G89.21	Chronic pain due to trauma
	G89.22	Chronic post-thoracotomy pain
	G89.28	Other chronic postprocedural pain
	G89.29	Other chronic pain
	G89.3	Neoplasm related pain (acute) (chronic)
⇄	G90.511	Complex regional pain syndrome I of right upper limb
⇄	G90.512	Complex regional pain syndrome I of left upper limb
⇄	G90.513	Complex regional pain syndrome I of upper limb, bilateral
⇄	G90.521	Complex regional pain syndrome I of right lower limb
⇄	G90.522	Complex regional pain syndrome I of left lower limb
⇄	G90.523	Complex regional pain syndrome I of lower limb, bilateral
	G96.12	Meningeal adhesions (cerebral) (spinal)
	M47.21	Other spondylosis with radiculopathy, occipito-atlanto-axial region
	M47.22	Other spondylosis with radiculopathy, cervical region
	M47.23	Other spondylosis with radiculopathy, cervicothoracic region
	M47.24	Other spondylosis with radiculopathy, thoracic region
	M47.25	Other spondylosis with radiculopathy, thoracolumbar region
	M47.26	Other spondylosis with radiculopathy, lumbar region
	M47.27	Other spondylosis with radiculopathy, lumbosacral region
	M47.28	Other spondylosis with radiculopathy, sacral and sacrococcygeal region
	M50.11	Cervical disc disorder with radiculopathy, high cervical region
	M50.121	Cervical disc disorder at C4-C5 level with radiculopathy
	M50.122	Cervical disc disorder at C5-C6 level with radiculopathy
	M50.123	Cervical disc disorder at C6-C7 level with radiculopathy
	M50.13	Cervical disc disorder with radiculopathy, cervicothoracic region
	M51.14	Intervertebral disc disorders with radiculopathy, thoracic region
	M51.15	Intervertebral disc disorders with radiculopathy, thoracolumbar region
	M51.16	Intervertebral disc disorders with radiculopathy, lumbar region
	M51.17	Intervertebral disc disorders with radiculopathy, lumbosacral region
	M54.11	Radiculopathy, occipito-atlanto-axial region
	M54.12	Radiculopathy, cervical region
	M54.13	Radiculopathy, cervicothoracic region
	M54.14	Radiculopathy, thoracic region
	M54.15	Radiculopathy, thoracolumbar region
	M54.16	Radiculopathy, lumbar region
	M54.17	Radiculopathy, lumbosacral region
	M54.18	Radiculopathy, sacral and sacrococcygeal region
	M54.2	Cervicalgia

⇄	M54.31	Sciatica, right side
⇄	M54.32	Sciatica, left side
⇄	M54.41	Lumbago with sciatica, right side
⇄	M54.42	Lumbago with sciatica, left side
	M54.5	Low back pain
	M54.6	Pain in thoracic spine
	M54.89	Other dorsalgia
	M96.1	Postlaminectomy syndrome, not elsewhere classified

CCI Edits

Refer to Appendix A for CCI edits.

Pub 100

63650: Pub 100-03, 1, 160.19, Pub 100-03, 1, 160.26, Pub 100-03, 1, 160.7-160.7.1

63655: Pub 100-03, 1, 160.26, Pub 100-03, 1, 160.7-160.7.1

Facility RVUs ▯

Code	Work	PE Facility	MP	Total Facility
63650	7.15	4.01	0.77	11.93
63655	10.92	9.64	3.45	24.01

Non-facility RVUs ▯

Code	Work	PE Non-Facility	MP	Total Non-Facility
63650	7.15	46.26	0.77	54.18
63655	10.92	9.64	3.45	24.01

Modifiers (PAR) ▯

Code	Mod 50	Mod 51	Mod 62	Mod 66	Mod 80
63650	0	2	0	0	1
63655	0	2	1	0	2

Global Period

Code	Days
63650	010
63655	090

63661-63662

63661 Removal of spinal neurostimulator electrode percutaneous array(s), including fluoroscopy, when performed

63662 Removal of spinal neurostimulator electrode plate/paddle(s) placed via laminotomy or laminectomy, including fluoroscopy, when performed

AMA Coding Guideline

Neurostimulators (Spinal) Procedures

For electronic analysis with programming, when performed, of spinal cord neurostimulator pulse generator/transmitters, see codes 95970, 95971, 95972. Test stimulation to confirm correct target site placement of the electrode array(s) and/or to confirm the functional status of the system is inherent to placement, and is not separately reported as electronic analysis or programming of the neurostimulator system. Electronic analysis (95970) at the time of implantation is not separately reported.

Codes 63650, 63655, and 63661-63664 describe the operative placement, revision, replacement, or removal of the spinal neurostimulator system components to provide spinal electrical stimulation. A neurostimulator system includes an implanted neurostimulator, external controller, extension, and collection of contacts. Multiple contacts or electrodes (4 or more) provide the actual electrical stimulation in the epidural space.

For percutaneously placed neurostimulator systems (63650, 63661, 63663), the contacts are on a catheter-like lead. An array defines the collection of contacts that are on one catheter.

For systems placed via an open surgical exposure (63655, 63662, 63664), the contacts are on a plate or paddle-shaped surface.

Do not report 63661 or 63663 when removing or replacing a temporary percutaneously placed array for an external generator.

AMA Coding Notes

Surgical Procedures on the Spine and Spinal Cord

(For application of caliper or tongs, use 20660)

(For treatment of fracture or dislocation of spine, see 22310-22327)

AMA *CPT Assistant* ☐

63661: Feb 10: 9, Aug 10: 8, Jan 11: 8, Apr 11: 10

63662: Feb 10: 9, Aug 10: 8, Apr 11: 10

Plain English Description

An implantable spinal cord stimulation system is used to treat chronic back and/or leg pain. Electrical stimulation of the spinal cord alleviates pain by activating pain-inhibiting neurons and inducing a tingling sensation that masks pain sensations. Typically, a temporary electrode array, plate, or paddle is placed to determine the effectiveness of the device in alleviating pain. The temporary device is eventually removed and if effective replaced with a permanent device or, if ineffective, it is removed without replacement. In 63661, percutaneous removal of an electrode array in the epidural space is performed. The subcutaneous pocket containing the generator/receiver is opened and the leads are disconnected. Using fluoroscopic guidance as needed, a small incision is made in the skin over the insertion site. The vertebra is exposed and the electrode array, also referred to as leads, is located and removed from the epidural space. The leads are dissected free of the subcutaneous tunnel and removed. If a permanent electrode array is to be placed, this is performed in a separately reportable procedure. If the electrode array is not being replaced, the incisions are closed. In 63662, an electrode plate or paddle that has been placed via a laminotomy or laminectomy is removed from the epidural space. The subcutaneous pocket containing the generator/receiver is opened and the leads are disconnected. Using fluoroscopic guidance as needed, an incision is made over the spine. Overlying soft tissue is dissected and the lamina exposed. The plate or paddle is located in the epidural space and removed. The leads are dissected free of the subcutaneous tunnel and removed. If a permanent electrode plate or paddle is to be placed, this is performed in a separately reportable procedure. If the electrode plate or paddle is not being replaced, the incisions are closed.

Removal of spinal neurostimulator electrode percutaneous array(s) including fluoroscopy

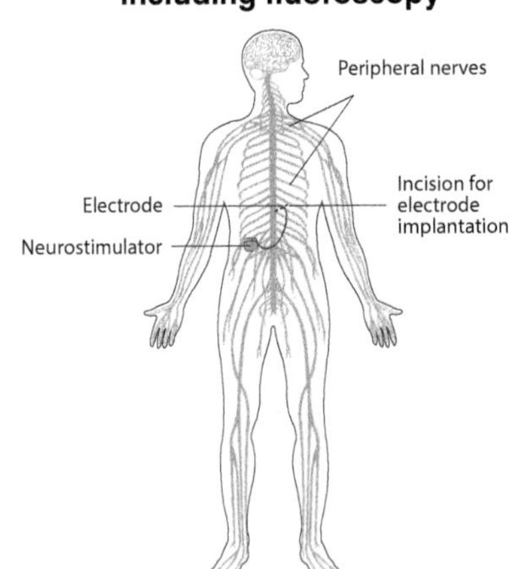

Percutaneous array(s) (63661); plate/paddle(s) placed via laminotomy/laminectomy (63662)

ICD-10-CM Diagnostic Codes

	Code	Description
➐	T85.112	Breakdown (mechanical) of implanted electronic neurostimulator of spinal cord electrode (lead)
➐	T85.122	Displacement of implanted electronic neurostimulator of spinal cord electrode (lead)
➐	T85.192	Other mechanical complication of implanted electronic neurostimulator of spinal cord electrode (lead)
➐	T85.733	Infection and inflammatory reaction due to implanted electronic neurostimulator of spinal cord, electrode (lead)
➐	T85.810	Embolism due to nervous system prosthetic devices, implants and grafts
➐	T85.820	Fibrosis due to nervous system prosthetic devices, implants and grafts
➐	T85.830	Hemorrhage due to nervous system prosthetic devices, implants and grafts
➐	T85.840	Pain due to nervous system prosthetic devices, implants and grafts
➐	T85.850	Stenosis due to nervous system prosthetic devices, implants and grafts
➐	T85.860	Thrombosis due to nervous system prosthetic devices, implants and grafts
➐	T85.890	Other specified complication of nervous system prosthetic devices, implants and grafts
	Z45.42	Encounter for adjustment and management of neurostimulator

ICD-10-CM Coding Notes

For codes requiring a 7th character extension, refer to your ICD-10-CM book. Review the character descriptions and coding guidelines for proper selection. For some procedures, only certain characters will apply.

CCI Edits

Refer to Appendix A for CCI edits.

Pub 100

63661: Pub 100-03, 1, 160.19, Pub 100-03, 1, 160.26, Pub 100-03, 1, 160.7-160.7.1

63662: Pub 100-03, 1, 160.19, Pub 100-03, 1, 160.26, Pub 100-03, 1, 160.7-160.7.1

Facility RVUs

Code	Work	PE Facility	MP	Total Facility
63661	5.08	3.40	0.85	9.33
63662	11.00	9.79	3.51	24.30

Non-facility RVUs

Code	Work	PE Non-Facility	MP	Total Non-Facility
63661	5.08	12.39	0.85	18.32
63662	11.00	9.79	3.51	24.30

Modifiers (PAR)

Code	Mod 50	Mod 51	Mod 62	Mod 66	Mod 80
63661	0	2	1	0	2
63662	0	2	1	0	2

Global Period

Code	Days
63661	010
63662	090

CPT® Procedural Coding

63663-63664

63663 Revision including replacement, when performed, of spinal neurostimulator electrode percutaneous array(s), including fluoroscopy, when performed

(Do not report 63663 in conjunction with 63661, 63662 for the same spinal level)

63664 Revision including replacement, when performed, of spinal neurostimulator electrode plate/ paddle(s) placed via laminotomy or laminectomy, including fluoroscopy, when performed

(Do not report 63664 in conjunction with 63661, 63662 for the same spinal level)

AMA Coding Guideline

Neurostimulators (Spinal) Procedures

For electronic analysis with programming, when performed, of spinal cord neurostimulator pulse generator/transmitters, see codes 95970, 95971, 95972. Test stimulation to confirm correct target site placement of the electrode array(s) and/ or to confirm the functional status of the system is inherent to placement, and is not separately reported as electronic analysis or programming of the neurostimulator system. Electronic analysis (95970) at the time of implantation is not separately reported.

Codes 63650, 63655, and 63661-63664 describe the operative placement, revision, replacement, or removal of the spinal neurostimulator system components to provide spinal electrical stimulation. A neurostimulator system includes an implanted neurostimulator, external controller, extension, and collection of contacts. Multiple contacts or electrodes (4 or more) provide the actual electrical stimulation in the epidural space.

For percutaneously placed neurostimulator systems (63650, 63661, 63663), the contacts are on a catheter-like lead. An array defines the collection of contacts that are on one catheter.

For systems placed via an open surgical exposure (63655, 63662, 63664), the contacts are on a plate or paddle-shaped surface.

Do not report 63661 or 63663 when removing or replacing a temporary percutaneously placed array for an external generator.

AMA Coding Notes

Surgical Procedures on the Spine and Spinal Cord

(For application of caliper or tongs, use 20660)

(For treatment of fracture or dislocation of spine, see 22310-22327)

AMA *CPT Assistant*

63663: Feb 10: 9, Aug 10: 8, Apr 11: 10

63664: Feb 10: 9, Aug 10: 8, Apr 11: 10

Plain English Description

An implantable spinal cord stimulation system is used to treat chronic back and/or leg pain. Electrical stimulation of the spinal cord alleviates pain by activating pain-inhibiting neurons and inducing a tingling sensation that masks pain sensations. In 63663, revision including replacement of an electrode array in the epidural space is performed. Using separately reportable fluoroscopic guidance, a small incision is made in the skin over the insertion site. The electrode array is located and explored to determine whether it needs to be repositioned or removed and replaced. If it needs to be repositioned, any sutures are removed and the array is then moved as needed to obtain optimal pain control. If the array needs to be replaced, it is removed in a separately reportable procedure. The new array is then advanced into the epidural space and secured with sutures. The patient is awakened and the revised or new array tested to ensure that the neurostimulator is properly placed and that there is no pain from the electrode array implant itself. The neurostimulator will be tested at various settings, and once the optimal settings are determined, they will be used to program the pulse generator or receiver that will be implanted in a separately reportable procedure. The lead wires are then tunneled to the pulse generator/receiver pocket where they are attached to the generator/receiver. In 63664, an electrode plate or paddle that has been placed via a laminotomy or laminectomy in the epidural space is revised and replaced as needed. An incision between 2 and 5 inches in length is made over the spine. Overlying soft tissue is dissected and the plate or paddle exposed and freed from the spine. If revision is performed, the plate or paddle is repositioned in the epidural space and secured to the spine. If the plate or paddle must be replaced, it is removed in a separately reportable procedure. A new plate or paddle is then placed in the epidural space and secured to the spine. Once the plate or paddle is in place, the patient is awakened and testing of the device, tunneling of the leads to the pulse generator/receiver pocket, and connection of the leads are performed as described above.

Revision including replacement, when performed, of spinal neurostimulator electrode percutaneous array(s)

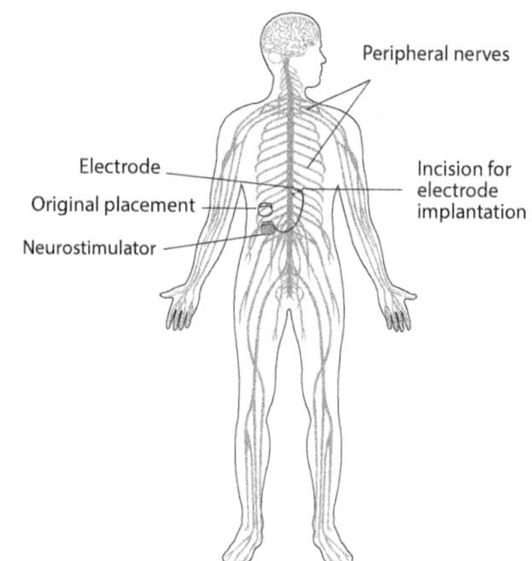

Percutaneous array(s) (63663); plate/paddle(s placed via laminotomy/laminectomy (63664)

ICD-10-CM Diagnostic Codes

	Code	Description
➐	T85.112	Breakdown (mechanical) of implanted electronic neurostimulator of spinal cord electrode (lead)
➐	T85.122	Displacement of implanted electronic neurostimulator of spinal cord electrode (lead)
➐	T85.192	Other mechanical complication of implanted electronic neurostimulator of spinal cord electrode (lead)
➐	T85.733	Infection and inflammatory reaction due to implanted electronic neurostimulator of spinal cord, electrode (lead)
➐	T85.810	Embolism due to nervous system prosthetic devices, implants and grafts
➐	T85.820	Fibrosis due to nervous system prosthetic devices, implants and grafts
➐	T85.830	Hemorrhage due to nervous system prosthetic devices, implants and grafts
➐	T85.840	Pain due to nervous system prosthetic devices, implants and grafts
➐	T85.850	Stenosis due to nervous system prosthetic devices, implants and grafts
➐	T85.860	Thrombosis due to nervous system prosthetic devices, implants and grafts
➐	T85.890	Other specified complication of nervous system prosthetic devices, implants and grafts
	Z45.42	Encounter for adjustment and management of neurostimulator

ICD-10-CM Coding Notes

For codes requiring a 7th character extension, refer to your ICD-10-CM book. Review the character descriptions and coding guidelines for proper selection. For some procedures, only certain characters will apply.

CCI Edits

Refer to Appendix A for CCI edits.

Pub 100

63663: Pub 100-03, 1, 160.19, Pub 100-03, 1, 160.26, Pub 100-03, 1, 160.7-160.7.1

63664: Pub 100-03, 1, 160.19, Pub 100-03, 1, 160.26, Pub 100-03, 1, 160.7-160.7.1

Facility RVUs

Code	Work	PE Facility	MP	Total Facility
63663	7.75	4.21	1.04	13.00
63664	11.52	10.04	3.73	25.29

Non-facility RVUs

Code	Work	PE Non-Facility	MP	Total Non-Facility
63663	7.75	15.59	1.04	24.38
63664	11.52	10.04	3.73	25.29

Modifiers (PAR)

Code	Mod 50	Mod 51	Mod 62	Mod 66	Mod 80
63663	0	2	1	0	2
63664	0	2	1	0	2

Global Period

Code	Days
63663	010
63664	090

63685-63688

63685 Insertion or replacement of spinal neurostimulator pulse generator or receiver, direct or inductive coupling

(Do not report 63685 in conjunction with 63688 for the same pulse generator or receiver)

63688 Revision or removal of implanted spinal neurostimulator pulse generator or receiver

(For electronic analysis with programming, when performed, of implanted spinal cord neurostimulator pulse generator/transmitter, see 95970, 95971, 95972)

AMA Coding Guideline

Neurostimulators (Spinal) Procedures

For electronic analysis with programming, when performed, of spinal cord neurostimulator pulse generator/transmitters, see codes 95970, 95971, 95972. Test stimulation to confirm correct target site placement of the electrode array(s) and/or to confirm the functional status of the system is inherent to placement, and is not separately reported as electronic analysis or programming of the neurostimulator system. Electronic analysis (95970) at the time of implantation is not separately reported.

Codes 63650, 63655, and 63661-63664 describe the operative placement, revision, replacement, or removal of the spinal neurostimulator system components to provide spinal electrical stimulation. A neurostimulator system includes an implanted neurostimulator, external controller, extension, and collection of contacts. Multiple contacts or electrodes (4 or more) provide the actual electrical stimulation in the epidural space.

For percutaneously placed neurostimulator systems (63650, 63661, 63663), the contacts are on a catheter-like lead. An array defines the collection of contacts that are on one catheter.

For systems placed via an open surgical exposure (63655, 63662, 63664), the contacts are on a plate or paddle-shaped surface.

Do not report 63661 or 63663 when removing or replacing a temporary percutaneously placed array for an external generator.

AMA Coding Notes

Surgical Procedures on the Spine and Spinal Cord

(For application of caliper or tongs, use 20660)

(For treatment of fracture or dislocation of spine, see 22310-22327)

AMA *CPT Assistant*

63685: Jun 98: 3, 4, Sep 99: 5, Feb 10: 9, Oct 10: 14, Dec 10: 14, Apr 11: 10, Dec 17: 16

63688: Jun 98: 3, 4, Sep 99: 5, Feb 10: 9, Apr 11: 11

Plain English Description

An implantable generator for spinal cord stimulation (SCS) generates electrical impulses to implanted electrodes in the spine. An implantable receiver receives electrical impulses from an external generator and then transmits those signals to the electrodes. In 63685, a pulse generator or receiver is inserted or replaced. For initial insertion, an incision is made in the skin overlying the planned insertion site for the neurostimulator pulse generator or receiver. A subcutaneous pocket is fashioned. The electrodes, which have been implanted and tunneled to the pocket in the separately reportable procedure, are connected to the generator or receiver and tested. Stimulation parameters are set and the device is placed in the skin pocket, which is closed with sutures. Replacement is performed in the same manner except that the existing generator or receiver is removed first by incising the skin over the existing generator or receiver. The skin pocket is opened and the existing device exposed. The electrodes are disconnected. The generator or receiver is dissected free of surrounding tissue and removed. The new generator or receiver is connected to the electrodes and tested. In 63688, an existing generator or receiver is revised or removed. Revision involves opening the skin pocket and removing the generator or receiver. The device is then evaluated and adjustments made as needed to ensure proper functioning. Removal is accomplished by exposing the device, disconnecting the electrodes (which are removed in a separate procedure), and closing the skin pocket.

Insertion or replacement of spinal neurostimulator pulse generator or receiver

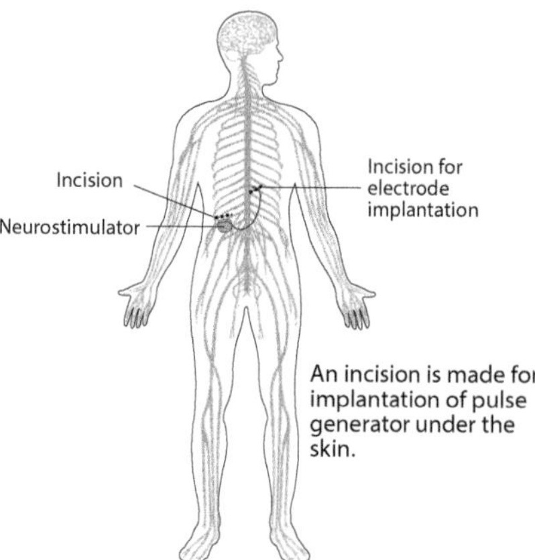

ICD-10-CM Diagnostic Codes

	Code	Description
	G03.1	Chronic meningitis
⇄	G56.41	Causalgia of right upper limb
⇄	G56.42	Causalgia of left upper limb
⇄	G56.43	Causalgia of bilateral upper limbs
⇄	G57.71	Causalgia of right lower limb
⇄	G57.72	Causalgia of left lower limb
⇄	G57.73	Causalgia of bilateral lower limbs
	G89.21	Chronic pain due to trauma
	G89.22	Chronic post-thoracotomy pain
	G89.28	Other chronic postprocedural pain
	G89.29	Other chronic pain
	G89.3	Neoplasm related pain (acute) (chronic)
⇄	G90.511	Complex regional pain syndrome I of right upper limb
⇄	G90.512	Complex regional pain syndrome I of left upper limb
⇄	G90.513	Complex regional pain syndrome I of upper limb, bilateral
⇄	G90.521	Complex regional pain syndrome I of right lower limb
⇄	G90.522	Complex regional pain syndrome I of left lower limb
⇄	G90.523	Complex regional pain syndrome I of lower limb, bilateral
	G96.12	Meningeal adhesions (cerebral) (spinal)
	M47.21	Other spondylosis with radiculopathy, occipito-atlanto-axial region
	M47.22	Other spondylosis with radiculopathy, cervical region
	M47.23	Other spondylosis with radiculopathy, cervicothoracic region
	M47.24	Other spondylosis with radiculopathy, thoracic region
	M47.25	Other spondylosis with radiculopathy, thoracolumbar region
	M47.26	Other spondylosis with radiculopathy, lumbar region
	M47.27	Other spondylosis with radiculopathy, lumbosacral region
	M47.28	Other spondylosis with radiculopathy, sacral and sacrococcygeal region
	M50.11	Cervical disc disorder with radiculopathy, high cervical region
	M50.121	Cervical disc disorder at C4-C5 level with radiculopathy
	M50.122	Cervical disc disorder at C5-C6 level with radiculopathy
	M50.123	Cervical disc disorder at C6-C7 level with radiculopathy
	M50.13	Cervical disc disorder with radiculopathy, cervicothoracic region
	M51.14	Intervertebral disc disorders with radiculopathy, thoracic region
	M51.15	Intervertebral disc disorders with radiculopathy, thoracolumbar region
	M51.16	Intervertebral disc disorders with radiculopathy, lumbar region
	M51.17	Intervertebral disc disorders with radiculopathy, lumbosacral region
	M54.11	Radiculopathy, occipito-atlanto-axial region
	M54.12	Radiculopathy, cervical region
	M54.13	Radiculopathy, cervicothoracic region
	M54.14	Radiculopathy, thoracic region
	M54.15	Radiculopathy, thoracolumbar region
	M54.16	Radiculopathy, lumbar region
	M54.17	Radiculopathy, lumbosacral region
	M54.18	Radiculopathy, sacral and sacrococcygeal region

	Code	Description
	M54.2	Cervicalgia
⇄	M54.31	Sciatica, right side
⇄	M54.32	Sciatica, left side
⇄	M54.41	Lumbago with sciatica, right side
⇄	M54.42	Lumbago with sciatica, left side
	M54.5	Low back pain
	M54.6	Pain in thoracic spine
	M54.89	Other dorsalgia
	M96.1	Postlaminectomy syndrome, not elsewhere classified
7	T85.113	Breakdown (mechanical) of implanted electronic neurostimulator, generator
7	T85.123	Displacement of implanted electronic neurostimulator, generator
7	T85.193	Other mechanical complication of implanted electronic neurostimulator, generator
7	T85.734	Infection and inflammatory reaction due to implanted electronic neurostimulator, generator
7	T85.810	Embolism due to nervous system prosthetic devices, implants and grafts
7	T85.820	Fibrosis due to nervous system prosthetic devices, implants and grafts
7	T85.830	Hemorrhage due to nervous system prosthetic devices, implants and grafts
7	T85.840	Pain due to nervous system prosthetic devices, implants and grafts
7	T85.850	Stenosis due to nervous system prosthetic devices, implants and grafts
7	T85.860	Thrombosis due to nervous system prosthetic devices, implants and grafts
7	T85.890	Other specified complication of nervous system prosthetic devices, implants and grafts
	Z45.42	Encounter for adjustment and management of neurostimulator

ICD-10-CM Coding Notes

For codes requiring a 7th character extension, refer to your ICD-10-CM book. Review the character descriptions and coding guidelines for proper selection. For some procedures, only certain characters will apply.

CCI Edits

Refer to Appendix A for CCI edits.

Pub 100

63685: Pub 100-03, 1, 160.19, Pub 100-03, 1, 160.26, Pub 100-03, 1, 160.7-160.7.1

63688: Pub 100-03, 1, 160.19, Pub 100-03, 1, 160.26, Pub 100-03, 1, 160.7-160.7.1

Facility RVUs

Code	Work	PE Facility	MP	Total Facility
63685	5.19	4.15	1.03	10.37
63688	5.30	4.28	1.12	10.70

Non-facility RVUs

Code	Work	PE Non-Facility	MP	Total Non-Facility
63685	5.19	4.15	1.03	10.37
63688	5.30	4.28	1.12	10.70

Modifiers (PAR)

Code	Mod 50	Mod 51	Mod 62	Mod 66	Mod 80
63685	0	2	1	0	2
63688	0	2	0	0	1

Global Period

Code	Days
63685	010
63688	010

63707-63709

63707 Repair of dural/cerebrospinal fluid leak, not requiring laminectomy

63709 Repair of dural/cerebrospinal fluid leak or pseudomeningocele, with laminectomy

AMA Coding Notes

Surgical Procedures on the Spine and Spinal Cord

(For application of caliper or tongs, use 20660)

(For treatment of fracture or dislocation of spine, see 22310-22327)

Plain English Description

A cerebrospinal fluid (CSF) leak in the spinal region may be due to trauma or a complication of a surgical procedure on the spine. The leak typically results from a tear or laceration of the spinal meninges that does not heal, resulting in cutaneous fistula formation. In some cases, fluid leaks into soft tissues without cutaneous fistula formation. A fibrous capsule forms in the soft tissue. If the dura has been lacerated but the arachnoid remains intact, it can herniate through the dural laceration forming a pseudomeningocele. In 63707, the leak is repaired without a laminectomy. Following a separately reportable imaging procedure to determine the exact location of the leak, the skin is incised over the affected spine segment. The area of the leak is located. A nonabsorbable suture is used for primary closure. Fibrin sealant may be used to reinforce the sutures and obtain a watertight seal. In 63709, a leak or pseudomeningocele is repaired with a laminectomy. The skin is incised over the cervical, thoracic, lumbar, or sacral region where the CSF leak is located and extended down to the spinous processes. Muscle is retracted off the lamina and facet joint. A bone drill is used to remove part or all of the lamina, and the spinal cord is exposed. If the leak is due to a rent, hole, or other defect in the meninges, it is repaired with suture. Alternatively, a muscle pledget may be used along with gelfoam and fibrin sealant. If a pseudomeningocele is present, the pseudomeningocele is incised. Any nerve roots present in the defect are freed and reduced into the dura. The dura is then sutured as described above.

ICD-10-CM Diagnostic Codes

G96.0	Cerebrospinal fluid leak
G96.11	Dural tear
G96.19	Other disorders of meninges, not elsewhere classified
G97.0	Cerebrospinal fluid leak from spinal puncture
G97.82	Other postprocedural complications and disorders of nervous system

CCI Edits

Refer to Appendix A for CCI edits.

Pub 100

63707: Pub 100-04, 12, 20.4.5

63709: Pub 100-04, 12, 20.4.5

Facility RVUs

Code	Work	PE Facility	MP	Total Facility
63707	12.65	10.37	3.80	26.82
63709	15.65	11.83	4.56	32.04

Non-facility RVUs

Code	Work	PE Non-Facility	MP	Total Non-Facility
63707	12.65	10.37	3.80	26.82
63709	15.65	11.83	4.56	32.04

Modifiers (PAR)

Code	Mod 50	Mod 51	Mod 62	Mod 66	Mod 80
63707	0	2	1	0	2
63709	0	2	1	0	2

Global Period

Code	Days
63707	090
63709	090

63710

63710 Dural graft, spinal

(For laminectomy and section of dentate ligaments, with or without dural graft, cervical, see 63180, 63182)

AMA Coding Notes

Surgical Procedures on the Spine and Spinal Cord

(For application of caliper or tongs, use 20660)

(For treatment of fracture or dislocation of spine, see 22310-22327)

Plain English Description

A dural graft is used to repair a defect in the dura mater of the spine. The defect is exposed and prepared for graft placement. Depending on the size of the defect, the physician may use an autologous tissue graft, bovine pericardium, dura from a cadaver, or synthetic material. The graft is configured to cover the defect and sutured into place. There are several choices for what to use as a dural graft: tissue taken from the patient's own body (autologous pericranium), bovine pericardium, dura taken from a cadaver, or a synthetic material.

Dural graft, spinal

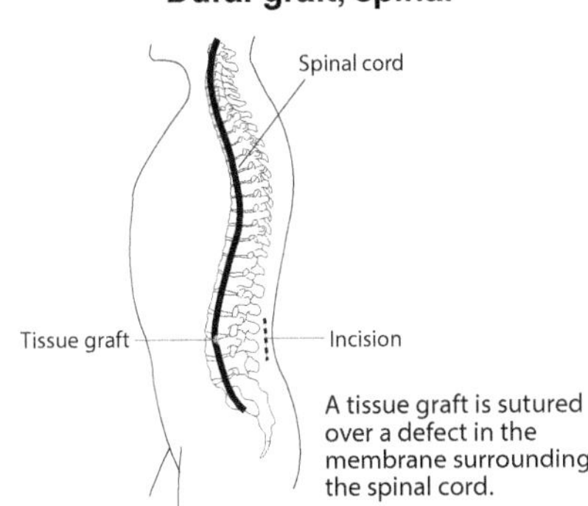

ICD-10-CM Diagnostic Codes

	Code	Description
	C70.1	Malignant neoplasm of spinal meninges
	G96.0	Cerebrospinal fluid leak
	G96.11	Dural tear
	G96.12	Meningeal adhesions (cerebral) (spinal)
	G96.19	Other disorders of meninges, not elsewhere classified
	G97.0	Cerebrospinal fluid leak from spinal puncture
	G97.41	Accidental puncture or laceration of dura during a procedure
	G97.82	Other postprocedural complications and disorders of nervous system
⑦	S14.101	Unspecified injury at C1 level of cervical spinal cord
⑦	S14.102	Unspecified injury at C2 level of cervical spinal cord
⑦	S14.103	Unspecified injury at C3 level of cervical spinal cord
⑦	S14.104	Unspecified injury at C4 level of cervical spinal cord
⑦	S14.105	Unspecified injury at C5 level of cervical spinal cord
⑦	S14.106	Unspecified injury at C6 level of cervical spinal cord
⑦	S14.107	Unspecified injury at C7 level of cervical spinal cord
⑦	S14.108	Unspecified injury at C8 level of cervical spinal cord
⑦	S24.101	Unspecified injury at T1 level of thoracic spinal cord
⑦	S24.102	Unspecified injury at T2-T6 level of thoracic spinal cord
⑦	S24.103	Unspecified injury at T7-T10 level of thoracic spinal cord
⑦	S24.104	Unspecified injury at T11-T12 level of thoracic spinal cord
⑦	S34.101	Unspecified injury to L1 level of lumbar spinal cord
⑦	S34.102	Unspecified injury to L2 level of lumbar spinal cord
⑦	S34.103	Unspecified injury to L3 level of lumbar spinal cord
⑦	S34.104	Unspecified injury to L4 level of lumbar spinal cord
⑦	S34.105	Unspecified injury to L5 level of lumbar spinal cord

ICD-10-CM Coding Notes

For codes requiring a 7th character extension, refer to your ICD-10-CM book. Review the character descriptions and coding guidelines for proper selection. For some procedures, only certain characters will apply.

CCI Edits

Refer to Appendix A for CCI edits.

Pub 100

63710: Pub 100-04, 12, 20.4.5

Facility RVUs ▢

Code	Work	PE Facility	MP	Total Facility
63710	15.40	11.67	4.33	31.40

Non-facility RVUs ▢

Code	Work	PE Non-Facility	MP	Total Non-Facility
63710	15.40	11.67	4.33	31.40

Modifiers (PAR) ▢

Code	Mod 50	Mod 51	Mod 62	Mod 66	Mod 80
63710	0	2	1	0	2

Global Period

Code	Days
63710	090

CPT® Procedural Coding

63740-63741

63740 Creation of shunt, lumbar, subarachnoid-peritoneal, -pleural, or other; including laminectomy

63741 Creation of shunt, lumbar, subarachnoid-peritoneal, -pleural, or other; percutaneous, not requiring laminectomy

AMA Coding Notes

Surgical Procedures on the Spine and Spinal Cord

(For application of caliper or tongs, use 20660)

(For treatment of fracture or dislocation of spine, see 22310-22327)

AMA *CPT Assistant*

63740: Winter 90: 8

63741: Winter 90: 8

Plain English Description

A lumbar subarachnoid shunt is used to treat communicating hydrocephalus. Cerebrospinal fluid (CSF) may be shunted to the peritoneal cavity, pleural cavity, or other location. In 63740, the spinal cord is exposed using a laminectomy, and a lumbar subarachnoid shunt is created. The skin is incised over the lumbar spine where the shunt will be created and extended down to the spinous processes. Muscle is retracted off the lamina and facet joint. A bone drill is used to remove part or all of the lamina, and the spinal cord is exposed. The meninges are opened and the catheter placed in the subarachnoid space. A tunnel is created from the laminectomy site to the peritoneum, pleura, or other site. The catheter is passed through the tunnel and into the selected terminal location. In 63741, the subarachnoid shunt is placed percutaneously. The skin over the planned puncture site is cleansed. A spinal needle with a Huber tip is inserted into through the selected intervertebral space and into the spinal canal using separately reportable imaging guidance. The meninges are punctured and a catheter is passed through the spinal needle into the subarachnoid space. A catheter passer and trocar are used to pass the terminal end of the catheter into the pleural or peritoneal space other termination site.

Creation of shunt, lumbar, subarachnoid-peritoneal, pleural, or other

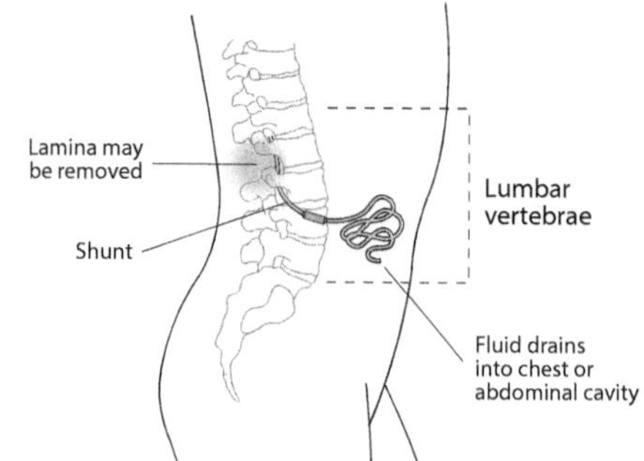

Including laminectomy (63740); percutaneous, not requiring laminectomy (63741)

ICD-10-CM Diagnostic Codes

G91.0	Communicating hydrocephalus
G91.2	(Idiopathic) normal pressure hydrocephalus
G91.3	Post-traumatic hydrocephalus, unspecified
G91.4	Hydrocephalus in diseases classified elsewhere
G91.8	Other hydrocephalus
G93.2	Benign intracranial hypertension
G95.0	Syringomyelia and syringobulbia
G96.0	Cerebrospinal fluid leak
G96.19	Other disorders of meninges, not elsewhere classified
G97.82	Other postprocedural complications and disorders of nervous system

CCI Edits

Refer to Appendix A for CCI edits.

Facility RVUs

Code	Work	PE Facility	MP	Total Facility
63740	12.63	10.89	4.64	28.16
63741	9.12	7.52	2.85	19.49

Non-facility RVUs

Code	Work	PE Non-Facility	MP	Total Non-Facility
63740	12.63	10.89	4.64	28.16
63741	9.12	7.52	2.85	19.49

Modifiers (PAR)

Code	Mod 50	Mod 51	Mod 62	Mod 66	Mod 80
63740	0	2	1	0	2
63741	0	2	1	0	2

Global Period

Code	Days
63740	090
63741	090

63744-63746

63744 Replacement, irrigation or revision of lumbosubarachnoid shunt

63746 Removal of entire lumbosubarachnoid shunt system without replacement

(For insertion of subarachnoid catheter with reservoir and/or pump for intermittent or continuous infusion of drug including laminectomy, see 62351 and 62360, 62361 or 62362)

(For insertion or replacement of subarachnoid or epidural catheter, with reservoir and/or pump for drug infusion without laminectomy, see 62350 and 62360, 62361 or 62362)

AMA Coding Notes

Surgical Procedures on the Spine and Spinal Cord

(For application of caliper or tongs, use 20660)

(For treatment of fracture or dislocation of spine, see 22310-22327)

Plain English Description

If a lumbar subarachnoid shunt becomes obstructed, infected, or other complications occur, the shunt may be replaced, irrigated, revised, or the entire shunt system may be removed. In 63744, the shunt is replaced, irrigated, or revised. To replace the shunt, the skin over the lumbar spine is incised. The catheter is opened and a guidewire advanced through the catheter into the subarachnoid space. The existing catheter is removed over the guidewire. A new catheter is advanced over the guidewire and into the subarachnoid space and the guidewire is removed. The guidewire is then passed through the distal portion of the catheter into the terminal end. The distal portion of the catheter is removed over the guidewire and the new catheter passed over the guidewire into the terminal site, in the peritoneal or pleural cavity, or other location. A connector is used to secure the proximal and distal catheter segments. To irrigate an obstructed shunt, the shunt is exposed and punctured with a needle. Sterile saline is then used to flush out the shunt. Once patency has been restored, the needle is removed and the skin closed over the shunt. To revise a shunt, a portion of the catheter is removed as described above. The removed segment is replaced and spliced together with the remaining segment of catheter using a connector. In 63746, the entire shunt system is completely removed. An incision is made in the skin over the lumbar spine at the level of the shunt. Overlying soft tissues are dissected and the shunt catheter is exposed. Any anchoring sutures are cut and the shunt is removed from the spinal canal. The subcutaneous tunnel is opened and the shunt is dissected free of the tunnel and the terminal end removed.

ICD-10-CM Diagnostic Codes

	G91.0	Communicating hydrocephalus
	G91.2	(Idiopathic) normal pressure hydrocephalus
	G91.3	Post-traumatic hydrocephalus, unspecified
	G91.4	Hydrocephalus in diseases classified elsewhere
	G91.8	Other hydrocephalus
	G93.2	Benign intracranial hypertension
	G95.0	Syringomyelia and syringobulbia
	G96.0	Cerebrospinal fluid leak
	G96.19	Other disorders of meninges, not elsewhere classified
	G97.82	Other postprocedural complications and disorders of nervous system
⑦	T85.615	Breakdown (mechanical) of other nervous system device, implant or graft
⑦	T85.625	Displacement of other nervous system device, implant or graft
⑦	T85.635	Leakage of other nervous system device, implant or graft
⑦	T85.695	Other mechanical complication of other nervous system device, implant or graft
⑦	T85.738	Infection and inflammatory reaction due to other nervous system device, implant or graft
	Z45.41	Encounter for adjustment and management of cerebrospinal fluid drainage device

ICD-10-CM Coding Notes

For codes requiring a 7th character extension, refer to your ICD-10-CM book. Review the character descriptions and coding guidelines for proper selection. For some procedures, only certain characters will apply.

CCI Edits

Refer to Appendix A for CCI edits.

Facility RVUs □

Code	Work	PE Facility	MP	Total Facility
63744	8.94	7.63	3.07	19.64
63746	7.33	7.35	2.72	17.40

Non-facility RVUs □

Code	Work	PE Non-Facility	MP	Total Non-Facility
63744	8.94	7.63	3.07	19.64
63746	7.33	7.35	2.72	17.40

Modifiers (PAR) □

Code	Mod 50	Mod 51	Mod 62	Mod 66	Mod 80
63744	0	2	1	0	2
63746	0	2	0	0	0

Global Period

Code	Days
63744	090
63746	090

64400-64405

▲ **64400 Injection(s), anesthetic agent(s) and/or steroid; trigeminal nerve, each branch (ie, ophthalmic, maxillary, mandibular)**

▲ **64405 Injection(s), anesthetic agent(s) and/or steroid; greater occipital nerve**

AMA Coding Guideline

Introduction/Injection of Anesthetic Agent (Nerve Block), Diagnostic or Therapeutic Procedures on the Somatic Nerves

Codes 64400-64489 describe the introduction/injection of an anesthetic agent and/or steroid into the somatic nervous system for diagnostic or therapeutic purposes. For injection or destruction of genicular nerve branches, see 64454, 64624, respectively.

Codes 64400-64450, 64454 describe the injection of an anesthetic agent(s) and/or steroid into a nerve plexus, nerve, or branch. These codes are reported once per nerve plexus, nerve, or branch as described in the descriptor regardless of the number of injections performed along the nerve plexus, nerve, or branch described by the code.

Imaging guidance and localization may be reported separately for 64400-64450. Imaging guidance and any injection of contrast are inclusive components of 64451 and 64454.

Codes 64455, 64479, 64480, 64483, 64484 are reported for single or multiple injections on the same site. For 64479, 64480, 64483, 64484, imaging guidance (fluoroscopy or CT) and any injection of contrast are inclusive components and are not reported separately. For 64455, imaging guidance (ultrasound, fluoroscopy, CT) and localization may be reported separately.

Codes 64461, 64462, 64463 describe injection of a paravertebral block (PVB). Codes 64486, 64487, 64488, 64489 describe injection of a transversus abdominis plane (TAP) block. Imaging guidance and any injection of contrast are inclusive components of 64461, 64462, 64463, 64486, 64487, 64488, 64489 and are not reported separately.

Please see the Surgical Guidelines section for the following table: The Central Venous Access Procedures Table

AMA Coding Notes

Introduction/Injection of Anesthetic Agent (Nerve Block), Diagnostic or Therapeutic Procedures on the Extracranial Nerves, Peripheral Nerves, and Autonomic Nervous System

(For destruction by neurolytic agent or chemodenervation, see 62280-62282, 64600-64681)

(For epidural or subarachnoid injection, see 62320, 62321, 62322, 62323, 62324, 62325, 62326, 62327)

(64400-64455, 64461, 64462, 64463, 64479, 64480, 64483, 64484, 64490-64495 are unilateral procedures. For bilateral procedures, report 64400, 64405, 64408, 64415, 64416, 64417, 64418, 64420, 64425-64455, 64461, 64463, 64479, 64483, 64490, 64493 with modifier 50. Report add-on codes 64421, 64462, 64480, 64484, 64491, 64492, 64494, 64495 twice, when performed bilaterally. Do not report modifier 50 in conjunction with 64421, 64462, 64480, 64484, 64491, 64492, 64494, 64495. Do not report modifier 50 in conjunction with 64421, 64462, 64480, 64484, 64491, 64492, 64494, 64495)

Surgical Procedures on the Extracranial Nerves, Peripheral Nerves, and Autonomic Nervous System

(For intracranial surgery on cranial nerves, see 61450, 61460, 61790)

AMA *CPT Assistant*

64400: Jul 98: 10, May 99: 8, Nov 99: 36, Apr 05: 13, Feb 10: 9, Jan 13: 13

64405: Jul 98: 10, Apr 05: 13, Jan 13: 13, Oct 16: 11

Plain English Description

Injection of an anesthetic agent, also referred to as a nerve block, may be performed as either a diagnostic or therapeutic measure. In 64400, any division or branch of the trigeminal nerve is injected. The most common indication for injection of the trigeminal nerve is trigeminal neuralgia, which is characterized by shock-like stabbing pain, also referred to as lancinating pain. The trigeminal nerve divisions or branches may be injected using an intraoral or transcutaneous approach depending on the division or branch being injected. A needle is introduced into the trigeminal nerve at the base of the skull or along any of the divisions or branches. An anesthetic agent such as glycol is injected. The patient is asked to assess the degree of pain relief. In 64402, the facial nerve is injected. The facial nerve, also referred to as cranial nerve VII (CN VII), is a mixed nerve with both motor and sensory components and assists with facial expression. The nerve may be injected to treat muscle spasms or to interrupt transmission of sensory stimuli. The skin is cleansed over the facial nerve and an anesthetic is injected. In 64405, the greater occipital nerve is injected. The greater occipital nerves originate between the second and third vertebrae of the spine and supply the top of the scalp and the region above the ears and over the salivary glands. Injecting the nerve near the base of the skull treats occipital neuralgia.

Injection, anesthetic agent

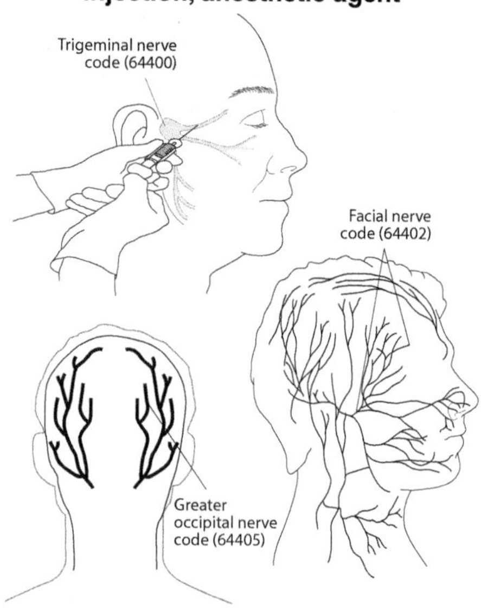

ICD-10-CM Diagnostic Codes

Code	Description
B02.22	Postherpetic trigeminal neuralgia
G43.811	Other migraine, intractable, with status migrainosus
G43.819	Other migraine, intractable, without status migrainosus
G44.001	Cluster headache syndrome, unspecified, intractable
G44.009	Cluster headache syndrome, unspecified, not intractable
G44.011	Episodic cluster headache, intractable
G44.019	Episodic cluster headache, not intractable
G44.021	Chronic cluster headache, intractable
G44.029	Chronic cluster headache, not intractable
G44.031	Episodic paroxysmal hemicrania, intractable
G44.039	Episodic paroxysmal hemicrania, not intractable
G44.041	Chronic paroxysmal hemicrania, intractable
G44.049	Chronic paroxysmal hemicrania, not intractable
G44.091	Other trigeminal autonomic cephalgias (TAC), intractable
G44.099	Other trigeminal autonomic cephalgias (TAC), not intractable
G44.89	Other headache syndrome
G50.0	Trigeminal neuralgia
G50.1	Atypical facial pain
G50.8	Other disorders of trigeminal nerve
G50.9	Disorder of trigeminal nerve, unspecified
G51.8	Other disorders of facial nerve
G51.9	Disorder of facial nerve, unspecified
G52.9	Cranial nerve disorder, unspecified
G58.8	Other specified mononeuropathies
G89.11	Acute pain due to trauma
G89.18	Other acute postprocedural pain
G89.21	Chronic pain due to trauma
G89.28	Other chronic postprocedural pain
G89.29	Other chronic pain

	Code	Description
	G89.3	Neoplasm related pain (acute) (chronic)
	G89.4	Chronic pain syndrome
	M53.0	Cervicocranial syndrome
	M54.11	Radiculopathy, occipito-atlanto-axial region
	M54.12	Radiculopathy, cervical region
	M54.81	Occipital neuralgia
	M62.838	Other muscle spasm
	M79.2	Neuralgia and neuritis, unspecified
➐⇄	S04.30	Injury of trigeminal nerve, unspecified side
➐⇄	S04.31	Injury of trigeminal nerve, right side
➐⇄	S04.32	Injury of trigeminal nerve, left side
➐⇄	S04.50	Injury of facial nerve, unspecified side
➐⇄	S04.51	Injury of facial nerve, right side
➐⇄	S04.52	Injury of facial nerve, left side
➐	S13.4	Sprain of ligaments of cervical spine
➐	S14.2	Injury of nerve root of cervical spine
➐	S14.8	Injury of other specified nerves of neck
➐	S16.1	Strain of muscle, fascia and tendon at neck level

ICD-10-CM Coding Notes

For codes requiring a 7th character extension, refer to your ICD-10-CM book. Review the character descriptions and coding guidelines for proper selection. For some procedures, only certain characters will apply.

CCI Edits

Refer to Appendix A for CCI edits.

Facility RVUs ▯

Code	Work	PE Facility	MP	Total Facility
64400	0.75	0.51	0.18	1.44
64405	0.94	0.40	0.21	1.55

Non-facility RVUs ▯

Code	Work	PE Non-Facility	MP	Total Non-Facility
64400	0.75	2.12	0.18	3.05
64405	0.94	0.92	0.21	2.07

Modifiers (PAR) ▯

Code	Mod 50	Mod 51	Mod 62	Mod 66	Mod 80
64400	1	2	0	0	1
64405	1	2	0	0	1

Global Period

Code	Days
64400	000
64405	000

64415-64416

▲ **64415 Injection(s), anesthetic agent(s) and/or steroid; brachial plexus**

▲ **64416 Injection(s), anesthetic agent(s) and/or steroid; brachial plexus, continuous infusion by catheter (including catheter placement)**

(Do not report 64416 in conjunction with 01996)

AMA Coding Guideline

Introduction/Injection of Anesthetic Agent (Nerve Block), Diagnostic or Therapeutic Procedures on the Somatic Nerves

Codes 64400-64489 describe the introduction/injection of an anesthetic agent and/or steroid into the somatic nervous system for diagnostic or therapeutic purposes. For injection or destruction of genicular nerve branches, see 64454, 64624, respectively.

Codes 64400-64450, 64454 describe the injection of an anesthetic agent(s) and/or steroid into a nerve plexus, nerve, or branch. These codes are reported once per nerve plexus, nerve, or branch as described in the descriptor regardless of the number of injections performed along the nerve plexus, nerve, or branch described by the code.

Imaging guidance and localization may be reported separately for 64400-64450. Imaging guidance and any injection of contrast are inclusive components of 64451 and 64454.

Codes 64455, 64479, 64480, 64483, 64484 are reported for single or multiple injections on the same site. For 64479, 64480, 64483, 64484, imaging guidance (fluoroscopy or CT) and any injection of contrast are inclusive components and are not reported separately. For 64455, imaging guidance (ultrasound, fluoroscopy, CT) and localization may be reported separately.

Codes 64461, 64462, 64463 describe injection of a paravertebral block (PVB). Codes 64486, 64487, 64488, 64489 describe injection of a transversus abdominis plane (TAP) block. Imaging guidance and any injection of contrast are inclusive components of 64461, 64462, 64463, 64486, 64487, 64488, 64489 and are not reported separately.

Please see the Surgical Guidelines section for the following table: The Central Venous Access Procedures Table

AMA Coding Notes

Introduction/Injection of Anesthetic Agent (Nerve Block), Diagnostic or Therapeutic Procedures on the Extracranial Nerves, Peripheral Nerves, and Autonomic Nervous System

(For destruction by neurolytic agent or chemodenervation, see 62280-62282, 64600-64681)

(For epidural or subarachnoid injection, see 62320, 62321, 62322, 62323, 62324, 62325, 62326, 62327)

(64400-64455, 64461, 64462, 64463, 64479, 64480, 64483, 64484, 64490-64495 are unilateral procedures. For bilateral procedures, report 64400, 64405, 64408, 64415, 64416, 64417, 64418, 64420, 64425-64455, 64461, 64463, 64479, 64483, 64490, 64493 with modifier 50. Report add-on codes 64421, 64462, 64480, 64484, 64491, 64492, 64494, 64495 twice, when performed bilaterally. Do not report modifier 50 in conjunction with 64421, 64462, 64480, 64484, 64491, 64492, 64494, 64495. Do not report modifier 50 in conjunction with 64421, 64462, 64480, 64484, 64491, 64492, 64494, 64495)

Surgical Procedures on the Extracranial Nerves, Peripheral Nerves, and Autonomic Nervous System

(For intracranial surgery on cranial nerves, see 61450, 61460, 61790)

AMA *CPT Assistant* ▯

64415: Fall 92: 17, Jul 98: 10, May 99: 8, Oct 01: 9, Feb 04: 7, Apr 05: 13, Nov 06: 23, Jan 13: 13

64416: Feb 04: 7, Apr 05: 13, Jan 13: 13

Plain English Description

The physician makes a single injection of a drug to numb the nerves in the arm. For code 64416, an anesthetic is injected into the brachial plexus by continuous infusion. The arm is abducted with the elbow flexed and the hand above the shoulder. The skin is cleansed and anesthetized before a needle is placed in the infraclavicular or supraclavicular region and advanced into position in the brachial plexus sheath. Proper placement of the needle is verified with electrical nerve stimulation and/or with the onset of numbness, tingling, or prickling sensations, or through separately reportable ultrasound imaging. The cannula for the nerve block is then threaded over the needle through the brachial plexus sheath. The needle is removed when the cannula is in position. Next, the epidural-type catheter for administering the anesthetic is threaded through the cannula into position in the brachial plexus sheath. The nerve block into the brachial plexus is then injected using a local anesthetic medication like lidocaine or bupivacaine. The function of the nerve block is determined, and the continuous infusion is started.

Injection, anesthetic and/or steroid; brachial plexus

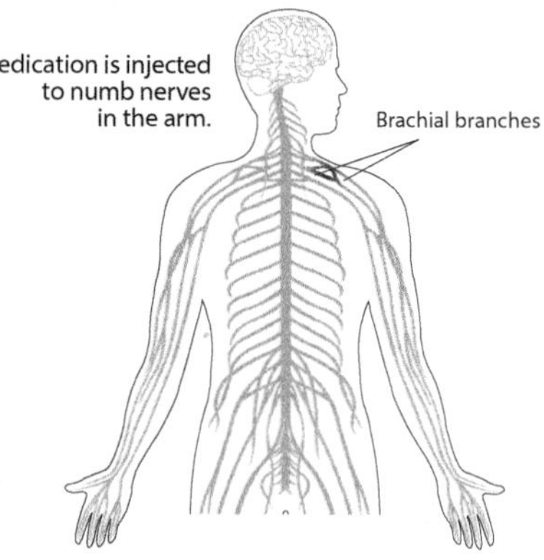

Use 64416 for continuous catheter infusion.

ICD-10-CM Diagnostic Codes

	Code	Description
	B02.29	Other postherpetic nervous system involvement
⇄	C40.01	Malignant neoplasm of scapula and long bones of right upper limb
⇄	C40.02	Malignant neoplasm of scapula and long bones of left upper limb
⇄	C47.11	Malignant neoplasm of peripheral nerves of right upper limb, including shoulder
⇄	C47.12	Malignant neoplasm of peripheral nerves of left upper limb, including shoulder
⇄	C49.11	Malignant neoplasm of connective and soft tissue of right upper limb, including shoulder
⇄	C49.12	Malignant neoplasm of connective and soft tissue of left upper limb, including shoulder
	C79.89	Secondary malignant neoplasm of other specified sites
	G54.0	Brachial plexus disorders
	G54.5	Neuralgic amyotrophy
	G54.6	Phantom limb syndrome with pain
⇄	G56.41	Causalgia of right upper limb
⇄	G56.42	Causalgia of left upper limb
	G89.11	Acute pain due to trauma
	G89.18	Other acute postprocedural pain
	G89.21	Chronic pain due to trauma
	G89.28	Other chronic postprocedural pain
	G89.29	Other chronic pain
	G89.3	Neoplasm related pain (acute) (chronic)
	G89.4	Chronic pain syndrome
⇄	G90.511	Complex regional pain syndrome I of right upper limb
⇄	G90.512	Complex regional pain syndrome I of left upper limb
⇄	G90.513	Complex regional pain syndrome I of upper limb, bilateral
⇄	M25.511	Pain in right shoulder
⇄	M25.512	Pain in left shoulder
	M54.13	Radiculopathy, cervicothoracic region
⇄	M79.601	Pain in right arm
⇄	M79.602	Pain in left arm
❼	S14.3	Injury of brachial plexus

ICD-10-CM Coding Notes

For codes requiring a 7th character extension, refer to your ICD-10-CM book. Review the character descriptions and coding guidelines for proper selection. For some procedures, only certain characters will apply.

CCI Edits

Refer to Appendix A for CCI edits.

Facility RVUs

Code	Work	PE Facility	MP	Total Facility
64415	1.35	0.37	0.11	1.83
64416	1.48	0.26	0.11	1.85

Non-facility RVUs

Code	Work	PE Non-Facility	MP	Total Non-Facility
64415	1.35	1.76	0.11	3.22
64416	1.48	0.26	0.11	1.85

Modifiers (PAR)

Code	Mod 50	Mod 51	Mod 62	Mod 66	Mod 80
64415	1	2	0	0	1
64416	1	2	0	0	1

Global Period

Code	Days
64415	000
64416	000

64417-64418

▲ **64417 Injection(s), anesthetic agent(s) and/or steroid; axillary nerve**

▲ **64418 Injection(s), anesthetic agent(s) and/or steroid; suprascapular nerve**

AMA Coding Guideline

Introduction/Injection of Anesthetic Agent (Nerve Block), Diagnostic or Therapeutic Procedures on the Somatic Nerves

Codes 64400-64489 describe the introduction/injection of an anesthetic agent and/or steroid into the somatic nervous system for diagnostic or therapeutic purposes. For injection or destruction of genicular nerve branches, see 64454, 64624, respectively.

Codes 64400-64450, 64454 describe the injection of an anesthetic agent(s) and/or steroid into a nerve plexus, nerve, or branch. These codes are reported once per nerve plexus, nerve, or branch as described in the descriptor regardless of the number of injections performed along the nerve plexus, nerve, or branch described by the code.

Imaging guidance and localization may be reported separately for 64400-64450. Imaging guidance and any injection of contrast are inclusive components of 64451 and 64454.

Codes 64455, 64479, 64480, 64483, 64484 are reported for single or multiple injections on the same site. For 64479, 64480, 64483, 64484, imaging guidance (fluoroscopy or CT) and any injection of contrast are inclusive components and are not reported separately. For 64455, imaging guidance (ultrasound, fluoroscopy, CT) and localization may be reported separately.

Codes 64461, 64462, 64463 describe injection of a paravertebral block (PVB). Codes 64486, 64487, 64488, 64489 describe injection of a transversus abdominis plane (TAP) block. Imaging guidance and any injection of contrast are inclusive components of 64461, 64462, 64463, 64486, 64487, 64488, 64489 and are not reported separately.

Please see the Surgical Guidelines section for the following table: The Central Venous Access Procedures Table

AMA Coding Notes

Introduction/Injection of Anesthetic Agent (Nerve Block), Diagnostic or Therapeutic Procedures on the Extracranial Nerves, Peripheral Nerves, and Autonomic Nervous System

(For destruction by neurolytic agent or chemodenervation, see 62280-62282, 64600-64681)

(For epidural or subarachnoid injection, see 62320, 62321, 62322, 62323, 62324, 62325, 62326, 62327)

(64400-64455, 64461, 64462, 64463, 64479, 64480, 64483, 64484, 64490-64495 are unilateral procedures. For bilateral procedures, report 64400, 64405, 64408, 64415, 64416, 64417, 64418, 64420, 64425-64455, 64461, 64463, 64479, 64483, 64490, 64493 with modifier 50. Report add-on codes 64421, 64462, 64480, 64484, 64491, 64492, 64494, 64495 twice, when performed bilaterally. Do not report modifier 50 in conjunction with 64421, 64462, 64480, 64484, 64491, 64492, 64494, 64495. Do not report modifier 50 in conjunction with 64421, 64462, 64480, 64484, 64491, 64492, 64494, 64495)

Surgical Procedures on the Extracranial Nerves, Peripheral Nerves, and Autonomic Nervous System

(For intracranial surgery on cranial nerves, see 61450, 61460, 61790)

AMA *CPT Assistant* □

64417: Jul 98: 10, Apr 05: 13, Jan 13: 13

64418: Jul 98: 10, Apr 05: 13, Aug 07: 15, Jan 13: 13

Plain English Description

Injection of an anesthetic agent, also referred to as a nerve block, may be performed as either a diagnostic or therapeutic measure. In 64417, an axillary nerve block is performed. The axillary nerve originates from the brachial plexus at the level of the axilla. It divides into anterior and posterior trunks. The anterior trunk branches and supplies the middle and anterior surface of the deltoid. The posterior trunk branches supply the teres minor and posterior deltoid muscle. In 64418, a subscapular nerve block is performed. The subscapular nerve arises from the brachial plexus and divides into upper and lower branches. The upper branch supplies the upper part of the subscapularis muscle and the lower part branches and one branch supplies the lower part of the subscapularis and another the teres major. The skin over the planned injection site is cleansed. A needle is inserted into the axillary or subscapular nerve, aspirated to ensure that it is not in a blood vessel, and an anesthetic is injected.

Injection, anesthetic and/or steroid

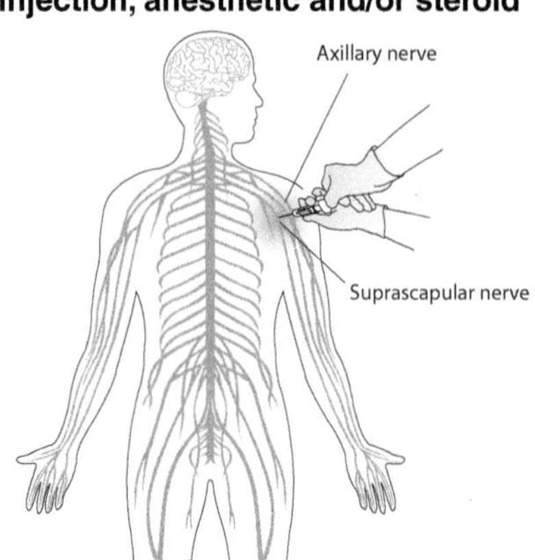

Axillary nerve (64417); suprascapular nerve (64418)

ICD-10-CM Diagnostic Codes

	Code	Description
	B02.29	Other postherpetic nervous system involvement
⇄	C40.01	Malignant neoplasm of scapula and long bones of right upper limb
⇄	C40.02	Malignant neoplasm of scapula and long bones of left upper limb
⇄	C47.11	Malignant neoplasm of peripheral nerves of right upper limb, including shoulder
⇄	C47.12	Malignant neoplasm of peripheral nerves of left upper limb, including shoulder
⇄	C49.11	Malignant neoplasm of connective and soft tissue of right upper limb, including shoulder
⇄	C49.12	Malignant neoplasm of connective and soft tissue of left upper limb, including shoulder
	C79.89	Secondary malignant neoplasm of other specified sites
	G54.6	Phantom limb syndrome with pain
⇄	G56.41	Causalgia of right upper limb
⇄	G56.42	Causalgia of left upper limb
⇄	G56.43	Causalgia of bilateral upper limbs
⇄	G56.81	Other specified mononeuropathies of right upper limb
⇄	G56.82	Other specified mononeuropathies of left upper limb
⇄	G56.83	Other specified mononeuropathies of bilateral upper limbs
	G89.11	Acute pain due to trauma
	G89.18	Other acute postprocedural pain
	G89.21	Chronic pain due to trauma
	G89.28	Other chronic postprocedural pain
	G89.29	Other chronic pain
	G89.3	Neoplasm related pain (acute) (chronic)
	G89.4	Chronic pain syndrome
⇄	G90.511	Complex regional pain syndrome I of right upper limb
⇄	G90.512	Complex regional pain syndrome I of left upper limb
⇄	G90.513	Complex regional pain syndrome I of upper limb, bilateral
⇄	M25.51	Pain in shoulder
⇄	M25.52	Pain in elbow
⇄	M75.01	Adhesive capsulitis of right shoulder
⇄	M75.02	Adhesive capsulitis of left shoulder
⇄	M75.11	Incomplete rotator cuff tear or rupture not specified as traumatic
⇄	M75.111	Incomplete rotator cuff tear or rupture of right shoulder, not specified as traumatic
⇄	M75.112	Incomplete rotator cuff tear or rupture of left shoulder, not specified as traumatic
⇄	M75.12	Complete rotator cuff tear or rupture not specified as traumatic
⇄	M75.121	Complete rotator cuff tear or rupture of right shoulder, not specified as traumatic
⇄	M75.122	Complete rotator cuff tear or rupture of left shoulder, not specified as traumatic
⇄	M75.31	Calcific tendinitis of right shoulder
⇄	M75.32	Calcific tendinitis of left shoulder

⇄	M75.41	Impingement syndrome of right shoulder
⇄	M75.42	Impingement syndrome of left shoulder
⇄	M75.81	Other shoulder lesions, right shoulder
⇄	M75.82	Other shoulder lesions, left shoulder
⇄	M79.621	Pain in right upper arm
⇄	M79.622	Pain in left upper arm
7⇄	S43.011	Anterior subluxation of right humerus
7⇄	S43.012	Anterior subluxation of left humerus
7⇄	S43.014	Anterior dislocation of right humerus
7⇄	S43.015	Anterior dislocation of left humerus
7⇄	S43.021	Posterior subluxation of right humerus
7⇄	S43.022	Posterior subluxation of left humerus
7⇄	S43.024	Posterior dislocation of right humerus
7⇄	S43.025	Posterior dislocation of left humerus
7⇄	S43.031	Inferior subluxation of right humerus
7⇄	S43.032	Inferior subluxation of left humerus
7⇄	S43.034	Inferior dislocation of right humerus
7⇄	S43.035	Inferior dislocation of left humerus
7⇄	S43.081	Other subluxation of right shoulder joint
7⇄	S43.082	Other subluxation of left shoulder joint
7⇄	S43.084	Other dislocation of right shoulder joint
7⇄	S43.085	Other dislocation of left shoulder joint
7⇄	S44.31	Injury of axillary nerve, right arm
7⇄	S44.32	Injury of axillary nerve, left arm
7⇄	S46.011	Strain of muscle(s) and tendon(s) of the rotator cuff of right shoulder
7⇄	S46.012	Strain of muscle(s) and tendon(s) of the rotator cuff of left shoulder

ICD-10-CM Coding Notes

For codes requiring a 7th character extension, refer to your ICD-10-CM book. Review the character descriptions and coding guidelines for proper selection. For some procedures, only certain characters will apply.

CCI Edits

Refer to Appendix A for CCI edits.

Facility RVUs

Code	Work	PE Facility	MP	Total Facility
64417	1.27	0.37	0.11	1.75
64418	1.10	0.42	0.12	1.64

Non-facility RVUs

Code	Work	PE Non-Facility	MP	Total Non-Facility
64417	1.27	2.51	0.11	3.89
64418	1.10	1.20	0.12	2.42

Modifiers (PAR)

Code	Mod 50	Mod 51	Mod 62	Mod 66	Mod 80
64417	1	2	0	0	1
64418	1	2	0	0	1

Global Period

Code	Days
64417	000
64418	000

64420-64421

▲ **64420 Injection(s), anesthetic agent(s) and/or steroid; intercostal nerve, single level**

+▲ **64421 Injection(s), anesthetic agent(s) and/or steroid; intercostal nerve, each additional level (List separately in addition to code for primary procedure)**

(Use 64421 in conjunction with 64420)

AMA Coding Guideline

Introduction/Injection of Anesthetic Agent (Nerve Block), Diagnostic or Therapeutic Procedures on the Somatic Nerves

Codes 64400-64489 describe the introduction/injection of an anesthetic agent and/or steroid into the somatic nervous system for diagnostic or therapeutic purposes. For injection or destruction of genicular nerve branches, see 64454, 64624, respectively.

Codes 64400-64450, 64454 describe the injection of an anesthetic agent(s) and/or steroid into a nerve plexus, nerve, or branch. These codes are reported once per nerve plexus, nerve, or branch as described in the descriptor regardless of the number of injections performed along the nerve plexus, nerve, or branch described by the code.

Imaging guidance and localization may be reported separately for 64400-64450. Imaging guidance and any injection of contrast are inclusive components of 64451 and 64454.

Codes 64455, 64479, 64480, 64483, 64484 are reported for single or multiple injections on the same site. For 64479, 64480, 64483, 64484, imaging guidance (fluoroscopy or CT) and any injection of contrast are inclusive components and are not reported separately. For 64455, imaging guidance (ultrasound, fluoroscopy, CT) and localization may be reported separately.

Codes 64461, 64462, 64463 describe injection of a paravertebral block (PVB). Codes 64486, 64487, 64488, 64489 describe injection of a transversus abdominis plane (TAP) block. Imaging guidance and any injection of contrast are inclusive components of 64461, 64462, 64463, 64486, 64487, 64488, 64489 and are not reported separately.

Please see the Surgical Guidelines section for the following table: The Central Venous Access Procedures Table

AMA Coding Notes

Introduction/Injection of Anesthetic Agent (Nerve Block), Diagnostic or Therapeutic Procedures on the Extracranial Nerves, Peripheral Nerves, and Autonomic Nervous System

(For destruction by neurolytic agent or chemodenervation, see 62280-62282, 64600-64681)

(For epidural or subarachnoid injection, see 62320, 62321, 62322, 62323, 62324, 62325, 62326, 62327)

(64400-64455, 64461, 64462, 64463, 64479, 64480, 64483, 64484, 64490-64495 are unilateral procedures. For bilateral procedures, report 64400, 64405, 64408, 64415, 64416, 64417, 64418, 64420, 64425-64455, 64461, 64463, 64479, 64483, 64490, 64493 with modifier 50. Report add-on codes 64421, 64462, 64480, 64484, 64491, 64492, 64494, 64495 twice, when performed bilaterally. Do not report modifier 50 in conjunction with 64421, 64462, 64480, 64484, 64491, 64492, 64494, 64495. Do not report modifier 50 in conjunction with 64421, 64462, 64480, 64484, 64491, 64492, 64494, 64495)

Surgical Procedures on the Extracranial Nerves, Peripheral Nerves, and Autonomic Nervous System

(For intracranial surgery on cranial nerves, see 61450, 61460, 61790)

AMA *CPT Assistant* □

64420: Jul 98: 10, Apr 05: 13, Aug 10: 12, Nov 10: 9, Jan 13: 13, Jun 15: 3

64421: Jul 98: 10, Apr 05: 13, Aug 10: 12, Nov 10: 9, Jan 13: 13, Jun 15: 3, May 18: 10

Plain English Description

The intercostal nerves are mixed nerves that supply the skin and muscles of the upper extremities, thorax, and abdominal wall. The intercostal nerves exit the posterior aspect of the intercostal membrane just distal to the intervertebral foramen and then enter the intercostal groove running parallel to the rib. Branches of the intercostal nerves may be found between the ribs. Intercostal nerves are most often blocked along the posterior axillary line or just lateral to the paraspinal muscles at the angle of the rib. The planned injection site(s) is identified and marked along the inferior border of the rib(s). The needle is introduced underneath the inferior border of the rib and advanced until it reaches the subcostal groove. The anesthetic agent is then injected. Use 64420 for injection of a single intercostal nerve. Use 64421 if multiple intercostal nerves are injected.

Injection, anesthetic and/or steroid; intercostal nerve

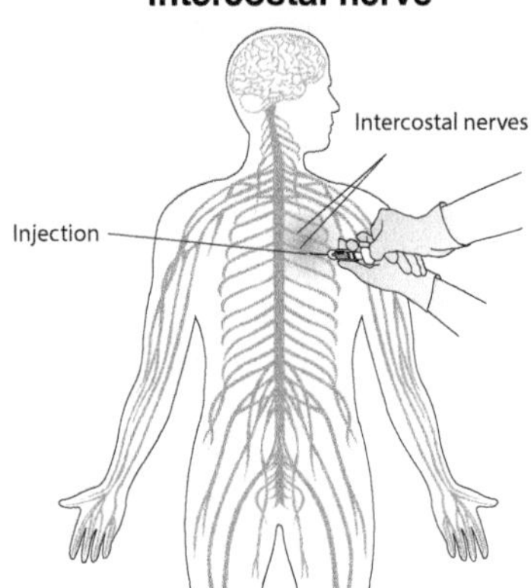

Single (64420); each additional (64421)

ICD-10-CM Diagnostic Codes

	Code	Description
	B02.29	Other postherpetic nervous system involvement
	C41.3	Malignant neoplasm of ribs, sternum and clavicle
	C47.3	Malignant neoplasm of peripheral nerves of thorax
	C76.1	Malignant neoplasm of thorax
	C79.51	Secondary malignant neoplasm of bone
	C79.89	Secondary malignant neoplasm of other specified sites
	G58.0	Intercostal neuropathy
	G89.11	Acute pain due to trauma
	G89.12	Acute post-thoracotomy pain
	G89.18	Other acute postprocedural pain
	G89.21	Chronic pain due to trauma
	G89.22	Chronic post-thoracotomy pain
	G89.28	Other chronic postprocedural pain
	G89.29	Other chronic pain
	G89.3	Neoplasm related pain (acute) (chronic)
	G89.4	Chronic pain syndrome
	M54.14	Radiculopathy, thoracic region
	M54.6	Pain in thoracic spine
	M54.9	Dorsalgia, unspecified
	M79.2	Neuralgia and neuritis, unspecified
	R07.82	Intercostal pain
	R10.10	Upper abdominal pain, unspecified
⇄	R10.11	Right upper quadrant pain
⇄	R10.12	Left upper quadrant pain
➐	S22.21	Fracture of manubrium
➐	S22.22	Fracture of body of sternum
➐	S22.23	Sternal manubrial dissociation
➐	S22.24	Fracture of xiphoid process
➐⇄	S22.31	Fracture of one rib, right side
➐⇄	S22.32	Fracture of one rib, left side
➐⇄	S22.41	Multiple fractures of ribs, right side
➐⇄	S22.42	Multiple fractures of ribs, left side
➐⇄	S22.43	Multiple fractures of ribs, bilateral
➐	S22.5	Flail chest
➐	S23.41	Sprain of ribs
➐	S23.421	Sprain of chondrosternal joint
➐	S23.428	Other sprain of sternum
➐	S23.8	Sprain of other specified parts of thorax
➐	S29.011	Strain of muscle and tendon of front wall of thorax
➐	S29.012	Strain of muscle and tendon of back wall of thorax

ICD-10-CM Coding Notes

For codes requiring a 7th character extension, refer to your ICD-10-CM book. Review the character descriptions and coding guidelines for proper selection. For some procedures, only certain characters will apply.

CCI Edits

Refer to Appendix A for CCI edits.

Facility RVUs

Code	Work	PE Facility	MP	Total Facility
64420	1.08	0.53	0.11	1.72
64421	0.50	0.18	0.05	0.73

Non-facility RVUs

Code	Work	PE Non-Facility	MP	Total Non-Facility
64420	1.08	1.66	0.11	2.85
64421	0.50	0.42	0.05	0.97

Modifiers (PAR)

Code	Mod 50	Mod 51	Mod 62	Mod 66	Mod 80
64420	1	2	0	0	1
64421	1	0	0	0	1

Global Period

Code	Days
64420	000
64421	ZZZ

64425

▲ **64425 Injection(s), anesthetic agent(s) and/or steroid; ilioinguinal, iliohypogastric nerves**

AMA Coding Guideline

Introduction/Injection of Anesthetic Agent (Nerve Block), Diagnostic or Therapeutic Procedures on the Somatic Nerves

Codes 64400-64489 describe the introduction/injection of an anesthetic agent and/or steroid into the somatic nervous system for diagnostic or therapeutic purposes. For injection or destruction of genicular nerve branches, see 64454, 64624, respectively.

Codes 64400-64450, 64454 describe the injection of an anesthetic agent(s) and/or steroid into a nerve plexus, nerve, or branch. These codes are reported once per nerve plexus, nerve, or branch as described in the descriptor regardless of the number of injections performed along the nerve plexus, nerve, or branch described by the code.

Imaging guidance and localization may be reported separately for 64400-64450. Imaging guidance and any injection of contrast are inclusive components of 64451 and 64454.

Codes 64455, 64479, 64480, 64483, 64484 are reported for single or multiple injections on the same site. For 64479, 64480, 64483, 64484, imaging guidance (fluoroscopy or CT) and any injection of contrast are inclusive components and are not reported separately. For 64455, imaging guidance (ultrasound, fluoroscopy, CT) and localization may be reported separately.

Codes 64461, 64462, 64463 describe injection of a paravertebral block (PVB). Codes 64486, 64487, 64488, 64489 describe injection of a transversus abdominis plane (TAP) block. Imaging guidance and any injection of contrast are inclusive components of 64461, 64462, 64463, 64486, 64487, 64488, 64489 and are not reported separately.

Please see the Surgical Guidelines section for the following table: The Central Venous Access Procedures Table

AMA Coding Notes

Introduction/Injection of Anesthetic Agent (Nerve Block), Diagnostic or Therapeutic Procedures on the Extracranial Nerves, Peripheral Nerves, and Autonomic Nervous System

(For destruction by neurolytic agent or chemodenervation, see 62280-62282, 64600-64681)

(For epidural or subarachnoid injection, see 62320, 62321, 62322, 62323, 62324, 62325, 62326, 62327)

(64400-64455, 64461, 64462, 64463, 64479, 64480, 64483, 64484, 64490-64495 are unilateral procedures. For bilateral procedures, report 64400, 64405, 64408, 64415, 64416, 64417, 64418, 64420, 64425-64455, 64461, 64463, 64479, 64483, 64490, 64493 with modifier 50. Report add-on codes 64421, 64462, 64480, 64484, 64491, 64492, 64494, 64495 twice, when performed bilaterally. Do not report modifier 50 in conjunction with 64421, 64462, 64480, 64484, 64491, 64492, 64494, 64495. Do not report modifier 50 in conjunction with 64421, 64462, 64480, 64484, 64491, 64492, 64494, 64495)

Surgical Procedures on the Extracranial Nerves, Peripheral Nerves, and Autonomic Nervous System

(For intracranial surgery on cranial nerves, see 61450, 61460, 61790)

AMA *CPT Assistant* □

64425: Jul 98: 10, Apr 05: 13, Jan 13: 13, Jun 15: 3

Plain English Description

The ilioinguinal and iliohypogastric nerves arise from L1. Both nerves emerge from the upper part of the lateral border of the psoas major muscle and then penetrate the transversus abdominus muscle just above and medial to the anterior superior iliac spine. The nerves run between the transversus abdominus and the internal oblique muscles for a short distance then penetrate the internal oblique. They run between the internal and external oblique muscles before branching and penetrating the external oblique muscle where branches provide skin sensation. The anterior superior iliac spine is located and the planned injection site medial and superior to it is marked. A needle is positioned perpendicular to the skin and the skin is punctured. The needle is advanced through the external oblique muscle and into the space between the internal and external oblique. The needle is aspirated to ensure that the needle is not in a blood vessel and the anesthetic agent is injected between the oblique muscles. The needle is then advanced through the internal oblique muscle into the space between the internal oblique and transversus abdominus. The space is aspirated and injected as described above. The needle is withdrawn and inserted at a 45-degree angle laterally and the procedure repeated.

Injection, anesthetic and/or steroid

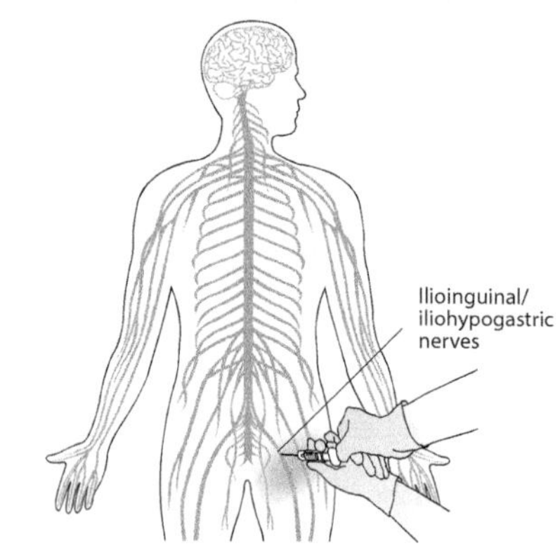

ICD-10-CM Diagnostic Codes

	Code	Description
	C76.3	Malignant neoplasm of pelvis
	C79.89	Secondary malignant neoplasm of other specified sites
⇄	G57.81	Other specified mononeuropathies of right lower limb
⇄	G57.82	Other specified mononeuropathies of left lower limb
	G89.11	Acute pain due to trauma
	G89.18	Other acute postprocedural pain
	G89.21	Chronic pain due to trauma
	G89.28	Other chronic postprocedural pain
	G89.29	Other chronic pain
	G89.3	Neoplasm related pain (acute) (chronic)
	G89.4	Chronic pain syndrome
⇄	M79.651	Pain in right thigh
⇄	M79.652	Pain in left thigh
	R10.2	Pelvic and perineal pain
	R10.30	Lower abdominal pain, unspecified
⇄	R10.31	Right lower quadrant pain
⇄	R10.32	Left lower quadrant pain
➐	S34.6	Injury of peripheral nerve(s) at abdomen, lower back and pelvis level
➐	S34.8	Injury of other nerves at abdomen, lower back and pelvis level
➐	S38.01	Crushing injury of penis
➐	S38.02	Crushing injury of scrotum and testis
➐	S38.03	Crushing injury of vulva
➐	S39.013	Strain of muscle, fascia and tendon of pelvis
➐	S39.093	Other injury of muscle, fascia and tendon of pelvis
➐	S39.83	Other specified injuries of pelvis
➐	S39.840	Fracture of corpus cavernosum penis
➐	S39.848	Other specified injuries of external genitals
➐⇄	S74.8X1	Injury of other nerves at hip and thigh level, right leg
➐⇄	S74.8X2	Injury of other nerves at hip and thigh level, left leg

ICD-10-CM Coding Notes

For codes requiring a 7th character extension, refer to your ICD-10-CM book. Review the character descriptions and coding guidelines for proper selection. For some procedures, only certain characters will apply.

● New ▲ Revised ✚ Add On ⊘Modifier 51 Exempt ★Telemedicine □ CPT QuickRef ✗FDA Pending ⇄ Laterality ➐ Seventh Character ♂Male ♀Female

CCI Edits

Refer to Appendix A for CCI edits.

Facility RVUs

Code	Work	PE Facility	MP	Total Facility
64425	1.00	0.49	0.11	1.60

Non-facility RVUs

Code	Work	PE Non-Facility	MP	Total Non-Facility
64425	1.00	2.08	0.11	3.19

Modifiers (PAR)

Code	Mod 50	Mod 51	Mod 62	Mod 66	Mod 80
64425	1	2	0	0	1

Global Period

Code	Days
64425	000

64445-64446

▲ **64445 Injection(s), anesthetic agent(s) and/or steroid; sciatic nerve**

▲ **64446 Injection(s), anesthetic agent(s) and/or steroid; sciatic nerve, continuous infusion by catheter (including catheter placement)**

(Do not report 64446 in conjunction with 01996)

AMA Coding Guideline

Introduction/Injection of Anesthetic Agent (Nerve Block), Diagnostic or Therapeutic Procedures on the Somatic Nerves

Codes 64400-64489 describe the introduction/injection of an anesthetic agent and/or steroid into the somatic nervous system for diagnostic or therapeutic purposes. For injection or destruction of genicular nerve branches, see 64454, 64624, respectively.

Codes 64400-64450, 64454 describe the injection of an anesthetic agent(s) and/or steroid into a nerve plexus, nerve, or branch. These codes are reported once per nerve plexus, nerve, or branch as described in the descriptor regardless of the number of injections performed along the nerve plexus, nerve, or branch described by the code.

Imaging guidance and localization may be reported separately for 64400-64450. Imaging guidance and any injection of contrast are inclusive components of 64451 and 64454.

Codes 64455, 64479, 64480, 64483, 64484 are reported for single or multiple injections on the same site. For 64479, 64480, 64483, 64484, imaging guidance (fluoroscopy or CT) and any injection of contrast are inclusive components and are not reported separately. For 64455, imaging guidance (ultrasound, fluoroscopy, CT) and localization may be reported separately.

Codes 64461, 64462, 64463 describe injection of a paravertebral block (PVB). Codes 64486, 64487, 64488, 64489 describe injection of a transversus abdominis plane (TAP) block. Imaging guidance and any injection of contrast are inclusive components of 64461, 64462, 64463, 64486, 64487, 64488, 64489 and are not reported separately.

Please see the Surgical Guidelines section for the following table: The Central Venous Access Procedures Table

AMA Coding Notes

Introduction/Injection of Anesthetic Agent (Nerve Block), Diagnostic or Therapeutic Procedures on the Extracranial Nerves, Peripheral Nerves, and Autonomic Nervous System

(For destruction by neurolytic agent or chemodenervation, see 62280-62282, 64600-64681)

(For epidural or subarachnoid injection, see 62320, 62321, 62322, 62323, 62324, 62325, 62326, 62327)

(64400-64455, 64461, 64462, 64463, 64479, 64480, 64483, 64484, 64490-64495 are unilateral procedures. For bilateral procedures, report 64400, 64405, 64408, 64415, 64416, 64417, 64418, 64420, 64425-64455, 64461, 64463, 64479, 64483, 64490, 64493 with modifier 50. Report add-on codes 64421, 64462, 64480, 64484, 64491, 64492, 64494, 64495 twice, when performed bilaterally. Do not report modifier 50 in conjunction with 64421, 64462, 64480, 64484, 64491, 64492, 64494, 64495. Do not report modifier 50 in conjunction with 64421, 64462, 64480, 64484, 64491, 64492, 64494, 64495)

Surgical Procedures on the Extracranial Nerves, Peripheral Nerves, and Autonomic Nervous System

(For intracranial surgery on cranial nerves, see 61450, 61460, 61790)

AMA *CPT Assistant* ▯

64445: Jul 98: 10, May 99: 8, Feb 04: 8, Apr 05: 13, Dec 11: 8, Apr 12: 19, Jan 13: 13

64446: Feb 04: 9, Apr 05: 13, Jan 13: 13

Plain English Description

The thigh is flexed at the hip. A line is marked from the back of the knee to a point between the greater trochanter and the ischial tuberosity. The skin is cleansed. A needle is introduced just above the marked line to test the sciatic nerve using electrical nerve stimulation. After a motor response in the ankle, foot, or toes has been elicited, a sciatic nerve block is performed using a single injection of an anesthetic agent.

Injection, anesthetic and/or steroid; femoral nerve

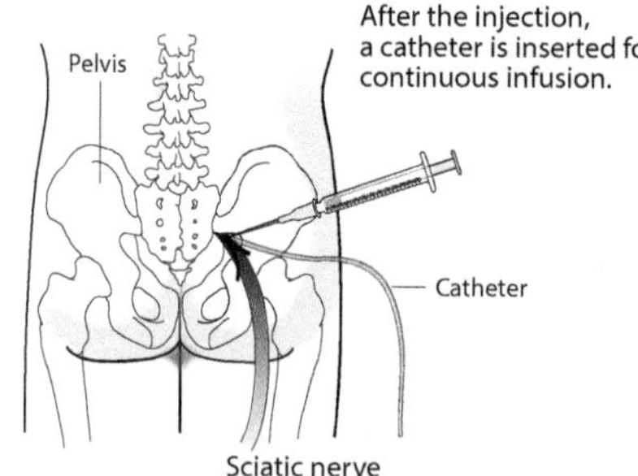

Use 64445 for injection only; use 64446 for continuous catheter infusion.

ICD-10-CM Diagnostic Codes

⇄	C47.21	Malignant neoplasm of peripheral nerves of right lower limb, including hip
⇄	C47.22	Malignant neoplasm of peripheral nerves of left lower limb, including hip
⇄	C49.21	Malignant neoplasm of connective and soft tissue of right lower limb, including hip
⇄	C49.22	Malignant neoplasm of connective and soft tissue of left lower limb, including hip
⇄	C76.51	Malignant neoplasm of right lower limb
⇄	C76.52	Malignant neoplasm of left lower limb
	C79.89	Secondary malignant neoplasm of other specified sites
⇄	G57.01	Lesion of sciatic nerve, right lower limb
⇄	G57.02	Lesion of sciatic nerve, left lower limb
	G58.8	Other specified mononeuropathies
	G89.11	Acute pain due to trauma
	G89.18	Other acute postprocedural pain
	G89.21	Chronic pain due to trauma
	G89.28	Other chronic postprocedural pain
	G89.29	Other chronic pain
	G89.3	Neoplasm related pain (acute) (chronic)
⇄	M54.31	Sciatica, right side
⇄	M54.32	Sciatica, left side
⇄	M79.661	Pain in right lower leg
⇄	M79.662	Pain in left lower leg
⇄	M79.671	Pain in right foot
⇄	M79.672	Pain in left foot
⇄	M79.674	Pain in right toe(s)
⇄	M79.675	Pain in left toe(s)
❼⇄	S74.01	Injury of sciatic nerve at hip and thigh level, right leg
❼⇄	S74.02	Injury of sciatic nerve at hip and thigh level, left leg

ICD-10-CM Coding Notes

For codes requiring a 7th character extension, refer to your ICD-10-CM book. Review the character descriptions and coding guidelines for proper selection. For some procedures, only certain characters will apply.

CCI Edits

Refer to Appendix A for CCI edits.

Facility RVUs

Code	Work	PE Facility	MP	Total Facility
64445	1.00	0.46	0.09	1.55
64446	1.36	0.24	0.11	1.71

Non-facility RVUs

Code	Work	PE Non-Facility	MP	Total Non-Facility
64445	1.00	2.48	0.09	3.57
64446	1.36	0.24	0.11	1.71

Modifiers (PAR)

Code	Mod 50	Mod 51	Mod 62	Mod 66	Mod 80
64445	1	2	0	0	1
64446	1	2	0	0	1

Global Period

Code	Days
64445	000
64446	000

64447-64448

▲ **64447 Injection(s), anesthetic agent(s) and/or steroid; femoral nerve**

(Do not report 64447 in conjunction with 01996)

▲ **64448 Injection(s), anesthetic agent(s) and/or steroid; femoral nerve, continuous infusion by catheter (including catheter placement)**

(Do not report 64448 in conjunction with 01996)

AMA Coding Guideline

Introduction/Injection of Anesthetic Agent (Nerve Block), Diagnostic or Therapeutic Procedures on the Somatic Nerves

Codes 64400-64489 describe the introduction/injection of an anesthetic agent and/or steroid into the somatic nervous system for diagnostic or therapeutic purposes. For injection or destruction of genicular nerve branches, see 64454, 64624, respectively.

Codes 64400-64450, 64454 describe the injection of an anesthetic agent(s) and/or steroid into a nerve plexus, nerve, or branch. These codes are reported once per nerve plexus, nerve, or branch as described in the descriptor regardless of the number of injections performed along the nerve plexus, nerve, or branch described by the code.

Imaging guidance and localization may be reported separately for 64400-64450. Imaging guidance and any injection of contrast are inclusive components of 64451 and 64454.

Codes 64455, 64479, 64480, 64483, 64484 are reported for single or multiple injections on the same site. For 64479, 64480, 64483, 64484, imaging guidance (fluoroscopy or CT) and any injection of contrast are inclusive components and are not reported separately. For 64455, imaging guidance (ultrasound, fluoroscopy, CT) and localization may be reported separately.

Codes 64461, 64462, 64463 describe injection of a paravertebral block (PVB). Codes 64486, 64487, 64488, 64489 describe injection of a transversus abdominis plane (TAP) block. Imaging guidance and any injection of contrast are inclusive components of 64461, 64462, 64463, 64486, 64487, 64488, 64489 and are not reported separately.

Please see the Surgical Guidelines section for the following table: The Central Venous Access Procedures Table

AMA Coding Notes

Introduction/Injection of Anesthetic Agent (Nerve Block), Diagnostic or Therapeutic Procedures on the Extracranial Nerves, Peripheral Nerves, and Autonomic Nervous System

(For destruction by neurolytic agent or chemodenervation, see 62280-62282, 64600-64681)

(For epidural or subarachnoid injection, see 62320, 62321, 62322, 62323, 62324, 62325, 62326, 62327)

(64400-64455, 64461, 64462, 64463, 64479, 64480, 64483, 64484, 64490-64495 are unilateral procedures. For bilateral procedures, report 64400, 64405, 64408, 64415, 64416, 64417, 64418, 64420, 64425-64455, 64461, 64463, 64479, 64483, 64490, 64493 with modifier 50. Report add-on codes 64421, 64462, 64480, 64484, 64491, 64492, 64494, 64495 twice, when performed bilaterally. Do not report modifier 50 in conjunction with 64421, 64462, 64480, 64484, 64491, 64492, 64494, 64495. Do not report modifier 50 in conjunction with 64421, 64462, 64480, 64484, 64491, 64492, 64494, 64495)

Surgical Procedures on the Extracranial Nerves, Peripheral Nerves, and Autonomic Nervous System

(For intracranial surgery on cranial nerves, see 61450, 61460, 61790)

AMA *CPT Assistant* ▯

64447: Feb 04: 9, Apr 05: 13, Jan 13: 13, Nov 14: 14, Dec 14: 16, Sep 15: 12

64448: Feb 04: 10, Apr 05: 13, Jan 13: 13, Nov 14: 14, Dec 14: 16, Sep 15: 12

Plain English Description

A femoral nerve block is performed using a single injection of an anesthetic agent in 64447 and by continuous infusion in 64448. The patient's groin is cleansed and prepped with a small amount of local anesthetic on the affected side. The planned injection site is marked. A needle for single use, or an insulated needle within a long cannula is placed through the anesthetized area of skin near the femoral artery and the inguinal ligament into the femoral nerve sheath. Proper placement of the needle is verified with electrical nerve stimulation and/or by the onset of numbness, tingling, or prickling sensations, or through separately reportable ultrasound imaging. Aspiration is performed to ensure there is no possibility of intravascular injection before the anesthetic is introduced in 64447. In 64448, the cannula is advanced over the needle into the femoral nerve sheath. A long-acting local anesthetic like bupivacaine with epinephrine is carefully injected through the cannula and monitored for nerve block function. Periodic aspiration is performed to ensure there is no possibility of intravascular injection. An epidural catheter is then threaded through the cannula and secured in position. The cannula is removed and continuous infusion is started.

Injection, anesthetic and/or steroid; femoral nerve

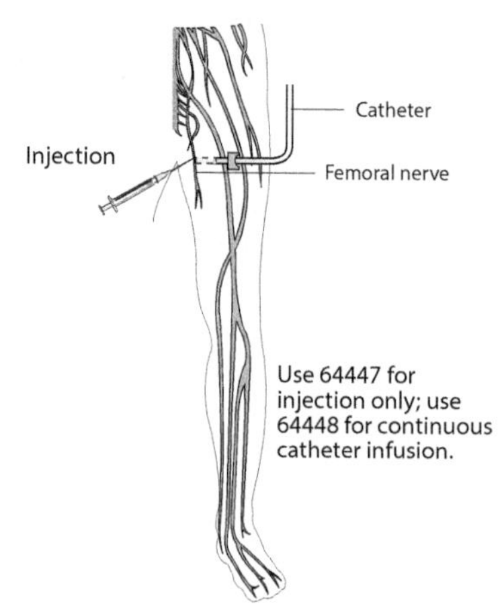

ICD-10-CM Diagnostic Codes

	Code	Description
⇄	C47.21	Malignant neoplasm of peripheral nerves of right lower limb, including hip
⇄	C47.22	Malignant neoplasm of peripheral nerves of left lower limb, including hip
⇄	C49.21	Malignant neoplasm of connective and soft tissue of right lower limb, including hip
⇄	C49.22	Malignant neoplasm of connective and soft tissue of left lower limb, including hip
⇄	C76.51	Malignant neoplasm of right lower limb
⇄	C76.52	Malignant neoplasm of left lower limb
	C79.89	Secondary malignant neoplasm of other specified sites
	E08.41	Diabetes mellitus due to underlying condition with diabetic mononeuropathy
	E09.41	Drug or chemical induced diabetes mellitus with neurological complications with diabetic mononeuropathy
	E10.41	Type 1 diabetes mellitus with diabetic mononeuropathy
	E11.41	Type 2 diabetes mellitus with diabetic mononeuropathy
	E13.41	Other specified diabetes mellitus with diabetic mononeuropathy
⇄	G57.21	Lesion of femoral nerve, right lower limb
⇄	G57.22	Lesion of femoral nerve, left lower limb
	G89.11	Acute pain due to trauma
	G89.18	Other acute postprocedural pain
	G89.21	Chronic pain due to trauma
	G89.28	Other chronic postprocedural pain
	G89.29	Other chronic pain
	G89.3	Neoplasm related pain (acute) (chronic)
⇄	M79.604	Pain in right leg
⇄	M79.605	Pain in left leg
⇄	M79.651	Pain in right thigh
⇄	M79.652	Pain in left thigh
⇄	M79.661	Pain in right lower leg

● New ▲ Revised ✚ Add On ⊘Modifier 51 Exempt ★Telemedicine ▯ CPT QuickRef ✗FDA Pending ⇄ Laterality ⓿ Seventh Character ♂Male ♀Female

⇄	M79.662	Pain in left lower leg
❼⇄	S74.11	Injury of femoral nerve at hip and thigh level, right leg
❼⇄	S74.12	Injury of femoral nerve at hip and thigh level, left leg

ICD-10-CM Coding Notes

For codes requiring a 7th character extension, refer to your ICD-10-CM book. Review the character descriptions and coding guidelines for proper selection. For some procedures, only certain characters will apply.

CCI Edits

Refer to Appendix A for CCI edits.

Facility RVUs ▯

Code	Work	PE Facility	MP	Total Facility
64447	1.10	0.34	0.09	1.53
64448	1.41	0.25	0.11	1.77

Non-facility RVUs ▯

Code	Work	PE Non-Facility	MP	Total Non-Facility
64447	1.10	1.34	0.09	2.53
64448	1.41	0.25	0.11	1.77

Modifiers **(PAR)** ▯

Code	Mod 50	Mod 51	Mod 62	Mod 66	Mod 80
64447	1	2	0	0	1
64448	1	2	0	0	1

Global Period

Code	Days
64447	000
64448	000

64449

▲ **64449 Injection(s), anesthetic agent(s) and/or steroid; lumbar plexus, posterior approach, continuous infusion by catheter (including catheter placement)**

(Do not report 64449 in conjunction with 01996)

AMA Coding Guideline

Introduction/Injection of Anesthetic Agent (Nerve Block), Diagnostic or Therapeutic Procedures on the Somatic Nerves

Codes 64400-64489 describe the introduction/injection of an anesthetic agent and/or steroid into the somatic nervous system for diagnostic or therapeutic purposes. For injection or destruction of genicular nerve branches, see 64454, 64624, respectively.

Codes 64400-64450, 64454 describe the injection of an anesthetic agent(s) and/or steroid into a nerve plexus, nerve, or branch. These codes are reported once per nerve plexus, nerve, or branch as described in the descriptor regardless of the number of injections performed along the nerve plexus, nerve, or branch described by the code.

Imaging guidance and localization may be reported separately for 64400-64450. Imaging guidance and any injection of contrast are inclusive components of 64451 and 64454.

Codes 64455, 64479, 64480, 64483, 64484 are reported for single or multiple injections on the same site. For 64479, 64480, 64483, 64484, imaging guidance (fluoroscopy or CT) and any injection of contrast are inclusive components and are not reported separately. For 64455, imaging guidance (ultrasound, fluoroscopy, CT) and localization may be reported separately.

Codes 64461, 64462, 64463 describe injection of a paravertebral block (PVB). Codes 64486, 64487, 64488, 64489 describe injection of a transversus abdominis plane (TAP) block. Imaging guidance and any injection of contrast are inclusive components of 64461, 64462, 64463, 64486, 64487, 64488, 64489 and are not reported separately.

Please see the Surgical Guidelines section for the following table: The Central Venous Access Procedures Table

AMA Coding Notes

Introduction/Injection of Anesthetic Agent (Nerve Block), Diagnostic or Therapeutic Procedures on the Extracranial Nerves, Peripheral Nerves, and Autonomic Nervous System

(For destruction by neurolytic agent or chemodenervation, see 62280-62282, 64600-64681)

(For epidural or subarachnoid injection, see 62320, 62321, 62322, 62323, 62324, 62325, 62326, 62327)

(64400-64455, 64461, 64462, 64463, 64479, 64480, 64483, 64484, 64490-64495 are unilateral procedures. For bilateral procedures, report 64400, 64405, 64408, 64415, 64416, 64417, 64418, 64420, 64425-64455, 64461, 64463, 64479, 64483, 64490, 64493 with modifier 50. Report add-on codes 64421, 64462, 64480, 64484, 64491, 64492, 64494, 64495 twice, when performed bilaterally. Do not report modifier 50 in conjunction with 64421, 64462, 64480, 64484, 64491, 64492, 64494, 64495. Do not report modifier 50 in conjunction with 64421, 64462, 64480, 64484, 64491, 64492, 64494, 64495)

Surgical Procedures on the Extracranial Nerves, Peripheral Nerves, and Autonomic Nervous System

(For intracranial surgery on cranial nerves, see 61450, 61460, 61790)

AMA *CPT Assistant* ▯

64449: Apr 05: 13, Jan 13: 13

Plain English Description

The needle insertion site is marked near the area between the iliac crests. The skin of the lower back is cleansed and prepped with a small amount of local anesthetic placed into deeper tissues. A special needle connected to a peripheral nerve stimulator is advanced into the psoas compartment. Proper positioning of the needle is verified by stimulating the lumbar plexus, which results in elevation of the patella and contraction of the quadriceps and sartorius. Aspiration is done to test for blood and cerebrospinal fluid, and a test dose of anesthesia is given to rule out intravenous or intrathecal injection. An infusion catheter is inserted through the needle after a small amount of local anesthetic is injected for the block. The function of the block is checked for analgesia of the left leg and hip. The correct catheter position is also verified for intravenous or intrathecal placement and secured in place. Continuous infusion of a dilute local anesthetic is started.

Injection, anesthetic/steroid; lumbar plexus, posterior approach, continuous infusion by catheter

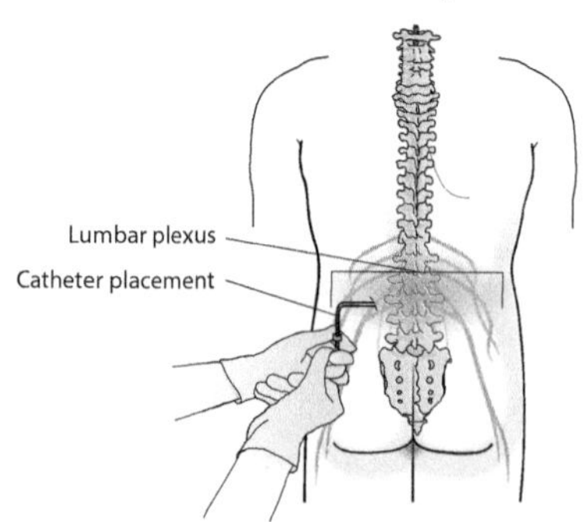

ICD-10-CM Diagnostic Codes

	Code	Description
	B02.29	Other postherpetic nervous system involvement
⇄	C47.21	Malignant neoplasm of peripheral nerves of right lower limb, including hip
⇄	C47.22	Malignant neoplasm of peripheral nerves of left lower limb, including hip
⇄	C49.21	Malignant neoplasm of connective and soft tissue of right lower limb, including hip
⇄	C49.22	Malignant neoplasm of connective and soft tissue of left lower limb, including hip
	C76.3	Malignant neoplasm of pelvis
⇄	C76.51	Malignant neoplasm of right lower limb
⇄	C76.52	Malignant neoplasm of left lower limb
	C79.49	Secondary malignant neoplasm of other parts of nervous system
	C79.89	Secondary malignant neoplasm of other specified sites
	G89.11	Acute pain due to trauma
	G89.18	Other acute postprocedural pain
	G89.21	Chronic pain due to trauma
	G89.28	Other chronic postprocedural pain
	G89.29	Other chronic pain
	G89.3	Neoplasm related pain (acute) (chronic)
⇄	M79.604	Pain in right leg
⇄	M79.605	Pain in left leg
⇄	M79.651	Pain in right thigh
⇄	M79.652	Pain in left thigh
⇄	M79.661	Pain in right lower leg
⇄	M79.662	Pain in left lower leg
⇄	R10.31	Right lower quadrant pain
⇄	R10.32	Left lower quadrant pain
❼⇄	S32.411	Displaced fracture of anterior wall of right acetabulum
❼⇄	S32.412	Displaced fracture of anterior wall of left acetabulum
❼⇄	S32.421	Displaced fracture of posterior wall of right acetabulum
❼⇄	S32.422	Displaced fracture of posterior wall of left acetabulum
❼⇄	S32.431	Displaced fracture of anterior column [iliopubic] of right acetabulum
❼⇄	S32.432	Displaced fracture of anterior column [iliopubic] of left acetabulum
❼⇄	S32.441	Displaced fracture of posterior column [ilioischial] of right acetabulum
❼⇄	S32.442	Displaced fracture of posterior column [ilioischial] of left acetabulum
❼⇄	S32.451	Displaced transverse fracture of right acetabulum
❼⇄	S32.452	Displaced transverse fracture of left acetabulum
❼⇄	S32.461	Displaced associated transverse-posterior fracture of right acetabulum
❼⇄	S32.462	Displaced associated transverse-posterior fracture of left acetabulum
❼⇄	S32.471	Displaced fracture of medial wall of right acetabulum

⑦⇄	S32.472	Displaced fracture of medial wall of left acetabulum
⑦⇄	S32.481	Displaced dome fracture of right acetabulum
⑦⇄	S32.482	Displaced dome fracture of left acetabulum

ICD-10-CM Coding Notes

For codes requiring a 7th character extension, refer to your ICD-10-CM book. Review the character descriptions and coding guidelines for proper selection. For some procedures, only certain characters will apply.

CCI Edits

Refer to Appendix A for CCI edits.

Facility RVUs ▯

Code	Work	PE Facility	MP	Total Facility
64449	1.27	0.40	0.12	1.79

Non-facility RVUs ▯

Code	Work	PE Non-Facility	MP	Total Non-Facility
64449	1.27	0.40	0.12	1.79

Modifiers (PAR) ▯

Code	Mod 50	Mod 51	Mod 62	Mod 66	Mod 80
64449	1	2	0	0	1

Global Period

Code	Days
64449	000

64450

▲ **64450 Injection(s), anesthetic agent(s) and/or steroid; other peripheral nerve or branch**

(For injection, anesthetic agent, nerves innervating the sacroiliac joint, use 64451)

AMA Coding Guideline

Introduction/Injection of Anesthetic Agent (Nerve Block), Diagnostic or Therapeutic Procedures on the Somatic Nerves

Codes 64400-64489 describe the introduction/injection of an anesthetic agent and/or steroid into the somatic nervous system for diagnostic or therapeutic purposes. For injection or destruction of genicular nerve branches, see 64454, 64624, respectively.

Codes 64400-64450, 64454 describe the injection of an anesthetic agent(s) and/or steroid into a nerve plexus, nerve, or branch. These codes are reported once per nerve plexus, nerve, or branch as described in the descriptor regardless of the number of injections performed along the nerve plexus, nerve, or branch described by the code.

Imaging guidance and localization may be reported separately for 64400-64450. Imaging guidance and any injection of contrast are inclusive components of 64451 and 64454.

Codes 64455, 64479, 64480, 64483, 64484 are reported for single or multiple injections on the same site. For 64479, 64480, 64483, 64484, imaging guidance (fluoroscopy or CT) and any injection of contrast are inclusive components and are not reported separately. For 64455, imaging guidance (ultrasound, fluoroscopy, CT) and localization may be reported separately.

Codes 64461, 64462, 64463 describe injection of a paravertebral block (PVB). Codes 64486, 64487, 64488, 64489 describe injection of a transversus abdominis plane (TAP) block. Imaging guidance and any injection of contrast are inclusive components of 64461, 64462, 64463, 64486, 64487, 64488, 64489 and are not reported separately.

Please see the Surgical Guidelines section for the following table: The Central Venous Access Procedures Table

AMA Coding Notes

Introduction/Injection of Anesthetic Agent (Nerve Block), Diagnostic or Therapeutic Procedures on the Extracranial Nerves, Peripheral Nerves, and Autonomic Nervous System

(For destruction by neurolytic agent or chemodenervation, see 62280-62282, 64600-64681)

(For epidural or subarachnoid injection, see 62320, 62321, 62322, 62323, 62324, 62325, 62326, 62327)

(64400-64455, 64461, 64462, 64463, 64479, 64480, 64483, 64484, 64490-64495 are unilateral procedures. For bilateral procedures, report 64400, 64405, 64408, 64415, 64416, 64417, 64418, 64420, 64425-64455, 64461, 64463, 64479, 64483, 64490, 64493 with modifier 50. Report add-on codes 64421, 64462, 64480, 64484, 64491, 64492, 64494, 64495 twice, when performed bilaterally. Do not report modifier 50 in conjunction with 64421, 64462, 64480, 64484, 64491, 64492, 64494, 64495. Do not report modifier 50 in conjunction with 64421, 64462, 64480, 64484, 64491, 64492, 64494, 64495)

Surgical Procedures on the Extracranial Nerves, Peripheral Nerves, and Autonomic Nervous System

(For intracranial surgery on cranial nerves, see 61450, 61460, 61790)

AMA *CPT Assistant* ▯

64450: Jul 98: 10, Nov 99: 37, Dec 99: 7, Oct 01: 9, Aug 03: 6, Apr 05: 13, Jan 09: 6, Jan 13: 13, Sep 15: 12, Nov 15: 11, Oct 16: 11, May 18: 10, Nov 18: 10

Plain English Description

An anesthetic agent is injected into a peripheral nerve or branch not specifically described by another code. This procedure may also be referred to as a peripheral nerve block. Generally, this is performed on peripheral nerves or branches in the arm or leg. The specific nerve or branch is identified. The skin over the planned puncture site is disinfected. The needle is inserted, aspirated to ensure it is not in a blood vessel, and the anesthetic is injected.

Injection, anesthetic/steroid; other peripheral nerve or branch

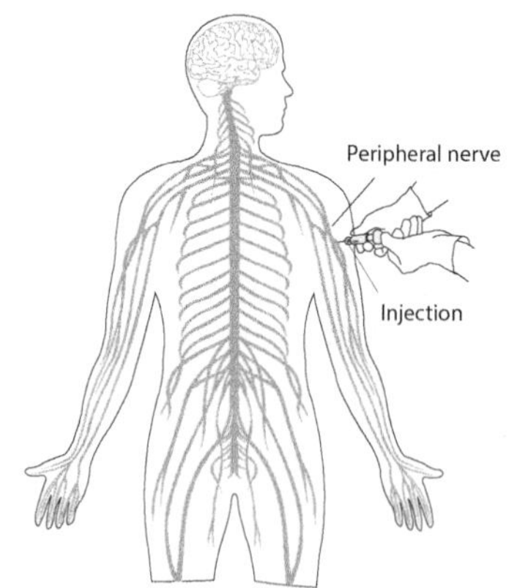

ICD-10-CM Diagnostic Codes

	Code	Description
⇄	G56.81	Other specified mononeuropathies of right upper limb
⇄	G56.82	Other specified mononeuropathies of left upper limb
⇄	G56.83	Other specified mononeuropathies of bilateral upper limbs
⇄	G57.51	Tarsal tunnel syndrome, right lower limb
⇄	G57.52	Tarsal tunnel syndrome, left lower limb
⇄	G57.53	Tarsal tunnel syndrome, bilateral lower limbs
⇄	G57.81	Other specified mononeuropathies of right lower limb
⇄	G57.82	Other specified mononeuropathies of left lower limb
⇄	G57.83	Other specified mononeuropathies of bilateral lower limbs
	G89.11	Acute pain due to trauma
	G89.18	Other acute postprocedural pain
	G89.21	Chronic pain due to trauma
	G89.28	Other chronic postprocedural pain
	G89.29	Other chronic pain
	G89.3	Neoplasm related pain (acute) (chronic)
⇄	M12.561	Traumatic arthropathy, right knee
⇄	M12.562	Traumatic arthropathy, left knee
	M17.0	Bilateral primary osteoarthritis of knee
⇄	M17.11	Unilateral primary osteoarthritis, right knee
⇄	M17.12	Unilateral primary osteoarthritis, left knee
	M17.2	Bilateral post-traumatic osteoarthritis of knee
⇄	M17.31	Unilateral post-traumatic osteoarthritis, right knee
⇄	M17.32	Unilateral post-traumatic osteoarthritis, left knee
	M17.4	Other bilateral secondary osteoarthritis of knee
	M17.5	Other unilateral secondary osteoarthritis of knee
⇄	M25.561	Pain in right knee
⇄	M25.562	Pain in left knee
	M79.2	Neuralgia and neuritis, unspecified

CCI Edits

Refer to Appendix A for CCI edits.

Facility RVUs ▯

Code	Work	PE Facility	MP	Total Facility
64450	0.75	0.39	0.09	1.23

Non-facility RVUs ▯

Code	Work	PE Non-Facility	MP	Total Non-Facility
64450	0.75	1.34	0.09	2.18

Modifiers (PAR) ▯

Code	Mod 50	Mod 51	Mod 62	Mod 66	Mod 80
64450	1	2	0	0	1

Global Period

Code	Days
64450	000

64451

● **64451 Injection(s), anesthetic agent(s) and/or steroid; nerves innervating the sacroiliac joint, with image guidance (ie, fluoroscopy or computed tomography)**

(Do not report 64451 in conjunction with 64493, 64494, 64495, 77002, 77003, 77012, 95873, 95874)

(For injection, anesthetic agent, nerves innervating the sacroiliac joint, with ultrasound, use 76999)

(For bilateral procedure, report 64451 with modifier 50)

AMA Coding Guideline

Introduction/Injection of Anesthetic Agent (Nerve Block), Diagnostic or Therapeutic Procedures on the Somatic Nerves

Codes 64400-64489 describe the introduction/ injection of an anesthetic agent and/or steroid into the somatic nervous system for diagnostic or therapeutic purposes. For injection or destruction of genicular nerve branches, see 64454, 64624, respectively.

Codes 64400-64450, 64454 describe the injection of an anesthetic agent(s) and/or steroid into a nerve plexus, nerve, or branch. These codes are reported once per nerve plexus, nerve, or branch as described in the descriptor regardless of the number of injections performed along the nerve plexus, nerve, or branch described by the code.

Imaging guidance and localization may be reported separately for 64400-64450. Imaging guidance and any injection of contrast are inclusive components of 64451 and 64454.

Codes 64455, 64479, 64480, 64483, 64484 are reported for single or multiple injections on the same site. For 64479, 64480, 64483, 64484, imaging guidance (fluoroscopy or CT) and any injection of contrast are inclusive components and are not reported separately. For 64455, imaging guidance (ultrasound, fluoroscopy, CT) and localization may be reported separately.

Codes 64461, 64462, 64463 describe injection of a paravertebral block (PVB). Codes 64486, 64487, 64488, 64489 describe injection of a transversus abdominis plane (TAP) block. Imaging guidance and any injection of contrast are inclusive components of 64461, 64462, 64463, 64486, 64487, 64488, 64489 and are not reported separately.

Please see the Surgical Guidelines section for the following table: The Central Venous Access Procedures Table

AMA Coding Notes

Introduction/Injection of Anesthetic Agent (Nerve Block), Diagnostic or Therapeutic Procedures on the Extracranial Nerves, Peripheral Nerves, and Autonomic Nervous System

(For destruction by neurolytic agent or chemodenervation, see 62280-62282, 64600-64681)

(For epidural or subarachnoid injection, see 62320, 62321, 62322, 62323, 62324, 62325, 62326, 62327)

(64400-64455, 64461, 64462, 64463, 64479, 64480, 64483, 64484, 64490-64495 are unilateral procedures. For bilateral procedures, report 64400, 64405, 64408, 64415, 64416, 64417, 64418, 64420, 64425-64455, 64461, 64463, 64479, 64483, 64490, 64493 with modifier 50. Report add-on codes 64421, 64462, 64480, 64484, 64491, 64492, 64494, 64495 twice, when performed bilaterally. Do not report modifier 50 in conjunction with 64421, 64462, 64480, 64484, 64491, 64492, 64494, 64495. Do not report modifier 50 in conjunction with 64421, 64462, 64480, 64484, 64491, 64492, 64494, 64495)

Surgical Procedures on the Extracranial Nerves, Peripheral Nerves, and Autonomic Nervous System

(For intracranial surgery on cranial nerves, see 61450, 61460, 61790)

Plain English Description

A sacroiliac (SI) joint nerve block is performed using injection of an anesthetic agent and/or steroid. This is performed primarily to treat or diagnose the source of low back pain and/or sciatic pain due to SI joint dysfunction. The SI joints connect the sacrum with the hip on either side of the spine. After the skin site is prepped, the needle is advanced into the SI joint, most commonly under fluoroscopy. Contrast is first injected to ensure accurate needle placement and observe how the medication spreads. The nerve blocking agent is then injected. When done for diagnostic purposes, a local anesthetic agent such as lidocaine may be injected first, and the patient tries to reproduce the pain. When 75-80% pain relief is achieved, a tentative diagnosis is made. This is followed by injection of a different anesthetic agent, such as Bupivicaine, to see if pain relief continues to confirm the diagnosis of SI joint dysfunction. When performed for therapeutic pain relief, an anesthetic agent in combination with an anti-inflammatory corticosteroid is injected in the same manner.

ICD-10-CM Diagnostic Codes

	A18.01	Tuberculosis of spine
	C41.4	Malignant neoplasm of pelvic bones, sacrum and coccyx
	C47.5	Malignant neoplasm of peripheral nerves of pelvis
	C49.5	Malignant neoplasm of connective and soft tissue of pelvis
	C79.51	Secondary malignant neoplasm of bone
	C79.89	Secondary malignant neoplasm of other specified sites
	G89.18	Other acute postprocedural pain
	G89.21	Chronic pain due to trauma
	G89.29	Other chronic pain
	G89.3	Neoplasm related pain (acute) (chronic)
	G89.4	Chronic pain syndrome
	M12.58	Traumatic arthropathy, other specified site
	M45.8	Ankylosing spondylitis sacral and sacrococcygeal region
	M46.1	Sacroiliitis, not elsewhere classified
	M47.28	Other spondylosis with radiculopathy, sacral and sacrococcygeal region
	M48.38	Traumatic spondylopathy, sacral and sacrococcygeal region
	M53.2	Spinal instabilities
	M53.3	Sacrococcygeal disorders, not elsewhere classified
	M99.14	Subluxation complex (vertebral) of sacral region
	M99.24	Subluxation stenosis of neural canal of sacral region
	M99.34	Osseous stenosis of neural canal of sacral region
	M99.44	Connective tissue stenosis of neural canal of sacral region
	M99.54	Intervertebral disc stenosis of neural canal of sacral region
	M99.84	Other biomechanical lesions of sacral region
	R10.2	Pelvic and perineal pain
⑦	S33.2	Dislocation of sacroiliac and sacrococcygeal joint
⑦	S33.6	Sprain of sacroiliac joint

ICD-10-CM Coding Notes

For codes requiring a 7th character extension, refer to your ICD-10-CM book. Review the character descriptions and coding guidelines for proper selection. For some procedures, only certain characters will apply.

CCI Edits

Refer to Appendix A for CCI edits.

Facility RVUs

Code	Work	PE Facility	MP	Total Facility
64451	1.52	0.62	0.15	2.29

Non-facility RVUs

Code	Work	PE Non-Facility	MP	Total Non-Facility
64451	1.52	4.32	0.15	5.99

Modifiers (PAR)

Code	Mod 50	Mod 51	Mod 62	Mod 66	Mod 80
64451	1	2	0	0	1

Global Period

Code	Days
64451	000

64479-64480

64479 Injection(s), anesthetic agent and/or steroid, transforaminal epidural, with imaging guidance (fluoroscopy or CT); cervical or thoracic, single level

(For transforaminal epidural injection under ultrasound guidance, use 0228T)

+ **64480 Injection(s), anesthetic agent and/or steroid, transforaminal epidural, with imaging guidance (fluoroscopy or CT); cervical or thoracic, each additional level (List separately in addition to code for primary procedure)**

(Use 64480 in conjunction with 64479)

(For transforaminal epidural injection under ultrasound guidance, use 0229T)

(For transforaminal epidural injection at the T12-L1 level, use 64479)

AMA Coding Guideline

Introduction/Injection of Anesthetic Agent (Nerve Block), Diagnostic or Therapeutic Procedures on the Somatic Nerves

Codes 64400-64489 describe the introduction/injection of an anesthetic agent and/or steroid into the somatic nervous system for diagnostic or therapeutic purposes. For injection or destruction of genicular nerve branches, see 64454, 64624, respectively.

Codes 64400-64450, 64454 describe the injection of an anesthetic agent(s) and/or steroid into a nerve plexus, nerve, or branch. These codes are reported once per nerve plexus, nerve, or branch as described in the descriptor regardless of the number of injections performed along the nerve plexus, nerve, or branch described by the code.

Imaging guidance and localization may be reported separately for 64400-64450. Imaging guidance and any injection of contrast are inclusive components of 64451 and 64454.

Codes 64455, 64479, 64480, 64483, 64484 are reported for single or multiple injections on the same site. For 64479, 64480, 64483, 64484, imaging guidance (fluoroscopy or CT) and any injection of contrast are inclusive components and are not reported separately. For 64455, imaging guidance (ultrasound, fluoroscopy, CT) and localization may be reported separately.

Codes 64461, 64462, 64463 describe injection of a paravertebral block (PVB). Codes 64486, 64487, 64488, 64489 describe injection of a transversus abdominis plane (TAP) block. Imaging guidance and any injection of contrast are inclusive components of 64461, 64462, 64463, 64486, 64487, 64488, 64489 and are not reported separately.

Please see the Surgical Guidelines section for the following table: The Central Venous Access Procedures Table

AMA Coding Notes

Introduction/Injection of Anesthetic Agent (Nerve Block), Diagnostic or Therapeutic Procedures on the Extracranial Nerves, Peripheral Nerves, and Autonomic Nervous System

(For destruction by neurolytic agent or chemodenervation, see 62280-62282, 64600-64681)

(For epidural or subarachnoid injection, see 62320, 62321, 62322, 62323, 62324, 62325, 62326, 62327)

(64400-64455, 64461, 64462, 64463, 64479, 64480, 64483, 64484, 64490-64495 are unilateral procedures. For bilateral procedures, report 64400, 64405, 64408, 64415, 64416, 64417, 64418, 64420, 64425-64455, 64461, 64463, 64479, 64483, 64490, 64493 with modifier 50. Report add-on codes 64421, 64462, 64480, 64484, 64491, 64492, 64494, 64495 twice, when performed bilaterally. Do not report modifier 50 in conjunction with 64421, 64462, 64480, 64484, 64491, 64492, 64494, 64495. Do not report modifier 50 in conjunction with 64421, 64462, 64480, 64484, 64491, 64492, 64494, 64495)

Surgical Procedures on the Extracranial Nerves, Peripheral Nerves, and Autonomic Nervous System

(For intracranial surgery on cranial nerves, see 61450, 61460, 61790)

AMA *CPT Assistant*

64479: Nov 99: 33, 37, Feb 00: 4, Jul 08: 9, Nov 08: 11, Feb 10: 9, Jan 11: 8, Feb 11: 4, Jul 11: 16, Jul 12: 5, Jan 16: 9

64480: Nov 99: 33, 37, Feb 00: 4, Feb 05: 14, Jul 08: 9, Feb 10: 9, Jan 11: 8, Feb 11: 4, Jul 11: 16, Jul 12: 5

Plain English Description

A transforaminal epidural injection allows for a very selective injection around a specific nerve root. Nerve roots exit the spinal canal through the foramina, which are small openings between the vertebrae. The skin is cleansed and prepared over the affected cervical or thoracic vertebra. Using computed tomography (CT) or fluoroscopic imaging, a needle is advanced through the skin and into the foramen. A small amount of radiopaque contrast material may be injected to enhance fluoroscopic images and to confirm proper placement of the spinal needle. The anesthetic and/or steroid is then injected around the nerve root. Use 64479 for transforaminal epidural injection at a single cervical or thoracic level. Use 64480 for each additional level injected.

Injection, anesthetic agent/steroid, transforaminal epidural; cervical/thoracic

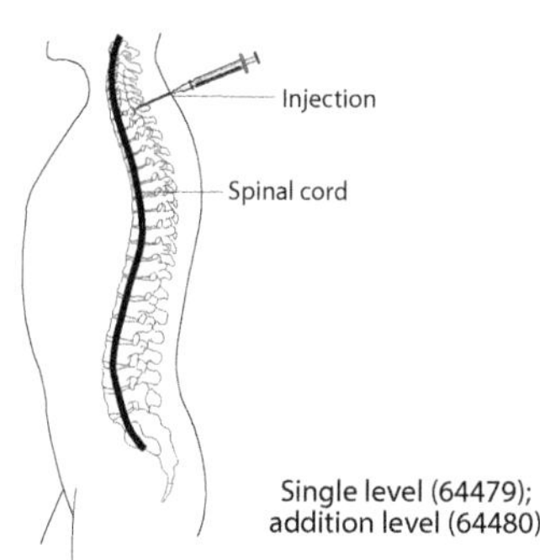

ICD-10-CM Diagnostic Codes

G54.2	Cervical root disorders, not elsewhere classified
G54.3	Thoracic root disorders, not elsewhere classified
G89.29	Other chronic pain
M43.02	Spondylolysis, cervical region
M43.03	Spondylolysis, cervicothoracic region
M43.04	Spondylolysis, thoracic region
M43.12	Spondylolisthesis, cervical region
M43.13	Spondylolisthesis, cervicothoracic region
M43.14	Spondylolisthesis, thoracic region
M43.22	Fusion of spine, cervical region
M43.23	Fusion of spine, cervicothoracic region
M43.24	Fusion of spine, thoracic region
M46.02	Spinal enthesopathy, cervical region
M46.03	Spinal enthesopathy, cervicothoracic region
M46.04	Spinal enthesopathy, thoracic region
M47.21	Other spondylosis with radiculopathy, occipito-atlanto-axial region
M47.22	Other spondylosis with radiculopathy, cervical region
M47.23	Other spondylosis with radiculopathy, cervicothoracic region
M47.24	Other spondylosis with radiculopathy, thoracic region
M48.02	Spinal stenosis, cervical region
M48.04	Spinal stenosis, thoracic region
M50.11	Cervical disc disorder with radiculopathy, high cervical region
M50.121	Cervical disc disorder at C4-C5 level with radiculopathy
M50.122	Cervical disc disorder at C5-C6 level with radiculopathy
M50.123	Cervical disc disorder at C6-C7 level with radiculopathy
M50.13	Cervical disc disorder with radiculopathy, cervicothoracic region
M54.11	Radiculopathy, occipito-atlanto-axial region
M54.12	Radiculopathy, cervical region
M54.13	Radiculopathy, cervicothoracic region

	M54.14	Radiculopathy, thoracic region
	M54.2	Cervicalgia
	M54.6	Pain in thoracic spine
⑦	S14.2	Injury of nerve root of cervical spine
⑦	S24.2	Injury of nerve root of thoracic spine

ICD-10-CM Coding Notes

For codes requiring a 7th character extension, refer to your ICD-10-CM book. Review the character descriptions and coding guidelines for proper selection. For some procedures, only certain characters will apply.

CCI Edits

Refer to Appendix A for CCI edits.

Facility RVUs

Code	Work	PE Facility	MP	Total Facility
64479	2.29	1.26	0.22	3.77
64480	1.20	0.48	0.12	1.80

Non-facility RVUs

Code	Work	PE Non-Facility	MP	Total Non-Facility
64479	2.29	4.75	0.22	7.26
64480	1.20	2.29	0.12	3.61

Modifiers (PAR)

Code	Mod 50	Mod 51	Mod 62	Mod 66	Mod 80
64479	1	2	0	0	1
64480	1	0	0	0	1

Global Period

Code	Days
64479	000
64480	ZZZ

64483-64484

64483 Injection(s), anesthetic agent and/or steroid, transforaminal epidural, with imaging guidance (fluoroscopy or CT); lumbar or sacral, single level

(For transforaminal epidural injection under ultrasound guidance, use 0230T)

+ **64484 Injection(s), anesthetic agent and/or steroid, transforaminal epidural, with imaging guidance (fluoroscopy or CT); lumbar or sacral, each additional level (List separately in addition to code for primary procedure)**

(Use 64484 in conjunction with 64483)

(For transforaminal epidural injection under ultrasound guidance, use 0231T)

(64479-64484 are unilateral procedures. For bilateral procedures, report 64479, 64483 with modifier 50. Report add-on codes 64480, 64484 twice, when performed bilaterally. Do not report modifier 50 in conjunction with 64480, 64484)

AMA Coding Guideline

Introduction/Injection of Anesthetic Agent (Nerve Block), Diagnostic or Therapeutic Procedures on the Somatic Nerves

Codes 64400-64489 describe the introduction/injection of an anesthetic agent and/or steroid into the somatic nervous system for diagnostic or therapeutic purposes. For injection or destruction of genicular nerve branches, see 64454, 64624, respectively.

Codes 64400-64450, 64454 describe the injection of an anesthetic agent(s) and/or steroid into a nerve plexus, nerve, or branch. These codes are reported once per nerve plexus, nerve, or branch as described in the descriptor regardless of the number of injections performed along the nerve plexus, nerve, or branch described by the code.

Imaging guidance and localization may be reported separately for 64400-64450. Imaging guidance and any injection of contrast are inclusive components of 64451 and 64454.

Codes 64455, 64479, 64480, 64483, 64484 are reported for single or multiple injections on the same site. For 64479, 64480, 64483, 64484, imaging guidance (fluoroscopy or CT) and any injection of contrast are inclusive components and are not reported separately. For 64455, imaging guidance (ultrasound, fluoroscopy, CT) and localization may be reported separately.

Codes 64461, 64462, 64463 describe injection of a paravertebral block (PVB). Codes 64486, 64487, 64488, 64489 describe injection of a transversus abdominis plane (TAP) block. Imaging guidance and any injection of contrast are inclusive components of 64461, 64462, 64463, 64486, 64487, 64488, 64489 and are not reported separately.

Please see the Surgical Guidelines section for the following table: The Central Venous Access Procedures Table

AMA Coding Notes

Introduction/Injection of Anesthetic Agent (Nerve Block), Diagnostic or Therapeutic Procedures on the Extracranial Nerves, Peripheral Nerves, and Autonomic Nervous System

(For destruction by neurolytic agent or chemodenervation, see 62280-62282, 64600-64681)

(For epidural or subarachnoid injection, see 62320, 62321, 62322, 62323, 62324, 62325, 62326, 62327)

(64400-64455, 64461, 64462, 64463, 64479, 64480, 64483, 64484, 64490-64495 are unilateral procedures. For bilateral procedures, report 64400, 64405, 64408, 64415, 64416, 64417, 64418, 64420, 64425-64455, 64461, 64463, 64479, 64483, 64490, 64493 with modifier 50. Report add-on codes 64421, 64462, 64480, 64484, 64491, 64492, 64494, 64495 twice, when performed bilaterally. Do not report modifier 50 in conjunction with 64421, 64462, 64480, 64484, 64491, 64492, 64494, 64495. Do not report modifier 50 in conjunction with 64421, 64462, 64480, 64484, 64491, 64492, 64494, 64495)

Surgical Procedures on the Extracranial Nerves, Peripheral Nerves, and Autonomic Nervous System

(For intracranial surgery on cranial nerves, see 61450, 61460, 61790)

AMA *CPT Assistant*

64483: Nov 99: 33, 37, Feb 00: 4, Jul 08: 9, Feb 10: 9, Jan 11: 8, Feb 11: 4, Jul 11: 16, May 12: 14, Jul 12: 5, Oct 16: 11

64484: Nov 99: 33, 37, Feb 00: 4, Feb 05: 14, Jul 08: 9, Nov 08: 11, Feb 10: 9, Feb 11: 4, Jul 11: 16, Jul 12: 5, Jan 16: 9

Plain English Description

A transforaminal epidural injection allows very selective injection around a specific nerve root. Nerve roots exit the spinal canal through the foramina, which are small openings between the vertebrae. The skin is cleansed and prepared over the affected lumbar or sacral vertebra. Using computed tomography (CT) or fluoroscopic imaging, a needle is advanced through the skin and into the foramen. A small amount of radiopaque contrast material may be injected to enhance fluoroscopic images and to confirm proper placement of the spinal needle. The anesthetic and/or steroid is then injected around the nerve root. Use 64483 for transforaminal epidural injection at a single lumbar or sacral level. Use 64484 for each additional level injected.

Injection, anesthetic agent/steroid, transforaminal epidural; lumbar/sacral

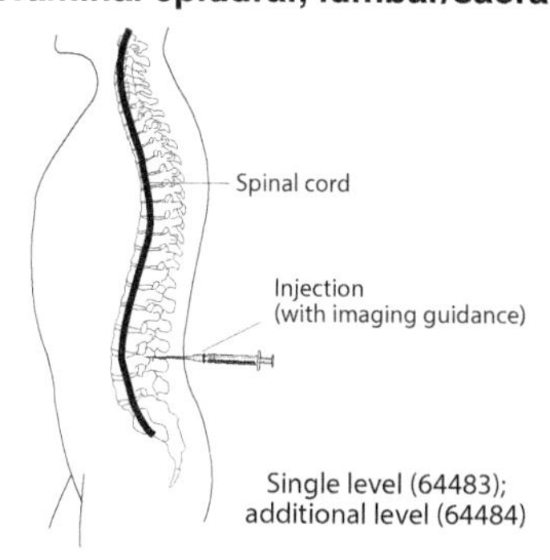

ICD-10-CM Diagnostic Codes

G54.1	Lumbosacral plexus disorders
G54.4	Lumbosacral root disorders, not elsewhere classified
G89.29	Other chronic pain
M43.06	Spondylolysis, lumbar region
M43.07	Spondylolysis, lumbosacral region
M43.08	Spondylolysis, sacral and sacrococcygeal region
M43.16	Spondylolisthesis, lumbar region
M43.17	Spondylolisthesis, lumbosacral region
M43.18	Spondylolisthesis, sacral and sacrococcygeal region
M47.25	Other spondylosis with radiculopathy, thoracolumbar region
M47.26	Other spondylosis with radiculopathy, lumbar region
M47.27	Other spondylosis with radiculopathy, lumbosacral region
M47.28	Other spondylosis with radiculopathy, sacral and sacrococcygeal region
M48.062	Spinal stenosis, lumbar region with neurogenic claudication
M51.15	Intervertebral disc disorders with radiculopathy, thoracolumbar region
M51.16	Intervertebral disc disorders with radiculopathy, lumbar region
M51.17	Intervertebral disc disorders with radiculopathy, lumbosacral region
M54.15	Radiculopathy, thoracolumbar region
M54.16	Radiculopathy, lumbar region
M54.17	Radiculopathy, lumbosacral region
M54.18	Radiculopathy, sacral and sacrococcygeal region
M54.5	Low back pain
M54.89	Other dorsalgia
⑦ S34.21	Injury of nerve root of lumbar spine
⑦ S34.22	Injury of nerve root of sacral spine

ICD-10-CM Coding Notes

For codes requiring a 7th character extension, refer to your ICD-10-CM book. Review the character descriptions and coding guidelines for proper selection. For some procedures, only certain characters will apply.

CCI Edits

Refer to Appendix A for CCI edits.

Facility RVUs

Code	Work	PE Facility	MP	Total Facility
64483	1.90	1.13	0.18	3.21
64484	1.00	0.41	0.09	1.50

Non-facility RVUs

Code	Work	PE Non-Facility	MP	Total Non-Facility
64483	1.90	4.65	0.18	6.73
64484	1.00	1.87	0.09	2.96

Modifiers (PAR)

Code	Mod 50	Mod 51	Mod 62	Mod 66	Mod 80
64483	1	2	0	0	1
64484	1	0	0	0	1

Global Period

Code	Days
64483	000
64484	ZZZ

64490-64492

64490 Injection(s), diagnostic or therapeutic agent, paravertebral facet (zygapophyseal) joint (or nerves innervating that joint) with image guidance (fluoroscopy or CT), cervical or thoracic; single level

✚ **64491 Injection(s), diagnostic or therapeutic agent, paravertebral facet (zygapophyseal) joint (or nerves innervating that joint) with image guidance (fluoroscopy or CT), cervical or thoracic; second level (List separately in addition to code for primary procedure)**

(Use 64491 in conjunction with 64490)

✚ **64492 Injection(s), diagnostic or therapeutic agent, paravertebral facet (zygapophyseal) joint (or nerves innervating that joint) with image guidance (fluoroscopy or CT), cervical or thoracic; third and any additional level(s) (List separately in addition to code for primary procedure)**

(Do not report 64492 more than once per day)

(Use 64492 in conjunction with 64490, 64491)

AMA Coding Notes

Introduction/Injection of Anesthetic Agent (Nerve Block), Diagnostic or Therapeutic Procedures on the Paravertebral Spinal Nerves and Branches

(Image guidance [fluoroscopy or CT] and any injection of contrast are inclusive components of 64490-64495. Imaging guidance and localization are required for the performance of paravertebral facet joint injections described by codes 64490-64495. If imaging is not used, report 20552-20553. If ultrasound guidance is used, report 0213T-0218T)

(For bilateral paravertebral facet injection procedures, report 64490, 64493 with modifier 50. Report add-on codes 64491, 64492, 64494, 64495 twice, when performed bilaterally. Do not report modifier 50 in conjunction with 64491, 64492, 64494, 64495)

(For paravertebral facet injection of the T12-L1 joint, or nerves innervating that joint, use 64490)

Introduction/Injection of Anesthetic Agent (Nerve Block), Diagnostic or Therapeutic Procedures on the Extracranial Nerves, Peripheral Nerves, and Autonomic Nervous System

(For destruction by neurolytic agent or chemodenervation, see 62280-62282, 64600-64681)

(For epidural or subarachnoid injection, see 62320, 62321, 62322, 62323, 62324, 62325, 62326, 62327)

(64400-64455, 64461, 64462, 64463, 64479, 64480, 64483, 64484, 64490-64495 are unilateral procedures. For bilateral procedures, report 64400, 64405, 64408, 64415, 64416, 64417, 64418, 64420, 64425-64455, 64461, 64463, 64479, 64483, 64490, 64493 with modifier 50. Report add-on codes 64421, 64462, 64480, 64484, 64491, 64492, 64494, 64495 twice, when performed bilaterally. Do not report modifier 50 in conjunction with 64421, 64462, 64480, 64484, 64491, 64492, 64494, 64495. Do not report modifier 50 in conjunction with 64421, 64462, 64480, 64484, 64491, 64492, 64494, 64495)

Surgical Procedures on the Extracranial Nerves, Peripheral Nerves, and Autonomic Nervous System

(For intracranial surgery on cranial nerves, see 61450, 61460, 61790)

AMA *CPT Assistant* ☐

64490: Feb 10: 9, Aug 10: 12, Dec 10: 13, Jan 11: 8, Feb 11: 4, Jun 12: 10, Oct 12: 15

64491: Aug 10: 12, Jun 12: 10, Oct 12: 15

64492: Feb 10: 9, Aug 10: 12, Jan 11: 8, Feb 11: 4, Jun 12: 10, Oct 12: 15

Plain English Description

Paravertebral facet joints, also called zygapophyseal joints, are located on the back (posterior) of the spine on each side of the vertebra at the point where one vertebra overlaps the next. Facet joint pain may be associated with post-laminectomy syndrome or other spine surgery due to destabilization of the spinal joints, scar tissue formation, or recurrent disc herniation. Other causes include spondylosis, spondylolisthesis, and arthritis. Using fluoroscopic or computed tomographic (CT) guidance, a diagnostic or therapeutic facet joint injection or injection of nerves innervating the joint is performed. The skin overlying the facet joint is prepared and a local anesthetic injected. A spinal needle is directed into the facet joint space until bone or cartilage is encountered. A small amount of contrast material is injected to verify that the needle is correctly positioned. This is followed by injection of a local anesthetic and/or steroid. Diagnostic facet joint injection uses a local anesthetic to identify the specific area generating the pain. If the patient experiences pain relief for a significant period of time following a diagnostic injection, the physician will perform a therapeutic injection on a subsequent date of service using a long-acting local anesthetic in conjunction with a steroid. Use 64490 for a single cervical or thoracic facet joint injection; use 64491 for the second level; and use 64492 for the third and any additional cervical or thoracic levels injected.

Paravertebral facet joint injection

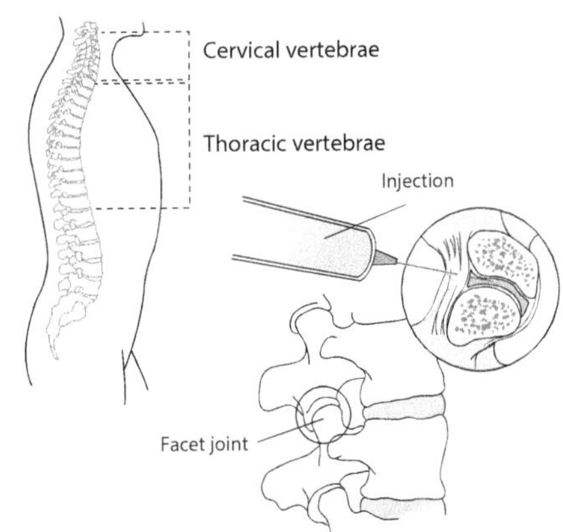

Single cervical or thoracic facet joint injection (64490); second level (64491); third and any additional cervical or thoracic levels (64492)

ICD-10-CM Diagnostic Codes

M46.81	Other specified inflammatory spondylopathies, occipito-atlanto-axial region
M46.82	Other specified inflammatory spondylopathies, cervical region
M46.83	Other specified inflammatory spondylopathies, cervicothoracic region
M46.84	Other specified inflammatory spondylopathies, thoracic region
M46.91	Unspecified inflammatory spondylopathy, occipito-atlanto-axial region
M46.92	Unspecified inflammatory spondylopathy, cervical region
M46.93	Unspecified inflammatory spondylopathy, cervicothoracic region
M46.94	Unspecified inflammatory spondylopathy, thoracic region
M47.11	Other spondylosis with myelopathy, occipito-atlanto-axial region
M47.12	Other spondylosis with myelopathy, cervical region
M47.13	Other spondylosis with myelopathy, cervicothoracic region
M47.14	Other spondylosis with myelopathy, thoracic region
M47.21	Other spondylosis with radiculopathy, occipito-atlanto-axial region
M47.22	Other spondylosis with radiculopathy, cervical region
M47.23	Other spondylosis with radiculopathy, cervicothoracic region
M47.24	Other spondylosis with radiculopathy, thoracic region
M54.11	Radiculopathy, occipito-atlanto-axial region
M54.12	Radiculopathy, cervical region
M54.13	Radiculopathy, cervicothoracic region
M54.14	Radiculopathy, thoracic region
M54.2	Cervicalgia
M54.6	Pain in thoracic spine

CCI Edits

Refer to Appendix A for CCI edits.

Facility RVUs □

Code	Work	PE Facility	MP	Total Facility
64490	1.82	1.04	0.18	3.04
64491	1.16	0.46	0.11	1.73
64492	1.16	0.48	0.11	1.75

Non-facility RVUs □

Code	Work	PE Non-Facility	MP	Total Non-Facility
64490	1.82	3.42	0.18	5.42
64491	1.16	1.45	0.11	2.72
64492	1.16	1.47	0.11	2.74

Modifiers (PAR) □

Code	Mod 50	Mod 51	Mod 62	Mod 66	Mod 80
64490	1	2	0	0	2
64491	1	0	0	0	2
64492	1	0	0	0	2

Global Period

Code	Days
64490	000
64491	ZZZ
64492	ZZZ

64493-64495

64493 Injection(s), diagnostic or therapeutic agent, paravertebral facet (zygapophyseal) joint (or nerves innervating that joint) with image guidance (fluoroscopy or CT), lumbar or sacral; single level

(For injection, anesthetic agent, nerves innervating the sacroiliac joint, use 64451)

+ 64494 Injection(s), diagnostic or therapeutic agent, paravertebral facet (zygapophyseal) joint (or nerves innervating that joint) with image guidance (fluoroscopy or CT), lumbar or sacral; second level (List separately in addition to code for primary procedure)

(Use 64494 in conjunction with 64493)

+ 64495 Injection(s), diagnostic or therapeutic agent, paravertebral facet (zygapophyseal) joint (or nerves innervating that joint) with image guidance (fluoroscopy or CT), lumbar or sacral; third and any additional level(s) (List separately in addition to code for primary procedure)

(Do not report 64495 more than once per day)

(Use 64495 in conjunction with 64493, 64494)

AMA Coding Notes

Introduction/Injection of Anesthetic Agent (Nerve Block), Diagnostic or Therapeutic Procedures on the Paravertebral Spinal Nerves and Branches

(Image guidance [fluoroscopy or CT] and any injection of contrast are inclusive components of 64490-64495. Imaging guidance and localization are required for the performance of paravertebral facet joint injections described by codes 64490-64495. If imaging is not used, report 20552-20553. If ultrasound guidance is used, report 0213T-0218T)

(For bilateral paravertebral facet injection procedures, report 64490, 64493 with modifier 50. Report add-on codes 64491, 64492, 64494, 64495 twice, when performed bilaterally. Do not report modifier 50 in conjunction with 64491, 64492, 64494, 64495)

(For paravertebral facet injection of the T12-L1 joint, or nerves innervating that joint, use 64490)

Introduction/Injection of Anesthetic Agent (Nerve Block), Diagnostic or Therapeutic Procedures on the Extracranial Nerves, Peripheral Nerves, and Autonomic Nervous System

(For destruction by neurolytic agent or chemodenervation, see 62280-62282, 64600-64681)

(For epidural or subarachnoid injection, see 62320, 62321, 62322, 62323, 62324, 62325, 62326, 62327)

(64400-64455, 64461, 64462, 64463, 64479, 64480, 64483, 64484, 64490-64495 are unilateral procedures. For bilateral procedures, report 64400, 64405, 64408, 64415, 64416, 64417, 64418, 64420, 64425-64455, 64461, 64463, 64479, 64483, 64490, 64493 with modifier 50. Report add-on codes 64421, 64462, 64480, 64484, 64491, 64492, 64494, 64495 twice, when performed bilaterally. Do not report modifier 50 in conjunction with 64421, 64462, 64480, 64484, 64491, 64492, 64494, 64495. Do not report modifier 50 in conjunction with 64421, 64462, 64480, 64484, 64491, 64492, 64494, 64495)

Surgical Procedures on the Extracranial Nerves, Peripheral Nerves, and Autonomic Nervous System

(For intracranial surgery on cranial nerves, see 61450, 61460, 61790)

AMA *CPT Assistant*

64493: Feb 10: 9, Aug 10: 12, Jan 11: 8, Feb 11: 4, Jun 12: 10, Oct 12: 15, May 18: 10

64494: Feb 10: 9, Aug 10: 12, Jan 11: 8, Feb 11: 4, Jun 12: 10, May 18: 10

64495: Feb 10: 9, Aug 10: 12, Jan 11: 8, Feb 11: 4, Jun 12: 10, Oct 12: 15, May 18: 10

Plain English Description

Paravertebral facet joints, also called zygapophyseal joints, are located on the back (posterior) of the spine on each side of the vertebra at the point where one vertebra overlaps the next. Facet joint pain may is associated with post-laminectomy syndrome or other spine surgery due to destabilization of the spinal joints, scar tissue formation, or recurrent disc herniation. Other causes include spondylosis, spondylolisthesis, and arthritis. Using fluoroscopic or computed tomographic (CT) guidance, a diagnostic or therapeutic facet joint injection or injection of nerves innervating the joint is performed. The skin overlying the facet joint is prepared and a local anesthetic injected. A spinal needle is directed into the facet joint space until bone or cartilage is encountered. A small amount of contrast material is injected to verify that the needle is correctly positioned. This is followed by injection of a local anesthetic and/or steroid. Diagnostic facet joint injection uses a local anesthetic to identify the specific area generating the pain. If the patient experiences pain relief for a significant period of time following a diagnostic injection, the physician will perform a therapeutic injection on a subsequent date of service using a long-acting local anesthetic in conjunction with a steroid. Use 64493 for a single lumbar or sacral facet joint injection; and use 64494 for the second level; use 64495 for the third and any additional lumbar or sacral levels injected.

Injection, diagnostic or therapeutic agent, paravertebral facet joint, lumbar or sacral

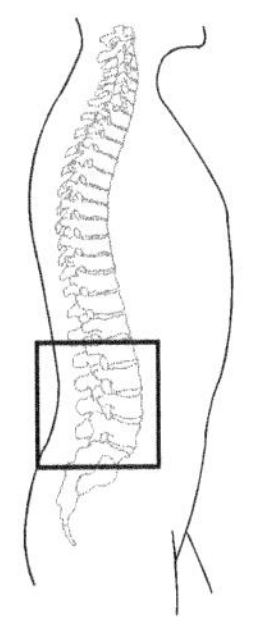

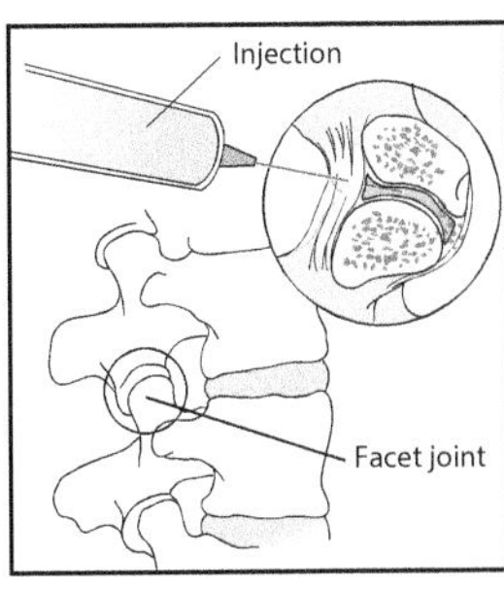

Single lumbar or sacral facet joint injection (64493); second level (64494); third and any additional levels (64495)

ICD-10-CM Diagnostic Codes

M46.86	Other specified inflammatory spondylopathies, lumbar region
M46.87	Other specified inflammatory spondylopathies, lumbosacral region
M46.96	Unspecified inflammatory spondylopathy, lumbar region
M46.97	Unspecified inflammatory spondylopathy, lumbosacral region
M47.16	Other spondylosis with myelopathy, lumbar region
M47.17	Other spondylosis with myelopathy, lumbosacral region
M47.26	Other spondylosis with radiculopathy, lumbar region
M47.27	Other spondylosis with radiculopathy, lumbosacral region
M54.16	Radiculopathy, lumbar region
M54.17	Radiculopathy, lumbosacral region
M54.5	Low back pain
M54.89	Other dorsalgia
M62.830	Muscle spasm of back

CCI Edits

Refer to Appendix A for CCI edits.

Facility RVUs

Code	Work	PE Facility	MP	Total Facility
64493	1.52	0.93	0.13	2.58
64494	1.00	0.40	0.09	1.49
64495	1.00	0.42	0.09	1.51

Non-facility RVUs

Code	Work	PE Non-Facility	MP	Total Non-Facility
64493	1.52	3.28	0.13	4.93
64494	1.00	1.44	0.09	2.53
64495	1.00	1.44	0.09	2.53

Modifiers (PAR)

Code	Mod 50	Mod 51	Mod 62	Mod 66	Mod 80
64493	1	2	0	0	2
64494	1	0	0	0	2
64495	1	0	0	0	2

Global Period

Code	Days
64493	000
64494	ZZZ
64495	ZZZ

64505

64505 Injection, anesthetic agent; sphenopalatine ganglion

AMA Coding Notes

Introduction/Injection of Anesthetic Agent (Nerve Block), Diagnostic or Therapeutic Procedures on the Extracranial Nerves, Peripheral Nerves, and Autonomic Nervous System

(For destruction by neurolytic agent or chemodenervation, see 62280-62282, 64600-64681)

(For epidural or subarachnoid injection, see 62320, 62321, 62322, 62323, 62324, 62325, 62326, 62327)

(64400-64455, 64461, 64462, 64463, 64479, 64480, 64483, 64484, 64490-64495 are unilateral procedures. For bilateral procedures, report 64400, 64405, 64408, 64415, 64416, 64417, 64418, 64420, 64425-64455, 64461, 64463, 64479, 64483, 64490, 64493 with modifier 50. Report add-on codes 64421, 64462, 64480, 64484, 64491, 64492, 64494, 64495 twice, when performed bilaterally. Do not report modifier 50 in conjunction with 64421, 64462, 64480, 64484, 64491, 64492, 64494, 64495. Do not report modifier 50 in conjunction with 64421, 64462, 64480, 64484, 64491, 64492, 64494, 64495)

Surgical Procedures on the Extracranial Nerves, Peripheral Nerves, and Autonomic Nervous System

(For intracranial surgery on cranial nerves, see 61450, 61460, 61790)

AMA *CPT Assistant*

64505: Jul 98: 10, Apr 05: 13, Jan 13: 13, Jun 13: 13, Jul 14: 8

Plain English Description

The sphenopalatine ganglion, also referred to as the pterygopalatine, nasal, Meckel's ganglion, or SPG, is a very small collection of nerves that includes sympathetic, parasympathetic, and sensory nerves. Blocking this ganglion has been proven to relieve headaches of varying etiology and ailments such as trigeminal neuralgia that cause facial pain. The ganglion is located behind the nose. In the procedure described by CPT code 64505, a needle is inserted through the cheek into the SPG and local anesthetic is injected. The coder should be cautioned that other techniques such as placing an anesthetic-coated cotton swab intra-nasally or the use of a catheter (e.g., the SphenoCath) to apply anesthetic are not injections and therefore do not meet the description of code 64505. In the case of the cotton swab, this procedure would be inclusive of an E/M service, or if not performed in addition to a visit, would be reported with the unlisted code 64999. The SphenoCath technique would also be reported with unlisted code 64999.

Injection, anesthetic agent; sphenopalatine ganglion

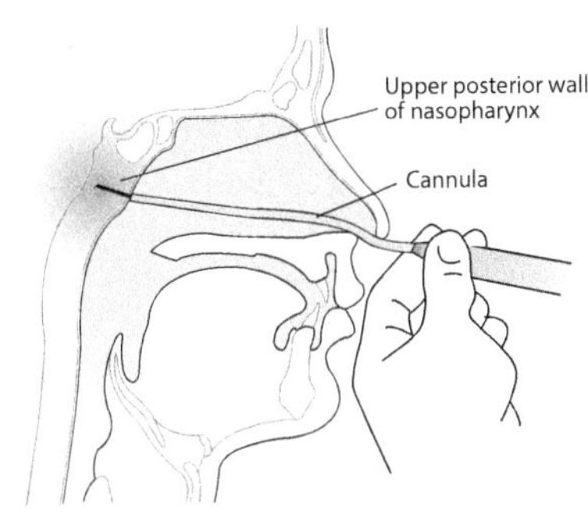

ICD-10-CM Diagnostic Codes

Code	Description
B02.29	Other postherpetic nervous system involvement
G43.001	Migraine without aura, not intractable, with status migrainosus
G43.009	Migraine without aura, not intractable, without status migrainosus
G43.011	Migraine without aura, intractable, with status migrainosus
G43.019	Migraine without aura, intractable, without status migrainosus
G43.101	Migraine with aura, not intractable, with status migrainosus
G43.109	Migraine with aura, not intractable, without status migrainosus
G43.111	Migraine with aura, intractable, with status migrainosus
G43.119	Migraine with aura, intractable, without status migrainosus
G43.401	Hemiplegic migraine, not intractable, with status migrainosus
G43.409	Hemiplegic migraine, not intractable, without status migrainosus
G43.411	Hemiplegic migraine, intractable, with status migrainosus
G43.419	Hemiplegic migraine, intractable, without status migrainosus
G43.501	Persistent migraine aura without cerebral infarction, not intractable, with status migrainosus
G43.509	Persistent migraine aura without cerebral infarction, not intractable, without status migrainosus
G43.511	Persistent migraine aura without cerebral infarction, intractable, with status migrainosus
G43.519	Persistent migraine aura without cerebral infarction, intractable, without status migrainosus
G43.701	Chronic migraine without aura, not intractable, with status migrainosus
G43.709	Chronic migraine without aura, not intractable, without status migrainosus
G43.711	Chronic migraine without aura, intractable, with status migrainosus
G43.719	Chronic migraine without aura, intractable, without status migrainosus
G43.801	Other migraine, not intractable, with status migrainosus
G43.809	Other migraine, not intractable, without status migrainosus
G43.811	Other migraine, intractable, with status migrainosus
G43.819	Other migraine, intractable, without status migrainosus
G43.901	Migraine, unspecified, not intractable, with status migrainosus
G43.909	Migraine, unspecified, not intractable, without status migrainosus
G43.911	Migraine, unspecified, intractable, with status migrainosus
G43.919	Migraine, unspecified, intractable, without status migrainosus
G44.001	Cluster headache syndrome, unspecified, intractable
G44.009	Cluster headache syndrome, unspecified, not intractable
G44.011	Episodic cluster headache, intractable
G44.019	Episodic cluster headache, not intractable
G44.021	Chronic cluster headache, intractable
G44.029	Chronic cluster headache, not intractable
G44.89	Other headache syndrome

CCI Edits

Refer to Appendix A for CCI edits.

Facility RVUs

Code	Work	PE Facility	MP	Total Facility
64505	1.36	1.15	0.28	2.79

Non-facility RVUs

Code	Work	PE Non-Facility	MP	Total Non-Facility
64505	1.36	1.98	0.28	3.62

Modifiers (PAR)

Code	Mod 50	Mod 51	Mod 62	Mod 66	Mod 80
64505	1	2	0	0	1

Global Period

Code	Days
64505	000

CPT® Procedural Coding

64520

64520 Injection, anesthetic agent; lumbar or thoracic (paravertebral sympathetic)

AMA Coding Notes

Introduction/Injection of Anesthetic Agent (Nerve Block), Diagnostic or Therapeutic Procedures on the Extracranial Nerves, Peripheral Nerves, and Autonomic Nervous System

(For destruction by neurolytic agent or chemodenervation, see 62280-62282, 64600-64681)

(For epidural or subarachnoid injection, see 62320, 62321, 62322, 62323, 62324, 62325, 62326, 62327)

(64400-64455, 64461, 64462, 64463, 64479, 64480, 64483, 64484, 64490-64495 are unilateral procedures. For bilateral procedures, report 64400, 64405, 64408, 64415, 64416, 64417, 64418, 64420, 64425-64455, 64461, 64463, 64479, 64483, 64490, 64493 with modifier 50. Report add-on codes 64421, 64462, 64480, 64484, 64491, 64492, 64494, 64495 twice, when performed bilaterally. Do not report modifier 50 in conjunction with 64421, 64462, 64480, 64484, 64491, 64492, 64494, 64495. Do not report modifier 50 in conjunction with 64421, 64462, 64480, 64484, 64491, 64492, 64494, 64495)

Surgical Procedures on the Extracranial Nerves, Peripheral Nerves, and Autonomic Nervous System

(For intracranial surgery on cranial nerves, see 61450, 61460, 61790)

AMA *CPT Assistant* ▢

64520: Jul 98: 10, Apr 05: 13, Dec 10: 14, Jan 13: 13

Plain English Description

Thoracic or lumbar paravertebral nerve block is used to treat acute or chronic pain in the thoracic or abdominal regions. The paravertebral space is a wedge-shaped area immediately adjacent to the vertebral bodies on either side of the spine where the spinal nerves emerge from the intervertebral foramen. Injection of a local anesthetic in this region produces unilateral motor, sensory, and sympathetic nerve blocks. The level of the blocks is determined, and the superior aspect of the spinous process is identified and marked. A needle entry site is marked approximately 2.5 cm lateral to the superior aspect of the spinous process. A local anesthetic is injected at the planned needle insertion site. A spinal epidural needle with tubing attached to a syringe is then inserted through the skin and advanced until contact is made with the transverse process. The needle is then withdrawn to the subcutaneous tissue and angled so that is can be walked off the lower (caudad) edge of the transverse process. The needle is reinserted and advanced into the paravertebral space. The needle is aspirated to ensure that it is not in the spinal canal or a blood vessel. The anesthetic is injected.

Injection, anesthetic agent; lumbar or thoracic

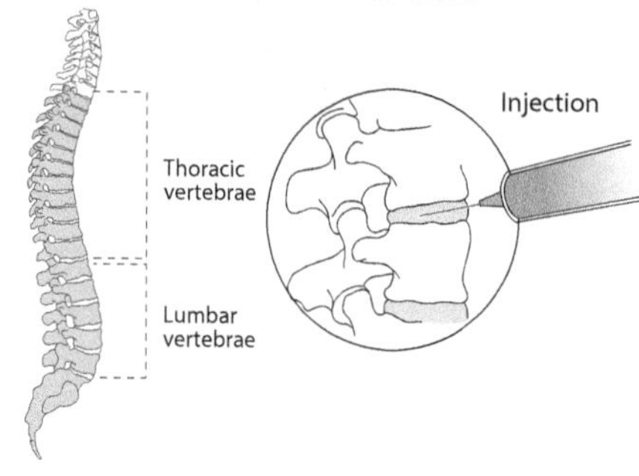

The physician injects a drug to numb the lumbar or thoracic sympathetic nerve to block pain to the pelvis, torso, and the legs.

ICD-10-CM Diagnostic Codes

	Code	Description
	B02.29	Other postherpetic nervous system involvement
	C41.2	Malignant neoplasm of vertebral column
	G89.11	Acute pain due to trauma
	G89.12	Acute post-thoracotomy pain
	G89.18	Other acute postprocedural pain
	G89.21	Chronic pain due to trauma
	G89.22	Chronic post-thoracotomy pain
	G89.28	Other chronic postprocedural pain
	G89.29	Other chronic pain
	G89.3	Neoplasm related pain (acute) (chronic)
➐	M48.54	Collapsed vertebra, not elsewhere classified, thoracic region
➐	M48.55	Collapsed vertebra, not elsewhere classified, thoracolumbar region
➐	M48.56	Collapsed vertebra, not elsewhere classified, lumbar region
⇄	M54.41	Lumbago with sciatica, right side
⇄	M54.42	Lumbago with sciatica, left side
	M54.5	Low back pain
	M54.6	Pain in thoracic spine
⇄	M79.604	Pain in right leg
⇄	M79.605	Pain in left leg
➐	M80.88	Other osteoporosis with current pathological fracture, vertebra(e)
➐	M84.58	Pathological fracture in neoplastic disease, other specified site
⇄	R10.11	Right upper quadrant pain
⇄	R10.12	Left upper quadrant pain
	R10.2	Pelvic and perineal pain
➐	S22.010	Wedge compression fracture of first thoracic vertebra
➐	S22.020	Wedge compression fracture of second thoracic vertebra
➐	S22.030	Wedge compression fracture of third thoracic vertebra
➐	S22.040	Wedge compression fracture of fourth thoracic vertebra
➐	S22.050	Wedge compression fracture of T5-T6 vertebra
➐	S22.060	Wedge compression fracture of T7-T8 vertebra
➐	S22.070	Wedge compression fracture of T9-T10 vertebra
➐	S22.080	Wedge compression fracture of T11-T12 vertebra
➐	S32.010	Wedge compression fracture of first lumbar vertebra
➐	S32.020	Wedge compression fracture of second lumbar vertebra
➐	S32.030	Wedge compression fracture of third lumbar vertebra
➐	S32.040	Wedge compression fracture of fourth lumbar vertebra
➐	S32.050	Wedge compression fracture of fifth lumbar vertebra

ICD-10-CM Coding Notes

For codes requiring a 7th character extension, refer to your ICD-10-CM book. Review the character descriptions and coding guidelines for proper selection. For some procedures, only certain characters will apply.

CCI Edits

Refer to Appendix A for CCI edits.

Facility RVUs ▢

Code	Work	PE Facility	MP	Total Facility
64520	1.35	0.90	0.13	2.38

Non-facility RVUs ▢

Code	Work	PE Non-Facility	MP	Total Non-Facility
64520	1.35	4.61	0.13	6.09

Modifiers (PAR) ▢

Code	Mod 50	Mod 51	Mod 62	Mod 66	Mod 80
64520	1	2	0	0	1

Global Period

Code	Days
64520	000

● New ▲ Revised ✚ Add On ⊘Modifier 51 Exempt ★Telemedicine ▢ CPT QuickRef ✗FDA Pending ⇄ Laterality ➐ Seventh Character ♂Male ♀Female

64553

64553 Percutaneous implantation of neurostimulator electrode array; cranial nerve

(For percutaneous electrical stimulation of a cranial nerve using needle[s] or needle electrode[s] [eg, PENS, PNT], use 64999)

(For open placement of cranial nerve (eg, vagus, trigeminal) neurostimulator pulse generator or receiver, see 61885, 61886, as appropriate)

AMA Coding Guideline

Neurostimulator Procedures on the Peripheral Nerves

For electronic analysis with programming, when performed, of peripheral nerve neurostimulator pulse generator/transmitters, see codes 95970, 95971, 95972. An electrode array is a catheter or other device with more than one contact. The function of each contact may be capable of being adjusted during programming services. Test stimulation to confirm correct target site placement of the electrode array(s) and/or to confirm the functional status of the system is inherent to placement, and is not separately reported as electronic analysis or programming of the neurostimulator system. Electronic analysis (95970) at the time of implantation is not separately reported.

Codes 64553, 64555, and 64561 may be used to report both temporary and permanent placement of percutaneous electrode arrays.

AMA Coding Notes

Neurostimulator Procedures on the Peripheral Nerves

(For transcutaneous nerve stimulation [TENS], use 97014 for electrical stimulation requiring supervision only or use 97032 for electrical stimulation requiring constant attendance)

(For percutaneous implantation or replacement of integrated neurostimulation system, posterior tibial nerve, use 0587T)

Surgical Procedures on the Extracranial Nerves, Peripheral Nerves, and Autonomic Nervous System

(For intracranial surgery on cranial nerves, see 61450, 61460, 61790)

AMA *CPT Assistant* □

64553: Nov 99: 38, Apr 01: 9, Oct 18: 8

Plain English Description

When implanting a neurostimulator electrode array, the exact procedure depends on which of the cranial nerves is being stimulated. One of the more common sites is the vagus nerve to help control epileptic seizures. For percutaneous vagus nerve neurostimulator electrode array placement, the planned insertion site in the neck is prepped. Anatomical landmarks are located and separately reportable ultrasound guidance is used as needed to facilitate correct placement of the electrodes. An electrically insulated needle is inserted into the side of the neck and advanced parallel to the vagus nerve until it is positioned near the carotid sheath. A power source is connected to the needle, stimulation is applied, and motor and sensory responses are evaluated as the position of the needle is changed until the desired response is achieved. The needle is disconnected from the power source. An electrode array is then passed through the lumen of the needle and positioned in the desired location next to the vagus nerve. The needle is removed, leaving the electrode array in place, which is then attached to an external generator/receiver.

Percutaneous implantation of neurostimulator electrode array; cranial nerve

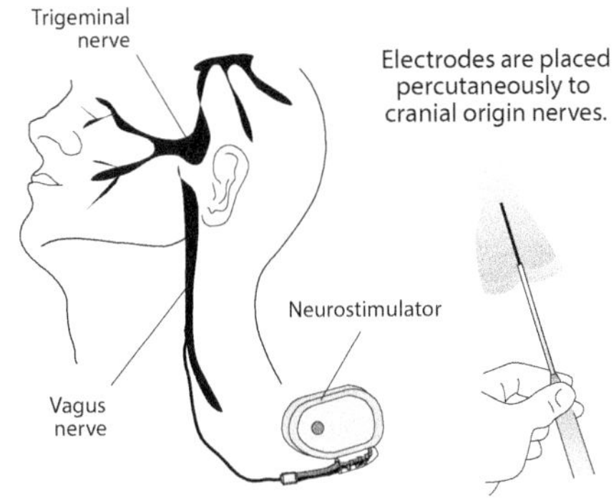

ICD-10-CM Diagnostic Codes

	Code	Description
	B02.21	Postherpetic geniculate ganglionitis
	B02.22	Postherpetic trigeminal neuralgia
	F31.32	Bipolar disorder, current episode depressed, moderate
	F31.4	Bipolar disorder, current episode depressed, severe, without psychotic features
	F31.75	Bipolar disorder, in partial remission, most recent episode depressed
	F32.1	Major depressive disorder, single episode, moderate
	F32.2	Major depressive disorder, single episode, severe without psychotic features
	F32.4	Major depressive disorder, single episode, in partial remission
	F33.1	Major depressive disorder, recurrent, moderate
	F33.2	Major depressive disorder, recurrent severe without psychotic features
	F33.41	Major depressive disorder, recurrent, in partial remission
	G40.011	Localization-related (focal) (partial) idiopathic epilepsy and epileptic syndromes with seizures of localized onset, intractable, with status epilepticus
	G40.019	Localization-related (focal) (partial) idiopathic epilepsy and epileptic syndromes with seizures of localized onset, intractable, without status epilepticus
	G40.111	Localization-related (focal) (partial) symptomatic epilepsy and epileptic syndromes with simple partial seizures, intractable, with status epilepticus
	G40.119	Localization-related (focal) (partial) symptomatic epilepsy and epileptic syndromes with simple partial seizures, intractable, without status epilepticus
	G40.211	Localization-related (focal) (partial) symptomatic epilepsy and epileptic syndromes with complex partial seizures, intractable, with status epilepticus
	G40.219	Localization-related (focal) (partial) symptomatic epilepsy and epileptic syndromes with complex partial seizures, intractable, without status epilepticus
	G47.33	Obstructive sleep apnea (adult) (pediatric)
	G50.0	Trigeminal neuralgia
	G50.1	Atypical facial pain
	G50.8	Other disorders of trigeminal nerve
	G50.9	Disorder of trigeminal nerve, unspecified
	G51.0	Bell's palsy
	G51.1	Geniculate ganglionitis
⇄	G51.31	Clonic hemifacial spasm, right
⇄	G51.32	Clonic hemifacial spasm, left
⇄	G51.33	Clonic hemifacial spasm, bilateral
	G52.1	Disorders of glossopharyngeal nerve
	G52.2	Disorders of vagus nerve
	G52.3	Disorders of hypoglossal nerve
	R56.9	Unspecified convulsions

CCI Edits

Refer to Appendix A for CCI edits.

Facility RVUs □

Code	Work	PE Facility	MP	Total Facility
64553	6.13	3.26	0.90	10.29

Non-facility RVUs □

Code	Work	PE Non-Facility	MP	Total Non-Facility
64553	6.13	50.47	0.90	57.50

Modifiers (PAR) □

Code	Mod 50	Mod 51	Mod 62	Mod 66	Mod 80
64553	0	2	0	0	0

Global Period

Code	Days
64553	010

64555

64555 Percutaneous implantation of neurostimulator electrode array; peripheral nerve (excludes sacral nerve)

(Do not report 64555 in conjunction with 64566)

(For percutaneous electrical stimulation of a peripheral nerve using needle[s] or needle electrode[s] [eg, PENS, PNT], use 64999)

AMA Coding Guideline

Neurostimulator Procedures on the Peripheral Nerves

For electronic analysis with programming, when performed, of peripheral nerve neurostimulator pulse generator/transmitters, see codes 95970, 95971, 95972. An electrode array is a catheter or other device with more than one contact. The function of each contact may be capable of being adjusted during programming services. Test stimulation to confirm correct target site placement of the electrode array(s) and/or to confirm the functional status of the system is inherent to placement, and is not separately reported as electronic analysis or programming of the neurostimulator system. Electronic analysis (95970) at the time of implantation is not separately reported.

Codes 64553, 64555, and 64561 may be used to report both temporary and permanent placement of percutaneous electrode arrays.

AMA Coding Notes

Neurostimulator Procedures on the Peripheral Nerves

(For transcutaneous nerve stimulation [TENS], use 97014 for electrical stimulation requiring supervision only or use 97032 for electrical stimulation requiring constant attendance)

(For percutaneous implantation or replacement of integrated neurostimulation system, posterior tibial nerve, use 0587T)

Surgical Procedures on the Extracranial Nerves, Peripheral Nerves, and Autonomic Nervous System

(For intracranial surgery on cranial nerves, see 61450, 61460, 61790)

AMA *CPT Assistant* ☐

64555: Jan 15: 14, Feb 16: 13, Dec 17: 16, Aug 18: 10, Oct 18: 8

Plain English Description

When implanting a neurostimulator electrode array, the exact procedure depends on which of the peripheral nerves is being stimulated. The planned insertion site is prepared. Anatomical landmarks are located and separately reportable ultrasound guidance is used as needed to facilitate correct placement of the electrodes. An electrically insulated needle is inserted into the skin and advanced parallel to the peripheral nerve. A power source is connected to the needle, stimulation is applied, and motor and sensory responses are evaluated as the position of the needle is changed until the desired response is achieved. The needle is disconnected from the power source. An electrode array is then passed through the lumen of the needle and positioned in the desired location next to the peripheral nerve. The needle is removed, leaving the electrode array in place, which is then attached to an external generator/receiver.

Percutaneous implantation of neurostimulator electrode array; peripheral nerve

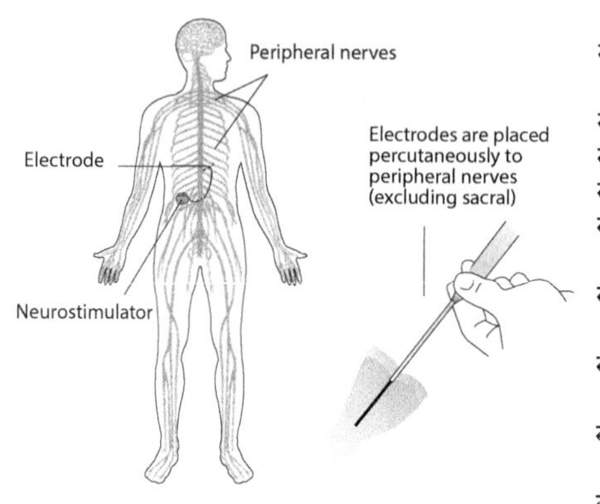

ICD-10-CM Diagnostic Codes

	Code	Description
	B02.29	Other postherpetic nervous system involvement
	G43.011	Migraine without aura, intractable, with status migrainosus
	G43.019	Migraine without aura, intractable, without status migrainosus
	G43.111	Migraine with aura, intractable, with status migrainosus
	G43.119	Migraine with aura, intractable, without status migrainosus
	G43.411	Hemiplegic migraine, intractable, with status migrainosus
	G43.419	Hemiplegic migraine, intractable, without status migrainosus
	G43.511	Persistent migraine aura without cerebral infarction, intractable, with status migrainosus
	G43.519	Persistent migraine aura without cerebral infarction, intractable, without status migrainosus
	G43.711	Chronic migraine without aura, intractable, with status migrainosus
	G43.719	Chronic migraine without aura, intractable, without status migrainosus
	G43.811	Other migraine, intractable, with status migrainosus
	G43.819	Other migraine, intractable, without status migrainosus
	G43.911	Migraine, unspecified, intractable, with status migrainosus
	G43.919	Migraine, unspecified, intractable, without status migrainosus
	G43.A1	Cyclical vomiting, in migraine, intractable
	G43.C1	Periodic headache syndromes in child or adult, intractable
	G44.001	Cluster headache syndrome, unspecified, intractable
	G44.011	Episodic cluster headache, intractable
	G44.021	Chronic cluster headache, intractable
	G44.031	Episodic paroxysmal hemicrania, intractable
	G44.041	Chronic paroxysmal hemicrania, intractable
	G54.6	Phantom limb syndrome with pain
⇄	G56.31	Lesion of radial nerve, right upper limb
⇄	G56.32	Lesion of radial nerve, left upper limb
⇄	G56.33	Lesion of radial nerve, bilateral upper limbs
⇄	G56.41	Causalgia of right upper limb
⇄	G56.42	Causalgia of left upper limb
⇄	G56.43	Causalgia of bilateral upper limbs
⇄	G56.81	Other specified mononeuropathies of right upper limb
⇄	G56.82	Other specified mononeuropathies of left upper limb
⇄	G56.83	Other specified mononeuropathies of bilateral upper limbs
⇄	G57.01	Lesion of sciatic nerve, right lower limb
⇄	G57.02	Lesion of sciatic nerve, left lower limb
⇄	G57.03	Lesion of sciatic nerve, bilateral lower limbs
⇄	G57.11	Meralgia paresthetica, right lower limb
⇄	G57.12	Meralgia paresthetica, left lower limb
⇄	G57.13	Meralgia paresthetica, bilateral lower limbs
⇄	G57.21	Lesion of femoral nerve, right lower limb
⇄	G57.22	Lesion of femoral nerve, left lower limb
⇄	G57.23	Lesion of femoral nerve, bilateral lower limbs
⇄	G57.31	Lesion of lateral popliteal nerve, right lower limb
⇄	G57.32	Lesion of lateral popliteal nerve, left lower limb
⇄	G57.33	Lesion of lateral popliteal nerve, bilateral lower limbs
⇄	G57.41	Lesion of medial popliteal nerve, right lower limb
⇄	G57.42	Lesion of medial popliteal nerve, left lower limb
⇄	G57.43	Lesion of medial popliteal nerve, bilateral lower limbs
⇄	G57.71	Causalgia of right lower limb
⇄	G57.72	Causalgia of left lower limb
⇄	G57.73	Causalgia of bilateral lower limbs
⇄	G57.81	Other specified mononeuropathies of right lower limb
⇄	G57.82	Other specified mononeuropathies of left lower limb
⇄	G57.83	Other specified mononeuropathies of bilateral lower limbs

	G58.0	Intercostal neuropathy
	G58.9	Mononeuropathy, unspecified
	G89.21	Chronic pain due to trauma
	G89.22	Chronic post-thoracotomy pain
	G89.28	Other chronic postprocedural pain
	G89.29	Other chronic pain
⇄	G90.511	Complex regional pain syndrome I of right upper limb
⇄	G90.512	Complex regional pain syndrome I of left upper limb
⇄	G90.513	Complex regional pain syndrome I of upper limb, bilateral
⇄	G90.521	Complex regional pain syndrome I of right lower limb
⇄	G90.522	Complex regional pain syndrome I of left lower limb
⇄	G90.523	Complex regional pain syndrome I of lower limb, bilateral
	M54.81	Occipital neuralgia
	M79.2	Neuralgia and neuritis, unspecified
⇄	M79.601	Pain in right arm
⇄	M79.602	Pain in left arm
⇄	M79.604	Pain in right leg
⇄	M79.605	Pain in left leg
7 ⇄	S54.21	Injury of radial nerve at forearm level, right arm
7 ⇄	S54.22	Injury of radial nerve at forearm level, left arm
7 ⇄	S64.21	Injury of radial nerve at wrist and hand level of right arm
7 ⇄	S64.22	Injury of radial nerve at wrist and hand level of left arm
7 ⇄	S74.01	Injury of sciatic nerve at hip and thigh level, right leg
7 ⇄	S74.02	Injury of sciatic nerve at hip and thigh level, left leg
7 ⇄	S74.11	Injury of femoral nerve at hip and thigh level, right leg
7 ⇄	S74.12	Injury of femoral nerve at hip and thigh level, left leg
7 ⇄	S84.01	Injury of tibial nerve at lower leg level, right leg
7 ⇄	S84.02	Injury of tibial nerve at lower leg level, left leg
7 ⇄	S84.11	Injury of peroneal nerve at lower leg level, right leg
7 ⇄	S84.12	Injury of peroneal nerve at lower leg level, left leg
7 ⇄	S94.21	Injury of deep peroneal nerve at ankle and foot level, right leg
7 ⇄	S94.22	Injury of deep peroneal nerve at ankle and foot level, left leg

ICD-10-CM Coding Notes

For codes requiring a 7th character extension, refer to your ICD-10-CM book. Review the character descriptions and coding guidelines for proper selection. For some procedures, only certain characters will apply.

CCI Edits

Refer to Appendix A for CCI edits.

Pub 100

64555: Pub 100-03, 1, 160.7-160.7.1

Facility RVUs ▯

Code	Work	PE Facility	MP	Total Facility
64555	5.76	3.32	0.79	9.87

Non-facility RVUs ▯

Code	Work	PE Non-Facility	MP	Total Non-Facility
64555	5.76	46.70	0.79	53.25

Modifiers (PAR) ▯

Code	Mod 50	Mod 51	Mod 62	Mod 66	Mod 80
64555	0	2	0	0	1

Global Period

Code	Days
64555	010

64566

64566 Posterior tibial neurostimulation, percutaneous needle electrode, single treatment, includes programming

(Do not report 64566 in conjunction with 64555, 95970-95972)

AMA Coding Guideline

Neurostimulator Procedures on the Peripheral Nerves

For electronic analysis with programming, when performed, of peripheral nerve neurostimulator pulse generator/transmitters, see codes 95970, 95971, 95972. An electrode array is a catheter or other device with more than one contact. The function of each contact may be capable of being adjusted during programming services. Test stimulation to confirm correct target site placement of the electrode array(s) and/or to confirm the functional status of the system is inherent to placement, and is not separately reported as electronic analysis or programming of the neurostimulator system. Electronic analysis (95970) at the time of implantation is not separately reported.

Codes 64553, 64555, and 64561 may be used to report both temporary and permanent placement of percutaneous electrode arrays.

AMA Coding Notes

Neurostimulator Procedures on the Peripheral Nerves

(For transcutaneous nerve stimulation [TENS], use 97014 for electrical stimulation requiring supervision only or use 97032 for electrical stimulation requiring constant attendance)

(For percutaneous implantation or replacement of integrated neurostimulation system, posterior tibial nerve, use 0587T)

Surgical Procedures on the Extracranial Nerves, Peripheral Nerves, and Autonomic Nervous System

(For intracranial surgery on cranial nerves, see 61450, 61460, 61790)

AMA *CPT Assistant* ▢

64566: Feb 11: 5, Sep 11: 8

Plain English Description

Posterior tibial neurostimulation is used to treat overactive bladder, urge incontinence, and the symptom of frequent urination in patients who have failed other treatment modalities. The posterior tibial nerve located near the ankle is a branch derived from the sacral nerve plexus, the nerves responsible for bladder and pelvic floor function. Neuromodulation of the posterior tibial nerve sends mild electrical impulses to stimulate the sacral nerve plexus, thereby improving voiding function and control. The patient's foot is comfortably elevated and supported. The skin just above the ankle over the tibial nerve is cleansed. The neurostimulator is programmed. A fine-needle electrode is inserted adjacent to the nerve and low-voltage electrical stimulation is delivered using the prescribed voltage for the prescribed amount of time. This code reports a single treatment session. Most patients receive once-a-week sessions over a 10- to 12-week period.

Posterior tibial neurostimulation, single treatment

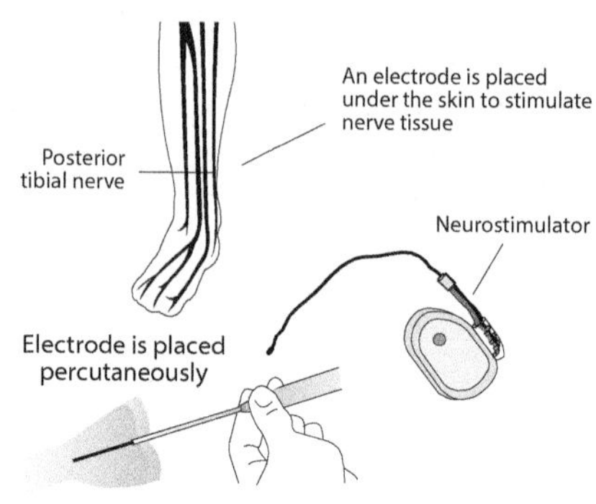

ICD-10-CM Diagnostic Codes

N32.81	Overactive bladder
N39.41	Urge incontinence
R35.0	Frequency of micturition
R39.15	Urgency of urination

CCI Edits

Refer to Appendix A for CCI edits.

Facility RVUs ▢

Code	Work	PE Facility	MP	Total Facility
64566	0.60	0.21	0.09	0.90

Non-facility RVUs ▢

Code	Work	PE Non-Facility	MP	Total Non-Facility
64566	0.60	2.90	0.09	3.59

Modifiers (PAR) ▢

Code	Mod 50	Mod 51	Mod 62	Mod 66	Mod 80
64566	0	2	0	0	0

Global Period

Code	Days
64566	000

64568

64568 Incision for implantation of cranial nerve (eg, vagus nerve) neurostimulator electrode array and pulse generator

(Do not report 64568 in conjunction with 61885, 61886, 64570)

(For insertion of chest wall respiratory sensor electrode or electrode array, including connection to pulse generator, use 0466T)

AMA Coding Guideline

Neurostimulator Procedures on the Peripheral Nerves

For electronic analysis with programming, when performed, of peripheral nerve neurostimulator pulse generator/transmitters, see codes 95970, 95971, 95972. An electrode array is a catheter or other device with more than one contact. The function of each contact may be capable of being adjusted during programming services. Test stimulation to confirm correct target site placement of the electrode array(s) and/or to confirm the functional status of the system is inherent to placement, and is not separately reported as electronic analysis or programming of the neurostimulator system. Electronic analysis (95970) at the time of implantation is not separately reported.

Codes 64553, 64555, and 64561 may be used to report both temporary and permanent placement of percutaneous electrode arrays.

AMA Coding Notes

Neurostimulator Procedures on the Peripheral Nerves

(For transcutaneous nerve stimulation [TENS], use 97014 for electrical stimulation requiring supervision only or use 97032 for electrical stimulation requiring constant attendance)

(For percutaneous implantation or replacement of integrated neurostimulation system, posterior tibial nerve, use 0587T)

Surgical Procedures on the Extracranial Nerves, Peripheral Nerves, and Autonomic Nervous System

(For intracranial surgery on cranial nerves, see 61450, 61460, 61790)

AMA *CPT Assistant*

64568: Feb 11: 5, Sep 11: 8, 10, 12, Nov 16: 6, Mar 18: 9

Plain English Description

For placement of a neurostimulator electrode array and pulse generator, the exact implantation procedure depends on which cranial nerve is being stimulated. One of the more common sites for electrode placement is the vagus nerve to help control epileptic seizures. For open vagus nerve neurostimulator electrode array placement, the planned insertion site in the neck is prepped. The skin is incised and soft tissues are dissected to expose the vagus nerve and carotid artery sheath. The electrode array is then positioned in the desired location next to the vagus nerve. The electrode array is connected to a power source; stimulation is applied; and motor responses are evaluated. The electrode array is repositioned and retested until the desired responses are attained. The electrodes are then secured in place. An incision is made in the skin and a subcutaneous pocket is developed. The pulse generator is placed in the subcutaneous pocket. The electrode array wires are tunneled to the generator and connected. The generator and leads are tested and the pocket is closed. Tissues in the neck are closed in layers over the electrode array.

Implantation of cranial nerve neurostimulator

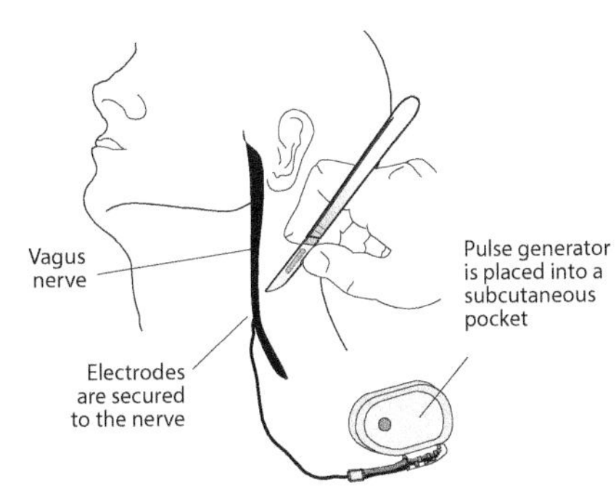

ICD-10-CM Diagnostic Codes

	Code	Description
	B02.21	Postherpetic geniculate ganglionitis
	B02.22	Postherpetic trigeminal neuralgia
	F31.32	Bipolar disorder, current episode depressed, moderate
	F31.4	Bipolar disorder, current episode depressed, severe, without psychotic features
	F31.75	Bipolar disorder, in partial remission, most recent episode depressed
	F32.1	Major depressive disorder, single episode, moderate
	F32.2	Major depressive disorder, single episode, severe without psychotic features
	F32.4	Major depressive disorder, single episode, in partial remission
	F33.1	Major depressive disorder, recurrent, moderate
	F33.2	Major depressive disorder, recurrent severe without psychotic features
	F33.41	Major depressive disorder, recurrent, in partial remission
	G40.011	Localization-related (focal) (partial) idiopathic epilepsy and epileptic syndromes with seizures of localized onset, intractable, with status epilepticus
	G40.019	Localization-related (focal) (partial) idiopathic epilepsy and epileptic syndromes with seizures of localized onset, intractable, without status epilepticus
	G40.111	Localization-related (focal) (partial) symptomatic epilepsy and epileptic syndromes with simple partial seizures, intractable, with status epilepticus
	G40.119	Localization-related (focal) (partial) symptomatic epilepsy and epileptic syndromes with simple partial seizures, intractable, without status epilepticus
	G40.211	Localization-related (focal) (partial) symptomatic epilepsy and epileptic syndromes with complex partial seizures, intractable, with status epilepticus
	G40.219	Localization-related (focal) (partial) symptomatic epilepsy and epileptic syndromes with complex partial seizures, intractable, without status epilepticus
	G47.33	Obstructive sleep apnea (adult) (pediatric)
	G50.0	Trigeminal neuralgia
	G50.1	Atypical facial pain
	G50.8	Other disorders of trigeminal nerve
	G50.9	Disorder of trigeminal nerve, unspecified
	G51.0	Bell's palsy
	G51.1	Geniculate ganglionitis
⇄	G51.31	Clonic hemifacial spasm, right
⇄	G51.32	Clonic hemifacial spasm, left
⇄	G51.33	Clonic hemifacial spasm, bilateral
	G52.1	Disorders of glossopharyngeal nerve
	G52.2	Disorders of vagus nerve
	G52.3	Disorders of hypoglossal nerve
	R56.9	Unspecified convulsions

CCI Edits

Refer to Appendix A for CCI edits.

Facility RVUs

Code	Work	PE Facility	MP	Total Facility
64568	9.00	6.73	2.33	18.06

Non-facility RVUs

Code	Work	PE Non-Facility	MP	Total Non-Facility
64568	9.00	6.73	2.33	18.06

Modifiers (PAR)

Code	Mod 50	Mod 51	Mod 62	Mod 66	Mod 80
64568	1	2	0	0	0

Global Period

Code	Days
64568	090

64569-64570

64569 Revision or replacement of cranial nerve (eg, vagus nerve) neurostimulator electrode array, including connection to existing pulse generator

(Do not report 64569 in conjunction with 64570 or 61888)

(For replacement of pulse generator, use 61885)

(For revision or replacement of chest wall respiratory sensor electrode or electrode array, including connection to existing pulse generator, use 0467T)

64570 Removal of cranial nerve (eg, vagus nerve) neurostimulator electrode array and pulse generator

(Do not report 64570 in conjunction with 61888)

(For laparoscopic implantation, revision, replacement, or removal of vagus nerve blocking neurostimulator electrode array and/or pulse generator at the esophagogastric junction, see 0312T-0317T)

(For removal of chest wall respiratory sensor electrode or electrode array, use 0468T)

AMA Coding Guideline

Neurostimulator Procedures on the Peripheral Nerves

For electronic analysis with programming, when performed, of peripheral nerve neurostimulator pulse generator/transmitters, see codes 95970, 95971, 95972. An electrode array is a catheter or other device with more than one contact. The function of each contact may be capable of being adjusted during programming services. Test stimulation to confirm correct target site placement of the electrode array(s) and/or to confirm the functional status of the system is inherent to placement, and is not separately reported as electronic analysis or programming of the neurostimulator system. Electronic analysis (95970) at the time of implantation is not separately reported.

Codes 64553, 64555, and 64561 may be used to report both temporary and permanent placement of percutaneous electrode arrays.

AMA Coding Notes

Neurostimulator Procedures on the Peripheral Nerves

(For transcutaneous nerve stimulation [TENS], use 97014 for electrical stimulation requiring supervision only or use 97032 for electrical stimulation requiring constant attendance)

(For percutaneous implantation or replacement of integrated neurostimulation system, posterior tibial nerve, use 0587T)

Surgical Procedures on the Extracranial Nerves, Peripheral Nerves, and Autonomic Nervous System

(For intracranial surgery on cranial nerves, see 61450, 61460, 61790)

AMA *CPT Assistant* ☐

64569: Feb 11: 5, Sep 11: 8, Nov 16: 6, Mar 18: 9

64570: Feb 11: 5, Sep 11: 10, Nov 16: 6, Mar 18: 9

Plain English Description

A neurostimulator electrode array is revised/replaced (64569) or removed along with the pulse generator (64570). The exact procedure depends on which cranial nerve is being stimulated. One of the more common sites for electrode placement is the vagus nerve to help control epileptic seizures. In 64569, the skin is incised and soft tissues are dissected to expose the electrode array and/or the pulse generator. Defective components are repaired or the array is replaced. The electrode array is then placed in the desired location next to the vagus nerve. The new or repaired electrode array is connected to the power source; stimulation is applied; and motor responses are evaluated. The electrode array is repositioned and retested until the desired responses are attained. The electrode array is then secured in place. If a new electrode array has been implanted, the electrode array wires are tunneled to the generator and connected. The generator and leads are tested and the pocket is then closed. Tissues in the neck are closed in layers over the electrode array. In 64570, the electrode array and pulse generator are exposed. The generator is detached from the array wires. The generator is removed and the subcutaneous pocket is closed. The electrode array is dissected free of surrounding tissues and the array and wires are removed. Incisions are closed.

Removal/revision/replacement, cranial neurostimulator

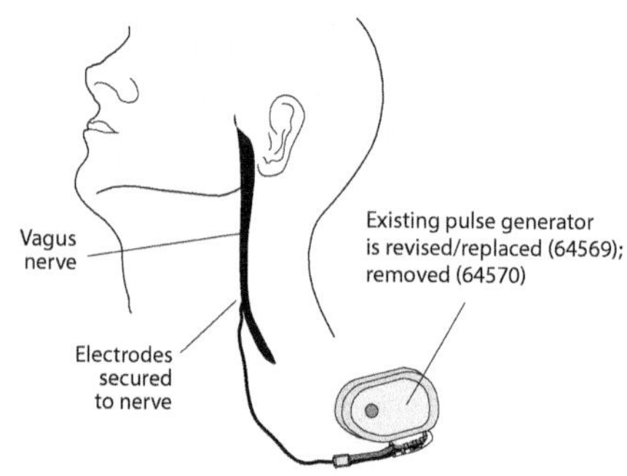

ICD-10-CM Diagnostic Codes

➐	T85.111	Breakdown (mechanical) of implanted electronic neurostimulator of peripheral nerve electrode (lead)
➐	T85.121	Displacement of implanted electronic neurostimulator of peripheral nerve electrode (lead)
➐	T85.191	Other mechanical complication of implanted electronic neurostimulator of peripheral nerve electrode (lead)
➐	T85.732	Infection and inflammatory reaction due to implanted electronic neurostimulator of peripheral nerve, electrode (lead)
➐	T85.820	Fibrosis due to nervous system prosthetic devices, implants and grafts
➐	T85.830	Hemorrhage due to nervous system prosthetic devices, implants and grafts
➐	T85.840	Pain due to nervous system prosthetic devices, implants and grafts
➐	T85.890	Other specified complication of nervous system prosthetic devices, implants and grafts
	Z45.42	Encounter for adjustment and management of neurostimulator
	Z45.49	Encounter for adjustment and management of other implanted nervous system device

ICD-10-CM Coding Notes

For codes requiring a 7th character extension, refer to your ICD-10-CM book. Review the character descriptions and coding guidelines for proper selection. For some procedures, only certain characters will apply.

CCI Edits

Refer to Appendix A for CCI edits.

Facility RVUs ☐

Code	Work	PE Facility	MP	Total Facility
64569	11.00	7.65	3.25	21.90
64570	9.10	8.62	3.36	21.08

Non-facility RVUs ☐

Code	Work	PE Non-Facility	MP	Total Non-Facility
64569	11.00	7.65	3.25	21.90
64570	9.10	8.62	3.36	21.08

Modifiers (PAR) ☐

Code	Mod 50	Mod 51	Mod 62	Mod 66	Mod 80
64569	1	2	1	1	0
64570	1	2	1	1	0

Global Period

Code	Days
64569	090
64570	090

64575

64575 Incision for implantation of neurostimulator electrode array; peripheral nerve (excludes sacral nerve)

AMA Coding Guideline

Neurostimulator Procedures on the Peripheral Nerves

For electronic analysis with programming, when performed, of peripheral nerve neurostimulator pulse generator/transmitters, see codes 95970, 95971, 95972. An electrode array is a catheter or other device with more than one contact. The function of each contact may be capable of being adjusted during programming services. Test stimulation to confirm correct target site placement of the electrode array(s) and/or to confirm the functional status of the system is inherent to placement, and is not separately reported as electronic analysis or programming of the neurostimulator system. Electronic analysis (95970) at the time of implantation is not separately reported.

Codes 64553, 64555, and 64561 may be used to report both temporary and permanent placement of percutaneous electrode arrays.

AMA Coding Notes

Neurostimulator Procedures on the Peripheral Nerves

(For transcutaneous nerve stimulation [TENS], use 97014 for electrical stimulation requiring supervision only or use 97032 for electrical stimulation requiring constant attendance)

(For percutaneous implantation or replacement of integrated neurostimulation system, posterior tibial nerve, use 0587T)

Surgical Procedures on the Extracranial Nerves, Peripheral Nerves, and Autonomic Nervous System

(For intracranial surgery on cranial nerves, see 61450, 61460, 61790)

Plain English Description

For placement of a neurostimulator electrode array, the exact procedure depends on which peripheral nerve is being stimulated. For open placement of a peripheral nerve neurostimulator electrode array, the planned insertion site is prepared and the skin is incised. Soft tissues are dissected to expose the targeted peripheral nerve. An electrode array is then positioned in the desired location next to the peripheral nerve and connected to a power source. Stimulation is applied and motor responses are evaluated. The electrode array is repositioned and retested until the desired responses are attained. The electrode array is then secured and tunneled to the generator/receiver, which is implanted in a separately reportable procedure. Tissues are closed in layers over the electrode array.

Incision for implantation of peripheral nerve neurostimulator electrode array (excludes sacral nerve)

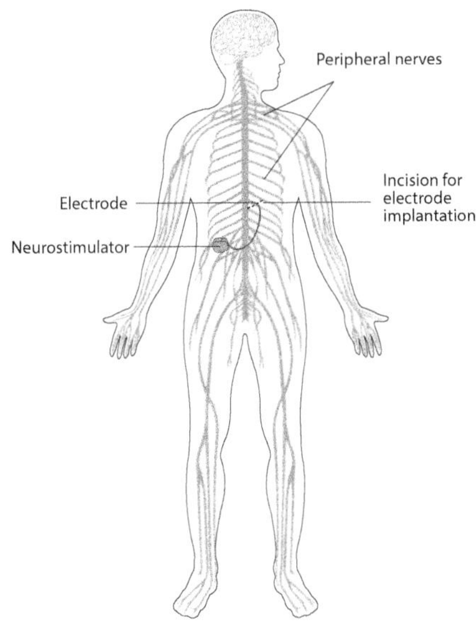

ICD-10-CM Diagnostic Codes

	Code	Description
	B02.29	Other postherpetic nervous system involvement
	G43.011	Migraine without aura, intractable, with status migrainosus
	G43.019	Migraine without aura, intractable, without status migrainosus
	G43.111	Migraine with aura, intractable, with status migrainosus
	G43.119	Migraine with aura, intractable, without status migrainosus
	G43.411	Hemiplegic migraine, intractable, with status migrainosus
	G43.419	Hemiplegic migraine, intractable, without status migrainosus
	G43.511	Persistent migraine aura without cerebral infarction, intractable, with status migrainosus
	G43.519	Persistent migraine aura without cerebral infarction, intractable, without status migrainosus
	G43.711	Chronic migraine without aura, intractable, with status migrainosus
	G43.719	Chronic migraine without aura, intractable, without status migrainosus
	G43.811	Other migraine, intractable, with status migrainosus
	G43.819	Other migraine, intractable, without status migrainosus
	G43.911	Migraine, unspecified, intractable, with status migrainosus
	G43.919	Migraine, unspecified, intractable, without status migrainosus
	G43.A1	Cyclical vomiting, in migraine, intractable
	G43.C1	Periodic headache syndromes in child or adult, intractable
	G44.001	Cluster headache syndrome, unspecified, intractable
	G44.011	Episodic cluster headache, intractable
	G44.021	Chronic cluster headache, intractable
	G44.031	Episodic paroxysmal hemicrania, intractable
	G44.041	Chronic paroxysmal hemicrania, intractable
	G54.6	Phantom limb syndrome with pain
⇄	G56.11	Other lesions of median nerve, right upper limb
⇄	G56.12	Other lesions of median nerve, left upper limb
⇄	G56.13	Other lesions of median nerve, bilateral upper limbs
⇄	G56.21	Lesion of ulnar nerve, right upper limb
⇄	G56.22	Lesion of ulnar nerve, left upper limb
⇄	G56.23	Lesion of ulnar nerve, bilateral upper limbs
⇄	G56.31	Lesion of radial nerve, right upper limb
⇄	G56.32	Lesion of radial nerve, left upper limb
⇄	G56.33	Lesion of radial nerve, bilateral upper limbs
⇄	G56.41	Causalgia of right upper limb
⇄	G56.42	Causalgia of left upper limb
⇄	G56.43	Causalgia of bilateral upper limbs
⇄	G56.81	Other specified mononeuropathies of right upper limb
⇄	G56.82	Other specified mononeuropathies of left upper limb
⇄	G56.83	Other specified mononeuropathies of bilateral upper limbs
⇄	G57.01	Lesion of sciatic nerve, right lower limb
⇄	G57.02	Lesion of sciatic nerve, left lower limb
⇄	G57.03	Lesion of sciatic nerve, bilateral lower limbs
⇄	G57.11	Meralgia paresthetica, right lower limb
⇄	G57.12	Meralgia paresthetica, left lower limb
⇄	G57.13	Meralgia paresthetica, bilateral lower limbs
⇄	G57.21	Lesion of femoral nerve, right lower limb
⇄	G57.22	Lesion of femoral nerve, left lower limb
⇄	G57.23	Lesion of femoral nerve, bilateral lower limbs
⇄	G57.31	Lesion of lateral popliteal nerve, right lower limb
⇄	G57.32	Lesion of lateral popliteal nerve, left lower limb
⇄	G57.33	Lesion of lateral popliteal nerve, bilateral lower limbs
⇄	G57.41	Lesion of medial popliteal nerve, right lower limb
⇄	G57.42	Lesion of medial popliteal nerve, left lower limb
⇄	G57.43	Lesion of medial popliteal nerve, bilateral lower limbs
⇄	G57.71	Causalgia of right lower limb
⇄	G57.72	Causalgia of left lower limb
⇄	G57.73	Causalgia of bilateral lower limbs
⇄	G57.81	Other specified mononeuropathies of right lower limb

CPT® Procedural Coding

⇄	G57.82	Other specified mononeuropathies of left lower limb
⇄	G57.83	Other specified mononeuropathies of bilateral lower limbs
	G58.0	Intercostal neuropathy
	G58.9	Mononeuropathy, unspecified
	G89.21	Chronic pain due to trauma
	G89.22	Chronic post-thoracotomy pain
	G89.28	Other chronic postprocedural pain
	G89.29	Other chronic pain
⇄	G90.511	Complex regional pain syndrome I of right upper limb
⇄	G90.512	Complex regional pain syndrome I of left upper limb
⇄	G90.513	Complex regional pain syndrome I of upper limb, bilateral
⇄	G90.521	Complex regional pain syndrome I of right lower limb
⇄	G90.522	Complex regional pain syndrome I of left lower limb
⇄	G90.523	Complex regional pain syndrome I of lower limb, bilateral
	G90.8	Other disorders of autonomic nervous system
	M54.81	Occipital neuralgia
	M79.2	Neuralgia and neuritis, unspecified
⇄	M79.601	Pain in right arm
⇄	M79.602	Pain in left arm
⇄	M79.604	Pain in right leg
⇄	M79.605	Pain in left leg
❼⇄	S54.21	Injury of radial nerve at forearm level, right arm
❼⇄	S54.22	Injury of radial nerve at forearm level, left arm
❼⇄	S64.21	Injury of radial nerve at wrist and hand level of right arm
❼⇄	S64.22	Injury of radial nerve at wrist and hand level of left arm
❼⇄	S74.01	Injury of sciatic nerve at hip and thigh level, right leg
❼⇄	S74.02	Injury of sciatic nerve at hip and thigh level, left leg
❼⇄	S74.11	Injury of femoral nerve at hip and thigh level, right leg
❼⇄	S74.12	Injury of femoral nerve at hip and thigh level, left leg
❼⇄	S84.01	Injury of tibial nerve at lower leg level, right leg
❼⇄	S84.02	Injury of tibial nerve at lower leg level, left leg
❼⇄	S84.11	Injury of peroneal nerve at lower leg level, right leg
❼⇄	S84.12	Injury of peroneal nerve at lower leg level, left leg
❼⇄	S94.21	Injury of deep peroneal nerve at ankle and foot level, right leg
❼⇄	S94.22	Injury of deep peroneal nerve at ankle and foot level, left leg

ICD-10-CM Coding Notes

For codes requiring a 7th character extension, refer to your ICD-10-CM book. Review the character descriptions and coding guidelines for proper selection. For some procedures, only certain characters will apply.

CCI Edits

Refer to Appendix A for CCI edits.

Pub 100

64575: Pub 100-03, 1, 160.19, Pub 100-03, 1, 160.26, Pub 100-03, 1, 160.7-160.7.1

Facility RVUs ☐

Code	Work	PE Facility	MP	Total Facility
64575	4.42	4.31	1.07	9.80

Non-facility RVUs ☐

Code	Work	PE Non-Facility	MP	Total Non-Facility
64575	4.42	4.31	1.07	9.80

Modifiers (PAR) ☐

Code	Mod 50	Mod 51	Mod 62	Mod 66	Mod 80
64575	0	2	0	0	1

Global Period

Code	Days
64575	090

64585

64585 Revision or removal of peripheral neurostimulator electrode array

AMA Coding Guideline

Neurostimulator Procedures on the Peripheral Nerves

For electronic analysis with programming, when performed, of peripheral nerve neurostimulator pulse generator/transmitters, see codes 95970, 95971, 95972. An electrode array is a catheter or other device with more than one contact. The function of each contact may be capable of being adjusted during programming services. Test stimulation to confirm correct target site placement of the electrode array(s) and/or to confirm the functional status of the system is inherent to placement, and is not separately reported as electronic analysis or programming of the neurostimulator system. Electronic analysis (95970) at the time of implantation is not separately reported.

Codes 64553, 64555, and 64561 may be used to report both temporary and permanent placement of percutaneous electrode arrays.

AMA Coding Notes

Neurostimulator Procedures on the Peripheral Nerves

(For transcutaneous nerve stimulation [TENS], use 97014 for electrical stimulation requiring supervision only or use 97032 for electrical stimulation requiring constant attendance)

(For percutaneous implantation or replacement of integrated neurostimulation system, posterior tibial nerve, use 0587T)

Surgical Procedures on the Extracranial Nerves, Peripheral Nerves, and Autonomic Nervous System

(For intracranial surgery on cranial nerves, see 61450, 61460, 61790)

Plain English Description

The exact revision or removal procedure depends on the location of the existing peripheral neurostimulator electrode array. A skin incision is made over the existing array. Soft tissues are dissected and the electrode array is exposed. The device is inspected and detached from the generator/receiver. The array is tested and any malfunctioning components are replaced. The array is then positioned in the desired location next to the peripheral nerve. Correct placement is verified by testing motor response to stimulation. The electrode array is reconnected to the generator/receiver. Alternatively, the array may be removed and the surgical wound closed in layers.

Revision or removal of peripheral neurostimulator electrode array

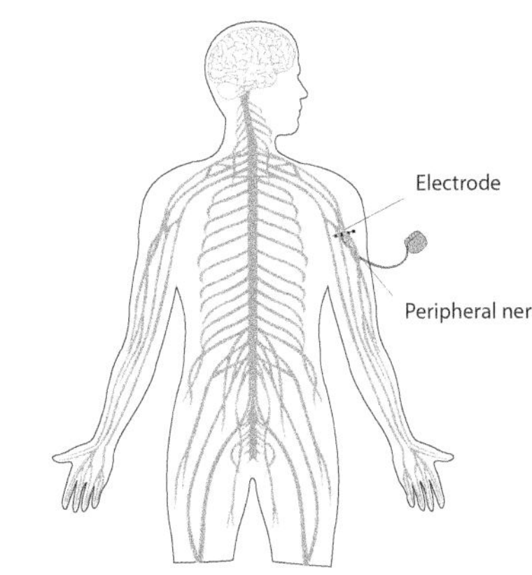

The electrodes used to stimulate the peripheral nervous tissues are removed or revised.

ICD-10-CM Diagnostic Codes

	Code	Description
⓻	T85.111	Breakdown (mechanical) of implanted electronic neurostimulator of peripheral nerve electrode (lead)
⓻	T85.121	Displacement of implanted electronic neurostimulator of peripheral nerve electrode (lead)
⓻	T85.191	Other mechanical complication of implanted electronic neurostimulator of peripheral nerve electrode (lead)
⓻	T85.732	Infection and inflammatory reaction due to implanted electronic neurostimulator of peripheral nerve, electrode (lead)
⓻	T85.820	Fibrosis due to nervous system prosthetic devices, implants and grafts
⓻	T85.830	Hemorrhage due to nervous system prosthetic devices, implants and grafts
⓻	T85.840	Pain due to nervous system prosthetic devices, implants and grafts
⓻	T85.890	Other specified complication of nervous system prosthetic devices, implants and grafts
	Z45.49	Encounter for adjustment and management of other implanted nervous system device

ICD-10-CM Coding Notes

For codes requiring a 7th character extension, refer to your ICD-10-CM book. Review the character descriptions and coding guidelines for proper selection. For some procedures, only certain characters will apply.

CCI Edits

Refer to Appendix A for CCI edits.

Pub 100

64585: Pub 100-03, 1, 160.19, Pub 100-03, 1, 160.7-160.7.1, Pub 100-04, 32, 40.2.1

Facility RVUs ▯

Code	Work	PE Facility	MP	Total Facility
64585	2.11	1.75	0.28	4.14

Non-facility RVUs ▯

Code	Work	PE Non-Facility	MP	Total Non-Facility
64585	2.11	4.66	0.28	7.05

Modifiers (PAR) ▯

Code	Mod 50	Mod 51	Mod 62	Mod 66	Mod 80
64585	0	2	0	0	1

Global Period

Code	Days
64585	010

64590-64595

64590 Insertion or replacement of peripheral or gastric neurostimulator pulse generator or receiver, direct or inductive coupling

(Do not report 64590 in conjunction with 64595)

64595 Revision or removal of peripheral or gastric neurostimulator pulse generator or receiver

AMA Coding Guideline

Neurostimulator Procedures on the Peripheral Nerves

For electronic analysis with programming, when performed, of peripheral nerve neurostimulator pulse generator/transmitters, see codes 95970, 95971, 95972. An electrode array is a catheter or other device with more than one contact. The function of each contact may be capable of being adjusted during programming services. Test stimulation to confirm correct target site placement of the electrode array(s) and/or to confirm the functional status of the system is inherent to placement, and is not separately reported as electronic analysis or programming of the neurostimulator system. Electronic analysis (95970) at the time of implantation is not separately reported.

Codes 64553, 64555, and 64561 may be used to report both temporary and permanent placement of percutaneous electrode arrays.

AMA Coding Notes

Neurostimulator Procedures on the Peripheral Nerves

(For transcutaneous nerve stimulation [TENS], use 97014 for electrical stimulation requiring supervision only or use 97032 for electrical stimulation requiring constant attendance)

(For percutaneous implantation or replacement of integrated neurostimulation system, posterior tibial nerve, use 0587T)

Surgical Procedures on the Extracranial Nerves, Peripheral Nerves, and Autonomic Nervous System

(For intracranial surgery on cranial nerves, see 61450, 61460, 61790)

AMA *CPT Assistant*

64590: Sep 99: 4, Apr 01: 8, Mar 07: 4, Apr 07: 7, Sep 11: 9, Dec 12: 14, Jan 15: 14, Dec 17: 16, Aug 18: 10

64595: Sep 99: 3, Mar 07: 4, Jan 08: 8

Plain English Description

To insert a peripheral or gastric neurostimulator pulse generator or receiver, an incision is made in the lower abdomen and carried through the subcutaneous tissue down to the muscle fascia. A small pocket is fashioned in the subcutaneous tissue for the device. To replace a peripheral or gastric neurostimulator pulse generator or receiver, an incision is made over the existing device and carried down to the subcutaneous pocket to expose the device. The electrode(s) is then disconnected and the device is dissected free of surrounding tissue and removed. The new neurostimulator pulse generator or receiver is then placed into the existing or newly fashioned subcutaneous pocket and connected to the peripheral or gastric electrode wire(s). The pulse generator or receiver is programmed and the incision is closed (64590). To revise or remove a peripheral or gastric neurostimulator pulse generator or receiver (64595), an incision is made over the existing device and carried down to the subcutaneous pocket to expose the device and the electrode wire(s). Revisions to the device are made and the electrode wire(s) are reconnected, or the device is dissected free of surrounding tissue and removed from the body.

Peripheral or gastric neurostimulator pulse

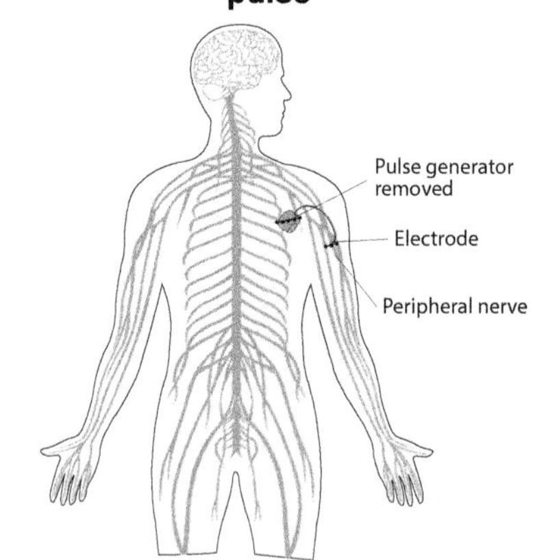

Use code 64590 for insertion or replacement; use code 64595 for revision or removal.

ICD-10-CM Diagnostic Codes

	Code	Description
	B02.23	Postherpetic polyneuropathy
	B02.24	Postherpetic myelitis
	B02.29	Other postherpetic nervous system involvement
	G54.6	Phantom limb syndrome with pain
⇄	G56.01	Carpal tunnel syndrome, right upper limb
⇄	G56.02	Carpal tunnel syndrome, left upper limb
⇄	G56.03	Carpal tunnel syndrome, bilateral upper limbs
⇄	G56.11	Other lesions of median nerve, right upper limb
⇄	G56.12	Other lesions of median nerve, left upper limb
⇄	G56.13	Other lesions of median nerve, bilateral upper limbs
⇄	G56.21	Lesion of ulnar nerve, right upper limb
⇄	G56.22	Lesion of ulnar nerve, left upper limb
⇄	G56.23	Lesion of ulnar nerve, bilateral upper limbs
⇄	G56.31	Lesion of radial nerve, right upper limb
⇄	G56.32	Lesion of radial nerve, left upper limb
⇄	G56.33	Lesion of radial nerve, bilateral upper limbs
⇄	G56.41	Causalgia of right upper limb
⇄	G56.42	Causalgia of left upper limb
⇄	G56.43	Causalgia of bilateral upper limbs
⇄	G56.81	Other specified mononeuropathies of right upper limb
⇄	G56.82	Other specified mononeuropathies of left upper limb
⇄	G56.83	Other specified mononeuropathies of bilateral upper limbs
⇄	G57.01	Lesion of sciatic nerve, right lower limb
⇄	G57.02	Lesion of sciatic nerve, left lower limb
⇄	G57.11	Meralgia paresthetica, right lower limb
⇄	G57.12	Meralgia paresthetica, left lower limb
⇄	G57.21	Lesion of femoral nerve, right lower limb
⇄	G57.22	Lesion of femoral nerve, left lower limb
⇄	G57.31	Lesion of lateral popliteal nerve, right lower limb
⇄	G57.32	Lesion of lateral popliteal nerve, left lower limb
⇄	G57.41	Lesion of medial popliteal nerve, right lower limb
⇄	G57.42	Lesion of medial popliteal nerve, left lower limb
⇄	G57.71	Causalgia of right lower limb
⇄	G57.72	Causalgia of left lower limb
⇄	G57.81	Other specified mononeuropathies of right lower limb
⇄	G57.82	Other specified mononeuropathies of left lower limb
	G58.0	Intercostal neuropathy
	G58.9	Mononeuropathy, unspecified
	G89.21	Chronic pain due to trauma
	G89.22	Chronic post-thoracotomy pain
	G89.28	Other chronic postprocedural pain
	G89.29	Other chronic pain
	G89.4	Chronic pain syndrome
⇄	G90.511	Complex regional pain syndrome I of right upper limb
⇄	G90.512	Complex regional pain syndrome I of left upper limb
⇄	G90.513	Complex regional pain syndrome I of upper limb, bilateral
⇄	G90.521	Complex regional pain syndrome I of right lower limb
⇄	G90.522	Complex regional pain syndrome I of left lower limb
⇄	G90.523	Complex regional pain syndrome I of lower limb, bilateral
	M79.2	Neuralgia and neuritis, unspecified
⇄	M79.601	Pain in right arm
⇄	M79.602	Pain in left arm
⇄	M79.604	Pain in right leg
⇄	M79.605	Pain in left leg
⇄	M79.621	Pain in right upper arm
⇄	M79.622	Pain in left upper arm
⇄	M79.631	Pain in right forearm
⇄	M79.632	Pain in left forearm

⇄	M79.651	Pain in right thigh
⇄	M79.652	Pain in left thigh
⇄	M79.661	Pain in right lower leg
⇄	M79.662	Pain in left lower leg
⑦	T85.113	Breakdown (mechanical) of implanted electronic neurostimulator, generator
⑦	T85.123	Displacement of implanted electronic neurostimulator, generator
⑦	T85.193	Other mechanical complication of implanted electronic neurostimulator, generator
⑦	T85.734	Infection and inflammatory reaction due to implanted electronic neurostimulator, generator
⑦	T85.820	Fibrosis due to nervous system prosthetic devices, implants and grafts
⑦	T85.830	Hemorrhage due to nervous system prosthetic devices, implants and grafts
⑦	T85.840	Pain due to nervous system prosthetic devices, implants and grafts
⑦	T85.850	Stenosis due to nervous system prosthetic devices, implants and grafts
⑦	T85.890	Other specified complication of nervous system prosthetic devices, implants and grafts
	Z45.42	Encounter for adjustment and management of neurostimulator
	Z45.49	Encounter for adjustment and management of other implanted nervous system device

ICD-10-CM Coding Notes

For codes requiring a 7th character extension, refer to your ICD-10-CM book. Review the character descriptions and coding guidelines for proper selection. For some procedures, only certain characters will apply.

CCI Edits

Refer to Appendix A for CCI edits.

Pub 100

64590: Pub 100-04, 32, 40.2.1
64595: Pub 100-04, 32, 40.2.1

Facility RVUs

Code	Work	PE Facility	MP	Total Facility
64590	2.45	1.84	0.34	4.63
64595	1.78	1.61	0.25	3.64

Non-facility RVUs

Code	Work	PE Non-Facility	MP	Total Non-Facility
64590	2.45	4.79	0.34	7.58
64595	1.78	4.77	0.25	6.80

Modifiers (PAR)

Code	Mod 50	Mod 51	Mod 62	Mod 66	Mod 80
64590	0	2	1	0	1
64595	0	2	0	0	1

Global Period

Code	Days
64590	010
64595	010

64600-64610

64600 Destruction by neurolytic agent, trigeminal nerve; supraorbital, infraorbital, mental, or inferior alveolar branch

64605 Destruction by neurolytic agent, trigeminal nerve; second and third division branches at foramen ovale

64610 Destruction by neurolytic agent, trigeminal nerve; second and third division branches at foramen ovale under radiologic monitoring

AMA Coding Guideline

Destruction by Neurolytic Agent (eg, Chemical, Thermal, Electrical or Radiofrequency) and Chemodenervation Procedures on the Extracranial Nerves, Peripheral Nerves, and Autonomic Nervous System

Codes 64600-64681 include the injection of other therapeutic agents (eg, corticosteroids). Do not report diagnostic/therapeutic injections separately. Do not report a code labeled as destruction when using therapies that are not destructive of the target nerve (eg, pulsed radiofrequency), use 64999. For codes labeled as chemodenervation, the supply of the chemodenervation agent is reported separately.

AMA Coding Notes

Destruction by Neurolytic Agent (eg, Chemical, Thermal, Electrical or Radiofrequency) and Chemodenervation Procedures on the Extracranial Nerves, Peripheral Nerves, and Autonomic Nervous System

(For chemodenervation of internal anal sphincter, use 46505)

(For chemodenervation of the bladder, use 52287)

(For chemodenervation for strabismus involving the extraocular muscles, use 67345)

(For chemodenervation guided by needle electromyography or muscle electrical stimulation, see 95873, 95874)

Surgical Procedures on the Extracranial Nerves, Peripheral Nerves, and Autonomic Nervous System

(For intracranial surgery on cranial nerves, see 61450, 61460, 61790)

AMA *CPT Assistant* ▢

64600: Aug 05: 13, Feb 10: 9, Sep 12: 14, Apr 19: 9

64605: Aug 05: 13, Feb 10: 9, Sep 12: 14, Apr 19: 9

64610: Aug 05: 13, Feb 10: 9, Sep 12: 14, Apr 17: 10, Apr 19: 9

Plain English Description

Destruction of a nerve is performed to treat chronic pain and may be performed by injection of a chemical neurolytic agent or using thermal, electrical, or radiofrequency techniques. The most common technique used today is radiofrequency destruction, although the other techniques may also be used for certain pain syndromes. Prior to the destruction procedure, an electrode needle is introduced through the skin and advanced toward the targeted neural tissue. The needle is connected to a generator for motor and sensory testing performed to ensure that the needle is correctly positioned at the nerve responsible for the pain. Once the correct nerve pathway has been identified, the nerve is destroyed. If a chemical agent is used, the chemical agent is injected along the nerve pathway. Neurolytic chemical agents include phenol, ethyl alcohol, glycerol, ammonium salt compounds, and hypertonic or hypotonic solutions. Thermal or electrical modalities involve the use of a probe or needle that is inserted through the skin and activated to produce heat and destroy nerve tissue. To perform radiofrequency nerve destruction, an electrode needle is introduced through the skin and advanced toward the targeted neural tissue. The electrode is adjusted as needed until correct positioning is achieved. The radiofrequency device is then activated and an electric current generated that produces heat at the tip of the electrode and destroys the targeted nerve tissue. Use 64600 for destruction of the supraorbital, infraorbital, mental, or inferior alveolar branch of the trigeminal nerve. For second or third division branches of the trigeminal nerve at the foramen ovale, use 64605 when the procedure is performed without the use of radiologic monitoring; use 64610 when the procedure is performed with radiologic monitoring.

Destruction by neurolytic agent, trigeminal nerve

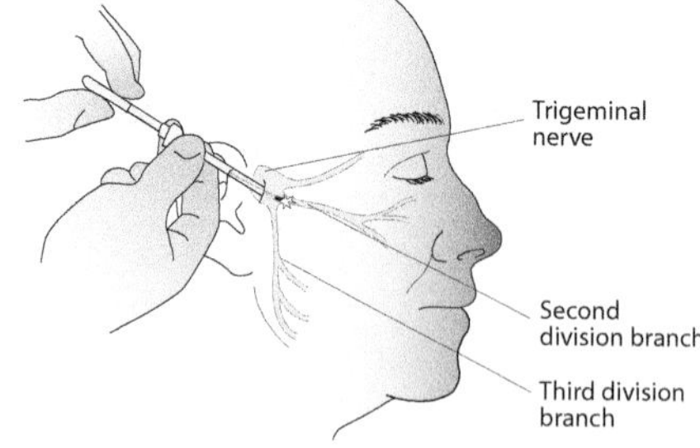

Second and third division branches at foramen ovale (64605); under radiologic monitoring (64610)

ICD-10-CM Diagnostic Codes

C03.0	Malignant neoplasm of upper gum
C03.1	Malignant neoplasm of lower gum
C04.0	Malignant neoplasm of anterior floor of mouth
C04.1	Malignant neoplasm of lateral floor of mouth
C04.8	Malignant neoplasm of overlapping sites of floor of mouth
C05.0	Malignant neoplasm of hard palate
C05.1	Malignant neoplasm of soft palate
C05.2	Malignant neoplasm of uvula
C05.8	Malignant neoplasm of overlapping sites of palate
C06.0	Malignant neoplasm of cheek mucosa
C06.1	Malignant neoplasm of vestibule of mouth
C06.2	Malignant neoplasm of retromolar area
C06.80	Malignant neoplasm of overlapping sites of unspecified parts of mouth
C07	Malignant neoplasm of parotid gland
C08.0	Malignant neoplasm of submandibular gland
C08.1	Malignant neoplasm of sublingual gland
C31.0	Malignant neoplasm of maxillary sinus
C41.0	Malignant neoplasm of bones of skull and face
C41.1	Malignant neoplasm of mandible
C76.0	Malignant neoplasm of head, face and neck
G50.0	Trigeminal neuralgia
G89.3	Neoplasm related pain (acute) (chronic)

CCI Edits

Refer to Appendix A for CCI edits.

Facility RVUs ▢

Code	Work	PE Facility	MP	Total Facility
64600	3.49	2.42	0.68	6.59
64605	5.65	3.47	1.07	10.19
64610	7.20	4.62	2.17	13.99

Non-facility RVUs ▢

Code	Work	PE Non-Facility	MP	Total Non-Facility
64600	3.49	8.57	0.68	12.74
64605	5.65	11.10	1.07	17.82
64610	7.20	12.93	2.17	22.30

Modifiers (PAR) ▢

Code	Mod 50	Mod 51	Mod 62	Mod 66	Mod 80
64600	2	2	0	0	1
64605	1	2	0	0	0
64610	1	2	0	0	1

Global Period

Code	Days
64600	010
64605	010
64610	010

64611

64611 Chemodenervation of parotid and submandibular salivary glands, bilateral

(Report 64611 with modifier 52 if fewer than four salivary glands are injected)

AMA Coding Guideline

Destruction by Neurolytic Agent (eg, Chemical, Thermal, Electrical or Radiofrequency) and Chemodenervation Procedures on the Extracranial Nerves, Peripheral Nerves, and Autonomic Nervous System

Codes 64600-64681 include the injection of other therapeutic agents (eg, corticosteroids). Do not report diagnostic/therapeutic injections separately. Do not report a code labeled as destruction when using therapies that are not destructive of the target nerve (eg, pulsed radiofrequency), use 64999. For codes labeled as chemodenervation, the supply of the chemodenervation agent is reported separately.

AMA Coding Notes

Destruction by Neurolytic Agent (eg, Chemical, Thermal, Electrical or Radiofrequency) and Chemodenervation Procedures on the Extracranial Nerves, Peripheral Nerves, and Autonomic Nervous System

(For chemodenervation of internal anal sphincter, use 46505)

(For chemodenervation of the bladder, use 52287)

(For chemodenervation for strabismus involving the extraocular muscles, use 67345)

(For chemodenervation guided by needle electromyography or muscle electrical stimulation, see 95873, 95874)

Surgical Procedures on the Extracranial Nerves, Peripheral Nerves, and Autonomic Nervous System

(For intracranial surgery on cranial nerves, see 61450, 61460, 61790)

AMA *CPT Assistant*

64611: Feb 11: 10, Sep 12: 14, Apr 19: 9

Plain English Description

Chemodenervation of the salivary glands is performed to treat excessive salivation and drooling, also referred to as sialorrhea. Sialorrhea can be a problem for individuals with some types of neurological conditions such as cerebral palsy, Parkinson's disease, and late effects of cerebrovascular accident (stroke). Imaging guidance is used as needed to locate the salivary glands. Type A botulinum toxin is injected directly into both the parotid and submandibular glands on each side. One or more injections may be required in each gland to accomplish the denervation.

Chemodenervation of parotid and submandibular glands, bilateral

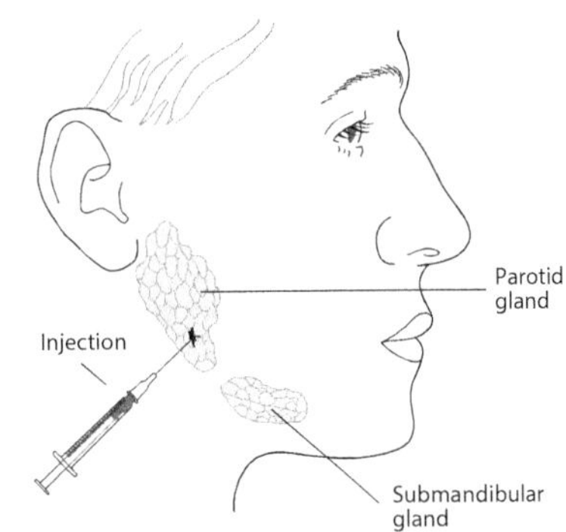

Type A botulinum toxin is injected into both glands on each side.

ICD-10-CM Diagnostic Codes

K11.1	Hypertrophy of salivary gland
K11.22	Acute recurrent sialoadenitis
K11.23	Chronic sialoadenitis
K11.4	Fistula of salivary gland
K11.6	Mucocele of salivary gland
K11.7	Disturbances of salivary secretion
K91.89	Other postprocedural complications and disorders of digestive system
M35.00	Sicca syndrome, unspecified

CCI Edits

Refer to Appendix A for CCI edits.

Facility RVUs

Code	Work	PE Facility	MP	Total Facility
64611	1.03	1.64	0.35	3.02

Non-facility RVUs

Code	Work	PE Non-Facility	MP	Total Non-Facility
64611	1.03	2.09	0.35	3.47

Modifiers (PAR)

Code	Mod 50	Mod 51	Mod 62	Mod 66	Mod 80
64611	2	2	0	0	0

Global Period

Code	Days
64611	010

64612

64612 Chemodenervation of muscle(s); muscle(s) innervated by facial nerve, unilateral (eg, for blepharospasm, hemifacial spasm)

(For bilateral procedure, report 64612 with modifier 50)

AMA Coding Guideline

Destruction by Neurolytic Agent (eg, Chemical, Thermal, Electrical or Radiofrequency) and Chemodenervation Procedures on the Extracranial Nerves, Peripheral Nerves, and Autonomic Nervous System

Codes 64600-64681 include the injection of other therapeutic agents (eg, corticosteroids). Do not report diagnostic/therapeutic injections separately. Do not report a code labeled as destruction when using therapies that are not destructive of the target nerve (eg, pulsed radiofrequency), use 64999. For codes labeled as chemodenervation, the supply of the chemodenervation agent is reported separately.

AMA Coding Notes

Destruction by Neurolytic Agent (eg, Chemical, Thermal, Electrical or Radiofrequency) and Chemodenervation Procedures on the Extracranial Nerves, Peripheral Nerves, and Autonomic Nervous System

(For chemodenervation of internal anal sphincter, use 46505)

(For chemodenervation of the bladder, use 52287)

(For chemodenervation for strabismus involving the extraocular muscles, use 67345)

(For chemodenervation guided by needle electromyography or muscle electrical stimulation, see 95873, 95874)

Surgical Procedures on the Extracranial Nerves, Peripheral Nerves, and Autonomic Nervous System

(For intracranial surgery on cranial nerves, see 61450, 61460, 61790)

AMA *CPT Assistant* □

64612: Oct 98: 10, Apr 01: 2, Aug 05: 13, Sep 06: 5, Dec 08: 9, Jan 09: 8, Feb 10: 9, 13, Dec 11: 19, Sep 12: 14, Apr 13: 5, Dec 13: 10, Jan 14: 6, May 14: 5, Apr 19: 9

Plain English Description

Chemodenervation is performed on muscles innervated by the facial nerve unilaterally to treat involuntary muscle contractions or muscle spasms, such as blepharospasm or for treatment of hemifacial pain. Injection of botulinum toxin (type A or B) directly into a muscle produces temporary muscle paralysis by blocking the release of acetylcholine at the peripheral nerve endings, which interrupts neuromuscular transmission of nerve impulses. The muscle and the specific muscle sites to be injected are determined either by use of electromyography or by examining and palpating the facial muscles and noting the location of the muscle spasm. The side of the face to be treated is prepared. The affected muscle or muscle group is then injected at carefully selected sites to accomplish the denervation.

Chemodenervation of muscle(s)

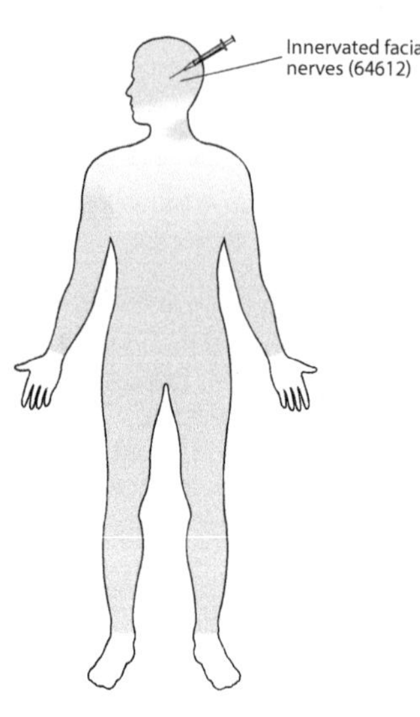

ICD-10-CM Diagnostic Codes

	Code	Description
	G11.4	Hereditary spastic paraplegia
	G20	Parkinson's disease
	G24.1	Genetic torsion dystonia
	G24.4	Idiopathic orofacial dystonia
	G24.5	Blepharospasm
	G35	Multiple sclerosis
⇄	G51.31	Clonic hemifacial spasm, right
⇄	G51.32	Clonic hemifacial spasm, left
⇄	G51.33	Clonic hemifacial spasm, bilateral
	G51.4	Facial myokymia
	G51.8	Other disorders of facial nerve
	G51.9	Disorder of facial nerve, unspecified
	P11.3	Birth injury to facial nerve

CCI Edits

Refer to Appendix A for CCI edits.

Facility RVUs □

Code	Work	PE Facility	MP	Total Facility
64612	1.41	1.67	0.27	3.35

Non-facility RVUs □

Code	Work	PE Non-Facility	MP	Total Non-Facility
64612	1.41	2.14	0.27	3.82

Modifiers (PAR) □

Code	Mod 50	Mod 51	Mod 62	Mod 66	Mod 80
64612	1	2	0	0	1

Global Period

Code	Days
64612	010

64615

64615 Chemodenervation of muscle(s); muscle(s) innervated by facial, trigeminal, cervical spinal and accessory nerves, bilateral (eg, for chronic migraine)

(Report 64615 only once per session)

(Do not report 64615 in conjunction with 64612, 64616, 64617, 64642, 64643, 64644, 64645, 64646, 64647)

(For guidance see 95873, 95874. Do not report more than one guidance code for 64615)

AMA Coding Guideline

Destruction by Neurolytic Agent (eg, Chemical, Thermal, Electrical or Radiofrequency) and Chemodenervation Procedures on the Extracranial Nerves, Peripheral Nerves, and Autonomic Nervous System

Codes 64600-64681 include the injection of other therapeutic agents (eg, corticosteroids). Do not report diagnostic/therapeutic injections separately. Do not report a code labeled as destruction when using therapies that are not destructive of the target nerve (eg, pulsed radiofrequency), use 64999. For codes labeled as chemodenervation, the supply of the chemodenervation agent is reported separately.

AMA Coding Notes

Destruction by Neurolytic Agent (eg, Chemical, Thermal, Electrical or Radiofrequency) and Chemodenervation Procedures on the Extracranial Nerves, Peripheral Nerves, and Autonomic Nervous System

(For chemodenervation of internal anal sphincter, use 46505)

(For chemodenervation of the bladder, use 52287)

(For chemodenervation for strabismus involving the extraocular muscles, use 67345)

(For chemodenervation guided by needle electromyography or muscle electrical stimulation, see 95873, 95874)

Surgical Procedures on the Extracranial Nerves, Peripheral Nerves, and Autonomic Nervous System

(For intracranial surgery on cranial nerves, see 61450, 61460, 61790)

AMA *CPT Assistant* ☐

64615: Apr 13: 5, Jan 14: 6, Apr 19: 9

Plain English Description

Chemical denervation involves the injection of a toxin (type A botulinum) directly into a muscle to produce temporary muscle paralysis by blocking the release of acetylcholine. Botulinum toxin injections have been shown to be effective in the prevention of migraines by blocking the neurotransmitter responsible for muscle contractions and pain. To perform chemical denervation of the muscles innervated by the facial, trigeminal, cervical spinal, and accessory nerves, small doses of botulinum toxin are injected bilaterally into muscles of the forehead, the side and back of the head, and the neck and shoulders.

ICD-10-CM Diagnostic Codes

Code	Description
G43.001	Migraine without aura, not intractable, with status migrainosus
G43.011	Migraine without aura, intractable, with status migrainosus
G43.019	Migraine without aura, intractable, without status migrainosus
G43.101	Migraine with aura, not intractable, with status migrainosus
G43.111	Migraine with aura, intractable, with status migrainosus
G43.119	Migraine with aura, intractable, without status migrainosus
G43.401	Hemiplegic migraine, not intractable, with status migrainosus
G43.411	Hemiplegic migraine, intractable, with status migrainosus
G43.419	Hemiplegic migraine, intractable, without status migrainosus
G43.501	Persistent migraine aura without cerebral infarction, not intractable, with status migrainosus
G43.511	Persistent migraine aura without cerebral infarction, intractable, with status migrainosus
G43.519	Persistent migraine aura without cerebral infarction, intractable, without status migrainosus
G43.701	Chronic migraine without aura, not intractable, with status migrainosus
G43.711	Chronic migraine without aura, intractable, with status migrainosus
G43.719	Chronic migraine without aura, intractable, without status migrainosus
G43.801	Other migraine, not intractable, with status migrainosus
G43.811	Other migraine, intractable, with status migrainosus
G43.819	Other migraine, intractable, without status migrainosus
G43.901	Migraine, unspecified, not intractable, with status migrainosus
G43.911	Migraine, unspecified, intractable, with status migrainosus
G43.919	Migraine, unspecified, intractable, without status migrainosus

CCI Edits

Refer to Appendix A for CCI edits.

Facility RVUs ☐

Code	Work	PE Facility	MP	Total Facility
64615	1.85	1.12	0.58	3.55

Non-facility RVUs ☐

Code	Work	PE Non-Facility	MP	Total Non-Facility
64615	1.85	1.89	0.58	4.32

Modifiers (PAR) ☐

Code	Mod 50	Mod 51	Mod 62	Mod 66	Mod 80
64615	2	2	0	0	1

Global Period

Code	Days
64615	010

64616

64616 Chemodenervation of muscle(s); neck muscle(s), excluding muscles of the larynx, unilateral (eg, for cervical dystonia, spasmodic torticollis)

(For bilateral procedure, report 64616 with modifier 50)

(For chemodenervation guided by needle electromyography or muscle electrical stimulation, see 95873, 95874. Do not report more than one guidance code for any unit of 64616)

AMA Coding Guideline

Destruction by Neurolytic Agent (eg, Chemical, Thermal, Electrical or Radiofrequency) and Chemodenervation Procedures on the Extracranial Nerves, Peripheral Nerves, and Autonomic Nervous System

Codes 64600-64681 include the injection of other therapeutic agents (eg, corticosteroids). Do not report diagnostic/therapeutic injections separately. Do not report a code labeled as destruction when using therapies that are not destructive of the target nerve (eg, pulsed radiofrequency), use 64999. For codes labeled as chemodenervation, the supply of the chemodenervation agent is reported separately.

AMA Coding Notes

Destruction by Neurolytic Agent (eg, Chemical, Thermal, Electrical or Radiofrequency) and Chemodenervation Procedures on the Extracranial Nerves, Peripheral Nerves, and Autonomic Nervous System

(For chemodenervation of internal anal sphincter, use 46505)

(For chemodenervation of the bladder, use 52287)

(For chemodenervation for strabismus involving the extraocular muscles, use 67345)

(For chemodenervation guided by needle electromyography or muscle electrical stimulation, see 95873, 95874)

Surgical Procedures on the Extracranial Nerves, Peripheral Nerves, and Autonomic Nervous System

(For intracranial surgery on cranial nerves, see 61450, 61460, 61790)

AMA *CPT Assistant* ▢

64616: Jan 14: 6, May 14: 5, Apr 19: 9

Plain English Description

Chemodenervation is performed on neck muscles unilaterally to treat involuntary muscle contractions or muscle spasms in the neck. This condition may be referred to as cervical dystonia or spasmodic torticollis. Injection of botulinum toxin (type A or B) directly into a muscle produces temporary muscle paralysis by blocking the release of acetylcholine at the peripheral nerve endings, which interrupts neuromuscular transmission of nerve impulses. The muscle and the specific muscle sites to be injected are determined either by use of electromyography or by examining the position of the head, palpating the neck muscles, and noting the location of the muscle spasm. The side of the neck to be treated is prepared. The affected muscle or muscle group is then injected at carefully selected sites to accomplish the denervation.

ICD-10-CM Diagnostic Codes

G24.02	Drug induced acute dystonia
G24.1	Genetic torsion dystonia
G24.2	Idiopathic nonfamilial dystonia
G24.3	Spasmodic torticollis
G24.8	Other dystonia
G89.21	Chronic pain due to trauma
G89.28	Other chronic postprocedural pain
G89.29	Other chronic pain
G89.3	Neoplasm related pain (acute) (chronic)
M54.2	Cervicalgia
M79.12	Myalgia of auxiliary muscles, head and neck

CCI Edits

Refer to Appendix A for CCI edits.

Facility RVUs ▢

Code	Work	PE Facility	MP	Total Facility
64616	1.53	1.13	0.48	3.14

Non-facility RVUs ▢

Code	Work	PE Non-Facility	MP	Total Non-Facility
64616	1.53	1.81	0.48	3.82

Modifiers (PAR) ▢

Code	Mod 50	Mod 51	Mod 62	Mod 66	Mod 80
64616	1	2	0	0	1

Global Period

Code	Days
64616	010

64617

64617 Chemodenervation of muscle(s); larynx, unilateral, percutaneous (eg, for spasmodic dysphonia), includes guidance by needle electromyography, when performed

(For bilateral procedure, report 64617 with modifier 50)

(Do not report 64617 in conjunction with 95873, 95874)

(For diagnostic needle electromyography of the larynx, use 95865)

(For chemodenervation of the larynx performed with direct laryngoscopy, see 31570, 31571)

AMA Coding Guideline

Destruction by Neurolytic Agent (eg, Chemical, Thermal, Electrical or Radiofrequency) and Chemodenervation Procedures on the Extracranial Nerves, Peripheral Nerves, and Autonomic Nervous System

Codes 64600-64681 include the injection of other therapeutic agents (eg, corticosteroids). Do not report diagnostic/therapeutic injections separately. Do not report a code labeled as destruction when using therapies that are not destructive of the target nerve (eg, pulsed radiofrequency), use 64999. For codes labeled as chemodenervation, the supply of the chemodenervation agent is reported separately.

AMA Coding Notes

Destruction by Neurolytic Agent (eg, Chemical, Thermal, Electrical or Radiofrequency) and Chemodenervation Procedures on the Extracranial Nerves, Peripheral Nerves, and Autonomic Nervous System

(For chemodenervation of internal anal sphincter, use 46505)

(For chemodenervation of the bladder, use 52287)

(For chemodenervation for strabismus involving the extraocular muscles, use 67345)

(For chemodenervation guided by needle electromyography or muscle electrical stimulation, see 95873, 95874)

Surgical Procedures on the Extracranial Nerves, Peripheral Nerves, and Autonomic Nervous System

(For intracranial surgery on cranial nerves, see 61450, 61460, 61790)

AMA *CPT Assistant*

64617: Jan 14: 6, Apr 19: 9

Plain English Description

Chemodenervation is performed to treat involuntary muscle contractions or muscle spasms in the vocal cord muscles of the larynx. These muscle spasms result from a neurological condition that manifests as spasmodic dysphonia, also referred to as laryngeal dystonia, or spastic dysphonia, which affects speech quality. Injection of botulinum toxin (type A or B) directly into a muscle produces temporary muscle paralysis by blocking the release of acetylcholine at the peripheral nerve endings, which interrupts neuromuscular transmission of nerve impulses. The muscle sites to be injected are determined by electromyography (EMG). A hollow EMG needle connected to the EMG recorder is used to perform the injection. The patient may be supine or seated with the head extended. The thyroid and cricoid cartilages are located by palpation and the midline of the cricothyroid membrane is identified. For abductor spasmodic dysphonia, the needle is placed percutaneously into the thyroarytenoid muscle and the desired amount of botulin toxin is injected. For adductor spasmodic dysphonia, the needle is placed percutaneously and botulinum toxin is injected into the posterior cricoarytenoid muscle. The injection is typically performed on one side at the first visit and then on the opposite side on a subsequent visit, with the visits spaced approximately two weeks apart. Code 64617 reports a unilateral procedure.

ICD-10-CM Diagnostic Codes

F44.4	Conversion disorder with motor symptom or deficit
J38.3	Other diseases of vocal cords
R49.0	Dysphonia
R49.8	Other voice and resonance disorders

CCI Edits

Refer to Appendix A for CCI edits.

Facility RVUs

Code	Work	PE Facility	MP	Total Facility
64617	1.90	0.96	0.27	3.13

Non-facility RVUs

Code	Work	PE Non-Facility	MP	Total Non-Facility
64617	1.90	2.46	0.27	4.63

Modifiers (PAR)

Code	Mod 50	Mod 51	Mod 62	Mod 66	Mod 80
64617	1	2	0	0	1

Global Period

Code	Days
64617	010

64625

● **64625 Radiofrequency ablation, nerves innervating the sacroiliac joint, with image guidance (ie, fluoroscopy or computed tomography)**

(Do not report 64625 in conjunction with 64635, 77002, 77003, 77012, 95873, 95874)

(For radiofrequency ablation, nerves innervating the sacroiliac joint, with ultrasound, use 76999)

(For bilateral procedure, report 64625 with modifier 50)

AMA Coding Guideline

Destruction by Neurolytic Agent (eg, Chemical, Thermal, Electrical or Radiofrequency) and Chemodenervation Procedures on the Extracranial Nerves, Peripheral Nerves, and Autonomic Nervous System

Codes 64600-64681 include the injection of other therapeutic agents (eg, corticosteroids). Do not report diagnostic/therapeutic injections separately. Do not report a code labeled as destruction when using therapies that are not destructive of the target nerve (eg, pulsed radiofrequency), use 64999. For codes labeled as chemodenervation, the supply of the chemodenervation agent is reported separately.

AMA Coding Notes

Destruction by Neurolytic Agent (eg, Chemical, Thermal, Electrical or Radiofrequency) and Chemodenervation Procedures on the Extracranial Nerves, Peripheral Nerves, and Autonomic Nervous System

(For chemodenervation of internal anal sphincter, use 46505)

(For chemodenervation of the bladder, use 52287)

(For chemodenervation for strabismus involving the extraocular muscles, use 67345)

(For chemodenervation guided by needle electromyography or muscle electrical stimulation, see 95873, 95874)

Surgical Procedures on the Extracranial Nerves, Peripheral Nerves, and Autonomic Nervous System

(For intracranial surgery on cranial nerves, see 61450, 61460, 61790)

Plain English Description

Radiofrequency ablation (RFA) of the nerves innervating the sacroiliac (SI) joint is performed. The SI joints connect the sacrum with the hip on either side of the spine. Radiofrequency nerve ablation is done to provide longer lasting relief of low back and/or sciatic pain due to SI joint dysfunction. In some cases, a lateral branch block of the smaller sacral spinal nerves innervating the joint may be carried out separately beforehand to determine the appropriateness of radiofrequency ablation. This minimally invasive procedure may be performed under mild sedation commonly using fluoroscopy for imaging guidance. With the patient positioned prone, an IV may be established for sedation. The skin is cleansed over the injection site and a small area is numbed first. The RFA needle is advanced to the lateral branching sacral spinal nerves transmitting pain signals from the SI joints. With the needle is position, an electrode is placed through the needle and a small electrical current is first run next to the target nerve to confirm placement by recreating the patient's pain. After the target nerve is confirmed, a lesion is created on the nerve by applying heat either by conventional, pulsed, or vapor radiofrequency.

ICD-10-CM Diagnostic Codes

	Code	Description
	A18.01	Tuberculosis of spine
	C41.4	Malignant neoplasm of pelvic bones, sacrum and coccyx
	C47.5	Malignant neoplasm of peripheral nerves of pelvis
	C49.5	Malignant neoplasm of connective and soft tissue of pelvis
	C79.51	Secondary malignant neoplasm of bone
	C79.89	Secondary malignant neoplasm of other specified sites
	G89.18	Other acute postprocedural pain
	G89.21	Chronic pain due to trauma
	G89.29	Other chronic pain
	G89.3	Neoplasm related pain (acute) (chronic)
	G89.4	Chronic pain syndrome
	M12.58	Traumatic arthropathy, other specified site
	M45.8	Ankylosing spondylitis sacral and sacrococcygeal region
	M46.1	Sacroiliitis, not elsewhere classified
	M47.28	Other spondylosis with radiculopathy, sacral and sacrococcygeal region
	M48.38	Traumatic spondylopathy, sacral and sacrococcygeal region
	M53.2	Spinal instabilities
	M53.3	Sacrococcygeal disorders, not elsewhere classified
	M99.14	Subluxation complex (vertebral) of sacral region
	M99.24	Subluxation stenosis of neural canal of sacral region
	M99.34	Osseous stenosis of neural canal of sacral region
	M99.44	Connective tissue stenosis of neural canal of sacral region
	M99.54	Intervertebral disc stenosis of neural canal of sacral region
	M99.84	Other biomechanical lesions of sacral region
	R10.2	Pelvic and perineal pain
❼	S33.2	Dislocation of sacroiliac and sacrococcygeal joint
❼	S33.6	Sprain of sacroiliac joint

ICD-10-CM Coding Notes

For codes requiring a 7th character extension, refer to your ICD-10-CM book. Review the character descriptions and coding guidelines for proper selection. For some procedures, only certain characters will apply.

CCI Edits

Refer to Appendix A for CCI edits.

Facility RVUs ▯

Code	Work	PE Facility	MP	Total Facility
64625	3.39	1.88	0.32	5.59

Non-facility RVUs ▯

Code	Work	PE Non-Facility	MP	Total Non-Facility
64625	3.39	10.43	0.32	14.14

Modifiers (PAR) ▯

Code	Mod 50	Mod 51	Mod 62	Mod 66	Mod 80
64625	1	2	0	0	1

Global Period

Code	Days
64625	010

64633-64636

64633 Destruction by neurolytic agent, paravertebral facet joint nerve(s), with imaging guidance (fluoroscopy or CT); cervical or thoracic, single facet joint

(For bilateral procedure, report 64633 with modifier 50)

✚ **64634 Destruction by neurolytic agent, paravertebral facet joint nerve(s), with imaging guidance (fluoroscopy or CT); cervical or thoracic, each additional facet joint (List separately in addition to code for primary procedure)**

(Use 64634 in conjunction with 64633)

(For bilateral procedure, report 64634 twice. Do not report modifier 50 in conjunction with 64634)

64635 Destruction by neurolytic agent, paravertebral facet joint nerve(s), with imaging guidance (fluoroscopy or CT); lumbar or sacral, single facet joint

(For bilateral procedure, report 64635 with modifier 50)

✚ **64636 Destruction by neurolytic agent, paravertebral facet joint nerve(s), with imaging guidance (fluoroscopy or CT); lumbar or sacral, each additional facet joint (List separately in addition to code for primary procedure)**

(Use 64636 in conjunction with 64635)

(For bilateral procedure, report 64636 twice. Do not report modifier 50 in conjunction with 64636)

(Do not report 64633-64636 in conjunction with 77003, 77012)

(For destruction by neurolytic agent, individual nerves, sacroiliac joint, use 64640)

AMA Coding Guideline

Destruction by Neurolytic Agent (eg, Chemical, Thermal, Electrical or Radiofrequency) and Chemodenervation Procedures on the Extracranial Nerves, Peripheral Nerves, and Autonomic Nervous System

Codes 64600-64681 include the injection of other therapeutic agents (eg, corticosteroids). Do not report diagnostic/therapeutic injections separately. Do not report a code labeled as destruction when using therapies that are not destructive of the target nerve (eg, pulsed radiofrequency), use 64999. For codes labeled as chemodenervation, the supply of the chemodenervation agent is reported separately.

AMA Coding Notes

Destruction by Neurolytic Agent (eg, Chemical, Thermal, Electrical or Radiofrequency) and Chemodenervation Procedures on the Extracranial Nerves, Peripheral Nerves, and Autonomic Nervous System

(For chemodenervation of internal anal sphincter, use 46505)

(For chemodenervation of the bladder, use 52287)

(For chemodenervation for strabismus involving the extraocular muscles, use 67345)

(For chemodenervation guided by needle electromyography or muscle electrical stimulation, see 95873, 95874)

Surgical Procedures on the Extracranial Nerves, Peripheral Nerves, and Autonomic Nervous System

(For intracranial surgery on cranial nerves, see 61450, 61460, 61790)

AMA *CPT Assistant* ☐

64633: Jun 12: 10, Jul 12: 6, Sep 12: 14, Apr 13: 10, Feb 15: 9, Apr 19: 9

64634: Jun 12: 10, Jul 12: 6, Sep 12: 14, Apr 13: 10, Feb 15: 9, Apr 19: 9

64635: Jun 12: 10, Jul 12: 6, 14, Sep 12: 14, Apr 13: 10, Feb 15: 9, Apr 19: 9

64636: Jun 12: 10, Jul 12: 6, 14, Sep 12: 14, Apr 13: 10, Feb 15: 9, Apr 19: 9

Plain English Description

Paravertebral facet joints, also called zygapophyseal joints, are located on the posterior aspect of the spine on each side of the vertebra at the point where one vertebra overlaps the next. Using fluoroscopic or computed tomographic (CT) guidance, the paravertebral facet joint nerve is destroyed using a neurolytic agent. The skin overlying the facet joint is prepared and a local anesthetic is injected. If a chemical neurolytic agent is used, a spinal needle is directed into the facet joint space until bone or cartilage is encountered. A small amount of contrast material is injected to verify that the needle is correctly positioned. This may be followed by injection of a local anesthetic and/or steroid. The selected chemical neurolytic agent is then injected along the nerve pathway. Neurolytic chemical agents include phenol, ethyl alcohol, glycerol, ammonium salt compounds, and hypertonic or hypotonic solutions. Thermal or electrical modalities for neurolysis involve the use of a probe, needle, or electrode inserted through the skin and activated to produce heat and destroy nerve tissue. Using fluoroscopic or CT guidance, an electrode needle is introduced through the skin and advanced toward the targeted neural tissue. The needle is connected to a generator for performing motor and sensory testing to ensure that the needle is correctly positioned along the facet joint nerve. Once the correct nerve pathway has been identified, the nerve is destroyed. The probe, needle, or electrode is activated and an electric current is generated that produces heat at the tip of the device and destroys the targeted nerve tissue. Use 64633 for a single cervical or thoracic facet joint nerve; use 64634 for each additional cervical or thoracic level. Use 64635 for a single lumbar or sacral facet joint nerve; use 64636 for each additional lumbar or sacral level.

ICD-10-CM Diagnostic Codes

	Code	Description
	C41.2	Malignant neoplasm of vertebral column
	C41.4	Malignant neoplasm of pelvic bones, sacrum and coccyx
	C76.0	Malignant neoplasm of head, face and neck
	C76.1	Malignant neoplasm of thorax
	C76.3	Malignant neoplasm of pelvis
	C79.51	Secondary malignant neoplasm of bone
	G89.29	Other chronic pain
	G89.3	Neoplasm related pain (acute) (chronic)
	M54.2	Cervicalgia
	M54.5	Low back pain
	M54.6	Pain in thoracic spine
	M54.9	Dorsalgia, unspecified
	R10.10	Upper abdominal pain, unspecified
⇄	R10.11	Right upper quadrant pain
⇄	R10.12	Left upper quadrant pain
	R10.2	Pelvic and perineal pain
⇄	R10.3	Pain localized to other parts of lower abdomen
⇄	R10.31	Right lower quadrant pain
⇄	R10.32	Left lower quadrant pain
	R10.9	Unspecified abdominal pain

CCI Edits

Refer to Appendix A for CCI edits.

Pub 100

64633: Pub 100-03, 1, 160.1

64634: Pub 100-03, 1, 160.1

64635: Pub 100-03, 1, 160.1

64636: Pub 100-03, 1, 160.1

Facility RVUs

Code	Work	PE Facility	MP	Total Facility
64633	3.84	2.25	0.37	6.46
64634	1.32	0.52	0.12	1.96
64635	3.78	2.24	0.35	6.37
64636	1.16	0.45	0.11	1.72

Non-facility RVUs

Code	Work	PE Non-Facility	MP	Total Non-Facility
64633	3.84	7.73	0.37	11.94
64634	1.32	3.90	0.12	5.34
64635	3.78	7.68	0.35	11.81
64636	1.16	3.60	0.11	4.87

Modifiers (PAR)

Code	Mod 50	Mod 51	Mod 62	Mod 66	Mod 80
64633	1	2	0	0	1
64634	1	0	0	0	1
64635	1	2	0	0	1
64636	1	0	0	0	1

Global Period

Code	Days
64633	010
64634	ZZZ
64635	010
64636	ZZZ

64640

64640 Destruction by neurolytic agent; other peripheral nerve or branch

AMA Coding Guideline

Destruction by Neurolytic Agent (eg, Chemical, Thermal, Electrical or Radiofrequency) and Chemodenervation Procedures on the Extracranial Nerves, Peripheral Nerves, and Autonomic Nervous System

Codes 64600-64681 include the injection of other therapeutic agents (eg, corticosteroids). Do not report diagnostic/therapeutic injections separately. Do not report a code labeled as destruction when using therapies that are not destructive of the target nerve (eg, pulsed radiofrequency), use 64999. For codes labeled as chemodenervation, the supply of the chemodenervation agent is reported separately.

AMA Coding Notes

Destruction by Neurolytic Agent (eg, Chemical, Thermal, Electrical or Radiofrequency) and Chemodenervation Procedures on the Extracranial Nerves, Peripheral Nerves, and Autonomic Nervous System

(For chemodenervation of internal anal sphincter, use 46505)

(For chemodenervation of the bladder, use 52287)

(For chemodenervation for strabismus involving the extraocular muscles, use 67345)

(For chemodenervation guided by needle electromyography or muscle electrical stimulation, see 95873, 95874)

Surgical Procedures on the Extracranial Nerves, Peripheral Nerves, and Autonomic Nervous System

(For intracranial surgery on cranial nerves, see 61450, 61460, 61790)

AMA *CPT Assistant* ▯

64640: Aug 05: 13, Dec 09: 11, Feb 10: 9, Jun 12: 15, Sep 12: 14, May 17: 10, Oct 17: 9, Jan 18: 7, Apr 19: 9

Plain English Description

Destruction of a nerve is performed to treat chronic pain and may be performed by injection of a chemical neurolytic agent or using thermal, electrical, or radiofrequency techniques. The most common technique used today is radiofrequency destruction, although the other techniques may also be used for certain pain syndromes. Prior to the destruction procedure, an electrode needle is introduced through the skin and advanced toward the targeted neural tissue. The needle is connected to a generator for motor and sensory testing performed to ensure that the needle is correctly positioned at the nerve responsible for the pain. Once the correct nerve pathway has been identified, the nerve is destroyed. If a chemical agent is used, the chemical agent is injected along the nerve pathway. Neurolytic chemical agents include phenol, ethyl alcohol, glycerol, ammonium salt compounds, and hypertonic or hypotonic solutions. Thermal or electrical modalities involve the use of a probe or needle that is inserted through the skin and activated to produce heat and destroy nerve tissue. To perform radiofrequency nerve destruction, an electrode needle is introduced through the skin and advanced toward the targeted neural tissue. The electrode is adjusted as needed until correct positioning is achieved. The radiofrequency device is then activated and an electric current generated that produces heat at the tip of the electrode and destroys the targeted nerve tissue. Use 64640 for destruction of a peripheral nerve or branch that does not have a more specific code listed.

Destruction by neurolytic agent; other peripheral nerve or branch

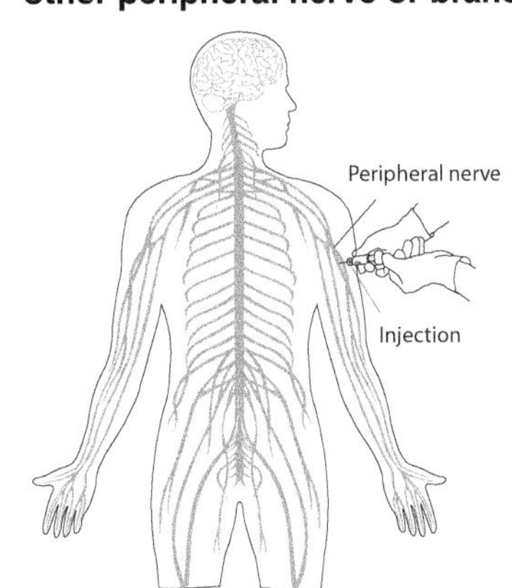

ICD-10-CM Diagnostic Codes

⇄	C76.51	Malignant neoplasm of right lower limb
⇄	C76.52	Malignant neoplasm of left lower limb
	C79.51	Secondary malignant neoplasm of bone
⇄	G57.11	Meralgia paresthetica, right lower limb
⇄	G57.12	Meralgia paresthetica, left lower limb
⇄	G57.21	Lesion of femoral nerve, right lower limb
⇄	G57.22	Lesion of femoral nerve, left lower limb
⇄	G57.31	Lesion of lateral popliteal nerve, right lower limb
⇄	G57.32	Lesion of lateral popliteal nerve, left lower limb
⇄	G57.33	Lesion of lateral popliteal nerve, bilateral lower limbs
⇄	G57.41	Lesion of medial popliteal nerve, right lower limb
⇄	G57.42	Lesion of medial popliteal nerve, left lower limb
⇄	G57.43	Lesion of medial popliteal nerve, bilateral lower limbs
⇄	G57.61	Lesion of plantar nerve, right lower limb
⇄	G57.62	Lesion of plantar nerve, left lower limb
⇄	G57.63	Lesion of plantar nerve, bilateral lower limbs
⇄	G57.71	Causalgia of right lower limb
⇄	G57.72	Causalgia of left lower limb
⇄	G57.73	Causalgia of bilateral lower limbs
⇄	G57.81	Other specified mononeuropathies of right lower limb
⇄	G57.82	Other specified mononeuropathies of left lower limb
⇄	G57.83	Other specified mononeuropathies of bilateral lower limbs
	G89.21	Chronic pain due to trauma
	G89.28	Other chronic postprocedural pain
	G89.29	Other chronic pain
	G89.3	Neoplasm related pain (acute) (chronic)
	G89.4	Chronic pain syndrome
⇄	G90.521	Complex regional pain syndrome I of right lower limb
⇄	G90.522	Complex regional pain syndrome I of left lower limb
⇄	G90.523	Complex regional pain syndrome I of lower limb, bilateral
⇄	M79.604	Pain in right leg
⇄	M79.605	Pain in left leg
⇄	M79.651	Pain in right thigh
⇄	M79.652	Pain in left thigh
⇄	M79.661	Pain in right lower leg
⇄	M79.662	Pain in left lower leg
❼⇄	S74.11	Injury of femoral nerve at hip and thigh level, right leg
❼⇄	S74.12	Injury of femoral nerve at hip and thigh level, left leg
❼⇄	S74.21	Injury of cutaneous sensory nerve at hip and high level, right leg
❼⇄	S74.22	Injury of cutaneous sensory nerve at hip and thigh level, left leg
❼⇄	S74.8X1	Injury of other nerves at hip and thigh level, right leg
❼⇄	S74.8X2	Injury of other nerves at hip and thigh level, left leg
❼⇄	S84.01	Injury of tibial nerve at lower leg level, right leg
❼⇄	S84.02	Injury of tibial nerve at lower leg level, left leg
❼⇄	S84.11	Injury of peroneal nerve at lower leg level, right leg
❼⇄	S84.12	Injury of peroneal nerve at lower leg level, left leg
❼⇄	S84.21	Injury of cutaneous sensory nerve at lower leg level, right leg
❼⇄	S84.22	Injury of cutaneous sensory nerve at lower leg level, left leg
❼⇄	S84.801	Injury of other nerves at lower leg level, right leg
❼⇄	S84.802	Injury of other nerves at lower leg level, left leg

ICD-10-CM Coding Notes

For codes requiring a 7th character extension, refer to your ICD-10-CM book. Review the character descriptions and coding guidelines for proper selection. For some procedures, only certain characters will apply.

CCI Edits

Refer to Appendix A for CCI edits.

Facility RVUs ▯

Code	Work	PE Facility	MP	Total Facility
64640	1.98	1.22	0.18	3.38

Non-facility RVUs ▯

Code	Work	PE Non-Facility	MP	Total Non-Facility
64640	1.98	4.89	0.18	7.05

Modifiers (PAR) ▯

Code	Mod 50	Mod 51	Mod 62	Mod 66	Mod 80
64640	1	2	0	0	1

Global Period

Code	Days
64640	010

64642-64643

64642 Chemodenervation of one extremity; 1-4 muscle(s)

✚ **64643 Chemodenervation of one extremity; each additional extremity, 1-4 muscle(s) (List separately in addition to code for primary procedure)**

(Use 64643 in conjunction with 64642, 64644)

AMA Coding Guideline

Destruction by Neurolytic Agent (eg, Chemical, Thermal, Electrical or Radiofrequency) and Chemodenervation Procedures on the Extracranial Nerves, Peripheral Nerves, and Autonomic Nervous System

Codes 64600-64681 include the injection of other therapeutic agents (eg, corticosteroids). Do not report diagnostic/therapeutic injections separately. Do not report a code labeled as destruction when using therapies that are not destructive of the target nerve (eg, pulsed radiofrequency), use 64999. For codes labeled as chemodenervation, the supply of the chemodenervation agent is reported separately.

AMA Coding Notes

Destruction by Neurolytic Agent (eg, Chemical, Thermal, Electrical or Radiofrequency) and Chemodenervation Procedures on the Extracranial Nerves, Peripheral Nerves, and Autonomic Nervous System

(For chemodenervation of internal anal sphincter, use 46505)

(For chemodenervation of the bladder, use 52287)

(For chemodenervation for strabismus involving the extraocular muscles, use 67345)

(For chemodenervation guided by needle electromyography or muscle electrical stimulation, see 95873, 95874)

Surgical Procedures on the Extracranial Nerves, Peripheral Nerves, and Autonomic Nervous System

(For intracranial surgery on cranial nerves, see 61450, 61460, 61790)

AMA *CPT Assistant* ▯

64642: Jan 14: 6, Oct 14: 15, Apr 19: 9, Aug 19: 10

64643: Jan 14: 6, Oct 14: 15, Apr 19: 9, Aug 19: 10

Plain English Description

Chemodenervation is performed on the muscles of one extremity to treat involuntary muscle contractions or muscle spasms such as those due to dystonia, cerebral palsy, or multiple sclerosis. Injection of botulinum toxin (type A or B) directly into a muscle produces temporary muscle paralysis by blocking the release of acetylcholine at the peripheral nerve endings, which interrupts neuromuscular transmission of nerve impulses. The muscle and muscle sites to be injected are determined either by use of electromyography or by examining the affected extremity, palpating the muscles, and noting the location of the muscle spasm. The extremity to be treated is prepared. The affected muscle or muscle group is then injected at carefully selected sites to accomplish the denervation. Use 64642 for 1-4 muscles of one extremity and 64643 for 1-4 muscles in each additional extremity.

ICD-10-CM Diagnostic Codes

	Code	Description
	G24.02	Drug induced acute dystonia
	G24.09	Other drug induced dystonia
	G24.1	Genetic torsion dystonia
	G24.2	Idiopathic nonfamilial dystonia
	G24.8	Other dystonia
	G24.9	Dystonia, unspecified
	G35	Multiple sclerosis
	G80.0	Spastic quadriplegic cerebral palsy
	G80.1	Spastic diplegic cerebral palsy
	G80.2	Spastic hemiplegic cerebral palsy
	G80.3	Athetoid cerebral palsy
	G80.4	Ataxic cerebral palsy
	G80.8	Other cerebral palsy
	G80.9	Cerebral palsy, unspecified
	G89.21	Chronic pain due to trauma
	G89.28	Other chronic postprocedural pain
	G89.29	Other chronic pain
	G89.3	Neoplasm related pain (acute) (chronic)
	M62.831	Muscle spasm of calf
	M62.838	Other muscle spasm
	M79.18	Myalgia, other site
⇄	M79.601	Pain in right arm
⇄	M79.602	Pain in left arm
⇄	M79.604	Pain in right leg
⇄	M79.605	Pain in left leg

CCI Edits

Refer to Appendix A for CCI edits.

Facility RVUs ▯

Code	Work	PE Facility	MP	Total Facility
64642	1.65	1.09	0.35	3.09
64643	1.22	0.62	0.22	2.06

Non-facility RVUs ▯

Code	Work	PE Non-Facility	MP	Total Non-Facility
64642	1.65	2.19	0.35	4.19
64643	1.22	1.21	0.22	2.65

Modifiers (PAR) ▯

Code	Mod 50	Mod 51	Mod 62	Mod 66	Mod 80
64642	0	2	0	0	1
64643	0	0	0	0	1

Global Period

Code	Days
64642	000
64643	ZZZ

64644-64645

64644 Chemodenervation of one extremity; 5 or more muscles

+ **64645 Chemodenervation of one extremity; each additional extremity, 5 or more muscles (List separately in addition to code for primary procedure)**

(Use 64645 in conjunction with 64644)

AMA Coding Guideline

Destruction by Neurolytic Agent (eg, Chemical, Thermal, Electrical or Radiofrequency) and Chemodenervation Procedures on the Extracranial Nerves, Peripheral Nerves, and Autonomic Nervous System

Codes 64600-64681 include the injection of other therapeutic agents (eg, corticosteroids). Do not report diagnostic/therapeutic injections separately. Do not report a code labeled as destruction when using therapies that are not destructive of the target nerve (eg, pulsed radiofrequency), use 64999. For codes labeled as chemodenervation, the supply of the chemodenervation agent is reported separately.

AMA Coding Notes

Destruction by Neurolytic Agent (eg, Chemical, Thermal, Electrical or Radiofrequency) and Chemodenervation Procedures on the Extracranial Nerves, Peripheral Nerves, and Autonomic Nervous System

(For chemodenervation of internal anal sphincter, use 46505)

(For chemodenervation of the bladder, use 52287)

(For chemodenervation for strabismus involving the extraocular muscles, use 67345)

(For chemodenervation guided by needle electromyography or muscle electrical stimulation, see 95873, 95874)

Surgical Procedures on the Extracranial Nerves, Peripheral Nerves, and Autonomic Nervous System

(For intracranial surgery on cranial nerves, see 61450, 61460, 61790)

AMA *CPT Assistant* ◻

64644: Jan 14: 6, Oct 14: 15, Apr 19: 9, Aug 19: 10

64645: Jan 14: 6, Oct 14: 15, Apr 19: 9, Aug 19: 10

Plain English Description

Chemodenervation is performed on the muscles of one extremity to treat involuntary muscle contractions or muscle spasms such as those due to dystonia, cerebral palsy, or multiple sclerosis. Injection of botulinum toxin (type A or B) directly into a muscle produces temporary muscle paralysis by blocking the release of acetylcholine at the peripheral nerve endings, which interrupts neuromuscular transmission of nerve impulses. The muscle and muscle sites to be injected are determined either by use of electromyography or by examining the affected extremity, palpating the muscles, and noting the location of the muscle spasm. The extremity to be treated is prepared. The affected muscles or muscle group(s) are then injected at carefully selected sites to accomplish the denervation. Use 64644 for 5 or more muscles of one extremity and 64645 for 5 or more muscles in each additional extremity.

ICD-10-CM Diagnostic Codes

	Code	Description
	G24.02	Drug induced acute dystonia
	G24.09	Other drug induced dystonia
	G24.1	Genetic torsion dystonia
	G24.2	Idiopathic nonfamilial dystonia
	G24.8	Other dystonia
	G24.9	Dystonia, unspecified
	G35	Multiple sclerosis
	G80.0	Spastic quadriplegic cerebral palsy
	G80.1	Spastic diplegic cerebral palsy
	G80.2	Spastic hemiplegic cerebral palsy
	G80.3	Athetoid cerebral palsy
	G80.4	Ataxic cerebral palsy
	G80.8	Other cerebral palsy
	G80.9	Cerebral palsy, unspecified
	G89.21	Chronic pain due to trauma
	G89.28	Other chronic postprocedural pain
	G89.29	Other chronic pain
	G89.3	Neoplasm related pain (acute) (chronic)
	M62.831	Muscle spasm of calf
	M62.838	Other muscle spasm
	M79.18	Myalgia, other site
⇄	M79.601	Pain in right arm
⇄	M79.602	Pain in left arm
⇄	M79.604	Pain in right leg
⇄	M79.605	Pain in left leg

CCI Edits

Refer to Appendix A for CCI edits.

Facility RVUs ◻

Code	Work	PE Facility	MP	Total Facility
64644	1.82	1.18	0.37	3.37
64645	1.39	0.70	0.28	2.37

Non-facility RVUs ◻

Code	Work	PE Non-Facility	MP	Total Non-Facility
64644	1.82	2.70	0.37	4.89
64645	1.39	1.68	0.28	3.35

Modifiers (PAR) ◻

Code	Mod 50	Mod 51	Mod 62	Mod 66	Mod 80
64644	0	2	0	0	1
64645	0	0	0	0	1

Global Period

Code	Days
64644	000
64645	ZZZ

64646-64647

64646 Chemodenervation of trunk muscle(s); 1-5 muscle(s)

64647 Chemodenervation of trunk muscle(s); 6 or more muscles

(Report either 64646 or 64647 only once per session)

AMA Coding Guideline

Destruction by Neurolytic Agent (eg, Chemical, Thermal, Electrical or Radiofrequency) and Chemodenervation Procedures on the Extracranial Nerves, Peripheral Nerves, and Autonomic Nervous System

Codes 64600-64681 include the injection of other therapeutic agents (eg, corticosteroids). Do not report diagnostic/therapeutic injections separately. Do not report a code labeled as destruction when using therapies that are not destructive of the target nerve (eg, pulsed radiofrequency), use 64999. For codes labeled as chemodenervation, the supply of the chemodenervation agent is reported separately.

AMA Coding Notes

Destruction by Neurolytic Agent (eg, Chemical, Thermal, Electrical or Radiofrequency) and Chemodenervation Procedures on the Extracranial Nerves, Peripheral Nerves, and Autonomic Nervous System

(For chemodenervation of internal anal sphincter, use 46505)

(For chemodenervation of the bladder, use 52287)

(For chemodenervation for strabismus involving the extraocular muscles, use 67345)

(For chemodenervation guided by needle electromyography or muscle electrical stimulation, see 95873, 95874)

Surgical Procedures on the Extracranial Nerves, Peripheral Nerves, and Autonomic Nervous System

(For intracranial surgery on cranial nerves, see 61450, 61460, 61790)

AMA *CPT Assistant* ☐

64646: Jan 14: 6, Apr 19: 9
64647: Jan 14: 6, Apr 19: 9

Plain English Description

Chemodenervation is performed on the muscles of the trunk to treat involuntary muscle contractions or muscle spasms such as those due to dystonia, cerebral palsy, or multiple sclerosis. Injection of botulinum toxin (type A or B) directly into a muscle produces temporary muscle paralysis by blocking the release of acetylcholine at the peripheral nerve endings, which interrupts neuromuscular transmission of nerve impulses. The muscle and muscle sites to be injected are determined either by use of electromyography or by examining the trunk, palpating the muscles, and noting the location of the muscle spasm. The trunk is prepared. The affected muscle(s) or muscle group is then injected at carefully selected sites to accomplish the denervation. Use 64646 for 1-5 muscles of the trunk and 64647 for 6 or more muscles in the trunk.

ICD-10-CM Diagnostic Codes

G24.02	Drug induced acute dystonia
G24.09	Other drug induced dystonia
G24.1	Genetic torsion dystonia
G24.2	Idiopathic nonfamilial dystonia
G24.8	Other dystonia
G24.9	Dystonia, unspecified
G35	Multiple sclerosis
G80.0	Spastic quadriplegic cerebral palsy
G80.1	Spastic diplegic cerebral palsy
G80.2	Spastic hemiplegic cerebral palsy
G80.3	Athetoid cerebral palsy
G80.4	Ataxic cerebral palsy
G80.8	Other cerebral palsy
G80.9	Cerebral palsy, unspecified
G89.21	Chronic pain due to trauma
G89.28	Other chronic postprocedural pain
G89.29	Other chronic pain
G89.3	Neoplasm related pain (acute) (chronic)
M54.5	Low back pain
M54.6	Pain in thoracic spine
M54.9	Dorsalgia, unspecified
M62.830	Muscle spasm of back
M62.838	Other muscle spasm

CCI Edits

Refer to Appendix A for CCI edits.

Facility RVUs ☐

Code	Work	PE Facility	MP	Total Facility
64646	1.80	1.11	0.41	3.32
64647	2.11	1.22	0.56	3.89

Non-facility RVUs ☐

Code	Work	PE Non-Facility	MP	Total Non-Facility
64646	1.80	2.20	0.41	4.41
64647	2.11	2.42	0.56	5.09

Modifiers (PAR) ☐

Code	Mod 50	Mod 51	Mod 62	Mod 66	Mod 80
64646	0	2	0	0	1
64647	0	2	0	0	1

Global Period

Code	Days
64646	000
64647	000

64650-64653

64650 Chemodenervation of eccrine glands; both axillae

64653 Chemodenervation of eccrine glands; other area(s) (eg, scalp, face, neck), per day

(Report the specific service in conjunction with code(s) for the specific substance(s) or drug(s) provided)

(For chemodenervation of extremities (eg, hands or feet), use 64999)

(For chemodenervation of bladder, use 52287)

AMA Coding Guideline

Destruction by Neurolytic Agent (eg, Chemical, Thermal, Electrical or Radiofrequency) and Chemodenervation Procedures on the Extracranial Nerves, Peripheral Nerves, and Autonomic Nervous System

Codes 64600-64681 include the injection of other therapeutic agents (eg, corticosteroids). Do not report diagnostic/therapeutic injections separately. Do not report a code labeled as destruction when using therapies that are not destructive of the target nerve (eg, pulsed radiofrequency), use 64999. For codes labeled as chemodenervation, the supply of the chemodenervation agent is reported separately.

AMA Coding Notes

Destruction by Neurolytic Agent (eg, Chemical, Thermal, Electrical or Radiofrequency) and Chemodenervation Procedures on the Extracranial Nerves, Peripheral Nerves, and Autonomic Nervous System

(For chemodenervation of internal anal sphincter, use 46505)

(For chemodenervation of the bladder, use 52287)

(For chemodenervation for strabismus involving the extraocular muscles, use 67345)

(For chemodenervation guided by needle electromyography or muscle electrical stimulation, see 95873, 95874)

Surgical Procedures on the Extracranial Nerves, Peripheral Nerves, and Autonomic Nervous System

(For intracranial surgery on cranial nerves, see 61450, 61460, 61790)

AMA *CPT Assistant*

64650: Jun 08: 9, Feb 10: 11, Sep 12: 14, Apr 19: 9

64653: Jun 08: 9, Sep 12: 14, Apr 19: 9

Plain English Description

The eccrine glands are sweat glands and are located over most parts of the body. Chemodenervation of the eccrine glands is performed to treat severe focal hyperhidrosis. Focal hyperhidrosis is profuse, localized sweating. Common sites for chemodenervation include the axillary region, scalp, face, neck, and palms of the hands. The locations of excessive sweating are identified by painting the region with an iodine solution and then dusting the area with starch powder. After 10-15 minutes, the presence of sweat causes the prepared areas to turn dark purple. The reactive area is then marked and the starch-iodine compound removed. The area is prepared with an antibacterial solution. The reconstituted botulinum toxin type A is then placed in syringes and injected into the dermis over the previously identified region at 1.5-2 cm intervals. Use 64650 for chemodenervation of eccrine glands in both axillae. Use 64653 for chemodenervation of eccrine glands in other areas. Code 64653 is reported once per day regardless of how many other areas are treated.

ICD-10-CM Diagnostic Codes

L74.510	Primary focal hyperhidrosis, axilla
L74.511	Primary focal hyperhidrosis, face
L74.512	Primary focal hyperhidrosis, palms
L74.513	Primary focal hyperhidrosis, soles
L74.519	Primary focal hyperhidrosis, unspecified
L74.52	Secondary focal hyperhidrosis
L74.8	Other eccrine sweat disorders
L74.9	Eccrine sweat disorder, unspecified
R61	Generalized hyperhidrosis

CCI Edits

Refer to Appendix A for CCI edits.

Facility RVUs

Code	Work	PE Facility	MP	Total Facility
64650	0.70	0.38	0.11	1.19
64653	0.88	0.46	0.19	1.53

Non-facility RVUs

Code	Work	PE Non-Facility	MP	Total Non-Facility
64650	0.70	1.49	0.11	2.30
64653	0.88	1.72	0.19	2.79

Modifiers (PAR)

Code	Mod 50	Mod 51	Mod 62	Mod 66	Mod 80
64650	0	2	0	0	0
64653	0	2	0	0	0

Global Period

Code	Days
64650	000
64653	000

64681

64681 Destruction by neurolytic agent, with or without radiologic monitoring; superior hypogastric plexus

AMA Coding Guideline

Destruction by Neurolytic Agent (eg, Chemical, Thermal, Electrical or Radiofrequency) and Chemodenervation Procedures on the Extracranial Nerves, Peripheral Nerves, and Autonomic Nervous System

Codes 64600-64681 include the injection of other therapeutic agents (eg, corticosteroids). Do not report diagnostic/therapeutic injections separately. Do not report a code labeled as destruction when using therapies that are not destructive of the target nerve (eg, pulsed radiofrequency), use 64999. For codes labeled as chemodenervation, the supply of the chemodenervation agent is reported separately.

AMA Coding Notes

Destruction by Neurolytic Agent (eg, Chemical, Thermal, Electrical or Radiofrequency) and Chemodenervation Procedures on the Extracranial Nerves, Peripheral Nerves, and Autonomic Nervous System

(For chemodenervation of internal anal sphincter, use 46505)

(For chemodenervation of the bladder, use 52287)

(For chemodenervation for strabismus involving the extraocular muscles, use 67345)

(For chemodenervation guided by needle electromyography or muscle electrical stimulation, see 95873, 95874)

Surgical Procedures on the Extracranial Nerves, Peripheral Nerves, and Autonomic Nervous System

(For intracranial surgery on cranial nerves, see 61450, 61460, 61790)

AMA *CPT Assistant*

64681: Aug 05: 13, Dec 07: 13, Sep 12: 14, Apr 19: 9

Plain English Description

The superior hypogastric plexus is a bilateral structure located in the retroperitoneum between the L5 and S1 vertebrae. Destruction of the superior hypogastric plexus is performed to treat pain due to a metastatic cancer in the pelvic region as well as nonmalignant chronic pain. Destruction may be performed by injection of a chemical neurolytic agent or using thermal, electrical, or radiofrequency techniques. This procedure may be performed with or without radiologic monitoring. If radiologic monitoring is used, a needle is inserted into the ventral lateral surface of the spine at the L5-S1 interspace. Contrast is then injected to confirm proper needle placement in the prevertebral space just ventral to the psoas fascia. If a chemical agent is used, the chemical agent is injected. Neurolytic chemical agents include phenol, ethyl alcohol, glycerol, ammonium salt compounds, and hypertonic or hypotonic solutions. Thermal or electrical modalities involve the use of a probe or needle that is inserted through the skin and activated to produce heat and destroy nerve tissue. To perform radiofrequency nerve destruction, an electrode needle is introduced through the skin and advanced toward the targeted neural tissue. The electrode is adjusted as needed until correct positioning is achieved. The radiofrequency device is then activated and an electric current generated that produces heat at the tip of the electrode and destroys the targeted nerve tissue.

Destruction by neurolytic agent, with or without radiologic monitoring; superior hypogastric plexus

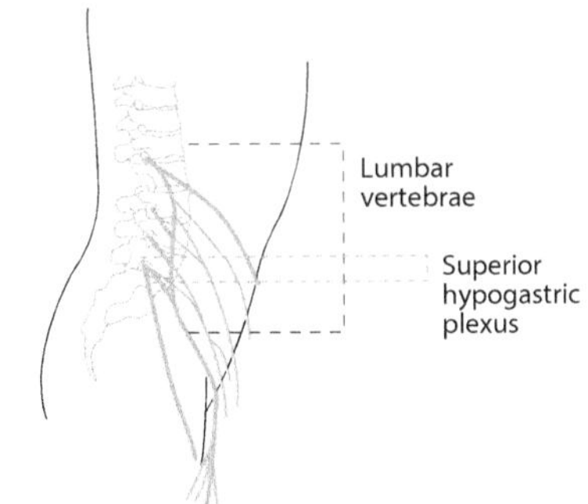

ICD-10-CM Diagnostic Codes

	C47.5	Malignant neoplasm of peripheral nerves of pelvis
	C48.0	Malignant neoplasm of retroperitoneum
	C48.1	Malignant neoplasm of specified parts of peritoneum
	C48.2	Malignant neoplasm of peritoneum, unspecified
	C48.8	Malignant neoplasm of overlapping sites of retroperitoneum and peritoneum
	C49.5	Malignant neoplasm of connective and soft tissue of pelvis
	C76.3	Malignant neoplasm of pelvis
	C78.6	Secondary malignant neoplasm of retroperitoneum and peritoneum
	C79.89	Secondary malignant neoplasm of other specified sites
	G89.21	Chronic pain due to trauma
	G89.28	Other chronic postprocedural pain
	G89.29	Other chronic pain
	G89.3	Neoplasm related pain (acute) (chronic)
	M54.16	Radiculopathy, lumbar region
	M54.17	Radiculopathy, lumbosacral region
	M54.18	Radiculopathy, sacral and sacrococcygeal region
	R10.2	Pelvic and perineal pain
7	S34.5	Injury of lumbar, sacral and pelvic sympathetic nerves

ICD-10-CM Coding Notes

For codes requiring a 7th character extension, refer to your ICD-10-CM book. Review the character descriptions and coding guidelines for proper selection. For some procedures, only certain characters will apply.

CCI Edits

Refer to Appendix A for CCI edits.

Facility RVUs

Code	Work	PE Facility	MP	Total Facility
64681	3.78	2.85	0.87	7.50

Non-facility RVUs

Code	Work	PE Non-Facility	MP	Total Non-Facility
64681	3.78	11.47	0.87	16.12

Modifiers (PAR)

Code	Mod 50	Mod 51	Mod 62	Mod 66	Mod 80
64681	0	2	0	0	1

Global Period

Code	Days
64681	010

64708-64712

64708 Neuroplasty, major peripheral nerve, arm or leg, open; other than specified

64712 Neuroplasty, major peripheral nerve, arm or leg, open; sciatic nerve

AMA Coding Guideline

Neuroplasty (Exploration, Neurolysis or Nerve Decompression) Procedures on the Extracranial Nerves, Peripheral Nerves, and Autonomic Nervous System

Neuroplasty is the surgical decompression or freeing of intact nerve from scar tissue, including external neurolysis and/or transposition to repair or restore the nerve.

AMA Coding Notes

Neuroplasty (Exploration, Neurolysis or Nerve Decompression) Procedures on the Extracranial Nerves, Peripheral Nerves, and Autonomic Nervous System

(For percutaneous neurolysis, see 62263, 62264, 62280-62282)

(For internal neurolysis requiring use of operating microscope, use 64727)

(For facial nerve decompression, use 69720)

(For neuroplasty with nerve wrapping, see 64702-64727, 64999)

Surgical Procedures on the Extracranial Nerves, Peripheral Nerves, and Autonomic Nervous System

(For intracranial surgery on cranial nerves, see 61450, 61460, 61790)

AMA *CPT Assistant* ◻

64708: Jun 01: 11, Jun 12: 12, Nov 17: 10
64712: Jun 01: 11, Jun 12: 12

Plain English Description

Neuroplasty is performed to treat nerve entrapment, which may be caused by inflammation of surrounding tissues, a tumor or mass, or scar tissue and adhesion formation. The skin over the nerve is incised and soft tissues are dissected. The nerve is identified and any scar tissue or adhesions are dissected free of the nerve. Other structures such as fascia or ligaments may be divided to release pressure on the nerve. Once the nerve is completely freed of surrounding tissue and impinging structures, the soft tissues are closed in layers. In 64708, neuroplasty is performed on a major peripheral nerve of the arm or leg other than one specified. In 64712, neuroplasty of the sciatic nerve is performed.

Neuroplasty, major peripheral nerve, arm or leg

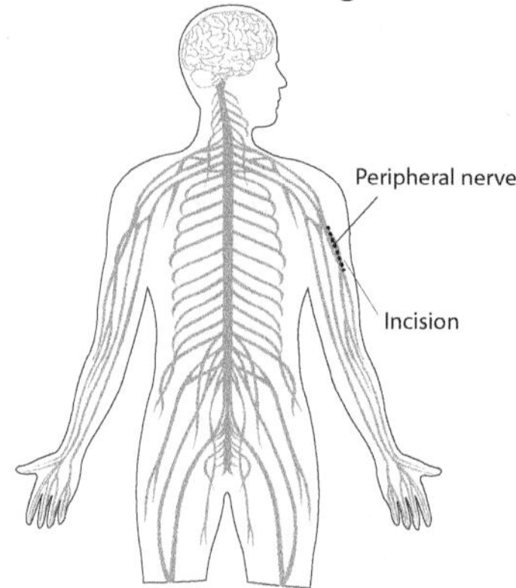

A major peripheral nerve is freed from the surrounding tissue.

ICD-10-CM Diagnostic Codes

	Code	Description
⇄	C47.11	Malignant neoplasm of peripheral nerves of right upper limb, including shoulder
⇄	C47.12	Malignant neoplasm of peripheral nerves of left upper limb, including shoulder
⇄	C47.21	Malignant neoplasm of peripheral nerves of right lower limb, including hip
⇄	C47.22	Malignant neoplasm of peripheral nerves of left lower limb, including hip
	C47.8	Malignant neoplasm of overlapping sites of peripheral nerves and autonomic nervous system
⇄	C49.11	Malignant neoplasm of connective and soft tissue of right upper limb, including shoulder
⇄	C49.12	Malignant neoplasm of connective and soft tissue of left upper limb, including shoulder
⇄	C49.21	Malignant neoplasm of connective and soft tissue of right lower limb, including hip
⇄	C49.22	Malignant neoplasm of connective and soft tissue of left lower limb, including hip
	D36.12	Benign neoplasm of peripheral nerves and autonomic nervous system, upper limb, including shoulder
	D36.13	Benign neoplasm of peripheral nerves and autonomic nervous system of lower limb, including hip
	D48.2	Neoplasm of uncertain behavior of peripheral nerves and autonomic nervous system
	G54.0	Brachial plexus disorders
⇄	G56.11	Other lesions of median nerve, right upper limb
⇄	G56.12	Other lesions of median nerve, left upper limb
⇄	G56.13	Other lesions of median nerve, bilateral upper limbs
⇄	G56.21	Lesion of ulnar nerve, right upper limb
⇄	G56.22	Lesion of ulnar nerve, left upper limb
⇄	G56.23	Lesion of ulnar nerve, bilateral upper limbs
⇄	G56.31	Lesion of radial nerve, right upper limb
⇄	G56.32	Lesion of radial nerve, left upper limb
⇄	G56.33	Lesion of radial nerve, bilateral upper limbs
⇄	G57.01	Lesion of sciatic nerve, right lower limb
⇄	G57.02	Lesion of sciatic nerve, left lower limb
⇄	G57.03	Lesion of sciatic nerve, bilateral lower limbs
⇄	G57.11	Meralgia paresthetica, right lower limb
⇄	G57.12	Meralgia paresthetica, left lower limb
⇄	G57.13	Meralgia paresthetica, bilateral lower limbs
⇄	G57.21	Lesion of femoral nerve, right lower limb
⇄	G57.22	Lesion of femoral nerve, left lower limb
⇄	G57.23	Lesion of femoral nerve, bilateral lower limbs
⇄	G57.31	Lesion of lateral popliteal nerve, right lower limb
⇄	G57.32	Lesion of lateral popliteal nerve, left lower limb
⇄	G57.33	Lesion of lateral popliteal nerve, bilateral lower limbs
⇄	G57.41	Lesion of medial popliteal nerve, right lower limb
⇄	G57.42	Lesion of medial popliteal nerve, left lower limb
⇄	G57.43	Lesion of medial popliteal nerve, bilateral lower limbs
⇄	G57.61	Lesion of plantar nerve, right lower limb
⇄	G57.62	Lesion of plantar nerve, left lower limb
⇄	G57.63	Lesion of plantar nerve, bilateral lower limbs
⇄	M79.601	Pain in right arm
⇄	M79.602	Pain in left arm
⇄	M79.604	Pain in right leg
⇄	M79.605	Pain in left leg
⇄	M79.621	Pain in right upper arm
⇄	M79.622	Pain in left upper arm
⇄	M79.631	Pain in right forearm
⇄	M79.632	Pain in left forearm
⇄	M79.651	Pain in right thigh
⇄	M79.652	Pain in left thigh
⇄	M79.661	Pain in right lower leg
⇄	M79.662	Pain in left lower leg
❼⇄	S44.01	Injury of ulnar nerve at upper arm level, right arm
❼⇄	S44.02	Injury of ulnar nerve at upper arm level, left arm
❼⇄	S44.11	Injury of median nerve at upper arm level, right arm
❼⇄	S44.12	Injury of median nerve at upper arm level, left arm
❼⇄	S44.21	Injury of radial nerve at upper arm level, right arm
❼⇄	S44.22	Injury of radial nerve at upper arm level, left arm
❼⇄	S44.31	Injury of axillary nerve, right arm

⑦⇄	S44.32	Injury of axillary nerve, left arm
⑦⇄	S44.41	Injury of musculocutaneous nerve, right arm
⑦⇄	S44.42	Injury of musculocutaneous nerve, left arm
⑦⇄	S54.11	Injury of median nerve at forearm level, right arm
⑦⇄	S54.12	Injury of median nerve at forearm level, left arm
⑦⇄	S54.21	Injury of radial nerve at forearm level, right arm
⑦⇄	S54.22	Injury of radial nerve at forearm level, left arm
⑦⇄	S74.01	Injury of sciatic nerve at hip and thigh level, right leg
⑦⇄	S74.02	Injury of sciatic nerve at hip and thigh level, left leg
⑦⇄	S74.11	Injury of femoral nerve at hip and thigh level, right leg
⑦⇄	S74.12	Injury of femoral nerve at hip and thigh level, left leg
⑦⇄	S84.01	Injury of tibial nerve at lower leg level, right leg
⑦⇄	S84.02	Injury of tibial nerve at lower leg level, left leg
⑦⇄	S84.11	Injury of peroneal nerve at lower leg level, right leg
⑦⇄	S84.12	Injury of peroneal nerve at lower leg level, left leg

ICD-10-CM Coding Notes

For codes requiring a 7th character extension, refer to your ICD-10-CM book. Review the character descriptions and coding guidelines for proper selection. For some procedures, only certain characters will apply.

CCI Edits

Refer to Appendix A for CCI edits.

Facility RVUs ▯

Code	Work	PE Facility	MP	Total Facility
64708	6.36	6.96	1.19	14.51
64712	8.07	7.30	1.58	16.95

Non-facility RVUs ▯

Code	Work	PE Non-Facility	MP	Total Non-Facility
64708	6.36	6.96	1.19	14.51
64712	8.07	7.30	1.58	16.95

Modifiers (PAR) ▯

Code	Mod 50	Mod 51	Mod 62	Mod 66	Mod 80
64708	0	2	1	0	2
64712	1	2	1	0	2

Global Period

Code	Days
64708	090
64712	090

64713

64713 Neuroplasty, major peripheral nerve, arm or leg, open; brachial plexus

AMA Coding Guideline

Neuroplasty (Exploration, Neurolysis or Nerve Decompression) Procedures on the Extracranial Nerves, Peripheral Nerves, and Autonomic Nervous System

Neuroplasty is the surgical decompression or freeing of intact nerve from scar tissue, including external neurolysis and/or transposition to repair or restore the nerve.

AMA Coding Notes

Neuroplasty (Exploration, Neurolysis or Nerve Decompression) Procedures on the Extracranial Nerves, Peripheral Nerves, and Autonomic Nervous System

(For percutaneous neurolysis, see 62263, 62264, 62280-62282)

(For internal neurolysis requiring use of operating microscope, use 64727)

(For facial nerve decompression, use 69720)

(For neuroplasty with nerve wrapping, see 64702-64727, 64999)

Surgical Procedures on the Extracranial Nerves, Peripheral Nerves, and Autonomic Nervous System

(For intracranial surgery on cranial nerves, see 61450, 61460, 61790)

AMA *CPT Assistant* ☐

64713: Jun 01: 11, Jun 12: 12, May 13: 12

Plain English Description

The brachial plexus is a network of nerves that sends signals from the spine to the shoulder, arm, and hand. Injury can occur as a result of blunt force, such as that occurring in contact sports, an auto accident, or a fall. The brachial plexus can also be damaged during the birth process or from inflammation, or a tumor. Damage to the brachial plexus can cause formation of scar tissue and adhesions that entrap and compress the nerves. A supraclavicular approach is used to expose the proximal aspect of the brachial plexus. The omohyoid muscle is divided. Electrophysiological tests are performed as needed to assess nerve function of exposed nerves and nerve roots as well as to determine which nerves are compressed. Compressed nerves in the brachial plexus are dissected free of scar tissue and other structures causing the compression. Once affected nerves are completely freed, the overlying soft tissues are closed in layers.

Brachial plexus neuroplasty

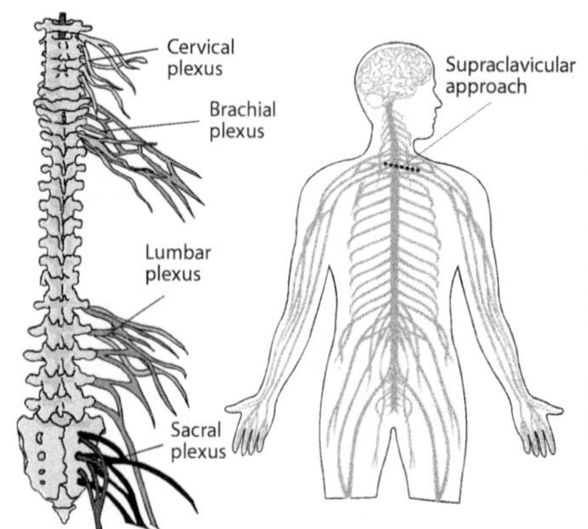

Compressed nerves in the brachial plexus are freed from the surrounding tissue.

ICD-10-CM Diagnostic Codes

⇄ C47.11 Malignant neoplasm of peripheral nerves of right upper limb, including shoulder
⇄ C47.12 Malignant neoplasm of peripheral nerves of left upper limb, including shoulder
⇄ C49.11 Malignant neoplasm of connective and soft tissue of right upper limb, including shoulder
⇄ C49.12 Malignant neoplasm of connective and soft tissue of left upper limb, including shoulder
C79.89 Secondary malignant neoplasm of other specified sites
⇄ D17.21 Benign lipomatous neoplasm of skin and subcutaneous tissue of right arm
⇄ D17.22 Benign lipomatous neoplasm of skin and subcutaneous tissue of left arm
D36.12 Benign neoplasm of peripheral nerves and autonomic nervous system, upper limb, including shoulder
D48.2 Neoplasm of uncertain behavior of peripheral nerves and autonomic nervous system
G54.0 Brachial plexus disorders
⇄ G83.21 Monoplegia of upper limb affecting right dominant side
⇄ G83.22 Monoplegia of upper limb affecting left dominant side
⇄ G83.23 Monoplegia of upper limb affecting right nondominant side
⇄ G83.24 Monoplegia of upper limb affecting left nondominant side
M62.81 Muscle weakness (generalized)
⇄ M79.601 Pain in right arm
⇄ M79.602 Pain in left arm
⇄ M79.621 Pain in right upper arm
⇄ M79.622 Pain in left upper arm
⇄ M79.631 Pain in right forearm
⇄ M79.632 Pain in left forearm
P14.3 Other brachial plexus birth injuries
Q07.8 Other specified congenital malformations of nervous system
R20.0 Anesthesia of skin
R20.2 Paresthesia of skin
R20.8 Other disturbances of skin sensation
R53.1 Weakness
⑦ S14.3 Injury of brachial plexus

ICD-10-CM Coding Notes

For codes requiring a 7th character extension, refer to your ICD-10-CM book. Review the character descriptions and coding guidelines for proper selection. For some procedures, only certain characters will apply.

CCI Edits

Refer to Appendix A for CCI edits.

Facility RVUs ☐

Code	Work	PE Facility	MP	Total Facility
64713	11.40	8.80	2.37	22.57

Non-facility RVUs ☐

Code	Work	PE Non-Facility	MP	Total Non-Facility
64713	11.40	8.80	2.37	22.57

Modifiers (PAR) ☐

Code	Mod 50	Mod 51	Mod 62	Mod 66	Mod 80
64713	1	2	1	0	2

Global Period

Code	Days
64713	090

● New ▲ Revised ✚ Add On ⊘Modifier 51 Exempt ★Telemedicine ☐ CPT QuickRef ⁄FDA Pending ⇄ Laterality ⑦Seventh Character ♂Male ♀Female

64714

64714 Neuroplasty, major peripheral nerve, arm or leg, open; lumbar plexus

AMA Coding Guideline

Neuroplasty (Exploration, Neurolysis or Nerve Decompression) Procedures on the Extracranial Nerves, Peripheral Nerves, and Autonomic Nervous System

Neuroplasty is the surgical decompression or freeing of intact nerve from scar tissue, including external neurolysis and/or transposition to repair or restore the nerve.

AMA Coding Notes

Neuroplasty (Exploration, Neurolysis or Nerve Decompression) Procedures on the Extracranial Nerves, Peripheral Nerves, and Autonomic Nervous System

(For percutaneous neurolysis, see 62263, 62264, 62280-62282)

(For internal neurolysis requiring use of operating microscope, use 64727)

(For facial nerve decompression, use 69720)

(For neuroplasty with nerve wrapping, see 64702-64727, 64999)

Surgical Procedures on the Extracranial Nerves, Peripheral Nerves, and Autonomic Nervous System

(For intracranial surgery on cranial nerves, see 61450, 61460, 61790)

AMA *CPT Assistant*

64714: Jun 97: 11, Sep 98: 16, Jun 01: 11, Jun 12: 12, Dec 13: 17

Plain English Description

The lumbar plexus is a network of nerves originating from the L1-L4 nerve roots that send signals to the back, abdomen, groin, thighs, knees, and calves. Injury can occur as a result of blunt force, such as that occurring in contact sports, an auto accident, or a fall. The lumbar plexus can also be damaged by an inflammatory process or a tumor. Injury or other disease processes can cause formation of scar tissue and adhesions that entrap and compress nerves contained in the lumbar plexus. An incision is made in the lower back over the affected side. Soft tissues are divided. The lumbar plexus is exposed. Electrophysiological tests are performed as needed to assess nerve function of exposed nerves and nerve roots as well as to determine which nerves are compressed. Compressed nerves in the lumbar plexus are dissected free of scar tissue and other structures causing the compression. Once affected nerves are completely freed, the overlying soft tissues are closed in layers.

Lumbar plexus neuroplasty

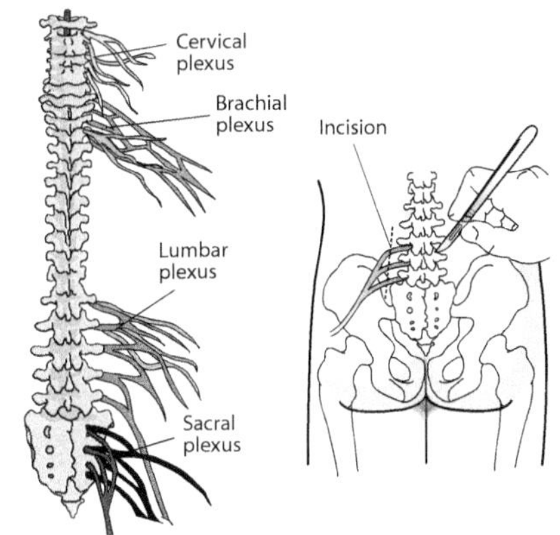

Compressed nerves in the lumbar plexus are freed from the surrounding tissue.

ICD-10-CM Diagnostic Codes

	Code	Description
⇄	C47.21	Malignant neoplasm of peripheral nerves of right lower limb, including hip
⇄	C47.22	Malignant neoplasm of peripheral nerves of left lower limb, including hip
	C47.6	Malignant neoplasm of peripheral nerves of trunk, unspecified
	C79.89	Secondary malignant neoplasm of other specified sites
	D36.13	Benign neoplasm of peripheral nerves and autonomic nervous system of lower limb, including hip
	D36.17	Benign neoplasm of peripheral nerves and autonomic nervous system of trunk, unspecified
	D48.2	Neoplasm of uncertain behavior of peripheral nerves and autonomic nervous system
	G54.1	Lumbosacral plexus disorders
⇄	G57.11	Meralgia paresthetica, right lower limb
⇄	G57.12	Meralgia paresthetica, left lower limb
⇄	G57.13	Meralgia paresthetica, bilateral lower limbs
⇄	G83.11	Monoplegia of lower limb affecting right dominant side
⇄	G83.12	Monoplegia of lower limb affecting left dominant side
⇄	G83.13	Monoplegia of lower limb affecting right nondominant side
⇄	G83.14	Monoplegia of lower limb affecting left nondominant side
⇄	M79.604	Pain in right leg
⇄	M79.605	Pain in left leg
➐	S34.21	Injury of nerve root of lumbar spine
➐	S34.22	Injury of nerve root of sacral spine
➐	S34.4	Injury of lumbosacral plexus

ICD-10-CM Coding Notes

For codes requiring a 7th character extension, refer to your ICD-10-CM book. Review the character descriptions and coding guidelines for proper selection. For some procedures, only certain characters will apply.

CCI Edits

Refer to Appendix A for CCI edits.

Facility RVUs

Code	Work	PE Facility	MP	Total Facility
64714	10.55	8.55	2.03	21.13

Non-facility RVUs

Code	Work	PE Non-Facility	MP	Total Non-Facility
64714	10.55	8.55	2.03	21.13

Modifiers (PAR)

Code	Mod 50	Mod 51	Mod 62	Mod 66	Mod 80
64714	1	2	1	0	2

Global Period

Code	Days
64714	090

64718-64719

64718 Neuroplasty and/or transposition; ulnar nerve at elbow

64719 Neuroplasty and/or transposition; ulnar nerve at wrist

AMA Coding Guideline

Neuroplasty (Exploration, Neurolysis or Nerve Decompression) Procedures on the Extracranial Nerves, Peripheral Nerves, and Autonomic Nervous System

Neuroplasty is the surgical decompression or freeing of intact nerve from scar tissue, including external neurolysis and/or transposition to repair or restore the nerve.

AMA Coding Notes

Neuroplasty (Exploration, Neurolysis or Nerve Decompression) Procedures on the Extracranial Nerves, Peripheral Nerves, and Autonomic Nervous System

(For percutaneous neurolysis, see 62263, 62264, 62280-62282)

(For internal neurolysis requiring use of operating microscope, use 64727)

(For facial nerve decompression, use 69720)

(For neuroplasty with nerve wrapping, see 64702-64727, 64999)

Surgical Procedures on the Extracranial Nerves, Peripheral Nerves, and Autonomic Nervous System

(For intracranial surgery on cranial nerves, see 61450, 61460, 61790)

AMA *CPT Assistant* ☐

64718: Jun 01: 11, Mar 09: 10

64719: Jun 01: 11, Mar 09: 10

Plain English Description

Neuroplasty and/or transposition of the ulnar nerve at the elbow or wrist is performed to treat nerve entrapment and compression of the nerve. The ulnar nerve passes under the collarbone, travels along the inner aspect of the arm, passes through the cubital tunnel in the inner aspect of the elbow, and then travels under the muscles of the inner arm and through Guyon's canal, which is another tunnel in the wrist before entering the hand. In 64718, the ulnar nerve is decompressed at the elbow. An incision is made along the inner aspect of the elbow over the ulnar nerve and soft tissues are dissected. The ulnar nerve is identified and any scar tissue or adhesions are dissected free of the nerve. An anterior transposition may also be performed. This involves relocating the ulnar nerve from its usual position behind the elbow to a position in front of the elbow. The nerve can be moved to a subcutaneous position beneath the skin and fat but above the muscle or it can be moved to a position under the muscle. Once the nerve is completely freed of surrounding tissue and impinging structures, the soft tissues are closed in layers. In 64719, the ulnar nerve is decompressed at the wrist. A zigzag incision is made at the base of the palm on the little finger side and extended over the wrist. The roof of Guyon's canal is incised and scar tissue, adhesions, or other impinging structures divided. Once the nerve is completely freed, overlying soft tissues are closed in layers.

Neuroplasty and/or transposition, ulnar nerve at elbow

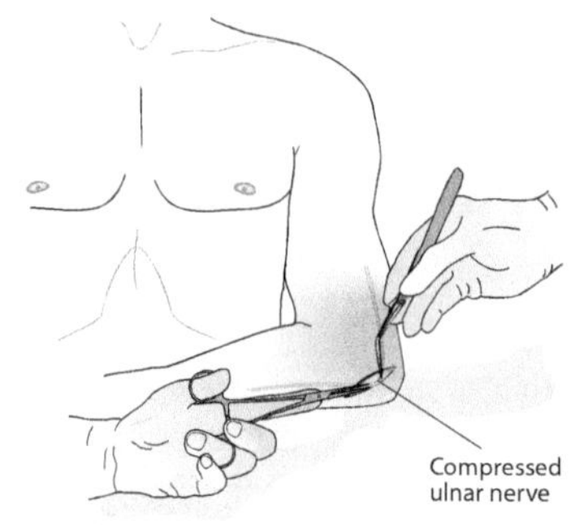

ICD-10-CM Diagnostic Codes

	Code	Description
⇄	G56.21	Lesion of ulnar nerve, right upper limb
⇄	G56.22	Lesion of ulnar nerve, left upper limb
⇄	G56.23	Lesion of ulnar nerve, bilateral upper limbs
⇄	M25.541	Pain in joints of right hand
⇄	M25.542	Pain in joints of left hand
⇄	M79.631	Pain in right forearm
⇄	M79.632	Pain in left forearm
⇄	M79.644	Pain in right finger(s)
⇄	M79.645	Pain in left finger(s)
❼⇄	S44.01	Injury of ulnar nerve at upper arm level, right arm
❼⇄	S44.02	Injury of ulnar nerve at upper arm level, left arm
❼⇄	S54.01	Injury of ulnar nerve at forearm level, right arm
❼⇄	S54.02	Injury of ulnar nerve at forearm level, left arm

ICD-10-CM Coding Notes

For codes requiring a 7th character extension, refer to your ICD-10-CM book. Review the character descriptions and coding guidelines for proper selection. For some procedures, only certain characters will apply.

CCI Edits

Refer to Appendix A for CCI edits.

Facility RVUs ☐

Code	Work	PE Facility	MP	Total Facility
64718	7.26	8.46	1.42	17.14
64719	4.97	5.72	0.90	11.59

Non-facility RVUs ☐

Code	Work	PE Non-Facility	MP	Total Non-Facility
64718	7.26	8.46	1.42	17.14
64719	4.97	5.72	0.90	11.59

Modifiers (PAR) ☐

Code	Mod 50	Mod 51	Mod 62	Mod 66	Mod 80
64718	1	2	0	0	0
64719	1	2	0	0	1

Global Period

Code	Days
64718	090
64719	090

64721

64721 Neuroplasty and/or transposition; median nerve at carpal tunnel

(For arthroscopic procedure, use 29848)

AMA Coding Guideline

Neuroplasty (Exploration, Neurolysis or Nerve Decompression) Procedures on the Extracranial Nerves, Peripheral Nerves, and Autonomic Nervous System

Neuroplasty is the surgical decompression or freeing of intact nerve from scar tissue, including external neurolysis and/or transposition to repair or restore the nerve.

AMA Coding Notes

Neuroplasty (Exploration, Neurolysis or Nerve Decompression) Procedures on the Extracranial Nerves, Peripheral Nerves, and Autonomic Nervous System

(For percutaneous neurolysis, see 62263, 62264, 62280-62282)

(For internal neurolysis requiring use of operating microscope, use 64727)

(For facial nerve decompression, use 69720)

(For neuroplasty with nerve wrapping, see 64702-64727, 64999)

Surgical Procedures on the Extracranial Nerves, Peripheral Nerves, and Autonomic Nervous System

(For intracranial surgery on cranial nerves, see 61450, 61460, 61790)

AMA *CPT Assistant*

64721: Fall 92: 17, Sep 97: 10, Jun 01: 11, Nov 06: 23, Aug 09: 11, Jun 12: 15, Sep 12: 16, Dec 13: 14, Jul 15: 10

Plain English Description

This procedure is performed to treat carpal tunnel syndrome (CTS), which results from median nerve compression within the carpal tunnel, a narrow passageway within the wrist between the carpal bones and carpal ligament. A regional or general anesthetic is administered. The skin is incised over the carpal tunnel in the palm of the hand and extended as needed over the wrist. The palmar fascia is exposed and incised. The carpal ligament is exposed. The median nerve and flexor tendons are identified and protected. The carpal ligament is then divided using scissors or a scalpel, which releases the pressure on the median nerve. The nerve may also be relocated within the carpal tunnel to relieve the compression. The palmar fascia and skin are closed in layers.

Neuroplasty and/or transposition; median nerve at carpal tunnel

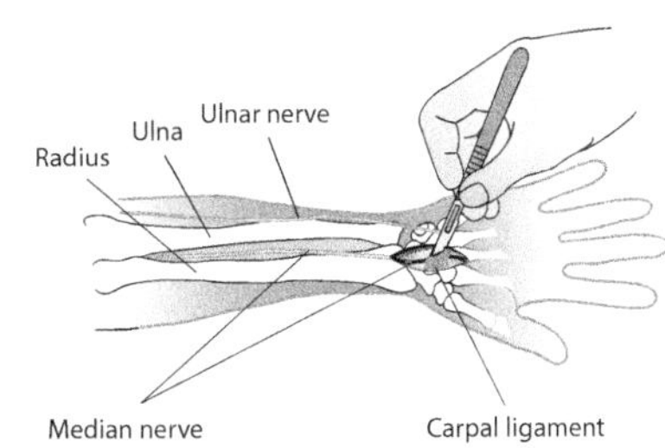

ICD-10-CM Diagnostic Codes

	Code	Description
⇄	G56.01	Carpal tunnel syndrome, right upper limb
⇄	G56.02	Carpal tunnel syndrome, left upper limb
⇄	G56.03	Carpal tunnel syndrome, bilateral upper limbs
⇄	G56.11	Other lesions of median nerve, right upper limb
⇄	G56.12	Other lesions of median nerve, left upper limb
⇄	M25.541	Pain in joints of right hand
⇄	M25.542	Pain in joints of left hand
⇄	M79.644	Pain in right finger(s)
⇄	M79.645	Pain in left finger(s)
➐⇄	S64.11	Injury of median nerve at wrist and hand level of right arm
➐⇄	S64.12	Injury of median nerve at wrist and hand level of left arm

ICD-10-CM Coding Notes

For codes requiring a 7th character extension, refer to your ICD-10-CM book. Review the character descriptions and coding guidelines for proper selection. For some procedures, only certain characters will apply.

CCI Edits

Refer to Appendix A for CCI edits.

Facility RVUs

Code	Work	PE Facility	MP	Total Facility
64721	4.97	6.44	0.96	12.37

Non-facility RVUs

Code	Work	PE Non-Facility	MP	Total Non-Facility
64721	4.97	6.61	0.96	12.54

Modifiers (PAR)

Code	Mod 50	Mod 51	Mod 62	Mod 66	Mod 80
64721	1	2	0	0	1

Global Period

Code	Days
64721	090

64722

64722 Decompression; unspecified nerve(s) (specify)

AMA Coding Guideline

Neuroplasty (Exploration, Neurolysis or Nerve Decompression) Procedures on the Extracranial Nerves, Peripheral Nerves, and Autonomic Nervous System

Neuroplasty is the surgical decompression or freeing of intact nerve from scar tissue, including external neurolysis and/or transposition to repair or restore the nerve.

AMA Coding Notes

Neuroplasty (Exploration, Neurolysis or Nerve Decompression) Procedures on the Extracranial Nerves, Peripheral Nerves, and Autonomic Nervous System

(For percutaneous neurolysis, see 62263, 62264, 62280-62282)

(For internal neurolysis requiring use of operating microscope, use 64727)

(For facial nerve decompression, use 69720)

(For neuroplasty with nerve wrapping, see 64702-64727, 64999)

Surgical Procedures on the Extracranial Nerves, Peripheral Nerves, and Autonomic Nervous System

(For intracranial surgery on cranial nerves, see 61450, 61460, 61790)

AMA *CPT Assistant* ▯

64722: Sep 98: 16, May 99: 11, Jun 01: 11, Oct 04: 12

Plain English Description

Decompression is performed to treat nerve entrapment, which may be caused by inflammation of surrounding tissues, a tumor or mass, or scar tissue and adhesion formation. The skin over the nerve is incised and soft tissues are dissected. The nerve is identified and any scar tissue or adhesions are dissected free of the nerve. Other structures such as fascia or ligaments may be divided to release pressure on the nerve. Once the nerve is completely freed of surrounding tissue and impinging structures, the soft tissues are closed in layers. Use 64722 for decompression of any nerve that does not have a more specific code.

Decompression; unspecified nerve(s)

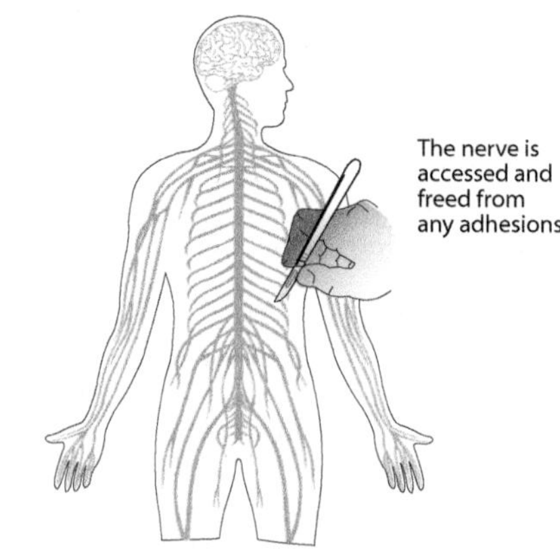

Decompression is performed on any nerve that does not have a specific code.

ICD-10-CM Diagnostic Codes

	Code	Description
	G54.0	Brachial plexus disorders
⇄	G57.11	Meralgia paresthetica, right lower limb
⇄	G57.12	Meralgia paresthetica, left lower limb
⇄	G57.13	Meralgia paresthetica, bilateral lower limbs
⇄	M25.541	Pain in joints of right hand
⇄	M25.542	Pain in joints of left hand
⇄	M79.601	Pain in right arm
⇄	M79.602	Pain in left arm
⇄	M79.604	Pain in right leg
⇄	M79.605	Pain in left leg
⇄	M79.621	Pain in right upper arm
⇄	M79.622	Pain in left upper arm
⇄	M79.631	Pain in right forearm
⇄	M79.632	Pain in left forearm
⇄	M79.644	Pain in right finger(s)
⇄	M79.645	Pain in left finger(s)
⇄	M79.651	Pain in right thigh
⇄	M79.652	Pain in left thigh
⇄	M79.661	Pain in right lower leg
⇄	M79.662	Pain in left lower leg
❼	S34.6	Injury of peripheral nerve(s) at abdomen, lower back and pelvis level
❼	S34.8	Injury of other nerves at abdomen, lower back and pelvis level
❼⇄	S44.8X1	Injury of other nerves at shoulder and upper arm level, right arm
❼⇄	S44.8X2	Injury of other nerves at shoulder and upper arm level, left arm
❼⇄	S54.8X1	Injury of other nerves at forearm level, right arm
❼⇄	S54.8X2	Injury of other nerves at forearm level, left arm
❼⇄	S64.8X1	Injury of other nerves at wrist and hand level of right arm
❼⇄	S64.8X2	Injury of other nerves at wrist and hand level of left arm
❼⇄	S74.8X1	Injury of other nerves at hip and thigh level, right leg
❼⇄	S74.8X2	Injury of other nerves at hip and thigh level, left leg
❼⇄	S84.21	Injury of cutaneous sensory nerve at lower leg level, right leg
❼⇄	S84.22	Injury of cutaneous sensory nerve at lower leg level, left leg
❼⇄	S84.801	Injury of other nerves at lower leg level, right leg
❼⇄	S84.802	Injury of other nerves at lower leg level, left leg
❼⇄	S94.31	Injury of cutaneous sensory nerve at ankle and foot level, right leg
❼⇄	S94.32	Injury of cutaneous sensory nerve at ankle and foot level, left leg
❼⇄	S94.8X1	Injury of other nerves at ankle and foot level, right leg
❼⇄	S94.8X2	Injury of other nerves at ankle and foot level, left leg

ICD-10-CM Coding Notes

For codes requiring a 7th character extension, refer to your ICD-10-CM book. Review the character descriptions and coding guidelines for proper selection. For some procedures, only certain characters will apply.

CCI Edits

Refer to Appendix A for CCI edits.

Facility RVUs ▯

Code	Work	PE Facility	MP	Total Facility
64722	4.82	4.68	0.85	10.35

Non-facility RVUs ▯

Code	Work	PE Non-Facility	MP	Total Non-Facility
64722	4.82	4.68	0.85	10.35

Modifiers (PAR) ▯

Code	Mod 50	Mod 51	Mod 62	Mod 66	Mod 80
64722	0	2	1	0	2

Global Period

Code	Days
64722	090

64727

✚ **64727 Internal neurolysis, requiring use of operating microscope (List separately in addition to code for neuroplasty) (Neuroplasty includes external neurolysis)**

(Do not report code 69990 in addition to code 64727)

AMA Coding Guideline

Neuroplasty (Exploration, Neurolysis or Nerve Decompression) Procedures on the Extracranial Nerves, Peripheral Nerves, and Autonomic Nervous System

Neuroplasty is the surgical decompression or freeing of intact nerve from scar tissue, including external neurolysis and/or transposition to repair or restore the nerve.

AMA Coding Notes

Neuroplasty (Exploration, Neurolysis or Nerve Decompression) Procedures on the Extracranial Nerves, Peripheral Nerves, and Autonomic Nervous System

(For percutaneous neurolysis, see 62263, 62264, 62280-62282)

(For internal neurolysis requiring use of operating microscope, use 64727)

(For facial nerve decompression, use 69720)

(For neuroplasty with nerve wrapping, see 64702-64727, 64999)

Surgical Procedures on the Extracranial Nerves, Peripheral Nerves, and Autonomic Nervous System

(For intracranial surgery on cranial nerves, see 61450, 61460, 61790)

AMA *CPT Assistant* ☐

64727: Nov 98: 19, Jun 01: 11, Jun 12: 13

Plain English Description

Internal neurolysis is performed to treat scarring and swelling occurring internally, that is within the outer nerve sheath. During a separately reportable neuroplasty procedure, the outer nerve sheath is incised using a microscope to improve visualization of the nerve. The nerve is inspected. If the nerve is swollen, opening the outer sheath alone will help relieve the nerve compression and promote blood flow to the nerve. If scar tissue is present within the outer sheath, it is carefully dissected. The outer sheath is left open.

ICD-10-CM Diagnostic Codes

See Primary Procedure code for crosswalks.

CCI Edits

Refer to Appendix A for CCI edits.

Facility RVUs ☐

Code	Work	PE Facility	MP	Total Facility
64727	3.10	1.55	0.62	5.27

Non-facility RVUs ☐

Code	Work	PE Non-Facility	MP	Total Non-Facility
64727	3.10	1.55	0.62	5.27

Modifiers (PAR) ☐

Code	Mod 50	Mod 51	Mod 62	Mod 66	Mod 80
64727	0	0	0	0	1

Global Period

Code	Days
64727	ZZZ

64771-64772

64771 Transection or avulsion of other cranial nerve, extradural

64772 Transection or avulsion of other spinal nerve, extradural

(For excision of tender scar, skin and subcutaneous tissue, with or without tiny neuroma, see 11400-11446, 13100-13153)

AMA Coding Notes

Transection or Avulsion Procedures on the Extracranial Nerves, Peripheral Nerves, and Autonomic Nervous System

(For stereotactic lesion of gasserian ganglion, use 61790)

Surgical Procedures on the Extracranial Nerves, Peripheral Nerves, and Autonomic Nervous System

(For intracranial surgery on cranial nerves, see 61450, 61460, 61790)

AMA *CPT Assistant*

64772: Apr 15: 10

Plain English Description

Transection or avulsion involves severing and/or removing a portion of the nerve and is performed to treat chronic pain. Transection or avulsion of a cranial or spinal nerve not described by a more specific code is performed. This procedure is performed outside the dural membrane that covers the brain and spinal cord. A skin incision is made and soft tissues dissected to access the cranial or spinal nerve. The nerve is isolated. Transection is performed by grasping the nerve and dividing it. The nerve may then be avulsed by twisting the nerve over a hemostat. Alternatively, the nerve may be stretched, ligated, and divided first distally and then proximally. The proximal end of the nerve will retract into deeper tissues. Soft tissues are closed in layers. Use 64771 for transection or avulsion of a cranial nerve and 64772 for a spinal nerve.

Transection or avulsion of other spinal nerve, extradural

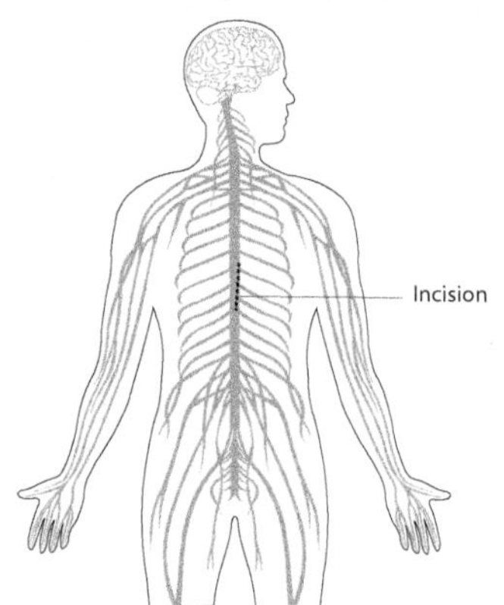

A spinal nerve is cut or removed.

CCI Edits

Refer to Appendix A for CCI edits.

Facility RVUs

Code	Work	PE Facility	MP	Total Facility
64771	8.15	7.95	1.42	17.52
64772	7.84	6.93	1.50	16.27

Non-facility RVUs

Code	Work	PE Non-Facility	MP	Total Non-Facility
64771	8.15	7.95	1.42	17.52
64772	7.84	6.93	1.50	16.27

Modifiers (PAR)

Code	Mod 50	Mod 51	Mod 62	Mod 66	Mod 80
64771	0	2	0	0	2
64772	0	2	1	0	2

Global Period

Code	Days
64771	090
64772	090

64788-64792

64788 Excision of neurofibroma or neurolemmoma; cutaneous nerve

64790 Excision of neurofibroma or neurolemmoma; major peripheral nerve

64792 Excision of neurofibroma or neurolemmoma; extensive (including malignant type)

(For destruction of extensive cutaneous neurofibroma, see 0419T, 0420T)

AMA Coding Notes

Excision and Implantation Procedures on the Somatic Nerves

(For Morton neurectomy, use 28080)

Surgical Procedures on the Extracranial Nerves, Peripheral Nerves, and Autonomic Nervous System

(For intracranial surgery on cranial nerves, see 61450, 61460, 61790)

AMA *CPT Assistant*

64788: Apr 16: 3
64790: Apr 16: 3
64792: Apr 16: 3

Plain English Description

Neurofibromas are tumors that involve nerve fibers. They arise from proliferation of Schwann cells and are one of the most common types of peripheral nerve tumors. While they sometimes occur as solitary tumors, the tumors more frequently occur in multiples as part of neurofibromatosis. Neurofibromatosis is a genetic disorder that varies greatly from very mild with limited tumors to severe with widespread debilitating tumor formation. Neurofibromas are typically benign, but plexiform neurofibromas do have the potential to transform into malignant neoplasms. Plexiform neurofibromas are large neurofibromas that involve a long segment of a nerve or nerves. Neurolemmas are neoplasms of the outermost sheath or neurolemma of Schwann cells. In 64788, a cutaneous nerve neurofibroma or neurolemma is excised. A skin incision is made over the site of the tumor. The tumor is exposed, dissected free of surrounding tissue, and excised. The incision is closed. In 64790, a neurofibroma or neurolemma is excised from a major peripheral nerve. The peripheral nerve is exposed. The segment of the nerve containing the tumor is dissected free of surrounding tissue. If the tumor is a neurofibroma, the nerve sheath is incised and the tumor is meticulously dissected from the nerve fibers. Following removal of the tumor, the nerve sheath is closed. If the tumor is a neurolemma, the involved segment of the nerve sheath is excised. In 64792, extensive or malignant tumors are excised. The technique is similar to that described for 64790, except that the procedure may involve multiple tumors in the same region or may require more extensive dissection for excision of a malignant lesion.

Excision of neurofibroma or neurolemmoma

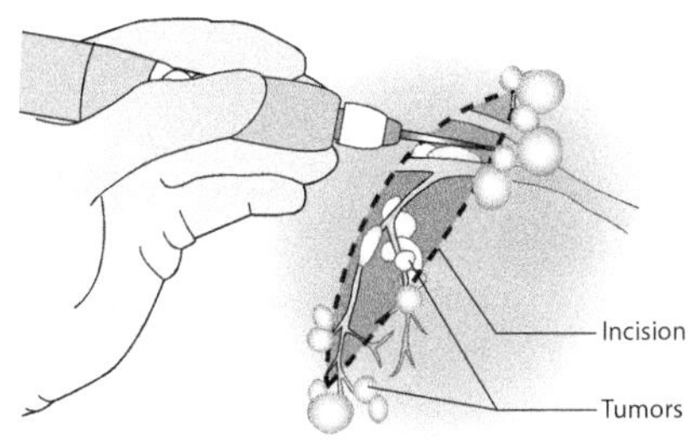

Cutaneous nerve (64788); major peripheral nerve (64790); extensive (including malignant type) (64792)

ICD-10-CM Diagnostic Codes

⇄	C47.11	Malignant neoplasm of peripheral nerves of right upper limb, including shoulder
⇄	C47.12	Malignant neoplasm of peripheral nerves of left upper limb, including shoulder
⇄	C47.21	Malignant neoplasm of peripheral nerves of right lower limb, including hip
⇄	C47.22	Malignant neoplasm of peripheral nerves of left lower limb, including hip
	C47.3	Malignant neoplasm of peripheral nerves of thorax
	C47.4	Malignant neoplasm of peripheral nerves of abdomen
	C47.8	Malignant neoplasm of overlapping sites of peripheral nerves and autonomic nervous system
	C79.89	Secondary malignant neoplasm of other specified sites
	D36.11	Benign neoplasm of peripheral nerves and autonomic nervous system of face, head, and neck
	D36.12	Benign neoplasm of peripheral nerves and autonomic nervous system, upper limb, including shoulder
	D36.13	Benign neoplasm of peripheral nerves and autonomic nervous system of lower limb, including hip
	D36.14	Benign neoplasm of peripheral nerves and autonomic nervous system of thorax
	D36.15	Benign neoplasm of peripheral nerves and autonomic nervous system of abdomen
⇄	G56.21	Lesion of ulnar nerve, right upper limb
⇄	G56.22	Lesion of ulnar nerve, left upper limb
⇄	G56.31	Lesion of radial nerve, right upper limb
⇄	G56.32	Lesion of radial nerve, left upper limb
⇄	G56.33	Lesion of radial nerve, bilateral upper limbs
⇄	G56.81	Other specified mononeuropathies of right upper limb
⇄	G56.82	Other specified mononeuropathies of left upper limb
⇄	G56.83	Other specified mononeuropathies of bilateral upper limbs
⇄	G56.91	Unspecified mononeuropathy of right upper limb
⇄	G56.92	Unspecified mononeuropathy of left upper limb
⇄	G56.93	Unspecified mononeuropathy of bilateral upper limbs
⇄	G57.01	Lesion of sciatic nerve, right lower limb
⇄	G57.02	Lesion of sciatic nerve, left lower limb
⇄	G57.03	Lesion of sciatic nerve, bilateral lower limbs
⇄	G57.11	Meralgia paresthetica, right lower limb
⇄	G57.12	Meralgia paresthetica, left lower limb
⇄	G57.13	Meralgia paresthetica, bilateral lower limbs
⇄	G57.21	Lesion of femoral nerve, right lower limb
⇄	G57.22	Lesion of femoral nerve, left lower limb
⇄	G57.23	Lesion of femoral nerve, bilateral lower limbs
⇄	G57.61	Lesion of plantar nerve, right lower limb
⇄	G57.62	Lesion of plantar nerve, left lower limb
⇄	G57.63	Lesion of plantar nerve, bilateral lower limbs
⇄	G57.81	Other specified mononeuropathies of right lower limb
⇄	G57.82	Other specified mononeuropathies of left lower limb
⇄	G57.83	Other specified mononeuropathies of bilateral lower limbs
⇄	G57.91	Unspecified mononeuropathy of right lower limb
⇄	G57.92	Unspecified mononeuropathy of left lower limb
⇄	G57.93	Unspecified mononeuropathy of bilateral lower limbs
	G58.8	Other specified mononeuropathies
	M79.2	Neuralgia and neuritis, unspecified
	Q85.00	Neurofibromatosis, unspecified
	Q85.01	Neurofibromatosis, type 1
	Q85.03	Schwannomatosis
	Q85.09	Other neurofibromatosis

CCI Edits

Refer to Appendix A for CCI edits.

Facility RVUs

Code	Work	PE Facility	MP	Total Facility
64788	5.24	5.31	1.05	11.60
64790	12.10	9.23	2.80	24.13
64792	15.86	11.04	3.65	30.55

Non-facility RVUs

Code	Work	PE Non-Facility	MP	Total Non-Facility
64788	5.24	5.31	1.05	11.60
64790	12.10	9.23	2.80	24.13
64792	15.86	11.04	3.65	30.55

Modifiers (PAR)

Code	Mod 50	Mod 51	Mod 62	Mod 66	Mod 80
64788	0	2	0	0	1
64790	0	2	1	0	0
64792	0	2	1	0	2

Global Period

Code	Days
64788	090
64790	090
64792	090

64795

64795 Biopsy of nerve

AMA Coding Notes

Excision and Implantation Procedures on the Somatic Nerves

(For Morton neurectomy, use 28080)

Surgical Procedures on the Extracranial Nerves, Peripheral Nerves, and Autonomic Nervous System

(For intracranial surgery on cranial nerves, see 61450, 61460, 61790)

Plain English Description

A nerve biopsy may be performed to evaluate a nerve lesion or to help diagnosis the cause of pain, weakness, or numbness when a definitive diagnosis cannot be made using other diagnostic modalities such as history and clinical examination, laboratory tests, and radiology studies. A skin incision is made over the nerve to be biopsied. Overlying soft tissues are dissected. A tissue sample is taken from the nerve lesion or a small segment of the nerve is excised and sent to the laboratory for separately reportable pathology examination. The overlying soft tissue and skin are closed in layers.

Biopsy of nerve

A tissue sample is taken from a nerve for examination and diagnosis.

A microscope is used to obtain biopsy.

Biopsy of nerve tumor

ICD-10-CM Diagnostic Codes

	Code	Description
	D86.89	Sarcoidosis of other sites
⇄	G56.81	Other specified mononeuropathies of right upper limb
⇄	G56.82	Other specified mononeuropathies of left upper limb
⇄	G56.83	Other specified mononeuropathies of bilateral upper limbs
⇄	G56.91	Unspecified mononeuropathy of right upper limb
⇄	G56.92	Unspecified mononeuropathy of left upper limb
⇄	G56.93	Unspecified mononeuropathy of bilateral upper limbs
⇄	G57.11	Meralgia paresthetica, right lower limb
⇄	G57.12	Meralgia paresthetica, left lower limb
⇄	G57.13	Meralgia paresthetica, bilateral lower limbs
⇄	G57.81	Other specified mononeuropathies of right lower limb
⇄	G57.82	Other specified mononeuropathies of left lower limb
⇄	G57.83	Other specified mononeuropathies of bilateral lower limbs
⇄	G57.91	Unspecified mononeuropathy of right lower limb
⇄	G57.92	Unspecified mononeuropathy of left lower limb
⇄	G57.93	Unspecified mononeuropathy of bilateral lower limbs
	G58.0	Intercostal neuropathy
	G58.7	Mononeuritis multiplex
	G58.8	Other specified mononeuropathies
	G58.9	Mononeuropathy, unspecified
	G59	Mononeuropathy in diseases classified elsewhere
	G60.0	Hereditary motor and sensory neuropathy
	G60.3	Idiopathic progressive neuropathy
	G60.8	Other hereditary and idiopathic neuropathies
	G61.81	Chronic inflammatory demyelinating polyneuritis
	G61.82	Multifocal motor neuropathy
	G61.89	Other inflammatory polyneuropathies
	G61.9	Inflammatory polyneuropathy, unspecified
	G62.0	Drug-induced polyneuropathy
	G62.1	Alcoholic polyneuropathy
	G62.2	Polyneuropathy due to other toxic agents
	G62.82	Radiation-induced polyneuropathy
	G62.89	Other specified polyneuropathies
	G62.9	Polyneuropathy, unspecified
	G63	Polyneuropathy in diseases classified elsewhere
	M31.8	Other specified necrotizing vasculopathies
⑦	S14.3	Injury of brachial plexus
⑦⇄	S44.01	Injury of ulnar nerve at upper arm level, right arm
⑦⇄	S44.02	Injury of ulnar nerve at upper arm level, left arm
⑦⇄	S44.11	Injury of median nerve at upper arm level, right arm
⑦⇄	S44.12	Injury of median nerve at upper arm level, left arm
⑦⇄	S44.21	Injury of radial nerve at upper arm level, right arm
⑦⇄	S44.22	Injury of radial nerve at upper arm level, left arm
⑦⇄	S44.31	Injury of axillary nerve, right arm
⑦⇄	S44.32	Injury of axillary nerve, left arm
⑦⇄	S44.41	Injury of musculocutaneous nerve, right arm
⑦⇄	S44.42	Injury of musculocutaneous nerve, left arm
⑦⇄	S44.8X1	Injury of other nerves at shoulder and upper arm level, right arm
⑦⇄	S44.8X2	Injury of other nerves at shoulder and upper arm level, left arm
⑦⇄	S84.01	Injury of tibial nerve at lower leg level, right leg
⑦⇄	S84.02	Injury of tibial nerve at lower leg level, left leg
⑦⇄	S84.11	Injury of peroneal nerve at lower leg level, right leg
⑦⇄	S84.12	Injury of peroneal nerve at lower leg level, left leg
⑦⇄	S84.801	Injury of other nerves at lower leg level, right leg
⑦⇄	S84.802	Injury of other nerves at lower leg level, left leg

ICD-10-CM Coding Notes

For codes requiring a 7th character extension, refer to your ICD-10-CM book. Review the character descriptions and coding guidelines for proper selection. For some procedures, only certain characters will apply.

CCI Edits

Refer to Appendix A for CCI edits.

Facility RVUs ▯

Code	Work	PE Facility	MP	Total Facility
64795	3.01	1.79	0.77	5.57

Non-facility RVUs ▯

Code	Work	PE Non-Facility	MP	Total Non-Facility
64795	3.01	1.79	0.77	5.57

Modifiers (PAR) ▯

Code	Mod 50	Mod 51	Mod 62	Mod 66	Mod 80
64795	0	2	0	0	1

Global Period

Code	Days
64795	000

64910-64911

64910 Nerve repair; with synthetic conduit or vein allograft (eg, nerve tube), each nerve

64911 Nerve repair; with autogenous vein graft (includes harvest of vein graft), each nerve

(Do not report 69990 in addition to 64910, 64911)

AMA Coding Notes

Surgical Procedures on the Extracranial Nerves, Peripheral Nerves, and Autonomic Nervous System

(For intracranial surgery on cranial nerves, see 61450, 61460, 61790)

AMA *CPT Assistant*

64910: Nov 07: 4, Apr 15: 10, Aug 15: 8, Dec 17: 12

64911: Nov 07: 4, Dec 17: 12

Plain English Description

Nerve repair using either a synthetic conduit or vein allograft (eg, nerve tube) is done on one nerve (64910). When nerve function is lost through injury, the distal nerve portion dies and degenerates. The proximal portion can regenerate to establish nerve function, but if the gap is too great, a graft must be inserted between the proximal and distal nerve stumps to guide the regenerating axons. This code reports the creation of either a biological nerve tube allograft from human vein or the placement of an artificial guidance channel between the ends of a severed peripheral nerve for regeneration and repair. A synthetic, tubular nerve guidance conduit is made from polymers like poly-L-lactic acid and plated with populations of cultured Schwann cells that adhere to the acidic polymer. Schwann cells compose the natural insulating myelin sheath wrapped around nerve axons. The impregnated synthetic guidance tube provides a biocompatible environment for promoting robust nerve regeneration in a specific direction. Harvested vein grafts are pulled through and turned inside out before being sutured between the severed nerve stumps because the inside layer of the vein wall is rich in collagen, which has the best success for regenerating nerves. New capillaries form in the vein graft and neurites from the proximal stump grow in around them to repair the connection. Report code 64911 for nerve repair on one nerve that is done using an autogenous piece of vein harvested from the patient first before being surgically planted between two severed nerve ends.

Nerve repair with synthetic conduit or vein allograft

Damaged nerve

Healthy nerve

Artificial nerve conduit

Synthetic bridge

ICD-10-CM Diagnostic Codes

	Code	Description
⇄	C47.11	Malignant neoplasm of peripheral nerves of right upper limb, including shoulder
⇄	C47.12	Malignant neoplasm of peripheral nerves of left upper limb, including shoulder
⇄	C47.21	Malignant neoplasm of peripheral nerves of right lower limb, including hip
⇄	C47.22	Malignant neoplasm of peripheral nerves of left lower limb, including hip
	D36.11	Benign neoplasm of peripheral nerves and autonomic nervous system of face, head, and neck
	D36.12	Benign neoplasm of peripheral nerves and autonomic nervous system, upper limb, including shoulder
	D36.13	Benign neoplasm of peripheral nerves and autonomic nervous system of lower limb, including hip
⑦	S14.4	Injury of peripheral nerves of neck
⑦	S24.3	Injury of peripheral nerves of thorax
⑦	S34.6	Injury of peripheral nerve(s) at abdomen, lower back and pelvis level
⑦⇄	S44.01	Injury of ulnar nerve at upper arm level, right arm
⑦⇄	S44.02	Injury of ulnar nerve at upper arm level, left arm
⑦⇄	S44.11	Injury of median nerve at upper arm level, right arm
⑦⇄	S44.12	Injury of median nerve at upper arm level, left arm
⑦⇄	S44.21	Injury of radial nerve at upper arm level, right arm
⑦⇄	S44.22	Injury of radial nerve at upper arm level, left arm
⑦⇄	S44.31	Injury of axillary nerve, right arm
⑦⇄	S44.32	Injury of axillary nerve, left arm
⑦⇄	S44.41	Injury of musculocutaneous nerve, right arm
⑦⇄	S44.42	Injury of musculocutaneous nerve, left arm
⑦⇄	S44.51	Injury of cutaneous sensory nerve at shoulder and upper arm level, right arm
⑦⇄	S44.52	Injury of cutaneous sensory nerve at shoulder and upper arm level, left arm
⑦⇄	S44.8X1	Injury of other nerves at shoulder and upper arm level, right arm
⑦⇄	S44.8X2	Injury of other nerves at shoulder and upper arm level, left arm
⑦⇄	S54.01	Injury of ulnar nerve at forearm level, right arm
⑦⇄	S54.02	Injury of ulnar nerve at forearm level, left arm
⑦⇄	S54.11	Injury of median nerve at forearm level, right arm
⑦⇄	S54.12	Injury of median nerve at forearm level, left arm
⑦⇄	S54.21	Injury of radial nerve at forearm level, right arm
⑦⇄	S54.22	Injury of radial nerve at forearm level, left arm
⑦⇄	S54.31	Injury of cutaneous sensory nerve at forearm level, right arm
⑦⇄	S54.32	Injury of cutaneous sensory nerve at forearm level, left arm
⑦⇄	S54.8X1	Injury of other nerves at forearm level, right arm
⑦⇄	S54.8X2	Injury of other nerves at forearm level, left arm
⑦⇄	S64.01	Injury of ulnar nerve at wrist and hand level of right arm
⑦⇄	S64.02	Injury of ulnar nerve at wrist and hand level of left arm
⑦⇄	S64.11	Injury of median nerve at wrist and hand level of right arm
⑦⇄	S64.12	Injury of median nerve at wrist and hand level of left arm
⑦⇄	S64.21	Injury of radial nerve at wrist and hand level of right arm
⑦⇄	S64.22	Injury of radial nerve at wrist and hand level of left arm
⑦⇄	S64.31	Injury of digital nerve of right thumb
⑦⇄	S64.32	Injury of digital nerve of left thumb
⑦⇄	S64.8X1	Injury of other nerves at wrist and hand level of right arm
⑦⇄	S64.8X2	Injury of other nerves at wrist and hand level of left arm
⑦⇄	S74.01	Injury of sciatic nerve at hip and thigh level, right leg
⑦⇄	S74.02	Injury of sciatic nerve at hip and thigh level, left leg
⑦⇄	S74.11	Injury of femoral nerve at hip and thigh level, right leg
⑦⇄	S74.12	Injury of femoral nerve at hip and thigh level, left leg
⑦⇄	S74.21	Injury of cutaneous sensory nerve at hip and high level, right leg
⑦⇄	S74.22	Injury of cutaneous sensory nerve at hip and thigh level, left leg
⑦⇄	S74.8X1	Injury of other nerves at hip and thigh level, right leg
⑦⇄	S74.8X2	Injury of other nerves at hip and thigh level, left leg
⑦⇄	S84.01	Injury of tibial nerve at lower leg level, right leg
⑦⇄	S84.02	Injury of tibial nerve at lower leg level, left leg
⑦⇄	S84.11	Injury of peroneal nerve at lower leg level, right leg

⇄ S84.12 Injury of peroneal nerve at lower leg level, left leg
⇄ S84.21 Injury of cutaneous sensory nerve at lower leg level, right leg
⇄ S84.22 Injury of cutaneous sensory nerve at lower leg level, left leg
⇄ S84.801 Injury of other nerves at lower leg level, right leg
⇄ S84.802 Injury of other nerves at lower leg level, left leg
⇄ S94.01 Injury of lateral plantar nerve, right leg
⇄ S94.02 Injury of lateral plantar nerve, left leg
⇄ S94.11 Injury of medial plantar nerve, right leg
⇄ S94.12 Injury of medial plantar nerve, left leg
⇄ S94.21 Injury of deep peroneal nerve at ankle and foot level, right leg
⇄ S94.22 Injury of deep peroneal nerve at ankle and foot level, left leg
⇄ S94.31 Injury of cutaneous sensory nerve at ankle and foot level, right leg
⇄ S94.32 Injury of cutaneous sensory nerve at ankle and foot level, left leg
⇄ S94.8X1 Injury of other nerves at ankle and foot level, right leg
⇄ S94.8X2 Injury of other nerves at ankle and foot level, left leg

ICD-10-CM Coding Notes

For codes requiring a 7th character extension, refer to your ICD-10-CM book. Review the character descriptions and coding guidelines for proper selection. For some procedures, only certain characters will apply.

CCI Edits

Refer to Appendix A for CCI edits.

Facility RVUs

Code	Work	PE Facility	MP	Total Facility
64910	10.52	10.43	1.78	22.73
64911	14.00	12.80	2.78	29.58

Non-facility RVUs

Code	Work	PE Non-Facility	MP	Total Non-Facility
64910	10.52	10.43	1.78	22.73
64911	14.00	12.80	2.78	29.58

Modifiers (PAR)

Code	Mod 50	Mod 51	Mod 62	Mod 66	Mod 80
64910	0	2	1	0	2
64911	0	2	1	0	2

Global Period

Code	Days
64910	090
64911	090

69990

✚ **69990 Microsurgical techniques, requiring use of operating microscope (List separately in addition to code for primary procedure)**

AMA Coding Guideline

Please see the Surgery Guidelines section for the following guidelines:

- *Operating Microscope Procedures*

AMA *CPT Assistant* ☐

69990: Nov 98: 20, Apr 99: 11, Jun 99: 11, Jul 99: 10, Oct 99: 10, Oct 00: 3, Oct 02: 8, Jan 04: 28, Mar 05: 11, Jul 05: 14, Aug 05: 1, Nov 07: 4, Sep 08: 10, Mar 09: 10, Dec 11: 14, Mar 12: 9, Jun 12: 17, Dec 12: 13, Oct 13: 14, Jan 14: 8, Apr 14: 10, Sep 14: 13, 14, Feb 16: 12, Dec 17: 13, Feb 18: 11

Plain English Description

The physician performs microsurgical techniques using an operating microscope during a separately reportable procedure. Microsurgery is typically used for anastomosis of small blood vessels and nerves as well as for tissue reconstruction. The surgeon visualizes the blood vessels, nerves or individual nerve fibers, or other tissue through the operating microscope. Using a foot pedal, the microscope is focused and manipulated during the course of the microscopic portion of the surgery. Using the operating microscope and microsurgical tools, the physician dissects and mobilizes blood vessels, nerves, or other tissues, meticulously controlling any bleeding. The physician then repairs the blood vessels, nerves, or other tissues using the operating microscope, which allows exact approximation of blood vessels, nerves, and tissue planes.

ICD-10-CM Diagnostic Codes

See Primary Procedure code for crosswalks.

CCI Edits

Refer to Appendix A for **CCI edits.**

Pub 100

69990: Pub 100-04, 12, 20.4.5

Facility RVUs ☐

Code	Work	PE Facility	MP	Total Facility
69990	3.46	1.59	1.25	6.30

Non-facility RVUs ☐

Code	Work	PE Non-Facility	MP	Total Non-Facility
69990	3.46	1.59	1.25	6.30

Modifiers (PAR) ☐

Code	Mod 50	Mod 51	Mod 62	Mod 66	Mod 80
69990	0	0	0	0	2

Global Period

Code	Days
69990	ZZZ

70015

70015 Cisternography, positive contrast, radiological supervision and interpretation

Plain English Description

Cisternography is a radiographic examination of the basal cisterns of the brain following the injection of contrast medium in the subarachnoid space. Positive contrast medium used in this procedure is iodinated. It has an increased absorption of X-rays and shows up as white-gray. This procedure is used to evaluate suspected cases of normal pressure hydrocephalus (NPH) or cerebral atrophy. The physician injects the contrast medium intrathecally through lumbar puncture. Radiographic images are then taken over a period of hours or even days, following the flow of the contrast agent. In a normal patient, the contrast medium will rise to the basal cisterns of the brain in 1-3 hours and then flow over and collect in the sagittal area in 12-24 hours. The cisterns are usually clear in 24 hours and the ventricles are not visualized during the series. In a patient with NPH, reabsorption of cerebral spinal fluid is impaired, the flow is reversed, and the ventricles are visualized early in the series, persisting for up to 48 hours, with almost no flow of the tracer into the sagittal area. Ventricular reflux also occurs in isolated cerebral atrophy.

RVUs

Code	Work	PE	PE Non-Facility	MP	Total Non-Facility	Total Facility	Global
70015	1.19	3.34	3.34	0.07	4.60	4.60	XXX

70250-70260

70250 Radiologic examination, skull; less than 4 views
70260 Radiologic examination, skull; complete, minimum of 4 views

Plain English Description

The physician performs a radiologic examination of the skull bones by taking up to three different X-ray images in 70250 or four or more images in 70260. Sponges or other supports may be placed around the head to keep it still as the head is turned various ways to obtain different views. X-ray uses indirect ionizing radiation to take pictures inside the body. X-rays work on non-uniform material, such as human tissue, because of the different density and composition of the object, which allows some of the X-rays to be absorbed and some to pass through and be captured behind the object on a detector. This produces a 2D image of the structures. The physician reviews the radiographs for developmental abnormalities, traumatic fractures or dislocations, bony projections or growths, and to detect progressive changes in skull dimensions.

RVUs

Code	Work	PE	PE Non-Facility	MP	Total Non-Facility	Total Facility	Global
70250	0.18	0.80	0.80	0.02	1.00	1.00	XXX
70260	0.28	0.94	0.94	0.02	1.24	1.24	XXX

70360

70360 Radiologic examination; neck, soft tissue

Plain English Description

X-rays are taken to evaluate the soft tissue of the neck. X-ray uses indirect ionizing radiation to take pictures inside the body. X-rays work on non-uniform material, such as human tissue, because of the different density and composition of the object, which allows some of the X-rays to be absorbed and some to pass through and be captured behind the object on a detector. This produces a 2D image of the structures. Frontal and lateral views of the neck may be taken for better evaluation. The physician reviews the radiographs to determine any asymmetry or enlargement on one side or the other, the caliber and contour of the trachea, and any soft tissue swelling that may involve the adenoids, tonsils, epiglottis, or aryepiglottic folds.

RVUs

Code	Work	PE	PE Non-Facility	MP	Total Non-Facility	Total Facility	Global
70360	0.18	0.66	0.66	0.02	0.86	0.86	XXX

70450-70470

70450 Computed tomography, head or brain; without contrast material
70460 Computed tomography, head or brain; with contrast material(s)
70470 Computed tomography, head or brain; without contrast material, followed by contrast material(s) and further sections

(To report 3D rendering, see 76376, 76377)

Plain English Description

Computerized tomography, also referred to as a CT scan, uses special X-ray equipment and computer technology to produce multiple cross-sectional images of the region being studied. In this study, CT scan of the head or brain is performed. The patient is positioned on the CT examination table. An initial pass is made through the CT scanner to determine the starting position of the scans after which the CT scan is performed. As the table moves slowly through the scanner, numerous X-ray beams and electronic X-ray detectors rotate around the body region being examined. The amount of radiation being absorbed is measured. As the beams and detectors rotate around the body, the table is moved through the scanner. A computer program processes the data and renders the data in 2D cross-sectional images of the body region being examined. These data are displayed on a monitor. The physician reviews the data as they are being obtained and may request additional sections to provide more detail of areas of interest. Use 70450 for CT of the head or brain without intravenous contrast material. Use 70460 when intravenous contrast material is administered before the CT scanning begins. Use 70470 when CT is first performed without intravenous contrast followed by administration of contrast and acquisition of additional sections. The physician reviews the CT scan, notes any abnormalities, and provides a written interpretation of the findings.

RVUs

Code	Work	PE	PE Non-Facility	MP	Total Non-Facility	Total Facility	Global
70450	0.85	2.34	2.34	0.06	3.25	3.25	XXX
70460	1.13	3.40	3.40	0.06	4.59	4.59	XXX
70470	1.27	4.04	4.04	0.07	5.38	5.38	XXX

70486-70488

70486 Computed tomography, maxillofacial area; without contrast material

70487 Computed tomography, maxillofacial area; with contrast material(s)

70488 Computed tomography, maxillofacial area; without contrast material, followed by contrast material(s) and further sections

(To report 3D rendering, see 76376, 76377)

Plain English Description

Computerized tomography, also referred to as a CT scan, uses special X-ray equipment and computer technology to produce multiple cross-sectional images of the region being studied. In this study, CT scan of the maxillofacial area is obtained. The maxillofacial area includes the forehead (frontal bone), sinuses, nose and nasal bones, and jaw (maxilla and mandible). The only facial region not included in this study is the orbit. The patient is positioned on the CT examination table. An initial pass is made through the CT scanner to determine the starting position of the scans, after which the CT scan is performed. As the table moves slowly through the scanner, numerous X-ray beams and electronic X-ray detectors rotate around the body region being examined. The amount of radiation being absorbed is measured. As the beams and detectors rotate around the body, the table is moved through the scanner. A computer program processes the data and renders the data in 2D cross-sectional images of the body region being examined. These data are displayed on a monitor. The physician reviews the data as they are being obtained and may request additional sections to provide more detail of areas of interest. Use 70486 for CT of the head or brain without intravenous contrast material. Use 70487 when intravenous contrast material is administered before the CT scanning begins. Use 70488 when CT is first performed without intravenous contrast followed by the administration of intravenous contrast and acquisition of additional sections. The physician reviews the CT scan, notes any abnormalities, and provides a written interpretation of the findings.

RVUs

Code	Work	PE	PE Non-Facility	MP	Total Non-Facility	Total Facility	Global
70486	0.85	3.01	3.01	0.06	3.92	3.92	XXX
70487	1.13	3.51	3.51	0.06	4.70	4.70	XXX
70488	1.27	4.39	4.39	0.07	5.73	5.73	XXX

70496

70496 Computed tomographic angiography, head, with contrast material(s), including noncontrast images, if performed, and image postprocessing

Plain English Description

A computed tomographic angiography (CTA) of the head is performed with contrast material including image postprocessing. Noncontrast images may also be obtained and are included when performed. CTA provides images of the blood vessels using a combination of computed tomography (CT) and angiography with contrast material. When angiography is performed using CT, multiple images are obtained and processed on a computer to create detailed, two-dimensional, cross-sectional views of the blood vessels. These images are then displayed on a computer monitor. The patient is positioned on the CT table. An intravenous line is inserted into a blood vessel, usually in the arm or hand. Non-contrast images may be obtained. A small dose of contrast is injected and test images are obtained to verify correct positioning. The CTA is then performed. Contrast is injected at a controlled rate and the CT table moves through the CT machine as the scanning is performed. After completion of the CTA, the radiologist reviews and interprets the CTA images of the head.

RVUs

Code	Work	PE	PE Non-Facility	MP	Total Non-Facility	Total Facility	Global
70496	1.75	6.49	6.49	0.11	8.35	8.35	XXX

70498

70498 Computed tomographic angiography, neck, with contrast material(s), including noncontrast images, if performed, and image postprocessing

Plain English Description

A computed tomographic angiography (CTA) of the neck is performed with contrast material including image postprocessing. Noncontrast images may also be obtained and are included when performed. CTA provides images of the blood vessels using a combination of computed tomography (CT) and angiography with contrast material. When angiography is performed using CT, multiple images are obtained and processed on a computer to create detailed, two-dimensional, cross-sectional views of the blood vessels. These images are then displayed on a computer monitor. The patient is positioned on the CT table. An intravenous line is inserted into a blood vessel, usually in the arm or hand. Non-contrast images may be obtained. A small dose of contrast is injected and test images are obtained to verify correct positioning. The CTA is then performed. Contrast is injected at a controlled rate and the CT table moves through the CT machine as the scanning is performed. After completion of the CTA, the radiologist reviews and interprets the CTA images of the neck.

RVUs

Code	Work	PE	PE Non-Facility	MP	Total Non-Facility	Total Facility	Global
70498	1.75	6.48	6.48	0.11	8.34	8.34	XXX

70540-70543

70540 Magnetic resonance (eg, proton) imaging, orbit, face, and/or neck; without contrast material(s)

(For head or neck magnetic resonance angiography studies, see 70544-70546, 70547-70549)

70542 Magnetic resonance (eg, proton) imaging, orbit, face, and/or neck; with contrast material(s)

70543 Magnetic resonance (eg, proton) imaging, orbit, face, and/or neck; without contrast material(s), followed by contrast material(s) and further sequences

(Report 70540-70543 once per imaging session)

Plain English Description

Magnetic resonance imaging (MRI) is done on the orbit, the face, and/or the neck. MRI is a noninvasive, non-radiating imaging technique that uses the magnetic properties of hydrogen atoms in the body. The patient is placed on a motorized table within a large MRI tunnel scanner that contains the magnet. The powerful magnetic field forces the hydrogen atoms to line up. Radiowaves are then transmitted within the strong magnetic field. Protons in the nuclei of different types of tissues emit a specific radiofrequency signal that bounces back to the computer, which processes the signals and converts the data into tomographic, 3D images with very high resolution. Orbital MRI provides reliable information for diagnosing tumors of the eye; infection or inflammation of the lacrimal glands and other soft tissues around the eye as well as osteomyelitis of nearby bone; damage or deterioration of the optic nerve; vascular edema or hemangioma of the eye area; and orbital muscular disorders. It is often performed in cases of trauma. MRI of the face and neck region is used to detect problems and abnormalities occurring outside the skull in the mouth, tongue, pharynx, nasal and sinus cavities, salivary glands, and vocal cords. MRI provides information on the presence and extent of tumors, masses, or lesions; infection, inflammation, and swelling of soft tissue; vascular edema or lesions; muscular abnormalities; and vocal cord paralysis. When MRI of the orbit, face, or neck is performed without intravenous contrast material, report 70540. When contrast dye such as gadolinium is injected before the imaging is done, report 70542; and use 70543 when MRI is first performed without intravenous contrast followed by the administration of intravenous contrast and acquisition of additional images. The physician reviews the MRI, notes any abnormalities, and provides a written interpretation of the findings.

RVUs

Code	Work	PE	PE Non-Facility	MP	Total Non-Facility	Total Facility	Global
70540	1.35	5.91	5.91	0.08	7.34	7.34	XXX
70542	1.62	6.99	6.99	0.11	8.72	8.72	XXX
70543	2.15	8.70	8.70	0.11	10.96	10.96	XXX

70544-70546

70544 Magnetic resonance angiography, head; without contrast material(s)

70545 Magnetic resonance angiography, head; with contrast material(s)

70546 Magnetic resonance angiography, head; without contrast material(s), followed by contrast material(s) and further sequences

Plain English Description

Magnetic resonance angiography (MRA) is performed on the head without contrast materials (70544), with contrast materials (70545), and without contrast materials followed by contrast materials (70546). MRA is a noninvasive radiology procedure used to evaluate arterial and venous vessels for conditions such as atherosclerotic stenosis, arterial dissection, acute thrombosis, aneurysms or pseudo-aneurysms, vascular loops, vascular malformations/tumors, or arterial causes of pulsatile tinnitus. MRA may be performed following vascular surgery on the intracranial vessels to assess vascular status. MRA uses a magnetic field and pulses of radiowave energy to provide images of the blood vessels. Multiple images, 1-2 mm in thickness, are obtained and then processed using an array algorithm to produce maximum intensity projections (MIPs). MIPs are similar to subtraction angiograms. Areas of interest are identified by the radiologist and coned down to produce detailed views of the arteries. This post-processing of the images is performed by a technologist. The MIPs are reviewed by the radiologist along with the initial MRA images. The radiologist provides a written interpretation of findings. In 70544, MRA is performed without contrast materials. In 70545, an intravenous line is placed and contrast material is administered prior to the MRA. In 70546, MRA is first performed without contrast, followed by contrast administered intravenously, and additional MRA images.

RVUs

Code	Work	PE	PE Non-Facility	MP	Total Non-Facility	Total Facility	Global
70544	1.20	5.62	5.62	0.08	6.90	6.90	XXX
70545	1.20	5.93	5.93	0.08	7.21	7.21	XXX
70546	1.48	8.87	8.87	0.11	10.46	10.46	XXX

70547-70549

70547 Magnetic resonance angiography, neck; without contrast material(s)

70548 Magnetic resonance angiography, neck; with contrast material(s)

70549 Magnetic resonance angiography, neck; without contrast material(s), followed by contrast material(s) and further sequences

Plain English Description

Magnetic resonance angiography (MRA) is performed on the neck without contrast materials (70547), with contrast materials (70548), and without contrast materials followed by contrast materials (70549). MRA is a noninvasive radiology procedure used to evaluate arterial and venous vessels for conditions such as atherosclerotic stenosis, arterial dissection, acute thrombosis, aneurysms or pseudo-aneurysms, vascular loops, vascular malformations/tumors, or arterial causes of pulsatile tinnitus. MRA may be performed following vascular surgery on the neck vessels to assess vascular status. MRA uses a magnetic field and pulses of radiowave energy to provide images of the blood vessels. Multiple images of 1-2 mm in thickness are obtained and then processed using an array algorithm to produce maximum intensity projections (MIPs). MIPs are similar to subtraction angiograms. Areas of interest are identified by the radiologist and coned down to produce detailed views of the arteries. This post-processing of the images is performed by a technologist. The MIPs are reviewed by the radiologist along with the initial MRA images. The radiologist provides a written interpretation of findings. In 70547, MRA is performed without contrast materials. In 70548, an intravenous line is placed and contrast material is administered prior to the MRA. In 70549, MRA is first performed without contrast, followed by contrast administered intravenously, and additional MRA images.

RVUs

Code	Work	PE	PE Non-Facility	MP	Total Non-Facility	Total Facility	Global
70547	1.20	5.65	5.65	0.08	6.93	6.93	XXX
70548	1.50	6.14	6.14	0.10	7.74	7.74	XXX
70549	1.80	9.05	9.05	0.12	10.97	10.97	XXX

70551-70553

70551 Magnetic resonance (eg, proton) imaging, brain (including brain stem); without contrast material

70552 Magnetic resonance (eg, proton) imaging, brain (including brain stem); with contrast material(s)

70553 Magnetic resonance (eg, proton) imaging, brain (including brain stem); without contrast material, followed by contrast material(s) and further sequences

(For magnetic spectroscopy, use 76390)

Plain English Description

Magnetic resonance imaging (MRI) is done on the brain. MRI is a noninvasive, non-radiating imaging technique that uses the magnetic properties of hydrogen atoms in the body. The patient is placed on a motorized table within a large MRI tunnel scanner that contains the magnet. The powerful magnetic field forces the hydrogen atoms to line up. Radiowaves are then transmitted within the strong magnetic field. Protons in the nuclei of different types of tissues emit a specific radiofrequency signal that bounces back to the computer, which processes the signals and converts the data into tomographic, 3D images with very high resolution. MRI of the brain provides reliable information for diagnosing the presence, location, and extent of tumors, cysts, or other masses; swelling and infection; vascular disorders or malformations, such as aneurysms and intracranial hemorrhage; disease of the pituitary gland; stroke; developmental and structural anomalies of the brain; hydrocephalus; and chronic conditions and diseases affecting the central nervous system such as headaches and multiple sclerosis. When MRI of the brain is performed without intravenous contrast material, report 70551. When contrast dye, such as gadolinium is injected before the imaging is done, report 70552; and use 70553 when MRI is first performed without contrast followed by the administration of intravenous contrast and acquisition of additional images. The physician reviews the MRI, notes any abnormalities, and provides a written interpretation of the findings.

RVUs

Code	Work	PE	PE Non-Facility	MP	Total Non-Facility	Total Facility	Global
70551	1.48	4.70	4.70	0.10	6.28	6.28	XXX
70552	1.78	6.80	6.80	0.11	8.69	8.69	XXX
70553	2.29	7.85	7.85	0.13	10.27	10.27	XXX

70557-70559

70557 Magnetic resonance (eg, proton) imaging, brain (including brain stem and skull base), during open intracranial procedure (eg, to assess for residual tumor or residual vascular malformation); without contrast material

70558 Magnetic resonance (eg, proton) imaging, brain (including brain stem and skull base), during open intracranial procedure (eg, to assess for residual tumor or residual vascular malformation); with contrast material(s)

70559 Magnetic resonance (eg, proton) imaging, brain (including brain stem and skull base), during open intracranial procedure (eg, to assess for residual tumor or residual vascular malformation); without contrast material(s), followed by contrast material(s) and further sequences

(For stereotactic biopsy of intracranial lesion with magnetic resonance guidance, use 61751,70557, 70558, or 70559 may be reported only if a separate report is generated. Report only 1 of the above codes once per operative session. Do not use these codes in conjunction with 61751, 77021, 77022)

Plain English Description

Magnetic resonance imaging (MRI) is done on the brain during open intracranial surgery. MRI is a noninvasive, non-radiating imaging technique that uses the magnetic properties of hydrogen atoms in the body. The patient is placed on a motorized table within a large MRI tunnel scanner that contains the magnet. The powerful magnetic field forces the hydrogen atoms to line up. Radiowaves are then transmitted within the strong magnetic field. Protons in the nuclei of different types of tissues emit a specific radiofrequency signal that bounces back to the computer, which processes the signals and converts the data into tomographic, 3D images with very high resolution. Intraoperative MRI of the brain is done during open intracranial procedures performed in a specialized operative imaging suite that has an MRI scanner in the room. This allows the neurosurgeon to rotate the patient into the tunnel scanner at any point during the surgery to see the brain tumor clearly, assess whether the tumor has been completely removed, or to help place deep brain neurostimulator systems. The use of MRI during intracranial surgery greatly enhances surgical accuracy and reduces the risk of damage to other parts of the brain while reaching and resecting the tumor, or placing a neurostimulator to treat conditions such as Parkinson's, epilepsy, dystonia, and essential tremor. Intraoperative MRI also helps ensure surgical success by helping the surgeon confirm complete removal of the brain lesion, vascular malformation, or pituitary tumor. When MRI is performed without contrast material, report 70557. When imaging is performed after injection of a contrast dye, such as gadolinium, report 70558; and use 70559 when intraoperative MRI is first performed without contrast followed by the administration of contrast and acquisition of additional images.

RVUs

Code	Work	PE	PE Non-Facility	MP	Total Non-Facility	Total Facility	Global
70557	0.00	0.00	0.00	0.00	0.00	0.00	XXX
70558	0.00	0.00	0.00	0.00	0.00	0.00	XXX
70559	0.00	0.00	0.00	0.00	0.00	0.00	XXX

71045-71048

71045 Radiologic examination, chest; single view

71046 Radiologic examination, chest; 2 views

71047 Radiologic examination, chest; 3 views

71048 Radiologic examination, chest; 4 or more views

(For complete acute abdomen series that includes 2 or more views of the abdomen [eg, supine, erect, decubitus], and a single view chest, use 74022)

(For concurrent computer-aided detection [CAD] performed in addition to 71045, 71046, 71047, 71048, use 0174T)

(Do not report 71045, 71046, 71047, 71048 in conjunction with 0175T for computer-aided detection [CAD] performed remotely from the primary interpretation)

Plain English Description

A radiologic examination of the chest is performed. Chest radiographs (X-rays) provide images of the heart, lungs, bronchi, major blood vessels (aorta, vena cava, pulmonary vessels), and bones, (sternum, ribs, clavicle, scapula, spine). In 71045, a single view of the chest is obtained; 2 views in 71056; 3 views in 71047; and 4 views in 71048. The most common views are frontal (also referred to as anteroposterior or AP), posteroanterior (PA), and lateral. To obtain a frontal view, the patient is positioned facing the X-ray machine. A PA view is obtained with the patient's back toward the X-ray machine. For a lateral view, the patient is positioned with side of the chest toward the machine. Other views that may be obtained include apical lordotic, oblique, and lateral decubitus. An apical lordotic image provides better visualization of the apical (top) regions of the lungs. The patient is positioned with the back arched so that the tops of the lungs can be X-rayed. Oblique views may be obtained to evaluate a pulmonary or mediastinal mass or opacity or to provide additional images of the heart and great vessels. There are four positions used for oblique views including right and left anterior oblique, and right and left posterior oblique. Anterior oblique views are obtained with the patient standing and the chest rotated 45 degrees. The arm closest to the X-ray cassette is flexed with the hand resting on the hip. The opposite arm is raised as high as possible. The part of the chest farthest away from the X-ray cassette is the area being studied. Posterior oblique views are typically obtained only when the patient is too ill to stand or lay prone for anterior oblique views. A lateral decubitus view is obtained with the patient lying on the side; the patient's head rests on one arm, and the other arm is raised over the head with the elbow bent. Images are recorded on hard copy film or stored electronically as digital images. The physician reviews the images, notes any abnormalities, and provides a written interpretation of the findings.

RVUs

Code	Work	PE	PE Non-Facility	MP	Total Non-Facility	Total Facility	Global
71045	0.18	0.52	0.52	0.02	0.72	0.72	XXX
71046	0.22	0.68	0.68	0.02	0.92	0.92	XXX
71047	0.27	0.87	0.87	0.02	1.16	1.16	XXX
71048	0.31	0.93	0.93	0.02	1.26	1.26	XXX

72020

72020 Radiologic examination, spine, single view, specify level

(For a single view that includes the entire thoracic and lumbar spine, use 72081)

Plain English Description

A diagnostic X-ray is taken of one area of the spine. X-ray uses indirect ionizing radiation to take pictures inside the body. X-rays work on non-uniform material, such as human tissue, because of the different density and composition of the object, which allows some of the X-rays to be absorbed and some to pass through and be captured behind the object on a detector. This produces a two-dimensional (2D) image of the structures. This code reports a single view of the spine to look for abnormalities or problems related to injury or pain and must be specified for the level.

RVUs

Code	Work	PE	PE Non-Facility	MP	Total Non-Facility	Total Facility	Global
72020	0.16	0.50	0.50	0.02	0.68	0.68	XXX

72040-72052

72040 Radiologic examination, spine, cervical; 2 or 3 views

72050 Radiologic examination, spine, cervical; 4 or 5 views

72052 Radiologic examination, spine, cervical; 6 or more views

Plain English Description

A radiologic exam is done of the cervical spine. Anteroposterior and lateral views are the most common projections taken. X-ray uses indirect ionizing radiation to take pictures inside the body. X-rays work on non-uniform material, such as human tissue, because of the different density and composition of the object, which allows some of the X-rays to be absorbed and some to pass through and be captured behind the object on a detector. This produces a two-dimensional (2D) image of the structures. When 2-3 views or less are taken of the cervical spine, report 72040. If 4 or 5 views are taken, report 72050. A cervical spine X-ray examination with 6 or more views is reported with 72052.

RVUs

Code	Work	PE	PE Non-Facility	MP	Total Non-Facility	Total Facility	Global
72040	0.22	0.83	0.83	0.02	1.07	1.07	XXX
72050	0.27	1.13	1.13	0.02	1.42	1.42	XXX
72052	0.30	1.35	1.35	0.02	1.67	1.67	XXX

72070-72074

72070 Radiologic examination, spine; thoracic, 2 views

72072 Radiologic examination, spine; thoracic, 3 views

72074 Radiologic examination, spine; thoracic, minimum of 4 views

Plain English Description

A radiologic exam is done of the thoracic spine. X-ray uses indirect ionizing radiation to take pictures inside the body. X-rays work on non-uniform material, such as human tissue, because of the different density and composition of the object, which allows some of the X-rays to be absorbed and some to pass through and be captured behind the object on a detector. This produces a two dimensional (2D) image of the structures. X-rays are taken of the thoracic spine to evaluate for back pain or suspected disease or injury. Films are taken from differing views that commonly include anteroposterior, lateral, posteroanterior, and a swimmer's view for the upper thoracic spine in which the patient reaches up with one arm and down with the other as if taking a swimming stroke. Report 72070 for 2 views of the thoracic spine; 72072 for 3 views; and 72074 for a minimum of 4 views of the thoracic spine.

RVUs

Code	Work	PE	PE Non-Facility	MP	Total Non-Facility	Total Facility	Global
72070	0.20	0.67	0.67	0.02	0.89	0.89	XXX
72072	0.23	0.83	0.83	0.02	1.08	1.08	XXX
72074	0.25	0.94	0.94	0.02	1.21	1.21	XXX

72080

72080 Radiologic examination, spine; thoracolumbar junction, minimum of 2 views

(For a single view examination of the thoracolumbar junction, use 72020)

Plain English Description

A radiologic X-ray exam is done of the thoracolumbar junction of the spine. X-ray uses indirect ionizing radiation to take pictures inside the body. X-rays work on non-uniform material, such as human tissue, because of the different density and composition of the object, which allows some of the X-rays to be absorbed and some to pass through and be captured behind the object on a detector. This produces a two dimensional (2D) image of the structures. A minimum of two views are taken of the thoracolumbar junction of the spine to evaluate for back pain or suspected disease or injury. X-ray films are commonly taken from frontal and lateral views or posteroanterior and lateral views.

RVUs

Code	Work	PE	PE Non-Facility	MP	Total Non-Facility	Total Facility	Global
72080	0.21	0.73	0.73	0.02	0.96	0.96	XXX

72081-72084

72081 Radiologic examination, spine, entire thoracic and lumbar, including skull, cervical and sacral spine if performed (eg, scoliosis evaluation); one view

72082 Radiologic examination, spine, entire thoracic and lumbar, including skull, cervical and sacral spine if performed (eg, scoliosis evaluation); 2 or 3 views

72083 Radiologic examination, spine, entire thoracic and lumbar, including skull, cervical and sacral spine if performed (eg, scoliosis evaluation); 4 or 5 views

72084 Radiologic examination, spine, entire thoracic and lumbar, including skull, cervical and sacral spine if performed (eg, scoliosis evaluation); minimum of 6 views

Plain English Description

A diagnostic radiographic examination is done of the entire thoracic and lumbar spine for a scoliosis evaluation. This study is done to assess scoliosis, such as the type of scoliosis, and the location and degree of curvature. X-ray uses indirect ionizing radiation to take pictures inside the body. X-rays work on non-uniform material, such as human tissue, because of the different density and composition of the object, which allows some of the X-rays to be absorbed and some to pass through and be captured behind the object on a detector. This produces a two-dimensional (2D) image of the structures. Code 72081 reports a single view X-ray of the entire thoracic and lumbar spine; code 72082 reports 2 or 3 views; code 72083 reports 4 or 5 views; and 72084 reports a spinal evaluation with a minimum of 6 views being taken. Posteroanterior, frontal, and lateral views are commonly taken of the spine while in an erect, standing, or upright position to help assess lateral curvature. The patient stands in front of a vertical grid with the knees together in full extension. The field of view includes the entire thoracic and lumbar spine and also the cervical and sacral spinal areas as well as the skull, whenever necessary. The vertebral bodies above and below the apex of the spinal curve that are the most tilted are measured by intersecting lines to give the degree of curvature. Lateral projections for viewing scoliosis may be taken with the patient's arms placed straight out in front for a better view of the curvature. Other views may also be taken of the spine while the patient is lying down face up.

RVUs

Code	Work	PE	PE Non-Facility	MP	Total Non-Facility	Total Facility	Global
72081	0.26	0.89	0.89	0.02	1.17	1.17	XXX
72082	0.31	1.56	1.56	0.03	1.90	1.90	XXX
72083	0.35	1.83	1.83	0.03	2.21	2.21	XXX
72084	0.41	2.18	2.18	0.03	2.62	2.62	XXX

72100-72114

72100 Radiologic examination, spine, lumbosacral; 2 or 3 views

72110 Radiologic examination, spine, lumbosacral; minimum of 4 views

72114 Radiologic examination, spine, lumbosacral; complete, including bending views, minimum of 6 views

Plain English Description

A radiologic exam is done of the lumbosacral spine. Frontal, posteroanterior, and lateral views are the most common projections taken. X-ray uses indirect ionizing radiation to take pictures inside the body. X-rays work on non-uniform material, such as human tissue, because of the different density and composition of the object, which allows some of the X-rays to be absorbed and some to pass through and be captured behind the object on a detector. This produces a two-dimensional (2D) image of the structures. When 2 or 3 views are taken of the lumbosacral spine, report 72100. If at least 4 views are taken, report 72110. A complete lumbosacral spine exam (72114) includes a minimum of 6 views, which may include views taken from oblique angles as well as in bending positions, flexion and extension. Lateral bending positions may also be taken with the patient sitting on a stool with the back against a contact to avoid moving the torso forward. The patient flexes the back over to each side as far as possible without losing contact with the stool. The complete exam is often done by taking anteroposterior and lateral views first, particularly to "clear" the spine before the technologist moves the patient into position for oblique angles and bending views if evaluating for trauma.

RVUs

Code	Work	PE	PE Non-Facility	MP	Total Non-Facility	Total Facility	Global
72100	0.22	0.83	0.83	0.02	1.07	1.07	XXX
72110	0.26	1.08	1.08	0.02	1.36	1.36	XXX
72114	0.30	1.35	1.35	0.02	1.67	1.67	XXX

72120

72120 Radiologic examination, spine, lumbosacral; bending views only, 2 or 3 views

(Contrast material in CT of spine is either by intrathecal or intravenous injection. For intrathecal injection, use also 61055 or 62284. IV injection of contrast material is part of the CT procedure)

Plain English Description

A radiologic exam of the lumbosacral spine is done taking 2 or 3 views with the patient in bending positions only. X-ray uses indirect ionizing radiation to take pictures inside the body. X-rays work on non-uniform material, such as human tissue, because of the different density and composition of the object, which allows some of the X-rays to be absorbed and some to pass through and be captured behind the object on a detector. This produces a two-dimensional (2D) image of the structures. Biomechanical dysfunction of the lumbar spine is revealed with lateral bending views. The patient is placed sitting on a stool with the back against a contact to avoid moving the torso forward. The patient flexes the back over to each side as far as possible without losing contact with the stool. Sitting instead of standing helps block out effects of gross musculature. These views are helpful when plain films seem normal and symptoms of dysfunction are not explained. Flexion or extension bending views may also be taken with the patient standing, such as bending over forward with the knees straight and the arms dangling.

RVUs

Code	Work	PE	PE Non-Facility	MP	Total Non-Facility	Total Facility	Global
72120	0.22	0.87	0.87	0.02	1.11	1.11	XXX

72125-72127

72125 Computed tomography, cervical spine; without contrast material

72126 Computed tomography, cervical spine; with contrast material

72127 Computed tomography, cervical spine; without contrast material, followed by contrast material(s) and further sections

(For intrathecal injection procedure, see 61055, 62284)

Plain English Description

Diagnostic computed tomography (CT) is done on the cervical spine. CT uses multiple, narrow X-ray beams aimed around a single rotational axis, taking a series of 2D images of the target structure from multiple angles. Contrast material is used to enhance the images. Computer software processes the data and produces several images of thin, cross-sectional 2D slices of the targeted organ or area. Three-dimensional (3D) models of the spine can be created by stacking multiple, individual 2D slices together. The patient is placed inside the CT scanner on the table and images are obtained of the cervical spine. In 72125, no contrast medium is used. In 72126, an iodine contrast dye is injected either intrathecally into the C1-C2 or other cervical level, or administered intravenously to see the target area better before images are taken. If intrathecal injection is performed, it is reported separately. In 72127, images are taken without contrast and again after the administration of the contrast. The physician reviews the images to look for suspected problems with the spine such as bone disease, fractures or other injuries, or birth defects of the spine in children.

RVUs

Code	Work	PE	PE Non-Facility	MP	Total Non-Facility	Total Facility	Global
72125	1.00	3.32	3.32	0.06	4.38	4.38	XXX
72126	1.22	4.21	4.21	0.07	5.50	5.50	XXX
72127	1.27	5.14	5.14	0.07	6.48	6.48	XXX

72128-72130

72128 Computed tomography, thoracic spine; without contrast material

72129 Computed tomography, thoracic spine; with contrast material

(For intrathecal injection procedure, see 61055, 62284)

72130 Computed tomography, thoracic spine; without contrast material, followed by contrast material(s) and further sections

(For intrathecal injection procedure, see 61055, 62284)

Plain English Description

Diagnostic computed tomography (CT) is done on the thoracic spine. CT uses multiple, narrow X-ray beams aimed around a single rotational axis, taking a series of 2D images of the target structure from multiple angles. Contrast material is used to enhance the images. Computer software processes the data and produces several images of thin, cross-sectional 2D slices of the targeted organ or area. Three-dimensional models of the spine can be created by stacking multiple, individual 2D slices together. The patient is placed inside the CT scanner on the table and images are obtained of the thoracic spine. In 72128, no contrast medium is used. In 72129, an iodine contrast dye is injected either intrathecally or administered intravenously to see the target area better before images are taken. If intrathecal injection is performed, it is reported separately. In 72130, images are taken without contrast and again after the administration of the contrast. The physician reviews the images to look for suspected problems with the spine such as bone disease and evaluates for fractures or other injuries as well as birth defects of the spine in children.

RVUs

Code	Work	PE	PE Non-Facility	MP	Total Non-Facility	Total Facility	Global
72128	1.00	3.32	3.32	0.06	4.38	4.38	XXX
72129	1.22	4.25	4.25	0.07	5.54	5.54	XXX
72130	1.27	5.15	5.15	0.07	6.49	6.49	XXX

72131-72133

72131 Computed tomography, lumbar spine; without contrast material

72132 Computed tomography, lumbar spine; with contrast material

72133 Computed tomography, lumbar spine; without contrast material, followed by contrast material(s) and further sections

(For intrathecal injection procedure, see 61055, 62284)

(To report 3D rendering, see 76376, 76377)

Plain English Description

Diagnostic computed tomography (CT) is done on the lumbar spine. CT uses multiple, narrow X-ray beams aimed around a single rotational axis, taking a series of 2D images of the target structure from multiple angles. Contrast material is used to enhance the images. Computer software processes the data and produces several images of thin, cross-sectional 2D slices of the targeted organ or area. Three-dimensional models of the spine can be created by stacking multiple, individual 2D slices together. The patient is placed inside the CT scanner on the table and images are obtained of the lumbar spine. In 72131, no contrast medium is used. In 72132, an iodine contrast dye is injected either intrathecally or administered intravenously to see the target area better before images are taken. If intrathecal injection is performed, it is reported separately. In 72133, images are taken without contrast and again after the administration of the contrast. The physician reviews the images to look for suspected problems with the spine such as bone disease and evaluates for fractures or other injuries as well as birth defects of the spine in children.

RVUs

Code	Work	PE	PE Non-Facility	MP	Total Non-Facility	Total Facility	Global
72131	1.00	3.30	3.30	0.06	4.36	4.36	XXX
72132	1.22	4.22	4.22	0.07	5.51	5.51	XXX
72133	1.27	5.11	5.11	0.07	6.45	6.45	XXX

72141-72142

72141 Magnetic resonance (eg, proton) imaging, spinal canal and contents, cervical; without contrast material

72142 Magnetic resonance (eg, proton) imaging, spinal canal and contents, cervical; with contrast material(s)

(For cervical spinal canal imaging without contrast material followed by contrast material, use 72156)

Plain English Description

Magnetic resonance imaging (MRI) is done on the cervical spinal canal and contents. MRI is a noninvasive, non-radiating imaging technique that uses the magnetic properties of nuclei within hydrogen atoms of the body. The powerful magnetic field forces the hydrogen atoms to line up. Radiowaves are then transmitted within the strong magnetic field. Protons in the nuclei of different types of tissues emit a specific radiofrequency signal that bounces back to the computer, which records the images. The computer processes the signals and converts the data into tomographic, 3D, sectional images in slices with very high resolution. The patient is placed on a motorized table within a large MRI tunnel scanner that contains the magnet. MRI scans of the spine are often done when conservative treatment of back/neck pain is unsuccessful and more aggressive treatments are considered or following surgery. In 72141, no contrast medium is used. In 72142, a contrast dye is administered first to see the spinal area better before images are taken. The physician reviews the images to look for specific information that may correlate to the patient's symptoms, such as abnormal spinal alignment; disease or injury of vertebral bodies; intervertebral disc herniation, degeneration, or dehydration; the size of the spinal canal to accommodate the cord and nerve roots; pinched or inflamed nerves; or any changes since surgery.

RVUs

Code	Work	PE	PE Non-Facility	MP	Total Non-Facility	Total Facility	Global
72141	1.48	4.54	4.54	0.09	6.11	6.11	XXX
72142	1.78	6.99	6.99	0.11	8.88	8.88	XXX

72146-72147

72146 Magnetic resonance (eg, proton) imaging, spinal canal and contents, thoracic; without contrast material

72147 Magnetic resonance (eg, proton) imaging, spinal canal and contents, thoracic; with contrast material(s)

(For thoracic spinal canal imaging without contrast material followed by contrast material, use 72157)

Plain English Description

Magnetic resonance imaging (MRI) is done on the thoracic spinal canal and contents. MRI is a noninvasive, non-radiating imaging technique that uses the magnetic properties of nuclei within hydrogen atoms of the body. The powerful magnetic field forces the hydrogen atoms to line up. Radiowaves are then transmitted within the strong magnetic field. Protons in the nuclei of different types of tissues emit a specific radiofrequency signal that bounces back to the computer, which records the images. The computer processes the signals and converts the data into tomographic, 3D, sectional images in slices with very high resolution. The patient is placed on a motorized table within a large MRI tunnel scanner that contains the magnet. MRI scans of the spine are often done when conservative treatment of back/neck pain is unsuccessful and more aggressive treatments are considered or following surgery. In 72146, no contrast medium is used. In 72147, a contrast dye is administered first to see the spinal area better before images are taken. The physician reviews the images to look for specific information that may correlate to the patient's symptoms, such as abnormal spinal alignment; disease or injury of vertebral bodies; intervertebral disc herniation, degeneration, or dehydration; the size of the spinal canal to accommodate the cord and nerve roots; pinched or inflamed nerves; or any changes since surgery.

RVUs

Code	Work	PE	PE Non-Facility	MP	Total Non-Facility	Total Facility	Global
72146	1.48	4.54	4.54	0.09	6.11	6.11	XXX
72147	1.78	6.93	6.93	0.11	8.82	8.82	XXX

72148-72149

72148 Magnetic resonance (eg, proton) imaging, spinal canal and contents, lumbar; without contrast material

72149 Magnetic resonance (eg, proton) imaging, spinal canal and contents, lumbar; with contrast material(s)

(For lumbar spinal canal imaging without contrast material followed by contrast material, use 72158)

Plain English Description

Magnetic resonance imaging (MRI) is done on the lumbar spinal canal and contents. MRI is a noninvasive, non-radiating imaging technique that uses the magnetic properties of nuclei within hydrogen atoms of the body. The powerful magnetic field forces the hydrogen atoms to line up. Radiowaves are then transmitted within the strong magnetic field. Protons in the nuclei of different types of tissues emit a specific radiofrequency signal that bounces back to the computer, which records the images. The computer processes the signals and coverts the data into tomographic, 3D, sectional images in slices with very high resolution. The patient is placed on a motorized table within a large MRI tunnel scanner that contains the magnet. MRI scans of the spine are often done when conservative treatment of back pain is unsuccessful and more aggressive treatments are considered or following surgery. In 72148, no contrast medium is used. In 72149, a contrast dye is administered first to see the spinal area better before images are taken. The physician reviews the images to look for specific information that may correlate to the patient's symptoms, such as abnormal spinal alignment; disease or injury of vertebral bodies; intervertebral disc herniation, degeneration, or dehydration; the size of the spinal canal to accommodate the cord and nerve roots; pinched or inflamed nerves; or any changes since surgery.

RVUs

Code	Work	PE	PE Non-Facility	MP	Total Non-Facility	Total Facility	Global
72148	1.48	4.55	4.55	0.09	6.12	6.12	XXX
72149	1.78	6.85	6.85	0.11	8.74	8.74	XXX

72156-72158

72156 Magnetic resonance (eg, proton) imaging, spinal canal and contents, without contrast material, followed by contrast material(s) and further sequences; cervical

72157 Magnetic resonance (eg, proton) imaging, spinal canal and contents, without contrast material, followed by contrast material(s) and further sequences; thoracic

72158 Magnetic resonance (eg, proton) imaging, spinal canal and contents, without contrast material, followed by contrast material(s) and further sequences; lumbar

Plain English Description

Magnetic resonance imaging (MRI) is done on the cervical, thoracic, or lumbar spinal canal and contents. MRI is a noninvasive, non-radiating imaging technique that uses the magnetic properties of nuclei within hydrogen atoms of the body. The powerful magnetic field forces the hydrogen atoms to line up. Radiowaves are then transmitted within the strong magnetic field. Protons in the nuclei of different types of tissues emit a specific radiofrequency signal that bounces back to the computer, which records the images. The computer processes the signals and coverts the data into tomographic, 3D, sectional images in slices with very high resolution. The patient is placed on a motorized table within a large MRI tunnel scanner that contains the magnet. MRI scans of the spine are often done when conservative treatment of back/neck pain is unsuccessful and more aggressive treatments are considered or following surgery. Images are taken first without contrast and again after the administration of contrast to see the spinal area better. The physician reviews the images to look for specific information that may correlate to the patient's symptoms, such as abnormal spinal alignment; disease or injury of vertebral bodies; intervertebral disc herniation, degeneration, or dehydration; the size of the spinal canal to accommodate the cord and nerve roots; pinched or inflamed nerves; or any changes since surgery. Use 72156 for MRI of the cervical spine, 72157 for the thoracic spine, and 72158 for the lumbar spine.

RVUs

Code	Work	PE	PE Non-Facility	MP	Total Non-Facility	Total Facility	Global
72156	2.29	7.93	7.93	0.13	10.35	10.35	XXX
72157	2.29	7.95	7.95	0.13	10.37	10.37	XXX
72158	2.29	7.91	7.91	0.13	10.33	10.33	XXX

72170-72190

72170 Radiologic examination, pelvis; 1 or 2 views

72190 Radiologic examination, pelvis; complete, minimum of 3 views

(For pelvimetry, use 74710)

(For a combined computed tomography [CT] or computed tomographic angiography abdomen and pelvis study, see 74174, 74176-74178)

Plain English Description

A diagnostic X-ray examination of the pelvis is performed. X-ray uses indirect ionizing radiation to take pictures inside the body. X-rays work on non-uniform material, such as human tissue, because of the different density and composition of the object, which allows some of the X-rays to be absorbed and some to pass through and be captured behind the object on a detector. This produces a 2D image of the structures. Bones appear white while soft tissue and fluids appear shades of gray. Pelvic X-rays are taken when the patient complains of pain and/or injury in the area of the pelvis or hip joints to assess for fractures and detect arthritis or bone disease. The patient is placed on a table and different views of the pelvis are taken by having the patient position the legs and feet differently, such as turning the feet inward to point at each other, or bending the knees outward with the soles of the feet together in a "frog-leg" position. Report 72170 for 1-2 views and 72190 for 3 or more views for a complete pelvic X-ray exam.

RVUs

Code	Work	PE	PE Non-Facility	MP	Total Non-Facility	Total Facility	Global
72170	0.17	0.61	0.61	0.02	0.80	0.80	XXX
72190	0.25	0.87	0.87	0.02	1.14	1.14	XXX

72195-72197

72195 Magnetic resonance (eg, proton) imaging, pelvis; without contrast material(s)

72196 Magnetic resonance (eg, proton) imaging, pelvis; with contrast material(s)

72197 Magnetic resonance (eg, proton) imaging, pelvis; without contrast material(s), followed by contrast material(s) and further sequences

(Do not report 72195, 72196, 72197 in conjunction with 74712, 74713)

(For magnetic resonance imaging of a fetus[es], see 74712, 74713)

Plain English Description

Magnetic resonance imaging (MRI) is performed on the pelvis and organs within the pelvic area. MRI is a noninvasive, non-radiating imaging technique that uses the magnetic properties of nuclei within hydrogen atoms of the body. The powerful magnetic field forces the hydrogen atoms to line up. Radio waves are then transmitted within the strong magnetic field. Protons in the nuclei of different types of tissues emit a specific radiofrequency signal that bounces back to the computer, which records the images. The computer processes the signals and converts the data into tomographic, 3D, sectional images in slices with very high resolution. The patient is placed on a motorized table within a large MRI tunnel scanner that contains the magnet. Small coils that help transmit and receive the radiowaves may be placed around the hip area. MRI scans of the pelvis are often performed for injury, trauma, birth defects, or unexplained hip or pelvic pain. In 72195, no contrast medium is used. In 72196, an iodine contrast dye is administered intravenously to see the target area better before images are taken. In 72197, images are taken without contrast and again after the administration of contrast. The physician reviews the images to look for information that may correlate to the patient's signs or symptoms. Pelvic MRI may be performed on males to evaluate lumps or swelling of the testicles or scrotum and locate an undescended testicle that does not appear on ultrasound. For females, an MRI scan may be used to evaluate abnormal vaginal bleeding, endometriosis, a pelvic mass, or unexplained infertility.

RVUs

Code	Work	PE	PE Non-Facility	MP	Total Non-Facility	Total Facility	Global
72195	1.46	5.93	5.93	0.10	7.49	7.49	XXX
72196	1.73	6.90	6.90	0.11	8.74	8.74	XXX
72197	2.20	8.68	8.68	0.11	10.99	10.99	XXX

72240-72270

72240 Myelography, cervical, radiological supervision and interpretation

(Do not report 72240 in conjunction with 62284, 62302, 62303, 62304, 62305)

(When both 62284 and 72240 are performed by the same physician or other qualified health care professional for cervical myelography, use 62302)

(For complete cervical myelography via injection procedure at C1-C2, see 61055, 72240)

72255 Myelography, thoracic, radiological supervision and interpretation

(Do not report 72255 in conjunction with 62284, 62302, 62303, 62304, 62305)

(When both 62284 and 72255 are performed by the same physician or other qualified health care professional for thoracic myelography, use 62303)

(For complete thoracic myelography via injection procedure at C1-C2, see 61055, 72255)

72265 Myelography, lumbosacral, radiological supervision and interpretation

(Do not report 72265 in conjunction with 62284, 62302, 62303, 62304, 62305)

(When both 62284 and 72265 are performed by the same physician or other qualified health care professional for lumbosacral myelography, use 62304)

(For complete lumbosacral myelography via injection procedure at C1-C2, see 61055, 72265)

72270 Myelography, 2 or more regions (eg, lumbar/thoracic, cervical/thoracic, lumbar/cervical, lumbar/thoracic/cervical), radiological supervision and interpretation

(Do not report 72270 in conjunction with 62284, 62302, 62303, 62304, 62305)

(When both 62284 and 72270 are performed by the same physician or other qualified health care professional for myelography of 2 or more regions, use 62305)

(For complete myelography of 2 or more regions via injection procedure at C1-C2, see 61055, 72270)

Plain English Description

Myelography is a type of diagnostic imaging that uses contrast material injected into the subarachnoid space and real-time fluoroscopic X-ray imaging. After introducing a needle into the spinal canal and injecting contrast material into the subarachnoid space, the radiologist evaluates the spinal cord, spinal canal, nerve roots, meninges, and blood vessels in real time as contrast flows through the space around the spinal cord and nerve roots. Permanent X-ray images may also be taken. Spinal myelography is used to diagnose intervertebral disc herniation, meningeal inflammation, spinal stenosis, tumors, and other spinal lesions caused by infection or previous trauma. Report 72240 for myelography of the cervical spine, 72255 for thoracic myelography, 72265 for lumbosacral myelography, and 72270 when two or more regions of the spine are examined together.

RVUs

Code	Work	PE	PE Non-Facility	MP	Total Non-Facility	Total Facility	Global
72240	0.91	2.17	2.17	0.06	3.14	3.14	XXX
72255	0.91	2.19	2.19	0.09	3.19	3.19	XXX
72265	0.83	2.01	2.01	0.06	2.90	2.90	XXX
72270	1.33	2.60	2.60	0.07	4.00	4.00	XXX

72275

72275 Epidurography, radiological supervision and interpretation

(72275 includes 77003)

(For injection procedure, see 62280, 62281, 62282, 62320, 62321, 62322, 62323, 62324, 62325, 62326, 62327, 64479, 64480, 64483, 64484)

(Use 72275 only when an epidurogram is performed, images documented, and a formal radiologic report is issued)

(Do not report 72275 in conjunction with 22586)

Plain English Description

Images of the epidural space surrounding the spinal cord are documented under radiological supervision while a therapeutic or diagnostic epidurography is performed. The radiologist also provides a formal radiologic report of the procedure after it is performed. The injection portion of the procedure to perform the epidurography is done by cleansing the skin over the targeted spinal region with an antiseptic solution and then injecting a local anesthetic. A spinal needle is inserted into the skin and advanced into the epidural space. Contrast may be injected to confirm proper needle placement or to perform the procedure itself. A diagnostic or therapeutic substance, such as an anesthetic, antispasmodic, opioid, steroid, or neurolytic substance, is injected into the epidural space. Images are taken. Following injection, the patient is monitored for 15-20 minutes to ensure that there are no adverse effects. Report 72275 for radiological supervision during the procedure that includes documented imaging and provision of a formal interpretation of the procedure by the radiologist.

RVUs

Code	Work	PE	PE Non-Facility	MP	Total Non-Facility	Total Facility	Global
72275	0.76	2.87	2.87	0.06	3.69	3.69	XXX

72295

72295 Discography, lumbar, radiological supervision and interpretation

Plain English Description

Images of a lumbar intervertebral disc are documented under radiological supervision while a discography is performed. A formal interpretation of the procedure is also provided. Discography is done to determine if an intervertebral disc abnormality is the cause of back pain. To perform the injection portion of the discography, the patient is positioned on the side and the site of the injection is cleansed with an antiseptic solution. A local anesthetic is injected. A large-bore needle is advanced through the skin to the targeted lumbar disc. A discography needle is advanced through the first needle and into the center of the disc. Contrast is injected and radiographs are obtained under supervision. Report 72295 for radiological supervision during the discography procedure and provision of a written interpretation after completion.

RVUs

Code	Work	PE	PE Non-Facility	MP	Total Non-Facility	Total Facility	Global
72295	0.83	2.13	2.13	0.06	3.02	3.02	XXX

73020-73030

73020 Radiologic examination, shoulder; 1 view

73030 Radiologic examination, shoulder; complete, minimum of 2 views

Plain English Description

A radiologic examination of the shoulder is done. The shoulder is the junction of the humeral head and the glenoid of the scapula. Standard views include the anteroposterior (AP) view and the lateral "Y" view, named because of the Y shape formed by the scapula when looking at it from the side. An axial view can also be obtained for further assessment when the patient is able to hold the arm in abduction. X-ray imaging uses indirect ionizing radiation to take pictures inside the body. X-rays work on non-uniform material, such as human tissue, because of the different density and composition of the object, which allows some of the X-rays to be absorbed and some to pass through and be captured behind the object on a detector. This produces a 2D image of the structures. Report 73020 for a single view and 73030 for a complete exam when a minimum of 2 views is taken.

RVUs

Code	Work	PE	PE Non-Facility	MP	Total Non-Facility	Total Facility	Global
73020	0.15	0.43	0.43	0.02	0.60	0.60	XXX
73030	0.18	0.73	0.73	0.02	0.93	0.93	XXX

73120-73130

73120 Radiologic examination, hand; 2 views

73130 Radiologic examination, hand; minimum of 3 views

Plain English Description

A radiologic examination of the hand is done. X-ray imaging uses indirect ionizing radiation to take pictures inside the body. X-rays work on non-uniform material, such as human tissue, because of the different density and composition of the object, which allows some of the X-rays to be absorbed and some to pass through and be captured behind the object on a detector. This produces a 2D image of the structures. The radiographs may be taken to look for conditions such as fractures, dislocations, deformities, degenerative bone conditions, osteomyelitis, arthritis, foreign body, or tumors. Hand X-rays are also used to help determine the "bone age" of children and assess whether any nutritional or metabolic disorders may be interfering with proper development. The posteroanterior projection is taken with the palm down flat and may show not only the metacarpals, phalanges, and interphalangeal joints, but the carpal bones, radius, and ulna as well. Lateral views may be taken with the hand placed upright, resting upon the ulnar side of the palm and little finger with the thumb on top, ideally with the fingers supported by a sponge and splayed to avoid overlap. Oblique views can be obtained with the hand placed palm down and rolled slightly to the outside with the fingertips still touching the film surface. The beam is angled perpendicular to the film cassette for oblique projections and aimed at the middle finger metacarpophalangeal joint. Report 73120 for a radiologic exam with 2 views taken of the hand and 73130 for an X-ray exam in which a minimum of 3 different projections is obtained.

RVUs

Code	Work	PE	PE Non-Facility	MP	Total Non-Facility	Total Facility	Global
73120	0.16	0.67	0.67	0.02	0.85	0.85	XXX
73130	0.17	0.79	0.79	0.02	0.98	0.98	XXX

73221-73223

73221 Magnetic resonance (eg, proton) imaging, any joint of upper extremity; without contrast material(s)

73222 Magnetic resonance (eg, proton) imaging, any joint of upper extremity; with contrast material(s)

73223 Magnetic resonance (eg, proton) imaging, any joint of upper extremity; without contrast material(s), followed by contrast material(s) and further sequences

Plain English Description

Magnetic resonance imaging is done on a joint of the upper or lower arm. Magnetic resonance is a noninvasive, non-radiating imaging technique that uses the magnetic properties of hydrogen atoms in the body. The patient is placed on a motorized table within a large MRI tunnel scanner that contains the magnet. The powerful magnetic field forces the hydrogen atoms to line up. Radiowaves are then transmitted within the strong magnetic field. Protons in the nuclei of different types of tissues emit a specific radiofrequency signal that bounces back to the computer, which processes the signals and converts the data into tomographic, 3D images with very high resolution. The patient is placed on a motorized table within a large MRI tunnel scanner that contains the magnet. Small coils that help transmit and receive the radiowaves may be placed around the joint. MRI scans on joints of the upper extremity are often done for injury, trauma, unexplained pain, redness, or swelling, and freezing of a joint with loss of motion. MRI scans provide clear images of areas that may be difficult to see on CT. In 73221, no contrast medium is used. In 73222, an iodine contrast dye is administered into the joint to see the target area better before images are taken. In 73223, images are taken without contrast and again after the administration of contrast. The physician reviews the images to look for information that may correlate to the patient's signs or symptoms. MRI provides reliable information on the presence and extent of tumors, masses, or lesions in the joint; infection, inflammation, and swelling of soft tissue; muscle atrophy and other anomalous muscular development; and joint effusion and vascular necrosis.

RVUs

Code	Work	PE	PE Non-Facility	MP	Total Non-Facility	Total Facility	Global
73221	1.35	5.02	5.02	0.10	6.47	6.47	XXX
73222	1.62	8.56	8.56	0.11	10.29	10.29	XXX
73223	2.15	10.46	10.46	0.11	12.72	12.72	XXX

73501-73503

73501 Radiologic examination, hip, unilateral, with pelvis when performed; 1 view

73502 Radiologic examination, hip, unilateral, with pelvis when performed; 2-3 views

73503 Radiologic examination, hip, unilateral, with pelvis when performed; minimum of 4 views

Plain English Description

A radiologic examination of the hip is done on either the left or the right side, which may also include the pelvis. X-ray imaging uses indirect ionizing radiation to take pictures inside the body. X-rays work on non-uniform material, such as human tissue, because of the different density and composition of the object, which allows some of the X-rays to be absorbed and some to pass through and be captured behind the object on a detector. This produces a 2D image of the structures. The radiographs may be taken to look for conditions such as fractures, dislocations, deformities, degenerative bone conditions, osteomyelitis, arthritis, foreign body, infection, or tumor. Hip standard views that are taken most frequently include the front to back anteroposterior view taken with the patient lying supine and the legs straight, rotated slightly inward; the lateral "frog-leg" view, taken with the hips flexed and abducted and the knees flexed with the soles of the feet placed together; a cross table view with the unaffected hip and knee flexed at a 90 degree angle out of the way and the beam aimed perpendicular to the long axis of the femur on the affected side. Another type of lateral view is taken with the hip flexed 45 degrees and abducted 45 degrees and the beam aimed perpendicular to the table. Report 73501 for an X-ray exam of either the left or the right hip consisting of only 1 view; report 73502 for a hip exam on one side only with 2-3 views and code 73503 for a hip exam with a minimum of 4 views taken.

RVUs

Code	Work	PE	PE Non-Facility	MP	Total Non-Facility	Total Facility	Global
73501	0.18	0.69	0.69	0.02	0.89	0.89	XXX
73502	0.22	1.03	1.03	0.02	1.27	1.27	XXX
73503	0.27	1.28	1.28	0.02	1.57	1.57	XXX

73521-73523

73521 Radiologic examination, hips, bilateral, with pelvis when performed; 2 views

73522 Radiologic examination, hips, bilateral, with pelvis when performed; 3-4 views

73523 Radiologic examination, hips, bilateral, with pelvis when performed; minimum of 5 views

Plain English Description

A radiologic examination is done on both the left and the right hip, which may also include the pelvis. X-ray imaging uses indirect ionizing radiation to take pictures inside the body. X-rays work on non-uniform material, such as human tissue, because of the different density and composition of the object, which allows some of the X-rays to be absorbed and some to pass through and be captured behind the object on a detector. This produces a 2D image of the structures. The radiographs may be taken to look for conditions such as fractures, dislocations, deformities, degenerative bone conditions, osteomyelitis, arthritis, foreign body, infection, or tumor. Hip standard views that are taken most frequently include the front to back anteroposterior view taken with the patient lying supine and the legs straight, rotated slightly inward; the lateral "frog-leg" view, taken with the hips flexed and abducted and the knees flexed with the soles of the feet placed together; a cross table view with the unaffected hip and knee flexed at a 90 degree angle out of the way and the beam aimed perpendicular to the long axis of the femur on the affected side. Another type of lateral view is taken with the hip flexed 45 degrees and abducted 45 degrees and the beam aimed perpendicular to the table. A front to back view of the hips in a pelvic view is often taken with the patient supine and both legs rotated slightly inward about 15 degrees. Report 73521 for an X-ray exam of both hips consisting of 2 projections; report 73522 for a bilateral hip X-ray exam with 3-4 views; and 73523 for a bilateral hip exam with a minimum of 5 views. The views taken may include a pelvic view.

RVUs

Code	Work	PE	PE Non-Facility	MP	Total Non-Facility	Total Facility	Global
73521	0.22	0.88	0.88	0.02	1.12	1.12	XXX
73522	0.29	1.15	1.15	0.02	1.46	1.46	XXX
73523	0.31	1.33	1.33	0.02	1.66	1.66	XXX

73560-73565

73560 Radiologic examination, knee; 1 or 2 views
73562 Radiologic examination, knee; 3 views
73564 Radiologic examination, knee; complete, 4 or more views
73565 Radiologic examination, knee; both knees, standing, anteroposterior

Plain English Description

A radiologic examination of the knee images the femur, tibia, fibula, patella, and soft tissue. X-ray imaging uses indirect ionizing radiation to take pictures inside the body. X-rays work on non-uniform material, such as human tissue, because of the different density and composition of the object, which allows some of the X-rays to be absorbed and some to pass through and be captured behind the object on a detector. This produces a 2D image of the structures. The radiographs may be taken to look for the cause of pain, limping, or swelling, or conditions such as fractures, dislocations, deformities, degenerative disease, osteomyelitis, arthritis, foreign body, and cysts or tumors. Knee X-rays may also be used to determine whether there is satisfactory alignment of lower extremity bones following fracture treatment. Standard views of the knee include front to back anteroposterior (AP), lateral (side), and back to front posteroanterior (PA) with variations in the flexion of the joint, and weight-bearing and nonweight-bearing postures. Code 73560 is used to report an X-ray exam of the knee in 1 or 2 views. Code 73562 is used for 3 views. Code 73564 is used to report a complete X-ray exam of the knee with 4 or more views. Code 73565 is used to report a weight-bearing X-ray exam of both knees, taken from front to back on a single film.

RVUs

Code	Work	PE	PE Non-Facility	MP	Total Non-Facility	Total Facility	Global
73560	0.16	0.76	0.76	0.02	0.94	0.94	XXX
73562	0.18	0.90	0.90	0.02	1.10	1.10	XXX
73564	0.22	0.99	0.99	0.02	1.23	1.23	XXX
73565	0.16	0.91	0.91	0.02	1.09	1.09	XXX

73620-73630

73620 Radiologic examination, foot; 2 views
73630 Radiologic examination, foot; complete, minimum of 3 views

Plain English Description

A radiologic examination of the foot images the bones of the distal lower extremity and may include the tibia, fibula, talus, calcaneus, cuboid, navicular, cuneiform, metatarsals, and phalanges. X-ray imaging uses indirect ionizing radiation to take pictures inside the body. X-rays work on non-uniform material, such as human tissue, because of the different density and composition of the object, which allows some of the X-rays to be absorbed and some to pass through and be captured behind the object on a detector. This produces a 2D image of the structures. The radiographs may be taken to look for the cause of pain, limping, or swelling, or conditions such as fractures, dislocations, deformities, degenerative disease, osteomyelitis, arthritis, foreign body, and cysts or tumors. Foot X-rays may also be used to determine whether there is satisfactory alignment of foot bones following fracture treatment. Standard views of the foot include top to bottom dorsal planter (DP), lateral (side), oblique (semi-prone position with body and leg partially rotated), and stress study with traction placed on the joint manually. Code 73620 is used to report an X-ray exam of the foot with 2 views. Code 73630 is used to report a complete X-ray exam of the foot with a minimum of 3 views included in the study.

RVUs

Code	Work	PE	PE Non-Facility	MP	Total Non-Facility	Total Facility	Global
73620	0.16	0.60	0.60	0.02	0.78	0.78	XXX
73630	0.17	0.73	0.73	0.02	0.92	0.92	XXX

73700-73702

73700 Computed tomography, lower extremity; without contrast material
73701 Computed tomography, lower extremity; with contrast material(s)
73702 Computed tomography, lower extremity; without contrast material, followed by contrast material(s) and further sections
(To report 3D rendering, see 76376, 76377)

Plain English Description

Diagnostic computed tomography (CT) is done on the lower extremity to provide detailed visualization of the tissues and bone structure of the leg. CT uses multiple, narrow X-ray beams aimed around a single rotational axis, taking a series of 2D images of the target structure from multiple angles. Contrast material is used to enhance the images. Computer software processes the data and produces several images of thin, cross-sectional 2D slices of the targeted organ or area. Three-dimensional models of the leg can be created by stacking multiple, individual 2D slices together. The patient is placed inside the CT scanner on the table and images are obtained of the lower extremity. In 73700, no contrast medium is used. In 73701, an iodine contrast dye is administered intravenously to see the target area better before images are taken. In 73702, CT is first performed without contrast followed by the administration of contrast and acquisition of additional sections. The physician reviews the CT scan, notes any abnormalities, and provides a written interpretation of the findings. The physician reviews the images to look for suspected problems with the leg such as locating tumors, abscesses, or masses; evaluating the bones for degenerative conditions, fractures, or other injury following trauma; and finding the cause of pain or swelling.

RVUs

Code	Work	PE	PE Non-Facility	MP	Total Non-Facility	Total Facility	Global
73700	1.00	3.30	3.30	0.06	4.36	4.36	XXX
73701	1.16	4.23	4.23	0.06	5.45	5.45	XXX
73702	1.22	5.27	5.27	0.07	6.56	6.56	XXX

73721-73723

73721 Magnetic resonance (eg, proton) imaging, any joint of lower extremity; without contrast material

73722 Magnetic resonance (eg, proton) imaging, any joint of lower extremity; with contrast material(s)

73723 Magnetic resonance (eg, proton) imaging, any joint of lower extremity; without contrast material(s), followed by contrast material(s) and further sequences

Plain English Description

Magnetic resonance imaging (MRI) is done on a joint of the upper or lower leg. Magnetic resonance is a noninvasive, non-radiating imaging technique that uses the magnetic properties of hydrogen atoms in the body. The patient is placed on a motorized table within a large MRI tunnel scanner that contains the magnet. The powerful magnetic field forces the hydrogen atoms to line up. Radiowaves are then transmitted within the strong magnetic field. Protons in the nuclei of different types of tissues emit a specific radiofrequency signal that bounces back to the computer, which processes the signals and converts the data into tomographic, 3D images with very high resolution. The patient is placed on a motorized table within a large MRI tunnel scanner that contains the magnet. Small coils that help transmit and receive the radiowaves may be placed around the joint. MRI scans on joints of the lower extremity are often done for injury, trauma, unexplained pain, redness, or swelling, and freezing of a joint with loss of motion. MRI scans provide clear images of areas that may be difficult to see on CT. In 73721, no contrast medium is used. In 73722, an iodine contrast dye is administered into the joint to see the target area better before images are taken. In 73723, images are taken without contrast and again after the administration of contrast. The physician reviews the images to look for information that may correlate to the patient's signs or symptoms. MRI provides reliable information on the presence and extent of tumors, masses, or lesions within the joint; infection, inflammation, and swelling of soft tissue; muscle atrophy and other anomalous muscular development; and joint effusion and vascular necrosis.

RVUs

Code	Work	PE	PE Non-Facility	MP	Total Non-Facility	Total Facility	Global
73721	1.35	5.01	5.01	0.08	6.44	6.44	XXX
73722	1.62	8.58	8.58	0.11	10.31	10.31	XXX
73723	2.15	10.44	10.44	0.11	12.70	12.70	XXX

74018-74022

74018 Radiologic examination, abdomen; 1 view

74019 Radiologic examination, abdomen; 2 views

74021 Radiologic examination, abdomen; 3 or more views

▲ **74022 Radiologic examination, complete acute abdomen series, including 2 or more views of the abdomen (eg, supine, erect, decubitus), and a single view chest**

Plain English Description

A radiologic examination of the abdomen images the internal organs, soft tissue (muscle, fat), and supporting skeleton. X-ray imaging uses indirect ionizing radiation to take pictures of non-uniform material, such as human tissue, because of its different density and composition, which allows some of the X-rays to be absorbed and some to pass through and be captured. This produces a 2D image of the structures. The radiographs may be taken to look for size, shape, and position of organs, pattern of air (bowel gas), obstruction, foreign objects, and calcification in the gallbladder, urinary tract, and aorta. A radiologic examination of the abdomen may be ordered to diagnose abdominal distention and pain, vomiting, diarrhea or constipation, and traumatic injury; it may also be obtained as a screening exam or scout film prior to other imagining procedures. Code 74018 is used to report a single view; code 74019 reports 2 views; 74021 reports 3 or more views. Code 74022 is used to report a complete acute abdomen series including supine, erect, and/or decubitus views and a single view of the chest. Common views of the abdomen include front to back anteroposterior (AP) with the patient lying supine or standing erect, back to front posteroanterior (PA) with the patient lying prone, lateral with the patient lying on the side, lateral decubitus AP (lying on the side, front to back view), lateral dorsal decubitus (lying supine, side view), oblique (anterior or posterior rotation), and coned (small collimated) views, which may be used to localize and differentiate lesions, calcifications, or herniations.

RVUs

Code	Work	PE	PE Non-Facility	MP	Total Non-Facility	Total Facility	Global
74018	0.18	0.62	0.62	0.02	0.82	0.82	XXX
74019	0.23	0.76	0.76	0.02	1.01	1.01	XXX
74021	0.27	0.88	0.88	0.02	1.17	1.17	XXX
74022	0.32	1.02	1.02	0.02	1.36	1.36	XXX

74176-74178

74176 Computed tomography, abdomen and pelvis; without contrast material

74177 Computed tomography, abdomen and pelvis; with contrast material(s)

74178 Computed tomography, abdomen and pelvis; without contrast material in one or both body regions, followed by contrast material(s) and further sections in one or both body regions

(Do not report 74176-74178 in conjunction with 72192-72194, 74150-74170)

(Report 74176, 74177, or 74178 only once per CT abdomen and pelvis examination)

Plain English Description

Computerized tomography, also referred to as a CT scan, uses special X-ray equipment and computer technology to produce multiple cross-sectional images of the abdomen and pelvis. The patient is positioned on the CT examination table. An initial pass is made through the CT scanner to determine the starting position of the scans. The CT scan is then performed. As the table moves slowly through the scanner, numerous X-ray beams and electronic X-ray detectors rotate around the abdomen and pelvis. The amount of radiation being absorbed is measured. As the beams and detectors rotate around the body, the table is moved through the scanner. A computer program processes the data that are then displayed on the monitor as 2D cross-sectional images of the abdomen or pelvis. The physician reviews the data and images as they are obtained and may request additional sections to provide more detail on areas of interest. Use 74176 for CT scan of the abdomen and pelvis without intravenous contrast material. Use 74177 for CT scan of the abdomen and pelvis in which intravenous contrast material is administered before CT scanning begins and contrast enhanced images are obtained. Use 74178 when CT is first performed without intravenous contrast followed by the administration of intravenous contrast and acquisition of additional sections. The physician reviews the CT scan, notes any abnormalities, and provides a written interpretation of the findings.

RVUs

Code	Work	PE	PE Non-Facility	MP	Total Non-Facility	Total Facility	Global
74176	1.74	3.79	3.79	0.10	5.63	5.63	XXX
74177	1.82	7.28	7.28	0.11	9.21	9.21	XXX
74178	2.01	8.23	8.23	0.11	10.35	10.35	XXX

74230

▲ **74230 Radiologic examination, swallowing function, with cineradiography/videoradiography, including scout neck radiograph(s) and delayed image(s), when performed, contrast (eg, barium) study**

(For otorhinolaryngologic services fluoroscopic evaluation of swallowing function, use 92611)

Plain English Description

A radiologic study with cineradiography/videoradiography may be performed to assess swallowing function in patients with dysphagia. A swallowing function study (modified barium swallow, MBS) may be indicated for patients with a history of stroke or other central nervous system (CNS) disorders, surgery or radiation to the head/neck, neuromuscular or rheumatologic disease, generalized debilitation and head/neck/throat injury including peripheral nerve injury. The patient is seated upright or semi-reclining with the fluoroscopy machine focused on the head and neck. Food and liquids of various texture and quantity are mixed or soaked in contrast medium (barium) and administered to the patient. A fluoroscopic recording is made of the food or fluid in the oral cavity, larynx, pharynx, and upper esophagus to document mastication and tongue mobility, elevation and retraction of the velum, tongue base retraction and movement of the hyoid bone and larynx, closure of the larynx, contraction of the pharynx, and the duration and extent of pharyngoesophageal segment opening. Observation and recording is made of any penetration or aspiration of food and fluid into the upper airways. The measurement of muscle sensation and strength may be inferred or calculated directly from the information obtained during the study.

RVUs

Code	Work	PE	PE Non-Facility	MP	Total Non-Facility	Total Facility	Global
74230	0.53	3.08	3.08	0.03	3.64	3.64	XXX

75705

75705 Angiography, spinal, selective, radiological supervision and interpretation

Plain English Description

A procedure is performed to study selective spinal arteries using radiopaque contrast medium and fluoroscopy. Selective spinal angiography images the blood flow to the spine and spinal cord and may be used to diagnose arteriovenous malformations and primary metastatic tumors of the vertebral bodies. A large bore needle is inserted into a blood vessel in the groin, a guidewire is introduced through the needle, and a catheter is advanced over the guidewire into the aorta using X-ray guidance. The catheter is then placed into the appropriate selective paired spinal arteries: intercostal, subclavian, thyrocervical, costocervical above the diaphragm and vertebral, internal iliac, lumbar, and median sacral below the diaphragm. Contrast medium is injected and X-ray images are obtained. The catheter is removed at the end of the procedure. Code 75705 reports the radiologist's supervision of the selective spinal angiography procedure, review of records and interpretation of the findings, and a written report.

RVUs

Code	Work	PE	PE Non-Facility	MP	Total Non-Facility	Total Facility	Global
75705	2.18	4.55	4.55	0.36	7.09	7.09	XXX

75710

75710 Angiography, extremity, unilateral, radiological supervision and interpretation

Plain English Description

A procedure is performed to study the integrity of the walls of an extremity's arteries and blood flow within the vessels using radiopaque contrast medium and fluoroscopy. To visualize lower extremity vessels, a large bore needle is inserted into the femoral artery in the groin and a guidewire is introduced through the needle. A catheter is advanced over the guidewire to the desired location for the study and dye is injected. To study an upper extremity, the needle may be inserted in the radial artery in the wrist or the brachial artery in the upper arm and a guidewire is introduced through the needle. A catheter is advanced over the guidewire to the desired location for the study and dye is injected. Blood flow is studied in real time with X-ray images obtained as the dye moves through the leg to the foot or through the arm to the hand. Images are recorded for more detailed study or to compare with previous examinations. Code 75710 reports the radiologist's supervision of the extremity imaging procedure on one side only; code 75716 reports supervision of extremity imaging done on both arms or both legs, along with review of records and interpretation of the image findings, and a written report.

RVUs

Code	Work	PE	PE Non-Facility	MP	Total Non-Facility	Total Facility	Global
75710	1.75	2.65	2.65	0.23	4.63	4.63	XXX

75774

✚ **75774 Angiography, selective, each additional vessel studied after basic examination, radiological supervision and interpretation (List separately in addition to code for primary procedure)**

(Use 75774 in addition to code for specific initial vessel studied)

(Do not report 75774 as part of diagnostic angiography of the extracranial and intracranial cervicocerebral vessels. It may be appropriate to report 75774 for diagnostic angiography of upper extremities and other vascular beds performed in the same session)

(For angiography, see 75600-75756)

(For catheterizations, see codes 36215-36248)

(For cardiac catheterization procedures, see 93452-93462, 93531-93533, 93563-93568)

(For radiological supervision and interpretation of dialysis circuit angiography performed through existing access[es] or catheter-based arterial access, use 36901 with modifier 52)Do not report 36218 or 75774 as part of diagnostic angiography of the extracranial and intracranial cervicocerebral vessels. It may be appropriate to report 36218 and 75774 for diagnostic angiography of upper extremities and other vascular beds of the neck and/or shoulder girdle performed in the same session as vertebral angiography (eg, workup of a neck tumor that requires catheterization and angiography of the vertebral artery as well as other brachiocephalic arteries).

Plain English Description

Selective angiography uses radiopaque contrast medium and fluoroscopy to study vessels located distal to the aorta. A large bore needle is inserted into a blood vessel in the groin; a guidewire is introduced through the needle and a catheter is advanced over the guidewire into the abdominal aorta using X-ray guidance. The catheter is manipulated to the area of suspected pathology and radiopaque contrast material is injected to visualize the vessels (basic exam). Additional selective catheterization and angiography of an artery/branch may be necessary when poor visualization, occlusive disease, or anatomical variances are encountered. The catheter is advanced beyond the area of the basic exam and contrast is injected to visualize the vessel(s). Code 75774 reports the radiological supervision of each additional vessel studied after the basic angiography imaging procedure, review of records and interpretation of the findings, with a written report. Code 75774 is reported in addition to the code for the basic angiography imaging procedure.

RVUs

Code	Work	PE	PE Non-Facility	MP	Total Non-Facility	Total Facility	Global
75774	1.01	1.93	1.93	0.10	3.04	3.04	ZZZ

75894

75894 Transcatheter therapy, embolization, any method, radiological supervision and interpretation

(Do not report 75894 in conjunction with 36475, 36476, 36478, 36479, 37241-37244)

Plain English Description

Radiological supervision is provided for a procedure performed to permanently or temporarily reduce or eliminate blood flow to a target area of the central nervous system, or the head or neck. Embolization therapy may be initiated for curative or palliative intent to manage hemorrhage caused by trauma and to treat neoplasms and congenital or acquired vascular anomalies. The appropriate blood vessel is accessed by needle puncture and a guidewire is inserted through the needle and threaded to the selected embolization site using fluoroscopic guidance. A catheter is then inserted over the guidewire, advanced to the targeted treatment area, and the guidewire is removed. Radiopaque contrast medium is injected and X-rays are obtained to confirm correct placement of the catheter. Embolization therapy is carried out using an appropriate method (eg, chemotherapeutic agent, radiofrequency, metallic coils, detachable balloon, autologous clot, absorbable gelatin sponge, microfibrillar collagen). At the conclusion of the procedure, the catheter is removed. Code 75894 reports only the radiological supervision of the transcatheter embolization procedure, review and interpretation of the images obtained of the procedure, and a written report of the findings.

RVUs

Code	Work	PE	PE Non-Facility	MP	Total Non-Facility	Total Facility	Global
75894	0.00	0.00	0.00	0.00	0.00	0.00	XXX

75898

75898 Angiography through existing catheter for follow-up study for transcatheter therapy, embolization or infusion, other than for thrombolysis

(For thrombolysis infusion management other than coronary, see 37211-37214, 61645)

(For non-thrombolysis infusion management other than coronary, see 61650, 61651)

(Do not report 75898 in conjunction with 37211-37214, 37241-37244, 61645, 61650, 61651)

Plain English Description

During a separately reportable transcatheter embolization or infusion procedure, follow-up angiograms are obtained to evaluate the outcome of the procedure. Using the existing catheter, contrast is injected and images obtained of the treatment site. If an embolization procedure has been performed, the images should show partial or complete occlusion of the desired blood vessel(s). If an infusion procedure has been performed, the images should identify whether the desired results have been obtained. A written interpretation of the follow-up angiography is provided.

RVUs

Code	Work	PE	PE Non-Facility	MP	Total Non-Facility	Total Facility	Global
75898	0.00	0.00	0.00	0.00	0.00	0.00	XXX

76000

76000 Fluoroscopy (separate procedure), up to 1 hour physician or other qualified health care professional time

(Do not report 76000 in conjunction with 33274, 33275, 33957, 33958, 33959, 33962, 33963, 33964, 0515T, 0516T, 0517T, 0518T, 0519T, 0520T)

Plain English Description

Fluoroscopic monitoring of a separately reportable procedure is performed. Fluoroscopy is an imaging technique used to obtain real-time moving images of internal structures using a device that consists of an X-ray source and a fluorescent screen. These devices include image intensifiers and video cameras that allow images to be recorded and displayed on a monitor. In 76000, the physician or other qualified health care professional provides fluoroscopic monitoring for up to 1 hour for a service or procedure that does not include the fluoroscopy service as part of the procedure.

RVUs

Code	Work	PE	PE Non-Facility	MP	Total Non-Facility	Total Facility	Global
76000	0.30	0.84	0.84	0.04	1.18	1.18	XXX

76120

76120 Cineradiography/videoradiography, except where specifically included

Plain English Description

Cineradiography/videoradiography combines cinematographic, fluoroscopic, and radiographic techniques to create a motion picture view of an anatomic area. Body motion is captured with a camera attached to the output port of a fluoroscopic image intensifier and converted into real-time video images that are viewed on a monitor and/or recorded for later analysis. The individual frames can be viewed in stop action or fast action by the radiologist for review and interpretation. Code 76120 reports cineradiography/videoradiography except where it is specifically included in an examination. Code 76125 reports cineradiography/videoradiography when it is performed to complement a routine examination and is listed separately and in addition to the code for the primary procedure.

RVUs

Code	Work	PE	PE Non-Facility	MP	Total Non-Facility	Total Facility	Global
76120	0.38	2.64	2.64	0.04	3.06	3.06	XXX

76125

+ 76125 Cineradiography/videoradiography to complement routine examination (List separately in addition to code for primary procedure)

Plain English Description

Cineradiography/videoradiography combines cinematographic, fluoroscopic, and radiographic techniques to create a motion picture view of an anatomic area. Body motion is captured with a camera attached to the output port of a fluoroscopic image intensifier and converted into real-time video images that are viewed on a monitor and/or recorded for later analysis. The individual frames can be viewed in stop action or fast action by the radiologist for review and interpretation. Code 76120 reports cineradiography/videoradiography except where it is specifically included in an examination. Code 76125 reports cineradiography/videoradiography when it is performed to complement a routine examination and is listed separately and in addition to the code for the primary procedure.

RVUs

Code	Work	PE	PE Non-Facility	MP	Total Non-Facility	Total Facility	Global
76125	0.00	0.00	0.00	0.00	0.00	0.00	ZZZ

76376-76377

76376 3D rendering with interpretation and reporting of computed tomography, magnetic resonance imaging, ultrasound, or other tomographic modality with image postprocessing under concurrent supervision; not requiring image postprocessing on an independent workstation

(Use 76376 in conjunction with code[s] for base imaging procedure[s])

(Do not report 76376 in conjunction with 31627, 34839, 70496, 70498, 70544, 70545, 70546, 70547, 70548, 70549, 71275, 71555, 72159, 72191, 72198, 73206, 73225, 73706, 73725, 74174, 74175, 74185, 74261, 74262, 74263, 75557, 75559, 75561, 75563, 75565, 75571, 75572, 75573, 75574, 75635, 76377, 77046, 77047, 77048, 77049, 77061, 77062, 77063, 78012-78999, 93355, 0523T, 0559T, 0560T, 0561T, 0562T)

76377 3D rendering with interpretation and reporting of computed tomography, magnetic resonance imaging, ultrasound, or other tomographic modality with image postprocessing under concurrent supervision; requiring image postprocessing on an independent workstation

(Use 76377 in conjunction with code[s] for base imaging procedure[s])

(Do not report 76377 in conjunction with 34839, 70496, 70498, 70544, 70545, 70546, 70547, 70548, 70549, 71275, 71555, 72159, 72191, 72198, 73206, 73225, 73706, 73725, 74174, 74175, 74185, 74261, 74262, 74263, 75557, 75559, 75561, 75563, 75565, 75571, 75572, 75573, 75574, 75635, 76376, 77046, 77047, 77048, 77049, 77061, 77062, 77063, 78012-78999, 93355, 0523T, 0559T, 0560T, 0561T, 0562T)

(76376, 76377 require concurrent supervision of image postprocessing 3D manipulation of volumetric data set and image rendering)

Plain English Description

Separately reportable ultrasound, MRI, CT scan, or other tomographic images are obtained. Using these images, complex 3D rendering is performed by a physician or a specially trained technologist. This may include shaded surface rendering, volumetric rendering, maximum intensity projections (MIPs), fusion imaging, and quantitative analysis of the images for treatment planning. If the 3D rendering and image postprocessing are performed by a technologist, concurrent physician supervision is required. An interpretation of the image postprocessing is provided in a written report. In 76376, complex 3D rendering is performed by the physician or a specially trained technologist under physician supervision without the use of an independent workstation. In 76377, complex 3D image rendering is performed by the physician or a specially trained technologist under physician supervision on an independent workstation.

RVUs

Code	Work	PE	PE Non-Facility	MP	Total Non-Facility	Total Facility	Global
76376	0.20	0.43	0.43	0.02	0.65	0.65	XXX
76377	0.79	1.18	1.18	0.06	2.03	2.03	XXX

76536

76536 Ultrasound, soft tissues of head and neck (eg, thyroid, parathyroid, parotid), real time with image documentation

Plain English Description

An ultrasound examination of soft tissues of the head and neck is performed with image documentation. The thyroid, parathyroid, or parotid glands and surrounding soft tissue may be examined. Ultrasound visualizes the body internally using sound waves far above human perception that bounce off interior anatomical structures. As the sound waves pass through different densities of tissue, they are reflected back to the receiving unit at varying speeds and converted into pictures displayed on screen. A linear scanner or mechanical sector scanner is used to evaluate the shape, size, border, internal architecture, distal enhancement, color flow, and echogenicity of the soft tissue structures of the head and neck as well as any lesions or masses. The echogenicity is compared to that of the surrounding muscle tissue. The physician reviews the images and provides a written interpretation.

RVUs

Code	Work	PE	PE Non-Facility	MP	Total Non-Facility	Total Facility	Global
76536	0.56	2.67	2.67	0.04	3.27	3.27	XXX

76700-76705

76700 Ultrasound, abdominal, real time with image documentation; complete

76705 Ultrasound, abdominal, real time with image documentation; limited (eg, single organ, quadrant, follow-up)

Plain English Description

A real-time abdominal ultrasound is performed with image documentation. The patient is placed supine. Acoustic coupling gel is applied to the skin of the abdomen. The transducer is pressed firmly against the skin and swept back and forth over the abdomen and images obtained. The ultrasonic wave pulses directed at the abdomen are imaged by recording the ultrasound echoes. Any abnormalities are evaluated to identify characteristics that might provide a definitive diagnosis. The physician reviews the ultrasound images of the abdomen and provides a written interpretation. Code 76700 is used for a complete abdominal ultrasound, which includes real-time scanning of the liver, gall bladder, common bile duct, pancreas, spleen, kidneys, upper abdominal aorta, and inferior vena cava. Code 76705 is used when a limited ultrasound examination is performed such as a single organ, single quadrant, or a follow-up scan.

RVUs

Code	Work	PE	PE Non-Facility	MP	Total Non-Facility	Total Facility	Global
76700	0.81	2.60	2.60	0.06	3.47	3.47	XXX
76705	0.59	1.94	1.94	0.04	2.57	2.57	XXX

76770-76775

76770 Ultrasound, retroperitoneal (eg, renal, aorta, nodes), real time with image documentation; complete

76775 Ultrasound, retroperitoneal (eg, renal, aorta, nodes), real time with image documentation; limited

Plain English Description

A real-time retroperitoneal ultrasound is performed with image documentation. The patient is placed supine. Acoustic coupling gel is applied to the skin of the abdomen. The transducer is pressed firmly against the skin and swept back and forth over the abdomen and images obtained of the retroperitoneal area. The ultrasonic wave pulses directed at the retroperitoneum are imaged by recording the ultrasound echoes. Any abnormalities are evaluated to identify characteristics that might provide a definitive diagnosis. The physician reviews the ultrasound images of the retroperitoneum and provides a written interpretation. Code 76770 is used for a complete retroperitoneal ultrasound, which includes real-time scanning of the kidneys, abdominal aorta, common iliac artery origins, and inferior vena cava. Alternatively, if ultrasonography is being performed to evaluate the urinary tract, examination of the kidneys and urinary bladder constitutes a complete exam. Code 76775 is used when a limited retroperitoneal ultrasound examination is performed.

RVUs

Code	Work	PE	PE Non-Facility	MP	Total Non-Facility	Total Facility	Global
76770	0.74	2.41	2.41	0.04	3.19	3.19	XXX
76775	0.58	1.04	1.04	0.04	1.66	1.66	XXX

76800

76800 Ultrasound, spinal canal and contents

Plain English Description

An ultrasound examination of the spinal canal and contents is performed. Ultrasound visualizes the body internally using sound waves far above human perception bounced off interior anatomical structures. As the sound waves pass through different densities of tissue, they are reflected back to the receiving unit at varying speeds and converted into pictures displayed on screen. Transdermal spinal ultrasound is used primarily in evaluation of newborns and infants because of the minimal ossification of the spine and the short distance between the skin and the spinal subarachnoid space. Spinal ultrasound may be used intraoperatively in adults and older children but is generally not considered an effective diagnostic tool in these patients. With the newborn or infant placed in a prone position, the neck is flexed. Acoustic coupling gel is applied to the skin along the spine. The spinal canal and contents are examined using a linear probe in both the sagittal and axial plane along the entire length of the spine. The physician reviews the images and provides a written interpretation.

RVUs

Code	Work	PE	PE Non-Facility	MP	Total Non-Facility	Total Facility	Global
76800	1.13	2.77	2.77	0.14	4.04	4.04	XXX

76881-76882

76881 Ultrasound, complete joint (ie, joint space and peri-articular soft-tissue structures), real-time with image documentation

76882 Ultrasound, limited, joint or other nonvascular extremity structure(s) (eg, joint space, peri-articular tendon[s], muscle[s], nerve[s], other soft-tissue structure[s], or soft-tissue mass[es]), real-time with image documentation

Plain English Description

Ultrasound, also referred to as sonography and echography, is a non-invasive imaging technique that uses high-frequency sound waves to evaluate tissues and structures. Nonvascular structures of the extremities that may be evaluated by ultrasound include periarticular soft tissue masses, muscles, tendons, nerves, ligaments, and joints. Common conditions that can be detected or evaluated by ultrasound include cystic lesions, solid tumors, abscesses, joint effusion, tendon tears, tendonitis, tenosynovitis, nerve compression, and stress fractures. Acoustic coupling gel is applied to the extremity to be examined. An ultrasound probe is placed against the skin and moved over the target joint area to be examined as sound waves pass through and bounce off extremity tissues and structures. The sound waves are reflected back to the receiving unit at varying speeds and converted into images. Longitudinal, transverse, and oblique images are obtained. The physician reviews the images and provides a written interpretation. Use 76881 for a complete ultrasound joint examination of a specific joint, such as the elbow or ankle. This includes assessment of the joint space and related periarticular soft tissue structures, such as the muscles, tendons, ligaments, nerve bundles, bursa, and synovium, to identify any tears, laxity, scarring, swelling, fluid collection, inflammation, or compression, as well as any structural abnormalities, subluxation, joint effusion, arthritis, or nearby growths, cysts, or lesions. Use 76882 for a limited examination of a joint space or other nonvascular extremity structure(s), such as an ultrasound focused on the Achilles tendon or gastrocnemius muscle, or an evaluation of a solitary soft tissue mass, cyst, or tumor.

RVUs

Code	Work	PE	PE Non-Facility	MP	Total Non-Facility	Total Facility	Global
76881	0.63	1.53	1.53	0.03	2.19	2.19	XXX
76882	0.49	1.09	1.09	0.03	1.61	1.61	XXX

76937

✚ **76937 Ultrasound guidance for vascular access requiring ultrasound evaluation of potential access sites, documentation of selected vessel patency, concurrent realtime ultrasound visualization of vascular needle entry, with permanent recording and reporting (List separately in addition to code for primary procedure)**

(Do not report 76937 in conjunction with 33274, 33275, 36568, 36569, 36572, 36573, 36584, 37191, 37192, 37193, 37760, 37761, 76942)

(Do not report 76937 in conjunction with 0505T for ultrasound guidance for vascular access)

(If extremity venous non-invasive vascular diagnostic study is performed separate from venous access guidance, see 93970, 93971)

Plain English Description

Using ultrasound (US) guidance prior to and during vascular access procedures can improve success rates and limit the number of needle puncture attempts, reduce incidence of iatrogenic injury and infection, and improve patient comfort and safety. US performed using 2-dimension (2D) or Doppler Color Flow (DCF) and real time (dynamic) technique can include short-axis (SAX) out of plane imaging or long-axis (LAX) in plane imaging. In SAX, the image plane is perpendicular to the vessel/needle. The vessel appears as an anechoic circle on the display screen, and the needle appears as a hyperechoic point in cross section. Using LAX, the imaging plane is parallel to the vessel and the direction of the vessel is viewed across the display screen with the shaft and point of needle visible as it advances. The patient should be interviewed and medical records reviewed to determine anatomic issues, prior procedures, and the potential for complications. US evaluation of the potential access site/vessel is then performed to differentiate arteries and veins, determine the size of the vessel, wall patency, its course (direction) and depth, identify surrounding structures, and adjacent pathology. Once the vessel has been chosen, the site is prepped in sterile fashion and ultrasound guidance provides concurrent real time visualization of needle entry for the vascular procedure reported separately.

RVUs

Code	Work	PE	PE Non-Facility	MP	Total Non-Facility	Total Facility	Global
76937	0.30	0.71	0.71	0.02	1.03	1.03	ZZZ

76942

76942 Ultrasonic guidance for needle placement (eg, biopsy, aspiration, injection, localization device), imaging supervision and interpretation

(Do not report 76942 in conjunction with 10004, 10005, 10006, 10021, 10030, 19083, 19285, 20604, 20606, 20611, 27096, 32554, 32555, 32556, 32557, 37760, 37761, 43232, 43237, 43242, 45341, 45342, 46948, 55874, 64479, 64480, 64483, 64484, 64490, 64491, 64493, 64494, 64495, 76975, 0213T, 0214T, 0215T, 0216T, 0217T, 0218T, 0228T, 0229T, 0230T, 0231T, 0232T, 0481T, 0582T)

(For harvesting, preparation, and injection[s] of platelet rich plasma, use 0232T)

Plain English Description

Ultrasound (US) guidance including imaging supervision and interpretation is performed for needle placement during a separately reportable biopsy, aspiration, injection, or placement of a localization device. A local anesthetic is injected at the site of the planned needle or localization device placement. A transducer is then used to locate the lesion, site of the planned injection, or site of the planned placement of the localization device. The radiologist constantly monitors needle placement with the US probe to ensure the needle is properly placed. The radiologist also uses US imaging to monitor separately reportable biopsy, aspiration, injection, or device localization procedures. Upon completion of the procedure, the needle is withdrawn and pressure applied to control bleeding. A dressing is applied as needed. The radiologist then provides a written report of the US imaging component of the procedure.

RVUs

Code	Work	PE	PE Non-Facility	MP	Total Non-Facility	Total Facility	Global
76942	0.67	0.91	0.91	0.04	1.62	1.62	XXX

76998

76998 Ultrasonic guidance, intraoperative

(Do not report 76998 in conjunction with 36475, 36479, 37760, 37761, 46948, 47370, 47371, 47380, 47381, 47382, 0515T, 0516T, 0517T, 0518T, 0519T, 0520T)

(For ultrasound guidance for open and laparoscopic radiofrequency tissue ablation, use 76940)

Plain English Description

Intraoperative sonographic guidance is used to aid visualization during surgical procedures and may be used in a number of different kinds of operations on different body locations. Ultrasound (US)is a noninvasive way of visualizing the body internally using sound waves far above human perception bounced off interior anatomical structures. As the sound waves pass through different densities of tissue, they are reflected back to the receiving unit at varying speeds. The waves are then converted into electrical pulses, which are instantly displayed as a picture on screen. This imaging helps the surgeon see target structures, determine location and depth of incisions, monitor surgical progression, etc. This code is not used for US guidance performed specifically for tissue ablation because that is reported elsewhere.

RVUs

Code	Work	PE	PE Non-Facility	MP	Total Non-Facility	Total Facility	Global
76998	0.00	0.00	0.00	0.00	0.00	0.00	XXX

77002

✚ **77002 Fluoroscopic guidance for needle placement (eg, biopsy, aspiration, injection, localization device) (List separately in addition to code for primary procedure)**

(See appropriate surgical code for procedure and anatomic location)

(Use 77002 in conjunction with 10160, 20206, 20220, 20225, 20520, 20525, 20526, 20550, 20551, 20552, 20553, 20555, 20600, 20605, 20610, 20612, 20615, 21116, 21550, 23350, 24220, 25246, 27093, 27095, 27369, 27648, 32400, 32405, 32553, 36002, 38220, 38221, 38222, 38505, 38794, 41019, 42400, 42405, 47000, 47001, 48102, 49180, 49411, 50200, 50390, 51100, 51101, 51102, 55700, 55876, 60100, 62268, 62269, 64505, 64600, 64605)

(77002 is included in all arthrography radiological supervision and interpretation codes. See Administration of Contrast Material[s] introductory guidelines for reporting of arthrography procedures)

Plain English Description

This code reports the radiological portion of fluoroscopic guidance used in needle placement for biopsy, aspiration, injection, or localization type procedures. Fluoroscopy is a continuous, X-ray beam passed through the body part being examined and projected onto a TV-like monitor to create a kind of X-ray movie. This uses more radiation than standard X-rays and can image many different body systems to study a specific structure or organ, localize a tumor or foreign body, and also study movement within the body. The area is identified with fluoroscopy and anesthetized. The appropriate type of needle is inserted under fluoroscopic guidance to perform the specified procedure such as removing aspirate or tissue samples for biopsy, injecting a therapeutic or diagnostic substance, or localizing a tumor or mass for further study. The primary procedural code reports the type of procedure and anatomic location.

RVUs

Code	Work	PE	PE Non-Facility	MP	Total Non-Facility	Total Facility	Global
77002	0.54	2.47	2.47	0.04	3.05	3.05	ZZZ

77003

✚ **77003 Fluoroscopic guidance and localization of needle or catheter tip for spine or paraspinous diagnostic or therapeutic injection procedures (epidural or subarachnoid) (List separately in addition to code for primary procedure)**

(Use 77003 in conjunction with 61050, 61055, 62267, 62273, 62280, 62281, 62282, 62284, 64510, 64517, 64520, 64610, 96450)

(Do not report 77003 in conjunction with 62270, 62272, 62320, 62321, 62322, 62323, 62324, 62325, 62326, 62327, 62328, 62329)

Plain English Description

Fluoroscopic guidance is used to locate the target site for inserting a needle or catheter tip for spinal or paraspinous diagnostic or therapeutic injection procedures. Fluoroscopy is a continuous, X-ray beam passed through the body part being examined and projected onto a TV-like monitor to create a kind of X-ray movie. This uses more radiation than standard X-rays and can image many different body systems to locate a specific structure or organ, as well as study movement within the body. The needle or catheter tip is inserted and a small amount of contrast material is injected and observed fluoroscopically to ensure correct positioning for an injection. The separately reportable primary injection procedure may be performed for diagnostic or therapeutic purposes, including injection of an anesthetic, a steroid, or destruction by neurolytic agent. Under fluoroscopic guidance, the physician monitors the injection procedure as it is carried out and provides a written report of the radiological component of the procedure.

RVUs

Code	Work	PE	PE Non-Facility	MP	Total Non-Facility	Total Facility	Global
77003	0.60	2.21	2.21	0.04	2.85	2.85	ZZZ

77011

77011 Computed tomography guidance for stereotactic localization

Plain English Description

This code reports computed tomography guidance for stereotactic localization. Stereotactic localization is a method of determining a lesion's unique location within a certain volume by describing it in terms of specific x, y, and z coordinates in relation to an original point of reference. The position of the lesion remains fixed while an initial image is made at 0 degrees angulation. Another pair of images is obtained relative to the 0 degree position by moving the imaging detector or beams in a controlled fashion around the center of rotation plus and minus specified degrees. Basic geometry is used to determine the lesion location in a 3D coordinate system by these paired images in relation to the fixed origin. CT imaging is the method used to locate the lesion and determine its coordinates.

RVUs

Code	Work	PE	PE Non-Facility	MP	Total Non-Facility	Total Facility	Global
77011	1.21	5.26	5.26	0.10	6.57	6.57	XXX

77012

77012 Computed tomography guidance for needle placement (eg, biopsy, aspiration, injection, localization device), radiological supervision and interpretation

(Do not report 77011, 77012 in conjunction with 22586)

(Do not report 77012 in conjunction with 10009, 10010, 10030, 27096, 32554, 32555, 32556, 32557, 62270, 62272, 62328, 62329, 64479, 64480, 64483, 64484, 64490, 64491, 64492, 64493, 64494, 64495, 64633, 64634, 64635, 64636, 0232T, 0481T)

(For harvesting, preparation, and injection[s] of platelet-rich plasma, use 0232T)

Plain English Description

This code reports the radiological supervision and interpretation portion of computed tomography (CT) guidance used in needle placement for biopsy, aspiration, injection, or localization procedures. The target area is localized using CT and then anesthetized. The appropriate type of needle is inserted under CT guidance to perform the specified procedure, such as removing aspirate or tissue samples for biopsy, injecting a therapeutic or diagnostic substance, or localizing a tumor or mass for further study. The surgical code reports the procedure and anatomic location. CT aims multiple, narrow X-ray beams around a single rotational axis, taking a large series of two-dimensional images of the target structure from multiple angles. The computer can digitally reconstruct the data into a 3D image and produce thin, cross-sectional 2D or 3D images (slices) of the test object.

RVUs

Code	Work	PE	PE Non-Facility	MP	Total Non-Facility	Total Facility	Global
77012	1.50	2.66	2.66	0.10	4.26	4.26	XXX

78600-78601

78600 Brain imaging, less than 4 static views

78601 Brain imaging, less than 4 static views; with vascular flow

Plain English Description

Static brain imaging with or without vascular flow imaging is performed using scintigraphy and a radiolabeled isotope tracer. This procedure is primarily used to document brain death. The patient is positioned on the imaging table with the gamma camera focused on the entire head and neck. An intravenous line is established and the radiolabeled isotope tracer is injected directly into the circulatory system. When vascular flow imaging is included, the imaging begins as soon as the isotope bolus arrives in the neck and continues to the end of the venous phase. A radiation detector (usually a scintillation detector) is used to record the spatial distribution of the radiopharmaceutical in the brain. Views are obtained from anterior, right lateral, and left lateral positions for this study. For static imaging, the camera captures images at a single point in time for about 5 minutes in each of the 3 view positions. Zoning and magnification of areas of interest may be included. The physician interprets the study and provides a written report of the findings. Code 78600 is used for brain imaging with less than 4 static views only. Code 78601 is used when vascular flow studies are obtained with the static views.

RVUs

Code	Work	PE	PE Non-Facility	MP	Total Non-Facility	Total Facility	Global
78600	0.44	4.75	4.75	0.07	5.26	5.26	XXX
78601	0.51	5.62	5.62	0.07	6.20	6.20	XXX

78605-78606

78605 Brain imaging, minimum 4 static views

78606 Brain imaging, minimum 4 static views; with vascular flow

Plain English Description

Static brain imaging with or without vascular flow imaging is performed using scintigraphy and a radiolabeled isotope tracer. This procedure is primarily used to document brain death. The patient is positioned on the imaging table with the gamma camera focused on the entire head and neck. An intravenous line is established and the radiolabeled isotope tracer is injected directly into the circulatory system. When vascular flow imaging is included, the imaging begins as soon as the isotope bolus arrives in the neck and continues to the end of the venous phase. A radiation detector (usually a scintillation detector) is used to record the spatial distribution of the radiopharmaceutical in the brain. Views are obtained from anterior, right lateral, left lateral, and posterior positions for this study. Other views may be included when appropriate. For static imaging, the camera captures images at a single point in time for about 5 minutes in each of the view positions. Zoning and magnification of areas of interest may be included. The physician interprets the study and provides a written report of the findings. Code 78605 is used for brain imaging with at least 4 static views only. Code 78606 is used when vascular flow studies are obtained with the static views.

RVUs

Code	Work	PE	PE Non-Facility	MP	Total Non-Facility	Total Facility	Global
78605	0.53	5.11	5.11	0.07	5.71	5.71	XXX
78606	0.64	8.73	8.73	0.08	9.45	9.45	XXX

78608

78608 Brain imaging, positron emission tomography (PET); metabolic evaluation

Plain English Description

Brain imaging is performed using positron emission tomography (PET) and a radiolabeled isotope tracer, such as fluorodeoxyglucose (FDG). PET is a diagnostic imaging procedure that uses a radioactive substance administered to the patient followed by acquisition of physiologic images that detect the emission of positrons from the radioactive substance in the body region being studied. This procedure provides a three dimensional (3-D) image of brain metabolism in action, derived from the regional uptake of the radiolabeled molecules or isotope tracer by the tissue at different rates and levels, displayed in the PET imaging as different colors or different levels of brightness. An intravenous line is established and the radiolabeled isotope tracer is injected directly into the circulatory system. After a prescribed period of time for the isotope to reach the target area, the patient is positioned on the imaging table with the PET scanner over the head and neck and tomographic views of the brain are obtained. The physician interprets the study and provides a written report of the findings.

RVUs

Code	Work	PE	PE Non-Facility	MP	Total Non-Facility	Total Facility	Global
78608	0.00	0.00	0.00	0.00	0.00	0.00	XXX

78610

78610 Brain imaging, vascular flow only

Plain English Description

Brain imaging with vascular flow only is performed using scintigraphy and a radiolabeled isotope tracer. This procedure may be helpful in the detection and evaluation of cerebrovascular disease or malformation, dementia, brain injury, or brain death. The patient is positioned on the imaging table with the gamma camera focused on the entire head and neck. An intravenous line is established and the radiolabeled isotope tracer is injected directly into the circulatory system. The imaging begins as soon as the isotope bolus arrives in the neck and continues to the end of the venous phase. Views are usually obtained in the anterior position to assess simultaneous blood flow to both sides of the brain. The physician interprets the study and provides a written report of the findings.

RVUs

Code	Work	PE	PE Non-Facility	MP	Total Non-Facility	Total Facility	Global
78610	0.30	4.63	4.63	0.04	4.97	4.97	XXX

78630-78635

78630 Cerebrospinal fluid flow, imaging (not including introduction of material); cisternography

(For injection procedure, see 61000-61070, 62270-62327)

78635 Cerebrospinal fluid flow, imaging (not including introduction of material); ventriculography

(For injection procedure, see 61000-61070, 62270-62294)

Plain English Description

Cerebrospinal fluid (CSF) flow imaging is performed using scintigraphy and a radiolabeled isotope tracer. This study may be used to detect abnormal CSF flow within the brain and spinal canal including communicating and non-communicating hydrocephalus and fistulas from a CSF reservoir (cistern) to the nasal cavity or ear. CSF is formed in the lateral ventricles and travels through the foramen of Monro into the 3rd ventricle and on to the 4th ventricle via the aqueduct of Sylvius. The small amount of CSF formed in the spinal canal joins the intraventricular supply in the 4th ventricle and moves on to the subarachnoid spaces by way of the medial foramen of Magendie and the two lateral foramina of Luschka. CSF is mobilized by bulk flow, circulation from high pressure area to lower pressure area, and pulsatile motion related to the cardiac cycle of the cerebral arteries. The radiolabeled isotope tracer is injected into the CSF via lumbar puncture. The patient is positioned on the imaging table, with the gamma camera over the area to be studied. Scanning is performed at specific intervals and the radioactive energy emitted is converted into an image. Code 78630 is used when the cisterns are the focus of the study (cisternography). Code 78635 is used when the ventricles are the focus of the study (ventriculography). The physician interprets the study and provides a written report of the findings.

RVUs

Code	Work	PE	PE Non-Facility	MP	Total Non-Facility	Total Facility	Global
78630	0.68	8.90	8.90	0.08	9.66	9.66	XXX
78635	0.61	8.97	8.97	0.08	9.66	9.66	XXX

78645

78645 Cerebrospinal fluid flow, imaging (not including introduction of material); shunt evaluation

(For injection procedure, see 61000-61070, 62270-62294)

Plain English Description

Cerebrospinal fluid (CSF) flow imaging is performed using scintigraphy and a radiolabeled isotope tracer to evaluate shunt patency. A shunt may be placed in the ventricle of the brain to drain CSF when there is a blockage somewhere along the pathway of CSF flow. The shunt is comprised of a proximal catheter (in the ventricles), a pressure sensitive valve with reservoir and a distal catheter positioned in one of three possible places. The most common distal site is the peritoneum (ventriculo-peritoneal or VP shunt); however, fluid may also be directed to a large vein in the neck (ventriculo-atrial or VA shunt) and less often into the chest around the lungs (ventriculo-pleural shunt). The radiolabeled isotope tracer is injected into the CSF via the shunt reservoir. The patient is positioned on the imaging table, with the gamma camera over the area to be studied. Scanning is performed at specific intervals and the radioactive energy emitted is converted into an image. The physician interprets the study and provides a written report of the findings.

RVUs

Code	Work	PE	PE Non-Facility	MP	Total Non-Facility	Total Facility	Global
78645	0.57	8.64	8.64	0.07	9.28	9.28	XXX

78650

78650 Cerebrospinal fluid leakage detection and localization

(For injection procedure, see 61000-61070, 62270-62294)

Plain English Description

Cerebrospinal fluid (CSF) leaks may be detected and localized using scintigraphy and a radiolabeled isotope tracer. CSF bathes the spinal cord and brain, cushioning and protecting the delicate tissue. Leaks can occur, or fistulas may form spontaneously, as a result of trauma or non-traumatic events that cause a bony defect in the skull and disrupt the underlying meningeal dura and pia-arachnoid mater. The most common sites of leakage are the nose (CSF rhinorrhea) and ear (CSF otorrhea). Following an intrathecal injection of the radiolabeled isotope tracer, the patient is positioned on the imaging table with the gamma camera over the area to be studied. Scanning is performed at specific intervals and the radioactive energy emitted is converted into an image. The physician interprets the study and provides a written report of the findings.

RVUs

Code	Work	PE	PE Non-Facility	MP	Total Non-Facility	Total Facility	Global
78650	0.61	7.22	7.22	0.06	7.89	7.89	XXX

78814

78814 Positron emission tomography (PET) with concurrently acquired computed tomography (CT) for attenuation correction and anatomical localization imaging; limited area (eg, chest, head/neck)

Plain English Description

A positron emission tomography (PET) scan may be paired with computed tomography (CT) to align accurately the functional and anatomical information derived from each. The PET scan images soft tissue structures and includes metabolic and chemical functioning. The CT scan images hard and soft tissue structures. Fusion of the two modalities can show bone structure, organs, and growing tissue or tumors. This technique is helpful for staging cancers and other types of tumors, localizing seizure foci in the brain, diagnosing infection and/or inflammatory processes, and for intermittent surveillance of medical conditions and diseases. The CT radiation dose is generally lower when used for attenuation correction and anatomical localization because of the limited diagnostic field of view. A higher level of radiation is used in a limited area of study (anatomical localization) and a lower dose is used in the remaining regions to provide attenuation correction for the entire PET study. An intravenous line is established and the radiolabeled isotope tracer is injected directly into the circulatory system. With the patient positioned on the imaging table, the PET scan is performed. The physician reviews the scan and details the areas for CT attenuation correction and anatomical localization. The CT scan is then performed. The physician interprets the studies and provides a written report of the combined findings.

RVUs

Code	Work	PE	PE Non-Facility	MP	Total Non-Facility	Total Facility	Global
78814	0.00	0.00	0.00	0.00	0.00	0.00	XXX

78815

78815 Positron emission tomography (PET) with concurrently acquired computed tomography (CT) for attenuation correction and anatomical localization imaging; skull base to mid-thigh

Plain English Description

Positron emission tomography (PET) imaging, also referred to as PET scan, is performed from the skull base to mid-thigh with a concurrently acquired computed tomography (CT) scan for correction and anatomical localization. PET imaging is a diagnostic imaging procedure that uses a radioactive substance (radioisotope) administered to the patient followed by acquisition of physiologic images that detect the emission of positrons from the radioactive substance in the body region being studied. PET imaging is used primarily for the detection of malignant lesions and to determine the effectiveness of treatment for malignancies. However, PET imaging is used for diagnosis and evaluation of other conditions as well. The radioisotopes used in PET imaging are short-lived and require the use of a cyclotron. The cyclotron produces the radioisotope immediately prior to the procedure and then the radioisotope is attached or tagged to a natural compound such as glucose. The radioisotope is administered intravenously or, less commonly, by inhalation. The radioisotope is then taken up by body tissues/organs. Normal and diseased tissues/organs accumulate the radioisotope at different rates and levels and so are displayed in the PET imaging as different colors or different levels of brightness. The patient is prepared for the PET imaging procedure. An intravenous line is placed. The radioisotope is administered. The patient is told to rest quietly until the radioisotope has been perfused to the body region(s) to be imaged. This may take 30 to 90 minutes. PET images are then obtained. CT images are obtained concurrently with the PET imaging to correct attenuation and localize anatomical structures. Attenuation of images occurs when the energy in a radiant source passes through body structures making the images less defined. Attenuation can diminish the intensity of the PET images. CT uses multiple x-ray beams combined with electronic detectors to produce a series of images (slices) that are processed on a computer and displayed as two-dimensional images on a computer monitor. CT is used to enhance the PET images and localize specific anatomic structures. The radiologist reviews the PET and CT images, noting variations in radioisotope accumulation in the body region(s) studied. The current PET/CT images are compared to any previously obtained radiological studies, interpreted, and a written report is provided.

RVUs

Code	Work	PE	PE Non-Facility	MP	Total Non-Facility	Total Facility	Global
78815	0.00	0.00	0.00	0.00	0.00	0.00	XXX

80047-80048

80047 Basic metabolic panel (Calcium, ionized)
This panel must include the following:
Calcium, ionized (82330); Carbon dioxide (bicarbonate) (82374); Chloride (82435); Creatinine (82565); Glucose (82947); Potassium (84132); Sodium (84295); Urea Nitrogen (BUN) (84520)

80048 Basic metabolic panel (Calcium, total)
This panel must include the following:
Calcium, total (82310); Carbon dioxide (bicarbonate) (82374); Chloride (82435); Creatinine (82565); Glucose (82947); Potassium (84132); Sodium (84295); Urea nitrogen (BUN) (84520)

Plain English Description

A basic metabolic blood panel is obtained that includes ionized calcium levels along with carbon dioxide (bicarbonate) (CO2), chloride, creatinine, glucose, potassium, sodium, and urea nitrogen (BUN). A basic metabolic panel with measurement of ionized calcium may be used to screen for or monitor overall metabolic function or identify imbalances. Ionized or free calcium flows freely in the blood, is not attached to any proteins, and represents the amount of calcium available to support metabolic processes such as, heart function, muscle contraction, nerve function, and blood clotting. Total carbon dioxide (bicarbonate) (CO2) level is composed of CO2, bicarbonate (HCO3), and carbonic acid (H2CO3) with the primary constituent being bicarbonate, a negatively charged electrolyte that works in conjunction with other electrolytes, such as potassium, sodium, and chloride, to maintain proper acid-base balance and electrical neutrality at the cellular level. Chloride is also a negatively charged electrolyte that helps regulate body fluid and maintain proper acid-base balance. Creatinine is a waste product excreted by the kidneys that is produced in the muscles while breaking down creatine, a compound used by the muscles to create energy. Blood levels of creatinine provide a good measurement of renal function. Glucose is a simple sugar and the main source of energy for the body, regulated by insulin. When more glucose is available than is required, it is stored in the liver as glycogen or stored in adipose tissue as fat. Glucose measurement determines whether the glucose/insulin metabolic process is functioning properly. Both potassium and sodium are positively charged electrolytes that work in conjunction with other electrolytes to regulate body fluid, stimulate muscle contraction, and maintain proper acid-base balance, and both are essential for maintaining normal metabolic processes. Urea is a waste product produced in the liver by the breakdown of protein from a sequence of chemical reactions referred to as the urea or Krebs-Henseleit cycle. Urea is taken up by the kidneys and excreted in the urine. Blood urea nitrogen, BUN, is a measure of renal function, and helps monitor renal disease and the effectiveness of dialysis. Report 80048 for the same basic metabolic panel, but with total calcium measured instead of ionized calcium. Total calcium is a measurement of the total amount of both ionized (free) calcium and calcium attached (bound) to proteins circulating in the blood. The measurement can screen for or monitor a number of conditions, including those affecting the bones, heart, nerves, kidneys, and teeth.

RVUs

Code	Work	PE	PE Non-Facility	MP	Total Non-Facility	Total Facility	Global
80047	0.00	0.00	0.00	0.00	0.00	0.00	XXX
80048	0.00	0.00	0.00	0.00	0.00	0.00	XXX

80053

80053 Comprehensive metabolic panel
This panel must include the following:
Albumin (82040); Bilirubin, total (82247); Calcium, total (82310); Carbon dioxide (bicarbonate) (82374); Chloride (82435); Creatinine (82565); Glucose (82947); Phosphatase, alkaline (84075); Potassium (84132); Protein, total (84155); Sodium (84295); Transferase, alanine amino (ALT) (SGPT) (84460); Transferase, aspartate amino (AST) (SGOT) (84450); Urea nitrogen (BUN) (84520)

Plain English Description

A comprehensive metabolic panel that includes albumin, bilirubin, total calcium, carbon dioxide, chloride, creatinine, glucose, alkaline phosphatase, potassium, total protein, sodium, alanine amino transferase (ALT) (SGPT), aspartate amino transferase (AST) (SGOT), and urea nitrogen (BUN) is obtained. This test is used to evaluate electrolytes and fluid balance as well as liver and kidney function. It is also used to help rule out conditions such as diabetes. Tests related to electrolytes and fluid balance include carbon dioxide, chloride, potassium, and sodium. Tests specific to liver function include albumin, bilirubin, alkaline phosphatase, ALT, AST, and total protein. Tests specific to kidney function include BUN and creatinine. Calcium is needed to support metabolic processes such as heart function, muscle contraction, nerve function, and blood clotting. Glucose is the main source of energy for the body and is regulated by insulin. Glucose measurement determines whether the glucose/insulin metabolic process is functioning properly.

RVUs

Code	Work	PE	PE Non-Facility	MP	Total Non-Facility	Total Facility	Global
80053	0.00	0.00	0.00	0.00	0.00	0.00	XXX

80061

80061 Lipid panel
This panel must include the following:
Cholesterol, serum, total (82465); Lipoprotein, direct measurement, high density cholesterol (HDL cholesterol) (83718); Triglycerides (84478)

Plain English Description

A lipid panel is obtained to assess the risk for cardiovascular disease and to monitor appropriate treatment. Lipids are comprised of cholesterol, protein, and triglycerides. They are stored in cells and circulate in the blood. Lipids are important for cell health and as an energy source. A lipid panel should include a measurement of triglycerides and total serum cholesterol and then calculated to find the measurement of high-density lipoprotein (HDL-C), low-density lipoprotein (LDL-C), and very low-density lipoprotein (VLDL-C). HDL contains the highest ratio of cholesterol and is often referred to as "good cholesterol" because it is capable of transporting excess cholesterol in the blood to the liver for removal. LDL contains the highest ratio of protein and is considered "bad cholesterol" because it transports and deposits cholesterol in the walls of blood vessels. VLDL contains the highest ratio of triglycerides and high levels are also considered "bad" because it converts to LDL after depositing triglyceride molecules in the walls of blood vessels. A blood sample is obtained by separately reportable venipuncture or finger stick. Serum/plasma is tested using quantitative enzymatic method.

RVUs

Code	Work	PE	PE Non-Facility	MP	Total Non-Facility	Total Facility	Global
80061	0.00	0.00	0.00	0.00	0.00	0.00	XXX

80069

80069 Renal function panel

This panel must include the following:

Albumin (82040); Calcium, total (82310); Carbon dioxide (bicarbonate) (82374); Chloride (82435); Creatinine (82565); Glucose (82947); Phosphorus inorganic (phosphate) (84100); Potassium (84132); Sodium (84295); Urea nitrogen (BUN) (84520)

Plain English Description

A renal panel is obtained for routine health screening and to monitor conditions such as diabetes, renal disease, liver disease, nutritional disorders, thyroid and parathyroid function, and interventional drug therapies. Tests in a renal panel include glucose or blood sugar; electrolytes and minerals as sodium, potassium, chloride, total calcium, and phosphorus; the waste products blood urea nitrogen (BUN) and creatinine; a protein called albumin; and bicarbonate (carbon dioxide, CO2) responsible for acid base balance. Glucose is the main source of energy for the body and is regulated by insulin. High levels may indicate diabetes or impaired kidney function. Sodium is found primarily outside cells and maintains water balance in the tissues, as well as nerve and muscle function. Potassium is primarily found inside cells and affects heart rhythm, cell metabolism, and muscle function. Chloride moves freely in and out of cells to regulate fluid levels and help maintain electrical neutrality. Calcium is needed to support metabolic processes, heart and nerve function, muscle contraction, and blood clotting. Phosphorus is essential for energy production, nerve and muscle function, and bone growth. Blood urea nitrogen (BUN) and creatinine are waste products from tissue breakdown that circulate in the blood and are filtered out by the kidneys. Albumin, a protein made by the liver, helps to nourish tissue and transport hormones, vitamins, drugs, and calcium throughout the body. Bicarbonate (HCO3) may also be referred to as carbon dioxide (CO2) maintains body pH or the acid/base balance. A specimen is obtained by separately reportable venipuncture. Serum/plasma is tested using quantitative chemiluminescent immunoassay or quantitative enzyme-linked immunosorbent assay.

RVUs

Code	Work	PE	PE Non-Facility	MP	Total Non-Facility	Total Facility	Global
80069	0.00	0.00	0.00	0.00	0.00	0.00	XXX

80076

80076 Hepatic function panel

This panel must include the following:

Albumin (82040); Bilirubin, total (82247); Bilirubin, direct (82248); Phosphatase, alkaline (84075); Protein, total (84155); Transferase, alanine amino (ALT) (SGPT) (84460); Transferase, aspartate amino (AST) (SGOT) (84450)

Plain English Description

A hepatic function panel is obtained to diagnose acute and chronic liver disease, inflammation, or scarring and to monitor hepatic function while taking certain medications. Tests in a hepatic function panel should include albumin (ALB), total and direct bilirubin, alkaline phosphatase (ALP), total protein (TP), alanine aminotransferase (ALT, SGPT), and aspartate aminotransferase (AST, SGOT). ALB is a protein made by the liver that helps to nourish tissue and transport hormones, vitamins, drugs, and calcium throughout the body. Bilirubin, a waste product from the breakdown of red blood cells, is removed by the liver in a conjugated state. Bilirubin is measured as total (all the bilirubin circulating in the blood) and direct (the conjugated amount only) to determine how well the liver is performing. ALP is an enzyme produced by the liver and other organs of the body. In the liver, cells along the bile duct produce ALP. Blockage of these ducts can cause elevated levels of ALP, whereas cirrhosis, cancer, and toxic drugs will decrease ALP levels. Circulating blood proteins include albumin (60 percent of total) and globulins (40 percent of total). By measuring total protein (TP) and albumin (ALB), the albumin/globulin (A/G) ratio can be determined and monitored. TP may decrease with malnutrition, congestive heart failure, hepatic disease, and renal disease and increase with inflammation and dehydration. Alanine aminotransferase (ALT, SGPT) is an enzyme produced primarily in the liver and kidneys. In healthy individuals ALT is normally low. ALT is released when the liver is damaged, especially with exposure to toxic substances such as drugs and alcohol. Aspartate aminotransferase (AST, SGOT) is an enzyme produced by the liver, heart, kidneys, and muscles. In healthy individuals AST is normally low. An AST/ALT ratio is often performed to determine if elevated levels are due to liver injury or damage to the heart or skeletal muscles. A specimen is obtained by separately reportable venipuncture. Serum/plasma is tested using quantitative enzymatic method or quantitative spectrophotometry.

RVUs

Code	Work	PE	PE Non-Facility	MP	Total Non-Facility	Total Facility	Global
80076	0.00	0.00	0.00	0.00	0.00	0.00	XXX

80156-80157

80156 Carbamazepine; total

80157 Carbamazepine; free

Plain English Description

A laboratory test is performed to determine total (80156) or free (80157) carbamazepine levels. Carbamazepine, also referred to as Tegretol, is an anticonvulsant used to treat epilepsy and may also be used as an analgesic to treat trigeminal neuralgia. Carbamazepine, carbamazepine metabolite (10,11-epoxide), and free carbamazepine are routinely measured to determine optimal doses in patients with epilepsy as well as to monitor for carbamazepine toxicity. A blood sample is obtained by separately reportable venipuncture. Blood serum is then tested using one of several techniques including high performance liquid chromatography or fluorescent polarization immunoassay. Total carbamazepine tests the total amount present in the blood. Under normal circumstances, circulating carbamazepine is 75% protein bound. In some patients carbamazepine may be displaced from protein resulting in higher levels of free carbamazepine circulating in the blood. In these patients, lower levels of the drug may result in toxicity, so the unbound (free) levels must be monitored.

RVUs

Code	Work	PE	PE Non-Facility	MP	Total Non-Facility	Total Facility	Global
80156	0.00	0.00	0.00	0.00	0.00	0.00	XXX
80157	0.00	0.00	0.00	0.00	0.00	0.00	XXX

80164-80165

80164 Valproic acid (dipropylacetic acid); total

80165 Valproic acid (dipropylacetic acid); free

Plain English Description

A laboratory test is performed to measure valproic acid (dipropylacetic acid, depakote). Valproic acid is an anticonvulsant that may be used to treat seizure disorders, manic phase of bipolar disorders, and migraine headaches. The drug works by changing certain chemicals neurotransmitters in the brain. The test for total valproic acid (80164) can be used to monitor drug therapy, assess patient compliance, and evaluate for potential toxicity. The test for free valproic acid (80165) may be used to evaluate the cause of toxicity when the total valproic acid concentration is within the normal range. Free valproic acid may be elevated in patients with an altered or unpredictable protein binding capacity. A blood sample is obtained by separately reportable venipuncture just prior to medication administration to obtain the trough level. Serum/plasma is tested for total valproic acid using fluorescence polarization immunoassay and for free valproic acid using quantitative enzyme multiplied immunoassay.

RVUs

Code	Work	PE	PE Non-Facility	MP	Total Non-Facility	Total Facility	Global
80164	0.00	0.00	0.00	0.00	0.00	0.00	XXX
80165	0.00	0.00	0.00	0.00	0.00	0.00	XXX

80168

80168 Ethosuximide

Plain English Description

A blood test is performed to measure ethosuximide levels. Ethosuximide also known as Zarontin, is an anticonvulsant drug and is prescribed to treat seizures. The drug is administered orally and blood concentration levels are monitored at the start of treatment, at regular intervals to maintain therapeutic levels and when symptoms/breakthrough seizure activity occurs, indicating possible low therapeutic blood levels. A blood sample is obtained by a separately reportable venipuncture. Blood serum is then tested using enzyme immunoassay.

RVUs

Code	Work	PE	PE Non-Facility	MP	Total Non-Facility	Total Facility	Global
80168	0.00	0.00	0.00	0.00	0.00	0.00	XXX

80173

80173 Haloperidol

Plain English Description

A blood test is performed to monitor haloperidol level. Haloperidol, also referred to as Haldol, is used to treat schizophrenia and may also be used to treat tics and vocal utterances in Tourette's syndrome. A blood specimen is obtained by separately reportable venipuncture. Blood serum or plasma is tested using high performance liquid chromatography or gas chromatography. This test is performed to monitor haloperidol for optimal dosing and to prevent toxicity.

RVUs

Code	Work	PE	PE Non-Facility	MP	Total Non-Facility	Total Facility	Global
80173	0.00	0.00	0.00	0.00	0.00	0.00	XXX

80175

80175 Lamotrigine

Plain English Description

A blood test is performed to measure lamotrigine levels. Lamotrigine (Lamictal) is an anticonvulsant from the phenyltriazine class of medications and is used to treat seizure disorders and bipolar disorders. The drug may also be prescribed off label for peripheral neuropathy, migraine headaches, and depression (without mania). A blood sample is obtained by separately reportable venipuncture. Serum and/or plasma is tested using quantitative enzyme immunoassay.

RVUs

Code	Work	PE	PE Non-Facility	MP	Total Non-Facility	Total Facility	Global
80175	0.00	0.00	0.00	0.00	0.00	0.00	XXX

80177

80177 Levetiracetam

Plain English Description

A blood test is performed to measure levetiracetam levels. Levetiracetam (Keppra) is an anticonvulsant medication used to treat seizure disorders. The drug may also be prescribed off label for neuropathic pain, Tourette's syndrome, autism, bipolar disorder, anxiety disorder, and Alzheimer's disease. A blood sample is obtained by separately reportable venipuncture. Serum and/or plasma is tested using quantitative enzyme immunoassay.

RVUs

Code	Work	PE	PE Non-Facility	MP	Total Non-Facility	Total Facility	Global
80177	0.00	0.00	0.00	0.00	0.00	0.00	XXX

80178

80178 Lithium

Plain English Description

A blood test is performed to measure lithium levels. Lithium (carbonate), also known as Eskalith or Lithobid, is a neurotransmitter that affects the flow of sodium through nerve and muscle cells. It is used to stabilize the manic phase in patients with bipolar disorder and may also be prescribed to treat cluster headaches and bipolar depression. Lithium has a very narrow therapeutic range and blood levels are monitored frequently at the beginning of therapy, when dose is being adjusted, for suspected high or low levels and then at regular intervals when on maintenance doses. Blood should be drawn 12 hours after the last dose. A blood sample is obtained by a separately reportable venipuncture. Blood serum is then tested using reflectance spectrophotometry.

RVUs

Code	Work	PE	PE Non-Facility	MP	Total Non-Facility	Total Facility	Global
80178	0.00	0.00	0.00	0.00	0.00	0.00	XXX

80183

80183 Oxcarbazepine

Plain English Description

A blood test is performed to measure Oxcarbazepine levels. Oxcarbazepine (Trileptal) is an anticonvulsant and mood stabilizing medication used to treat seizure disorders. The drug may also be prescribed off label for anxiety, mood disorders, and benign motor tics. A blood sample is obtained by separately reportable venipuncture. Serum/plasma is tested for oxcarbazepine metabolite using quantitative liquid chromatography-tandem mass spectrometry.

RVUs

Code	Work	PE	PE Non-Facility	MP	Total Non-Facility	Total Facility	Global
80183	0.00	0.00	0.00	0.00	0.00	0.00	XXX

80184

80184 Phenobarbital

Plain English Description

A blood test is performed to measure phenobarbital levels. Phenobarbital, also known as Luminal, is an anticonvulsant/hypnotic prescribed to treat seizures and insomnia by decreasing electrical activity in the brain. The drug may be administered orally or by injection. Blood concentration levels are monitored at regular intervals and also when breakthrough seizure activity or over sedation occurs, indicating possible high/low therapeutic blood levels. A blood sample is obtained by a separately reportable venipuncture. Blood serum is then tested using high performance liquid chromatography.

RVUs

Code	Work	PE	PE Non-Facility	MP	Total Non-Facility	Total Facility	Global
80184	0.00	0.00	0.00	0.00	0.00	0.00	XXX

80185-80186

80185 Phenytoin; total
80186 Phenytoin; free

Plain English Description

A blood test is performed to measure phenytoin total (80185) and phenytoin free (80186) levels. Phenytoin also known as Dilantin, Phenytek or Prompt, is an anticonvulsant prescribed to treat seizures and works by decreasing electrical activity in the brain. The drug may be administered orally or by injection. Phenytoin has a narrow therapeutic range and the patient should be monitored for both total and free phenytoin levels. Total phenytoin reflects the total serum concentration of the drug while free phenytoin levels reflect the unbound levels. Only the unbound levels are biologically active. Ninety (90) percent of the drug is typically highly bound and biologically inactive, but bound phenytoin is sensitive to displacement by other protein binding drugs which can elevate levels of free phenytoin in the blood. Blood concentration levels are monitored at regular intervals and also when breakthrough seizures occur, indicating possible low therapeutic levels. A blood sample is obtained by a separately reportable venipuncture. Blood serum is then tested using immunoassay.

RVUs

Code	Work	PE	PE Non-Facility	MP	Total Non-Facility	Total Facility	Global
80185	0.00	0.00	0.00	0.00	0.00	0.00	XXX
80186	0.00	0.00	0.00	0.00	0.00	0.00	XXX

80188

80188 Primidone

Plain English Description

A blood test is performed to measure primidone levels. Primidone, also known as Mysoline is an anticonvulsant prescribed to treat seizures and essential tremor and works by decreasing electrical activity in the brain. The drug is administered orally. Blood concentration levels are monitored at regular intervals and also when breakthrough seizures occur, indicating possible low therapeutic levels. A blood sample is obtained by a separately reportable venipuncture. Blood serum is then tested using fluorescence polarization immunoassay.

RVUs

Code	Work	PE	PE Non-Facility	MP	Total Non-Facility	Total Facility	Global
80188	0.00	0.00	0.00	0.00	0.00	0.00	XXX

80235

● **80235 Lacosamide**

Plain English Description

A laboratory test is performed to monitor therapeutic drug levels of lacosamide, an anti-epileptic used to treat partial-onset seizures in patients age 4 and older and peripheral neuropathy. The drug selectively enhances a slow inactivation of sodium channels in brain synapses while interacting with the neuroplasticity-relevant target collapsin-response mediator protein-2 (CRMP-2). Peak levels of lacosamide are achieved about 1 hour after intravenous infusion and 4 hours after oral administration with a drug half-life of approximately 13 hours which necessitates a twice daily dosing regimen to prevent breakthrough seizures. The drug is metabolized by the liver and excreted in urine. A blood sample is obtained by separately reported procedure. Serum is tested for peak levels 1-4 hours after dose administration and trough levels 12 hours after last administration using liquid chromatography/tandem mass spectrometry (LC/MS-MS).

RVUs

Code	Work	PE	PE Non-Facility	MP	Total Non-Facility	Total Facility	Global
80235	0.00	0.00	0.00	0.00	0.00	0.00	XXX

80305-80307

80305 Drug test(s), presumptive, any number of drug classes, any number of devices or procedures; capable of being read by direct optical observation only (eg, utilizing immunoassay [eg, dipsticks, cups, cards, or cartridges]), includes sample validation when performed, per date of service

80306 Drug test(s), presumptive, any number of drug classes, any number of devices or procedures; read by instrument assisted direct optical observation (eg, utilizing immunoassay [eg, dipsticks, cups, cards, or cartridges]), includes sample validation when performed, per date of service

80307 Drug test(s), presumptive, any number of drug classes, any number of devices or procedures; by instrument chemistry analyzers (eg, utilizing immunoassay [eg, EIA, ELISA, EMIT, FPIA, IA, KIMS, RIA]), chromatography (eg, GC, HPLC), and mass spectrometry either with or without chromatography, (eg, DART, DESI, GC-MS, GC-MS/MS, LC-MS, LC-MS/MS, LDTD, MALDI, TOF) includes sample validation when performed, per date of service

Plain English Description

A laboratory test is performed to detect the presence or absence of drug classes in a patient's system during a specific encounter. Presumptive screening is commonly done first, followed by test(s) for definitive drug identification because presumptive testing will not provide qualitative identification of individual drugs, or quantitative levels present. A sample of blood or urine is obtained by separately reported procedure. Methods used include immunoassays, chromatography, and mass spectrometry. Code 80305 reports presumptive drug testing for any number of drug classes, any number of drug device,s or procedures using CLIA-waived methodologies for direct optical observation only, including dipsticks, cups, cards, or cartridges with sample validation, such as pH, nitrite, and specific gravity, when performed.

Code 80306 reports presumptive drug testing using FDA-specified equipment for moderate complexity testing methodologies with instrument-assisted direct optical observation, including dipstick, cups, cards, and cartridges with sample validation, when performed. Code 80307 reports presumptive drug testing using FDA-specified equipment for high complexity testing methodologies by instrument chemistry analyzers for immunoassay, chromatography, and mass spectrometry including sample validation when performed.

RVUs

Code	Work	PE	PE Non-Facility	MP	Total Non-Facility	Total Facility	Global
80305	0.00	0.00	0.00	0.00	0.00	0.00	XXX
80306	0.00	0.00	0.00	0.00	0.00	0.00	XXX
80307	0.00	0.00	0.00	0.00	0.00	0.00	XXX

80339-80341

80339 Antiepileptics, not otherwise specified; 1-3

80340 Antiepileptics, not otherwise specified; 4-6

80341 Antiepileptics, not otherwise specified; 7 or more

(To report definitive drug testing for antihistamines, see 80375, 80376, 80377)

Plain English Description

A laboratory test is performed to measure antiepileptics, not otherwise specified. Antiepileptics are used to treat seizure disorders and may also be prescribed to patients with chronic pain conditions like migraine or fibromyalgia. The mechanism of action can vary substantially between drugs in this category but they all function to change brain chemicals such as sodium channels, GABA receptors, NMDA receptors, calcium channels, AMPA receptors, and potassium channels, and to decrease the incidence of unusual electrical discharges that may trigger seizure activity or pain sensation. Primary analytical methods for testing urine, serum, or plasma for antiepileptics include high performance liquid chromatography, gas chromatography, liquid chromatography-tandem mass spectrometry, and immunoassays. Code 80339 is used when testing for 1-3 antiepileptics; code 80340 is used when testing for 4-6 compounds; and code 80341 is used when evaluating a sample for 7 or more antiepileptic drugs.

RVUs

Code	Work	PE	PE Non-Facility	MP	Total Non-Facility	Total Facility	Global
80339	0.00	0.00	0.00	0.00	0.00	0.00	XXX
80340	0.00	0.00	0.00	0.00	0.00	0.00	XXX
80341	0.00	0.00	0.00	0.00	0.00	0.00	XXX

80349

80349 Cannabinoids, natural

Plain English Description

A laboratory test is performed to measure natural cannabinoids in meconium stool, urine, serum, or plasma. Cannabinoids occur naturally in the marijuana plant (Cannabis sativa). Tetrahydrocannabinol, or THC, is the principal mind-altering constituent of cannabis. When smoked or ingested, THC primarily affects the limbic system responsible for memory, cognition, and psychomotor performance, and the mesolimbic pathways responsible for the feeling of reward and pain perception. The chemical is fat soluble with a long elimination half-life. Cannabinoids may be detected in urine for several weeks and in serum or plasma for up to 12 hours. A blood sample is obtained by separately reportable venipuncture, urine sample by random void or catheterization, and meconium stool collected from a diaper. Samples are tested for THC and its metabolite 9-carboxy-THC using quantitative liquid chromatography-tandem mass spectrometry.

RVUs

Code	Work	PE	PE Non-Facility	MP	Total Non-Facility	Total Facility	Global
80349	0.00	0.00	0.00	0.00	0.00	0.00	XXX

80350-80352

80350 Cannabinoids, synthetic; 1-3

80351 Cannabinoids, synthetic; 4-6

80352 Cannabinoids, synthetic; 7 or more

Plain English Description

A laboratory test is performed to measure synthetic cannabinoids in urine, saliva, or blood. Synthetic cannabinoids include the designer drugs "spice" and "K2." They may be referred to as "herbal incense," "potpourri," or "legal" marijuana. These chemicals affect the same receptors in the central nervous system as THC to produce similar psychoactive effects but are more likely to cause anxiety, agitation, and hallucinations in addition. Synthetic cannabinoids are usually assigned to three classes that include classical cannabinoids (HU-210), cyclohexylphenols, and aminoalkylindoles. These designer drugs are manufactured with continually changing chemical structures to avoid detection in commercially available tests. Synthetic cannabinoids will not be detected in immunoassay tests for THC. A blood sample is obtained by separately reportable venipuncture, a urine sample by random void or catheterization, and saliva is collected by swab or in a sample cup. Blood and saliva are tested using liquid chromatography-tandem mass spectrometry. Urine is screened using enzyme-linked immunosorbent assay and confirmed using high performance liquid chromatography-tandem mass spectrometry. Code 80350 is used when testing for 1-3 synthetic cannabinoids; code 80351 is used for 4-6 compounds; and code 80352 is used for 7 or more synthetic cannabinoids.

RVUs

Code	Work	PE	PE Non-Facility	MP	Total Non-Facility	Total Facility	Global
80350	0.00	0.00	0.00	0.00	0.00	0.00	XXX
80351	0.00	0.00	0.00	0.00	0.00	0.00	XXX
80352	0.00	0.00	0.00	0.00	0.00	0.00	XXX

81000-81003

81000 Urinalysis, by dip stick or tablet reagent for bilirubin, glucose, hemoglobin, ketones, leukocytes, nitrite, pH, protein, specific gravity, urobilinogen, any number of these constituents; non-automated, with microscopy

81001 Urinalysis, by dip stick or tablet reagent for bilirubin, glucose, hemoglobin, ketones, leukocytes, nitrite, pH, protein, specific gravity, urobilinogen, any number of these constituents; automated, with microscopy

81002 Urinalysis, by dip stick or tablet reagent for bilirubin, glucose, hemoglobin, ketones, leukocytes, nitrite, pH, protein, specific gravity, urobilinogen, any number of these constituents; non-automated, without microscopy

81003 Urinalysis, by dip stick or tablet reagent for bilirubin, glucose, hemoglobin, ketones, leukocytes, nitrite, pH, protein, specific gravity, urobilinogen, any number of these constituents; automated, without microscopy

Plain English Description

A urinalysis is performed with dip stick or tablet reagent for bilirubin, glucose, hemoglobin, ketones, leukocytes, nitrite, pH, protein, specific gravity, and/or urobilinogen. Urinalysis can quickly screen for conditions that do not immediately produce symptoms, such as diabetes mellitus, kidney disease, or urinary tract infection. A dip stick allows qualitative and semi-quantitative analysis using a paper or plastic stick with color strips for each agent being tested. The stick is dipped in the urine specimen and the color strips are then compared to a color chart to determine the presence or absence and/or a rough estimate of the concentration of each agent tested. Reagent tablets use an absorbent mat with a few drops of urine placed on the mat followed by a reagent tablet. A drop of distilled, deionized water is then placed on the tablet and the color change is observed. Bilirubin is a byproduct of the breakdown of red blood cells by the liver. Normally bilirubin is excreted through the bowel, but in patients with liver disease, bilirubin is filtered by the kidneys and excreted in the urine. Glucose is a sugar that is normally filtered by the glomerulus and excreted only in small quantities in the urine. Excess sugar in the urine (glycosuria) is indicative of diabetes mellitus. The peroxidase activity of erythrocytes is used to detect hemoglobin in the urine, which may be indicative of hematuria, myoglobinuria, or hemoglobinuria. Ketones in the urine are the result of diabetic ketoacidosis or calorie deprivation (starvation). A leukocyte esterase test identifies the presence of white blood cells in the urine. The presence of nitrites in the urine is indicative of bacteria. The pH identifies the acid-base levels in the urine. The presence of excessive amounts of protein (proteinuria) may be indicative of nephrotic syndrome. Specific gravity measures urine density and is indicative of the kidneys' ability to concentrate and dilute urine. Following dip stick or reagent testing, the urine sample may be examined under a microscope. The urine sample is placed in a test tube and centrifuged. The sediment is resuspended. A drop of the resuspended sediment is then placed on a glass slide, cover-slipped, and examined under a microscope for crystals, casts, squamous cells, blood (white, red) cells, and bacteria. Use 81000 for a non-automated test with microscopy and 81001 for an automated test with microscopy. Use 81002 for a non-automated test without microscopy and 81003 for an automated test without microscopy.

RVUs

Code	Work	PE	PE Non-Facility	MP	Total Non-Facility	Total Facility	Global
81000	0.00	0.00	0.00	0.00	0.00	0.00	XXX
81001	0.00	0.00	0.00	0.00	0.00	0.00	XXX
81002	0.00	0.00	0.00	0.00	0.00	0.00	XXX
81003	0.00	0.00	0.00	0.00	0.00	0.00	XXX

81271

81271 HTT (huntingtin) (eg, Huntington disease) gene analysis; evaluation to detect abnormal (eg, expanded) alleles

Plain English Description

Molecular genetic testing is performed to identify abnormal (expanded) alleles and specific characterization of alleles on the HTT (huntingtin) gene associated with Huntington disease, a progressive neurodegenerative disorder. The HTT gene is located on the short (p) arm of chromosome 4 at position 16.3 (4p16.3) and codes a protein responsible for nerve cell function essential to normal brain development. It may also be a factor in chemical signaling, binding of proteins and other structures, and protecting cells from self-destruction. Symptoms of Huntington disease include cognitive impairment, dementia, apathy, depression, anxiety and extrapyramidal body movements. Onset of symptoms may occur in childhood or adolescence in the juvenile form, or in mid-adulthood. The HTT gene has a unique DNA allele with a trinucleotide building block pattern of 3 amino acids: cysteine, alanine, glycine (CAG) that usually repeats 10-35 times. An elongated protein with expanded alleles is fragile and breaks easily into fragments that bind together and accumulate in nerve cells. When the allele has 27-35 CAG repeats, it is considered a pre-mutation. Individuals will be asymptomatic, but due to the instability of the allele, the risk of further expansion increases with each generation. An allele with 36-39 CAG repeats may cause no symptoms or very mild symptoms. Individuals with 40-50 CAG repeats will usually manifest symptoms in adulthood and those with >60 CAG repeats will be symptomatic in childhood or adolescence. Code 81271 reports HTT gene analysis for evaluation of expanded alleles. Code 81274 reports HTT gene analysis to pinpoint characteristics of the expanded alleles, such as determining their expanded size, similarities, or differences.

RVUs

Code	Work	PE	PE Non-Facility	MP	Total Non-Facility	Total Facility	Global
81271	0.00	0.00	0.00	0.00	0.00	0.00	XXX

81274

81274 HTT (huntingtin) (eg, Huntington disease) gene analysis; characterization of alleles (eg, expanded size)

Plain English Description

Molecular genetic testing is performed to identify abnormal (expanded) alleles and specific characterization of alleles on the HTT (huntingtin) gene associated with Huntington disease, a progressive neurodegenerative disorder. The HTT gene is located on the short (p) arm of chromosome 4 at position 16.3 (4p16.3) and codes a protein responsible for nerve cell function essential to normal brain development. It may also be a factor in chemical signaling, binding of proteins and other structures, and protecting cells from self-destruction. Symptoms of Huntington disease include cognitive impairment, dementia, apathy, depression, anxiety and extrapyramidal body movements. Onset of symptoms may occur in childhood or adolescence in the juvenile form, or in mid-adulthood. The HTT gene has a unique DNA allele with a trinucleotide building block pattern of 3 amino acids: cysteine, alanine, glycine (CAG) that usually repeats 10-35 times. An elongated protein with expanded alleles is fragile and breaks easily into fragments that bind together and accumulate in nerve cells. When the allele has 27-35 CAG repeats, it is considered a pre-mutation. Individuals will be asymptomatic, but due to the instability of the allele, the risk of further expansion increases with each generation. An allele with 36-39 CAG repeats may cause no symptoms or very mild symptoms. Individuals with 40-50 CAG repeats will usually manifest symptoms in adulthood and those with >60 CAG repeats will be symptomatic in childhood or adolescence. Code 81271 reports HTT gene analysis for evaluation of expanded alleles. Code 81274 reports HTT gene analysis to pinpoint characteristics of the expanded alleles, such as determining their expanded size, similarities, or differences.

RVUs

Code	Work	PE	PE Non-Facility	MP	Total Non-Facility	Total Facility	Global
81274	0.00	0.00	0.00	0.00	0.00	0.00	XXX

81448

81448 Hereditary peripheral neuropathies (eg, Charcot-Marie-Tooth, spastic paraplegia), genomic sequence analysis panel, must include sequencing of at least 5 peripheral neuropathy-related genes (eg, BSCL2, GJB1, MFN2, MPZ, REEP1, SPAST, SPG11, SPTLC1)

Plain English Description

Gene analysis may be performed on a panel of genes associated with hereditary peripheral neuropathies including Charcot-Marie-Tooth (CMT) and spastic paraplegia to identify gene variants and mutations. Hereditary peripheral neuropathies are the most commonly inherited neuromuscular diseases, falling into two categories, primary axonopathies or primary myelinopathies depending on the affected portion of the nerve fiber. Further anatomic classification of peripheral neuropathies includes sensory vs. motor fiber, large vs. small nerve fiber, and the gross distribution of nerve(s) affected including symmetry and length dependency. Symptoms of peripheral neuropathies affecting motor and sensory nerves can include progressive distal muscle weakness, paresthesia and/or loss of sensation, foot drop, decreased deep tendon reflexes, hammer toe, and high arches. Symptoms of neuropathies affecting only motor nerves may include progressive weakness and atrophy of distal muscles, decreased or absent deep tendon reflexes, foot deformities, and vocal cord or diaphragm paralysis. Symptoms of sensory and autonomic neuropathies can include decreasing sensation of pain, temperature, and touch, distal muscle weakness, decreased reflexes, excessive sweating, gastroesophageal reflux, postural hypotension, apnea, incontinence, and hearing loss. This test may be used to establish a genetic cause for symptoms and confirm inheritance patterns; identify at risk pregnancies; and provide accurate genetic counseling and family planning. A blood sample is obtained by separately reported procedure. The sample is tested using Next Generation Sequencing (NGS) with confirmation by Sanger Sequencing for the presence of mutations.

RVUs

Code	Work	PE	PE Non-Facility	MP	Total Non-Facility	Total Facility	Global
81448	0.00	0.00	0.00	0.00	0.00	0.00	XXX

82043-82044

82043 Albumin; urine (eg, microalbumin), quantitative

82044 Albumin; urine (eg, microalbumin), semiquantitative (eg, reagent strip assay)

(For prealbumin, use 84134)

Plain English Description

A test on urine is used to measure microalbumin levels and is routinely performed annually on diabetic patients with stable blood glucose levels to assess for early onset nephropathy. The quantitative test (82043), which measures the actual amount of microalbumin present in the urine, may be performed on a random urine sample, with a notation of total volume and voiding time, or a 24-hour urine sample using immunoturbidimetric technique. The semi-quantitative test (82044) identifies the presence of elevated microalbumin levels in the urine within a general range and involves a chemical dipstick placed into the urine sample which reacts and changes color when albumin is present.

RVUs

Code	Work	PE	PE Non-Facility	MP	Total Non-Facility	Total Facility	Global
82043	0.00	0.00	0.00	0.00	0.00	0.00	XXX
82044	0.00	0.00	0.00	0.00	0.00	0.00	XXX

82306

82306 Vitamin D; 25 hydroxy, includes fraction(s), if performed

Plain English Description

Blood levels of 25-hydroxyvitamin D are used to determine whether a deficiency of Vitamin D or abnormal metabolism of calcium is the cause of bone weakness or malformation. Vitamin D is a fat-soluble vitamin that is absorbed from the intestine like fat, and 25-hydroxyvitamin D levels are also evaluated in individuals with conditions or diseases that interfere with fat absorption, such as cystic fibrosis, Crohns disease, or in patients who have undergone gastric bypass surgery. A blood sample is obtained. Levels of 25-hydroxyvitamin D3 and 25-hydroxyvitamin D2 are evaluated using chemiluminescent immunoassay. The test results may be the sum of vitamin D3 and D2 or the results may include fractions of D3 and D2 as well as the sum of these values.

RVUs

Code	Work	PE	PE Non-Facility	MP	Total Non-Facility	Total Facility	Global
82306	0.00	0.00	0.00	0.00	0.00	0.00	XXX

82550-82554

82550 Creatine kinase (CK), (CPK); total

82552 Creatine kinase (CK), (CPK); isoenzymes

82553 Creatine kinase (CK), (CPK); MB fraction only

82554 Creatine kinase (CK), (CPK); isoforms

Plain English Description

Creatine kinase (CK) also known as, creatine phosphokinase (CPK), is an enzyme found in the heart, brain, skeletal muscle and certain other tissue. The subtypes are known as CK-MM found primarily in skeletal and heart muscle, CK-MB found in heart muscle and CK-BB located in the brain. CK circulating in blood rarely contains CK-BB but is largely comprised of CK-MM or CK-MB. Levels may be elevated following heart muscle damage (heart attack/ myocardial infarction) and skeletal muscle injury (trauma, vigorous exercise). Statin drugs that lower cholesterol level and alcohol intake may cause elevated CK blood levels. In 82550, a blood test is performed to measure total creatine kinase (CK) levels. A blood specimen is obtained by separately reportable venipuncture. Serum or plasma is tested using quantitative enzymatic methodology. In 82552, creatine kinase (CK) isoenzyme levels are measured. Testing for isoenzymes can help determine the exact location of muscle damage when total CK is elevated. A blood specimen is obtained by separately reportable venipuncture. Serum is tested using quantitative enzymatic methodology. In 82553, only creatine kinase (CK) MB fraction is measured. Testing for this isoenzyme can help identify heart muscle damage following a heart attack (myocardial infarction). A blood test is obtained by separately reportable venipuncture. Serum is tested using chemiluminescent immunoassay. In 82554, creatine kinase (CK) isoforms of the isoenzymes CK-MM and CK-MB are measured. Following their release, CK isoenzymes continue to break down into more distinct isoforms. The CK-MM contains at least three major isoform subtypes and CK-MB has at least two. Identifying isoform subtypes of the isoenzymes, can help identify and define the time as well as the location of muscle injury. A blood specimen is obtained by separately reportable venipuncture. Serum may be tested using a number of techniques including high resolution electrophoresis, isoelectric and chromatofocusing and liquid chromatography.

RVUs

Code	Work	PE	PE Non-Facility	MP	Total Non-Facility	Total Facility	Global
82550	0.00	0.00	0.00	0.00	0.00	0.00	XXX
82552	0.00	0.00	0.00	0.00	0.00	0.00	XXX
82553	0.00	0.00	0.00	0.00	0.00	0.00	XXX
82554	0.00	0.00	0.00	0.00	0.00	0.00	XXX

82565

82565 Creatinine; blood

Plain English Description

A blood sample is taken to measure creatinine levels. Creatinine is a waste product produced by the muscles in the breakdown of creatine, which is a compound used by the muscles to create energy for contraction. The waste product, creatinine, is excreted by the kidneys and blood levels provide a good measurement of renal function. Creatinine may be checked to screen for or monitor treatment of renal disease. Creatinine levels may also be monitored in patients with acute or chronic illnesses that may impair renal function and in patients on medications that affect renal function. Creatinine is measured using spectrophotometry.

RVUs

Code	Work	PE	PE Non-Facility	MP	Total Non-Facility	Total Facility	Global
82565	0.00	0.00	0.00	0.00	0.00	0.00	XXX

82570

82570 Creatinine; other source

Plain English Description

A sample other than blood is taken to measure creatinine levels in 82570. Creatinine is a waste product produced by the muscles in the breakdown of creatine, which is a compound used by the muscles to create energy for contraction. The waste product, creatinine, is excreted by the kidneys and blood levels provide a good measurement of renal function. Creatinine may be checked to screen for or monitor treatment of renal disease. Creatinine levels may also be monitored in patients with acute or chronic illnesses that may impair renal function and in patients on medications that affect renal function. Creatinine clearance (82575), also known as urea or urea nitrogen clearance tests both blood and urine samples for a calculation of creatinine content adjusted for urine volume and physical size as a general indicator of glomerular filtration function.

RVUs

Code	Work	PE	PE Non-Facility	MP	Total Non-Facility	Total Facility	Global
82570	0.00	0.00	0.00	0.00	0.00	0.00	XXX

82575

82575 Creatinine; clearance

Plain English Description

A sample other than blood is taken to measure creatinine levels in 82570. Creatinine is a waste product produced by the muscles in the breakdown of creatine, which is a compound used by the muscles to create energy for contraction. The waste product, creatinine, is excreted by the kidneys and blood levels provide a good measurement of renal function. Creatinine may be checked to screen for or monitor treatment of renal disease. Creatinine levels may also be monitored in patients with acute or chronic illnesses that may impair renal function and in patients on medications that affect renal function. Creatinine clearance (82575), also known as urea or urea nitrogen clearance tests both blood and urine samples for a calculation of creatinine content adjusted for urine volume and physical size as a general indicator of glomerular filtration function.

RVUs

Code	Work	PE	PE Non-Facility	MP	Total Non-Facility	Total Facility	Global
82575	0.00	0.00	0.00	0.00	0.00	0.00	XXX

82607-82608

82607 Cyanocobalamin (Vitamin B-12)

82608 Cyanocobalamin (Vitamin B-12); unsaturated binding capacity

(Cyclic AMP, use 82030)

(Cyclosporine, use 80158)

Plain English Description

Cyanocobalamin is a vitamer of the B-12 vitamin family and plays an important role in metabolism, red blood cell production and nervous system function. In 82607 blood levels of cyanocobalamin are measured. Blood levels may be reduced with pernicious and other forms of anemia, and in individuals who follow a strict vegan diet, have chronic infections (such as HIV) and during pregnancy. A blood sample is obtained by separately reportable venipuncture. Serum is tested using quantitative chemiluminescent immunoassay. In 82608, a blood test is performed to measure cyanocobalamin unsaturated binding capacity. The unsaturated binding capacity of cyanocobalamin may be elevated in diseases such as myelocytic leukemia, polycythemia vera, some liver disorders and in Gaucher disease. Levels may be decreased with megaloblastic anemia from congenital transcobalamin II deficiency and from other causes. A blood sample is obtained by separately reportable venipuncture. Serum is tested using quantitative radioimmunoassay.

RVUs

Code	Work	PE	PE Non-Facility	MP	Total Non-Facility	Total Facility	Global
82607	0.00	0.00	0.00	0.00	0.00	0.00	XXX
82608	0.00	0.00	0.00	0.00	0.00	0.00	XXX

82728

82728 Ferritin

(Fetal hemoglobin, see hemoglobin 83030, 83033, and 85460)

(Fetoprotein, alpha-1, see 82105, 82106)

Plain English Description

A blood test is performed to measure ferritin levels. Ferritin is an intracellular protein that stores iron and releases it into circulation in a controlled manner to protect the body against iron overload and iron deficiency. Ferritin levels may be obtained to evaluate for elevated levels caused by excess storage diseases such as hemochromatosis and following multiple transfusions. Levels may also be obtained to evaluate for decreased levels due to iron deficiency. A blood sample is obtained by separately reportable venipuncture. Serum is tested using quantitative chemiluminescent immunoassay.

RVUs

Code	Work	PE	PE Non-Facility	MP	Total Non-Facility	Total Facility	Global
82728	0.00	0.00	0.00	0.00	0.00	0.00	XXX

82746-82747

82746 Folic acid; serum

82747 Folic acid; RBC

(Follicle stimulating hormone [FSH], use 83001)

Plain English Description

A blood test is performed to measure folic acid (folate) levels in serum or red blood cells (RBCs). Folic acid (folate) may also be referred to as Vitamin B9 and is essential for the growth, division, and repair of cells, especially fetal growth during pregnancy and in early infancy. It is also necessary for the production of healthy RBCs and to prevent anemia at all ages. The test may be used to diagnose anemia or certain neuropathies and to monitor the effectiveness of treatment for these conditions. A blood sample is obtained by separately reportable venipuncture. Use 82746 when serum is tested. Use 82747 when RBCs are tested. The amount of folic acid in RBCs measures the level when the cell was made, up to 2 months earlier. Both tests are typically performed using quantitative chemiluminescent immunoassay.

RVUs

Code	Work	PE	PE Non-Facility	MP	Total Non-Facility	Total Facility	Global
82746	0.00	0.00	0.00	0.00	0.00	0.00	XXX
82747	0.00	0.00	0.00	0.00	0.00	0.00	XXX

82947-82948

82947 Glucose; quantitative, blood (except reagent strip)

82948 Glucose; blood, reagent strip

Plain English Description

A blood sample is obtained to measure total (quantitative) blood glucose level. Glucose is a simple sugar that is the main source of energy for the body. Carbohydrates are broken down into simple sugars, primarily glucose, absorbed by the intestine, and circulated in the blood. Insulin, a hormone produced by the pancreas, regulates glucose level in the blood and transports glucose to cells in other tissues and organs. When more glucose is available in the blood than is required, it is converted to glycogen and stored in the liver or converted to fat and stored in adipose (fat) tissue. If the glucose/insulin metabolic process is working properly, blood glucose will remain at a fairly constant, healthy level. Glucose is measured to determine whether the glucose/insulin metabolic process is functioning properly. It is used to monitor glucose levels and determine whether they are too low (hypoglycemia) or too high (hyperglycemia) as well as test for diabetes and to monitor blood sugar control in diabetics. Use 82947 for quantitative blood glucose determination by enzymatic methodology or any method other than reagent strip. Use 82948 for blood glucose determination by reagent strip. A drop of blood is placed on a reagent strip, which is then compared to a calibrated color scale, and a visual determination is made as to the amount of glucose present in the specimen.

RVUs

Code	Work	PE	PE Non-Facility	MP	Total Non-Facility	Total Facility	Global
82947	0.00	0.00	0.00	0.00	0.00	0.00	XXX
82948	0.00	0.00	0.00	0.00	0.00	0.00	XXX

82962

82962 Glucose, blood by glucose monitoring device(s) cleared by the FDA specifically for home use

Plain English Description

A portable testing device called a glucometer is used at the patient's home or a physician's office to monitor glucose levels in the blood. Glucose is a monosaccharide (single sugar) used for energy by the body. Certain diseases, such as diabetes, and medications may cause glucose levels to be abnormally high or low. A blood sample is obtained by fingerstick and placed on a test strip. Most commercial glucometers use a chemically treated test strip that produces a small electric current when blood is introduced. The strength of the electrical charge is dependent on the level of glucose in the sample. The glucose level is displayed on the monitoring device in a numeric measurement as mg/dL. This code is only reported when the physician or other healthcare professional uses this type of device in the office or other setting to check glucose levels, not when the patient self-administers the test.

RVUs

Code	Work	PE	PE Non-Facility	MP	Total Non-Facility	Total Facility	Global
82962	0.00	0.00	0.00	0.00	0.00	0.00	XXX

83036-83037

83036 Hemoglobin; glycosylated (A1C)

(For glycosylated [A1C] hemoglobin analysis, by electrophoresis or chromatography, in the setting of an identified hemoglobin variant, see 83020, 83021)

(For fecal hemoglobin detection by immunoassay, use 82274)

83037 Hemoglobin; glycosylated (A1C) by device cleared by FDA for home use

Plain English Description

A blood test is performed to measure glycosylated hemoglobin (HbA1C) levels. Plasma glucose binds to hemoglobin and the HbA1C test measures the average plasma glucose concentration over the life of red blood cells (approximately 90-120 days). HbA1C levels may be used as a diagnostic reference for patients with suspected diabetes mellitus (DM) and to monitor blood glucose control in patients with known DM. HbA1C levels should be monitored at least every 6 months in patients with DM and more frequently when the level is >7.0%. In 83036, a blood sample is obtained by separately reportable venipuncture. Whole blood is tested using quantitative high performance liquid chromatography/boronate affinity. In 83037, the HbA1C test is performed using a FDA approved testing device for home use. A capillary or venous blood sample is obtained. A drop of blood is placed in buffer solution and shaken to lyse the red blood cells. The sample is then transferred to the testing device where the HbAIC levels are measured and results displayed on the device.

RVUs

Code	Work	PE	PE Non-Facility	MP	Total Non-Facility	Total Facility	Global
83036	0.00	0.00	0.00	0.00	0.00	0.00	XXX
83037	0.00	0.00	0.00	0.00	0.00	0.00	XXX

83090

83090 Homocysteine

Plain English Description

A blood test is performed to measure homocysteine levels. Homocysteine is a non-protein homologue of the amino acid cysteine. It is biosynthesized in the body by a multi-step process from methionine. Elevated levels of homocysteine are a risk factor for cardiovascular disease. Other conditions that may cause elevated homocysteine levels include: Vitamin B deficiency, intense (prolonged) exercise, alcoholism, genetically inherited diseases. A blood sample is obtained by separately reportable venipuncture. Serum or plasma is tested using quantitative enzymatic technique.

RVUs

Code	Work	PE	PE Non-Facility	MP	Total Non-Facility	Total Facility	Global
83090	0.00	0.00	0.00	0.00	0.00	0.00	XXX

83540

83540 Iron

Plain English Description

A blood, urine, or liver test is performed to measure iron levels. Iron (Fe) is an essential element that circulates in the blood attached to the protein transferrin. Iron is a necessary component of hemoglobin, found in red blood cells (RBCs) and myoglobin found in muscle cells. Low iron levels may cause a decrease in red blood cells and iron deficiency anemia. High iron levels may be caused by excessive intake of iron supplements or a hereditary genetic condition such as hemochromatosis from a mutation of the RGMc gene or HAMP gene. A blood sample is obtained by separately reportable venipuncture. Serum or plasma is tested using quantitative spectrophotometry. A random voided or 24-hour urine specimen is obtained and tested using quantitative inductively coupled plasma/emission spectrometry. Patient should wait 2-4 days after receiving iodine or gadolinium contrast media to collect a urine specimen. A liver sample is obtained by a separately reportable procedure. Liver tissue is tested using quantitative inductively coupled plasma-mass spectrometry.

RVUs

Code	Work	PE	PE Non-Facility	MP	Total Non-Facility	Total Facility	Global
83540	0.00	0.00	0.00	0.00	0.00	0.00	XXX

83550

83550 Iron binding capacity

Plain English Description

A blood test is performed to measure the iron binding capacity of transferrin. Transferrin, a protein found in circulating blood is responsible for carrying iron molecules. This test measures the ability of transferrin to carry iron. A blood sample is obtained by separately reportable venipuncture. Serum or plasma is tested using quantitative spectrophotometry/calculation.

RVUs

Code	Work	PE	PE Non-Facility	MP	Total Non-Facility	Total Facility	Global
83550	0.00	0.00	0.00	0.00	0.00	0.00	XXX

83735

83735 Magnesium

Plain English Description

A blood, urine, or fecal test is performed to measure magnesium levels. Magnesium is an essential dietary mineral responsible for enzyme function, energy production, and contraction and relaxation of muscle fibers. Decreased levels may result from severe burns, metabolic disorders, certain medications, and low blood calcium levels. A blood sample is obtained by separately reportable venipuncture. Red blood cells (RBCs) are tested using quantitative inductively coupled plasma-mass spectrometry. Serum/plasma is tested using quantitative spectrophotometry. A 24-hour voided urine specimen is tested using quantitative spectrophotometry. A random or 24-hour fecal sample is tested using quantitative spectrophotometry.

RVUs

Code	Work	PE	PE Non-Facility	MP	Total Non-Facility	Total Facility	Global
83735	0.00	0.00	0.00	0.00	0.00	0.00	XXX

83970

83970 Parathormone (parathyroid hormone)

(Pesticide, quantitative, see code for specific method. For screen for chlorinated hydrocarbons, usc 82441)

Plain English Description

A blood or tissue test is performed to measure parathormone (parathyroid hormone, parathyrin) levels. Parathyroid hormone (PTH) is produced by chief cells in the parathyroid gland. The hormone helps to regulate blood calcium levels, absorption/excretion of phosphate by the kidneys and in vitamin D synthesis in the body. Elevated levels (hyperparathyroidism) may be caused by parathyroid gland tumors or chronic renal failure. Decreased levels (hypoparathyroidism) may result from inadvertent removal (during thyroid gland surgery), autoimmune disorders or genetic inborn errors of metabolism. A blood sample is obtained by separately reportable venipuncture. Parathyroid gland tissue is obtained by separately reportable fine needle aspirate. Serum/plasma or tissue sample are tested using quantitative electrochemiluminescent immunoassay. Plasma is tested for parathyroid hormone, CAP (cyclase activating parathyroid hormone) using immunoradiometric assay.

RVUs

Code	Work	PE	PE Non-Facility	MP	Total Non-Facility	Total Facility	Global
83970	0.00	0.00	0.00	0.00	0.00	0.00	XXX

84100-84105

84100 Phosphorus inorganic (phosphate)

84105 Phosphorus inorganic (phosphate); urine

(Pituitary gonadotropins, see 83001-83002)

(PKU, see 84030, 84035)

Plain English Description

A blood or urine test is performed to measure inorganic phosphorus (phosphate) levels. Phosphate is an intracellular anion, found primarily in bone and soft tissue. It plays an important role in cellular energy (nerve and muscle function) and the building/repair of bone and teeth. Decreased levels are most often caused by malnutrition and lead to muscle and neurological dysfunction. Elevated levels may be due to kidney or parathyroid gland problems. In 84100, a blood sample is obtained by separately reportable venipuncture. Serum/

plasma is tested using quantitative spectrophotometry. In 84105, a 24-hour or random urine sample is obtained. Urine is tested using quantitative spectrophotometry.

RVUs

Code	Work	PE	PE Non-Facility	MP	Total Non-Facility	Total Facility	Global
84100	0.00	0.00	0.00	0.00	0.00	0.00	XXX
84105	0.00	0.00	0.00	0.00	0.00	0.00	XXX

84156

84156 Protein, total, except by refractometry; urine

Plain English Description

A urine test is performed to measure total protein levels. Protein is not normally found in urine and usually indicates damage or disease in the kidneys. Elevated levels are often present in patients with diabetes, hypertension, and multiple myeloma. A 24-hour or random urine sample is obtained and tested using quantitative spectrophotometry.

RVUs

Code	Work	PE	PE Non-Facility	MP	Total Non-Facility	Total Facility	Global
84156	0.00	0.00	0.00	0.00	0.00	0.00	XXX

84165

84165 Protein; electrophoretic fractionation and quantitation, serum

Plain English Description

A blood test is performed to measure protein levels in serum. This test is often performed in conjunction with total protein (84155) to detect pathophysiologic states such as inflammation, gammopathies, and dysproteinemias. There are more sensitive tests available to detect these and similar disorders. A blood sample is obtained by separately reportable venipuncture. Serum is tested using electrophoretic fractionation and quantitation.

RVUs

Code	Work	PE	PE Non-Facility	MP	Total Non-Facility	Total Facility	Global
84165	0.00	0.00	0.00	0.00	0.00	0.00	XXX

84436-84439

84436 Thyroxine; total
84437 Thyroxine; requiring elution (eg, neonatal)
84439 Thyroxine; free

Plain English Description

A blood sample is obtained and levels of total thyroxin (84436), thyroxine requiring elution as for testing in neonates (84437), or free thyroxine (84439) are evaluated. Thyroxine, also referred to as T4, is tested to determine whether the thyroid is functioning properly and is used to aid in the diagnosis of overactive (hyperthyroidism) or underactive (hypothyroidism) thyroid function. In 84436, total thyroxine levels are evaluated. Total thyroxine measures the total amount of both bound and unbound (free) thyroxine in the blood. In 84437, a thyroxine level requiring elution is performed. This test is typically performed on neonates using cord blood to diagnose congenital hypothyroidism. In 84439, free thyroxine levels are tested. Free thyroxine is the amount of active thyroxine in the blood. Free thyroxine levels are considered to be a more accurate indicator of thyroid function. All thyroxine tests use electrochemiluminescent immunoassay methodology.

RVUs

Code	Work	PE	PE Non-Facility	MP	Total Non-Facility	Total Facility	Global
84436	0.00	0.00	0.00	0.00	0.00	0.00	XXX
84437	0.00	0.00	0.00	0.00	0.00	0.00	XXX
84439	0.00	0.00	0.00	0.00	0.00	0.00	XXX

84443

84443 Thyroid stimulating hormone (TSH)

Plain English Description

A blood test is performed to determine levels of thyroid stimulating hormone (TSH). TSH is produced in the pituitary and helps to regulate two other thyroid hormones, triiodothyronine (T3) and thyroxin (T4), which in turn help regulate the body's metabolic processes. TSH levels are tested to determine whether the thyroid is functioning properly. Patients with symptoms of weight gain, tiredness, dry skin, constipation, or menstrual irregularities may have an underactive thyroid (hypothyroidism). Patients with symptoms of weight loss, rapid heart rate, nervousness, diarrhea, feeling of being too hot, or menstrual irregularities may have an overactive thyroid (hyperthyroidism). TSH levels are also periodically tested in individuals on thyroid medications. The test is performed by electrochemiluminescent immunoassay.

RVUs

Code	Work	PE	PE Non-Facility	MP	Total Non-Facility	Total Facility	Global
84443	0.00	0.00	0.00	0.00	0.00	0.00	XXX

84450

84450 Transferase; aspartate amino (AST) (SGOT)

Plain English Description

A blood test is performed to measure aspartate aminotransferase (AST) levels. This enzyme was previously referred to as serum glutamic oxaloacetic transaminase (SGOT). AST is an enzyme found primarily in liver and muscle cells. Elevated levels may result from liver disease or damage, such as hepatitis, cirrhosis, ischemia, drug toxicity, and/or muscle damage, especially cardiac muscle (myocardial infarction). This test is often ordered in conjunction with alanine transferase, ALT (84460) or other liver function tests to diagnose disease and monitor individuals taking cholesterol lowering medications. A blood sample is obtained by separately reportable venipuncture. Serum and/or plasma is tested using quantitative enzymatic method.

RVUs

Code	Work	PE	PE Non-Facility	MP	Total Non-Facility	Total Facility	Global
84450	0.00	0.00	0.00	0.00	0.00	0.00	XXX

84460

84460 Transferase; alanine amino (ALT) (SGPT)

Plain English Description

A blood test is performed to measure alanine aminotransferase (ALT) levels. This enzyme was previously referred to as serum glutamic pyruvic transaminase (SGPT). ALT is an enzyme found primarily in liver and muscle cells. Elevated levels may result from liver disease or damage, such as hepatitis, cirrhosis, ischemia, drug toxicity, and/or muscle damage, especially cardiac muscle (myocardial infarction). This test is often ordered in conjunction with aspartate transferase, AST (84450) or other liver function tests to diagnose disease and monitor individuals taking cholesterol lowering medications. A blood sample is obtained by separately reportable venipuncture. Serum and/or plasma is tested using quantitative enzymatic method.

RVUs

Code	Work	PE	PE Non-Facility	MP	Total Non-Facility	Total Facility	Global
84460	0.00	0.00	0.00	0.00	0.00	0.00	XXX

84520

84520 Urea nitrogen; quantitative

Plain English Description

A blood sample is obtained to measure total (quantitative) urea nitrogen (BUN) level. Urea is a waste product produced in the liver by the breakdown of protein from a sequence of chemical reactions referred to as the urea or Krebs-Henseleit cycle. Urea then enters the bloodstream, is taken up by the kidneys, and excreted in the urine. Blood BUN is measured to evaluate renal function, to monitor patients with renal disease, and to evaluate effectiveness of dialysis. BUN may also be measured in patients with acute or chronic illnesses that affect renal function. BUN is measured using spectrophotometry.

RVUs

Code	Work	PE	PE Non-Facility	MP	Total Non-Facility	Total Facility	Global
84520	0.00	0.00	0.00	0.00	0.00	0.00	XXX

84550

84550 Uric acid; blood

Plain English Description

A blood test is performed to measure uric acid levels. Uric acid forms from the natural breakdown of body cells and the food we ingest. Uric acid is normally filtered by the kidneys and excreted in urine. Elevated blood levels may result from kidney disease, certain cancers and/or cancer therapies, hemolytic or sickle cell anemia, heart failure, cirrhosis, lead poisoning, and low levels of thyroid or parathyroid hormones. Levels may be decreased in Wilson's disease, poor dietary intake of protein, and with the use of certain drugs. A blood sample is obtained by separately reportable venipuncture. Serum/plasma is tested using quantitative spectrophotometry.

RVUs

Code	Work	PE	PE Non-Facility	MP	Total Non-Facility	Total Facility	Global
84550	0.00	0.00	0.00	0.00	0.00	0.00	XXX

85025-85027

85025 Blood count; complete (CBC), automated (Hgb, Hct, RBC, WBC and platelet count) and automated differential WBC count

85027 Blood count; complete (CBC), automated (Hgb, Hct, RBC, WBC and platelet count)

Plain English Description

An automated complete blood count (CBC) is performed with or without automated differential white blood cell (WBC) count. A CBC is used as a screening test to evaluate overall health and symptoms such as fatigue, bruising, bleeding, and inflammation, or to help diagnose infection. A CBC includes measurement of Hgb and Hct, RBC count, WBC count with or without differential, and platelet count. Hgb measures the amount of oxygen-carrying protein in the blood. Hct refers to the volume of red blood cells (erythrocytes) in a given volume of blood and is usually expressed as a percentage of total blood volume. RBC count is the number of red blood cells (erythrocytes) in a specific volume of blood. WBC count is the number of white blood cells (leukocytes) in a specific volume of blood. There are five types of WBCs: neutrophils, eosinophils, basophils, monocytes, and lymphocytes. If a differential is performed, each of the five types is counted separately. Platelet count is the number of platelets (thrombocytes) in the blood. Platelets are responsible for blood clotting. The CBC is performed with an automated blood cell-counting instrument that can also be programmed to provide an automated WBC differential count. Use 85025 for CBC with automated differential WBC count or 85027 for CBC without differential WBC count.

RVUs

Code	Work	PE	PE Non-Facility	MP	Total Non-Facility	Total Facility	Global
85025	0.00	0.00	0.00	0.00	0.00	0.00	XXX
85027	0.00	0.00	0.00	0.00	0.00	0.00	XXX

85576

85576 Platelet, aggregation (in vitro), each agent

(For thromboxane metabolite[s], including thromboxane, if performed, measurement[s] in urine, use 84431)

Plain English Description

A laboratory test is performed to measure platelet aggregation, the ability of platelets to clump together and form a blood clot. In vitro aggregation adds known platelet activators such as ADP, arachidonic acid, thrombin, epinephrine, or ristocetin to whole blood samples and monitors the platelet response. This test may be used to screen at risk patients prior to surgery, monitor platelet function during surgery, detect aspirin resistance, diagnose and evaluate excessive bruising/bleeding disorders, and monitor effectiveness of anti-platelet therapy. Ristocetin activator testing may help subtype von Willebrand syndrome. A blood sample is obtained by separately reportable venipuncture. Whole blood is tested using aggregation, quantitative aggregation, or light transmission aggregometry.

RVUs

Code	Work	PE	PE Non-Facility	MP	Total Non-Facility	Total Facility	Global
85576	0.00	0.00	0.00	0.00	0.00	0.00	XXX

85610-85611

85610 Prothrombin time

85611 Prothrombin time; substitution, plasma fractions, each

Plain English Description

Prothrombin time (PT) measures how long it takes for blood to clot. Prothrombin, also called factor II, is one of the clotting factors made by the liver and adequate levels of vitamin K are needed for the liver to produce sufficient prothrombin. Prothrombin time is used to help identify the cause of abnormal bleeding or bruising; to check whether blood-thinning medication, such as warfarin (Coumadin), is working; to check for low levels of blood-clotting factors I, II, V, VII, and X; and to check for low levels of vitamin K; to check liver function, to see how quickly the body is using up its clotting factors. The test is performed using electromagnetic mechanical clot detection. If prothrombin time is elevated and the patient is not on a blood-thinning medication, a second prothrombin time using substitution plasma fractions (85611), also referred to as a prothrombin time mixing study, may be performed. This is performed by mixing patient plasma with normal plasma using a 1:1 mix. The mixture is incubated and the clotting time is again measured. If the result does not correct, it may be indicative that the patient has an inhibitor, such as lupus anticoagulant. If the result does correct, the patient may have a coagulation factor deficiency. Code 85611 is reported for each prothrombin time mixing study performed.

RVUs

Code	Work	PE	PE Non-Facility	MP	Total Non-Facility	Total Facility	Global
85610	0.00	0.00	0.00	0.00	0.00	0.00	XXX
85611	0.00	0.00	0.00	0.00	0.00	0.00	XXX

85651-85652

85651 Sedimentation rate, erythrocyte; non-automated

85652 Sedimentation rate, erythrocyte; automated

Plain English Description

A blood sample is obtained and a non-automated erythrocyte sedimentation rate (ESR) performed. This test may also be referred to as a Westergren ESR. ESR is a non-specific test used to identify conditions associated with acute and chronic inflammation, such as infection, cancer, and autoimmune diseases. ESR is typically used in conjunction with other tests that can more specifically identify the cause of the inflammatory process. The blood sample is anti-coagulated and placed in a tall thin tube. The distance erythrocytes (red blood cells) have fallen in one hour in a vertical column under the influence of gravity is then measured. In 85652, an automated ESR is performed. The blood sample is anti-coagulated, aspirated, and put into the automated system. An automated sedimentation rate reading is provided after the required sedimentation time has elapsed. There are a number of different automated systems available and the technique varies slightly depending on the automated system used.

RVUs

Code	Work	PE	PE Non-Facility	MP	Total Non-Facility	Total Facility	Global
85651	0.00	0.00	0.00	0.00	0.00	0.00	XXX
85652	0.00	0.00	0.00	0.00	0.00	0.00	XXX

86038-86039

86038 Antinuclear antibodies (ANA)

86039 Antinuclear antibodies (ANA); titer

(Antistreptococcal antibody, ie, anti-DNAse, use 86215)

(Antistreptokinase titer, use 86590)

Plain English Description

A blood sample is obtained to screen for the presence of antinuclear antibodies (ANA) (86038) or to measure the concentration of antinuclear antibody in the blood, which is referred to as an ANA titer (86039). Antinuclear antibodies are auto-antibodies that bind to structures within the nucleus of cells. Auto-antibodies are a type of antibody that is directed against the body's own tissues. The presence and concentration of antinuclear antibodies may indicate one of several autoimmune disorders that cause inflammation of body tissues, including systemic lupus erythematosus, Sjogrens syndrome, rheumatoid arthritis, polymyositis, scleroderma, Hashimoto's thyroiditis, juvenile diabetes mellitus, Addison disease, vitiligo, pernicious anemia, glomerulonephritis, and pulmonary fibrosis. When testing for antinuclear antibodies, the specimen is typically screened first (86038) using an enzyme-linked immunosorbent assay (ELISA) If the screening test is positive, that is if antinuclear antibodies are detected, a titer (86039) is then obtained. An antinuclear antibody titer is performed by diluting the blood sample with increasing amounts of a saline solution and retesting until antinuclear antibodies are no longer detectable. ANA titer is expressed as 1:10, 1:20, 1:40, 1:80, etc., with the "1" indicating "one" part blood and the second number indicating the parts of saline solution. A higher second number indicates a higher concentration of antinuclear antibodies in the blood.

RVUs

Code	Work	PE	PE Non-Facility	MP	Total Non-Facility	Total Facility	Global
86038	0.00	0.00	0.00	0.00	0.00	0.00	XXX
86039	0.00	0.00	0.00	0.00	0.00	0.00	XXX

86140

86140 C-reactive protein

(Candidiasis, use 86628)

Plain English Description

A blood test is performed to measure C-reactive protein (CRP) levels. This standard test has a wide value range. CRP is an acute phase protein, synthesized by the liver and released in response to inflammation and infection. The test is not diagnostic for any specific disease or condition but can be used as a marker to monitor the body's response to treatment(s) or to evaluate the need for further testing. Elevation of CRP levels may be found during pregnancy, with the use of oral contraceptives, or hormone replacement therapy. Diseases/conditions that cause an elevation of CRP include: lymphoma, arteritis/vasculitis, osteomyelitis, inflammatory bowel disease, rheumatoid arthritis, pelvic inflammatory disease (PID), systemic lupus erythematosus (SLE), acute infections, burns, surgical procedures, and organ transplants. A blood sample is obtained by separately reportable venipuncture. Serum in neonates is tested using immunoassay. Serum/plasma in all other patients is tested using quantitative immunoturbidimetric method.

RVUs

Code	Work	PE	PE Non-Facility	MP	Total Non-Facility	Total Facility	Global
86140	0.00	0.00	0.00	0.00	0.00	0.00	XXX

86235

86235 Extractable nuclear antigen, antibody to, any method (eg, nRNP, SS-A, SS-B, Sm, RNP, Sc170, J01), each antibody

Plain English Description

A blood test is performed to measure extractable nuclear antigen or antibody to it. One or more of these antibodies are typically elevated in autoimmune diseases such as Sjogren yndrome, polymyositis, systemic lupus erythematosus, and progressive systemic sclerosis. Many are included in comprehensive panels that screen for multiple antibodies at one time. A blood sample is obtained by separately reportable venipuncture and tested by any method, particularly semiquantitative multi-analyte fluorescent detection. Report once for each antibody, such as SSA (Ro) (ENA) Antibody, IgG; Jo-1 Antibody, IgG; scleroderma (Scl-70) (ENA) Antibody, IgG; Smith (ENA) Antibody, IgG; SSB (La) (ENA) Antibody, IgG; and RNP (U1) (Ribonucleic Protein) (ENA) Antibody, IgG.

RVUs

Code	Work	PE	PE Non-Facility	MP	Total Non-Facility	Total Facility	Global
86235	0.00	0.00	0.00	0.00	0.00	0.00	XXX

86592-86593

86592 Syphilis test, non-treponemal antibody; qualitative (eg, VDRL, RPR, ART)

(For antibodies to infectious agents, see 86602-86804)

86593 Syphilis test, non-treponemal antibody; quantitative

(For antibodies to infectious agents, see 86602-86804)

(Tetanus antibody, use 86774)

(Thyroglobulin antibody, use 86800)

(Thyroglobulin, use 84432)

(Thyroid microsomal antibody, use 86376)

(For toxoplasma antibody, see 86777-86778)

Plain English Description

A test for syphilis is performed. Syphilis is a sexually transmitted disease (STD) caused by the bacterium Treponema pallidum. During the primary stage, a sore called a chancre appears at the site where the syphilis bacterium entered the body. The chancre resolves without treatment in 3-6 weeks but the patient remains infected. Without treatment, the infection will progress to a secondary stage in which a skin rash and mucous membrane lesions appear. The most common site of the rash is the palms of the hands and soles of the feet. Other symptoms during the secondary stage include fever, swollen lymph nodes, sore throat, hair loss, headaches, weight loss, muscle aches, and fatigue. Symptoms of secondary syphilis also resolve spontaneously but the patient remains infected. The patient then enters the late or latent stage of the disease. Symptoms of this stage may not appear for 10-20 years. Symptoms of late stage syphilis include difficulty coordinating muscle movements, paralysis, numbness, gradual blindness, and dementia. These symptoms occur as the disease damages internal organs including the brain, nerves, eyes, heart, blood vessels, liver, bones, and joints. Of particular concern is undiagnosed syphilis infection during pregnancy as the infection can be passed to the baby in utero. This increases the risk of stillbirth or death shortly after birth. Untreated infants who survive often experience developmental delays or seizures. In 86592, a qualitative syphilis test, such as the venereal disease research laboratory (VDRL) test, rapid plasma reagin (RPR) test, or automated reagin test (ART) is used. The VDRL, RPR, and ART are nontreponemal tests that measure antibody response to lipoidal antigen from T. pallidum and/or antibody interaction with host tissues. If a screening test is positive and the result is confirmed with a second confirmatory test, quantitative testing is then performed to determine disease activity and monitor response to treatment. Quantitative testing may be performed by enzyme linked immunosorbent assay (ELISA). Use 86593 for quantitative testing. Both qualitative and quantitative tests can be performed on blood or, in the case of suspected central nervous system involvement, the test may be performed on cerebral spinal fluid (CSF).

RVUs

Code	Work	PE	PE Non-Facility	MP	Total Non-Facility	Total Facility	Global
86592	0.00	0.00	0.00	0.00	0.00	0.00	XXX
86593	0.00	0.00	0.00	0.00	0.00	0.00	XXX

86618

86618 Antibody; Borrelia burgdorferi (Lyme disease)

Plain English Description

A laboratory test is performed to measure Borrelia burgdorferi (Lyme disease) antibodies in serum and/or cerebral spinal fluid (CSF). This test is used for first line screening when a patient has symptoms of Lyme disease infection and lives or has visited an area endemic to black legged ticks. It is most reliable when performed within four weeks of a tick bite and the appearance of erythema migrans (bull's eye) rash. The presence of C6 peptide antibodies to B. burgdorferi is considered a stand-alone diagnostic test for Lyme disease. IgM antibodies will be positive within 2-3 weeks of exposure and may also be used to diagnose early disease. IgG antibodies rise with early exposure but do not peak until 4-6 months after the initial infection. A positive test for C6 peptide antibodies is often followed with screening for IgG and IgM antibodies. Positive or equivocal test results for C6 peptide, IgM and IgG antibodies should always be reflexed for a Western Blot or immunoblot confirmation test. A blood sample is obtained by separately reportable venipuncture; CSF by separately reportable lumbar puncture. Serum and CSF are tested using semi-quantitative enzyme-linked immunosorbent assay (ELISA).

RVUs

Code	Work	PE	PE Non-Facility	MP	Total Non-Facility	Total Facility	Global
86618	0.00	0.00	0.00	0.00	0.00	0.00	XXX

86780

86780 Antibody; Treponema pallidum

(For syphilis testing by non-treponemal antibody analysis, see 86592-86593)

Plain English Description

An antibody test for Treponema pallidum, the causative agent of syphilis, is performed using a technique such as fluorescent treponemal antibody absorption (FTA-ABS), T. pallidum particle agglutination (TP-PA), or indirect fluorescent antibody (IFA). Syphilis is a sexually transmitted disease (STD). During the primary stage of syphilis, a sore called a chancre appears at the site where the syphilis bacterium entered the body. The chancre resolves without treatment in three to six weeks but the patient remains infected and without treatment the infection will progress to a secondary stage. During the second stage, a skin rash and mucous membrane lesions appear. The most common site of the rash is the palms of the hands and soles of the feet. Other symptoms during the secondary stage include fever, swollen lymph nodes, sore throat, hair loss, headaches, weight loss, muscle aches, and fatigue. Symptoms of secondary syphilis also resolve spontaneously but the patient remains infected. The patient then enters the late or latent stage of the disease and symptoms of this stage may not appear for 10-20 years. Symptoms of late stage syphilis include difficulty coordinating muscle movements, paralysis, numbness, gradual blindness, and dementia. These symptoms occur as the disease damages internal organs including the brain, nerves, eyes, heart, blood vessels, liver, bones, and joints. Of particular concern is undiagnosed syphilis infection during pregnancy as the infection can be passed to the baby in utero. This increases the risk of stillbirth or of a live born infant dying shortly after birth. Untreated infants who survive often experience developmental delays or seizures. The FTA-ABS and IFA tests can be performed on blood or cerebral spinal fluid (CSF) samples. TP-PA is used only on blood samples.

RVUs

Code	Work	PE	PE Non-Facility	MP	Total Non-Facility	Total Facility	Global
86780	0.00	0.00	0.00	0.00	0.00	0.00	XXX

88302-88309

88302 Level II - Surgical pathology, gross and microscopic examination

Appendix, incidental; Fallopian tube, sterilization; Fingers/toes, amputation, traumatic; Foreskin, newborn; Hernia sac, any location; Hydrocele sac; Nerve; Skin, plastic repair; Sympathetic ganglion; Testis, castration; Vaginal mucosa, incidental; Vas deferens, sterilization

88304 Level III - Surgical pathology, gross and microscopic examination

Abortion, induced; Abscess; Aneurysm - arterial/ventricular; Anus, tag; Appendix, other than incidental; Artery, atheromatous plaque; Bartholin's gland cyst; Bone fragment(s), other than pathologic fracture; Bursa/synovial cyst; Carpal tunnel tissue; Cartilage, shavings; Cholesteatoma; Colon, colostomy stoma; Conjunctiva - biopsy/pterygium; Cornea; Diverticulum - esophagus/small intestine; Dupuytren's contracture tissue; Femoral head, other than fracture; Fissure/fistula; Foreskin, other than newborn; Gallbladder; Ganglion cyst; Hematoma; Hemorrhoids; Hydatid of Morgagni; Intervertebral disc; Joint, loose body; Meniscus; Mucocele, salivary; Neuroma - Morton's/traumatic; Pilonidal cyst/sinus; Polyps, inflammatory - nasal/sinusoidal; Skin - cyst/tag/debridement; Soft tissue, debridement; Soft tissue, lipoma; Spermatocele; Tendon/tendon sheath; Testicular appendage; Thrombus or embolus; Tonsil and/or adenoids; Varicocele; Vas deferens, other than sterilization; Vein, varicosity

88305 Level IV - Surgical pathology, gross and microscopic examination

Abortion - spontaneous/missed; Artery, biopsy; Bone marrow, biopsy; Bone exostosis; Brain/meninges, other than for tumor resection; Breast, biopsy, not requiring microscopic evaluation of surgical margins; Breast, reduction mammoplasty; Bronchus, biopsy; Cell block, any source; Cervix, biopsy; Colon, biopsy; Duodenum, biopsy; Endocervix, curettings/biopsy; Endometrium, curettings/biopsy; Esophagus, biopsy; Extremity, amputation, traumatic; Fallopian tube, biopsy; Fallopian tube, ectopic pregnancy; Femoral head, fracture; Fingers/toes, amputation, non-traumatic; Gingiva/oral mucosa, biopsy; Heart valve; Joint, resection; Kidney, biopsy; Larynx, biopsy; Leiomyoma(s), uterine myomectomy - without uterus; Lip, biopsy/wedge resection; Lung, transbronchial biopsy; Lymph node, biopsy; Muscle, biopsy; Nasal mucosa, biopsy; Nasopharynx/oropharynx, biopsy; Nerve, biopsy; Odontogenic/dental cyst; Omentum, biopsy; Ovary with or without tube, non-neoplastic; Ovary, biopsy/wedge resection; Parathyroid gland; Peritoneum, biopsy; Pituitary tumor; Placenta, other than third trimester; Pleura/pericardium - biopsy/tissue; Polyp, cervical/endometrial; Polyp, colorectal; Polyp, stomach/small intestine; Prostate, needle biopsy; Prostate, TUR; Salivary gland, biopsy; Sinus, paranasal biopsy; Skin, other than cyst/tag/debridement/plastic repair; Small intestine, biopsy; Soft tissue, other than tumor/mass/lipoma/debridement; Spleen; Stomach, biopsy; Synovium; Testis, other than tumor/biopsy/castration; Thyroglossal duct/brachial cleft cyst; Tongue, biopsy; Tonsil, biopsy; Trachea, biopsy; Ureter, biopsy; Urethra, biopsy; Urinary bladder, biopsy; Uterus, with or without tubes and ovaries, for prolapse; Vagina, biopsy; Vulva/labia, biopsy

88307 Level V - Surgical pathology, gross and microscopic examination

Adrenal, resection; Bone - biopsy/curettings; Bone fragment(s), pathologic fracture; Brain, biopsy; Brain/meninges, tumor resection; Breast, excision of lesion, requiring microscopic evaluation of surgical margins; Breast, mastectomy - partial/simple; Cervix, conization; Colon, segmental resection, other than for tumor; Extremity, amputation, non-traumatic; Eye, enucleation; Kidney, partial/total nephrectomy; Larynx, partial/total resection; Liver, biopsy - needle/wedge; Liver, partial resection; Lung, wedge biopsy; Lymph nodes, regional resection; Mediastinum, mass; Myocardium, biopsy; Odontogenic tumor; Ovary with or without tube, neoplastic; Pancreas, biopsy; Placenta, third trimester; Prostate, except radical resection; Salivary gland; Sentinel lymph node; Small intestine, resection, other than for tumor; Soft tissue mass (except lipoma) - biopsy/simple excision; Stomach - subtotal/total resection, other than for tumor; Testis, biopsy; Thymus, tumor; Thyroid, total/lobe; Ureter, resection; Urinary bladder, TUR; Uterus, with or without tubes and ovaries, other than neoplastic/prolapse

88309 Level VI - Surgical pathology, gross and microscopic examination

Bone resection; Breast, mastectomy - with regional lymph nodes; Colon, segmental resection for tumor; Colon, total resection; Esophagus, partial/total resection; Extremity, disarticulation; Fetus, with dissection; Larynx, partial/total resection - with regional lymph nodes; Lung - total/lobe/segment resection; Pancreas, total/subtotal resection; Prostate, radical resection; Small intestine, resection for tumor; Soft tissue tumor, extensive resection; Stomach - subtotal/total resection for tumor; Testis, tumor; Tongue/tonsil -resection for tumor; Urinary bladder, partial/total resection; Uterus, with or without tubes and ovaries, neoplastic; Vulva, total/subtotal resection

(For fine needle aspiration biopsy, see 10004, 10005, 10006, 10007, 10008, 10009, 10010, 10011, 10012, 10021)

(For evaluation of fine needle aspirate, see 88172-88173)

(Do not report 88302-88309 on the same specimen as part of Mohs surgery)

Plain English Description

Tissue removed during a surgical procedure, such as a biopsy, excision, or resection, is examined macroscopically (gross or visual examination) and then under a microscope. The cells, tissues, or organ are transported from the surgical suite to the pathologist. The pathologist first visually examines the specimen and notes any defining characteristics. The specimen is then prepared for microscopic evaluation. The physician carefully analyzes the specimens to help establish a diagnosis, identify the presence or absence of malignant neoplasm, identify the exact type of malignancy if present, and examine the margins of the specimen to determine whether or not the entire diseased area was removed. A written report of findings is then prepared and a copy sent to the treating physician. Pathology services are reported based on the type of tissue examined, whether or not the tissue is expected to be normal or diseased, the difficulty of the pathology exam, and the time required to complete the exam. Use 88302 for a Level II pathology examination; 88304 for a Level III exam; 88305 for a Level IV exam; 88307 for a Level V exam; and 88309 for a Level VI exam.

RVUs

Code	Work	PE	PE Non-Facility	MP	Total Non-Facility	Total Facility	Global
88302	0.13	0.72	0.72	0.02	0.87	0.87	XXX
88304	0.22	0.92	0.92	0.02	1.16	1.16	XXX
88305	0.75	1.21	1.21	0.02	1.98	1.98	XXX
88307	1.59	6.15	6.15	0.06	7.80	7.80	XXX
88309	2.80	8.97	8.97	0.08	11.85	11.85	XXX

88312-88313

88312 Special stain including interpretation and report; Group I for microorganisms (eg, acid fast, methenamine silver)

(Report one unit of 88312 for each special stain, on each surgical pathology block, cytologic specimen, or hematologic smear)

88313 Special stain including interpretation and report; Group II, all other (eg, iron, trichrome), except stain for microorganisms, stains for enzyme constituents, or immunocytochemistry and immunohistochemistry

(Report one unit of 88313 for each special stain, on each surgical pathology block, cytologic specimen, or hematologic smear)

(For immunocytochemistry and immunohistochemistry, use 88342)

Plain English Description

Special staining techniques are sometimes required to visualize micro-organisms or cell and tissue structures. Staining is composed of a number of steps beginning with fixation of the specimen using a fixative or by freezing to prevent damage to the internal structure of the organism, cell, or tissue. If tissue is being evaluated, the tissue must be prepared for slicing and then sliced into very thin sections using a vibratome. The specimen is then treated with a variety of reagents, solutions, and stains designed to highlight specific features or components of the micro-organism, cell, or tissue. The specimen is then examined under a microscope. The staining results are interpreted and a written report of findings is provided. Use code 88312 for Group I special stains for micro-organisms; use 88313 for Group II special stains for all other specimens excluding stains for micro-organisms, stains for enzyme constituents, and immunohistochemistry.

RVUs

Code	Work	PE	PE Non-Facility	MP	Total Non-Facility	Total Facility	Global
88312	0.54	2.41	2.41	0.02	2.97	2.97	XXX
88313	0.24	1.88	1.88	0.02	2.14	2.14	XXX

88314

✚ **88314 Special stain including interpretation and report; histochemical stain on frozen tissue block (List separately in addition to code for primary procedure)**

(Use 88314 in conjunction with 17311-17315, 88302-88309, 88331, 88332)

(Do not report 88314 with 17311-17315 for routine frozen section stain [eg, hematoxylin and eosin, toluidine blue], performed during Mohs surgery. When a nonroutine histochemical stain on frozen tissue during Mohs surgery is utilized, report 88314 with modifier 59)

(Report one unit of 88314 for each special stain on each frozen surgical pathology block)

(For a special stain performed on frozen tissue section material to identify enzyme constituents, use 88319)

(For determinative histochemistry to identify chemical components, use 88313)

Plain English Description

Histochemical staining of tissue involves the use of one or more stains that add color to the tissue components making it easier to evaluate the tissue and cell structure. Frozen blocks are used because freezing stabilizes the internal structure of the tissue and prevents cell lysis. The tissue may be embedded in epoxy resin so that it can be sliced into thin sections. A vibratome is used to slice the tissue, which may be treated with a variety of reagents or solutions prior to staining. The tissue is stained. Two examples of histochemical staining techniques are Golgi silver impregnation staining and Nissl staining using cresyl violet. The specimen is examined under a microscope. The staining results are interpreted and a written report of findings is provided. Use 88314 for each tissue block examined using histochemical stains.

RVUs

Code	Work	PE	PE Non-Facility	MP	Total Non-Facility	Total Facility	Global
88314	0.45	2.26	2.26	0.02	2.73	2.73	XXX

88319

88319 Special stain including interpretation and report; Group III, for enzyme constituents

(For each stain on each surgical pathology block, cytologic specimen, or hematologic smear, use one unit of 88319)

(For detection of enzyme constituents by immunohistochemical or immunocytochemical technique, use 88342)

Plain English Description

Special stains of blood, bone marrow, or tissue are performed to identify enzyme constituents. Cytochemical stains for enzyme constituents are used to aid in identification of abnormal cells and to provide additional diagnostic information about normal appearing cells. Staining of blood or bone marrow, or organ imprints for enzyme constituents is performed using a fresh specimen that is smeared onto a slide. A fixative is applied to adhere the specimen to the slide. The slide is then washed and the staining reagent is applied. The slide is washed again and additional counterstaining is performed as needed to enhance detail. A control sample of normal cells is also stained at the same time for quality control purposes. The presence or absence of enzyme activity for the specific enzyme being tested is represented by the presence or absence and relative intensity of the stain in various constituents of blood, bone marrow, or tissue cells. Examples of some types of stains for enzyme constituents include tartrate resistant acid phosphatase stain, myeloperoxidase (MPO) stain, and chloroacetate esterase stain.

RVUs

Code	Work	PE	PE Non-Facility	MP	Total Non-Facility	Total Facility	Global
88319	0.53	2.60	2.60	0.02	3.15	3.15	XXX

88341-88344

88342 Immunohistochemistry or immunocytochemistry, per specimen; initial single antibody stain procedure

(For quantitative or semiquantitative immunohistochemistry, see 88360, 88361)

88344 Immunohistochemistry or immunocytochemistry, per specimen; each multiplex antibody stain procedure

(Do not use more than one unit of 88341, 88342, or 88344 for the same separately identifiable antibody per specimen)

(Do not report 88341, 88342, 88344 in conjunction with 88360, 88361 unless each procedure is for a different antibody)

(When multiple separately identifiable antibodies are applied to the same specimen [ie, multiplex antibody stain procedure], use one unit of 88344)

(When multiple antibodies are applied to the same slide that are not separately identifiable, [eg, antibody cocktails], use 88342, unless an additional separately identifiable antibody is also used, then use 88344)

Plain English Description

Immunohistochemistry or immunocytochemistry identifies a certain antigen by using an antibody specific to that antigen when examining cells contained in a specimen, such as a tissue block, brushed cell samples, blood smear, or fine needle biopsy (FNB). The specimen is prepped for histological or cytological examination on a glass slide that has been fixed with a commercially available antibody. Enzymes and/or special stains are then applied to the specimen slide. The characteristic changes to the cells in the sample can help determine the antigenic profile of morphologically undifferentiated cells, and aid in the diagnosis of malignant neoplasms. The prepped slide specimen may be used to identify a single antibody or multiple antibodies. Use code 88342 for the first identifiable single antibody per slide/stain procedure. Use code 88341 for each additional single antibody. Use code 88344 when multiple separately identifiable antibodies are applied to the same slide/stain specimen.

RVUs

Code	Work	PE	PE Non-Facility	MP	Total Non-Facility	Total Facility	Global
88342	0.70	2.25	2.25	0.02	2.97	2.97	XXX
88344	0.77	4.07	4.07	0.02	4.86	4.86	XXX

88356

88356 Morphometric analysis; nerve

Plain English Description

A laboratory test is performed for pathological analysis and calculation of intraepidermal nerve fiber (IENF) density and/or sweat gland nerve fiber (SGNF) density in a skin punch biopsy to diagnose peripheral nerve disease targeting small nerve fibers. Small fiber neuropathy (SFN) is characterized by sensory pain in the extremities with normal electromyography and nerve conduction studies and no evidence of large fiber neuropathic disease. Conditions associated with SFN include diabetes, HIV, systemic lupus erythematosus, and neurosarcoidosis. A skin punch biopsy is obtained from the lower extremity, preferably the calf. The tissue is sectioned by microtome and immunostained with anti-protein-gene-product 9.5 antibodies. The tissue is visually examined using immunohistochemical or immunofluorescent technique to identify the morphology of small sensory fibers innervating the skin. The number of intraepidermally originating nerve fibers crossing the basement membrane between the dermis and epidermis are counted in several sections, the total length of the epidermis is measured, and a calculation is performed to find the number of nerve fibers/mm. This number is compared to normative data of nerve fiber density to support or rule out a diagnosis of SFN.

RVUs

Code	Work	PE	PE Non-Facility	MP	Total Non-Facility	Total Facility	Global
88356	2.80	3.76	3.76	0.10	6.66	6.66	XXX

90662

90662 Influenza virus vaccine (IIV), split virus, preservative free, enhanced immunogenicity via increased antigen content, for intramuscular use

Plain English Description

Unlike immune globulins that provide short-term, passive immunity, a vaccine provides active, long-term immunity by exposing the recipient's immune system to altered versions of specific viruses or bacteria that induce the immune system to produce its own antibodies against the invading micro-organism. The body then remembers how to make antibodies when exposed to the antigen again. A preservative-free, split-virus influenza vaccine with increased antigen content for enhanced immunogenicity has significantly more hemagglutinin per influenza strain in each vaccine and provides an improved immune response. The preservative-free formulation trace amount is either thimerosal-free or thimerosal-reduced. The FDA considers both to be preservative-free and both are labeled as such. Like other split-virus influenza vaccines, this formulation is developed in embryonated chicken eggs. The fluid containing the virus is harvested and inactivated with formaldehyde. The influenza virus is concentrated using a technique that increases antigen content and purified. This is followed by chemical disruption to create a split virus and further purification. The enhanced immunogenicity split-virus influenza vaccine is indicated for use in the elderly, where immune responsiveness is reduced. A preservative-free, enhanced immunogenicity, split-virus influenza vaccine is administered by intramuscular injection, which is reported separately. This code reports only the product (vaccine) used.

RVUs

Code	Work	PE	PE Non-Facility	MP	Total Non-Facility	Total Facility	Global
90662	0.00	0.00	0.00	0.00	0.00	0.00	XXX

90674

90674 Influenza virus vaccine, quadrivalent (ccIIV4), derived from cell cultures, subunit, preservative and antibiotic free, 0.5 mL dosage, for intramuscular use

Plain English Description

Unlike immune globulins which provide short-term, passive immunity, a vaccine provides active, long-term immunity by exposing the recipient's immune system to altered versions of specific viruses or bacteria that induce the immune system to produce its own antibodies against the invading micro-organism. The body then remembers how to make antibodies when exposed to the antigen again. A preservative and antibiotic-free influenza virus vaccine derived from cell cultures (ccIIV4) is different from other influenza vaccine formulations in that it is produced from cell cultures in master and working cell banks in a sterile, controlled environment. Influenza vaccine produced in this manner does not require embryonated eggs, antibiotics, or preservatives, and is a non-allergenic, preservative-free, antibiotic-free formulation. Quadrivalent influenza vaccines are formulated with four influenza viruses, which include two different influenza type A strains and two influenza type B strains. Code

90674 reports a 0.5mL dosage of a quadrivalent, preservative and antibiotic-free, influenza virus vaccine derived from cell cultures to be administered intramuscularly. This code reports only the product (vaccine) used.

RVUs

Code	Work	PE	PE Non-Facility	MP	Total Non-Facility	Total Facility	Global
90674	0.00	0.00	0.00	0.00	0.00	0.00	XXX

90685-90686

90685 Influenza virus vaccine, quadrivalent (IIV4), split virus, preservative free, 0.25 mL dosage, for intramuscular use

90686 Influenza virus vaccine, quadrivalent (IIV4), split virus, preservative free, 0.5 mL dosage, for intramuscular use

Plain English Description

A quadrivalent, split virus, preservative-free influenza vaccine (IIV4) product for intramuscular use is provided. Unlike immune globulins which provide short-term, passive immunity, a vaccine provides active, long-term immunity by exposing the recipient's immune system to altered versions of specific viruses or bacteria that induce the immune system to produce its own antibodies against the invading micro-organism. The body then remembers how to make antibodies when exposed to the antigen again. A preservative-free formulation does not contain the preservative thimerosal, or contains only trace amounts, and is either thimerosal-free or thimerosal-reduced. The FDA considers both to be preservative-free and both are labeled as such. This vaccine is administered by intramuscular injection, which is reported separately. Influenza vaccine is developed in embryonated chicken eggs. Fluid containing the virus is then harvested and inactivated with formaldehyde. The influenza virus is concentrated and purified, followed by chemical disruption to create a split virus and further purification. Quadrivalent influenza vaccines are formulated for protection against 4 influenza viruses, which include two different influenza type A strains and two influenza type B strains. Report code 90685 for a 0.25 mL dosage of the vaccine to be administered intramuscularly and code 90686 for a 0.5 mL dosage. These codes report only the product (vaccine) used. Report the intramuscular injection separately.

RVUs

Code	Work	PE	PE Non-Facility	MP	Total Non-Facility	Total Facility	Global
90685	0.00	0.00	0.00	0.00	0.00	0.00	XXX
90686	0.00	0.00	0.00	0.00	0.00	0.00	XXX

90791-90792

★ **90791 Psychiatric diagnostic evaluation**

★ **90792 Psychiatric diagnostic evaluation with medical services**

(Do not report 90791 or 90792 in conjunction with 99201-99337, 99341-99350, 99366-99368, 99401-99443, 97151, 97152, 97153, 97154, 97155, 97156, 97157, 97158, 0362T, 0373T)

(Use 90785 in conjunction with 90791, 90792 when the diagnostic evaluation includes interactive complexity services)

Plain English Description

Code 90791 reports a psychiatric diagnostic interview exam including a complete medical and psychiatric history, a mental status exam, ordering of laboratory and other diagnostic studies with interpretation, and communication with other sources or informants. The psychiatrist then establishes a tentative diagnosis and determines the patient's capacity to benefit from psychotherapy treatment. The patient's condition will determine the extent of the mental status exam needed during the diagnostic interview. In determining mental status, the doctor looks for symptoms of psychopathology in appearance, attitude, behavior, speech, stream of talk, emotional reactions, mood, and content of thoughts, perceptions, and sometimes cognition. The diagnostic interview exam is done when the provider first sees a patient, but may also be utilized again for a new episode of illness, or for re-admission as an inpatient due to underlying complications. When a psychiatric diagnostic evaluation is performed alone, report code 90791. When medical services are provided in conjunction with the psychiatric diagnostic evaluation, report code 90792.

RVUs

Code	Work	PE	PE Non-Facility	MP	Total Non-Facility	Total Facility	Global
90791	3.00	0.43	0.92	0.11	4.03	3.54	XXX
90792	3.25	0.60	1.10	0.11	4.46	3.96	XXX

90832-90838

★ **90832 Psychotherapy, 30 minutes with patient**

★+ **90833 Psychotherapy, 30 minutes with patient when performed with an evaluation and management service (List separately in addition to the code for primary procedure)**

(Use 90833 in conjunction with 99201-99255, 99304-99337, 99341-99350)

★ **90834 Psychotherapy, 45 minutes with patient**

★+ **90836 Psychotherapy, 45 minutes with patient when performed with an evaluation and management service (List separately in addition to the code for primary procedure)**

(Use 90836 in conjunction with 99201-99255, 99304-99337, 99341-99350)

★ **90837 Psychotherapy, 60 minutes with patient**

(Use the appropriate prolonged services code [99354, 99355, 99356, 99357] for psychotherapy services not performed with an E/M service of 90 minutes or longer face-to-face with the patient)

Plain English Description

Individual psychotherapy is provided to a patient utilizing re-education, support and reassurance, insight discussions, and occasionally medication to affect behavior modification through self-understanding, or to evaluate and improve family relationship dynamics as they relate to the patient's condition. If psychotherapy alone is provided, report 90832 for 30 minutes, 90834 for 45 minutes, and 90837 for 60 minutes. If medical evaluation and management services are performed with the psychotherapy, report code 90833 for 30 minutes, 90836 for 45 minutes, and 90838 for 60 minutes.

RVUs

Code	Work	PE	PE Non-Facility	MP	Total Non-Facility	Total Facility	Global
90832	1.50	0.21	0.41	0.06	1.97	1.77	XXX
90833	1.50	0.28	0.46	0.06	2.02	1.84	ZZZ
90834	2.00	0.28	0.54	0.08	2.62	2.36	XXX
90836	1.90	0.35	0.58	0.08	2.56	2.33	ZZZ
90837	3.00	0.42	0.81	0.11	3.92	3.53	XXX

90867-90869

90867 Therapeutic repetitive transcranial magnetic stimulation (TMS) treatment; initial, including cortical mapping, motor threshold determination, delivery and management

(Report only once per course of treatment)

(Do not report 90867 in conjunction with 90868, 90869, 95860, 95870, 95928, 95929, 95939)

90868 Therapeutic repetitive transcranial magnetic stimulation (TMS) treatment; subsequent delivery and management, per session

90869 Therapeutic repetitive transcranial magnetic stimulation (TMS) treatment; subsequent motor threshold re-determination with delivery and management

(Do not report 90869 in conjunction with 90867, 90868, 95860-95870, 95928, 95929, 95939)

(If a significant, separately identifiable evaluation and management, medication management, or psychotherapy service is performed, the appropriate E/M or psychotherapy code may be reported in addition to 90867-90869. Evaluation and management activities directly related to cortical mapping, motor threshold determination, delivery and management of TMS are not separately reported)

Plain English Description

Repetitive transcranial magnetic stimulation (rTMS) is used primarily to treat depression in individuals who have not responded to other treatment modalities. rTMS may also be used as a treatment for anxiety, obsessive compulsive disorder, auditory hallucinations, and migraines. In these disorders, one part of the brain is overactive or sluggish. For example, the left prefrontal cortex is less active in people with depression. The procedure involves the use of magnetic fields to stimulate nerve cells in the region of the brain associated with the mood or other disorder. A large electromagnetic coil is placed against the scalp over the appropriate region of the brain. The electromagnetic coil delivers painless electric currents that stimulate the nerve cells. This therapy alters the brain's biochemistry, the firing patterns of neurons in the cortex, and the levels of neurotransmitters, such as serotonin. In 90867, in an initial planning, treatment, and management session, the physician determines the best sites on the forehead for placement of the magnets, the optimal rate of stimulating pulses, and the optimal dose of magnetic energy for treatment. The electromagnetic coil is placed against the forehead and switched on and off at a rate of up to 10 times per second. When the device is on, it delivers stimulating pulses that result in a tapping or clicking sound and a tapping sensation on the head. During the mapping process, the optimal site is identified by moving the electromagnetic coils and the optimal rate of the pulses is determined by varying the pulse rate. The physician then determines the optimal dose. The energy delivered is increased until the fingers or hands twitch to determine the motor threshold. Once the motor threshold has been determined, the physician calculates the optimal dose. During the course of treatment, the optimal dose may be adjusted depending on the response to treatment and side effects. Use 90868 for each subsequent delivery and management session when motor threshold does not require adjustment. During each subsequent treatment session, the magnets are placed on the head and the optimal level and duration of stimulation is delivered. Use 90869 for each subsequent delivery and management session requiring motor threshold re-determination. During each subsequent treatment session following re-determination of motor threshold, the magnets are placed on the head and the optimal level and duration of stimulation is delivered.

RVUs

Code	Work	PE	PE Non-Facility	MP	Total Non-Facility	Total Facility	Global
90867	0.00	0.00	0.00	0.00	0.00	0.00	000
90868	0.00	0.00	0.00	0.00	0.00	0.00	000
90869	0.00	0.00	0.00	0.00	0.00	0.00	000

90901

90901 Biofeedback training by any modality

Plain English Description

Biofeedback training is provided to help a patient learn to control automatic bodily responses. While biofeedback cannot cure disease, it can help patients learn to control physical responses that influence their health. Biofeedback is used by a variety of specialists to treat physical conditions, such as migraine headaches and other types of pain, digestive system disorders, high or low blood pressure, cardiac arrhythmias, Raynaud's disease, epilepsy, paralysis due to stroke, or cerebral palsy. Biofeedback includes identification of triggers that bring on symptoms and the use of relaxation techniques to help control symptoms. A clinician places electrical sensors on different parts of the body that monitor muscle tension, increased heart rate, temperature, or other physiologic signs. The sensors are attached to a biofeedback machine that provides cues such as a beeping sound or flashing light to indicate physiologic changes, such as increased muscle tension or heart rate, changes in temperature, or other physiological responses. The patient then responds by concentrating on reducing muscle tension, slowing heart rate, modifying temperature, or providing another appropriate response to the biofeedback information. A typical biofeedback training session lasts from 30 to 60 minutes. The patient is also required to practice biofeedback methods at home on a day-to-day basis to help modify and control physiological responses.

RVUs

Code	Work	PE	PE Non-Facility	MP	Total Non-Facility	Total Facility	Global
90901	0.41	0.14	0.72	0.02	1.15	0.57	000

90935-90937

90935 Hemodialysis procedure with single evaluation by a physician or other qualified health care professional

90937 Hemodialysis procedure requiring repeated evaluation(s) with or without substantial revision of dialysis prescription

Plain English Description

A nurse or technician inserts two needles into a previously created vascular access site. The vascular access site may be a surgically created internal fistula or shunt, an internal graft, or less commonly a central venous catheter. Each needle is attached to a separate piece of flexible plastic tubing that is connected to the dialysis machine. One tube removes blood from the body. The blood is circulated through the dialysis machine and then returned to the body through the second tube. The blood circulating through the dialysis machine passes on one side of a membrane and dialysis fluid passes on the other. The wastes and excess fluid pass from the blood through the membrane and into the dialysis fluid. These wastes are discarded with the dialysis fluid. The cleansed blood is returned to the bloodstream through the second tube. The hemodialysis procedure includes all evaluation and management services performed on the date of the dialysis procedure that are related to the patient's renal disease. Code 90935 is used when a single evaluation and management service is performed on the date of the hemodialysis procedure. Code 90937 is used when repeated evaluation and management services are required during the course of the hemodialysis procedure.

RVUs

Code	Work	PE	PE Non-Facility	MP	Total Non-Facility	Total Facility	Global
90935	1.48	0.51	0.51	0.09	2.08	2.08	000
90937	2.11	0.74	0.74	0.12	2.97	2.97	000

90945-90947

90945 Dialysis procedure other than hemodialysis (eg, peritoneal dialysis, hemofiltration, or other continuous renal replacement therapies), with single evaluation by a physician or other qualified health care professional

(For home infusion of peritoneal dialysis, use 99601, 99602)

90947 Dialysis procedure other than hemodialysis (eg, peritoneal dialysis, hemofiltration, or other continuous renal replacement therapies) requiring repeated evaluations by a physician or other qualified health care professional, with or without substantial revision of dialysis prescription

Plain English Description

A dialysis procedure other than hemodialysis with related evaluation services is performed. Types of dialysis procedures performed include peritoneal dialysis, hemofiltration, or other continuous renal replacement therapies. Peritoneal dialysis, hemofiltration, and other continuous renal replacement therapies filter blood continuously without interruption. If peritoneal dialysis is performed, a nurse or technician instills dialysis fluid through a previously placed abdominal catheter. The dialysis solution contains the sugar dextrose, which pulls wastes and extra fluid out of the blood through the peritoneal membrane and into the abdominal cavity. The dialysis fluid remains in the abdominal cavity for a period of four to six hours after which the dialysis solution along with the wastes and excess fluid is removed from the abdomen through the catheter. This process of filling and draining the abdomen may be repeated several times during the day. Hemofiltration may be performed by an arteriovenous or venovenous procedure. In an arteriovenous procedure, the femoral artery is cannulated. Arterial pressure forces blood through a filter into the femoral vein. Water and soluble waste products filter from the blood through a permeable membrane and are discarded. The cleansed blood is returned to the body with replacement fluid of physiologically balanced water and electrolytes. The procedure for venovenous filtration is similar. A double lumen catheter is placed in the femoral, subclavian, or internal jugular vein. A pump is used to push blood from the vein through the dialysis circuit. The cleansed blood is then pushed back into the same vein. Code 90945 is used when a single evaluation and management service is performed on the date of the peritoneal dialysis, hemofiltration, or other continuous renal replacement therapy. Code 90947 is used when repeated evaluation and management services are required during the course of the peritoneal dialysis procedure, hemofiltration procedure, or other continuous renal replacement therapy procedure.

RVUs

Code	Work	PE	PE Non-Facility	MP	Total Non-Facility	Total Facility	Global
90945	1.56	0.79	0.79	0.09	2.44	2.44	000
90947	2.52	0.87	0.87	0.15	3.54	3.54	000

90960-90962

★ **90960 End-stage renal disease (ESRD) related services monthly, for patients 20 years of age and older; with 4 or more face-to-face visits by a physician or other qualified health care professional per month**

★ **90961 End-stage renal disease (ESRD) related services monthly, for patients 20 years of age and older; with 2-3 face-to-face visits by a physician or other qualified health care professional per month**

90962 End-stage renal disease (ESRD) related services monthly, for patients 20 years of age and older; with 1 face-to-face visit by a physician or other qualified health care professional per month

Plain English Description

End-stage renal disease (ESRD) related services are provided per one full month in an outpatient setting to a patient 20 years of age and older. The physician or other qualified health care professional establishes the dialyzing cycle, performs outpatient evaluation and management services related to the dialysis services, and provides oversight and management of the patient during the dialysis service as well as telephone follow-up as needed for the entire month. The patient is examined on a routine basis for existing and potential medical problems, and is seen as needed when new symptoms or problems develop. The physician or other qualified health care professional ensures that dialysis services are being provided as prescribed and makes adjustments to the dialysis prescription as needed. Laboratory data are reviewed. Medications and nutritional supplements are monitored, and changes are made as needed. The physician or other qualified health care professional also establishes, monitors, and coordinates care, which may include social service interventions, nutritional support, kidney transplant planning, and services provided by other medical and/or surgical specialists. These ESRD services are included in one code, which is reported only once per month based on the number of face-to-face visits. Code 90960 is for 4 or more face-to-face visits per month; code 90961 is for 2-3 face-to-face visits per month; and code 90962 reports 1 face-to-face visit per month.

RVUs

Code	Work	PE	PE Non-Facility	MP	Total Non-Facility	Total Facility	Global
90960	5.18	2.58	2.58	0.31	8.07	8.07	XXX
90961	4.26	2.26	2.26	0.26	6.78	6.78	XXX
90962	3.15	1.89	1.89	0.19	5.23	5.23	XXX

90966

90966 End-stage renal disease (ESRD) related services for home dialysis per full month, for patients 20 years of age and older

Plain English Description

End-stage renal disease (ESRD) related services are provided for one full month for home dialysis for patients 20 years of age and older. The physician establishes the dialyzing cycle, performs outpatient evaluation and management services related to the home dialysis services, and provides oversight and management of the patient during the dialysis as well as telephone follow-up as needed for the entire month. The physician examines the patient on a routine basis for existing and potential medical problems. The patient is seen as needed when new symptoms or problems develop. The physician ensures that dialysis services are being provided as prescribed and makes adjustments to the dialysis prescription as needed. Laboratory data are reviewed. Medications and nutritional supplements are monitored, and changes are made as needed. The physician also establishes, monitors, and coordinates care, which may include social service interventions, nutritional support, kidney transplant planning, and services provided by other medical and/or surgical specialists.

RVUs

Code	Work	PE	PE Non-Facility	MP	Total Non-Facility	Total Facility	Global
90966	4.26	2.25	2.25	0.26	6.77	6.77	XXX

90967-90970

90967 End-stage renal disease (ESRD) related services for dialysis less than a full month of service, per day; for patients younger than 2 years of age

90968 End-stage renal disease (ESRD) related services for dialysis less than a full month of service, per day; for patients 2-11 years of age

90969 End-stage renal disease (ESRD) related services for dialysis less than a full month of service, per day; for patients 12-19 years of age

90970 End-stage renal disease (ESRD) related services for dialysis less than a full month of service, per day; for patients 20 years of age and older

Plain English Description

End-stage renal disease (ESRD) services are provided per day in an outpatient setting when less than a full month of service is required. Outpatient ESRD services may be provided for only part of a month due to inpatient hospitalization or initiation of the services after the first of the month. The physician establishes the dialyzing cycle, performs outpatient evaluation and management services related to the dialysis services, and provides oversight and management of the patient during the dialysis as well as telephone follow-up as needed. The physician examines the patient on a routine basis for existing and potential medical problems. The patient is seen as needed when new symptoms or problems develop. The physician ensures that dialysis services are being provided as prescribed and makes adjustments to the dialysis prescription as needed. The physician monitors the patient's weight, makes recommendations regarding the patient's diet and fluid intake, and prescribes special renal supplement formula as needed. Laboratory data are reviewed. Medications and nutritional supplements are monitored and changes are made as needed. The physician also establishes, monitors, and coordinates care, which may include social service interventions, nutritional support, kidney transplant planning, and services provided by other medical and/or surgical specialists. For younger patients, the physician initiates the necessary interventions for delays in growth or development, which may include injection of growth hormones. Social development is monitored and any behavioral or school problems are addressed by making referrals and intervening as needed. The physician counsels the parents and/or caregivers and responds to questions and concerns. These ESRD services are age-specific and reported on a daily basis. Code 90967 is for patients younger than 2; code 90968 is for patients aged 2-11; code 90969 is for patients 12-19 years of age; and code 90970 is for patients aged 20 or older.

RVUs

Code	Work	PE	PE Non-Facility	MP	Total Non-Facility	Total Facility	Global
90967	0.35	0.14	0.14	0.02	0.51	0.51	XXX
90968	0.30	0.13	0.13	0.02	0.45	0.45	XXX
90969	0.29	0.12	0.12	0.02	0.43	0.43	XXX
90970	0.14	0.08	0.08	0.01	0.23	0.23	XXX

92060

92060 Sensorimotor examination with multiple measurements of ocular deviation (eg, restrictive or paretic muscle with diplopia) with interpretation and report (separate procedure)

Plain English Description

An extended sensorimotor examination is performed to evaluate eye movement. The test is performed bilaterally. Motor function is tested by taking ocular alignment measurements as the eyes focus on different locations. More than one field of gaze is tested at distance and/or near. In adults and children who are old enough and able to respond, at least one sensory test, such as Titmus fly, Worth 4 dot, Maddox rod, or Bagolini lens test, is also performed. Any deviations in normal eye movements are documented. Test results are interpreted and a report of findings provided.

RVUs

Code	Work	PE	PE Non-Facility	MP	Total Non-Facility	Total Facility	Global
92060	0.69	1.08	1.08	0.02	1.79	1.79	XXX

92083

92083 Visual field examination, unilateral or bilateral, with interpretation and report; extended examination (eg, Goldmann visual fields with at least 3 isopters plotted and static determination within the central 30°, or quantitative, automated threshold perimetry, Octopus program G-1, 32 or 42, Humphrey visual field analyzer full threshold programs 30-2, 24-2, or 30/60-2)

(Gross visual field testing (eg, confrontation testing) is a part of general ophthalmological services and is not reported separately)

(For visual field assessment by patient activated data transmission to a remote surveillance center, see 0378T, 0379T)

Plain English Description

A visual field examination tests the total area in which the patient can see objects within the peripheral vision while focusing on a central point. One or both eyes are tested for loss of peripheral vision and causative conditions, such as glaucomatous optic nerve damage and retinal disease. One eye is completely covered while the other is tested. An extended examination includes more comprehensive quantitative automated perimetry tests with multilevel threshold testing or manual perimetry tests with 3 isopters on Goldman visual field and static determination within central 30 degrees. The Octopus and the Humphrey-Zeiss field analyzer are popular automated devices that test static perimetry running a choice of programs (such as Octopus program G-1, 32, or 42 or Humphrey full threshold programs 30-2, 24-2, or 30/60-2) by an onboard computer. They employ stationary pinpoint light sources or dots projected within a large, white bowl. The patient focuses on a central point and pushes a button when he/she sees the light or movement in different locations or at different intensities. The computer stores the data and generates a vision field report. The traditional Goldman perimeter is a kinetic perimetry test process that utilizes moving light sources. A trained technician moves the light source and monitors that the patient maintains central focus fixation throughout the test. A map of peripheral vision perception intensity within specified degrees is then produced. Interpretation and report is included.

RVUs

Code	Work	PE	PE Non-Facility	MP	Total Non-Facility	Total Facility	Global
92083	0.50	1.26	1.26	0.02	1.78	1.78	XXX

92133-92134

92133 Scanning computerized ophthalmic diagnostic imaging, posterior segment, with interpretation and report, unilateral or bilateral; optic nerve

92134 Scanning computerized ophthalmic diagnostic imaging, posterior segment, with interpretation and report, unilateral or bilateral; retina

(Do not report 92133 and 92134 at the same patient encounter)

(For scanning computerized ophthalmic diagnostic imaging of the optic nerve and retina, see 92133, 92134)

Plain English Description

These tests may be performed on one or both eyes to evaluate diseases affecting the optic nerve or retina. Two different types of laser scanning devices are available, confocal laser scanning ophthalmoscopy (topography) and scanning laser polarimetry. Confocal laser scanning topography uses stereoscopic videographic digitized images to calculate measurements of anterior or posterior eye structures. Scanning laser polarimetry measures the change in linear polarization of light. This device employs a polarimeter, an optical device, and a scanning laser ophthalmoscope. The patient is told to fixate on an internal target generated by the computer. Multiple radial scans of the posterior segment of the eye are obtained. Scans may be obtained of the optic nerve head (92133) or the retina (92134). Digitized images are displayed on a monitor. The computer calculates optic nerve head measurements, retinal thickness, or other measurements. The digitized images and measurements are evaluated by the physician and then interpreted, with a written report provided.

RVUs

Code	Work	PE	PE Non-Facility	MP	Total Non-Facility	Total Facility	Global
92133	0.40	0.63	0.63	0.02	1.05	1.05	XXX
92134	0.45	0.68	0.68	0.02	1.15	1.15	XXX

92250

92250 Fundus photography with interpretation and report

Plain English Description

Fundus photography is the use of a retinal camera to take pictures of the inside of the back of the eye. Fundus photography may look at the optic nerve, macula, vitreous, the retina, and its vasculature. The highly specialized retinal camera is mounted on a microscope that contains high-powered, intricate lenses and mirrors. The lenses capture images of the back of the eye when light is focused through the cornea, the pupil, and the lens. The pupils are dilated with drops to prevent them from constricting at the bright light. The patient is instructed to stare at one fixation point to keep the eyes still. Pictures are then taken as a series of flashes of bright light are focused through the eye and camera lens. Fundus photography is performed to evaluate abnormalities, follow the progress of a disease, assess therapeutic effects and surgical treatments, and plan for future treatment. Diseases that indicate a need for fundus photography include retinal neoplasms, macular degeneration, diabetic retinopathy, glaucoma, multiple sclerosis, and other central nervous system problems.

RVUs

Code	Work	PE	PE Non-Facility	MP	Total Non-Facility	Total Facility	Global
92250	0.40	0.85	0.85	0.02	1.27	1.27	XXX

92507-92508

92507 Treatment of speech, language, voice, communication, and/or auditory processing disorder; individual

(Do not report 92507 in conjunction with 97153, 97155)

92508 Treatment of speech, language, voice, communication, and/or auditory processing disorder; group, 2 or more individuals

(Do not report 92508 in conjunction with 97154, 97158)

(For auditory rehabilitation, prelingual hearing loss, use 92630)

(For auditory rehabilitation, postlingual hearing loss, use 92633)

(For cochlear implant programming, see 92601-92604)

Plain English Description

A speech-language pathologist treats a speech, language, voice, communication, and/or auditory processing disorder. Using the information obtained from a separately reportable screening and in-depth evaluation of a speech or language disorder, the clinician develops an individualized treatment plan for the patient. The clinician defines specific treatment goals and sets baseline measures with which to assess the patient's progress. These goals are continuously monitored and fine-tuned throughout the treatment period. Once the goals and baseline measures have been established the clinician uses a number of intervention activities to correct the specific speech or language disorder identified. These can include games, stories, rhymes, drills, and other tasks. If the patient has a speech disorder, the clinician may demonstrate the sounds and have the patient copy the way the clinician moves the lips, mouth, and tongue to make the right sound. A mirror may be used so that the patient can practice making the sound while observing himself or herself in the mirror. Treatment of a language disorder might include help with grammar. If the patient is having difficulty with auditory processing, a game like Simon Says might be used to help improve understanding of verbal instructions. Code 92507 is used for individual treatment of speech, language, voice, communication, and/or auditory processing disorder. Code 92508 is used when these services are provided to a group of two or more individuals.

RVUs

Code	Work	PE	PE Non-Facility	MP	Total Non-Facility	Total Facility	Global
92507	1.30	0.90	0.90	0.05	2.25	2.25	XXX
92508	0.33	0.34	0.34	0.01	0.68	0.68	XXX

92522

92522 Evaluation of speech sound production (eg, articulation, phonological process, apraxia, dysarthria)

Plain English Description

Speech sound production disorders affect an individual's ability to communicate. There may be an organic cause for the problem (hearing impairment, cleft lip/palate, cerebral palsy, ankyloglossia) or it may be functional with no known cause. Articulation disorders are characterized by substitution, distortion, omission or addition of sounds and words. Phonological processing disorders are characterized by a set pattern of sound errors. Although small mistakes are common and normal in young children who are developing language skills, when articulation disorders persist past the age of 8 or phonological processing mistakes continue past the age of 5, an evaluation by a speech-language pathologist (SLP) that includes an audiogram to assess hearing, formal and informal observation of speech and standardized testing with tools such as the Clinical Assessment of Articulation and Phonology (CAAP) is typically performed. Verbal apraxia is a condition in which an individual who does not have a diagnosed weakness or paralysis of the speech muscles has difficulty stating what he/she wants to communicate correctly and consistently. Acquired verbal apraxia can occur at any age and is due to changes in an area of the brain. Stroke, head injury, tumor or illness/infection can cause this type of change. Developmental verbal apraxia is present from birth. It can manifest as an overall language disorder or a neurologic disorder affecting signals to and movement of the muscles involved with speech. There may be a genetic link to developmental apraxia as it is often occurs in multiple family members. Dysarthria is a speech disturbance that may be caused by a brain injury or by paralysis, spasticity or lack of coordination of the speech muscles. Evaluation by a speech-language pathologist (SLP) typically includes an audiogram to assess hearing (reported separately), formal and informal observation of speech and assessment using standardized testing tools such as Screening Test for Developmental Apraxia of Speech.

RVUs

Code	Work	PE	PE Non-Facility	MP	Total Non-Facility	Total Facility	Global
92522	1.50	1.04	1.04	0.08	2.62	2.62	XXX

92537

92537 Caloric vestibular test with recording, bilateral; bithermal (ie, one warm and one cool irrigation in each ear for a total of four irrigations)

(Do not report 92537 in conjunction with 92270, 92538)

(For three irrigations, use modifier 52)

(For monothermal caloric vestibular testing, use 92538)

Plain English Description

A procedure is performed to measure vestibulo-ocular reflex (nystagmus) to validate a diagnosis of asymmetrical functioning of the peripheral vestibular system in patients with dizziness and/or balance problems. The patient is positioned supine at a 30 degree incline to bring the horizontal semi-circular canals located in the ear into a vertical plane. To measure the corneo-retinal potential using electrodes (electro-nystagmography, ENG), electrodes are placed on the skin around the forehead and eyes and the recording device is calibrated with the tracking software. To measure pupil eye movement using video-nystagmography (VNG), infra-red goggles are placed over the eyes and the recording device is calibrated with the tracking software. Each external auditory canal is then irrigated with water using a nozzle or syringe. Eye movement is recorded while the patient does "tasking" such as counting or naming to allow natural eye movements to occur. For bithermal caloric vestibular testing (92537), warm water irrigation followed by cold water irrigation is done in each ear sequentially with at least a 5 minute rest period between irrigations. For monothermal caloric vestibular testing (92538), a single bolus of ice water is infused into the external auditory canal of one ear and then the other.

RVUs

Code	Work	PE	PE Non-Facility	MP	Total Non-Facility	Total Facility	Global
92537	0.60	0.56	0.56	0.02	1.18	1.18	XXX

92538

92538 Caloric vestibular test with recording, bilateral; monothermal (ie, one irrigation in each ear for a total of two irrigations)

(Do not report 92538 in conjunction with 92270, 92537)

(For one irrigation, use modifier 52)

(For bilateral, bithermal caloric vestibular testing, use 92537)

Plain English Description

A procedure is performed to measure vestibulo-ocular reflex (nystagmus) to validate a diagnosis of asymmetrical functioning of the peripheral vestibular system in patients with dizziness and/or balance problems. The patient is positioned supine at a 30 degree incline to bring the horizontal semi-circular canals located in the ear into a vertical plane. To measure the corneo-retinal potential using electrodes (electro-nystagmography, ENG), electrodes are placed on the skin around the forehead and eyes and the recording device is calibrated with the tracking software. To measure pupil eye movement using video-nystagmography (VNG), infra-red goggles are placed over the eyes and the recording device is calibrated with the tracking software. Each external auditory canal is then irrigated with water using a nozzle or syringe. Eye movement is recorded while the patient does "tasking" such as counting or naming to allow natural eye movements to occur. For bithermal caloric vestibular testing (92537), warm water irrigation followed by cold water irrigation is done in each ear sequentially with at least a 5 minute rest period between irrigations. For monothermal caloric vestibular testing (92538), a single bolus of ice water is infused into the external auditory canal of one ear and then the other.

RVUs

Code	Work	PE	PE Non-Facility	MP	Total Non-Facility	Total Facility	Global
92538	0.30	0.32	0.32	0.02	0.64	0.64	XXX

92540

92540 Basic vestibular evaluation, includes spontaneous nystagmus test with eccentric gaze fixation nystagmus, with recording, positional nystagmus test, minimum of 4 positions, with recording, optokinetic nystagmus test, bidirectional foveal and peripheral stimulation, with recording, and oscillating tracking test, with recording

(Do not report 92540 in conjunction with 92270, 92541, 92542, 92544, 92545)

Plain English Description

A vestibular evaluation is performed for nystagmus, which is a rapid, involuntary movement of the eye. Nystagmus tests are performed to identify the presence of a vestibular disorder characterized by vertigo (dizziness) and balance disturbance including the inability to maintain balance, to stand upright, or to walk with a normal gait. The physician first observes eye movement with the naked eye. The tests are performed with recording using electronystagmography (ENG). Horizontal electrodes are placed on the skin at the inner and outer aspect of each eye. A spontaneous nystagmus test with eccentric gaze and fixation is performed. For gaze testing, the patient first looks straight ahead for 30 seconds and then fixates on a target 30 degrees to the right for 10 seconds. The gaze is then returned to center. This is repeated with gaze directed to the left, up, and down. A positional nystagmus test is performed in a minimum of four positions to identify vertigo and nystagmus associated with certain movements of the head or body. Positional nystagmus is associated with disorders of function of the semicircular canals of the middle ear. Standard testing positions include head hanging forward, supine, supine with head turned to right, supine with head turned to left, lateral left, lateral right, or any other position that causes dizziness. Eye movement is recorded. A minimum of four positions are tested and any abnormal eye movement noted. An optokinetic nystagmus (OKN) test with bidirectional, foveal, or peripheral stimulation is performed. Eye movements are recorded and measured as the patient watches a series of targets moving simultaneously to the right and then to the left. The types of targets used include stripes on a rotating drum, a stream of lighted dots across a light bar, or a full-field array of moving stars or trees. The targets are moved at a rate of 300, 400, or 600 feet per second. This test generates eye movements that resemble nystagmus. The physician evaluates the symmetry of the response. If the response is not symmetrical it may be indicative of central nervous system pathology. An oscillating tracking test is performed. The test evaluates the patient's ability to keep a moving visual target registered on the fovea. The patient tracks a pendulum, metronome, light, or computer generated stimulus as it moves back and forth along a smooth arc or path. Eye movement is recorded. A computer is used to calculate the gain, expressed as target velocity divided by eye velocity. This calculation is compared to age-matched norms. Upon completion of the vestibular evaluation, the recordings are reviewed and interpreted, and the physician provides a written report of findings.

RVUs

Code	Work	PE	PE Non-Facility	MP	Total Non-Facility	Total Facility	Global
92540	1.50	1.48	1.48	0.06	3.04	3.04	XXX

92541

92541 Spontaneous nystagmus test, including gaze and fixation nystagmus, with recording

(Do not report 92541 in conjunction with 92270, 92540 or the set of 92542, 92544, and 92545)

Plain English Description

A spontaneous nystagmus test with gaze evoked nystagmus (GEN) and fixation nystagmus is performed with recording using electronystagmography (ENG). Nystagmus is a rapid, involuntary movement of the eye. Nystagmus tests are performed to identify the presence of a vestibular disorder characterized by vertigo (dizziness) and balance disturbance including the inability to maintain balance, stand upright, or walk with a normal gait. The physician first observes eye movement with the naked eye. Tests are then conducted using a recording device. Horizontal electrodes are placed on the skin at the inner and outer aspect of each eye. Each eye is tested separately. For gaze testing, the patient first looks straight ahead for 30 seconds and then fixates on a target 30 degrees to the right for 10 seconds. The gaze is then returned to center. This is repeated with gaze directed to the left, up, and down. The test is conducted using targets placed on the wall or ceiling or with computer generated targets. To test spontaneous nystagmus, it is important to eliminate any suppression of eye movement in order to note abnormal movements. The physician reviews the ENG, and analyzes and interprets the results of the tests.

RVUs

Code	Work	PE	PE Non-Facility	MP	Total Non-Facility	Total Facility	Global
92541	0.40	0.30	0.30	0.02	0.72	0.72	XXX

92542

92542 Positional nystagmus test, minimum of 4 positions, with recording

(Do not report 92542 in conjunction with 92270, 92540 or the set of 92541, 92544, and 92545)

Plain English Description

A positional nystagmus test is performed in a minimum of four positions with recording using electronystagmography (ENG). Nystagmus is a rapid, involuntary movement of the eye. Nystagmus tests are performed to identify the presence of a vestibular disorder characterized by vertigo (dizziness) and balance disturbance, including the inability to maintain balance, stand upright, or walk with a normal gait. Positional nystagmus tests are performed to identify vertigo and nystagmus associated with certain movements of the head or body due to functional disorders of the semicircular canals of the middle ear. The physician first observes eye movement with the naked eye. Tests are then conducted using a recording device. Horizontal electrodes are placed on the skin at the inner and outer aspect of each eye. Standard testing positions include head hanging forward, supine, supine with head turned to the right, supine with head turned to the left, lateral left, lateral right, or any other position that causes dizziness. Eye movement is then recorded. A minimum of four positions are tested and any abnormal eye movement is noted. The physician reviews the ENG recording, and analyzes and interprets the results.

RVUs

Code	Work	PE	PE Non-Facility	MP	Total Non-Facility	Total Facility	Global
92542	0.48	0.34	0.34	0.02	0.84	0.84	XXX

92546

92546 Sinusoidal vertical axis rotational testing

(Do not report 92546 in conjunction with 92270)

Plain English Description

A sinusoidal vertical axis rotational test is performed with recording using electronystagmography (ENG). The test evaluates the integrity of the vestibular-ocular system. The test reflects the relationship between natural head and eye movements involved in the balance mechanism. Horizontal electrodes are placed on the skin at the inner and outer aspect of each eye. The patient sits in a rotational chair. A slow, harmonic acceleration rotation lasting 30-40 minutes is typically performed under computer control and eye movement is recorded. The physician reviews the recording and analyzes and interprets the results.

RVUs

Code	Work	PE	PE Non-Facility	MP	Total Non-Facility	Total Facility	Global
92546	0.29	2.83	2.83	0.03	3.15	3.15	XXX

92547

✚ **92547 Use of vertical electrodes (List separately in addition to code for primary procedure)**

(Use 92547 in conjunction with 92540-92546)

(For unlisted vestibular tests, use 92700)

(Do not report 92547 in conjunction with 92270)

Plain English Description

Nystagmus tests are performed using electronystagmography (ENG) with vertical electrodes (leads). Electrodes with a vertical channel are placed around each eye. Eye movement is recorded. The physician reviews the recording and analyzes and interprets the results. The use of vertical electrodes is reported in addition to the code for the horizontal ENG recording of the primary procedure.

RVUs

Code	Work	PE	PE Non-Facility	MP	Total Non-Facility	Total Facility	Global
92547	0.00	0.24	0.24	0.00	0.24	0.24	ZZZ

92548-92549

▲ **92548 Computerized dynamic posturography sensory organization test (CDP-SOT), 6 conditions (ie, eyes open, eyes closed, visual sway, platform sway, eyes closed platform sway, platform and visual sway), including interpretation and report**

● **92549 Computerized dynamic posturography sensory organization test (CDP-SOT), 6 conditions (ie, eyes open, eyes closed, visual sway, platform sway, eyes closed platform sway, platform and visual sway), including interpretation and report; with motor control test (MCT) and adaptation test (ADT)**

(Do not report 92548, 92549 in conjunction with 92270)

Plain English Description

A computerized dynamic posturography (CDP) test is performed. CDP is used to evaluate balance impairments and differentiate between sensory, motor, and central adaptive causes of impaired balance. The patient stands on a moveable support surface inside a moveable enclosure. A computer is used to move the support surface and the enclosure. A sensory organization test (SOT), motor control test (MCT), and adaptation test (ADT) are performed. Sensory organization tests the patient's vestibular balance control and the adaptive responses of the central nervous system to perceived changes in the support surface resulting from changes in the visual display. Sensory conflict is created by eliminating useful visual and support surface information. SOT is performed with eyes open and closed, on a fixed and sway referenced surface, using fixed and sway referenced visual inputs. Motor control tests the patient's ability to quickly and automatically recover from unexpected movement in the support surface. During MCT. the support surface is moved backwards and forwards and the patient's postural responses are assessed for timing, strength, and lateral symmetry of the response. Adaptation tests the patient's ability to modify posture and minimize sway as the support surface is tilted in toes up and toes down positions. Measures are controlled and calibrated based on the patient's height and weight. Results are displayed using standardized graphical summaries that are compared to age-based norms.

RVUs

Code	Work	PE	PE Non-Facility	MP	Total Non-Facility	Total Facility	Global
92548	0.67	0.71	0.71	0.03	1.41	1.41	XXX
92549	0.87	0.90	0.90	0.03	1.80	1.80	XXX

92585-92586

92585 Auditory evoked potentials for evoked response audiometry and/or testing of the central nervous system; comprehensive

92586 Auditory evoked potentials for evoked response audiometry and/or testing of the central nervous system; limited

Plain English Description

Auditory evoked potentials for evoked response audiometry and/or testing of the central nervous system is performed to evaluate hearing loss and help identify conditions such as acoustic neuroma or vestibular schwannoma. In 92585, a comprehensive auditory evoked response (AER) examination is performed, which includes brainstem response with middle latency and late cortical responses. AER tests brainstem response to auditory (click) stimuli. The click is transmitted from an acoustic transducer by an earphone or headphone. The elicited waveform response is measured by surface electrodes typically placed on the forehead (vertex of the scalp) and earlobes. Another electrode configuration is placement on the forehead, nape of the neck (inverting), and either the shoulder or cheek. The amplitude of the signal is averaged and charted against time, similar to an EEG recording. The recording is then interpreted and a written report of findings is provided. In 92586, a limited audiometry examination is performed which tests only brainstem response and may also be referred to as an auditory brainstem response (ABR).

RVUs

Code	Work	PE	PE Non-Facility	MP	Total Non-Facility	Total Facility	Global
92585	0.50	3.28	3.28	0.04	3.82	3.82	XXX
92586	0.00	2.66	2.66	0.02	2.68	2.68	XXX

92610

92610 Evaluation of oral and pharyngeal swallowing function

(For motion fluoroscopic evaluation of swallowing function, use 92611)

(For flexible endoscopic examination, use 92612-92617)

Plain English Description

An evaluation of the oral and pharyngeal phase of the swallowing function is performed in a patient who is suspected of having oropharyngeal dysphagia. The initial evaluation represented by code 92610 is typically performed by a dysphagia specialist, usually a speech-language pathologist. This evaluation is performed to determine whether more extensive studies are warranted. Swallowing function is divided into oral, pharyngeal, and esophageal phases. The oral and pharyngeal phases are made up of oral preparation for solid foods (not required for liquids or pureed foods), oral transfer, and initiation of the swallow. Both oral and pharyngeal movements are necessary in preparing, transferring, and swallowing food. The patient is given both solids and liquids to swallow. During oral preparation of solid food the ability of the tongue to move the food from side-to-side so that the solid can be chewed and prepared for swallowing is evaluated. Once the solid food is prepared and transferred to the back of the throat, the swallowing movements are evaluated. Propelling solids or liquids requires a complex set of movements including retraction of the base of the tongue, elevation of the hyolaryngeal complex, closure of the velopharyngeal communication between the nasal cavity and the mouth, contraction of the pharynx, opening of the upper esophageal sphincter, and closure of the airway. The speech-language pathologist observes the patient to determine whether solids and liquids are being prepared, transferred, and propelled from the pharynx into the esophagus. A written report of findings is provided.

RVUs

Code	Work	PE	PE Non-Facility	MP	Total Non-Facility	Total Facility	Global
92610	1.30	0.71	1.11	0.06	2.47	2.07	XXX

93000-93010

93000 Electrocardiogram, routine ECG with at least 12 leads; with interpretation and report

93005 Electrocardiogram, routine ECG with at least 12 leads; tracing only, without interpretation and report

93010 Electrocardiogram, routine ECG with at least 12 leads; interpretation and report only

(For ECG monitoring, see 99354-99360)

(Do not report 93000, 93005, 93010 in conjunction with, 0525T, 0526T, 0527T, 0528T, 0529T, 0530T, 0531T, 0532T)

Plain English Description

An electrocardiogram (ECG) is used to evaluate the electrical activity of the heart. The test is performed with the patient lying prone on the exam table. Small plastic patches are attached at specific locations on the chest, abdomen, arms, and/or legs. Leads (wires) from the ECG tracing device are then attached to the patches. A tracing is obtained of the electrical signals from the heart. Electrical activity begins in the sinoatrial node, which generates an electrical stimulus at regular intervals, usually 60 to 100 times per minute. This stimulus travels through the conduction pathways to the sinoatrial node causing the atria to contract. The stimulus then travels along the bundle of His, which divides into right and left pathways providing electrical stimulation of the ventricles causing them to contract. Each contraction of the ventricles represents one heart beat. The ECG tracing includes the following elements: P wave, QRS complex, ST segment, and T wave. The P wave, a small upward notch in the tracing, indicates electrical stimulation of the atria. This is followed by the QRS complex, which indicates the ventricles are electrically stimulated to contract. The short flat ST segment follows and indicates the time between the end of the ventricular contraction and the T wave. The T wave represents the recovery period of the ventricles. The physician reviews, interprets, and provides a written report of the ECG recording taking care to note any abnormalities. Use 93000 to report the complete procedure, including ECG tracing with physician review, interpretation, and report; use 93005 to report the tracing only; and use 93010 to report physician interpretation and written report only.

RVUs

Code	Work	PE	PE Non-Facility	MP	Total Non-Facility	Total Facility	Global
93000	0.17	0.29	0.29	0.02	0.48	0.48	XXX
93005	0.00	0.23	0.23	0.01	0.24	0.24	XXX
93010	0.17	0.06	0.06	0.01	0.24	0.24	XXX

93040-93042

93040 Rhythm ECG, 1-3 leads; with interpretation and report

93041 Rhythm ECG, 1-3 leads; tracing only without interpretation and report

93042 Rhythm ECG, 1-3 leads; interpretation and report only

Plain English Description

Electrocardiography (ECG) is an interpretation of the electrical activity of the heart over time captured and externally recorded by skin electrodes placed in the thoracic area. It is a noninvasive recording produced by an electrocardiographic device that transmits information, displayed on a report, which indicates the overall rhythm of the heart and weaknesses in different parts of the heart muscle. It measures and diagnoses abnormal rhythms of the heart. In 93040, 1-3 leads are used and a report is generated. In 93041, only the procedure is reported. In 93042, only a physician report is generated without the procedure portion.

RVUs

Code	Work	PE	PE Non-Facility	MP	Total Non-Facility	Total Facility	Global
93040	0.15	0.19	0.19	0.02	0.36	0.36	XXX
93041	0.00	0.15	0.15	0.01	0.16	0.16	XXX
93042	0.15	0.04	0.04	0.01	0.20	0.20	XXX

93224-93227

93224 External electrocardiographic recording up to 48 hours by continuous rhythm recording and storage; includes recording, scanning analysis with report, review and interpretation by a physician or other qualified health care professional

93225 External electrocardiographic recording up to 48 hours by continuous rhythm recording and storage; recording (includes connection, recording, and disconnection)

93226 External electrocardiographic recording up to 48 hours by continuous rhythm recording and storage; scanning analysis with report

93227 External electrocardiographic recording up to 48 hours by continuous rhythm recording and storage; review and interpretation by a physician or other qualified health care professional

(For less than 12 hours of continuous recording, use modifier 52)

(For greater than 48 hours of monitoring, see Category III codes 0295T-0298T)

Plain English Description

Electrocardiographic (ECG) rhythm-derived data is gathered for up to 48 hours of monitoring as the patient goes about regular daily activity while wearing an external ECG recording device, also called a Holter monitor. Electrodes or leads are placed on the patient's chest, and the patient is instructed on the use of the monitor. The recording device makes continuous, original ECG wave recordings for a 12 to 48 hour period. The recordings are captured on magnetic tape or digitized medium to be reviewed later. At the end of the recording period, the patient returns to the office with the device. Stored data derived from the continuous recordings of the electrical activity of the heart include heart rhythm and rate, ST analysis, variability in heart rate and T-wave alternans. Visual superimposition scanning is performed to give a 'page review' of the entire recording, identifying different ECG waveforms with selective samples of rhythm strips. A report is made after analysis of the scanning, and the physician or other qualified health care professional reviews and interprets the data for heart arrhythmias. Report 93224 for the complete procedure, including recording, scanning with report, review and interpretation. Report 93225 for the recording portion only, which includes connection, recording, and disconnection. Report 93226 for analysis of the scanning with report only. Report 93227 for the review and interpretation only.

RVUs

Code	Work	PE	PE Non-Facility	MP	Total Non-Facility	Total Facility	Global
93224	0.52	1.93	1.93	0.04	2.49	2.49	XXX
93225	0.00	0.71	0.71	0.01	0.72	0.72	XXX
93226	0.00	1.01	1.01	0.01	1.02	1.02	XXX
93227	0.52	0.21	0.21	0.02	0.75	0.75	XXX

93228-93229

★ **93228 External mobile cardiovascular telemetry with electrocardiographic recording, concurrent computerized real time data analysis and greater than 24 hours of accessible ECG data storage (retrievable with query) with ECG triggered and patient selected events transmitted to a remote attended surveillance center for up to 30 days; review and interpretation with report by a physician or other qualified health care professional**

(Report 93228 only once per 30 days)

(Do not report 93228 in conjunction with 93224, 93227)

★ **93229 External mobile cardiovascular telemetry with electrocardiographic recording, concurrent computerized real time data analysis and greater than 24 hours of accessible ECG data storage (retrievable with query) with ECG triggered and patient selected events transmitted to a remote attended surveillance center for up to 30 days; technical support for connection and patient instructions for use, attended surveillance, analysis and transmission of daily and emergent data reports as prescribed by a physician or other qualified health care professional**

(Report 93229 only once per 30 days)

(Do not report 93229 in conjunction with 93224, 93226)

(For external cardiovascular monitors that do not perform automatic ECG triggered transmissions to an attended surveillance center, see 93224-93227, 93268-93272)

Plain English Description

The patient is fitted with a telemetry transmitter connected to an external cardiovascular monitoring system. The telemetry transmitter receives data from the external monitoring system and transmits the data via a wireless connection such as a radio frequency link to a telemetry receiver at a monitoring station. Clinical personnel at the monitoring station acquire and analyze the data transmissions and notify the physician or other qualified health care professional of cardiac events requiring immediate review. Monitoring software may also be used to alert the clinician to these cardiac events. The transmitted ECG and other data is reviewed using either a printed readout or on a computer screen. The data may include periodic ECGs, stored cardiac episodes, paced and sensed events from heart chambers, and histograms. Device function, such as battery voltage and impedance, pacing and shocking lead impedance, and sensed ECG voltage amplitude are reviewed. Programmed parameters are also evaluated and changes are made as needed. The patient may be monitored for up to 30 days. Previously generated data and current data are compared and any changes noted. The data is interpreted and a report is provided that includes medical findings and recommended treatment. Use code 93228 for physician or other qualified health care professional review and interpretation with report. Use code 93229 for technical support including fitting and connection of the external system, patient instructions related to use, attended surveillance at the monitoring station, and analysis and acquisition of physician prescribed daily and emergent data reports.

RVUs

Code	Work	PE	PE Non-Facility	MP	Total Non-Facility	Total Facility	Global
93228	0.52	0.19	0.19	0.05	0.76	0.76	XXX
93229	0.00	19.75	19.75	0.08	19.83	19.83	XXX

93268-93272

★ **93268 External patient and, when performed, auto activated electrocardiographic rhythm derived event recording with symptom-related memory loop with remote download capability up to 30 days, 24-hour attended monitoring; includes transmission, review and interpretation by a physician or other qualified health care professional**

★ **93270 External patient and, when performed, auto activated electrocardiographic rhythm derived event recording with symptom-related memory loop with remote download capability up to 30 days, 24-hour attended monitoring; recording (includes connection, recording, and disconnection)**

★ **93271 External patient and, when performed, auto activated electrocardiographic rhythm derived event recording with symptom-related memory loop with remote download capability up to 30 days, 24-hour attended monitoring; transmission and analysis**

★ **93272 External patient and, when performed, auto activated electrocardiographic rhythm derived event recording with symptom-related memory loop with remote download capability up to 30 days, 24-hour attended monitoring; review and interpretation by a physician or other qualified health care professional**

(For subcutaneous cardiac rhythm monitoring, see 33285, 93285, 93291, 93298)

Plain English Description

Electrocardiographic (ECG) rhythm derived data is gathered with 24-hour attended monitoring as the patient goes about regular daily activity while wearing an external ECG recording device. Electrodes or leads are placed on the patient's chest and the patient is instructed in the use of the monitoring device. The monitor records in a continuous loop mechanism and is capable of storing a single channel of ECG data in refreshed memory. When symptoms occur, the patient activates the monitor. The ECG data is then permanently saved from the memory loop including the 60-90 seconds prior to the episode, the symptomatic period, and a period of time following cessation of the episode. This allows capture and recording of the onset of arrhythmias or other transient event. The patient then transmits the data to a receiving station where a printout is generated and the physician or other qualified health care professional reviews and interprets the ECG data. Report 93268 for transmission and professional review and interpretation. Report 93270 for recording only, including connection and disconnection. Report 93271 for receipt of transmissions and analysis only. Report 93272 for physician or other qualified health care professional review and interpretation only. These codes are reported only once per 30-day time period.

RVUs

Code	Work	PE	PE Non-Facility	MP	Total Non-Facility	Total Facility	Global
93268	0.52	5.08	5.08	0.04	5.64	5.64	XXX
93270	0.00	0.24	0.24	0.01	0.25	0.25	XXX
93271	0.00	4.66	4.66	0.01	4.67	4.67	XXX
93272	0.52	0.18	0.18	0.02	0.72	0.72	XXX

93306

93306 Echocardiography, transthoracic, real-time with image documentation (2D), includes M-mode recording, when performed, complete, with spectral Doppler echocardiography, and with color flow Doppler echocardiography

(For transthoracic echocardiography without spectral and color Doppler, use 93307)

Plain English Description

The physician performs complete transthoracic real-time echocardiography with image documentation (2-D) including M-mode recording, if performed, with spectral Doppler and color flow Doppler echocardiography. Cardiac structure and dynamics are evaluated using a series of real-time tomographic images with multiple views recorded digitally or on videotape. Time-motion (M-mode) recordings are made as needed to allow dimensional measurement. Blood flow and velocity patterns within the heart, across valves and within the great vessels are evaluated by color flow Doppler. Normal blood flow patterns through these regions have a characteristic pattern defined by direction, velocity, duration, and timing throughout the cardiac cycle. Spectral Doppler by pulsed or continuous wave technique is used to evaluate antegrade flow through inflow and outflow tracts and cardiac valves. Multiple transducer positions or orientations may be required. The physician reviews the echocardiography images and orders additional images as needed to allow evaluation of any abnormalities. Digital or videotaped images are then reviewed by the physician. Abnormalities of cardiac structure or dynamics are noted. The extent of the abnormalities is evaluated and quantified. Any previous cardiac studies are compared to the current study and any quantitative or qualitative changes are identified. The physician provides an interpretation of the echocardiography with a written report of findings.

RVUs

Code	Work	PE	PE Non-Facility	MP	Total Non-Facility	Total Facility	Global
93306	1.50	4.29	4.29	0.07	5.86	5.86	XXX

93660

93660 Evaluation of cardiovascular function with tilt table evaluation, with continuous ECG monitoring and intermittent blood pressure monitoring, with or without pharmacological intervention

(For testing of autonomic nervous system function, see 95921, 95924, 95943)

Plain English Description

Cardiovascular function is evaluated using a tilt table with continuous ECG and intermittent blood pressure monitoring. Tilt table testing is used to diagnose the cause of syncope (fainting). Following placement of ECG electrodes and a blood pressure monitor, the patient is placed supine on a tilt table with restraints attached to keep the patient in position when the tilt table is raised and lowered. The table is then rapidly raised to a 60 degree angle and kept at that angle while heart rate and blood pressure are monitored and any resulting syncope is observed. If the test does not induce syncope, a pharmacological agent that causes venous pooling or increases adrenergic stimulation is administered intravenously and the test is repeated. Any hypotensive changes in blood pressure, heart rate slowing (bradycardia), or syncope is noted and monitored.

RVUs

Code	Work	PE	PE Non-Facility	MP	Total Non-Facility	Total Facility	Global
93660	1.89	2.52	2.52	0.09	4.50	4.50	000

93880-93882

93880 Duplex scan of extracranial arteries; complete bilateral study

(Do not report 93880 in conjunction with 93895, 0126T)

93882 Duplex scan of extracranial arteries; unilateral or limited study

(Do not report 93882 in conjunction with 93895, 0126T)

(To report common carotid intima-media thickness (IMT) study for evaluation of atherosclerotic burden or coronary heart disease risk factor assessment, use Category III code 0126T)

Plain English Description

A vascular ultrasound study is performed to evaluate the extracranial arteries which include the common carotid and external carotid arteries. A duplex scan uses both B-mode and Doppler studies. A clear gel is placed on the skin over the arteries to be studied. A B-mode transducer is placed on the skin and real-time images of the artery are obtained. A Doppler probe within the B-mode transducer provides information on pattern and direction of blood flow in the artery. The B-mode transducer produces ultrasonic sound waves that move through the skin and bounce off the arteries when the probe is placed over the arteries at various locations and angles. The Doppler probe produces sound waves that bounce off blood cells moving within the artery. The reflected sound waves are sent to an amplifier that makes the sound waves audible. The pitch of the sound waves changes if there is reduced blood flow, or ceases altogether if a vessel is completely obstructed. A computer converts the sound waves to images that are overlaid with colors to produce video images showing the speed and direction of blood flow as well as any obstruction. Spectral Doppler analysis is performed to provide information on anatomy and hemodynamic function, including information on the presence of narrowing and plaque formation within the arteries. The physician reviews the duplex scan and provides a written interpretation of findings. Use code 93880 for a complete bilateral study of the common and external carotid arteries. Use code 93882 for a unilateral or limited study.

RVUs

Code	Work	PE	PE Non-Facility	MP	Total Non-Facility	Total Facility	Global
93880	0.80	4.76	4.76	0.08	5.64	5.64	XXX
93882	0.50	3.04	3.04	0.10	3.64	3.64	XXX

93886-93888

93886 Transcranial Doppler study of the intracranial arteries; complete study

93888 Transcranial Doppler study of the intracranial arteries; limited study

Plain English Description

A transcranial vascular Doppler ultrasound study is performed to evaluate the intracranial arteries. The intracranial arteries are divided into three regions which include the right and left anterior circulation territories, and the posterior circulation territory. Doppler studies provide information on the pattern and direction of blood flow within the region being studied. For a complete transcranial Doppler study, clear gel is placed on the skin on the back of the neck, above each cheek bone, in front of both ears and over both eyelids. The Doppler probe is placed on the skin over each site. The probe produces sound waves that bounce off blood cells moving within the artery. The reflected sound waves are sent to an amplifier that makes the sound waves audible. The pitch of the sound waves changes if there is reduced blood flow, or ceases altogether if a vessel is completely obstructed. A computer converts the sound waves to images that are overlaid with colors to produce video images showing the speed and direction of blood flow as well as any obstruction.

Spectral Doppler analysis is performed to provide information on anatomy and hemodynamic function, including information on the presence of narrowing and plaque formation within the intracranial arteries. The physician reviews the Doppler study and provides a written interpretation of findings. Use code 93886 for a complete study of all three regions. Use code 93888 for a limited study which includes two regions or less.

RVUs

Code	Work	PE	PE Non-Facility	MP	Total Non-Facility	Total Facility	Global
93886	0.91	6.71	6.71	0.08	7.70	7.70	XXX
93888	0.50	4.02	4.02	0.07	4.59	4.59	XXX

93890

93890 Transcranial Doppler study of the intracranial arteries; vasoreactivity study

Plain English Description

A transcranial Doppler study is performed to evaluate cerebrovascular reactivity which provides information on the reserve capacity of the cerebrovascular system in a patient with known cerebrovascular disease of the carotid and/or vertebrobasilar arteries. The study may also be performed prior to surgery affecting blood flow to the brain to assess cerebrovascular reserve. Vasoreactivity studies measure the change in intracranial blood flow velocity resulting from a change in the level of carbon dioxide following inhalation of a gas mixture higher in carbon dioxide than normal room air and/or with breath holding or hyperventilation. Alternatively, intracranial blood flow velocity can be evaluated following injection of acetazolamide or another drug that alters blood flow to the brain. Gel is applied to the skin. A hand-held Doppler probe is positioned on the skin and directed at the middle cerebral arteries (MCA) bilaterally. Continuous monitoring of the MCAs is performed during the rest phase and following the physiological challenge (breath holding, hyperventilation, and/or administration of CO_2 or medication) altering blood flow velocity to the brain. A computer program determines the blood flow reserve by calculating the change in blood flow from the baseline to following the physiological challenge. The physician reviews the images and the computer calculations and provides a written report detailing the findings, including whether there are adequate collateral blood flow channels that can maintain blood flow to the brain in the event of an interruption caused by stroke or a procedure that would temporarily alter blood flow to the brain.

RVUs

Code	Work	PE	PE Non-Facility	MP	Total Non-Facility	Total Facility	Global
93890	1.00	6.75	6.75	0.07	7.82	7.82	XXX

93892-93893

93892 Transcranial Doppler study of the intracranial arteries; emboli detection without intravenous microbubble injection

93893 Transcranial Doppler study of the intracranial arteries; emboli detection with intravenous microbubble injection

Plain English Description

A transcranial Doppler study is performed for emboli detection. Emboli are identified by short-duration, high-intensity signals on Doppler studies. The intensity of the signal is dependent on the density difference between the embolus and the blood cells with gaseous emboli showing the highest intensity signals and solid emboli (thrombotic, platelet, or atheromatous) showing slightly lower high intensity signals. Gel is applied to the skin. A hand-held Doppler probe is positioned on the skin and directed at the middle cerebral arteries (MCA) bilaterally. Continuous transcranial Doppler monitoring of the MCAs is performed through the temporal bone window. These are recorded on a designated computer system that provides both sound and visual images. A computer algorithm provides an analysis of the recording. Following completion of the recording, the physician reviews it for embolic signals, which are differentiated from artifacts. The physician then provides a written report detailing the findings. Use 93892 when emboli detection is performed without intravenous microbubble injection. Use 93893 when emboli detection is performed with an intravenous injection of agitated saline. Intravenous access is obtained and agitated saline is rapidly injected as a contrast agent. Monitoring begins immediately prior to the injection and is continued until after the agitated saline clears the MCAs. The physician reviews the contrast studies and provides a written report of findings.

RVUs

Code	Work	PE	PE Non-Facility	MP	Total Non-Facility	Total Facility	Global
93892	1.15	7.55	7.55	0.11	8.81	8.81	XXX
93893	1.15	8.86	8.86	0.09	10.10	10.10	XXX

93922-93923

93922 Limited bilateral noninvasive physiologic studies of upper or lower extremity arteries, (eg, for lower extremity: ankle/brachial indices at distal posterior tibial and anterior tibial/dorsalis pedis arteries plus bidirectional, Doppler waveform recording and analysis at 1-2 levels, or ankle/brachial indices at distal posterior tibial and anterior tibial/dorsalis pedis arteries plus volume plethysmography at 1-2 levels, or ankle/brachial indices at distal posterior tibial and anterior tibial/dorsalis pedis arteries with, transcutaneous oxygen tension measurement at 1-2 levels)

(When only 1 arm or leg is available for study, report 93922 with modifier 52 for a unilateral study when recording 1-2 levels. Report 93922 when recording 3 or more levels or performing provocative functional maneuvers)

(Report 93922 only once in the upper extremity(s) and/or once in the lower extremity(s). When both the upper and lower extremities are evaluated in the same setting, 93922 may be reported twice by adding modifier 59 to the second procedure)

(For transcutaneous oxyhemoglobin measurement in a lower extremity wound by near infrared spectroscopy, use 0493T)

93923 Complete bilateral noninvasive physiologic studies of upper or lower extremity arteries, 3 or more levels (eg, for lower extremity: ankle/brachial indices at distal posterior tibial and anterior tibial/dorsalis pedis arteries plus segmental blood pressure measurements with bidirectional Doppler waveform recording and analysis, at 3 or more levels, or ankle/brachial indices at distal posterior tibial and anterior tibial/dorsalis pedis arteries plus segmental volume plethysmography at 3 or more levels, or ankle/brachial indices at distal posterior tibial and anterior tibial/dorsalis pedis arteries plus segmental transcutaneous oxygen tension measurements at 3 or more levels), or single level study with provocative functional maneuvers (eg, measurements with postural provocative tests, or measurements with reactive hyperemia)

(When only 1 arm or leg is available for study, report 93922 for a unilateral study when recording 3 or more levels or when performing provocative functional maneuvers)

(Report 93923 only once in the upper extremity(s) and/or once in the lower extremity(s). When both the upper and lower extremities are evaluated in the same setting, 93923 may be reported twice by adding modifier 59 to the second procedure)

Plain English Description

Noninvasive physiologic studies of the upper or lower extremity arteries are performed to evaluate arterial disease and may include Doppler ultrasound waveform bidirectional studies, plethysmography, oxygen tension measurements, and/or provocative functional maneuvers. To perform Doppler ultrasound waveform bidirectional studies, a Doppler probe is placed on the skin over the vessel to be studied. The probe detects blood flow signals from the artery that are recorded and displayed on a computer monitor. The Doppler waveform system is also able to detect forward and reverse (bidirectional) blood flow during the various phases of the cardiac cycle. Plethysmography measures the amount of blood flow present or passing through a body region and is helpful in identifying deep vein thrombosis and arterial occlusive disease. There are two common types of plethysmography used to evaluate extremity arteries -- electrical impedance plethysmography and segmental plethysmography. To perform segmental plethysmography, pneumatic cuffs are placed at several levels along the extremity. A measured volume of air is injected into the cuffs and pulsatile volume change is measured and recorded at each level. Oxygen tension measurements are taken transcutaneously using an oximetry device to measure oxygen saturation in capillaries at various levels along the extremity. Provocative functional maneuvers provoke changes in blood flow using postural changes or temporary occlusion of blood vessels using a tourniquet placed around the extremity at various levels. Changes in blood flow are measured before and after the provocative maneuver. Which studies are performed and at what levels is dependent upon the type, site, and extent of the arterial disease. Use 93922 for limited noninvasive studies generally defined as bilateral studies at 1-2 levels. Use 93923 for complete noninvasive physiologic studies generally defined as bilateral studies at 3 or more levels or provocative functional maneuvers at a single level. The studies are evaluated by a physician and a written report of findings is provided.

RVUs

Code	Work	PE	PE Non-Facility	MP	Total Non-Facility	Total Facility	Global
93922	0.25	2.11	2.11	0.04	2.40	2.40	XXX
93923	0.45	3.22	3.22	0.07	3.74	3.74	XXX

93925-93926

93925 Duplex scan of lower extremity arteries or arterial bypass grafts; complete bilateral study

(Do not report 93925 in conjunction with 93985 for the same extremities)

93926 Duplex scan of lower extremity arteries or arterial bypass grafts; unilateral or limited study

(Do not report 93926 in conjunction with 93986 for the same extremity)

Plain English Description

A vascular ultrasound study is performed to evaluate the lower extremity arteries or arterial bypass grafts. A duplex scan uses both B-mode and Doppler studies. A clear gel is placed on the skin of the lower extremity over the region to be studied. A B-mode transducer is placed on the skin and real-time images of the arteries or arterial bypass grafts are obtained. A Doppler probe within the B-mode transducer provides information on the pattern and direction of blood flow in the artery. The B-mode transducer produces ultrasonic sound waves that move through the skin and bounce off the arteries when the probe is moved over the region being studied. The Doppler probe produces sound waves that bounce off blood cells moving within the artery. The reflected sound waves are sent to an amplifier that makes the sound waves audible. The pitch of the sound waves changes if there is reduced blood flow, or ceases altogether if a vessel is completely obstructed. A computer converts the sound waves to images that are overlaid with colors to produce video images showing the speed and direction of blood flow as well as any obstruction. Spectral Doppler analysis is performed to provide information on anatomy and hemodynamic function, including information on the presence of narrowing and plaque formation within the arteries. The physician reviews the duplex scan and provides a written interpretation of findings. Use code 93925 for a complete bilateral study. Use code 93926 for a unilateral or limited study.

RVUs

Code	Work	PE	PE Non-Facility	MP	Total Non-Facility	Total Facility	Global
93925	0.80	6.28	6.28	0.09	7.17	7.17	XXX
93926	0.50	3.67	3.67	0.07	4.24	4.24	XXX

93970-93971

93970 Duplex scan of extremity veins including responses to compression and other maneuvers; complete bilateral study

(Do not report 93970 in conjunction with 93985, 93986 for the same extremity[ies])

93971 Duplex scan of extremity veins including responses to compression and other maneuvers; unilateral or limited study

(Do not report 93970, 93971 in conjunction with 36475, 36476, 36478, 36479)

(Do not report 93971 in conjunction with 93985, 93986 for the same extremity)

Plain English Description

A vascular ultrasound study is performed to evaluate veins in the extremities. A duplex scan uses both B-mode and Doppler studies. A clear gel is placed on the skin of the extremity over the region to be studied. A B-mode transducer is placed on the skin and real-time images of the veins are obtained. A Doppler probe within the B-mode transducer provides information on the pattern and direction of blood flow in the veins. The B-mode transducer produces ultrasonic sound waves that move through the skin and bounce off the veins when the probe is moved over the region being studied. The Doppler probe produces sound waves that bounce off blood cells moving within the veins. The reflected sound waves are sent to an amplifier that makes the sound waves audible. The pitch of the sound waves changes if there is reduced blood flow, or ceases altogether if a vessel is completely obstructed. A computer converts the sound waves to images that are overlaid with colors to produce video images showing the speed and direction of blood flow as well as any obstruction. Spectral Doppler analysis is performed to provide information on anatomy and hemodynamic function. The duplex scan may include a baseline evaluation followed by additional scans obtained with compression or using other maneuvers that alter blood flow. The physician reviews the duplex scan and provides a written interpretation of findings. Use code 93970 for a complete bilateral study of the upper or lower extremity veins. Use code 93971 for a unilateral or limited study.

RVUs

Code	Work	PE	PE Non-Facility	MP	Total Non-Facility	Total Facility	Global
93970	0.70	4.73	4.73	0.08	5.51	5.51	XXX
93971	0.45	2.95	2.95	0.04	3.44	3.44	XXX

94010

94010 Spirometry, including graphic record, total and timed vital capacity, expiratory flow rate measurement(s), with or without maximal voluntary ventilation

(Do not report 94010 in conjunction with 94150, 94200, 94375, 94728)

Plain English Description

Spirometry is a pulmonary function test that is used to help diagnose the cause of shortness of breath and to monitor existing pulmonary disease, such as chronic bronchitis, emphysema, pulmonary fibrosis, chronic obstructive pulmonary disease (COPD), and asthma. A spirometry device consisting of a mouthpiece and tubing connected to a machine that records and displays results is used to perform the test. The patient inhales deeply and then exhales through the mouthpiece. Inhalation and exhalation measurements are first taken with the patient breathing normally. The patient is then instructed to perform rapid, forceful inhalation and exhalation. The spirometer records the volume of air inhaled, exhaled, and the length of time each breath takes. The test results are displayed on a graph that the physician reviews and interprets in a written report.

RVUs

Code	Work	PE	PE Non-Facility	MP	Total Non-Facility	Total Facility	Global
94010	0.17	0.81	0.81	0.02	1.00	1.00	XXX

94660

94660 Continuous positive airway pressure ventilation (CPAP), initiation and management

Plain English Description

Continuous positive airway pressure (CPAP) ventilation is used primarily to treat sleep apnea. It may also be prescribed to treat preterm infants whose lungs have not fully developed. CPAP uses a mask or other breathing device that fits over the nose and mouth which is connected via a tube to a CPAP device. The CPAP machine delivers an air mixture at a continuous low level of pressure. The continuous positive airway pressure keeps the airways open and prevents mechanical obstruction of the flow of air caused by relaxation and collapse of airway structures during sleep. This code is used for initial set-up and management. A durable medical device provider delivers the CPAP device and other required equipment to the home or a residential facility. The device is set up and programmed to the settings indicated by the written prescription obtained from the physician or other qualified health care professional. The patient or caregiver is instructed on correct use of the CPAP and then is asked to demonstrate understanding by placing the mask over the mouth and nose and turning on the machine.

RVUs

Code	Work	PE	PE Non-Facility	MP	Total Non-Facility	Total Facility	Global
94660	0.76	0.27	0.99	0.06	1.81	1.09	XXX

94760-94762

94760 Noninvasive ear or pulse oximetry for oxygen saturation; single determination

(For blood gases, see 82803-82810)

94761 Noninvasive ear or pulse oximetry for oxygen saturation; multiple determinations (eg, during exercise)

(Do not report 94760, 94761 in conjunction with 94617, 94618, 94621)

94762 Noninvasive ear or pulse oximetry for oxygen saturation; by continuous overnight monitoring (separate procedure)

(For other in vivo laboratory procedures, see 88720-88741)

Plain English Description

Ear or pulse oximetry measures the percentage of hemoglobin (Hb) that is saturated with oxygen and is used to monitor oxygen saturation of blood and detect lower than normal levels of oxygen in the blood. Oximeters also record pulse rate and provide a graphical display of blood flow past the probe. A probe is attached to the patient's ear lobe or finger. The probe is connected to a computerized unit. A light source from the probe is emitted at two wavelengths. The light is partially absorbed by Hb in amounts that differ based on whether the Hb is saturated or desaturated with oxygen. The absorption of the two wavelengths is then computed by the oximeter processer and the percentage of oxygenated Hb is displayed. The oximeter can be programmed to sound an audible alarm when the oxygen saturation of blood falls below a certain level. Use code 94760 for a single oxygen saturation determination, 94761 for multiple determinations, such as that obtained during exercise, or 94762 for continuous overnight monitoring.

RVUs

Code	Work	PE	PE Non-Facility	MP	Total Non-Facility	Total Facility	Global
94760	0.00	0.06	0.06	0.01	0.07	0.07	XXX
94761	0.00	0.10	0.10	0.01	0.11	0.11	XXX
94762	0.00	0.73	0.73	0.01	0.74	0.74	XXX

95700

- ● **95700 Electroencephalogram (EEG) continuous recording, with video when performed, setup, patient education, and takedown when performed, administered in person by EEG technologist, minimum of 8 channels**

  (95700 should be reported once per recording period)

  (For EEG using patient-placed electrode sets, use 95999)

  (For setup performed by non-EEG technologist or remotely supervised by an EEG technologist, use 95999)

Plain English Description

Long-term electroencephalogram (EEG) continuous recording including video (VEEG), when performed, is done to capture brain wave activity for a period of 2 hours or more. Time is counted when actual recording begins and for as long as recording is taking place. An extended EEG service may be done to diagnose the specific type and location of seizures, monitor current treatment, diagnose a seizure disorder versus another abnormality, and determine if the patient's epilepsy may be treated surgically. Extended EEG services may also be done on seriously ill patients to screen for new, adverse neurological changes. An EEG technician applies a minimum of 8 electrodes in different positions on the scalp using a sticky paste. More than 15 channels are generally used for older children or adults, while 15 or less may be used on infants. The electrodes are connected by wires to an amplifier and recording machine. The patient is instructed to lie still with the eyes closed. The machine is activated, and the recording period begins. The machine converts electrical signals from the brain into visible wavy lines. This code reports the services of an EEG technician performing the setup and takedown in person for EEG or VEEG continuous recording services done with at least 8 channels.

RVUs

Code	Work	PE	PE Non-Facility	MP	Total Non-Facility	Total Facility	Global
95700	0.00	0.00	0.00	0.00	0.00	0.00	XXX

95705-95710

- ● **95705 Electroencephalogram (EEG), without video, review of data, technical description by EEG technologist, 2-12 hours; unmonitored**
- ● **95706 Electroencephalogram (EEG), without video, review of data, technical description by EEG technologist, 2-12 hours; with intermittent monitoring and maintenance**
- ● **95707 Electroencephalogram (EEG), without video, review of data, technical description by EEG technologist, 2-12 hours; with continuous, real-time monitoring and maintenance**
- ● **95708 Electroencephalogram (EEG), without video, review of data, technical description by EEG technologist, each increment of 12-26 hours; unmonitored**
- ● **95709 Electroencephalogram (EEG), without video, review of data, technical description by EEG technologist, each increment of 12-26 hours; with intermittent monitoring and maintenance**
- ● **95710 Electroencephalogram (EEG), without video, review of data, technical description by EEG technologist, each increment of 12-26 hours; with continuous, real-time monitoring and maintenance**

Plain English Description

Long-term electroencephalogram (EEG) continuous recording without video is done to capture brain wave activity for a period of 2 hours or more. Time is counted when actual recording begins and for as long as recording is taking place. An extended EEG service may be done to diagnose the specific type and location of seizures, monitor current treatment, diagnose a seizure disorder versus another abnormality, and determine if the patient's epilepsy may be treated surgically. Extended EEG services may also be done on seriously ill patients to screen for new, adverse neurological changes. These codes report the technical portion for extended EEG services based on time and monitoring given. This includes the EEG technician's uploading of the data generated by the EEG equipment; review of the raw data with annotations and edits of recognized events, both patient generated and machine detected; storing or archiving the reviewed data for further review by the physician or other qualified personnel; and a written report documenting his/her review of the data, including any technical interventions. For unmonitored technician services, report 95705 for 2-12 hours and 95708 for 12-26 hours. Report 95706 (2-12 hours) and 95709 (12-26 hours) when provided with intermittent monitoring and maintenance in which the technician also oversees the quality of the EEG recording and provides real-time data review at least every 2 hours during the entire period. Report 95707 (2-12 hours) and 95710 (12-26 hours) when provided with continuous, real-time concurrent monitoring and maintenance during the entire recording period that provides documentation of the monitoring, event recognition, and notification of the physician, per instruction.

RVUs

Code	Work	PE	PE Non-Facility	MP	Total Non-Facility	Total Facility	Global
95705	0.00	0.00	0.00	0.00	0.00	0.00	XXX
95706	0.00	0.00	0.00	0.00	0.00	0.00	XXX
95707	0.00	0.00	0.00	0.00	0.00	0.00	XXX
95708	0.00	0.00	0.00	0.00	0.00	0.00	XXX
95709	0.00	0.00	0.00	0.00	0.00	0.00	XXX
95710	0.00	0.00	0.00	0.00	0.00	0.00	XXX

95711-95716

- **95711 Electroencephalogram with video (VEEG), review of data, technical description by EEG technologist, 2-12 hours; unmonitored**
- **95712 Electroencephalogram with video (VEEG), review of data, technical description by EEG technologist, 2-12 hours; with intermittent monitoring and maintenance**
- **95713 Electroencephalogram with video (VEEG), review of data, technical description by EEG technologist, 2-12 hours; with continuous, real-time monitoring and maintenance**
- **95714 Electroencephalogram with video (VEEG), review of data, technical description by EEG technologist, each increment of 12-26 hours; unmonitored**
- **95715 Electroencephalogram with video (VEEG), review of data, technical description by EEG technologist, each increment of 12-26 hours; with intermittent monitoring and maintenance**
- **95716 Electroencephalogram with video (VEEG), review of data, technical description by EEG technologist, each increment of 12-26 hours; with continuous, real-time monitoring and maintenance**

(95705, 95706, 95707, 95711, 95712, 95713 may be reported a maximum of once for an entire longer-term EEG service to capture either the entire time of service or the final 2-12 hour increment of a service extending beyond 26 hours)

Plain English Description

Long-term electroencephalogram (EEG) continuous recording is done with video (VEEG) to capture brain wave activity for a period of 2 hours or more while the patient is monitored over a video screen concurrently for at least 80% of the time that the diagnostic EEG is recording. This allows the physician to observe brain wave activity right when the seizure is occurring. Time is counted when actual EEG recording begins and for as long as recording is taking place. An extended EEG service may be done to diagnose the specific type and location of seizures, monitor current treatment, diagnose a seizure disorder versus another abnormality, and determine if the patient's epilepsy may be treated surgically. Extended EEG services may also be done on seriously ill patients to screen for new, adverse neurological changes. These codes report the technical portion for extended EEG services based on time and monitoring given. This includes the EEG technician's uploading of the data generated by the EEG equipment; review of the raw data with annotations and edits of recognized events, both patient generated and machine detected; storing or archiving the reviewed data for further review by the physician or other qualified personnel; and a written report documenting his/her review of the data, including any technical interventions. For unmonitored technician services, report 95711 for 2-12 hours and 95714 for 12-26 hours. Report 95712 (2-12 hours) and 95715 (12-26 hours) when provided with intermittent monitoring and maintenance in which the technician also oversees the quality of the EEG recording and provides real-time data review at least every 2 hours during the entire period. Report 95713 (2-12 hours) and 95716 (12-26 hours) when provided with continuous, real-time concurrent monitoring and maintenance during the entire recording period that provides documentation of the monitoring, event recognition, and notification of the physician, per instruction.

RVUs

Code	Work	PE	PE Non-Facility	MP	Total Non-Facility	Total Facility	Global
95711	0.00	0.00	0.00	0.00	0.00	0.00	XXX
95712	0.00	0.00	0.00	0.00	0.00	0.00	XXX
95713	0.00	0.00	0.00	0.00	0.00	0.00	XXX
95714	0.00	0.00	0.00	0.00	0.00	0.00	XXX
95715	0.00	0.00	0.00	0.00	0.00	0.00	XXX
95716	0.00	0.00	0.00	0.00	0.00	0.00	XXX

95717-95720

- **95717 Electroencephalogram (EEG), continuous recording, physician or other qualified health care professional review of recorded events, analysis of spike and seizure detection, interpretation and report, 2-12 hours of EEG recording; without video**
- **95718 Electroencephalogram (EEG), continuous recording, physician or other qualified health care professional review of recorded events, analysis of spike and seizure detection, interpretation and report, 2-12 hours of EEG recording; with video (VEEG)**

(For recording greater than 12 hours, see 95719, 95720, 95721, 95722, 95723, 95724, 95725, 95726)

(95717, 95718 may be reported a maximum of once for an entire long-term EEG service to capture either the entire time of service or the final 2-12 hour increment of a service extending beyond 24 hours)

- **95719 Electroencephalogram (EEG), continuous recording, physician or other qualified health care professional review of recorded events, analysis of spike and seizure detection, each increment of greater than 12 hours, up to 26 hours of EEG recording, interpretation and report after each 24-hour period; without video**
- **95720 Electroencephalogram (EEG), continuous recording, physician or other qualified health care professional review of recorded events, analysis of spike and seizure detection, each increment of greater than 12 hours, up to 26 hours of EEG recording, interpretation and report after each 24-hour period; with video (VEEG)**

(95719, 95720 may be reported only once for a recording period greater than 12 hours up to 26 hours. For multiple-day studies, 95719, 95720 may be reported after each 24-hour period during the extended recording period. 95719, 95720 describe reporting for a 26-hour recording period, whether done as a single report or as multiple reports during the same time)

(95717, 95718 may be reported in conjunction with 95719, 95720 for studies lasting greater than 26 hours)

(Do not report 95717, 95718, 95719, 95720 for professional interpretation of long-term EEG studies when the recording is greater than 36 hours and the entire professional report is retroactively generated, even if separate daily reports are rendered after the completion of recording)

(When the entire study includes recording greater than 36 hours, and the professional interpretation is performed after the entire recording is completed, see 95721, 95722, 95723, 95724, 95725, 95726)

Plain English Description

Long-term electroencephalogram (EEG) continuous recording is done to capture brain wave activity for a period of 2 hours or more. This may be done with video (VEEG) as the patient is monitored over a video screen concurrently for at least 80% of the time that the diagnostic EEG is recording. This allows the physician to observe brain wave activity right when the seizure is occurring. Time is counted when actual EEG recording begins and for as long as recording is taking place. An extended EEG service may be done to diagnose the specific type and location of seizures, monitor current treatment, diagnose a seizure disorder versus another abnormality, and determine if the patient's epilepsy may be treated surgically. Extended EEG services may also be done on seriously ill patients to screen for new, adverse neurological changes. These codes report the professional component for extended EEG services based on the time of the recording the professional is reviewing, and video provision. The physician or other qualified professional reviews the data from the EEG/VEEG and provides a written report. The professional review includes a diagnostic analysis of spikes, generated events, and seizure detection, with a diagnostic interpretation of the recorded results, and recommendations based on the findings. Report 95717 for these professional services for 2-12 hours of EEG recording without video and 95718 with video. Report 95719 when the professional generates a report daily for continuous EEG recording for each increment of greater than 12 hours up to 26 hours without video and 95720 with video.

RVUs

Code	Work	PE	PE Non-Facility	MP	Total Non-Facility	Total Facility	Global
95717	2.00	0.78	0.82	0.12	2.94	2.90	XXX
95718	2.50	1.13	1.19	0.18	3.87	3.81	XXX
95719	3.00	1.29	1.34	0.21	4.55	4.50	XXX
95720	3.86	1.76	1.85	0.28	5.99	5.90	XXX

95721-95726

● **95721 Electroencephalogram (EEG), continuous recording, physician or other qualified health care professional review of recorded events, analysis of spike and seizure detection, interpretation, and summary report, complete study; greater than 36 hours, up to 60 hours of EEG recording, without video**

● **95722 Electroencephalogram (EEG), continuous recording, physician or other qualified health care professional review of recorded events, analysis of spike and seizure detection, interpretation, and summary report, complete study; greater than 36 hours, up to 60 hours of EEG recording, with video (VEEG)**

● **95723 Electroencephalogram (EEG), continuous recording, physician or other qualified health care professional review of recorded events, analysis of spike and seizure detection, interpretation, and summary report, complete study; greater than 60 hours, up to 84 hours of EEG recording, without video**

● **95724 Electroencephalogram (EEG), continuous recording, physician or other qualified health care professional review of recorded events, analysis of spike and seizure detection, interpretation, and summary report, complete study; greater than 60 hours, up to 84 hours of EEG recording, with video (VEEG)**

● **95725 Electroencephalogram (EEG), continuous recording, physician or other qualified health care professional review of recorded events, analysis of spike and seizure detection, interpretation, and summary report, complete study; greater than 84 hours of EEG recording, without video**

● **95726 Electroencephalogram (EEG), continuous recording, physician or other qualified health care professional review of recorded events, analysis of spike and seizure detection, interpretation, and summary report, complete study; greater than 84 hours of EEG recording, with video (VEEG)**

(When the entire study includes recording greater than 36 hours, and the professional interpretation is performed after the entire recording is completed, see 95721, 95722, 95723, 95724, 95725, 95726)

(Do not report 95721, 95722, 95723, 95724, 95725, 95726 in conjunction with 95717, 95718, 95719, 95720)

Plain English Description

Long-term electroencephalogram (EEG) continuous recording is done to capture brain wave activity for a period of 2 hours or more. This may be done with video (VEEG) as the patient is monitored over a video screen concurrently for at least 80% of the time that the diagnostic EEG is recording. This allows the physician to observe brain wave activity right when the seizure is occurring. Time is counted when actual EEG recording begins and for as long as recording is taking place. An extended EEG service may be done to diagnose the specific type and location of seizures, monitor current treatment, diagnose a seizure disorder versus another abnormality, and determine if the patient's epilepsy may be treated surgically. Extended EEG services may also be done on seriously ill patients to screen for new, adverse neurological changes. These codes report the professional component for extended EEG services based on the time of the recording the professional is reviewing, and video provision. The physician or other qualified professional reviews the data from the EEG/VEEG and provides one summary written report with the entire professional interpretation after study completion. The professional review includes a diagnostic analysis of spikes, generated events, and seizure detection, with a diagnostic interpretation of the recorded results, and recommendations based on the findings. Report 95721 for these professional services for more than 36 hours, up to 60 hours of EEG recording, without video and 95722 with video. Report 95723 for these professional services for more than 60 hours, up to 84 hours of EEG recording, without video and 95724 with video. Report 95725 for these professional services for more than 84 hours of EEG recording, without video and 95726 with video.

RVUs

Code	Work	PE	PE Non-Facility	MP	Total Non-Facility	Total Facility	Global
95721	3.86	1.78	1.90	0.28	6.04	5.92	XXX
95722	4.70	2.15	2.28	0.35	7.33	7.20	XXX
95723	4.75	2.21	2.37	0.37	7.49	7.33	XXX
95724	6.00	2.74	2.92	0.44	9.36	9.18	XXX
95725	5.40	2.52	2.73	0.42	8.55	8.34	XXX
95726	7.58	3.46	3.69	0.56	11.83	11.60	XXX

95806

95806 Sleep study, unattended, simultaneous recording of, heart rate, oxygen saturation, respiratory airflow, and respiratory effort (eg, thoracoabdominal movement)

(Do not report 95806 in conjunction with 93041-93227, 93228, 93229, 93268-93272, 95800, 95801)

(For unattended sleep study that measures heart rate, oxygen saturation, respiratory analysis, and sleep time, use 95800)

(For unattended sleep study that measures a minimum heart rate, oxygen saturation, and respiratory analysis, use 95801)

Plain English Description

Sleep studies are performed to evaluate and diagnose a variety of sleep disorders including sleep apnea, narcolepsy, insomnia, sleep walking, restless leg syndrome, and other periodic movements during sleep. An unattended sleep study may be performed as an outpatient procedure or at the patient's home. If a home sleep study is performed, the necessary sleep study equipment is delivered to the patient. A heart monitor is used to measure heart rate. A band is placed over the chest to monitor respiratory effort as indicated by thoracoabdominal movement. An oxygen probe is attached to the finger to monitor oxygen saturation of the blood. An airflow measurement device is placed over the nose and mouth to monitor respiratory airflow. The room is darkened and heart rate, ventilation, respiratory effort, oxygen saturation of the blood, and air flow through the nose and mouth are monitored and recorded. If the study has been performed at the patient's home, the testing equipment is picked up at the patient's home and the recorded data delivered to the physician. The physician analyzes the recorded data obtained during the sleep study and provides a written interpretation of the test results.

RVUs

Code	Work	PE	PE Non-Facility	MP	Total Non-Facility	Total Facility	Global
95806	0.93	2.33	2.33	0.04	3.30	3.30	XXX

95808-95811

95810 Polysomnography; age 6 years or older, sleep staging with 4 or more additional parameters of sleep, attended by a technologist

95811 Polysomnography; age 6 years or older, sleep staging with 4 or more additional parameters of sleep, with initiation of continuous positive airway pressure therapy or bilevel ventilation, attended by a technologist

Plain English Description

Polysomnography is performed with sleep staging by a sleep technologist. Sleep studies are performed to evaluate and diagnose a variety of sleep disorders including sleep apnea, narcolepsy, insomnia, sleep walking, restless leg syndrome, and other periodic movements during sleep. The patient presents to the sleep study center in the evening. Sleep staging is accomplished using electroencephalography (EEG), electro-oculogram (EOG), and electromyogram (EMG). EEG is performed using one to four electrodes attached to the scalp. Electrodes are attached around the eyes and an EOG performed to monitor eye movement. A submental EMG is performed by placing an electrode under the chin to record muscle tone. One or more additional parameters of sleep are recorded and analyzed including: heart rate and rhythm; airflow; ventilation and respiratory effort; gas exchange by oximetry, transcutaneous monitoring, or end tidal gas analysis; extremity muscle activity or motor activity-movement; extended EEG monitoring; penile tumescence; gastroesophageal reflux; continuous blood pressure monitoring; snoring; and/or body position. The room is darkened and brain activity, eye and muscle movement are recorded. Other parameters of sleep are monitored and recorded as needed. The physician analyzes the recorded data obtained during the polysomnography and provides a written interpretation of the test results. Use code 95808 when one to three additional parameters of sleep are measured on a patient of any age. Use code 95810 when four or more additional parameters of sleep are measured on a patient age 6 years or older. Use code 95811 when four or more additional parameters of sleep are measured and continuous positive airway pressure therapy or bilevel ventilation is performed on a patient age 6 years or older. If CPAP is performed a nasal mask is applied to the nose to keep the airway open during inhalation. If bi-level ventilation is performed, a ventilator is used to augment respiration while still allowing spontaneous unassisted respiration.

RVUs

Code	Work	PE	PE Non-Facility	MP	Total Non-Facility	Total Facility	Global
95810	2.50	14.51	14.51	0.20	17.21	17.21	XXX
95811	2.60	15.18	15.18	0.20	17.98	17.98	XXX

95812-95813

95812 Electroencephalogram (EEG) extended monitoring; 41-60 minutes

(Do not report 95812 in conjunction with 95700-95726)

▲ **95813 Electroencephalogram (EEG) extended monitoring; 61-119 minutes**

(Do not report 95813 in conjunction with 95700-95726)

(For long-term EEG services [2 hours or more], see 95700-95726)

Plain English Description

An electroencephalogram (EEG) with extended monitoring is performed. An EEG may be performed to diagnose a seizure disorder, to determine the cause of confusion, to investigate periods of unconsciousness, to evaluate a head injury, or to identify other conditions affecting the brain such as a tumor, infection, degenerative disease, or metabolic disturbance. An EEG may also be used to evaluate a sleep disorder. An EEG technician applies sixteen or more electrodes in different positions on the scalp using a sticky paste. The electrodes are connected by wires to an amplifier and recording machine. The patient is instructed to lie still with the eyes closed. The machine is activated and the recording period begins. The machine converts electrical signals from the brain to wavy lines that are recorded on a moving piece of graph paper. During the recording the patient may be asked to hyperventilate or photic stimulation may be used in an attempt to trigger seizure activity. The physician reviews the EEG and provides a written interpretation of the test results. Use code 95812 for extended EEG monitoring lasting 41 to 60 minutes. Use code 95813 when the extended monitoring is for more than an hour.

RVUs

Code	Work	PE	PE Non-Facility	MP	Total Non-Facility	Total Facility	Global
95812	1.08	8.13	8.13	0.08	9.29	9.29	XXX
95813	1.63	9.79	9.79	0.13	11.55	11.55	XXX

95816-95822

95816 Electroencephalogram (EEG); including recording awake and drowsy

(Do not report 95816 in conjunction with 95700-95726)

95819 Electroencephalogram (EEG); including recording awake and asleep

(Do not report 95819 in conjunction with 95700-95726)

95822 Electroencephalogram (EEG); recording in coma or sleep only

(Do not report 95822 in conjunction with 95700-95726)

Plain English Description

An EEG may be performed to diagnose a seizure disorder, to determine the cause of confusion, to investigate periods of unconsciousness, to evaluate a head injury, or to identify other conditions affecting the brain such as a tumor, infection, degenerative disease, or metabolic disturbance. An EEG may also be used to evaluate a sleep disorder. An EEG technician applies sixteen or more electrodes to different positions on the scalp using a sticky paste. The electrodes are connected by wires to an amplifier and recording machine. The patient is instructed to lie still with the eyes closed. The machine is activated and the recording period begins. The machine converts electrical signals from the brain to wavy lines that are recorded on a moving piece of graph paper. During the awake portion of the recording the patient may be asked to hyperventilate or photic stimulation may be used in an attempt to trigger seizure activity. To identify some types of abnormal electrical activity of the brain, the patient must be drowsy or asleep. In order to accomplish the asleep or drowsy portion of the test, the patient should sleep less than normal the night before the EEG. The patient is tested while drowsy or asleep and brain activity recorded. An EEG may also be performed on a patient in a coma to evaluate the presence of brain activity. The physician reviews the EEG and provides a written interpretation of the test results. Use 95816 for EEG recording with the patient awake and drowsy. Use 95819 for EEG recording with the patient awake and asleep. Use 95822 for EEG recording for a patient who is in a coma or asleep.

RVUs

Code	Work	PE	PE Non-Facility	MP	Total Non-Facility	Total Facility	Global
95816	1.08	9.14	9.14	0.08	10.30	10.30	XXX
95819	1.08	11.05	11.05	0.10	12.23	12.23	XXX
95822	1.08	9.91	9.91	0.10	11.09	11.09	XXX

95829

95829 Electrocorticogram at surgery (separate procedure)

Plain English Description

Electrocorticogram (ECoG) is an electroencephalogram (EEG) that is performed directly on the exposed cerebral cortex during a surgical procedure. ECoG is typically performed to identify critical regions in the sensory cortex. ECoG allows the surgeon to identify the limits of a surgical resection in a patient with a neoplasm or brain injury or in a patient with epilepsy where the epileptogenic regions are to be resected. Following exposure of the brain in a separately reportable procedure, ECoG electrodes are placed on the brain, either on the outside of the dura (epidural) or under the dura (subdural). The electrodes may be configured in arrays, strips, or grids and are positioned based on the results of separately reportable preoperative EEGs and imaging procedures. Brain activity is continuously monitored as the surgical procedure is performed. A written report of the intraoperative ECoG is provided.

RVUs

Code	Work	PE	PE Non-Facility	MP	Total Non-Facility	Total Facility	Global
95829	6.20	46.16	46.16	0.56	52.92	52.92	XXX

95830

95830 Insertion by physician or other qualified health care professional of sphenoidal electrodes for electroencephalographic (EEG) recording

Plain English Description

Placement of sphenoidal electrodes is performed to capture an electroencephalogram (EEG) recording of the temporal lobe of the brain in a patient with a seizure disorder. The patient is placed on his/her back and the skin of one side of the face is cleaned with an antiseptic. A local anesthetic is injected into the deeper tissues of the face. Using X-ray guidance, a needle with an electrode is placed into the soft tissues at the base of the skull underneath the temporal lobe of the brain. The needle is removed and the electrode remains in place. The electrode is secured with tape and bandage. The same procedure is repeated on the opposite side. X-ray images are obtained to verify correct placement of the electrodes. A separately reportable EEG recording is obtained. Upon completion of the EEG, the sphenoidal electrodes are removed.

RVUs

Code	Work	PE	PE Non-Facility	MP	Total Non-Facility	Total Facility	Global
95830	1.70	0.82	12.40	0.13	14.23	2.65	XXX

95860-95864

95860 Needle electromyography; 1 extremity with or without related paraspinal areas

95861 Needle electromyography; 2 extremities with or without related paraspinal areas

(For dynamic electromyography performed during motion analysis studies, see 96002-96003)

95863 Needle electromyography; 3 extremities with or without related paraspinal areas

95864 Needle electromyography; 4 extremities with or without related paraspinal areas

Plain English Description

Needle electromyography (EMG) is a diagnostic test used to evaluate pain, weakness, numbness, or tingling in the upper or lower extremities. The test records the electrical activity of the muscles. Abnormal electrical activity of muscles can be caused by a number of diseases or conditions including inflammation of the muscles, pinched nerves, intervertebral disc herniation, peripheral nerve damage, muscular dystrophy, amyotrophic lateral sclerosis (ALS), myasthenia gravis, as well as other conditions. One or more pin electrodes are inserted through the skin and into the muscle. The electrode cable is attached to a recording device with a visual display. Electrical activity of the muscle is recorded. The patient may be asked to move the extremity so that electrical recordings can be obtained with the muscle flexed and extended. The ability of muscle fibers to respond to nervous stimulation, called the action potential, is displayed graphically as a wave form. The test includes any EMG recordings of related paraspinal areas. The physician reviews the EMG recordings and provides a written report of findings. Use 95860 for needle EMG of one extremity; 95861 for two extremities; 95863 for three extremities; and 95864 for four extremities.

RVUs

Code	Work	PE	PE Non-Facility	MP	Total Non-Facility	Total Facility	Global
95860	0.96	2.38	2.38	0.06	3.40	3.40	XXX
95861	1.54	3.24	3.24	0.09	4.87	4.87	XXX
95863	1.87	4.06	4.06	0.09	6.02	6.02	XXX
95864	1.99	4.98	4.98	0.10	7.07	7.07	XXX

95865

95865 Needle electromyography; larynx

(Do not report modifier 50 in conjunction with 95865)

(For unilateral procedure, report modifier 52 in conjunction with 95865)

Plain English Description

Needle electromyography (EMG) is performed on the larynx to diagnose and evaluate laryngeal nerve and muscle disorders. It may also be used when Botox injections in the larynx are performed, or intraoperatively during procedures on the larynx. Small EMG needles are advanced through the skin and cricothyroid membrane and positioned in the muscles that move the vocal cords. The patient then performs a series of vocal exercises which cause movement of the vocal cords. Electrical responses are recorded. Upon completion of the test, the EMG needles are removed and pressure is applied at the puncture sites. The physician reviews the EMG recording and provides a written report of findings.

RVUs

Code	Work	PE	PE Non-Facility	MP	Total Non-Facility	Total Facility	Global
95865	1.57	2.68	2.68	0.09	4.34	4.34	XXX

95867-95868

95867 Needle electromyography; cranial nerve supplied muscle(s), unilateral

95868 Needle electromyography; cranial nerve supplied muscles, bilateral

Plain English Description

Needle electromyography (EMG) is performed to evaluate muscle and nerve function of cranial nerve supplied muscles. Cranial nerves and their branches that can be tested by EMG include CN III Oculomotor, CN IV Trochlear, CN V Trigeminal, CN VI Abducens, CN VII Facial, CN IX Glossopharyngeal, CN X Vagus, CN XI Spinal, and CN XII Hypoglossal. An EMG electrode needle is advanced through the skin and into the targeted muscle supplied by the cranial nerve. Electrical responses are recorded. The physician reviews the EMG recording and provides a written report of findings. Use code 95867 when the EMG is performed on one of the paired cranial nerves on only one side of the body. Use code 95868 when both of the paired cranial nerves are tested.

RVUs

Code	Work	PE	PE Non-Facility	MP	Total Non-Facility	Total Facility	Global
95867	0.79	2.20	2.20	0.06	3.05	3.05	XXX
95868	1.18	2.76	2.76	0.06	4.00	4.00	XXX

95869

95869 Needle electromyography; thoracic paraspinal muscles (excluding T1 or T12)

Plain English Description

Needle electromyography (EMG) is performed to evaluate muscle and nerve function of the thoracic paraspinal muscles, excluding those at levels T1 and T12. The paravertebral level where there is pain or other nerve or muscle symptoms is palpated. An EMG electrode needle is advanced through the skin and into the paravertebral gutter and positioned in the targeted thoracic paravertebral muscles. Electrical responses are recorded. The physician reviews the EMG recording and provides a written report of findings.

RVUs

Code	Work	PE	PE Non-Facility	MP	Total Non-Facility	Total Facility	Global
95869	0.37	2.31	2.31	0.03	2.71	2.71	XXX

95870

95870 Needle electromyography; limited study of muscles in 1 extremity or non-limb (axial) muscles (unilateral or bilateral), other than thoracic paraspinal, cranial nerve supplied muscles, or sphincters

(To report a complete study of the extremities, see 95860-95864)

(For anal or urethral sphincter, detrusor, urethra, perineum musculature, see 51785-51792)

(For eye muscles, use 92265)

Plain English Description

Needle electromyography (EMG) is a diagnostic test used to evaluate pain, weakness, numbness, or tingling in the muscles. In this procedure a limited study is performed on one extremity or the axial muscles excluding thoracic paraspinal muscles, cranial nerve supplied muscles, or sphincters. The test records the electrical activity of the muscles. Abnormal electrical activity of muscles can be caused by a number of diseases or conditions including inflammation of the muscles, pinched nerves, intervertebral disc herniation, peripheral nerve damage, muscular dystrophy, amyotrophic lateral sclerosis (ALS), myasthenia gravis, as well as other conditions. One or more pin electrodes are inserted through the skin and into the muscle. The electrode cable is attached to a recording device with a visual display. Electrical activity of the muscle is recorded. The patient may be asked to move the extremity so that electrical recordings can be obtained with the muscle flexed and extended. The ability of muscle fibers to respond to nervous stimulation, called the action potential, is displayed graphically as a wave form. The physician reviews the EMG recordings and provides a written report of findings.

RVUs

Code	Work	PE	PE Non-Facility	MP	Total Non-Facility	Total Facility	Global
95870	0.37	2.16	2.16	0.03	2.56	2.56	XXX

95873

✚ **95873 Electrical stimulation for guidance in conjunction with chemodenervation (List separately in addition to code for primary procedure)**

(Do not report 95873 in conjunction with 64451, 64617, 64625, 95860-95870, 95874)

Plain English Description

Electrical stimulation is performed prior to chemodenervation to allow more precise localization of the chemodenervation injection site. A combination stimulation needle electrode and hypodermic containing the chemodenervation toxin is advanced through the skin and into the targeted injection site in the muscle. The stimulating device is activated and the stimulation needle is repositioned as needed until muscle contraction is observed or palpated by the physician. The position of the stimulation needle is manipulated until maximal contraction with a low level stimulus is achieved to ensure that the needle is in the most optimal position closest to the motor endplate of the nerve. The chemodenervation toxin is then injected in a separately reportable procedure. The stimulation and injection needle may be advanced along the muscle or may be withdrawn and reinserted at different sites in the muscle and the process repeated until the desired results are achieved.

RVUs

Code	Work	PE	PE Non-Facility	MP	Total Non-Facility	Total Facility	Global
95873	0.37	1.79	1.79	0.01	2.17	2.17	ZZZ

95874

✚ **95874 Needle electromyography for guidance in conjunction with chemodenervation (List separately in addition to code for primary procedure)**

(Use 95873, 95874 in conjunction with 64612, 64615, 64616, 64642, 64643, 64644, 64645, 64646, 64647)

(Do not report more than one guidance code for each corresponding chemodenervation code)

(Do not report 95874 in conjunction with 64451, 64617, 64625, 95860-95870, 95873)

Plain English Description

Needle electromyography (EMG) is performed prior to chemodenervation to allow more precise localization of the chemodenervation injection site. A combination recording needle electrode and hypodermic containing the chemodenervation toxin is advanced through the skin and into the targeted injection site in the muscle. The recording device is activated to ensure that the needle is positioned in the spastic muscle and not in nearby blood vessels. The chemodenervation toxin is then injected in a separately reportable procedure. The recording and injection needle may be advanced along the muscle or may be withdrawn and reinserted at different sites in the muscle and additional injections performed until the desired results are achieved.

RVUs

Code	Work	PE	PE Non-Facility	MP	Total Non-Facility	Total Facility	Global
95874	0.37	1.85	1.85	0.01	2.23	2.23	ZZZ

95885-95886

✚ **95885 Needle electromyography, each extremity, with related paraspinal areas, when performed, done with nerve conduction, amplitude and latency/velocity study; limited (List separately in addition to code for primary procedure)**

✚ **95886 Needle electromyography, each extremity, with related paraspinal areas, when performed, done with nerve conduction, amplitude and latency/velocity study; complete, five or more muscles studied, innervated by three or more nerves or four or more spinal levels (List separately in addition to code for primary procedure)**

(Use 95885, 95886 in conjunction with 95907-95913)

(Do not report 95885, 95886 in conjunction with 95860-95864, 95870, 95905)

Plain English Description

Needle electromyography (EMG) is a diagnostic test used to evaluate pain, weakness, numbness, or tingling in the extremities. EMG is often performed in conjunction with nerve conduction studies. Needle EMG records the electrical activity of the muscles. Abnormal electrical activity of muscles can be caused by a number of diseases or conditions including inflammation of the muscles, pinched nerves, intervertebral disc herniation, peripheral nerve damage, muscular dystrophy, amyotrophic lateral sclerosis (ALS), myasthenia gravis, and other conditions. Nerve conduction studies are performed to diagnose and evaluate damage to nerves, nerve disorders, and symptoms such as numbness, tingling, or other abnormal sensations. Needle EMG is performed using one or more pin electrodes inserted through the skin and into the muscle. The electrode cable is attached to a recording device with a visual display. Electrical activity of the muscle is recorded. The patient may be asked to move the extremity so that electrical recordings can be obtained with the muscle flexed and extended. The ability of muscle fibers to respond to nerve stimulation, called the action potential, is displayed graphically as a wave form. The test includes any EMG recordings of related paraspinal areas. Nerve conduction studies are performed using several flat metal disc electrodes that are attached to the skin with paste or tape. A shock-emitting electrode is placed over the nerve to be studied and a recording electrode is placed over the muscles innervated by that nerve. Electrical pulses are sent through the shock-emitting electrode. The conduction time, which is the time it takes for the muscle to contract in response to the shock, is recorded. The amplitude or strength of the response and the speed as reflected by latency or velocity of the response is also recorded. The physician reviews the needle EMG and nerve conduction recordings and provides a written report of findings. Use 95885 and 95886 when EMG and nerve conduction studies are performed with another separately reportable diagnostic neuromuscular procedure. Use 95885 for a limited study of each extremity. Use 95886 for a complete study of each extremity.

RVUs

Code	Work	PE	PE Non-Facility	MP	Total Non-Facility	Total Facility	Global
95885	0.35	1.41	1.41	0.01	1.77	1.77	ZZZ
95886	0.86	1.86	1.86	0.03	2.75	2.75	ZZZ

95887

✚ **95887 Needle electromyography, non-extremity (cranial nerve supplied or axial) muscle(s) done with nerve conduction, amplitude and latency/velocity study (List separately in addition to code for primary procedure)**

(Use 95887 in conjunction with 95907-95913)

(Do not report 95887 in conjunction with 95867-95870, 95905)

Plain English Description

Needle electromyography (EMG) is a diagnostic test used to evaluate pain, weakness, numbness, or tingling in the muscles. EMG is often performed in conjunction with nerve conduction studies. This test is performed on non-extremity muscles, such as cranial nerve supplied or axial muscles. Needle EMG records the electrical activity of the muscles. Nerve conduction studies are performed to diagnose and evaluate damage to nerves, nerve disorders, and symptoms such as numbness, tingling, or other abnormal sensations. Needle EMG is performed using one or more pin electrodes inserted through the skin and into the muscle. The electrode cable is attached to a recording device with a visual display. Electrical activity of the muscle is recorded. The ability of muscle fibers to respond to nerve stimulation, called the action potential, is displayed graphically as a wave form. Nerve conduction studies are performed using several flat metal disc electrodes that are attached to the skin with paste or tape. A shock-emitting electrode is placed over the nerve to be studied and a recording electrode is placed over the muscles innervated by the nerve. Electrical pulses are sent through the shock-emitting electrode. The conduction time, which is the time it takes for the muscle to contract in response to the shock, is recorded. The amplitude or strength of the response as well as the speed as reflected by latency or velocity of the response is also recorded. The physician reviews the needle EMG and nerve conduction recordings and provides a written report of findings. Use 95887 when EMG and nerve conduction studies are performed with another separately reportable diagnostic neuromuscular procedure.

RVUs

Code	Work	PE	PE Non-Facility	MP	Total Non-Facility	Total Facility	Global
95887	0.71	1.66	1.66	0.03	2.40	2.40	ZZZ

95907-95913

95907 Nerve conduction studies; 1-2 studies
95908 Nerve conduction studies; 3-4 studies
95909 Nerve conduction studies; 5-6 studies
95910 Nerve conduction studies; 7-8 studies
95911 Nerve conduction studies; 9-10 studies
95912 Nerve conduction studies; 11-12 studies
95913 Nerve conduction studies; 13 or more studies

Plain English Description

Nerve conduction studies are performed to diagnose and evaluate damage to nerves, nerve disorders such as carpal tunnel syndrome, and symptoms such as numbness, tingling, or other abnormal sensations. Several flat metal disc electrodes are attached to the skin with paste or tape. A shock-emitting electrode is placed over the nerve to be studied and a recording electrode over the muscles innervated by the nerve. Electrical pulses are sent through the shock-emitting electrode. The conduction time, which is the time it takes for the muscle to contract in response to the shock, is recorded. The amplitude or strength of the response as well as the speed as reflected by latency or velocity of the response is also recorded. The physician reviews the recordings and provides a written report of findings. Use 95907 for 1-2 nerve conduction studies; 95908 for 3-4 nerve conduction studies; 95909 for 5-6 studies; 95910 for 7-8 studies; 95911 for 9-10 studies; 95912 for 11-12 studies; and 95913 for 13 studies or more.

RVUs

Code	Work	PE	PE Non-Facility	MP	Total Non-Facility	Total Facility	Global
95907	1.00	1.65	1.65	0.06	2.71	2.71	XXX
95908	1.25	2.13	2.13	0.06	3.44	3.44	XXX
95909	1.50	2.55	2.55	0.07	4.12	4.12	XXX
95910	2.00	3.32	3.32	0.10	5.42	5.42	XXX
95911	2.50	3.89	3.89	0.10	6.49	6.49	XXX
95912	3.00	4.30	4.30	0.13	7.43	7.43	XXX
95913	3.56	4.89	4.89	0.15	8.60	8.60	XXX

95921-95922

95921 Testing of autonomic nervous system function; cardiovagal innervation (parasympathetic function), including 2 or more of the following: heart rate response to deep breathing with recorded R-R interval, Valsalva ratio, and 30:15 ratio

95922 Testing of autonomic nervous system function; vasomotor adrenergic innervation (sympathetic adrenergic function), including beat-to-beat blood pressure and R-R interval changes during Valsalva maneuver and at least 5 minutes of passive tilt

(Do not report 95922 in conjunction with 95921)

Plain English Description

The autonomic nervous system (ANS) is divided into two parts, the sympathetic and parasympathetic nervous system. The sympathetic nervous system helps control blood pressure while the parasympathetic nervous system helps control heart rate. In 95921, cardiovagal innervation (parasympathetic function) is tested. An electrocardiographic (ECG) rhythm strip is used to record heart rate, which varies in response to deep breathing, the Valsalva maneuver, and moving from a lying to standing position if parasympathetic function is normal. The patient performs deep breathing and the recorded R-R interval on the ECG is evaluated. The Valsalva maneuver, which involves attempting to forcibly exhale with the glottis closed so that no air escapes from the nose or mouth, is also evaluated using the R-R interval on the ECG. The last test involves having the patient lie quietly on an exam table. The patient is then told to stand and the ratio of the longest R-R interval around 30th beat to the shortest R-R interval around the 15th beat is calculated (30:15 ratio). The physician reviews the tests and provides a written report of findings. In 95922, vasomotor adrenergic innervation (sympathetic adrenergic function) is tested. An ECG rhythm strip is used to record heart rate and R-R intervals and a blood pressure monitor is used to track changes in blood pressure. During the Valsalva maneuver beat-to-beat blood pressure and R-R intervals are recorded. The Valsalva maneuver increases intrathoracic pressure and reduces venous return, which in turn should cause BP changes and reflex vasoconstriction if sympathetic adrenergic function is normal. A tilt test is also performed. The patient is placed on a tilt table in head-down position for five minutes. The tilt table is then moved to a head-up position, which causes blood to shift from the head to the extremities. If sympathetic adrenergic function is normal, reflex responses occur in blood pressure.

RVUs

Code	Work	PE	PE Non-Facility	MP	Total Non-Facility	Total Facility	Global
95921	0.90	1.49	1.49	0.04	2.43	2.43	XXX
95922	0.96	1.76	1.76	0.07	2.79	2.79	XXX

95923

95923 Testing of autonomic nervous system function; sudomotor, including 1 or more of the following: quantitative sudomotor axon reflex test (QSART), silastic sweat imprint, thermoregulatory sweat test, and changes in sympathetic skin potential

Plain English Description

Sudomotor autonomic nervous system function is performed to evaluate small nerve fibers linked to sweat glands. There are a number of test methods available and the physician may use one or more of these methods. Quantitative sudomotor axon reflex test (QSART) begins by first measuring resting skin temperature and sweat output. Measurements are taken on the arms and/or legs. A plastic cup-shaped device is placed on the skin and the resting temperature and sweat output are measured. The patient is then given a chemical to stimulate sweat production, which is delivered electrically through, the skin to the sweat gland. Sweat production is measured. A computer is used to analyze the data to determine function of the portion of the autonomic nervous system that controls the sweat glands. Silastic sweat imprint uses silastic material placed on the skin, a device that records the imprint of the sweat droplets on the silastic material. The thermoregulatory sweat test is performed by dusting the skin with an indicator powder. The patient is then placed in a heat cabinet to stimulate sweat production. The indicator powder changes color in response to sweat production. Changes in sympathetic peripheral autonomic skin potentials (PASP) are evoked using electrical stimulation of the skin. Electrical potential recordings are then made over the palms and soles of the feet to evaluate whether autonomic nerve fibers are functioning normally. The physician reviews the test results and provides a written report of findings.

RVUs

Code	Work	PE	PE Non-Facility	MP	Total Non-Facility	Total Facility	Global
95923	0.90	2.68	2.68	0.06	3.64	3.64	XXX

95924

95924 Testing of autonomic nervous system function; combined parasympathetic and sympathetic adrenergic function testing with at least 5 minutes of passive tilt

(Do not report 95924 in conjunction with 95921 or 95922)

Plain English Description

The autonomic nervous system (ANS) is divided into two parts, the sympathetic and parasympathetic nervous system. The sympathetic nervous system helps control blood pressure while the parasympathetic nervous system helps control heart rate. Testing of the parasympathetic nervous system typically includes two or more of the following tests: heart rate response to deep breathing with R-R interval, Valsalva ratio, and 30:15 ratio. An ECG rhythm strip is used to record heart rate, which varies in response to deep breathing, the Valsalva maneuver and moving from a lying to standing position if parasympathetic function is normal. The patient performs deep breathing and the recorded R-R interval on the ECG is evaluated. The Valsalva maneuver which involves attempting to forcibly exhale with the glottis closed so that no air escapes from the nose or mouth is also evaluated using the R-R interval on the ECG. The last test involves having the patient lie quietly on an exam table. The patient is then told to stand and the ratio of the longest R-R interval around 30th beat to the shortest R-R interval around the 15th beat is calculated (30:15 ratio). Testing of the sympathetic nervous system typically includes: vasomotor adrenergic innervation with beat-to-beat blood pressure and R-R interval changes during Valsalva maneuver and at least 5 minutes of passive tilt. An ECG rhythm strip is used to record heart rate and R-R intervals and a blood pressure monitor is used to track changes in blood pressure. During the Valsalva maneuver beat-to-beat blood pressure and R-R intervals are recorded. The Valsalva maneuver increases intrathoracic pressure and reduces venous return which in turn should cause BP changes and reflex vasoconstriction if sympathetic adrenergic function is normal. A tilt test is also performed. The patient is placed on a tilt table in head down position for five minutes. The tilt table is then moved to a head-up position which causes blood to shift from the head to the extremities. If sympathetic adrenergic function is normal reflex responses occur in blood pressure.

RVUs

Code	Work	PE	PE Non-Facility	MP	Total Non-Facility	Total Facility	Global
95924	1.73	2.42	2.42	0.11	4.26	4.26	XXX

95925-95927

95925 Short-latency somatosensory evoked potential study, stimulation of any/all peripheral nerves or skin sites, recording from the central nervous system; in upper limbs

(Do not report 95925 in conjunction with 95926)

95926 Short-latency somatosensory evoked potential study, stimulation of any/all peripheral nerves or skin sites, recording from the central nervous system; in lower limbs

(Do not report 95926 in conjunction with 95925)

95927 Short-latency somatosensory evoked potential study, stimulation of any/all peripheral nerves or skin sites, recording from the central nervous system; in the trunk or head

(To report a unilateral study, use modifier 52)

(For auditory evoked potentials, use 92585)

Plain English Description

Somatosensory evoked potentials (SEPs) are electrical signals generated by afferent peripheral nerve fibers in response to sensory stimuli. SEPs are divided into three categories: short-latency, middle-latency, and long-latency. Short-latency SEPs refers to the portion of the SEP waveform that has the shortest delay (latency) time. The latency time varies depending on which nerve is being tested. Short-latency SEPs for the upper extremity nerves are the portion of the waveform occurring within 25 milliseconds of stimulation, while stimulation of the tibial nerve refers to the portion of the SEP waveform occurring within 50 milliseconds of stimulation. An abnormal SEP result indicates that there is dysfunction within the somatosensory pathways. Testing SEPs involves the use of electrical stimulation. Electrodes are placed on the skin over the selected peripheral nerve. A ground electrode is placed on the selected limb or other site to reduce stimulus artifact. Recording electrodes are placed over the scalp, spine, and peripheral nerves proximal to the stimulation site. Monophasic rectangular pulses are delivered using either constant voltage or a constant current stimulator. The stimulus causes the muscle to twitch and generates a SEP waveform. SEPs are recorded in a series of waves that reflect sequential activation of neural structures along the somatosensory pathways. The physician reviews the SEP recording and provides a written report of findings. Use 95925 for a short-latency SEP study of the upper limbs; use 95926 for the lower limbs; use 95927 for the trunk and head.

RVUs

Code	Work	PE	PE Non-Facility	MP	Total Non-Facility	Total Facility	Global
95925	0.54	3.36	3.36	0.05	3.95	3.95	XXX
95926	0.54	3.18	3.18	0.04	3.76	3.76	XXX
95927	0.54	3.16	3.16	0.05	3.75	3.75	XXX

95928-95929

95928 Central motor evoked potential study (transcranial motor stimulation); upper limbs

(Do not report 95928 in conjunction with 95929)

95929 Central motor evoked potential study (transcranial motor stimulation); lower limbs

(Do not report 95929 in conjunction with 95928)

Plain English Description

A central motor evoked potential (MEP) study uses electrical stimulation of the motor area of the cerebral cortex with recording from peripheral muscles in the extremities to evaluate motor pathway function. In 95928, motor pathway function in the upper extremities is evaluated. Prior to MEP recording, baseline nerve conduction studies of the upper extremities are performed. Electrodes are placed on the skin over the appropriate muscles, usually the biceps, triceps, abductor pollicis brevis, and abductor digiti minimi muscles. Impedances are checked and the electrodes are adjusted as needed. Beginning with the abductor digiti minimi muscles, and for each additional muscle tested, the optimal scalp location for electrical stimulation is identified. The MEP threshold is then determined. The motor area of the cerebral cortex is stimulated and MEPs are recorded. Transcranial MEP amplitude or strength of response as well as the speed of response as reflected by onset latency is measured and compared to the baseline nerve conduction study. Next, compound muscle action potential (CMAP) is tested. For the abductor digiti minimi CMAP, the ulnar nerve is stimulated. The relative abductor digiti minimi MEP strength of response reflected as a percentage of CMAP strength of response is measured. The central motor conduction time (CMCT) is calculated. Stimulator output is reduced in 5% increments so that the dissociation between MEP threshold and the cortical stimulation silent period (CSSP) can be measured. Stimulator output is reduced until stimulation no longer alters the appearance of the average EMG for the muscle being tested. Dissociation between excitory and inhibitory effects of transcranial stimulation is defined as EMG inhibition without a preceding MEP at 2 or more stimulus intensities. The data is replicated and the signals are stored. The procedure is repeated on 3-4 muscles on the ipsilateral upper extremity and then the contralateral upper extremity is tested in the same manner. The physician reviews the recordings and provides a written report of findings. In 95929, motor pathway function of the lower extremities is evaluated. The procedure is performed as described above except that electrodes are placed over selected muscles in the legs.

RVUs

Code	Work	PE	PE Non-Facility	MP	Total Non-Facility	Total Facility	Global
95928	1.50	4.81	4.81	0.07	6.38	6.38	XXX
95929	1.50	5.00	5.00	0.07	6.57	6.57	XXX

95930

95930 Visual evoked potential (VEP) checkerboard or flash testing, central nervous system except glaucoma, with interpretation and report

(For visual evoked potential testing for glaucoma, use 0464T)

(For screening of visual acuity using automated visual evoked potential devices, use 0333T)

Plain English Description

Visual evoked potential (VEP) tests, also called visually evoked response (VER) and visually evoked cortical potential (VECP), are performed to evaluate the function of the visual pathways. The visual pathways originate in the retina, travel along the optic nerves, and terminate in the visual cortex. VEPs use scalp electrodes to record electrical potentials that result from brief visual stimuli. The VEP waveforms are recorded and extracted from an electroencephalogram recording using signal averaging. The planned electrode sites on the scalp are cleansed and recording and grounding electrodes are placed. Either a flash or checkerboard stimulus is used to evoke a response from the visual cortex. Flash uses strobe light that rapidly flashes on and off. The most common stimulus uses the checkerboard reversal pattern. The patient looks at a black and white checkerboard stimulus where the black and white boxes reverse colors every half second. The patient focuses on the stimulus as the VEP waveforms are recorded. The waveforms are displayed on a computer screen and may be printed out on paper. The physician reviews the waveform and provides a written interpretation and report of the test results.

RVUs

Code	Work	PE	PE Non-Facility	MP	Total Non-Facility	Total Facility	Global
95930	0.35	1.51	1.51	0.02	1.88	1.88	XXX

95933

95933 Orbicularis oculi (blink) reflex, by electrodiagnostic testing

Plain English Description

Electrodiagnostic studies of the blink reflex, also called the orbicularis oculi reflex, are performed to help diagnose and localize pathology in the trigeminal cranial nerve (CN V), facial nerve (CN VII), or brainstem. The neural circuit of the blink reflex begins in the nerve endings in the cornea. From the cornea the nerve impulse travels along the trigeminal nerve and ganglion to the spinal trigeminal tract and nucleus to the interneurons in the reticular formation and then to the motor neurons in the facial nucleus and nerve, ending in the orbicularis oculi muscles. Electrodiagnostic studies of the blink reflex use a brief electrical shock, usually to the supraorbital nerve, to elicit a blink response. Electrodes are placed on the skin around the eyes. The supraorbital nerve is stimulated using an electrode placed above each eyebrow. The responses to the electrical stimuli applied to the supraorbital nerves above each eye are recorded and displayed on a computer screen. The recordings are printed out and reviewed by the physician who provides a written interpretation of the test results.

RVUs

Code	Work	PE	PE Non-Facility	MP	Total Non-Facility	Total Facility	Global
95933	0.59	1.70	1.70	0.04	2.33	2.33	XXX

95937

95937 Neuromuscular junction testing (repetitive stimulation, paired stimuli), each nerve, any 1 method

Plain English Description

The neuromuscular junction is the site where neurotransmitters are released from the end of the nerve, cross the synapse, a small gap between the end of the nerve and the muscle surface, to the receptors in the muscle which then cause the muscle to contract. To test neuromuscular junction function, either repetitive or paired stimuli are used to stimulate muscle contraction. A shock-emitting electrode is placed over or inserted percutaneously near the motor nerve to be studied. Recording surface or percutaneous electrodes are placed in the muscle innervated by that nerve. Repetitive electrical pulses are then sent through the shock-emitting electrode. The corresponding surface electrode records the evoked muscle action potentials and the recording is displayed on a computer screen. The conduction time, which is the time it takes for the muscle to contract in response to the shock, is recorded. The amplitude or strength of the response, as well as the speed reflected by latency or velocity of the response, are recorded. The physician reviews the recordings and provides a written report of findings.

RVUs

Code	Work	PE	PE Non-Facility	MP	Total Non-Facility	Total Facility	Global
95937	0.65	1.97	1.97	0.04	2.66	2.66	XXX

95938

95938 Short-latency somatosensory evoked potential study, stimulation of any/all peripheral nerves or skin sites, recording from the central nervous system; in upper and lower limbs

(Do not report 95938 in conjunction with 95925, 95926)

Plain English Description

Somatosensory evoked potentials (SEPs) are electrical signals generated by afferent peripheral nerve fibers in response to sensory stimuli. SEPs are divided into three categories: short-latency, middle-latency, and long-latency. Short-latency SEPs refers to the portion of the SEP waveform that has the shortest delay (latency) time. The short-latency time varies depending on which nerve is being tested. Short-latency SEPs for the upper extremity nerves comprise the portion of the waveform occurring within 25 milliseconds of stimulation, while stimulation of the tibial nerve refers to the portion of the SEP waveform occurring within 50 milliseconds of stimulation. An abnormal SEP result indicates that there is dysfunction within the somatosensory pathways. Testing SEPs involves the use of electrical stimulation. Electrodes are placed on the skin over the selected peripheral nerve. A ground electrode is placed on the selected limb or other site to reduce stimulus artifacts. Recording electrodes are placed over the scalp, spine, and peripheral nerves proximal to the stimulation site. Monophasic rectangular pulses are delivered using either constant voltage or a constant current stimulator. The stimulus causes the muscle to twitch and generates a SEP waveform. SEPs are recorded in a series of waves that reflect sequential activation of neural structures along the somatosensory pathways. The physician reviews the recording and provides a written report of findings. Use 95938 for a short-latency SEP study of the upper limbs and lower limbs.

RVUs

Code	Work	PE	PE Non-Facility	MP	Total Non-Facility	Total Facility	Global
95938	0.86	8.92	8.92	0.10	9.88	9.88	XXX

95939

95939 Central motor evoked potential study (transcranial motor stimulation); in upper and lower limbs

(Do not report 95939 in conjunction with 95928, 95929)

Plain English Description

A central motor evoked potential (MEP) study uses electrical stimulation of the motor area of the cerebral cortex with recording from peripheral muscles in the extremities to evaluate motor pathway function. In 95939, motor pathway function in the upper and lower extremities is evaluated. Prior to MEP recording, baseline nerve conduction studies of the upper and lower extremities are performed. Electrodes are placed on the skin over the appropriate muscles. For the upper extremity, response is usually tested in the biceps, triceps, abductor pollicis brevis, and abductor digiti minimi muscles. Impedances are checked and the electrodes are adjusted as needed. Beginning with the abductor digiti minimi muscles, and for each additional muscle tested, the optimal scalp location for electrical stimulation is identified. The MEP threshold is then determined. The motor area of the cerebral cortex is stimulated and MEPs are recorded. Transcranial MEP amplitude or strength of response and the speed of response as reflected by onset latency is measured and compared to the baseline nerve conduction study. Next compound muscle action potential (CMAP) is tested. For the abductor digiti minimi CMAP, the ulnar nerve is stimulated. The relative abductor digiti minimi MEP strength of response reflected as a percentage of CMAP strength of response is measured. The central motor conduction time (CMCT) is calculated. Stimulator output is reduced in 5% increments so that the dissociation between MEP threshold and the cortical stimulation silent period (CSSP) can be measured.

Stimulator output is reduced until stimulation no longer alters the appearance of the average EMG for the muscle being tested. Dissociation between excitatory and inhibitory effects of transcranial stimulation is defined as EMG inhibition without a preceding MEP at 2 or more stimulus intensities. The data is replicated and the signals are stored. The procedure is repeated on 3-4 muscles on the ipsilateral upper extremity and then the contralateral upper extremity is tested in the same manner. Motor pathway function of the lower extremities is then evaluated. The procedure is performed as described above except that electrodes are placed over selected muscles in the legs. The physician reviews the recordings for the upper and lower extremities and provides a written report of findings.

RVUs

Code	Work	PE	PE Non-Facility	MP	Total Non-Facility	Total Facility	Global
95939	2.25	12.45	12.45	0.14	14.84	14.84	XXX

95940-95941

✚ **95940 Continuous intraoperative neurophysiology monitoring in the operating room, one on one monitoring requiring personal attendance, each 15 minutes (List separately in addition to code for primary procedure)**

(Use 95940 in conjunction with the study performed, 92585, 95822, 95860-95870, 95907-95913, 95925, 95926, 95927, 95928, 95929, 95930-95937, 95938, 95939)

✚ **95941 Continuous intraoperative neurophysiology monitoring, from outside the operating room (remote or nearby) or for monitoring of more than one case while in the operating room, per hour (List separately in addition to code for primary procedure)**

(Use 95941 in conjunction with the study performed, 92585, 95822, 95860-95870, 95907-95913, 95925, 95926, 95927, 95928, 95929, 95930-95937, 95938, 95939)

(For time spent waiting on standby before monitoring, use 99360)

(For electrocorticography, use 95829)

(For intraoperative EEG during nonintracranial surgery, use 95955)

(For intraoperative functional cortical or subcortical mapping, see 95961-95962)

(For intraoperative neurostimulator programming, see 95971, 95972, 95976, 95977, 95983, 95984)

Plain English Description

Neurophysiology monitoring is performed during the course of a procedure which includes ongoing electrophysiological monitoring of sensory evoked potentials and EMG potentials performed intraoperatively to reduce permanent postoperative neurological deficits. Report code 95940 for each 15 minutes of one-on-one continuous intraoperative neurophysiology monitoring. Code 95941 is reported per hour of continuous intraoperative neurophysiology monitoring of more than one case in the operating room.

RVUs

Code	Work	PE	PE Non-Facility	MP	Total Non-Facility	Total Facility	Global
95940	0.60	0.29	0.29	0.05	0.94	0.94	XXX
95941	0.00	0.00	0.00	0.00	0.00	0.00	XXX

95943

95943 Simultaneous, independent, quantitative measures of both parasympathetic function and sympathetic function, based on time-frequency analysis of heart rate variability concurrent with time-frequency analysis of continuous respiratory activity, with mean heart rate and blood pressure measures, during rest, paced (deep) breathing, Valsalva maneuvers, and head-up postural change

(Do not report 95943 in conjunction with 93040, 95921, 95922, 95924)

Plain English Description

The autonomic nervous system (ANS) is divided into two parts, the sympathetic and parasympathetic nervous system. The sympathetic nervous system helps control blood pressure while the parasympathetic nervous system helps control heart rate. Measurement of heart rate variability (HRV) obtained during deep breathing and Valsalva is a non-invasive technique that can be used to investigate the functioning of the autonomic nervous system. HRV combined with concurrent analysis of respiratory activity is performed to obtain quantitative, independent, simultaneous, noninvasive measures of both autonomic branches. This test is typically performed using automated equipment.

RVUs

Code	Work	PE	PE Non-Facility	MP	Total Non-Facility	Total Facility	Global
95943	0.00	0.00	0.00	0.00	0.00	0.00	XXX

95954

95954 Pharmacological or physical activation requiring physician or other qualified health care professional attendance during EEG recording of activation phase (eg, thiopental activation test)

Plain English Description

During a separately reportable EEG recording, seizure activity is stimulated using a drug such as thiopental or another form of physical activation. The physician or other qualified health care professional administers the medication or supervises other forms of physical activation and remains in attendance to monitor the patient during the activation phase of the EEG recording.

RVUs

Code	Work	PE	PE Non-Facility	MP	Total Non-Facility	Total Facility	Global
95954	2.45	8.41	8.41	0.17	11.03	11.03	XXX

95955

95955 Electroencephalogram (EEG) during nonintracranial surgery (eg, carotid surgery)

Plain English Description

An electroencephalogram is performed during a non-intracranial procedure, such as carotid endarterectomy, aneurysm repair requiring clamping of the carotid artery, or cardiac surgery requiring hypothermic cardiac arrest. Electrodes are secured to the scalp. Typically 10-20 electrodes are applied and an 8-32 channel EEG is used. Electrical activity of the brain is recorded and continuously monitored during the surgical procedure. Any changes indicating decreased blood flow to the brain are communicated to the surgical team so that necessary interventions can be initiated. The physician provides a written report of the EEG monitoring.

RVUs

Code	Work	PE	PE Non-Facility	MP	Total Non-Facility	Total Facility	Global
95955	1.01	4.87	4.87	0.06	5.94	5.94	XXX

95957

95957 Digital analysis of electroencephalogram (EEG) (eg, for epileptic spike analysis)

(Do not report 95957 for use of automated software. For use of automated spike and seizure detection and trending software when performed with long-term EEG, see 95700-95726)

Plain English Description

An electroencephalogram is analyzed digitally using tools that allow changes in filtering, horizontal and vertical display scales, and montage reformatting. The digital EEG is recorded using only minimally restrictive analog filtering and a single common reference for all electrodes. The technician uses a computer to reformat the EEG recording to the desired referential or bipolar montage. The EEG is also digitally filtered as needed. Segments of the EEG showing abnormalities may be reformatted multiple times using different montages and filters. Digital reformatting allows better display of abnormalities and helps the physician differentiate epileptiform brain wave patterns from nonepileptiform patterns. The physician reviews the original EEG and the digitally reformatted EEG and provides a written report of findings.

RVUs

Code	Work	PE	PE Non-Facility	MP	Total Non-Facility	Total Facility	Global
95957	1.98	5.14	5.14	0.12	7.24	7.24	XXX

95958

95958 Wada activation test for hemispheric function, including electroencephalographic (EEG) monitoring

Plain English Description

The Wada test determines which hemisphere (right or left) of the brain controls language function and how important each side of the brain is with regard to memory. Typically, language is controlled by the left side of the brain and memory function is controlled by both sides but one side is dominant. However, there are variations between individuals so for patients who are considering surgical interventions for epilepsy or other conditions, the Wada activation test is performed prior to surgery. Electroencephalogram (EEG) monitoring is used during the procedure. Electrodes are placed on the scalp and connected to the recording device. The physician then injects an anesthetic into the right or left internal carotid artery to put one side of the brain to sleep. EEG recordings are analyzed to ensure that the brain on the side that was injected is asleep. The physician then tests the patient's ability to speak and also shows the patient cards with individual pictures and words. The side of the brain that is awake will try to speak and will try to recognize and remember the pictures and words. After the anesthetic wears off and the side of the brain that was anesthetized wakes up, the physician queries the patient about the cards to determine if the patient can remember the pictures and words that were displayed. The patient's responses are recorded. The opposite internal carotid artery is then injected with anesthetic and the test is repeated with the opposite side of the brain anesthetized. The results for each side of the brain are compared and the physician determines which side of the brain is dominant for language and memory and provides a written report of findings.

RVUs

Code	Work	PE	PE Non-Facility	MP	Total Non-Facility	Total Facility	Global
95958	4.24	11.85	11.85	0.40	16.49	16.49	XXX

95961-95962

95961 Functional cortical and subcortical mapping by stimulation and/or recording of electrodes on brain surface, or of depth electrodes, to provoke seizures or identify vital brain structures; initial hour of attendance by a physician or other qualified health care professional

✚ **95962 Functional cortical and subcortical mapping by stimulation and/or recording of electrodes on brain surface, or of depth electrodes, to provoke seizures or identify vital brain structures; each additional hour of attendance by a physician or other qualified health care professional (List separately in addition to code for primary procedure)**

(Use 95962 in conjunction with 95961)

Plain English Description

Functional and cortical mapping of the brain is performed during a separately reportable neurosurgical procedure to identify regions of the brain cortex responsible for eloquent motor and sensory functions or to provoke seizures. The patient is sedated and a craniotomy is performed to expose the region of the brain were the surgical procedure will be performed. The patient is awakened. Electrodes are placed on the surface of the brain and or depth electrodes are placed in deeper brain tissue. Regions of the brain responsible for vital functions are stimulated and mapped. The separately reportable surgical procedure is then carried out using the mapping information to avoid as much as possible vital regions of the brain. Code 95961 is reported the first hour of attendance and mapping by a physician or other qualified health care professional and code 95962 reports each additional hour.

RVUs

Code	Work	PE	PE Non-Facility	MP	Total Non-Facility	Total Facility	Global
95961	2.97	5.55	5.55	0.27	8.79	8.79	XXX
95962	3.21	4.03	4.03	0.20	7.44	7.44	ZZZ

95970-95972

95970 Electronic analysis of implanted neurostimulator pulse generator/transmitter (eg, contact group[s], interleaving, amplitude, pulse width, frequency [Hz], on/off cycling, burst, magnet mode, dose lockout, patient selectable parameters, responsive neurostimulation, detection algorithms, closed loop parameters, and passive parameters) by physician or other qualified health care professional; with brain, cranial nerve, spinal cord, peripheral nerve, or sacral nerve, neurostimulator pulse generator/transmitter, without programming

(Do not report 95970 in conjunction with 43647, 43648, 43881, 43882, 61850, 61860, 61863, 61864, 61867, 61868, 61870, 61880, 61885, 61886, 61888, 63650, 63655, 63661, 63662, 63663, 63664, 63685, 63688, 64553, 64555, 64561, 64566, 64568, 64569, 64570, 64575, 64580, 64581, 64585, 64590, 64595, during the same operative session)

(Do not report 95970 in conjunction with 95971, 95972, 95976, 95977, 95983, 95984)

95971 Electronic analysis of implanted neurostimulator pulse generator/transmitter (eg, contact group[s], interleaving, amplitude, pulse width, frequency [Hz], on/off cycling, burst, magnet mode, dose lockout, patient selectable parameters, responsive neurostimulation, detection algorithms, closed loop parameters, and passive parameters) by physician or other qualified health care professional; with simple spinal cord or peripheral nerve (eg, sacral nerve) neurostimulator pulse generator/ transmitter programming by physician or other qualified health care professional

(Do not report 95971 in conjunction with 95972)

95972 Electronic analysis of implanted neurostimulator pulse generator/transmitter (eg, contact group[s], interleaving, amplitude, pulse width, frequency [Hz], on/off cycling, burst, magnet mode, dose lockout, patient selectable parameters, responsive neurostimulation, detection algorithms, closed loop parameters, and passive parameters) by physician or other qualified health care professional; with complex spinal cord or peripheral nerve (eg, sacral nerve) neurostimulator pulse generator/ transmitter programming by physician or other qualified health care professional

(For percutaneous implantation or replacement of integrated neurostimulation system, posterior tibial nerve, use 0587T)

Plain English Description

An implanted neurostimulator pulse generator system consists of a generator/ transmitter placed in a subcutaneous pocket and electrical leads connected from the nerve or area being stimulated to the transmitter. Electrical impulses from the generator/transmitter stimulate target regions of the brain, spinal cord, or fibers of a cranial nerve, peripheral nerve, or sacral nerve to treat a variety of conditions such as pain, epilepsy, and even depression. Neurostimulators are commonly used to treat chronic, intractable pain when other treatment modalities have failed or are contraindicated. The pulse generator/transmitter is analyzed and programmed at the time of implantation. Electronic analysis with or without reprogramming is then performed at regular intervals by the health care professional to ensure optimal functioning of the device. Electronic analysis involves documenting the values, settings, and impedances of the system's parameters prior to programming. Not all parameters are available in all systems. Stored data from the implanted device is downloaded to a computer software program. Some or all of the following parameters may be evaluated during routine electronic analysis: contact of the stimulator wires to target area(s) or group(s), interleaving, amplitude, pulse width, frequency (Hz), on/off cycling, burst, magnet mode, dose lockout, patient selectable parameters, responsive neurostimulation, detection algorithms, closed loop parameters, and passive parameters. Code 95970 is used to report electronic analysis only without reprogramming of the device. In 95971, the physician or other qualified professional performs simple programming of a spinal cord or peripheral nerve pulse generator/transmitter. which involves adjusting 1-3 of the system parameters to improve therapy and address the patient's symptoms. Any parameter that needs to be adjusted at least two or more times during a session is counted. Report 95972 for complex programming of a spinal cord or peripheral nerve pulse generator/transmitter involving adjustment of more than three parameters.

RVUs

Code	Work	PE	PE Non-Facility	MP	Total Non-Facility	Total Facility	Global
95970	0.35	0.16	0.17	0.03	0.55	0.54	XXX
95971	0.78	0.31	0.58	0.08	1.44	1.17	XXX
95972	0.80	0.30	0.73	0.09	1.62	1.19	XXX

95976-95977

95976 Electronic analysis of implanted neurostimulator pulse generator/transmitter (eg, contact group[s], interleaving, amplitude, pulse width, frequency [Hz], on/off cycling, burst, magnet mode, dose lockout, patient selectable parameters, responsive neurostimulation, detection algorithms, closed loop parameters, and passive parameters) by physician or other qualified health care professional; with simple cranial nerve neurostimulator pulse generator/transmitter programming by physician or other qualified health care professional

(Do not report 95976 in conjunction with 95977)

95977 Electronic analysis of implanted neurostimulator pulse generator/transmitter (eg, contact group[s], interleaving, amplitude, pulse width, frequency [Hz], on/off cycling, burst, magnet mode, dose lockout, patient selectable parameters, responsive neurostimulation, detection algorithms, closed loop parameters, and passive parameters) by physician or other qualified health care professional; with complex cranial nerve neurostimulator pulse generator/transmitter programming by physician or other qualified health care professional

Plain English Description

Electronic analysis is performed on a simple or complex cranial nerve neurostimulator generator/transmitter with programming. An implanted neurostimulator pulse generator system consists of a generator placed in a subcutaneous pocket and leads tunneled from the nerve being stimulated to the generator. Electrical impulses are sent from the generator to cranial nerves to treat conditions such as pain, epilepsy, and depression. Electronic analysis is then performed at regular intervals to ensure optimal functioning of the device. Diagnostic analysis of contact group[s], interleaving, amplitude, pulse width, frequency [Hz], on/off cycling, burst, magnet mode, dose lockout, patient selectable parameters, responsive neurostimulation, detection algorithms, closed loop parameters, and passive parameters is performed and documented by the physician or other qualified health care professional. Any logged events from the equipment as well as battery status, electrode impedance, and current programmed settings are also documented. For cranial nerve neurostimulator pulse generator programming, the parameters for achieving optimal therapeutic stimulation are adjusted, which may include frequency, pulse width, current, duration, magnetic mode, or sensing. Multiple trials stimulating the nerve are carried out, adjusting three or fewer of these parameters for a simple cranial nerve neurostimulator pulse generator/transmitter (95976) and four or more parameters for a complex one (95977), until optimal therapeutic stimulation is achieved.

RVUs

Code	Work	PE	PE Non-Facility	MP	Total Non-Facility	Total Facility	Global
95976	0.73	0.35	0.37	0.08	1.18	1.16	XXX
95977	0.97	0.46	0.48	0.09	1.54	1.52	XXX

95983-95984

95983 Electronic analysis of implanted neurostimulator pulse generator/transmitter (eg, contact group[s], interleaving, amplitude, pulse width, frequency [Hz], on/off cycling, burst, magnet mode, dose lockout, patient selectable parameters, responsive neurostimulation, detection algorithms, closed loop parameters, and passive parameters) by physician or other qualified health care professional; with brain neurostimulator pulse generator/transmitter programming, first 15 minutes face-to-face time with physician or other qualified health care professional

+ **95984 Electronic analysis of implanted neurostimulator pulse generator/transmitter (eg, contact group[s], interleaving, amplitude, pulse width, frequency [Hz], on/off cycling, burst, magnet mode, dose lockout, patient selectable parameters, responsive neurostimulation, detection algorithms, closed loop parameters, and passive parameters) by physician or other qualified health care professional; with brain neurostimulator pulse generator/transmitter programming, each additional 15 minutes face-to-face time with physician or other qualified health care professional (List separately in addition to code for primary procedure)**

(Use 95984 in conjunction with 95983)

(Do not report 95970, 95971, 95972, 95976, 95977, 95983, 95984 in conjunction with 0587T, 0588T, 0589T, 0590T)

(For percutaneous implantation or replacement of integrated neurostimulation system, posterior tibial nerve, use 0587T)

Plain English Description

Electronic analysis is performed on a brain neurostimulator generator/transmitter with programming. An implanted brain neurostimulator pulse generator system consists of a generator placed in a subcutaneous pocket with a tunneled wire connecting electrode array(s) inserted into the target area—either the brain surface area for cortical stimulation or deep brain structures to treat movement conditions such as Parkinson's, essential tremor, dystonia, and refractory epilepsy, to stimulate injured brain regions, or to treat neuropathic pain disorders. Electronic analysis is then performed at regular intervals to ensure optimal functioning of the device. Diagnostic analysis of contact group[s], interleaving, amplitude, pulse width, frequency [Hz], on/off cycling, burst, magnet mode, dose lockout, patient selectable parameters, responsive neurostimulation, detection algorithms, closed loop parameters, and passive parameters is performed and documented by the physician or other qualified health care professional. Any logged events from the equipment as well as battery status, electrode impedance, and current programmed settings are also documented. For brain neurostimulator pulse generator programming, stimulating parameters and electrode mapping is checked for achieving optimal therapeutic stimulation. Each electrode array is activated systematically one at a time in monopolar mode while observing the neurologic effects such as bradykinesia, twitching, rigidity, or face pulling. After this electrode mapping, the final, adjusted combination of parameters is determined and selected that will result in optimal stimulation while minimizing adverse effects. Code 95983 reports the initial 15 minutes face-to-face time with the physician or other qualified professional for analysis and programming; code 95984 reports each additional 15 minutes.

RVUs

Code	Work	PE	PE Non-Facility	MP	Total Non-Facility	Total Facility	Global
95983	0.91	0.44	0.46	0.09	1.46	1.44	XXX
95984	0.80	0.38	0.40	0.09	1.29	1.27	ZZZ

95990-95991

95990 Refilling and maintenance of implantable pump or reservoir for drug delivery, spinal (intrathecal, epidural) or brain (intraventricular), includes electronic analysis of pump, when performed

95991 Refilling and maintenance of implantable pump or reservoir for drug delivery, spinal (intrathecal, epidural) or brain (intraventricular), includes electronic analysis of pump, when performed; requiring skill of a physician or other qualified health care professional

(Do not report 95990, 95991 in conjunction with 62367-62370. For analysis and/or reprogramming of implantable infusion pump, see 62367-62370)

(For refill and maintenance of implanted infusion pump or reservoir for systemic drug therapy [eg, chemotherapy], use 96522)

Plain English Description

An implantable spinal or brain infusion pump provides long-term continuous or intermittent drug infusion. Because drugs are infused over an extended period of time, the pump or reservoir must be periodically refilled. When the pump is refilled, any pump or reservoir maintenance is performed and an electronic analysis may also be done. The drug is received from the pharmacy and the prescription and patient information are verified. An external needle is used to inject the drug into the pump or reservoir through a self-septum in the implantable infusion pump. Electronic analysis is performed as needed using an interrogation device. A connection is established between the programmable pump and the interrogation device, which provides information on reservoir status, alarm status, and drug flow rates, which are evaluated to ensure that they are all within normal parameters. Use 95991 when refilling and maintenance requires the skill of a physician or other qualified health care professional.

RVUs

Code	Work	PE	PE Non-Facility	MP	Total Non-Facility	Total Facility	Global
95990	0.00	2.50	2.50	0.05	2.55	2.55	XXX
95991	0.77	0.30	2.38	0.09	3.24	1.16	XXX

95992

95992 Canalith repositioning procedure(s) (eg, Epley maneuver, Semont maneuver), per day

(Do not report 95992 in conjunction with 92531, 92532)

Plain English Description

One or more canalith repositioning procedures, such as the Epley or Semont maneuver, are performed to alleviate vertigo (dizziness) caused by calcium crystal debris in the semicircular canal. This type of vertigo is referred to as benign paroxysmal positional vertigo (BPPV). The repositioning procedure redeposits the debris into a neutral area where it no longer causes vertigo. The Epley maneuver is performed by placing the patient in a series of positions that change the orientation of the head. The patient is placed upright in a sitting position. The patient then quickly lies on the back with the head turned to the symptomatic side at a 45-degree angle. The head is also slightly hyperextended. This position is held for 30 to 60 seconds. The patient's eyes are observed for nystagmus, which indicates that the patient is experiencing vertigo. When the vertigo subsides, the head is turned and placed at a 45-degree angle on the opposite side. This position is maintained for another 30 to 60 seconds and the eyes again observed for nystagmus. The patient's body is then turned in the same direction as the head and the patient lies on the side with the head maintained at the 45-degree angle from the body for 30 seconds. The patient may experience another episode of dizziness. The patient is then returned to a sitting position with the head tilted slightly forward. The patient may be very dizzy at this point and may need support to maintain the sitting position. The maneuver is repeated one or more times as needed to alleviate the dizziness. The Semont maneuver is not as popular in the United States. The maneuver begins in a sitting position as described for the Epley maneuver. The patient then lies down on the affected side and is rapidly moved to the opposite side and then returned to sitting position. The maneuver is repeated one or more times. Canalith repositioning may require several treatment sessions over several days and is reported on a per day basis.

RVUs

Code	Work	PE	PE Non-Facility	MP	Total Non-Facility	Total Facility	Global
95992	0.75	0.28	0.47	0.05	1.27	1.08	XXX

96105

96105 Assessment of aphasia (includes assessment of expressive and receptive speech and language function, language comprehension, speech production ability, reading, spelling, writing, eg, by Boston Diagnostic Aphasia Examination) with interpretation and report, per hour

Plain English Description

Aphasia is defined as a disturbance in the comprehension or production of speech caused by a neurological condition or brain injury, such as atherosclerotic disease leading to a cerebral infarction or a skull fracture with intracranial bleeding due to a blow to the head. Assessment of aphasia involves an evaluation of spontaneous speech; word, phrase, and sentence repetition; speech comprehension; recognition and naming of objects; reading; and writing. Assessment involves both the use of an aphasia assessment tool such as the Boston Diagnostic Aphasia Examination and the training, knowledge, and skill of the medical professional performing the assessment. The medical professional administers the test using appropriate testing protocols. The medical professional then reviews the test results and provides a written interpretation of the results. The interpretation will generally identify the specific type of aphasia, such as expressive aphasia or receptive aphasia and will further describe the patient's specific speech and language deficits, such as receptive aphasia with the inability to recognize spoken words (pure word deafness) and the inability to comprehend the meaning of words (transcortical sensory aphasia) or expressive aphasia with the inability to translate thoughts into spoken language. Code 96105 is reported per hour for the assessment, interpretation, and written report.

RVUs

Code	Work	PE	PE Non-Facility	MP	Total Non-Facility	Total Facility	Global
96105	1.75	1.09	1.09	0.09	2.93	2.93	XXX

96116

★ **96116 Neurobehavioral status exam (clinical assessment of thinking, reasoning and judgment, [eg, acquired knowledge, attention, language, memory, planning and problem solving, and visual spatial abilities]), by physician or other qualified health care professional, both face-to-face time with the patient and time interpreting test results and preparing the report; first hour**

(To report neuropsychological testing evaluation and administration and scoring services, see 96132, 96133, 96136, 96137, 96138, 96139, 96146)

(To report psychological test administration using a single automated instrument, use 96146)

Plain English Description

A neurobehavioral status exam is performed by a physician or other qualified professional to assess brain dysfunction. The causes of brain dysfunction and the resulting neurobehavioral changes are diverse and include conditions such as vascular or metabolic disorders, head injuries, infections, toxins, brain tumors, developmental disorders such as autism spectrum disorders, and degeneration of the nervous system. Neurobehavioral status exams often involve lengthy observation and evaluation of the patient's development and behavior without the use of direct testing tools. The neurobehavioral status exam can be used as an initial assessment tool to help diagnose and characterize brain dysfunction, or following diagnosis to assess the progression of brain dysfunction and evaluate changes in symptoms over time. The physician or other professional evaluates thinking, reasoning, and judgment. Examples of areas assessed include acquired knowledge, attention, language, memory, the ability to plan and problem solve, and visual spatial abilities. Following the exam, the physician or other qualified professional interprets the test results and provides a written report. Code 96116 is reported for the first hour and 96121 is reported for each additional hour.

RVUs

Code	Work	PE	PE Non-Facility	MP	Total Non-Facility	Total Facility	Global
96116	1.86	0.45	0.81	0.09	2.76	2.40	XXX

96121

✚ **96121 Neurobehavioral status exam (clinical assessment of thinking, reasoning and judgment, [eg, acquired knowledge, attention, language, memory, planning and problem solving, and visual spatial abilities]), by physician or other qualified health care professional, both face-to-face time with the patient and time interpreting test results and preparing the report; each additional hour (List separately in addition to code for primary procedure)**

(Use 96121 in conjunction with 96116)

Plain English Description

A neurobehavioral status exam is performed by a physician or other qualified professional to assess brain dysfunction. The causes of brain dysfunction and the resulting neurobehavioral changes are diverse and include conditions such as vascular or metabolic disorders, head injuries, infections, toxins, brain tumors, developmental disorders such as autism spectrum disorders, and degeneration of the nervous system. Neurobehavioral status exams often involve lengthy observation and evaluation of the patient's development and behavior without the use of direct testing tools. The neurobehavioral status exam can be used as an initial assessment tool to help diagnose and characterize brain dysfunction, or following diagnosis to assess the progression of brain dysfunction and evaluate changes in symptoms over time. The physician or other professional evaluates thinking, reasoning, and judgment. Examples of areas assessed include acquired knowledge, attention, language, memory, the ability to plan and problem solve, and visual spatial abilities. Following the exam, the physician or other qualified professional interprets the test results and provides a written report. Code 96116 is reported for the first hour and 96121 is reported for each additional hour.

RVUs

Code	Work	PE	PE Non-Facility	MP	Total Non-Facility	Total Facility	Global
96121	1.71	0.42	0.59	0.09	2.39	2.22	ZZZ

96127

96127 Brief emotional/behavioral assessment (eg, depression inventory, attention-deficit/hyperactivity disorder [ADHD] scale), with scoring and documentation, per standardized instrument

(For developmental screening, use 96110)

Plain English Description

Emotional/behavioral assessments may be performed by medical and mental health professionals in the clinical setting and also by trained professionals in the educational setting. These assessments gather information regarding feelings and emotions and problem behaviors through direct observation of the individual and/or questionnaires completed by the individual, caregivers, teachers, and others. Areas assessed can include activities of daily living (ADL), relationships, attitude, adaptability, aggression, anxiety, attention, atypicality, conduct problems, depression, functional communication, hyperactivity, social skills, somatization, withdrawal, and self-esteem. Assessment tools may include the Behavior Assessment System for Children-Second Edition (BASC-2), Behavior Rating Profile-Second Edition (BRP-2), Child Behavior Checklist (CBCL), Conners Rating Scale, Pervasive Developmental Disorder Behavior Inventory (PDDBI), Brief Infant Toddler Social Emotional Assessment (BITSEA) and the Patient Health Questionnaire for Depression and Anxiety (PHQ-4, PHQ-9). The individual tests can take from 10-45 minutes to complete with additional time allocated for the results to be compiled and scored. Code 96127 can be applied for each standardized test that is administered, scored, and reported.

RVUs

Code	Work	PE	PE Non-Facility	MP	Total Non-Facility	Total Facility	Global
96127	0.00	0.13	0.13	0.01	0.14	0.14	XXX

96132

96132 Neuropsychological testing evaluation services by physician or other qualified health care professional, including integration of patient data, interpretation of standardized test results and clinical data, clinical decision making, treatment planning and report, and interactive feedback to the patient, family member(s) or caregiver(s), when performed; first hour

Plain English Description

Neuropsychological testing evaluation may include neuropsychological diagnostic assessment of several different and overlapping domains including intellectual and executive function, language and communication as well as attention capabilities and memory, visual-spatial and sensorimotor functioning, personality and emotional characteristics and adaptive behavior using standardized tests. These codes report time-based evaluation services reported per hour of physician or other qualified health care professional time spent interpreting test results and patient data, preparing the report and treatment plan, with incorporated clinical decision making. Raw and standardized scores may be analyzed with any additional test data acquired from computer or technician testing. Evaluation services usually include integration of the patient's data with other sources of clinical data and may also include interactive feedback to the patient, family member(s), or caregiver(s). Report 96132 for the first hour and 96133 for each additional hour.

RVUs

Code	Work	PE	PE Non-Facility	MP	Total Non-Facility	Total Facility	Global
96132	2.56	0.39	1.13	0.09	3.78	3.04	XXX

96133

✚ **96133 Neuropsychological testing evaluation services by physician or other qualified health care professional, including integration of patient data, interpretation of standardized test results and clinical data, clinical decision making, treatment planning and report, and interactive feedback to the patient, family member(s) or caregiver(s), when performed; each additional hour (List separately in addition to code for primary procedure)**

Plain English Description

Neuropsychological testing evaluation may include neuropsychological diagnostic assessment of several different and overlapping domains including intellectual and executive function, language and communication as well as attention capabilities and memory, visual-spatial and sensorimotor functioning, personality and emotional characteristics and adaptive behavior using standardized tests. These codes report time-based evaluation services reported per hour of physician or other qualified health care professional time spent interpreting test results and patient data, preparing the report and treatment plan, with incorporated clinical decision making. Raw and standardized scores may be analyzed with any additional test data acquired from computer or technician testing. Evaluation services usually include integration of the patient's data with other sources of clinical data and may also include interactive feedback to the patient, family member(s), or caregiver(s). Report 96132 for the first hour and 96133 for each additional hour.

RVUs

Code	Work	PE	PE Non-Facility	MP	Total Non-Facility	Total Facility	Global
96133	1.96	0.30	0.80	0.08	2.84	2.34	ZZZ

96136

96136 Psychological or neuropsychological test administration and scoring by physician or other qualified health care professional, two or more tests, any method; first 30 minutes

Plain English Description

Psychological or neuropsychological testing is performed to evaluate brain and mental function and impairment using standardized tests such as Halstead-Reitan Neuropsychological Battery, Wechsler Memory Scales, and Wisconsin Card Sorting Test. These codes report time-based testing services for two or more tests administered and are reported per 30 minutes of face-to-face time spent administering and scoring the tests. The psychologist, neuropsychologist, neurologist, or other qualified professional identifies and selects the appropriate tests to be administered. In a face-to-face encounter, the tests are administered. Raw and standardized scores are derived. Report 96136 for the first 30 minutes of test administration and scoring done by a physician or other qualified health care professional and 96137 for each additional 30 minutes. Report 96138 for the first 30 minutes of test administration and scoring done by a technician and 96139 for each additional 30 minutes. Report 96146 when the test is given and scored by a single automated, standardized instrument via electronic platform. The test data is returned to a qualified health care professional for interpretation, evaluation, and written report.

RVUs

Code	Work	PE	PE Non-Facility	MP	Total Non-Facility	Total Facility	Global
96136	0.55	0.12	0.75	0.03	1.33	0.70	XXX

96137

✚ **96137 Psychological or neuropsychological test administration and scoring by physician or other qualified health care professional, two or more tests, any method; each additional 30 minutes (List separately in addition to code for primary procedure)**

(96136, 96137 may be reported in conjunction with 96130, 96131, 96132, 96133 on the same or different days)

Plain English Description

Psychological or neuropsychological testing is performed to evaluate brain and mental function and impairment using standardized tests such as Halstead-Reitan Neuropsychological Battery, Wechsler Memory Scales, and Wisconsin Card Sorting Test. These codes report time-based testing services for two or more tests administered and are reported per 30 minutes of face-to-face time spent administering and scoring the tests. The psychologist, neuropsychologist, neurologist, or other qualified professional identifies and selects the appropriate tests to be administered. In a face-to-face encounter, the tests are administered. Raw and standardized scores are derived. Report 96136 for the first 30 minutes of test administration and scoring done by a physician or other qualified health care professional and 96137 for each additional 30 minutes. Report 96138 for the first 30 minutes of test administration and scoring done by a technician and 96139 for each additional 30 minutes. Report 96146 when the test is given and scored by a single automated, standardized instrument via electronic platform. The test data is returned to a qualified health care professional for interpretation, evaluation, and written report.

RVUs

Code	Work	PE	PE Non-Facility	MP	Total Non-Facility	Total Facility	Global
96137	0.46	0.07	0.74	0.02	1.22	0.55	ZZZ

96138

96138 Psychological or neuropsychological test administration and scoring by technician, two or more tests, any method; first 30 minutes

Plain English Description

Psychological or neuropsychological testing is performed to evaluate brain and mental function and impairment using standardized tests such as Halstead-Reitan Neuropsychological Battery, Wechsler Memory Scales, and Wisconsin Card Sorting Test. These codes report time-based testing services for two or more tests administered and are reported per 30 minutes of face-to-face time spent administering and scoring the tests. The psychologist, neuropsychologist, neurologist, or other qualified professional identifies and selects the appropriate tests to be administered. In a face-to-face encounter, the tests are administered. Raw and standardized scores are derived. Report 96136 for the first 30 minutes of test administration and scoring done by a physician or other qualified health care professional and 96137 for each additional 30 minutes. Report 96138 for the first 30 minutes of test administration and scoring done by a technician and 96139 for each additional 30 minutes. Report 96146 when the test is given and scored by a single automated, standardized instrument via electronic platform. The test data is returned to a qualified health care professional for interpretation, evaluation, and written report.

RVUs

Code	Work	PE	PE Non-Facility	MP	Total Non-Facility	Total Facility	Global
96138	0.00	1.06	1.06	0.01	1.07	1.07	XXX

96139

✚ **96139 Psychological or neuropsychological test administration and scoring by technician, two or more tests, any method; each additional 30 minutes (List separately in addition to code for primary procedure)**

(96138, 96139 may be reported in conjunction with 96130, 96131, 96132, 96133 on the same or different days)

(For 96136, 96137, 96138, 96139, do not include time for evaluation services [eg, integration of patient data or interpretation of test results]. This time is included in 96130, 96131, 96132, 96133)

Plain English Description

Psychological or neuropsychological testing is performed to evaluate brain and mental function and impairment using standardized tests such as Halstead-Reitan Neuropsychological Battery, Wechsler Memory Scales, and Wisconsin Card Sorting Test. These codes report time-based testing services for two or more tests administered and are reported per 30 minutes of face-to-face time spent administering and scoring the tests. The psychologist, neuropsychologist, neurologist, or other qualified professional identifies and selects the appropriate tests to be administered. In a face-to-face encounter, the tests are administered. Raw and standardized scores are derived. Report 96136 for the first 30 minutes of test administration and scoring done by a physician or other qualified health care professional and 96137 for each additional 30 minutes. Report 96138 for the first 30 minutes of test administration and scoring done by a technician and 96139 for each additional 30 minutes. Report 96146 when the test is given and scored by a single automated, standardized instrument via electronic platform. The test data is returned to a qualified health care professional for interpretation, evaluation, and written report.

RVUs

Code	Work	PE	PE Non-Facility	MP	Total Non-Facility	Total Facility	Global
96139	0.00	1.06	1.06	0.01	1.07	1.07	ZZZ

96146

96146 Psychological or neuropsychological test administration, with single automated, standardized instrument via electronic platform, with automated result only

(If test is administered by physician, other qualified health care professional, or technician, do not report 96146. To report, see 96127, 96136, 96137, 96138, 96139)

Plain English Description

Psychological or neuropsychological testing is performed to evaluate brain and mental function and impairment using standardized tests such as Halstead-Reitan Neuropsychological Battery, Wechsler Memory Scales, and Wisconsin Card Sorting Test. These codes report time-based testing services for two or more tests administered and are reported per 30 minutes of face-to-face time spent administering and scoring the tests. The psychologist, neuropsychologist, neurologist, or other qualified professional identifies and selects the appropriate tests to be administered. In a face-to-face encounter, the tests are administered. Raw and standardized scores are derived. Report 96136 for the first 30 minutes of test administration and scoring done by a physician or other qualified health care professional and 96137 for each additional 30 minutes. Report 96138 for the first 30 minutes of test administration and scoring done by a technician and 96139 for each additional 30 minutes. Report 96146 when the test is given and scored by a single automated, standardized instrument via electronic platform. The test data is returned to a qualified health care professional for interpretation, evaluation, and written report.

RVUs

Code	Work	PE	PE Non-Facility	MP	Total Non-Facility	Total Facility	Global
96146	0.00	0.05	0.05	0.01	0.06	0.06	XXX

96164-96171

● **96164 Health behavior intervention, group (2 or more patients), face-to-face; initial 30 minutes**

+● **96165 Health behavior intervention, group (2 or more patients), face-to-face; each additional 15 minutes (List separately in addition to code for primary service)**

(Use 96165 in conjunction with 96164)

● **96167 Health behavior intervention, family (with the patient present), face-to-face; initial 30 minutes**

+● **96168 Health behavior intervention, family (with the patient present), face-to-face; each additional 15 minutes (List separately in addition to code for primary service)**

(Use 96168 in conjunction with 96167)

● **96170 Health behavior intervention, family (without the patient present), face-to-face; initial 30 minutes**

+● **96171 Health behavior intervention, family (without the patient present), face-to-face; each additional 15 minutes (List separately in addition to code for primary service)**

(Use 96171 in conjunction with 96170)

Plain English Description

Health behavior intervention services are performed that may include cognitive, behavioral, social, psychophysiological, or other techniques designed to improve health, function, and treatment outcomes; reduce the frequency and severity of disease-related problems; minimize psychological stumbling blocks to managing the condition; and improve overall well-being. The intervention services may be provided by any health care professional with specialized training in health and behavior interventions including physicians, psychologists, advanced practice nurses, or clinical social workers. Intervention services are designed for the specific individual(s) based on a separately reportable assessment. Techniques used might include education related to biopsychosocial factors influencing health; stress reduction techniques including relaxation and guided imagery; seeking social support and participating in group discussions; developing needed social skills; and training in new management and coping strategies. Services focus on active patient participation in interventions aimed to improve the specific challenges related to the condition. Report 96164 for the first 30 minutes of face-to-face intervention services held in a group of 2 or more and 96165 for each additional 15 minutes.

RVUs

Code	Work	PE	PE Non-Facility	MP	Total Non-Facility	Total Facility	Global
96164	0.21	0.03	0.06	0.01	0.28	0.25	XXX
96165	0.10	0.01	0.03	0.00	0.13	0.11	ZZZ
96167	1.55	0.22	0.42	0.06	2.03	1.83	XXX
96168	0.55	0.08	0.15	0.02	0.72	0.65	ZZZ
96170	1.50	0.58	0.69	0.11	2.30	2.19	XXX
96171	0.54	0.21	0.25	0.05	0.84	0.80	ZZZ

96360-96361

96360 Intravenous infusion, hydration; initial, 31 minutes to 1 hour

(Do not report 96360 if performed as a concurrent infusion service)

(Do not report intravenous infusion for hydration of 30 minutes or less)

+ **96361 Intravenous infusion, hydration; each additional hour (List separately in addition to code for primary procedure)**

(Use 96361 in conjunction with 96360)

(Report 96361 for hydration infusion intervals of greater than 30 minutes beyond 1 hour increments)

(Report 96361 to identify hydration if provided as a secondary or subsequent service after a different initial service [96360, 96365, 96374, 96409, 96413] is administered through the same IV access)

Plain English Description

An intravenous infusion is administered for hydration. An intravenous line is placed into a vein, usually in the arm, and fluid is administered to provide additional fluid levels and electrolytes to counteract the effects of dehydration or supplement deficient oral fluid intake. The physician provides direct supervision of the fluid administration and is immediately available to intervene should complications arise. The physician provides periodic assessments of the patient and documentation of the patient's response to treatment. Use 96360 for the initial 31 minutes to 1 hour of hydration. Use 96361 for each additional hour.

RVUs

Code	Work	PE	PE Non-Facility	MP	Total Non-Facility	Total Facility	Global
96360	0.17	0.77	0.77	0.02	0.96	0.96	XXX
96361	0.09	0.28	0.28	0.01	0.38	0.38	ZZZ

96365-96368

96365 Intravenous infusion, for therapy, prophylaxis, or diagnosis (specify substance or drug); initial, up to 1 hour

+ **96366 Intravenous infusion, for therapy, prophylaxis, or diagnosis (specify substance or drug); each additional hour (List separately in addition to code for primary procedure)**

(Report 96366 in conjunction with 96365, 96367)

(Report 96366 for additional hour[s] of sequential infusion)

(Report 96366 for infusion intervals of greater than 30 minutes beyond 1 hour increments)

(Report 96366 in conjunction with 96365 to identify each second and subsequent infusions of the same drug/substance)

+ **96367 Intravenous infusion, for therapy, prophylaxis, or diagnosis (specify substance or drug); additional sequential infusion of a new drug/substance, up to 1 hour (List separately in addition to code for primary procedure)**

(Report 96367 in conjunction with 96365, 96374, 96409, 96413 to identify the infusion of a new drug/substance provided as a secondary or subsequent service after a different initial service is administered through the same IV access. Report 96367 only once per sequential infusion of same infusate mix)

+ **96368 Intravenous infusion, for therapy, prophylaxis, or diagnosis (specify substance or drug); concurrent infusion (List separately in addition to code for primary procedure)**

(Report 96368 only once per date of service)

(Report 96368 in conjunction with 96365, 96366, 96413, 96415, 96416)

Plain English Description

An intravenous infusion of a specified substance or drug is administered for therapy, prophylaxis, or diagnosis. An intravenous line is placed into a vein, usually in the arm, and the specified substance or drug is administered. The physician provides direct supervision of the administration and is immediately available to intervene should complications arise. The physician provides periodic assessments of the patient and documentation of the patient's response to treatment. Use code 96365 for an intravenous infusion up to 1 hour. Use add-on code 96366 for each additional hour of the same infusion. Use add-on code 96367 for another, sequential infusion of a different substance or drug for up to 1 hour. Use add-on code 96368 when a different substance or drug is administered at the same time as another drug in a concurrent infusion.

RVUs

Code	Work	PE	PE Non-Facility	MP	Total Non-Facility	Total Facility	Global
96365	0.21	1.74	1.74	0.05	2.00	2.00	XXX
96366	0.18	0.42	0.42	0.01	0.61	0.61	ZZZ
96367	0.19	0.66	0.66	0.02	0.87	0.87	ZZZ
96368	0.17	0.41	0.41	0.01	0.59	0.59	ZZZ

96372

96372 Therapeutic, prophylactic, or diagnostic injection (specify substance or drug); subcutaneous or intramuscular

(For administration of vaccines/toxoids, see 90460, 90461, 90471, 90472)

(Report 96372 for non-antineoplastic hormonal therapy injections)

(Report 96401 for anti-neoplastic nonhormonal injection therapy)

(Report 96402 for anti-neoplastic hormonal injection therapy)

(Do not report 96372 for injections given without direct physician or other qualified health care professional supervision. To report, use 99211. Hospitals may report 96372 when the physician or other qualified health care professional is not present)

(96372 does not include injections for allergen immunotherapy. For allergen immunotherapy injections, see 95115-95117)

Plain English Description

A subcutaneous or intramuscular injection of a therapeutic, prophylactic, or diagnostic substance or drug is given. A subcutaneous injection is administered just under the skin in the fatty tissue of the abdomen, upper arm, upper leg, or buttocks. The skin is cleansed. A 2-inch fold of skin is pinched between the thumb and forefinger. The needle is inserted completely under the skin at a 45- to 90-degree angle using a quick, sharp thrust. The plunger is retracted to check for blood. If blood is present, a new site is selected. If no blood is present, the medication is injected slowly into the tissue. The needle is withdrawn and mild pressure is applied. An intramuscular injection is administered in a similar fashion deep into muscle tissue, differing only in the sites of administration and the angle of needle insertion. Common sites include the gluteal muscles of the buttocks, the vastus lateralis muscle of the thigh, or the deltoid muscle of the upper arm. The angle of insertion is 90 degrees. Intramuscular administration provides rapid systemic absorption and can be used for administration of relatively large doses of medication.

RVUs

Code	Work	PE	PE Non-Facility	MP	Total Non-Facility	Total Facility	Global
96372	0.17	0.22	0.22	0.01	0.40	0.40	XXX

96374-96376

96374 Therapeutic, prophylactic, or diagnostic injection (specify substance or drug); intravenous push, single or initial substance/drug

+ **96375 Therapeutic, prophylactic, or diagnostic injection (specify substance or drug); each additional sequential intravenous push of a new substance/drug (List separately in addition to code for primary procedure)**

(Use 96375 in conjunction with 96365, 96374, 96409, 96413)

(Report 96375 to identify intravenous push of a new substance/drug if provided as a secondary or subsequent service after a different initial service is administered through the same IV access)

+ **96376 Therapeutic, prophylactic, or diagnostic injection (specify substance or drug); each additional sequential intravenous push of the same substance/drug provided in a facility (List separately in addition to code for primary procedure)**

(Do not report 96376 for a push performed within 30 minutes of a reported push of the same substance or drug)

(96376 may be reported by facilities only)

(Report 96376 in conjunction with 96365, 96374, 96409, 96413)

Plain English Description

A therapeutic, prophylactic, or diagnostic injection is administered by intravenous push (IVP) technique. The specified substance or drug is injected using a syringe directly into an injection site of an existing intravenous line or intermittent infusion set (saline lock). The injection is given over a short period of time, usually less than 15 minutes. Use 96374 for a single or initial substance or drug. Use 96375 as an add-on code for each additional sequential push of a new substance or drug provided through the same venous access site. Use 96376 for the facility component for each additional sequential intravenous push of the same substance/drug when the interval between each administration is 30 minutes or more.

RVUs

Code	Work	PE	PE Non-Facility	MP	Total Non-Facility	Total Facility	Global
96374	0.18	0.91	0.91	0.02	1.11	1.11	XXX
96375	0.10	0.35	0.35	0.01	0.46	0.46	ZZZ
96376	0.00	0.00	0.00	0.00	0.00	0.00	ZZZ

96413-96417

96413 Chemotherapy administration, intravenous infusion technique; up to 1 hour, single or initial substance/drug

(Report 96361 to identify hydration if administered as a secondary or subsequent service in association with 96413 through the same IV access)

(Report 96366, 96367, 96375 to identify therapeutic, prophylactic, or diagnostic drug infusion or injection, if administered as a secondary or subsequent service in association with 96413 through the same IV access)

+ **96415 Chemotherapy administration, intravenous infusion technique; each additional hour (List separately in addition to code for primary procedure)**

(Use 96415 in conjunction with 96413)

(Report 96415 for infusion intervals of greater than 30 minutes beyond 1-hour increments)

96416 Chemotherapy administration, intravenous infusion technique; initiation of prolonged chemotherapy infusion (more than 8 hours), requiring use of a portable or implantable pump

(For refilling and maintenance of a portable pump or an implantable infusion pump or reservoir for drug delivery, see 96521-96523)

+ **96417 Chemotherapy administration, intravenous infusion technique; each additional sequential infusion (different substance/drug), up to 1 hour (List separately in addition to code for primary procedure)**

(Use 96417 in conjunction with 96413)

(Report only once per sequential infusion. Report 96415 for additional hour(s) of sequential infusion)

Plain English Description

An intravenous infusion of a chemotherapy substance or drug is administered for treatment of a malignant neoplasm. An intravenous line is placed into a vein, usually in the arm, and the specified chemotherapy agent is administered. The physician provides direct supervision of the administration of the chemotherapy agent and is immediately available to intervene should complications arise. The physician provides periodic assessments of the patient and documentation of the patient's response to treatment. Use code 96413 for an intravenous infusion up to one hour of a single or initial chemotherapy substance or drug. Use add-on code 96415 for each additional hour of the chemotherapy substance or drug. Use 96416 for prolonged chemotherapy intravenous infusion of more than eight hours requiring the use of a portable or implantable pump. Use add-on code 96417 for an additional sequential infusion of a different substance or drug for up to one hour.

RVUs

Code	Work	PE	PE Non-Facility	MP	Total Non-Facility	Total Facility	Global
96413	0.28	3.58	3.58	0.09	3.95	3.95	XXX
96415	0.19	0.64	0.64	0.02	0.85	0.85	ZZZ
96416	0.21	3.65	3.65	0.09	3.95	3.95	XXX
96417	0.21	1.66	1.66	0.05	1.92	1.92	ZZZ

96450

96450 Chemotherapy administration, into CNS (eg, intrathecal), requiring and including spinal puncture

(For intravesical (bladder) chemotherapy administration, use 51720)

(For insertion of subarachnoid catheter and reservoir for infusion of drug, see 62350, 62351, 62360-62362; for insertion of intraventricular catheter and reservoir, see 61210, 61215)

(If fluoroscopic guidance is performed, use 77003)

Plain English Description

One or a combination of antineoplastic drugs is injected into the central nervous system. This procedure is also referred to as intrathecal chemotherapy. The skin over the lumbar spine is disinfected and a local anesthetic is administered. A lumbar puncture needle is then inserted into the spinal canal. CSF specimens are collected as needed. A spinal catheter is advanced through the lumbar puncture needle. The antineoplastic drugs are then injected into the spinal fluid in the spinal canal. The spinal fluid containing the antineoplastic drugs then circulates around the spinal canal and brain delivering the drugs to the central nervous system. Upon completion of the procedure, the spinal catheter is removed and pressure is applied at the puncture site as needed.

RVUs

Code	Work	PE	PE Non-Facility	MP	Total Non-Facility	Total Facility	Global
96450	1.53	0.61	3.43	0.12	5.08	2.26	000

96542

96542 Chemotherapy injection, subarachnoid or intraventricular via subcutaneous reservoir, single or multiple agents

(For radioactive isotope therapy, use 79005)

Plain English Description

One or a combination of antineoplastic drugs is injected into the subarachnoid or intraventricular spaces of the central nervous system via a previously placed subcutaneous reservoir. A subcutaneous reservoir is used for injection of chemotherapy drugs, monoclonal antibody agents, other biologic response modifiers, and other antineoplastic substances. The skin is prepped over the reservoir site. A special needle is used to puncture the skin and the needle is then advanced into the reservoir. The reservoir is filled with the prescribed amount of the chemotherapy drug or other highly complex drug or biologic agent. The reservoir may then be manually compressed to deliver the drug to the subarachnoid space or ventricles or a pump may be used to deliver the drug. The drug circulates with the cerebrospinal fluid and is delivered to the site of the neoplasm.

RVUs

Code	Work	PE	PE Non-Facility	MP	Total Non-Facility	Total Facility	Global
96542	0.75	0.38	2.89	0.08	3.72	1.21	XXX

97032

97032 Application of a modality to 1 or more areas; electrical stimulation (manual), each 15 minutes

(For transcutaneous electrical modulation pain reprocessing [TEMPR/scrambler therapy], use 0278T)

Plain English Description

Electrical stimulation involves the use of a transcutaneous electrical nerve stimulation device (TENS), functional electrical stimulation device (FES), or a neuromuscular electrical stimulation device (NMES). The physical therapist or other physical therapy aid places the electrodes of the selected device over the region to be stimulated. The electrical impulse is set to the desired strength and the control unit is turned on. Electrical impulses are transmitted to the skin. The electrical stimulation device causes the muscles to contract. The muscle contraction stimulates both muscle and nerve tissues to relieve pain and promote healing. Electrical stimulation may be provided as a supervised modality that does not require direct (one-on-one) patient contact or it may be provided under constant attendance with direct (one-on-one) patient contact. Code 97032 reports electrical stimulation with constant attendance and direct (one-on-one) patient contact per 15 minutes.

RVUs

Code	Work	PE	PE Non-Facility	MP	Total Non-Facility	Total Facility	Global
97032	0.25	0.16	0.16	0.01	0.42	0.42	XXX

97110

97110 Therapeutic procedure, 1 or more areas, each 15 minutes; therapeutic exercises to develop strength and endurance, range of motion and flexibility

Plain English Description

Therapeutic exercise is the application of careful, graduated force to the body to increase strength, endurance, range of motion, and flexibility. Increased muscle strength is achieved by the deliberate overloading of a targeted muscle or muscle group and improved endurance is achieved by raising the intensity of the strengthening exercise to the targeted area(s) over a prolonged period of time. To maintain range of motion (ROM) and flexibility requires the careful movement and stretching of contractile and non-contractile tissue that may tighten with injury or neurological disease, causing weakness and/or spasticity. Therapeutic exercise can increase blood flow to the targeted area, reduce pain and inflammation, reduce the risk of blood clots from venous stasis, decrease muscle atrophy, and improve coordination and motor control. Therapeutic exercise may be prescribed following acute illness or injury and for chronic conditions that affect physical activity or function.

RVUs

Code	Work	PE	PE Non-Facility	MP	Total Non-Facility	Total Facility	Global
97110	0.45	0.40	0.40	0.02	0.87	0.87	XXX

97112

97112 Therapeutic procedure, 1 or more areas, each 15 minutes; neuromuscular reeducation of movement, balance, coordination, kinesthetic sense, posture, and/or proprioception for sitting and/or standing activities

Plain English Description

Therapeutic procedures for neuromuscular reeducation are used to develop conscious control of a single muscle or muscle group and heighten the awareness of the body's position in space, especially the position of the extremities when sitting or standing. Neuromuscular reeducation is employed during the recovery or regeneration stage following severe injury or trauma, cerebral vascular accident, or systemic neurological disease. The goal of therapy is improved range of motion (ROM), balance, coordination, posture, and spatial awareness. Techniques may include proprioceptive neuromuscular facilitation which uses diagonal contract-relax patterns of skeletal muscles to stimulate receptors in the joints that communicate body position to the brain via motor and sensory nerves. Feldenkrais is a method which observes the patient's habitual movement patterns and teaches new patterns based on efficient active or passive repetitive conditioning. Additional techniques that may be useful for neuromuscular reeducation are Bobath concept, which promotes motor learning and efficient motor control, and biomechanical ankle platform system (BAPS) boards.

RVUs

Code	Work	PE	PE Non-Facility	MP	Total Non-Facility	Total Facility	Global
97112	0.50	0.48	0.48	0.02	1.00	1.00	XXX

97116

97116 Therapeutic procedure, 1 or more areas, each 15 minutes; gait training (includes stair climbing)

(Use 96000-96003 to report comprehensive gait and motion analysis procedures)

Plain English Description

Gait training is a therapeutic procedure that observes and educates an individual in the manner of walking including the rhythm, cadence, step, stride, and speed. The objective of gait training is to strengthen muscles and joints, improve balance and posture, and develop muscle memory. As the lower extremities are retrained for repetitive motion, the body also benefits from the exercise with increased endurance, improved heart/lung function, and reduced or improved osteoporosis. Gait training is an appropriate therapeutic procedure following brain and/or spinal cord injury, stroke, fracture of the pelvis and/or lower extremity, joint injury or replacement of the knee, hip, or ankle, amputation, and for certain musculoskeletal and/or neurological diseases. A treadmill fitted with a safety harness is initially used to ensure safe walking. As the patient gains strength and balance, step training and stair climbing is added to the treatment modality.

RVUs

Code	Work	PE	PE Non-Facility	MP	Total Non-Facility	Total Facility	Global
97116	0.45	0.39	0.39	0.02	0.86	0.86	XXX

97124

97124 Therapeutic procedure, 1 or more areas, each 15 minutes; massage, including effleurage, petrissage and/or tapotement (stroking, compression, percussion)

(For myofascial release, use 97140)

Plain English Description

Therapeutic massage uses pressure on the skin and underlying tissues to redirect venous and lymphatic flow back toward the heart. Massage techniques include effleurage—a smooth, rhythmic pressure applied continuously to the skin either superficially or deeply; petrissage—a technique in which skin is lifted, pressed down, squeezed, pinched, rolled, wrung, or shaken to stimulate local circulation; and tapotement—a technique that includes rapid, repetitive, rhythmic blows to skin and soft tissue. Massage increases blood flow to the skin, muscle, and connective tissue and facilitates vasodilation. It may help to reduce pain and inflammation, reduce the formation of scar tissue or adhesions, mobilize fluids, relax muscles, and promote a feeling of relaxation and sedation.

RVUs

Code	Work	PE	PE Non-Facility	MP	Total Non-Facility	Total Facility	Global
97124	0.35	0.47	0.47	0.01	0.83	0.83	XXX

97140

97140 Manual therapy techniques (eg, mobilization/manipulation, manual lymphatic drainage, manual traction), 1 or more regions, each 15 minutes

(For needle insertion[s] without injection[s] [eg, dry needling, trigger-point acupuncture], see 20560, 20561)

Plain English Description

Manual therapies are skilled, specific, hands-on techniques usually performed by physical therapists, occupational therapists, chiropractors, osteopaths, and/or physiatrists to diagnose and treat soft tissue and joint problems. The goal of manual therapy is to modulate pain and induce relaxation, increase range of motion (ROM), facilitate movement, function, and stability, decrease inflammation, and improve muscle tone and extensibility. Tissue mobilization involves slow, controlled myofascial stretching using deep pressure to break up fibrous muscle tissue and/or connective tissue adhesions. Manipulation is a more forceful stretching of the myofascial tissue that takes the joint just beyond its restricted barrier. Manual lymphatic drainage is a type of light massage employed to reduce swelling by gentle movement of the skin in the direction of lymphatic flow. Manual traction involves the controlled counterforce of the therapist to induce asymptomatic strain by gently stretching muscle and/or connective tissue.

RVUs

Code	Work	PE	PE Non-Facility	MP	Total Non-Facility	Total Facility	Global
97140	0.43	0.35	0.35	0.02	0.80	0.80	XXX

97161-97164

97161 Physical therapy evaluation: low complexity, requiring these components:

A history with no personal factors and/or comorbidities that impact the plan of care;

An examination of body system(s) using standardized tests and measures addressing 1-2 elements from any of the following: body structures and functions, activity limitations, and/or participation restrictions;

A clinical presentation with stable and/or uncomplicated characteristics; and

Clinical decision making of low complexity using standardized patient assessment instrument and/or measurable assessment of functional outcome.

Typically, 20 minutes are spent face-to-face with the patient and/or family.

97162 Physical therapy evaluation: moderate complexity, requiring these components:

A history of present problem with 1-2 personal factors and/or comorbidities that impact the plan of care;

An examination of body systems using standardized tests and measures in addressing a total of 3 or more elements from any of the following: body structures and functions, activity limitations, and/or participation restrictions;

An evolving clinical presentation with changing characteristics; and

Clinical decision making of moderate complexity using standardized patient assessment instrument and/or measurable assessment of functional outcome.

Typically, 30 minutes are spent face-to-face with the patient and/or family.

97163 Physical therapy evaluation: high complexity, requiring these components:

A history of present problem with 3 or more personal factors and/or comorbidities that impact the plan of care;

An examination of body systems using standardized tests and measures addressing a total of 4 or more elements from any of the following: body structures and functions, activity limitations, and/or participation restrictions;

A clinical presentation with unstable and unpredictable characteristics; and

Clinical decision making of high complexity using standardized patient assessment instrument and/or measurable assessment of functional outcome.

Typically, 45 minutes are spent face-to-face with the patient and/or family.

97164 Re-evaluation of physical therapy established plan of care, requiring these components:

An examination including a review of history and use of standardized tests and measures is required; and

Revised plan of care using a standardized patient assessment instrument and/or measurable assessment of functional outcome

Typically, 20 minutes are spent face-to-face with the patient and/or family.

Plain English Description

A physical therapy evaluation or re-evaluation is performed. The physical therapist takes a history of the current complaint, including onset of symptoms, comorbidities, changes since the onset, treatment received for the symptoms or condition, medications prescribed for it, and any other medications the patient is taking. A physical examination of body systems is done to assess physical structure and function, any activities or movements that exacerbate the symptoms, limit activity, or restrict participation in movement, as well as anything that helps to relieve the symptoms. The evaluation may involve provocative maneuvers or positions that increase symptoms; tests for joint flexibility and muscle strength; assessments of general mobility, posture, and core strength; evaluation of muscle tone; and tests for restrictions of movement caused by myofascial disorders. Following the history and physical, the therapist determines the patient's clinical presentation characteristics, provides a detailed explanation of the condition, identifies physical therapy treatment options, and explains how often and how long physical therapy modalities should be applied. The physical therapist will then develop a plan of care with clinical decision making based on patient assessment and/or measurable functional outcome. The plan of care may include both physical therapy in the clinic and exercises or changes in the home environment. Upon re-evaluation, the established care plan is reviewed and an interim history is taken requiring the use of standardized tests and measures. The patient's response to treatment is evaluated and the plan of care is revised based on the patient's measurable response. Report code 97161 for physical therapy evaluation of low complexity; 97162 for moderate complexity; 97163 for high complexity; and 97164 for re-evaluation.

RVUs

Code	Work	PE	PE Non-Facility	MP	Total Non-Facility	Total Facility	Global
97161	1.20	1.18	1.18	0.05	2.43	2.43	XXX
97162	1.20	1.18	1.18	0.05	2.43	2.43	XXX
97163	1.20	1.18	1.18	0.05	2.43	2.43	XXX
97164	0.75	0.89	0.89	0.03	1.67	1.67	XXX

97530

97530 Therapeutic activities, direct (one-on-one) patient contact (use of dynamic activities to improve functional performance), each 15 minutes

Plain English Description

In a one-on-one physical therapy session, the provider instructs and assists the patient in therapeutic activities designed to address specific functional limitations. The therapeutic activities are specifically developed and modified for the patient. Dynamic/movement activities, also called kinetic activities, that are designed to improve functional performance such as lifting, bending, pushing, pulling, jumping, and reaching are included in this service. For example, the patient may be given therapeutic activities to perform to improve the ability to sit, stand, and get out of bed after an injury without straining or risking reinjury. This code is reported for each 15 minutes of one-on-one therapeutic activity provided.

RVUs

Code	Work	PE	PE Non-Facility	MP	Total Non-Facility	Total Facility	Global
97530	0.44	0.66	0.66	0.02	1.12	1.12	XXX

97597-97598

97597 Debridement (eg, high pressure waterjet with/without suction, sharp selective debridement with scissors, scalpel and forceps), open wound, (eg, fibrin, devitalized epidermis and/or dermis, exudate, debris, biofilm), including topical application(s), wound assessment, use of a whirlpool, when performed and instruction(s) for ongoing care, per session, total wound(s) surface area; first 20 sq cm or less

+ **97598 Debridement (eg, high pressure waterjet with/without suction, sharp selective debridement with scissors, scalpel and forceps), open wound, (eg, fibrin, devitalized epidermis and/or dermis, exudate, debris, biofilm), including topical application(s), wound assessment, use of a whirlpool, when performed and instruction(s) for ongoing care, per session, total wound(s) surface area; each additional 20 sq cm, or part thereof (List separately in addition to code for primary procedure)**

(Use 97598 in conjunction with 97597)

Plain English Description

An open wound is evaluated for size, depth, and evidence of inflammation, ulceration, or necrosis. Whirlpool is used as needed prior to the debridement procedure. The involved tissue, including fibrin, devitalized epidermis and/ or dermis, exudate, debris, or biofilm, is selectively debrided using a high-pressure waterjet or sharp debridement. A high-pressure waterjet system consists of a power console, foot pedal, disposable hand-held waterjet/ aspirator, sterile water, tubing, and evacuation receptacle. The target tissue is identified. A high-pressure stream of water is projected at the target tissue, which is simultaneously cut and aspirated into an evacuation receptacle. Sharp debridement involves using scissors, scalpel, and/or forceps to selectively remove devitalized tissue and debris. Topical agents to promote healing and dressings are applied as needed following the debridement. The patient or caregiver is instructed on dressing changes and wound evaluation. Use 97597 for debridement of the first 20 sq cm of wound surface area. Use 97598 for each additional 20 sq cm debrided or portion thereof.

RVUs

Code	Work	PE	PE Non-Facility	MP	Total Non-Facility	Total Facility	Global
97597	0.77	0.22	1.91	0.06	2.74	1.05	000
97598	0.50	0.18	0.75	0.06	1.31	0.74	ZZZ

97750

97750 Physical performance test or measurement (eg, musculoskeletal, functional capacity), with written report, each 15 minutes

Plain English Description

The physical performance test (PPT) provides a direct, objective, quantitative assessment of the functional capacity of an individual. Using a stopwatch, pen, paper, 5 kidney beans, 1 teaspoon, an empty coffee can, a heavy book, a shelf, a jacket, sweater, or coat, and a penny, the individual is observed performing tasks that simulate activities of daily living. The test is most often performed on the elderly and/or cognitively impaired. PPT may include a 7 item scale or a 9 item scale. Each item is scored 0-4, with a minimum possible score of 0 (both 7 and 9 item) and maximum score of 28 (7 item) or 36 (9 item). The higher the score, the better the performance and lower the incidence of cognitive impairment. In a 7 item test, the individual is scored on writing a sentence, simulating eating, turning 360 degrees, putting on and taking off a jacket, sweater, or coat, lifting a book and placing it on a shelf, picking up a penny from the floor and walking 50 feet. For a 9 item test, stair climbing is also included and scored as 2 items. An evaluator monitors and times the test and provides a written report of the findings.

RVUs

Code	Work	PE	PE Non-Facility	MP	Total Non-Facility	Total Facility	Global
97750	0.45	0.52	0.52	0.02	0.99	0.99	XXX

97810-97814

97810 Acupuncture, 1 or more needles; without electrical stimulation, initial 15 minutes of personal one-on-one contact with the patient

(Do not report 97810 in conjunction with 97813)

+ **97811 Acupuncture, 1 or more needles; without electrical stimulation, each additional 15 minutes of personal one-on-one contact with the patient, with re-insertion of needle(s) (List separately in addition to code for primary procedure)**

(Use 97811 in conjunction with 97810, 97813)

97813 Acupuncture, 1 or more needles; with electrical stimulation, initial 15 minutes of personal one-on-one contact with the patient

(Do not report 97813 in conjunction with 97810)

+ **97814 Acupuncture, 1 or more needles; with electrical stimulation, each additional 15 minutes of personal one-on-one contact with the patient, with re-insertion of needle(s) (List separately in addition to code for primary procedure)**

(Use 97814 in conjunction with 97810, 97813)

(Do not report 97810, 97811, 97813, 97814 in conjunction with 20560, 20561. When both time-based acupuncture services and needle insertion[s] without injection[s] are performed, report only the time-based acupuncture codes)

Plain English Description

Acupuncture is a traditional Chinese medicine technique used most commonly for pain relief in which the practitioner stimulates specific acupuncture points on the body by inserting thin, sterile needles through the skin. Stimulation of the acupuncture points opens the flow of chi through the meridian pathways and corrects the imbalance of energy flow through the body. Traditional acupuncture may be used together with moxibustion or cupping therapy. Moxibustion is the burning of prepared cones of moxa, a dried, spongy herb known as mugwort, on or near the skin to facilitate healing. Cupping is the creation of local areas of suction to increase blood flow and facilitate healing. Acupuncture is done with or without electrical stimulation in which the needles that are inserted into the skin are then connected to a small generator device, which sends continuous pulses of electrical stimulation through the needle into the tissue. Report 97810 for the first 15 minutes of acupuncture without electrical stimulation and 97811 for each additional 15 minutes without electrical stimulation including re-insertion of needles. Report 97813 for the first 15 minutes of acupuncture with electrical stimulation and 97814 for each additional 15 minutes with electrical stimulation including re-insertion of needles.

RVUs

Code	Work	PE	PE Non-Facility	MP	Total Non-Facility	Total Facility	Global
97810	0.60	0.23	0.40	0.05	1.05	0.88	XXX
97811	0.50	0.19	0.25	0.05	0.80	0.74	ZZZ
97813	0.65	0.25	0.47	0.05	1.17	0.95	XXX
97814	0.55	0.21	0.36	0.05	0.96	0.81	ZZZ

99151-99153

⊘ **99151 Moderate sedation services provided by the same physician or other qualified health care professional performing the diagnostic or therapeutic service that the sedation supports, requiring the presence of an independent trained observer to assist in the monitoring of the patient's level of consciousness and physiological status; initial 15 minutes of intraservice time, patient younger than 5 years of age**

⊘ **99152 Moderate sedation services provided by the same physician or other qualified health care professional performing the diagnostic or therapeutic service that the sedation supports, requiring the presence of an independent trained observer to assist in the monitoring of the patient's level of consciousness and physiological status; initial 15 minutes of intraservice time, patient age 5 years or older**

+ **99153 Moderate sedation services provided by the same physician or other qualified health care professional performing the diagnostic or therapeutic service that the sedation supports, requiring the presence of an independent trained observer to assist in the monitoring of the patient's level of consciousness and physiological status; each additional 15 minutes intraservice time (List separately in addition to code for primary service)**

(Use 99153 in conjunction with 99151, 99152)

(Do not report 99153 in conjunction with 99155, 99156)

Plain English Description

Moderate sedation services are provided by the same physician or other qualified health care professional who is performing the diagnostic or therapeutic service requiring the sedation with an independent trained observer to assist in monitoring the patient. A patient assessment is performed. An intravenous line is inserted and fluids are administered as needed. A sedative agent is then administered. The patient is maintained under moderate sedation, with monitoring of the patient's consciousness level and physiological status that includes oxygen saturation, heart rate, and blood pressure. Following completion of the procedure, the physician or other qualified health care professional continues to monitor the patient until he/she has recovered from the sedation and can be turned over to nursing staff for continued care. Use 99151 for the first 15 minutes of intraservice time for a patient younger than 5 years old; 99152 for the first 15 minutes of intraservice time for a patient age 5 years or older; and 99153 for each additional 15 minutes.

RVUs

Code	Work	PE	PE Non-Facility	MP	Total Non-Facility	Total Facility	Global
99151	0.50	0.12	1.55	0.05	2.10	0.67	XXX
99152	0.25	0.08	1.16	0.02	1.43	0.35	XXX
99153	0.00	0.29	0.29	0.01	0.30	0.30	ZZZ

99183

99183 Physician or other qualified health care professional attendance and supervision of hyperbaric oxygen therapy, per session

(Evaluation and Management services and/or procedures [eg, wound debridement] provided in a hyperbaric oxygen treatment facility in conjunction with a hyperbaric oxygen therapy session should be reported separately)

Plain English Description

Hyperbaric oxygen therapy is performed to treat decompression sickness, also referred to as "the bends," which is caused by surfacing too quickly when scuba diving. It may also be performed for air embolism or to treat serious infections, severe anemia, and wounds that won't heal, such as those seen in diabetics or in patients with radiation injuries. The patient is placed in a special chamber or room where the air pressure is raised to a level up to 3 times higher than normal air pressure. The increased air pressure causes the lungs to take in more oxygen than is possible under normal air pressure. The increased levels of oxygen in the lungs then enter the blood increasing oxygen levels and restoring normal blood gases. Adequate oxygen levels in the blood are essential for normal tissue function and also for healing of injured tissues. The patient may remain in the hyperbaric oxygen chamber or room for up to 2 hours. During the treatment period, the patient is observed and the response to treatment monitored by a physician or other qualified health care professional.

RVUs

Code	Work	PE	PE Non-Facility	MP	Total Non-Facility	Total Facility	Global
99183	2.11	0.78	0.78	0.27	3.16	3.16	XXX

0075T-0076T

0075T Transcatheter placement of extracranial vertebral artery stent(s), including radiologic supervision and interpretation, open or percutaneous; initial vessel

+ **0076T Transcatheter placement of extracranial vertebral artery stent(s), including radiologic supervision and interpretation, open or percutaneous; each additional vessel (List separately in addition to code for primary procedure)**

(Use 0076T in conjunction with 0075T)

(When the ipsilateral extracranial vertebral arteriogram (including imaging and selective catheterization) confirms the need for stenting, then 0075T and 0076T include all ipsilateral extracranial vertebral catheterization, all diagnostic imaging for ipsilateral extracranial vertebral artery stenting, and all related radiologic supervision and interpretation. If stenting is not indicated, then the appropriate codes for selective catheterization and imaging should be reported in lieu of 0075T or 0076T)

Plain English Description

The transcatheter placement of an extracranial vertebral artery stent(s) is a minimally invasive procedure that may be performed on patients with atherosclerotic stenosis, dissection, or aneurysm of the vessel. The vertebral artery originates from the subclavian artery and can be divided into four sections, V1-V4. V1-V3 lie extracranially in the area of the cervical vertebra and V4 begins at the dura mater, becoming intracranial. V1 is the most common site for sclerotic disease to form; and V3 near the dura mater is a common location for dissection to occur. The placement of an extracranial vertebral artery stent(s) is usually performed under local anesthesia with the patient pretreated with antiplatelet medication to reduce the risk of stent thrombosis. A sheath or guide approach is carried out in the femoral artery or ipsilateral brachial or radial arteries. For open cut down technique, an incision is made in the skin, carried down though the fascia to locate the vessel, and a catheter is inserted. For percutaneous technique, the vessel is cannulated using a large bore needle inserted through the skin into the vessel, and a catheter is inserted though the needle into the artery. Under fluoroscopy, the catheter is threaded into the subclavian artery and advanced to a point just proximal to where the vertebral artery originates. Biplane road maps are obtained to identify the area of disease which is then bypassed with a guidewire. Balloon angioplasty may be performed before deployment of the stent. After satisfactory placement of the stent is confirmed, the catheter is removed. Code 0075T is used for treatment of the first vessel. Code 0076T is reported for each additional vessel.

RVUs

Code	Work	PE	PE Non-Facility	MP	Total Non-Facility	Total Facility	Global
0075T	0.00	0.00	0.00	0.00	0.00	0.00	XXX
0076T	0.00	0.00	0.00	0.00	0.00	0.00	XXX

0106T-0110T

0106T Quantitative sensory testing (QST), testing and interpretation per extremity; using touch pressure stimuli to assess large diameter sensation

0107T Quantitative sensory testing (QST), testing and interpretation per extremity; using vibration stimuli to assess large diameter fiber sensation

0108T Quantitative sensory testing (QST), testing and interpretation per extremity; using cooling stimuli to assess small nerve fiber sensation and hyperalgesia

0109T Quantitative sensory testing (QST), testing and interpretation per extremity; using heat-pain stimuli to assess small nerve fiber sensation and hyperalgesia

0110T Quantitative sensory testing (QST), testing and interpretation per extremity; using other stimuli to assess sensation

Plain English Description

A device is used that provides specific sensory stimulation to test the sensory response of one of the patient's limbs. If the physician tests pressure stimulation, use 0106T. If vibration sensation is tested, use 0107T. If the patient's sensory response to cool temperatures is tested, use 0108T. For the testing of heat and/or pain stimuli, use 0109T. If other stimuli not found in codes 0106T-0109T are used to test sensation, use 0110T.

RVUs

Code	Work	PE	PE Non-Facility	MP	Total Non-Facility	Total Facility	Global
0106T	0.00	0.00	0.00	0.00	0.00	0.00	XXX
0107T	0.00	0.00	0.00	0.00	0.00	0.00	XXX
0108T	0.00	0.00	0.00	0.00	0.00	0.00	XXX
0109T	0.00	0.00	0.00	0.00	0.00	0.00	XXX
0110T	0.00	0.00	0.00	0.00	0.00	0.00	XXX

0213T-0215T

0213T Injection(s), diagnostic or therapeutic agent, paravertebral facet (zygapophyseal) joint (or nerves innervating that joint) with ultrasound guidance, cervical or thoracic; single level

(To report bilateral procedure, use 0213T with modifier 50)

✚ **0214T Injection(s), diagnostic or therapeutic agent, paravertebral facet (zygapophyseal) joint (or nerves innervating that joint) with ultrasound guidance, cervical or thoracic; second level (List separately in addition to code for primary procedure)**

(Use 0214T in conjunction with 0213T)

(For bilateral procedure, report 0214T twice. Do not report modifier 50 in conjunction with 0214T)

✚ **0215T Injection(s), diagnostic or therapeutic agent, paravertebral facet (zygapophyseal) joint (or nerves innervating that joint) with ultrasound guidance, cervical or thoracic; third and any additional level(s) (List separately in addition to code for primary procedure)**

(Do not report 0215T more than once per day)

(Use 0215T in conjunction with 0213T, 0214T)

(For bilateral procedure, report 0215T twice. Do not report modifier 50 in conjunction with 0215T)

Plain English Description

Paravertebral facet joints, also called zygapophyseal joints, are located on the back (posterior) of the spine on each side of the vertebra at the point where one vertebra overlaps the next. Facet joint pain may be associated with post-laminectomy syndrome or other spinal surgery with destabilization of the spinal joints, scar tissue formation, or recurrent disc herniation. Other causes include spondylosis, spondylolisthesis, and arthritis. Using ultrasound guidance, a diagnostic or therapeutic facet joint injection or injection of nerves innervating the joint is performed. The skin overlying the facet joint is prepared and a local anesthetic is injected. A spinal needle is directed into the facet joint space until bone or cartilage is encountered. A small amount of contrast material is injected to verify that the needle is correctly positioned. This is followed by injection of a local anesthetic and/or steroid. Diagnostic facet joint injection uses a local anesthetic to identify the specific area generating the pain. If the patient experiences pain relief for a significant period of time following a diagnostic injection, the physician will perform a therapeutic injection on a subsequent date of service using a long-acting local anesthetic in conjunction with a steroid. Use 0213T for a single cervical or thoracic facet joint injection; use 0214T for the second level; and use 0215T for the third and any additional cervical or thoracic levels injected.

RVUs

Code	Work	PE	PE Non-Facility	MP	Total Non-Facility	Total Facility	Global
0213T	0.00	0.00	0.00	0.00	0.00	0.00	XXX
0214T	0.00	0.00	0.00	0.00	0.00	0.00	ZZZ
0215T	0.00	0.00	0.00	0.00	0.00	0.00	ZZZ

0216T-0218T

0216T Injection(s), diagnostic or therapeutic agent, paravertebral facet (zygapophyseal) joint (or nerves innervating that joint) with ultrasound guidance, lumbar or sacral; single level

(To report bilateral procedure, use 0216T with modifier 50)

+ **0217T Injection(s), diagnostic or therapeutic agent, paravertebral facet (zygapophyseal) joint (or nerves innervating that joint) with ultrasound guidance, lumbar or sacral; second level (List separately in addition to code for primary procedure)**

(Use 0217T in conjunction with 0216T)

(For bilateral procedure, report 0217T twice. Do not report modifier 50 in conjunction with 0217T)

+ **0218T Injection(s), diagnostic or therapeutic agent, paravertebral facet (zygapophyseal) joint (or nerves innervating that joint) with ultrasound guidance, lumbar or sacral; third and any additional level(s) (List separately in addition to code for primary procedure)**

(Do not report 0218T more than once per day)

(Use 0218T in conjunction with 0216T, 0217T)

(If injection(s) are performed using fluoroscopy or CT, see 64490-64495)

(For bilateral procedure, report 0218T twice. Do not report modifier 50 in conjunction with 0218T)

Plain English Description

Paravertebral facet joints, also called zygapophyseal joints, are located on the back (posterior) of the spine on each side of the vertebra at the point where one vertebra overlaps the next. Facet joint pain may be associated with post-laminectomy syndrome or other spinal surgery with destabilization of the spinal joints, scar tissue formation, or recurrent disc herniation. Other causes include spondylosis, spondylolisthesis, and arthritis. Using ultrasound guidance, a diagnostic or therapeutic facet joint injection or injection of nerves innervating the joint is performed. The skin overlying the facet joint is prepared and a local anesthetic is injected. A spinal needle is directed into the facet joint space until bone or cartilage is encountered. A small amount of contrast material is injected to verify that the needle is correctly positioned. This is followed by injection of a local anesthetic and/or steroid. Diagnostic facet joint injection uses a local anesthetic to identify the specific area generating the pain. If the patient experiences pain relief for a significant period of time following a diagnostic injection, the physician will perform a therapeutic injection on a subsequent date of service using a long-acting local anesthetic in conjunction with a steroid. Use 0216T for a single lumbar or sacral facet joint injection; use 0217T for the second level; and use 0218T for the third and any additional lumbar or sacral levels injected.

RVUs

Code	Work	PE	PE Non-Facility	MP	Total Non-Facility	Total Facility	Global
0216T	0.00	0.00	0.00	0.00	0.00	0.00	XXX
0217T	0.00	0.00	0.00	0.00	0.00	0.00	ZZZ
0218T	0.00	0.00	0.00	0.00	0.00	0.00	ZZZ

0274T-0275T

0274T Percutaneous laminotomy/laminectomy (interlaminar approach) for decompression of neural elements, (with or without ligamentous resection, discectomy, facetectomy and/or foraminotomy), any method, under indirect image guidance (eg, fluoroscopic, CT), single or multiple levels, unilateral or bilateral; cervical or thoracic

0275T Percutaneous laminotomy/laminectomy (interlaminar approach) for decompression of neural elements, (with or without ligamentous resection, discectomy, facetectomy and/or foraminotomy), any method, under indirect image guidance (eg, fluoroscopic, CT), single or multiple levels, unilateral or bilateral; lumbar

(For percutaneous decompression of the nucleus pulposus of intervertebral disc utilizing needle based technique, use 62287)

Plain English Description

A percutaneous laminotomy or laminectomy is performed for neural decompression. Separately reportable preoperative MRI, CT, or myelography is performed to identify the target entry site over the spine. CT or C-arm fluoroscopy is used intraoperatively to visualize the spine. Percutaneous devices are designed to access the interlaminar space using a posterior approach. Contrast is injected as needed into the epidural space to facilitate better visualization of surrounding structures and to evaluate the degree of decompression achieved. A guiding portal and inner trocar are inserted percutaneously inferior to the vertebral segment being decompressed and lateral to the spinous process margin. The guiding portal and inner trocar are advanced to the inferior vertebral segment lamina toward the border of the interlaminar space using imaging guidance. The inner trocar is removed leaving the hollow access portal in the interlaminar space. The portal is secured against the skin surface using plate and guide devices, which are used to ensure proper placement of the surgical instruments. A bone sculptor is advanced through the portal to the free edge of the lamina. Small pieces of bone are removed from the superior and inferior lamina (laminotomy/laminectomy). Once the interlaminar space has been enlarged, the bone sculptor is removed and a tissue sculptor is advanced through the portal. The ligamentum flavum is resected as needed. The openings under the facet joints where the nerve runs through are checked and a portion of the bone around the opening may be removed for additional pressure relief, if necessary (foraminotomy). Ruptured disc fragments or bulging nucleus pulposus is also removed to decompress the nerve(s). Decompression is then visually confirmed by changes in the epidurogram and flow of contrast. The procedure may be performed as a unilateral or bilateral procedure at each vertebral level and it may be performed at one or more levels. Use 0274T for percutaneous decompression of neural elements in the cervical or thoracic spine, unilateral or bilateral, single or multiple levels. Use 0275T for percutaneous decompression of neural elements in the lumbar spine, unilateral or bilateral, single or multiple levels.

RVUs

Code	Work	PE	PE Non-Facility	MP	Total Non-Facility	Total Facility	Global
0274T	0.00	0.00	0.00	0.00	0.00	0.00	YYY
0275T	0.00	0.00	0.00	0.00	0.00	0.00	YYY

A9575

A9575 Injection, gadoterate meglumine, 0.1 ml

RVUs

Global: XXX

	Work	PE	MP	Total
Facility	0.00	0.00	0.00	0.00
Non-facility	0.00	0.00	0.00	0.00

Modifiers (PAR)

Mod 50	Mod 51	Mod 62	Mod 80
9	9	9	9

CCI Edits

Refer to Appendix A for CCI edits.

A9585

A9585 Injection, gadobutrol, 0.1 ml

RVUs

Global: XXX

	Work	PE	MP	Total
Facility	0.00	0.00	0.00	0.00
Non-facility	0.00	0.00	0.00	0.00

Modifiers (PAR)

Mod 50	Mod 51	Mod 62	Mod 80
9	9	9	9

CCI Edits

Refer to Appendix A for CCI edits.

G0453

G0453 Continuous intraoperative neurophysiology monitoring, from outside the operating room (remote or nearby), per patient, (attention directed exclusively to one patient) each 15 minutes (list in addition to primary procedure)

RVUs

Global: XXX

	Work	PE	MP	Total
Facility	0.60	0.29	0.05	0.94
Non-facility	0.60	0.29	0.05	0.94

Modifiers (PAR)

Mod 50	Mod 51	Mod 62	Mod 80
0	0	0	0

CCI Edits

Refer to Appendix A for CCI edits.

J0585

ⓘJ0585 Injection, onabotulinumtoxina, 1 unit

RVUs

Global: XXX

	Work	PE	MP	Total
Facility	0.00	0.00	0.00	0.00
Non-facility	0.00	0.00	0.00	0.00

Modifiers (PAR)

Mod 50	Mod 51	Mod 62	Mod 80
9	9	9	9

CCI Edits

Refer to Appendix A for CCI edits.

J0586

J0586 Injection, abobotulinumtoxina, 5 units

RVUs

Global: XXX

	Work	PE	MP	Total
Facility	0.00	0.00	0.00	0.00
Non-facility	0.00	0.00	0.00	0.00

Modifiers (PAR)

Mod 50	Mod 51	Mod 62	Mod 80
9	9	9	9

CCI Edits

Refer to Appendix A for CCI edits.

J0587

ⓘJ0587 Injection, rimabotulinumtoxinb, 100 units

RVUs

Global: XXX

	Work	PE	MP	Total
Facility	0.00	0.00	0.00	0.00
Non-facility	0.00	0.00	0.00	0.00

Modifiers (PAR)

Mod 50	Mod 51	Mod 62	Mod 80
9	9	9	9

CCI Edits

Refer to Appendix A for CCI edits.

J0588

J0588 Injection, incobotulinumtoxin a, 1 unit

RVUs

Global: XXX

	Work	PE	MP	Total
Facility	0.00	0.00	0.00	0.00
Non-facility	0.00	0.00	0.00	0.00

Modifiers (PAR)

Mod 50	Mod 51	Mod 62	Mod 80
9	9	9	9

CCI Edits

Refer to Appendix A for CCI edits.

J0897

J0897 Injection, denosumab, 1 mg

RVUs

Global: XXX

	Work	PE	MP	Total
Facility	0.00	0.00	0.00	0.00
Non-facility	0.00	0.00	0.00	0.00

Modifiers (PAR)

Mod 50	Mod 51	Mod 62	Mod 80
9	9	9	9

CCI Edits

Refer to Appendix A for CCI edits.

J1100

ⓘJ1100 Injection, dexamethasone sodium phosphate, 1 mg

RVUs

Global: XXX

	Work	PE	MP	Total
Facility	0.00	0.00	0.00	0.00
Non-facility	0.00	0.00	0.00	0.00

Modifiers (PAR)

Mod 50	Mod 51	Mod 62	Mod 80
9	9	9	9

Pub 100

J1100: Pub 100-04, 17, 20

CCI Edits

Refer to Appendix A for CCI edits.

J1459

J1459 Injection, immune globulin (privigen), intravenous, non-lyophilized (e.g., liquid), 500 mg

RVUs

Global: XXX

	Work	PE	MP	Total
Facility	0.00	0.00	0.00	0.00
Non-facility	0.00	0.00	0.00	0.00

Modifiers (PAR)

Mod 50	Mod 51	Mod 62	Mod 80
9	9	9	9

CCI Edits

Refer to Appendix A for CCI edits.

J1557

J1557 Injection, immune globulin, (gammaplex), intravenous, non-lyophilized (e.g., liquid), 500 mg

RVUs

Global: XXX

	Work	PE	MP	Total
Facility	0.00	0.00	0.00	0.00
Non-facility	0.00	0.00	0.00	0.00

Modifiers (PAR)

Mod 50	Mod 51	Mod 62	Mod 80
9	9	9	9

CCI Edits

Refer to Appendix A for CCI edits.

J1561

ⓘJ1561 Injection, immune globulin, (gamunex-c/gammaked), non-lyophilized (e.g., liquid), 500 mg

RVUs

Global: XXX

	Work	PE	MP	Total
Facility	0.00	0.00	0.00	0.00
Non-facility	0.00	0.00	0.00	0.00

Modifiers (PAR)

Mod 50	Mod 51	Mod 62	Mod 80
9	9	9	9

Pub 100

J1561: Pub 100-04, 17, 20

CCI Edits

Refer to Appendix A for CCI edits.

J1566

ⓘJ1566 Injection, immune globulin, intravenous, lyophilized (e.g., powder), not otherwise specified, 500 mg

RVUs

Global: XXX

	Work	PE	MP	Total
Facility	0.00	0.00	0.00	0.00
Non-facility	0.00	0.00	0.00	0.00

Modifiers (PAR)

Mod 50	Mod 51	Mod 62	Mod 80
9	9	9	9

CCI Edits

Refer to Appendix A for CCI edits.

J1568

J1568 Injection, immune globulin, (octagam), intravenous, non-lyophilized (e.g., liquid), 500 mg

RVUs

Global: XXX

	Work	PE	MP	Total
Facility	0.00	0.00	0.00	0.00
Non-facility	0.00	0.00	0.00	0.00

Modifiers (PAR)

Mod 50	Mod 51	Mod 62	Mod 80
9	9	9	9

CCI Edits

Refer to Appendix A for CCI edits.

J1569

ⓘJ1569 Injection, immune globulin, (gammagard liquid), non-lyophilized, (e.g., liquid), 500 mg

RVUs

Global: XXX

	Work	PE	MP	Total
Facility	0.00	0.00	0.00	0.00
Non-facility	0.00	0.00	0.00	0.00

Modifiers (PAR)

Mod 50	Mod 51	Mod 62	Mod 80
9	9	9	9

CCI Edits

Refer to Appendix A for CCI edits.

J2323

J2323 Injection, natalizumab, 1 mg

RVUs

Global: XXX

	Work	PE	MP	Total
Facility	0.00	0.00	0.00	0.00
Non-facility	0.00	0.00	0.00	0.00

Modifiers (PAR)

Mod 50	Mod 51	Mod 62	Mod 80
9	9	9	9

CCI Edits

Refer to Appendix A for CCI edits.

J3301

ⓘJ3301 Injection, triamcinolone acetonide, not otherwise specified, 10 mg

RVUs

Global: XXX

	Work	PE	MP	Total
Facility	0.00	0.00	0.00	0.00
Non-facility	0.00	0.00	0.00	0.00

Modifiers (PAR)

Mod 50	Mod 51	Mod 62	Mod 80
9	9	9	9

AHA: 2Q 2013, 4CCI Edits

Refer to Appendix A for CCI edits.

Q9967

ⓘQ9967 Low osmolar contrast material, 300-399 mg/ml iodine concentration, per ml

RVUs

Global: XXX

	Work	PE	MP	Total
Facility	0.00	0.00	0.00	0.00
Non-facility	0.00	0.00	0.00	0.00

Modifiers (PAR)

Mod 50	Mod 51	Mod 62	Mod 80
9	9	9	9

CCI Edits

Refer to Appendix A for CCI edits.

Modifiers

The CPT® code selected must be the one that most closely describes the service(s) and/or procedure(s) documented by the physician. However, sometimes certain services or procedures go above and beyond the definition of the assigned CPT code definition and require further clarification. For these and other reasons, modifiers were developed and implemented by the American Medical Association (AMA), the Centers for Medicare & Medicaid Services (CMS), and local Part B Medicare Administrative Contractors (MACs). These modifiers give health care providers a way to indicate that a service or procedure has been modified by some circumstance but still meets the code definition. Modifiers were designed to expand on the information already provided by the current CPT coding system and to assist in the prompt processing of claims. A CPT modifier is a two-digit numeric character reported with the appropriate CPT code, and is intended to transfer specific information regarding a certain procedure or service.

Modifiers are used to ensure payment accuracy, coding consistency, and editing under the outpatient prospective payment system (OPPS), and are also mandated for private practitioners (solo and multiple), ambulatory surgery centers (ASCs), and other outpatient hospital services.

Modifier Usage

Modifiers are indicated when:

- A service/procedure contains a professional and technical component but only one is applicable
- A service/procedure was performed by more than one physician and/or in more than one location
- The service reported was increased or decreased from that of the original definition
- Unusual events occurred during the service/procedure
- A service/procedure was performed more than once
- A bilateral procedure was performed
- Only part of a service was performed
- An adjunctive service was performed

If a modifier is to be utilized, the following must be documented in the patient's medical record:

- The special circumstances indicating the need to add that modifier
- All pertinent information and an adequate definition of the service/procedure performed supporting the use of the assigned modifier

CPT Modifiers

CPT modifiers are attached to the end of the appropriate CPT code. For professional services, modifiers will be reported as an attachment to the CPT code as reported on the CMS-1500 form, and for outpatient services, modifiers will be reported as an attachment to the CPT code as reported in the UB-04 form locator FL 44.

Some modifiers are strictly informational:

- Modifier 57, identifying a decision for surgery at the time of an evaluation and management service

Other modifiers are informational and indicate additional reimbursement may be warranted:

- Modifier 22, identifying an unusual service that is greater than what is typical for that code

Placement of a modifier after a CPT code does not always ensure additional reimbursement. A special report may be required if the service is rarely provided, unusual, variable, or new. The report should include pertinent information and an adequate definition or description of the nature, extent, and need for the service/procedure. It should also describe the complexity of the patient's symptoms, pertinent history and physical findings, diagnostic and therapeutic procedures, final diagnosis and associated conditions, and follow-up care.

Like CPT codes, the use of modifiers requires understanding of the purpose of each modifier. It is also important to identify when a modifier has been expanded or restricted by a payer prior to submission of a claim. There will also be times when the coding and modifier information issued by the CMS differs from that of CPT's coding guidelines on the usage of modifiers.

Note: For the purposes of this Modifier chapter, payer-specific information is indicated with the symbol ⓘ. It is good to check with individual payers to determine modifier acceptance.

The following is a list of CPT modifiers:

22 Increased Procedural Services

When the work required to provide a service is substantially greater than typically required, it may be identified by adding modifier 22 to the usual procedure code. Documentation must support the substantial additional work and the reason for the additional work (i.e., increased intensity, time, technical difficulty of procedure, severity of patient's condition, physical and mental effort required).

Note: This modifier should not be appended to an E/M service.

ⓘ Claims submitted to Medicare, Medicaid, and other payers containing modifier 22 for unusual procedural services that do not have attached supporting documentation that illustrates the unusual distinction of the services will be processed as if the procedure codes were not appended with this modifier. Some payers might suspend the claims and request additional information from the provider, but this is the exception rather than the rule. For most payers, this modifier includes additional reimbursement to the provider for the additional work.

23 Unusual Anesthesia

Occasionally, a procedure which usually requires either no anesthesia or local anesthesia, because of unusual circumstances must be done under general anesthesia. This circumstance may be reported by adding modifier 23 to the procedure code of the basic service.

24 Unrelated Evaluation and Management Service by the Same Physician or Other Qualified Health Care Professional During a Postoperative Period

The physician or other qualified health care professional may need to indicate that an evaluation and management service was performed during a postoperative period for a reason(s) unrelated to the original procedure. This circumstance may be reported by adding modifier 24 to the appropriate level of E/M service.

ⓘ By payer definition, a postoperative period is one that has been determined to be included in the payment for the procedure that was performed. During this time, the provider offers treatment for the procedure in follow-up visits, which is not reimbursed. Medicare has postoperative periods for procedures of 0, 10, or 90 days (number of days applicable for each procedure can be found in the Federal Register or Physician Fee Schedule (RBRVS) put out by CMS.) Commercial payers may vary the postoperative days; check with each to determine the appropriate number of days for a given procedure.

25 Significant, Separately Identifiable Evaluation and Management Service by the Same Physician or Other Qualified Health Care Professional on the Same Day of the Procedure or Other Service

It may be necessary to indicate that on the day a procedure or service identified by a CPT code was performed, the patient's condition required a significant, separately identifiable E/M service above and beyond the other service provided or beyond the usual preoperative or postoperative care associated with the procedure that was performed. A significant, separately identifiable E/M service is defined or substantiated by documentation that satisfies the relevant criteria for the respective E/M service to be reported (see **Evaluation and Management Services Guidelines** for instructions on determining level of E/M service). The E/M service may be prompted by the symptom or condition for which the procedure and/or service was provided. As such, different diagnoses are not required for reporting of the E/M service on the same date. This circumstance may be reported by adding modifier 25 to the appropriate level of E/M service.

Note: This modifier is not used to report an E/M service that resulted in a decision to perform surgery. See modifier 57. For significant, separately identifiable non-E/M services, see modifier 59.

ⓘ Modifier 25 Guidelines

1. Modifier 25 should be used only when a visit is separately payable when billed in addition to a minor surgical procedure (any surgery with a 0- or 10-day postoperative period per Medicare). Payment for pre- and postoperative work in minor procedures is included in the payment for the procedure. Where the decision to perform the minor procedure is typically made immediately before the service (e.g., sutures are needed to close a wound), it is considered to be a routine preoperative service and an E/M service should not be billed in addition to the minor procedure. In circumstances in which the physician provides an E/M service that is beyond the usual pre- and postoperative work for the service, the visit may be billed with a modifier 25. A modifier is not needed if the visit was performed the day before a minor surgery because the global period for minor procedures does not include the day prior to the surgery.
2. The global surgery policy does not apply to services of other physicians who may be rendering services during the pre- or postoperative period unless the physician is a member of the same group as the operating physician.
3. The provider must determine if the E/M service for which they are billing is clearly distinct from the surgical service. When the decision to perform the minor procedure is typically done immediately before the procedure is rendered, the visit should not be billed separately.

26 Professional Component

Certain procedures are a combination of a physician or other qualified health care professional component and a technical component. When the physician or other qualified health care professional component is reported separately, the service may be identified by adding modifier 26 to the usual procedure number.

ⓘ To determine which codes have both a professional and technical component for CMS, review the Federal Register and/or the Physician Fee Schedule for a breakdown. Usually commercial payers go along with CMS determinations of professional and technical components. Some CPT codes are already broken down into professional and technical components. Examples of these are:

93005 Electrocardiography, routine ECG with at least 12 leads; tracing only, without interpretation and report (technical component)

93010 Electrocardiography, routine ECG with at least 12 leads; interpretation and report only

Modifier 26 should not be appended to either of the codes because the nomenclature itself has determined that they are already technical or professional components.

32 Mandated Services

Services related to *mandated* consultation and/or related services (e.g., third-party payer, governmental, legislative, or regulatory requirement) may be identified by adding modifier 32 to the basic procedure.

33 Preventive Services

When the primary purpose of the service is the delivery of an evidence based service in accordance with the US Preventive Services Task Force A or B rating in effect and other preventive services identified in preventive services mandates (legislative or regulatory), the service may be identified by adding 33 to the procedure. For separately reported services specifically identified as preventive, the modifier should not be used.

47 Anesthesia by Surgeon

Regional or general anesthesia provided by the surgeon may be reported by adding modifier 47 to the basic service. (This does not include local anesthesia.)

Note: Modifier 47 would not be used as a modifier for the anesthesia procedures.

ⓘ This service is not covered by Medicare and many state Medicaid programs. Commercial payers and managed care organizations may cover this additional service.

50 Bilateral Procedure

Unless otherwise identified in the listings, bilateral procedures that are performed at the same session should be identified by adding modifier 50 to the appropriate 5-digit code.

Note: This modifier should not be appended to designated "add-on" codes (see Appendix D*).

ⓘ Reported as a one-line item for Medicare claims with modifier 50 appended to the end of the code. Some carriers or payers may request that bilateral procedures be reported with the LT and RT HCPCS Level II modifiers as two-line items.

51 Multiple Procedures

When multiple procedures, other than E/M Services, Physical Medicine and Rehabilitation services, or provision of supplies (e.g., vaccines), are performed at the same session by the same individual, the primary procedure or service may be reported as listed. The additional procedure(s) or service(s) may be identified by appending modifier 51 to the additional procedure or service code(s).

Note: This modifier should not be appended to designated "add-on" codes (see Appendix D*).

52 Reduced Services

Under certain circumstances a service or procedure is partially reduced or eliminated at the discretion of the physician or other qualified health care professional. Under these circumstances the service provided can be identified by its usual procedure number and the addition of modifier 52, signifying that the service is reduced. This provides a means of reporting reduced services without disturbing the identification of the basic service.

Note: For hospital outpatient reporting of a previously scheduled procedure/service that is partially reduced or cancelled as a result of extenuating circumstances or those that threaten the well-being of the patient prior to or after administration of anesthesia, see modifiers 73 and 74 (see modifiers approved for ASC hospital outpatient use in the CPT codebook).

ⓘ Procedures reported with modifier 52 are typically billed at a reduced amount. Most payers do not require documentation to support the use of modifier 52 and will reimburse the procedure at a reduced level.

53 Discontinued Procedure

Under certain circumstances, the physician or other qualified health care professional may elect to terminate a surgical or diagnostic procedure. Due to extenuating circumstances or those that threaten the well being of the patient, it may be necessary to indicate that a surgical or diagnostic procedure was started but discontinued. This circumstance may be reported by adding modifier 53 to the code reported by the individual for the discontinued procedure.

Note: This modifier is not used to report the elective cancellation of a procedure prior to the patient's anesthesia induction and/or surgical preparation in the operating suite. For outpatient hospital/ambulatory surgery center (ASC) reporting of a previously scheduled procedure/service that is partially reduced or cancelled as a result of extenuating circumstances or those that threaten the well being of the patient prior to or after administration of anesthesia, see modifiers 73 and 74 (see modifiers approved for ASC hospital outpatient use in the CPT codebook).

54 Surgical Care Only

When 1 physician or other qualified health care professional performs a surgical procedure and another provides preoperative and/or postoperative management, surgical services may be identified by adding modifier 54 to the usual procedure number.

ⓘ Both claims submitted by the surgeon and the other provider must report the date patient care was assumed and relinquished in block 19 of the CMS-1500 or electronic equivalent. Both the surgeon and the other provider must keep a copy of the written transfer agreement in the patient's medical record. Both providers will use the same CPT code, but they will use different modifiers that identify which portion of care they provided.

55 Postoperative Management Only

When 1 physician or other qualified health care professional performed the postoperative management and another performed the surgical procedure, the postoperative component may be identified by adding modifier 55 to the usual procedure number.

ⓘ Both providers will use the same CPT code, but they will use different modifiers that identify which portion of care they provided.

56 Preoperative Management Only

When 1 physician or other qualified health care professional performed the preoperative care and evaluation and another performed the surgical procedure, the preoperative component may be identified by adding modifier 56 to the usual procedure number.

ⓘ Both providers will use the same CPT code, but will they will use different modifiers that identify which portion of care they provided. Some payers do not allow modifier 56 as by their definition the pre-operative care is included in the surgical component.

57 Decision for Surgery

An evaluation and management service that resulted in the initial decision to perform the surgery may be identified by adding modifier 57 to the appropriate level of E/M service.

ⓘ Major Surgical Procedures

Major Surgery with a global period of 90 days (as defined by Medicare) include the day before and the day of surgery. For example, a visit the day before or the same day could be properly billed in addition to a cholecystotomy if the need for the surgery was found during the encounter. Modifier 57 should be added to the E/M code. Billing for a visit would not be appropriate if the physician was only discussing the upcoming surgical procedure.

Procedures with a 90 day global period are considered to be major surgery, as categorized by CMS. The RBRVS (Resource-Based Relative Value Scale) manual or Federal Register lists the global period for all procedure codes eligible for payment by Medicare.

ⓘ Minor Surgical Procedures

Procedures with a 0 or 10 day global period are considered to be minor or endoscopic surgeries, as categorized by CMS. E/M visits by the same physician on the same day as a minor surgery or endoscopy are included in the payment for the procedure, unless a significant, separately identifiable service is also performed.

58 Staged or Related Procedure or Service by the Same Physician or Other Qualified Health Care Professional During the Postoperative Period

It may be necessary to indicate that the performance of a procedure or service during the postoperative period was: (a) planned or anticipated (staged); (b) more extensive than the original procedure; or (c) for therapy following a diagnostic surgical procedure. This circumstance may be reported by adding modifier 58 to the staged or related procedure.

Note: For treatment of a problem that requires a return to the operating/procedure room (eg, unanticipated clinical condition), see modifier 78.

ⓘ Modifier 58 must be used for purposes of identifying procedures performed by the original physician during the postoperative period of the original procedure, within the constraints of the modifier's definition. These procedures cannot be repeat operations (unless the procedures are more extensive than the original procedure) and cannot be for the treatment of complications requiring a return trip to the operating room.

*Pages in this section refer to the AMA *CPT® 2020 Professional Edition*

The existence of modifier 58 does not negate the global fee concept. Services that are included in CPT as multiple sessions or are defined as including multiple services or events may not be billed with this modifier. This modifier is designed to allow a method of reporting additional, related surgeries that are due to a progression of the disease and are not to be used to avoid global surgery edits applicable to staged procedures.

Modifier 58 should be used on surgical codes only and has no effect on the payment amount. It should not be used with the following codes because the codes are defined as "one or more sessions or stages":

65855	67031	67108	67145	67220
66762	67101	67110	67208	67227
66821	67105	67112	67210	67228
66840	67107	67141	67218	67229

59 Distinct Procedural Service

Under certain circumstances, it may be necessary to indicate that a procedure or service was distinct or independent from other non-E/M services performed on the same day. Modifier 59 is used to identify procedures/services, other than E/M services, that are not normally reported together, but are appropriate under the circumstances. Documentation must support a different session, different procedure or surgery, different site or organ system, separate incision/excision, separate lesions, or separate injury (or area of injury in extensive injuries) not ordinarily encountered or performed on the same day by the same individual. However, when another already established modifier is more appropriate, it should be used rather than modifier 59. Only if no more descriptive modifier is available, and the use of modifier 59 best explains the circumstances, should modifier 59 be used.

Note: Modifier 59 should not be appended to an E/M service. To report a separate and distinct E/M service with a non-E/M service performed on the same date, see modifier 25.

ⓘ Modifier 59 was established to demonstrate that multiple, yet distinct, services were provided to a patient on the same date of service by the same provider. Because distinct procedures or services rendered on the same day by the same physician cannot be easily identified and properly adjudicated by simply listing the CPT procedure codes, modifier 59 assists the payer or Medicare carrier in applying the appropriate reimbursement protocol. If the modifier is not used in these circumstances, services may be denied, with the explanation of benefits stating that the payer does not reimburse for this service because it is part of another service that was performed at the same time.

62 Two Surgeons

When 2 surgeons work together as primary surgeons performing distinct part(s) of a procedure, each surgeon should report his/her distinct operative work by adding modifier 62 to the procedure code and any associated add-on code(s) for that procedure as long as both surgeons continue to work together as primary surgeons. Each surgeon should report the co-surgery once using the same procedure code. If additional procedure(s) (including add-on procedures[s]) are performed during the same surgical session, separate code(s) may also be reported with modifier 62 added.

Note: If a co-surgeon acts as an assistant in the performance of additional procedure(s), other than those reported with the modifier 62, during the same surgical session, those services may be reported using separate procedure code(s) with modifier 80 or modifier 82 added, as appropriate.

ⓘ According to Medicare, payment for the two physicians is based on the two physicians splitting 125% of the allowed charge(s). Check with other payers to determine payment based on this modifier. This modifier should not be confused with modifier 80 (assistant surgeon).

63 Procedure Performed on Infants Less Than 4 kg

Procedures performed on neonates and infants up to a present body weight of 4 kg may involve significantly increased complexity and physician or other qualified health care professional work commonly associated with these patients. This circumstance may be reported by adding modifier 63 to the procedure number.

Note: Unless otherwise designated, this modifier may only be appended to procedures/services listed in the 20100-69990 code series and 92920, 92928, 92953, 92960, 92986, 92987, 92990, 92997, 92998, 93312, 93313, 93314, 93315, 93316, 93317, 93318, 93452, 93505, 93530, 93531, 93532, 93533, 93561, 93562, 93563, 93564, 93568, 93580, 93582, 93590, 93591, 93592, 93615, 93616 from the Medicine/Cardiovascular section. Modifier 63 should not be appended to any CPT codes listed in the **Evaluation and Management Services, Anesthesia, Radiology, Pathology/Laboratory,** or **Medicine** sections (other than those identified above from the Medicine/Cardiovascular section).

66 Surgical Team

Under some circumstances, highly complex procedures (requiring the concomitant services of several physicians or other qualified health care professionals, often of different specialties, plus other highly skilled, specially trained personnel, various types of complex equipment) are carried out under the "surgical team" concept (e.g., organ transplants). Such circumstances may be identified by each participating individual with the addition of modifier 66 to the basic procedure code used for reporting services.

ⓘ Each surgeon that participates in the procedure would report the same CPT code with modifier 66. Only surgical CPT codes (10021-69990) should be used with modifier 66 unless otherwise stated by the payer.

76 Repeat Procedure or Service by Same Physician or Other Qualified Health Care Professional

It may be necessary to indicate that a procedure or service was repeated by the same physician or other qualified health care professional subsequent to the original procedure or service. This circumstance may be reported by adding modifier 76 to the repeated procedure or service.

Note: This modifier should not be appended to an E/M service.

77 Repeat Procedure or Service by Another Physician or Other Qualified Health Care Professional

It may be necessary to indicate that a basic procedure or service was repeated by another physician or other qualified health care professional subsequent to the original procedure or service. This circumstance may be reported by adding modifier 77 to the repeated procedure or service.

Note: This modifier should not be appended to an E/M service.

ⓘ Appending this modifier does not guarantee payment of the repeat procedure, but will assist in determining duplicate billings for the procedure.

78 Unplanned Return to the Operating/Procedure Room by the Same Physician or Other Qualified Health Care Professional Following Initial Procedure for a Related Procedure During the Postoperative Period

It may be necessary to indicate that another procedure was performed during the postoperative period of the initial procedure (unplanned procedure following initial procedure). When this procedure is related to the first, and requires the use of an operating/procedure room, it may be reported by adding modifier 78 to the related procedure. (For repeat procedures, see modifier 76.)

ⓘ Medicare includes specific medical and/or surgical care for postoperative complications within the global surgical package and does not allow additional payment. Included in the global surgical package are "additional medical and surgical services required of the surgeon during the postoperative period of the surgery because of complications which do not require additional trips to the operating room."

79 Unrelated Procedure or Service by the Same Physician or Other Qualified Health Care Professional During the Postoperative Period

The individual may need to indicate that the performance of a procedure or service during the postoperative period was unrelated to the original procedure. This circumstance may be reported by using modifier 79. (For repeat procedures on the same day, see modifier 76.)

ⓘ When billing for an unrelated procedure by the same physician during the postoperative period of an original procedure, a new postoperative period will begin with the subsequent procedure. A different ICD-10-CM diagnosis should be indicated on the claim.

80 Assistant Surgeon

Surgical assistant services may be identified by adding modifier 80 to the usual procedure number(s).

ⓘ Some surgical procedures are not eligible for this modifier; check the Medicare physician fee schedule or with other payers to determine payment eligibility

81 Minimum Assistant Surgeon

Minimum surgical assistant services are identified by adding modifier 81 to the usual procedure number.

ⓘ Check with payers to determine if payment is allowed for this modifier.

82 Assistant Surgeon (When a Qualified Resident Is Not Available)

The unavailability of a qualified resident surgeon is a prerequisite for use of modifier 82 appended to the usual procedure code number(s).

ⓘ In some hospitals with residency programs, Medicare pays through the medical program or graduate medical education (GME) program. Because of this, they will not reimburse for a resident when they are used as an assistant surgeon. Although under special circumstances, payment may be made if there is a emergent situation that is life-threatening.

90 Reference (Outside) Laboratory

When laboratory procedures are performed by a party other than the treating or reporting physician or other qualified health care professional, the procedure may be identified by adding modifier 90 to the usual procedure number.

ⓘ Check with payers to determine if the provider may bill for the laboratory procedure if not performed by the provider.

91 Repeat Clinical Diagnostic Laboratory Test

In the course of treatment of the patient, it may be necessary to repeat the same laboratory test on the same day to obtain subsequent (multiple) test results. Under these circumstances, the laboratory test performed can be identified by its usual procedure number and the addition of modifier 91.

Note: This modifier may not be used when tests are rerun to confirm initial results; due to testing problems with specimens or equipment; or for any other reason when a normal, one-time, reportable result is all that is required. This modifier may not be used when other code(s) describe a series of test results (eg, glucose tolerance tests, evocative/suppression testing). This modifier may only be used for laboratory test(s) performed more than once on the same day on the same patient.

92 Alternative Laboratory Platform Testing

When laboratory testing is performed using a kit or transportable instrument that wholly or in part consists of a single use, disposable analytical chamber, the service may be identified by adding modifier 92 to the usual laboratory procedure code (HIV testing 86701-86703, and 87389). The test does not require permanent dedicated space, hence by its design may be hand carried or transported to the vicinity of the patient for immediate testing at that site, although location of testing is not in itself determinative of the use of this modifier.

95 Synchronous Telemedicine Service Rendered Via a Real-Time Interactive Audio and Video Telecommunications System

Synchronous telemedicine service is defined as a real-time interaction between a physician or other qualified health care professional and a patient who is located at a distant site from the physician or other qualified health care professional. The totality of the communication of information exchanged between the physician or other qualified health care professional and the patient during the course of the synchronous telemedicine service must be of an amount and nature that would be sufficient to meet the key components and/or requirements of the same services when rendered via a face-to-face interaction. Modifier 95 may only be appended to the services listed in Appendix P*. Appendix P is the list of the CPT codes for services that are typically performed face-to-face, but may be rendered via a real-time (synchronous) interactive audio and video telecommunications system.

96 Habilitative Services

When a service or procedure that may be either habilitative or rehabilitative in nature is provided for habilitative purposes, the physician or other qualified health care professional may add modifier 96 to the service or procedure code to indicate that the service or procedure provided was a habilitative service. Habilitative services help an individual learn skills and functioning for daily living that the individual has not yet developed, and then keep and/or improve those learned skills. Habilitative services also help an individual keep, learn, or improve skills and functioning for daily living.

97 Rehabilitative Services

When a service or procedure that may be either habilitative or rehabilitative in nature is provided for rehabilitative purposes, the physician or other qualified health care professional may add modifier 97 to the service or procedure code to indicate that the service or procedure provided was a rehabilitative service. Rehabilitative services help an individual keep, get back, or improve skills and functioning for daily living that have been lost or impaired because the individual was sick, hurt, or disabled.

99 Multiple Modifiers

Under certain circumstances 2 or more modifiers may be necessary to completely delineate a service. In such situations modifier 99 should be added to the basic procedure, and other applicable modifiers may be listed as part of the description of the service.

ⓘ Check with payers to determine if this modifier is necessary when reporting multiple modifiers.

*Pages in this section refer to the AMA *CPT® 2020 Professional Edition*

Modifiers Approved for Ambulatory Surgery Center (ASC) Hospital Outpatient Use

There are some differences in modifiers for professional and ASC hospital use. The following list consists of the only approved modifiers that can be used in an ASC/hospital setting:

25 Significant, Separately Identifiable Evaluation and Management Service by the Same Physician or Other Qualified Health Care Professional on the Same Day of the Procedure or Other Service

It may be necessary to indicate that on the day a procedure or service identified by a CPT code was performed, the patient's condition required a significant, separately identifiable E/M service above and beyond the other service provided or beyond the usual preoperative and postoperative care associated with the procedure that was performed. A significant, separately identifiable E/M service is defined or substantiated by documentation that satisfies the relevant criteria for the respective E/M service to be reported (see **Evaluation and Management Services Guidelines** for instructions on determining level of E/M service). The E/M service may be prompted by the symptom or condition for which the procedure and/or service was provided. As such, different diagnoses are not required for reporting of the E/M services on the same date. This circumstance may be reported by adding modifier 25 to the appropriate level of E/M service.

Note: This modifier is not used to report an E/M service that resulted in a decision to perform surgery. See modifier 57. For significant, separately identifiable non-E/M services, see modifier 59.

ⓘ According to Medicare, modifier 25 may be appended to an Emergency Department Services E/M code (99281-99285) if provided on the same day as a diagnostic or therapeutic procedure.

27 Multiple Outpatient Hospital E/M Encounters on the Same Date

For hospital outpatient reporting purposes, utilization of hospital resources related to separate and distinct E/M encounters performed in multiple outpatient hospital settings on the same date may be reported by adding the modifier 27 to each appropriate level outpatient and/or emergency department E/M code(s). This modifier provides a means of reporting circumstances involving E/M services provided by physician(s) in more than one (multiple) outpatient hospital setting(s) (e.g., hospital emergency department, clinic).

Note: This modifier is not to be used for physician reporting of multiple E/M services performed by the same physician on the same date. For physician reporting of all outpatient E/M services provided by the same physician on the same date and performed in multiple outpatient setting(s) (eg, hospital emergency department, clinic), see **Evaluation and Management, Emergency Department**, or **Preventive Medicine Services** codes.

33 Preventive Services

When the primary purpose of the service is the delivery of evidence based service in accordance with a US Preventive Services Task Force A or B rating in effect and other preventive services identified in preventive services mandates (legislative or regulatory), the services may be identified by adding 33 to the procedure. For separately reported services specifically identified as preventive, the modifier should not be used.

50 Bilateral Procedure

Unless otherwise identified in the listings, bilateral procedures that are performed at the same session should be identified by adding modifier 50 to the appropriate 5-digit code.

Note: This modifier should not be appended to designated "add-on" codes (see Appendix D*)

ⓘ Reported on procedures performed at the same operative session, this modifier should be reported only once as a one-line item for Medicare, with the modifier appended to the end of the code.

ⓘ Some payers may accept the bilateral procedures as two-line items, with HCPCS Level II modifiers LT and RT appended to the end of the codes.

52 Reduced Services

Under certain circumstances a service or procedure is partially reduced or eliminated at the discretion of the physician or other qualified health care professional. Under these circumstances the service provided can be identified by its usual procedure number and the addition of modifier 52, signifying that the service is reduced. This provides a means of reporting reduced services without disturbing the identification of the basic service.

Note: For hospital outpatient reporting of a previously scheduled procedure/service that is partially reduced or cancelled as a result of extenuating circumstances or those that threaten the well-being of the patient prior to or after administration of anesthesia, see modifiers 73 and 74.

ⓘ Procedures reported with modifier 52 are typically billed at a reduced amount. Most payers do not require documentation to support the use of modifier 52 and will reimburse the procedure at a reduced level.

58 Staged or Related Procedure or Service by the Same Physician or Other Qualified Health Care Professional During the Postoperative Period

It may be necessary to indicate that the performance of a procedure or service during the postoperative period was: (a) planned or anticipated (staged); (b) more extensive than the original procedure; or (c) for therapy following a diagnostic surgical procedure. This circumstance may be reported by adding modifier 58 to the staged or related procedure.

Note: For treatment of a problem that requires a return to the operating/procedure room (e.g., unanticipated clinical condition), see modifier 78.

ⓘ Modifier 58 must be used for purposes of identifying procedures performed by the original physician during the postoperative period of the original procedure, within the constraints of the modifier's definition. These procedures cannot be repeat operations (unless the procedures are more extensive than the original procedure) and cannot be for the treatment of complications requiring a return trip to the operating room.

The existence of modifier 58 does not negate the global fee concept. Services that are included in CPT as multiple sessions or are defined as including multiple services or events may not be billed with this modifier. This modifier is designed to allow a method of reporting additional, related surgeries that are due to a progression of the disease and are not to be used to avoid global surgery edits applicable to staged procedures.

Modifier 58 should be used on surgical codes only and has no effect on the payment amount.

59 Distinct Procedural Service

Under certain circumstances, it may be necessary to indicate that a procedure or service was distinct or independent from other non-E/M services performed on the same day. Modifier 59 is used to identify procedures/services, other than E/M services, that are not normally reported together, but are appropriate under the circumstances. Documentation must support a different session, different procedure or surgery, different site or organ system, separate incision/excision, separate lesions, or separate injury (or area of injury in extensive injuries) not ordinarily encountered or performed on the same day by the same individual. However, when another already established modifier is appropriate, it should be used rather than modifier 59. Only if no more descriptive modifier is available, and the use of modifier 59 best explains the circumstances, should modifier 59 be used.

Note: Modifier 59 should not be appended to an E/M service. To report a separate and distinct E/M service with a non-E/M service performed on the same date, see modifier 25.

ⓘ Modifier 59 was established to demonstrate that multiple, yet distinct, services were provided to a patient on the same date of service by the same provider. Because distinct procedures or services rendered on the same day by the same physician cannot be easily identified and properly adjudicated by simply listing the CPT procedure codes, modifier 59 assists the payer or Medicare carrier in applying the appropriate reimbursement protocol. If the modifier is not used in these circumstances, services may be denied, with the explanation of benefits stating that the payer does not reimburse for this service because it is part of another service that was performed at the same time.

73 Discontinued Out-Patient Hospital/Ambulatory Surgery Center (ASC) Procedure Prior to Administration of Anesthesia

Due to extenuating circumstances or those that threaten the well being of the patient, the physician may cancel a surgical or diagnostic procedure subsequent to the patient's surgical preparation (including sedation when provided, and being taken to the room where the procedure is to be performed), but prior to the administration of anesthesia (local, regional block(s), or general). Under these circumstances, the intended service that is prepared for but cancelled can be reported by its usual procedure number and the addition of modifier 73.

Note: The elective cancellation of a service prior to the administration of anesthesia and/or surgical preparation of the patient should not be reported. For physician reporting of a discontinued procedure, see modifier 53.

74 Discontinued Out-Patient Hospital/Ambulatory Surgery Center (ASC) Procedure After Administration of Anesthesia

Due to extenuating circumstances or those that threaten the well being of the patient, the physician may terminate a surgical or diagnostic procedure after the administration of anesthesia (local, regional block(s), or general) or after the procedure was started (e.g., incision made, intubation started, scope inserted). Under these circumstances, the intended service that is prepared for but cancelled can be reported by its usual procedure number and the addition of modifier 74.

Note: The elective cancellation of a service prior to the administration of anesthesia and/or surgical preparation of the patient should not be reported. For physician reporting of a discontinued procedure, see modifier 53.

76 Repeat Procedure or Service by Same Physician or Other Qualified Health Care Professional

It may be necessary to indicate that a procedure or service was repeated subsequent to the original procedure or service. This circumstance may be reported by adding modifier 76 to the repeated procedure or service.

Note: This modifier should not be appended to an E/M service.

77 Repeat Procedure by Another Physician or Other Qualified Health Care Professional

It may be necessary to indicate that a basic procedure or service was repeated by another physician or other qualified health care professional subsequent to the original procedure or service. This circumstance may be reported by adding modifier 77 to the repeated procedure or service.

Note: This modifier should not be appended to an E/M service.

ⓘ Appending this modifier does not guarantee payment of the repeat procedure, but will assist in determining duplicate billings for the procedure.

78 Unplanned Return to the Operating/Procedure Room by the Same Physician or Other Qualified Health Care Professional Following Initial Procedure for a Related Procedure During the Postoperative Period

It may be necessary to indicate that another procedure was performed during the postoperative period of the initial procedure (unplanned procedure following initial procedure). When this procedure is related to the first, and requires the use of an operating/procedure room, it may be reported by adding modifier 78 to the related procedure. (For repeat procedures, see modifier 76.)

ⓘ Medicare includes specific medical and/or surgical care for postoperative complications within the global surgical package and does not allow additional payment. Included in the global surgical package are "additional medical and surgical services required of the surgeon during the postoperative period of the surgery because of complications which do not require additional trips to the operating room."

79 Unrelated Procedure or Service by the Same Physician or Other Qualified Health Care Professional During the Postoperative Period

The individual may need to indicate that the performance of a procedure or service during the postoperative period was unrelated to the original procedure. This circumstance may be reported by using modifier 79. (For repeat procedures on the same day, see modifier 76.)

ⓘ When billing for an unrelated procedure by the same physician during the postoperative period of an original procedure, a new postoperative period will begin with the subsequent procedure. A different diagnosis should be indicated on the claim to identify the unrelated procedure.

91 Repeat Clinical Diagnostic Laboratory Test

In the course of treatment of the patient, it may be necessary to repeat the same laboratory test on the same day to obtain subsequent (multiple) test results. Under these circumstances, the laboratory test performed can be identified by its usual procedure number and the addition of the modifier 91.

Note: This modifier may not be used when tests are rerun to confirm initial results; due to testing problems with specimens or equipment; or for any other reason when a normal, one-time, reportable result is all that is required. This modifier may not be used when other code(s) describe a series of test results (e.g., glucose tolerance tests, evocative/suppression testing). This modifier may only be used for laboratory test(s) performed more than once on the same day on the same patient.

Category II Modifiers

The following performance measurement modifiers may be used for Category II codes to indicate that a service specified in the associated measure(s) was considered but, due to either medical, patient, or system circumstance(s) documented in the medical record, the service was not provided. These modifiers serve as denominator exclusions from the performance measure. The user should note that not all listed measures provide for exclusions (see Alphabetical Clinical Topics Listing for more discussion regarding exclusion criteria).

Category II modifiers should only be reported with Category II codes—they should not be reported with Category I or Category III codes. In addition, the modifiers in the Category II section should only be used where specified in the guidelines,

Modifiers

reporting instructions, parenthetic notes, or code descriptor language listed in the Category II section (code listing and the Alphabetical Clinical Topics Listing).

1P Performance Measure Exclusion Modifier due to Medical Reasons

Reasons include:

- Not indicated (absence of organ/limb, already received/performed, other)
- Contraindicated (patient allergic history, potential adverse drug interaction, other)
- Other medical reasons

2P Performance Measure Exclusion Modifier due to Patient Reasons

Reasons include:

- Patient declined
- Economic, social, or religious reasons
- Other patient reasons

3P Performance Measure Exclusion Modifier due to System Reasons

Reasons include:

- Resources to perform the services not available
- Insurance coverage/payor-related limitations
- Other reasons attributable to health care delivery system

Modifier 8P is intended to be used as a "reporting modifier" to allow the reporting of circumstances when an action described in a measure's numerator is not performed and the reason is not otherwise specified.

8P Performance measure reporting modifier–action not performed, reason not otherwise specified

Level II (HCPCS/National) Modifiers

E1 Upper left, eyelid

E2 Lower left, eyelid

E3 Upper right, eyelid

E4 Lower right, eyelid

F1 Left hand, second digit

F2 Left hand, third digit

F3 Left hand, fourth digit

F4 Left hand, fifth digit

F5 Right hand, thumb

F6 Right hand, second digit

F7 Right hand, third digit

F8 Right hand, fourth digit

F9 Right hand, fifth digit

FA Left hand, thumb

GG Performance and payment of a screening mammogram and diagnostic mammogram on the same patient, same day

GH Diagnostic mammogram converted from screening mammogram on same day

LC Left circumflex coronary artery

LD Left anterior descending coronary artery

LM Left main coronary artery

LT Left side (used to identify procedures performed on the left side of the body)

QM Ambulance service provided under arrangement by a provider of services

QN Ambulance service furnished directly by a provider of services

RC Right coronary artery

RI Ramus intermedius coronary artery

RT Right side (used to identify procedures performed on the right side of the body)

T1 Left foot, second digit

T2 Left foot, third digit

T3 Left foot, fourth digit

T4 Left foot, fifth digit

T5 Right foot, great toe

T6 Right foot, second digit

T7 Right foot, third digit

T8 Right foot, fourth digit

T9 Right foot, fifth digit

TA Left foot, great toe

XE Separate Encounter *

XS Separate Structure *

XP Separate Practitioner *

XU Unusual Non-Overlapping Service *

(*HCPCS modifiers for selective identification of subsets of Distinct Procedural Services [59 modifier])

Modifier Rules

Mult Proc = Multiple Procedure (Modifier 51)

Indicates applicable payment-adjustment rule for multiple procedures:

0 No payment-adjustment rules for multiple procedures apply. If procedure is reported on the same day as another procedure, base the payment on the lower of (a) the actual charge, or (b) the fee-schedule amount for the procedure.

1 Standard payment-adjustment rules in effect before January 1, 1995 for multiple procedures apply. In the 1995 file, this indicator only applies to codes with a status code of "D." If procedure is reported on the same day as another procedure that has an indicator of 1, 2, or 3, rank the procedures by fee-schedule amount and apply the appropriate reduction to this code (100%, 50%, 25%, 25%, 25%, and by report). Base the payment on the lower of (a) the actual charge, or (b) the fee-schedule amount reduced by the appropriate percentage.

2 Standard payment-adjustment rules for multiple procedures apply. If procedure is reported on the same day as another procedure with an indicator of 1, 2, or 3, rank the procedures by fee-schedule amount and apply the appropriate reduction to this code (100%, 50%, 50%, 50%, 50% and by report). Base the payment on the lower of (a) the actual charge, or (b) the fee-schedule amount reduced by the appropriate percentage.

3 Special rules for multiple endoscopic procedures apply if procedure is billed with another endoscopy in the same family (i.e., another endoscopy that has the same base procedure). The base procedure for each code with this indicator is identified in the ENDO BASE field of this file. Apply the multiple endoscopy rules to a family before ranking the family with the other procedures performed on the same day (for example, if multiple endoscopies in the same family are reported on the same day as endoscopies in another family or on the same day as a non-endoscopic procedure). If an endoscopic procedure is reported with only its base procedure, do not pay separately for the base procedure. Payment for the base procedure is included in the payment for the other endoscopy.

5 Subject to 20% of the practice expense component for certain therapy services (25% reduction for services rendered in an institutional setting - effective for services January 1, 2012 and after).

9 Concept does not apply.

Bilat Surg = Bilateral Surgery (Modifier 50)

Indicates services subject to payment adjustment.

0 150% payment adjustment for bilateral procedures does not apply. If procedure is reported with modifier 50 or with modifiers RT and LT, base the payment for the two sides on the lower of: (a) the total actual charge for both sides or (b) 100% of the fee-schedule amount for a single code. Example: The fee-schedule amount for code XXXXX is $125. The physician reports code XXXXX-LT with an actual charge of $100 and XXXXX-RT with an actual charge of $100. Payment should be based on the fee-schedule amount ($125) since it is lower than the total actual charges for the left and right sides ($200). The bilateral adjustment is inappropriate for codes in this category (a) because of physiology or anatomy, or (b) because the code description specifically states that it is a unilateral procedure and there is an existing code for the bilateral procedure.

1 150% payment adjustment for bilateral procedures applies. If the code is billed with the bilateral modifier or is reported twice on the same day by any other means (e.g., with RT and LT modifiers, or with a "2" in the units field), base the payment for these codes when reported as bilateral procedures on the lower of: (a) the total actual charge for both sides or (b) 150% of the fee-schedule amount for a single code. If the code is reported as a bilateral procedure and is reported with other procedure codes on the same day, apply the bilateral adjustment before applying any multiple procedure rules.

2 150% payment adjustment does not apply. RVUs are already based on the procedure being performed as a bilateral procedure. If the procedure is reported with modifier 50 or is reported twice on the same day by any other means (e.g., with RT and LT modifiers or with a "2" in the units field), base the payment for both sides on the lower of (a) the total actual charge by the physician for both sides, or (b) 100% of the fee-schedule for a single code. Example: The fee-schedule amount for code YYYYY is $125. The physician reports code YYYYY-LT with an actual charge of $100 and YYYYY-RT with an actual charge of $100. Payment should be based on the fee-schedule amount ($125) since it is lower than the total actual charges for the left and right sides ($200). The RVUs are based on a bilateral procedure because (a) the code descriptor specifically states that the procedure is bilateral,
(b) the code descriptor states that the procedure may be performed either unilaterally or bilaterally, or (c) the procedure is usually performed as a bilateral procedure.

3 The usual payment adjustment for bilateral procedures does not apply. If the procedure is reported with modifier 50 or is reported for both sides on the same day by any other means (e.g., with RT and LT modifiers or with a "2" in the units field), base the payment for each side or organ or site of a paired organ on the lower of (a) the actual charge for each side or (b) 100% of the fee-schedule amount for each side. If the procedure is reported as a bilateral procedure and with other procedure codes on the same day, determine the fee-schedule amount for a bilateral procedure before applying any multiple procedure rules. Services in this category are generally radiology procedures or other diagnostic tests, which are not subject to the special payment rules for other bilateral surgeries.

9 Concept does not apply.

Asst Surg = Assistant at Surgery (Modifier 80)

Indicates services where an assistant at surgery is never paid for per Medicare Claims Manual.

0 Payment restriction for assistants at surgery applies to this procedure unless supporting documentation is submitted to establish medical necessity.

1 Statutory payment restriction for assistants at surgery applies to this procedure. Assistant at surgery may not be paid.

2 Payment restriction for assistants at surgery does not apply to this procedure. Assistant at surgery may be paid.

9 Concept does not apply.

Co Surg = Co-surgeons (Modifier 62)

Indicates services for which two surgeons, each in a different specialty, may be paid.

0 Co-surgeons not permitted for this procedure.

1 Co-surgeons could be paid, though supporting documentation is required to establish the medical necessity of two surgeons for the procedure.

2 Co-surgeons permitted and no documentation required if the two-specialty requirement is met.

9 Concept does not apply.

Team Surg = Team Surgery (Modifier 66)

Indicates services for which team surgeons may be paid.

0 Team surgeons not permitted for this procedure.

1 Team surgeons could be paid, though supporting documentation required to establish medical necessity of a team; pay by report.

2 Team surgeons permitted; pay by report.

9 Concept does not apply.

National Correct Coding Initiative

A. Introduction

The principles of correct coding apply to the CPT codes in the range 40000-49999. Several general guidelines are repeated in this Chapter.

Physicians should report the HCPCS/CPT code that describes the procedure performed to the greatest specificity possible. A HCPCS/CPT code should be reported only if all services described by the code are performed. A physician should not report multiple HCPCS/CPT codes if a single HCPCS/CPT code exists that describes the services. This type of unbundling is incorrect coding.

HCPCS/CPT codes include all services usually performed as part of the procedure as a standard of medical/surgical practice. A physician should not separately report these services simply because HCPCS/CPT codes exist for them.

Specific issues unique to this section of CPT are clarified in this Chapter.

B. Evaluation and Management (E/M) Services

Medicare Global Surgery Rules define the rules for reporting evaluation and management (E/M) services with procedures covered by these rules. This section summarizes some of the rules.

All procedures on the Medicare Physician Fee Schedule are assigned a global period of 000, 010, 090, XXX, YYY, ZZZ, or MMM. The global concept does not apply to XXX procedures. The global period for YYY procedures is defined by the Carrier (A/B MAC processing practitioner service claims). All procedures with a global period of ZZZ are related to another procedure, and the applicable global period for the ZZZ code is determined by the related procedure. Procedures with a global period of MMM are maternity procedures.

Since NCCI PTP edits are applied to same day services by the same provider to the same beneficiary, certain Global Surgery Rules are applicable to NCCI. An E/M service is separately reportable on the same date of service as a procedure with a global period of 000, 010, or 090 under limited circumstances.

If a procedure has a global period of 090 days, it is defined as a major surgical procedure. If an E/M is performed on the same date of service as a major surgical procedure for the purpose of deciding whether to perform this surgical procedure, the E/M service is separately reportable with modifier 57. Other preoperative E/M services on the same date of service as a major surgical procedure are included in the global payment for the procedure and are not separately reportable. NCCI does not contain edits based on this rule because Medicare Carriers (A/B MACs processing practitioner service claims) have separate edits.

If a procedure has a global period of 000 or 010 days, it is defined as a minor surgical procedure. In general E/M services on the same date of service as the minor surgical procedure are included in the payment for the procedure. The decision to perform a minor surgical procedure is included in the payment for the minor surgical procedure and should not be reported separately as an E/M service. However, a significant and separately identifiable E/M service unrelated to the decision to perform the minor surgical procedure is separately reportable with modifier 25. The E/M service and minor surgical procedure do not require different diagnoses. If a minor surgical procedure is performed on a new patient, the same rules for reporting E/M services apply. The fact that the patient is "new" to the provider is not sufficient alone to justify reporting an E/M service on the same date of service as a minor surgical procedure. NCCI contains many, but not all, possible edits based on these principles.

Example: If a physician determines that a new patient with head trauma requires sutures, confirms the allergy and immunization status, obtains informed consent, and performs the repair, an E/M service is not separately reportable. However, if the physician also performs a medically reasonable and necessary full neurological examination, an E/M service may be separately reportable.

For major and minor surgical procedures, postoperative E/M services related to recovery from the surgical procedure during the postoperative period are included in the global surgical package as are E/M services related to complications of the surgery. Postoperative visits unrelated to the diagnosis for which the surgical procedure was performed unless related to a complication of surgery may be reported separately on the same day as a surgical procedure with modifier 24 ("Unrelated Evaluation and Management Service by the Same Physician or Other Qualified Health Care Professional During a Postoperative Period").

Procedures with a global surgery indicator of "XXX" are not covered by these rules. Many of these "XXX" procedures are performed by physicians and have inherent pre-procedure, intra-procedure, and post-procedure work usually performed each time the procedure is completed. This work should never be reported as a separate E/M code. Other "XXX" procedures are not usually performed by a physician and have no physician work relative value units associated with them. A physician should never report a separate E/M code with these procedures for the supervision of others performing the procedure or for the interpretation of the procedure. With most "XXX" procedures, the physician may, however, perform a significant and separately identifiable E/M service on the same date of service which may be reported by appending modifier 25 to the E/M code. This E/M service may be related to the same diagnosis necessitating performance of the "XXX" procedure but cannot include any work inherent in the

"XXX" procedure, supervision of others performing the "XXX" procedure, or time for interpreting the result of the "XXX" procedure. Appending modifier 25 to a significant, separately identifiable E/M service when performed on the same date of service as an "XXX" procedure is correct coding.

C. Endoscopic Services

Endoscopic services may be performed in many places of service (e.g., office, outpatient, ambulatory surgical centers (ASC)). Services that are an integral component of an endoscopic procedure are not separately reportable. These services include, but are not limited to, venous access (e.g., CPT code 36000), infusion/injection (e.g., CPT codes 96360-96376), non-invasive oximetry (e.g., CPT codes 94760 and 94761), and anesthesia provided by the surgeon.

1. Per CPT Manual instructions, surgical endoscopy includes diagnostic endoscopy. A diagnostic endoscopy HCPCS/CPT code should not be reported with a surgical endoscopy code.
2. If multiple endoscopic services are performed, the most comprehensive code describing the service(s) rendered should be reported. If multiple services are performed and not adequately described by a single HCPCS/CPT code, more than one code may be reported. The multiple procedure modifier 51 should be appended to the secondary HCPCS/CPT code. Only medically necessary services may be reported. Incidental examination of other areas should not be reported separately.
3. If the same endoscopic procedure (e.g., polypectomy) is performed multiple times at a single patient encounter in the same region as defined by the CPT Manual narrative, only one CPT code may be reported with one unit of service.
4. Gastroenterological procedures included in CPT code ranges 43753-43757 and 91000-91299 are frequently complementary to endoscopic procedures. Esophageal and gastric washings for cytology when performed are integral components of an esophagogastroduodenoscopy (e.g., CPT code 43235). Gastric or duodenal intubation with or without aspiration (e.g., CPT codes 43753, 43754, 43756) should not be separately reported when performed as part of an upper gastrointestinal endoscopic procedure. Gastric or duodenal stimulation testing (e.g., CPT codes 43755, 43757) may be facilitated by gastrointestinal endoscopy (e.g., procurement of gastric or duodenal specimens). When performed concurrent with an upper gastrointestinal endoscopy, CPT code 43755 or 43757 should be reported with modifier 52 indicating a reduced level of service was performed.
5. If an endoscopy or enteroscopy is performed as a common standard of practice when performing another service, the endoscopy or enteroscopy is not separately reportable. For example, if a small intestinal endoscopy or enteroscopy is performed during the creation or revision of an enterostomy, the small intestinal endoscopy or enteroscopy is not separately reportable.
6. A "scout" endoscopy to assess anatomic landmarks or assess extent of disease preceding another surgical procedure at the same patient encounter is not separately reportable. However, an endoscopic procedure for diagnostic purposes to decide whether a more extensive open procedure needs to be performed is separately reportable. In the latter situation, modifier 58 may be utilized to indicate that the diagnostic endoscopy and more extensive open procedure were staged procedures.
   If an endoscopic procedure is performed at the same patient encounter as a non-endoscopic procedure to ensure no intraoperative injury occurred or verify the procedure was performed correctly, the endoscopic procedure is not separately reportable with the non-endoscopic procedure.
7. If a non-endoscopic esophageal dilation (e.g., CPT codes 43450, 43453) fails and is followed by an endoscopic esophageal dilation procedure (e.g., CPT codes 43213, 43214, 43233), only the endoscopic esophageal dilation procedure may be reported. The physician should not report the failed procedure.
8. If it is necessary to perform diagnostic or surgical endoscopy of the hepatic/biliary/pancreatic system utilizing different methodologies (e.g., biliary T-tube endoscopy, ERCP) multiple CPT codes may be reported. Modifier 51 indicating multiple procedures were performed at the same patient encounter should be appended.
9. Intubation of the gastrointestinal tract (e.g., percutaneous placement of G-tube) includes subsequent removal of the tube. CPT codes such as 43247 (upper gastrointestinal endoscopic removal of foreign body(s)) should not be reported for removal of previously placed therapeutic devices. If a previously placed therapeutic device must be removed endoscopically because it cannot be removed by a non-endoscopic procedure, a CPT code such as 43247 may be reported for the endoscopic removal.
10. Rules for reporting biopsies performed at the same patient encounter as an excision, destruction, or other type of removal are discussed in Section H (General Policy Statements) (paragraph 21).
11. Control of bleeding is an integral component of endoscopic procedures and is not separately reportable. For example, if a provider performs endoscopic band ligation(s) by flexible sigmoidoscopy (CPT code 45350) or colonoscopy (CPT code 45398), control of bleeding is not separately reportable with CPT codes 45334 (flexible sigmoidoscopic control of bleeding) or 45382 (colonoscopic control of bleeding) respectively. If it is necessary to repeat an endoscopy to control bleeding at a separate patient encounter on the same date of service, the HCPCS/CPT code for endoscopy for control of bleeding is separately reportable with modifier 78 indicating that the procedure required return to the operating room (or endoscopy suite) for a related procedure during the postoperative period.
12. Only the more extensive endoscopic procedure may be reported for a patient encounter. For example if a sigmoidoscopy is completed and the physician also performs a colonoscopy during the same patient encounter, only the colonoscopy may be reported.
13. If an endoscopic procedure fails and is converted into an open procedure at the same patient encounter, only the open procedure is reportable. Neither a surgical endoscopy nor

diagnostic endoscopy procedure code should be reported with the open procedure code when an endoscopic procedure is converted to an open procedure.

14. If a transabdominal colonoscopy via colostomy and/or standard sigmoidoscopy or colonoscopy is performed as a necessary part of an open procedure (e.g., colectomy), the endoscopic procedure(s) is (are) not separately reportable. However, if either endoscopic procedure is performed as a diagnostic procedure upon which the decision to perform the open procedure is made, the endoscopic procedure may be reported separately. Modifier 58 may be utilized to indicate that the diagnostic endoscopy and the open procedure were staged or planned services. (CPT code 45355 was deleted January 1, 2015.)
15. If the larynx is viewed through an esophagoscope or upper gastrointestinal endoscope during endoscopy, a laryngoscopy CPT code cannot be reported separately. However, if a medically necessary laryngoscopy is performed with a separate laryngoscope, both the laryngoscopy and esophagoscopy (or upper gastro- intestinal endoscopy) CPT codes may be reported with NCCI- associated modifiers.
16. Fluoroscopy (CPT codes 76000 and 76001) is an integral component of all endoscopic procedures when performed. CPT codes 76000 and/or 76001 should not be reported separately with an endoscopic procedure. For example, fluoroscopy (e.g., CPT code 76000) is not separately reportable with CPT codes describing gastrointestinal endoscopy for foreign body removal (e.g., 43194, 43215, 43247, 44390, 45332, 45379).

D. Esophageal Procedures

1. CPT codes 39000 and 39010 describe mediastinotomy by cervical or thoracic approach respectively with "exploration, drainage, removal of foreign body, or biopsy." Exploration of the surgical field is not separately reportable with another procedure performed in the surgical field. CPT codes 39000 and 39010 should not be reported separately for exploration of the mediastinum when performed with an esophageal procedure. These codes may be reported separately if mediastinal drainage, removal of foreign body, or biopsy is performed. However, these codes should not be reported separately for removal of foreign body with CPT code 43020 (esophagotomy, cervical approach, with removal of foreign body) or CPT code 43045 (esophagotomy, thoracic approach, with removal of foreign body).

E. Abdominal Procedures

1. During an open abdominal procedure exploration of the surgical field is routinely performed to identify anatomic structures and disease. An exploratory laparotomy (CPT code 49000) is not separately reportable with an open abdominal procedure.
2. Hepatectomy procedures (e.g., CPT codes 47120-47130, 47133-47142) include removal of the gallbladder based on anatomic considerations and standards of practice. A cholecystectomy CPT code is not separately reportable with a hepatectomy CPT code.
3. A medically necessary appendectomy may be reported separately. However, an incidental appendectomy of a normal appendix during another abdominal procedure is not separately reportable.
4. If a hernia repair is performed at the site of an incision for an open or laparoscopic abdominal procedure, the hernia repair (e.g., CPT codes 49560-49566, 49652-49657) is not separately reportable. The hernia repair is separately reportable if it is performed at a site other than the incision and is medically reasonable and necessary. An incidental hernia repair is not medically reasonable and necessary and should not be reported separately.
5. If a recurrent hernia requires repair, a recurrent hernia repair code may be reported. A code for incisional hernia repair should not be reported in addition to the recurrent hernia repair code unless a medically necessary incisional hernia repair is performed at a different site. In the latter case, modifier 59 should be appended to the incisional hernia repair code.
6. CPT code 49568 is an add-on code describing implantation of mesh or other prosthesis for incisional or ventral hernia repair. This code may be reported with incisional or ventral hernia repair CPT codes 49560-49566. Although mesh or other prosthesis may be implanted with other types of hernia repairs, CPT code 49568 should not be reported with these other hernia repair codes. If a provider performs an incisional or ventral hernia repair with mesh/prosthesis implantation as well as another type of hernia repair at the same patient encounter, CPT code 49568 may be reported with modifier 59 to bypass edits bundling CPT code 49568 into all hernia repair codes other than the incisional or ventral hernia repair codes.
7. Removal of excessive skin and subcutaneous tissue (panniculectomy) at the site of an abdominal incision for an open procedure including hernia repair is not separately reportable. CPT code 15830 should not be reported for this type of panniculectomy. However, an abdominoplasty which requires significantly more work than a panniculectomy is separately reportable. In order to report an abdominoplasty in 2007, CPT requires the physician to report an infraumbilical abdominal panniculectomy (CPT code 15830 in 2007) plus the add-on CPT code 15847 for the abdominoplasty. Since NCCI bundles CPT code 15830 (in 2007) into abdominal wall hernia repair CPT codes, a provider should report CPT codes 15830 plus 15847 with modifier 59 appended to CPT code 15830 in order to report an abdominoplasty with an abdominal hernia repair CPT code.
8. Open enterolysis (CPT code 44005) and laparoscopic enterolysis (CPT code 44180) are defined by the CPT Manual as "separate procedures." They are not separately reportable with other intra-abdominal or pelvic procedures. However, if a provider performs an extensive and time-consuming enterolysis in conjunction with another intra-abdominal or pelvic procedure, the provider may append modifier 22 to the CPT code describing the latter procedure. The local carrier (A/B MAC processing practitioner service claims) will determine whether additional payment is appropriate.
9. If an iatrogenic laceration/perforation of the small or large intestine occurs during the course of another procedure, repair

of the laceration/perforation is not separately reportable. Treatment of an iatrogenic complication of surgery such as an intestinal laceration/perforation is not a separately reportable service. For example CPT codes describing suture of the small intestine (CPT codes 44602, 44603) or suture of large intestine (CPT codes 44604, 44605) should not be reported for repair of an intestinal laceration/perforation during an enterectomy, colectomy, gastrectomy, pancreatectomy, hysterectomy, or oophorectomy procedure.

10. A Whipple type pancreatectomy procedure (CPT codes 48150-48154) includes removal of the gallbladder. A cholecystectomy (e.g., CPT codes 47562-47564, 47600-47620) should not be reported separately.
11. If closure of a fistula requires excision of a portion of an organ into which the fistula passes, excision of that tissue should not be reported separately. For example, if closure of an enterocolic fistula requires removal of a portion of adjacent small intestinal tissue and a portion of adjacent colonic tissue, closure of the enterocolic fistula (CPT code 44650) includes the removal of the small and large intestinal tissue. The excision of the small intestinal or colonic tissue should not be reported separately.
12. Pelvic exenteration procedures (CPT codes 45126, 51597, 58240) include extensive removal of structures from the pelvis. Physicians should not separately report codes for the removal of pelvic structures (e.g., colon, rectum, urinary bladder, uterine body and/or cervix, fallopian tubes, ovaries, lymph nodes, prostate gland).
13. Liver allotransplantation procedures include, if performed, biliary tract T-tube insertion/conversion/exchange/ removal, drainage, or stent procedures (e.g., CPT codes 47533-47540). CPT codes such as 47510, 47511, 47525, 47530, or 47801 should not be reported with a liver allotransplantation procedure. (CPT codes 47510, 47511, 47525, and 47530 were deleted January 1, 2016.)
14. CPT code 49321 describes a laparoscopic biopsy. If this procedure is performed for diagnostic purposes and the decision to proceed with an open or laparoscopic –ectomy procedure is based on this biopsy, CPT code 49321 may be reported in addition to the CPT code for the –ectomy procedure. However, if the laparoscopic biopsy is performed for a different purpose such as assessing the margins of resection, CPT code 49321 is not separately reportable.

F. Laparoscopy

1. Surgical laparoscopy includes diagnostic laparoscopy which is not separately reportable. If a diagnostic laparoscopy leads to a surgical laparoscopy at the same patient encounter, only the surgical laparoscopy may be reported.
2. If a laparoscopy is performed as a "scout" procedure to assess the surgical field or extent of disease, it is not separately reportable. If the findings of a diagnostic laparoscopy lead to the decision to perform an open procedure, the diagnostic laparoscopy may be separately reportable. Modifier 58 may be reported to indicate that the diagnostic laparoscopy and non-laparoscopic therapeutic procedures were staged or planned procedures. The medical record must indicate the medical necessity for the diagnostic laparoscopy.
3. CPT code 49321 describes a laparoscopic biopsy. If this procedure is performed for diagnostic purposes and the decision to proceed with an open or laparoscopic –ectomy procedure is based on this biopsy, CPT code 49321 may be reported in addition to the CPT code for the –ectomy procedure. However, if the laparoscopic biopsy is performed for a different purpose such as assessing the margins of resection, CPT code 49321 is not separately reportable.
4. If a laparoscopic procedure is converted to an open procedure, only the open procedure may be reported. Neither a surgical laparoscopy nor a diagnostic laparoscopy code should be reported with the open procedure code when a laparoscopic procedure is converted to an open procedure.
5. Laparoscopic lysis of adhesions (CPT codes 44180 or 58660) is not separately reportable with other surgical laparoscopic procedures.
6. CPT code 44970 describes a laparoscopic appendectomy and may be reported separately with another laparoscopic procedure code when a diseased appendix is removed. Since removal of a normal appendix with another laparoscopic procedure is not separately reportable, this code should not be reported for an incidental laparoscopic appendectomy.
7. Fluoroscopy (CPT codes 76000 and 76001) is an integral component of all laparoscopic procedures when performed. CPT codes 76000 and/or 76001 should not be reported separately with a laparoscopic procedure.
8. A diagnostic laparoscopy includes "washing," infusion and/or removal of fluid from the body cavity. A physician should not report CPT codes 49082-49083 (abdominal paracentesis) or 49084 (peritoneal lavage) for infusion and/or removal of fluid from the body cavity performed during a diagnostic or surgical laparoscopic procedure.
9. Injection of air into the abdominal or pelvic cavity is integral to many laparoscopic procedures. Physicians should not separately report CPT code 49400 (injection of air or contrast into peritoneal cavity (separate procedure)) for this service.
10. CPT codes 43281 and 43282 describe laparoscopic paraesophageal hernia repair with fundoplasty, if performed, without or with mesh implantation respectively. These codes should not be reported for a figure-of-eight suture often performed during gastric restrictive procedures.

G. Medically Unlikely Edits

1. MUEs are described in Chapter I, Section V.
2. Providers/suppliers should be cautious about reporting services on multiple lines of a claim utilizing modifiers to bypass MUEs. MUEs were set so that such occurrences should be uncommon. If a provider/supplier does this frequently for any HCPCS/ CPT code, the provider/supplier may be coding units of service incorrectly. The provider/supplier should consider contacting his/her national health care organization or the national medical/ surgical society whose members commonly perform the procedure to clarify the correct reporting of units of service. A national healthcare organization, provider/supplier, or other interested third party may request a reconsideration of the MUE value of a HCPCS/CPT code by CMS by writing

the MUE contractor, Correct Coding Solutions, LLC, at the address indicated in Chapter I, Section V.

3. The CMS Internet-Only Manual (Publication 100-04 Medicare Claims Processing Manual, Chapter 12 (Physicians/ Nonphysician Practitioners), Section 40.7.B. and Chapter 4 (Part B Hospital (Including Inpatient Hospital Part B and OPPS)), Section 20.6.2 requires that practitioners and outpatient hospitals report bilateral surgical procedures with modifier 50 and one (1) UOS on a single claim line. MUE values for surgical procedures that may be performed bilaterally are based on this reporting requirement. Since this reporting requirement does not apply to an ambulatory surgical center (ASC), an ASC should report a bilateral surgical procedure on two claim lines, each with one (1) UOS using modifiers LT and RT on different claim lines. This reporting requirement does not apply to non-surgical diagnostic procedures.
4. Gastrointestinal endoscopy CPT codes describing dilation of stricture(s) (e.g., CPT codes 43213, 45340, 45386) include dilation of all strictures dilated during the endoscopic procedure. These codes should not be reported with more than one (1) unit of service if more than one stricture is dilated.
5. The unit of service (UOS) for CPT code 43277 (Endoscopic retrograde cholangiopancreatography (ERCP); with transendoscopic balloon dilation of biliary/pancreatic duct(s) or of ampulla (sphincteroplasty), including sphincterotomy, when performed, each duct) is each duct. One UOS includes transendoscopic balloon dilation of one or more strictures within each duct. Dilation of one or more strictures in the pancreatic duct including the major and minor ductal branches is reported as a single UOS. Similarly, dilation of one or more strictures in each of the following ducts may be reported as a single UOS for each duct: common bile duct, cystic duct, right hepatic duct, and left hepatic duct.

H. General Policy Statements

1. MUE and NCCI PTP edits are based on services provided by the same physician to the same beneficiary on the same date of service. Physicians should not inconvenience beneficiaries nor increase risks to beneficiaries by performing services on different dates of service to avoid MUE or NCCI PTP edits.
2. In this Manual many policies are described utilizing the term "physician." Unless indicated differently the usage of this term does not restrict the policies to physicians only but applies to all practitioners, hospitals, providers, or suppliers eligible to bill the relevant HCPCS/CPT codes pursuant to applicable portions of the Social Security Act (SSA) of 1965, the Code of Federal Regulations (CFR), and Medicare rules. In some sections of this Manual, the term "physician" would not include some of these entities because specific rules do not apply to them. For example, Anesthesia Rules [e.g., CMS Internet-Only Manual, Publication 100-04 (Medicare Claims Processing Manual), Chapter 12 (Physician/Nonphysician Practitioners), Section 50 (Payment for Anesthesiology Services)] and Global Surgery Rules [e.g., CMS Internet-Only Manual, Publication 100-04 (Medicare Claims Processing Manual), Chapter 12 (Physician/ Nonphysician Practitioners), Section 40 (Surgeons and Global Surgery)] do not apply to hospitals.
3. Providers reporting services under Medicare's hospital outpatient prospective payment system (OPPS) should report all services in accordance with appropriate Medicare Internet-Only Manual (IOM) instructions.
4. In 2010 the CPT Manual modified the numbering of codes so that the sequence of codes as they appear in the CPT Manual does not necessarily correspond to a sequential numbering of codes. In the National Correct Coding Initiative Policy Manual for Medicare Services, use of a numerical range of codes reflects all codes that numerically fall within the range regardless of their sequential order in the CPT Manual.
5. With few exceptions the payment for a surgical procedure includes payment for dressings, supplies, and local anesthesia. These items are not separately reportable under their own HCPCS/CPT codes. Wound closures utilizing adhesive strips or tape alone are not separately reportable. In the absence of an operative procedure, these types of wound closures are included in an E/M service. Under limited circumstances wound closure utilizing tissue adhesive may be reported separately. If a practitioner utilizes a tissue adhesive alone for a wound closure, it may be reported separately with HCPCS code G0168 (wound closure utilizing tissue adhesive(s) only). If a practitioner utilizes tissue adhesive in addition to staples or sutures to close a wound, HCPCS code G0168 is not separately reportable but is included in the tissue repair. Under OPPS HCPCS code G0168 is not recognized and paid. Facilities may report wound closure utilizing sutures, staples, or tissue adhesives, either singly or in combination with each other, with the appropriate CPT code in the "Repair (Closure)" section of the CPT Manual.
6. The vagotomy CPT codes (e.g., 43635-43641, 64755-64760) are not separately reportable with esophageal or gastric procedures that include vagotomy as part of the service. For example, the esophagogastrostomy procedure described by CPT code 43320 includes a vagotomy if performed. The vagotomy procedures are mutually exclusive, and only one vagotomy procedure code may be reported at a patient encounter.
7. If closure of an enterostomy or fistula involving the intestine requires resection and anastomosis of a segment of intestine, the resection and anastomosis of the intestine are not separately reportable.
8. If multiple services are utilized to treat hemorrhoids at the same patient encounter, only one HCPCS/CPT code describing the most extensive procedure may be reported. If an abscess is drained during the treatment of hemorrhoids, the incision and drainage is not separately reportable unless the incision and drainage is at a separate site unrelated to the hemorrhoids. In the latter case, the incision and drainage code may be reported appending an anatomic modifier or modifier 59.
9. Diagnostic anoscopy (CPT code 46600) is not separately reportable with an open or endoscopic procedure of the anus (e.g., 46020-46942, 0184T, 0249T, 0377T). The diagnostic anoscopy (CPT code 46600) is an included service that is not separately reportable. It is a misuse of CPT codes describing diagnostic proctosigmoidoscopy (CPT code 45300), sigmoidoscopy (CPT code 45330), or colonoscopy

(CPT code 45378) to report an examination limited to the anus. If the physician performs a complete diagnostic proctosigmoidoscopy, sigmoidoscopy, or colonoscopy, the procedure may be reported separately.

10. The CPT Manual contains groups of codes describing different approaches or methods to accomplish similar results. These codes are generally mutually exclusive of one another. For example CPT codes 45110-45123 describe different proctectomy procedures and are mutually exclusive of one another. Other examples include groups of codes for colectomy (CPT codes 44140- 44160), gastrectomy (CPT codes 43620-43635), and pancreatectomy (CPT codes 48140-48155).
11. An enterostomy closure HCPCS/CPT code should not be reported with a code for creation or revision of a colostomy. Closure of an enterostomy is mutually exclusive with the creation or revision of the colostomy.
12. If an excised section of intestine includes a fistula tract, a fistula closure code should not be reported separately. Closure of the fistula is included in the excision of intestine.
13. The mouth and anus have mucocutaneous margins. Numerous procedures (e.g., biopsy, destruction, excision) have CPT codes that describe the procedure as an integumentary procedure (CPT codes 10000-19999) or as a digestive system procedure (CPT codes 40000-49999). If a procedure is performed on a lesion at or near a mucocutaneous margin, only one CPT code which best describes the procedure may be reported. If the code descriptor of a CPT code from the digestive system (or any other system) includes a tissue transfer service (e.g., flap, graft), the CPT codes for such services (e.g., transfer, graft, flap) from the integumentary system (e.g., CPT codes 14000-15770) should not be reported separately.
14. If a physician must drain an abscess in order to complete a sialolithotomy procedure, the drainage of the abscess is not separately reportable. If a definitive surgical procedure requires access through diseased tissue, treatment of the diseased tissue for this access is not separately reportable.
15. An open cholecystectomy includes an examination of the abdomen through the abdominal wall incision. If this examination is performed laparoscopically, it is not separately reportable as CPT code 49320 (diagnostic laparoscopy).
16. CPT code 92502 (otolaryngologic examination under general anesthesia) is not separately reportable with any other otolaryngologic procedure performed under general anesthesia.
17. CPT codes 43770-43774 describe laparoscopic gastric restrictive procedures. Only one of these procedure codes may be reported for a single patient encounter. If a patient develops a complication during the postoperative period of the initial procedure requiring return to the operating room for a different laparoscopic gastric restrictive procedure to treat the complication, the second procedure should be reported with modifier 78.
18. With limited exceptions Medicare Anesthesia Rules prevent separate payment for anesthesia for a medical or surgical procedure when provided by the physician performing the procedure. The physician should not report CPT codes 00100-01999, 62320-62327, or 64400-64530 for anesthesia for a procedure. Additionally, the physician should not unbundle the anesthesia procedure and report component codes individually. For example, introduction of a needle or intracatheter into a vein (CPT code 36000), venipuncture (CPT code 36410), drug administration (CPT codes 96360-96377) or cardiac assessment (e.g., CPT codes 93000-93010, 93040-93042) should not be reported when these procedures are related to the delivery of an anesthetic agent.
19. Medicare allows separate reporting for moderate conscious sedation services (CPT codes 99151-99153) when provided by the same physician performing a medical or surgical procedure.
20. Under Medicare Global Surgery Rules, drug administration services (CPT codes 96360-96377) are not separately reportable by the physician performing a procedure for drug administration services related to the procedure.
21. Under the OPPS drug administration services related to operative procedures are included in the associated procedural HCPCS/CPT codes. Examples of such drug administration services include, but are not limited to, anesthesia (local or other), hydration, and medications such as anxiolytics or antibiotics. Providers should not report CPT codes 96360-96377 for these services.
22. Medicare Global Surgery Rules prevent separate payment for postoperative pain management when provided by the physician performing an operative procedure. CPT codes 36000, 36410, 62320-62327, 64400-64489, and 96360-96377 describe some services that may be utilized for postoperative pain management. The services described by these codes may be reported by the physician performing the operative procedure only if provided for purposes unrelated to the postoperative pain management, the operative procedure, or anesthesia for the procedure.
23. If a physician performing an operative procedure provides a drug administration service (CPT codes 96360-96375) for a purpose unrelated to anesthesia, intra-operative care, or post-procedure pain management, the drug administration service (CPT codes 96360-96375) may be reported with an NCCI-associated modifier if performed in a non-facility site of service.
24. The Medicare global surgery package includes insertion of urinary catheters. CPT codes 51701-51703 (insertion of bladder catheters) should not be reported with any procedure with a global period of 000, 010, or 090 days nor with some procedures with a global period of MMM.
25. Closure/repair of a surgical incision is included in the global surgical package. Wound repair CPT codes 12001-13153 should not be reported separately to describe closure of surgical incisions for procedures with global surgery indicators of 000, 010, 090, or MMM.
26. Control of bleeding during an operative procedure is an integral component of a surgical procedure and is not separately reportable. Postoperative control of bleeding not requiring return to the operating room is included in the global surgical package and is not separately reportable. However, control of bleeding requiring return to the operating room in the postoperative period is separately reportable utilizing modifier 78.
27. A biopsy performed at the time of another more extensive procedure (e.g., excision, destruction, removal) is separately

reportable under specific circumstances. If the biopsy is performed on a separate lesion, it is separately reportable. This situation may be reported with anatomic modifiers or modifier 59. If the biopsy is performed on the same lesion on which a more extensive procedure is performed, it is separately reportable only if the biopsy is utilized for immediate pathologic diagnosis prior to the more extensive procedure, and the decision to proceed with the more extensive procedure is based on the diagnosis established by the pathologic examination. The biopsy is not separately reportable if the pathologic examination at the time of surgery is for the purpose of assessing margins of resection or verifying resectability. When separately reportable modifier 58 may be reported to indicate that the biopsy and the more extensive procedure were planned or staged procedures. If a biopsy is performed and submitted for pathologic evaluation that will be completed after the more extensive procedure is performed, the biopsy is not separately reportable with the more extensive procedure.

28. Fine needle aspiration (FNA) (CPT codes 10021, 10022) should not be reported with another biopsy procedure code for the same lesion unless one specimen is inadequate for diagnosis. For example, an FNA specimen is usually examined for adequacy when the specimen is aspirated. If the specimen is adequate for diagnosis, it is not necessary to obtain an additional biopsy specimen. However, if the specimen is not adequate and another type of biopsy (e.g., needle, open) is subsequently performed at the same patient encounter, the other biopsy procedure code may also be reported with an NCCI-associated modifier.
29. The NCCI PTP edit with column one CPT code 45385 (Flexible colonoscopy with removal of tumor(s), polyp(s), or lesion(s) by snare technique) and column two CPT code 45380 (Flexible colonoscopy with single or multiple biopsies) is often bypassed by utilizing modifier 59. Use of modifier 59 with the column two CPT code 45380 of this NCCI PTP edit is only appropriate if the two procedures are performed on separate lesions or at separate patient encounters.
30. If the code descriptor of a HCPCS/CPT code includes the phrase, "separate procedure," the procedure is subject to NCCI PTP edits based on this designation. CMS does not allow separate reporting of a procedure designated as a "separate procedure" when it is performed at the same patient encounter as another procedure in an anatomically related area through the same skin incision, orifice, or surgical approach.
31. Most NCCI PTP edits for codes describing procedures that may be performed on bilateral organs or structures (e.g., arms, eyes, kidneys, lungs) allow use of NCCI-associated modifiers (modifier indicator of "1") because the two codes of the code pair edit may be reported if the two procedures are performed on contralateral organs or structures. Most of these code pairs should not be reported with NCCI-associated modifiers when the corresponding procedures are performed on the ipsilateral organ or structure unless there is a specific coding rationale to bypass the edit. The existence of the NCCI PTP edit indicates that the two codes generally should not be reported together unless the two corresponding procedures are performed at two separate patient encounters or two separate anatomic sites. However, if the corresponding procedures are performed at the same patient encounter and in contiguous structures, NCCI-associated modifiers should generally not be utilized.
32. If fluoroscopy is performed during an endoscopic procedure, it is integral to the procedure. This principle applies to all endoscopic procedures including, but not limited to, laparoscopy, hysteroscopy, thoracoscopy, arthroscopy, esophagoscopy, colonoscopy, other GI endoscopy, laryngoscopy, bronchoscopy, and cystourethroscopy.
33. If the code descriptor for a HCPCS/CPT code, CPT Manual instruction for a code, or CMS instruction for a code indicates that the procedure includes radiologic guidance, a physician should not separately report a HCPCS/CPT code for radiologic guidance including, but not limited to, fluoroscopy, ultrasound, computed tomography, or magnetic resonance imaging codes. If the physician performs an additional procedure on the same date of service for which a radiologic guidance or imaging code may be separately reported, the radiologic guidance or imaging code appropriate for that additional procedure may be reported separately with an NCCI-associated modifier if appropriate.
34. A cystourethroscopy (CPT code 52000) performed near the termination of an intra-abdominal, intra-pelvic, or retroperitoneal surgical procedure to assure that there was no intraoperative injury to the ureters or urinary bladder and that they are functioning properly is not separately reportable with the surgical procedure.

CCI Table Information

The CCI Modification indicator is noted with superscript letters and is also located in the footer of each page for reference purposes. The codes are suffixed as **0** or **1**.

- **0** indicates there is no circumstance in which a modifier would be allowed or appropriate, meaning services represented by the code combination will not be paid separately.
- **1** signifies a modifier is allowed in order to differentiate between the services provided.

Note: The responsibility for the content of this product is the Centers for Medicare and Medicaid Services (CMS) and no endorsement by the American Medical Association (AMA) is intended or should be implied. The AMA disclaims responsibility for any consequences or liability attributable to or related to any uses, non-use, or interpretation of information contained or not contained in this product.

The NCCI edits on the following tables represent only the codes contained in this book. There are NCCI edits for CPT codes not found in this guide. The edits herein represent all active edits as of 1/1/2020. NCCI edits are updated quarterly. To view all NCCI edits, as well as quarterly updates, visit www.cms.gov/nationalcorrectcodeinited/.

Code 1	Code 2
10140	0213T[0], 0216T[0], 0228T[0], 0230T[0], 11055[1], 11056[1], 11057[1], 11719[1], 11720[1], 11721[1], 12001[1], 12002[1], 12004[1], 12005[1], 12006[1], 12007[1], 12011[1], 12013[1], 12014[1], 12015[1], 12016[1], 12017[1], 12018[1], 12020[1], 12021[1], 12031[1], 12032[1], 12034[1], 12035[1], 12036[1], 12037[1], 12041[1], 12042[1], 12044[1], 12045[1], 12046[1], 12047[1], 12051[1], 12052[1], 12053[1], 12054[1], 12055[1], 12056[1], 12057[1], 13100[1], 13101[1], 13102[1], 13120[1], 13121[1], 13122[1], 13131[1], 13132[1], 13133[1], 13151[1], 13152[1], 13153[1], 29580[1], 29581[1], 36000[1], 36400[1], 36405[1], 36406[1], 36410[1], 36420[1], 36425[1], 36430[1], 36440[1], 36591[0], 36592[0], 36600[1], 36640[1], 43752[1], 51701[1], 51702[1], 51703[1], 62320[0], 62321[0], 62322[0], 62323[0], 62324[0], 62325[0], 62326[0], 62327[0], 64400[0], 64405[0], 64408[0], 64415[0], 64416[0], 64417[0], 64418[0], 64420[0], 64421[0], 64425[0], 64430[0], 64435[0], 64445[0], 64446[0], 64447[0], 64448[0], 64449[0], 64450[1], 64451[0], 64454[1], 64461[0], 64462[0], 64463[0], 64479[0], 64480[0], 64483[0], 64484[0], 64486[0], 64487[0], 64488[0], 64489[0], 64490[0], 64491[0], 64492[0], 64493[0], 64494[0], 64495[0], 64505[0], 64510[0], 64517[0], 64520[0], 64530[0], 69990[0], 76000[1], 76942[1], 76998[1], 77002[1], 77012[1], 77021[1], 92012[1], 92014[1], 93000[1], 93005[1], 93010[1], 93040[1], 93041[1], 93042[1], 93318[1], 93355[1], 94002[1], 94200[1], 94250[1], 94680[1], 94681[1], 94690[1], 94770[1], 95812[1], 95813[1], 95816[1], 95819[1], 95822[1], 95829[1], 95955[1], 96360[1], 96361[1], 96365[1], 96366[1], 96367[1], 96368[1], 96372[1], 96374[1], 96375[1], 96376[1], 96377[1], 96523[0], 99155[0], 99156[0], 99157[0], 99211[1], 99212[1], 99213[1], 99214[1], 99215[1], 99217[1], 99218[1], 99219[1], 99220[1], 99221[1], 99222[1], 99223[1], 99231[1], 99232[1], 99233[1], 99234[1], 99235[1], 99236[1], 99238[1], 99239[1], 99241[1], 99242[1], 99243[1], 99244[1], 99245[1], 99251[1], 99252[1], 99253[1], 99254[1], 99255[1], 99291[1], 99292[1], 99304[1], 99305[1], 99306[1], 99307[1], 99308[1], 99309[1], 99310[1], 99315[1], 99316[1], 99334[1], 99335[1], 99336[1], 99337[1], 99347[1], 99348[1], 99349[1], 99350[1], 99374[1], 99375[1], 99377[1], 99378[1], 99446[0], 99447[0], 99448[0], 99449[0], 99451[0], 99452[0], 99495[0], 99496[0], G0127[1], G0463[1], G0471[1], J0670[1], J2001[1]
10160	0213T[0], 0216T[0], 0228T[0], 0230T[0], 10061[1], 10140[1], 11055[1], 11056[1], 11057[1], 11719[1], 11720[1], 11721[1], 12001[1], 12002[1], 12004[1], 12005[1], 12006[1], 12007[1], 12011[1], 12013[1], 12014[1], 12015[1], 12016[1], 12017[1], 12018[1], 12020[1], 12021[1], 12031[1], 12032[1], 12034[1], 12035[1], 12036[1], 12037[1], 12041[1], 12042[1], 12044[1], 12045[1], 12046[1], 12047[1], 12051[1], 12052[1], 12053[1], 12054[1], 12055[1], 12056[1], 12057[1], 13100[1], 13101[1], 13102[1], 13120[1], 13121[1], 13122[1], 13131[1], 13132[1], 13133[1], 13151[1], 13152[1], 13153[1], 29580[1], 29581[1], 36000[1], 36400[1], 36405[1], 36406[1], 36410[1], 36420[1], 36425[1], 36430[1], 36440[1], 36591[0], 36592[0], 36600[1], 36640[1], 43752[1], 51701[1], 51702[1], 51703[1], 62320[0], 62321[0], 62322[0], 62323[0], 62324[0], 62325[0], 62326[0], 62327[0], 64400[0], 64405[0], 64408[0], 64415[0], 64416[0], 64417[0], 64418[0], 64420[0], 64421[0], 64425[0], 64430[0], 64435[0], 64445[0], 64446[0], 64447[0], 64448[0], 64449[0], 64450[1], 64451[0], 64454[1], 64461[0], 64462[0], 64463[0], 64479[0], 64480[0], 64483[0], 64484[0], 64486[0], 64487[0], 64488[0], 64489[0], 64490[0], 64491[0], 64492[0], 64493[0], 64494[0], 64495[0], 64505[0], 64510[0], 64517[0], 64520[0], 64530[0], 69990[0], 92012[1], 92014[1], 93000[1], 93005[1], 93010[1], 93040[1], 93041[1], 93042[1], 93318[1], 93355[1], 94002[1], 94200[1], 94250[1], 94680[1], 94681[1], 94690[1], 94770[1], 95812[1], 95813[1], 95816[1], 95819[1], 95822[1], 95829[1], 95955[1], 96360[1], 96361[1], 96365[1], 96366[1], 96367[1], 96368[1], 96372[1], 96374[1], 96375[1], 96376[1], 96377[1], 96523[0], 99155[0], 99156[0], 99157[0], 99211[1], 99212[1], 99213[1], 99214[1], 99215[1], 99217[1], 99218[1], 99219[1], 99220[1], 99221[1], 99222[1], 99223[1], 99231[1], 99232[1], 99233[1], 99234[1], 99235[1], 99236[1], 99238[1], 99239[1], 99241[1], 99242[1], 99243[1], 99244[1], 99245[1], 99251[1], 99252[1], 99253[1], 99254[1], 99255[1], 99291[1], 99292[1], 99304[1], 99305[1], 99306[1], 99307[1], 99308[1], 99309[1], 99310[1], 99315[1], 99316[1], 99334[1], 99335[1], 99336[1], 99337[1], 99347[1], 99348[1], 99349[1], 99350[1], 99374[1], 99375[1], 99377[1], 99378[1], 99446[0], 99447[0], 99448[0], 99449[0], 99451[0], 99452[0], 99495[0], 99496[0], G0127[1], G0463[1], G0471[1], J0670[1], J2001[1]
10180	0213T[0], 0216T[0], 0228T[0], 0230T[0], 11720[1], 11721[1], 12001[1], 12002[1], 12004[1], 12005[1], 12006[1], 12007[1], 12011[1], 12013[1], 12014[1], 12015[1], 12016[1], 12017[1], 12018[1], 12020[1], 12021[1], 12031[1], 12032[1], 12034[1], 12035[1], 12036[1], 12037[1], 12041[1], 12042[1], 12044[1], 12045[1], 12046[1], 12047[1], 12051[1], 12052[1], 12053[1], 12054[1], 12055[1], 12056[1], 12057[1], 13100[1], 13101[1], 13102[1], 13120[1], 13121[1], 13122[1], 13131[1], 13132[1], 13133[1], 13151[1], 13152[1], 13153[1], 20500[1], 36000[1], 36400[1], 36405[1], 36406[1], 36410[1], 36420[1], 36425[1], 36430[1], 36440[1], 36591[0], 36592[0], 36600[1], 36640[1], 43752[1], 51701[1], 51702[1], 51703[1], 62320[0], 62321[0], 62322[0], 62323[0], 62324[0], 62325[0], 62326[0], 62327[0], 64400[0], 64405[0], 64408[0], 64415[0], 64416[0], 64417[0], 64418[0], 64420[0], 64421[0], 64425[0], 64430[0], 64435[0], 64445[0], 64446[0], 64447[0], 64448[0], 64449[0], 64450[1], 64451[0], 64454[1], 64461[0], 64462[0], 64463[0], 64479[0], 64480[0], 64483[0], 64484[0], 64486[0], 64487[0], 64488[0], 64489[0], 64490[0], 64491[0], 64492[0], 64493[0], 64494[0], 64495[0], 64505[0], 64510[0], 64517[0], 64520[0], 64530[0], 69990[0], 92012[1], 92014[1], 93000[1], 93005[1], 93010[1], 93040[1], 93041[1], 93042[1], 93318[1], 93355[1], 94002[1], 94200[1], 94250[1], 94680[1], 94681[1], 94690[1], 94770[1], 95812[1], 95813[1], 95816[1], 95819[1], 95822[1], 95829[1], 95955[1], 96360[1], 96361[1], 96365[1], 96366[1], 96367[1], 96368[1], 96372[1], 96374[1], 96375[1], 96376[1], 96377[1], 96523[0], 99155[0], 99156[0], 99157[0], 99211[1], 99212[1], 99213[1], 99214[1], 99215[1], 99217[1], 99218[1], 99219[1], 99220[1], 99221[1], 99222[1], 99223[1], 99231[1], 99232[1], 99233[1], 99234[1], 99235[1], 99236[1], 99238[1], 99239[1], 99241[1], 99242[1], 99243[1], 99244[1], 99245[1], 99251[1], 99252[1], 99253[1], 99254[1], 99255[1], 99291[1], 99292[1], 99304[1], 99305[1], 99306[1], 99307[1], 99308[1], 99309[1], 99310[1], 99315[1], 99316[1], 99334[1], 99335[1], 99336[1], 99337[1], 99347[1], 99348[1], 99349[1], 99350[1], 99374[1], 99375[1], 99377[1], 99378[1], 99446[0], 99447[0], 99448[0], 99449[0], 99451[0], 99452[0], 99495[0], 99496[0], G0463[1], G0471[1], J0670[1], J2001[1]
11042	0213T[0], 0216T[0], 0228T[0], 0230T[0], 0552T[1], 10030[1], 10060[1], 11000[1], 11008[1], 11010[1], 11011[1], 11719[1], 11720[1], 11721[1], 12007[1], 12014[1], 12016[1], 12017[1], 12018[1], 12036[1], 12037[1], 12041[1], 12044[1], 12046[1], 12047[1], 12053[1], 12055[1], 12056[1], 12057[1], 13102[1], 13122[1], 13133[1], 13153[1], 15852[1], 17000[1], 17250[1], 20526[1], 20552[1], 20553[1], 20560[1], 20561[1], 24300[1], 25259[1], 26340[1], 29000[1], 29010[1], 29015[1], 29035[1], 29040[1], 29044[1], 29046[1], 29049[1], 29055[1], 29058[1], 29065[1], 29075[1], 29085[1], 29086[1], 29105[1], 29125[1], 29126[1], 29130[1], 29131[1], 29200[1], 29240[1], 29260[1], 29280[1], 29305[1], 29325[1], 29345[1], 29355[1], 29358[1], 29365[1], 29405[1], 29425[1], 29435[1], 29440[1], 29445[1], 29450[1], 29505[1], 29515[1], 29520[1], 29530[1], 29540[1], 29550[1], 29580[1], 29581[1], 29584[1], 29730[1], 35702[1], 35703[1], 36000[1], 36400[1], 36405[1], 36406[1], 36410[1], 36420[1], 36425[1], 36430[1], 36440[1], 36591[0], 36592[0], 36600[1], 36640[1], 43752[1], 62320[0], 62321[0], 62322[0], 62323[0], 62324[0], 62325[0], 62326[0], 62327[0], 64400[0], 64405[0], 64408[0], 64415[0], 64416[0], 64417[0], 64418[0], 64420[0], 64421[0], 64425[0], 64430[0], 64435[0], 64445[0], 64446[0], 64447[0], 64448[0], 64449[0], 64450[1], 64451[0], 64454[1], 64461[0], 64462[0], 64463[0], 64479[0], 64480[0], 64483[0], 64484[0], 64486[0], 64487[0], 64488[0], 64489[0], 64490[0], 64491[0], 64492[0], 64493[0], 64494[0], 64495[0], 64505[0], 64510[0], 64517[0], 64520[0], 64530[0], 64553[1], 66987[1], 66988[1], 69990[0], 72295[1], 76000[1], 77001[1], 77002[1], 92012[1], 92014[1], 93000[1], 93005[1], 93010[1], 93040[1], 93041[1], 93042[1], 93318[1], 93355[1], 94002[1], 94200[1], 94250[1], 94680[1], 94681[1], 94690[1], 94770[1], 95812[1], 95813[1], 95816[1], 95819[1], 95822[1], 95829[1], 95955[1], 96360[1], 96361[1], 96365[1], 96366[1], 96367[1], 96368[1], 96372[1], 96374[1], 96375[1], 96376[1], 96377[1], 96523[0], 97022[1], 97597[1], 97598[1], 97602[1], 97610[1], 99155[0], 99156[0], 99157[0], 99211[1], 99212[1], 99213[1], 99214[1], 99215[1], 99217[1], 99218[1], 99219[1], 99220[1], 99221[1], 99222[1], 99223[1], 99231[1], 99232[1], 99233[1], 99234[1], 99235[1], 99236[1], 99238[1], 99239[1], 99241[1], 99242[1], 99243[1], 99244[1], 99245[1], 99251[1], 99252[1], 99253[1], 99254[1], 99255[1], 99291[1], 99292[1], 99304[1], 99305[1], 99306[1], 99307[1], 99308[1], 99309[1], 99310[1], 99315[1], 99316[1], 99334[1], 99335[1], 99336[1], 99337[1], 99347[1], 99348[1], 99349[1], 99350[1], 99374[1], 99375[1], 99377[1], 99378[1], 99446[0], 99447[0], 99448[0], 99449[0], 99451[0], 99452[0], 99495[1], 99496[1], G0463[1], G0471[1]
11043	0213T[0], 0216T[0], 0228T[0], 0230T[0], 0552T[1], 10030[1], 10060[1], 10061[1], 11000[1], 11008[1], 11010[1], 11011[1], 11012[1], 11042[1], 11719[1], 11720[1], 11721[1], 12001[1], 12002[1], 12004[1], 12007[1], 12011[1], 12013[1], 12014[1], 12015[1], 12016[1], 12017[1], 12018[1], 12021[1], 12031[1], 12041[1], 12042[1], 12045[1], 12047[1], 12051[1], 12052[1], 12053[1], 12054[1], 12055[1], 12056[1], 12057[1], 13102[1], 13122[1], 13133[1], 13153[1], 15852[1], 17250[1], 20552[1], 20553[1], 20560[1], 20561[1], 24300[1], 25001[1], 29000[1], 29010[1], 29015[1], 29035[1], 29040[1], 29044[1], 29046[1], 29049[1], 29055[1], 29058[1], 29065[1], 29075[1], 29085[1], 29086[1], 29105[1], 29125[1], 29126[1], 29130[1], 29131[1], 29200[1], 29240[1], 29260[1], 29280[1], 29305[1], 29325[1], 29345[1], 29355[1], 29358[1], 29365[1], 29405[1], 29425[1], 29435[1], 29440[1], 29445[1], 29450[1], 29505[1], 29515[1], 29520[1], 29530[1], 29540[1], 29550[1], 29580[1], 29581[1], 29584[1], 35702[1], 35703[1], 36000[1], 36400[1], 36405[1], 36406[1], 36410[1], 36420[1], 36425[1], 36430[1], 36440[1], 36591[0], 36592[0], 36600[1], 36640[1], 43752[1], 62320[0], 62321[0], 62322[0], 62323[0], 62324[0], 62325[0], 62326[0], 62327[0], 64400[0], 64405[0], 64408[0], 64415[0], 64416[0], 64417[0], 64418[0], 64420[0], 64421[0], 64425[0], 64430[0], 64435[0], 64445[0], 64446[0], 64447[0], 64448[0], 64449[0], 64450[1], 64451[0], 64454[1], 64461[0], 64462[0], 64463[0], 64479[0], 64480[0], 64483[0], 64484[0], 64486[0], 64487[0], 64488[0], 64489[0], 64490[0], 64491[0], 64492[0], 64493[0], 64494[0], 64495[0], 64505[0], 64510[0], 64517[0], 64520[0], 64530[0], 66987[1], 66988[1], 69990[0], 75710[1], 75820[1], 76000[1], 77001[1], 77002[1], 92012[1], 92014[1], 93000[1], 93005[1], 93010[1], 93040[1], 93041[1], 93042[1], 93318[1], 93355[1], 94002[1], 94200[1], 94250[1], 94680[1], 94681[1], 94690[1], 94770[1], 95812[1], 95813[1], 95816[1], 95819[1], 95822[1], 95829[1], 95955[1], 96360[1], 96361[1], 96365[1], 96366[1], 96367[1], 96368[1], 96372[1], 96374[1], 96375[1], 96376[1], 96377[1], 96523[0], 97597[1], 97598[1], 97602[1], 97610[1], 99155[0], 99156[0], 99157[0], 99211[1], 99212[1], 99213[1], 99214[1], 99215[1], 99217[1], 99218[1], 99219[1], 99220[1], 99221[1], 99222[1], 99223[1], 99231[1], 99232[1], 99233[1], 99234[1], 99235[1], 99236[1], 99238[1], 99239[1], 99241[1], 99242[1], 99243[1], 99244[1], 99245[1], 99251[1], 99252[1], 99253[1], 99254[1], 99255[1], 99291[1], 99292[1], 99304[1], 99305[1], 99306[1], 99307[1], 99308[1], 99309[1], 99310[1], 99315[1], 99316[1], 99334[1], 99335[1], 99336[1], 99337[1], 99347[1], 99348[1], 99349[1], 99350[1], 99374[1], 99375[1], 99377[1], 99378[1], 99446[0], 99447[0], 99448[0], 99449[0], 99451[0], 99452[0], 99495[1], 99496[1], G0127[1], G0463[1], G0471[1], J0670[1], J2001[1]
11044	0213T[0], 0216T[0], 0228T[0], 0230T[0], 0552T[1], 10030[1], 10060[1], 10061[1], 11000[1], 11008[1], 11010[1], 11011[1], 11012[1], 11042[1], 11043[1], 11719[1], 11720[1], 11721[1], 12001[1], 12002[1], 12004[1], 12005[1], 12006[1], 12007[1], 12011[1], 12013[1], 12014[1], 12015[1], 12016[1], 12017[1], 12018[1], 12021[1], 12031[1], 12032[1], 12034[1], 12036[1], 12041[1], 12042[1], 12045[1], 12047[1], 12051[1], 12052[1], 12053[1], 12054[1], 12055[1], 12056[1], 12057[1], 13102[1], 13122[1], 13133[1],

0 = Modifier usage not allowed or inappropriate 1 = Modifier usage allowed

Code 1	Code 2
	13153[1], 15852[1], 17250[1], 20552[1], 20553[1], 20560[1], 20561[1], 24300[1], 25001[1], 29000[1], 29010[1], 29015[1], 29035[1], 29040[1], 29044[1], 29046[1], 29049[1], 29055[1], 29058[1], 29065[1], 29075[1], 29085[1], 29086[1], 29105[1], 29125[1], 29126[1], 29130[1], 29131[1], 29200[1], 29240[1], 29260[1], 29280[1], 29305[1], 29325[1], 29345[1], 29355[1], 29358[1], 29365[1], 29405[1], 29425[1], 29435[1], 29440[1], 29445[1], 29450[1], 29505[1], 29515[1], 29520[1], 29530[1], 29540[1], 29550[1], 29580[1], 29581[1], 29584[1], 35702[1], 35703[1], 36000[1], 36400[1], 36405[1], 36406[1], 36410[1], 36420[1], 36425[1], 36430[1], 36440[1], 36591[0], 36592[0], 36600[1], 36640[1], 43752[1], 62320[0], 62321[0], 62322[0], 62323[0], 62324[0], 62325[0], 62326[0], 62327[0], 64400[0], 64405[0], 64408[0], 64415[0], 64416[0], 64417[0], 64418[0], 64420[0], 64421[0], 64425[0], 64430[0], 64435[0], 64445[0], 64446[0], 64447[0], 64448[0], 64449[0], 64450[1], 64451[0], 64454[1], 64461[0], 64462[0], 64463[0], 64479[0], 64480[0], 64483[0], 64484[0], 64486[0], 64487[0], 64488[0], 64489[0], 64490[0], 64491[0], 64492[0], 64493[0], 64494[0], 64495[0], 64505[0], 64510[0], 64517[0], 64520[0], 64530[0], 66987[1], 66988[1], 69990[0], 75710[1], 75716[1], 92012[1], 92014[1], 93000[1], 93005[1], 93010[1], 93040[1], 93041[1], 93042[1], 93318[1], 93355[1], 94002[1], 94200[1], 94250[1], 94680[1], 94681[1], 94690[1], 94770[1], 95812[1], 95813[1], 95816[1], 95819[1], 95822[1], 95829[1], 95955[1], 96360[1], 96361[1], 96365[1], 96366[1], 96367[1], 96368[1], 96372[1], 96374[1], 96375[1], 96376[1], 96377[1], 96523[0], 97597[1], 97598[1], 97602[1], 97610[1], 99155[0], 99156[0], 99157[0], 99211[1], 99212[1], 99213[1], 99214[1], 99215[1], 99217[1], 99218[1], 99219[1], 99220[1], 99221[1], 99222[1], 99223[1], 99231[1], 99232[1], 99233[1], 99234[1], 99235[1], 99236[1], 99238[1], 99239[1], 99241[1], 99242[1], 99243[1], 99244[1], 99245[1], 99251[1], 99252[1], 99253[1], 99254[1], 99255[1], 99291[1], 99292[1], 99304[1], 99305[1], 99306[1], 99307[1], 99308[1], 99309[1], 99310[1], 99315[1], 99316[1], 99334[1], 99335[1], 99336[1], 99337[1], 99347[1], 99348[1], 99349[1], 99350[1], 99374[1], 99375[1], 99377[1], 99378[1], 99446[0], 99447[0], 99448[0], 99449[0], 99451[0], 99452[0], 99495[1], 99496[1], G0463[1], G0471[1], J0670[1], J2001[1]
11045	20560[1], 20561[1], 29000[1], 29010[1], 29015[1], 29035[1], 29040[1], 29044[1], 29046[1], 29049[1], 29055[1], 29058[1], 29065[1], 29075[1], 29085[1], 29086[1], 29105[1], 29125[1], 29126[1], 29130[1], 29131[1], 29200[1], 29240[1], 29260[1], 29280[1], 29305[1], 29325[1], 29345[1], 29355[1], 29358[1], 29365[1], 29405[1], 29425[1], 29435[1], 29440[1], 29445[1], 29450[1], 29505[1], 29515[1], 29520[1], 29530[1], 29540[1], 29550[1], 29580[1], 29581[1], 29584[1], 36591[0], 36592[0], 66987[1], 66988[1], 96523[0], 97597[1], 97598[1], 97602[1]
11047	20560[1], 20561[1], 29000[1], 29010[1], 29015[1], 29035[1], 29040[1], 29044[1], 29046[1], 29049[1], 29055[1], 29058[1], 29065[1], 29075[1], 29085[1], 29086[1], 29105[1], 29125[1], 29126[1], 29130[1], 29131[1], 29200[1], 29240[1], 29260[1], 29280[1], 29305[1], 29325[1], 29345[1], 29355[1], 29358[1], 29365[1], 29405[1], 29425[1], 29435[1], 29440[1], 29445[1], 29450[1], 29505[1], 29515[1], 29520[1], 29530[1], 29540[1], 29550[1], 29580[1], 29581[1], 29584[1], 36591[0], 36592[0], 66987[1], 66988[1], 96523[0], 97597[1], 97598[1], 97602[1], J0670[1], J2001[1]
11104	00170[0], 0213T[0], 0216T[0], 0228T[0], 0230T[0], 0470T[1], 0471T[1], 10011[1], 11000[1], 11001[1], 11042[1], 11043[1], 11044[1], 11045[1], 11046[1], 11047[1], 11055[1], 11056[1], 11057[1], 11102[0], 11200[1], 11300[1], 11301[1], 11305[1], 11306[1], 11310[1], 11719[1], 12001[1], 12002[1], 12004[1], 12005[1], 12006[1], 12007[1], 12011[1], 12013[1], 12014[1], 12015[1], 12016[1], 12017[1], 12018[1], 12020[1], 12021[1], 12031[1], 12032[1], 12034[1], 12035[1], 12036[1], 12037[1], 12041[1], 12042[1], 12044[1], 12045[1], 12046[1], 12047[1], 12051[1], 12052[1], 12053[1], 12054[1], 12055[1], 12056[1], 12057[1], 13100[1], 13101[1], 13102[1], 13120[1], 13121[1], 13122[1], 13131[1], 13132[1], 13133[1], 13151[1], 13152[1], 13153[1], 15824[1], 15825[1], 15826[1], 15828[1], 15829[1], 16000[1], 16020[1], 17000[1], 17110[1], 17250[1], 17260[1], 36000[1], 36400[1], 36405[1], 36406[1], 36410[1], 36420[1], 36425[1], 36430[1], 36440[1], 36591[0], 36592[0], 36600[1], 36640[1], 43752[1], 51701[1], 51702[1], 51703[1], 62320[0], 62321[0], 62322[0], 62323[0], 62324[0], 62325[0], 62326[0], 62327[0], 64400[0], 64405[0], 64408[0], 64415[0], 64416[0], 64417[0], 64418[0], 64420[0], 64421[0], 64425[0], 64430[0], 64435[0], 64445[0], 64446[0], 64447[0], 64448[0], 64449[0], 64450[0], 64451[0], 64454[0], 64461[0], 64462[0], 64463[0], 64479[0], 64480[0], 64483[0], 64484[0], 64486[0], 64487[0], 64488[0], 64489[0], 64490[0], 64491[0], 64492[0], 64493[0], 64494[0], 64495[0], 64505[0], 64510[0], 64517[0], 64520[0], 64530[0], 69100[1], 69990[0], 92012[1], 92014[1], 93000[1], 93005[1], 93010[1], 93040[1], 93041[1], 93042[1], 93318[1], 93355[1], 94002[1], 94200[1], 94250[1], 94680[1], 94681[1], 94690[1], 94770[1], 95812[1], 95813[1], 95816[1], 95819[1], 95822[1], 95829[1], 95955[1], 96360[1], 96361[1], 96365[1], 96366[1], 96367[1], 96368[1], 96372[1], 96374[1], 96375[1], 96376[1], 96377[1], 96523[0], 96931[1], 96932[1], 96933[1], 96934[1], 96935[1], 96936[1], 97597[1], 97598[1], 97602[1], 99155[0], 99156[0], 99157[0], 99211[1], 99212[1], 99213[1], 99214[1], 99215[1], 99217[1], 99218[1], 99219[1], 99220[1], 99221[1], 99222[1], 99223[1], 99231[1], 99232[1], 99233[1], 99234[1], 99235[1], 99236[1], 99238[1], 99239[1], 99241[1], 99242[1], 99243[1], 99244[1], 99245[1], 99251[1], 99252[1], 99253[1], 99254[1], 99255[1], 99291[1], 99292[1], 99304[1], 99305[1], 99306[1], 99307[1], 99308[1], 99309[1], 99310[1], 99315[1], 99316[1], 99334[1], 99335[1], 99336[1], 99337[1], 99347[1], 99348[1], 99349[1], 99350[1], 99374[1], 99375[1], 99377[1], 99378[1], 99446[0], 99447[0], 99448[0], 99449[0], 99451[0], 99495[1], 99496[1], G0127[1], G0168[1], G0463[1], G0471[1], J0670[1], J2001[1]
11105	00170[0], 0213T[0], 0216T[0], 0228T[0], 0230T[0], 0470T[1], 0471T[1], 10011[1], 11000[1], 11001[1], 11042[1], 11043[1], 11044[1], 11045[1], 11046[1], 11047[1], 11719[1], 12001[1], 12002[1], 12004[1], 12005[1], 12006[1], 12007[1], 12011[1], 12013[1], 12014[1], 12015[1], 12016[1], 12017[1], 12018[1], 12020[1], 12021[1], 12031[1], 12032[1], 12034[1], 12035[1], 12036[1], 12037[1], 12041[1], 12042[1], 12044[1], 12045[1], 12046[1], 12047[1], 12051[1], 12052[1], 12053[1], 12054[1], 12055[1], 12056[1], 12057[1], 13100[1], 13101[1], 13102[1], 13120[1], 13121[1], 13122[1], 13131[1], 13132[1], 13133[1], 13151[1], 13152[1], 13153[1], 36000[1], 36400[1], 36405[1], 36406[1], 36410[1], 36420[1], 36425[1], 36430[1], 36440[1], 36591[0], 36592[0], 36600[1], 36640[1], 43752[1], 51701[1], 51702[1], 51703[1], 62320[0], 62321[0], 62322[0], 62323[0], 62324[0], 62325[0], 62326[0], 62327[0], 64400[0], 64405[0], 64408[0], 64415[0], 64416[0], 64417[0], 64418[0], 64420[0], 64421[0], 64425[0], 64430[0], 64435[0], 64445[0], 64446[0], 64447[0], 64448[0], 64449[0], 64450[0], 64451[0], 64454[0], 64461[0], 64462[0], 64463[0], 64479[0], 64480[0], 64483[0], 64484[0], 64486[0], 64487[0], 64488[0], 64489[0], 64490[0], 64491[0], 64492[0], 64493[0], 64494[0], 64495[0], 64505[0], 64510[0], 64517[0], 64520[0], 64530[0], 69990[0], 92012[1], 92014[1], 93000[1], 93005[1], 93010[1], 93040[1], 93041[1], 93042[1], 93318[1], 93355[1], 94002[1], 94200[1], 94250[1], 94680[1], 94681[1], 94690[1], 94770[1], 95812[1], 95813[1], 95816[1], 95819[1], 95822[1], 95829[1], 95955[1], 96360[1], 96361[1], 96365[1], 96366[1], 96367[1], 96368[1], 96372[1], 96374[1], 96375[1], 96376[1], 96377[1], 96523[0], 96931[1], 96932[1], 96933[1], 96934[1], 96935[1], 96936[1], 97597[1], 97598[1], 97602[1], 99155[0], 99156[0], 99157[0], 99211[1], 99212[1], 99213[1], 99214[1], 99215[1], 99217[1], 99218[1], 99219[1], 99220[1], 99221[1], 99222[1], 99223[1], 99231[1], 99232[1], 99233[1], 99234[1], 99235[1], 99236[1], 99238[1], 99239[1], 99241[1], 99242[1], 99243[1], 99244[1], 99245[1], 99251[1], 99252[1], 99253[1], 99254[1], 99255[1], 99291[1], 99292[1], 99304[1], 99305[1], 99306[1], 99307[1], 99308[1], 99309[1], 99310[1], 99315[1], 99316[1], 99334[1], 99335[1], 99336[1], 99337[1], 99347[1], 99348[1], 99349[1], 99350[1], 99374[1], 99375[1], 99377[1], 99378[1], 99446[0], 99447[0], 99448[0], 99449[0], 99451[0], 99495[1], 99496[1], G0127[1], G0168[1], G0463[1], G0471[1], J0670[1], J2001[1]
13160	0213T[0], 0216T[0], 0228T[0], 0230T[0], 10180[1], 11000[1], 11001[1], 11004[1], 11005[1], 11006[1], 11010[1], 11011[1], 11012[1], 11042[1], 11043[1], 11044[1], 11045[1], 11046[1], 11047[1], 11102[1], 11104[1], 11106[1], 11900[1], 11901[1], 12001[1], 12002[1], 12004[1], 12005[1], 12006[1], 12007[1], 12011[1], 12013[1], 12014[1], 12015[1], 12016[1], 12017[1], 12018[1], 12020[1], 12021[1], 12031[1], 12032[1], 12034[1], 12035[1], 12036[1], 12037[1], 12041[1], 12042[1], 12044[1], 12045[1], 12046[1], 12047[1], 12051[1], 12052[1], 12053[1], 12054[1], 12055[1], 12056[1], 12057[1], 36000[1], 36400[1], 36405[1], 36406[1], 36410[1], 36420[1], 36425[1], 36430[1], 36440[1], 36591[0], 36592[0], 36600[1], 36640[1], 43752[1], 51701[1], 51702[1], 51703[1], 62320[0], 62321[0], 62322[0], 62323[0], 62324[0], 62325[0], 62326[0], 62327[0], 64400[0], 64405[0], 64408[0], 64415[0], 64416[0], 64417[0], 64418[0], 64420[0], 64421[0], 64425[0], 64430[0], 64435[0], 64445[0], 64446[0], 64447[0], 64448[0], 64449[0], 64450[1], 64451[0], 64454[1], 64461[0], 64462[0], 64463[0], 64479[0], 64480[0], 64483[0], 64484[0], 64486[0], 64487[0], 64488[0], 64489[0], 64490[0], 64491[0], 64492[0], 64493[0], 64494[0], 64495[0], 64505[0], 64510[0], 64517[0], 64520[0], 64530[0], 69990[0], 92012[1], 92014[1], 93000[1], 93005[1], 93010[1], 93040[1], 93041[1], 93042[1], 93318[1], 93355[1], 94002[1], 94200[1], 94250[1], 94680[1], 94681[1], 94690[1], 94770[1], 95812[1], 95813[1], 95816[1], 95819[1], 95822[1], 95829[1], 95955[1], 96360[1], 96361[1], 96365[1], 96366[1], 96367[1], 96368[1], 96372[1], 96374[1], 96375[1], 96376[1], 96377[1], 96523[0], 97597[1], 97598[1], 97602[1], 97605[1], 97606[1], 97607[1], 97608[1], 99155[0], 99156[0], 99157[0], 99211[1], 99212[1], 99213[1], 99214[1], 99215[1], 99217[1], 99218[1], 99219[1], 99220[1], 99221[1], 99222[1], 99223[1], 99231[1], 99232[1], 99233[1], 99234[1], 99235[1], 99236[1], 99238[1], 99239[1], 99241[1], 99242[1], 99243[1], 99244[1], 99245[1], 99251[1], 99252[1], 99253[1], 99254[1], 99255[1], 99291[1], 99292[1], 99304[1], 99305[1], 99306[1], 99307[1], 99308[1], 99309[1], 99310[1], 99315[1], 99316[1], 99334[1], 99335[1], 99336[1], 99337[1], 99347[1], 99348[1], 99349[1], 99350[1], 99374[1], 99375[1], 99377[1], 99378[1], 99446[0], 99447[0], 99448[0], 99449[0], 99451[0], 99452[0], 99495[0], 99496[0], G0168[1], G0463[1], G0471[1]
20200	0213T[0], 0216T[0], 0228T[0], 0230T[0], 10005[1], 10007[1], 10009[1], 10011[1], 10021[1], 12001[1], 12002[1], 12004[1], 12005[1], 12006[1], 12007[1], 12011[1], 12013[1], 12014[1], 12015[1], 12016[1], 12017[1], 12018[1], 12020[1], 12021[1], 12031[1], 12032[1], 12034[1], 12035[1], 12036[1], 12037[1], 12041[1], 12042[1], 12044[1], 12045[1], 12046[1], 12047[1], 12051[1], 12052[1], 12053[1], 12054[1], 12055[1], 12056[1], 12057[1], 13100[1], 13101[1], 13102[1], 13120[1], 13121[1], 13122[1], 13131[1], 13132[1], 13133[1], 13151[1], 13152[1], 13153[1], 20103[1], 20206[1], 24300[1], 25259[1], 26340[1], 36000[1], 36400[1], 36405[1], 36406[1], 36410[1], 36420[1], 36425[1], 36430[1], 36440[1], 36591[0], 36592[0], 36600[1], 36640[1], 43752[1], 51701[1], 51702[1], 51703[1], 62320[0], 62321[0], 62322[0], 62323[0], 62324[0], 62325[0], 62326[0], 62327[0], 64400[0], 64405[0], 64408[0], 64415[0], 64416[0], 64417[0], 64418[0], 64420[0], 64421[0], 64425[0], 64430[0], 64435[0], 64445[0], 64446[0], 64447[0], 64448[0], 64449[0], 64450[1], 64451[0], 64454[1], 64461[0], 64462[0], 64463[0], 64479[0], 64480[0], 64483[0], 64484[0], 64486[0], 64487[0], 64488[0], 64489[0], 64490[0], 64491[0], 64492[0], 64493[0], 64494[0], 64495[0], 64505[0], 64510[0], 64517[0], 64520[0], 64530[0], 69990[0], 92012[1], 92014[1], 93000[1], 93005[1], 93010[1], 93040[1], 93041[1], 93042[1], 93318[1], 93355[1], 94002[1], 94200[1], 94250[1], 94680[1], 94681[1], 94690[1], 94770[1], 95812[1], 95813[1], 95816[1], 95819[1], 95822[1], 95829[1], 95955[1], 96360[1], 96361[1], 96365[1], 96366[1], 96367[1], 96368[1], 96372[1], 96374[1], 96375[1], 96376[1], 96377[1], 96523[0], 99155[0], 99156[0], 99157[0], 99211[1], 99212[1], 99213[1], 99214[1], 99215[1], 99217[1], 99218[1], 99219[1], 99220[1], 99221[1], 99222[1], 99223[1], 99231[1], 99232[1], 99233[1], 99234[1], 99235[1], 99236[1], 99238[1], 99239[1], 99241[1], 99242[1], 99243[1],

0 = Modifier usage not allowed or inappropriate　　1 = Modifier usage allowed

Code 1	Code 2
	99244[1], 99245[1], 99251[1], 99252[1], 99253[1], 99254[1], 99255[1], 99291[1], 99292[1], 99304[1], 99305[1], 99306[1], 99307[1], 99308[1], 99309[1], 99310[1], 99315[1], 99316[1], 99334[1], 99335[1], 99336[1], 99337[1], 99347[1], 99348[1], 99349[1], 99350[1], 99374[1], 99375[1], 99377[1], 99378[1], 99446[0], 99447[0], 99448[0], 99449[0], 99451[0], 99452[0], 99495[1], 99496[1], G0463[1], G0471[1], J0670[1], J2001[1]
20205	0213T[0], 0216T[0], 0228T[0], 0230T[0], 10005[1], 10007[1], 10009[1], 10011[1], 10021[1], 12001[1], 12002[1], 12004[1], 12005[1], 12006[1], 12007[1], 12011[1], 12013[1], 12014[1], 12015[1], 12016[1], 12017[1], 12018[1], 12020[1], 12021[1], 12031[1], 12032[1], 12034[1], 12035[1], 12036[1], 12037[1], 12041[1], 12042[1], 12044[1], 12045[1], 12046[1], 12047[1], 12051[1], 12052[1], 12053[1], 12054[1], 12055[1], 12056[1], 12057[1], 13100[1], 13101[1], 13102[1], 13120[1], 13121[1], 13122[1], 13131[1], 13132[1], 13133[1], 13151[1], 13152[1], 13153[1], 20103[1], 20200[1], 20206[1], 24300[1], 25259[1], 26340[1], 36000[1], 36400[1], 36405[1], 36406[1], 36410[1], 36420[1], 36425[1], 36430[1], 36440[1], 36591[0], 36592[0], 36600[1], 36640[1], 43752[1], 49000[0], 49002[1], 51701[1], 51702[1], 51703[1], 62320[0], 62321[0], 62322[0], 62323[0], 62324[0], 62325[0], 62326[0], 62327[0], 64400[0], 64405[0], 64408[0], 64415[0], 64416[0], 64417[0], 64418[0], 64420[0], 64421[0], 64425[0], 64430[0], 64435[0], 64445[0], 64446[0], 64447[0], 64448[0], 64449[0], 64450[1], 64451[0], 64454[1], 64461[0], 64462[0], 64463[0], 64479[0], 64480[0], 64483[0], 64484[0], 64486[0], 64487[0], 64488[0], 64489[0], 64490[0], 64491[0], 64492[0], 64493[0], 64494[0], 64495[0], 64505[0], 64510[0], 64517[0], 64520[0], 64530[0], 69990[0], 92012[1], 92014[1], 93000[1], 93005[1], 93010[1], 93040[1], 93041[1], 93042[1], 93318[1], 93355[1], 94002[1], 94200[1], 94250[1], 94680[1], 94681[1], 94690[1], 94770[1], 95812[1], 95813[1], 95816[1], 95819[1], 95822[1], 95829[1], 95907[1], 95908[1], 95909[1], 95910[1], 95911[1], 95912[1], 95913[1], 95955[1], 96360[1], 96361[1], 96365[1], 96366[1], 96367[1], 96368[1], 96372[1], 96374[1], 96375[1], 96376[1], 96377[1], 96523[0], 99155[0], 99156[0], 99157[0], 99211[1], 99212[1], 99213[1], 99214[1], 99215[1], 99217[1], 99218[1], 99219[1], 99220[1], 99221[1], 99222[1], 99223[1], 99231[1], 99232[1], 99233[1], 99234[1], 99235[1], 99236[1], 99238[1], 99239[1], 99241[1], 99242[1], 99243[1], 99244[1], 99245[1], 99251[1], 99252[1], 99253[1], 99254[1], 99255[1], 99291[1], 99292[1], 99304[1], 99305[1], 99306[1], 99307[1], 99308[1], 99309[1], 99310[1], 99315[1], 99316[1], 99334[1], 99335[1], 99336[1], 99337[1], 99347[1], 99348[1], 99349[1], 99350[1], 99374[1], 99375[1], 99377[1], 99378[1], 99446[0], 99447[0], 99448[0], 99449[0], 99451[0], 99452[0], 99495[1], 99496[1], G0463[1], G0471[1], J0670[1], J2001[1]
20526	0213T[1], 0216T[1], 0228T[1], 0230T[1], 10030[1], 10160[1], 11900[1], 11901[1], 20500[1], 29075[1], 29105[1], 29125[1], 29260[1], 29584[1], 36000[1], 36400[1], 36405[1], 36406[1], 36410[1], 36420[1], 36425[1], 36430[1], 36440[1], 36591[0], 36592[0], 36600[1], 36640[1], 43752[1], 51701[1], 51702[1], 51703[1], 64400[1], 64405[1], 64408[1], 64415[1], 64416[1], 64417[1], 64418[1], 64420[1], 64421[1], 64425[1], 64430[1], 64435[1], 64445[1], 64446[1], 64447[1], 64448[1], 64449[1], 64461[0], 64462[0], 64463[0], 64479[1], 64480[0], 64483[1], 64484[0], 64486[0], 64487[0], 64488[0], 64489[0], 64490[1], 64491[0], 64492[0], 64493[1], 64494[0], 64495[0], 64505[1], 64510[1], 64517[1], 64520[1], 64530[1], 69990[0], 76000[1], 77001[1], 92012[1], 92014[1], 93000[1], 93005[1], 93010[1], 93040[1], 93041[1], 93042[1], 93318[1], 93355[1], 94002[1], 94200[1], 94250[1], 94680[1], 94681[1], 94690[1], 94770[1], 95812[1], 95813[1], 95816[1], 95819[1], 95822[1], 95829[1], 95955[1], 96360[1], 96361[1], 96365[1], 96366[1], 96367[1], 96368[1], 96372[1], 96374[1], 96375[1], 96376[1], 96377[1], 96523[0], 99155[0], 99156[0], 99157[0], 99211[1], 99212[1], 99213[1], 99214[1], 99215[1], 99217[1], 99218[1], 99219[1], 99220[1], 99221[1], 99222[1], 99223[1], 99231[1], 99232[1], 99233[1], 99234[1], 99235[1], 99236[1], 99238[1], 99239[1], 99241[1], 99242[1], 99243[1], 99244[1], 99245[1], 99251[1], 99252[1], 99253[1], 99254[1], 99255[1], 99291[1], 99292[1], 99304[1], 99305[1], 99306[1], 99307[1], 99308[1], 99309[1], 99310[1], 99315[1], 99316[1], 99334[1], 99335[1], 99336[1], 99337[1], 99347[1], 99348[1], 99349[1], 99350[1], 99374[1], 99375[1], 99377[1], 99378[1], 99446[0], 99447[0], 99448[0], 99449[0], 99451[0], 99452[0], 99495[1], 99496[1], G0463[1], G0471[1], J0670[1], J2001[1]
20550	0232T[1], 0481T[1], 0490T[1], 10030[1], 10160[1], 11010[1], 11900[1], 11901[1], 12032[1], 12042[1], 20500[1], 20526[1], 20551[1], 20552[1], 20553[1], 20560[1], 20561[1], 29075[1], 29105[1], 29125[1], 29130[1], 29260[1], 29405[1], 29425[1], 29450[1], 29515[1], 29530[1], 29540[1], 29550[1], 29580[1], 29581[1], 29584[1], 36000[1], 36400[1], 36405[1], 36406[1], 36410[1], 36420[1], 36425[1], 36430[1], 36440[1], 36591[0], 36592[0], 36600[1], 36640[1], 43752[1], 51701[1], 51702[1], 51703[1], 62320[1], 62321[1], 62322[1], 62323[1], 62324[1], 62325[1], 62326[1], 62327[1], 64408[1], 64435[1], 64455[1], 64461[0], 64463[0], 64480[0], 64484[0], 64486[0], 64487[0], 64488[0], 64489[0], 64494[0], 64495[0], 64505[1], 64510[1], 64517[1], 64520[1], 64530[1], 64714[1], 69990[0], 72240[1], 72265[1], 72295[1], 76000[1], 77001[1], 87076[0], 87077[0], 87102[0], 92012[1], 92014[1], 93000[1], 93005[1], 93010[1], 93040[1], 93041[1], 93042[1], 93318[1], 93355[1], 94002[1], 94200[1], 94250[1], 94680[1], 94681[1], 94690[1], 94770[1], 95812[1], 95813[1], 95816[1], 95819[1], 95822[1], 95829[1], 95907[1], 95908[1], 95909[1], 95910[1], 95911[1], 95912[1], 95913[1], 95955[1], 96360[1], 96361[1], 96365[1], 96366[1], 96367[1], 96368[1], 96372[1], 96374[1], 96375[1], 96376[1], 96377[1], 96523[0], 99155[0], 99156[0], 99157[0], 99211[1], 99212[1], 99213[1], 99214[1], 99215[1], 99217[1], 99218[1], 99219[1], 99220[1], 99221[1], 99222[1], 99223[1], 99231[1], 99232[1], 99233[1], 99234[1], 99235[1], 99236[1], 99238[1], 99239[1], 99241[1], 99242[1], 99243[1], 99244[1], 99245[1], 99251[1], 99252[1], 99253[1], 99254[1], 99255[1], 99291[1], 99292[1], 99304[1], 99305[1], 99306[1], 99307[1], 99308[1], 99309[1], 99310[1], 99315[1], 99316[1], 99334[1], 99335[1], 99336[1], 99337[1], 99347[1], 99348[1], 99349[1], 99350[1], 99374[1], 99375[1], 99377[1], 99378[1], 99446[0], 99447[0], 99448[0], 99449[0], 99451[0], 99452[0], 99495[1], 99496[1], G0463[1], G0471[1], J0670[1], J2001[1]
20551	0232T[1], 0481T[1], 0490T[1], 10030[1], 10160[1], 11000[1], 11001[1], 11004[1], 11005[1], 11006[1], 11042[1], 11043[1], 11044[1], 11045[1], 11046[1], 11047[1], 11900[1], 11901[1], 20500[1], 20526[1], 20552[1], 20553[1], 20560[1], 20561[1], 29075[1], 29105[1], 29125[1], 29130[1], 29260[1], 29405[1], 29425[1], 29450[1], 29515[1], 29530[1], 29540[1], 29550[1], 29580[1], 29581[1], 29584[1], 36000[1], 36400[1], 36405[1], 36406[1], 36410[1], 36420[1], 36425[1], 36430[1], 36440[1], 36591[0], 36592[0], 36600[1], 36640[1], 43752[1], 51701[1], 51702[1], 51703[1], 62320[1], 62321[1], 62322[1], 62323[1], 62324[1], 62325[1], 62326[1], 62327[1], 64408[1], 64435[1], 64455[1], 64461[0], 64463[0], 64480[0], 64484[0], 64486[0], 64487[0], 64488[0], 64489[0], 64494[0], 64495[0], 64505[1], 64510[1], 64517[1], 64520[1], 64530[1], 69990[0], 76000[1], 77001[1], 92012[1], 92014[1], 93000[1], 93005[1], 93010[1], 93040[1], 93041[1], 93042[1], 93318[1], 93355[1], 94002[1], 94200[1], 94250[1], 94680[1], 94681[1], 94690[1], 94770[1], 95812[1], 95813[1], 95816[1], 95819[1], 95822[1], 95829[1], 95955[1], 96360[1], 96361[1], 96365[1], 96366[1], 96367[1], 96368[1], 96372[1], 96374[1], 96375[1], 96376[1], 96377[1], 96523[0], 97597[1], 97598[1], 97602[1], 99155[0], 99156[0], 99157[0], 99211[1], 99212[1], 99213[1], 99214[1], 99215[1], 99217[1], 99218[1], 99219[1], 99220[1], 99221[1], 99222[1], 99223[1], 99231[1], 99232[1], 99233[1], 99234[1], 99235[1], 99236[1], 99238[1], 99239[1], 99241[1], 99242[1], 99243[1], 99244[1], 99245[1], 99251[1], 99252[1], 99253[1], 99254[1], 99255[1], 99291[1], 99292[1], 99304[1], 99305[1], 99306[1], 99307[1], 99308[1], 99309[1], 99310[1], 99315[1], 99316[1], 99334[1], 99335[1], 99336[1], 99337[1], 99347[1], 99348[1], 99349[1], 99350[1], 99374[1], 99375[1], 99377[1], 99378[1], 99446[0], 99447[0], 99448[0], 99449[0], 99451[0], 99452[0], 99495[1], 99496[1], G0463[1], G0471[1], J0670[1], J2001[1]
20552	01991[0], 01992[0], 0213T[1], 0216T[1], 0228T[1], 0230T[1], 0490T[1], 10030[1], 10160[1], 11900[1], 11901[1], 20500[1], 20526[1], 29075[1], 29105[1], 29125[1], 29130[1], 29260[1], 29405[1], 29425[1], 29450[1], 29515[1], 29530[1], 29540[1], 29550[1], 29580[1], 29581[1], 29584[1], 36000[1], 36400[1], 36405[1], 36406[1], 36410[1], 36420[1], 36425[1], 36430[1], 36440[1], 36591[0], 36592[0], 36600[1], 36640[1], 43752[1], 51701[1], 51702[1], 51703[1], 64400[1], 64405[1], 64408[1], 64415[1], 64416[1], 64417[1], 64418[1], 64420[1], 64421[1], 64425[1], 64430[1], 64435[1], 64445[1], 64446[1], 64447[1], 64448[1], 64449[1], 64450[1], 64451[1], 64454[1], 64455[1], 64461[1], 64462[1], 64463[1], 64479[1], 64480[1], 64483[1], 64484[1], 64486[0], 64487[0], 64488[0], 64489[0], 64490[1], 64491[1], 64492[1], 64493[1], 64494[1], 64495[1], 64505[1], 64510[1], 64517[1], 64520[1], 64530[1], 69990[0], 76000[1], 76970[1], 76998[1], 77001[1], 77012[1], 92012[1], 92014[1], 93000[1], 93005[1], 93010[1], 93040[1], 93041[1], 93042[1], 93318[1], 93355[1], 94002[1], 94200[1], 94250[1], 94680[1], 94681[1], 94690[1], 94770[1], 95812[1], 95813[1], 95816[1], 95819[1], 95822[1], 95829[1], 95955[1], 96360[1], 96361[1], 96365[1], 96366[1], 96367[1], 96368[1], 96372[1], 96374[1], 96375[1], 96376[1], 96377[1], 96523[0], 99155[0], 99156[0], 99157[0], 99211[1], 99212[1], 99213[1], 99214[1], 99215[1], 99217[1], 99218[1], 99219[1], 99220[1], 99221[1], 99222[1], 99223[1], 99231[1], 99232[1], 99233[1], 99234[1], 99235[1], 99236[1], 99238[1], 99239[1], 99241[1], 99242[1], 99243[1], 99244[1], 99245[1], 99251[1], 99252[1], 99253[1], 99254[1], 99255[1], 99291[1], 99292[1], 99304[1], 99305[1], 99306[1], 99307[1], 99308[1], 99309[1], 99310[1], 99315[1], 99316[1], 99334[1], 99335[1], 99336[1], 99337[1], 99347[1], 99348[1], 99349[1], 99350[1], 99374[1], 99375[1], 99377[1], 99378[1], 99446[0], 99447[0], 99448[0], 99449[0], 99451[0], 99452[0], 99495[1], 99496[1], G0463[1], G0471[1], J0670[1], J2001[1]
20553	01991[0], 01992[0], 0213T[1], 0216T[1], 0228T[1], 0230T[1], 0490T[1], 10030[1], 10160[1], 11900[1], 11901[1], 20500[1], 20526[1], 20552[0], 29075[1], 29105[1], 29125[1], 29130[1], 29260[1], 29405[1], 29425[1], 29450[1], 29515[1], 29530[1], 29540[1], 29550[1], 29580[1], 29581[1], 29584[1], 36000[1], 36400[1], 36405[1], 36406[1], 36410[1], 36420[1], 36425[1], 36430[1], 36440[1], 36591[0], 36592[0], 36600[1], 36640[1], 43752[1], 51701[1], 51702[1], 51703[1], 64400[1], 64405[1], 64408[1], 64415[1], 64416[1], 64417[1], 64418[1], 64420[1], 64421[1], 64425[1], 64430[1], 64435[1], 64445[1], 64446[1], 64447[1], 64448[1], 64449[1], 64450[1], 64451[1], 64454[1], 64455[1], 64461[1], 64462[1], 64463[1], 64479[1], 64480[1], 64483[1], 64484[1], 64486[0], 64487[0], 64488[0], 64489[0], 64490[1], 64491[1], 64492[1], 64493[1], 64494[1], 64495[1], 64505[1], 64510[1], 64517[1], 64520[1], 64530[1], 69990[0], 76000[1], 76970[1], 76998[1], 77001[1], 77012[1], 92012[1], 92014[1], 93000[1], 93005[1], 93010[1], 93040[1], 93041[1], 93042[1], 93318[1], 93355[1], 94002[1], 94200[1], 94250[1], 94680[1], 94681[1], 94690[1], 94770[1], 95812[1], 95813[1], 95816[1], 95819[1], 95822[1], 95829[1], 95955[1], 96360[1], 96361[1], 96365[1], 96366[1], 96367[1], 96368[1], 96372[1], 96374[1], 96375[1], 96376[1], 96377[1], 96523[0], 99155[0], 99156[0], 99157[0], 99211[1], 99212[1], 99213[1], 99214[1], 99215[1], 99217[1], 99218[1], 99219[1], 99220[1], 99221[1], 99222[1], 99223[1], 99231[1], 99232[1], 99233[1], 99234[1], 99235[1], 99236[1], 99238[1], 99239[1], 99241[1], 99242[1], 99243[1], 99244[1], 99245[1], 99251[1], 99252[1], 99253[1], 99254[1], 99255[1], 99291[1], 99292[1], 99304[1], 99305[1], 99306[1], 99307[1], 99308[1], 99309[1], 99310[1], 99315[1], 99316[1], 99334[1], 99335[1], 99336[1], 99337[1], 99347[1], 99348[1], 99349[1], 99350[1], 99374[1], 99375[1], 99377[1], 99378[1], 99446[0], 99447[0], 99448[0], 99449[0], 99451[0], 99452[0], 99495[1], 99496[1], G0463[1], G0471[1], J0670[1], J2001[1]
20660	0213T[0], 0216T[0], 0228T[0], 0230T[0], 0333T[0], 0464T[0], 11000[1], 11001[1], 11004[1], 11005[1], 11006[1], 11010[1], 11042[1], 11043[1], 11044[1], 11045[1], 11046[1], 11047[1], 12001[1], 12002[1],

Appendix A: NCCI - CPT Codes

0 = Modifier usage not allowed or inappropriate 1 = Modifier usage allowed

Code 1	Code 2
	12004[1], 12005[1], 12006[1], 12007[1], 12011[1], 12013[1], 12014[1], 12015[1], 12016[1], 12017[1], 12018[1], 12020[1], 12021[1], 12031[1], 12032[1], 12034[1], 12035[1], 12036[1], 12037[1], 12041[1], 12042[1], 12044[1], 12045[1], 12046[1], 12047[1], 12051[1], 12052[1], 12053[1], 12054[1], 12055[1], 12056[1], 12057[1], 13100[1], 13101[1], 13102[1], 13120[1], 13121[1], 13122[1], 13131[1], 13132[1], 13133[1], 13151[1], 13152[1], 13153[1], 29540[1], 36000[1], 36400[1], 36405[1], 36406[1], 36410[1], 36420[1], 36425[1], 36430[1], 36440[1], 36591[0], 36592[0], 36600[1], 36640[1], 43752[1], 51701[1], 51702[1], 51703[1], 62320[0], 62321[0], 62322[0], 62323[0], 62324[0], 62325[0], 62326[0], 62327[0], 64400[0], 64405[0], 64408[0], 64415[0], 64416[0], 64417[0], 64418[0], 64420[0], 64421[0], 64425[0], 64430[0], 64435[0], 64445[0], 64446[0], 64447[0], 64448[0], 64449[0], 64450[1], 64451[0], 64454[1], 64461[0], 64462[0], 64463[0], 64479[0], 64480[0], 64483[0], 64484[0], 64486[0], 64487[0], 64488[0], 64489[0], 64490[0], 64491[0], 64492[0], 64493[0], 64494[0], 64495[0], 64505[0], 64510[0], 64517[0], 64520[0], 64530[0], 69990[0], 92012[1], 92014[1], 92585[0], 93000[1], 93005[1], 93010[1], 93040[1], 93041[1], 93042[1], 93318[1], 93355[1], 94002[1], 94200[1], 94250[1], 94680[1], 94681[1], 94690[1], 94770[1], 95812[1], 95813[1], 95816[1], 95819[1], 95822[0], 95829[1], 95860[0], 95861[0], 95863[0], 95864[0], 95865[0], 95866[0], 95867[0], 95868[0], 95869[0], 95870[0], 95907[0], 95908[0], 95909[0], 95910[0], 95911[0], 95912[0], 95913[0], 95925[0], 95926[0], 95927[0], 95928[0], 95929[0], 95930[0], 95933[0], 95937[0], 95938[0], 95939[0], 95940[0], 95955[1], 96360[1], 96361[1], 96365[1], 96366[1], 96367[1], 96368[1], 96372[1], 96374[1], 96375[1], 96376[1], 96377[1], 96523[0], 97597[1], 97598[1], 97602[1], 99155[0], 99156[0], 99157[0], 99211[1], 99212[1], 99213[1], 99214[1], 99215[1], 99217[1], 99218[1], 99219[1], 99220[1], 99221[1], 99222[1], 99223[1], 99231[1], 99232[1], 99233[1], 99234[1], 99235[1], 99236[1], 99238[1], 99239[1], 99241[1], 99242[1], 99243[1], 99244[1], 99245[1], 99251[1], 99252[1], 99253[1], 99254[1], 99255[1], 99291[1], 99292[1], 99304[1], 99305[1], 99306[1], 99307[1], 99308[1], 99309[1], 99310[1], 99315[1], 99316[1], 99334[1], 99335[1], 99336[1], 99337[1], 99347[1], 99348[1], 99349[1], 99350[1], 99374[1], 99375[1], 99377[1], 99378[1], 99446[0], 99447[0], 99448[0], 99449[0], 99451[0], 99452[0], 99495[1], 99496[1], G0453[0], G0463[1], G0471[1]
20930	36591[0], 36592[0], 96523[0]
20931	0333T[0], 0464T[0], 11010[1], 36591[0], 36592[0], 92585[0], 95822[0], 95860[0], 95861[0], 95863[0], 95864[0], 95865[0], 95866[0], 95867[0], 95868[0], 95869[0], 95870[0], 95907[0], 95908[0], 95909[0], 95910[0], 95911[0], 95912[0], 95913[0], 95925[0], 95926[0], 95927[0], 95928[0], 95929[0], 95930[0], 95933[0], 95937[0], 95938[0], 95939[0], 95940[0], 96523[0], G0453[0]
20936	36591[0], 36592[0], 96523[0]
20937	0333T[0], 0464T[0], 11010[1], 36591[0], 36592[0], 38220[0], 38221[1], 38222[0], 92585[0], 95822[0], 95860[0], 95861[0], 95863[0], 95864[0], 95865[0], 95866[0], 95867[0], 95868[0], 95869[0], 95870[0], 95907[0], 95908[0], 95909[0], 95910[0], 95911[0], 95912[0], 95913[0], 95925[0], 95926[0], 95927[0], 95928[0], 95929[0], 95930[0], 95933[0], 95937[0], 95938[0], 95939[0], 95940[0], 96523[0], G0453[0]
20938	11010[1], 11011[1], 11012[1], 36591[0], 36592[0], 38220[0], 38221[1], 38222[0], 96523[0]
20939	01112[0], 01120[0], 0213T[0], 0216T[0], 0228T[0], 0230T[0], 0232T[1], 0481T[1], 12001[1], 12002[1], 12004[1], 12005[1], 12006[1], 12007[1], 12011[1], 12013[1], 12014[1], 12015[1], 12016[1], 12017[1], 12018[1], 12020[1], 12021[1], 12031[1], 12032[1], 12034[1], 12035[1], 12036[1], 12037[1], 12041[1], 12042[1], 12044[1], 12045[1], 12046[1], 12047[1], 12051[1], 12052[1], 12053[1], 12054[1], 12055[1], 12056[1], 12057[1], 13100[1], 13101[1], 13102[1], 13120[1], 13121[1], 13122[1], 13131[1], 13132[1], 13133[1], 13151[1], 13152[1], 13153[1], 36000[1], 36400[1], 36405[1], 36406[1], 36410[1], 36420[1], 36425[1], 36430[1], 36440[1], 36591[0], 36592[0], 36600[1], 36640[1], 43752[1], 51701[1], 51702[1], 51703[1], 61650[1], 62320[0], 62321[0], 62322[0], 62323[0], 62324[0], 62325[0], 62326[0], 62327[0], 64400[0], 64405[0], 64408[0], 64415[0], 64416[0], 64417[0], 64418[0], 64420[0], 64421[0], 64425[0], 64430[0], 64435[0], 64445[0], 64446[0], 64447[0], 64448[0], 64449[0], 64450[1], 64451[0], 64454[1], 64461[0], 64462[0], 64463[0], 64479[0], 64480[0], 64483[0], 64484[0], 64486[0], 64487[0], 64488[0], 64489[0], 64490[0], 64491[0], 64492[0], 64493[0], 64494[0], 64495[0], 64505[0], 64510[0], 64517[0], 64520[0], 64530[0], 69990[0], 80500[1], 80502[1], 92012[1], 92014[1], 93000[1], 93005[1], 93010[1], 93040[1], 93041[1], 93042[1], 93318[1], 94002[1], 94200[1], 94250[1], 94680[1], 94681[1], 94690[1], 94770[1], 95812[1], 95813[1], 95816[1], 95819[1], 95822[1], 95829[1], 95955[1], 96360[1], 96361[1], 96365[1], 96366[1], 96367[1], 96368[1], 96372[1], 96374[1], 96375[1], 96376[1], 96377[1], 96523[0], 99155[0], 99156[0], 99157[0], 99211[1], 99212[1], 99213[1], 99214[1], 99215[1], 99217[1], 99218[1], 99219[1], 99220[1], 99221[1], 99222[1], 99223[1], 99231[1], 99232[1], 99233[1], 99234[1], 99235[1], 99236[1], 99238[1], 99239[1], 99241[1], 99242[1], 99243[1], 99244[1], 99245[1], 99251[1], 99252[1], 99253[1], 99254[1], 99255[1], 99291[1], 99292[1], 99304[1], 99305[1], 99306[1], 99307[1], 99308[1], 99309[1], 99310[1], 99315[1], 99316[1], 99334[1], 99335[1], 99336[1], 99337[1], 99347[1], 99348[1], 99349[1], 99350[1], 99374[1], 99375[1], 99377[1], 99378[1], J0670[1], J2001[1]
22010	00600[0], 00604[0], 00620[0], 00625[0], 00626[0], 0213T[0], 0216T[0], 0228T[0], 0230T[0], 10030[1], 10060[1], 10140[1], 10160[1], 10180[1], 12001[1], 12002[1], 12004[1], 12005[1], 12006[1], 12007[1], 12011[1], 12013[1], 12014[1], 12015[1], 12016[1], 12017[1], 12018[1], 12020[1], 12021[1], 12031[1], 12032[1], 12034[1], 12035[1], 12036[1], 12037[1], 12041[1], 12042[1], 12044[1], 12045[1], 12046[1], 12047[1], 12051[1], 12052[1], 12053[1], 12054[1], 12055[1], 12056[1], 12057[1], 13100[1], 13101[1], 13102[1], 13120[1], 13121[1], 13122[1], 13131[1], 13132[1], 13133[1], 13151[1], 13152[1], 13153[1], 22015[1], 22505[0], 36000[1], 36400[1], 36405[1], 36406[1], 36410[1], 36420[1], 36425[1], 36430[1], 36440[1], 36591[0], 36592[0], 36600[1], 36640[1], 43752[1], 51701[1], 51702[1], 51703[1], 62320[0], 62321[0], 62322[0], 62323[0], 62324[0], 62325[0], 62326[0], 62327[0], 63707[1], 63709[1], 64400[0], 64405[0], 64408[0], 64415[0], 64416[0], 64417[0], 64418[0], 64420[0], 64421[0], 64425[0], 64430[0], 64435[0], 64445[0], 64446[0], 64447[0], 64448[0], 64449[0], 64450[1], 64451[0], 64454[1], 64461[0], 64462[0], 64463[0], 64479[0], 64480[0], 64483[0], 64484[0], 64486[0], 64487[0], 64488[0], 64489[0], 64490[0], 64491[0], 64492[0], 64493[0], 64494[0], 64495[0], 64505[0], 64510[0], 64517[0], 64520[0], 64530[0], 69990[0], 76000[1], 77001[1], 77002[1], 92012[1], 92014[1], 93000[1], 93005[1], 93010[1], 93040[1], 93041[1], 93042[1], 93318[1], 93355[1], 94002[1], 94200[1], 94250[1], 94680[1], 94681[1], 94690[1], 94770[1], 95812[1], 95813[1], 95816[1], 95819[1], 95822[1], 95829[1], 95955[1], 96360[1], 96361[1], 96365[1], 96366[1], 96367[1], 96368[1], 96372[1], 96374[1], 96375[1], 96376[1], 96377[1], 96523[0], 97597[1], 97598[1], 97602[1], 97605[1], 97606[1], 97607[1], 97608[1], 99155[0], 99156[0], 99157[0], 99211[1], 99212[1], 99213[1], 99214[1], 99215[1], 99217[1], 99218[1], 99219[1], 99220[1], 99221[1], 99222[1], 99223[1], 99231[1], 99232[1], 99233[1], 99234[1], 99235[1], 99236[1], 99238[1], 99239[1], 99241[1], 99242[1], 99243[1], 99244[1], 99245[1], 99251[1], 99252[1], 99253[1], 99254[1], 99255[1], 99291[1], 99292[1], 99304[1], 99305[1], 99306[1], 99307[1], 99308[1], 99309[1], 99310[1], 99315[1], 99316[1], 99334[1], 99335[1], 99336[1], 99337[1], 99347[1], 99348[1], 99349[1], 99350[1], 99374[1], 99375[1], 99377[1], 99378[1], 99446[0], 99447[0], 99448[0], 99449[0], 99451[0], 99452[0], 99495[0], 99496[0], G0463[1], G0471[1]
22015	00600[0], 00604[0], 00620[0], 00625[0], 00626[0], 0213T[0], 0216T[0], 0228T[0], 0230T[0], 10030[1], 10060[1], 10140[1], 10160[1], 10180[1], 12001[1], 12002[1], 12004[1], 12005[1], 12006[1], 12007[1], 12011[1], 12013[1], 12014[1], 12015[1], 12016[1], 12017[1], 12018[1], 12020[1], 12021[1], 12031[1], 12032[1], 12034[1], 12035[1], 12036[1], 12037[1], 12041[1], 12042[1], 12044[1], 12045[1], 12046[1], 12047[1], 12051[1], 12052[1], 12053[1], 12054[1], 12055[1], 12056[1], 12057[1], 13100[1], 13101[1], 13102[1], 13120[1], 13121[1], 13122[1], 13131[1], 13132[1], 13133[1], 13151[1], 13152[1], 13153[1], 22505[0], 36000[1], 36400[1], 36405[1], 36406[1], 36410[1], 36420[1], 36425[1], 36430[1], 36440[1], 36591[0], 36592[0], 36600[1], 36640[1], 43752[1], 51701[1], 51702[1], 51703[1], 62320[0], 62321[0], 62322[0], 62323[0], 62324[0], 62325[0], 62326[0], 62327[0], 63707[1], 63709[1], 64400[0], 64405[0], 64408[0], 64415[0], 64416[0], 64417[0], 64418[0], 64420[0], 64421[0], 64425[0], 64430[0], 64435[0], 64445[0], 64446[0], 64447[0], 64448[0], 64449[0], 64450[1], 64451[0], 64454[1], 64461[0], 64462[0], 64463[0], 64479[0], 64480[0], 64483[0], 64484[0], 64486[0], 64487[0], 64488[0], 64489[0], 64490[0], 64491[0], 64492[0], 64493[0], 64494[0], 64495[0], 64505[0], 64510[0], 64517[0], 64520[0], 64530[0], 69990[0], 76000[1], 77001[1], 77002[1], 92012[1], 92014[1], 93000[1], 93005[1], 93010[1], 93040[1], 93041[1], 93042[1], 93318[1], 93355[1], 94002[1], 94200[1], 94250[1], 94680[1], 94681[1], 94690[1], 94770[1], 95812[1], 95813[1], 95816[1], 95819[1], 95822[1], 95829[1], 95955[1], 96360[1], 96361[1], 96365[1], 96366[1], 96367[1], 96368[1], 96372[1], 96374[1], 96375[1], 96376[1], 96377[1], 96523[0], 97597[1], 97598[1], 97602[1], 97605[1], 97606[1], 97607[1], 97608[1], 99155[0], 99156[0], 99157[0], 99211[1], 99212[1], 99213[1], 99214[1], 99215[1], 99217[1], 99218[1], 99219[1], 99220[1], 99221[1], 99222[1], 99223[1], 99231[1], 99232[1], 99233[1], 99234[1], 99235[1], 99236[1], 99238[1], 99239[1], 99241[1], 99242[1], 99243[1], 99244[1], 99245[1], 99251[1], 99252[1], 99253[1], 99254[1], 99255[1], 99291[1], 99292[1], 99304[1], 99305[1], 99306[1], 99307[1], 99308[1], 99309[1], 99310[1], 99315[1], 99316[1], 99334[1], 99335[1], 99336[1], 99337[1], 99347[1], 99348[1], 99349[1], 99350[1], 99374[1], 99375[1], 99377[1], 99378[1], 99446[0], 99447[0], 99448[0], 99449[0], 99451[0], 99452[0], 99495[0], 99496[0], G0463[1], G0471[1]
22206	0213T[0], 0216T[0], 0228T[0], 0230T[0], 0274T[1], 0333T[0], 0464T[0], 0565T[1], 11000[1], 11001[1], 11004[1], 11005[1], 11006[1], 11010[1], 11011[1], 11012[1], 11042[1], 11043[1], 11044[1], 11045[1], 11046[1], 11047[1], 12001[1], 12002[1], 12004[1], 12005[1], 12006[1], 12007[1], 12011[1], 12013[1], 12014[1], 12015[1], 12016[1], 12017[1], 12018[1], 12020[1], 12021[1], 12031[1], 12032[1], 12034[1], 12035[1], 12036[1], 12037[1], 12041[1], 12042[1], 12044[1], 12045[1], 12046[1], 12047[1], 12051[1], 12052[1], 12053[1], 12054[1], 12055[1], 12056[1], 12057[1], 13100[1], 13101[1], 13102[1], 13120[1], 13121[1], 13122[1], 13131[1], 13132[1], 13133[1], 13151[1], 13152[1], 13153[1], 15769[1], 22100[1], 22101[1], 22112[1], 22114[1], 22207[0], 22212[1], 22214[1], 22216[1], 22220[1], 22222[1], 22224[1], 22226[1], 22327[1], 22505[0], 22551[1], 22830[1], 36000[1], 36400[1], 36405[1], 36406[1], 36410[1], 36420[1], 36425[1], 36430[1], 36440[1], 36591[0], 36592[0], 36600[1], 36640[1], 38220[0], 38222[0], 38230[0], 38232[0], 43752[1], 62320[0], 62321[0], 62322[0], 62323[0], 62324[0], 62325[0], 62326[0], 62327[0], 62380[1], 63001[1], 63003[1], 63005[1], 63011[1], 63012[1], 63015[1], 63016[1], 63017[1], 63020[1], 63030[1], 63035[1], 63040[1], 63042[1], 63043[1], 63044[1], 63045[1], 63046[1], 63048[1], 63055[1], 63056[1], 63057[1], 63064[1], 63066[1], 63075[1], 63076[1], 63077[1], 63078[1], 63081[1], 63082[1], 63085[1], 63086[1], 63087[1], 63088[1], 63090[1], 63091[1], 63101[1], 63102[1], 63103[1], 63170[1], 63172[1], 63173[1], 63180[1], 63182[1], 63185[1], 63190[1], 63191[1], 63194[1], 63195[1], 63196[1], 63197[1], 63198[1], 63199[1], 63200[1], 63265[1], 63266[1], 63267[1], 63268[1], 63270[1], 63271[1], 63272[1], 63273[1], 63275[1], 63276[1], 63277[1], 63278[1], 63280[1], 63281[1], 63282[1], 63283[1], 63295[1], 63300[1], 63301[1], 63302[1], 63303[1], 63304[1], 63305[1], 63307[1], 63707[1], 63709[1], 64400[0], 64405[0], 64408[0], 64415[0], 64416[0], 64417[0], 64418[0], 64420[0], 64421[0], 64425[0], 64430[0], 64435[0], 64445[0], 64446[0], 64447[0], 64448[0], 64449[0], 64450[1], 64451[0], 64454[1], 64461[0], 64462[0], 64463[0], 64479[0], 64480[0], 64483[0], 64484[0], 64486[0], 64487[0],

0 = Modifier usage not allowed or inappropriate 1 = Modifier usage allowed

Code 1	Code 2
	64488[0], 64489[0], 64490[0], 64491[0], 64492[0], 64493[0], 64494[0], 64495[0], 64505[0], 64510[0], 64517[0], 64520[0], 64530[0], 69990[0], 76000[1], 77001[1], 77002[1], 92012[1], 92014[1], 92585[0], 93000[1], 93005[1], 93010[1], 93040[1], 93041[1], 93042[1], 93318[1], 93355[1], 94002[1], 94200[1], 94250[1], 94680[1], 94681[1], 94690[1], 94770[1], 95812[1], 95813[1], 95816[1], 95819[1], 95822[0], 95829[1], 95860[0], 95861[0], 95863[0], 95864[0], 95865[0], 95866[0], 95867[0], 95868[0], 95869[0], 95870[0], 95907[0], 95908[0], 95909[0], 95910[0], 95911[0], 95912[0], 95913[0], 95925[0], 95926[0], 95927[0], 95928[0], 95929[0], 95930[0], 95933[0], 95937[0], 95938[0], 95939[0], 95940[0], 95955[1], 96360[1], 96361[1], 96365[1], 96366[1], 96367[1], 96368[1], 96372[1], 96374[1], 96375[1], 96376[1], 96377[1], 96523[0], 97597[1], 97598[1], 97602[1], 99155[0], 99156[0], 99157[0], 99211[1], 99212[1], 99213[1], 99214[1], 99215[1], 99217[1], 99218[1], 99219[1], 99220[1], 99221[1], 99222[1], 99223[1], 99231[1], 99232[1], 99233[1], 99234[1], 99235[1], 99236[1], 99238[1], 99239[1], 99241[1], 99242[1], 99243[1], 99244[1], 99245[1], 99251[1], 99252[1], 99253[1], 99254[1], 99255[1], 99291[1], 99292[1], 99304[1], 99305[1], 99306[1], 99307[1], 99308[1], 99309[1], 99310[1], 99315[1], 99316[1], 99334[1], 99335[1], 99336[1], 99337[1], 99347[1], 99348[1], 99349[1], 99350[1], 99374[1], 99375[1], 99377[1], 99378[1], 99446[0], 99447[0], 99448[0], 99449[0], 99451[0], 99452[0], 99495[0], 99496[0], G0453[0], G0463[1]
22207	0202T[1], 0213T[0], 0216T[0], 0228T[0], 0230T[0], 0274T[1], 0275T[1], 0333T[0], 0464T[0], 0565T[1], 11000[1], 11001[1], 11004[1], 11005[1], 11006[1], 11010[1], 11011[1], 11012[1], 11042[1], 11043[1], 11044[1], 11045[1], 11046[1], 11047[1], 12001[1], 12002[1], 12004[1], 12005[1], 12006[1], 12007[1], 12011[1], 12013[1], 12014[1], 12015[1], 12016[1], 12017[1], 12018[1], 12020[1], 12021[1], 12031[1], 12032[1], 12034[1], 12035[1], 12036[1], 12037[1], 12041[1], 12042[1], 12044[1], 12045[1], 12046[1], 12047[1], 12051[1], 12052[1], 12053[1], 12054[1], 12055[1], 12056[1], 12057[1], 13100[1], 13101[1], 13102[1], 13120[1], 13121[1], 13122[1], 13131[1], 13132[1], 13133[1], 13151[1], 13152[1], 13153[1], 15769[1], 22100[1], 22102[1], 22112[1], 22114[1], 22210[1], 22212[1], 22214[1], 22216[1], 22220[1], 22222[1], 22224[1], 22226[1], 22325[1], 22505[0], 22551[1], 22830[1], 36000[1], 36400[1], 36405[1], 36406[1], 36410[1], 36420[1], 36425[1], 36430[1], 36440[1], 36591[0], 36592[0], 36600[1], 36640[1], 38220[0], 38222[0], 38230[0], 38232[0], 43752[1], 62320[0], 62321[0], 62322[0], 62323[0], 62324[0], 62325[0], 62326[0], 62327[0], 62380[1], 63001[1], 63003[1], 63005[1], 63011[1], 63012[1], 63015[1], 63016[1], 63017[1], 63020[1], 63030[1], 63035[1], 63040[1], 63042[1], 63043[1], 63044[1], 63045[1], 63046[1], 63047[1], 63048[1], 63055[1], 63056[1], 63057[1], 63064[1], 63066[1], 63075[1], 63076[1], 63077[1], 63078[1], 63081[1], 63082[1], 63085[1], 63086[1], 63087[1], 63088[1], 63090[1], 63091[1], 63101[1], 63102[1], 63103[1], 63170[1], 63172[1], 63173[1], 63180[1], 63182[1], 63185[1], 63190[1], 63191[1], 63194[1], 63195[1], 63196[1], 63197[1], 63198[1], 63199[1], 63200[1], 63265[1], 63266[1], 63267[1], 63268[1], 63270[1], 63271[1], 63272[1], 63273[1], 63275[1], 63276[1], 63277[1], 63278[1], 63280[1], 63281[1], 63282[1], 63283[1], 63295[1], 63300[1], 63301[1], 63302[1], 63303[1], 63304[1], 63305[1], 63306[1], 63307[1], 63707[1], 63709[1], 64400[0], 64405[0], 64408[0], 64415[0], 64416[0], 64417[0], 64418[0], 64420[0], 64421[0], 64425[0], 64430[0], 64435[0], 64445[0], 64446[0], 64447[0], 64448[0], 64449[0], 64450[1], 64451[0], 64454[1], 64461[0], 64462[0], 64463[0], 64479[0], 64480[0], 64483[0], 64484[0], 64486[0], 64487[0], 64488[0], 64489[0], 64490[0], 64491[0], 64492[0], 64493[0], 64494[0], 64495[0], 64505[0], 64510[0], 64517[0], 64520[0], 64530[0], 69990[0], 76000[1], 77001[1], 77002[1], 92012[1], 92014[1], 92585[0], 93000[1], 93005[1], 93010[1], 93040[1], 93041[1], 93042[1], 93318[1], 93355[1], 94002[1], 94200[1], 94250[1], 94680[1], 94681[1], 94690[1], 94770[1], 95812[1], 95813[1], 95816[1], 95819[1], 95822[0], 95829[1], 95860[0], 95861[0], 95863[0], 95864[0], 95865[0], 95866[0], 95867[0], 95868[0], 95869[0], 95870[0], 95907[0], 95908[0], 95909[0], 95910[0], 95911[0], 95912[0], 95913[0], 95925[0], 95926[0], 95927[0], 95928[0], 95929[0], 95930[0], 95933[0], 95937[0], 95938[0], 95939[0], 95940[0], 95955[1], 96360[1], 96361[1], 96365[1], 96366[1], 96367[1], 96368[1], 96372[1], 96374[1], 96375[1], 96376[1], 96377[1], 96523[0], 97597[1], 97598[1], 97602[1], 99155[0], 99156[0], 99157[0], 99211[1], 99212[1], 99213[1], 99214[1], 99215[1], 99217[1], 99218[1], 99219[1], 99220[1], 99221[1], 99222[1], 99223[1], 99231[1], 99232[1], 99233[1], 99234[1], 99235[1], 99236[1], 99238[1], 99239[1], 99241[1], 99242[1], 99243[1], 99244[1], 99245[1], 99251[1], 99252[1], 99253[1], 99254[1], 99255[1], 99291[1], 99292[1], 99304[1], 99305[1], 99306[1], 99307[1], 99308[1], 99309[1], 99310[1], 99315[1], 99316[1], 99334[1], 99335[1], 99336[1], 99337[1], 99347[1], 99348[1], 99349[1], 99350[1], 99374[1], 99375[1], 99377[1], 99378[1], 99446[0], 99447[0], 99448[0], 99449[0], 99451[0], 99452[0], 99495[0], 99496[0], G0276[1], G0453[0], G0463[1]
22208	11000[1], 11001[1], 11004[1], 11005[1], 11006[1], 11042[1], 11043[1], 11044[1], 11045[1], 11046[1], 11047[1], 22210[1], 22212[1], 22214[1], 22216[1], 22226[1], 36591[0], 36592[0], 38220[0], 38222[0], 38230[0], 38232[0], 63035[1], 63043[1], 63044[1], 63048[1], 63057[1], 63066[1], 63076[1], 63078[1], 63082[1], 63086[1], 63088[1], 63091[1], 63103[1], 63707[1], 63709[1], 95863[0], 95864[0], 95865[0], 95866[0], 95869[0], 96523[0], 97597[1], 97598[1], 97602[1]
22210	0213T[0], 0216T[0], 0228T[0], 0230T[0], 0274T[1], 0333T[0], 0464T[0], 0565T[1], 11000[1], 11001[1], 11004[1], 11005[1], 11006[1], 11042[1], 11043[1], 11044[1], 11045[1], 11046[1], 11047[1], 12001[1], 12002[1], 12004[1], 12005[1], 12006[1], 12007[1], 12011[1], 12013[1], 12014[1], 12015[1], 12016[1], 12017[1], 12018[1], 12020[1], 12021[1], 12031[1], 12032[1], 12034[1], 12035[1], 12036[1], 12037[1], 12041[1], 12042[1], 12044[1], 12045[1], 12046[1], 12047[1], 12051[1], 12052[1], 12053[1], 12054[1], 12055[1], 12056[1], 12057[1], 13100[1], 13101[1], 13102[1], 13120[1], 13121[1], 13122[1], 13131[1], 13132[1], 13133[1], 13151[1], 13152[1], 13153[1], 15769[1], 22100[1], 22110[1], 22212[1], 22326[1], 22505[0], 36000[1], 36400[1], 36405[1], 36406[1], 36410[1], 36420[1], 36425[1], 36430[1], 36440[1], 36591[0], 36592[0], 36600[1], 36640[1], 38220[0], 38222[0], 38230[0], 38232[0], 43752[1], 51701[1], 51702[1], 51703[1], 62320[0], 62321[0], 62322[0], 62323[0], 62324[0], 62325[0], 62326[0], 62327[0], 63001[1], 63015[1], 63020[1], 63045[1], 63707[1], 63709[1], 64400[0], 64405[0], 64408[0], 64415[0], 64416[0], 64417[0], 64418[0], 64420[0], 64421[0], 64425[0], 64430[0], 64435[0], 64445[0], 64446[0], 64447[0], 64448[0], 64449[0], 64450[1], 64451[0], 64454[1], 64461[0], 64462[0], 64463[0], 64479[0], 64480[0], 64483[0], 64484[0], 64486[0], 64487[0], 64488[0], 64489[0], 64490[0], 64491[0], 64492[0], 64493[0], 64494[0], 64495[0], 64505[0], 64510[0], 64517[0], 64520[0], 64530[0], 69990[0], 76000[1], 77001[1], 77002[1], 92012[1], 92014[1], 92585[0], 93000[1], 93005[1], 93010[1], 93040[1], 93041[1], 93042[1], 93318[1], 93355[1], 94002[1], 94200[1], 94250[1], 94680[1], 94681[1], 94690[1], 94770[1], 95812[1], 95813[1], 95816[1], 95819[1], 95822[0], 95829[1], 95860[0], 95861[0], 95863[0], 95864[0], 95865[0], 95866[0], 95867[0], 95868[0], 95869[0], 95870[0], 95907[0], 95908[0], 95909[0], 95910[0], 95911[0], 95912[0], 95913[0], 95925[0], 95926[0], 95927[0], 95928[0], 95929[0], 95930[0], 95933[0], 95937[0], 95938[0], 95939[0], 95940[0], 95955[1], 96360[1], 96361[1], 96365[1], 96366[1], 96367[1], 96368[1], 96372[1], 96374[1], 96375[1], 96376[1], 96377[1], 96523[0], 97597[1], 97598[1], 97602[1], 99155[0], 99156[0], 99157[0], 99211[1], 99212[1], 99213[1], 99214[1], 99215[1], 99217[1], 99218[1], 99219[1], 99220[1], 99221[1], 99222[1], 99223[1], 99231[1], 99232[1], 99233[1], 99234[1], 99235[1], 99236[1], 99238[1], 99239[1], 99241[1], 99242[1], 99243[1], 99244[1], 99245[1], 99251[1], 99252[1], 99253[1], 99254[1], 99255[1], 99291[1], 99292[1], 99304[1], 99305[1], 99306[1], 99307[1], 99308[1], 99309[1], 99310[1], 99315[1], 99316[1], 99334[1], 99335[1], 99336[1], 99337[1], 99347[1], 99348[1], 99349[1], 99350[1], 99374[1], 99375[1], 99377[1], 99378[1], 99446[0], 99447[0], 99448[0], 99449[0], 99451[0], 99452[0], 99495[0], 99496[0], G0453[0], G0463[1], G0471[1]
22212	0213T[0], 0216T[0], 0228T[0], 0230T[0], 0333T[0], 0464T[0], 0565T[1], 11000[1], 11001[1], 11004[1], 11005[1], 11006[1], 11042[1], 11043[1], 11044[1], 11045[1], 11046[1], 11047[1], 12001[1], 12002[1], 12004[1], 12005[1], 12006[1], 12007[1], 12011[1], 12013[1], 12014[1], 12015[1], 12016[1], 12017[1], 12018[1], 12020[1], 12021[1], 12031[1], 12032[1], 12034[1], 12035[1], 12036[1], 12037[1], 12041[1], 12042[1], 12044[1], 12045[1], 12046[1], 12047[1], 12051[1], 12052[1], 12053[1], 12054[1], 12055[1], 12056[1], 12057[1], 13100[1], 13101[1], 13102[1], 13120[1], 13121[1], 13122[1], 13131[1], 13132[1], 13133[1], 13151[1], 13152[1], 13153[1], 15769[1], 22101[1], 22112[1], 22222[1], 22327[1], 22505[0], 36000[1], 36400[1], 36405[1], 36406[1], 36410[1], 36420[1], 36425[1], 36430[1], 36440[1], 36591[0], 36592[0], 36600[1], 36640[1], 38220[0], 38222[0], 38230[0], 38232[0], 43752[1], 51701[1], 51702[1], 51703[1], 62320[0], 62321[0], 62322[0], 62323[0], 62324[0], 62325[0], 62326[0], 62327[0], 63003[1], 63016[1], 63707[1], 63709[1], 64400[0], 64405[0], 64408[0], 64415[0], 64416[0], 64417[0], 64418[0], 64420[0], 64421[0], 64425[0], 64430[0], 64435[0], 64445[0], 64446[0], 64447[0], 64448[0], 64449[0], 64450[1], 64451[0], 64454[1], 64461[0], 64462[0], 64463[0], 64479[0], 64480[0], 64483[0], 64484[0], 64486[0], 64487[0], 64488[0], 64489[0], 64490[0], 64491[0], 64492[0], 64493[0], 64494[0], 64495[0], 64505[0], 64510[0], 64517[0], 64520[0], 64530[0], 76000[1], 77001[1], 77002[1], 92012[1], 92014[1], 92585[0], 93000[1], 93005[1], 93010[1], 93040[1], 93041[1], 93042[1], 93318[1], 93355[1], 94002[1], 94200[1], 94250[1], 94680[1], 94681[1], 94690[1], 94770[1], 95812[1], 95813[1], 95816[1], 95819[1], 95822[0], 95829[1], 95860[0], 95861[0], 95863[0], 95864[0], 95865[0], 95866[0], 95867[0], 95868[0], 95869[0], 95870[0], 95907[0], 95908[0], 95909[0], 95910[0], 95911[0], 95912[0], 95913[0], 95925[0], 95926[0], 95927[0], 95928[0], 95929[0], 95930[0], 95933[0], 95937[0], 95938[0], 95939[0], 95940[0], 95955[1], 96360[1], 96361[1], 96365[1], 96366[1], 96367[1], 96368[1], 96372[1], 96374[1], 96375[1], 96376[1], 96377[1], 96523[0], 97597[1], 97598[1], 97602[1], 99155[0], 99156[0], 99157[0], 99211[1], 99212[1], 99213[1], 99214[1], 99215[1], 99217[1], 99218[1], 99219[1], 99220[1], 99221[1], 99222[1], 99223[1], 99231[1], 99232[1], 99233[1], 99234[1], 99235[1], 99236[1], 99238[1], 99239[1], 99241[1], 99242[1], 99243[1], 99244[1], 99245[1], 99251[1], 99252[1], 99253[1], 99254[1], 99255[1], 99291[1], 99292[1], 99304[1], 99305[1], 99306[1], 99307[1], 99308[1], 99309[1], 99310[1], 99315[1], 99316[1], 99334[1], 99335[1], 99336[1], 99337[1], 99347[1], 99348[1], 99349[1], 99350[1], 99374[1], 99375[1], 99377[1], 99378[1], 99446[0], 99447[0], 99448[0], 99449[0], 99451[0], 99452[0], 99495[0], 99496[0], G0453[0], G0463[1], G0471[1]
22214	0213T[0], 0216T[0], 0228T[0], 0230T[0], 0275T[1], 0333T[0], 0464T[0], 0565T[1], 11000[1], 11001[1], 11004[1], 11005[1], 11006[1], 11042[1], 11043[1], 11044[1], 11045[1], 11046[1], 11047[1], 12001[1], 12002[1], 12004[1], 12005[1], 12006[1], 12007[1], 12011[1], 12013[1], 12014[1], 12015[1], 12016[1], 12017[1], 12018[1], 12020[1], 12021[1], 12031[1], 12032[1], 12034[1], 12035[1], 12036[1], 12037[1], 12041[1], 12042[1], 12044[1], 12045[1], 12046[1], 12047[1], 12051[1], 12052[1], 12053[1], 12054[1], 12055[1], 12056[1], 12057[1], 13100[1], 13101[1], 13102[1], 13120[1], 13121[1], 13122[1], 13131[1], 13132[1], 13133[1], 13151[1], 13152[1], 13153[1], 15769[1], 22102[1], 22114[1], 22212[1], 22224[1], 22325[1], 22505[0], 22867[1], 22868[1], 22869[1], 22870[1], 36000[1], 36400[1], 36405[1], 36406[1], 36410[1], 36420[1], 36425[1], 36430[1], 36440[1], 36591[0], 36592[0], 36600[1], 36640[1], 38220[0], 38222[0], 38230[0], 38232[0], 43752[1], 51701[1], 51702[1], 51703[1], 62320[0], 62321[0], 62322[0], 62323[0], 62324[0], 62325[0], 62326[0], 62327[0], 62380[1], 63005[1], 63017[1], 63030[1], 63047[1], 63707[1], 63709[1], 64400[0], 64405[0], 64408[0], 64415[0], 64416[0], 64417[0], 64418[0], 64420[0], 64421[0], 64425[0], 64430[0], 64435[0], 64445[0], 64446[0], 64447[0], 64448[0], 64449[0], 64450[1], 64451[0], 64454[1], 64461[0], 64462[0], 64463[0], 64479[0], 64480[0], 64483[0], 64484[0], 64486[0],

Code 1	Code 2
	64487^0, 64488^0, 64489^0, 64490^0, 64491^0, 64492^0, 64493^0, 64494^0, 64495^0, 64505^0, 64510^0, 64517^0, 64520^0, 64530^0, 69990^0, 76000^1, 77001^1, 77002^1, 92012^1, 92014^1, 92585^0, 93000^1, 93005^1, 93010^1, 93040^1, 93041^1, 93042^1, 93318^1, 93355^1, 94002^1, 94200^1, 94250^1, 94680^1, 94681^1, 94690^1, 94770^1, 95812^1, 95813^1, 95816^1, 95819^1, 95822^0, 95829^1, 95860^0, 95861^0, 95863^0, 95864^0, 95865^0, 95866^0, 95867^0, 95868^0, 95869^0, 95870^0, 95907^0, 95908^0, 95909^0, 95910^0, 95911^0, 95912^0, 95913^0, 95925^0, 95926^0, 95927^0, 95928^0, 95929^0, 95930^0, 95933^0, 95937^0, 95938^0, 95939^0, 95940^0, 95955^1, 96360^1, 96361^1, 96365^1, 96366^1, 96367^1, 96368^1, 96372^1, 96374^1, 96375^1, 96376^1, 96377^1, 96523^0, 97597^1, 97598^1, 97602^1, 99155^0, 99156^0, 99157^0, 99211^1, 99212^1, 99213^1, 99214^1, 99215^1, 99217^1, 99218^1, 99219^1, 99220^1, 99221^1, 99222^1, 99223^1, 99231^1, 99232^1, 99233^1, 99234^1, 99235^1, 99236^1, 99238^1, 99239^1, 99241^1, 99242^1, 99243^1, 99244^1, 99245^1, 99251^1, 99252^1, 99253^1, 99254^1, 99255^1, 99291^1, 99292^1, 99304^1, 99305^1, 99306^1, 99307^1, 99308^1, 99309^1, 99310^1, 99315^1, 99316^1, 99334^1, 99335^1, 99336^1, 99337^1, 99347^1, 99348^1, 99349^1, 99350^1, 99374^1, 99375^1, 99377^1, 99378^1, 99446^0, 99447^0, 99448^0, 99449^0, 99451^0, 99452^0, 99495^0, 99496^0, G0276^1, G0453^0, G0463^1, G0471^1
22216	0333T^0, 0464T^0, 11000^1, 11001^1, 11004^1, 11005^1, 11006^1, 11042^1, 11043^1, 11044^1, 11045^1, 11046^1, 11047^1, 36591^0, 36592^0, 38220^0, 38222^0, 38230^0, 38232^0, 63707^1, 63709^1, 92585^0, 95822^0, 95860^0, 95861^0, 95863^0, 95864^0, 95865^0, 95866^0, 95867^0, 95868^0, 95869^0, 95907^0, 95908^0, 95909^0, 95910^0, 95911^0, 95912^0, 95913^0, 95925^0, 95926^0, 95927^0, 95930^0, 95933^0, 95937^0, 95938^0, 95939^0, 95940^0, 96523^0, 97597^1, 97598^1, 97602^1, G0453^0
22220	0213T^0, 0216T^0, 0228T^0, 0230T^0, 0333T^0, 0464T^0, 0565T^1, 11000^1, 11001^1, 11004^1, 11005^1, 11006^1, 11042^1, 11043^1, 11044^1, 11045^1, 11046^1, 11047^1, 12001^1, 12002^1, 12004^1, 12005^1, 12006^1, 12007^1, 12011^1, 12013^1, 12014^1, 12015^1, 12016^1, 12017^1, 12018^1, 12020^1, 12021^1, 12031^1, 12032^1, 12034^1, 12035^1, 12036^1, 12037^1, 12041^1, 12042^1, 12044^1, 12045^1, 12046^1, 12047^1, 12051^1, 12052^1, 12053^1, 12054^1, 12055^1, 12056^1, 12057^1, 13100^1, 13101^1, 13102^1, 13120^1, 13121^1, 13122^1, 13131^1, 13132^1, 13133^1, 13151^1, 13152^1, 13153^1, 15769^1, 22110^1, 22208^1, 22210^1, 22318^1, 22319^1, 22326^1, 22505^0, 22551^1, 22858^1, 36000^1, 36400^1, 36405^1, 36406^1, 36410^1, 36420^1, 36425^1, 36430^1, 36440^1, 36591^0, 36592^0, 36600^1, 36640^1, 38220^0, 38222^0, 38230^0, 38232^0, 43752^1, 51701^1, 51702^1, 51703^1, 62291^1, 62320^0, 62321^0, 62322^0, 62323^0, 62324^0, 62325^0, 62326^0, 62327^0, 63075^1, 63081^1, 63707^1, 63709^1, 64400^0, 64405^0, 64408^0, 64415^0, 64416^0, 64417^0, 64418^0, 64420^0, 64421^0, 64425^0, 64430^0, 64435^0, 64445^0, 64446^0, 64447^0, 64448^0, 64449^0, 64450^1, 64451^0, 64454^1, 64461^0, 64462^0, 64463^0, 64479^0, 64480^0, 64483^0, 64484^0, 64486^0, 64487^0, 64488^0, 64489^0, 64490^0, 64491^0, 64492^0, 64493^0, 64494^0, 64495^0, 64505^0, 64510^0, 64517^0, 64520^0, 64530^0, 69990^0, 72285^1, 76000^1, 77001^1, 77002^1, 92012^1, 92014^1, 92585^0, 93000^1, 93005^1, 93010^1, 93040^1, 93041^1, 93042^1, 93318^1, 93355^1, 94002^1, 94200^1, 94250^1, 94680^1, 94681^1, 94690^1, 94770^1, 95812^1, 95813^1, 95816^1, 95819^1, 95822^0, 95829^1, 95860^0, 95861^0, 95863^0, 95864^0, 95865^0, 95866^0, 95867^0, 95868^0, 95869^0, 95870^0, 95907^0, 95908^0, 95909^0, 95910^0, 95911^0, 95912^0, 95913^0, 95925^0, 95926^0, 95927^0, 95928^0, 95929^0, 95930^0, 95933^0, 95937^0, 95938^0, 95939^0, 95940^0, 95955^1, 96360^1, 96361^1, 96365^1, 96366^1, 96367^1, 96368^1, 96372^1, 96374^1, 96375^1, 96376^1, 96377^1, 96523^0, 97597^1, 97598^1, 97602^1, 99155^0, 99156^0, 99157^0, 99211^1, 99212^1, 99213^1, 99214^1, 99215^1, 99217^1, 99218^1, 99219^1, 99220^1, 99221^1, 99222^1, 99223^1, 99231^1, 99232^1, 99233^1, 99234^1, 99235^1, 99236^1, 99238^1, 99239^1, 99241^1, 99242^1, 99243^1, 99244^1, 99245^1, 99251^1, 99252^1, 99253^1, 99254^1, 99255^1, 99291^1, 99292^1, 99304^1, 99305^1, 99306^1, 99307^1, 99308^1, 99309^1, 99310^1, 99315^1, 99316^1, 99334^1, 99335^1, 99336^1, 99337^1, 99347^1, 99348^1, 99349^1, 99350^1, 99374^1, 99375^1, 99377^1, 99378^1, 99446^0, 99447^0, 99448^0, 99449^0, 99451^0, 99452^0, 99495^0, 99496^0, G0453^0, G0463^1, G0471^1
22222	0213T^0, 0216T^0, 0228T^0, 0230T^0, 0333T^0, 0464T^0, 0565T^1, 11000^1, 11001^1, 11004^1, 11005^1, 11006^1, 11042^1, 11043^1, 11044^1, 11045^1, 11046^1, 11047^1, 12001^1, 12002^1, 12004^1, 12005^1, 12006^1, 12007^1, 12011^1, 12013^1, 12014^1, 12015^1, 12016^1, 12017^1, 12018^1, 12020^1, 12021^1, 12031^1, 12032^1, 12034^1, 12035^1, 12036^1, 12037^1, 12041^1, 12042^1, 12044^1, 12045^1, 12046^1, 12047^1, 12051^1, 12052^1, 12053^1, 12054^1, 12055^1, 12056^1, 12057^1, 13100^1, 13101^1, 13102^1, 13120^1, 13121^1, 13122^1, 13131^1, 13132^1, 13133^1, 13151^1, 13152^1, 13153^1, 15769^1, 22112^1, 22208^1, 22220^1, 22327^1, 22505^0, 32100^1, 36000^1, 36400^1, 36405^1, 36406^1, 36410^1, 36420^1, 36425^1, 36430^1, 36440^1, 36591^0, 36592^0, 36600^1, 36640^1, 38220^0, 38222^0, 38230^0, 38232^0, 43752^1, 49010^0, 51701^1, 51702^1, 51703^1, 62291^1, 62320^0, 62321^0, 62322^0, 62323^0, 62324^0, 62325^0, 62326^0, 62327^0, 63077^1, 63085^1, 63087^1, 63101^1, 63707^1, 63709^1, 64400^0, 64405^0, 64408^0, 64415^0, 64416^0, 64417^0, 64418^0, 64420^0, 64421^0, 64425^0, 64430^0, 64435^0, 64445^0, 64446^0, 64447^0, 64448^0, 64449^0, 64450^1, 64451^0, 64454^1, 64461^0, 64462^0, 64463^0, 64479^0, 64480^0, 64483^0, 64484^0, 64486^0, 64487^0, 64488^0, 64489^0, 64490^0, 64491^0, 64492^0, 64493^0, 64494^0, 64495^0, 64505^0, 64510^0, 64517^0, 64520^0, 64530^0, 69990^0, 72285^1, 76000^1, 77001^1, 77002^1, 92012^1, 92014^1, 92585^0, 93000^1, 93005^1, 93010^1, 93040^1, 93041^1, 93042^1, 93318^1, 93355^1, 94002^1, 94200^1, 94250^1, 94680^1, 94681^1, 94690^1, 94770^1, 95812^1, 95813^1, 95816^1, 95819^1, 95822^0, 95829^1, 95860^0, 95861^0, 95863^0, 95864^0, 95865^0, 95866^0, 95867^0, 95868^0, 95869^0, 95870^0, 95907^0, 95908^0, 95909^0, 95910^0, 95911^0, 95912^0, 95913^0, 95925^0, 95926^0, 95927^0, 95928^0, 95929^0, 95930^0, 95933^0, 95937^0, 95938^0, 95939^0, 95940^0, 95955^1, 96360^1, 96361^1, 96365^1, 96366^1, 96367^1, 96368^1, 96372^1, 96374^1, 96375^1, 96376^1, 96377^1, 96523^0, 97597^1, 97598^1, 97602^1, 99155^0, 99156^0, 99157^0, 99211^1, 99212^1, 99213^1, 99214^1, 99215^1, 99217^1, 99218^1, 99219^1, 99220^1, 99221^1, 99222^1, 99223^1, 99231^1, 99232^1, 99233^1, 99234^1, 99235^1, 99236^1, 99238^1, 99239^1, 99241^1, 99242^1, 99243^1, 99244^1, 99245^1, 99251^1, 99252^1, 99253^1, 99254^1, 99255^1, 99291^1, 99292^1, 99304^1, 99305^1, 99306^1, 99307^1, 99308^1, 99309^1, 99310^1, 99315^1, 99316^1, 99334^1, 99335^1, 99336^1, 99337^1, 99347^1, 99348^1, 99349^1, 99350^1, 99374^1, 99375^1, 99377^1, 99378^1, 99446^0, 99447^0, 99448^0, 99449^0, 99451^0, 99452^0, 99495^0, 99496^0, G0453^0, G0463^1, G0471^1
22224	0213T^0, 0216T^0, 0228T^0, 0230T^0, 0333T^0, 0464T^0, 0565T^1, 11000^1, 11001^1, 11004^1, 11005^1, 11006^1, 11042^1, 11043^1, 11044^1, 11045^1, 11046^1, 11047^1, 12001^1, 12002^1, 12004^1, 12005^1, 12006^1, 12007^1, 12011^1, 12013^1, 12014^1, 12015^1, 12016^1, 12017^1, 12018^1, 12020^1, 12021^1, 12031^1, 12032^1, 12034^1, 12035^1, 12036^1, 12037^1, 12041^1, 12042^1, 12044^1, 12045^1, 12046^1, 12047^1, 12051^1, 12052^1, 12053^1, 12054^1, 12055^1, 12056^1, 12057^1, 13100^1, 13101^1, 13102^1, 13120^1, 13121^1, 13122^1, 13131^1, 13132^1, 13133^1, 13151^1, 13152^1, 13153^1, 15769^1, 22114^1, 22208^1, 22222^1, 22325^1, 22505^0, 22857^1, 36000^1, 36400^1, 36405^1, 36406^1, 36410^1, 36420^1, 36425^1, 36430^1, 36440^1, 36591^0, 36592^0, 36600^1, 36640^1, 38220^0, 38222^0, 38230^0, 38232^0, 43752^1, 49000^0, 49002^1, 49010^0, 51701^1, 51702^1, 51703^1, 62267^1, 62290^1, 62320^0, 62321^0, 62322^0, 62323^0, 62324^0, 62325^0, 62326^0, 62327^0, 63087^1, 63090^1, 63102^1, 63707^1, 63709^1, 64400^0, 64405^0, 64408^0, 64415^0, 64416^0, 64417^0, 64418^0, 64420^0, 64421^0, 64425^0, 64430^0, 64435^0, 64445^0, 64446^0, 64447^0, 64448^0, 64449^0, 64450^1, 64451^0, 64454^1, 64461^0, 64462^0, 64463^0, 64479^0, 64480^0, 64483^0, 64484^0, 64486^0, 64487^0, 64488^0, 64489^0, 64490^0, 64491^0, 64492^0, 64493^0, 64494^0, 64495^0, 64505^0, 64510^0, 64517^0, 64520^0, 64530^0, 69990^0, 72295^1, 76000^1, 77001^1, 77002^1, 92012^1, 92014^1, 92585^0, 93000^1, 93005^1, 93010^1, 93040^1, 93041^1, 93042^1, 93318^1, 93355^1, 94002^1, 94200^1, 94250^1, 94680^1, 94681^1, 94690^1, 94770^1, 95812^1, 95813^1, 95816^1, 95819^1, 95822^0, 95829^1, 95860^0, 95861^0, 95863^0, 95864^0, 95865^0, 95866^0, 95867^0, 95868^0, 95869^0, 95870^0, 95907^0, 95908^0, 95909^0, 95910^0, 95911^0, 95912^0, 95913^0, 95925^0, 95926^0, 95927^0, 95928^0, 95929^0, 95930^0, 95933^0, 95937^0, 95938^0, 95939^0, 95940^0, 95955^1, 96360^1, 96361^1, 96365^1, 96366^1, 96367^1, 96368^1, 96372^1, 96374^1, 96375^1, 96376^1, 96377^1, 96523^0, 97597^1, 97598^1, 97602^1, 99155^0, 99156^0, 99157^0, 99211^1, 99212^1, 99213^1, 99214^1, 99215^1, 99217^1, 99218^1, 99219^1, 99220^1, 99221^1, 99222^1, 99223^1, 99231^1, 99232^1, 99233^1, 99234^1, 99235^1, 99236^1, 99238^1, 99239^1, 99241^1, 99242^1, 99243^1, 99244^1, 99245^1, 99251^1, 99252^1, 99253^1, 99254^1, 99255^1, 99291^1, 99292^1, 99304^1, 99305^1, 99306^1, 99307^1, 99308^1, 99309^1, 99310^1, 99315^1, 99316^1, 99334^1, 99335^1, 99336^1, 99337^1, 99347^1, 99348^1, 99349^1, 99350^1, 99374^1, 99375^1, 99377^1, 99378^1, 99446^0, 99447^0, 99448^0, 99449^0, 99451^0, 99452^0, 99495^0, 99496^0, G0453^0, G0463^1, G0471^1
22226	0333T^0, 0464T^0, 11000^1, 11001^1, 11004^1, 11005^1, 11006^1, 11042^1, 11043^1, 11044^1, 11045^1, 11046^1, 11047^1, 36591^0, 36592^0, 38220^0, 38222^0, 38230^0, 38232^0, 63707^1, 63709^1, 92585^0, 95822^0, 95860^0, 95861^0, 95863^0, 95864^0, 95865^0, 95866^0, 95867^0, 95868^0, 95869^0, 95907^0, 95908^0, 95909^0, 95910^0, 95911^0, 95912^0, 95913^0, 95925^0, 95926^0, 95927^0, 95930^0, 95933^0, 95937^0, 95938^0, 95939^0, 95940^0, 96523^0, 97597^1, 97598^1, 97602^1, G0453^0
22310	00640^0, 0213T^0, 0216T^0, 0228T^0, 0230T^0, 0333T^0, 0464T^0, 12001^1, 12002^1, 12004^1, 12005^1, 12006^1, 12007^1, 12011^1, 12013^1, 12014^1, 12015^1, 12016^1, 12017^1, 12018^1, 12020^1, 12021^1, 12031^1, 12032^1, 12034^1, 12035^1, 12036^1, 12037^1, 12041^1, 12042^1, 12044^1, 12045^1, 12046^1, 12047^1, 12051^1, 12052^1, 12053^1, 12054^1, 12055^1, 12056^1, 12057^1, 13100^1, 13101^1, 13102^1, 13120^1, 13121^1, 13122^1, 13131^1, 13132^1, 13133^1, 13151^1, 13152^1, 13153^1, 22505^0, 29010^0, 29035^0, 29200^0, 29700^1, 29705^1, 29710^1, 36000^1, 36400^1, 36405^1, 36406^1, 36410^1, 36420^1, 36425^1, 36430^1, 36440^1, 36591^0, 36592^0, 36600^1, 36640^1, 38220^0, 38222^0, 38230^0, 38232^0, 43752^1, 51701^1, 51702^1, 51703^1, 62320^0, 62321^0, 62322^0, 62323^0, 62324^0, 62325^0, 62326^0, 62327^0, 64400^0, 64405^0, 64408^0, 64415^0, 64416^0, 64417^0, 64418^0, 64420^0, 64421^0, 64425^0, 64430^0, 64435^0, 64445^0, 64446^0, 64447^0, 64448^0, 64449^0, 64450^1, 64451^0, 64454^1, 64461^0, 64462^0, 64463^0, 64479^0, 64480^0, 64483^0, 64484^0, 64486^0, 64487^0, 64488^0, 64489^0, 64490^0, 64491^0, 64492^0, 64493^0, 64494^0, 64495^0, 64505^0, 64510^0, 64517^0, 64520^0, 64530^0, 69990^0, 76000^1, 77001^1, 77002^1, 92012^1, 92014^1, 92585^0, 93000^1, 93005^1,

0 = Modifier usage not allowed or inappropriate 1 = Modifier usage allowed

Code 1	Code 2
	93010[1], 93040[1], 93041[1], 93042[1], 93318[1], 93355[1], 94002[1], 94200[1], 94250[1], 94680[1], 94681[1], 94690[1], 94770[1], 95812[1], 95813[1], 95816[1], 95819[1], 95822[0], 95829[1], 95860[0], 95861[0], 95863[0], 95864[0], 95865[0], 95866[0], 95867[0], 95868[0], 95869[0], 95870[0], 95907[0], 95908[0], 95909[0], 95910[0], 95911[0], 95912[0], 95913[0], 95925[0], 95926[0], 95927[0], 95928[0], 95929[0], 95930[0], 95933[0], 95937[0], 95938[0], 95939[0], 95940[0], 95955[1], 96360[1], 96361[1], 96365[1], 96366[1], 96367[1], 96368[1], 96372[1], 96374[1], 96375[1], 96376[1], 96377[1], 96523[0], 97597[1], 97598[1], 97602[1], 97605[1], 97606[1], 97607[1], 97608[1], 99155[0], 99156[0], 99157[0], 99211[1], 99212[1], 99213[1], 99214[1], 99215[1], 99217[1], 99218[1], 99219[1], 99220[1], 99221[1], 99222[1], 99223[1], 99231[1], 99232[1], 99233[1], 99234[1], 99235[1], 99236[1], 99238[1], 99239[1], 99241[1], 99242[1], 99243[1], 99244[1], 99245[1], 99251[1], 99252[1], 99253[1], 99254[1], 99255[1], 99291[1], 99292[1], 99304[1], 99305[1], 99306[1], 99307[1], 99308[1], 99309[1], 99310[1], 99315[1], 99316[1], 99334[1], 99335[1], 99336[1], 99337[1], 99347[1], 99348[1], 99349[1], 99350[1], 99374[1], 99375[1], 99377[1], 99378[1], 99446[0], 99447[0], 99448[0], 99449[0], 99451[0], 99452[0], 99495[0], 99496[0], G0453[0], G0463[1], G0471[1]
22315	00640[0], 0213T[0], 0216T[0], 0228T[0], 0230T[0], 0333T[0], 0464T[0], 12001[1], 12002[1], 12004[1], 12005[1], 12006[1], 12007[1], 12011[1], 12013[1], 12014[1], 12015[1], 12016[1], 12017[1], 12018[1], 12020[1], 12021[1], 12031[1], 12032[1], 12034[1], 12035[1], 12036[1], 12037[1], 12041[1], 12042[1], 12044[1], 12045[1], 12046[1], 12047[1], 12051[1], 12052[1], 12053[1], 12054[1], 12055[1], 12056[1], 12057[1], 13100[1], 13101[1], 13102[1], 13120[1], 13121[1], 13122[1], 13131[1], 13132[1], 13133[1], 13151[1], 13152[1], 13153[1], 20650[1], 20690[1], 22310[1], 22505[0], 22510[1], 22511[1], 22512[1], 22513[1], 22514[1], 22515[1], 29010[0], 29035[0], 29200[0], 29700[1], 29705[1], 29710[1], 36000[1], 36400[1], 36405[1], 36406[1], 36410[1], 36420[1], 36425[1], 36430[1], 36440[1], 36591[0], 36592[0], 36600[1], 36640[1], 38220[0], 38222[0], 38230[0], 38232[0], 43752[1], 51701[1], 51702[1], 51703[1], 62320[0], 62321[0], 62322[0], 62323[0], 62324[0], 62325[0], 62326[0], 62327[0], 64400[0], 64405[0], 64408[0], 64415[0], 64416[0], 64417[0], 64418[0], 64420[0], 64421[0], 64425[0], 64430[0], 64435[0], 64445[0], 64446[0], 64447[0], 64448[0], 64449[0], 64450[1], 64451[0], 64454[1], 64461[0], 64462[0], 64463[0], 64479[0], 64480[0], 64483[0], 64484[0], 64486[0], 64487[0], 64488[0], 64489[0], 64490[0], 64491[0], 64492[0], 64493[0], 64494[0], 64495[0], 64505[0], 64510[0], 64517[0], 64520[0], 64530[0], 69990[0], 76000[1], 77001[1], 77002[1], 92012[1], 92014[1], 92585[0], 93000[1], 93005[1], 93010[1], 93040[1], 93041[1], 93042[1], 93318[1], 93355[1], 94002[1], 94200[1], 94250[1], 94680[1], 94681[1], 94690[1], 94770[1], 95812[1], 95813[1], 95816[1], 95819[1], 95822[0], 95829[1], 95860[0], 95861[0], 95863[0], 95864[0], 95865[0], 95866[0], 95867[0], 95868[0], 95869[0], 95870[0], 95907[0], 95908[0], 95909[0], 95910[0], 95911[0], 95912[0], 95913[0], 95925[0], 95926[0], 95927[0], 95928[0], 95929[0], 95930[0], 95933[0], 95937[0], 95938[0], 95939[0], 95940[0], 95955[1], 96360[1], 96361[1], 96365[1], 96366[1], 96367[1], 96368[1], 96372[1], 96374[1], 96375[1], 96376[1], 96377[1], 96523[0], 97597[1], 97598[1], 97602[1], 97605[1], 97606[1], 97607[1], 97608[1], 99155[0], 99156[0], 99157[0], 99211[1], 99212[1], 99213[1], 99214[1], 99215[1], 99217[1], 99218[1], 99219[1], 99220[1], 99221[1], 99222[1], 99223[1], 99231[1], 99232[1], 99233[1], 99234[1], 99235[1], 99236[1], 99238[1], 99239[1], 99241[1], 99242[1], 99243[1], 99244[1], 99245[1], 99251[1], 99252[1], 99253[1], 99254[1], 99255[1], 99291[1], 99292[1], 99304[1], 99305[1], 99306[1], 99307[1], 99308[1], 99309[1], 99310[1], 99315[1], 99316[1], 99334[1], 99335[1], 99336[1], 99337[1], 99347[1], 99348[1], 99349[1], 99350[1], 99374[1], 99375[1], 99377[1], 99378[1], 99446[0], 99447[0], 99448[0], 99449[0], 99451[0], 99452[0], 99495[0], 99496[0], G0453[0], G0463[1], G0471[1], J2001[1]
22318	0213T[0], 0216T[0], 0228T[0], 0230T[0], 0333T[0], 0464T[0], 12001[1], 12002[1], 12004[1], 12005[1], 12006[1], 12007[1], 12011[1], 12013[1], 12014[1], 12015[1], 12016[1], 12017[1], 12018[1], 12020[1], 12021[1], 12031[1], 12032[1], 12034[1], 12035[1], 12036[1], 12037[1], 12041[1], 12042[1], 12044[1], 12045[1], 12046[1], 12047[1], 12051[1], 12052[1], 12053[1], 12054[1], 12055[1], 12056[1], 12057[1], 13100[1], 13101[1], 13102[1], 13120[1], 13121[1], 13122[1], 13131[1], 13132[1], 13133[1], 13151[1], 13152[1], 13153[1], 20100[1], 20650[1], 20661[1], 20931[1], 20932[1], 20933[1], 20934[1], 20937[1], 20938[1], 22310[1], 22315[1], 22319[1], 22505[0], 29000[1], 29015[1], 29040[1], 29700[1], 29705[1], 29710[1], 36000[1], 36400[1], 36405[1], 36406[1], 36410[1], 36420[1], 36425[1], 36430[1], 36440[1], 36591[0], 36592[0], 36600[1], 36640[1], 38220[0], 38222[0], 38230[0], 38232[0], 43752[1], 51701[1], 51702[1], 51703[1], 62320[0], 62321[0], 62322[0], 62323[0], 62324[0], 62325[0], 62326[0], 62327[0], 63707[1], 63709[1], 64400[0], 64405[0], 64408[0], 64415[0], 64416[0], 64417[0], 64418[0], 64420[0], 64421[0], 64425[0], 64430[0], 64435[0], 64445[0], 64446[0], 64447[0], 64448[0], 64449[0], 64450[1], 64451[0], 64454[1], 64461[0], 64462[0], 64463[0], 64479[0], 64480[0], 64483[0], 64484[0], 64486[0], 64487[0], 64488[0], 64489[0], 64490[0], 64491[0], 64492[0], 64493[0], 64494[0], 64495[0], 64505[0], 64510[0], 64517[0], 64520[0], 64530[0], 69990[0], 76000[1], 77001[1], 77002[1], 92012[1], 92014[1], 92585[0], 93000[1], 93005[1], 93010[1], 93040[1], 93041[1], 93042[1], 93318[1], 93355[1], 94002[1], 94200[1], 94250[1], 94680[1], 94681[1], 94690[1], 94770[1], 95812[1], 95813[1], 95816[1], 95819[1], 95822[0], 95829[1], 95860[0], 95861[0], 95863[0], 95864[0], 95865[0], 95866[0], 95867[0], 95868[0], 95869[0], 95870[0], 95907[0], 95908[0], 95909[0], 95910[0], 95911[0], 95912[0], 95913[0], 95925[0], 95926[0], 95927[0], 95928[0], 95929[0], 95930[0], 95933[0], 95937[0], 95938[0], 95939[0], 95940[0], 95955[1], 96360[1], 96361[1], 96365[1], 96366[1], 96367[1], 96368[1], 96372[1], 96374[1], 96375[1], 96376[1], 96377[1], 96523[0], 97597[1], 97598[1], 97602[1], 97605[1], 97606[1], 97607[1], 97608[1], 99155[0], 99156[0], 99157[0], 99211[1], 99212[1], 99213[1], 99214[1], 99215[1], 99217[1], 99218[1], 99219[1], 99220[1], 99221[1], 99222[1], 99223[1], 99231[1], 99232[1], 99233[1], 99234[1], 99235[1], 99236[1], 99238[1], 99239[1], 99241[1], 99242[1], 99243[1], 99244[1], 99245[1], 99251[1], 99252[1], 99253[1], 99254[1], 99255[1], 99291[1], 99292[1], 99304[1], 99305[1], 99306[1], 99307[1], 99308[1], 99309[1], 99310[1], 99315[1], 99316[1], 99334[1], 99335[1], 99336[1], 99337[1], 99347[1], 99348[1], 99349[1], 99350[1], 99374[1], 99375[1], 99377[1], 99378[1], 99446[0], 99447[0], 99448[0], 99449[0], 99451[0], 99452[0], 99495[0], 99496[0], G0453[0], G0463[1], G0471[1]
22319	0213T[0], 0216T[0], 0228T[0], 0230T[0], 0333T[0], 0464T[0], 12001[1], 12002[1], 12004[1], 12005[1], 12006[1], 12007[1], 12011[1], 12013[1], 12014[1], 12015[1], 12016[1], 12017[1], 12018[1], 12020[1], 12021[1], 12031[1], 12032[1], 12034[1], 12035[1], 12036[1], 12037[1], 12041[1], 12042[1], 12044[1], 12045[1], 12046[1], 12047[1], 12051[1], 12052[1], 12053[1], 12054[1], 12055[1], 12056[1], 12057[1], 13100[1], 13101[1], 13102[1], 13120[1], 13121[1], 13122[1], 13131[1], 13132[1], 13133[1], 13151[1], 13152[1], 13153[1], 20100[1], 20650[1], 20661[1], 22310[1], 22315[1], 22505[0], 29000[1], 29015[1], 29040[1], 29700[1], 29705[1], 29710[1], 36000[1], 36400[1], 36405[1], 36406[1], 36410[1], 36420[1], 36425[1], 36430[1], 36440[1], 36591[0], 36592[0], 36600[1], 36640[1], 38220[0], 38222[0], 38230[0], 38232[0], 43752[1], 51701[1], 51702[1], 51703[1], 62320[0], 62321[0], 62322[0], 62323[0], 62324[0], 62325[0], 62326[0], 62327[0], 63707[1], 63709[1], 64400[0], 64405[0], 64408[0], 64415[0], 64416[0], 64417[0], 64418[0], 64420[0], 64421[0], 64425[0], 64430[0], 64435[0], 64445[0], 64446[0], 64447[0], 64448[0], 64449[0], 64450[1], 64451[0], 64454[1], 64461[0], 64462[0], 64463[0], 64479[0], 64480[0], 64483[0], 64484[0], 64486[0], 64487[0], 64488[0], 64489[0], 64490[0], 64491[0], 64492[0], 64493[0], 64494[0], 64495[0], 64505[0], 64510[0], 64517[0], 64520[0], 64530[0], 69990[0], 76000[1], 77001[1], 77002[1], 92012[1], 92014[1], 92585[0], 93000[1], 93005[1], 93010[1], 93040[1], 93041[1], 93042[1], 93318[1], 93355[1], 94002[1], 94200[1], 94250[1], 94680[1], 94681[1], 94690[1], 94770[1], 95812[1], 95813[1], 95816[1], 95819[1], 95822[0], 95829[1], 95860[0], 95861[0], 95863[0], 95864[0], 95865[0], 95866[0], 95867[0], 95868[0], 95869[0], 95870[0], 95907[0], 95908[0], 95909[0], 95910[0], 95911[0], 95912[0], 95913[0], 95925[0], 95926[0], 95927[0], 95928[0], 95929[0], 95930[0], 95933[0], 95937[0], 95938[0], 95939[0], 95940[0], 95955[1], 96360[1], 96361[1], 96365[1], 96366[1], 96367[1], 96368[1], 96372[1], 96374[1], 96375[1], 96376[1], 96377[1], 96523[0], 97597[1], 97598[1], 97602[1], 97605[1], 97606[1], 97607[1], 97608[1], 99155[0], 99156[0], 99157[0], 99211[1], 99212[1], 99213[1], 99214[1], 99215[1], 99217[1], 99218[1], 99219[1], 99220[1], 99221[1], 99222[1], 99223[1], 99231[1], 99232[1], 99233[1], 99234[1], 99235[1], 99236[1], 99238[1], 99239[1], 99241[1], 99242[1], 99243[1], 99244[1], 99245[1], 99251[1], 99252[1], 99253[1], 99254[1], 99255[1], 99291[1], 99292[1], 99304[1], 99305[1], 99306[1], 99307[1], 99308[1], 99309[1], 99310[1], 99315[1], 99316[1], 99334[1], 99335[1], 99336[1], 99337[1], 99347[1], 99348[1], 99349[1], 99350[1], 99374[1], 99375[1], 99377[1], 99378[1], 99446[0], 99447[0], 99448[0], 99449[0], 99451[0], 99452[0], 99495[0], 99496[0], G0453[0], G0463[1], G0471[1]
22325	0213T[0], 0216T[0], 0228T[0], 0230T[0], 0333T[0], 0464T[0], 12001[1], 12002[1], 12004[1], 12005[1], 12006[1], 12007[1], 12011[1], 12013[1], 12014[1], 12015[1], 12016[1], 12017[1], 12018[1], 12020[1], 12021[1], 12031[1], 12032[1], 12034[1], 12035[1], 12036[1], 12037[1], 12041[1], 12042[1], 12044[1], 12045[1], 12046[1], 12047[1], 12051[1], 12052[1], 12053[1], 12054[1], 12055[1], 12056[1], 12057[1], 13100[1], 13101[1], 13102[1], 13120[1], 13121[1], 13122[1], 13131[1], 13132[1], 13133[1], 13151[1], 13152[1], 13153[1], 20102[1], 20650[1], 22310[1], 22315[1], 22505[0], 22510[1], 22511[0], 22512[1], 22513[1], 22514[1], 22515[1], 29010[0], 29035[0], 29700[1], 29705[1], 29710[1], 36000[1], 36400[1], 36405[1], 36406[1], 36410[1], 36420[1], 36425[1], 36430[1], 36440[1], 36591[0], 36592[0], 36600[1], 36640[1], 38220[0], 38222[0], 38230[0], 38232[0], 43752[1], 49013[1], 49014[1], 51701[1], 51702[1], 51703[1], 62320[0], 62321[0], 62322[0], 62323[0], 62324[0], 62325[0], 62326[0], 62327[0], 63707[1], 63709[1], 64400[0], 64405[0], 64408[0], 64415[0], 64416[0], 64417[0], 64418[0], 64420[0], 64421[0], 64425[0], 64430[0], 64435[0], 64445[0], 64446[0], 64447[0], 64448[0], 64449[0], 64450[1], 64451[0], 64454[1], 64461[0], 64462[0], 64463[0], 64479[0], 64480[0], 64483[0], 64484[0], 64486[0], 64487[0], 64488[0], 64489[0], 64490[0], 64491[0], 64492[0], 64493[0], 64494[0], 64495[0], 64505[0], 64510[0], 64517[0], 64520[0], 64530[0], 69990[0], 75822[1], 76000[1], 77001[1], 77002[1], 92012[1], 92014[1], 92585[0], 93000[1], 93005[1], 93010[1], 93040[1], 93041[1], 93042[1], 93318[1], 93355[1], 94002[1], 94200[1], 94250[1], 94680[1], 94681[1], 94690[1], 94770[1], 95812[1], 95813[1], 95816[1], 95819[1], 95822[0], 95829[1], 95860[0], 95861[0], 95863[0], 95864[0], 95865[0], 95866[0], 95867[0], 95868[0], 95869[0], 95870[0], 95907[0], 95908[0], 95909[0], 95910[0], 95911[0], 95912[0], 95913[0], 95925[0], 95926[0], 95927[0], 95928[0], 95929[0], 95930[0], 95933[0], 95937[0], 95938[0], 95939[0], 95940[0], 95955[1], 96360[1], 96361[1], 96365[1], 96366[1], 96367[1], 96368[1], 96372[1], 96374[1], 96375[1], 96376[1], 96377[1], 96523[0], 97597[1], 97598[1], 97602[1], 97605[1], 97606[1], 97607[1], 97608[1], 99155[0], 99156[0], 99157[0], 99211[1], 99212[1], 99213[1], 99214[1], 99215[1], 99217[1], 99218[1], 99219[1], 99220[1], 99221[1], 99222[1], 99223[1], 99231[1], 99232[1], 99233[1], 99234[1], 99235[1], 99236[1], 99238[1], 99239[1], 99241[1], 99242[1], 99243[1], 99244[1], 99245[1], 99251[1], 99252[1], 99253[1], 99254[1], 99255[1], 99291[1], 99292[1], 99304[1], 99305[1], 99306[1], 99307[1], 99308[1], 99309[1], 99310[1], 99315[1], 99316[1], 99334[1], 99335[1], 99336[1], 99337[1], 99347[1], 99348[1], 99349[1], 99350[1], 99374[1], 99375[1], 99377[1], 99378[1], 99446[0], 99447[0], 99448[0], 99449[0], 99451[0], 99452[0], 99495[0], 99496[0], G0453[0], G0463[1], G0471[1]
22326	0213T[0], 0216T[0], 0228T[0], 0230T[0], 0333T[0], 0464T[0], 12001[1], 12002[1], 12004[1], 12005[1], 12006[1], 12007[1], 12011[1], 12013[1], 12014[1], 12015[1], 12016[1], 12017[1], 12018[1], 12020[1],

Appendix A: NCCI - CPT Codes

0 = Modifier usage not allowed or inappropriate 1 = Modifier usage allowed

Code 1	Code 2
	12021[1], 12031[1], 12032[1], 12034[1], 12035[1], 12036[1], 12037[1], 12041[1], 12042[1], 12044[1], 12045[1], 12046[1], 12047[1], 12051[1], 12052[1], 12053[1], 12054[1], 12055[1], 12056[1], 12057[1], 13100[1], 13101[1], 13102[1], 13120[1], 13121[1], 13122[1], 13131[1], 13132[1], 13133[1], 13151[1], 13152[1], 13153[1], 20100[1], 20102[1], 20650[1], 22310[1], 22315[1], 22318[1], 22319[1], 22327[1], 22505[0], 22510[1], 22512[1], 29700[1], 29705[1], 29710[1], 36000[1], 36400[1], 36405[1], 36406[1], 36410[1], 36420[1], 36425[1], 36430[1], 36440[1], 36591[0], 36592[0], 36600[1], 36640[1], 38220[0], 38222[0], 38230[0], 38232[0], 43752[1], 49013[1], 49014[1], 51701[1], 51702[1], 51703[1], 62320[0], 62321[0], 62322[0], 62323[0], 62324[0], 62325[0], 62326[0], 62327[0], 63045[1], 63707[1], 63709[1], 64400[0], 64405[0], 64408[0], 64415[0], 64416[0], 64417[0], 64418[0], 64420[0], 64421[0], 64425[0], 64430[0], 64435[0], 64445[0], 64446[0], 64447[0], 64448[0], 64449[0], 64450[1], 64451[0], 64454[1], 64461[0], 64462[0], 64463[0], 64479[0], 64480[0], 64483[0], 64484[0], 64486[0], 64487[0], 64488[0], 64489[0], 64490[0], 64491[0], 64492[0], 64493[0], 64494[0], 64495[0], 64505[0], 64510[0], 64517[0], 64520[0], 64530[0], 69990[0], 76000[1], 77001[1], 77002[1], 92012[1], 92014[1], 92585[0], 93000[1], 93005[1], 93010[1], 93040[1], 93041[1], 93042[1], 93318[1], 93355[1], 94002[1], 94200[1], 94250[1], 94680[1], 94681[1], 94690[1], 94770[1], 95812[1], 95813[1], 95816[1], 95819[1], 95822[0], 95829[1], 95860[0], 95861[0], 95863[0], 95864[0], 95865[0], 95866[0], 95867[0], 95868[0], 95869[0], 95870[0], 95907[0], 95908[0], 95909[0], 95910[0], 95911[0], 95912[0], 95913[0], 95925[0], 95926[0], 95927[0], 95928[0], 95929[0], 95930[0], 95933[0], 95937[0], 95938[0], 95939[0], 95940[0], 95955[1], 96360[1], 96361[1], 96365[1], 96366[1], 96367[1], 96368[1], 96372[1], 96374[1], 96375[1], 96376[1], 96377[1], 96523[0], 97597[1], 97598[1], 97602[1], 97605[1], 97606[1], 97607[1], 97608[1], 99155[0], 99156[0], 99157[0], 99211[1], 99212[1], 99213[1], 99214[1], 99215[1], 99217[1], 99218[1], 99219[1], 99220[1], 99221[1], 99222[1], 99223[1], 99231[1], 99232[1], 99233[1], 99234[1], 99235[1], 99236[1], 99238[1], 99239[1], 99241[1], 99242[1], 99243[1], 99244[1], 99245[1], 99251[1], 99252[1], 99253[1], 99254[1], 99255[1], 99291[1], 99292[1], 99304[1], 99305[1], 99306[1], 99307[1], 99308[1], 99309[1], 99310[1], 99315[1], 99316[1], 99334[1], 99335[1], 99336[1], 99337[1], 99347[1], 99348[1], 99349[1], 99350[1], 99374[1], 99375[1], 99377[1], 99378[1], 99446[0], 99447[0], 99448[0], 99449[0], 99451[0], 99452[0], 99495[0], 99496[0], G0453[0], G0463[1], G0471[1]
22327	0213T[0], 0216T[0], 0228T[0], 0230T[0], 0333T[0], 0464T[0], 12001[1], 12002[1], 12004[1], 12005[1], 12006[1], 12007[1], 12011[1], 12013[1], 12014[1], 12015[1], 12016[1], 12017[1], 12018[1], 12020[1], 12021[1], 12031[1], 12032[1], 12034[1], 12035[1], 12036[1], 12037[1], 12041[1], 12042[1], 12044[1], 12045[1], 12046[1], 12047[1], 12051[1], 12052[1], 12053[1], 12054[1], 12055[1], 12056[1], 12057[1], 13100[1], 13101[1], 13102[1], 13120[1], 13121[1], 13122[1], 13131[1], 13132[1], 13133[1], 13151[1], 13152[1], 13153[1], 20102[1], 20650[1], 22310[1], 22315[1], 22325[1], 22505[0], 22510[0], 22511[1], 22512[1], 22513[1], 22514[1], 22515[1], 29010[0], 29035[0], 29200[0], 29700[1], 29705[1], 29710[1], 36000[1], 36400[1], 36405[1], 36406[1], 36410[1], 36420[1], 36425[1], 36430[1], 36440[1], 36591[0], 36592[0], 36600[1], 36640[1], 38220[0], 38222[0], 38230[0], 38232[0], 43752[1], 49013[1], 49014[1], 51701[1], 51702[1], 51703[1], 62320[0], 62321[0], 62322[0], 62323[0], 62324[0], 62325[0], 62326[0], 62327[0], 63046[1], 63707[1], 63709[1], 64400[0], 64405[0], 64408[0], 64415[0], 64416[0], 64417[0], 64418[0], 64420[0], 64421[0], 64425[0], 64430[0], 64435[0], 64445[0], 64446[0], 64447[0], 64448[0], 64449[0], 64450[1], 64451[0], 64454[1], 64461[0], 64462[0], 64463[0], 64479[0], 64480[0], 64483[0], 64484[0], 64486[0], 64487[0], 64488[0], 64489[0], 64490[0], 64491[0], 64492[0], 64493[0], 64494[0], 64495[0], 64505[0], 64510[0], 64517[0], 64520[0], 64530[0], 69990[0], 76000[1], 77001[1], 77002[1], 92012[1], 92014[1], 92585[0], 93000[1], 93005[1], 93010[1], 93040[1], 93041[1], 93042[1], 93318[1], 93355[1], 94002[1], 94200[1], 94250[1], 94680[1], 94681[1], 94690[1], 94770[1], 95812[1], 95813[1], 95816[1], 95819[1], 95822[0], 95829[1], 95860[0], 95861[0], 95863[0], 95864[0], 95865[0], 95866[0], 95867[0], 95868[0], 95869[0], 95870[0], 95907[0], 95908[0], 95909[0], 95910[0], 95911[0], 95912[0], 95913[0], 95925[0], 95926[0], 95927[0], 95928[0], 95929[0], 95930[0], 95933[0], 95937[0], 95938[0], 95939[0], 95940[0], 95955[1], 96360[1], 96361[1], 96365[1], 96366[1], 96367[1], 96368[1], 96372[1], 96374[1], 96375[1], 96376[1], 96377[1], 96523[0], 97597[1], 97598[1], 97602[1], 97605[1], 97606[1], 97607[1], 97608[1], 99155[0], 99156[0], 99157[0], 99211[1], 99212[1], 99213[1], 99214[1], 99215[1], 99217[1], 99218[1], 99219[1], 99220[1], 99221[1], 99222[1], 99223[1], 99231[1], 99232[1], 99233[1], 99234[1], 99235[1], 99236[1], 99238[1], 99239[1], 99241[1], 99242[1], 99243[1], 99244[1], 99245[1], 99251[1], 99252[1], 99253[1], 99254[1], 99255[1], 99291[1], 99292[1], 99304[1], 99305[1], 99306[1], 99307[1], 99308[1], 99309[1], 99310[1], 99315[1], 99316[1], 99334[1], 99335[1], 99336[1], 99337[1], 99347[1], 99348[1], 99349[1], 99350[1], 99374[1], 99375[1], 99377[1], 99378[1], 99446[0], 99447[0], 99448[0], 99449[0], 99451[0], 99452[0], 99495[0], 99496[0], G0453[0], G0463[1], G0471[1]
22328	0333T[0], 0464T[0], 20650[1], 36591[0], 36592[0], 38220[0], 38222[0], 38230[0], 38232[0], 63707[1], 63709[1], 92585[0], 95822[0], 95860[0], 95861[0], 95863[0], 95864[0], 95865[0], 95866[0], 95867[0], 95868[0], 95869[0], 95907[0], 95908[0], 95909[0], 95910[0], 95911[0], 95912[0], 95913[0], 95925[0], 95926[0], 95927[0], 95930[0], 95933[0], 95937[0], 95938[0], 95939[0], 95940[0], 96523[0], G0453[0]
22513	01935[0], 01936[0], 0213T[0], 0216T[0], 0228T[0], 0230T[0], 0333T[0], 0464T[0], 10005[1], 10007[1], 10009[1], 10011[1], 10021[1], 11000[1], 11001[1], 11004[1], 11005[1], 11006[1], 11042[1], 11043[1], 11044[1], 11045[1], 11046[1], 11047[1], 12001[1], 12002[1], 12004[1], 12005[1], 12006[1], 12007[1], 12011[1], 12013[1], 12014[1], 12015[1], 12016[1], 12017[1], 12018[1], 12020[1], 12021[1], 12031[1], 12032[1], 12034[1], 12035[1], 12036[1], 12037[1], 12041[1], 12042[1], 12044[1], 12045[1], 12046[1], 12047[1], 12051[1], 12052[1], 12053[1], 12054[1], 12055[1], 12056[1], 12057[1], 13100[1], 13101[1], 13102[1], 13120[1], 13121[1], 13122[1], 13131[1], 13132[1], 13133[1], 13151[1], 13152[1], 13153[1], 20220[1], 20225[1], 20240[1], 20250[1], 20650[1], 20939[1], 22310[1], 22505[0], 22510[1], 22514[0], 22853[1], 22854[1], 22859[1], 36000[1], 36400[1], 36405[1], 36406[1], 36410[1], 36420[1], 36425[1], 36430[1], 36440[1], 36591[0], 36592[0], 36600[1], 36640[1], 38220[1], 38221[1], 38222[1], 43752[1], 51701[1], 51702[1], 51703[1], 62292[0], 62320[0], 62321[0], 62322[0], 62323[0], 62324[0], 62325[0], 62326[0], 62327[0], 63707[1], 63709[1], 64400[0], 64405[0], 64408[0], 64415[0], 64416[0], 64417[0], 64418[0], 64420[0], 64421[0], 64425[0], 64430[0], 64435[0], 64445[0], 64446[0], 64447[0], 64448[0], 64449[0], 64450[1], 64451[0], 64454[1], 64461[0], 64462[0], 64463[0], 64479[0], 64480[0], 64483[0], 64484[0], 64486[0], 64487[0], 64488[0], 64489[0], 64490[0], 64491[0], 64492[0], 64493[0], 64494[0], 64495[0], 64505[0], 64510[0], 64517[0], 64520[0], 64530[0], 69990[0], 72128[1], 72129[1], 72130[1], 75872[1], 76000[1], 76380[1], 76942[1], 76970[1], 76998[1], 77001[1], 77002[1], 77003[1], 77012[1], 77021[1], 92012[1], 92014[1], 92585[0], 93000[1], 93005[1], 93010[1], 93040[1], 93041[1], 93042[1], 93318[1], 93355[1], 94002[1], 94200[1], 94250[1], 94680[1], 94681[1], 94690[1], 94770[1], 95812[1], 95813[1], 95816[1], 95819[1], 95822[0], 95829[1], 95860[0], 95861[0], 95863[0], 95864[0], 95865[0], 95866[0], 95867[0], 95868[0], 95869[0], 95870[0], 95907[0], 95908[0], 95909[0], 95910[0], 95911[0], 95912[0], 95913[0], 95925[0], 95926[0], 95927[0], 95928[0], 95929[0], 95930[0], 95933[0], 95937[0], 95938[0], 95939[0], 95940[0], 95941[0], 95955[1], 96360[1], 96361[1], 96365[1], 96366[1], 96367[1], 96368[1], 96372[1], 96374[1], 96375[1], 96376[1], 96377[1], 96523[0], 97597[1], 97598[1], 97602[1], 99155[0], 99156[0], 99157[0], 99211[1], 99212[1], 99213[1], 99214[1], 99215[1], 99217[1], 99218[1], 99219[1], 99220[1], 99221[1], 99222[1], 99223[1], 99231[1], 99232[1], 99233[1], 99234[1], 99235[1], 99236[1], 99238[1], 99239[1], 99241[1], 99242[1], 99243[1], 99244[1], 99245[1], 99251[1], 99252[1], 99253[1], 99254[1], 99255[1], 99291[1], 99292[1], 99304[1], 99305[1], 99306[1], 99307[1], 99308[1], 99309[1], 99310[1], 99315[1], 99316[1], 99334[1], 99335[1], 99336[1], 99337[1], 99347[1], 99348[1], 99349[1], 99350[1], 99374[1], 99375[1], 99377[1], 99378[1], 99446[0], 99447[0], 99448[0], 99449[0], 99451[0], 99452[0], 99495[0], 99496[0], G0453[0], G0463[1], G0471[1], J0670[1], J2001[1]
22514	01935[0], 01936[0], 0213T[0], 0216T[0], 0228T[0], 0230T[0], 0333T[0], 0464T[0], 10005[1], 10007[1], 10009[1], 10011[1], 10021[1], 11000[1], 11001[1], 11004[1], 11005[1], 11006[1], 11042[1], 11043[1], 11044[1], 11045[1], 11046[1], 11047[1], 12001[1], 12002[1], 12004[1], 12005[1], 12006[1], 12007[1], 12011[1], 12013[1], 12014[1], 12015[1], 12016[1], 12017[1], 12018[1], 12020[1], 12021[1], 12031[1], 12032[1], 12034[1], 12035[1], 12036[1], 12037[1], 12041[1], 12042[1], 12044[1], 12045[1], 12046[1], 12047[1], 12051[1], 12052[1], 12053[1], 12054[1], 12055[1], 12056[1], 12057[1], 13100[1], 13101[1], 13102[1], 13120[1], 13121[1], 13122[1], 13131[1], 13132[1], 13133[1], 13151[1], 13152[1], 13153[1], 20220[1], 20225[1], 20240[1], 20250[1], 20650[1], 20939[1], 22310[1], 22505[0], 22511[1], 22853[1], 22854[1], 22859[1], 36000[1], 36400[1], 36405[1], 36406[1], 36410[1], 36420[1], 36425[1], 36430[1], 36440[1], 36591[0], 36592[0], 36600[1], 36640[1], 38220[1], 38221[1], 38222[1], 43752[1], 51701[1], 51702[1], 51703[1], 62292[0], 62320[0], 62321[0], 62322[0], 62323[0], 62324[0], 62325[0], 62326[0], 62327[0], 63707[1], 63709[1], 64400[0], 64405[0], 64408[0], 64415[0], 64416[0], 64417[0], 64418[0], 64420[0], 64421[0], 64425[0], 64430[0], 64435[0], 64445[0], 64446[0], 64447[0], 64448[0], 64449[0], 64450[1], 64451[0], 64454[1], 64461[0], 64462[0], 64463[0], 64479[0], 64480[0], 64483[0], 64484[0], 64486[0], 64487[0], 64488[0], 64489[0], 64490[0], 64491[0], 64492[0], 64493[0], 64494[0], 64495[0], 64505[0], 64510[0], 64517[0], 64520[0], 64530[0], 69990[0], 72131[1], 72132[1], 72133[1], 75872[1], 76000[1], 76380[1], 76942[1], 76970[1], 76998[1], 77001[1], 77002[1], 77003[1], 77012[1], 77021[1], 92012[1], 92014[1], 92585[0], 93000[1], 93005[1], 93010[1], 93040[1], 93041[1], 93042[1], 93318[1], 93355[1], 94002[1], 94200[1], 94250[1], 94680[1], 94681[1], 94690[1], 94770[1], 95812[1], 95813[1], 95816[1], 95819[1], 95822[0], 95829[1], 95860[0], 95861[0], 95863[0], 95864[0], 95865[0], 95866[0], 95867[0], 95868[0], 95869[0], 95870[0], 95907[0], 95908[0], 95909[0], 95910[0], 95911[0], 95912[0], 95913[0], 95925[0], 95926[0], 95927[0], 95928[0], 95929[0], 95930[0], 95933[0], 95937[0], 95938[0], 95939[0], 95940[0], 95941[0], 95955[1], 96360[1], 96361[1], 96365[1], 96366[1], 96367[1], 96368[1], 96372[1], 96374[1], 96375[1], 96376[1], 96377[1], 96523[0], 97597[1], 97598[1], 97602[1], 99155[0], 99156[0], 99157[0], 99211[1], 99212[1], 99213[1], 99214[1], 99215[1], 99217[1], 99218[1], 99219[1], 99220[1], 99221[1], 99222[1], 99223[1], 99231[1], 99232[1], 99233[1], 99234[1], 99235[1], 99236[1], 99238[1], 99239[1], 99241[1], 99242[1], 99243[1], 99244[1], 99245[1], 99251[1], 99252[1], 99253[1], 99254[1], 99255[1], 99291[1], 99292[1], 99304[1], 99305[1], 99306[1], 99307[1], 99308[1], 99309[1], 99310[1], 99315[1], 99316[1], 99334[1], 99335[1], 99336[1], 99337[1], 99347[1], 99348[1], 99349[1], 99350[1], 99374[1], 99375[1], 99377[1], 99378[1], 99446[0], 99447[0], 99448[0], 99449[0], 99451[0], 99452[0], 99495[0], 99496[0], G0453[0], G0463[1], G0471[1], J0670[1], J2001[1]
22515	10005[1], 10007[1], 10009[1], 10011[1], 10021[1], 11000[1], 11001[1], 11004[1], 11005[1], 11006[1], 11042[1], 11043[1], 11044[1], 11045[1], 11046[1], 11047[1], 20220[1], 20225[1], 20240[1], 20650[1], 20939[1], 22310[1], 36591[0], 36592[0], 38220[1], 38221[1], 38222[1], 63707[1], 63709[1], 76000[1], 76380[1], 76942[1], 76970[1], 76998[1], 77001[1], 77002[1], 77003[1], 77012[1], 77021[1], 95863[0], 95864[0], 95865[0], 95866[0], 95869[0], 96523[0], 97597[1], 97598[1], 97602[1]
22532	0213T[0], 0216T[0], 0228T[0], 0230T[0], 0333T[0], 0464T[0], 0566T[1], 11000[1], 11001[1], 11004[1], 11005[1], 11006[1], 11010[1], 11011[1], 11012[1], 11042[1], 11043[1], 11044[1], 11045[1], 11046[1], 11047[1], 12001[1], 12002[1], 12004[1], 12005[1], 12006[1], 12007[1], 12011[1], 12013[1], 12014[1],

0 = Modifier usage not allowed or inappropriate   1 = Modifier usage allowed

Code 1	Code 2
	12015[1], 12016[1], 12017[1], 12018[1], 12020[1], 12021[1], 12031[1], 12032[1], 12034[1], 12035[1], 12036[1], 12037[1], 12041[1], 12042[1], 12044[1], 12045[1], 12046[1], 12047[1], 12051[1], 12052[1], 12053[1], 12054[1], 12055[1], 12056[1], 12057[1], 13100[1], 13101[1], 13102[1], 13120[1], 13121[1], 13122[1], 13131[1], 13132[1], 13133[1], 13151[1], 13152[1], 13153[1], 20600[1], 20604[1], 20605[1], 20606[1], 20610[1], 20611[1], 20660[0], 20704[1], 22505[0], 22830[1], 22849[1], 22850[1], 22852[1], 22855[1], 22867[1], 22868[1], 22869[1], 22870[1], 29000[0], 29010[0], 29015[0], 29035[0], 29040[0], 29044[0], 29046[0], 29200[0], 32100[1], 36000[1], 36400[1], 36405[1], 36406[1], 36410[1], 36420[1], 36425[1], 36430[1], 36440[1], 36591[0], 36592[0], 36600[1], 36640[1], 37616[1], 38220[0], 38222[0], 38230[0], 38232[0], 43752[1], 51701[1], 51702[1], 51703[1], 62291[1], 62320[0], 62321[0], 62322[0], 62323[0], 62324[0], 62325[0], 62326[0], 62327[0], 63046[1], 63055[1], 63707[1], 63709[1], 64400[0], 64405[0], 64408[0], 64415[0], 64416[0], 64417[0], 64418[0], 64420[0], 64421[0], 64425[0], 64430[0], 64435[0], 64445[0], 64446[0], 64447[0], 64448[0], 64449[0], 64450[1], 64451[0], 64454[1], 64461[0], 64462[0], 64463[0], 64479[0], 64480[0], 64483[0], 64484[0], 64486[0], 64487[0], 64488[0], 64489[0], 64490[0], 64491[0], 64492[0], 64493[0], 64494[0], 64495[0], 64505[0], 64510[0], 64517[0], 64520[0], 64530[0], 69990[0], 72285[1], 76000[1], 77001[1], 77002[1], 92012[1], 92014[1], 92585[0], 93000[1], 93005[1], 93010[1], 93040[1], 93041[1], 93042[1], 93318[1], 93355[1], 94002[1], 94200[1], 94250[1], 94680[1], 94681[1], 94690[1], 94770[1], 95812[1], 95813[1], 95816[1], 95819[1], 95822[0], 95829[1], 95860[0], 95861[0], 95863[0], 95864[0], 95865[0], 95866[0], 95867[0], 95868[0], 95869[0], 95870[0], 95907[0], 95908[0], 95909[0], 95910[0], 95911[0], 95912[0], 95913[0], 95925[0], 95926[0], 95927[0], 95928[0], 95929[0], 95930[0], 95933[0], 95937[0], 95938[0], 95939[0], 95940[0], 95955[1], 96360[1], 96361[1], 96365[1], 96366[1], 96367[1], 96368[1], 96372[1], 96374[1], 96375[1], 96376[1], 96377[1], 96523[0], 97597[1], 97598[1], 97602[1], 99155[0], 99156[0], 99157[0], 99211[1], 99212[1], 99213[1], 99214[1], 99215[1], 99217[1], 99218[1], 99219[1], 99220[1], 99221[1], 99222[1], 99223[1], 99231[1], 99232[1], 99233[1], 99234[1], 99235[1], 99236[1], 99238[1], 99239[1], 99241[1], 99242[1], 99243[1], 99244[1], 99245[1], 99251[1], 99252[1], 99253[1], 99254[1], 99255[1], 99291[1], 99292[1], 99304[1], 99305[1], 99306[1], 99307[1], 99308[1], 99309[1], 99310[1], 99315[1], 99316[1], 99334[1], 99335[1], 99336[1], 99337[1], 99347[1], 99348[1], 99349[1], 99350[1], 99374[1], 99375[1], 99377[1], 99378[1], 99446[0], 99447[0], 99448[0], 99449[0], 99451[0], 99452[0], 99495[0], 99496[0], G0453[0], G0463[1], G0471[1]
22533	0213T[0], 0216T[0], 0228T[0], 0230T[0], 0333T[0], 0464T[0], 0566T[1], 11000[1], 11001[1], 11004[1], 11005[1], 11006[1], 11010[1], 11011[1], 11012[1], 11042[1], 11043[1], 11044[1], 11045[1], 11046[1], 11047[1], 12001[1], 12002[1], 12004[1], 12005[1], 12006[1], 12007[1], 12011[1], 12013[1], 12014[1], 12015[1], 12016[1], 12017[1], 12018[1], 12020[1], 12021[1], 12031[1], 12032[1], 12034[1], 12035[1], 12036[1], 12037[1], 12041[1], 12042[1], 12044[1], 12045[1], 12046[1], 12047[1], 12051[1], 12052[1], 12053[1], 12054[1], 12055[1], 12056[1], 12057[1], 13100[1], 13101[1], 13102[1], 13120[1], 13121[1], 13122[1], 13131[1], 13132[1], 13133[1], 13151[1], 13152[1], 13153[1], 20600[1], 20604[1], 20605[1], 20606[1], 20610[1], 20611[1], 20660[0], 20704[1], 22505[0], 22830[1], 22849[1], 22850[1], 22852[1], 22855[1], 22867[1], 22868[1], 22869[1], 22870[1], 29044[0], 29046[0], 32100[1], 36000[1], 36400[1], 36405[1], 36406[1], 36410[1], 36420[1], 36425[1], 36430[1], 36440[1], 36591[0], 36592[0], 36600[1], 36640[1], 37616[1], 37617[1], 38220[0], 38222[0], 38230[0], 38232[0], 43752[1], 49000[0], 49002[1], 49010[0], 51701[1], 51702[1], 51703[1], 62267[1], 62287[1], 62290[1], 62320[0], 62321[0], 62322[0], 62323[0], 62324[0], 62325[0], 62326[0], 62327[0], 63047[1], 63056[1], 63707[1], 63709[1], 64400[0], 64405[0], 64408[0], 64415[0], 64416[0], 64417[0], 64418[0], 64420[0], 64421[0], 64425[0], 64430[0], 64435[0], 64445[0], 64446[0], 64447[0], 64448[0], 64449[0], 64450[1], 64451[0], 64454[1], 64461[0], 64462[0], 64463[0], 64479[0], 64480[0], 64483[0], 64484[0], 64486[0], 64487[0], 64488[0], 64489[0], 64490[0], 64491[0], 64492[0], 64493[0], 64494[0], 64495[0], 64505[0], 64510[0], 64517[0], 64520[0], 64530[0], 69990[0], 72295[1], 76000[1], 77001[1], 77002[1], 92012[1], 92014[1], 92585[0], 93000[1], 93005[1], 93010[1], 93040[1], 93041[1], 93042[1], 93318[1], 93355[1], 94002[1], 94200[1], 94250[1], 94680[1], 94681[1], 94690[1], 94770[1], 95812[1], 95813[1], 95816[1], 95819[1], 95822[0], 95829[1], 95860[0], 95861[0], 95863[0], 95864[0], 95865[0], 95866[0], 95867[0], 95868[0], 95869[0], 95870[0], 95907[0], 95908[0], 95909[0], 95910[0], 95911[0], 95912[0], 95913[0], 95925[0], 95926[0], 95927[0], 95928[0], 95929[0], 95930[0], 95933[0], 95937[0], 95938[0], 95939[0], 95940[0], 95955[1], 96360[1], 96361[1], 96365[1], 96366[1], 96367[1], 96368[1], 96372[1], 96374[1], 96375[1], 96376[1], 96377[1], 96523[0], 97597[1], 97598[1], 97602[1], 99155[0], 99156[0], 99157[0], 99211[1], 99212[1], 99213[1], 99214[1], 99215[1], 99217[1], 99218[1], 99219[1], 99220[1], 99221[1], 99222[1], 99223[1], 99231[1], 99232[1], 99233[1], 99234[1], 99235[1], 99236[1], 99238[1], 99239[1], 99241[1], 99242[1], 99243[1], 99244[1], 99245[1], 99251[1], 99252[1], 99253[1], 99254[1], 99255[1], 99291[1], 99292[1], 99304[1], 99305[1], 99306[1], 99307[1], 99308[1], 99309[1], 99310[1], 99315[1], 99316[1], 99334[1], 99335[1], 99336[1], 99337[1], 99347[1], 99348[1], 99349[1], 99350[1], 99374[1], 99375[1], 99377[1], 99378[1], 99446[0], 99447[0], 99448[0], 99449[0], 99451[0], 99452[0], 99495[0], 99496[0], G0453[0], G0463[1], G0471[1]
22534	0333T[0], 0464T[0], 11000[1], 11001[1], 11004[1], 11005[1], 11006[1], 11042[1], 11043[1], 11044[1], 11045[1], 11046[1], 11047[1], 22867[1], 22868[1], 22869[1], 22870[1], 36591[0], 36592[0], 38220[0], 38222[0], 38230[0], 38232[0], 63707[1], 63709[1], 92585[0], 95822[0], 95860[0], 95861[0], 95863[0], 95864[0], 95865[0], 95866[0], 95867[0], 95868[0], 95869[0], 95907[0], 95908[0], 95909[0], 95910[0], 95911[0], 95912[0], 95913[0], 95925[0], 95926[0], 95927[0], 95930[0], 95933[0], 95937[0], 95938[0], 95939[0], 95940[0], 96523[0], 97597[1], 97598[1], 97602[1], G0453[0]
22551	0213T[0], 0216T[0], 0333T[0], 0464T[0], 11000[1], 11001[1], 11004[1], 11005[1], 11006[1], 11042[1], 11043[1], 11044[1], 11045[1], 11046[1], 11047[1], 12001[1], 12002[1], 12004[1], 12005[1], 12006[1], 12007[1], 12011[1], 12013[1], 12014[1], 12015[1], 12016[1], 12017[1], 12018[1], 12020[1], 12021[1], 12031[1], 12032[1], 12034[1], 12035[1], 12036[1], 12037[1], 12041[1], 12042[1], 12044[1], 12045[1], 12046[1], 12047[1], 12051[1], 12052[1], 12053[1], 12054[1], 12055[1], 12056[1], 12057[1], 13100[1], 13101[1], 13102[1], 13120[1], 13121[1], 13122[1], 13131[1], 13132[1], 13133[1], 13151[1], 13152[1], 13153[1], 20660[0], 22554[1], 22585[1], 36000[1], 36400[1], 36405[1], 36406[1], 36410[1], 36420[1], 36425[1], 36430[1], 36440[1], 36591[0], 36592[0], 36600[1], 36640[1], 38220[0], 38222[0], 38230[0], 38232[0], 43752[1], 51701[1], 51702[1], 51703[1], 62291[1], 62320[0], 62321[0], 62322[0], 62323[0], 62324[0], 62325[0], 62326[0], 62327[0], 63075[1], 63076[1], 63077[1], 63707[1], 63709[1], 64400[0], 64405[0], 64408[0], 64415[0], 64416[0], 64417[0], 64418[0], 64420[0], 64421[0], 64425[0], 64430[0], 64435[0], 64445[0], 64446[0], 64447[0], 64448[0], 64449[0], 64450[1], 64451[0], 64454[1], 64461[0], 64462[0], 64463[0], 64479[0], 64480[0], 64483[0], 64484[0], 64486[0], 64487[0], 64488[0], 64489[0], 64490[0], 64491[0], 64492[0], 64493[0], 64494[0], 64495[0], 64505[0], 64510[0], 64517[0], 64520[0], 64530[0], 69990[0], 72285[1], 76000[1], 92012[1], 92014[1], 92585[0], 93000[1], 93005[1], 93010[1], 93040[1], 93041[1], 93042[1], 93318[1], 93355[1], 94002[1], 94200[1], 94250[1], 94680[1], 94681[1], 94690[1], 94770[1], 95812[1], 95813[1], 95816[1], 95819[1], 95822[0], 95829[1], 95860[0], 95861[0], 95863[0], 95864[0], 95865[0], 95866[0], 95867[0], 95868[0], 95869[0], 95870[0], 95907[0], 95908[0], 95909[0], 95910[0], 95911[0], 95912[0], 95913[0], 95925[0], 95926[0], 95927[0], 95928[0], 95929[0], 95930[0], 95933[0], 95937[0], 95938[0], 95939[0], 95940[0], 95955[1], 96360[1], 96361[1], 96365[1], 96366[1], 96367[1], 96368[1], 96372[1], 96374[1], 96375[1], 96376[1], 96377[1], 96523[0], 97597[1], 97598[1], 97602[1], 99155[0], 99156[0], 99157[0], 99211[1], 99212[1], 99213[1], 99214[1], 99215[1], 99217[1], 99218[1], 99219[1], 99220[1], 99221[1], 99222[1], 99223[1], 99231[1], 99232[1], 99233[1], 99234[1], 99235[1], 99236[1], 99238[1], 99239[1], 99241[1], 99242[1], 99243[1], 99244[1], 99245[1], 99251[1], 99252[1], 99253[1], 99254[1], 99255[1], 99291[1], 99292[1], 99304[1], 99305[1], 99306[1], 99307[1], 99308[1], 99309[1], 99310[1], 99315[1], 99316[1], 99334[1], 99335[1], 99336[1], 99337[1], 99347[1], 99348[1], 99349[1], 99350[1], 99374[1], 99375[1], 99377[1], 99378[1], 99446[0], 99447[0], 99448[0], 99449[0], 99451[0], 99452[0], 99495[0], 99496[0], G0453[0], G0463[1], G0471[1]
22552	11000[1], 11001[1], 11004[1], 11005[1], 11006[1], 11042[1], 11043[1], 11044[1], 11045[1], 11046[1], 11047[1], 36591[0], 36592[0], 38220[0], 38222[0], 38230[0], 38232[0], 63707[1], 63709[1], 69990[0], 95863[0], 95864[0], 95865[0], 95866[0], 95869[0], 96523[0], 97597[1], 97598[1], 97602[1]
22554	0213T[0], 0216T[0], 0228T[0], 0230T[0], 0333T[0], 0464T[0], 0566T[1], 11000[1], 11001[1], 11004[1], 11005[1], 11006[1], 11042[1], 11043[1], 11044[1], 11045[1], 11046[1], 11047[1], 12001[1], 12002[1], 12004[1], 12005[1], 12006[1], 12007[1], 12011[1], 12013[1], 12014[1], 12015[1], 12016[1], 12017[1], 12018[1], 12020[1], 12021[1], 12031[1], 12032[1], 12034[1], 12035[1], 12036[1], 12037[1], 12041[1], 12042[1], 12044[1], 12045[1], 12046[1], 12047[1], 12051[1], 12052[1], 12053[1], 12054[1], 12055[1], 12056[1], 12057[1], 13100[1], 13101[1], 13102[1], 13120[1], 13121[1], 13122[1], 13131[1], 13132[1], 13133[1], 13151[1], 13152[1], 13153[1], 20600[1], 20604[1], 20605[1], 20606[1], 20610[1], 20611[1], 20660[0], 20704[1], 22505[0], 22552[1], 22830[1], 29000[0], 29015[0], 29040[0], 36000[1], 36400[1], 36405[1], 36406[1], 36410[1], 36420[1], 36425[1], 36430[1], 36440[1], 36591[0], 36592[0], 36600[1], 36640[1], 38220[0], 38222[0], 38230[0], 38232[0], 43752[1], 51701[1], 51702[1], 51703[1], 62291[1], 62320[0], 62321[0], 62322[0], 62323[0], 62324[0], 62325[0], 62326[0], 62327[0], 63076[1], 63707[1], 63709[1], 64400[0], 64405[0], 64408[0], 64415[0], 64416[0], 64417[0], 64418[0], 64420[0], 64421[0], 64425[0], 64430[0], 64435[0], 64445[0], 64446[0], 64447[0], 64448[0], 64449[0], 64450[1], 64451[0], 64454[1], 64461[0], 64462[0], 64463[0], 64479[0], 64480[0], 64483[0], 64484[0], 64486[0], 64487[0], 64488[0], 64489[0], 64490[0], 64491[0], 64492[0], 64493[0], 64494[0], 64495[0], 64505[0], 64510[0], 64517[0], 64520[0], 64530[0], 64718[1], 64722[1], 69990[0], 72285[1], 76000[1], 77001[1], 77002[1], 92012[1], 92014[1], 92585[0], 93000[1], 93005[1], 93010[1], 93040[1], 93041[1], 93042[1], 93318[1], 93355[1], 94002[1], 94200[1], 94250[1], 94680[1], 94681[1], 94690[1], 94770[1], 95812[1], 95813[1], 95816[1], 95819[1], 95822[0], 95829[1], 95860[0], 95861[0], 95863[0], 95864[0], 95865[0], 95866[0], 95867[0], 95868[0], 95869[0], 95870[0], 95907[0], 95908[0], 95909[0], 95910[0], 95911[0], 95912[0], 95913[0], 95925[0], 95926[0], 95927[0], 95928[0], 95929[0], 95930[0], 95933[0], 95937[0], 95938[0], 95939[0], 95940[0], 95955[1], 96360[1], 96361[1], 96365[1], 96366[1], 96367[1], 96368[1], 96372[1], 96374[1], 96375[1], 96376[1], 96377[1], 96523[0], 97597[1], 97598[1], 97602[1], 99155[0], 99156[0], 99157[0], 99211[1], 99212[1], 99213[1], 99214[1], 99215[1], 99217[1], 99218[1], 99219[1], 99220[1], 99221[1], 99222[1], 99223[1], 99231[1], 99232[1], 99233[1], 99234[1], 99235[1], 99236[1], 99238[1], 99239[1], 99241[1], 99242[1], 99243[1], 99244[1], 99245[1], 99251[1], 99252[1], 99253[1], 99254[1], 99255[1], 99291[1], 99292[1], 99304[1], 99305[1], 99306[1], 99307[1], 99308[1], 99309[1], 99310[1], 99315[1], 99316[1], 99334[1], 99335[1], 99336[1], 99337[1], 99347[1], 99348[1], 99349[1], 99350[1], 99374[1], 99375[1], 99377[1], 99378[1], 99446[0], 99447[0], 99448[0], 99449[0], 99451[0], 99452[0], 99495[0], 99496[0], G0453[0], G0463[1], G0471[1]
22558	0213T[0], 0216T[0], 0228T[0], 0230T[0], 0333T[0], 0464T[0], 0566T[1], 11000[1], 11001[1], 11004[1], 11005[1], 11006[1], 11042[1], 11043[1], 11044[1], 11045[1], 11046[1], 11047[1], 12001[1], 12002[1],

0 = Modifier usage not allowed or inappropriate 1 = Modifier usage allowed

Code 1	Code 2
	12004[1], 12005[1], 12006[1], 12007[1], 12011[1], 12013[1], 12014[1], 12015[1], 12016[1], 12017[1], 12018[1], 12020[1], 12021[1], 12031[1], 12032[1], 12034[1], 12035[1], 12036[1], 12037[1], 12041[1], 12042[1], 12044[1], 12045[1], 12046[1], 12047[1], 12051[1], 12052[1], 12053[1], 12054[1], 12055[1], 12056[1], 12057[1], 13100[1], 13101[1], 13102[1], 13120[1], 13121[1], 13122[1], 13131[1], 13132[1], 13133[1], 13151[1], 13152[1], 13153[1], 20600[1], 20604[1], 20605[1], 20606[1], 20610[1], 20611[1], 20660[0], 20704[1], 22505[0], 22634[1], 22830[1], 22867[1], 22868[1], 22869[1], 22870[1], 29044[0], 29046[0], 32100[1], 36000[1], 36400[1], 36405[1], 36406[1], 36410[1], 36420[1], 36425[1], 36430[1], 36440[1], 36591[0], 36592[0], 36600[1], 36640[1], 37617[1], 38220[0], 38222[0], 38230[0], 38232[0], 43752[1], 49000[0], 49002[1], 49010[0], 51701[1], 51702[1], 51703[1], 62267[1], 62290[1], 62320[0], 62321[0], 62322[0], 62323[0], 62324[0], 62325[0], 62326[0], 62327[0], 63707[1], 63709[1], 64400[0], 64405[0], 64408[0], 64415[0], 64416[0], 64417[0], 64418[0], 64420[0], 64421[0], 64425[0], 64430[0], 64435[0], 64445[0], 64446[0], 64447[0], 64448[0], 64449[0], 64450[1], 64451[0], 64454[1], 64461[0], 64462[0], 64463[0], 64479[0], 64480[0], 64483[0], 64484[0], 64486[0], 64487[0], 64488[0], 64489[0], 64490[0], 64491[0], 64492[0], 64493[0], 64494[0], 64495[0], 64505[0], 64510[0], 64517[0], 64520[0], 64530[0], 69990[0], 72295[1], 76000[1], 77001[1], 77002[1], 92012[1], 92014[1], 92585[0], 93000[1], 93005[1], 93010[1], 93040[1], 93041[1], 93042[1], 93318[1], 93355[1], 94002[1], 94200[1], 94250[1], 94680[1], 94681[1], 94690[1], 94770[1], 95812[1], 95813[1], 95816[1], 95819[1], 95822[0], 95829[1], 95860[0], 95861[0], 95863[0], 95864[0], 95865[0], 95866[0], 95867[0], 95868[0], 95869[0], 95870[0], 95907[0], 95908[0], 95909[0], 95910[0], 95911[0], 95912[0], 95913[0], 95925[0], 95926[0], 95927[0], 95928[0], 95929[0], 95930[0], 95933[0], 95937[0], 95938[0], 95939[0], 95940[0], 95955[1], 96360[1], 96361[1], 96365[1], 96366[1], 96367[1], 96368[1], 96372[1], 96374[1], 96375[1], 96376[1], 96377[1], 96523[0], 97597[1], 97598[1], 97602[1], 99155[0], 99156[0], 99157[0], 99211[1], 99212[1], 99213[1], 99214[1], 99215[1], 99217[1], 99218[1], 99219[1], 99220[1], 99221[1], 99222[1], 99223[1], 99231[1], 99232[1], 99233[1], 99234[1], 99235[1], 99236[1], 99238[1], 99239[1], 99241[1], 99242[1], 99243[1], 99244[1], 99245[1], 99251[1], 99252[1], 99253[1], 99254[1], 99255[1], 99291[1], 99292[1], 99304[1], 99305[1], 99306[1], 99307[1], 99308[1], 99309[1], 99310[1], 99315[1], 99316[1], 99334[1], 99335[1], 99336[1], 99337[1], 99347[1], 99348[1], 99349[1], 99350[1], 99374[1], 99375[1], 99377[1], 99378[1], 99446[0], 99447[0], 99448[0], 99449[0], 99451[0], 99452[0], 99495[0], 99496[0], G0453[0], G0463[1], G0471[1]
22585	0333T[0], 0464T[0], 11000[1], 11001[1], 11004[1], 11005[1], 11006[1], 11042[1], 11043[1], 11044[1], 11045[1], 11046[1], 11047[1], 20660[0], 36591[0], 36592[0], 38220[0], 38222[0], 38230[0], 38232[0], 63707[1], 63709[1], 92585[0], 95822[0], 95860[0], 95861[0], 95863[0], 95864[0], 95865[0], 95866[0], 95867[0], 95868[0], 95869[0], 95907[0], 95908[0], 95909[0], 95910[0], 95911[0], 95912[0], 95913[0], 95925[0], 95926[0], 95927[0], 95930[0], 95933[0], 95937[0], 95938[0], 95939[0], 95940[0], 96523[0], 97597[1], 97598[1], 97602[1], G0453[0]
22600	0213T[0], 0216T[0], 0219T[1], 0228T[0], 0230T[0], 0333T[0], 0464T[0], 0566T[1], 12001[1], 12002[1], 12004[1], 12005[1], 12006[1], 12007[1], 12011[1], 12013[1], 12014[1], 12015[1], 12016[1], 12017[1], 12018[1], 12020[1], 12021[1], 12031[1], 12032[1], 12034[1], 12035[1], 12036[1], 12037[1], 12041[1], 12042[1], 12044[1], 12045[1], 12046[1], 12047[1], 12051[1], 12052[1], 12053[1], 12054[1], 12055[1], 12056[1], 12057[1], 13100[1], 13101[1], 13102[1], 13120[1], 13121[1], 13122[1], 13131[1], 13132[1], 13133[1], 13151[1], 13152[1], 13153[1], 20600[1], 20604[1], 20605[1], 20606[1], 20610[1], 20611[1], 20660[0], 20704[1], 22505[0], 22610[1], 22804[1], 22808[1], 22830[1], 22858[1], 29000[0], 29015[0], 29040[0], 36000[1], 36400[1], 36405[1], 36406[1], 36410[1], 36420[1], 36425[1], 36430[1], 36440[1], 36591[0], 36592[0], 36600[1], 36640[1], 38220[0], 38222[0], 38230[0], 38232[0], 43752[1], 51701[1], 51702[1], 51703[1], 61250[1], 61253[1], 62320[0], 62321[0], 62322[0], 62323[0], 62324[0], 62325[0], 62326[0], 62327[0], 63295[1], 63707[1], 63709[1], 64400[0], 64405[0], 64408[0], 64415[0], 64416[0], 64417[0], 64418[0], 64420[0], 64421[0], 64425[0], 64430[0], 64435[0], 64445[0], 64446[0], 64447[0], 64448[0], 64449[0], 64450[1], 64451[0], 64454[1], 64461[0], 64462[0], 64463[0], 64479[0], 64480[0], 64483[0], 64484[0], 64486[0], 64487[0], 64488[0], 64489[0], 64490[0], 64491[0], 64492[0], 64493[0], 64494[0], 64495[0], 64505[0], 64510[0], 64517[0], 64520[0], 64530[0], 69990[0], 76000[1], 77001[1], 77002[1], 92012[1], 92014[1], 92585[0], 93000[1], 93005[1], 93010[1], 93040[1], 93041[1], 93042[1], 93318[1], 93355[1], 94002[1], 94200[1], 94250[1], 94680[1], 94681[1], 94690[1], 94770[1], 95812[1], 95813[1], 95816[1], 95819[1], 95822[0], 95829[1], 95860[0], 95861[0], 95863[0], 95864[0], 95865[0], 95866[0], 95867[0], 95868[0], 95869[0], 95870[0], 95907[0], 95908[0], 95909[0], 95910[0], 95911[0], 95912[0], 95913[0], 95925[0], 95926[0], 95927[0], 95928[0], 95929[0], 95930[0], 95933[0], 95937[0], 95938[0], 95939[0], 95940[0], 95955[1], 96360[1], 96361[1], 96365[1], 96366[1], 96367[1], 96368[1], 96372[1], 96374[1], 96375[1], 96376[1], 96377[1], 96523[0], 99155[0], 99156[0], 99157[0], 99211[1], 99212[1], 99213[1], 99214[1], 99215[1], 99217[1], 99218[1], 99219[1], 99220[1], 99221[1], 99222[1], 99223[1], 99231[1], 99232[1], 99233[1], 99234[1], 99235[1], 99236[1], 99238[1], 99239[1], 99241[1], 99242[1], 99243[1], 99244[1], 99245[1], 99251[1], 99252[1], 99253[1], 99254[1], 99255[1], 99291[1], 99292[1], 99304[1], 99305[1], 99306[1], 99307[1], 99308[1], 99309[1], 99310[1], 99315[1], 99316[1], 99334[1], 99335[1], 99336[1], 99337[1], 99347[1], 99348[1], 99349[1], 99350[1], 99374[1], 99375[1], 99377[1], 99378[1], 99446[0], 99447[0], 99448[0], 99449[0], 99451[0], 99452[0], 99495[0], 99496[0], G0453[0], G0463[1], G0471[1]
22610	0213T[0], 0216T[0], 0219T[1], 0220T[1], 0221T[1], 0228T[0], 0230T[0], 0333T[0], 0464T[0], 0566T[1], 12001[1], 12002[1], 12004[1], 12005[1], 12006[1], 12007[1], 12011[1], 12013[1], 12014[1], 12015[1], 12016[1], 12017[1], 12018[1], 12020[1], 12021[1], 12031[1], 12032[1], 12034[1], 12035[1], 12036[1], 12037[1], 12041[1], 12042[1], 12044[1], 12045[1], 12046[1], 12047[1], 12051[1], 12052[1], 12053[1], 12054[1], 12055[1], 12056[1], 12057[1], 13100[1], 13101[1], 13102[1], 13120[1], 13121[1], 13122[1], 13131[1], 13132[1], 13133[1], 13151[1], 13152[1], 13153[1], 20600[1], 20604[1], 20605[1], 20606[1], 20610[1], 20611[1], 20660[0], 20704[1], 22505[0], 22804[1], 22808[1], 22830[1], 29000[0], 29010[0], 29015[0], 29035[0], 29040[0], 29044[0], 29046[0], 29200[0], 36000[1], 36400[1], 36405[1], 36406[1], 36410[1], 36420[1], 36425[1], 36430[1], 36440[1], 36591[0], 36592[0], 36600[1], 36640[1], 38220[0], 38222[0], 38230[0], 38232[0], 43752[1], 51701[1], 51702[1], 51703[1], 62320[0], 62321[0], 62322[0], 62323[0], 62324[0], 62325[0], 62326[0], 62327[0], 63050[1], 63051[1], 63295[1], 63707[1], 63709[1], 64400[0], 64405[0], 64408[0], 64415[0], 64416[0], 64417[0], 64418[0], 64420[0], 64421[0], 64425[0], 64430[0], 64435[0], 64445[0], 64446[0], 64447[0], 64448[0], 64449[0], 64450[1], 64451[0], 64454[1], 64461[0], 64462[0], 64463[0], 64479[0], 64480[0], 64483[0], 64484[0], 64486[0], 64487[0], 64488[0], 64489[0], 64490[0], 64491[0], 64492[0], 64493[0], 64494[0], 64495[0], 64505[0], 64510[0], 64517[0], 64520[0], 64530[0], 69990[0], 76000[1], 77001[1], 77002[1], 92012[1], 92014[1], 92585[0], 93000[1], 93005[1], 93010[1], 93040[1], 93041[1], 93042[1], 93318[1], 93355[1], 94002[1], 94200[1], 94250[1], 94680[1], 94681[1], 94690[1], 94770[1], 95812[1], 95813[1], 95816[1], 95819[1], 95822[0], 95829[1], 95860[0], 95861[0], 95863[0], 95864[0], 95865[0], 95866[0], 95867[0], 95868[0], 95869[0], 95870[0], 95907[0], 95908[0], 95909[0], 95910[0], 95911[0], 95912[0], 95913[0], 95925[0], 95926[0], 95927[0], 95928[0], 95929[0], 95930[0], 95933[0], 95937[0], 95938[0], 95939[0], 95940[0], 95955[1], 96360[1], 96361[1], 96365[1], 96366[1], 96367[1], 96368[1], 96372[1], 96374[1], 96375[1], 96376[1], 96377[1], 96523[0], 99155[0], 99156[0], 99157[0], 99211[1], 99212[1], 99213[1], 99214[1], 99215[1], 99217[1], 99218[1], 99219[1], 99220[1], 99221[1], 99222[1], 99223[1], 99231[1], 99232[1], 99233[1], 99234[1], 99235[1], 99236[1], 99238[1], 99239[1], 99241[1], 99242[1], 99243[1], 99244[1], 99245[1], 99251[1], 99252[1], 99253[1], 99254[1], 99255[1], 99291[1], 99292[1], 99304[1], 99305[1], 99306[1], 99307[1], 99308[1], 99309[1], 99310[1], 99315[1], 99316[1], 99334[1], 99335[1], 99336[1], 99337[1], 99347[1], 99348[1], 99349[1], 99350[1], 99374[1], 99375[1], 99377[1], 99378[1], 99446[0], 99447[0], 99448[0], 99449[0], 99451[0], 99452[0], 99495[0], 99496[0], G0453[0], G0463[1], G0471[1]
22612	0213T[0], 0216T[0], 0219T[1], 0220T[1], 0221T[1], 0228T[0], 0230T[0], 0333T[0], 0464T[0], 0566T[1], 12001[1], 12002[1], 12004[1], 12005[1], 12006[1], 12007[1], 12011[1], 12013[1], 12014[1], 12015[1], 12016[1], 12017[1], 12018[1], 12020[1], 12021[1], 12031[1], 12032[1], 12034[1], 12035[1], 12036[1], 12037[1], 12041[1], 12042[1], 12044[1], 12045[1], 12046[1], 12047[1], 12051[1], 12052[1], 12053[1], 12054[1], 12055[1], 12056[1], 12057[1], 13100[1], 13101[1], 13102[1], 13120[1], 13121[1], 13122[1], 13131[1], 13132[1], 13133[1], 13151[1], 13152[1], 13153[1], 20600[1], 20604[1], 20605[1], 20606[1], 20610[1], 20611[1], 20660[0], 20704[1], 22505[0], 22610[1], 22630[1], 22804[1], 22808[1], 22830[1], 22857[1], 22867[1], 22868[1], 22869[1], 22870[1], 29044[0], 29046[0], 36000[1], 36400[1], 36405[1], 36406[1], 36410[1], 36420[1], 36425[1], 36430[1], 36440[1], 36591[0], 36592[0], 36600[1], 36640[1], 38220[0], 38222[0], 38230[0], 38232[0], 43752[1], 49000[0], 49002[1], 51701[1], 51702[1], 51703[1], 62320[0], 62321[0], 62322[0], 62323[0], 62324[0], 62325[0], 62326[0], 62327[0], 63050[1], 63051[1], 63295[1], 63707[1], 63709[1], 64400[0], 64405[0], 64408[0], 64415[0], 64416[0], 64417[0], 64418[0], 64420[0], 64421[0], 64425[0], 64430[0], 64435[0], 64445[0], 64446[0], 64447[0], 64448[0], 64449[0], 64450[1], 64451[0], 64454[1], 64461[0], 64462[0], 64463[0], 64479[0], 64480[0], 64483[0], 64484[0], 64486[0], 64487[0], 64488[0], 64489[0], 64490[0], 64491[0], 64492[0], 64493[0], 64494[0], 64495[0], 64505[0], 64510[0], 64517[0], 64520[0], 64530[0], 64712[1], 64714[1], 69990[0], 76000[1], 77001[1], 77002[1], 92012[1], 92014[1], 92585[0], 93000[1], 93005[1], 93010[1], 93040[1], 93041[1], 93042[1], 93318[1], 93355[1], 94002[1], 94200[1], 94250[1], 94680[1], 94681[1], 94690[1], 94770[1], 95812[1], 95813[1], 95816[1], 95819[1], 95822[0], 95829[1], 95860[0], 95861[0], 95863[0], 95864[0], 95865[0], 95866[0], 95867[0], 95868[0], 95869[0], 95870[0], 95907[0], 95908[0], 95909[0], 95910[0], 95911[0], 95912[0], 95913[0], 95925[0], 95926[0], 95927[0], 95928[0], 95929[0], 95930[0], 95933[0], 95937[0], 95938[0], 95939[0], 95940[0], 95955[1], 96360[1], 96361[1], 96365[1], 96366[1], 96367[1], 96368[1], 96372[1], 96374[1], 96375[1], 96376[1], 96377[1], 96523[0], 99155[0], 99156[0], 99157[0], 99211[1], 99212[1], 99213[1], 99214[1], 99215[1], 99217[1], 99218[1], 99219[1], 99220[1], 99221[1], 99222[1], 99223[1], 99231[1], 99232[1], 99233[1], 99234[1], 99235[1], 99236[1], 99238[1], 99239[1], 99241[1], 99242[1], 99243[1], 99244[1], 99245[1], 99251[1], 99252[1], 99253[1], 99254[1], 99255[1], 99291[1], 99292[1], 99304[1], 99305[1], 99306[1], 99307[1], 99308[1], 99309[1], 99310[1], 99315[1], 99316[1], 99334[1], 99335[1], 99336[1], 99337[1], 99347[1], 99348[1], 99349[1], 99350[1], 99374[1], 99375[1], 99377[1], 99378[1], 99446[0], 99447[0], 99448[0], 99449[0], 99451[0], 99452[0], 99495[0], 99496[0], G0453[0], G0463[1], G0471[1]
22614	0333T[0], 0464T[0], 22867[1], 22868[1], 22869[1], 22870[1], 36591[0], 36592[0], 38220[0], 38222[0], 38230[0], 38232[0], 63707[1], 63709[1], 92585[0], 95822[0], 95860[0], 95861[0], 95863[0], 95864[0], 95865[0], 95866[0], 95867[0], 95868[0], 95869[0], 95907[0], 95908[0], 95909[0], 95910[0], 95911[0], 95912[0], 95913[0], 95925[0], 95926[0], 95927[0], 95930[0], 95933[0], 95937[0], 95938[0], 95939[0], 95940[0], 96523[0], G0453[0]

0 = Modifier usage not allowed or inappropriate 1 = Modifier usage allowed

Code 1	Code 2
22630	0202T[1], 0213T[0], 0216T[0], 0228T[0], 0230T[0], 0275T[1], 0333T[0], 0464T[0], 0566T[1], 11000[1], 11001[1], 11004[1], 11005[1], 11006[1], 11042[1], 11043[1], 11044[1], 11045[1], 11046[1], 11047[1], 12001[1], 12002[1], 12004[1], 12005[1], 12006[1], 12007[1], 12011[1], 12013[1], 12014[1], 12015[1], 12016[1], 12017[1], 12018[1], 12020[1], 12021[1], 12031[1], 12032[1], 12034[1], 12035[1], 12036[1], 12037[1], 12041[1], 12042[1], 12044[1], 12045[1], 12046[1], 12047[1], 12051[1], 12052[1], 12053[1], 12054[1], 12055[1], 12056[1], 12057[1], 13100[1], 13101[1], 13102[1], 13120[1], 13121[1], 13122[1], 13131[1], 13132[1], 13133[1], 13151[1], 13152[1], 13153[1], 20600[1], 20604[1], 20605[1], 20606[1], 20610[1], 20611[1], 20660[0], 20704[1], 22224[1], 22505[0], 22558[1], 22610[1], 22804[1], 22808[1], 22830[1], 22857[1], 22867[1], 22868[1], 22869[1], 22870[1], 29044[0], 29046[0], 36000[1], 36400[1], 36405[1], 36406[1], 36410[1], 36420[1], 36425[1], 36430[1], 36440[1], 36591[0], 36592[0], 36600[1], 36640[1], 38220[0], 38222[0], 38230[0], 38232[0], 43752[1], 51701[1], 51702[1], 51703[1], 62267[1], 62287[1], 62320[0], 62321[0], 62322[0], 62323[0], 62324[0], 62325[0], 62326[0], 62327[0], 62380[1], 63005[1], 63012[1], 63017[1], 63030[1], 63042[1], 63047[1], 63056[1], 63170[1], 63185[1], 63190[1], 63191[1], 63200[1], 63267[1], 63277[1], 63707[1], 63709[1], 64400[0], 64405[0], 64408[0], 64415[0], 64416[0], 64417[0], 64418[0], 64420[0], 64421[0], 64425[0], 64430[0], 64435[0], 64445[0], 64446[0], 64447[0], 64448[0], 64449[0], 64450[1], 64451[0], 64454[1], 64461[0], 64462[0], 64463[0], 64479[0], 64480[0], 64483[0], 64484[0], 64486[0], 64487[0], 64488[0], 64489[0], 64490[0], 64491[0], 64492[0], 64493[0], 64494[0], 64495[0], 64505[0], 64510[0], 64517[0], 64520[0], 64530[0], 69990[0], 76000[1], 77001[1], 77002[1], 92012[1], 92014[1], 92585[0], 93000[1], 93005[1], 93010[1], 93040[1], 93041[1], 93042[1], 93318[1], 93355[1], 94002[1], 94200[1], 94250[1], 94680[1], 94681[1], 94690[1], 94770[1], 95812[1], 95813[1], 95816[1], 95819[1], 95822[0], 95829[1], 95860[0], 95861[0], 95863[0], 95864[0], 95865[0], 95866[0], 95867[0], 95868[0], 95869[0], 95870[0], 95907[0], 95908[0], 95909[0], 95910[0], 95911[0], 95912[0], 95913[0], 95925[0], 95926[0], 95927[0], 95928[0], 95929[0], 95930[0], 95933[0], 95937[0], 95938[0], 95939[0], 95940[0], 95955[1], 96360[1], 96361[1], 96365[1], 96366[1], 96367[1], 96368[1], 96372[1], 96374[1], 96375[1], 96376[1], 96377[1], 96523[0], 97597[1], 97598[1], 97602[1], 99155[0], 99156[0], 99157[0], 99211[1], 99212[1], 99213[1], 99214[1], 99215[1], 99217[1], 99218[1], 99219[1], 99220[1], 99221[1], 99222[1], 99223[1], 99231[1], 99232[1], 99233[1], 99234[1], 99235[1], 99236[1], 99238[1], 99239[1], 99241[1], 99242[1], 99243[1], 99244[1], 99245[1], 99251[1], 99252[1], 99253[1], 99254[1], 99255[1], 99291[1], 99292[1], 99304[1], 99305[1], 99306[1], 99307[1], 99308[1], 99309[1], 99310[1], 99315[1], 99316[1], 99334[1], 99335[1], 99336[1], 99337[1], 99347[1], 99348[1], 99349[1], 99350[1], 99374[1], 99375[1], 99377[1], 99378[1], 99446[0], 99447[0], 99448[0], 99449[0], 99451[0], 99452[0], 99495[0], 99496[0], G0276[1], G0453[0], G0463[1], G0471[1]
22632	0333T[0], 0464T[0], 11000[1], 11001[1], 11004[1], 11005[1], 11006[1], 11042[1], 11043[1], 11044[1], 11045[1], 11046[1], 11047[1], 22867[1], 22868[1], 22869[1], 22870[1], 36591[0], 36592[0], 38220[0], 38222[0], 38230[0], 38232[0], 63707[1], 63709[1], 92585[0], 95822[0], 95860[0], 95861[0], 95863[0], 95864[0], 95865[0], 95866[0], 95867[0], 95868[0], 95869[0], 95907[0], 95908[0], 95909[0], 95910[0], 95911[0], 95912[0], 95913[0], 95925[0], 95926[0], 95927[0], 95930[0], 95933[0], 95937[0], 95938[0], 95939[0], 95940[0], 96523[0], 97597[1], 97598[1], 97602[1], G0453[0]
22633	0202T[1], 0213T[0], 0216T[0], 0221T[1], 0228T[0], 0230T[0], 0275T[1], 0333T[0], 0464T[0], 0566T[1], 11000[1], 11001[1], 11004[1], 11005[1], 11006[1], 11010[1], 11011[1], 11012[1], 11042[1], 11043[1], 11044[1], 11045[1], 11046[1], 11047[1], 12001[1], 12002[1], 12004[1], 12005[1], 12006[1], 12007[1], 12011[1], 12013[1], 12014[1], 12015[1], 12016[1], 12017[1], 12018[1], 12020[1], 12021[1], 12031[1], 12032[1], 12034[1], 12035[1], 12036[1], 12037[1], 12041[1], 12042[1], 12044[1], 12045[1], 12046[1], 12047[1], 12051[1], 12052[1], 12053[1], 12054[1], 12055[1], 12056[1], 12057[1], 13100[1], 13101[1], 13102[1], 13120[1], 13121[1], 13122[1], 13131[1], 13132[1], 13133[1], 13151[1], 13152[1], 13153[1], 20600[1], 20604[1], 20605[1], 20606[1], 20610[1], 20611[1], 20660[0], 20704[1], 22224[1], 22505[0], 22558[1], 22586[1], 22610[1], 22612[0], 22630[0], 22808[1], 22830[1], 22857[1], 22867[1], 22868[1], 22869[1], 22870[1], 29044[0], 29046[0], 36000[1], 36400[1], 36405[1], 36406[1], 36410[1], 36420[1], 36425[1], 36430[1], 36440[1], 36591[0], 36592[0], 36600[1], 36640[1], 38220[0], 38222[0], 38230[0], 38232[0], 43752[1], 49000[0], 49002[1], 51701[1], 51702[1], 51703[1], 62267[1], 62287[1], 62320[0], 62321[0], 62322[0], 62323[0], 62324[0], 62325[0], 62326[0], 62327[0], 62380[1], 63005[1], 63012[1], 63017[1], 63030[1], 63042[1], 63047[1], 63050[1], 63051[1], 63056[1], 63170[1], 63185[1], 63190[1], 63191[1], 63200[1], 63267[1], 63277[1], 63295[1], 63707[1], 63709[1], 64400[0], 64405[0], 64408[0], 64415[0], 64416[0], 64417[0], 64418[0], 64420[0], 64421[0], 64425[0], 64430[0], 64435[0], 64445[0], 64446[0], 64447[0], 64448[0], 64449[0], 64450[1], 64451[0], 64454[1], 64461[0], 64462[0], 64463[0], 64479[0], 64480[0], 64483[0], 64484[0], 64486[0], 64487[0], 64488[0], 64489[0], 64490[0], 64491[0], 64492[0], 64493[0], 64494[0], 64495[0], 64505[0], 64510[0], 64517[0], 64520[0], 64530[0], 64712[1], 64714[1], 69990[0], 76000[1], 77001[1], 77002[1], 92012[1], 92014[1], 92585[0], 93000[1], 93005[1], 93010[1], 93040[1], 93041[1], 93042[1], 93318[1], 93355[1], 94002[1], 94200[1], 94250[1], 94680[1], 94681[1], 94690[1], 94770[1], 95812[1], 95813[1], 95816[1], 95819[1], 95822[0], 95829[1], 95861[0], 95863[0], 95864[0], 95865[0], 95866[0], 95868[0], 95869[0], 95870[0], 95887[0], 95907[0], 95908[0], 95909[0], 95910[0], 95911[0], 95912[0], 95913[0], 95925[0], 95926[0], 95927[0], 95928[0], 95929[0], 95930[0], 95933[0], 95937[0], 95938[0], 95939[0], 95955[1], 96360[1], 96361[1], 96365[1], 96366[1], 96367[1], 96368[1], 96372[1], 96374[1], 96375[1], 96376[1], 96377[1], 96523[0], 97597[1], 97598[1], 97602[1], 99155[0], 99156[0], 99157[0], 99211[1], 99212[1], 99213[1], 99214[1], 99215[1], 99217[1], 99218[1], 99219[1], 99220[1], 99221[1], 99222[1], 99223[1], 99231[1], 99232[1], 99233[1], 99234[1], 99235[1], 99236[1], 99238[1], 99239[1], 99241[1], 99242[1], 99243[1], 99244[1], 99245[1], 99251[1], 99252[1], 99253[1], 99254[1], 99255[1], 99291[1], 99292[1], 99304[1], 99305[1], 99306[1], 99307[1], 99308[1], 99309[1], 99310[1], 99315[1], 99316[1], 99334[1], 99335[1], 99336[1], 99337[1], 99347[1], 99348[1], 99349[1], 99350[1], 99374[1], 99375[1], 99377[1], 99378[1], 99446[0], 99447[0], 99448[0], 99449[0], 99451[0], 99452[0], 99495[0], 99496[0], G0276[1], G0463[1], G0471[1]
22634	0202T[1], 0213T[0], 0216T[0], 0221T[1], 0228T[0], 0230T[0], 0275T[1], 0333T[0], 0464T[0], 0566T[1], 11000[1], 11001[1], 11004[1], 11005[1], 11006[1], 11042[1], 11043[1], 11044[1], 11045[1], 11046[1], 11047[1], 12001[1], 12002[1], 12004[1], 12005[1], 12006[1], 12007[1], 12020[1], 12021[1], 12031[1], 12032[1], 12034[1], 12035[1], 12036[1], 12037[1], 13100[1], 13101[1], 20600[1], 20604[1], 20605[1], 20606[1], 20610[1], 20611[1], 20704[1], 22224[1], 22505[0], 22610[1], 22830[1], 22867[1], 22868[1], 22869[1], 22870[1], 29044[0], 29046[0], 36000[1], 36400[1], 36405[1], 36406[1], 36410[1], 36420[1], 36425[1], 36430[1], 36440[1], 36591[0], 36592[0], 36600[1], 36640[1], 38220[0], 38222[0], 38230[0], 38232[0], 43752[1], 49000[0], 49002[1], 51701[1], 51702[1], 51703[1], 61650[1], 62267[1], 62287[1], 62320[0], 62321[0], 62322[0], 62323[0], 62324[0], 62325[0], 62326[0], 62327[0], 62380[1], 63005[1], 63012[1], 63017[1], 63030[1], 63047[1], 63050[1], 63051[1], 63056[1], 63170[1], 63185[1], 63190[1], 63191[1], 63200[1], 63267[1], 63277[1], 63295[1], 63707[1], 63709[1], 64400[0], 64405[0], 64408[0], 64415[0], 64416[0], 64417[0], 64418[0], 64420[0], 64421[0], 64425[0], 64430[0], 64435[0], 64445[0], 64446[0], 64447[0], 64448[0], 64449[0], 64450[1], 64451[0], 64454[1], 64461[0], 64463[0], 64479[0], 64483[0], 64486[1], 64487[1], 64488[1], 64489[1], 64490[0], 64493[0], 64505[0], 64510[0], 64517[0], 64520[0], 64530[0], 64712[1], 64714[1], 69990[0], 76000[1], 77001[1], 77002[1], 92585[0], 93000[1], 93005[1], 93010[1], 93040[1], 93041[1], 93042[1], 93318[1], 93355[1], 94002[1], 94200[1], 94250[1], 94680[1], 94681[1], 94690[1], 94770[1], 95812[1], 95813[1], 95816[1], 95819[1], 95822[0], 95829[1], 95861[0], 95863[0], 95864[0], 95865[0], 95866[0], 95868[0], 95869[0], 95870[0], 95887[0], 95907[0], 95908[0], 95909[0], 95910[0], 95911[0], 95912[0], 95913[0], 95925[0], 95926[0], 95927[0], 95928[0], 95929[0], 95930[0], 95933[0], 95937[0], 95938[0], 95939[0], 95955[1], 96360[1], 96365[1], 96372[1], 96374[1], 96375[1], 96376[1], 96377[1], 96523[0], 97597[1], 97598[1], 97602[1], 99155[0], 99156[0], 99157[0], G0276[1], G0471[1]
22830	0213T[0], 0216T[0], 0228T[0], 0230T[0], 0333T[0], 0464T[0], 12001[1], 12002[1], 12004[1], 12005[1], 12006[1], 12007[1], 12011[1], 12013[1], 12014[1], 12015[1], 12016[1], 12017[1], 12018[1], 12020[1], 12021[1], 12031[1], 12032[1], 12034[1], 12035[1], 12036[1], 12037[1], 12041[1], 12042[1], 12044[1], 12045[1], 12046[1], 12047[1], 12051[1], 12052[1], 12053[1], 12054[1], 12055[1], 12056[1], 12057[1], 13100[1], 13101[1], 13102[1], 13120[1], 13121[1], 13122[1], 13131[1], 13132[1], 13133[1], 13151[1], 13152[1], 13153[1], 20660[0], 22208[1], 22505[0], 29000[0], 29010[0], 29015[0], 29035[0], 29040[0], 29044[0], 29046[0], 29200[0], 36000[1], 36400[1], 36405[1], 36406[1], 36410[1], 36420[1], 36425[1], 36430[1], 36440[1], 36591[0], 36592[0], 36600[1], 36640[1], 38220[0], 38222[0], 38230[0], 38232[0], 43752[1], 51701[1], 51702[1], 51703[1], 62320[0], 62321[0], 62322[0], 62323[0], 62324[0], 62325[0], 62326[0], 62327[0], 63707[1], 63709[1], 64400[0], 64405[0], 64408[0], 64415[0], 64416[0], 64417[0], 64418[0], 64420[0], 64421[0], 64425[0], 64430[0], 64435[0], 64445[0], 64446[0], 64447[0], 64448[0], 64449[0], 64450[1], 64451[0], 64454[1], 64461[0], 64462[0], 64463[0], 64479[0], 64480[0], 64483[0], 64484[0], 64486[0], 64487[0], 64488[0], 64489[0], 64490[0], 64491[0], 64492[0], 64493[0], 64494[0], 64495[0], 64505[0], 64510[0], 64517[0], 64520[0], 64530[0], 69990[0], 76000[1], 77001[1], 77002[1], 92012[1], 92014[1], 92585[0], 93000[1], 93005[1], 93010[1], 93040[1], 93041[1], 93042[1], 93318[1], 93355[1], 94002[1], 94200[1], 94250[1], 94680[1], 94681[1], 94690[1], 94770[1], 95812[1], 95813[1], 95816[1], 95819[1], 95822[0], 95829[1], 95860[0], 95861[0], 95863[0], 95864[0], 95865[0], 95866[0], 95867[0], 95868[0], 95869[0], 95870[0], 95907[0], 95908[0], 95909[0], 95910[0], 95911[0], 95912[0], 95913[0], 95925[0], 95926[0], 95927[0], 95928[0], 95929[0], 95930[0], 95933[0], 95937[0], 95938[0], 95939[0], 95940[0], 95955[1], 96360[1], 96361[1], 96365[1], 96366[1], 96367[1], 96368[1], 96372[1], 96374[1], 96375[1], 96376[1], 96377[1], 96523[0], 99155[0], 99156[0], 99157[0], 99211[1], 99212[1], 99213[1], 99214[1], 99215[1], 99217[1], 99218[1], 99219[1], 99220[1], 99221[1], 99222[1], 99223[1], 99231[1], 99232[1], 99233[1], 99234[1], 99235[1], 99236[1], 99238[1], 99239[1], 99241[1], 99242[1], 99243[1], 99244[1], 99245[1], 99251[1], 99252[1], 99253[1], 99254[1], 99255[1], 99291[1], 99292[1], 99304[1], 99305[1], 99306[1], 99307[1], 99308[1], 99309[1], 99310[1], 99315[1], 99316[1], 99334[1], 99335[1], 99336[1], 99337[1], 99347[1], 99348[1], 99349[1], 99350[1], 99374[1], 99375[1], 99377[1], 99378[1], 99446[0], 99447[0], 99448[0], 99449[0], 99451[0], 99452[0], 99495[0], 99496[0], G0453[0], G0463[1], G0471[1]
22840	0202T[1], 0228T[1], 0333T[0], 0464T[0], 20650[1], 22505[0], 22841[1], 22850[1], 22852[1], 22869[1], 22870[1], 36591[0], 36592[0], 38220[0], 38222[0], 38230[0], 38232[0], 51701[1], 51702[1], 51703[1], 62320[0], 62321[0], 62324[0], 62325[0], 63295[1], 63707[1], 63709[1], 64479[1], 92585[0], 95822[0], 95860[0], 95861[0], 95863[0], 95864[0], 95865[0], 95866[0], 95867[0], 95868[0], 95869[0], 95870[0], 95907[0], 95908[0], 95909[0], 95910[0], 95911[0], 95912[0], 95913[0], 95925[0], 95926[0], 95927[0], 95928[0], 95929[0], 95930[0], 95933[0], 95937[0], 95938[0], 95939[0], 95940[0], 96523[0], G0453[0], G0471[1]
22842	0228T[1], 0230T[1], 0333T[0], 0464T[0], 20650[1], 22505[0], 22840[1], 22841[1], 22850[1], 22852[1], 22869[1], 22870[1], 36591[0], 36592[0], 38220[0], 38222[0], 38230[0], 38232[0], 51701[1], 51702[1], 51703[1], 62320[0], 62321[0], 62322[0], 62323[0], 62324[0], 62325[0], 62326[0], 62327[0], 63295[1],

Appendix A: NCCI - CPT Codes

0 = Modifier usage not allowed or inappropriate 1 = Modifier usage allowed

Code 1	Code 2
	63707^1, 63709^1, 64479^1, 64483^1, 76000^1, 77001^1, 77002^1, 92585^0, 95822^0, 95860^0, 95861^0, 95863^0, 95864^0, 95865^0, 95866^0, 95867^0, 95868^0, 95869^0, 95870^0, 95907^0, 95908^0, 95909^0, 95910^0, 95911^0, 95912^0, 95913^0, 95925^0, 95926^0, 95927^0, 95928^0, 95929^0, 95930^0, 95933^0, 95937^0, 95938^0, 95939^0, 95940^0, 96523^0, G0453^0, G0471^1
22843	0228T^1, 0230T^1, 0333T^0, 0464T^0, 20650^1, 22505^0, 22840^1, 22841^1, 22842^1, 22850^1, 22852^1, 36591^0, 36592^0, 38220^0, 38222^0, 38230^0, 38232^0, 51701^1, 51702^1, 51703^1, 62320^0, 62321^0, 62322^0, 62323^0, 62324^0, 62325^0, 62326^0, 62327^0, 63295^1, 63707^1, 63709^1, 64479^1, 64483^1, 92585^0, 95822^0, 95860^0, 95861^0, 95863^0, 95864^0, 95865^0, 95866^0, 95867^0, 95868^0, 95869^0, 95870^0, 95907^0, 95908^0, 95909^0, 95910^0, 95911^0, 95912^0, 95913^0, 95925^0, 95926^0, 95927^0, 95928^0, 95929^0, 95930^0, 95933^0, 95937^0, 95938^0, 95939^0, 95940^0, 96523^0, G0453^0, G0471^1
22844	0228T^1, 0230T^1, 0333T^0, 0464T^0, 20650^1, 22505^0, 22840^1, 22841^1, 22842^1, 22843^1, 22850^1, 22852^1, 22855^1, 36591^0, 36592^0, 38220^0, 38222^0, 38230^0, 38232^0, 51701^1, 51702^1, 51703^1, 62320^0, 62321^0, 62322^0, 62323^0, 62324^0, 62325^0, 62326^0, 62327^0, 63295^1, 63707^1, 63709^1, 64479^1, 64483^1, 92585^0, 95822^0, 95860^0, 95861^0, 95863^0, 95864^0, 95865^0, 95866^0, 95867^0, 95868^0, 95869^0, 95870^0, 95907^0, 95908^0, 95909^0, 95910^0, 95911^0, 95912^0, 95913^0, 95925^0, 95926^0, 95927^0, 95928^0, 95929^0, 95930^0, 95933^0, 95937^0, 95938^0, 95939^0, 95940^0, 96523^0, G0453^0, G0471^1
22845	0228T^1, 0230T^1, 0333T^0, 0464T^0, 20650^1, 22505^0, 22850^1, 22852^1, 32100^1, 36591^0, 36592^0, 38220^0, 38222^0, 38230^0, 38232^0, 49000^0, 49002^1, 51701^1, 51702^1, 51703^1, 62320^0, 62321^0, 62322^0, 62323^0, 62324^0, 62325^0, 62326^0, 62327^0, 64479^1, 64483^1, 92585^0, 95822^0, 95860^0, 95861^0, 95863^0, 95864^0, 95865^0, 95866^0, 95867^0, 95868^0, 95869^0, 95870^0, 95907^0, 95908^0, 95909^0, 95910^0, 95911^0, 95912^0, 95913^0, 95925^0, 95926^0, 95927^0, 95928^0, 95929^0, 95930^0, 95933^0, 95937^0, 95938^0, 95939^0, 95940^0, 96523^0, G0453^0, G0471^1
22846	0228T^1, 0230T^1, 0333T^0, 0464T^0, 20650^1, 22505^0, 22845^1, 22850^1, 22852^1, 32100^1, 36591^0, 36592^0, 38220^0, 38222^0, 38230^0, 38232^0, 49000^0, 49002^1, 51701^1, 51702^1, 51703^1, 62320^0, 62321^0, 62322^0, 62323^0, 62324^0, 62325^0, 62326^0, 62327^0, 64479^1, 64483^1, 92585^0, 95822^0, 95860^0, 95861^0, 95863^0, 95864^0, 95865^0, 95866^0, 95867^0, 95868^0, 95869^0, 95870^0, 95907^0, 95908^0, 95909^0, 95910^0, 95911^0, 95912^0, 95913^0, 95925^0, 95926^0, 95927^0, 95928^0, 95929^0, 95930^0, 95933^0, 95937^0, 95938^0, 95939^0, 95940^0, 96523^0, G0453^0, G0471^1
22847	0228T^1, 0230T^1, 0333T^0, 0464T^0, 20650^1, 22505^0, 22845^1, 22846^1, 22850^1, 22852^1, 32100^1, 36591^0, 36592^0, 38220^0, 38222^0, 38230^0, 38232^0, 49000^0, 49002^1, 51701^1, 51702^1, 51703^1, 62320^0, 62321^0, 62322^0, 62323^0, 62324^0, 62325^0, 62326^0, 62327^0, 64479^1, 64483^1, 92585^0, 95822^0, 95860^0, 95861^0, 95863^0, 95864^0, 95865^0, 95866^0, 95867^0, 95868^0, 95869^0, 95870^0, 95907^0, 95908^0, 95909^0, 95910^0, 95911^0, 95912^0, 95913^0, 95925^0, 95926^0, 95927^0, 95928^0, 95929^0, 95930^0, 95933^0, 95937^0, 95938^0, 95939^0, 95940^0, 96523^0, G0453^0, G0471^1
22849	0213T^0, 0216T^0, 0228T^0, 0230T^0, 0333T^0, 0464T^0, 11000^1, 11001^1, 11004^1, 11005^1, 11006^1, 11042^1, 11043^1, 11044^1, 11045^1, 11046^1, 11047^1, 12001^1, 12002^1, 12004^1, 12005^1, 12006^1, 12007^1, 12011^1, 12013^1, 12014^1, 12015^1, 12016^1, 12017^1, 12018^1, 12020^1, 12021^1, 12031^1, 12032^1, 12034^1, 12035^1, 12036^1, 12037^1, 12041^1, 12042^1, 12044^1, 12045^1, 12046^1, 12047^1, 12051^1, 12052^1, 12053^1, 12054^1, 12055^1, 12056^1, 12057^1, 13100^1, 13101^1, 13102^1, 13120^1, 13121^1, 13122^1, 13131^1, 13132^1, 13133^1, 13151^1, 13152^1, 13153^1, 20650^1, 22505^0, 22840^1, 22841^0, 22842^1, 22843^1, 22844^1, 22845^1, 22846^1, 22847^1, 22848^1, 22850^1, 22852^1, 22853^1, 22854^1, 22855^1, 22859^1, 29000^0, 29010^0, 29015^0, 29035^0, 29040^0, 29044^0, 29046^0, 29200^0, 36000^1, 36400^1, 36405^1, 36406^1, 36410^1, 36420^1, 36425^1, 36430^1, 36440^1, 36591^0, 36592^0, 36600^1, 36640^1, 38220^0, 38222^0, 38230^0, 38232^0, 43752^1, 51701^1, 51702^1, 51703^1, 62320^0, 62321^0, 62322^0, 62323^0, 62324^0, 62325^0, 62326^0, 62327^0, 63707^1, 63709^1, 64400^0, 64405^0, 64408^0, 64415^0, 64416^0, 64417^0, 64418^0, 64420^0, 64421^0, 64425^0, 64430^0, 64435^0, 64445^0, 64446^0, 64447^0, 64448^0, 64449^0, 64450^1, 64451^0, 64454^1, 64461^0, 64462^0, 64463^0, 64479^0, 64480^0, 64483^0, 64484^0, 64486^0, 64487^0, 64488^0, 64489^0, 64490^0, 64491^0, 64492^0, 64493^0, 64494^0, 64495^0, 64505^0, 64510^0, 64517^0, 64520^0, 64530^0, 76000^1, 77001^1, 77002^1, 92012^1, 92014^1, 92585^0, 93000^1, 93005^1, 93010^1, 93040^1, 93041^1, 93042^1, 93318^1, 93355^1, 94002^1, 94200^1, 94250^1, 94680^1, 94681^1, 94690^1, 94770^1, 95812^1, 95813^1, 95816^1, 95819^1, 95822^0, 95829^1, 95860^0, 95861^0, 95863^0, 95864^0, 95865^0, 95866^0, 95867^0, 95868^0, 95869^0, 95870^0, 95907^0, 95908^0, 95909^0, 95910^0, 95911^0, 95912^0, 95913^0, 95925^0, 95926^0, 95927^0, 95928^0, 95929^0, 95930^0, 95933^0, 95937^0, 95938^0, 95939^0, 95940^0, 95955^1, 96360^1, 96361^1, 96365^1, 96366^1, 96367^1, 96368^1, 96372^1, 96374^1, 96375^1, 96376^1, 96377^1, 96523^0, 97597^1, 97598^1, 97602^1, 99155^0, 99156^0, 99157^0, 99211^1, 99212^1, 99213^1, 99214^1, 99215^1, 99217^1, 99218^1, 99219^1, 99220^1, 99221^1, 99222^1, 99223^1, 99231^1, 99232^1, 99233^1, 99234^1, 99235^1, 99236^1, 99238^1, 99239^1, 99241^1, 99242^1, 99243^1, 99244^1, 99245^1, 99251^1, 99252^1, 99253^1, 99254^1, 99255^1, 99291^1, 99292^1, 99304^1, 99305^1, 99306^1, 99307^1, 99308^1, 99309^1, 99310^1, 99315^1, 99316^1, 99334^1, 99335^1, 99336^1, 99337^1, 99347^1, 99348^1, 99349^1, 99350^1, 99374^1, 99375^1, 99377^1, 99378^1, 99446^0, 99447^0, 99448^0, 99449^0, 99451^0, 99452^0, 99495^0, 99496^0, G0453^0, G0463^1, G0471^1
22850	0213T^0, 0216T^0, 0228T^0, 0230T^0, 0333T^0, 0464T^0, 11000^1, 11001^1, 11004^1, 11005^1, 11006^1, 11042^1, 11043^1, 11044^1, 11045^1, 11046^1, 11047^1, 12001^1, 12002^1, 12004^1, 12005^1, 12006^1, 12007^1, 12011^1, 12013^1, 12014^1, 12015^1, 12016^1, 12017^1, 12018^1, 12020^1, 12021^1, 12031^1, 12032^1, 12034^1, 12035^1, 12036^1, 12037^1, 12041^1, 12042^1, 12044^1, 12045^1, 12046^1, 12047^1, 12051^1, 12052^1, 12053^1, 12054^1, 12055^1, 12056^1, 12057^1, 13100^1, 13101^1, 13102^1, 13120^1, 13121^1, 13122^1, 13131^1, 13132^1, 13133^1, 13151^1, 13152^1, 13153^1, 20650^1, 22010^1, 22015^1, 22505^0, 22830^1, 22841^0, 22848^1, 29000^0, 29010^0, 29015^0, 29035^0, 29040^0, 29044^0, 29046^0, 29200^0, 36000^1, 36400^1, 36405^1, 36406^1, 36410^1, 36420^1, 36425^1, 36430^1, 36440^1, 36591^0, 36592^0, 36600^1, 36640^1, 38220^0, 38222^0, 38230^0, 38232^0, 43752^1, 51701^1, 51702^1, 51703^1, 62320^0, 62321^0, 62322^0, 62323^0, 62324^0, 62325^0, 62326^0, 62327^0, 63707^1, 63709^1, 64400^0, 64405^0, 64408^0, 64415^0, 64416^0, 64417^0, 64418^0, 64420^0, 64421^0, 64425^0, 64430^0, 64435^0, 64445^0, 64446^0, 64447^0, 64448^0, 64449^0, 64450^1, 64451^0, 64454^1, 64461^0, 64462^0, 64463^0, 64479^0, 64480^0, 64483^0, 64484^0, 64486^0, 64487^0, 64488^0, 64489^0, 64490^0, 64491^0, 64492^0, 64493^0, 64494^0, 64495^0, 64505^0, 64510^0, 64517^0, 64520^0, 64530^0, 76000^1, 77001^1, 77002^1, 92012^1, 92014^1, 92585^0, 93000^1, 93005^1, 93010^1, 93040^1, 93041^1, 93042^1, 93318^1, 93355^1, 94002^1, 94200^1, 94250^1, 94680^1, 94681^1, 94690^1, 94770^1, 95812^1, 95813^1, 95816^1, 95819^1, 95822^0, 95829^1, 95860^0, 95861^0, 95863^0, 95864^0, 95865^0, 95866^0, 95867^0, 95868^0, 95869^0, 95870^0, 95907^0, 95908^0, 95909^0, 95910^0, 95911^0, 95912^0, 95913^0, 95925^0, 95926^0, 95927^0, 95928^0, 95929^0, 95930^0, 95933^0, 95937^0, 95938^0, 95939^0, 95940^0, 95955^1, 96360^1, 96361^1, 96365^1, 96366^1, 96367^1, 96368^1, 96372^1, 96374^1, 96375^1, 96376^1, 96377^1, 96523^0, 97597^1, 97598^1, 97602^1, 99155^0, 99156^0, 99157^0, 99211^1, 99212^1, 99213^1, 99214^1, 99215^1, 99217^1, 99218^1, 99219^1, 99220^1, 99221^1, 99222^1, 99223^1, 99231^1, 99232^1, 99233^1, 99234^1, 99235^1, 99236^1, 99238^1, 99239^1, 99241^1, 99242^1, 99243^1, 99244^1, 99245^1, 99251^1, 99252^1, 99253^1, 99254^1, 99255^1, 99291^1, 99292^1, 99304^1, 99305^1, 99306^1, 99307^1, 99308^1, 99309^1, 99310^1, 99315^1, 99316^1, 99334^1, 99335^1, 99336^1, 99337^1, 99347^1, 99348^1, 99349^1, 99350^1, 99374^1, 99375^1, 99377^1, 99378^1, 99446^0, 99447^0, 99448^0, 99449^0, 99451^0, 99452^0, 99495^0, 99496^0, G0453^0, G0463^1, G0471^1
22852	0213T^0, 0216T^0, 0228T^0, 0230T^0, 0333T^0, 0464T^0, 11000^1, 11001^1, 11004^1, 11005^1, 11006^1, 11042^1, 11043^1, 11044^1, 11045^1, 11046^1, 11047^1, 12001^1, 12002^1, 12004^1, 12005^1, 12006^1, 12007^1, 12011^1, 12013^1, 12014^1, 12015^1, 12016^1, 12017^1, 12018^1, 12020^1, 12021^1, 12031^1, 12032^1, 12034^1, 12035^1, 12036^1, 12037^1, 12041^1, 12042^1, 12044^1, 12045^1, 12046^1, 12047^1, 12051^1, 12052^1, 12053^1, 12054^1, 12055^1, 12056^1, 12057^1, 13100^1, 13101^1, 13102^1, 13120^1, 13121^1, 13122^1, 13131^1, 13132^1, 13133^1, 13151^1, 13152^1, 13153^1, 20650^1, 22010^1, 22015^1, 22505^0, 22830^1, 22841^0, 22848^1, 29000^0, 29010^0, 29015^0, 29035^0, 29040^0, 29044^0, 29046^0, 29200^0, 32100^1, 36000^1, 36400^1, 36405^1, 36406^1, 36410^1, 36420^1, 36425^1, 36430^1, 36440^1, 36591^0, 36592^0, 36600^1, 36640^1, 38220^0, 38222^0, 38230^0, 38232^0, 43752^1, 49010^0, 51701^1, 51702^1, 51703^1, 62320^0, 62321^0, 62322^0, 62323^0, 62324^0, 62325^0, 62326^0, 62327^0, 63707^1, 63709^1, 64400^0, 64405^0, 64408^0, 64415^0, 64416^0, 64417^0, 64418^0, 64420^0, 64421^0, 64425^0, 64430^0, 64435^0, 64445^0, 64446^0, 64447^0, 64448^0, 64449^0, 64450^1, 64451^0, 64454^1, 64461^0, 64462^0, 64463^0, 64479^0, 64480^0, 64483^0, 64484^0, 64486^0, 64487^0, 64488^0, 64489^0, 64490^0, 64491^0, 64492^0, 64493^0, 64494^0, 64495^0, 64505^0, 64510^0, 64517^0, 64520^0, 64530^0, 76000^1, 77001^1, 77002^1, 92012^1, 92014^1, 92585^0, 93000^1, 93005^1, 93010^1, 93040^1, 93041^1, 93042^1, 93318^1, 93355^1, 94002^1, 94200^1, 94250^1, 94680^1, 94681^1, 94690^1, 94770^1, 95812^1, 95813^1, 95816^1, 95819^1, 95822^0, 95829^1, 95860^0, 95861^0, 95863^0, 95864^0, 95865^0, 95866^0, 95867^0, 95868^0, 95869^0, 95870^0, 95907^0, 95908^0, 95909^0, 95910^0, 95911^0, 95912^0, 95913^0, 95925^0, 95926^0, 95927^0, 95928^0, 95929^0, 95930^0, 95933^0, 95937^0, 95938^0, 95939^0, 95940^0, 95955^1, 96360^1, 96361^1, 96365^1, 96366^1, 96367^1, 96368^1, 96372^1, 96374^1, 96375^1, 96376^1, 96377^1, 96523^0, 97597^1, 97598^1, 97602^1, 99155^0, 99156^0, 99157^0, 99211^1, 99212^1, 99213^1, 99214^1, 99215^1, 99217^1, 99218^1, 99219^1, 99220^1, 99221^1, 99222^1, 99223^1, 99231^1, 99232^1, 99233^1, 99234^1, 99235^1, 99236^1, 99238^1, 99239^1, 99241^1, 99242^1, 99243^1, 99244^1, 99245^1, 99251^1, 99252^1, 99253^1, 99254^1, 99255^1, 99291^1, 99292^1, 99304^1, 99305^1, 99306^1, 99307^1, 99308^1, 99309^1, 99310^1, 99315^1, 99316^1, 99334^1, 99335^1, 99336^1, 99337^1, 99347^1, 99348^1, 99349^1, 99350^1, 99374^1, 99375^1, 99377^1, 99378^1, 99446^0, 99447^0, 99448^0, 99449^0, 99451^0, 99452^0, 99495^0, 99496^0, G0453^0, G0463^1, G0471^1
22853	01935^0, 01936^0, 0213T^0, 0216T^0, 0228T^0, 0230T^0, 0333T^0, 0464T^0, 11010^1, 11011^1, 11012^1, 12001^1, 12002^1, 12004^1, 12005^1, 12006^1, 12007^1, 12011^1, 12013^1, 12014^1,

0 = Modifier usage not allowed or inappropriate   1 = Modifier usage allowed

Code 1	Code 2
	12015[1], 12016[1], 12017[1], 12018[1], 12020[1], 12021[1], 12031[1], 12032[1], 12034[1], 12035[1], 12036[1], 12037[1], 12041[1], 12042[1], 12044[1], 12045[1], 12046[1], 12047[1], 12051[1], 12052[1], 12053[1], 12054[1], 12055[1], 12056[1], 12057[1], 13100[1], 13101[1], 13102[1], 13120[1], 13121[1], 13122[1], 13131[1], 13132[1], 13133[1], 13151[1], 13152[1], 13153[1], 20650[1], 22505[0], 22845[1], 22846[1], 22847[1], 36000[1], 36400[1], 36405[1], 36406[1], 36410[1], 36420[1], 36425[1], 36430[1], 36440[1], 36591[0], 36592[0], 36600[1], 36640[1], 38220[0], 38222[0], 38230[0], 38232[0], 43752[1], 49000[0], 49002[1], 51701[1], 51702[1], 51703[1], 62320[0], 62321[0], 62322[0], 62323[0], 62324[0], 62325[0], 62326[0], 62327[0], 64400[0], 64405[0], 64408[0], 64415[0], 64416[0], 64417[0], 64418[0], 64420[0], 64421[0], 64425[0], 64430[0], 64435[0], 64445[0], 64446[0], 64447[0], 64448[0], 64449[0], 64450[1], 64451[0], 64454[1], 64461[0], 64462[0], 64463[0], 64479[0], 64480[0], 64483[0], 64484[0], 64486[0], 64487[0], 64488[0], 64489[0], 64490[0], 64491[0], 64492[0], 64493[0], 64494[0], 64495[0], 64505[0], 64510[0], 64517[0], 64520[0], 64530[0], 69990[0], 76000[1], 77001[1], 77002[1], 92012[1], 92014[1], 92585[0], 93000[1], 93005[1], 93010[1], 93040[1], 93041[1], 93042[1], 93318[1], 94002[1], 94200[1], 94250[1], 94680[1], 94681[1], 94690[1], 94770[1], 95812[1], 95813[1], 95816[1], 95819[1], 95822[0], 95829[1], 95860[0], 95861[0], 95863[0], 95864[0], 95865[0], 95866[0], 95867[0], 95868[0], 95869[0], 95870[0], 95907[0], 95908[0], 95909[0], 95910[0], 95911[0], 95912[0], 95913[0], 95925[0], 95926[0], 95927[0], 95928[0], 95929[0], 95930[0], 95933[0], 95937[0], 95938[0], 95939[0], 95940[0], 95941[0], 95955[1], 96360[1], 96361[1], 96365[1], 96366[1], 96367[1], 96368[1], 96372[1], 96374[1], 96375[1], 96376[1], 96377[1], 96523[0], 99155[0], 99156[0], 99157[0], 99211[1], 99212[1], 99213[1], 99214[1], 99215[1], 99217[1], 99218[1], 99219[1], 99220[1], 99221[1], 99222[1], 99223[1], 99231[1], 99232[1], 99233[1], 99234[1], 99235[1], 99236[1], 99238[1], 99239[1], 99241[1], 99242[1], 99243[1], 99244[1], 99245[1], 99251[1], 99252[1], 99253[1], 99254[1], 99255[1], 99291[1], 99292[1], 99304[1], 99305[1], 99306[1], 99307[1], 99308[1], 99309[1], 99310[1], 99315[1], 99316[1], 99334[1], 99335[1], 99336[1], 99337[1], 99347[1], 99348[1], 99349[1], 99350[1], 99374[1], 99375[1], 99377[1], 99378[1], G0453[0], G0471[1]
22854	01935[0], 01936[0], 0213T[0], 0216T[0], 0228T[0], 0230T[0], 0333T[0], 0464T[0], 11010[1], 11011[1], 11012[1], 12001[1], 12002[1], 12004[1], 12005[1], 12006[1], 12007[1], 12011[1], 12013[1], 12014[1], 12015[1], 12016[1], 12017[1], 12018[1], 12020[1], 12021[1], 12031[1], 12032[1], 12034[1], 12035[1], 12036[1], 12037[1], 12041[1], 12042[1], 12044[1], 12045[1], 12046[1], 12047[1], 12051[1], 12052[1], 12053[1], 12054[1], 12055[1], 12056[1], 12057[1], 13100[1], 13101[1], 13102[1], 13120[1], 13121[1], 13122[1], 13131[1], 13132[1], 13133[1], 13151[1], 13152[1], 13153[1], 20650[1], 22505[0], 22845[1], 22846[1], 22847[1], 36000[1], 36400[1], 36405[1], 36406[1], 36410[1], 36420[1], 36425[1], 36430[1], 36440[1], 36591[0], 36592[0], 36600[1], 36640[1], 38220[0], 38222[0], 38230[0], 38232[0], 43752[1], 49000[0], 49002[1], 51701[1], 51702[1], 51703[1], 62320[0], 62321[0], 62322[0], 62323[0], 62324[0], 62325[0], 62326[0], 62327[0], 64400[0], 64405[0], 64408[0], 64415[0], 64416[0], 64417[0], 64418[0], 64420[0], 64421[0], 64425[0], 64430[0], 64435[0], 64445[0], 64446[0], 64447[0], 64448[0], 64449[0], 64450[1], 64451[0], 64454[1], 64461[0], 64462[0], 64463[0], 64479[0], 64480[0], 64483[0], 64484[0], 64486[0], 64487[0], 64488[0], 64489[0], 64490[0], 64491[0], 64492[0], 64493[0], 64494[0], 64495[0], 64505[0], 64510[0], 64517[0], 64520[0], 64530[0], 69990[0], 76000[1], 77001[1], 77002[1], 92012[1], 92014[1], 92585[0], 93000[1], 93005[1], 93010[1], 93040[1], 93041[1], 93042[1], 93318[1], 94002[1], 94200[1], 94250[1], 94680[1], 94681[1], 94690[1], 94770[1], 95812[1], 95813[1], 95816[1], 95819[1], 95822[0], 95829[1], 95860[0], 95861[0], 95863[0], 95864[0], 95865[0], 95866[0], 95867[0], 95868[0], 95869[0], 95870[0], 95907[0], 95908[0], 95909[0], 95910[0], 95911[0], 95912[0], 95913[0], 95925[0], 95926[0], 95927[0], 95928[0], 95929[0], 95930[0], 95933[0], 95937[0], 95938[0], 95939[0], 95940[0], 95941[0], 95955[1], 96360[1], 96361[1], 96365[1], 96366[1], 96367[1], 96368[1], 96372[1], 96374[1], 96375[1], 96376[1], 96377[1], 96523[0], 99155[0], 99156[0], 99157[0], 99211[1], 99212[1], 99213[1], 99214[1], 99215[1], 99217[1], 99218[1], 99219[1], 99220[1], 99221[1], 99222[1], 99223[1], 99231[1], 99232[1], 99233[1], 99234[1], 99235[1], 99236[1], 99238[1], 99239[1], 99241[1], 99242[1], 99243[1], 99244[1], 99245[1], 99251[1], 99252[1], 99253[1], 99254[1], 99255[1], 99291[1], 99292[1], 99304[1], 99305[1], 99306[1], 99307[1], 99308[1], 99309[1], 99310[1], 99315[1], 99316[1], 99334[1], 99335[1], 99336[1], 99337[1], 99347[1], 99348[1], 99349[1], 99350[1], 99374[1], 99375[1], 99377[1], 99378[1], G0453[0], G0471[1]
22855	0213T[0], 0216T[0], 0228T[0], 0230T[0], 0333T[0], 0464T[0], 11000[1], 11001[1], 11004[1], 11005[1], 11006[1], 11042[1], 11043[1], 11044[1], 11045[1], 11046[1], 11047[1], 12001[1], 12002[1], 12004[1], 12005[1], 12006[1], 12007[1], 12011[1], 12013[1], 12014[1], 12015[1], 12016[1], 12017[1], 12018[1], 12020[1], 12021[1], 12031[1], 12032[1], 12034[1], 12035[1], 12036[1], 12037[1], 12041[1], 12042[1], 12044[1], 12045[1], 12046[1], 12047[1], 12051[1], 12052[1], 12053[1], 12054[1], 12055[1], 12056[1], 12057[1], 13100[1], 13101[1], 13102[1], 13120[1], 13121[1], 13122[1], 13131[1], 13132[1], 13133[1], 13151[1], 13152[1], 13153[1], 20650[1], 22505[0], 22830[1], 22840[1], 22841[0], 22842[1], 22843[1], 22845[1], 22846[1], 22847[1], 22848[1], 29000[0], 29010[0], 29015[0], 29035[0], 29040[0], 29044[0], 29046[0], 29200[0], 32100[1], 36000[1], 36400[1], 36405[1], 36406[1], 36410[1], 36420[1], 36425[1], 36430[1], 36440[1], 36591[0], 36592[0], 36600[1], 36640[1], 38220[0], 38222[0], 38230[0], 38232[0], 43752[1], 49000[0], 49002[1], 49010[0], 51701[1], 51702[1], 51703[1], 62320[0], 62321[0], 62322[0], 62323[0], 62324[0], 62325[0], 62326[0], 62327[0], 64400[0], 64405[0], 64408[0], 64415[0], 64416[0], 64417[0], 64418[0], 64420[0], 64421[0], 64425[0], 64430[0], 64435[0], 64445[0], 64446[0], 64447[0], 64448[0], 64449[0], 64450[1], 64451[0], 64454[1], 64461[0], 64462[0], 64463[0], 64479[0], 64480[0], 64483[0], 64484[0], 64486[0], 64487[0], 64488[0], 64489[0], 64490[0], 64491[0], 64492[0], 64493[0], 64494[0], 64495[0], 64505[0], 64510[0], 64517[0], 64520[0], 64530[0], 76000[1], 77001[1], 77002[1], 92012[1], 92014[1], 92585[0], 93000[1], 93005[1], 93010[1], 93040[1], 93041[1], 93042[1], 93318[1], 93355[1], 94002[1], 94200[1], 94250[1], 94680[1], 94681[1], 94690[1], 94770[1], 95812[1], 95813[1], 95816[1], 95819[1], 95822[0], 95829[1], 95860[0], 95861[0], 95863[0], 95864[0], 95865[0], 95866[0], 95867[0], 95868[0], 95869[0], 95870[0], 95907[0], 95908[0], 95909[0], 95910[0], 95911[0], 95912[0], 95913[0], 95925[0], 95926[0], 95927[0], 95928[0], 95929[0], 95930[0], 95933[0], 95937[0], 95938[0], 95939[0], 95940[0], 95955[1], 96360[1], 96361[1], 96365[1], 96366[1], 96367[1], 96368[1], 96372[1], 96374[1], 96375[1], 96376[1], 96377[1], 96523[0], 97597[1], 97598[1], 97602[1], 99155[0], 99156[0], 99157[0], 99211[1], 99212[1], 99213[1], 99214[1], 99215[1], 99217[1], 99218[1], 99219[1], 99220[1], 99221[1], 99222[1], 99223[1], 99231[1], 99232[1], 99233[1], 99234[1], 99235[1], 99236[1], 99238[1], 99239[1], 99241[1], 99242[1], 99243[1], 99244[1], 99245[1], 99251[1], 99252[1], 99253[1], 99254[1], 99255[1], 99291[1], 99292[1], 99304[1], 99305[1], 99306[1], 99307[1], 99308[1], 99309[1], 99310[1], 99315[1], 99316[1], 99334[1], 99335[1], 99336[1], 99337[1], 99347[1], 99348[1], 99349[1], 99350[1], 99374[1], 99375[1], 99377[1], 99378[1], 99446[0], 99447[0], 99448[0], 99449[0], 99451[0], 99452[0], 99495[0], 99496[0], G0453[0], G0463[1], G0471[1]
22859	01935[0], 01936[0], 0213T[0], 0216T[0], 0228T[0], 0230T[0], 0333T[0], 0464T[0], 11010[1], 11011[1], 11012[1], 12001[1], 12002[1], 12004[1], 12005[1], 12006[1], 12007[1], 12011[1], 12013[1], 12014[1], 12015[1], 12016[1], 12017[1], 12018[1], 12020[1], 12021[1], 12031[1], 12032[1], 12034[1], 12035[1], 12036[1], 12037[1], 12041[1], 12042[1], 12044[1], 12045[1], 12046[1], 12047[1], 12051[1], 12052[1], 12053[1], 12054[1], 12055[1], 12056[1], 12057[1], 13100[1], 13101[1], 13102[1], 13120[1], 13121[1], 13122[1], 13131[1], 13132[1], 13133[1], 13151[1], 13152[1], 13153[1], 20650[1], 22505[0], 36000[1], 36400[1], 36405[1], 36406[1], 36410[1], 36420[1], 36425[1], 36430[1], 36440[1], 36591[0], 36592[0], 36600[1], 36640[1], 38220[0], 38222[0], 38230[0], 38232[0], 43752[1], 49000[0], 49002[1], 51701[1], 51702[1], 51703[1], 62320[0], 62321[0], 62322[0], 62323[0], 62324[0], 62325[0], 62326[0], 62327[0], 64400[0], 64405[0], 64408[0], 64415[0], 64416[0], 64417[0], 64418[0], 64420[0], 64421[0], 64425[0], 64430[0], 64435[0], 64445[0], 64446[0], 64447[0], 64448[0], 64449[0], 64450[1], 64451[0], 64454[1], 64461[0], 64462[0], 64463[0], 64479[0], 64480[0], 64483[0], 64484[0], 64486[0], 64487[0], 64488[0], 64489[0], 64490[0], 64491[0], 64492[0], 64493[0], 64494[0], 64495[0], 64505[0], 64510[0], 64517[0], 64520[0], 64530[0], 69990[0], 76000[1], 77001[1], 77002[1], 92012[1], 92014[1], 92585[0], 93000[1], 93005[1], 93010[1], 93040[1], 93041[1], 93042[1], 93318[1], 94002[1], 94200[1], 94250[1], 94680[1], 94681[1], 94690[1], 94770[1], 95812[1], 95813[1], 95816[1], 95819[1], 95822[0], 95829[1], 95860[0], 95861[0], 95863[0], 95864[0], 95865[0], 95866[0], 95867[0], 95868[0], 95869[0], 95870[0], 95907[0], 95908[0], 95909[0], 95910[0], 95911[0], 95912[0], 95913[0], 95925[0], 95926[0], 95927[0], 95928[0], 95929[0], 95930[0], 95933[0], 95937[0], 95938[0], 95939[0], 95940[0], 95941[0], 95955[1], 96360[1], 96361[1], 96365[1], 96366[1], 96367[1], 96368[1], 96372[1], 96374[1], 96375[1], 96376[1], 96377[1], 96523[0], 99155[0], 99156[0], 99157[0], 99211[1], 99212[1], 99213[1], 99214[1], 99215[1], 99217[1], 99218[1], 99219[1], 99220[1], 99221[1], 99222[1], 99223[1], 99231[1], 99232[1], 99233[1], 99234[1], 99235[1], 99236[1], 99238[1], 99239[1], 99241[1], 99242[1], 99243[1], 99244[1], 99245[1], 99251[1], 99252[1], 99253[1], 99254[1], 99255[1], 99291[1], 99292[1], 99304[1], 99305[1], 99306[1], 99307[1], 99308[1], 99309[1], 99310[1], 99315[1], 99316[1], 99334[1], 99335[1], 99336[1], 99337[1], 99347[1], 99348[1], 99349[1], 99350[1], 99374[1], 99375[1], 99377[1], 99378[1], G0453[0], G0471[1]
22867	0202T[1], 0213T[0], 0216T[0], 0221T[1], 0228T[0], 0230T[0], 0275T[1], 0333T[0], 0464T[0], 11000[1], 11001[1], 11004[1], 11005[1], 11006[1], 11042[1], 11043[1], 11044[1], 11045[1], 11046[1], 11047[1], 12001[1], 12002[1], 12004[1], 12005[1], 12006[1], 12007[1], 12011[1], 12013[1], 12014[1], 12015[1], 12016[1], 12017[1], 12018[1], 12020[1], 12021[1], 12031[1], 12032[1], 12034[1], 12035[1], 12036[1], 12037[1], 12041[1], 12042[1], 12044[1], 12045[1], 12046[1], 12047[1], 12051[1], 12052[1], 12053[1], 12054[1], 12055[1], 12056[1], 12057[1], 13100[1], 13101[1], 13102[1], 13120[1], 13121[1], 13122[1], 13131[1], 13132[1], 13133[1], 13151[1], 13152[1], 13153[1], 20220[1], 20225[1], 20240[1], 20245[1], 20250[1], 20251[1], 22102[1], 22505[0], 22511[1], 22514[1], 22840[1], 22841[1], 22842[1], 22869[1], 22870[1], 36000[1], 36400[1], 36405[1], 36406[1], 36410[1], 36420[1], 36425[1], 36430[1], 36440[1], 36591[0], 36592[0], 36600[1], 36640[1], 38220[0], 38222[0], 38230[0], 38232[0], 43752[1], 51701[1], 51702[1], 51703[1], 61650[1], 62320[0], 62321[0], 62322[0], 62323[0], 62324[0], 62325[0], 62326[0], 62327[0], 62380[1], 63030[1], 63035[1], 64400[0], 64405[0], 64408[0], 64415[0], 64416[0], 64417[0], 64418[0], 64420[0], 64421[0], 64425[0], 64430[0], 64435[0], 64445[0], 64446[0], 64447[0], 64448[0], 64449[0], 64450[1], 64451[0], 64454[1], 64461[0], 64462[0], 64463[0], 64479[0], 64480[0], 64483[0], 64484[0], 64486[0], 64487[0], 64488[0], 64489[0], 64490[0], 64491[0], 64492[0], 64493[0], 64494[0], 64495[0], 64505[0], 64510[0], 64517[0], 64520[0], 64530[0], 69990[0], 76000[1], 76800[1], 76942[1], 76998[1], 77001[1], 77002[1], 77003[1], 92012[1], 92014[1], 92585[0], 93000[1], 93005[1], 93010[1], 93040[1], 93041[1], 93042[1], 93318[1], 94002[1], 94200[1], 94250[1], 94680[1], 94681[1], 94690[1], 94770[1], 95812[1], 95813[1], 95816[1], 95819[1], 95822[0], 95829[1], 95860[0], 95861[0], 95863[0], 95864[0], 95865[0], 95866[0], 95867[0], 95868[0], 95869[0], 95870[0], 95907[0], 95908[0], 95909[0], 95910[0], 95911[0], 95912[0], 95913[0], 95925[0], 95926[0], 95927[0], 95928[0], 95929[0], 95930[0], 95933[0], 95937[0], 95938[0], 95939[0], 95940[0], 95941[0], 95955[1], 96360[1], 96361[1], 96365[1], 96366[1], 96367[1], 96368[1], 96372[1], 96374[1], 96375[1], 96376[1], 96377[1], 96523[0], 97597[1], 97598[1], 97602[1], 99155[0], 99156[0], 99157[0], 99211[1], 99212[1], 99213[1], 99214[1], 99215[1],

0 = Modifier usage not allowed or inappropriate 1 = Modifier usage allowed

Code 1	Code 2
	99217[1], 99218[1], 99219[1], 99220[1], 99221[1], 99222[1], 99223[1], 99231[1], 99232[1], 99233[1], 99234[1], 99235[1], 99236[1], 99238[1], 99239[1], 99241[1], 99242[1], 99243[1], 99244[1], 99245[1], 99251[1], 99252[1], 99253[1], 99254[1], 99255[1], 99291[1], 99292[1], 99304[1], 99305[1], 99306[1], 99307[1], 99308[1], 99309[1], 99310[1], 99315[1], 99316[1], 99334[1], 99335[1], 99336[1], 99337[1], 99347[1], 99348[1], 99349[1], 99350[1], 99374[1], 99375[1], 99377[1], 99378[1], 99446[0], 99447[0], 99448[0], 99449[0], 99451[0], 99452[0], G0276[1], G0453[0]
22868	0202T[1], 0213T[0], 0216T[0], 0221T[1], 0228T[0], 0230T[0], 0275T[1], 0333T[0], 0464T[0], 11000[1], 11001[1], 11004[1], 11005[1], 11006[1], 11042[1], 11043[1], 11044[1], 11045[1], 11046[1], 11047[1], 12001[1], 12002[1], 12004[1], 12005[1], 12006[1], 12007[1], 12011[1], 12013[1], 12014[1], 12015[1], 12016[1], 12017[1], 12018[1], 12020[1], 12021[1], 12031[1], 12032[1], 12034[1], 12035[1], 12036[1], 12037[1], 12041[1], 12042[1], 12044[1], 12045[1], 12046[1], 12047[1], 12051[1], 12052[1], 12053[1], 12054[1], 12055[1], 12056[1], 12057[1], 13100[1], 13101[1], 13102[1], 13120[1], 13121[1], 13122[1], 13131[1], 13132[1], 13133[1], 13151[1], 13152[1], 13153[1], 20220[1], 20225[1], 20240[1], 20245[1], 20250[1], 20251[1], 22102[1], 22505[0], 22511[1], 22514[1], 22840[1], 22841[1], 22842[1], 22869[1], 22870[1], 36000[1], 36400[1], 36405[1], 36406[1], 36410[1], 36420[1], 36425[1], 36430[1], 36440[1], 36591[0], 36592[0], 36600[1], 36640[1], 38220[0], 38222[0], 38230[0], 38232[0], 43752[1], 51701[1], 51702[1], 51703[1], 61650[1], 62320[0], 62321[0], 62322[0], 62323[0], 62324[0], 62325[0], 62326[0], 62327[0], 62380[1], 63030[1], 63035[1], 64400[0], 64405[0], 64408[0], 64415[0], 64416[0], 64417[0], 64418[0], 64420[0], 64421[0], 64425[0], 64430[0], 64435[0], 64445[0], 64446[0], 64447[0], 64448[0], 64449[0], 64450[1], 64451[0], 64454[1], 64461[0], 64462[0], 64463[0], 64479[0], 64480[0], 64483[0], 64484[0], 64486[0], 64487[0], 64488[0], 64489[0], 64490[0], 64491[0], 64492[0], 64493[0], 64494[0], 64495[0], 64505[0], 64510[0], 64517[0], 64520[0], 64530[0], 69990[0], 76000[1], 76800[1], 76942[1], 76998[1], 77001[1], 77002[1], 77003[1], 92012[1], 92014[1], 92585[0], 93000[1], 93005[1], 93010[1], 93040[1], 93041[1], 93042[1], 93318[1], 94002[1], 94200[1], 94250[1], 94680[1], 94681[1], 94690[1], 94770[1], 95812[1], 95813[1], 95816[1], 95819[1], 95822[0], 95829[1], 95860[0], 95861[0], 95863[0], 95864[0], 95865[0], 95866[0], 95867[0], 95868[0], 95869[0], 95870[0], 95907[0], 95908[0], 95909[0], 95910[0], 95911[0], 95912[0], 95913[0], 95925[0], 95926[0], 95927[0], 95928[0], 95929[0], 95930[0], 95933[0], 95937[0], 95938[0], 95939[0], 95940[0], 95941[0], 95955[1], 96360[1], 96361[1], 96365[1], 96366[1], 96367[1], 96368[1], 96372[1], 96374[1], 96375[1], 96376[1], 96377[1], 96523[0], 97597[1], 97598[1], 97602[1], 99155[0], 99156[0], 99157[0], 99211[1], 99212[1], 99213[1], 99214[1], 99215[1], 99217[1], 99218[1], 99219[1], 99220[1], 99221[1], 99222[1], 99223[1], 99231[1], 99232[1], 99233[1], 99234[1], 99235[1], 99236[1], 99238[1], 99239[1], 99241[1], 99242[1], 99243[1], 99244[1], 99245[1], 99251[1], 99252[1], 99253[1], 99254[1], 99255[1], 99291[1], 99292[1], 99304[1], 99305[1], 99306[1], 99307[1], 99308[1], 99309[1], 99310[1], 99315[1], 99316[1], 99334[1], 99335[1], 99336[1], 99337[1], 99347[1], 99348[1], 99349[1], 99350[1], 99374[1], 99375[1], 99377[1], 99378[1], 99446[0], 99447[0], 99448[0], 99449[0], 99451[0], 99452[0], G0276[1], G0453[0]
27096	0216T[0], 0230T[1], 0566T[1], 12001[1], 12002[1], 12004[1], 12005[1], 12006[1], 12007[1], 12011[1], 12013[1], 12014[1], 12015[1], 12016[1], 12017[1], 12018[1], 12020[1], 12021[1], 12031[1], 12032[1], 12034[1], 12035[1], 12036[1], 12037[1], 12041[1], 12042[1], 12044[1], 12045[1], 12046[1], 12047[1], 12051[1], 12052[1], 12053[1], 12054[1], 12055[1], 12056[1], 12057[1], 13100[1], 13101[1], 13102[1], 13120[1], 13121[1], 13122[1], 13131[1], 13132[1], 13133[1], 13151[1], 13152[1], 13153[1], 20552[1], 20553[1], 20560[1], 20561[1], 20600[1], 20604[1], 20605[1], 20606[1], 20610[1], 20611[1], 20704[1], 36000[1], 36400[1], 36405[1], 36406[1], 36410[1], 36420[1], 36425[1], 36430[1], 36440[1], 36591[0], 36592[0], 36600[1], 36640[1], 43752[1], 51701[1], 51702[1], 51703[1], 62322[1], 62323[1], 62326[1], 62327[1], 64449[1], 64450[1], 64454[1], 64483[1], 64484[0], 64486[0], 64487[0], 64488[0], 64489[0], 69990[0], 76000[1], 76380[1], 76942[1], 76970[1], 76998[1], 77001[1], 77002[1], 77003[1], 77012[1], 92012[1], 92014[1], 93000[1], 93005[1], 93010[1], 93040[1], 93041[1], 93042[1], 93318[1], 93355[1], 94002[1], 94200[1], 94250[1], 94680[1], 94681[1], 94690[1], 94770[1], 95812[1], 95813[1], 95816[1], 95819[1], 95822[1], 95829[1], 95955[1], 96360[1], 96361[1], 96365[1], 96366[1], 96367[1], 96368[1], 96372[1], 96374[1], 96375[1], 96376[1], 96377[1], 96523[0], 99155[0], 99156[0], 99157[0], 99211[1], 99212[1], 99213[1], 99214[1], 99215[1], 99217[1], 99218[1], 99219[1], 99220[1], 99221[1], 99222[1], 99223[1], 99231[1], 99232[1], 99233[1], 99234[1], 99235[1], 99236[1], 99238[1], 99239[1], 99241[1], 99242[1], 99243[1], 99244[1], 99245[1], 99251[1], 99252[1], 99253[1], 99254[1], 99255[1], 99291[1], 99292[1], 99304[1], 99305[1], 99306[1], 99307[1], 99308[1], 99309[1], 99310[1], 99315[1], 99316[1], 99334[1], 99335[1], 99336[1], 99337[1], 99347[1], 99348[1], 99349[1], 99350[1], 99374[1], 99375[1], 99377[1], 99378[1], 99446[0], 99447[0], 99448[0], 99449[0], 99451[0], 99452[0], 99495[1], 99496[1], G0463[1], G0471[1], J0670[1], J1644[1], J2001[1]
27279	0213T[0], 0216T[0], 0228T[0], 0230T[0], 11010[1], 11011[1], 11012[1], 12001[1], 12002[1], 12004[1], 12005[1], 12006[1], 12007[1], 12011[1], 12013[1], 12014[1], 12015[1], 12016[1], 12017[1], 12018[1], 12020[1], 12021[1], 12031[1], 12032[1], 12034[1], 12035[1], 12036[1], 12037[1], 12041[1], 12042[1], 12044[1], 12045[1], 12046[1], 12047[1], 12051[1], 12052[1], 12053[1], 12054[1], 12055[1], 12056[1], 12057[1], 13100[1], 13101[1], 13102[1], 13120[1], 13121[1], 13122[1], 13131[1], 13132[1], 13133[1], 13151[1], 13152[1], 13153[1], 20650[1], 20690[1], 20692[1], 20696[1], 20900[1], 20902[1], 22848[1], 27218[1], 36000[1], 36400[1], 36405[1], 36406[1], 36410[1], 36420[1], 36425[1], 36430[1], 36440[1], 36591[0], 36592[0], 36600[1], 36640[1], 43752[1], 51701[1], 51702[1], 51703[1], 62320[0], 62321[0], 62322[0], 62323[0], 62324[0], 62325[0], 62326[0], 62327[0], 64400[0], 64405[0], 64408[0], 64415[0], 64416[0], 64417[0], 64418[0], 64420[0], 64421[0], 64425[0], 64430[0], 64435[0], 64445[0], 64446[0], 64447[0], 64448[0], 64449[0], 64450[1], 64451[0], 64454[1], 64461[0], 64462[0], 64463[0], 64479[0], 64480[0], 64483[0], 64484[0], 64486[0], 64487[0], 64488[0], 64489[0], 64490[0], 64491[0], 64492[0], 64493[0], 64494[0], 64495[0], 64505[0], 64510[0], 64517[0], 64520[0], 64530[0], 69990[0], 76000[1], 76380[1], 76942[1], 76970[1], 76998[1], 77002[1], 77003[1], 77012[1], 77021[1], 92012[1], 92014[1], 93000[1], 93005[1], 93010[1], 93040[1], 93041[1], 93042[1], 93318[1], 93355[1], 94002[1], 94200[1], 94250[1], 94680[1], 94681[1], 94690[1], 94770[1], 95812[1], 95813[1], 95816[1], 95819[1], 95822[1], 95829[1], 95955[1], 96360[1], 96361[1], 96365[1], 96366[1], 96367[1], 96368[1], 96372[1], 96374[1], 96375[1], 96376[1], 96377[1], 96523[0], 99155[0], 99156[0], 99157[0], 99211[1], 99212[1], 99213[1], 99214[1], 99215[1], 99217[1], 99218[1], 99219[1], 99220[1], 99221[1], 99222[1], 99223[1], 99231[1], 99232[1], 99233[1], 99234[1], 99235[1], 99236[1], 99238[1], 99239[1], 99241[1], 99242[1], 99243[1], 99244[1], 99245[1], 99251[1], 99252[1], 99253[1], 99254[1], 99255[1], 99291[1], 99292[1], 99304[1], 99305[1], 99306[1], 99307[1], 99308[1], 99309[1], 99310[1], 99315[1], 99316[1], 99334[1], 99335[1], 99336[1], 99337[1], 99347[1], 99348[1], 99349[1], 99350[1], 99374[1], 99375[1], 99377[1], 99378[1], 99446[0], 99447[0], 99448[0], 99449[0], 99451[0], 99452[0], 99495[0], 99496[0], G0463[1], G0471[1]
35301	0213T[0], 0216T[0], 0228T[0], 0230T[0], 11000[1], 11001[1], 11004[1], 11005[1], 11006[1], 11042[1], 11043[1], 11044[1], 11045[1], 11046[1], 11047[1], 12001[1], 12002[1], 12004[1], 12005[1], 12006[1], 12007[1], 12011[1], 12013[1], 12014[1], 12015[1], 12016[1], 12017[1], 12018[1], 12020[1], 12021[1], 12031[1], 12032[1], 12034[1], 12035[1], 12036[1], 12037[1], 12041[1], 12042[1], 12044[1], 12045[1], 12046[1], 12047[1], 12051[1], 12052[1], 12053[1], 12054[1], 12055[1], 12056[1], 12057[1], 13100[1], 13101[1], 13102[1], 13120[1], 13121[1], 13122[1], 13131[1], 13132[1], 13133[1], 13151[1], 13152[1], 13153[1], 34001[1], 35231[1], 35261[1], 35701[1], 35702[1], 35703[1], 35800[1], 36000[1], 36002[1], 36100[1], 36140[1], 36215[1], 36216[1], 36400[1], 36405[1], 36406[1], 36410[1], 36420[1], 36425[1], 36430[1], 36440[1], 36591[0], 36592[0], 36595[1], 36596[1], 36600[1], 36640[1], 36831[1], 36833[1], 36904[1], 36905[1], 36906[1], 37700[1], 37718[1], 37722[1], 38510[1], 43752[1], 51701[1], 51702[1], 51703[1], 62320[0], 62321[0], 62322[0], 62323[0], 62324[0], 62325[0], 62326[0], 62327[0], 64400[0], 64405[0], 64408[0], 64415[0], 64416[0], 64417[0], 64418[0], 64420[0], 64421[0], 64425[0], 64430[0], 64435[0], 64445[0], 64446[0], 64447[0], 64448[0], 64449[0], 64450[0], 64451[0], 64454[0], 64461[0], 64462[0], 64463[0], 64479[0], 64480[0], 64483[0], 64484[0], 64486[0], 64487[0], 64488[0], 64489[0], 64490[0], 64491[0], 64492[0], 64493[0], 64494[0], 64495[0], 64505[0], 64510[0], 64517[0], 64520[0], 64530[0], 69990[0], 75600[1], 75605[1], 92012[1], 92014[1], 93000[1], 93005[1], 93010[1], 93040[1], 93041[1], 93042[1], 93318[1], 93355[1], 94002[1], 94200[1], 94250[1], 94680[1], 94681[1], 94690[1], 94770[1], 95812[1], 95813[1], 95816[1], 95819[1], 95822[1], 95829[1], 95955[1], 96360[1], 96361[1], 96365[1], 96366[1], 96367[1], 96368[1], 96372[1], 96374[1], 96375[1], 96376[1], 96377[1], 96523[0], 97597[1], 97598[1], 97602[1], 99155[0], 99156[0], 99157[0], 99211[1], 99212[1], 99213[1], 99214[1], 99215[1], 99217[1], 99218[1], 99219[1], 99220[1], 99221[1], 99222[1], 99223[1], 99231[1], 99232[1], 99233[1], 99234[1], 99235[1], 99236[1], 99238[1], 99239[1], 99241[1], 99242[1], 99243[1], 99244[1], 99245[1], 99251[1], 99252[1], 99253[1], 99254[1], 99255[1], 99291[1], 99292[1], 99304[1], 99305[1], 99306[1], 99307[1], 99308[1], 99309[1], 99310[1], 99315[1], 99316[1], 99334[1], 99335[1], 99336[1], 99337[1], 99347[1], 99348[1], 99349[1], 99350[1], 99374[1], 99375[1], 99377[1], 99378[1], 99446[0], 99447[0], 99448[0], 99449[0], 99451[0], 99452[0], 99495[0], 99496[0], G0463[1], G0471[1]
36000	0543T[1], 0544T[1], 0548T[1], 0567T[1], 0568T[1], 0569T[1], 0570T[1], 0571T[1], 0572T[1], 0573T[1], 0574T[1], 0580T[1], 0581T[1], 0582T[1], 36591[0], 36592[0], 66987[1], 66988[1], 69990[0], 77001[1], 77002[1], 96523[0]
36215	01916[0], 01924[0], 01925[0], 01926[0], 35201[1], 35206[1], 35226[1], 35231[1], 35236[1], 35256[1], 35261[1], 35266[1], 35286[1], 36002[1], 36100[1], 36140[1], 36200[1], 36500[1], 36591[0], 36592[0], 69990[1], 75893[1], 76000[1], 77001[1], 77002[1], 93050[0], 96523[0], J0670[1], J1642[1], J1644[1], J2001[1]
36216	01916[0], 01924[0], 01925[0], 01926[0], 35201[1], 35206[1], 35226[1], 35231[1], 35236[1], 35256[1], 35261[1], 35266[1], 35286[1], 36002[1], 36100[1], 36140[1], 36200[1], 36215[1], 36500[1], 36591[0], 36592[0], 69990[1], 75893[1], 76000[1], 77001[1], 77002[1], 93050[0], 96523[0], J0670[1], J1642[1], J1644[1], J2001[1]
36217	01916[0], 01924[0], 01925[0], 01926[0], 35201[1], 35206[1], 35226[1], 35231[1], 35236[1], 35256[1], 35261[1], 35266[1], 35286[1], 36002[1], 36100[1], 36140[1], 36200[1], 36215[1], 36216[1], 36500[1], 36591[0], 36592[0], 69990[1], 75893[1], 76000[1], 77001[1], 77002[1], 93050[0], 96523[0], J0670[1], J1642[1], J1644[1], J2001[1]
36218	01916[0], 36002[1], 36591[0], 36592[0], 93050[0], 96523[0]
36222	01916[0], 01924[0], 01925[0], 01926[0], 12001[1], 12002[1], 12004[1], 12005[1], 12006[1], 12007[1], 12011[1], 12013[1], 12014[1], 12015[1], 12016[1], 12017[1], 12018[1], 12020[1], 12021[1], 12031[1], 12032[1], 12034[1], 12035[1], 12036[1], 12037[1], 12041[1], 12042[1], 12044[1], 12045[1], 12046[1], 12047[1], 12051[1], 12052[1], 12053[1], 12054[1], 12055[1], 12056[1], 12057[1], 13100[1], 13101[1], 13102[1], 13120[1], 13121[1], 13122[1], 13131[1], 13132[1], 13133[1], 13151[1], 13152[1], 13153[1], 35201[1], 35206[1], 35226[1], 35231[1], 35236[1], 35256[1], 35261[1], 35266[1], 35286[1], 36000[1],

0 = Modifier usage not allowed or inappropriate 1 = Modifier usage allowed

Code 1	Code 2
	36002[1], 36005[1], 36100[1], 36140[1], 36160[1], 36200[1], 36215[1], 36216[1], 36217[1], 36218[1], 36221[0], 36400[1], 36405[1], 36406[1], 36410[1], 36420[1], 36425[1], 36430[1], 36440[1], 36500[1], 36591[0], 36592[0], 36600[1], 36640[1], 43752[1], 51701[1], 51702[1], 51703[1], 62320[0], 62321[0], 62322[0], 62323[0], 62324[0], 62325[0], 62326[0], 62327[0], 64400[0], 64405[0], 64408[0], 64415[0], 64416[0], 64417[0], 64418[0], 64420[0], 64421[0], 64425[0], 64430[0], 64435[0], 64445[0], 64446[0], 64447[0], 64448[0], 64449[0], 64450[0], 64451[0], 64454[0], 64461[0], 64462[0], 64463[0], 64479[0], 64480[0], 64483[0], 64484[0], 64486[0], 64487[0], 64488[0], 64489[0], 64490[0], 64491[0], 64492[0], 64493[0], 64494[0], 64495[0], 64505[0], 64510[0], 64517[0], 64520[0], 64530[0], 69990[0], 75600[1], 75605[1], 75774[1], 75860[1], 75870[1], 75872[1], 75893[1], 76000[1], 76942[1], 76970[1], 76998[1], 77001[1], 77002[1], 92012[1], 92014[1], 93000[1], 93005[1], 93010[1], 93040[1], 93041[1], 93042[1], 93050[0], 93318[1], 93355[1], 94002[1], 94200[1], 94250[1], 94680[1], 94681[1], 94690[1], 94770[1], 95812[1], 95813[1], 95816[1], 95819[1], 95822[1], 95829[1], 95955[1], 96360[1], 96361[1], 96365[1], 96366[1], 96367[1], 96368[1], 96372[1], 96374[1], 96375[1], 96376[1], 96377[1], 96523[0], 99155[0], 99156[0], 99157[0], 99211[1], 99212[1], 99213[1], 99214[1], 99215[1], 99217[1], 99218[1], 99219[1], 99220[1], 99221[1], 99222[1], 99223[1], 99231[1], 99232[1], 99233[1], 99234[1], 99235[1], 99236[1], 99238[1], 99239[1], 99241[1], 99242[1], 99243[1], 99244[1], 99245[1], 99251[1], 99252[1], 99253[1], 99254[1], 99255[1], 99291[1], 99292[1], 99304[1], 99305[1], 99306[1], 99307[1], 99308[1], 99309[1], 99310[1], 99315[1], 99316[1], 99334[1], 99335[1], 99336[1], 99337[1], 99347[1], 99348[1], 99349[1], 99350[1], 99374[1], 99375[1], 99377[1], 99378[1], 99446[0], 99447[0], 99448[0], 99449[0], 99451[0], 99452[0], 99495[1], 99496[1], G0269[1], G0463[1], G0471[1], J0670[1], J1642[1], J1644[1], J2001[1]
36223	01916[0], 01924[0], 01925[0], 01926[0], 12001[1], 12002[1], 12004[1], 12005[1], 12006[1], 12007[1], 12011[1], 12013[1], 12014[1], 12015[1], 12016[1], 12017[1], 12018[1], 12020[1], 12021[1], 12031[1], 12032[1], 12034[1], 12035[1], 12036[1], 12037[1], 12041[1], 12042[1], 12044[1], 12045[1], 12046[1], 12047[1], 12051[1], 12052[1], 12053[1], 12054[1], 12055[1], 12056[1], 12057[1], 13100[1], 13101[1], 13102[1], 13120[1], 13121[1], 13122[1], 13131[1], 13132[1], 13133[1], 13151[1], 13152[1], 13153[1], 35201[1], 35206[1], 35226[1], 35231[1], 35236[1], 35256[1], 35261[1], 35266[1], 35286[1], 36000[1], 36002[1], 36005[1], 36100[1], 36140[1], 36160[1], 36200[1], 36215[1], 36216[1], 36217[1], 36218[1], 36221[0], 36222[1], 36400[1], 36405[1], 36406[1], 36410[1], 36420[1], 36425[1], 36430[1], 36440[1], 36500[1], 36591[0], 36592[0], 36600[1], 36640[1], 43752[1], 51701[1], 51702[1], 51703[1], 62320[0], 62321[0], 62322[0], 62323[0], 62324[0], 62325[0], 62326[0], 62327[0], 64400[0], 64405[0], 64408[0], 64415[0], 64416[0], 64417[0], 64418[0], 64420[0], 64421[0], 64425[0], 64430[0], 64435[0], 64445[0], 64446[0], 64447[0], 64448[0], 64449[0], 64450[0], 64451[0], 64454[0], 64461[0], 64462[0], 64463[0], 64479[0], 64480[0], 64483[0], 64484[0], 64486[0], 64487[0], 64488[0], 64489[0], 64490[0], 64491[0], 64492[0], 64493[0], 64494[0], 64495[0], 64505[0], 64510[0], 64517[0], 64520[0], 64530[0], 69990[0], 75600[1], 75605[1], 75774[1], 75860[1], 75870[1], 75872[1], 75893[1], 76000[1], 76942[1], 76970[1], 76998[1], 77001[1], 77002[1], 92012[1], 92014[1], 93000[1], 93005[1], 93010[1], 93040[1], 93041[1], 93042[1], 93050[0], 93318[1], 93355[1], 94002[1], 94200[1], 94250[1], 94680[1], 94681[1], 94690[1], 94770[1], 95812[1], 95813[1], 95816[1], 95819[1], 95822[1], 95829[1], 95955[1], 96360[1], 96361[1], 96365[1], 96366[1], 96367[1], 96368[1], 96372[1], 96374[1], 96375[1], 96376[1], 96377[1], 96523[0], 99155[0], 99156[0], 99157[0], 99211[1], 99212[1], 99213[1], 99214[1], 99215[1], 99217[1], 99218[1], 99219[1], 99220[1], 99221[1], 99222[1], 99223[1], 99231[1], 99232[1], 99233[1], 99234[1], 99235[1], 99236[1], 99238[1], 99239[1], 99241[1], 99242[1], 99243[1], 99244[1], 99245[1], 99251[1], 99252[1], 99253[1], 99254[1], 99255[1], 99291[1], 99292[1], 99304[1], 99305[1], 99306[1], 99307[1], 99308[1], 99309[1], 99310[1], 99315[1], 99316[1], 99334[1], 99335[1], 99336[1], 99337[1], 99347[1], 99348[1], 99349[1], 99350[1], 99374[1], 99375[1], 99377[1], 99378[1], 99446[0], 99447[0], 99448[0], 99449[0], 99451[0], 99452[0], 99495[1], 99496[1], G0269[1], G0463[1], G0471[1], J0670[1], J1642[1], J1644[1], J2001[1]
36224	01916[0], 01924[0], 01925[0], 01926[0], 12001[1], 12002[1], 12004[1], 12005[1], 12006[1], 12007[1], 12011[1], 12013[1], 12014[1], 12015[1], 12016[1], 12017[1], 12018[1], 12020[1], 12021[1], 12031[1], 12032[1], 12034[1], 12035[1], 12036[1], 12037[1], 12041[1], 12042[1], 12044[1], 12045[1], 12046[1], 12047[1], 12051[1], 12052[1], 12053[1], 12054[1], 12055[1], 12056[1], 12057[1], 13100[1], 13101[1], 13102[1], 13120[1], 13121[1], 13122[1], 13131[1], 13132[1], 13133[1], 13151[1], 13152[1], 13153[1], 35201[1], 35206[1], 35226[1], 35231[1], 35236[1], 35256[1], 35261[1], 35266[1], 35286[1], 36000[1], 36002[1], 36005[1], 36100[1], 36140[1], 36160[1], 36200[1], 36215[1], 36216[1], 36217[1], 36218[1], 36221[0], 36222[1], 36223[1], 36400[1], 36405[1], 36406[1], 36410[1], 36420[1], 36425[1], 36430[1], 36440[1], 36500[1], 36591[0], 36592[0], 36600[1], 36640[1], 43752[1], 51701[1], 51702[1], 51703[1], 62320[0], 62321[0], 62322[0], 62323[0], 62324[0], 62325[0], 62326[0], 62327[0], 64400[0], 64405[0], 64408[0], 64415[0], 64416[0], 64417[0], 64418[0], 64420[0], 64421[0], 64425[0], 64430[0], 64435[0], 64445[0], 64446[0], 64447[0], 64448[0], 64449[0], 64450[0], 64451[0], 64454[0], 64461[0], 64462[0], 64463[0], 64479[0], 64480[0], 64483[0], 64484[0], 64486[0], 64487[0], 64488[0], 64489[0], 64490[0], 64491[0], 64492[0], 64493[0], 64494[0], 64495[0], 64505[0], 64510[0], 64517[0], 64520[0], 64530[0], 69990[0], 75600[1], 75605[1], 75774[1], 75860[1], 75870[1], 75872[1], 75893[1], 76000[1], 76942[1], 76970[1], 76998[1], 77001[1], 77002[1], 92012[1], 92014[1], 93000[1], 93005[1], 93010[1], 93040[1], 93041[1], 93042[1], 93050[0], 93318[1], 93355[1], 94002[1], 94200[1], 94250[1], 94680[1], 94681[1], 94690[1], 94770[1], 95812[1], 95813[1], 95816[1], 95819[1], 95822[1], 95829[1], 95955[1], 96360[1], 96361[1], 96365[1], 96366[1], 96367[1], 96368[1], 96372[1], 96374[1], 96375[1], 96376[1], 96377[1], 96523[0], 99155[0], 99156[0], 99157[0], 99211[1], 99212[1], 99213[1], 99214[1], 99215[1], 99217[1], 99218[1], 99219[1], 99220[1], 99221[1], 99222[1], 99223[1], 99231[1], 99232[1], 99233[1], 99234[1], 99235[1], 99236[1], 99238[1], 99239[1], 99241[1], 99242[1], 99243[1], 99244[1], 99245[1], 99251[1], 99252[1], 99253[1], 99254[1], 99255[1], 99291[1], 99292[1], 99304[1], 99305[1], 99306[1], 99307[1], 99308[1], 99309[1], 99310[1], 99315[1], 99316[1], 99334[1], 99335[1], 99336[1], 99337[1], 99347[1], 99348[1], 99349[1], 99350[1], 99374[1], 99375[1], 99377[1], 99378[1], 99446[0], 99447[0], 99448[0], 99449[0], 99451[0], 99452[0], 99495[1], 99496[1], G0269[1], G0463[1], G0471[1], J0670[1], J1642[1], J1644[1], J2001[1]
36225	01916[0], 01924[0], 01925[0], 01926[0], 12001[1], 12002[1], 12004[1], 12005[1], 12006[1], 12007[1], 12011[1], 12013[1], 12014[1], 12015[1], 12016[1], 12017[1], 12018[1], 12020[1], 12021[1], 12031[1], 12032[1], 12034[1], 12035[1], 12036[1], 12037[1], 12041[1], 12042[1], 12044[1], 12045[1], 12046[1], 12047[1], 12051[1], 12052[1], 12053[1], 12054[1], 12055[1], 12056[1], 12057[1], 13100[1], 13101[1], 13102[1], 13120[1], 13121[1], 13122[1], 13131[1], 13132[1], 13133[1], 13151[1], 13152[1], 13153[1], 35201[1], 35206[1], 35226[1], 35231[1], 35236[1], 35256[1], 35261[1], 35266[1], 35286[1], 36000[1], 36002[1], 36005[1], 36100[1], 36140[1], 36160[1], 36200[1], 36215[1], 36216[1], 36217[1], 36221[0], 36400[1], 36405[1], 36406[1], 36410[1], 36420[1], 36425[1], 36430[1], 36440[1], 36500[1], 36591[0], 36592[0], 36600[1], 36640[1], 43752[1], 51701[1], 51702[1], 51703[1], 62320[0], 62321[0], 62322[0], 62323[0], 62324[0], 62325[0], 62326[0], 62327[0], 64400[0], 64405[0], 64408[0], 64415[0], 64416[0], 64417[0], 64418[0], 64420[0], 64421[0], 64425[0], 64430[0], 64435[0], 64445[0], 64446[0], 64447[0], 64448[0], 64449[0], 64450[0], 64451[0], 64454[0], 64461[0], 64462[0], 64463[0], 64479[0], 64480[0], 64483[0], 64484[0], 64486[0], 64487[0], 64488[0], 64489[0], 64490[0], 64491[0], 64492[0], 64493[0], 64494[0], 64495[0], 64505[0], 64510[0], 64517[0], 64520[0], 64530[0], 69990[0], 75600[1], 75605[1], 75774[1], 75860[1], 75870[1], 75872[1], 75893[1], 76000[1], 76942[1], 76970[1], 76998[1], 77001[1], 77002[1], 92012[1], 92014[1], 93000[1], 93005[1], 93010[1], 93040[1], 93041[1], 93042[1], 93050[0], 93318[1], 93355[1], 94002[1], 94200[1], 94250[1], 94680[1], 94681[1], 94690[1], 94770[1], 95812[1], 95813[1], 95816[1], 95819[1], 95822[1], 95829[1], 95955[1], 96360[1], 96361[1], 96365[1], 96366[1], 96367[1], 96368[1], 96372[1], 96374[1], 96375[1], 96376[1], 96377[1], 96523[0], 99155[0], 99156[0], 99157[0], 99211[1], 99212[1], 99213[1], 99214[1], 99215[1], 99217[1], 99218[1], 99219[1], 99220[1], 99221[1], 99222[1], 99223[1], 99231[1], 99232[1], 99233[1], 99234[1], 99235[1], 99236[1], 99238[1], 99239[1], 99241[1], 99242[1], 99243[1], 99244[1], 99245[1], 99251[1], 99252[1], 99253[1], 99254[1], 99255[1], 99291[1], 99292[1], 99304[1], 99305[1], 99306[1], 99307[1], 99308[1], 99309[1], 99310[1], 99315[1], 99316[1], 99334[1], 99335[1], 99336[1], 99337[1], 99347[1], 99348[1], 99349[1], 99350[1], 99374[1], 99375[1], 99377[1], 99378[1], 99446[0], 99447[0], 99448[0], 99449[0], 99451[0], 99452[0], 99495[1], 99496[1], G0269[1], G0463[1], G0471[1], J0670[1], J1642[1], J1644[1], J2001[1]
36226	01916[0], 01924[0], 01925[0], 01926[0], 12001[1], 12002[1], 12004[1], 12005[1], 12006[1], 12007[1], 12011[1], 12013[1], 12014[1], 12015[1], 12016[1], 12017[1], 12018[1], 12020[1], 12021[1], 12031[1], 12032[1], 12034[1], 12035[1], 12036[1], 12037[1], 12041[1], 12042[1], 12044[1], 12045[1], 12046[1], 12047[1], 12051[1], 12052[1], 12053[1], 12054[1], 12055[1], 12056[1], 12057[1], 13100[1], 13101[1], 13102[1], 13120[1], 13121[1], 13122[1], 13131[1], 13132[1], 13133[1], 13151[1], 13152[1], 13153[1], 35201[1], 35206[1], 35226[1], 35231[1], 35236[1], 35256[1], 35261[1], 35266[1], 35286[1], 36000[1], 36002[1], 36005[1], 36100[1], 36140[1], 36160[1], 36200[1], 36215[1], 36216[1], 36217[1], 36221[0], 36225[1], 36400[1], 36405[1], 36406[1], 36410[1], 36420[1], 36425[1], 36430[1], 36440[1], 36500[1], 36591[0], 36592[0], 36600[1], 36640[1], 43752[1], 51701[1], 51702[1], 51703[1], 62320[0], 62321[0], 62322[0], 62323[0], 62324[0], 62325[0], 62326[0], 62327[0], 64400[0], 64405[0], 64408[0], 64415[0], 64416[0], 64417[0], 64418[0], 64420[0], 64421[0], 64425[0], 64430[0], 64435[0], 64445[0], 64446[0], 64447[0], 64448[0], 64449[0], 64450[0], 64451[0], 64454[0], 64461[0], 64462[0], 64463[0], 64479[0], 64480[0], 64483[0], 64484[0], 64486[0], 64487[0], 64488[0], 64489[0], 64490[0], 64491[0], 64492[0], 64493[0], 64494[0], 64495[0], 64505[0], 64510[0], 64517[0], 64520[0], 64530[0], 69990[0], 75600[1], 75605[1], 75774[1], 75860[1], 75870[1], 75872[1], 75893[1], 76000[1], 76942[1], 76970[1], 76998[1], 77001[1], 77002[1], 92012[1], 92014[1], 93000[1], 93005[1], 93010[1], 93040[1], 93041[1], 93042[1], 93050[0], 93318[1], 93355[1], 94002[1], 94200[1], 94250[1], 94680[1], 94681[1], 94690[1], 94770[1], 95812[1], 95813[1], 95816[1], 95819[1], 95822[1], 95829[1], 95955[1], 96360[1], 96361[1], 96365[1], 96366[1], 96367[1], 96368[1], 96372[1], 96374[1], 96375[1], 96376[1], 96377[1], 96523[0], 99155[0], 99156[0], 99157[0], 99211[1], 99212[1], 99213[1], 99214[1], 99215[1], 99217[1], 99218[1], 99219[1], 99220[1], 99221[1], 99222[1], 99223[1], 99231[1], 99232[1], 99233[1], 99234[1], 99235[1], 99236[1], 99238[1], 99239[1], 99241[1], 99242[1], 99243[1], 99244[1], 99245[1], 99251[1], 99252[1], 99253[1], 99254[1], 99255[1], 99291[1], 99292[1], 99304[1], 99305[1], 99306[1], 99307[1], 99308[1], 99309[1], 99310[1], 99315[1], 99316[1], 99334[1], 99335[1], 99336[1], 99337[1], 99347[1], 99348[1], 99349[1], 99350[1], 99374[1], 99375[1], 99377[1], 99378[1], 99446[0], 99447[0], 99448[0], 99449[0], 99451[0], 99452[0], 99495[1], 99496[1], G0269[1], G0463[1], G0471[1], J0670[1], J1642[1], J1644[1], J2001[1]
36227	35201[1], 35206[1], 35226[1], 35231[1], 35236[1], 35256[1], 35261[1], 35266[1], 35286[1], 36160[1], 36200[1], 36215[1], 36216[1], 36217[1], 36218[1], 36221[0], 36591[0], 36592[0], 51702[1], 75774[1], 76000[1], 93050[0], 96523[0], G0269[1], G0471[1]

Appendix A: NCCI - CPT Codes

0 = Modifier usage not allowed or inappropriate   1 = Modifier usage allowed

Code 1	Code 2
36228	35201[1], 35206[1], 35226[1], 35231[1], 35236[1], 35256[1], 35261[1], 35266[1], 35286[1], 36160[1], 36200[1], 36215[1], 36216[1], 36217[1], 36218[1], 36221[0], 36591[0], 36592[0], 51702[1], 75774[1], 76000[1], 93050[0], 96523[0], G0269[1], G0471[1]
36415	36591[0], 36592[0], 96523[0], 99211[1]
36416	36591[0], 36592[0], 96523[0]
37215	0075T[1], 01924[0], 01925[0], 01926[0], 0213T[0], 0216T[0], 0228T[0], 0230T[0], 11000[1], 11001[1], 11004[1], 11005[1], 11006[1], 11042[1], 11043[1], 11044[1], 11045[1], 11046[1], 11047[1], 12001[1], 12002[1], 12004[1], 12005[1], 12006[1], 12007[1], 12011[1], 12013[1], 12014[1], 12015[1], 12016[1], 12017[1], 12018[1], 12020[1], 12021[1], 12031[1], 12032[1], 12034[1], 12035[1], 12036[1], 12037[1], 12041[1], 12042[1], 12044[1], 12045[1], 12046[1], 12047[1], 12051[1], 12052[1], 12053[1], 12054[1], 12055[1], 12056[1], 12057[1], 13100[1], 13101[1], 13102[1], 13120[1], 13121[1], 13122[1], 13131[1], 13132[1], 13133[1], 13151[1], 13152[1], 13153[1], 34713[1], 34714[1], 34715[1], 34716[1], 34812[1], 34820[1], 34834[1], 35201[1], 35206[1], 35226[1], 35231[1], 35236[1], 35256[1], 35261[1], 35266[1], 35286[1], 36000[1], 36100[1], 36140[1], 36200[1], 36215[1], 36216[1], 36217[1], 36222[1], 36223[1], 36224[1], 36245[1], 36400[1], 36405[1], 36406[1], 36410[1], 36420[1], 36425[1], 36430[1], 36440[1], 36500[1], 36591[0], 36592[0], 36600[1], 36620[1], 36625[1], 36640[1], 37184[1], 37217[1], 37218[1], 37236[1], 37246[1], 37247[1], 43752[1], 51701[1], 51702[1], 51703[1], 61645[1], 62320[0], 62321[0], 62322[0], 62323[0], 62324[0], 62325[0], 62326[0], 62327[0], 64400[0], 64405[0], 64408[0], 64415[0], 64416[0], 64417[0], 64418[0], 64420[0], 64421[0], 64425[0], 64430[0], 64435[0], 64445[0], 64446[0], 64447[0], 64448[0], 64449[0], 64450[0], 64451[0], 64454[0], 64461[0], 64462[0], 64463[0], 64479[0], 64480[0], 64483[0], 64484[0], 64486[0], 64487[0], 64488[0], 64489[0], 64490[0], 64491[0], 64492[0], 64493[0], 64494[0], 64495[0], 64505[0], 64510[0], 64517[0], 64520[0], 64530[0], 69990[0], 75605[1], 75893[1], 76000[1], 76380[1], 76942[1], 76970[1], 76998[1], 77001[1], 77002[1], 77012[1], 77021[1], 92012[1], 92014[1], 93000[1], 93005[1], 93010[1], 93040[1], 93041[1], 93042[1], 93050[0], 93318[1], 93355[1], 94002[1], 94200[1], 94250[1], 94680[1], 94681[1], 94690[1], 94770[1], 95812[1], 95813[1], 95816[1], 95819[1], 95822[1], 95829[1], 95955[1], 96360[1], 96361[1], 96365[1], 96366[1], 96367[1], 96368[1], 96372[1], 96374[1], 96375[1], 96376[1], 96377[1], 96523[0], 97597[1], 97598[1], 97602[1], 99155[0], 99156[0], 99157[0], 99211[1], 99212[1], 99213[1], 99214[1], 99215[1], 99217[1], 99218[1], 99219[1], 99220[1], 99221[1], 99222[1], 99223[1], 99231[1], 99232[1], 99233[1], 99234[1], 99235[1], 99236[1], 99238[1], 99239[1], 99241[1], 99242[1], 99243[1], 99244[1], 99245[1], 99251[1], 99252[1], 99253[1], 99254[1], 99255[1], 99291[1], 99292[1], 99304[1], 99305[1], 99306[1], 99307[1], 99308[1], 99309[1], 99310[1], 99315[1], 99316[1], 99334[1], 99335[1], 99336[1], 99337[1], 99347[1], 99348[1], 99349[1], 99350[1], 99374[1], 99375[1], 99377[1], 99378[1], 99446[0], 99447[0], 99448[0], 99449[0], 99451[0], 99452[0], 99495[0], 99496[0], G0463[1], G0471[1]
37216	11000[1], 11001[1], 11004[1], 11005[1], 11006[1], 11042[1], 11043[1], 11044[1], 11045[1], 11046[1], 11047[1], 12001[1], 12002[1], 12004[1], 12005[1], 12006[1], 12007[1], 12011[1], 12013[1], 12014[1], 12015[1], 12016[1], 12017[1], 12018[1], 12020[1], 12021[1], 12031[1], 12032[1], 12034[1], 12035[1], 12036[1], 12037[1], 12041[1], 12042[1], 12044[1], 12045[1], 12046[1], 12047[1], 12051[1], 12052[1], 12053[1], 12054[1], 12055[1], 12056[1], 12057[1], 13100[1], 13101[1], 13102[1], 13120[1], 13121[1], 13122[1], 13131[1], 13132[1], 13133[1], 13151[1], 13152[1], 13153[1], 36222[1], 36223[1], 36224[1], 36400[1], 36405[1], 36406[1], 36420[1], 36425[1], 36430[1], 36440[1], 36591[0], 36592[0], 36600[1], 36640[1], 37236[1], 43752[1], 62320[0], 62321[0], 62322[0], 62323[0], 64400[0], 64405[0], 64408[0], 64418[0], 64420[0], 64421[0], 64425[0], 64430[0], 64435[0], 64445[0], 64446[0], 64447[0], 64448[0], 64449[0], 64451[0], 64461[0], 64462[0], 64463[0], 64479[0], 64480[0], 64483[0], 64484[0], 64486[0], 64487[0], 64488[0], 64489[0], 64490[0], 64491[0], 64492[0], 64493[0], 64494[0], 64495[0], 64505[0], 64510[0], 64517[0], 64520[0], 64530[0], 92012[1], 92014[1], 93000[1], 93005[1], 93010[1], 93040[1], 93041[1], 93042[1], 93050[0], 93318[1], 93355[1], 94002[1], 94200[1], 94250[1], 94680[1], 94681[1], 94690[1], 94770[1], 95812[1], 95813[1], 95816[1], 95819[1], 95822[1], 95829[1], 95955[1], 96360[1], 96361[1], 96365[1], 96366[1], 96367[1], 96368[1], 96372[1], 96374[1], 96375[1], 96376[1], 96377[1], 96523[0], 97597[1], 97598[1], 97602[1], 99155[0], 99156[0], 99157[0], 99211[1], 99212[1], 99213[1], 99214[1], 99215[1], 99217[1], 99218[1], 99219[1], 99220[1], 99221[1], 99222[1], 99223[1], 99231[1], 99232[1], 99233[1], 99234[1], 99235[1], 99236[1], 99238[1], 99239[1], 99241[1], 99242[1], 99243[1], 99244[1], 99245[1], 99251[1], 99252[1], 99253[1], 99254[1], 99255[1], 99291[1], 99292[1], 99304[1], 99305[1], 99306[1], 99307[1], 99308[1], 99309[1], 99310[1], 99315[1], 99316[1], 99334[1], 99335[1], 99336[1], 99337[1], 99347[1], 99348[1], 99349[1], 99350[1], 99374[1], 99375[1], 99377[1], 99378[1], 99446[0], 99447[0], 99448[0], 99449[0], 99451[0], 99452[0], 99495[0], 99496[0], G0463[1]
51784	00910[0], 0213T[0], 0216T[0], 0228T[0], 0230T[0], 0333T[1], 0464T[1], 12001[1], 12002[1], 12004[1], 12005[1], 12006[1], 12007[1], 12011[1], 12013[1], 12014[1], 12015[1], 12016[1], 12017[1], 12018[1], 12020[1], 12021[1], 12031[1], 12032[1], 12034[1], 12035[1], 12036[1], 12037[1], 12041[1], 12042[1], 12044[1], 12045[1], 12046[1], 12047[1], 12051[1], 12052[1], 12053[1], 12054[1], 12055[1], 12056[1], 12057[1], 13100[1], 13101[1], 13102[1], 13120[1], 13121[1], 13122[1], 13131[1], 13132[1], 13133[1], 13151[1], 13152[1], 13153[1], 36000[1], 36400[1], 36405[1], 36406[1], 36410[1], 36420[1], 36425[1], 36430[1], 36440[1], 36591[0], 36592[0], 36600[1], 36640[1], 43752[1], 50715[1], 51701[0], 51703[1], 51785[1], 62320[0], 62321[0], 62322[0], 62323[0], 62324[0], 62325[0], 62326[0], 62327[0], 64400[0], 64405[0], 64408[0], 64415[0], 64416[0], 64417[0], 64418[0], 64420[0], 64421[0], 64425[0], 64430[0], 64435[0], 64445[0], 64446[0], 64447[0], 64448[0], 64449[0], 64450[0], 64451[0], 64454[0], 64461[0], 64463[0], 64479[0], 64483[0], 64486[0], 64487[0], 64488[0], 64489[0], 64490[0], 64493[0], 64505[0], 64510[0], 64517[0], 64520[0], 64530[0], 69990[0], 92012[1], 92014[1], 92585[1], 93000[1], 93005[1], 93010[1], 93040[1], 93041[1], 93042[1], 93318[1], 93355[1], 94002[1], 94200[1], 94250[1], 94680[1], 94681[1], 94690[1], 94770[1], 95812[1], 95813[1], 95816[1], 95819[1], 95822[1], 95829[1], 95860[1], 95861[1], 95867[1], 95868[1], 95870[1], 95907[1], 95908[1], 95909[1], 95910[1], 95911[1], 95912[1], 95913[1], 95925[1], 95926[1], 95927[1], 95930[1], 95933[1], 95937[1], 95940[1], 95955[1], 96360[1], 96361[1], 96365[1], 96366[1], 96367[1], 96368[1], 96372[1], 96374[1], 96375[1], 96376[1], 96377[1], 96523[0], 99155[0], 99156[0], 99157[0], 99211[1], 99212[1], 99213[1], 99214[1], 99215[1], 99217[1], 99218[1], 99219[1], 99220[1], 99221[1], 99222[1], 99223[1], 99231[1], 99232[1], 99233[1], 99234[1], 99235[1], 99236[1], 99238[1], 99239[1], 99241[1], 99242[1], 99243[1], 99244[1], 99245[1], 99251[1], 99252[1], 99253[1], 99254[1], 99255[1], 99291[1], 99292[1], 99304[1], 99305[1], 99306[1], 99307[1], 99308[1], 99309[1], 99310[1], 99315[1], 99316[1], 99334[1], 99335[1], 99336[1], 99337[1], 99347[1], 99348[1], 99349[1], 99350[1], 99374[1], 99375[1], 99377[1], 99378[1], 99446[0], 99447[0], 99448[0], 99449[0], 99451[0], 99452[0], 99495[1], 99496[1], G0453[1], G0463[1]
51785	00910[0], 0213T[0], 0216T[0], 0228T[0], 0230T[0], 0333T[1], 0464T[1], 12001[1], 12002[1], 12004[1], 12005[1], 12006[1], 12007[1], 12011[1], 12013[1], 12014[1], 12015[1], 12016[1], 12017[1], 12018[1], 12020[1], 12021[1], 12031[1], 12032[1], 12034[1], 12035[1], 12036[1], 12037[1], 12041[1], 12042[1], 12044[1], 12045[1], 12046[1], 12047[1], 12051[1], 12052[1], 12053[1], 12054[1], 12055[1], 12056[1], 12057[1], 13100[1], 13101[1], 13102[1], 13120[1], 13121[1], 13122[1], 13131[1], 13132[1], 13133[1], 13151[1], 13152[1], 13153[1], 36000[1], 36400[1], 36405[1], 36406[1], 36410[1], 36420[1], 36425[1], 36430[1], 36440[1], 36591[0], 36592[0], 36600[1], 36640[1], 43752[1], 50715[1], 51701[0], 51702[0], 51703[0], 62320[0], 62321[0], 62322[0], 62323[0], 62324[0], 62325[0], 62326[0], 62327[0], 64400[0], 64405[0], 64408[0], 64415[0], 64416[0], 64417[0], 64418[0], 64420[0], 64421[0], 64425[0], 64430[0], 64435[0], 64445[0], 64446[0], 64447[0], 64448[0], 64449[0], 64450[0], 64451[0], 64454[0], 64461[0], 64463[0], 64479[0], 64483[0], 64486[0], 64487[0], 64488[0], 64489[0], 64490[0], 64493[0], 64505[0], 64510[0], 64517[0], 64520[0], 64530[0], 69990[0], 92012[1], 92014[1], 92585[1], 93000[1], 93005[1], 93010[1], 93040[1], 93041[1], 93042[1], 93318[1], 93355[1], 94002[1], 94200[1], 94250[1], 94680[1], 94681[1], 94690[1], 94770[1], 95812[1], 95813[1], 95816[1], 95819[1], 95822[1], 95829[1], 95860[1], 95861[1], 95867[1], 95868[1], 95870[1], 95907[1], 95908[1], 95909[1], 95910[1], 95911[1], 95912[1], 95913[1], 95925[1], 95926[1], 95927[1], 95930[1], 95933[1], 95937[1], 95940[1], 95955[1], 96360[1], 96361[1], 96365[1], 96366[1], 96367[1], 96368[1], 96372[1], 96374[1], 96375[1], 96376[1], 96377[1], 96523[0], 99155[0], 99156[0], 99157[0], 99211[1], 99212[1], 99213[1], 99214[1], 99215[1], 99217[1], 99218[1], 99219[1], 99220[1], 99221[1], 99222[1], 99223[1], 99231[1], 99232[1], 99233[1], 99234[1], 99235[1], 99236[1], 99238[1], 99239[1], 99241[1], 99242[1], 99243[1], 99244[1], 99245[1], 99251[1], 99252[1], 99253[1], 99254[1], 99255[1], 99291[1], 99292[1], 99304[1], 99305[1], 99306[1], 99307[1], 99308[1], 99309[1], 99310[1], 99315[1], 99316[1], 99334[1], 99335[1], 99336[1], 99337[1], 99347[1], 99348[1], 99349[1], 99350[1], 99374[1], 99375[1], 99377[1], 99378[1], 99446[0], 99447[0], 99448[0], 99449[0], 99451[0], 99452[0], 99495[1], 99496[1], G0453[1], G0463[1], G0471[0], P9612[0]
61020	0213T[0], 0216T[0], 0228T[0], 0230T[0], 0333T[0], 0464T[0], 12001[1], 12002[1], 12004[1], 12005[1], 12006[1], 12007[1], 12011[1], 12013[1], 12014[1], 12015[1], 12016[1], 12017[1], 12018[1], 12020[1], 12021[1], 12031[1], 12032[1], 12034[1], 12035[1], 12036[1], 12037[1], 12041[1], 12042[1], 12044[1], 12045[1], 12046[1], 12047[1], 12051[1], 12052[1], 12053[1], 12054[1], 12055[1], 12056[1], 12057[1], 13100[1], 13101[1], 13102[1], 13120[1], 13121[1], 13122[1], 13131[1], 13132[1], 13133[1], 13151[1], 13152[1], 13153[1], 36000[1], 36400[1], 36405[1], 36406[1], 36410[1], 36420[1], 36425[1], 36430[1], 36440[1], 36591[0], 36592[0], 36600[1], 36640[1], 43752[1], 51701[1], 51702[1], 51703[1], 61000[1], 61001[1], 61070[1], 62100[1], 62320[0], 62321[0], 62322[0], 62323[0], 62324[0], 62325[0], 62326[0], 62327[0], 64400[0], 64405[0], 64408[0], 64415[0], 64416[0], 64417[0], 64418[0], 64420[0], 64421[0], 64425[0], 64430[0], 64435[0], 64445[0], 64446[0], 64447[0], 64448[0], 64449[0], 64450[0], 64451[0], 64454[0], 64461[0], 64462[0], 64463[0], 64479[0], 64480[0], 64483[0], 64484[0], 64486[0], 64487[0], 64488[0], 64489[0], 64490[0], 64491[0], 64492[0], 64493[0], 64494[0], 64495[0], 64505[0], 64510[0], 64517[0], 64520[0], 64530[0], 69990[0], 92012[1], 92014[1], 92585[0], 93000[1], 93005[1], 93010[1], 93040[1], 93041[1], 93042[1], 93318[1], 93355[1], 94002[1], 94200[1], 94250[1], 94680[1], 94681[1], 94690[1], 94770[1], 95812[1], 95813[1], 95816[1], 95819[1], 95822[0], 95829[1], 95860[0], 95861[0], 95863[0], 95864[0], 95865[0], 95866[0], 95867[0], 95868[0], 95869[0], 95870[0], 95907[0], 95908[0], 95909[0], 95910[0], 95911[0], 95912[0], 95913[0], 95925[0], 95926[0], 95927[0], 95928[0], 95929[0], 95930[0], 95933[0], 95937[0], 95938[0], 95939[0], 95940[0], 95955[1], 96360[1], 96361[1], 96365[1], 96366[1], 96367[1], 96368[1], 96372[1], 96374[1], 96375[1], 96376[1], 96377[1], 96523[0], 99155[0], 99156[0], 99157[0], 99211[1], 99212[1], 99213[1], 99214[1], 99215[1], 99217[1], 99218[1], 99219[1], 99220[1], 99221[1], 99222[1], 99223[1], 99231[1], 99232[1], 99233[1], 99234[1], 99235[1], 99236[1], 99238[1], 99239[1], 99241[1], 99242[1], 99243[1], 99244[1], 99245[1], 99251[1], 99252[1], 99253[1], 99254[1], 99255[1], 99291[1], 99292[1], 99304[1], 99305[1], 99306[1], 99307[1], 99308[1], 99309[1], 99310[1], 99315[1], 99316[1], 99334[1], 99335[1], 99336[1], 99337[1], 99347[1], 99348[1], 99349[1], 99350[1], 99374[1], 99375[1], 99377[1], 99378[1], 99446[0], 99447[0], 99448[0], 99449[0], 99451[0], 99452[0], 99495[1], 99496[1], G0453[0], G0463[1], G0471[1], J2001[1]

0 = Modifier usage not allowed or inappropriate 1 = Modifier usage allowed

Code 1	Code 2
61026	0213T^0, 0216T^0, 0228T^0, 0230T^0, 0333T^0, 0464T^0, 12001^1, 12002^1, 12004^1, 12005^1, 12006^1, 12007^1, 12011^1, 12013^1, 12014^1, 12015^1, 12016^1, 12017^1, 12018^1, 12020^1, 12021^1, 12031^1, 12032^1, 12034^1, 12035^1, 12036^1, 12037^1, 12041^1, 12042^1, 12044^1, 12045^1, 12046^1, 12047^1, 12051^1, 12052^1, 12053^1, 12054^1, 12055^1, 12056^1, 12057^1, 13100^1, 13101^1, 13102^1, 13120^1, 13121^1, 13122^1, 13131^1, 13132^1, 13133^1, 13151^1, 13152^1, 13153^1, 36000^1, 36400^1, 36405^1, 36406^1, 36410^1, 36420^1, 36425^1, 36430^1, 36440^1, 36591^0, 36592^0, 36600^1, 36640^1, 43752^1, 51701^1, 51702^1, 51703^1, 61000^1, 61001^1, 61020^1, 61070^1, 62100^1, 62320^0, 62321^0, 62322^0, 62323^0, 62324^0, 62325^0, 62326^0, 62327^0, 64400^0, 64405^0, 64408^0, 64415^0, 64416^0, 64417^0, 64418^0, 64420^0, 64421^0, 64425^0, 64430^0, 64435^0, 64445^0, 64446^0, 64447^0, 64448^0, 64449^0, 64450^0, 64451^0, 64454^0, 64461^0, 64462^0, 64463^0, 64479^0, 64480^0, 64483^0, 64484^0, 64486^0, 64487^0, 64488^0, 64489^0, 64490^0, 64491^0, 64492^0, 64493^0, 64494^0, 64495^0, 64505^0, 64510^0, 64517^0, 64520^0, 64530^0, 69990^0, 92012^1, 92014^1, 92585^0, 93000^1, 93005^1, 93010^1, 93040^1, 93041^1, 93042^1, 93318^1, 93355^1, 94002^1, 94200^1, 94250^1, 94680^1, 94681^1, 94690^1, 94770^1, 95812^1, 95813^1, 95816^1, 95819^1, 95822^0, 95829^1, 95860^0, 95861^0, 95863^0, 95864^0, 95865^0, 95866^0, 95867^0, 95868^0, 95869^0, 95870^0, 95907^0, 95908^0, 95909^0, 95910^0, 95911^0, 95912^0, 95913^0, 95925^0, 95926^0, 95927^0, 95928^0, 95929^0, 95930^0, 95933^0, 95937^0, 95938^0, 95939^0, 95940^0, 95955^1, 96360^1, 96361^1, 96365^1, 96366^1, 96367^1, 96368^1, 96372^1, 96374^1, 96375^1, 96376^1, 96377^1, 96523^0, 99155^0, 99156^0, 99157^0, 99211^1, 99212^1, 99213^1, 99214^1, 99215^1, 99217^1, 99218^1, 99219^1, 99220^1, 99221^1, 99222^1, 99223^1, 99231^1, 99232^1, 99233^1, 99234^1, 99235^1, 99236^1, 99238^1, 99239^1, 99241^1, 99242^1, 99243^1, 99244^1, 99245^1, 99251^1, 99252^1, 99253^1, 99254^1, 99255^1, 99291^1, 99292^1, 99304^1, 99305^1, 99306^1, 99307^1, 99308^1, 99309^1, 99310^1, 99315^1, 99316^1, 99334^1, 99335^1, 99336^1, 99337^1, 99347^1, 99348^1, 99349^1, 99350^1, 99374^1, 99375^1, 99377^1, 99378^1, 99446^0, 99447^0, 99448^0, 99449^0, 99451^0, 99452^0, 99495^1, 99496^1, G0453^0, G0463^1, G0471^1, J2001^1
61070	0213T^0, 0216T^0, 0228T^0, 0230T^0, 0333T^0, 0464T^0, 12001^1, 12002^1, 12004^1, 12005^1, 12006^1, 12007^1, 12011^1, 12013^1, 12014^1, 12015^1, 12016^1, 12017^1, 12018^1, 12020^1, 12021^1, 12031^1, 12032^1, 12034^1, 12035^1, 12036^1, 12037^1, 12041^1, 12042^1, 12044^1, 12045^1, 12046^1, 12047^1, 12051^1, 12052^1, 12053^1, 12054^1, 12055^1, 12056^1, 12057^1, 13100^1, 13101^1, 13102^1, 13120^1, 13121^1, 13122^1, 13131^1, 13132^1, 13133^1, 13151^1, 13152^1, 13153^1, 36000^1, 36400^1, 36405^1, 36406^1, 36410^1, 36420^1, 36425^1, 36430^1, 36440^1, 36591^0, 36592^0, 36600^1, 36640^1, 43752^1, 51701^1, 51702^1, 51703^1, 62320^0, 62321^0, 62322^0, 62323^0, 62324^0, 62325^0, 62326^0, 62327^0, 64400^0, 64405^0, 64408^0, 64415^0, 64416^0, 64417^0, 64418^0, 64420^0, 64421^0, 64425^0, 64430^0, 64435^0, 64445^0, 64446^0, 64447^0, 64448^0, 64449^0, 64450^0, 64451^0, 64454^0, 64461^0, 64462^0, 64463^0, 64479^0, 64480^0, 64483^0, 64484^0, 64486^0, 64487^0, 64488^0, 64489^0, 64490^0, 64491^0, 64492^0, 64493^0, 64494^0, 64495^0, 64505^0, 64510^0, 64517^0, 64520^0, 64530^0, 69990^0, 76000^1, 76942^1, 76970^1, 76998^1, 77001^1, 77002^1, 92012^1, 92014^1, 92585^0, 93000^1, 93005^1, 93010^1, 93040^1, 93041^1, 93042^1, 93318^1, 93355^1, 94002^1, 94200^1, 94250^1, 94680^1, 94681^1, 94690^1, 94770^1, 95812^1, 95813^1, 95816^1, 95819^1, 95822^0, 95829^1, 95860^0, 95861^0, 95863^0, 95864^0, 95865^0, 95866^0, 95867^0, 95868^0, 95869^0, 95870^0, 95907^0, 95908^0, 95909^0, 95910^0, 95911^0, 95912^0, 95913^0, 95925^0, 95926^0, 95927^0, 95928^0, 95929^0, 95930^0, 95933^0, 95937^0, 95938^0, 95939^0, 95940^0, 95955^1, 96360^1, 96361^1, 96365^1, 96366^1, 96367^1, 96368^1, 96372^1, 96374^1, 96375^1, 96376^1, 96377^1, 96523^0, 99155^0, 99156^0, 99157^0, 99211^1, 99212^1, 99213^1, 99214^1, 99215^1, 99217^1, 99218^1, 99219^1, 99220^1, 99221^1, 99222^1, 99223^1, 99231^1, 99232^1, 99233^1, 99234^1, 99235^1, 99236^1, 99238^1, 99239^1, 99241^1, 99242^1, 99243^1, 99244^1, 99245^1, 99251^1, 99252^1, 99253^1, 99254^1, 99255^1, 99291^1, 99292^1, 99304^1, 99305^1, 99306^1, 99307^1, 99308^1, 99309^1, 99310^1, 99315^1, 99316^1, 99334^1, 99335^1, 99336^1, 99337^1, 99347^1, 99348^1, 99349^1, 99350^1, 99374^1, 99375^1, 99377^1, 99378^1, 99446^0, 99447^0, 99448^0, 99449^0, 99451^0, 99452^0, 99495^1, 99496^1, G0453^0, G0463^1, G0471^1, J2001^1
61105	0213T^0, 0216T^0, 0228T^0, 0230T^0, 0333T^0, 0464T^0, 12001^1, 12002^1, 12004^1, 12005^1, 12006^1, 12007^1, 12011^1, 12013^1, 12014^1, 12015^1, 12016^1, 12017^1, 12018^1, 12020^1, 12021^1, 12031^1, 12032^1, 12034^1, 12035^1, 12036^1, 12037^1, 12041^1, 12042^1, 12044^1, 12045^1, 12046^1, 12047^1, 12051^1, 12052^1, 12053^1, 12054^1, 12055^1, 12056^1, 12057^1, 13100^1, 13101^1, 13102^1, 13120^1, 13121^1, 13122^1, 13131^1, 13132^1, 13133^1, 13151^1, 13152^1, 13153^1, 36000^1, 36400^1, 36405^1, 36406^1, 36410^1, 36420^1, 36425^1, 36430^1, 36440^1, 36591^0, 36592^0, 36600^1, 36640^1, 43752^1, 51701^1, 51702^1, 51703^1, 61796^1, 61798^1, 62320^0, 62321^0, 62322^0, 62323^0, 62324^0, 62325^0, 62326^0, 62327^0, 63620^1, 64400^0, 64405^0, 64408^0, 64415^0, 64416^0, 64417^0, 64418^0, 64420^0, 64421^0, 64425^0, 64430^0, 64435^0, 64445^0, 64446^0, 64447^0, 64448^0, 64449^0, 64450^0, 64451^0, 64454^0, 64461^0, 64462^0, 64463^0, 64479^0, 64480^0, 64483^0, 64484^0, 64486^0, 64487^0, 64488^0, 64489^0, 64490^0, 64491^0, 64492^0, 64493^0, 64494^0, 64495^0, 64505^0, 64510^0, 64517^0, 64520^0, 64530^0, 69990^1, 92012^1, 92014^1, 92585^0, 93000^1, 93005^1, 93010^1, 93040^1, 93041^1, 93042^1, 93318^1, 93355^1, 94002^1, 94200^1, 94250^1, 94680^1, 94681^1, 94690^1, 94770^1, 95812^1, 95813^1, 95816^1, 95819^1, 95822^0, 95829^1, 95860^0, 95861^0, 95863^0, 95864^0, 95865^0, 95866^0, 95867^0, 95868^0, 95869^0, 95870^0, 95907^0, 95908^0, 95909^0, 95910^0, 95911^0, 95912^0, 95913^0, 95925^0, 95926^0, 95927^0, 95928^0, 95929^0, 95930^0, 95933^0, 95937^0, 95938^0, 95939^0, 95940^0, 95955^1, 96360^1, 96361^1, 96365^1, 96366^1, 96367^1, 96368^1, 96372^1, 96374^1, 96375^1, 96376^1, 96377^1, 96523^0, 99155^0, 99156^0, 99157^0, 99211^1, 99212^1, 99213^1, 99214^1, 99215^1, 99217^1, 99218^1, 99219^1, 99220^1, 99221^1, 99222^1, 99223^1, 99231^1, 99232^1, 99233^1, 99234^1, 99235^1, 99236^1, 99238^1, 99239^1, 99241^1, 99242^1, 99243^1, 99244^1, 99245^1, 99251^1, 99252^1, 99253^1, 99254^1, 99255^1, 99291^1, 99292^1, 99304^1, 99305^1, 99306^1, 99307^1, 99308^1, 99309^1, 99310^1, 99315^1, 99316^1, 99334^1, 99335^1, 99336^1, 99337^1, 99347^1, 99348^1, 99349^1, 99350^1, 99374^1, 99375^1, 99377^1, 99378^1, 99446^0, 99447^0, 99448^0, 99449^0, 99451^0, 99452^0, 99495^0, 99496^0, G0339^1, G0340^1, G0453^0, G0463^1, G0471^1
61107	0213T^0, 0216T^0, 0228T^0, 0230T^0, 0333T^0, 0464T^0, 12001^1, 12002^1, 12004^1, 12005^1, 12006^1, 12007^1, 12011^1, 12013^1, 12014^1, 12015^1, 12016^1, 12017^1, 12018^1, 12020^1, 12021^1, 12031^1, 12032^1, 12034^1, 12035^1, 12036^1, 12037^1, 12041^1, 12042^1, 12044^1, 12045^1, 12046^1, 12047^1, 12051^1, 12052^1, 12053^1, 12054^1, 12055^1, 12056^1, 12057^1, 13100^1, 13101^1, 13102^1, 13120^1, 13121^1, 13122^1, 13131^1, 13132^1, 13133^1, 13151^1, 13152^1, 13153^1, 36000^1, 36400^1, 36405^1, 36406^1, 36410^1, 36420^1, 36425^1, 36430^1, 36440^1, 36591^0, 36592^0, 36600^1, 36640^1, 43752^1, 51701^1, 51702^1, 51703^1, 61105^1, 61796^1, 61798^1, 62320^0, 62321^0, 62322^0, 62323^0, 62324^0, 62325^0, 62326^0, 62327^0, 63620^1, 64400^0, 64405^0, 64408^0, 64415^0, 64416^0, 64417^0, 64418^0, 64420^0, 64421^0, 64425^0, 64430^0, 64435^0, 64445^0, 64446^0, 64447^0, 64448^0, 64449^0, 64450^0, 64451^0, 64454^0, 64461^0, 64462^0, 64463^0, 64479^0, 64480^0, 64483^0, 64484^0, 64486^0, 64487^0, 64488^0, 64489^0, 64490^0, 64491^0, 64492^0, 64493^0, 64494^0, 64495^0, 64505^0, 64510^0, 64517^0, 64520^0, 64530^0, 69990^1, 92012^1, 92014^1, 92585^0, 93000^1, 93005^1, 93010^1, 93040^1, 93041^1, 93042^1, 93318^1, 93355^1, 94002^1, 94200^1, 94250^1, 94680^1, 94681^1, 94690^1, 94770^1, 95812^1, 95813^1, 95816^1, 95819^1, 95822^0, 95829^1, 95860^0, 95861^0, 95863^0, 95864^0, 95865^0, 95866^0, 95867^0, 95868^0, 95869^0, 95870^0, 95907^0, 95908^0, 95909^0, 95910^0, 95911^0, 95912^0, 95913^0, 95925^0, 95926^0, 95927^0, 95928^0, 95929^0, 95930^0, 95933^0, 95937^0, 95938^0, 95939^0, 95940^0, 95955^1, 96360^1, 96361^1, 96365^1, 96366^1, 96367^1, 96368^1, 96372^1, 96374^1, 96375^1, 96376^1, 96377^1, 96523^0, 99155^0, 99156^0, 99157^0, 99211^1, 99212^1, 99213^1, 99214^1, 99215^1, 99217^1, 99218^1, 99219^1, 99220^1, 99221^1, 99222^1, 99223^1, 99231^1, 99232^1, 99233^1, 99234^1, 99235^1, 99236^1, 99238^1, 99239^1, 99241^1, 99242^1, 99243^1, 99244^1, 99245^1, 99251^1, 99252^1, 99253^1, 99254^1, 99255^1, 99291^1, 99292^1, 99304^1, 99305^1, 99306^1, 99307^1, 99308^1, 99309^1, 99310^1, 99315^1, 99316^1, 99334^1, 99335^1, 99336^1, 99337^1, 99347^1, 99348^1, 99349^1, 99350^1, 99374^1, 99375^1, 99377^1, 99378^1, 99446^0, 99447^0, 99448^0, 99449^0, 99451^0, 99452^0, 99495^1, 99496^1, G0339^1, G0340^1, G0453^0, G0463^1, G0471^1
61108	0213T^0, 0216T^0, 0228T^0, 0230T^0, 0333T^0, 0464T^0, 12001^1, 12002^1, 12004^1, 12005^1, 12006^1, 12007^1, 12011^1, 12013^1, 12014^1, 12015^1, 12016^1, 12017^1, 12018^1, 12020^1, 12021^1, 12031^1, 12032^1, 12034^1, 12035^1, 12036^1, 12037^1, 12041^1, 12042^1, 12044^1, 12045^1, 12046^1, 12047^1, 12051^1, 12052^1, 12053^1, 12054^1, 12055^1, 12056^1, 12057^1, 13100^1, 13101^1, 13102^1, 13120^1, 13121^1, 13122^1, 13131^1, 13132^1, 13133^1, 13151^1, 13152^1, 13153^1, 36000^1, 36400^1, 36405^1, 36406^1, 36410^1, 36420^1, 36425^1, 36430^1, 36440^1, 36591^0, 36592^0, 36600^1, 36640^1, 43752^1, 51701^1, 51702^1, 51703^1, 61105^1, 61107^1, 62320^0, 62321^0, 62322^0, 62323^0, 62324^0, 62325^0, 62326^0, 62327^0, 64400^0, 64405^0, 64408^0, 64415^0, 64416^0, 64417^0, 64418^0, 64420^0, 64421^0, 64425^0, 64430^0, 64435^0, 64445^0, 64446^0, 64447^0, 64448^0, 64449^0, 64450^0, 64451^0, 64454^0, 64461^0, 64462^0, 64463^0, 64479^0, 64480^0, 64483^0, 64484^0, 64486^0, 64487^0, 64488^0, 64489^0, 64490^0, 64491^0, 64492^0, 64493^0, 64494^0, 64495^0, 64505^0, 64510^0, 64517^0, 64520^0, 64530^0, 69990^1, 92012^1, 92014^1, 92585^0, 93000^1, 93005^1, 93010^1, 93040^1, 93041^1, 93042^1, 93318^1, 93355^1, 94002^1, 94200^1, 94250^1, 94680^1, 94681^1, 94690^1, 94770^1, 95812^1, 95813^1, 95816^1, 95819^1, 95822^0, 95829^1, 95860^0, 95861^0, 95863^0, 95864^0, 95865^0, 95866^0, 95867^0, 95868^0, 95869^0, 95870^0, 95907^0, 95908^0, 95909^0, 95910^0, 95911^0, 95912^0, 95913^0, 95925^0, 95926^0, 95927^0, 95928^0, 95929^0, 95930^0, 95933^0, 95937^0, 95938^0, 95939^0, 95940^0, 95955^1, 96360^1, 96361^1, 96365^1, 96366^1, 96367^1, 96368^1, 96372^1, 96374^1, 96375^1, 96376^1, 96377^1, 96523^0, 99155^0, 99156^0, 99157^0, 99211^1, 99212^1, 99213^1, 99214^1, 99215^1, 99217^1, 99218^1, 99219^1, 99220^1, 99221^1, 99222^1, 99223^1, 99231^1, 99232^1, 99233^1, 99234^1, 99235^1, 99236^1, 99238^1, 99239^1, 99241^1, 99242^1, 99243^1, 99244^1, 99245^1, 99251^1, 99252^1, 99253^1, 99254^1, 99255^1, 99291^1, 99292^1, 99304^1, 99305^1, 99306^1, 99307^1, 99308^1, 99309^1, 99310^1, 99315^1, 99316^1, 99334^1, 99335^1, 99336^1, 99337^1, 99347^1, 99348^1, 99349^1, 99350^1, 99374^1, 99375^1, 99377^1, 99378^1, 99446^0, 99447^0, 99448^0, 99449^0, 99451^0, 99452^0, 99495^0, 99496^0, G0453^0, G0463^1, G0471^1

Code 1	Code 2
61140	0213T[0], 0216T[0], 0228T[0], 0230T[0], 0333T[0], 0464T[0], 10005[1], 10007[1], 10009[1], 10011[1], 10021[1], 12001[1], 12002[1], 12004[1], 12005[1], 12006[1], 12007[1], 12011[1], 12013[1], 12014[1], 12015[1], 12016[1], 12017[1], 12018[1], 12020[1], 12021[1], 12031[1], 12032[1], 12034[1], 12035[1], 12036[1], 12037[1], 12041[1], 12042[1], 12044[1], 12045[1], 12046[1], 12047[1], 12051[1], 12052[1], 12053[1], 12054[1], 12055[1], 12056[1], 12057[1], 13100[1], 13101[1], 13102[1], 13120[1], 13121[1], 13122[1], 13131[1], 13132[1], 13133[1], 13151[1], 13152[1], 13153[1], 36000[1], 36400[1], 36405[1], 36406[1], 36410[1], 36420[1], 36425[1], 36430[1], 36440[1], 36591[0], 36592[0], 36600[1], 36640[1], 43752[1], 51701[1], 51702[1], 51703[1], 61150[1], 61156[1], 61796[1], 61798[1], 62100[1], 62320[0], 62321[0], 62322[0], 62323[0], 62324[0], 62325[0], 62326[0], 62327[0], 63620[1], 64400[0], 64405[0], 64408[0], 64415[0], 64416[0], 64417[0], 64418[0], 64420[0], 64421[0], 64425[0], 64430[0], 64435[0], 64445[0], 64446[0], 64447[0], 64448[0], 64449[0], 64450[0], 64451[0], 64454[0], 64461[0], 64462[0], 64463[0], 64479[0], 64480[0], 64483[0], 64484[0], 64486[0], 64487[0], 64488[0], 64489[0], 64490[0], 64491[0], 64492[0], 64493[0], 64494[0], 64495[0], 64505[0], 64510[0], 64517[0], 64520[0], 64530[0], 69990[1], 92012[1], 92014[1], 92585[0], 93000[1], 93005[1], 93010[1], 93040[1], 93041[1], 93042[1], 93318[1], 93355[1], 94002[1], 94200[1], 94250[1], 94680[1], 94681[1], 94690[1], 94770[1], 95812[1], 95813[1], 95816[1], 95819[1], 95822[0], 95829[1], 95860[0], 95861[0], 95863[0], 95864[0], 95865[0], 95866[0], 95867[0], 95868[0], 95869[0], 95870[0], 95907[0], 95908[0], 95909[0], 95910[0], 95911[0], 95912[0], 95913[0], 95925[0], 95926[0], 95927[0], 95928[0], 95929[0], 95930[0], 95933[0], 95937[0], 95938[0], 95939[0], 95940[0], 95955[1], 96360[1], 96361[1], 96365[1], 96366[1], 96367[1], 96368[1], 96372[1], 96374[1], 96375[1], 96376[1], 96377[1], 96523[0], 99155[0], 99156[0], 99157[0], 99211[1], 99212[1], 99213[1], 99214[1], 99215[1], 99217[1], 99218[1], 99219[1], 99220[1], 99221[1], 99222[1], 99223[1], 99231[1], 99232[1], 99233[1], 99234[1], 99235[1], 99236[1], 99238[1], 99239[1], 99241[1], 99242[1], 99243[1], 99244[1], 99245[1], 99251[1], 99252[1], 99253[1], 99254[1], 99255[1], 99291[1], 99292[1], 99304[1], 99305[1], 99306[1], 99307[1], 99308[1], 99309[1], 99310[1], 99315[1], 99316[1], 99334[1], 99335[1], 99336[1], 99337[1], 99347[1], 99348[1], 99349[1], 99350[1], 99374[1], 99375[1], 99377[1], 99378[1], 99446[0], 99447[0], 99448[0], 99449[0], 99451[0], 99452[0], 99495[0], 99496[0], G0339[1], G0340[1], G0453[0], G0463[1], G0471[1]
61150	0213T[0], 0216T[0], 0228T[0], 0230T[0], 0333T[0], 0464T[0], 12001[1], 12002[1], 12004[1], 12005[1], 12006[1], 12007[1], 12011[1], 12013[1], 12014[1], 12015[1], 12016[1], 12017[1], 12018[1], 12020[1], 12021[1], 12031[1], 12032[1], 12034[1], 12035[1], 12036[1], 12037[1], 12041[1], 12042[1], 12044[1], 12045[1], 12046[1], 12047[1], 12051[1], 12052[1], 12053[1], 12054[1], 12055[1], 12056[1], 12057[1], 13100[1], 13101[1], 13102[1], 13120[1], 13121[1], 13122[1], 13131[1], 13132[1], 13133[1], 13151[1], 13152[1], 13153[1], 36000[1], 36400[1], 36405[1], 36406[1], 36410[1], 36420[1], 36425[1], 36430[1], 36440[1], 36591[0], 36592[0], 36600[1], 36640[1], 43752[1], 51701[1], 51702[1], 51703[1], 61796[1], 61798[1], 62100[1], 62320[0], 62321[0], 62322[0], 62323[0], 62324[0], 62325[0], 62326[0], 62327[0], 63620[1], 64400[0], 64405[0], 64408[0], 64415[0], 64416[0], 64417[0], 64418[0], 64420[0], 64421[0], 64425[0], 64430[0], 64435[0], 64445[0], 64446[0], 64447[0], 64448[0], 64449[0], 64450[0], 64451[0], 64454[0], 64461[0], 64462[0], 64463[0], 64479[0], 64480[0], 64483[0], 64484[0], 64486[0], 64487[0], 64488[0], 64489[0], 64490[0], 64491[0], 64492[0], 64493[0], 64494[0], 64495[0], 64505[0], 64510[0], 64517[0], 64520[0], 64530[0], 69990[1], 92012[1], 92014[1], 92585[0], 93000[1], 93005[1], 93010[1], 93040[1], 93041[1], 93042[1], 93318[1], 93355[1], 94002[1], 94200[1], 94250[1], 94680[1], 94681[1], 94690[1], 94770[1], 95812[1], 95813[1], 95816[1], 95819[1], 95822[0], 95829[1], 95860[0], 95861[0], 95863[0], 95864[0], 95865[0], 95866[0], 95867[0], 95868[0], 95869[0], 95870[0], 95907[0], 95908[0], 95909[0], 95910[0], 95911[0], 95912[0], 95913[0], 95925[0], 95926[0], 95927[0], 95928[0], 95929[0], 95930[0], 95933[0], 95937[0], 95938[0], 95939[0], 95940[0], 95955[1], 96360[1], 96361[1], 96365[1], 96366[1], 96367[1], 96368[1], 96372[1], 96374[1], 96375[1], 96376[1], 96377[1], 96523[0], 99155[0], 99156[0], 99157[0], 99211[1], 99212[1], 99213[1], 99214[1], 99215[1], 99217[1], 99218[1], 99219[1], 99220[1], 99221[1], 99222[1], 99223[1], 99231[1], 99232[1], 99233[1], 99234[1], 99235[1], 99236[1], 99238[1], 99239[1], 99241[1], 99242[1], 99243[1], 99244[1], 99245[1], 99251[1], 99252[1], 99253[1], 99254[1], 99255[1], 99291[1], 99292[1], 99304[1], 99305[1], 99306[1], 99307[1], 99308[1], 99309[1], 99310[1], 99315[1], 99316[1], 99334[1], 99335[1], 99336[1], 99337[1], 99347[1], 99348[1], 99349[1], 99350[1], 99374[1], 99375[1], 99377[1], 99378[1], 99446[0], 99447[0], 99448[0], 99449[0], 99451[0], 99452[0], 99495[0], 99496[0], G0339[1], G0340[1], G0453[0], G0463[1], G0471[1]
61151	0213T[0], 0216T[0], 0228T[0], 0230T[0], 0333T[0], 0464T[0], 12001[1], 12002[1], 12004[1], 12005[1], 12006[1], 12007[1], 12011[1], 12013[1], 12014[1], 12015[1], 12016[1], 12017[1], 12018[1], 12020[1], 12021[1], 12031[1], 12032[1], 12034[1], 12035[1], 12036[1], 12037[1], 12041[1], 12042[1], 12044[1], 12045[1], 12046[1], 12047[1], 12051[1], 12052[1], 12053[1], 12054[1], 12055[1], 12056[1], 12057[1], 13100[1], 13101[1], 13102[1], 13120[1], 13121[1], 13122[1], 13131[1], 13132[1], 13133[1], 13151[1], 13152[1], 13153[1], 36000[1], 36400[1], 36405[1], 36406[1], 36410[1], 36420[1], 36425[1], 36430[1], 36440[1], 36591[0], 36592[0], 36600[1], 36640[1], 43752[1], 51701[1], 51702[1], 51703[1], 61140[1], 61150[1], 61154[1], 61156[1], 61253[1], 61796[1], 61798[1], 62100[1], 62320[0], 62321[0], 62322[0], 62323[0], 62324[0], 62325[0], 62326[0], 62327[0], 63620[1], 64400[0], 64405[0], 64408[0], 64415[0], 64416[0], 64417[0], 64418[0], 64420[0], 64421[0], 64425[0], 64430[0], 64435[0], 64445[0], 64446[0], 64447[0], 64448[0], 64449[0], 64450[0], 64451[0], 64454[0], 64461[0], 64462[0], 64463[0], 64479[0], 64480[0], 64483[0], 64484[0], 64486[0], 64487[0], 64488[0], 64489[0], 64490[0], 64491[0], 64492[0], 64493[0], 64494[0], 64495[0], 64505[0], 64510[0], 64517[0], 64520[0], 64530[0], 69990[1], 92012[1], 92014[1], 92585[0], 93000[1], 93005[1], 93010[1], 93040[1], 93041[1], 93042[1], 93318[1], 93355[1], 94002[1], 94200[1], 94250[1], 94680[1], 94681[1], 94690[1], 94770[1], 95812[1], 95813[1], 95816[1], 95819[1], 95822[0], 95829[1], 95860[0], 95861[0], 95863[0], 95864[0], 95865[0], 95866[0], 95867[0], 95868[0], 95869[0], 95870[0], 95907[0], 95908[0], 95909[0], 95910[0], 95911[0], 95912[0], 95913[0], 95925[0], 95926[0], 95927[0], 95928[0], 95929[0], 95930[0], 95933[0], 95937[0], 95938[0], 95939[0], 95940[0], 95955[1], 96360[1], 96361[1], 96365[1], 96366[1], 96367[1], 96368[1], 96372[1], 96374[1], 96375[1], 96376[1], 96377[1], 96523[0], 99155[0], 99156[0], 99157[0], 99211[1], 99212[1], 99213[1], 99214[1], 99215[1], 99217[1], 99218[1], 99219[1], 99220[1], 99221[1], 99222[1], 99223[1], 99231[1], 99232[1], 99233[1], 99234[1], 99235[1], 99236[1], 99238[1], 99239[1], 99241[1], 99242[1], 99243[1], 99244[1], 99245[1], 99251[1], 99252[1], 99253[1], 99254[1], 99255[1], 99291[1], 99292[1], 99304[1], 99305[1], 99306[1], 99307[1], 99308[1], 99309[1], 99310[1], 99315[1], 99316[1], 99334[1], 99335[1], 99336[1], 99337[1], 99347[1], 99348[1], 99349[1], 99350[1], 99374[1], 99375[1], 99377[1], 99378[1], 99446[0], 99447[0], 99448[0], 99449[0], 99451[0], 99452[0], 99495[0], 99496[0], G0339[1], G0340[1], G0453[0], G0463[1], G0471[1]
61154	0213T[0], 0216T[0], 0228T[0], 0230T[0], 0333T[0], 0464T[0], 10030[1], 10140[1], 12001[1], 12002[1], 12004[1], 12005[1], 12006[1], 12007[1], 12011[1], 12013[1], 12014[1], 12015[1], 12016[1], 12017[1], 12018[1], 12020[1], 12021[1], 12031[1], 12032[1], 12034[1], 12035[1], 12036[1], 12037[1], 12041[1], 12042[1], 12044[1], 12045[1], 12046[1], 12047[1], 12051[1], 12052[1], 12053[1], 12054[1], 12055[1], 12056[1], 12057[1], 13100[1], 13101[1], 13102[1], 13120[1], 13121[1], 13122[1], 13131[1], 13132[1], 13133[1], 13151[1], 13152[1], 13153[1], 36000[1], 36400[1], 36405[1], 36406[1], 36410[1], 36420[1], 36425[1], 36430[1], 36440[1], 36591[0], 36592[0], 36600[1], 36640[1], 43752[1], 51701[1], 51702[1], 51703[1], 61140[1], 61150[1], 62100[1], 62320[0], 62321[0], 62322[0], 62323[0], 62324[0], 62325[0], 62326[0], 62327[0], 64400[0], 64405[0], 64408[0], 64415[0], 64416[0], 64417[0], 64418[0], 64420[0], 64421[0], 64425[0], 64430[0], 64435[0], 64445[0], 64446[0], 64447[0], 64448[0], 64449[0], 64450[0], 64451[0], 64454[0], 64461[0], 64462[0], 64463[0], 64479[0], 64480[0], 64483[0], 64484[0], 64486[0], 64487[0], 64488[0], 64489[0], 64490[0], 64491[0], 64492[0], 64493[0], 64494[0], 64495[0], 64505[0], 64510[0], 64517[0], 64520[0], 64530[0], 69990[1], 92012[1], 92014[1], 92585[0], 93000[1], 93005[1], 93010[1], 93040[1], 93041[1], 93042[1], 93318[1], 93355[1], 94002[1], 94200[1], 94250[1], 94680[1], 94681[1], 94690[1], 94770[1], 95812[1], 95813[1], 95816[1], 95819[1], 95822[0], 95829[1], 95860[0], 95861[0], 95863[0], 95864[0], 95865[0], 95866[0], 95867[0], 95868[0], 95869[0], 95870[0], 95907[0], 95908[0], 95909[0], 95910[0], 95911[0], 95912[0], 95913[0], 95925[0], 95926[0], 95927[0], 95928[0], 95929[0], 95930[0], 95933[0], 95937[0], 95938[0], 95939[0], 95940[0], 95955[1], 96360[1], 96361[1], 96365[1], 96366[1], 96367[1], 96368[1], 96372[1], 96374[1], 96375[1], 96376[1], 96377[1], 96523[0], 99155[0], 99156[0], 99157[0], 99211[1], 99212[1], 99213[1], 99214[1], 99215[1], 99217[1], 99218[1], 99219[1], 99220[1], 99221[1], 99222[1], 99223[1], 99231[1], 99232[1], 99233[1], 99234[1], 99235[1], 99236[1], 99238[1], 99239[1], 99241[1], 99242[1], 99243[1], 99244[1], 99245[1], 99251[1], 99252[1], 99253[1], 99254[1], 99255[1], 99291[1], 99292[1], 99304[1], 99305[1], 99306[1], 99307[1], 99308[1], 99309[1], 99310[1], 99315[1], 99316[1], 99334[1], 99335[1], 99336[1], 99337[1], 99347[1], 99348[1], 99349[1], 99350[1], 99374[1], 99375[1], 99377[1], 99378[1], 99446[0], 99447[0], 99448[0], 99449[0], 99451[0], 99452[0], 99495[0], 99496[0], G0453[0], G0463[1], G0471[1]
61156	0213T[0], 0216T[0], 0228T[0], 0230T[0], 0333T[0], 0464T[0], 10030[1], 10140[1], 12001[1], 12002[1], 12004[1], 12005[1], 12006[1], 12007[1], 12011[1], 12013[1], 12014[1], 12015[1], 12016[1], 12017[1], 12018[1], 12020[1], 12021[1], 12031[1], 12032[1], 12034[1], 12035[1], 12036[1], 12037[1], 12041[1], 12042[1], 12044[1], 12045[1], 12046[1], 12047[1], 12051[1], 12052[1], 12053[1], 12054[1], 12055[1], 12056[1], 12057[1], 13100[1], 13101[1], 13102[1], 13120[1], 13121[1], 13122[1], 13131[1], 13132[1], 13133[1], 13151[1], 13152[1], 13153[1], 36000[1], 36400[1], 36405[1], 36406[1], 36410[1], 36420[1], 36425[1], 36430[1], 36440[1], 36591[0], 36592[0], 36600[1], 36640[1], 43752[1], 51701[1], 51702[1], 51703[1], 61150[1], 61154[1], 62100[1], 62320[0], 62321[0], 62322[0], 62323[0], 62324[0], 62325[0], 62326[0], 62327[0], 64400[0], 64405[0], 64408[0], 64415[0], 64416[0], 64417[0], 64418[0], 64420[0], 64421[0], 64425[0], 64430[0], 64435[0], 64445[0], 64446[0], 64447[0], 64448[0], 64449[0], 64450[0], 64451[0], 64454[0], 64461[0], 64462[0], 64463[0], 64479[0], 64480[0], 64483[0], 64484[0], 64486[0], 64487[0], 64488[0], 64489[0], 64490[0], 64491[0], 64492[0], 64493[0], 64494[0], 64495[0], 64505[0], 64510[0], 64517[0], 64520[0], 64530[0], 69990[1], 92012[1], 92014[1], 92585[0], 93000[1], 93005[1], 93010[1], 93040[1], 93041[1], 93042[1], 93318[1], 93355[1], 94002[1], 94200[1], 94250[1], 94680[1], 94681[1], 94690[1], 94770[1], 95812[1], 95813[1], 95816[1], 95819[1], 95822[0], 95829[1], 95860[0], 95861[0], 95863[0], 95864[0], 95865[0], 95866[0], 95867[0], 95868[0], 95869[0], 95870[0], 95907[0], 95908[0], 95909[0], 95910[0], 95911[0], 95912[0], 95913[0], 95925[0], 95926[0], 95927[0], 95928[0], 95929[0], 95930[0], 95933[0], 95937[0], 95938[0], 95939[0], 95940[0], 95955[1], 96360[1], 96361[1], 96365[1], 96366[1], 96367[1], 96368[1], 96372[1], 96374[1], 96375[1], 96376[1], 96377[1], 96523[0], 99155[0], 99156[0], 99157[0], 99211[1], 99212[1], 99213[1], 99214[1], 99215[1], 99217[1], 99218[1], 99219[1], 99220[1], 99221[1], 99222[1], 99223[1], 99231[1], 99232[1], 99233[1], 99234[1], 99235[1], 99236[1], 99238[1], 99239[1], 99241[1], 99242[1], 99243[1], 99244[1], 99245[1], 99251[1], 99252[1], 99253[1], 99254[1], 99255[1], 99291[1], 99292[1], 99304[1], 99305[1], 99306[1], 99307[1], 99308[1], 99309[1], 99310[1], 99315[1], 99316[1], 99334[1], 99335[1], 99336[1], 99337[1], 99347[1], 99348[1], 99349[1], 99350[1], 99374[1], 99375[1], 99377[1], 99378[1], 99446[0], 99447[0], 99448[0], 99449[0], 99451[0], 99452[0], 99495[0], 99496[0], G0453[0], G0463[1], G0471[1]

0 = Modifier usage not allowed or inappropriate 1 = Modifier usage allowed

Code 1	Code 2
61210	0213T[0], 0216T[0], 0228T[0], 0230T[0], 0333T[0], 0464T[0], 12001[1], 12002[1], 12004[1], 12005[1], 12006[1], 12007[1], 12011[1], 12013[1], 12014[1], 12015[1], 12016[1], 12017[1], 12018[1], 12020[1], 12021[1], 12031[1], 12032[1], 12034[1], 12035[1], 12036[1], 12037[1], 12041[1], 12042[1], 12044[1], 12045[1], 12046[1], 12047[1], 12051[1], 12052[1], 12053[1], 12054[1], 12055[1], 12056[1], 12057[1], 13100[1], 13101[1], 13102[1], 13120[1], 13121[1], 13122[1], 13131[1], 13132[1], 13133[1], 13151[1], 13152[1], 13153[1], 36000[1], 36400[1], 36405[1], 36406[1], 36410[1], 36420[1], 36425[1], 36430[1], 36440[1], 36591[0], 36592[0], 36600[1], 36640[1], 43752[1], 51701[1], 51702[1], 51703[1], 61107[1], 61120[1], 61140[1], 61150[1], 61151[1], 61154[1], 61156[1], 61215[1], 61250[1], 61253[1], 62100[1], 62320[0], 62321[0], 62322[0], 62323[0], 62324[0], 62325[0], 62326[0], 62327[0], 64400[0], 64405[0], 64408[0], 64415[0], 64416[0], 64417[0], 64418[0], 64420[0], 64421[0], 64425[0], 64430[0], 64435[0], 64445[0], 64446[0], 64447[0], 64448[0], 64449[0], 64450[0], 64451[0], 64454[0], 64461[0], 64462[0], 64463[0], 64479[0], 64480[0], 64483[0], 64484[0], 64486[0], 64487[0], 64488[0], 64489[0], 64490[0], 64491[0], 64492[0], 64493[0], 64494[0], 64495[0], 64505[0], 64510[0], 64517[0], 64520[0], 64530[0], 69990[1], 92012[1], 92014[1], 92585[0], 93000[1], 93005[1], 93010[1], 93040[1], 93041[1], 93042[1], 93318[1], 93355[1], 94002[1], 94200[1], 94250[1], 94680[1], 94681[1], 94690[1], 94770[1], 95812[1], 95813[1], 95816[1], 95819[1], 95822[0], 95829[1], 95860[0], 95861[0], 95863[0], 95864[0], 95865[0], 95866[0], 95867[0], 95868[0], 95869[0], 95870[0], 95907[0], 95908[0], 95909[0], 95910[0], 95911[0], 95912[0], 95913[0], 95925[0], 95926[0], 95927[0], 95928[0], 95929[0], 95930[0], 95933[0], 95937[0], 95938[0], 95939[0], 95940[0], 95955[1], 96360[1], 96361[1], 96365[1], 96366[1], 96367[1], 96368[1], 96372[1], 96374[1], 96375[1], 96376[1], 96377[1], 96523[0], 99155[0], 99156[0], 99157[0], 99211[1], 99212[1], 99213[1], 99214[1], 99215[1], 99217[1], 99218[1], 99219[1], 99220[1], 99221[1], 99222[1], 99223[1], 99231[1], 99232[1], 99233[1], 99234[1], 99235[1], 99236[1], 99238[1], 99239[1], 99241[1], 99242[1], 99243[1], 99244[1], 99245[1], 99251[1], 99252[1], 99253[1], 99254[1], 99255[1], 99291[1], 99292[1], 99304[1], 99305[1], 99306[1], 99307[1], 99308[1], 99309[1], 99310[1], 99315[1], 99316[1], 99334[1], 99335[1], 99336[1], 99337[1], 99347[1], 99348[1], 99349[1], 99350[1], 99374[1], 99375[1], 99377[1], 99378[1], 99446[0], 99447[0], 99448[0], 99449[0], 99451[0], 99452[0], 99495[1], 99496[1], G0453[0], G0463[1], G0471[1]
61215	0213T[0], 0216T[0], 0228T[0], 0230T[0], 0333T[0], 0464T[0], 11000[1], 11001[1], 11004[1], 11005[1], 11006[1], 11042[1], 11043[1], 11044[1], 11045[1], 11046[1], 11047[1], 12001[1], 12002[1], 12004[1], 12005[1], 12006[1], 12007[1], 12011[1], 12013[1], 12014[1], 12015[1], 12016[1], 12017[1], 12018[1], 12020[1], 12021[1], 12031[1], 12032[1], 12034[1], 12035[1], 12036[1], 12037[1], 12041[1], 12042[1], 12044[1], 12045[1], 12046[1], 12047[1], 12051[1], 12052[1], 12053[1], 12054[1], 12055[1], 12056[1], 12057[1], 13100[1], 13101[1], 13102[1], 13120[1], 13121[1], 13122[1], 13131[1], 13132[1], 13133[1], 13151[1], 13152[1], 13153[1], 36000[1], 36400[1], 36405[1], 36406[1], 36410[1], 36420[1], 36425[1], 36430[1], 36440[1], 36591[0], 36592[0], 36600[1], 36640[1], 43752[1], 51701[1], 51702[1], 51703[1], 61140[1], 61150[1], 61151[1], 61154[1], 61156[1], 61250[1], 61253[1], 62320[0], 62321[0], 62322[0], 62323[0], 62324[0], 62325[0], 62326[0], 62327[0], 64400[0], 64405[0], 64408[0], 64415[0], 64416[0], 64417[0], 64418[0], 64420[0], 64421[0], 64425[0], 64430[0], 64435[0], 64445[0], 64446[0], 64447[0], 64448[0], 64449[0], 64450[0], 64451[0], 64454[0], 64461[0], 64462[0], 64463[0], 64479[0], 64480[0], 64483[0], 64484[0], 64486[0], 64487[0], 64488[0], 64489[0], 64490[0], 64491[0], 64492[0], 64493[0], 64494[0], 64495[0], 64505[0], 64510[0], 64517[0], 64520[0], 64530[0], 69990[0], 92012[1], 92014[1], 92585[0], 93000[1], 93005[1], 93010[1], 93040[1], 93041[1], 93042[1], 93318[1], 93355[1], 94002[1], 94200[1], 94250[1], 94680[1], 94681[1], 94690[1], 94770[1], 95812[1], 95813[1], 95816[1], 95819[1], 95822[0], 95829[1], 95860[0], 95861[0], 95863[0], 95864[0], 95865[0], 95866[0], 95867[0], 95868[0], 95869[0], 95870[0], 95907[0], 95908[0], 95909[0], 95910[0], 95911[0], 95912[0], 95913[0], 95925[0], 95926[0], 95927[0], 95928[0], 95929[0], 95930[0], 95933[0], 95937[0], 95938[0], 95939[0], 95940[0], 95955[1], 95990[1], 95991[1], 96360[1], 96361[1], 96365[1], 96366[1], 96367[1], 96368[1], 96372[1], 96374[1], 96375[1], 96376[1], 96377[1], 96522[1], 96523[0], 97597[1], 97598[1], 97602[1], 99155[0], 99156[0], 99157[0], 99211[1], 99212[1], 99213[1], 99214[1], 99215[1], 99217[1], 99218[1], 99219[1], 99220[1], 99221[1], 99222[1], 99223[1], 99231[1], 99232[1], 99233[1], 99234[1], 99235[1], 99236[1], 99238[1], 99239[1], 99241[1], 99242[1], 99243[1], 99244[1], 99245[1], 99251[1], 99252[1], 99253[1], 99254[1], 99255[1], 99291[1], 99292[1], 99304[1], 99305[1], 99306[1], 99307[1], 99308[1], 99309[1], 99310[1], 99315[1], 99316[1], 99334[1], 99335[1], 99336[1], 99337[1], 99347[1], 99348[1], 99349[1], 99350[1], 99374[1], 99375[1], 99377[1], 99378[1], 99446[0], 99447[0], 99448[0], 99449[0], 99451[0], 99452[0], 99495[0], 99496[0], G0453[0], G0463[1], G0471[1]
61304	0213T[0], 0216T[0], 0228T[0], 0230T[0], 0333T[0], 0464T[0], 11000[1], 11001[1], 11004[1], 11005[1], 11006[1], 11042[1], 11043[1], 11044[1], 11045[1], 11046[1], 11047[1], 12001[1], 12002[1], 12004[1], 12005[1], 12006[1], 12007[1], 12011[1], 12013[1], 12014[1], 12015[1], 12016[1], 12017[1], 12018[1], 12020[1], 12021[1], 12031[1], 12032[1], 12034[1], 12035[1], 12036[1], 12037[1], 12041[1], 12042[1], 12044[1], 12045[1], 12046[1], 12047[1], 12051[1], 12052[1], 12053[1], 12054[1], 12055[1], 12056[1], 12057[1], 13100[1], 13101[1], 13102[1], 13120[1], 13121[1], 13122[1], 13131[1], 13132[1], 13133[1], 13151[1], 13152[1], 13153[1], 36000[1], 36400[1], 36405[1], 36406[1], 36410[1], 36420[1], 36425[1], 36430[1], 36440[1], 36591[0], 36592[0], 36600[1], 36640[1], 43752[1], 51701[1], 51702[1], 51703[1], 61107[1], 61210[1], 61250[1], 61535[0], 61796[1], 61798[1], 62100[1], 62140[0], 62141[0], 62320[0], 62321[0], 62322[0], 62323[0], 62324[0], 62325[0], 62326[0], 62327[0], 64400[0], 64405[0], 64408[0], 64415[0], 64416[0], 64417[0], 64418[0], 64420[0], 64421[0], 64425[0], 64430[0], 64435[0], 64445[0], 64446[0], 64447[0], 64448[0], 64449[0], 64450[0], 64451[0], 64454[0], 64461[0], 64462[0], 64463[0], 64479[0], 64480[0], 64483[0], 64484[0], 64486[0], 64487[0], 64488[0], 64489[0], 64490[0], 64491[0], 64492[0], 64493[0], 64494[0], 64495[0], 64505[0], 64510[0], 64517[0], 64520[0], 64530[0], 92012[1], 92014[1], 92585[0], 93000[1], 93005[1], 93010[1], 93040[1], 93041[1], 93042[1], 93318[1], 93355[1], 94002[1], 94200[1], 94250[1], 94680[1], 94681[1], 94690[1], 94770[1], 95812[1], 95813[1], 95816[1], 95819[1], 95822[0], 95829[1], 95860[0], 95861[0], 95863[0], 95864[0], 95865[0], 95866[0], 95867[0], 95868[0], 95869[0], 95870[0], 95907[0], 95908[0], 95909[0], 95910[0], 95911[0], 95912[0], 95913[0], 95925[0], 95926[0], 95927[0], 95928[0], 95929[0], 95930[0], 95933[0], 95937[0], 95938[0], 95939[0], 95940[0], 95955[1], 96360[1], 96361[1], 96365[1], 96366[1], 96367[1], 96368[1], 96372[1], 96374[1], 96375[1], 96376[1], 96377[1], 96523[0], 97597[1], 97598[1], 97602[1], 99155[0], 99156[0], 99157[0], 99211[1], 99212[1], 99213[1], 99214[1], 99215[1], 99217[1], 99218[1], 99219[1], 99220[1], 99221[1], 99222[1], 99223[1], 99231[1], 99232[1], 99233[1], 99234[1], 99235[1], 99236[1], 99238[1], 99239[1], 99241[1], 99242[1], 99243[1], 99244[1], 99245[1], 99251[1], 99252[1], 99253[1], 99254[1], 99255[1], 99291[1], 99292[1], 99304[1], 99305[1], 99306[1], 99307[1], 99308[1], 99309[1], 99310[1], 99315[1], 99316[1], 99334[1], 99335[1], 99336[1], 99337[1], 99347[1], 99348[1], 99349[1], 99350[1], 99374[1], 99375[1], 99377[1], 99378[1], 99446[0], 99447[0], 99448[0], 99449[0], 99451[0], 99452[0], 99495[0], 99496[0], G0453[0], G0463[1], G0471[1]
61305	0213T[0], 0216T[0], 0228T[0], 0230T[0], 0333T[0], 0464T[0], 11000[1], 11001[1], 11004[1], 11005[1], 11006[1], 11042[1], 11043[1], 11044[1], 11045[1], 11046[1], 11047[1], 12001[1], 12002[1], 12004[1], 12005[1], 12006[1], 12007[1], 12011[1], 12013[1], 12014[1], 12015[1], 12016[1], 12017[1], 12018[1], 12020[1], 12021[1], 12031[1], 12032[1], 12034[1], 12035[1], 12036[1], 12037[1], 12041[1], 12042[1], 12044[1], 12045[1], 12046[1], 12047[1], 12051[1], 12052[1], 12053[1], 12054[1], 12055[1], 12056[1], 12057[1], 13100[1], 13101[1], 13102[1], 13120[1], 13121[1], 13122[1], 13131[1], 13132[1], 13133[1], 13151[1], 13152[1], 13153[1], 36000[1], 36400[1], 36405[1], 36406[1], 36410[1], 36420[1], 36425[1], 36430[1], 36440[1], 36591[0], 36592[0], 36600[1], 36640[1], 43752[1], 51701[1], 51702[1], 51703[1], 61107[1], 61210[1], 61253[1], 61535[1], 61796[1], 61798[1], 62100[1], 62140[0], 62141[0], 62320[0], 62321[0], 62322[0], 62323[0], 62324[0], 62325[0], 62326[0], 62327[0], 64400[0], 64405[0], 64408[0], 64415[0], 64416[0], 64417[0], 64418[0], 64420[0], 64421[0], 64425[0], 64430[0], 64435[0], 64445[0], 64446[0], 64447[0], 64448[0], 64449[0], 64450[0], 64451[0], 64454[0], 64461[0], 64462[0], 64463[0], 64479[0], 64480[0], 64483[0], 64484[0], 64486[0], 64487[0], 64488[0], 64489[0], 64490[0], 64491[0], 64492[0], 64493[0], 64494[0], 64495[0], 64505[0], 64510[0], 64517[0], 64520[0], 64530[0], 92012[1], 92014[1], 92585[0], 93000[1], 93005[1], 93010[1], 93040[1], 93041[1], 93042[1], 93318[1], 93355[1], 94002[1], 94200[1], 94250[1], 94680[1], 94681[1], 94690[1], 94770[1], 95812[1], 95813[1], 95816[1], 95819[1], 95822[0], 95829[1], 95860[0], 95861[0], 95863[0], 95864[0], 95865[0], 95866[0], 95867[0], 95868[0], 95869[0], 95870[0], 95907[0], 95908[0], 95909[0], 95910[0], 95911[0], 95912[0], 95913[0], 95925[0], 95926[0], 95927[0], 95928[0], 95929[0], 95930[0], 95933[0], 95937[0], 95938[0], 95939[0], 95940[0], 95955[1], 96360[1], 96361[1], 96365[1], 96366[1], 96367[1], 96368[1], 96372[1], 96374[1], 96375[1], 96376[1], 96377[1], 96523[0], 97597[1], 97598[1], 97602[1], 99155[0], 99156[0], 99157[0], 99211[1], 99212[1], 99213[1], 99214[1], 99215[1], 99217[1], 99218[1], 99219[1], 99220[1], 99221[1], 99222[1], 99223[1], 99231[1], 99232[1], 99233[1], 99234[1], 99235[1], 99236[1], 99238[1], 99239[1], 99241[1], 99242[1], 99243[1], 99244[1], 99245[1], 99251[1], 99252[1], 99253[1], 99254[1], 99255[1], 99291[1], 99292[1], 99304[1], 99305[1], 99306[1], 99307[1], 99308[1], 99309[1], 99310[1], 99315[1], 99316[1], 99334[1], 99335[1], 99336[1], 99337[1], 99347[1], 99348[1], 99349[1], 99350[1], 99374[1], 99375[1], 99377[1], 99378[1], 99446[0], 99447[0], 99448[0], 99449[0], 99451[0], 99452[0], 99495[0], 99496[0], G0453[0], G0463[1], G0471[1]
61312	0213T[0], 0216T[0], 0228T[0], 0230T[0], 0333T[0], 0464T[0], 10030[1], 10140[1], 11000[1], 11001[1], 11004[1], 11005[1], 11006[1], 11042[1], 11043[1], 11044[1], 11045[1], 11046[1], 11047[1], 12001[1], 12002[1], 12004[1], 12005[1], 12006[1], 12007[1], 12011[1], 12013[1], 12014[1], 12015[1], 12016[1], 12017[1], 12018[1], 12020[1], 12021[1], 12031[1], 12032[1], 12034[1], 12035[1], 12036[1], 12037[1], 12041[1], 12042[1], 12044[1], 12045[1], 12046[1], 12047[1], 12051[1], 12052[1], 12053[1], 12054[1], 12055[1], 12056[1], 12057[1], 13100[1], 13101[1], 13102[1], 13120[1], 13121[1], 13122[1], 13131[1], 13132[1], 13133[1], 13151[1], 13152[1], 13153[1], 36000[1], 36400[1], 36405[1], 36406[1], 36410[1], 36420[1], 36425[1], 36430[1], 36440[1], 36591[0], 36592[0], 36600[1], 36640[1], 43752[1], 51701[1], 51702[1], 51703[1], 61107[1], 61108[1], 61154[1], 61210[1], 61304[1], 61305[1], 61535[0], 61796[1], 61798[1], 62100[1], 62140[0], 62141[0], 62320[0], 62321[0], 62322[0], 62323[0], 62324[0], 62325[0], 62326[0], 62327[0], 64400[0], 64405[0], 64408[0], 64415[0], 64416[0], 64417[0], 64418[0], 64420[0], 64421[0], 64425[0], 64430[0], 64435[0], 64445[0], 64446[0], 64447[0], 64448[0], 64449[0], 64450[0], 64451[0], 64454[0], 64461[0], 64462[0], 64463[0], 64479[0], 64480[0], 64483[0], 64484[0], 64486[0], 64487[0], 64488[0], 64489[0], 64490[0], 64491[0], 64492[0], 64493[0], 64494[0], 64495[0], 64505[0], 64510[0], 64517[0], 64520[0], 64530[0], 92012[1], 92014[1], 92585[0], 93000[1], 93005[1], 93010[1], 93040[1], 93041[1], 93042[1], 93318[1], 93355[1], 94002[1], 94200[1], 94250[1], 94680[1], 94681[1], 94690[1], 94770[1], 95812[1], 95813[1], 95816[1], 95819[1], 95822[0], 95829[1], 95860[0], 95861[0], 95863[0], 95864[0], 95865[0], 95866[0], 95867[0], 95868[0], 95869[0], 95870[0], 95907[0], 95908[0], 95909[0], 95910[0], 95911[0], 95912[0], 95913[0], 95925[0], 95926[0], 95927[0], 95928[0], 95929[0], 95930[0], 95933[0], 95937[0], 95938[0], 95939[0], 95940[0], 95955[1], 96360[1], 96361[1], 96365[1], 96366[1], 96367[1], 96368[1], 96372[1], 96374[1], 96375[1], 96376[1], 96377[1], 96523[0], 97597[1],

0 = Modifier usage not allowed or inappropriate 1 = Modifier usage allowed

Code 1	Code 2
	97598[1], 97602[1], 99155[0], 99156[0], 99157[0], 99211[1], 99212[1], 99213[1], 99214[1], 99215[1], 99217[1], 99218[1], 99219[1], 99220[1], 99221[1], 99222[1], 99223[1], 99231[1], 99232[1], 99233[1], 99234[1], 99235[1], 99236[1], 99238[1], 99239[1], 99241[1], 99242[1], 99243[1], 99244[1], 99245[1], 99251[1], 99252[1], 99253[1], 99254[1], 99255[1], 99291[1], 99292[1], 99304[1], 99305[1], 99306[1], 99307[1], 99308[1], 99309[1], 99310[1], 99315[1], 99316[1], 99334[1], 99335[1], 99336[1], 99337[1], 99347[1], 99348[1], 99349[1], 99350[1], 99374[1], 99375[1], 99377[1], 99378[1], 99446[0], 99447[0], 99448[0], 99449[0], 99451[0], 99452[0], 99495[0], 99496[0], G0453[0], G0463[1], G0471[1]
61313	0213T[0], 0216T[0], 0228T[0], 0230T[0], 0333T[0], 0464T[0], 10030[1], 10140[1], 11000[1], 11001[1], 11004[1], 11005[1], 11006[1], 11042[1], 11043[1], 11044[1], 11045[1], 11046[1], 11047[1], 12001[1], 12002[1], 12004[1], 12005[1], 12006[1], 12007[1], 12011[1], 12013[1], 12014[1], 12015[1], 12016[1], 12017[1], 12018[1], 12020[1], 12021[1], 12031[1], 12032[1], 12034[1], 12035[1], 12036[1], 12037[1], 12041[1], 12042[1], 12044[1], 12045[1], 12046[1], 12047[1], 12051[1], 12052[1], 12053[1], 12054[1], 12055[1], 12056[1], 12057[1], 13100[1], 13101[1], 13102[1], 13120[1], 13121[1], 13122[1], 13131[1], 13132[1], 13133[1], 13151[1], 13152[1], 13153[1], 36000[1], 36400[1], 36405[1], 36406[1], 36410[1], 36420[1], 36425[1], 36430[1], 36440[1], 36591[0], 36592[0], 36600[1], 36640[1], 43752[1], 51701[1], 51702[1], 51703[1], 61107[1], 61304[1], 61305[1], 61312[1], 61535[1], 61796[1], 61798[1], 62100[1], 62140[0], 62141[0], 62320[0], 62321[0], 62322[0], 62323[0], 62324[0], 62325[0], 62326[0], 62327[0], 64400[0], 64405[0], 64408[0], 64415[0], 64416[0], 64417[0], 64418[0], 64420[0], 64421[0], 64425[0], 64430[0], 64435[0], 64445[0], 64446[0], 64447[0], 64448[0], 64449[0], 64450[0], 64451[0], 64454[0], 64461[0], 64462[0], 64463[0], 64479[0], 64480[0], 64483[0], 64484[0], 64486[0], 64487[0], 64488[0], 64489[0], 64490[0], 64491[0], 64492[0], 64493[0], 64494[0], 64495[0], 64505[0], 64510[0], 64517[0], 64520[0], 64530[0], 92012[1], 92014[1], 92585[0], 93000[1], 93005[1], 93010[1], 93040[1], 93041[1], 93042[1], 93318[1], 93355[1], 94002[1], 94200[1], 94250[1], 94680[1], 94681[1], 94690[1], 94770[1], 95812[1], 95813[1], 95816[1], 95819[1], 95822[0], 95829[1], 95860[0], 95861[0], 95863[0], 95864[0], 95865[0], 95866[0], 95867[0], 95868[0], 95869[0], 95870[0], 95907[0], 95908[0], 95909[0], 95910[0], 95911[0], 95912[0], 95913[0], 95925[0], 95926[0], 95927[0], 95928[0], 95929[0], 95930[0], 95933[0], 95937[0], 95938[0], 95939[0], 95940[0], 95955[1], 96360[1], 96361[1], 96365[1], 96366[1], 96367[1], 96368[1], 96372[1], 96374[1], 96375[1], 96376[1], 96377[1], 96523[0], 97597[1], 97598[1], 97602[1], 99155[0], 99156[0], 99157[0], 99211[1], 99212[1], 99213[1], 99214[1], 99215[1], 99217[1], 99218[1], 99219[1], 99220[1], 99221[1], 99222[1], 99223[1], 99231[1], 99232[1], 99233[1], 99234[1], 99235[1], 99236[1], 99238[1], 99239[1], 99241[1], 99242[1], 99243[1], 99244[1], 99245[1], 99251[1], 99252[1], 99253[1], 99254[1], 99255[1], 99291[1], 99292[1], 99304[1], 99305[1], 99306[1], 99307[1], 99308[1], 99309[1], 99310[1], 99315[1], 99316[1], 99334[1], 99335[1], 99336[1], 99337[1], 99347[1], 99348[1], 99349[1], 99350[1], 99374[1], 99375[1], 99377[1], 99378[1], 99446[0], 99447[0], 99448[0], 99449[0], 99451[0], 99452[0], 99495[0], 99496[0], G0453[0], G0463[1], G0471[1]
61314	0213T[0], 0216T[0], 0228T[0], 0230T[0], 0333T[0], 0464T[0], 10030[1], 10140[1], 11000[1], 11001[1], 11004[1], 11005[1], 11006[1], 11042[1], 11043[1], 11044[1], 11045[1], 11046[1], 11047[1], 12001[1], 12002[1], 12004[1], 12005[1], 12006[1], 12007[1], 12011[1], 12013[1], 12014[1], 12015[1], 12016[1], 12017[1], 12018[1], 12020[1], 12021[1], 12031[1], 12032[1], 12034[1], 12035[1], 12036[1], 12037[1], 12041[1], 12042[1], 12044[1], 12045[1], 12046[1], 12047[1], 12051[1], 12052[1], 12053[1], 12054[1], 12055[1], 12056[1], 12057[1], 13100[1], 13101[1], 13102[1], 13120[1], 13121[1], 13122[1], 13131[1], 13132[1], 13133[1], 13151[1], 13152[1], 13153[1], 36000[1], 36400[1], 36405[1], 36406[1], 36410[1], 36420[1], 36425[1], 36430[1], 36440[1], 36591[0], 36592[0], 36600[1], 36640[1], 43752[1], 51701[1], 51702[1], 51703[1], 61107[1], 61210[1], 61304[1], 61305[1], 61315[1], 61535[1], 61796[1], 61798[1], 62100[1], 62140[0], 62141[0], 62320[0], 62321[0], 62322[0], 62323[0], 62324[0], 62325[0], 62326[0], 62327[0], 64400[0], 64405[0], 64408[0], 64415[0], 64416[0], 64417[0], 64418[0], 64420[0], 64421[0], 64425[0], 64430[0], 64435[0], 64445[0], 64446[0], 64447[0], 64448[0], 64449[0], 64450[0], 64451[0], 64454[0], 64461[0], 64462[0], 64463[0], 64479[0], 64480[0], 64483[0], 64484[0], 64486[0], 64487[0], 64488[0], 64489[0], 64490[0], 64491[0], 64492[0], 64493[0], 64494[0], 64495[0], 64505[0], 64510[0], 64517[0], 64520[0], 64530[0], 92012[1], 92014[1], 92585[0], 93000[1], 93005[1], 93010[1], 93040[1], 93041[1], 93042[1], 93318[1], 93355[1], 94002[1], 94200[1], 94250[1], 94680[1], 94681[1], 94690[1], 94770[1], 95812[1], 95813[1], 95816[1], 95819[1], 95822[0], 95829[1], 95860[0], 95861[0], 95863[0], 95864[0], 95865[0], 95866[0], 95867[0], 95868[0], 95869[0], 95870[0], 95907[0], 95908[0], 95909[0], 95910[0], 95911[0], 95912[0], 95913[0], 95925[0], 95926[0], 95927[0], 95928[0], 95929[0], 95930[0], 95933[0], 95937[0], 95938[0], 95939[0], 95940[0], 95955[1], 96360[1], 96361[1], 96365[1], 96366[1], 96367[1], 96368[1], 96372[1], 96374[1], 96375[1], 96376[1], 96377[1], 96523[0], 97597[1], 97598[1], 97602[1], 99155[0], 99156[0], 99157[0], 99211[1], 99212[1], 99213[1], 99214[1], 99215[1], 99217[1], 99218[1], 99219[1], 99220[1], 99221[1], 99222[1], 99223[1], 99231[1], 99232[1], 99233[1], 99234[1], 99235[1], 99236[1], 99238[1], 99239[1], 99241[1], 99242[1], 99243[1], 99244[1], 99245[1], 99251[1], 99252[1], 99253[1], 99254[1], 99255[1], 99291[1], 99292[1], 99304[1], 99305[1], 99306[1], 99307[1], 99308[1], 99309[1], 99310[1], 99315[1], 99316[1], 99334[1], 99335[1], 99336[1], 99337[1], 99347[1], 99348[1], 99349[1], 99350[1], 99374[1], 99375[1], 99377[1], 99378[1], 99446[0], 99447[0], 99448[0], 99449[0], 99451[0], 99452[0], 99495[0], 99496[0], G0453[0], G0463[1], G0471[1]
61315	0213T[0], 0216T[0], 0228T[0], 0230T[0], 0333T[0], 0464T[0], 10030[1], 10140[1], 11000[1], 11001[1], 11004[1], 11005[1], 11006[1], 11042[1], 11043[1], 11044[1], 11045[1], 11046[1], 11047[1], 12001[1], 12002[1], 12004[1], 12005[1], 12006[1], 12007[1], 12011[1], 12013[1], 12014[1], 12015[1], 12016[1], 12017[1], 12018[1], 12020[1], 12021[1], 12031[1], 12032[1], 12034[1], 12035[1], 12036[1], 12037[1], 12041[1], 12042[1], 12044[1], 12045[1], 12046[1], 12047[1], 12051[1], 12052[1], 12053[1], 12054[1], 12055[1], 12056[1], 12057[1], 13100[1], 13101[1], 13102[1], 13120[1], 13121[1], 13122[1], 13131[1], 13132[1], 13133[1], 13151[1], 13152[1], 13153[1], 36000[1], 36400[1], 36405[1], 36406[1], 36410[1], 36420[1], 36425[1], 36430[1], 36440[1], 36591[0], 36592[0], 36600[1], 36640[1], 43752[1], 51701[1], 51702[1], 51703[1], 61107[1], 61210[1], 61304[1], 61305[1], 61535[1], 61796[1], 61798[1], 62100[1], 62140[0], 62141[0], 62320[0], 62321[0], 62322[0], 62323[0], 62324[0], 62325[0], 62326[0], 62327[0], 64400[0], 64405[0], 64408[0], 64415[0], 64416[0], 64417[0], 64418[0], 64420[0], 64421[0], 64425[0], 64430[0], 64435[0], 64445[0], 64446[0], 64447[0], 64448[0], 64449[0], 64450[0], 64451[0], 64454[0], 64461[0], 64462[0], 64463[0], 64479[0], 64480[0], 64483[0], 64484[0], 64486[0], 64487[0], 64488[0], 64489[0], 64490[0], 64491[0], 64492[0], 64493[0], 64494[0], 64495[0], 64505[0], 64510[0], 64517[0], 64520[0], 64530[0], 92012[1], 92014[1], 92585[0], 93000[1], 93005[1], 93010[1], 93040[1], 93041[1], 93042[1], 93318[1], 93355[1], 94002[1], 94200[1], 94250[1], 94680[1], 94681[1], 94690[1], 94770[1], 95812[1], 95813[1], 95816[1], 95819[1], 95822[0], 95829[1], 95860[0], 95861[0], 95863[0], 95864[0], 95865[0], 95866[0], 95867[0], 95868[0], 95869[0], 95870[0], 95907[0], 95908[0], 95909[0], 95910[0], 95911[0], 95912[0], 95913[0], 95925[0], 95926[0], 95927[0], 95928[0], 95929[0], 95930[0], 95933[0], 95937[0], 95938[0], 95939[0], 95940[0], 95955[1], 96360[1], 96361[1], 96365[1], 96366[1], 96367[1], 96368[1], 96372[1], 96374[1], 96375[1], 96376[1], 96377[1], 96523[0], 97597[1], 97598[1], 97602[1], 99155[0], 99156[0], 99157[0], 99211[1], 99212[1], 99213[1], 99214[1], 99215[1], 99217[1], 99218[1], 99219[1], 99220[1], 99221[1], 99222[1], 99223[1], 99231[1], 99232[1], 99233[1], 99234[1], 99235[1], 99236[1], 99238[1], 99239[1], 99241[1], 99242[1], 99243[1], 99244[1], 99245[1], 99251[1], 99252[1], 99253[1], 99254[1], 99255[1], 99291[1], 99292[1], 99304[1], 99305[1], 99306[1], 99307[1], 99308[1], 99309[1], 99310[1], 99315[1], 99316[1], 99334[1], 99335[1], 99336[1], 99337[1], 99347[1], 99348[1], 99349[1], 99350[1], 99374[1], 99375[1], 99377[1], 99378[1], 99446[0], 99447[0], 99448[0], 99449[0], 99451[0], 99452[0], 99495[0], 99496[0], G0453[0], G0463[1], G0471[1]
61316	0213T[1], 0216T[1], 0333T[0], 0464T[0], 36000[1], 36410[1], 36591[0], 36592[0], 61107[1], 61650[1], 62324[0], 62325[0], 62326[0], 62327[0], 64415[1], 64417[1], 64450[1], 64454[1], 64486[1], 64487[1], 64488[1], 64489[1], 64490[1], 64493[1], 92585[0], 95822[0], 95860[0], 95861[0], 95863[0], 95864[0], 95865[0], 95866[0], 95867[0], 95868[0], 95869[0], 95907[0], 95908[0], 95909[0], 95910[0], 95911[0], 95912[0], 95913[0], 95925[0], 95926[0], 95927[0], 95930[0], 95933[0], 95937[0], 95938[0], 95939[0], 95940[0], 96523[0], G0453[0]
61320	0213T[0], 0216T[0], 0228T[0], 0230T[0], 0333T[0], 0464T[0], 11000[1], 11001[1], 11004[1], 11005[1], 11006[1], 11042[1], 11043[1], 11044[1], 11045[1], 11046[1], 11047[1], 12001[1], 12002[1], 12004[1], 12005[1], 12006[1], 12007[1], 12011[1], 12013[1], 12014[1], 12015[1], 12016[1], 12017[1], 12018[1], 12020[1], 12021[1], 12031[1], 12032[1], 12034[1], 12035[1], 12036[1], 12037[1], 12041[1], 12042[1], 12044[1], 12045[1], 12046[1], 12047[1], 12051[1], 12052[1], 12053[1], 12054[1], 12055[1], 12056[1], 12057[1], 13100[1], 13101[1], 13102[1], 13120[1], 13121[1], 13122[1], 13131[1], 13132[1], 13133[1], 13151[1], 13152[1], 13153[1], 36000[1], 36400[1], 36405[1], 36406[1], 36410[1], 36420[1], 36425[1], 36430[1], 36440[1], 36591[0], 36592[0], 36600[1], 36640[1], 43752[1], 51701[1], 51702[1], 51703[1], 61107[1], 61210[1], 61304[1], 61305[1], 61321[1], 61535[0], 61796[1], 61798[1], 62100[1], 62140[0], 62141[0], 62320[0], 62321[0], 62322[0], 62323[0], 62324[0], 62325[0], 62326[0], 62327[0], 64400[0], 64405[0], 64408[0], 64415[0], 64416[0], 64417[0], 64418[0], 64420[0], 64421[0], 64425[0], 64430[0], 64435[0], 64445[0], 64446[0], 64447[0], 64448[0], 64449[0], 64450[0], 64451[0], 64454[0], 64461[0], 64462[0], 64463[0], 64479[0], 64480[0], 64483[0], 64484[0], 64486[0], 64487[0], 64488[0], 64489[0], 64490[0], 64491[0], 64492[0], 64493[0], 64494[0], 64495[0], 64505[0], 64510[0], 64517[0], 64520[0], 64530[0], 92012[1], 92014[1], 92585[0], 93000[1], 93005[1], 93010[1], 93040[1], 93041[1], 93042[1], 93318[1], 93355[1], 94002[1], 94200[1], 94250[1], 94680[1], 94681[1], 94690[1], 94770[1], 95812[1], 95813[1], 95816[1], 95819[1], 95822[0], 95829[1], 95860[0], 95861[0], 95863[0], 95864[0], 95865[0], 95866[0], 95867[0], 95868[0], 95869[0], 95870[0], 95907[0], 95908[0], 95909[0], 95910[0], 95911[0], 95912[0], 95913[0], 95925[0], 95926[0], 95927[0], 95928[0], 95929[0], 95930[0], 95933[0], 95937[0], 95938[0], 95939[0], 95940[0], 95955[1], 96360[1], 96361[1], 96365[1], 96366[1], 96367[1], 96368[1], 96372[1], 96374[1], 96375[1], 96376[1], 96377[1], 96523[0], 97597[1], 97598[1], 97602[1], 99155[0], 99156[0], 99157[0], 99211[1], 99212[1], 99213[1], 99214[1], 99215[1], 99217[1], 99218[1], 99219[1], 99220[1], 99221[1], 99222[1], 99223[1], 99231[1], 99232[1], 99233[1], 99234[1], 99235[1], 99236[1], 99238[1], 99239[1], 99241[1], 99242[1], 99243[1], 99244[1], 99245[1], 99251[1], 99252[1], 99253[1], 99254[1], 99255[1], 99291[1], 99292[1], 99304[1], 99305[1], 99306[1], 99307[1], 99308[1], 99309[1], 99310[1], 99315[1], 99316[1], 99334[1], 99335[1], 99336[1], 99337[1], 99347[1], 99348[1], 99349[1], 99350[1], 99374[1], 99375[1], 99377[1], 99378[1], 99446[0], 99447[0], 99448[0], 99449[0], 99451[0], 99452[0], 99495[0], 99496[0], G0453[0], G0463[1], G0471[1]
61321	0213T[0], 0216T[0], 0228T[0], 0230T[0], 0333T[0], 0464T[0], 11000[1], 11001[1], 11004[1], 11005[1], 11006[1], 11042[1], 11043[1], 11044[1], 11045[1], 11046[1], 11047[1], 12001[1], 12002[1], 12004[1], 12005[1], 12006[1], 12007[1], 12011[1], 12013[1], 12014[1], 12015[1], 12016[1], 12017[1], 12018[1], 12020[1], 12021[1], 12031[1], 12032[1], 12034[1], 12035[1], 12036[1], 12037[1], 12041[1], 12042[1], 12044[1], 12045[1], 12046[1], 12047[1], 12051[1], 12052[1], 12053[1], 12054[1], 12055[1], 12056[1],

0 = Modifier usage not allowed or inappropriate 1 = Modifier usage allowed

Code 1	Code 2
	12057[1], 13100[1], 13101[1], 13102[1], 13120[1], 13121[1], 13122[1], 13131[1], 13132[1], 13133[1], 13151[1], 13152[1], 13153[1], 36000[1], 36400[1], 36405[1], 36406[1], 36410[1], 36420[1], 36425[1], 36430[1], 36440[1], 36591[0], 36592[0], 36600[1], 36640[1], 43752[1], 51701[1], 51702[1], 51703[1], 61107[1], 61210[1], 61304[1], 61305[1], 61535[1], 61796[1], 61798[1], 62100[1], 62140[0], 62141[0], 62320[0], 62321[0], 62322[0], 62323[0], 62324[0], 62325[0], 62326[0], 62327[0], 64400[0], 64405[0], 64408[0], 64415[0], 64416[0], 64417[0], 64418[0], 64420[0], 64421[0], 64425[0], 64430[0], 64435[0], 64445[0], 64446[0], 64447[0], 64448[0], 64449[0], 64450[0], 64451[0], 64454[0], 64461[0], 64462[0], 64463[0], 64479[0], 64480[0], 64483[0], 64484[0], 64486[0], 64487[0], 64488[0], 64489[0], 64490[0], 64491[0], 64492[0], 64493[0], 64494[0], 64495[0], 64505[0], 64510[0], 64517[0], 64520[0], 64530[0], 92012[1], 92014[1], 92585[0], 93000[1], 93005[1], 93010[1], 93040[1], 93041[1], 93042[1], 93318[1], 93355[1], 94002[1], 94200[1], 94250[1], 94680[1], 94681[1], 94690[1], 94770[1], 95812[1], 95813[1], 95816[1], 95819[1], 95822[0], 95829[1], 95860[0], 95861[0], 95863[0], 95864[0], 95865[0], 95866[0], 95867[0], 95868[0], 95869[0], 95870[0], 95907[0], 95908[0], 95909[0], 95910[0], 95911[0], 95912[0], 95913[0], 95925[0], 95926[0], 95927[0], 95928[0], 95929[0], 95930[0], 95933[0], 95937[0], 95938[0], 95939[0], 95940[0], 95955[1], 96360[1], 96361[1], 96365[1], 96366[1], 96367[1], 96368[1], 96372[1], 96374[1], 96375[1], 96376[1], 96377[1], 96523[0], 97597[1], 97598[1], 97602[1], 99155[0], 99156[0], 99157[0], 99211[1], 99212[1], 99213[1], 99214[1], 99215[1], 99217[1], 99218[1], 99219[1], 99220[1], 99221[1], 99222[1], 99223[1], 99231[1], 99232[1], 99233[1], 99234[1], 99235[1], 99236[1], 99238[1], 99239[1], 99241[1], 99242[1], 99243[1], 99244[1], 99245[1], 99251[1], 99252[1], 99253[1], 99254[1], 99255[1], 99291[1], 99292[1], 99304[1], 99305[1], 99306[1], 99307[1], 99308[1], 99309[1], 99310[1], 99315[1], 99316[1], 99334[1], 99335[1], 99336[1], 99337[1], 99347[1], 99348[1], 99349[1], 99350[1], 99374[1], 99375[1], 99377[1], 99378[1], 99446[0], 99447[0], 99448[0], 99449[0], 99451[0], 99452[0], 99495[0], 99496[0], G0453[0], G0463[1], G0471[1]
61322	0213T[0], 0216T[0], 0228T[0], 0230T[0], 0333T[0], 0464T[0], 11000[1], 11001[1], 11004[1], 11005[1], 11006[1], 11042[1], 11043[1], 11044[1], 11045[1], 11046[1], 11047[1], 12001[1], 12002[1], 12004[1], 12005[1], 12006[1], 12007[1], 12011[1], 12013[1], 12014[1], 12015[1], 12016[1], 12017[1], 12018[1], 12020[1], 12021[1], 12031[1], 12032[1], 12034[1], 12035[1], 12036[1], 12037[1], 12041[1], 12042[1], 12044[1], 12045[1], 12046[1], 12047[1], 12051[1], 12052[1], 12053[1], 12054[1], 12055[1], 12056[1], 12057[1], 13100[1], 13101[1], 13102[1], 13120[1], 13121[1], 13122[1], 13131[1], 13132[1], 13133[1], 13151[1], 13152[1], 13153[1], 36000[1], 36400[1], 36405[1], 36406[1], 36410[1], 36420[1], 36425[1], 36430[1], 36440[1], 36591[0], 36592[0], 36600[1], 36640[1], 43752[1], 51701[1], 51702[1], 51703[1], 61107[1], 61304[1], 61312[1], 61313[0], 61535[1], 61543[1], 62100[1], 62140[0], 62141[0], 62320[0], 62321[0], 62322[0], 62323[0], 62324[0], 62325[0], 62326[0], 62327[0], 64400[0], 64405[0], 64408[0], 64415[0], 64416[0], 64417[0], 64418[0], 64420[0], 64421[0], 64425[0], 64430[0], 64435[0], 64445[0], 64446[0], 64447[0], 64448[0], 64449[0], 64450[0], 64451[0], 64454[0], 64461[0], 64462[0], 64463[0], 64479[0], 64480[0], 64483[0], 64484[0], 64486[0], 64487[0], 64488[0], 64489[0], 64490[0], 64491[0], 64492[0], 64493[0], 64494[0], 64495[0], 64505[0], 64510[0], 64517[0], 64520[0], 64530[0], 92012[1], 92014[1], 92585[0], 93000[1], 93005[1], 93010[1], 93040[1], 93041[1], 93042[1], 93318[1], 93355[1], 94002[1], 94200[1], 94250[1], 94680[1], 94681[1], 94690[1], 94770[1], 95812[1], 95813[1], 95816[1], 95819[1], 95822[0], 95829[1], 95860[0], 95861[0], 95863[0], 95864[0], 95865[0], 95866[0], 95867[0], 95868[0], 95869[0], 95870[0], 95907[0], 95908[0], 95909[0], 95910[0], 95911[0], 95912[0], 95913[0], 95925[0], 95926[0], 95927[0], 95928[0], 95929[0], 95930[0], 95933[0], 95937[0], 95938[0], 95939[0], 95940[0], 95955[1], 96360[1], 96361[1], 96365[1], 96366[1], 96367[1], 96368[1], 96372[1], 96374[1], 96375[1], 96376[1], 96377[1], 96523[0], 97597[1], 97598[1], 97602[1], 99155[0], 99156[0], 99157[0], 99211[1], 99212[1], 99213[1], 99214[1], 99215[1], 99217[1], 99218[1], 99219[1], 99220[1], 99221[1], 99222[1], 99223[1], 99231[1], 99232[1], 99233[1], 99234[1], 99235[1], 99236[1], 99238[1], 99239[1], 99241[1], 99242[1], 99243[1], 99244[1], 99245[1], 99251[1], 99252[1], 99253[1], 99254[1], 99255[1], 99291[1], 99292[1], 99304[1], 99305[1], 99306[1], 99307[1], 99308[1], 99309[1], 99310[1], 99315[1], 99316[1], 99334[1], 99335[1], 99336[1], 99337[1], 99347[1], 99348[1], 99349[1], 99350[1], 99374[1], 99375[1], 99377[1], 99378[1], 99446[0], 99447[0], 99448[0], 99449[0], 99451[0], 99452[0], 99495[0], 99496[0], G0453[0], G0463[1], G0471[1]
61323	0213T[0], 0216T[0], 0228T[0], 0230T[0], 0333T[0], 0464T[0], 11000[1], 11001[1], 11004[1], 11005[1], 11006[1], 11042[1], 11043[1], 11044[1], 11045[1], 11046[1], 11047[1], 12001[1], 12002[1], 12004[1], 12005[1], 12006[1], 12007[1], 12011[1], 12013[1], 12014[1], 12015[1], 12016[1], 12017[1], 12018[1], 12020[1], 12021[1], 12031[1], 12032[1], 12034[1], 12035[1], 12036[1], 12037[1], 12041[1], 12042[1], 12044[1], 12045[1], 12046[1], 12047[1], 12051[1], 12052[1], 12053[1], 12054[1], 12055[1], 12056[1], 12057[1], 13100[1], 13101[1], 13102[1], 13120[1], 13121[1], 13122[1], 13131[1], 13132[1], 13133[1], 13151[1], 13152[1], 13153[1], 36000[1], 36400[1], 36405[1], 36406[1], 36410[1], 36420[1], 36425[1], 36430[1], 36440[1], 36591[0], 36592[0], 36600[1], 36640[1], 43752[1], 51701[1], 51702[1], 51703[1], 61107[1], 61304[1], 61312[1], 61313[0], 61322[1], 61535[1], 61543[1], 62100[1], 62140[0], 62141[0], 62320[0], 62321[0], 62322[0], 62323[0], 62324[0], 62325[0], 62326[0], 62327[0], 64400[0], 64405[0], 64408[0], 64415[0], 64416[0], 64417[0], 64418[0], 64420[0], 64421[0], 64425[0], 64430[0], 64435[0], 64445[0], 64446[0], 64447[0], 64448[0], 64449[0], 64450[0], 64451[0], 64454[0], 64461[0], 64462[0], 64463[0], 64479[0], 64480[0], 64483[0], 64484[0], 64486[0], 64487[0], 64488[0], 64489[0], 64490[0], 64491[0], 64492[0], 64493[0], 64494[0], 64495[0], 64505[0], 64510[0], 64517[0], 64520[0], 64530[0], 92012[1], 92014[1], 92585[0], 93000[1], 93005[1], 93010[1], 93040[1], 93041[1], 93042[1], 93318[1], 93355[1], 94002[1], 94200[1], 94250[1], 94680[1], 94681[1], 94690[1], 94770[1], 95812[1], 95813[1], 95816[1], 95819[1], 95822[0], 95829[1], 95860[0], 95861[0], 95863[0], 95864[0], 95865[0], 95866[0], 95867[0], 95868[0], 95869[0], 95870[0], 95907[0], 95908[0], 95909[0], 95910[0], 95911[0], 95912[0], 95913[0], 95925[0], 95926[0], 95927[0], 95928[0], 95929[0], 95930[0], 95933[0], 95937[0], 95938[0], 95939[0], 95940[0], 95955[1], 96360[1], 96361[1], 96365[1], 96366[1], 96367[1], 96368[1], 96372[1], 96374[1], 96375[1], 96376[1], 96377[1], 96523[0], 97597[1], 97598[1], 97602[1], 99155[0], 99156[0], 99157[0], 99211[1], 99212[1], 99213[1], 99214[1], 99215[1], 99217[1], 99218[1], 99219[1], 99220[1], 99221[1], 99222[1], 99223[1], 99231[1], 99232[1], 99233[1], 99234[1], 99235[1], 99236[1], 99238[1], 99239[1], 99241[1], 99242[1], 99243[1], 99244[1], 99245[1], 99251[1], 99252[1], 99253[1], 99254[1], 99255[1], 99291[1], 99292[1], 99304[1], 99305[1], 99306[1], 99307[1], 99308[1], 99309[1], 99310[1], 99315[1], 99316[1], 99334[1], 99335[1], 99336[1], 99337[1], 99347[1], 99348[1], 99349[1], 99350[1], 99374[1], 99375[1], 99377[1], 99378[1], 99446[0], 99447[0], 99448[0], 99449[0], 99451[0], 99452[0], 99495[0], 99496[0], G0453[0], G0463[1], G0471[1]
61343	0213T[0], 0216T[0], 0228T[0], 0230T[0], 0333T[0], 0464T[0], 0565T[1], 11000[1], 11001[1], 11004[1], 11005[1], 11006[1], 11042[1], 11043[1], 11044[1], 11045[1], 11046[1], 11047[1], 12001[1], 12002[1], 12004[1], 12005[1], 12006[1], 12007[1], 12011[1], 12013[1], 12014[1], 12015[1], 12016[1], 12017[1], 12018[1], 12020[1], 12021[1], 12031[1], 12032[1], 12034[1], 12035[1], 12036[1], 12037[1], 12041[1], 12042[1], 12044[1], 12045[1], 12046[1], 12047[1], 12051[1], 12052[1], 12053[1], 12054[1], 12055[1], 12056[1], 12057[1], 13100[1], 13101[1], 13102[1], 13120[1], 13121[1], 13122[1], 13131[1], 13132[1], 13133[1], 13151[1], 13152[1], 13153[1], 15769[1], 36000[1], 36400[1], 36405[1], 36406[1], 36410[1], 36420[1], 36425[1], 36430[1], 36440[1], 36591[0], 36592[0], 36600[1], 36640[1], 43752[1], 51701[1], 51702[1], 51703[1], 61107[1], 61210[1], 61304[1], 61305[1], 62100[1], 62140[0], 62141[0], 62320[0], 62321[0], 62322[0], 62323[0], 62324[0], 62325[0], 62326[0], 62327[0], 63001[0], 63015[0], 64400[0], 64405[0], 64408[0], 64415[0], 64416[0], 64417[0], 64418[0], 64420[0], 64421[0], 64425[0], 64430[0], 64435[0], 64445[0], 64446[0], 64447[0], 64448[0], 64449[0], 64450[0], 64451[0], 64454[0], 64461[0], 64462[0], 64463[0], 64479[0], 64480[0], 64483[0], 64484[0], 64486[0], 64487[0], 64488[0], 64489[0], 64490[0], 64491[0], 64492[0], 64493[0], 64494[0], 64495[0], 64505[0], 64510[0], 64517[0], 64520[0], 64530[0], 92012[1], 92014[1], 92585[0], 93000[1], 93005[1], 93010[1], 93040[1], 93041[1], 93042[1], 93318[1], 93355[1], 94002[1], 94200[1], 94250[1], 94680[1], 94681[1], 94690[1], 94770[1], 95812[1], 95813[1], 95816[1], 95819[1], 95822[0], 95829[1], 95860[0], 95861[0], 95863[0], 95864[0], 95865[0], 95866[0], 95867[0], 95868[0], 95869[0], 95870[0], 95907[0], 95908[0], 95909[0], 95910[0], 95911[0], 95912[0], 95913[0], 95925[0], 95926[0], 95927[0], 95928[0], 95929[0], 95930[0], 95933[0], 95937[0], 95938[0], 95939[0], 95940[0], 95955[1], 96360[1], 96361[1], 96365[1], 96366[1], 96367[1], 96368[1], 96372[1], 96374[1], 96375[1], 96376[1], 96377[1], 96523[0], 97597[1], 97598[1], 97602[1], 99155[0], 99156[0], 99157[0], 99211[1], 99212[1], 99213[1], 99214[1], 99215[1], 99217[1], 99218[1], 99219[1], 99220[1], 99221[1], 99222[1], 99223[1], 99231[1], 99232[1], 99233[1], 99234[1], 99235[1], 99236[1], 99238[1], 99239[1], 99241[1], 99242[1], 99243[1], 99244[1], 99245[1], 99251[1], 99252[1], 99253[1], 99254[1], 99255[1], 99291[1], 99292[1], 99304[1], 99305[1], 99306[1], 99307[1], 99308[1], 99309[1], 99310[1], 99315[1], 99316[1], 99334[1], 99335[1], 99336[1], 99337[1], 99347[1], 99348[1], 99349[1], 99350[1], 99374[1], 99375[1], 99377[1], 99378[1], 99446[0], 99447[0], 99448[0], 99449[0], 99451[0], 99452[0], 99495[0], 99496[0], G0453[0], G0463[1], G0471[1]
61345	0213T[0], 0216T[0], 0228T[0], 0230T[0], 0333T[0], 0464T[0], 12001[1], 12002[1], 12004[1], 12005[1], 12006[1], 12007[1], 12011[1], 12013[1], 12014[1], 12015[1], 12016[1], 12017[1], 12018[1], 12020[1], 12021[1], 12031[1], 12032[1], 12034[1], 12035[1], 12036[1], 12037[1], 12041[1], 12042[1], 12044[1], 12045[1], 12046[1], 12047[1], 12051[1], 12052[1], 12053[1], 12054[1], 12055[1], 12056[1], 12057[1], 13100[1], 13101[1], 13102[1], 13120[1], 13121[1], 13122[1], 13131[1], 13132[1], 13133[1], 13151[1], 13152[1], 13153[1], 36000[1], 36400[1], 36405[1], 36406[1], 36410[1], 36420[1], 36425[1], 36430[1], 36440[1], 36591[0], 36592[0], 36600[1], 36640[1], 43752[1], 51701[1], 51702[1], 51703[1], 61107[1], 61304[1], 61305[1], 61535[1], 62140[0], 62141[0], 62320[0], 62321[0], 62322[0], 62323[0], 62324[0], 62325[0], 62326[0], 62327[0], 64400[0], 64405[0], 64408[0], 64415[0], 64416[0], 64417[0], 64418[0], 64420[0], 64421[0], 64425[0], 64430[0], 64435[0], 64445[0], 64446[0], 64447[0], 64448[0], 64449[0], 64450[0], 64451[0], 64454[0], 64461[0], 64462[0], 64463[0], 64479[0], 64480[0], 64483[0], 64484[0], 64486[0], 64487[0], 64488[0], 64489[0], 64490[0], 64491[0], 64492[0], 64493[0], 64494[0], 64495[0], 64505[0], 64510[0], 64517[0], 64520[0], 64530[0], 92012[1], 92014[1], 92585[0], 93000[1], 93005[1], 93010[1], 93040[1], 93041[1], 93042[1], 93318[1], 93355[1], 94002[1], 94200[1], 94250[1], 94680[1], 94681[1], 94690[1], 94770[1], 95812[1], 95813[1], 95816[1], 95819[1], 95822[0], 95829[1], 95860[0], 95861[0], 95863[0], 95864[0], 95865[0], 95866[0], 95867[0], 95868[0], 95869[0], 95870[0], 95907[0], 95908[0], 95909[0], 95910[0], 95911[0], 95912[0], 95913[0], 95925[0], 95926[0], 95927[0], 95928[0], 95929[0], 95930[0], 95933[0], 95937[0], 95938[0], 95939[0], 95940[0], 95955[1], 96360[1], 96361[1], 96365[1], 96366[1], 96367[1], 96368[1], 96372[1], 96374[1], 96375[1], 96376[1], 96377[1], 96523[0], 99155[0], 99156[0], 99157[0], 99211[1], 99212[1], 99213[1], 99214[1], 99215[1], 99217[1], 99218[1], 99219[1], 99220[1], 99221[1], 99222[1], 99223[1], 99231[1], 99232[1], 99233[1], 99234[1], 99235[1], 99236[1], 99238[1], 99239[1], 99241[1], 99242[1], 99243[1], 99244[1], 99245[1], 99251[1], 99252[1], 99253[1], 99254[1], 99255[1], 99291[1], 99292[1], 99304[1], 99305[1], 99306[1], 99307[1], 99308[1], 99309[1], 99310[1], 99315[1], 99316[1], 99334[1], 99335[1], 99336[1], 99337[1], 99347[1], 99348[1],

Appendix A: NCCI - CPT Codes

0 = Modifier usage not allowed or inappropriate 1 = Modifier usage allowed

Code 1	Code 2
	99349[1], 99350[1], 99374[1], 99375[1], 99377[1], 99378[1], 99446[0], 99447[0], 99448[0], 99449[0], 99451[0], 99452[0], 99495[0], 99496[0], G0453[0], G0463[1], G0471[1]
61450	0213T[0], 0216T[0], 0228T[0], 0230T[0], 0333T[0], 0464T[0], 11000[1], 11001[1], 11004[1], 11005[1], 11006[1], 11042[1], 11043[1], 11044[1], 11045[1], 11046[1], 11047[1], 12001[1], 12002[1], 12004[1], 12005[1], 12006[1], 12007[1], 12011[1], 12013[1], 12014[1], 12015[1], 12016[1], 12017[1], 12018[1], 12020[1], 12021[1], 12031[1], 12032[1], 12034[1], 12035[1], 12036[1], 12037[1], 12041[1], 12042[1], 12044[1], 12045[1], 12046[1], 12047[1], 12051[1], 12052[1], 12053[1], 12054[1], 12055[1], 12056[1], 12057[1], 13100[1], 13101[1], 13102[1], 13120[1], 13121[1], 13122[1], 13131[1], 13132[1], 13133[1], 13151[1], 13152[1], 13153[1], 36000[1], 36400[1], 36405[1], 36406[1], 36410[1], 36420[1], 36425[1], 36430[1], 36440[1], 36591[0], 36592[0], 36600[1], 36640[1], 43752[1], 51701[1], 51702[1], 51703[1], 61107[1], 61210[1], 61304[1], 61305[1], 61340[1], 61535[1], 61796[1], 61798[1], 62100[1], 62140[0], 62141[0], 62320[0], 62321[0], 62322[0], 62323[0], 62324[0], 62325[0], 62326[0], 62327[0], 64400[0], 64405[0], 64408[0], 64415[0], 64416[0], 64417[0], 64418[0], 64420[0], 64421[0], 64425[0], 64430[0], 64435[0], 64445[0], 64446[0], 64447[0], 64448[0], 64449[0], 64450[0], 64451[0], 64454[0], 64461[0], 64462[0], 64463[0], 64479[0], 64480[0], 64483[0], 64484[0], 64486[0], 64487[0], 64488[0], 64489[0], 64490[0], 64491[0], 64492[0], 64493[0], 64494[0], 64495[0], 64505[0], 64510[0], 64517[0], 64520[0], 64530[0], 92012[1], 92014[1], 92585[0], 93000[1], 93005[1], 93010[1], 93040[1], 93041[1], 93042[1], 93318[1], 93355[1], 94002[1], 94200[1], 94250[1], 94680[1], 94681[1], 94690[1], 94770[1], 95812[1], 95813[1], 95816[1], 95819[1], 95822[0], 95829[1], 95860[0], 95861[0], 95863[0], 95864[0], 95865[0], 95866[0], 95867[0], 95868[0], 95869[0], 95870[0], 95907[0], 95908[0], 95909[0], 95910[0], 95911[0], 95912[0], 95913[0], 95925[0], 95926[0], 95927[0], 95928[0], 95929[0], 95930[0], 95933[0], 95937[0], 95938[0], 95939[0], 95940[0], 95955[1], 96360[1], 96361[1], 96365[1], 96366[1], 96367[1], 96368[1], 96372[1], 96374[1], 96375[1], 96376[1], 96377[1], 96523[0], 97597[1], 97598[1], 97602[1], 99155[0], 99156[0], 99157[0], 99211[1], 99212[1], 99213[1], 99214[1], 99215[1], 99217[1], 99218[1], 99219[1], 99220[1], 99221[1], 99222[1], 99223[1], 99231[1], 99232[1], 99233[1], 99234[1], 99235[1], 99236[1], 99238[1], 99239[1], 99241[1], 99242[1], 99243[1], 99244[1], 99245[1], 99251[1], 99252[1], 99253[1], 99254[1], 99255[1], 99291[1], 99292[1], 99304[1], 99305[1], 99306[1], 99307[1], 99308[1], 99309[1], 99310[1], 99315[1], 99316[1], 99334[1], 99335[1], 99336[1], 99337[1], 99347[1], 99348[1], 99349[1], 99350[1], 99374[1], 99375[1], 99377[1], 99378[1], 99446[0], 99447[0], 99448[0], 99449[0], 99451[0], 99452[0], 99495[0], 99496[0], G0453[0], G0463[1], G0471[1]
61458	0213T[0], 0216T[0], 0228T[0], 0230T[0], 0333T[0], 0464T[0], 11000[1], 11001[1], 11004[1], 11005[1], 11006[1], 11042[1], 11043[1], 11044[1], 11045[1], 11046[1], 11047[1], 12001[1], 12002[1], 12004[1], 12005[1], 12006[1], 12007[1], 12011[1], 12013[1], 12014[1], 12015[1], 12016[1], 12017[1], 12018[1], 12020[1], 12021[1], 12031[1], 12032[1], 12034[1], 12035[1], 12036[1], 12037[1], 12041[1], 12042[1], 12044[1], 12045[1], 12046[1], 12047[1], 12051[1], 12052[1], 12053[1], 12054[1], 12055[1], 12056[1], 12057[1], 13100[1], 13101[1], 13102[1], 13120[1], 13121[1], 13122[1], 13131[1], 13132[1], 13133[1], 13151[1], 13152[1], 13153[1], 36000[1], 36400[1], 36405[1], 36406[1], 36410[1], 36420[1], 36425[1], 36430[1], 36440[1], 36591[0], 36592[0], 36600[1], 36640[1], 43752[1], 51701[1], 51702[1], 51703[1], 61107[1], 61210[1], 61304[1], 61796[1], 61798[1], 62100[1], 62140[0], 62141[0], 62320[0], 62321[0], 62322[0], 62323[0], 62324[0], 62325[0], 62326[0], 62327[0], 64400[0], 64405[0], 64408[0], 64415[0], 64416[0], 64417[0], 64418[0], 64420[0], 64421[0], 64425[0], 64430[0], 64435[0], 64445[0], 64446[0], 64447[0], 64448[0], 64449[0], 64450[0], 64451[0], 64454[0], 64461[0], 64462[0], 64463[0], 64479[0], 64480[0], 64483[0], 64484[0], 64486[0], 64487[0], 64488[0], 64489[0], 64490[0], 64491[0], 64492[0], 64493[0], 64494[0], 64495[0], 64505[0], 64510[0], 64517[0], 64520[0], 64530[0], 92012[1], 92014[1], 92585[0], 93000[1], 93005[1], 93010[1], 93040[1], 93041[1], 93042[1], 93318[1], 93355[1], 94002[1], 94200[1], 94250[1], 94680[1], 94681[1], 94690[1], 94770[1], 95812[1], 95813[1], 95816[1], 95819[1], 95822[0], 95829[1], 95860[0], 95861[0], 95863[0], 95864[0], 95865[0], 95866[0], 95867[0], 95868[0], 95869[0], 95870[0], 95907[0], 95908[0], 95909[0], 95910[0], 95911[0], 95912[0], 95913[0], 95925[0], 95926[0], 95927[0], 95928[0], 95929[0], 95930[0], 95933[0], 95937[0], 95938[0], 95939[0], 95940[0], 95955[1], 96360[1], 96361[1], 96365[1], 96366[1], 96367[1], 96368[1], 96372[1], 96374[1], 96375[1], 96376[1], 96377[1], 96523[0], 97597[1], 97598[1], 97602[1], 99155[0], 99156[0], 99157[0], 99211[1], 99212[1], 99213[1], 99214[1], 99215[1], 99217[1], 99218[1], 99219[1], 99220[1], 99221[1], 99222[1], 99223[1], 99231[1], 99232[1], 99233[1], 99234[1], 99235[1], 99236[1], 99238[1], 99239[1], 99241[1], 99242[1], 99243[1], 99244[1], 99245[1], 99251[1], 99252[1], 99253[1], 99254[1], 99255[1], 99291[1], 99292[1], 99304[1], 99305[1], 99306[1], 99307[1], 99308[1], 99309[1], 99310[1], 99315[1], 99316[1], 99334[1], 99335[1], 99336[1], 99337[1], 99347[1], 99348[1], 99349[1], 99350[1], 99374[1], 99375[1], 99377[1], 99378[1], 99446[0], 99447[0], 99448[0], 99449[0], 99451[0], 99452[0], 99495[0], 99496[0], G0453[0], G0463[1], G0471[1]
61460	0213T[0], 0216T[0], 0228T[0], 0230T[0], 0333T[0], 0464T[0], 11000[1], 11001[1], 11004[1], 11005[1], 11006[1], 11042[1], 11043[1], 11044[1], 11045[1], 11046[1], 11047[1], 12001[1], 12002[1], 12004[1], 12005[1], 12006[1], 12007[1], 12011[1], 12013[1], 12014[1], 12015[1], 12016[1], 12017[1], 12018[1], 12020[1], 12021[1], 12031[1], 12032[1], 12034[1], 12035[1], 12036[1], 12037[1], 12041[1], 12042[1], 12044[1], 12045[1], 12046[1], 12047[1], 12051[1], 12052[1], 12053[1], 12054[1], 12055[1], 12056[1], 12057[1], 13100[1], 13101[1], 13102[1], 13120[1], 13121[1], 13122[1], 13131[1], 13132[1], 13133[1], 13151[1], 13152[1], 13153[1], 36000[1], 36400[1], 36405[1], 36406[1], 36410[1], 36420[1], 36425[1], 36430[1], 36440[1], 36591[0], 36592[0], 36600[1], 36640[1], 43752[1], 51701[1], 51702[1], 51703[1], 61107[1], 61210[1], 61304[1], 61305[1], 61458[1], 61796[1], 61798[1], 62100[1], 62140[0], 62141[0], 62320[0], 62321[0], 62322[0], 62323[0], 62324[0], 62325[0], 62326[0], 62327[0], 64400[0], 64405[0], 64408[0], 64415[0], 64416[0], 64417[0], 64418[0], 64420[0], 64421[0], 64425[0], 64430[0], 64435[0], 64445[0], 64446[0], 64447[0], 64448[0], 64449[0], 64450[0], 64451[0], 64454[0], 64461[0], 64462[0], 64463[0], 64479[0], 64480[0], 64483[0], 64484[0], 64486[0], 64487[0], 64488[0], 64489[0], 64490[0], 64491[0], 64492[0], 64493[0], 64494[0], 64495[0], 64505[0], 64510[0], 64517[0], 64520[0], 64530[0], 92012[1], 92014[1], 92585[0], 93000[1], 93005[1], 93010[1], 93040[1], 93041[1], 93042[1], 93318[1], 93355[1], 94002[1], 94200[1], 94250[1], 94680[1], 94681[1], 94690[1], 94770[1], 95812[1], 95813[1], 95816[1], 95819[1], 95822[0], 95829[1], 95860[0], 95861[0], 95863[0], 95864[0], 95865[0], 95866[0], 95867[0], 95868[0], 95869[0], 95870[0], 95907[0], 95908[0], 95909[0], 95910[0], 95911[0], 95912[0], 95913[0], 95925[0], 95926[0], 95927[0], 95928[0], 95929[0], 95930[0], 95933[0], 95937[0], 95938[0], 95939[0], 95940[0], 95955[1], 96360[1], 96361[1], 96365[1], 96366[1], 96367[1], 96368[1], 96372[1], 96374[1], 96375[1], 96376[1], 96377[1], 96523[0], 97597[1], 97598[1], 97602[1], 99155[0], 99156[0], 99157[0], 99211[1], 99212[1], 99213[1], 99214[1], 99215[1], 99217[1], 99218[1], 99219[1], 99220[1], 99221[1], 99222[1], 99223[1], 99231[1], 99232[1], 99233[1], 99234[1], 99235[1], 99236[1], 99238[1], 99239[1], 99241[1], 99242[1], 99243[1], 99244[1], 99245[1], 99251[1], 99252[1], 99253[1], 99254[1], 99255[1], 99291[1], 99292[1], 99304[1], 99305[1], 99306[1], 99307[1], 99308[1], 99309[1], 99310[1], 99315[1], 99316[1], 99334[1], 99335[1], 99336[1], 99337[1], 99347[1], 99348[1], 99349[1], 99350[1], 99374[1], 99375[1], 99377[1], 99378[1], 99446[0], 99447[0], 99448[0], 99449[0], 99451[0], 99452[0], 99495[0], 99496[0], G0453[0], G0463[1], G0471[1]
61500	0213T[0], 0216T[0], 0228T[0], 0230T[0], 0333T[0], 0464T[0], 11000[1], 11001[1], 11004[1], 11005[1], 11006[1], 11042[1], 11043[1], 11044[1], 11045[1], 11046[1], 11047[1], 12001[1], 12002[1], 12004[1], 12005[1], 12006[1], 12007[1], 12011[1], 12013[1], 12014[1], 12015[1], 12016[1], 12017[1], 12018[1], 12020[1], 12021[1], 12031[1], 12032[1], 12034[1], 12035[1], 12036[1], 12037[1], 12041[1], 12042[1], 12044[1], 12045[1], 12046[1], 12047[1], 12051[1], 12052[1], 12053[1], 12054[1], 12055[1], 12056[1], 12057[1], 13100[1], 13101[1], 13102[1], 13120[1], 13121[1], 13122[1], 13131[1], 13132[1], 13133[1], 13151[1], 13152[1], 13153[1], 36000[1], 36400[1], 36405[1], 36406[1], 36410[1], 36420[1], 36425[1], 36430[1], 36440[1], 36591[0], 36592[0], 36600[1], 36640[1], 43752[1], 51701[1], 51702[1], 51703[1], 61107[1], 61210[1], 61304[1], 61305[1], 61535[1], 61796[1], 61798[1], 62100[1], 62320[0], 62321[0], 62322[0], 62323[0], 62324[0], 62325[0], 62326[0], 62327[0], 64400[0], 64405[0], 64408[0], 64415[0], 64416[0], 64417[0], 64418[0], 64420[0], 64421[0], 64425[0], 64430[0], 64435[0], 64445[0], 64446[0], 64447[0], 64448[0], 64449[0], 64450[0], 64451[0], 64454[0], 64461[0], 64462[0], 64463[0], 64479[0], 64480[0], 64483[0], 64484[0], 64486[0], 64487[0], 64488[0], 64489[0], 64490[0], 64491[0], 64492[0], 64493[0], 64494[0], 64495[0], 64505[0], 64510[0], 64517[0], 64520[0], 64530[0], 92012[1], 92014[1], 92585[0], 93000[1], 93005[1], 93010[1], 93040[1], 93041[1], 93042[1], 93318[1], 93355[1], 94002[1], 94200[1], 94250[1], 94680[1], 94681[1], 94690[1], 94770[1], 95812[1], 95813[1], 95816[1], 95819[1], 95822[0], 95829[1], 95860[0], 95861[0], 95863[0], 95864[0], 95865[0], 95866[0], 95867[0], 95868[0], 95869[0], 95870[0], 95907[0], 95908[0], 95909[0], 95910[0], 95911[0], 95912[0], 95913[0], 95925[0], 95926[0], 95927[0], 95928[0], 95929[0], 95930[0], 95933[0], 95937[0], 95938[0], 95939[0], 95940[0], 95955[1], 96360[1], 96361[1], 96365[1], 96366[1], 96367[1], 96368[1], 96372[1], 96374[1], 96375[1], 96376[1], 96377[1], 96523[0], 97597[1], 97598[1], 97602[1], 99155[0], 99156[0], 99157[0], 99211[1], 99212[1], 99213[1], 99214[1], 99215[1], 99217[1], 99218[1], 99219[1], 99220[1], 99221[1], 99222[1], 99223[1], 99231[1], 99232[1], 99233[1], 99234[1], 99235[1], 99236[1], 99238[1], 99239[1], 99241[1], 99242[1], 99243[1], 99244[1], 99245[1], 99251[1], 99252[1], 99253[1], 99254[1], 99255[1], 99291[1], 99292[1], 99304[1], 99305[1], 99306[1], 99307[1], 99308[1], 99309[1], 99310[1], 99315[1], 99316[1], 99334[1], 99335[1], 99336[1], 99337[1], 99347[1], 99348[1], 99349[1], 99350[1], 99374[1], 99375[1], 99377[1], 99378[1], 99446[0], 99447[0], 99448[0], 99449[0], 99451[0], 99452[0], 99495[0], 99496[0], G0453[0], G0463[1], G0471[1]
61501	0213T[0], 0216T[0], 0228T[0], 0230T[0], 0333T[0], 0464T[0], 11000[1], 11001[1], 11004[1], 11005[1], 11006[1], 11042[1], 11043[1], 11044[1], 11045[1], 11046[1], 11047[1], 12001[1], 12002[1], 12004[1], 12005[1], 12006[1], 12007[1], 12011[1], 12013[1], 12014[1], 12015[1], 12016[1], 12017[1], 12018[1], 12020[1], 12021[1], 12031[1], 12032[1], 12034[1], 12035[1], 12036[1], 12037[1], 12041[1], 12042[1], 12044[1], 12045[1], 12046[1], 12047[1], 12051[1], 12052[1], 12053[1], 12054[1], 12055[1], 12056[1], 12057[1], 13100[1], 13101[1], 13102[1], 13120[1], 13121[1], 13122[1], 13131[1], 13132[1], 13133[1], 13151[1], 13152[1], 13153[1], 36000[1], 36400[1], 36405[1], 36406[1], 36410[1], 36420[1], 36425[1], 36430[1], 36440[1], 36591[0], 36592[0], 36600[1], 36640[1], 43752[1], 51701[1], 51702[1], 51703[1], 61107[1], 61210[1], 61304[1], 61305[1], 61500[1], 61535[1], 61796[1], 61798[1], 62100[1], 62320[0], 62321[0], 62322[0], 62323[0], 62324[0], 62325[0], 62326[0], 62327[0], 63620[1], 64400[0], 64405[0], 64408[0], 64415[0], 64416[0], 64417[0], 64418[0], 64420[0], 64421[0], 64425[0], 64430[0], 64435[0], 64445[0], 64446[0], 64447[0], 64448[0], 64449[0], 64450[0], 64451[0], 64454[0], 64461[0], 64462[0], 64463[0], 64479[0], 64480[0], 64483[0], 64484[0], 64486[0], 64487[0], 64488[0], 64489[0], 64490[0], 64491[0], 64492[0], 64493[0], 64494[0], 64495[0], 64505[0], 64510[0], 64517[0], 64520[0], 64530[0], 92012[1], 92014[1], 92585[0], 93000[1], 93005[1], 93010[1], 93040[1], 93041[1], 93042[1], 93318[1], 93355[1], 94002[1], 94200[1], 94250[1], 94680[1], 94681[1], 94690[1], 94770[1], 95812[1], 95813[1], 95816[1], 95819[1], 95822[0], 95829[1], 95860[0], 95861[0], 95863[0], 95864[0], 95865[0], 95866[0],

0 = Modifier usage not allowed or inappropriate 1 = Modifier usage allowed

Code 1	Code 2
	95867[0], 95868[0], 95869[0], 95870[0], 95907[0], 95908[0], 95909[0], 95910[0], 95911[0], 95912[0], 95913[0], 95925[0], 95926[0], 95927[0], 95928[0], 95929[0], 95930[0], 95933[0], 95937[0], 95938[0], 95939[0], 95940[0], 95955[1], 96360[1], 96361[1], 96365[1], 96366[1], 96367[1], 96368[1], 96372[1], 96374[1], 96375[1], 96376[1], 96377[1], 96523[0], 97597[1], 97598[1], 97602[1], 99155[0], 99156[0], 99157[0], 99211[1], 99212[1], 99213[1], 99214[1], 99215[1], 99217[1], 99218[1], 99219[1], 99220[1], 99221[1], 99222[1], 99223[1], 99231[1], 99232[1], 99233[1], 99234[1], 99235[1], 99236[1], 99238[1], 99239[1], 99241[1], 99242[1], 99243[1], 99244[1], 99245[1], 99251[1], 99252[1], 99253[1], 99254[1], 99255[1], 99291[1], 99292[1], 99304[1], 99305[1], 99306[1], 99307[1], 99308[1], 99309[1], 99310[1], 99315[1], 99316[1], 99334[1], 99335[1], 99336[1], 99337[1], 99347[1], 99348[1], 99349[1], 99350[1], 99374[1], 99375[1], 99377[1], 99378[1], 99446[0], 99447[0], 99448[0], 99449[0], 99451[0], 99452[0], 99495[0], 99496[0], G0339[1], G0340[1], G0453[0], G0463[1], G0471[1]
61510	0213T[0], 0216T[0], 0228T[0], 0230T[0], 0333T[0], 0464T[0], 11000[1], 11001[1], 11004[1], 11005[1], 11006[1], 11042[1], 11043[1], 11044[1], 11045[1], 11046[1], 11047[1], 12001[1], 12002[1], 12004[1], 12005[1], 12006[1], 12007[1], 12011[1], 12013[1], 12014[1], 12015[1], 12016[1], 12017[1], 12018[1], 12020[1], 12021[1], 12031[1], 12032[1], 12034[1], 12035[1], 12036[1], 12037[1], 12041[1], 12042[1], 12044[1], 12045[1], 12046[1], 12047[1], 12051[1], 12052[1], 12053[1], 12054[1], 12055[1], 12056[1], 12057[1], 13100[1], 13101[1], 13102[1], 13120[1], 13121[1], 13122[1], 13131[1], 13132[1], 13133[1], 13151[1], 13152[1], 13153[1], 36000[1], 36400[1], 36405[1], 36406[1], 36410[1], 36420[1], 36425[1], 36430[1], 36440[1], 36591[0], 36592[0], 36600[1], 36640[1], 43752[1], 51701[1], 51702[1], 51703[1], 61107[1], 61140[0], 61210[1], 61304[1], 61305[1], 61312[1], 61313[1], 61512[1], 61535[0], 61796[1], 61798[1], 62100[1], 62140[1], 62141[1], 62164[1], 62320[0], 62321[0], 62322[0], 62323[0], 62324[0], 62325[0], 62326[0], 62327[0], 64400[0], 64405[0], 64408[0], 64415[0], 64416[0], 64417[0], 64418[0], 64420[0], 64421[0], 64425[0], 64430[0], 64435[0], 64445[0], 64446[0], 64447[0], 64448[0], 64449[0], 64450[0], 64451[0], 64454[0], 64461[0], 64462[0], 64463[0], 64479[0], 64480[0], 64483[0], 64484[0], 64486[0], 64487[0], 64488[0], 64489[0], 64490[0], 64491[0], 64492[0], 64493[0], 64494[0], 64495[0], 64505[0], 64510[0], 64517[0], 64520[0], 64530[0], 92012[1], 92014[1], 92585[0], 93000[1], 93005[1], 93010[1], 93040[1], 93041[1], 93042[1], 93318[1], 93355[1], 94002[1], 94200[1], 94250[1], 94680[1], 94681[1], 94690[1], 94770[1], 95812[1], 95813[1], 95816[1], 95819[1], 95822[0], 95829[1], 95860[0], 95861[0], 95863[0], 95864[0], 95865[0], 95866[0], 95867[0], 95868[0], 95869[0], 95870[0], 95907[0], 95908[0], 95909[0], 95910[0], 95911[0], 95912[0], 95913[0], 95925[0], 95926[0], 95927[0], 95928[0], 95929[0], 95930[0], 95933[0], 95937[0], 95938[0], 95939[0], 95940[0], 95955[1], 96360[1], 96361[1], 96365[1], 96366[1], 96367[1], 96368[1], 96372[1], 96374[1], 96375[1], 96376[1], 96377[1], 96523[0], 97597[1], 97598[1], 97602[1], 99155[0], 99156[0], 99157[0], 99211[1], 99212[1], 99213[1], 99214[1], 99215[1], 99217[1], 99218[1], 99219[1], 99220[1], 99221[1], 99222[1], 99223[1], 99231[1], 99232[1], 99233[1], 99234[1], 99235[1], 99236[1], 99238[1], 99239[1], 99241[1], 99242[1], 99243[1], 99244[1], 99245[1], 99251[1], 99252[1], 99253[1], 99254[1], 99255[1], 99291[1], 99292[1], 99304[1], 99305[1], 99306[1], 99307[1], 99308[1], 99309[1], 99310[1], 99315[1], 99316[1], 99334[1], 99335[1], 99336[1], 99337[1], 99347[1], 99348[1], 99349[1], 99350[1], 99374[1], 99375[1], 99377[1], 99378[1], 99446[0], 99447[0], 99448[0], 99449[0], 99451[0], 99452[0], 99495[0], 99496[0], G0453[0], G0463[1], G0471[1]
61512	0213T[0], 0216T[0], 0228T[0], 0230T[0], 0333T[0], 0464T[0], 11000[1], 11001[1], 11004[1], 11005[1], 11006[1], 11042[1], 11043[1], 11044[1], 11045[1], 11046[1], 11047[1], 12001[1], 12002[1], 12004[1], 12005[1], 12006[1], 12007[1], 12011[1], 12013[1], 12014[1], 12015[1], 12016[1], 12017[1], 12018[1], 12020[1], 12021[1], 12031[1], 12032[1], 12034[1], 12035[1], 12036[1], 12037[1], 12041[1], 12042[1], 12044[1], 12045[1], 12046[1], 12047[1], 12051[1], 12052[1], 12053[1], 12054[1], 12055[1], 12056[1], 12057[1], 13100[1], 13101[1], 13102[1], 13120[1], 13121[1], 13122[1], 13131[1], 13132[1], 13133[1], 13151[1], 13152[1], 13153[1], 36000[1], 36400[1], 36405[1], 36406[1], 36410[1], 36420[1], 36425[1], 36430[1], 36440[1], 36591[0], 36592[0], 36600[1], 36640[1], 43752[1], 51701[1], 51702[1], 51703[1], 61107[1], 61210[1], 61304[1], 61305[1], 61312[1], 61535[0], 61796[1], 61798[1], 62100[1], 62140[1], 62141[1], 62164[1], 62320[0], 62321[0], 62322[0], 62323[0], 62324[0], 62325[0], 62326[0], 62327[0], 64400[0], 64405[0], 64408[0], 64415[0], 64416[0], 64417[0], 64418[0], 64420[0], 64421[0], 64425[0], 64430[0], 64435[0], 64445[0], 64446[0], 64447[0], 64448[0], 64449[0], 64450[0], 64451[0], 64454[0], 64461[0], 64462[0], 64463[0], 64479[0], 64480[0], 64483[0], 64484[0], 64486[0], 64487[0], 64488[0], 64489[0], 64490[0], 64491[0], 64492[0], 64493[0], 64494[0], 64495[0], 64505[0], 64510[0], 64517[0], 64520[0], 64530[0], 92012[1], 92014[1], 92585[0], 93000[1], 93005[1], 93010[1], 93040[1], 93041[1], 93042[1], 93318[1], 93355[1], 94002[1], 94200[1], 94250[1], 94680[1], 94681[1], 94690[1], 94770[1], 95812[1], 95813[1], 95816[1], 95819[1], 95822[0], 95829[1], 95860[0], 95861[0], 95863[0], 95864[0], 95865[0], 95866[0], 95867[0], 95868[0], 95869[0], 95870[0], 95907[0], 95908[0], 95909[0], 95910[0], 95911[0], 95912[0], 95913[0], 95925[0], 95926[0], 95927[0], 95928[0], 95929[0], 95930[0], 95933[0], 95937[0], 95938[0], 95939[0], 95940[0], 95955[1], 96360[1], 96361[1], 96365[1], 96366[1], 96367[1], 96368[1], 96372[1], 96374[1], 96375[1], 96376[1], 96377[1], 96523[0], 97597[1], 97598[1], 97602[1], 99155[0], 99156[0], 99157[0], 99211[1], 99212[1], 99213[1], 99214[1], 99215[1], 99217[1], 99218[1], 99219[1], 99220[1], 99221[1], 99222[1], 99223[1], 99231[1], 99232[1], 99233[1], 99234[1], 99235[1], 99236[1], 99238[1], 99239[1], 99241[1], 99242[1], 99243[1], 99244[1], 99245[1], 99251[1], 99252[1], 99253[1], 99254[1], 99255[1], 99291[1], 99292[1], 99304[1], 99305[1], 99306[1], 99307[1], 99308[1], 99309[1], 99310[1], 99315[1], 99316[1], 99334[1], 99335[1], 99336[1], 99337[1], 99347[1], 99348[1], 99349[1], 99350[1], 99374[1], 99375[1], 99377[1], 99378[1], 99446[0], 99447[0], 99448[0], 99449[0], 99451[0], 99452[0], 99495[0], 99496[0], G0453[0], G0463[1], G0471[1]
61514	0213T[0], 0216T[0], 0228T[0], 0230T[0], 0333T[0], 0464T[0], 11000[1], 11001[1], 11004[1], 11005[1], 11006[1], 11042[1], 11043[1], 11044[1], 11045[1], 11046[1], 11047[1], 12001[1], 12002[1], 12004[1], 12005[1], 12006[1], 12007[1], 12011[1], 12013[1], 12014[1], 12015[1], 12016[1], 12017[1], 12018[1], 12020[1], 12021[1], 12031[1], 12032[1], 12034[1], 12035[1], 12036[1], 12037[1], 12041[1], 12042[1], 12044[1], 12045[1], 12046[1], 12047[1], 12051[1], 12052[1], 12053[1], 12054[1], 12055[1], 12056[1], 12057[1], 13100[1], 13101[1], 13102[1], 13120[1], 13121[1], 13122[1], 13131[1], 13132[1], 13133[1], 13151[1], 13152[1], 13153[1], 36000[1], 36400[1], 36405[1], 36406[1], 36410[1], 36420[1], 36425[1], 36430[1], 36440[1], 36591[0], 36592[0], 36600[1], 36640[1], 43752[1], 51701[1], 51702[1], 51703[1], 61107[1], 61210[1], 61304[1], 61305[1], 61320[1], 61535[0], 61796[1], 61798[1], 62100[1], 62140[0], 62141[0], 62320[0], 62321[0], 62322[0], 62323[0], 62324[0], 62325[0], 62326[0], 62327[0], 64400[0], 64405[0], 64408[0], 64415[0], 64416[0], 64417[0], 64418[0], 64420[0], 64421[0], 64425[0], 64430[0], 64435[0], 64445[0], 64446[0], 64447[0], 64448[0], 64449[0], 64450[0], 64451[0], 64454[0], 64461[0], 64462[0], 64463[0], 64479[0], 64480[0], 64483[0], 64484[0], 64486[0], 64487[0], 64488[0], 64489[0], 64490[0], 64491[0], 64492[0], 64493[0], 64494[0], 64495[0], 64505[0], 64510[0], 64517[0], 64520[0], 64530[0], 92012[1], 92014[1], 92585[0], 93000[1], 93005[1], 93010[1], 93040[1], 93041[1], 93042[1], 93318[1], 93355[1], 94002[1], 94200[1], 94250[1], 94680[1], 94681[1], 94690[1], 94770[1], 95812[1], 95813[1], 95816[1], 95819[1], 95822[0], 95829[1], 95860[0], 95861[0], 95863[0], 95864[0], 95865[0], 95866[0], 95867[0], 95868[0], 95869[0], 95870[0], 95907[0], 95908[0], 95909[0], 95910[0], 95911[0], 95912[0], 95913[0], 95925[0], 95926[0], 95927[0], 95928[0], 95929[0], 95930[0], 95933[0], 95937[0], 95938[0], 95939[0], 95940[0], 95955[1], 96360[1], 96361[1], 96365[1], 96366[1], 96367[1], 96368[1], 96372[1], 96374[1], 96375[1], 96376[1], 96377[1], 96523[0], 97597[1], 97598[1], 97602[1], 99155[0], 99156[0], 99157[0], 99211[1], 99212[1], 99213[1], 99214[1], 99215[1], 99217[1], 99218[1], 99219[1], 99220[1], 99221[1], 99222[1], 99223[1], 99231[1], 99232[1], 99233[1], 99234[1], 99235[1], 99236[1], 99238[1], 99239[1], 99241[1], 99242[1], 99243[1], 99244[1], 99245[1], 99251[1], 99252[1], 99253[1], 99254[1], 99255[1], 99291[1], 99292[1], 99304[1], 99305[1], 99306[1], 99307[1], 99308[1], 99309[1], 99310[1], 99315[1], 99316[1], 99334[1], 99335[1], 99336[1], 99337[1], 99347[1], 99348[1], 99349[1], 99350[1], 99374[1], 99375[1], 99377[1], 99378[1], 99446[0], 99447[0], 99448[0], 99449[0], 99451[0], 99452[0], 99495[0], 99496[0], G0453[0], G0463[1], G0471[1]
61516	0213T[0], 0216T[0], 0228T[0], 0230T[0], 0333T[0], 0464T[0], 11000[1], 11001[1], 11004[1], 11005[1], 11006[1], 11042[1], 11043[1], 11044[1], 11045[1], 11046[1], 11047[1], 12001[1], 12002[1], 12004[1], 12005[1], 12006[1], 12007[1], 12011[1], 12013[1], 12014[1], 12015[1], 12016[1], 12017[1], 12018[1], 12020[1], 12021[1], 12031[1], 12032[1], 12034[1], 12035[1], 12036[1], 12037[1], 12041[1], 12042[1], 12044[1], 12045[1], 12046[1], 12047[1], 12051[1], 12052[1], 12053[1], 12054[1], 12055[1], 12056[1], 12057[1], 13100[1], 13101[1], 13102[1], 13120[1], 13121[1], 13122[1], 13131[1], 13132[1], 13133[1], 13151[1], 13152[1], 13153[1], 36000[1], 36400[1], 36405[1], 36406[1], 36410[1], 36420[1], 36425[1], 36430[1], 36440[1], 36591[0], 36592[0], 36600[1], 36640[1], 43752[1], 51701[1], 51702[1], 51703[1], 61107[1], 61140[1], 61210[1], 61304[1], 61305[1], 61535[0], 61796[1], 61798[1], 62100[1], 62140[1], 62141[1], 62161[1], 62320[0], 62321[0], 62322[0], 62323[0], 62324[0], 62325[0], 62326[0], 62327[0], 64400[0], 64405[0], 64408[0], 64415[0], 64416[0], 64417[0], 64418[0], 64420[0], 64421[0], 64425[0], 64430[0], 64435[0], 64445[0], 64446[0], 64447[0], 64448[0], 64449[0], 64450[0], 64451[0], 64454[0], 64461[0], 64462[0], 64463[0], 64479[0], 64480[0], 64483[0], 64484[0], 64486[0], 64487[0], 64488[0], 64489[0], 64490[0], 64491[0], 64492[0], 64493[0], 64494[0], 64495[0], 64505[0], 64510[0], 64517[0], 64520[0], 64530[0], 92012[1], 92014[1], 92585[0], 93000[1], 93005[1], 93010[1], 93040[1], 93041[1], 93042[1], 93318[1], 93355[1], 94002[1], 94200[1], 94250[1], 94680[1], 94681[1], 94690[1], 94770[1], 95812[1], 95813[1], 95816[1], 95819[1], 95822[0], 95829[1], 95860[0], 95861[0], 95863[0], 95864[0], 95865[0], 95866[0], 95867[0], 95868[0], 95869[0], 95870[0], 95907[0], 95908[0], 95909[0], 95910[0], 95911[0], 95912[0], 95913[0], 95925[0], 95926[0], 95927[0], 95928[0], 95929[0], 95930[0], 95933[0], 95937[0], 95938[0], 95939[0], 95940[0], 95955[1], 96360[1], 96361[1], 96365[1], 96366[1], 96367[1], 96368[1], 96372[1], 96374[1], 96375[1], 96376[1], 96377[1], 96523[0], 97597[1], 97598[1], 97602[1], 99155[0], 99156[0], 99157[0], 99211[1], 99212[1], 99213[1], 99214[1], 99215[1], 99217[1], 99218[1], 99219[1], 99220[1], 99221[1], 99222[1], 99223[1], 99231[1], 99232[1], 99233[1], 99234[1], 99235[1], 99236[1], 99238[1], 99239[1], 99241[1], 99242[1], 99243[1], 99244[1], 99245[1], 99251[1], 99252[1], 99253[1], 99254[1], 99255[1], 99291[1], 99292[1], 99304[1], 99305[1], 99306[1], 99307[1], 99308[1], 99309[1], 99310[1], 99315[1], 99316[1], 99334[1], 99335[1], 99336[1], 99337[1], 99347[1], 99348[1], 99349[1], 99350[1], 99374[1], 99375[1], 99377[1], 99378[1], 99446[0], 99447[0], 99448[0], 99449[0], 99451[0], 99452[0], 99495[0], 99496[0], G0453[0], G0463[1], G0471[1]
61517	0213T[1], 0216T[1], 0333T[0], 0464T[0], 36000[1], 36410[1], 36591[0], 36592[0], 61107[1], 61650[1], 62324[0], 62325[0], 62326[0], 62327[0], 64415[1], 64417[1], 64450[1], 64454[1], 64486[1], 64487[1], 64488[1], 64489[1], 64490[1], 64493[1], 92585[0], 95822[0], 95860[0], 95861[0], 95863[0], 95864[0], 95865[0], 95866[0], 95867[0], 95868[0], 95869[0], 95907[0], 95908[0], 95909[0], 95910[0], 95911[0], 95912[0], 95913[0], 95925[0], 95926[0], 95927[0], 95930[0], 95933[0], 95937[0], 95938[0], 95939[0], 95940[0], 96523[0], G0453[0]

0 = Modifier usage not allowed or inappropriate 1 = Modifier usage allowed

Code 1	Code 2
61518	0213T[0], 0216T[0], 0228T[0], 0230T[0], 0333T[0], 0464T[0], 11000[1], 11001[1], 11004[1], 11005[1], 11006[1], 11042[1], 11043[1], 11044[1], 11045[1], 11046[1], 11047[1], 12001[1], 12002[1], 12004[1], 12005[1], 12006[1], 12007[1], 12011[1], 12013[1], 12014[1], 12015[1], 12016[1], 12017[1], 12018[1], 12020[1], 12021[1], 12031[1], 12032[1], 12034[1], 12035[1], 12036[1], 12037[1], 12041[1], 12042[1], 12044[1], 12045[1], 12046[1], 12047[1], 12051[1], 12052[1], 12053[1], 12054[1], 12055[1], 12056[1], 12057[1], 13100[1], 13101[1], 13102[1], 13120[1], 13121[1], 13122[1], 13131[1], 13132[1], 13133[1], 13151[1], 13152[1], 13153[1], 36000[1], 36400[1], 36405[1], 36406[1], 36410[1], 36420[1], 36425[1], 36430[1], 36440[1], 36591[0], 36592[0], 36600[1], 36640[1], 43752[1], 51701[1], 51702[1], 51703[1], 61107[1], 61140[0], 61210[1], 61304[1], 61305[1], 61519[1], 61535[1], 61796[1], 61798[1], 62100[1], 62140[1], 62141[1], 62164[1], 62320[0], 62321[0], 62322[0], 62323[0], 62324[0], 62325[0], 62326[0], 62327[0], 63285[1], 64400[0], 64405[0], 64408[0], 64415[0], 64416[0], 64417[0], 64418[0], 64420[0], 64421[0], 64425[0], 64430[0], 64435[0], 64445[0], 64446[0], 64447[0], 64448[0], 64449[0], 64450[0], 64451[0], 64454[0], 64461[0], 64462[0], 64463[0], 64479[0], 64480[0], 64483[0], 64484[0], 64486[0], 64487[0], 64488[0], 64489[0], 64490[0], 64491[0], 64492[0], 64493[0], 64494[0], 64495[0], 64505[0], 64510[0], 64517[0], 64520[0], 64530[0], 92012[1], 92014[1], 92585[0], 93000[1], 93005[1], 93010[1], 93040[1], 93041[1], 93042[1], 93318[1], 93355[1], 94002[1], 94200[1], 94250[1], 94680[1], 94681[1], 94690[1], 94770[1], 95812[1], 95813[1], 95816[1], 95819[1], 95822[0], 95829[1], 95860[0], 95861[0], 95863[0], 95864[0], 95865[0], 95866[0], 95867[0], 95868[0], 95869[0], 95870[0], 95907[0], 95908[0], 95909[0], 95910[0], 95911[0], 95912[0], 95913[0], 95925[0], 95926[0], 95927[0], 95928[0], 95929[0], 95930[0], 95933[0], 95937[0], 95938[0], 95939[0], 95940[0], 95955[1], 96360[1], 96361[1], 96365[1], 96366[1], 96367[1], 96368[1], 96372[1], 96374[1], 96375[1], 96376[1], 96377[1], 96523[0], 97597[1], 97598[1], 97602[1], 99155[0], 99156[0], 99157[0], 99211[1], 99212[1], 99213[1], 99214[1], 99215[1], 99217[1], 99218[1], 99219[1], 99220[1], 99221[1], 99222[1], 99223[1], 99231[1], 99232[1], 99233[1], 99234[1], 99235[1], 99236[1], 99238[1], 99239[1], 99241[1], 99242[1], 99243[1], 99244[1], 99245[1], 99251[1], 99252[1], 99253[1], 99254[1], 99255[1], 99291[1], 99292[1], 99304[1], 99305[1], 99306[1], 99307[1], 99308[1], 99309[1], 99310[1], 99315[1], 99316[1], 99334[1], 99335[1], 99336[1], 99337[1], 99347[1], 99348[1], 99349[1], 99350[1], 99374[1], 99375[1], 99377[1], 99378[1], 99446[0], 99447[0], 99448[0], 99449[0], 99451[0], 99452[0], 99495[0], 99496[0], G0453[0], G0463[1], G0471[1]
61519	0213T[0], 0216T[0], 0228T[0], 0230T[0], 0333T[0], 0464T[0], 11000[1], 11001[1], 11004[1], 11005[1], 11006[1], 11042[1], 11043[1], 11044[1], 11045[1], 11046[1], 11047[1], 12001[1], 12002[1], 12004[1], 12005[1], 12006[1], 12007[1], 12011[1], 12013[1], 12014[1], 12015[1], 12016[1], 12017[1], 12018[1], 12020[1], 12021[1], 12031[1], 12032[1], 12034[1], 12035[1], 12036[1], 12037[1], 12041[1], 12042[1], 12044[1], 12045[1], 12046[1], 12047[1], 12051[1], 12052[1], 12053[1], 12054[1], 12055[1], 12056[1], 12057[1], 13100[1], 13101[1], 13102[1], 13120[1], 13121[1], 13122[1], 13131[1], 13132[1], 13133[1], 13151[1], 13152[1], 13153[1], 36000[1], 36400[1], 36405[1], 36406[1], 36410[1], 36420[1], 36425[1], 36430[1], 36440[1], 36591[0], 36592[0], 36600[1], 36640[1], 43752[1], 51701[1], 51702[1], 51703[1], 61107[1], 61140[0], 61210[1], 61304[1], 61305[1], 61535[1], 61796[1], 61798[1], 62100[1], 62140[1], 62141[1], 62164[1], 62320[0], 62321[0], 62322[0], 62323[0], 62324[0], 62325[0], 62326[0], 62327[0], 64400[0], 64405[0], 64408[0], 64415[0], 64416[0], 64417[0], 64418[0], 64420[0], 64421[0], 64425[0], 64430[0], 64435[0], 64445[0], 64446[0], 64447[0], 64448[0], 64449[0], 64450[0], 64451[0], 64454[0], 64461[0], 64462[0], 64463[0], 64479[0], 64480[0], 64483[0], 64484[0], 64486[0], 64487[0], 64488[0], 64489[0], 64490[0], 64491[0], 64492[0], 64493[0], 64494[0], 64495[0], 64505[0], 64510[0], 64517[0], 64520[0], 64530[0], 92012[1], 92014[1], 92585[0], 93000[1], 93005[1], 93010[1], 93040[1], 93041[1], 93042[1], 93318[1], 93355[1], 94002[1], 94200[1], 94250[1], 94680[1], 94681[1], 94690[1], 94770[1], 95812[1], 95813[1], 95816[1], 95819[1], 95822[0], 95829[1], 95860[0], 95861[0], 95863[0], 95864[0], 95865[0], 95866[0], 95867[0], 95868[0], 95869[0], 95870[0], 95907[0], 95908[0], 95909[0], 95910[0], 95911[0], 95912[0], 95913[0], 95925[0], 95926[0], 95927[0], 95928[0], 95929[0], 95930[0], 95933[0], 95937[0], 95938[0], 95939[0], 95940[0], 95955[1], 96360[1], 96361[1], 96365[1], 96366[1], 96367[1], 96368[1], 96372[1], 96374[1], 96375[1], 96376[1], 96377[1], 96523[0], 97597[1], 97598[1], 97602[1], 99155[0], 99156[0], 99157[0], 99211[1], 99212[1], 99213[1], 99214[1], 99215[1], 99217[1], 99218[1], 99219[1], 99220[1], 99221[1], 99222[1], 99223[1], 99231[1], 99232[1], 99233[1], 99234[1], 99235[1], 99236[1], 99238[1], 99239[1], 99241[1], 99242[1], 99243[1], 99244[1], 99245[1], 99251[1], 99252[1], 99253[1], 99254[1], 99255[1], 99291[1], 99292[1], 99304[1], 99305[1], 99306[1], 99307[1], 99308[1], 99309[1], 99310[1], 99315[1], 99316[1], 99334[1], 99335[1], 99336[1], 99337[1], 99347[1], 99348[1], 99349[1], 99350[1], 99374[1], 99375[1], 99377[1], 99378[1], 99446[0], 99447[0], 99448[0], 99449[0], 99451[0], 99452[0], 99495[0], 99496[0], G0453[0], G0463[1], G0471[1]
61520	0213T[0], 0216T[0], 0228T[0], 0230T[0], 0333T[0], 0464T[0], 11000[1], 11001[1], 11004[1], 11005[1], 11006[1], 11042[1], 11043[1], 11044[1], 11045[1], 11046[1], 11047[1], 12001[1], 12002[1], 12004[1], 12005[1], 12006[1], 12007[1], 12011[1], 12013[1], 12014[1], 12015[1], 12016[1], 12017[1], 12018[1], 12020[1], 12021[1], 12031[1], 12032[1], 12034[1], 12035[1], 12036[1], 12037[1], 12041[1], 12042[1], 12044[1], 12045[1], 12046[1], 12047[1], 12051[1], 12052[1], 12053[1], 12054[1], 12055[1], 12056[1], 12057[1], 13100[1], 13101[1], 13102[1], 13120[1], 13121[1], 13122[1], 13131[1], 13132[1], 13133[1], 13151[1], 13152[1], 13153[1], 36000[1], 36400[1], 36405[1], 36406[1], 36410[1], 36420[1], 36425[1], 36430[1], 36440[1], 36591[0], 36592[0], 36600[1], 36640[1], 43752[1], 51701[1], 51702[1], 51703[1], 61107[1], 61140[0], 61210[1], 61304[1], 61305[1], 61535[1], 61796[1], 61798[1], 62100[1], 62140[1], 62141[1], 62164[1], 62320[0], 62321[0], 62322[0], 62323[0], 62324[0], 62325[0], 62326[0], 62327[0], 64400[0], 64405[0], 64408[0], 64415[0], 64416[0], 64417[0], 64418[0], 64420[0], 64421[0], 64425[0], 64430[0], 64435[0], 64445[0], 64446[0], 64447[0], 64448[0], 64449[0], 64450[0], 64451[0], 64454[0], 64461[0], 64462[0], 64463[0], 64479[0], 64480[0], 64483[0], 64484[0], 64486[0], 64487[0], 64488[0], 64489[0], 64490[0], 64491[0], 64492[0], 64493[0], 64494[0], 64495[0], 64505[0], 64510[0], 64517[0], 64520[0], 64530[0], 92012[1], 92014[1], 92585[0], 93000[1], 93005[1], 93010[1], 93040[1], 93041[1], 93042[1], 93318[1], 93355[1], 94002[1], 94200[1], 94250[1], 94680[1], 94681[1], 94690[1], 94770[1], 95812[1], 95813[1], 95816[1], 95819[1], 95822[0], 95829[1], 95860[0], 95861[0], 95863[0], 95864[0], 95865[0], 95866[0], 95867[0], 95868[0], 95869[0], 95870[0], 95907[0], 95908[0], 95909[0], 95910[0], 95911[0], 95912[0], 95913[0], 95925[0], 95926[0], 95927[0], 95928[0], 95929[0], 95930[0], 95933[0], 95937[0], 95938[0], 95939[0], 95940[0], 95955[1], 96360[1], 96361[1], 96365[1], 96366[1], 96367[1], 96368[1], 96372[1], 96374[1], 96375[1], 96376[1], 96377[1], 96523[0], 97597[1], 97598[1], 97602[1], 99155[0], 99156[0], 99157[0], 99211[1], 99212[1], 99213[1], 99214[1], 99215[1], 99217[1], 99218[1], 99219[1], 99220[1], 99221[1], 99222[1], 99223[1], 99231[1], 99232[1], 99233[1], 99234[1], 99235[1], 99236[1], 99238[1], 99239[1], 99241[1], 99242[1], 99243[1], 99244[1], 99245[1], 99251[1], 99252[1], 99253[1], 99254[1], 99255[1], 99291[1], 99292[1], 99304[1], 99305[1], 99306[1], 99307[1], 99308[1], 99309[1], 99310[1], 99315[1], 99316[1], 99334[1], 99335[1], 99336[1], 99337[1], 99347[1], 99348[1], 99349[1], 99350[1], 99374[1], 99375[1], 99377[1], 99378[1], 99446[0], 99447[0], 99448[0], 99449[0], 99451[0], 99452[0], 99495[0], 99496[0], G0453[0], G0463[1], G0471[1]
61521	0213T[0], 0216T[0], 0228T[0], 0230T[0], 0333T[0], 0464T[0], 11000[1], 11001[1], 11004[1], 11005[1], 11006[1], 11042[1], 11043[1], 11044[1], 11045[1], 11046[1], 11047[1], 12001[1], 12002[1], 12004[1], 12005[1], 12006[1], 12007[1], 12011[1], 12013[1], 12014[1], 12015[1], 12016[1], 12017[1], 12018[1], 12020[1], 12021[1], 12031[1], 12032[1], 12034[1], 12035[1], 12036[1], 12037[1], 12041[1], 12042[1], 12044[1], 12045[1], 12046[1], 12047[1], 12051[1], 12052[1], 12053[1], 12054[1], 12055[1], 12056[1], 12057[1], 13100[1], 13101[1], 13102[1], 13120[1], 13121[1], 13122[1], 13131[1], 13132[1], 13133[1], 13151[1], 13152[1], 13153[1], 36000[1], 36400[1], 36405[1], 36406[1], 36410[1], 36420[1], 36425[1], 36430[1], 36440[1], 36591[0], 36592[0], 36600[1], 36640[1], 43752[1], 51701[1], 51702[1], 51703[1], 61107[1], 61140[0], 61210[1], 61304[1], 61305[1], 61535[1], 61796[1], 61798[1], 62100[1], 62140[1], 62141[1], 62164[1], 62320[0], 62321[0], 62322[0], 62323[0], 62324[0], 62325[0], 62326[0], 62327[0], 64400[0], 64405[0], 64408[0], 64415[0], 64416[0], 64417[0], 64418[0], 64420[0], 64421[0], 64425[0], 64430[0], 64435[0], 64445[0], 64446[0], 64447[0], 64448[0], 64449[0], 64450[0], 64451[0], 64454[0], 64461[0], 64462[0], 64463[0], 64479[0], 64480[0], 64483[0], 64484[0], 64486[0], 64487[0], 64488[0], 64489[0], 64490[0], 64491[0], 64492[0], 64493[0], 64494[0], 64495[0], 64505[0], 64510[0], 64517[0], 64520[0], 64530[0], 92012[1], 92014[1], 92585[0], 93000[1], 93005[1], 93010[1], 93040[1], 93041[1], 93042[1], 93318[1], 93355[1], 94002[1], 94200[1], 94250[1], 94680[1], 94681[1], 94690[1], 94770[1], 95812[1], 95813[1], 95816[1], 95819[1], 95822[0], 95829[1], 95860[0], 95861[0], 95863[0], 95864[0], 95865[0], 95866[0], 95867[0], 95868[0], 95869[0], 95870[0], 95907[0], 95908[0], 95909[0], 95910[0], 95911[0], 95912[0], 95913[0], 95925[0], 95926[0], 95927[0], 95928[0], 95929[0], 95930[0], 95933[0], 95937[0], 95938[0], 95939[0], 95940[0], 95955[1], 96360[1], 96361[1], 96365[1], 96366[1], 96367[1], 96368[1], 96372[1], 96374[1], 96375[1], 96376[1], 96377[1], 96523[0], 97597[1], 97598[1], 97602[1], 99155[0], 99156[0], 99157[0], 99211[1], 99212[1], 99213[1], 99214[1], 99215[1], 99217[1], 99218[1], 99219[1], 99220[1], 99221[1], 99222[1], 99223[1], 99231[1], 99232[1], 99233[1], 99234[1], 99235[1], 99236[1], 99238[1], 99239[1], 99241[1], 99242[1], 99243[1], 99244[1], 99245[1], 99251[1], 99252[1], 99253[1], 99254[1], 99255[1], 99291[1], 99292[1], 99304[1], 99305[1], 99306[1], 99307[1], 99308[1], 99309[1], 99310[1], 99315[1], 99316[1], 99334[1], 99335[1], 99336[1], 99337[1], 99347[1], 99348[1], 99349[1], 99350[1], 99374[1], 99375[1], 99377[1], 99378[1], 99446[0], 99447[0], 99448[0], 99449[0], 99451[0], 99452[0], 99495[0], 99496[0], G0453[0], G0463[1], G0471[1]
61522	0213T[0], 0216T[0], 0228T[0], 0230T[0], 0333T[0], 0464T[0], 11000[1], 11001[1], 11004[1], 11005[1], 11006[1], 11042[1], 11043[1], 11044[1], 11045[1], 11046[1], 11047[1], 12001[1], 12002[1], 12004[1], 12005[1], 12006[1], 12007[1], 12011[1], 12013[1], 12014[1], 12015[1], 12016[1], 12017[1], 12018[1], 12020[1], 12021[1], 12031[1], 12032[1], 12034[1], 12035[1], 12036[1], 12037[1], 12041[1], 12042[1], 12044[1], 12045[1], 12046[1], 12047[1], 12051[1], 12052[1], 12053[1], 12054[1], 12055[1], 12056[1], 12057[1], 13100[1], 13101[1], 13102[1], 13120[1], 13121[1], 13122[1], 13131[1], 13132[1], 13133[1], 13151[1], 13152[1], 13153[1], 36000[1], 36400[1], 36405[1], 36406[1], 36410[1], 36420[1], 36425[1], 36430[1], 36440[1], 36591[0], 36592[0], 36600[1], 36640[1], 43752[1], 51701[1], 51702[1], 51703[1], 61107[1], 61210[1], 61304[1], 61305[1], 61321[1], 61526[1], 61530[1], 61535[1], 61796[1], 61798[1], 62100[1], 62140[0], 62141[0], 62320[0], 62321[0], 62322[0], 62323[0], 62324[0], 62325[0], 62326[0], 62327[0], 64400[0], 64405[0], 64408[0], 64415[0], 64416[0], 64417[0], 64418[0], 64420[0], 64421[0], 64425[0], 64430[0], 64435[0], 64445[0], 64446[0], 64447[0], 64448[0], 64449[0], 64450[0], 64451[0], 64454[0], 64461[0], 64462[0], 64463[0], 64479[0], 64480[0], 64483[0], 64484[0], 64486[0], 64487[0], 64488[0], 64489[0], 64490[0], 64491[0], 64492[0], 64493[0], 64494[0], 64495[0], 64505[0], 64510[0], 64517[0], 64520[0], 64530[0], 92012[1], 92014[1], 92585[0], 93000[1], 93005[1], 93010[1], 93040[1], 93041[1], 93042[1], 93318[1], 93355[1], 94002[1], 94200[1], 94250[1], 94680[1], 94681[1], 94690[1], 94770[1], 95812[1], 95813[1], 95816[1], 95819[1], 95822[0], 95829[1], 95860[0], 95861[0], 95863[0], 95864[0], 95865[0], 95866[0], 95867[0], 95868[0], 95869[0], 95870[0], 95907[0], 95908[0], 95909[0], 95910[0], 95911[0], 95912[0], 95913[0], 95925[0], 95926[0], 95927[0], 95928[0], 95929[0], 95930[0], 95933[0], 95937[0], 95938[0], 95939[0], 95940[0], 95955[1], 96360[1], 96361[1], 96365[1], 96366[1],

0 = Modifier usage not allowed or inappropriate   1 = Modifier usage allowed

Appendix A: NCCI - CPT Codes

Code 1	Code 2
	96367[1], 96368[1], 96372[1], 96374[1], 96375[1], 96376[1], 96377[1], 96523[0], 97597[1], 97598[1], 97602[1], 99155[0], 99156[0], 99157[0], 99211[1], 99212[1], 99213[1], 99214[1], 99215[1], 99217[1], 99218[1], 99219[1], 99220[1], 99221[1], 99222[1], 99223[1], 99231[1], 99232[1], 99233[1], 99234[1], 99235[1], 99236[1], 99238[1], 99239[1], 99241[1], 99242[1], 99243[1], 99244[1], 99245[1], 99251[1], 99252[1], 99253[1], 99254[1], 99255[1], 99291[1], 99292[1], 99304[1], 99305[1], 99306[1], 99307[1], 99308[1], 99309[1], 99310[1], 99315[1], 99316[1], 99334[1], 99335[1], 99336[1], 99337[1], 99347[1], 99348[1], 99349[1], 99350[1], 99374[1], 99375[1], 99377[1], 99378[1], 99446[0], 99447[0], 99448[0], 99449[0], 99451[0], 99452[0], 99495[0], 99496[0], G0453[0], G0463[1], G0471[1]
61524	0213T[0], 0216T[0], 0228T[0], 0230T[0], 0333T[0], 0464T[0], 11000[1], 11001[1], 11004[1], 11005[1], 11006[1], 11042[1], 11043[1], 11044[1], 11045[1], 11046[1], 11047[1], 12001[1], 12002[1], 12004[1], 12005[1], 12006[1], 12007[1], 12011[1], 12013[1], 12014[1], 12015[1], 12016[1], 12017[1], 12018[1], 12020[1], 12021[1], 12031[1], 12032[1], 12034[1], 12035[1], 12036[1], 12037[1], 12041[1], 12042[1], 12044[1], 12045[1], 12046[1], 12047[1], 12051[1], 12052[1], 12053[1], 12054[1], 12055[1], 12056[1], 12057[1], 13100[1], 13101[1], 13102[1], 13120[1], 13121[1], 13122[1], 13131[1], 13132[1], 13133[1], 13151[1], 13152[1], 13153[1], 36000[1], 36400[1], 36405[1], 36406[1], 36410[1], 36420[1], 36425[1], 36430[1], 36440[1], 36591[0], 36592[0], 36600[1], 36640[1], 43752[1], 51701[1], 51702[1], 51703[1], 61107[1], 61140[1], 61210[1], 61304[1], 61305[1], 61522[1], 61530[1], 61535[1], 61796[1], 61798[1], 62100[1], 62140[0], 62141[0], 62161[1], 62162[1], 62320[0], 62321[0], 62322[0], 62323[0], 62324[0], 62325[0], 62326[0], 62327[0], 64400[0], 64405[0], 64408[0], 64415[0], 64416[0], 64417[0], 64418[0], 64420[0], 64421[0], 64425[0], 64430[0], 64435[0], 64445[0], 64446[0], 64447[0], 64448[0], 64449[0], 64450[0], 64451[0], 64454[0], 64461[0], 64462[0], 64463[0], 64479[0], 64480[0], 64483[0], 64484[0], 64486[0], 64487[0], 64488[0], 64489[0], 64490[0], 64491[0], 64492[0], 64493[0], 64494[0], 64495[0], 64505[0], 64510[0], 64517[0], 64520[0], 64530[0], 92012[1], 92014[1], 92585[0], 93000[1], 93005[1], 93010[1], 93040[1], 93041[1], 93042[1], 93318[1], 93355[1], 94002[1], 94200[1], 94250[1], 94680[1], 94681[1], 94690[1], 94770[1], 95812[1], 95813[1], 95816[1], 95819[1], 95822[0], 95829[1], 95860[0], 95861[0], 95863[0], 95864[0], 95865[0], 95866[0], 95867[0], 95868[0], 95869[0], 95870[0], 95907[0], 95908[0], 95909[0], 95910[0], 95911[0], 95912[0], 95913[0], 95925[0], 95926[0], 95927[0], 95928[0], 95929[0], 95930[0], 95933[0], 95937[0], 95938[0], 95939[0], 95940[0], 95955[1], 96360[1], 96361[1], 96365[1], 96366[1], 96367[1], 96368[1], 96372[1], 96374[1], 96375[1], 96376[1], 96377[1], 96523[0], 97597[1], 97598[1], 97602[1], 99155[0], 99156[0], 99157[0], 99211[1], 99212[1], 99213[1], 99214[1], 99215[1], 99217[1], 99218[1], 99219[1], 99220[1], 99221[1], 99222[1], 99223[1], 99231[1], 99232[1], 99233[1], 99234[1], 99235[1], 99236[1], 99238[1], 99239[1], 99241[1], 99242[1], 99243[1], 99244[1], 99245[1], 99251[1], 99252[1], 99253[1], 99254[1], 99255[1], 99291[1], 99292[1], 99304[1], 99305[1], 99306[1], 99307[1], 99308[1], 99309[1], 99310[1], 99315[1], 99316[1], 99334[1], 99335[1], 99336[1], 99337[1], 99347[1], 99348[1], 99349[1], 99350[1], 99374[1], 99375[1], 99377[1], 99378[1], 99446[0], 99447[0], 99448[0], 99449[0], 99451[0], 99452[0], 99495[0], 99496[0], G0453[0], G0463[1], G0471[1]
61526	0213T[0], 0216T[0], 0228T[0], 0230T[0], 0333T[0], 0464T[0], 11000[1], 11001[1], 11004[1], 11005[1], 11006[1], 11042[1], 11043[1], 11044[1], 11045[1], 11046[1], 11047[1], 12001[1], 12002[1], 12004[1], 12005[1], 12006[1], 12007[1], 12011[1], 12013[1], 12014[1], 12015[1], 12016[1], 12017[1], 12018[1], 12020[1], 12021[1], 12031[1], 12032[1], 12034[1], 12035[1], 12036[1], 12037[1], 12041[1], 12042[1], 12044[1], 12045[1], 12046[1], 12047[1], 12051[1], 12052[1], 12053[1], 12054[1], 12055[1], 12056[1], 12057[1], 13100[1], 13101[1], 13102[1], 13120[1], 13121[1], 13122[1], 13131[1], 13132[1], 13133[1], 13151[1], 13152[1], 13153[1], 36000[1], 36400[1], 36405[1], 36406[1], 36410[1], 36420[1], 36425[1], 36430[1], 36440[1], 36591[0], 36592[0], 36600[1], 36640[1], 43752[1], 51701[1], 51702[1], 51703[1], 61107[1], 61140[0], 61210[1], 61304[1], 61305[1], 61518[1], 61796[1], 61798[1], 62100[1], 62140[1], 62141[1], 62164[1], 62320[0], 62321[0], 62322[0], 62323[0], 62324[0], 62325[0], 62326[0], 62327[0], 64400[0], 64405[0], 64408[0], 64415[0], 64416[0], 64417[0], 64418[0], 64420[0], 64421[0], 64425[0], 64430[0], 64435[0], 64445[0], 64446[0], 64447[0], 64448[0], 64449[0], 64450[0], 64451[0], 64454[0], 64461[0], 64462[0], 64463[0], 64479[0], 64480[0], 64483[0], 64484[0], 64486[0], 64487[0], 64488[0], 64489[0], 64490[0], 64491[0], 64492[0], 64493[0], 64494[0], 64495[0], 64505[0], 64510[0], 64517[0], 64520[0], 64530[0], 92012[1], 92014[1], 92585[0], 93000[1], 93005[1], 93010[1], 93040[1], 93041[1], 93042[1], 93318[1], 93355[1], 94002[1], 94200[1], 94250[1], 94680[1], 94681[1], 94690[1], 94770[1], 95812[1], 95813[1], 95816[1], 95819[1], 95822[0], 95829[1], 95860[0], 95861[0], 95863[0], 95864[0], 95865[0], 95866[0], 95867[0], 95868[0], 95869[0], 95870[0], 95907[0], 95908[0], 95909[0], 95910[0], 95911[0], 95912[0], 95913[0], 95925[0], 95926[0], 95927[0], 95928[0], 95929[0], 95930[0], 95933[0], 95937[0], 95938[0], 95939[0], 95940[0], 95955[1], 96360[1], 96361[1], 96365[1], 96366[1], 96367[1], 96368[1], 96372[1], 96374[1], 96375[1], 96376[1], 96377[1], 96523[0], 97597[1], 97598[1], 97602[1], 99155[0], 99156[0], 99157[0], 99211[1], 99212[1], 99213[1], 99214[1], 99215[1], 99217[1], 99218[1], 99219[1], 99220[1], 99221[1], 99222[1], 99223[1], 99231[1], 99232[1], 99233[1], 99234[1], 99235[1], 99236[1], 99238[1], 99239[1], 99241[1], 99242[1], 99243[1], 99244[1], 99245[1], 99251[1], 99252[1], 99253[1], 99254[1], 99255[1], 99291[1], 99292[1], 99304[1], 99305[1], 99306[1], 99307[1], 99308[1], 99309[1], 99310[1], 99315[1], 99316[1], 99334[1], 99335[1], 99336[1], 99337[1], 99347[1], 99348[1], 99349[1], 99350[1], 99374[1], 99375[1], 99377[1], 99378[1], 99446[0], 99447[0], 99448[0], 99449[0], 99451[0], 99452[0], 99495[0], 99496[0], G0453[0], G0463[1], G0471[1]
61530	0213T[0], 0216T[0], 0228T[0], 0230T[0], 0333T[0], 0464T[0], 11000[1], 11001[1], 11004[1], 11005[1], 11006[1], 11042[1], 11043[1], 11044[1], 11045[1], 11046[1], 11047[1], 12001[1], 12002[1], 12004[1], 12005[1], 12006[1], 12007[1], 12011[1], 12013[1], 12014[1], 12015[1], 12016[1], 12017[1], 12018[1], 12020[1], 12021[1], 12031[1], 12032[1], 12034[1], 12035[1], 12036[1], 12037[1], 12041[1], 12042[1], 12044[1], 12045[1], 12046[1], 12047[1], 12051[1], 12052[1], 12053[1], 12054[1], 12055[1], 12056[1], 12057[1], 13100[1], 13101[1], 13102[1], 13120[1], 13121[1], 13122[1], 13131[1], 13132[1], 13133[1], 13151[1], 13152[1], 13153[1], 36000[1], 36400[1], 36405[1], 36406[1], 36410[1], 36420[1], 36425[1], 36430[1], 36440[1], 36591[0], 36592[0], 36600[1], 36640[1], 43752[1], 51701[1], 51702[1], 51703[1], 61107[1], 61140[0], 61210[1], 61304[1], 61305[1], 61526[1], 61534[1], 61535[1], 61796[1], 61798[1], 62100[1], 62140[1], 62141[1], 62164[1], 62320[0], 62321[0], 62322[0], 62323[0], 62324[0], 62325[0], 62326[0], 62327[0], 64400[0], 64405[0], 64408[0], 64415[0], 64416[0], 64417[0], 64418[0], 64420[0], 64421[0], 64425[0], 64430[0], 64435[0], 64445[0], 64446[0], 64447[0], 64448[0], 64449[0], 64450[0], 64451[0], 64454[0], 64461[0], 64462[0], 64463[0], 64479[0], 64480[0], 64483[0], 64484[0], 64486[0], 64487[0], 64488[0], 64489[0], 64490[0], 64491[0], 64492[0], 64493[0], 64494[0], 64495[0], 64505[0], 64510[0], 64517[0], 64520[0], 64530[0], 92012[1], 92014[1], 92585[0], 93000[1], 93005[1], 93010[1], 93040[1], 93041[1], 93042[1], 93318[1], 93355[1], 94002[1], 94200[1], 94250[1], 94680[1], 94681[1], 94690[1], 94770[1], 95812[1], 95813[1], 95816[1], 95819[1], 95822[0], 95829[1], 95860[0], 95861[0], 95863[0], 95864[0], 95865[0], 95866[0], 95867[0], 95868[0], 95869[0], 95870[0], 95907[0], 95908[0], 95909[0], 95910[0], 95911[0], 95912[0], 95913[0], 95925[0], 95926[0], 95927[0], 95928[0], 95929[0], 95930[0], 95933[0], 95937[0], 95938[0], 95939[0], 95940[0], 95955[1], 96360[1], 96361[1], 96365[1], 96366[1], 96367[1], 96368[1], 96372[1], 96374[1], 96375[1], 96376[1], 96377[1], 96523[0], 97597[1], 97598[1], 97602[1], 99155[0], 99156[0], 99157[0], 99211[1], 99212[1], 99213[1], 99214[1], 99215[1], 99217[1], 99218[1], 99219[1], 99220[1], 99221[1], 99222[1], 99223[1], 99231[1], 99232[1], 99233[1], 99234[1], 99235[1], 99236[1], 99238[1], 99239[1], 99241[1], 99242[1], 99243[1], 99244[1], 99245[1], 99251[1], 99252[1], 99253[1], 99254[1], 99255[1], 99291[1], 99292[1], 99304[1], 99305[1], 99306[1], 99307[1], 99308[1], 99309[1], 99310[1], 99315[1], 99316[1], 99334[1], 99335[1], 99336[1], 99337[1], 99347[1], 99348[1], 99349[1], 99350[1], 99374[1], 99375[1], 99377[1], 99378[1], 99446[0], 99447[0], 99448[0], 99449[0], 99451[0], 99452[0], 99495[0], 99496[0], G0453[0], G0463[1], G0471[1]
61531	0213T[0], 0216T[0], 0228T[0], 0230T[0], 0333T[0], 0464T[0], 12001[1], 12002[1], 12004[1], 12005[1], 12006[1], 12007[1], 12011[1], 12013[1], 12014[1], 12015[1], 12016[1], 12017[1], 12018[1], 12020[1], 12021[1], 12031[1], 12032[1], 12034[1], 12035[1], 12036[1], 12037[1], 12041[1], 12042[1], 12044[1], 12045[1], 12046[1], 12047[1], 12051[1], 12052[1], 12053[1], 12054[1], 12055[1], 12056[1], 12057[1], 13100[1], 13101[1], 13102[1], 13120[1], 13121[1], 13122[1], 13131[1], 13132[1], 13133[1], 13151[1], 13152[1], 13153[1], 36000[1], 36400[1], 36405[1], 36406[1], 36410[1], 36420[1], 36425[1], 36430[1], 36440[1], 36591[0], 36592[0], 36600[1], 36640[1], 43752[1], 51701[1], 51702[1], 51703[1], 61107[1], 61210[1], 61304[1], 61305[1], 62140[0], 62141[0], 62320[0], 62321[0], 62322[0], 62323[0], 62324[0], 62325[0], 62326[0], 62327[0], 64400[0], 64405[0], 64408[0], 64415[0], 64416[0], 64417[0], 64418[0], 64420[0], 64421[0], 64425[0], 64430[0], 64435[0], 64445[0], 64446[0], 64447[0], 64448[0], 64449[0], 64450[0], 64451[0], 64454[0], 64461[0], 64462[0], 64463[0], 64479[0], 64480[0], 64483[0], 64484[0], 64486[0], 64487[0], 64488[0], 64489[0], 64490[0], 64491[0], 64492[0], 64493[0], 64494[0], 64495[0], 64505[0], 64510[0], 64517[0], 64520[0], 64530[0], 92012[1], 92014[1], 92585[0], 93000[1], 93005[1], 93010[1], 93040[1], 93041[1], 93042[1], 93318[1], 93355[1], 94002[1], 94200[1], 94250[1], 94680[1], 94681[1], 94690[1], 94770[1], 95812[1], 95813[1], 95816[1], 95819[1], 95822[0], 95829[1], 95860[0], 95861[0], 95863[0], 95864[0], 95865[0], 95866[0], 95867[0], 95868[0], 95869[0], 95870[0], 95907[0], 95908[0], 95909[0], 95910[0], 95911[0], 95912[0], 95913[0], 95925[0], 95926[0], 95927[0], 95928[0], 95929[0], 95930[0], 95933[0], 95937[0], 95938[0], 95939[0], 95940[0], 95955[1], 96360[1], 96361[1], 96365[1], 96366[1], 96367[1], 96368[1], 96372[1], 96374[1], 96375[1], 96376[1], 96377[1], 96523[0], 99155[0], 99156[0], 99157[0], 99211[1], 99212[1], 99213[1], 99214[1], 99215[1], 99217[1], 99218[1], 99219[1], 99220[1], 99221[1], 99222[1], 99223[1], 99231[1], 99232[1], 99233[1], 99234[1], 99235[1], 99236[1], 99238[1], 99239[1], 99241[1], 99242[1], 99243[1], 99244[1], 99245[1], 99251[1], 99252[1], 99253[1], 99254[1], 99255[1], 99291[1], 99292[1], 99304[1], 99305[1], 99306[1], 99307[1], 99308[1], 99309[1], 99310[1], 99315[1], 99316[1], 99334[1], 99335[1], 99336[1], 99337[1], 99347[1], 99348[1], 99349[1], 99350[1], 99374[1], 99375[1], 99377[1], 99378[1], 99446[0], 99447[0], 99448[0], 99449[0], 99451[0], 99452[0], 99495[0], 99496[0], G0453[0], G0463[1], G0471[1]
61533	0213T[0], 0216T[0], 0228T[0], 0230T[0], 0333T[0], 0464T[0], 11000[1], 11001[1], 11004[1], 11005[1], 11006[1], 11042[1], 11043[1], 11044[1], 11045[1], 11046[1], 11047[1], 12001[1], 12002[1], 12004[1], 12005[1], 12006[1], 12007[1], 12011[1], 12013[1], 12014[1], 12015[1], 12016[1], 12017[1], 12018[1], 12020[1], 12021[1], 12031[1], 12032[1], 12034[1], 12035[1], 12036[1], 12037[1], 12041[1], 12042[1], 12044[1], 12045[1], 12046[1], 12047[1], 12051[1], 12052[1], 12053[1], 12054[1], 12055[1], 12056[1], 12057[1], 13100[1], 13101[1], 13102[1], 13120[1], 13121[1], 13122[1], 13131[1], 13132[1], 13133[1], 13151[1], 13152[1], 13153[1], 36000[1], 36400[1], 36405[1], 36406[1], 36410[1], 36420[1], 36425[1], 36430[1], 36440[1], 36591[0], 36592[0], 36600[1], 36640[1], 43752[1], 51701[1], 51702[1], 51703[1], 61107[1], 61210[1], 61304[1], 61305[1], 61531[1], 62100[1], 62140[0], 62141[0], 62320[0], 62321[0], 62322[0], 62323[0], 62324[0], 62325[0], 62326[0], 62327[0], 64400[0], 64405[0], 64408[0], 64415[0], 64416[0], 64417[0], 64418[0], 64420[0], 64421[0], 64425[0], 64430[0], 64435[0], 64445[0], 64446[0], 64447[0], 64448[0], 64449[0], 64450[0], 64451[0], 64454[0], 64461[0], 64462[0], 64463[0], 64479[0],

0 = Modifier usage not allowed or inappropriate 1 = Modifier usage allowed

Code 1	Code 2
	64480[0], 64483[0], 64484[0], 64486[0], 64487[0], 64488[0], 64489[0], 64490[0], 64491[0], 64492[0], 64493[0], 64494[0], 64495[0], 64505[0], 64510[0], 64517[0], 64520[0], 64530[0], 92012[1], 92014[1], 92585[0], 93000[1], 93005[1], 93010[1], 93040[1], 93041[1], 93042[1], 93318[1], 93355[1], 94002[1], 94200[1], 94250[1], 94680[1], 94681[1], 94690[1], 94770[1], 95812[1], 95813[1], 95816[1], 95819[1], 95822[0], 95829[1], 95860[0], 95861[0], 95863[0], 95864[0], 95865[0], 95866[0], 95867[0], 95868[0], 95869[0], 95870[0], 95907[0], 95908[0], 95909[0], 95910[0], 95911[0], 95912[0], 95913[0], 95925[0], 95926[0], 95927[0], 95928[0], 95929[0], 95930[0], 95933[0], 95937[0], 95938[0], 95939[0], 95940[0], 95955[1], 96360[1], 96361[1], 96365[1], 96366[1], 96367[1], 96368[1], 96372[1], 96374[1], 96375[1], 96376[1], 96377[1], 96523[0], 97597[1], 97598[1], 97602[1], 99155[0], 99156[0], 99157[0], 99211[1], 99212[1], 99213[1], 99214[1], 99215[1], 99217[1], 99218[1], 99219[1], 99220[1], 99221[1], 99222[1], 99223[1], 99231[1], 99232[1], 99233[1], 99234[1], 99235[1], 99236[1], 99238[1], 99239[1], 99241[1], 99242[1], 99243[1], 99244[1], 99245[1], 99251[1], 99252[1], 99253[1], 99254[1], 99255[1], 99291[1], 99292[1], 99304[1], 99305[1], 99306[1], 99307[1], 99308[1], 99309[1], 99310[1], 99315[1], 99316[1], 99334[1], 99335[1], 99336[1], 99337[1], 99347[1], 99348[1], 99349[1], 99350[1], 99374[1], 99375[1], 99377[1], 99378[1], 99446[0], 99447[0], 99448[0], 99449[0], 99451[0], 99452[0], 99495[0], 99496[0], G0453[0], G0463[1], G0471[1]
61534	0213T[0], 0216T[0], 0228T[0], 0230T[0], 0333T[0], 0464T[0], 11000[1], 11001[1], 11004[1], 11005[1], 11006[1], 11042[1], 11043[1], 11044[1], 11045[1], 11046[1], 11047[1], 12001[1], 12002[1], 12004[1], 12005[1], 12006[1], 12007[1], 12011[1], 12013[1], 12014[1], 12015[1], 12016[1], 12017[1], 12018[1], 12020[1], 12021[1], 12031[1], 12032[1], 12034[1], 12035[1], 12036[1], 12037[1], 12041[1], 12042[1], 12044[1], 12045[1], 12046[1], 12047[1], 12051[1], 12052[1], 12053[1], 12054[1], 12055[1], 12056[1], 12057[1], 13100[1], 13101[1], 13102[1], 13120[1], 13121[1], 13122[1], 13131[1], 13132[1], 13133[1], 13151[1], 13152[1], 13153[1], 36000[1], 36400[1], 36405[1], 36406[1], 36410[1], 36420[1], 36425[1], 36430[1], 36440[1], 36591[0], 36592[0], 36600[1], 36640[1], 43752[1], 51701[1], 51702[1], 51703[1], 61107[1], 61210[1], 61304[1], 61305[1], 61533[1], 62100[1], 62140[0], 62141[0], 62320[0], 62321[0], 62322[0], 62323[0], 62324[0], 62325[0], 62326[0], 62327[0], 64400[0], 64405[0], 64408[0], 64415[0], 64416[0], 64417[0], 64418[0], 64420[0], 64421[0], 64425[0], 64430[0], 64435[0], 64445[0], 64446[0], 64447[0], 64448[0], 64449[0], 64450[0], 64451[0], 64454[0], 64461[0], 64462[0], 64463[0], 64479[0], 64480[0], 64483[0], 64484[0], 64486[0], 64487[0], 64488[0], 64489[0], 64490[0], 64491[0], 64492[0], 64493[0], 64494[0], 64495[0], 64505[0], 64510[0], 64517[0], 64520[0], 64530[0], 92012[1], 92014[1], 92585[0], 93000[1], 93005[1], 93010[1], 93040[1], 93041[1], 93042[1], 93318[1], 93355[1], 94002[1], 94200[1], 94250[1], 94680[1], 94681[1], 94690[1], 94770[1], 95812[1], 95813[1], 95816[1], 95819[1], 95822[0], 95829[1], 95860[0], 95861[0], 95863[0], 95864[0], 95865[0], 95866[0], 95867[0], 95868[0], 95869[0], 95870[0], 95907[0], 95908[0], 95909[0], 95910[0], 95911[0], 95912[0], 95913[0], 95925[0], 95926[0], 95927[0], 95928[0], 95929[0], 95930[0], 95933[0], 95937[0], 95938[0], 95939[0], 95940[0], 95955[1], 95961[0], 95962[0], 96360[1], 96361[1], 96365[1], 96366[1], 96367[1], 96368[1], 96372[1], 96374[1], 96375[1], 96376[1], 96377[1], 96523[0], 97597[1], 97598[1], 97602[1], 99155[0], 99156[0], 99157[0], 99211[1], 99212[1], 99213[1], 99214[1], 99215[1], 99217[1], 99218[1], 99219[1], 99220[1], 99221[1], 99222[1], 99223[1], 99231[1], 99232[1], 99233[1], 99234[1], 99235[1], 99236[1], 99238[1], 99239[1], 99241[1], 99242[1], 99243[1], 99244[1], 99245[1], 99251[1], 99252[1], 99253[1], 99254[1], 99255[1], 99291[1], 99292[1], 99304[1], 99305[1], 99306[1], 99307[1], 99308[1], 99309[1], 99310[1], 99315[1], 99316[1], 99334[1], 99335[1], 99336[1], 99337[1], 99347[1], 99348[1], 99349[1], 99350[1], 99374[1], 99375[1], 99377[1], 99378[1], 99446[0], 99447[0], 99448[0], 99449[0], 99451[0], 99452[0], 99495[0], 99496[0], G0453[0], G0463[1], G0471[1]
61535	0213T[0], 0216T[0], 0228T[0], 0230T[0], 0333T[0], 0464T[0], 11000[1], 11001[1], 11004[1], 11005[1], 11006[1], 11042[1], 11043[1], 11044[1], 11045[1], 11046[1], 11047[1], 12001[1], 12002[1], 12004[1], 12005[1], 12006[1], 12007[1], 12011[1], 12013[1], 12014[1], 12015[1], 12016[1], 12017[1], 12018[1], 12020[1], 12021[1], 12031[1], 12032[1], 12034[1], 12035[1], 12036[1], 12037[1], 12041[1], 12042[1], 12044[1], 12045[1], 12046[1], 12047[1], 12051[1], 12052[1], 12053[1], 12054[1], 12055[1], 12056[1], 12057[1], 13100[1], 13101[1], 13102[1], 13120[1], 13121[1], 13122[1], 13131[1], 13132[1], 13133[1], 13151[1], 13152[1], 13153[1], 36000[1], 36400[1], 36405[1], 36406[1], 36410[1], 36420[1], 36425[1], 36430[1], 36440[1], 36591[0], 36592[0], 36600[1], 36640[1], 43752[1], 51701[1], 51702[1], 51703[1], 61107[1], 61210[1], 61531[0], 61533[0], 61534[0], 62100[1], 62140[0], 62141[0], 62320[0], 62321[0], 62322[0], 62323[0], 62324[0], 62325[0], 62326[0], 62327[0], 64400[0], 64405[0], 64408[0], 64415[0], 64416[0], 64417[0], 64418[0], 64420[0], 64421[0], 64425[0], 64430[0], 64435[0], 64445[0], 64446[0], 64447[0], 64448[0], 64449[0], 64450[0], 64451[0], 64454[0], 64461[0], 64462[0], 64463[0], 64479[0], 64480[0], 64483[0], 64484[0], 64486[0], 64487[0], 64488[0], 64489[0], 64490[0], 64491[0], 64492[0], 64493[0], 64494[0], 64495[0], 64505[0], 64510[0], 64517[0], 64520[0], 64530[0], 92012[1], 92014[1], 92585[0], 93000[1], 93005[1], 93010[1], 93040[1], 93041[1], 93042[1], 93318[1], 93355[1], 94002[1], 94200[1], 94250[1], 94680[1], 94681[1], 94690[1], 94770[1], 95812[1], 95813[1], 95816[1], 95819[1], 95822[0], 95829[1], 95860[0], 95861[0], 95863[0], 95864[0], 95865[0], 95866[0], 95867[0], 95868[0], 95869[0], 95870[0], 95907[0], 95908[0], 95909[0], 95910[0], 95911[0], 95912[0], 95913[0], 95925[0], 95926[0], 95927[0], 95928[0], 95929[0], 95930[0], 95933[0], 95937[0], 95938[0], 95939[0], 95940[0], 95955[1], 95961[0], 95962[0], 96360[1], 96361[1], 96365[1], 96366[1], 96367[1], 96368[1], 96372[1], 96374[1], 96375[1], 96376[1], 96377[1], 96523[0], 97597[1], 97598[1], 97602[1], 99155[0], 99156[0], 99157[0], 99211[1], 99212[1], 99213[1], 99214[1], 99215[1], 99217[1], 99218[1], 99219[1], 99220[1], 99221[1], 99222[1], 99223[1], 99231[1], 99232[1], 99233[1], 99234[1], 99235[1], 99236[1], 99238[1], 99239[1], 99241[1], 99242[1], 99243[1], 99244[1], 99245[1], 99251[1], 99252[1], 99253[1], 99254[1], 99255[1], 99291[1], 99292[1], 99304[1], 99305[1], 99306[1], 99307[1], 99308[1], 99309[1], 99310[1], 99315[1], 99316[1], 99334[1], 99335[1], 99336[1], 99337[1], 99347[1], 99348[1], 99349[1], 99350[1], 99374[1], 99375[1], 99377[1], 99378[1], 99446[0], 99447[0], 99448[0], 99449[0], 99451[0], 99452[0], 99495[0], 99496[0], G0453[0], G0463[1], G0471[1]
61536	0213T[0], 0216T[0], 0228T[0], 0230T[0], 0333T[0], 0464T[0], 11000[1], 11001[1], 11004[1], 11005[1], 11006[1], 11042[1], 11043[1], 11044[1], 11045[1], 11046[1], 11047[1], 12001[1], 12002[1], 12004[1], 12005[1], 12006[1], 12007[1], 12011[1], 12013[1], 12014[1], 12015[1], 12016[1], 12017[1], 12018[1], 12020[1], 12021[1], 12031[1], 12032[1], 12034[1], 12035[1], 12036[1], 12037[1], 12041[1], 12042[1], 12044[1], 12045[1], 12046[1], 12047[1], 12051[1], 12052[1], 12053[1], 12054[1], 12055[1], 12056[1], 12057[1], 13100[1], 13101[1], 13102[1], 13120[1], 13121[1], 13122[1], 13131[1], 13132[1], 13133[1], 13151[1], 13152[1], 13153[1], 36000[1], 36400[1], 36405[1], 36406[1], 36410[1], 36420[1], 36425[1], 36430[1], 36440[1], 36591[0], 36592[0], 36600[1], 36640[1], 43752[1], 51701[1], 51702[1], 51703[1], 61107[1], 61210[1], 61304[1], 61305[1], 61535[0], 62100[1], 62140[0], 62141[0], 62320[0], 62321[0], 62322[0], 62323[0], 62324[0], 62325[0], 62326[0], 62327[0], 64400[0], 64405[0], 64408[0], 64415[0], 64416[0], 64417[0], 64418[0], 64420[0], 64421[0], 64425[0], 64430[0], 64435[0], 64445[0], 64446[0], 64447[0], 64448[0], 64449[0], 64450[0], 64451[0], 64454[0], 64461[0], 64462[0], 64463[0], 64479[0], 64480[0], 64483[0], 64484[0], 64486[0], 64487[0], 64488[0], 64489[0], 64490[0], 64491[0], 64492[0], 64493[0], 64494[0], 64495[0], 64505[0], 64510[0], 64517[0], 64520[0], 64530[0], 92012[1], 92014[1], 92585[0], 93000[1], 93005[1], 93010[1], 93040[1], 93041[1], 93042[1], 93318[1], 93355[1], 94002[1], 94200[1], 94250[1], 94680[1], 94681[1], 94690[1], 94770[1], 95812[1], 95813[1], 95816[1], 95819[1], 95822[0], 95829[1], 95860[0], 95861[0], 95863[0], 95864[0], 95865[0], 95866[0], 95867[0], 95868[0], 95869[0], 95870[0], 95907[0], 95908[0], 95909[0], 95910[0], 95911[0], 95912[0], 95913[0], 95925[0], 95926[0], 95927[0], 95928[0], 95929[0], 95930[0], 95933[0], 95937[0], 95938[0], 95939[0], 95940[0], 95955[1], 95961[0], 95962[0], 96360[1], 96361[1], 96365[1], 96366[1], 96367[1], 96368[1], 96372[1], 96374[1], 96375[1], 96376[1], 96377[1], 96523[0], 97597[1], 97598[1], 97602[1], 99155[0], 99156[0], 99157[0], 99211[1], 99212[1], 99213[1], 99214[1], 99215[1], 99217[1], 99218[1], 99219[1], 99220[1], 99221[1], 99222[1], 99223[1], 99231[1], 99232[1], 99233[1], 99234[1], 99235[1], 99236[1], 99238[1], 99239[1], 99241[1], 99242[1], 99243[1], 99244[1], 99245[1], 99251[1], 99252[1], 99253[1], 99254[1], 99255[1], 99291[1], 99292[1], 99304[1], 99305[1], 99306[1], 99307[1], 99308[1], 99309[1], 99310[1], 99315[1], 99316[1], 99334[1], 99335[1], 99336[1], 99337[1], 99347[1], 99348[1], 99349[1], 99350[1], 99374[1], 99375[1], 99377[1], 99378[1], 99446[0], 99447[0], 99448[0], 99449[0], 99451[0], 99452[0], 99495[0], 99496[0], G0453[0], G0463[1], G0471[1]
61537	0213T[0], 0216T[0], 0228T[0], 0230T[0], 0333T[0], 0464T[0], 11000[1], 11001[1], 11004[1], 11005[1], 11006[1], 11042[1], 11043[1], 11044[1], 11045[1], 11046[1], 11047[1], 12001[1], 12002[1], 12004[1], 12005[1], 12006[1], 12007[1], 12011[1], 12013[1], 12014[1], 12015[1], 12016[1], 12017[1], 12018[1], 12020[1], 12021[1], 12031[1], 12032[1], 12034[1], 12035[1], 12036[1], 12037[1], 12041[1], 12042[1], 12044[1], 12045[1], 12046[1], 12047[1], 12051[1], 12052[1], 12053[1], 12054[1], 12055[1], 12056[1], 12057[1], 13100[1], 13101[1], 13102[1], 13120[1], 13121[1], 13122[1], 13131[1], 13132[1], 13133[1], 13151[1], 13152[1], 13153[1], 36000[1], 36400[1], 36405[1], 36406[1], 36410[1], 36420[1], 36425[1], 36430[1], 36440[1], 36591[0], 36592[0], 36600[1], 36640[1], 43752[1], 51701[1], 51702[1], 51703[1], 61107[1], 61210[1], 61304[1], 61533[1], 61535[1], 62100[1], 62140[0], 62141[0], 62320[0], 62321[0], 62322[0], 62323[0], 62324[0], 62325[0], 62326[0], 62327[0], 64400[0], 64405[0], 64408[0], 64415[0], 64416[0], 64417[0], 64418[0], 64420[0], 64421[0], 64425[0], 64430[0], 64435[0], 64445[0], 64446[0], 64447[0], 64448[0], 64449[0], 64450[0], 64451[0], 64454[0], 64461[0], 64462[0], 64463[0], 64479[0], 64480[0], 64483[0], 64484[0], 64486[0], 64487[0], 64488[0], 64489[0], 64490[0], 64491[0], 64492[0], 64493[0], 64494[0], 64495[0], 64505[0], 64510[0], 64517[0], 64520[0], 64530[0], 92012[1], 92014[1], 92585[0], 93000[1], 93005[1], 93010[1], 93040[1], 93041[1], 93042[1], 93318[1], 93355[1], 94002[1], 94200[1], 94250[1], 94680[1], 94681[1], 94690[1], 94770[1], 95812[1], 95813[1], 95816[1], 95819[1], 95822[0], 95829[1], 95860[0], 95861[0], 95863[0], 95864[0], 95865[0], 95866[0], 95867[0], 95868[0], 95869[0], 95870[0], 95907[0], 95908[0], 95909[0], 95910[0], 95911[0], 95912[0], 95913[0], 95925[0], 95926[0], 95927[0], 95928[0], 95929[0], 95930[0], 95933[0], 95937[0], 95938[0], 95939[0], 95940[0], 95955[0], 95961[0], 95962[0], 96360[1], 96361[1], 96365[1], 96366[1], 96367[1], 96368[1], 96372[1], 96374[1], 96375[1], 96376[1], 96377[1], 96523[0], 97597[1], 97598[1], 97602[1], 99155[0], 99156[0], 99157[0], 99211[1], 99212[1], 99213[1], 99214[1], 99215[1], 99217[1], 99218[1], 99219[1], 99220[1], 99221[1], 99222[1], 99223[1], 99231[1], 99232[1], 99233[1], 99234[1], 99235[1], 99236[1], 99238[1], 99239[1], 99241[1], 99242[1], 99243[1], 99244[1], 99245[1], 99251[1], 99252[1], 99253[1], 99254[1], 99255[1], 99291[1], 99292[1], 99304[1], 99305[1], 99306[1], 99307[1], 99308[1], 99309[1], 99310[1], 99315[1], 99316[1], 99334[1], 99335[1], 99336[1], 99337[1], 99347[1], 99348[1], 99349[1], 99350[1], 99374[1], 99375[1], 99377[1], 99378[1], 99446[0], 99447[0], 99448[0], 99449[0], 99451[0], 99452[0], 99495[0], 99496[0], G0453[0], G0463[1], G0471[1]
61538	0213T[0], 0216T[0], 0228T[0], 0230T[0], 0333T[0], 0464T[0], 11000[1], 11001[1], 11004[1], 11005[1], 11006[1], 11042[1], 11043[1], 11044[1], 11045[1], 11046[1], 11047[1], 12001[1], 12002[1], 12004[1], 12005[1], 12006[1], 12007[1], 12011[1], 12013[1], 12014[1], 12015[1], 12016[1], 12017[1], 12018[1],

0 = Modifier usage not allowed or inappropriate 1 = Modifier usage allowed

Code 1	Code 2
	12020[1], 12021[1], 12031[1], 12032[1], 12034[1], 12035[1], 12036[1], 12037[1], 12041[1], 12042[1], 12044[1], 12045[1], 12046[1], 12047[1], 12051[1], 12052[1], 12053[1], 12054[1], 12055[1], 12056[1], 12057[1], 13100[1], 13101[1], 13102[1], 13120[1], 13121[1], 13122[1], 13131[1], 13132[1], 13133[1], 13151[1], 13152[1], 13153[1], 36000[1], 36400[1], 36405[1], 36406[1], 36410[1], 36420[1], 36425[1], 36430[1], 36440[1], 36591[0], 36592[0], 36600[1], 36640[1], 43752[1], 51701[1], 51702[1], 51703[1], 61107[1], 61210[1], 61304[1], 61305[1], 61535[0], 61537[1], 61539[1], 62100[1], 62140[0], 62141[0], 62320[0], 62321[0], 62322[0], 62323[0], 62324[0], 62325[0], 62326[0], 62327[0], 64400[0], 64405[0], 64408[0], 64415[0], 64416[0], 64417[0], 64418[0], 64420[0], 64421[0], 64425[0], 64430[0], 64435[0], 64445[0], 64446[0], 64447[0], 64448[0], 64449[0], 64450[0], 64451[0], 64454[0], 64461[0], 64462[0], 64463[0], 64479[0], 64480[0], 64483[0], 64484[0], 64486[0], 64487[0], 64488[0], 64489[0], 64490[0], 64491[0], 64492[0], 64493[0], 64494[0], 64495[0], 64505[0], 64510[0], 64517[0], 64520[0], 64530[0], 92012[1], 92014[1], 92585[0], 93000[1], 93005[1], 93010[1], 93040[1], 93041[1], 93042[1], 93318[1], 93355[1], 94002[1], 94200[1], 94250[1], 94680[1], 94681[1], 94690[1], 94770[1], 95812[1], 95813[1], 95816[1], 95819[1], 95822[0], 95829[1], 95860[0], 95861[0], 95863[0], 95864[0], 95865[0], 95866[0], 95867[0], 95868[0], 95869[0], 95870[0], 95907[0], 95908[0], 95909[0], 95910[0], 95911[0], 95912[0], 95913[0], 95925[0], 95926[0], 95927[0], 95928[0], 95929[0], 95930[0], 95933[0], 95937[0], 95938[0], 95939[0], 95940[0], 95955[1], 95961[0], 95962[0], 96360[1], 96361[1], 96365[1], 96366[1], 96367[1], 96368[1], 96372[1], 96374[1], 96375[1], 96376[1], 96377[1], 96523[0], 97597[1], 97598[1], 97602[1], 99155[0], 99156[0], 99157[0], 99211[1], 99212[1], 99213[1], 99214[1], 99215[1], 99217[1], 99218[1], 99219[1], 99220[1], 99221[1], 99222[1], 99223[1], 99231[1], 99232[1], 99233[1], 99234[1], 99235[1], 99236[1], 99238[1], 99239[1], 99241[1], 99242[1], 99243[1], 99244[1], 99245[1], 99251[1], 99252[1], 99253[1], 99254[1], 99255[1], 99291[1], 99292[1], 99304[1], 99305[1], 99306[1], 99307[1], 99308[1], 99309[1], 99310[1], 99315[1], 99316[1], 99334[1], 99335[1], 99336[1], 99337[1], 99347[1], 99348[1], 99349[1], 99350[1], 99374[1], 99375[1], 99377[1], 99378[1], 99446[0], 99447[0], 99448[0], 99449[0], 99451[0], 99452[0], 99495[0], 99496[0], G0453[0], G0463[1], G0471[1]
61539	0213T[0], 0216T[0], 0228T[0], 0230T[0], 0333T[0], 0464T[0], 11000[1], 11001[1], 11004[1], 11005[1], 11006[1], 11042[1], 11043[1], 11044[1], 11045[1], 11046[1], 11047[1], 12001[1], 12002[1], 12004[1], 12005[1], 12006[1], 12007[1], 12011[1], 12013[1], 12014[1], 12015[1], 12016[1], 12017[1], 12018[1], 12020[1], 12021[1], 12031[1], 12032[1], 12034[1], 12035[1], 12036[1], 12037[1], 12041[1], 12042[1], 12044[1], 12045[1], 12046[1], 12047[1], 12051[1], 12052[1], 12053[1], 12054[1], 12055[1], 12056[1], 12057[1], 13100[1], 13101[1], 13102[1], 13120[1], 13121[1], 13122[1], 13131[1], 13132[1], 13133[1], 13151[1], 13152[1], 13153[1], 36000[1], 36400[1], 36405[1], 36406[1], 36410[1], 36420[1], 36425[1], 36430[1], 36440[1], 36591[0], 36592[0], 36600[1], 36640[1], 43752[1], 51701[1], 51702[1], 51703[1], 61107[1], 61210[1], 61304[1], 61305[1], 61535[0], 61536[1], 61537[1], 61540[1], 61567[1], 62100[1], 62140[0], 62141[0], 62320[0], 62321[0], 62322[0], 62323[0], 62324[0], 62325[0], 62326[0], 62327[0], 64400[0], 64405[0], 64408[0], 64415[0], 64416[0], 64417[0], 64418[0], 64420[0], 64421[0], 64425[0], 64430[0], 64435[0], 64445[0], 64446[0], 64447[0], 64448[0], 64449[0], 64450[0], 64451[0], 64454[0], 64461[0], 64462[0], 64463[0], 64479[0], 64480[0], 64483[0], 64484[0], 64486[0], 64487[0], 64488[0], 64489[0], 64490[0], 64491[0], 64492[0], 64493[0], 64494[0], 64495[0], 64505[0], 64510[0], 64517[0], 64520[0], 64530[0], 92012[1], 92014[1], 92585[0], 93000[1], 93005[1], 93010[1], 93040[1], 93041[1], 93042[1], 93318[1], 93355[1], 94002[1], 94200[1], 94250[1], 94680[1], 94681[1], 94690[1], 94770[1], 95812[1], 95813[1], 95816[1], 95819[1], 95822[0], 95829[1], 95860[0], 95861[0], 95863[0], 95864[0], 95865[0], 95866[0], 95867[0], 95868[0], 95869[0], 95870[0], 95907[0], 95908[0], 95909[0], 95910[0], 95911[0], 95912[0], 95913[0], 95925[0], 95926[0], 95927[0], 95928[0], 95929[0], 95930[0], 95933[0], 95937[0], 95938[0], 95939[0], 95940[0], 95955[0], 95961[0], 95962[0], 96360[1], 96361[1], 96365[1], 96366[1], 96367[1], 96368[1], 96372[1], 96374[1], 96375[1], 96376[1], 96377[1], 96523[0], 97597[1], 97598[1], 97602[1], 99155[0], 99156[0], 99157[0], 99211[1], 99212[1], 99213[1], 99214[1], 99215[1], 99217[1], 99218[1], 99219[1], 99220[1], 99221[1], 99222[1], 99223[1], 99231[1], 99232[1], 99233[1], 99234[1], 99235[1], 99236[1], 99238[1], 99239[1], 99241[1], 99242[1], 99243[1], 99244[1], 99245[1], 99251[1], 99252[1], 99253[1], 99254[1], 99255[1], 99291[1], 99292[1], 99304[1], 99305[1], 99306[1], 99307[1], 99308[1], 99309[1], 99310[1], 99315[1], 99316[1], 99334[1], 99335[1], 99336[1], 99337[1], 99347[1], 99348[1], 99349[1], 99350[1], 99374[1], 99375[1], 99377[1], 99378[1], 99446[0], 99447[0], 99448[0], 99449[0], 99451[0], 99452[0], 99495[0], 99496[0], G0453[0], G0463[1], G0471[1]
61540	0213T[0], 0216T[0], 0228T[0], 0230T[0], 0333T[0], 0464T[0], 11000[1], 11001[1], 11004[1], 11005[1], 11006[1], 11042[1], 11043[1], 11044[1], 11045[1], 11046[1], 11047[1], 12001[1], 12002[1], 12004[1], 12005[1], 12006[1], 12007[1], 12011[1], 12013[1], 12014[1], 12015[1], 12016[1], 12017[1], 12018[1], 12020[1], 12021[1], 12031[1], 12032[1], 12034[1], 12035[1], 12036[1], 12037[1], 12041[1], 12042[1], 12044[1], 12045[1], 12046[1], 12047[1], 12051[1], 12052[1], 12053[1], 12054[1], 12055[1], 12056[1], 12057[1], 13100[1], 13101[1], 13102[1], 13120[1], 13121[1], 13122[1], 13131[1], 13132[1], 13133[1], 13151[1], 13152[1], 13153[1], 36000[1], 36400[1], 36405[1], 36406[1], 36410[1], 36420[1], 36425[1], 36430[1], 36440[1], 36591[0], 36592[0], 36600[1], 36640[1], 43752[1], 51701[1], 51702[1], 51703[1], 61107[1], 61304[1], 61533[1], 61535[1], 61537[1], 61538[1], 62100[1], 62140[0], 62141[0], 62320[0], 62321[0], 62322[0], 62323[0], 62324[0], 62325[0], 62326[0], 62327[0], 64400[0], 64405[0], 64408[0], 64415[0], 64416[0], 64417[0], 64418[0], 64420[0], 64421[0], 64425[0], 64430[0], 64435[0], 64445[0], 64446[0], 64447[0], 64448[0], 64449[0], 64450[0], 64451[0], 64454[0], 64461[0], 64462[0], 64463[0], 64479[0], 64480[0], 64483[0], 64484[0], 64486[0], 64487[0], 64488[0], 64489[0], 64490[0], 64491[0], 64492[0], 64493[0], 64494[0], 64495[0], 64505[0], 64510[0], 64517[0], 64520[0], 64530[0], 92012[1], 92014[1], 92585[0], 93000[1], 93005[1], 93010[1], 93040[1], 93041[1], 93042[1], 93318[1], 93355[1], 94002[1], 94200[1], 94250[1], 94680[1], 94681[1], 94690[1], 94770[1], 95812[1], 95813[1], 95816[1], 95819[1], 95822[0], 95829[1], 95860[0], 95861[0], 95863[0], 95864[0], 95865[0], 95866[0], 95867[0], 95868[0], 95869[0], 95870[0], 95907[0], 95908[0], 95909[0], 95910[0], 95911[0], 95912[0], 95913[0], 95925[0], 95926[0], 95927[0], 95928[0], 95929[0], 95930[0], 95933[0], 95937[0], 95938[0], 95939[0], 95940[0], 95955[1], 95961[0], 95962[0], 96360[1], 96361[1], 96365[1], 96366[1], 96367[1], 96368[1], 96372[1], 96374[1], 96375[1], 96376[1], 96377[1], 96523[0], 97597[1], 97598[1], 97602[1], 99155[0], 99156[0], 99157[0], 99211[1], 99212[1], 99213[1], 99214[1], 99215[1], 99217[1], 99218[1], 99219[1], 99220[1], 99221[1], 99222[1], 99223[1], 99231[1], 99232[1], 99233[1], 99234[1], 99235[1], 99236[1], 99238[1], 99239[1], 99241[1], 99242[1], 99243[1], 99244[1], 99245[1], 99251[1], 99252[1], 99253[1], 99254[1], 99255[1], 99291[1], 99292[1], 99304[1], 99305[1], 99306[1], 99307[1], 99308[1], 99309[1], 99310[1], 99315[1], 99316[1], 99334[1], 99335[1], 99336[1], 99337[1], 99347[1], 99348[1], 99349[1], 99350[1], 99374[1], 99375[1], 99377[1], 99378[1], 99446[0], 99447[0], 99448[0], 99449[0], 99451[0], 99452[0], 99495[0], 99496[0], G0453[0], G0463[1], G0471[1]
61541	0213T[0], 0216T[0], 0228T[0], 0230T[0], 0333T[0], 0464T[0], 11000[1], 11001[1], 11004[1], 11005[1], 11006[1], 11042[1], 11043[1], 11044[1], 11045[1], 11046[1], 11047[1], 12001[1], 12002[1], 12004[1], 12005[1], 12006[1], 12007[1], 12011[1], 12013[1], 12014[1], 12015[1], 12016[1], 12017[1], 12018[1], 12020[1], 12021[1], 12031[1], 12032[1], 12034[1], 12035[1], 12036[1], 12037[1], 12041[1], 12042[1], 12044[1], 12045[1], 12046[1], 12047[1], 12051[1], 12052[1], 12053[1], 12054[1], 12055[1], 12056[1], 12057[1], 13100[1], 13101[1], 13102[1], 13120[1], 13121[1], 13122[1], 13131[1], 13132[1], 13133[1], 13151[1], 13152[1], 13153[1], 36000[1], 36400[1], 36405[1], 36406[1], 36410[1], 36420[1], 36425[1], 36430[1], 36440[1], 36591[0], 36592[0], 36600[1], 36640[1], 43752[1], 51701[1], 51702[1], 51703[1], 61107[1], 61210[1], 61304[1], 61305[1], 61533[1], 61535[0], 62100[1], 62140[0], 62141[0], 62320[0], 62321[0], 62322[0], 62323[0], 62324[0], 62325[0], 62326[0], 62327[0], 64400[0], 64405[0], 64408[0], 64415[0], 64416[0], 64417[0], 64418[0], 64420[0], 64421[0], 64425[0], 64430[0], 64435[0], 64445[0], 64446[0], 64447[0], 64448[0], 64449[0], 64450[0], 64451[0], 64454[0], 64461[0], 64462[0], 64463[0], 64479[0], 64480[0], 64483[0], 64484[0], 64486[0], 64487[0], 64488[0], 64489[0], 64490[0], 64491[0], 64492[0], 64493[0], 64494[0], 64495[0], 64505[0], 64510[0], 64517[0], 64520[0], 64530[0], 92012[1], 92014[1], 92585[0], 93000[1], 93005[1], 93010[1], 93040[1], 93041[1], 93042[1], 93318[1], 93355[1], 94002[1], 94200[1], 94250[1], 94680[1], 94681[1], 94690[1], 94770[1], 95812[1], 95813[1], 95816[1], 95819[1], 95822[0], 95829[1], 95860[0], 95861[0], 95863[0], 95864[0], 95865[0], 95866[0], 95867[0], 95868[0], 95869[0], 95870[0], 95907[0], 95908[0], 95909[0], 95910[0], 95911[0], 95912[0], 95913[0], 95925[0], 95926[0], 95927[0], 95928[0], 95929[0], 95930[0], 95933[0], 95937[0], 95938[0], 95939[0], 95940[0], 95955[1], 95961[0], 95962[0], 96360[1], 96361[1], 96365[1], 96366[1], 96367[1], 96368[1], 96372[1], 96374[1], 96375[1], 96376[1], 96377[1], 96523[0], 97597[1], 97598[1], 97602[1], 99155[0], 99156[0], 99157[0], 99211[1], 99212[1], 99213[1], 99214[1], 99215[1], 99217[1], 99218[1], 99219[1], 99220[1], 99221[1], 99222[1], 99223[1], 99231[1], 99232[1], 99233[1], 99234[1], 99235[1], 99236[1], 99238[1], 99239[1], 99241[1], 99242[1], 99243[1], 99244[1], 99245[1], 99251[1], 99252[1], 99253[1], 99254[1], 99255[1], 99291[1], 99292[1], 99304[1], 99305[1], 99306[1], 99307[1], 99308[1], 99309[1], 99310[1], 99315[1], 99316[1], 99334[1], 99335[1], 99336[1], 99337[1], 99347[1], 99348[1], 99349[1], 99350[1], 99374[1], 99375[1], 99377[1], 99378[1], 99446[0], 99447[0], 99448[0], 99449[0], 99451[0], 99452[0], 99495[0], 99496[0], G0453[0], G0463[1], G0471[1]
61545	0213T[0], 0216T[0], 0228T[0], 0230T[0], 0333T[0], 0464T[0], 11000[1], 11001[1], 11004[1], 11005[1], 11006[1], 11042[1], 11043[1], 11044[1], 11045[1], 11046[1], 11047[1], 12001[1], 12002[1], 12004[1], 12005[1], 12006[1], 12007[1], 12011[1], 12013[1], 12014[1], 12015[1], 12016[1], 12017[1], 12018[1], 12020[1], 12021[1], 12031[1], 12032[1], 12034[1], 12035[1], 12036[1], 12037[1], 12041[1], 12042[1], 12044[1], 12045[1], 12046[1], 12047[1], 12051[1], 12052[1], 12053[1], 12054[1], 12055[1], 12056[1], 12057[1], 13100[1], 13101[1], 13102[1], 13120[1], 13121[1], 13122[1], 13131[1], 13132[1], 13133[1], 13151[1], 13152[1], 13153[1], 36000[1], 36400[1], 36405[1], 36406[1], 36410[1], 36420[1], 36425[1], 36430[1], 36440[1], 36591[0], 36592[0], 36600[1], 36640[1], 43752[1], 51701[1], 51702[1], 51703[1], 61107[1], 61210[1], 61304[1], 61305[1], 61535[1], 62100[1], 62140[0], 62141[0], 62164[1], 62320[0], 62321[0], 62322[0], 62323[0], 62324[0], 62325[0], 62326[0], 62327[0], 64400[0], 64405[0], 64408[0], 64415[0], 64416[0], 64417[0], 64418[0], 64420[0], 64421[0], 64425[0], 64430[0], 64435[0], 64445[0], 64446[0], 64447[0], 64448[0], 64449[0], 64450[0], 64451[0], 64454[0], 64461[0], 64462[0], 64463[0], 64479[0], 64480[0], 64483[0], 64484[0], 64486[0], 64487[0], 64488[0], 64489[0], 64490[0], 64491[0], 64492[0], 64493[0], 64494[0], 64495[0], 64505[0], 64510[0], 64517[0], 64520[0], 64530[0], 92012[1], 92014[1], 92585[0], 93000[1], 93005[1], 93010[1], 93040[1], 93041[1], 93042[1], 93318[1], 93355[1], 94002[1], 94200[1], 94250[1], 94680[1], 94681[1], 94690[1], 94770[1], 95812[1], 95813[1], 95816[1], 95819[1], 95822[0], 95829[1], 95860[0], 95861[0], 95863[0], 95864[0], 95865[0], 95866[0], 95867[0], 95868[0], 95869[0], 95870[0], 95907[0], 95908[0], 95909[0], 95910[0], 95911[0], 95912[0], 95913[0], 95925[0], 95926[0], 95927[0], 95928[0], 95929[0], 95930[0], 95933[0], 95937[0], 95938[0], 95939[0], 95940[0], 95955[1], 96360[1], 96361[1], 96365[1], 96366[1], 96367[1], 96368[1], 96372[1], 96374[1], 96375[1], 96376[1], 96377[1], 96523[0], 97597[1], 97598[1], 97602[1], 99155[0], 99156[0], 99157[0], 99211[1], 99212[1], 99213[1], 99214[1], 99215[1], 99217[1], 99218[1], 99219[1], 99220[1], 99221[1], 99222[1], 99223[1], 99231[1], 99232[1], 99233[1], 99234[1], 99235[1], 99236[1], 99238[1], 99239[1],

0 = Modifier usage not allowed or inappropriate 1 = Modifier usage allowed

Appendix A: NCCI - CPT Codes

Code 1	Code 2
	99241[1], 99242[1], 99243[1], 99244[1], 99245[1], 99251[1], 99252[1], 99253[1], 99254[1], 99255[1], 99291[1], 99292[1], 99304[1], 99305[1], 99306[1], 99307[1], 99308[1], 99309[1], 99310[1], 99315[1], 99316[1], 99334[1], 99335[1], 99336[1], 99337[1], 99347[1], 99348[1], 99349[1], 99350[1], 99374[1], 99375[1], 99377[1], 99378[1], 99446[0], 99447[0], 99448[0], 99449[0], 99451[0], 99452[0], 99495[0], 99496[0], G0453[0], G0463[1], G0471[1]
61546	0213T[0], 0216T[0], 0228T[0], 0230T[0], 0333T[0], 0464T[0], 11000[1], 11001[1], 11004[1], 11005[1], 11006[1], 11042[1], 11043[1], 11044[1], 11045[1], 11046[1], 11047[1], 12001[1], 12002[1], 12004[1], 12005[1], 12006[1], 12007[1], 12011[1], 12013[1], 12014[1], 12015[1], 12016[1], 12017[1], 12018[1], 12020[1], 12021[1], 12031[1], 12032[1], 12034[1], 12035[1], 12036[1], 12037[1], 12041[1], 12042[1], 12044[1], 12045[1], 12046[1], 12047[1], 12051[1], 12052[1], 12053[1], 12054[1], 12055[1], 12056[1], 12057[1], 13100[1], 13101[1], 13102[1], 13120[1], 13121[1], 13122[1], 13131[1], 13132[1], 13133[1], 13151[1], 13152[1], 13153[1], 36000[1], 36400[1], 36405[1], 36406[1], 36410[1], 36420[1], 36425[1], 36430[1], 36440[1], 36591[0], 36592[0], 36600[1], 36640[1], 43752[1], 51701[1], 51702[1], 51703[1], 61107[1], 61210[1], 61304[1], 61305[1], 61535[1], 62100[1], 62140[0], 62141[0], 62165[1], 62320[0], 62321[0], 62322[0], 62323[0], 62324[0], 62325[0], 62326[0], 62327[0], 64400[0], 64405[0], 64408[0], 64415[0], 64416[0], 64417[0], 64418[0], 64420[0], 64421[0], 64425[0], 64430[0], 64435[0], 64445[0], 64446[0], 64447[0], 64448[0], 64449[0], 64450[0], 64451[0], 64454[0], 64461[0], 64462[0], 64463[0], 64479[0], 64480[0], 64483[0], 64484[0], 64486[0], 64487[0], 64488[0], 64489[0], 64490[0], 64491[0], 64492[0], 64493[0], 64494[0], 64495[0], 64505[0], 64510[0], 64517[0], 64520[0], 64530[0], 92012[1], 92014[1], 92585[0], 93000[1], 93005[1], 93010[1], 93040[1], 93041[1], 93042[1], 93318[1], 93355[1], 94002[1], 94200[1], 94250[1], 94680[1], 94681[1], 94690[1], 94770[1], 95812[1], 95813[1], 95816[1], 95819[1], 95822[0], 95829[1], 95860[0], 95861[0], 95863[0], 95864[0], 95865[0], 95866[0], 95867[0], 95868[0], 95869[0], 95870[0], 95907[0], 95908[0], 95909[0], 95910[0], 95911[0], 95912[0], 95913[0], 95925[0], 95926[0], 95927[0], 95928[0], 95929[0], 95930[0], 95933[0], 95937[0], 95938[0], 95939[0], 95940[0], 95955[1], 96360[1], 96361[1], 96365[1], 96366[1], 96367[1], 96368[1], 96372[1], 96374[1], 96375[1], 96376[1], 96377[1], 96523[0], 97597[1], 97598[1], 97602[1], 99155[0], 99156[0], 99157[0], 99211[1], 99212[1], 99213[1], 99214[1], 99215[1], 99217[1], 99218[1], 99219[1], 99220[1], 99221[1], 99222[1], 99223[1], 99231[1], 99232[1], 99233[1], 99234[1], 99235[1], 99236[1], 99238[1], 99239[1], 99241[1], 99242[1], 99243[1], 99244[1], 99245[1], 99251[1], 99252[1], 99253[1], 99254[1], 99255[1], 99291[1], 99292[1], 99304[1], 99305[1], 99306[1], 99307[1], 99308[1], 99309[1], 99310[1], 99315[1], 99316[1], 99334[1], 99335[1], 99336[1], 99337[1], 99347[1], 99348[1], 99349[1], 99350[1], 99374[1], 99375[1], 99377[1], 99378[1], 99446[0], 99447[0], 99448[0], 99449[0], 99451[0], 99452[0], 99495[0], 99496[0], G0453[0], G0463[1], G0471[1]
61548	0213T[0], 0216T[0], 0228T[0], 0230T[0], 0333T[0], 0464T[0], 11000[1], 11001[1], 11004[1], 11005[1], 11006[1], 11042[1], 11043[1], 11044[1], 11045[1], 11046[1], 11047[1], 12001[1], 12002[1], 12004[1], 12005[1], 12006[1], 12007[1], 12011[1], 12013[1], 12014[1], 12015[1], 12016[1], 12017[1], 12018[1], 12020[1], 12021[1], 12031[1], 12032[1], 12034[1], 12035[1], 12036[1], 12037[1], 12041[1], 12042[1], 12044[1], 12045[1], 12046[1], 12047[1], 12051[1], 12052[1], 12053[1], 12054[1], 12055[1], 12056[1], 12057[1], 13100[1], 13101[1], 13102[1], 13120[1], 13121[1], 13122[1], 13131[1], 13132[1], 13133[1], 13151[1], 13152[1], 13153[1], 30520[0], 30930[0], 36000[1], 36400[1], 36405[1], 36406[1], 36410[1], 36420[1], 36425[1], 36430[1], 36440[1], 36591[0], 36592[0], 36600[1], 36640[1], 43752[1], 51701[1], 51702[1], 51703[1], 61304[1], 61305[1], 61546[1], 62140[0], 62141[0], 62320[0], 62321[0], 62322[0], 62323[0], 62324[0], 62325[0], 62326[0], 62327[0], 64400[0], 64405[0], 64408[0], 64415[0], 64416[0], 64417[0], 64418[0], 64420[0], 64421[0], 64425[0], 64430[0], 64435[0], 64445[0], 64446[0], 64447[0], 64448[0], 64449[0], 64450[0], 64451[0], 64454[0], 64461[0], 64462[0], 64463[0], 64479[0], 64480[0], 64483[0], 64484[0], 64486[0], 64487[0], 64488[0], 64489[0], 64490[0], 64491[0], 64492[0], 64493[0], 64494[0], 64495[0], 64505[0], 64510[0], 64517[0], 64520[0], 64530[0], 69990[0], 92012[1], 92014[1], 92585[0], 93000[1], 93005[1], 93010[1], 93040[1], 93041[1], 93042[1], 93318[1], 93355[1], 94002[1], 94200[1], 94250[1], 94680[1], 94681[1], 94690[1], 94770[1], 95812[1], 95813[1], 95816[1], 95819[1], 95822[0], 95829[1], 95860[0], 95861[0], 95863[0], 95864[0], 95865[0], 95866[0], 95867[0], 95868[0], 95869[0], 95870[0], 95907[0], 95908[0], 95909[0], 95910[0], 95911[0], 95912[0], 95913[0], 95925[0], 95926[0], 95927[0], 95928[0], 95929[0], 95930[0], 95933[0], 95937[0], 95938[0], 95939[0], 95940[0], 95955[1], 96360[1], 96361[1], 96365[1], 96366[1], 96367[1], 96368[1], 96372[1], 96374[1], 96375[1], 96376[1], 96377[1], 96523[0], 97597[1], 97598[1], 97602[1], 99155[0], 99156[0], 99157[0], 99211[1], 99212[1], 99213[1], 99214[1], 99215[1], 99217[1], 99218[1], 99219[1], 99220[1], 99221[1], 99222[1], 99223[1], 99231[1], 99232[1], 99233[1], 99234[1], 99235[1], 99236[1], 99238[1], 99239[1], 99241[1], 99242[1], 99243[1], 99244[1], 99245[1], 99251[1], 99252[1], 99253[1], 99254[1], 99255[1], 99291[1], 99292[1], 99304[1], 99305[1], 99306[1], 99307[1], 99308[1], 99309[1], 99310[1], 99315[1], 99316[1], 99334[1], 99335[1], 99336[1], 99337[1], 99347[1], 99348[1], 99349[1], 99350[1], 99374[1], 99375[1], 99377[1], 99378[1], 99446[0], 99447[0], 99448[0], 99449[0], 99451[0], 99452[0], 99495[0], 99496[0], G0453[0], G0463[1], G0471[1]
61566	0213T[0], 0216T[0], 0228T[0], 0230T[0], 0333T[0], 0464T[0], 11000[1], 11001[1], 11004[1], 11005[1], 11006[1], 11042[1], 11043[1], 11044[1], 11045[1], 11046[1], 11047[1], 12001[1], 12002[1], 12004[1], 12005[1], 12006[1], 12007[1], 12011[1], 12013[1], 12014[1], 12015[1], 12016[1], 12017[1], 12018[1], 12020[1], 12021[1], 12031[1], 12032[1], 12034[1], 12035[1], 12036[1], 12037[1], 12041[1], 12042[1], 12044[1], 12045[1], 12046[1], 12047[1], 12051[1], 12052[1], 12053[1], 12054[1], 12055[1], 12056[1], 12057[1], 13100[1], 13101[1], 13102[1], 13120[1], 13121[1], 13122[1], 13131[1], 13132[1], 13133[1], 13151[1], 13152[1], 13153[1], 36000[1], 36400[1], 36405[1], 36406[1], 36410[1], 36420[1], 36425[1], 36430[1], 36440[1], 36591[0], 36592[0], 36600[1], 36640[1], 43752[1], 51701[1], 51702[1], 51703[1], 61107[1], 61304[1], 61533[1], 61535[1], 61537[0], 61538[0], 62100[1], 62140[0], 62141[0], 62320[0], 62321[0], 62322[0], 62323[0], 62324[0], 62325[0], 62326[0], 62327[0], 64400[0], 64405[0], 64408[0], 64415[0], 64416[0], 64417[0], 64418[0], 64420[0], 64421[0], 64425[0], 64430[0], 64435[0], 64445[0], 64446[0], 64447[0], 64448[0], 64449[0], 64450[0], 64451[0], 64454[0], 64461[0], 64462[0], 64463[0], 64479[0], 64480[0], 64483[0], 64484[0], 64486[0], 64487[0], 64488[0], 64489[0], 64490[0], 64491[0], 64492[0], 64493[0], 64494[0], 64495[0], 64505[0], 64510[0], 64517[0], 64520[0], 64530[0], 92012[1], 92014[1], 92585[0], 93000[1], 93005[1], 93010[1], 93040[1], 93041[1], 93042[1], 93318[1], 93355[1], 94002[1], 94200[1], 94250[1], 94680[1], 94681[1], 94690[1], 94770[1], 95812[1], 95813[1], 95816[1], 95819[1], 95822[0], 95829[1], 95860[0], 95861[0], 95863[0], 95864[0], 95865[0], 95866[0], 95867[0], 95868[0], 95869[0], 95870[0], 95907[0], 95908[0], 95909[0], 95910[0], 95911[0], 95912[0], 95913[0], 95925[0], 95926[0], 95927[0], 95928[0], 95929[0], 95930[0], 95933[0], 95937[0], 95938[0], 95939[0], 95940[0], 95955[1], 95961[0], 95962[0], 96360[1], 96361[1], 96365[1], 96366[1], 96367[1], 96368[1], 96372[1], 96374[1], 96375[1], 96376[1], 96377[1], 96523[0], 97597[1], 97598[1], 97602[1], 99155[0], 99156[0], 99157[0], 99211[1], 99212[1], 99213[1], 99214[1], 99215[1], 99217[1], 99218[1], 99219[1], 99220[1], 99221[1], 99222[1], 99223[1], 99231[1], 99232[1], 99233[1], 99234[1], 99235[1], 99236[1], 99238[1], 99239[1], 99241[1], 99242[1], 99243[1], 99244[1], 99245[1], 99251[1], 99252[1], 99253[1], 99254[1], 99255[1], 99291[1], 99292[1], 99304[1], 99305[1], 99306[1], 99307[1], 99308[1], 99309[1], 99310[1], 99315[1], 99316[1], 99334[1], 99335[1], 99336[1], 99337[1], 99347[1], 99348[1], 99349[1], 99350[1], 99374[1], 99375[1], 99377[1], 99378[1], 99446[0], 99447[0], 99448[0], 99449[0], 99451[0], 99452[0], 99495[0], 99496[0], G0453[0], G0463[1], G0471[1]
61567	0213T[0], 0216T[0], 0228T[0], 0230T[0], 0333T[0], 0464T[0], 11000[1], 11001[1], 11004[1], 11005[1], 11006[1], 11042[1], 11043[1], 11044[1], 11045[1], 11046[1], 11047[1], 12001[1], 12002[1], 12004[1], 12005[1], 12006[1], 12007[1], 12011[1], 12013[1], 12014[1], 12015[1], 12016[1], 12017[1], 12018[1], 12020[1], 12021[1], 12031[1], 12032[1], 12034[1], 12035[1], 12036[1], 12037[1], 12041[1], 12042[1], 12044[1], 12045[1], 12046[1], 12047[1], 12051[1], 12052[1], 12053[1], 12054[1], 12055[1], 12056[1], 12057[1], 13100[1], 13101[1], 13102[1], 13120[1], 13121[1], 13122[1], 13131[1], 13132[1], 13133[1], 13151[1], 13152[1], 13153[1], 36000[1], 36400[1], 36405[1], 36406[1], 36410[1], 36420[1], 36425[1], 36430[1], 36440[1], 36591[0], 36592[0], 36600[1], 36640[1], 43752[1], 51701[1], 51702[1], 51703[1], 61107[1], 61304[1], 61535[1], 62100[1], 62140[0], 62141[0], 62320[0], 62321[0], 62322[0], 62323[0], 62324[0], 62325[0], 62326[0], 62327[0], 64400[0], 64405[0], 64408[0], 64415[0], 64416[0], 64417[0], 64418[0], 64420[0], 64421[0], 64425[0], 64430[0], 64435[0], 64445[0], 64446[0], 64447[0], 64448[0], 64449[0], 64450[0], 64451[0], 64454[0], 64461[0], 64462[0], 64463[0], 64479[0], 64480[0], 64483[0], 64484[0], 64486[0], 64487[0], 64488[0], 64489[0], 64490[0], 64491[0], 64492[0], 64493[0], 64494[0], 64495[0], 64505[0], 64510[0], 64517[0], 64520[0], 64530[0], 92012[1], 92014[1], 92585[0], 93000[1], 93005[1], 93010[1], 93040[1], 93041[1], 93042[1], 93318[1], 93355[1], 94002[1], 94200[1], 94250[1], 94680[1], 94681[1], 94690[1], 94770[1], 95812[1], 95813[1], 95816[1], 95819[1], 95822[0], 95829[1], 95860[0], 95861[0], 95863[0], 95864[0], 95865[0], 95866[0], 95867[0], 95868[0], 95869[0], 95870[0], 95907[0], 95908[0], 95909[0], 95910[0], 95911[0], 95912[0], 95913[0], 95925[0], 95926[0], 95927[0], 95928[0], 95929[0], 95930[0], 95933[0], 95937[0], 95938[0], 95939[0], 95940[0], 95955[1], 95961[0], 95962[0], 96360[1], 96361[1], 96365[1], 96366[1], 96367[1], 96368[1], 96372[1], 96374[1], 96375[1], 96376[1], 96377[1], 96523[0], 97597[1], 97598[1], 97602[1], 99155[0], 99156[0], 99157[0], 99211[1], 99212[1], 99213[1], 99214[1], 99215[1], 99217[1], 99218[1], 99219[1], 99220[1], 99221[1], 99222[1], 99223[1], 99231[1], 99232[1], 99233[1], 99234[1], 99235[1], 99236[1], 99238[1], 99239[1], 99241[1], 99242[1], 99243[1], 99244[1], 99245[1], 99251[1], 99252[1], 99253[1], 99254[1], 99255[1], 99291[1], 99292[1], 99304[1], 99305[1], 99306[1], 99307[1], 99308[1], 99309[1], 99310[1], 99315[1], 99316[1], 99334[1], 99335[1], 99336[1], 99337[1], 99347[1], 99348[1], 99349[1], 99350[1], 99374[1], 99375[1], 99377[1], 99378[1], 99446[0], 99447[0], 99448[0], 99449[0], 99451[0], 99452[0], 99495[0], 99496[0], G0453[0], G0463[1], G0471[1]
61580	0213T[0], 0216T[0], 0228T[0], 0230T[0], 0333T[0], 0464T[0], 11000[1], 11001[1], 11004[1], 11005[1], 11006[1], 11042[1], 11043[1], 11044[1], 11045[1], 11046[1], 11047[1], 12001[1], 12002[1], 12004[1], 12005[1], 12006[1], 12007[1], 12011[1], 12013[1], 12014[1], 12015[1], 12016[1], 12017[1], 12018[1], 12020[1], 12021[1], 12031[1], 12032[1], 12034[1], 12035[1], 12036[1], 12037[1], 12041[1], 12042[1], 12044[1], 12045[1], 12046[1], 12047[1], 12051[1], 12052[1], 12053[1], 12054[1], 12055[1], 12056[1], 12057[1], 13100[1], 13101[1], 13102[1], 13120[1], 13121[1], 13122[1], 13131[1], 13132[1], 13133[1], 13151[1], 13152[1], 13153[1], 36000[1], 36400[1], 36405[1], 36406[1], 36410[1], 36420[1], 36425[1], 36430[1], 36440[1], 36591[0], 36592[0], 36600[1], 36640[1], 43752[1], 51701[1], 51702[1], 51703[1], 61586[0], 61618[0], 61619[0], 62320[0], 62321[0], 62322[0], 62323[0], 62324[0], 62325[0], 62326[0], 62327[0], 64400[0], 64405[0], 64408[0], 64415[0], 64416[0], 64417[0], 64418[0], 64420[0], 64421[0], 64425[0], 64430[0], 64435[0], 64445[0], 64446[0], 64447[0], 64448[0], 64449[0], 64450[0], 64451[0], 64454[0], 64461[0], 64462[0], 64463[0], 64479[0], 64480[0], 64483[0], 64484[0], 64486[0], 64487[0], 64488[0], 64489[0], 64490[0], 64491[0], 64492[0], 64493[0], 64494[0], 64495[0], 64505[0], 64510[0], 64517[0], 64520[0], 64530[0], 92012[1], 92014[1], 92585[0], 93000[1], 93005[1], 93010[1], 93040[1],

0 = Modifier usage not allowed or inappropriate 1 = Modifier usage allowed

Code 1	Code 2
	93041[1], 93042[1], 93318[1], 93355[1], 94002[1], 94200[1], 94250[1], 94680[1], 94681[1], 94690[1], 94770[1], 95812[1], 95813[1], 95816[1], 95819[1], 95822[0], 95829[1], 95860[0], 95861[0], 95863[0], 95864[0], 95865[0], 95866[0], 95867[0], 95868[0], 95869[0], 95870[0], 95907[0], 95908[0], 95909[0], 95910[0], 95911[0], 95912[0], 95913[0], 95925[0], 95926[0], 95927[0], 95928[0], 95929[0], 95930[0], 95933[0], 95937[0], 95938[0], 95939[0], 95940[0], 95955[1], 96360[1], 96361[1], 96365[1], 96366[1], 96367[1], 96368[1], 96372[1], 96374[1], 96375[1], 96376[1], 96377[1], 96523[0], 97597[1], 97598[1], 97602[1], 99155[0], 99156[0], 99157[0], 99211[1], 99212[1], 99213[1], 99214[1], 99215[1], 99217[1], 99218[1], 99219[1], 99220[1], 99221[1], 99222[1], 99223[1], 99231[1], 99232[1], 99233[1], 99234[1], 99235[1], 99236[1], 99238[1], 99239[1], 99241[1], 99242[1], 99243[1], 99244[1], 99245[1], 99251[1], 99252[1], 99253[1], 99254[1], 99255[1], 99291[1], 99292[1], 99304[1], 99305[1], 99306[1], 99307[1], 99308[1], 99309[1], 99310[1], 99315[1], 99316[1], 99334[1], 99335[1], 99336[1], 99337[1], 99347[1], 99348[1], 99349[1], 99350[1], 99374[1], 99375[1], 99377[1], 99378[1], 99446[0], 99447[0], 99448[0], 99449[0], 99451[0], 99452[0], 99495[0], 99496[0], G0453[0], G0463[1], G0471[1], J0670[1], J2001[1]
61581	0213T[0], 0216T[0], 0228T[0], 0230T[0], 0333T[0], 0464T[0], 11000[1], 11001[1], 11004[1], 11005[1], 11006[1], 11042[1], 11043[1], 11044[1], 11045[1], 11046[1], 11047[1], 12001[1], 12002[1], 12004[1], 12005[1], 12006[1], 12007[1], 12011[1], 12013[1], 12014[1], 12015[1], 12016[1], 12017[1], 12018[1], 12020[1], 12021[1], 12031[1], 12032[1], 12034[1], 12035[1], 12036[1], 12037[1], 12041[1], 12042[1], 12044[1], 12045[1], 12046[1], 12047[1], 12051[1], 12052[1], 12053[1], 12054[1], 12055[1], 12056[1], 12057[1], 13100[1], 13101[1], 13102[1], 13120[1], 13121[1], 13122[1], 13131[1], 13132[1], 13133[1], 13151[1], 13152[1], 13153[1], 36000[1], 36400[1], 36405[1], 36406[1], 36410[1], 36420[1], 36425[1], 36430[1], 36440[1], 36591[0], 36592[0], 36600[1], 36640[1], 43752[1], 51701[1], 51702[1], 51703[1], 61580[0], 61586[0], 61618[0], 61619[0], 62320[0], 62321[0], 62322[0], 62323[0], 62324[0], 62325[0], 62326[0], 62327[0], 64400[0], 64405[0], 64408[0], 64415[0], 64416[0], 64417[0], 64418[0], 64420[0], 64421[0], 64425[0], 64430[0], 64435[0], 64445[0], 64446[0], 64447[0], 64448[0], 64449[0], 64450[0], 64451[0], 64454[0], 64461[0], 64462[0], 64463[0], 64479[0], 64480[0], 64483[0], 64484[0], 64486[0], 64487[0], 64488[0], 64489[0], 64490[0], 64491[0], 64492[0], 64493[0], 64494[0], 64495[0], 64505[0], 64510[0], 64517[0], 64520[0], 64530[0], 92012[1], 92014[1], 92585[0], 93000[1], 93005[1], 93010[1], 93040[1], 93041[1], 93042[1], 93318[1], 93355[1], 94002[1], 94200[1], 94250[1], 94680[1], 94681[1], 94690[1], 94770[1], 95812[1], 95813[1], 95816[1], 95819[1], 95822[0], 95829[1], 95860[0], 95861[0], 95863[0], 95864[0], 95865[0], 95866[0], 95867[0], 95868[0], 95869[0], 95870[0], 95907[0], 95908[0], 95909[0], 95910[0], 95911[0], 95912[0], 95913[0], 95925[0], 95926[0], 95927[0], 95928[0], 95929[0], 95930[0], 95933[0], 95937[0], 95938[0], 95939[0], 95940[0], 95955[1], 96360[1], 96361[1], 96365[1], 96366[1], 96367[1], 96368[1], 96372[1], 96374[1], 96375[1], 96376[1], 96377[1], 96523[0], 97597[1], 97598[1], 97602[1], 99155[0], 99156[0], 99157[0], 99211[1], 99212[1], 99213[1], 99214[1], 99215[1], 99217[1], 99218[1], 99219[1], 99220[1], 99221[1], 99222[1], 99223[1], 99231[1], 99232[1], 99233[1], 99234[1], 99235[1], 99236[1], 99238[1], 99239[1], 99241[1], 99242[1], 99243[1], 99244[1], 99245[1], 99251[1], 99252[1], 99253[1], 99254[1], 99255[1], 99291[1], 99292[1], 99304[1], 99305[1], 99306[1], 99307[1], 99308[1], 99309[1], 99310[1], 99315[1], 99316[1], 99334[1], 99335[1], 99336[1], 99337[1], 99347[1], 99348[1], 99349[1], 99350[1], 99374[1], 99375[1], 99377[1], 99378[1], 99446[0], 99447[0], 99448[0], 99449[0], 99451[0], 99452[0], 99495[0], 99496[0], G0453[0], G0463[1], G0471[1], J0670[1], J2001[1]
61582	0213T[0], 0216T[0], 0228T[0], 0230T[0], 0333T[0], 0464T[0], 11000[1], 11001[1], 11004[1], 11005[1], 11006[1], 11042[1], 11043[1], 11044[1], 11045[1], 11046[1], 11047[1], 12001[1], 12002[1], 12004[1], 12005[1], 12006[1], 12007[1], 12011[1], 12013[1], 12014[1], 12015[1], 12016[1], 12017[1], 12018[1], 12020[1], 12021[1], 12031[1], 12032[1], 12034[1], 12035[1], 12036[1], 12037[1], 12041[1], 12042[1], 12044[1], 12045[1], 12046[1], 12047[1], 12051[1], 12052[1], 12053[1], 12054[1], 12055[1], 12056[1], 12057[1], 13100[1], 13101[1], 13102[1], 13120[1], 13121[1], 13122[1], 13131[1], 13132[1], 13133[1], 13151[1], 13152[1], 13153[1], 36000[1], 36400[1], 36405[1], 36406[1], 36410[1], 36420[1], 36425[1], 36430[1], 36440[1], 36591[0], 36592[0], 36600[1], 36640[1], 43752[1], 51701[1], 51702[1], 51703[1], 61580[0], 61581[0], 61583[0], 61584[0], 61586[0], 61618[0], 61619[0], 62100[1], 62320[0], 62321[0], 62322[0], 62323[0], 62324[0], 62325[0], 62326[0], 62327[0], 64400[0], 64405[0], 64408[0], 64415[0], 64416[0], 64417[0], 64418[0], 64420[0], 64421[0], 64425[0], 64430[0], 64435[0], 64445[0], 64446[0], 64447[0], 64448[0], 64449[0], 64450[0], 64451[0], 64454[0], 64461[0], 64462[0], 64463[0], 64479[0], 64480[0], 64483[0], 64484[0], 64486[0], 64487[0], 64488[0], 64489[0], 64490[0], 64491[0], 64492[0], 64493[0], 64494[0], 64495[0], 64505[0], 64510[0], 64517[0], 64520[0], 64530[0], 92012[1], 92014[1], 92585[0], 93000[1], 93005[1], 93010[1], 93040[1], 93041[1], 93042[1], 93318[1], 93355[1], 94002[1], 94200[1], 94250[1], 94680[1], 94681[1], 94690[1], 94770[1], 95812[1], 95813[1], 95816[1], 95819[1], 95822[0], 95829[1], 95860[0], 95861[0], 95863[0], 95864[0], 95865[0], 95866[0], 95867[0], 95868[0], 95869[0], 95870[0], 95907[0], 95908[0], 95909[0], 95910[0], 95911[0], 95912[0], 95913[0], 95925[0], 95926[0], 95927[0], 95928[0], 95929[0], 95930[0], 95933[0], 95937[0], 95938[0], 95939[0], 95940[0], 95955[1], 96360[1], 96361[1], 96365[1], 96366[1], 96367[1], 96368[1], 96372[1], 96374[1], 96375[1], 96376[1], 96377[1], 96523[0], 97597[1], 97598[1], 97602[1], 99155[0], 99156[0], 99157[0], 99211[1], 99212[1], 99213[1], 99214[1], 99215[1], 99217[1], 99218[1], 99219[1], 99220[1], 99221[1], 99222[1], 99223[1], 99231[1], 99232[1], 99233[1], 99234[1], 99235[1], 99236[1], 99238[1], 99239[1], 99241[1], 99242[1], 99243[1], 99244[1], 99245[1], 99251[1], 99252[1], 99253[1], 99254[1], 99255[1], 99291[1], 99292[1], 99304[1], 99305[1], 99306[1], 99307[1], 99308[1], 99309[1], 99310[1], 99315[1], 99316[1], 99334[1], 99335[1], 99336[1], 99337[1], 99347[1], 99348[1], 99349[1], 99350[1], 99374[1], 99375[1], 99377[1], 99378[1], 99446[0], 99447[0], 99448[0], 99449[0], 99451[0], 99452[0], 99495[0], 99496[0], G0453[0], G0463[1], G0471[1], J0670[1], J2001[1]
61583	0213T[0], 0216T[0], 0228T[0], 0230T[0], 0333T[0], 0464T[0], 11000[1], 11001[1], 11004[1], 11005[1], 11006[1], 11042[1], 11043[1], 11044[1], 11045[1], 11046[1], 11047[1], 12001[1], 12002[1], 12004[1], 12005[1], 12006[1], 12007[1], 12011[1], 12013[1], 12014[1], 12015[1], 12016[1], 12017[1], 12018[1], 12020[1], 12021[1], 12031[1], 12032[1], 12034[1], 12035[1], 12036[1], 12037[1], 12041[1], 12042[1], 12044[1], 12045[1], 12046[1], 12047[1], 12051[1], 12052[1], 12053[1], 12054[1], 12055[1], 12056[1], 12057[1], 13100[1], 13101[1], 13102[1], 13120[1], 13121[1], 13122[1], 13131[1], 13132[1], 13133[1], 13151[1], 13152[1], 13153[1], 36000[1], 36400[1], 36405[1], 36406[1], 36410[1], 36420[1], 36425[1], 36430[1], 36440[1], 36591[0], 36592[0], 36600[1], 36640[1], 43752[1], 51701[1], 51702[1], 51703[1], 61580[0], 61581[0], 61584[0], 61586[0], 61618[0], 61619[0], 62100[1], 62320[0], 62321[0], 62322[0], 62323[0], 62324[0], 62325[0], 62326[0], 62327[0], 64400[0], 64405[0], 64408[0], 64415[0], 64416[0], 64417[0], 64418[0], 64420[0], 64421[0], 64425[0], 64430[0], 64435[0], 64445[0], 64446[0], 64447[0], 64448[0], 64449[0], 64450[0], 64451[0], 64454[0], 64461[0], 64462[0], 64463[0], 64479[0], 64480[0], 64483[0], 64484[0], 64486[0], 64487[0], 64488[0], 64489[0], 64490[0], 64491[0], 64492[0], 64493[0], 64494[0], 64495[0], 64505[0], 64510[0], 64517[0], 64520[0], 64530[0], 92012[1], 92014[1], 92585[0], 93000[1], 93005[1], 93010[1], 93040[1], 93041[1], 93042[1], 93318[1], 93355[1], 94002[1], 94200[1], 94250[1], 94680[1], 94681[1], 94690[1], 94770[1], 95812[1], 95813[1], 95816[1], 95819[1], 95822[0], 95829[1], 95860[0], 95861[0], 95863[0], 95864[0], 95865[0], 95866[0], 95867[0], 95868[0], 95869[0], 95870[0], 95907[0], 95908[0], 95909[0], 95910[0], 95911[0], 95912[0], 95913[0], 95925[0], 95926[0], 95927[0], 95928[0], 95929[0], 95930[0], 95933[0], 95937[0], 95938[0], 95939[0], 95940[0], 95955[1], 96360[1], 96361[1], 96365[1], 96366[1], 96367[1], 96368[1], 96372[1], 96374[1], 96375[1], 96376[1], 96377[1], 96523[0], 97597[1], 97598[1], 97602[1], 99155[0], 99156[0], 99157[0], 99211[1], 99212[1], 99213[1], 99214[1], 99215[1], 99217[1], 99218[1], 99219[1], 99220[1], 99221[1], 99222[1], 99223[1], 99231[1], 99232[1], 99233[1], 99234[1], 99235[1], 99236[1], 99238[1], 99239[1], 99241[1], 99242[1], 99243[1], 99244[1], 99245[1], 99251[1], 99252[1], 99253[1], 99254[1], 99255[1], 99291[1], 99292[1], 99304[1], 99305[1], 99306[1], 99307[1], 99308[1], 99309[1], 99310[1], 99315[1], 99316[1], 99334[1], 99335[1], 99336[1], 99337[1], 99347[1], 99348[1], 99349[1], 99350[1], 99374[1], 99375[1], 99377[1], 99378[1], 99446[0], 99447[0], 99448[0], 99449[0], 99451[0], 99452[0], 99495[0], 99496[0], G0453[0], G0463[1], G0471[1], J0670[1], J2001[1]
61584	0213T[0], 0216T[0], 0228T[0], 0230T[0], 0333T[0], 0464T[0], 11000[1], 11001[1], 11004[1], 11005[1], 11006[1], 11042[1], 11043[1], 11044[1], 11045[1], 11046[1], 11047[1], 12001[1], 12002[1], 12004[1], 12005[1], 12006[1], 12007[1], 12011[1], 12013[1], 12014[1], 12015[1], 12016[1], 12017[1], 12018[1], 12020[1], 12021[1], 12031[1], 12032[1], 12034[1], 12035[1], 12036[1], 12037[1], 12041[1], 12042[1], 12044[1], 12045[1], 12046[1], 12047[1], 12051[1], 12052[1], 12053[1], 12054[1], 12055[1], 12056[1], 12057[1], 13100[1], 13101[1], 13102[1], 13120[1], 13121[1], 13122[1], 13131[1], 13132[1], 13133[1], 13151[1], 13152[1], 13153[1], 36000[1], 36400[1], 36405[1], 36406[1], 36410[1], 36420[1], 36425[1], 36430[1], 36440[1], 36591[0], 36592[0], 36600[1], 36640[1], 43752[1], 51701[1], 51702[1], 51703[1], 61580[0], 61581[0], 61586[0], 61618[0], 61619[0], 62320[0], 62321[0], 62322[0], 62323[0], 62324[0], 62325[0], 62326[0], 62327[0], 64400[0], 64405[0], 64408[0], 64415[0], 64416[0], 64417[0], 64418[0], 64420[0], 64421[0], 64425[0], 64430[0], 64435[0], 64445[0], 64446[0], 64447[0], 64448[0], 64449[0], 64450[0], 64451[0], 64454[0], 64461[0], 64462[0], 64463[0], 64479[0], 64480[0], 64483[0], 64484[0], 64486[0], 64487[0], 64488[0], 64489[0], 64490[0], 64491[0], 64492[0], 64493[0], 64494[0], 64495[0], 64505[0], 64510[0], 64517[0], 64520[0], 64530[0], 92012[1], 92014[1], 92585[0], 93000[1], 93005[1], 93010[1], 93040[1], 93041[1], 93042[1], 93318[1], 93355[1], 94002[1], 94200[1], 94250[1], 94680[1], 94681[1], 94690[1], 94770[1], 95812[1], 95813[1], 95816[1], 95819[1], 95822[0], 95829[1], 95860[0], 95861[0], 95863[0], 95864[0], 95865[0], 95866[0], 95867[0], 95868[0], 95869[0], 95870[0], 95907[0], 95908[0], 95909[0], 95910[0], 95911[0], 95912[0], 95913[0], 95925[0], 95926[0], 95927[0], 95928[0], 95929[0], 95930[0], 95933[0], 95937[0], 95938[0], 95939[0], 95940[0], 95955[1], 96360[1], 96361[1], 96365[1], 96366[1], 96367[1], 96368[1], 96372[1], 96374[1], 96375[1], 96376[1], 96377[1], 96523[0], 97597[1], 97598[1], 97602[1], 99155[0], 99156[0], 99157[0], 99211[1], 99212[1], 99213[1], 99214[1], 99215[1], 99217[1], 99218[1], 99219[1], 99220[1], 99221[1], 99222[1], 99223[1], 99231[1], 99232[1], 99233[1], 99234[1], 99235[1], 99236[1], 99238[1], 99239[1], 99241[1], 99242[1], 99243[1], 99244[1], 99245[1], 99251[1], 99252[1], 99253[1], 99254[1], 99255[1], 99291[1], 99292[1], 99304[1], 99305[1], 99306[1], 99307[1], 99308[1], 99309[1], 99310[1], 99315[1], 99316[1], 99334[1], 99335[1], 99336[1], 99337[1], 99347[1], 99348[1], 99349[1], 99350[1], 99374[1], 99375[1], 99377[1], 99378[1], 99446[0], 99447[0], 99448[0], 99449[0], 99451[0], 99452[0], 99495[0], 99496[0], G0453[0], G0463[1], G0471[1], J0670[1], J2001[1]
61585	0213T[0], 0216T[0], 0228T[0], 0230T[0], 0333T[0], 0464T[0], 11000[1], 11001[1], 11004[1], 11005[1], 11006[1], 11042[1], 11043[1], 11044[1], 11045[1], 11046[1], 11047[1], 12001[1], 12002[1], 12004[1], 12005[1], 12006[1], 12007[1], 12011[1], 12013[1], 12014[1], 12015[1], 12016[1], 12017[1], 12018[1], 12020[1], 12021[1], 12031[1], 12032[1], 12034[1], 12035[1], 12036[1], 12037[1], 12041[1], 12042[1], 12044[1], 12045[1], 12046[1], 12047[1], 12051[1], 12052[1], 12053[1], 12054[1], 12055[1], 12056[1], 12057[1], 13100[1], 13101[1], 13102[1], 13120[1], 13121[1], 13122[1], 13131[1], 13132[1], 13133[1],

Appendix A: NCCI - CPT Codes

0 = Modifier usage not allowed or inappropriate 1 = Modifier usage allowed

Code 1	Code 2
	13151[1], 13152[1], 13153[1], 36000[1], 36400[1], 36405[1], 36406[1], 36410[1], 36420[1], 36425[1], 36430[1], 36440[1], 36591[0], 36592[0], 36600[1], 36640[1], 43752[1], 51701[1], 51702[1], 51703[1], 61580[0], 61581[0], 61582[0], 61583[0], 61584[0], 61586[0], 61618[0], 61619[0], 62320[0], 62321[0], 62322[0], 62323[0], 62324[0], 62325[0], 62326[0], 62327[0], 64400[0], 64405[0], 64408[0], 64415[0], 64416[0], 64417[0], 64418[0], 64420[0], 64421[0], 64425[0], 64430[0], 64435[0], 64445[0], 64446[0], 64447[0], 64448[0], 64449[0], 64450[0], 64451[0], 64454[0], 64461[0], 64462[0], 64463[0], 64479[0], 64480[0], 64483[0], 64484[0], 64486[0], 64487[0], 64488[0], 64489[0], 64490[0], 64491[0], 64492[0], 64493[0], 64494[0], 64495[0], 64505[0], 64510[0], 64517[0], 64520[0], 64530[0], 92012[1], 92014[1], 92585[0], 93000[1], 93005[1], 93010[1], 93040[1], 93041[1], 93042[1], 93318[1], 93355[1], 94002[1], 94200[1], 94250[1], 94680[1], 94681[1], 94690[1], 94770[1], 95812[1], 95813[1], 95816[1], 95819[1], 95822[0], 95829[1], 95860[0], 95861[0], 95863[0], 95864[0], 95865[0], 95866[0], 95867[0], 95868[0], 95869[0], 95870[0], 95907[0], 95908[0], 95909[0], 95910[0], 95911[0], 95912[0], 95913[0], 95925[0], 95926[0], 95927[0], 95928[0], 95929[0], 95930[0], 95933[0], 95937[0], 95938[0], 95939[0], 95940[0], 95955[1], 96360[1], 96361[1], 96365[1], 96366[1], 96367[1], 96368[1], 96372[1], 96374[1], 96375[1], 96376[1], 96377[1], 96523[0], 97597[1], 97598[1], 97602[1], 99155[0], 99156[0], 99157[0], 99211[1], 99212[1], 99213[1], 99214[1], 99215[1], 99217[1], 99218[1], 99219[1], 99220[1], 99221[1], 99222[1], 99223[1], 99231[1], 99232[1], 99233[1], 99234[1], 99235[1], 99236[1], 99238[1], 99239[1], 99241[1], 99242[1], 99243[1], 99244[1], 99245[1], 99251[1], 99252[1], 99253[1], 99254[1], 99255[1], 99291[1], 99292[1], 99304[1], 99305[1], 99306[1], 99307[1], 99308[1], 99309[1], 99310[1], 99315[1], 99316[1], 99334[1], 99335[1], 99336[1], 99337[1], 99347[1], 99348[1], 99349[1], 99350[1], 99374[1], 99375[1], 99377[1], 99378[1], 99446[0], 99447[0], 99448[0], 99449[0], 99451[0], 99452[0], 99495[0], 99496[0], G0453[0], G0463[1], G0471[1], J0670[1], J2001[1]
61590	0213T[0], 0216T[0], 0228T[0], 0230T[0], 0333T[0], 0464T[0], 11000[1], 11001[1], 11004[1], 11005[1], 11006[1], 11042[1], 11043[1], 11044[1], 11045[1], 11046[1], 11047[1], 12001[1], 12002[1], 12004[1], 12005[1], 12006[1], 12007[1], 12011[1], 12013[1], 12014[1], 12015[1], 12016[1], 12017[1], 12018[1], 12020[1], 12021[1], 12031[1], 12032[1], 12034[1], 12035[1], 12036[1], 12037[1], 12041[1], 12042[1], 12044[1], 12045[1], 12046[1], 12047[1], 12051[1], 12052[1], 12053[1], 12054[1], 12055[1], 12056[1], 12057[1], 13100[1], 13101[1], 13102[1], 13120[1], 13121[1], 13122[1], 13131[1], 13132[1], 13133[1], 13151[1], 13152[1], 13153[1], 36000[1], 36400[1], 36405[1], 36406[1], 36410[1], 36420[1], 36425[1], 36430[1], 36440[1], 36591[0], 36592[0], 36600[1], 36640[1], 43752[1], 51701[1], 51702[1], 51703[1], 61618[0], 61619[0], 62100[1], 62320[0], 62321[0], 62322[0], 62323[0], 62324[0], 62325[0], 62326[0], 62327[0], 64400[0], 64405[0], 64408[0], 64415[0], 64416[0], 64417[0], 64418[0], 64420[0], 64421[0], 64425[0], 64430[0], 64435[0], 64445[0], 64446[0], 64447[0], 64448[0], 64449[0], 64450[0], 64451[0], 64454[0], 64461[0], 64462[0], 64463[0], 64479[0], 64480[0], 64483[0], 64484[0], 64486[0], 64487[0], 64488[0], 64489[0], 64490[0], 64491[0], 64492[0], 64493[0], 64494[0], 64495[0], 64505[0], 64510[0], 64517[0], 64520[0], 64530[0], 92012[1], 92014[1], 92585[0], 93000[1], 93005[1], 93010[1], 93040[1], 93041[1], 93042[1], 93318[1], 93355[1], 94002[1], 94200[1], 94250[1], 94680[1], 94681[1], 94690[1], 94770[1], 95812[1], 95813[1], 95816[1], 95819[1], 95822[0], 95829[1], 95860[0], 95861[0], 95863[0], 95864[0], 95865[0], 95866[0], 95867[0], 95868[0], 95869[0], 95870[0], 95907[0], 95908[0], 95909[0], 95910[0], 95911[0], 95912[0], 95913[0], 95925[0], 95926[0], 95927[0], 95928[0], 95929[0], 95930[0], 95933[0], 95937[0], 95938[0], 95939[0], 95940[0], 95955[1], 96360[1], 96361[1], 96365[1], 96366[1], 96367[1], 96368[1], 96372[1], 96374[1], 96375[1], 96376[1], 96377[1], 96523[0], 97597[1], 97598[1], 97602[1], 99155[0], 99156[0], 99157[0], 99211[1], 99212[1], 99213[1], 99214[1], 99215[1], 99217[1], 99218[1], 99219[1], 99220[1], 99221[1], 99222[1], 99223[1], 99231[1], 99232[1], 99233[1], 99234[1], 99235[1], 99236[1], 99238[1], 99239[1], 99241[1], 99242[1], 99243[1], 99244[1], 99245[1], 99251[1], 99252[1], 99253[1], 99254[1], 99255[1], 99291[1], 99292[1], 99304[1], 99305[1], 99306[1], 99307[1], 99308[1], 99309[1], 99310[1], 99315[1], 99316[1], 99334[1], 99335[1], 99336[1], 99337[1], 99347[1], 99348[1], 99349[1], 99350[1], 99374[1], 99375[1], 99377[1], 99378[1], 99446[0], 99447[0], 99448[0], 99449[0], 99451[0], 99452[0], 99495[0], 99496[0], G0453[0], G0463[1], G0471[1]
61591	0213T[0], 0216T[0], 0228T[0], 0230T[0], 0333T[0], 0464T[0], 11000[1], 11001[1], 11004[1], 11005[1], 11006[1], 11042[1], 11043[1], 11044[1], 11045[1], 11046[1], 11047[1], 12001[1], 12002[1], 12004[1], 12005[1], 12006[1], 12007[1], 12011[1], 12013[1], 12014[1], 12015[1], 12016[1], 12017[1], 12018[1], 12020[1], 12021[1], 12031[1], 12032[1], 12034[1], 12035[1], 12036[1], 12037[1], 12041[1], 12042[1], 12044[1], 12045[1], 12046[1], 12047[1], 12051[1], 12052[1], 12053[1], 12054[1], 12055[1], 12056[1], 12057[1], 13100[1], 13101[1], 13102[1], 13120[1], 13121[1], 13122[1], 13131[1], 13132[1], 13133[1], 13151[1], 13152[1], 13153[1], 35701[1], 36000[1], 36400[1], 36405[1], 36406[1], 36410[1], 36420[1], 36425[1], 36430[1], 36440[1], 36591[0], 36592[0], 36600[1], 36640[1], 43752[1], 51701[1], 51702[1], 51703[1], 61590[1], 61618[0], 61619[0], 62320[0], 62321[0], 62322[0], 62323[0], 62324[0], 62325[0], 62326[0], 62327[0], 64400[0], 64405[0], 64408[0], 64415[0], 64416[0], 64417[0], 64418[0], 64420[0], 64421[0], 64425[0], 64430[0], 64435[0], 64445[0], 64446[0], 64447[0], 64448[0], 64449[0], 64450[0], 64451[0], 64454[0], 64461[0], 64462[0], 64463[0], 64479[0], 64480[0], 64483[0], 64484[0], 64486[0], 64487[0], 64488[0], 64489[0], 64490[0], 64491[0], 64492[0], 64493[0], 64494[0], 64495[0], 64505[0], 64510[0], 64517[0], 64520[0], 64530[0], 69960[1], 92012[1], 92014[1], 92585[0], 93000[1], 93005[1], 93010[1], 93040[1], 93041[1], 93042[1], 93318[1], 93355[1], 94002[1], 94200[1], 94250[1], 94680[1], 94681[1], 94690[1], 94770[1], 95812[1], 95813[1], 95816[1], 95819[1], 95822[0], 95829[1], 95860[0], 95861[0], 95863[0], 95864[0], 95865[0], 95866[0], 95867[0], 95868[0], 95869[0], 95870[0], 95907[0], 95908[0], 95909[0], 95910[0], 95911[0], 95912[0], 95913[0], 95925[0], 95926[0], 95927[0], 95928[0], 95929[0], 95930[0], 95933[0], 95937[0], 95938[0], 95939[0], 95940[0], 95955[1], 96360[1], 96361[1], 96365[1], 96366[1], 96367[1], 96368[1], 96372[1], 96374[1], 96375[1], 96376[1], 96377[1], 96523[0], 97597[1], 97598[1], 97602[1], 99155[0], 99156[0], 99157[0], 99211[1], 99212[1], 99213[1], 99214[1], 99215[1], 99217[1], 99218[1], 99219[1], 99220[1], 99221[1], 99222[1], 99223[1], 99231[1], 99232[1], 99233[1], 99234[1], 99235[1], 99236[1], 99238[1], 99239[1], 99241[1], 99242[1], 99243[1], 99244[1], 99245[1], 99251[1], 99252[1], 99253[1], 99254[1], 99255[1], 99291[1], 99292[1], 99304[1], 99305[1], 99306[1], 99307[1], 99308[1], 99309[1], 99310[1], 99315[1], 99316[1], 99334[1], 99335[1], 99336[1], 99337[1], 99347[1], 99348[1], 99349[1], 99350[1], 99374[1], 99375[1], 99377[1], 99378[1], 99446[0], 99447[0], 99448[0], 99449[0], 99451[0], 99452[0], 99495[0], 99496[0], G0453[0], G0463[1], G0471[1]
61592	0213T[0], 0216T[0], 0228T[0], 0230T[0], 0333T[0], 0464T[0], 11000[1], 11001[1], 11004[1], 11005[1], 11006[1], 11042[1], 11043[1], 11044[1], 11045[1], 11046[1], 11047[1], 12001[1], 12002[1], 12004[1], 12005[1], 12006[1], 12007[1], 12011[1], 12013[1], 12014[1], 12015[1], 12016[1], 12017[1], 12018[1], 12020[1], 12021[1], 12031[1], 12032[1], 12034[1], 12035[1], 12036[1], 12037[1], 12041[1], 12042[1], 12044[1], 12045[1], 12046[1], 12047[1], 12051[1], 12052[1], 12053[1], 12054[1], 12055[1], 12056[1], 12057[1], 13100[1], 13101[1], 13102[1], 13120[1], 13121[1], 13122[1], 13131[1], 13132[1], 13133[1], 13151[1], 13152[1], 13153[1], 36000[1], 36400[1], 36405[1], 36406[1], 36410[1], 36420[1], 36425[1], 36430[1], 36440[1], 36591[0], 36592[0], 36600[1], 36640[1], 43752[1], 51701[1], 51702[1], 51703[1], 61590[0], 61591[0], 61618[0], 61619[0], 62100[1], 62320[0], 62321[0], 62322[0], 62323[0], 62324[0], 62325[0], 62326[0], 62327[0], 64400[0], 64405[0], 64408[0], 64415[0], 64416[0], 64417[0], 64418[0], 64420[0], 64421[0], 64425[0], 64430[0], 64435[0], 64445[0], 64446[0], 64447[0], 64448[0], 64449[0], 64450[0], 64451[0], 64454[0], 64461[0], 64462[0], 64463[0], 64479[0], 64480[0], 64483[0], 64484[0], 64486[0], 64487[0], 64488[0], 64489[0], 64490[0], 64491[0], 64492[0], 64493[0], 64494[0], 64495[0], 64505[0], 64510[0], 64517[0], 64520[0], 64530[0], 92012[1], 92014[1], 92585[0], 93000[1], 93005[1], 93010[1], 93040[1], 93041[1], 93042[1], 93318[1], 93355[1], 94002[1], 94200[1], 94250[1], 94680[1], 94681[1], 94690[1], 94770[1], 95812[1], 95813[1], 95816[1], 95819[1], 95822[0], 95829[1], 95860[0], 95861[0], 95863[0], 95864[0], 95865[0], 95866[0], 95867[0], 95868[0], 95869[0], 95870[0], 95907[0], 95908[0], 95909[0], 95910[0], 95911[0], 95912[0], 95913[0], 95925[0], 95926[0], 95927[0], 95928[0], 95929[0], 95930[0], 95933[0], 95937[0], 95938[0], 95939[0], 95940[0], 95955[1], 96360[1], 96361[1], 96365[1], 96366[1], 96367[1], 96368[1], 96372[1], 96374[1], 96375[1], 96376[1], 96377[1], 96523[0], 97597[1], 97598[1], 97602[1], 99155[0], 99156[0], 99157[0], 99211[1], 99212[1], 99213[1], 99214[1], 99215[1], 99217[1], 99218[1], 99219[1], 99220[1], 99221[1], 99222[1], 99223[1], 99231[1], 99232[1], 99233[1], 99234[1], 99235[1], 99236[1], 99238[1], 99239[1], 99241[1], 99242[1], 99243[1], 99244[1], 99245[1], 99251[1], 99252[1], 99253[1], 99254[1], 99255[1], 99291[1], 99292[1], 99304[1], 99305[1], 99306[1], 99307[1], 99308[1], 99309[1], 99310[1], 99315[1], 99316[1], 99334[1], 99335[1], 99336[1], 99337[1], 99347[1], 99348[1], 99349[1], 99350[1], 99374[1], 99375[1], 99377[1], 99378[1], 99446[0], 99447[0], 99448[0], 99449[0], 99451[0], 99452[0], 99495[0], 99496[0], G0453[0], G0463[1], G0471[1]
61595	0213T[0], 0216T[0], 0228T[0], 0230T[0], 0333T[0], 0464T[0], 11000[1], 11001[1], 11004[1], 11005[1], 11006[1], 11042[1], 11043[1], 11044[1], 11045[1], 11046[1], 11047[1], 12001[1], 12002[1], 12004[1], 12005[1], 12006[1], 12007[1], 12011[1], 12013[1], 12014[1], 12015[1], 12016[1], 12017[1], 12018[1], 12020[1], 12021[1], 12031[1], 12032[1], 12034[1], 12035[1], 12036[1], 12037[1], 12041[1], 12042[1], 12044[1], 12045[1], 12046[1], 12047[1], 12051[1], 12052[1], 12053[1], 12054[1], 12055[1], 12056[1], 12057[1], 13100[1], 13101[1], 13102[1], 13120[1], 13121[1], 13122[1], 13131[1], 13132[1], 13133[1], 13151[1], 13152[1], 13153[1], 36000[1], 36400[1], 36405[1], 36406[1], 36410[1], 36420[1], 36425[1], 36430[1], 36440[1], 36591[0], 36592[0], 36600[1], 36640[1], 43752[1], 51701[1], 51702[1], 51703[1], 61618[0], 61619[0], 62320[0], 62321[0], 62322[0], 62323[0], 62324[0], 62325[0], 62326[0], 62327[0], 64400[0], 64405[0], 64408[0], 64415[0], 64416[0], 64417[0], 64418[0], 64420[0], 64421[0], 64425[0], 64430[0], 64435[0], 64445[0], 64446[0], 64447[0], 64448[0], 64449[0], 64450[0], 64451[0], 64454[0], 64461[0], 64462[0], 64463[0], 64479[0], 64480[0], 64483[0], 64484[0], 64486[0], 64487[0], 64488[0], 64489[0], 64490[0], 64491[0], 64492[0], 64493[0], 64494[0], 64495[0], 64505[0], 64510[0], 64517[0], 64520[0], 64530[0], 92012[1], 92014[1], 92585[0], 93000[1], 93005[1], 93010[1], 93040[1], 93041[1], 93042[1], 93318[1], 93355[1], 94002[1], 94200[1], 94250[1], 94680[1], 94681[1], 94690[1], 94770[1], 95812[1], 95813[1], 95816[1], 95819[1], 95822[0], 95829[1], 95860[0], 95861[0], 95863[0], 95864[0], 95865[0], 95866[0], 95867[0], 95868[0], 95869[0], 95870[0], 95907[0], 95908[0], 95909[0], 95910[0], 95911[0], 95912[0], 95913[0], 95925[0], 95926[0], 95927[0], 95928[0], 95929[0], 95930[0], 95933[0], 95937[0], 95938[0], 95939[0], 95940[0], 95955[1], 96360[1], 96361[1], 96365[1], 96366[1], 96367[1], 96368[1], 96372[1], 96374[1], 96375[1], 96376[1], 96377[1], 96523[0], 97597[1], 97598[1], 97602[1], 99155[0], 99156[0], 99157[0], 99211[1], 99212[1], 99213[1], 99214[1], 99215[1], 99217[1], 99218[1], 99219[1], 99220[1], 99221[1], 99222[1], 99223[1], 99231[1], 99232[1], 99233[1], 99234[1], 99235[1], 99236[1], 99238[1], 99239[1], 99241[1], 99242[1], 99243[1], 99244[1], 99245[1], 99251[1], 99252[1], 99253[1], 99254[1], 99255[1], 99291[1], 99292[1], 99304[1], 99305[1], 99306[1], 99307[1], 99308[1], 99309[1], 99310[1], 99315[1], 99316[1], 99334[1], 99335[1], 99336[1], 99337[1], 99347[1], 99348[1], 99349[1], 99350[1], 99374[1], 99375[1], 99377[1], 99378[1], 99446[0], 99447[0], 99448[0], 99449[0], 99451[0], 99452[0], 99495[0], 99496[0], G0453[0], G0463[1], G0471[1]

0 = Modifier usage not allowed or inappropriate 1 = Modifier usage allowed

Code 1	Code 2
61597	0213T[0], 0216T[0], 0228T[0], 0230T[0], 0333T[0], 0464T[0], 11000[1], 11001[1], 11004[1], 11005[1], 11006[1], 11042[1], 11043[1], 11044[1], 11045[1], 11046[1], 11047[1], 12001[1], 12002[1], 12004[1], 12005[1], 12006[1], 12007[1], 12011[1], 12013[1], 12014[1], 12015[1], 12016[1], 12017[1], 12018[1], 12020[1], 12021[1], 12031[1], 12032[1], 12034[1], 12035[1], 12036[1], 12037[1], 12041[1], 12042[1], 12044[1], 12045[1], 12046[1], 12047[1], 12051[1], 12052[1], 12053[1], 12054[1], 12055[1], 12056[1], 12057[1], 13100[1], 13101[1], 13102[1], 13120[1], 13121[1], 13122[1], 13131[1], 13132[1], 13133[1], 13151[1], 13152[1], 13153[1], 36000[1], 36400[1], 36405[1], 36406[1], 36410[1], 36420[1], 36425[1], 36430[1], 36440[1], 36591[0], 36592[0], 36600[1], 36640[1], 43752[1], 51701[1], 51702[1], 51703[1], 61595[0], 61596[0], 61598[0], 61618[0], 61619[0], 62320[0], 62321[0], 62322[0], 62323[0], 62324[0], 62325[0], 62326[0], 62327[0], 64400[0], 64405[0], 64408[0], 64415[0], 64416[0], 64417[0], 64418[0], 64420[0], 64421[0], 64425[0], 64430[0], 64435[0], 64445[0], 64446[0], 64447[0], 64448[0], 64449[0], 64450[0], 64451[0], 64454[0], 64461[0], 64462[0], 64463[0], 64479[0], 64480[0], 64483[0], 64484[0], 64486[0], 64487[0], 64488[0], 64489[0], 64490[0], 64491[0], 64492[0], 64493[0], 64494[0], 64495[0], 64505[0], 64510[0], 64517[0], 64520[0], 64530[0], 92012[1], 92014[1], 92585[0], 93000[1], 93005[1], 93010[1], 93040[1], 93041[1], 93042[1], 93318[1], 93355[1], 94002[1], 94200[1], 94250[1], 94680[1], 94681[1], 94690[1], 94770[1], 95812[1], 95813[1], 95816[1], 95819[1], 95822[0], 95829[1], 95860[0], 95861[0], 95863[0], 95864[0], 95865[0], 95866[0], 95867[0], 95868[0], 95869[0], 95870[0], 95907[0], 95908[0], 95909[0], 95910[0], 95911[0], 95912[0], 95913[0], 95925[0], 95926[0], 95927[0], 95928[0], 95929[0], 95930[0], 95933[0], 95937[0], 95938[0], 95939[0], 95940[0], 95955[1], 96360[1], 96361[1], 96365[1], 96366[1], 96367[1], 96368[1], 96372[1], 96374[1], 96375[1], 96376[1], 96377[1], 96523[0], 97597[1], 97598[1], 97602[1], 99155[0], 99156[0], 99157[0], 99211[1], 99212[1], 99213[1], 99214[1], 99215[1], 99217[1], 99218[1], 99219[1], 99220[1], 99221[1], 99222[1], 99223[1], 99231[1], 99232[1], 99233[1], 99234[1], 99235[1], 99236[1], 99238[1], 99239[1], 99241[1], 99242[1], 99243[1], 99244[1], 99245[1], 99251[1], 99252[1], 99253[1], 99254[1], 99255[1], 99291[1], 99292[1], 99304[1], 99305[1], 99306[1], 99307[1], 99308[1], 99309[1], 99310[1], 99315[1], 99316[1], 99334[1], 99335[1], 99336[1], 99337[1], 99347[1], 99348[1], 99349[1], 99350[1], 99374[1], 99375[1], 99377[1], 99378[1], 99446[0], 99447[0], 99448[0], 99449[0], 99451[0], 99452[0], 99495[0], 99496[0], G0453[0], G0463[1], G0471[1]
61598	0213T[0], 0216T[0], 0228T[0], 0230T[0], 0333T[0], 0464T[0], 12001[1], 12002[1], 12004[1], 12005[1], 12006[1], 12007[1], 12011[1], 12013[1], 12014[1], 12015[1], 12016[1], 12017[1], 12018[1], 12020[1], 12021[1], 12031[1], 12032[1], 12034[1], 12035[1], 12036[1], 12037[1], 12041[1], 12042[1], 12044[1], 12045[1], 12046[1], 12047[1], 12051[1], 12052[1], 12053[1], 12054[1], 12055[1], 12056[1], 12057[1], 13100[1], 13101[1], 13102[1], 13120[1], 13121[1], 13122[1], 13131[1], 13132[1], 13133[1], 13151[1], 13152[1], 13153[1], 36000[1], 36400[1], 36405[1], 36406[1], 36410[1], 36420[1], 36425[1], 36430[1], 36440[1], 36591[0], 36592[0], 36600[1], 36640[1], 43752[1], 51701[1], 51702[1], 51703[1], 61595[0], 61596[0], 61618[0], 61619[0], 62320[0], 62321[0], 62322[0], 62323[0], 62324[0], 62325[0], 62326[0], 62327[0], 64400[0], 64405[0], 64408[0], 64415[0], 64416[0], 64417[0], 64418[0], 64420[0], 64421[0], 64425[0], 64430[0], 64435[0], 64445[0], 64446[0], 64447[0], 64448[0], 64449[0], 64450[0], 64451[0], 64454[0], 64461[0], 64462[0], 64463[0], 64479[0], 64480[0], 64483[0], 64484[0], 64486[0], 64487[0], 64488[0], 64489[0], 64490[0], 64491[0], 64492[0], 64493[0], 64494[0], 64495[0], 64505[0], 64510[0], 64517[0], 64520[0], 64530[0], 92012[1], 92014[1], 92585[0], 93000[1], 93005[1], 93010[1], 93040[1], 93041[1], 93042[1], 93318[1], 93355[1], 94002[1], 94200[1], 94250[1], 94680[1], 94681[1], 94690[1], 94770[1], 95812[1], 95813[1], 95816[1], 95819[1], 95822[0], 95829[1], 95860[0], 95861[0], 95863[0], 95864[0], 95865[0], 95866[0], 95867[0], 95868[0], 95869[0], 95870[0], 95907[0], 95908[0], 95909[0], 95910[0], 95911[0], 95912[0], 95913[0], 95925[0], 95926[0], 95927[0], 95928[0], 95929[0], 95930[0], 95933[0], 95937[0], 95938[0], 95939[0], 95940[0], 95955[1], 96360[1], 96361[1], 96365[1], 96366[1], 96367[1], 96368[1], 96372[1], 96374[1], 96375[1], 96376[1], 96377[1], 96523[0], 99155[0], 99156[0], 99157[0], 99211[1], 99212[1], 99213[1], 99214[1], 99215[1], 99217[1], 99218[1], 99219[1], 99220[1], 99221[1], 99222[1], 99223[1], 99231[1], 99232[1], 99233[1], 99234[1], 99235[1], 99236[1], 99238[1], 99239[1], 99241[1], 99242[1], 99243[1], 99244[1], 99245[1], 99251[1], 99252[1], 99253[1], 99254[1], 99255[1], 99291[1], 99292[1], 99304[1], 99305[1], 99306[1], 99307[1], 99308[1], 99309[1], 99310[1], 99315[1], 99316[1], 99334[1], 99335[1], 99336[1], 99337[1], 99347[1], 99348[1], 99349[1], 99350[1], 99374[1], 99375[1], 99377[1], 99378[1], 99446[0], 99447[0], 99448[0], 99449[0], 99451[0], 99452[0], 99495[0], 99496[0], G0453[0], G0463[1], G0471[1]
61600	0213T[0], 0216T[0], 0228T[0], 0230T[0], 0333T[0], 0464T[0], 11000[1], 11001[1], 11004[1], 11005[1], 11006[1], 11042[1], 11043[1], 11044[1], 11045[1], 11046[1], 11047[1], 12001[1], 12002[1], 12004[1], 12005[1], 12006[1], 12007[1], 12011[1], 12013[1], 12014[1], 12015[1], 12016[1], 12017[1], 12018[1], 12020[1], 12021[1], 12031[1], 12032[1], 12034[1], 12035[1], 12036[1], 12037[1], 12041[1], 12042[1], 12044[1], 12045[1], 12046[1], 12047[1], 12051[1], 12052[1], 12053[1], 12054[1], 12055[1], 12056[1], 12057[1], 13100[1], 13101[1], 13102[1], 13120[1], 13121[1], 13122[1], 13131[1], 13132[1], 13133[1], 13151[1], 13152[1], 13153[1], 36000[1], 36400[1], 36405[1], 36406[1], 36410[1], 36420[1], 36425[1], 36430[1], 36440[1], 36591[0], 36592[0], 36600[1], 36640[1], 43752[1], 51701[1], 51702[1], 51703[1], 61601[1], 61618[0], 61619[0], 62320[0], 62321[0], 62322[0], 62323[0], 62324[0], 62325[0], 62326[0], 62327[0], 64400[0], 64405[0], 64408[0], 64415[0], 64416[0], 64417[0], 64418[0], 64420[0], 64421[0], 64425[0], 64430[0], 64435[0], 64445[0], 64446[0], 64447[0], 64448[0], 64449[0], 64450[0], 64451[0], 64454[0], 64461[0], 64462[0], 64463[0], 64479[0], 64480[0], 64483[0], 64484[0], 64486[0], 64487[0], 64488[0], 64489[0], 64490[0], 64491[0], 64492[0], 64493[0], 64494[0], 64495[0], 64505[0], 64510[0], 64517[0], 64520[0], 64530[0], 92012[1], 92014[1], 92585[0], 93000[1], 93005[1], 93010[1], 93040[1], 93041[1], 93042[1], 93318[1], 93355[1], 94002[1], 94200[1], 94250[1], 94680[1], 94681[1], 94690[1], 94770[1], 95812[1], 95813[1], 95816[1], 95819[1], 95822[0], 95829[1], 95860[0], 95861[0], 95863[0], 95864[0], 95865[0], 95866[0], 95867[0], 95868[0], 95869[0], 95870[0], 95907[0], 95908[0], 95909[0], 95910[0], 95911[0], 95912[0], 95913[0], 95925[0], 95926[0], 95927[0], 95928[0], 95929[0], 95930[0], 95933[0], 95937[0], 95938[0], 95939[0], 95940[0], 95955[1], 96360[1], 96361[1], 96365[1], 96366[1], 96367[1], 96368[1], 96372[1], 96374[1], 96375[1], 96376[1], 96377[1], 96523[0], 97597[1], 97598[1], 97602[1], 99155[0], 99156[0], 99157[0], 99211[1], 99212[1], 99213[1], 99214[1], 99215[1], 99217[1], 99218[1], 99219[1], 99220[1], 99221[1], 99222[1], 99223[1], 99231[1], 99232[1], 99233[1], 99234[1], 99235[1], 99236[1], 99238[1], 99239[1], 99241[1], 99242[1], 99243[1], 99244[1], 99245[1], 99251[1], 99252[1], 99253[1], 99254[1], 99255[1], 99291[1], 99292[1], 99304[1], 99305[1], 99306[1], 99307[1], 99308[1], 99309[1], 99310[1], 99315[1], 99316[1], 99334[1], 99335[1], 99336[1], 99337[1], 99347[1], 99348[1], 99349[1], 99350[1], 99374[1], 99375[1], 99377[1], 99378[1], 99446[0], 99447[0], 99448[0], 99449[0], 99451[0], 99452[0], 99495[0], 99496[0], G0453[0], G0463[1], G0471[1]
61601	0213T[0], 0216T[0], 0228T[0], 0230T[0], 0333T[0], 0464T[0], 11000[1], 11001[1], 11004[1], 11005[1], 11006[1], 11042[1], 11043[1], 11044[1], 11045[1], 11046[1], 11047[1], 12001[1], 12002[1], 12004[1], 12005[1], 12006[1], 12007[1], 12011[1], 12013[1], 12014[1], 12015[1], 12016[1], 12017[1], 12018[1], 12020[1], 12021[1], 12031[1], 12032[1], 12034[1], 12035[1], 12036[1], 12037[1], 12041[1], 12042[1], 12044[1], 12045[1], 12046[1], 12047[1], 12051[1], 12052[1], 12053[1], 12054[1], 12055[1], 12056[1], 12057[1], 13100[1], 13101[1], 13102[1], 13120[1], 13121[1], 13122[1], 13131[1], 13132[1], 13133[1], 13151[1], 13152[1], 13153[1], 36000[1], 36400[1], 36405[1], 36406[1], 36410[1], 36420[1], 36425[1], 36430[1], 36440[1], 36591[0], 36592[0], 36600[1], 36640[1], 43752[1], 51701[1], 51702[1], 51703[1], 61618[0], 61619[0], 62164[1], 62320[0], 62321[0], 62322[0], 62323[0], 62324[0], 62325[0], 62326[0], 62327[0], 64400[0], 64405[0], 64408[0], 64415[0], 64416[0], 64417[0], 64418[0], 64420[0], 64421[0], 64425[0], 64430[0], 64435[0], 64445[0], 64446[0], 64447[0], 64448[0], 64449[0], 64450[0], 64451[0], 64454[0], 64461[0], 64462[0], 64463[0], 64479[0], 64480[0], 64483[0], 64484[0], 64486[0], 64487[0], 64488[0], 64489[0], 64490[0], 64491[0], 64492[0], 64493[0], 64494[0], 64495[0], 64505[0], 64510[0], 64517[0], 64520[0], 64530[0], 92012[1], 92014[1], 92585[0], 93000[1], 93005[1], 93010[1], 93040[1], 93041[1], 93042[1], 93318[1], 93355[1], 94002[1], 94200[1], 94250[1], 94680[1], 94681[1], 94690[1], 94770[1], 95812[1], 95813[1], 95816[1], 95819[1], 95822[0], 95829[1], 95860[0], 95861[0], 95863[0], 95864[0], 95865[0], 95866[0], 95867[0], 95868[0], 95869[0], 95870[0], 95907[0], 95908[0], 95909[0], 95910[0], 95911[0], 95912[0], 95913[0], 95925[0], 95926[0], 95927[0], 95928[0], 95929[0], 95930[0], 95933[0], 95937[0], 95938[0], 95939[0], 95940[0], 95955[1], 96360[1], 96361[1], 96365[1], 96366[1], 96367[1], 96368[1], 96372[1], 96374[1], 96375[1], 96376[1], 96377[1], 96523[0], 97597[1], 97598[1], 97602[1], 99155[0], 99156[0], 99157[0], 99211[1], 99212[1], 99213[1], 99214[1], 99215[1], 99217[1], 99218[1], 99219[1], 99220[1], 99221[1], 99222[1], 99223[1], 99231[1], 99232[1], 99233[1], 99234[1], 99235[1], 99236[1], 99238[1], 99239[1], 99241[1], 99242[1], 99243[1], 99244[1], 99245[1], 99251[1], 99252[1], 99253[1], 99254[1], 99255[1], 99291[1], 99292[1], 99304[1], 99305[1], 99306[1], 99307[1], 99308[1], 99309[1], 99310[1], 99315[1], 99316[1], 99334[1], 99335[1], 99336[1], 99337[1], 99347[1], 99348[1], 99349[1], 99350[1], 99374[1], 99375[1], 99377[1], 99378[1], 99446[0], 99447[0], 99448[0], 99449[0], 99451[0], 99452[0], 99495[0], 99496[0], G0453[0], G0463[1], G0471[1]
61605	0213T[0], 0216T[0], 0228T[0], 0230T[0], 0333T[0], 0464T[0], 11000[1], 11001[1], 11004[1], 11005[1], 11006[1], 11042[1], 11043[1], 11044[1], 11045[1], 11046[1], 11047[1], 12001[1], 12002[1], 12004[1], 12005[1], 12006[1], 12007[1], 12011[1], 12013[1], 12014[1], 12015[1], 12016[1], 12017[1], 12018[1], 12020[1], 12021[1], 12031[1], 12032[1], 12034[1], 12035[1], 12036[1], 12037[1], 12041[1], 12042[1], 12044[1], 12045[1], 12046[1], 12047[1], 12051[1], 12052[1], 12053[1], 12054[1], 12055[1], 12056[1], 12057[1], 13100[1], 13101[1], 13102[1], 13120[1], 13121[1], 13122[1], 13131[1], 13132[1], 13133[1], 13151[1], 13152[1], 13153[1], 36000[1], 36400[1], 36405[1], 36406[1], 36410[1], 36420[1], 36425[1], 36430[1], 36440[1], 36591[0], 36592[0], 36600[1], 36640[1], 43752[1], 51701[1], 51702[1], 51703[1], 61606[1], 61618[0], 61619[0], 62320[0], 62321[0], 62322[0], 62323[0], 62324[0], 62325[0], 62326[0], 62327[0], 64400[0], 64405[0], 64408[0], 64415[0], 64416[0], 64417[0], 64418[0], 64420[0], 64421[0], 64425[0], 64430[0], 64435[0], 64445[0], 64446[0], 64447[0], 64448[0], 64449[0], 64450[0], 64451[0], 64454[0], 64461[0], 64462[0], 64463[0], 64479[0], 64480[0], 64483[0], 64484[0], 64486[0], 64487[0], 64488[0], 64489[0], 64490[0], 64491[0], 64492[0], 64493[0], 64494[0], 64495[0], 64505[0], 64510[0], 64517[0], 64520[0], 64530[0], 92012[1], 92014[1], 92585[0], 93000[1], 93005[1], 93010[1], 93040[1], 93041[1], 93042[1], 93318[1], 93355[1], 94002[1], 94200[1], 94250[1], 94680[1], 94681[1], 94690[1], 94770[1], 95812[1], 95813[1], 95816[1], 95819[1], 95822[0], 95829[1], 95860[0], 95861[0], 95863[0], 95864[0], 95865[0], 95866[0], 95867[0], 95868[0], 95869[0], 95870[0], 95907[0], 95908[0], 95909[0], 95910[0], 95911[0], 95912[0], 95913[0], 95925[0], 95926[0], 95927[0], 95928[0], 95929[0], 95930[0], 95933[0], 95937[0], 95938[0], 95939[0], 95940[0], 95955[1], 96360[1], 96361[1], 96365[1], 96366[1], 96367[1], 96368[1], 96372[1], 96374[1], 96375[1], 96376[1], 96377[1], 96523[0], 97597[1], 97598[1], 97602[1], 99155[0], 99156[0], 99157[0], 99211[1], 99212[1], 99213[1], 99214[1], 99215[1], 99217[1], 99218[1], 99219[1], 99220[1], 99221[1], 99222[1], 99223[1], 99231[1], 99232[1], 99233[1], 99234[1], 99235[1], 99236[1], 99238[1], 99239[1], 99241[1], 99242[1], 99243[1], 99244[1], 99245[1], 99251[1], 99252[1], 99253[1], 99254[1], 99255[1], 99291[1], 99292[1], 99304[1], 99305[1], 99306[1], 99307[1], 99308[1], 99309[1], 99310[1], 99315[1], 99316[1], 99334[1], 99335[1], 99336[1], 99337[1], 99347[1],

0 = Modifier usage not allowed or inappropriate 1 = Modifier usage allowed

Code 1	Code 2
	99348[1], 99349[1], 99350[1], 99374[1], 99375[1], 99377[1], 99378[1], 99446[0], 99447[0], 99448[0], 99449[0], 99451[0], 99452[0], 99495[0], 99496[0], G0453[0], G0463[1], G0471[1]
61606	0213T[0], 0216T[0], 0228T[0], 0230T[0], 0333T[0], 0464T[0], 11000[1], 11001[1], 11004[1], 11005[1], 11006[1], 11042[1], 11043[1], 11044[1], 11045[1], 11046[1], 11047[1], 12001[1], 12002[1], 12004[1], 12005[1], 12006[1], 12007[1], 12011[1], 12013[1], 12014[1], 12015[1], 12016[1], 12017[1], 12018[1], 12020[1], 12021[1], 12031[1], 12032[1], 12034[1], 12035[1], 12036[1], 12037[1], 12041[1], 12042[1], 12044[1], 12045[1], 12046[1], 12047[1], 12051[1], 12052[1], 12053[1], 12054[1], 12055[1], 12056[1], 12057[1], 13100[1], 13101[1], 13102[1], 13120[1], 13121[1], 13122[1], 13131[1], 13132[1], 13133[1], 13151[1], 13152[1], 13153[1], 36000[1], 36400[1], 36405[1], 36406[1], 36410[1], 36420[1], 36425[1], 36430[1], 36440[1], 36591[0], 36592[0], 36600[1], 36640[1], 43752[1], 51701[1], 51702[1], 51703[1], 61618[0], 61619[0], 62164[1], 62320[0], 62321[0], 62322[0], 62323[0], 62324[0], 62325[0], 62326[0], 62327[0], 64400[0], 64405[0], 64408[0], 64415[0], 64416[0], 64417[0], 64418[0], 64420[0], 64421[0], 64425[0], 64430[0], 64435[0], 64445[0], 64446[0], 64447[0], 64448[0], 64449[0], 64450[0], 64451[0], 64454[0], 64461[0], 64462[0], 64463[0], 64479[0], 64480[0], 64483[0], 64484[0], 64486[0], 64487[0], 64488[0], 64489[0], 64490[0], 64491[0], 64492[0], 64493[0], 64494[0], 64495[0], 64505[0], 64510[0], 64517[0], 64520[0], 64530[0], 92012[1], 92014[1], 92585[0], 93000[1], 93005[1], 93010[1], 93040[1], 93041[1], 93042[1], 93318[1], 93355[1], 94002[1], 94200[1], 94250[1], 94680[1], 94681[1], 94690[1], 94770[1], 95812[1], 95813[1], 95816[1], 95819[1], 95822[0], 95829[1], 95860[0], 95861[0], 95863[0], 95864[0], 95865[0], 95866[0], 95867[0], 95868[0], 95869[0], 95870[0], 95907[0], 95908[0], 95909[0], 95910[0], 95911[0], 95912[0], 95913[0], 95925[0], 95926[0], 95927[0], 95928[0], 95929[0], 95930[0], 95933[0], 95937[0], 95938[0], 95939[0], 95940[0], 95955[1], 96360[1], 96361[1], 96365[1], 96366[1], 96367[1], 96368[1], 96372[1], 96374[1], 96375[1], 96376[1], 96377[1], 96523[0], 97597[1], 97598[1], 97602[1], 99155[0], 99156[0], 99157[0], 99211[1], 99212[1], 99213[1], 99214[1], 99215[1], 99217[1], 99218[1], 99219[1], 99220[1], 99221[1], 99222[1], 99223[1], 99231[1], 99232[1], 99233[1], 99234[1], 99235[1], 99236[1], 99238[1], 99239[1], 99241[1], 99242[1], 99243[1], 99244[1], 99245[1], 99251[1], 99252[1], 99253[1], 99254[1], 99255[1], 99291[1], 99292[1], 99304[1], 99305[1], 99306[1], 99307[1], 99308[1], 99309[1], 99310[1], 99315[1], 99316[1], 99334[1], 99335[1], 99336[1], 99337[1], 99347[1], 99348[1], 99349[1], 99350[1], 99374[1], 99375[1], 99377[1], 99378[1], 99446[0], 99447[0], 99448[0], 99449[0], 99451[0], 99452[0], 99495[0], 99496[0], G0453[0], G0463[1], G0471[1]
61607	0213T[0], 0216T[0], 0228T[0], 0230T[0], 0333T[0], 0464T[0], 11000[1], 11001[1], 11004[1], 11005[1], 11006[1], 11042[1], 11043[1], 11044[1], 11045[1], 11046[1], 11047[1], 12001[1], 12002[1], 12004[1], 12005[1], 12006[1], 12007[1], 12011[1], 12013[1], 12014[1], 12015[1], 12016[1], 12017[1], 12018[1], 12020[1], 12021[1], 12031[1], 12032[1], 12034[1], 12035[1], 12036[1], 12037[1], 12041[1], 12042[1], 12044[1], 12045[1], 12046[1], 12047[1], 12051[1], 12052[1], 12053[1], 12054[1], 12055[1], 12056[1], 12057[1], 13100[1], 13101[1], 13102[1], 13120[1], 13121[1], 13122[1], 13131[1], 13132[1], 13133[1], 13151[1], 13152[1], 13153[1], 36000[1], 36400[1], 36405[1], 36406[1], 36410[1], 36420[1], 36425[1], 36430[1], 36440[1], 36591[0], 36592[0], 36600[1], 36640[1], 43752[1], 51701[1], 51702[1], 51703[1], 61608[1], 61618[0], 61619[0], 62164[1], 62320[0], 62321[0], 62322[0], 62323[0], 62324[0], 62325[0], 62326[0], 62327[0], 64400[0], 64405[0], 64408[0], 64415[0], 64416[0], 64417[0], 64418[0], 64420[0], 64421[0], 64425[0], 64430[0], 64435[0], 64445[0], 64446[0], 64447[0], 64448[0], 64449[0], 64450[0], 64451[0], 64454[0], 64461[0], 64462[0], 64463[0], 64479[0], 64480[0], 64483[0], 64484[0], 64486[0], 64487[0], 64488[0], 64489[0], 64490[0], 64491[0], 64492[0], 64493[0], 64494[0], 64495[0], 64505[0], 64510[0], 64517[0], 64520[0], 64530[0], 92012[1], 92014[1], 92585[0], 93000[1], 93005[1], 93010[1], 93040[1], 93041[1], 93042[1], 93318[1], 93355[1], 94002[1], 94200[1], 94250[1], 94680[1], 94681[1], 94690[1], 94770[1], 95812[1], 95813[1], 95816[1], 95819[1], 95822[0], 95829[1], 95860[0], 95861[0], 95863[0], 95864[0], 95865[0], 95866[0], 95867[0], 95868[0], 95869[0], 95870[0], 95907[0], 95908[0], 95909[0], 95910[0], 95911[0], 95912[0], 95913[0], 95925[0], 95926[0], 95927[0], 95928[0], 95929[0], 95930[0], 95933[0], 95937[0], 95938[0], 95939[0], 95940[0], 95955[1], 96360[1], 96361[1], 96365[1], 96366[1], 96367[1], 96368[1], 96372[1], 96374[1], 96375[1], 96376[1], 96377[1], 96523[0], 97597[1], 97598[1], 97602[1], 99155[0], 99156[0], 99157[0], 99211[1], 99212[1], 99213[1], 99214[1], 99215[1], 99217[1], 99218[1], 99219[1], 99220[1], 99221[1], 99222[1], 99223[1], 99231[1], 99232[1], 99233[1], 99234[1], 99235[1], 99236[1], 99238[1], 99239[1], 99241[1], 99242[1], 99243[1], 99244[1], 99245[1], 99251[1], 99252[1], 99253[1], 99254[1], 99255[1], 99291[1], 99292[1], 99304[1], 99305[1], 99306[1], 99307[1], 99308[1], 99309[1], 99310[1], 99315[1], 99316[1], 99334[1], 99335[1], 99336[1], 99337[1], 99347[1], 99348[1], 99349[1], 99350[1], 99374[1], 99375[1], 99377[1], 99378[1], 99446[0], 99447[0], 99448[0], 99449[0], 99451[0], 99452[0], 99495[0], 99496[0], G0453[0], G0463[1], G0471[1]
61608	0213T[0], 0216T[0], 0228T[0], 0230T[0], 0333T[0], 0464T[0], 11000[1], 11001[1], 11004[1], 11005[1], 11006[1], 11042[1], 11043[1], 11044[1], 11045[1], 11046[1], 11047[1], 12001[1], 12002[1], 12004[1], 12005[1], 12006[1], 12007[1], 12011[1], 12013[1], 12014[1], 12015[1], 12016[1], 12017[1], 12018[1], 12020[1], 12021[1], 12031[1], 12032[1], 12034[1], 12035[1], 12036[1], 12037[1], 12041[1], 12042[1], 12044[1], 12045[1], 12046[1], 12047[1], 12051[1], 12052[1], 12053[1], 12054[1], 12055[1], 12056[1], 12057[1], 13100[1], 13101[1], 13102[1], 13120[1], 13121[1], 13122[1], 13131[1], 13132[1], 13133[1], 13151[1], 13152[1], 13153[1], 36000[1], 36400[1], 36405[1], 36406[1], 36410[1], 36420[1], 36425[1], 36430[1], 36440[1], 36591[0], 36592[0], 36600[1], 36640[1], 43752[1], 51701[1], 51702[1], 51703[1], 61618[0], 61619[0], 62164[1], 62320[0], 62321[0], 62322[0], 62323[0], 62324[0], 62325[0], 62326[0], 62327[0], 64400[0], 64405[0], 64408[0], 64415[0], 64416[0], 64417[0], 64418[0], 64420[0], 64421[0], 64425[0], 64430[0], 64435[0], 64445[0], 64446[0], 64447[0], 64448[0], 64449[0], 64450[0], 64451[0], 64454[0], 64461[0], 64462[0], 64463[0], 64479[0], 64480[0], 64483[0], 64484[0], 64486[0], 64487[0], 64488[0], 64489[0], 64490[0], 64491[0], 64492[0], 64493[0], 64494[0], 64495[0], 64505[0], 64510[0], 64517[0], 64520[0], 64530[0], 92012[1], 92014[1], 92585[0], 93000[1], 93005[1], 93010[1], 93040[1], 93041[1], 93042[1], 93318[1], 93355[1], 94002[1], 94200[1], 94250[1], 94680[1], 94681[1], 94690[1], 94770[1], 95812[1], 95813[1], 95816[1], 95819[1], 95822[0], 95829[1], 95860[0], 95861[0], 95863[0], 95864[0], 95865[0], 95866[0], 95867[0], 95868[0], 95869[0], 95870[0], 95907[0], 95908[0], 95909[0], 95910[0], 95911[0], 95912[0], 95913[0], 95925[0], 95926[0], 95927[0], 95928[0], 95929[0], 95930[0], 95933[0], 95937[0], 95938[0], 95939[0], 95940[0], 95955[1], 96360[1], 96361[1], 96365[1], 96366[1], 96367[1], 96368[1], 96372[1], 96374[1], 96375[1], 96376[1], 96377[1], 96523[0], 97597[1], 97598[1], 97602[1], 99155[0], 99156[0], 99157[0], 99211[1], 99212[1], 99213[1], 99214[1], 99215[1], 99217[1], 99218[1], 99219[1], 99220[1], 99221[1], 99222[1], 99223[1], 99231[1], 99232[1], 99233[1], 99234[1], 99235[1], 99236[1], 99238[1], 99239[1], 99241[1], 99242[1], 99243[1], 99244[1], 99245[1], 99251[1], 99252[1], 99253[1], 99254[1], 99255[1], 99291[1], 99292[1], 99304[1], 99305[1], 99306[1], 99307[1], 99308[1], 99309[1], 99310[1], 99315[1], 99316[1], 99334[1], 99335[1], 99336[1], 99337[1], 99347[1], 99348[1], 99349[1], 99350[1], 99374[1], 99375[1], 99377[1], 99378[1], 99446[0], 99447[0], 99448[0], 99449[0], 99451[0], 99452[0], 99495[0], 99496[0], G0453[0], G0463[1], G0471[1]
61615	0213T[0], 0216T[0], 0228T[0], 0230T[0], 0333T[0], 0464T[0], 11000[1], 11001[1], 11004[1], 11005[1], 11006[1], 11042[1], 11043[1], 11044[1], 11045[1], 11046[1], 11047[1], 12001[1], 12002[1], 12004[1], 12005[1], 12006[1], 12007[1], 12011[1], 12013[1], 12014[1], 12015[1], 12016[1], 12017[1], 12018[1], 12020[1], 12021[1], 12031[1], 12032[1], 12034[1], 12035[1], 12036[1], 12037[1], 12041[1], 12042[1], 12044[1], 12045[1], 12046[1], 12047[1], 12051[1], 12052[1], 12053[1], 12054[1], 12055[1], 12056[1], 12057[1], 13100[1], 13101[1], 13102[1], 13120[1], 13121[1], 13122[1], 13131[1], 13132[1], 13133[1], 13151[1], 13152[1], 13153[1], 36000[1], 36400[1], 36405[1], 36406[1], 36410[1], 36420[1], 36425[1], 36430[1], 36440[1], 36591[0], 36592[0], 36600[1], 36640[1], 43752[1], 51701[1], 51702[1], 51703[1], 61616[1], 61618[0], 61619[0], 62164[1], 62320[0], 62321[0], 62322[0], 62323[0], 62324[0], 62325[0], 62326[0], 62327[0], 64400[0], 64405[0], 64408[0], 64415[0], 64416[0], 64417[0], 64418[0], 64420[0], 64421[0], 64425[0], 64430[0], 64435[0], 64445[0], 64446[0], 64447[0], 64448[0], 64449[0], 64450[0], 64451[0], 64454[0], 64461[0], 64462[0], 64463[0], 64479[0], 64480[0], 64483[0], 64484[0], 64486[0], 64487[0], 64488[0], 64489[0], 64490[0], 64491[0], 64492[0], 64493[0], 64494[0], 64495[0], 64505[0], 64510[0], 64517[0], 64520[0], 64530[0], 92012[1], 92014[1], 92585[0], 93000[1], 93005[1], 93010[1], 93040[1], 93041[1], 93042[1], 93318[1], 93355[1], 94002[1], 94200[1], 94250[1], 94680[1], 94681[1], 94690[1], 94770[1], 95812[1], 95813[1], 95816[1], 95819[1], 95822[0], 95829[1], 95860[0], 95861[0], 95863[0], 95864[0], 95865[0], 95866[0], 95867[0], 95868[0], 95869[0], 95870[0], 95907[0], 95908[0], 95909[0], 95910[0], 95911[0], 95912[0], 95913[0], 95925[0], 95926[0], 95927[0], 95928[0], 95929[0], 95930[0], 95933[0], 95937[0], 95938[0], 95939[0], 95940[0], 95955[1], 96360[1], 96361[1], 96365[1], 96366[1], 96367[1], 96368[1], 96372[1], 96374[1], 96375[1], 96376[1], 96377[1], 96523[0], 97597[1], 97598[1], 97602[1], 99155[0], 99156[0], 99157[0], 99211[1], 99212[1], 99213[1], 99214[1], 99215[1], 99217[1], 99218[1], 99219[1], 99220[1], 99221[1], 99222[1], 99223[1], 99231[1], 99232[1], 99233[1], 99234[1], 99235[1], 99236[1], 99238[1], 99239[1], 99241[1], 99242[1], 99243[1], 99244[1], 99245[1], 99251[1], 99252[1], 99253[1], 99254[1], 99255[1], 99291[1], 99292[1], 99304[1], 99305[1], 99306[1], 99307[1], 99308[1], 99309[1], 99310[1], 99315[1], 99316[1], 99334[1], 99335[1], 99336[1], 99337[1], 99347[1], 99348[1], 99349[1], 99350[1], 99374[1], 99375[1], 99377[1], 99378[1], 99446[0], 99447[0], 99448[0], 99449[0], 99451[0], 99452[0], 99495[0], 99496[0], G0453[0], G0463[1], G0471[1]
61616	0213T[0], 0216T[0], 0228T[0], 0230T[0], 0333T[0], 0464T[0], 11000[1], 11001[1], 11004[1], 11005[1], 11006[1], 11042[1], 11043[1], 11044[1], 11045[1], 11046[1], 11047[1], 12001[1], 12002[1], 12004[1], 12005[1], 12006[1], 12007[1], 12011[1], 12013[1], 12014[1], 12015[1], 12016[1], 12017[1], 12018[1], 12020[1], 12021[1], 12031[1], 12032[1], 12034[1], 12035[1], 12036[1], 12037[1], 12041[1], 12042[1], 12044[1], 12045[1], 12046[1], 12047[1], 12051[1], 12052[1], 12053[1], 12054[1], 12055[1], 12056[1], 12057[1], 13100[1], 13101[1], 13102[1], 13120[1], 13121[1], 13122[1], 13131[1], 13132[1], 13133[1], 13151[1], 13152[1], 13153[1], 36000[1], 36400[1], 36405[1], 36406[1], 36410[1], 36420[1], 36425[1], 36430[1], 36440[1], 36591[0], 36592[0], 36600[1], 36640[1], 43752[1], 51701[1], 51702[1], 51703[1], 61618[0], 61619[0], 62164[1], 62320[0], 62321[0], 62322[0], 62323[0], 62324[0], 62325[0], 62326[0], 62327[0], 64400[0], 64405[0], 64408[0], 64415[0], 64416[0], 64417[0], 64418[0], 64420[0], 64421[0], 64425[0], 64430[0], 64435[0], 64445[0], 64446[0], 64447[0], 64448[0], 64449[0], 64450[0], 64451[0], 64454[0], 64461[0], 64462[0], 64463[0], 64479[0], 64480[0], 64483[0], 64484[0], 64486[0], 64487[0], 64488[0], 64489[0], 64490[0], 64491[0], 64492[0], 64493[0], 64494[0], 64495[0], 64505[0], 64510[0], 64517[0], 64520[0], 64530[0], 92012[1], 92014[1], 92585[0], 93000[1], 93005[1], 93010[1], 93040[1], 93041[1], 93042[1], 93318[1], 93355[1], 94002[1], 94200[1], 94250[1], 94680[1], 94681[1], 94690[1], 94770[1], 95812[1], 95813[1], 95816[1], 95819[1], 95822[0], 95829[1], 95860[0], 95861[0], 95863[0], 95864[0], 95865[0], 95866[0], 95867[0], 95868[0], 95869[0], 95870[0], 95907[0], 95908[0], 95909[0], 95910[0], 95911[0], 95912[0], 95913[0], 95925[0], 95926[0], 95927[0], 95928[0], 95929[0], 95930[0], 95933[0], 95937[0], 95938[0], 95939[0], 95940[0], 95955[1], 96360[1], 96361[1], 96365[1], 96366[1], 96367[1], 96368[1], 96372[1], 96374[1], 96375[1], 96376[1], 96377[1], 96523[0], 97597[1], 97598[1], 97602[1], 99155[0], 99156[0], 99157[0], 99211[1], 99212[1], 99213[1], 99214[1], 99215[1], 99217[1],

0 = Modifier usage not allowed or inappropriate 1 = Modifier usage allowed

Code 1	Code 2
	99218^1, 99219^1, 99220^1, 99221^1, 99222^1, 99223^1, 99231^1, 99232^1, 99233^1, 99234^1, 99235^1, 99236^1, 99238^1, 99239^1, 99241^1, 99242^1, 99243^1, 99244^1, 99245^1, 99251^1, 99252^1, 99253^1, 99254^1, 99255^1, 99291^1, 99292^1, 99304^1, 99305^1, 99306^1, 99307^1, 99308^1, 99309^1, 99310^1, 99315^1, 99316^1, 99334^1, 99335^1, 99336^1, 99337^1, 99347^1, 99348^1, 99349^1, 99350^1, 99374^1, 99375^1, 99377^1, 99378^1, 99446^0, 99447^0, 99448^0, 99449^0, 99451^0, 99452^0, 99495^0, 99496^0, G0453^0, G0463^1, G0471^1
61618	0213T^0, 0216T^0, 0228T^0, 0230T^0, 0333T^0, 0464T^0, 12001^1, 12002^1, 12004^1, 12005^1, 12006^1, 12007^1, 12011^1, 12013^1, 12014^1, 12015^1, 12016^1, 12017^1, 12018^1, 12020^1, 12021^1, 12031^1, 12032^1, 12034^1, 12035^1, 12036^1, 12037^1, 12041^1, 12042^1, 12044^1, 12045^1, 12046^1, 12047^1, 12051^1, 12052^1, 12053^1, 12054^1, 12055^1, 12056^1, 12057^1, 13100^1, 13101^1, 13102^1, 13120^1, 13121^1, 13122^1, 13131^1, 13132^1, 13133^1, 13151^1, 13152^1, 13153^1, 36000^1, 36400^1, 36405^1, 36406^1, 36410^1, 36420^1, 36425^1, 36430^1, 36440^1, 36591^0, 36592^0, 36600^1, 36640^1, 43752^1, 51701^1, 51702^1, 51703^1, 61619^1, 62320^0, 62321^0, 62322^0, 62323^0, 62324^0, 62325^0, 62326^0, 62327^0, 64400^0, 64405^0, 64408^0, 64415^0, 64416^0, 64417^0, 64418^0, 64420^0, 64421^0, 64425^0, 64430^0, 64435^0, 64445^0, 64446^0, 64447^0, 64448^0, 64449^0, 64450^0, 64451^0, 64454^0, 64461^0, 64462^0, 64463^0, 64479^0, 64480^0, 64483^0, 64484^0, 64486^0, 64487^0, 64488^0, 64489^0, 64490^0, 64491^0, 64492^0, 64493^0, 64494^0, 64495^0, 64505^0, 64510^0, 64517^0, 64520^0, 64530^0, 92012^1, 92014^1, 92585^0, 93000^1, 93005^1, 93010^1, 93040^1, 93041^1, 93042^1, 93318^1, 93355^1, 94002^1, 94200^1, 94250^1, 94680^1, 94681^1, 94690^1, 94770^1, 95812^1, 95813^1, 95816^1, 95819^1, 95822^0, 95829^1, 95860^0, 95861^0, 95863^0, 95864^0, 95865^0, 95866^0, 95867^0, 95868^0, 95869^0, 95870^0, 95907^0, 95908^0, 95909^0, 95910^0, 95911^0, 95912^0, 95913^0, 95925^0, 95926^0, 95927^0, 95928^0, 95929^0, 95930^0, 95933^0, 95937^0, 95938^0, 95939^0, 95940^0, 95955^1, 96360^1, 96361^1, 96365^1, 96366^1, 96367^1, 96368^1, 96372^1, 96374^1, 96375^1, 96376^1, 96377^1, 96523^0, 99155^0, 99156^0, 99157^0, 99211^1, 99212^1, 99213^1, 99214^1, 99215^1, 99217^1, 99218^1, 99219^1, 99220^1, 99221^1, 99222^1, 99223^1, 99231^1, 99232^1, 99233^1, 99234^1, 99235^1, 99236^1, 99238^1, 99239^1, 99241^1, 99242^1, 99243^1, 99244^1, 99245^1, 99251^1, 99252^1, 99253^1, 99254^1, 99255^1, 99291^1, 99292^1, 99304^1, 99305^1, 99306^1, 99307^1, 99308^1, 99309^1, 99310^1, 99315^1, 99316^1, 99334^1, 99335^1, 99336^1, 99337^1, 99347^1, 99348^1, 99349^1, 99350^1, 99374^1, 99375^1, 99377^1, 99378^1, 99446^0, 99447^0, 99448^0, 99449^0, 99451^0, 99452^0, 99495^0, 99496^0, G0453^0, G0463^1, G0471^1
61619	0213T^0, 0216T^0, 0228T^0, 0230T^0, 0333T^0, 0464T^0, 12001^1, 12002^1, 12004^1, 12005^1, 12006^1, 12007^1, 12011^1, 12013^1, 12014^1, 12015^1, 12016^1, 12017^1, 12018^1, 12020^1, 12021^1, 12031^1, 12032^1, 12034^1, 12035^1, 12036^1, 12037^1, 12041^1, 12042^1, 12044^1, 12045^1, 12046^1, 12047^1, 12051^1, 12052^1, 12053^1, 12054^1, 12055^1, 12056^1, 12057^1, 13100^1, 13101^1, 13102^1, 13120^1, 13121^1, 13122^1, 13131^1, 13132^1, 13133^1, 13151^1, 13152^1, 13153^1, 36000^1, 36400^1, 36405^1, 36406^1, 36410^1, 36420^1, 36425^1, 36430^1, 36440^1, 36591^0, 36592^0, 36600^1, 36640^1, 43752^1, 51701^1, 51702^1, 51703^1, 62320^0, 62321^0, 62322^0, 62323^0, 62324^0, 62325^0, 62326^0, 62327^0, 64400^0, 64405^0, 64408^0, 64415^0, 64416^0, 64417^0, 64418^0, 64420^0, 64421^0, 64425^0, 64430^0, 64435^0, 64445^0, 64446^0, 64447^0, 64448^0, 64449^0, 64450^0, 64451^0, 64454^0, 64461^0, 64462^0, 64463^0, 64479^0, 64480^0, 64483^0, 64484^0, 64486^0, 64487^0, 64488^0, 64489^0, 64490^0, 64491^0, 64492^0, 64493^0, 64494^0, 64495^0, 64505^0, 64510^0, 64517^0, 64520^0, 64530^0, 92012^1, 92014^1, 92585^0, 93000^1, 93005^1, 93010^1, 93040^1, 93041^1, 93042^1, 93318^1, 93355^1, 94002^1, 94200^1, 94250^1, 94680^1, 94681^1, 94690^1, 94770^1, 95812^1, 95813^1, 95816^1, 95819^1, 95822^0, 95829^1, 95860^0, 95861^0, 95863^0, 95864^0, 95865^0, 95866^0, 95867^0, 95868^0, 95869^0, 95870^0, 95907^0, 95908^0, 95909^0, 95910^0, 95911^0, 95912^0, 95913^0, 95925^0, 95926^0, 95927^0, 95928^0, 95929^0, 95930^0, 95933^0, 95937^0, 95938^0, 95939^0, 95940^0, 95955^1, 96360^1, 96361^1, 96365^1, 96366^1, 96367^1, 96368^1, 96372^1, 96374^1, 96375^1, 96376^1, 96377^1, 96523^0, 99155^0, 99156^0, 99157^0, 99211^1, 99212^1, 99213^1, 99214^1, 99215^1, 99217^1, 99218^1, 99219^1, 99220^1, 99221^1, 99222^1, 99223^1, 99231^1, 99232^1, 99233^1, 99234^1, 99235^1, 99236^1, 99238^1, 99239^1, 99241^1, 99242^1, 99243^1, 99244^1, 99245^1, 99251^1, 99252^1, 99253^1, 99254^1, 99255^1, 99291^1, 99292^1, 99304^1, 99305^1, 99306^1, 99307^1, 99308^1, 99309^1, 99310^1, 99315^1, 99316^1, 99334^1, 99335^1, 99336^1, 99337^1, 99347^1, 99348^1, 99349^1, 99350^1, 99374^1, 99375^1, 99377^1, 99378^1, 99446^0, 99447^0, 99448^0, 99449^0, 99451^0, 99452^0, 99495^0, 99496^0, G0453^0, G0463^1, G0471^1
61623	01924^0, 01925^0, 01926^0, 0213T^0, 0216T^0, 0228T^0, 0230T^0, 0333T^0, 0464T^0, 12001^1, 12002^1, 12004^1, 12005^1, 12006^1, 12007^1, 12011^1, 12013^1, 12014^1, 12015^1, 12016^1, 12017^1, 12018^1, 12020^1, 12021^1, 12031^1, 12032^1, 12034^1, 12035^1, 12036^1, 12037^1, 12041^1, 12042^1, 12044^1, 12045^1, 12046^1, 12047^1, 12051^1, 12052^1, 12053^1, 12054^1, 12055^1, 12056^1, 12057^1, 13100^1, 13101^1, 13102^1, 13120^1, 13121^1, 13122^1, 13131^1, 13132^1, 13133^1, 13151^1, 13152^1, 13153^1, 36000^1, 36100^1, 36140^1, 36215^1, 36216^1, 36217^1, 36400^1, 36405^1, 36406^1, 36410^1, 36420^1, 36425^1, 36430^1, 36440^1, 36591^0, 36592^0, 36600^1, 36640^1, 37606^1, 37607^1, 37609^1, 43752^1, 51701^1, 51702^1, 51703^1, 62320^0, 62321^0, 62322^0, 62323^0, 62324^0, 62325^0, 62326^0, 62327^0, 64400^0, 64405^0, 64408^0, 64415^0, 64416^0, 64417^0, 64418^0, 64420^0, 64421^0, 64425^0, 64430^0, 64435^0, 64445^0, 64446^0, 64447^0, 64448^0, 64449^0, 64450^0, 64451^0, 64454^0, 64461^0, 64462^0, 64463^0, 64479^0, 64480^0, 64483^0, 64484^0, 64486^0, 64487^0, 64488^0, 64489^0, 64490^0, 64491^0, 64492^0, 64493^0, 64494^0, 64495^0, 64505^0, 64510^0, 64517^0, 64520^0, 64530^0, 92012^1, 92014^1, 92585^0, 93000^1, 93005^1, 93010^1, 93040^1, 93041^1, 93042^1, 93318^1, 93355^1, 94002^1, 94200^1, 94250^1, 94680^1, 94681^1, 94690^1, 94770^1, 95812^1, 95813^1, 95816^1, 95819^1, 95822^0, 95829^1, 95860^0, 95861^0, 95863^0, 95864^0, 95865^0, 95866^0, 95867^0, 95868^0, 95869^0, 95870^0, 95907^0, 95908^0, 95909^0, 95910^0, 95911^0, 95912^0, 95913^0, 95925^0, 95926^0, 95927^0, 95928^0, 95929^0, 95930^0, 95933^0, 95937^0, 95938^0, 95939^0, 95940^0, 95955^1, 96360^1, 96361^1, 96365^1, 96366^1, 96367^1, 96368^1, 96372^1, 96374^1, 96375^1, 96376^1, 96377^1, 96523^0, 99155^0, 99156^0, 99157^0, 99211^1, 99212^1, 99213^1, 99214^1, 99215^1, 99217^1, 99218^1, 99219^1, 99220^1, 99221^1, 99222^1, 99223^1, 99231^1, 99232^1, 99233^1, 99234^1, 99235^1, 99236^1, 99238^1, 99239^1, 99241^1, 99242^1, 99243^1, 99244^1, 99245^1, 99251^1, 99252^1, 99253^1, 99254^1, 99255^1, 99291^1, 99292^1, 99304^1, 99305^1, 99306^1, 99307^1, 99308^1, 99309^1, 99310^1, 99315^1, 99316^1, 99334^1, 99335^1, 99336^1, 99337^1, 99347^1, 99348^1, 99349^1, 99350^1, 99374^1, 99375^1, 99377^1, 99378^1, 99446^0, 99447^0, 99448^0, 99449^0, 99451^0, 99452^0, 99495^1, 99496^1, G0453^0, G0463^1, G0471^1
61624	01924^0, 01926^0, 0213T^0, 0216T^0, 0228T^0, 0230T^0, 0333T^0, 0464T^0, 12001^1, 12002^1, 12004^1, 12005^1, 12006^1, 12007^1, 12011^1, 12013^1, 12014^1, 12015^1, 12016^1, 12017^1, 12018^1, 12020^1, 12021^1, 12031^1, 12032^1, 12034^1, 12035^1, 12036^1, 12037^1, 12041^1, 12042^1, 12044^1, 12045^1, 12046^1, 12047^1, 12051^1, 12052^1, 12053^1, 12054^1, 12055^1, 12056^1, 12057^1, 13100^1, 13101^1, 13102^1, 13120^1, 13121^1, 13122^1, 13131^1, 13132^1, 13133^1, 13151^1, 13152^1, 13153^1, 36000^1, 36400^1, 36405^1, 36406^1, 36410^1, 36420^1, 36425^1, 36430^1, 36440^1, 36591^0, 36592^0, 36600^1, 36640^1, 37236^1, 37238^1, 37241^1, 37242^1, 37243^1, 37244^1, 37600^1, 37605^1, 37606^1, 37607^1, 37609^1, 43752^1, 51701^1, 51702^1, 51703^1, 62320^0, 62321^0, 62322^0, 62323^0, 62324^0, 62325^0, 62326^0, 62327^0, 64400^0, 64405^0, 64408^0, 64415^0, 64416^0, 64417^0, 64418^0, 64420^0, 64421^0, 64425^0, 64430^0, 64435^0, 64445^0, 64446^0, 64447^0, 64448^0, 64449^0, 64450^0, 64451^0, 64454^0, 64461^0, 64462^0, 64463^0, 64479^0, 64480^0, 64483^0, 64484^0, 64486^0, 64487^0, 64488^0, 64489^0, 64490^0, 64491^0, 64492^0, 64493^0, 64494^0, 64495^0, 64505^0, 64510^0, 64517^0, 64520^0, 64530^0, 92012^1, 92014^1, 92585^0, 93000^1, 93005^1, 93010^1, 93040^1, 93041^1, 93042^1, 93318^1, 93355^1, 94002^1, 94200^1, 94250^1, 94680^1, 94681^1, 94690^1, 94770^1, 95812^1, 95813^1, 95816^1, 95819^1, 95822^0, 95829^1, 95860^0, 95861^0, 95863^0, 95864^0, 95865^0, 95866^0, 95867^0, 95868^0, 95869^0, 95870^0, 95907^0, 95908^0, 95909^0, 95910^0, 95911^0, 95912^0, 95913^0, 95925^0, 95926^0, 95927^0, 95928^0, 95929^0, 95930^0, 95933^0, 95937^0, 95938^0, 95939^0, 95940^0, 95955^1, 96360^1, 96361^1, 96365^1, 96366^1, 96367^1, 96368^1, 96372^1, 96374^1, 96375^1, 96376^1, 96377^1, 96523^0, 99155^0, 99156^0, 99157^0, 99211^1, 99212^1, 99213^1, 99214^1, 99215^1, 99217^1, 99218^1, 99219^1, 99220^1, 99221^1, 99222^1, 99223^1, 99231^1, 99232^1, 99233^1, 99234^1, 99235^1, 99236^1, 99238^1, 99239^1, 99241^1, 99242^1, 99243^1, 99244^1, 99245^1, 99251^1, 99252^1, 99253^1, 99254^1, 99255^1, 99291^1, 99292^1, 99304^1, 99305^1, 99306^1, 99307^1, 99308^1, 99309^1, 99310^1, 99315^1, 99316^1, 99334^1, 99335^1, 99336^1, 99337^1, 99347^1, 99348^1, 99349^1, 99350^1, 99374^1, 99375^1, 99377^1, 99378^1, 99446^0, 99447^0, 99448^0, 99449^0, 99451^0, 99452^0, 99495^1, 99496^1, G0453^0, G0463^1, G0471^1
61626	01924^0, 0213T^0, 0216T^0, 0228T^0, 0230T^0, 0333T^0, 0464T^0, 12001^1, 12002^1, 12004^1, 12005^1, 12006^1, 12007^1, 12011^1, 12013^1, 12014^1, 12015^1, 12016^1, 12017^1, 12018^1, 12020^1, 12021^1, 12031^1, 12032^1, 12034^1, 12035^1, 12036^1, 12037^1, 12041^1, 12042^1, 12044^1, 12045^1, 12046^1, 12047^1, 12051^1, 12052^1, 12053^1, 12054^1, 12055^1, 12056^1, 12057^1, 13100^1, 13101^1, 13102^1, 13120^1, 13121^1, 13122^1, 13131^1, 13132^1, 13133^1, 13151^1, 13152^1, 13153^1, 36000^1, 36400^1, 36405^1, 36406^1, 36410^1, 36420^1, 36425^1, 36430^1, 36440^1, 36591^0, 36592^0, 36600^1, 36640^1, 37236^1, 37238^1, 37241^1, 37242^1, 37243^1, 37244^1, 37600^1, 37605^1, 37606^1, 37607^1, 37609^1, 43752^1, 51701^1, 51702^1, 51703^1, 62320^0, 62321^0, 62322^0, 62323^0, 62324^0, 62325^0, 62326^0, 62327^0, 64400^0, 64405^0, 64408^0, 64415^0, 64416^0, 64417^0, 64418^0, 64420^0, 64421^0, 64425^0, 64430^0, 64435^0, 64445^0, 64446^0, 64447^0, 64448^0, 64449^0, 64450^0, 64451^0, 64454^0, 64461^0, 64462^0, 64463^0, 64479^0, 64480^0, 64483^0, 64484^0, 64486^0, 64487^0, 64488^0, 64489^0, 64490^0, 64491^0, 64492^0, 64493^0, 64494^0, 64495^0, 64505^0, 64510^0, 64517^0, 64520^0, 64530^0, 92012^1, 92014^1, 92585^0, 93000^1, 93005^1, 93010^1, 93040^1, 93041^1, 93042^1, 93318^1, 93355^1, 94002^1, 94200^1, 94250^1, 94680^1, 94681^1, 94690^1, 94770^1, 95812^1, 95813^1, 95816^1, 95819^1, 95822^0, 95829^1, 95860^0, 95861^0, 95863^0, 95864^0, 95865^0, 95866^0, 95867^0, 95868^0, 95869^0, 95870^0, 95907^0, 95908^0, 95909^0, 95910^0, 95911^0, 95912^0, 95913^0, 95925^0, 95926^0, 95927^0, 95928^0, 95929^0, 95930^0, 95933^0, 95937^0, 95938^0, 95939^0, 95940^0, 95955^1, 96360^1, 96361^1, 96365^1, 96366^1, 96367^1, 96368^1,

Code 1	Code 2
	96372[1], 96374[1], 96375[1], 96376[1], 96377[1], 96523[0], 99155[0], 99156[0], 99157[0], 99211[1], 99212[1], 99213[1], 99214[1], 99215[1], 99217[1], 99218[1], 99219[1], 99220[1], 99221[1], 99222[1], 99223[1], 99231[1], 99232[1], 99233[1], 99234[1], 99235[1], 99236[1], 99238[1], 99239[1], 99241[1], 99242[1], 99243[1], 99244[1], 99245[1], 99251[1], 99252[1], 99253[1], 99254[1], 99255[1], 99291[1], 99292[1], 99304[1], 99305[1], 99306[1], 99307[1], 99308[1], 99309[1], 99310[1], 99315[1], 99316[1], 99334[1], 99335[1], 99336[1], 99337[1], 99347[1], 99348[1], 99349[1], 99350[1], 99374[1], 99375[1], 99377[1], 99378[1], 99446[0], 99447[0], 99448[0], 99449[0], 99451[0], 99452[0], 99495[1], 99496[1], G0453[0], G0463[1], G0471[1]
61630	01924[0], 01926[0], 01930[0], 01933[0], 0213T[1], 0216T[1], 0333T[0], 0464T[0], 11000[1], 11001[1], 11004[1], 11005[1], 11006[1], 11042[1], 11043[1], 11044[1], 11045[1], 11046[1], 11047[1], 35201[1], 35206[1], 35226[1], 35231[1], 35236[1], 35256[1], 35261[1], 35266[1], 35286[1], 36000[1], 36100[1], 36140[1], 36200[1], 36215[1], 36216[1], 36217[1], 36410[1], 36591[0], 36592[0], 36620[1], 36625[1], 37215[1], 37217[1], 37218[1], 37236[1], 37238[1], 37246[1], 37247[1], 51701[1], 51702[1], 51703[1], 61645[1], 61650[1], 62324[1], 62325[1], 62326[1], 62327[1], 64415[1], 64416[1], 64417[1], 64450[1], 64454[1], 64486[1], 64487[1], 64488[1], 64489[1], 64490[1], 64493[1], 76000[1], 76380[1], 76942[1], 76970[1], 76998[1], 77001[1], 77002[1], 77012[1], 77021[1], 92585[0], 95822[0], 95860[0], 95861[0], 95863[0], 95864[0], 95865[0], 95866[0], 95867[0], 95868[0], 95869[0], 95870[0], 95907[0], 95908[0], 95909[0], 95910[0], 95911[0], 95912[0], 95913[0], 95925[0], 95926[0], 95927[0], 95928[0], 95929[0], 95930[0], 95933[0], 95937[0], 95938[0], 95939[0], 95940[0], 96360[1], 96365[1], 96372[1], 96374[1], 96375[1], 96376[1], 96377[1], 96523[0], 97597[1], 97598[1], 97602[1], G0453[0], G0471[1]
61635	01924[0], 01926[0], 01930[0], 01933[0], 0213T[1], 0216T[1], 0333T[0], 0464T[0], 11000[1], 11001[1], 11004[1], 11005[1], 11006[1], 11042[1], 11043[1], 11044[1], 11045[1], 11046[1], 11047[1], 35201[1], 35206[1], 35226[1], 35231[1], 35236[1], 35256[1], 35261[1], 35266[1], 35286[1], 36000[1], 36100[1], 36140[1], 36200[1], 36215[1], 36216[1], 36217[1], 36410[1], 36591[0], 36592[0], 36620[1], 36625[1], 37215[1], 37217[1], 37218[1], 37236[1], 37238[1], 37246[1], 37247[1], 51701[1], 51702[1], 51703[1], 61630[0], 61645[1], 61650[1], 62324[1], 62325[1], 62326[1], 62327[1], 64415[1], 64416[1], 64417[1], 64450[1], 64454[1], 64486[1], 64487[1], 64488[1], 64489[1], 64490[1], 64493[1], 76000[1], 76380[1], 76942[1], 76970[1], 76998[1], 77001[1], 77002[1], 77012[1], 77021[1], 92585[0], 95822[0], 95860[0], 95861[0], 95863[0], 95864[0], 95865[0], 95866[0], 95867[0], 95868[0], 95869[0], 95870[0], 95907[0], 95908[0], 95909[0], 95910[0], 95911[0], 95912[0], 95913[0], 95925[0], 95926[0], 95927[0], 95928[0], 95929[0], 95930[0], 95933[0], 95937[0], 95938[0], 95939[0], 95940[0], 96360[1], 96365[1], 96372[1], 96374[1], 96375[1], 96376[1], 96377[1], 96523[0], 97597[1], 97598[1], 97602[1], G0453[0], G0471[1]
61640	12001[1], 12002[1], 12004[1], 12005[1], 12006[1], 12007[1], 12011[1], 12013[1], 12014[1], 12015[1], 12016[1], 12017[1], 12018[1], 12020[1], 12021[1], 12031[1], 12032[1], 12034[1], 12035[1], 12036[1], 12037[1], 12041[1], 12042[1], 12044[1], 12045[1], 12046[1], 12047[1], 12051[1], 12052[1], 12053[1], 12054[1], 12055[1], 12056[1], 12057[1], 13100[1], 13101[1], 13102[1], 13120[1], 13121[1], 13122[1], 13131[1], 13132[1], 13133[1], 13151[1], 13152[1], 13153[1], 36000[1], 36400[1], 36405[1], 36406[1], 36410[1], 36420[1], 36425[1], 36430[1], 36440[1], 36591[0], 36592[0], 36600[1], 36640[1], 43752[1], 61650[1], 61651[1], 62320[0], 62321[0], 62322[0], 62323[0], 62324[0], 62325[0], 62326[0], 62327[0], 64400[0], 64405[0], 64408[0], 64415[0], 64416[0], 64417[0], 64418[0], 64420[0], 64421[0], 64425[0], 64430[0], 64435[0], 64445[0], 64446[0], 64447[0], 64448[0], 64449[0], 64450[0], 64451[0], 64454[0], 64461[0], 64462[0], 64463[0], 64479[0], 64480[0], 64483[0], 64484[0], 64486[0], 64487[0], 64488[0], 64489[0], 64490[0], 64491[0], 64492[0], 64493[0], 64494[0], 64495[0], 64505[0], 64510[0], 64517[0], 64520[0], 64530[0], 92012[1], 92014[1], 93000[1], 93005[1], 93010[1], 93040[1], 93041[1], 93042[1], 93318[1], 93355[1], 94002[1], 94200[1], 94250[1], 94680[1], 94681[1], 94690[1], 94770[1], 95812[1], 95813[1], 95816[1], 95819[1], 95822[1], 95829[1], 95955[1], 96360[1], 96361[1], 96365[1], 96366[1], 96367[1], 96368[1], 96372[1], 96374[1], 96375[1], 96376[1], 96377[1], 96523[0], 99155[0], 99156[0], 99157[0], 99211[1], 99212[1], 99213[1], 99214[1], 99215[1], 99217[1], 99218[1], 99219[1], 99220[1], 99221[1], 99222[1], 99223[1], 99231[1], 99232[1], 99233[1], 99234[1], 99235[1], 99236[1], 99238[1], 99239[1], 99241[1], 99242[1], 99243[1], 99244[1], 99245[1], 99251[1], 99252[1], 99253[1], 99254[1], 99255[1], 99291[1], 99292[1], 99304[1], 99305[1], 99306[1], 99307[1], 99308[1], 99309[1], 99310[1], 99315[1], 99316[1], 99334[1], 99335[1], 99336[1], 99337[1], 99347[1], 99348[1], 99349[1], 99350[1], 99374[1], 99375[1], 99377[1], 99378[1], 99446[0], 99447[0], 99448[0], 99449[0], 99451[0], 99452[0], 99495[1], 99496[1], G0463[1]
61641	36591[0], 36592[0], 61651[1], 96523[0]
61642	36591[0], 36592[0], 61651[1], 96523[0]
61645	0075T[1], 01916[0], 01924[0], 01925[0], 01926[0], 01930[0], 01931[0], 01932[0], 01933[0], 0213T[0], 0216T[0], 0228T[0], 0230T[0], 11000[1], 11001[1], 11004[1], 11005[1], 11006[1], 11042[1], 11043[1], 11044[1], 11045[1], 11046[1], 11047[1], 12001[1], 12002[1], 12004[1], 12005[1], 12006[1], 12007[1], 12011[1], 12013[1], 12014[1], 12015[1], 12016[1], 12017[1], 12018[1], 12020[1], 12021[1], 12031[1], 12032[1], 12034[1], 12035[1], 12036[1], 12037[1], 12041[1], 12042[1], 12044[1], 12045[1], 12046[1], 12047[1], 12051[1], 12052[1], 12053[1], 12054[1], 12055[1], 12056[1], 12057[1], 13100[1], 13101[1], 13102[1], 13120[1], 13121[1], 13122[1], 13131[1], 13132[1], 13133[1], 13151[1], 13152[1], 13153[1], 34101[1], 34111[1], 34713[1], 34714[1], 34812[1], 34813[1], 35201[1], 35206[1], 35226[1], 35231[1], 35236[1], 35256[1], 35261[1], 35266[1], 35286[1], 36000[1], 36005[1], 36221[1], 36222[1], 36223[1], 36224[1], 36225[1], 36226[1], 36227[1], 36228[1], 36400[1], 36405[1], 36406[1], 36410[1], 36420[1], 36425[1], 36430[1], 36440[1], 36500[1], 36591[0], 36592[0], 36593[1], 36600[1], 36620[1], 36625[1], 36640[1], 36860[1], 36861[1], 36904[1], 36905[1], 36906[1], 37195[0], 37211[1], 37212[1], 37213[0], 37214[0], 37217[1], 37218[1], 43752[1], 51701[1], 51702[1], 51703[1], 61650[1], 61651[1], 62320[0], 62321[0], 62322[0], 62323[0], 62324[0], 62325[0], 62326[0], 62327[0], 64400[0], 64405[0], 64408[0], 64415[0], 64416[0], 64417[0], 64418[0], 64420[0], 64421[0], 64425[0], 64430[0], 64435[0], 64445[0], 64446[0], 64447[0], 64448[0], 64449[0], 64450[0], 64451[0], 64454[0], 64461[0], 64462[0], 64463[0], 64479[0], 64480[0], 64483[0], 64484[0], 64486[0], 64487[0], 64488[0], 64489[0], 64490[0], 64491[0], 64492[0], 64493[0], 64494[0], 64495[0], 64505[0], 64510[0], 64517[0], 64520[0], 64530[0], 69990[0], 75600[1], 75605[1], 75625[1], 75630[1], 75635[1], 75705[1], 75710[1], 75716[1], 75726[1], 75731[1], 75733[1], 75736[1], 75741[1], 75743[1], 75746[1], 75756[1], 75774[1], 75809[1], 75810[1], 75820[1], 75822[1], 75825[1], 75827[1], 75831[1], 75833[1], 75840[1], 75842[1], 75860[1], 75870[1], 75872[1], 75880[1], 75885[1], 75887[1], 75889[1], 75891[1], 75893[1], 75894[1], 75898[1], 76000[1], 76380[1], 76942[1], 76970[1], 76998[1], 77001[1], 77002[1], 77012[1], 77021[1], 92012[1], 92014[1], 92585[0], 92977[1], 93000[1], 93005[1], 93010[1], 93040[1], 93041[1], 93042[1], 93318[1], 93355[1], 94002[1], 94200[1], 94250[1], 94680[1], 94681[1], 94690[1], 94770[1], 95812[1], 95813[1], 95816[1], 95819[1], 95822[1], 95829[1], 95860[0], 95861[0], 95863[0], 95864[0], 95865[0], 95866[0], 95867[0], 95868[0], 95869[0], 95870[0], 95907[0], 95908[0], 95909[0], 95910[0], 95911[0], 95912[0], 95913[0], 95925[0], 95926[0], 95927[0], 95928[0], 95929[0], 95930[0], 95933[0], 95937[0], 95938[0], 95939[0], 95940[0], 95941[0], 95955[1], 96360[1], 96361[1], 96365[1], 96366[1], 96367[1], 96368[1], 96372[1], 96374[1], 96375[1], 96376[1], 96377[1], 96523[0], 97597[1], 97598[1], 97602[1], 99155[0], 99156[0], 99157[0], 99201[1], 99202[1], 99203[1], 99204[1], 99205[1], 99211[1], 99212[1], 99213[1], 99214[1], 99215[1], 99217[1], 99218[1], 99219[1], 99220[1], 99221[1], 99222[1], 99223[1], 99224[1], 99225[1], 99226[1], 99231[1], 99232[1], 99233[1], 99234[1], 99235[1], 99236[1], 99238[1], 99239[1], 99241[1], 99242[1], 99243[1], 99244[1], 99245[1], 99251[1], 99252[1], 99253[1], 99254[1], 99255[1], 99291[1], 99292[1], 99304[1], 99305[1], 99306[1], 99307[1], 99308[1], 99309[1], 99310[1], 99315[1], 99316[1], 99318[1], 99324[1], 99325[1], 99326[1], 99327[1], 99328[1], 99334[1], 99335[1], 99336[1], 99337[1], 99339[1], 99340[1], 99341[1], 99342[1], 99343[1], 99344[1], 99345[1], 99347[1], 99348[1], 99349[1], 99350[1], 99354[1], 99355[1], 99356[1], 99357[1], 99358[1], 99359[1], 99360[1], 99374[1], 99375[1], 99377[1], 99378[1], 99415[1], 99416[1], 99446[0], 99447[0], 99448[0], 99449[0], 99451[0], 99452[0], 99460[1], 99461[1], 99462[1], 99463[1], 99483[1], 99495[1], 99496[1], 99497[1], G0453[0], G0463[1], G0471[1]
61650	0213T[0], 0216T[0], 0228T[0], 0230T[0], 12001[1], 12002[1], 12004[1], 12005[1], 12006[1], 12007[1], 12011[1], 12013[1], 12014[1], 12015[1], 12016[1], 12017[1], 12018[1], 12020[1], 12021[1], 12031[1], 12032[1], 12034[1], 12035[1], 12036[1], 12037[1], 12041[1], 12042[1], 12044[1], 12045[1], 12046[1], 12047[1], 12051[1], 12052[1], 12053[1], 12054[1], 12055[1], 12056[1], 12057[1], 13100[1], 13101[1], 13102[1], 13120[1], 13121[1], 13122[1], 13131[1], 13132[1], 13133[1], 13151[1], 13152[1], 13153[1], 34713[1], 34714[1], 34812[1], 36000[1], 36005[1], 36010[1], 36011[1], 36012[1], 36013[1], 36014[1], 36015[1], 36100[1], 36140[1], 36160[1], 36200[1], 36215[1], 36216[1], 36221[1], 36222[1], 36223[1], 36224[1], 36225[1], 36226[1], 36228[1], 36245[1], 36246[1], 36400[1], 36405[1], 36406[1], 36410[1], 36420[1], 36425[1], 36430[1], 36440[1], 36591[0], 36592[0], 36600[1], 36620[1], 36625[1], 36640[1], 36800[1], 36810[1], 36815[1], 36821[1], 36825[1], 36830[1], 36831[1], 36832[1], 36833[1], 36835[1], 36860[1], 36861[1], 37200[1], 37211[1], 37212[1], 37213[1], 37214[1], 43752[1], 51701[1], 51702[1], 51703[1], 61641[1], 61642[1], 62320[0], 62321[0], 62322[0], 62323[0], 62324[0], 62325[0], 62326[0], 62327[0], 64400[0], 64405[0], 64408[0], 64415[0], 64416[0], 64417[0], 64418[0], 64420[0], 64421[0], 64425[0], 64430[0], 64435[0], 64445[0], 64446[0], 64447[0], 64448[0], 64449[0], 64450[0], 64451[0], 64454[0], 64479[0], 64480[0], 64483[0], 64484[0], 64486[0], 64487[0], 64488[0], 64489[0], 64490[0], 64491[0], 64492[0], 64493[0], 64494[0], 64495[0], 64505[0], 64510[0], 64517[0], 64520[0], 64530[0], 69990[0], 75600[1], 75605[1], 75625[1], 75630[1], 75635[1], 75705[1], 75710[1], 75716[1], 75726[1], 75731[1], 75733[1], 75736[1], 75741[1], 75743[1], 75746[1], 75756[1], 75774[1], 75810[1], 75820[1], 75822[1], 75825[1], 75827[1], 75831[1], 75833[1], 75840[1], 75842[1], 75860[1], 75870[1], 75872[1], 75880[1], 75885[1], 75887[1], 75889[1], 75891[1], 75893[1], 75898[1], 76000[1], 76380[1], 76942[1], 76970[1], 76998[1], 77001[1], 77002[1], 77012[1], 77021[1], 92012[1], 92014[1], 92585[0], 93000[1], 93005[1], 93010[1], 93040[1], 93041[1], 93042[1], 93318[1], 93355[1], 94002[1], 94200[1], 94250[1], 94680[1], 94681[1], 94690[1], 94770[1], 95812[1], 95813[1], 95816[1], 95819[1], 95822[1], 95829[1], 95860[0], 95861[0], 95863[0], 95864[0], 95865[0], 95866[0], 95867[0], 95868[0], 95869[0], 95870[0], 95907[0], 95908[0], 95909[0], 95910[0], 95911[0], 95912[0], 95913[0], 95925[0], 95926[0], 95927[0], 95928[0], 95929[0], 95930[0], 95933[0], 95937[0], 95938[0], 95939[0], 95940[0], 95941[0], 95955[1], 96360[1], 96365[1], 96372[1], 96373[1], 96374[1], 96375[1], 96376[1], 96377[1], 96420[1], 96422[1], 96423[1], 96425[1], 96523[0], 99155[0], 99156[0], 99157[0], 99211[1], 99212[1], 99213[1], 99214[1], 99215[1], 99217[1], 99218[1], 99219[1], 99220[1], 99221[1], 99222[1], 99223[1], 99231[1], 99232[1], 99233[1], 99234[1], 99235[1], 99236[1], 99238[1], 99239[1], 99241[1], 99242[1], 99243[1], 99244[1], 99245[1], 99251[1], 99252[1], 99253[1], 99254[1], 99255[1], 99291[1], 99292[1], 99304[1], 99305[1], 99306[1], 99307[1], 99308[1], 99309[1], 99310[1], 99315[1], 99316[1], 99334[1], 99335[1], 99336[1], 99337[1], 99347[1], 99348[1], 99349[1], 99350[1], 99374[1], 99375[1], 99377[1], 99378[1], 99446[0], 99447[0], 99448[0], 99449[0], 99451[0], 99452[0], 99495[1], 99496[1], G0453[0], G0463[1], G0471[1]

0 = Modifier usage not allowed or inappropriate   1 = Modifier usage allowed

Code 1	Code 2
61651	0213T[0], 0216T[0], 0228T[0], 0230T[0], 12001[0], 12002[1], 12004[1], 12005[1], 12006[1], 12007[1], 12011[1], 12013[1], 12014[1], 12015[1], 12016[1], 12017[1], 12018[1], 12020[1], 12021[1], 12031[1], 12032[1], 12034[1], 12035[1], 12036[1], 12037[1], 12041[1], 12042[1], 12044[1], 12045[1], 12046[1], 12047[1], 12051[1], 12052[1], 12053[1], 12054[1], 12055[1], 12056[1], 12057[1], 13100[1], 13101[1], 13102[1], 13120[1], 13121[1], 13122[1], 13131[1], 13132[1], 13133[1], 13151[1], 13152[1], 13153[1], 34713[1], 34714[1], 34812[1], 36000[1], 36005[1], 36010[1], 36011[1], 36012[1], 36013[1], 36014[1], 36015[1], 36100[1], 36140[1], 36160[1], 36200[1], 36215[1], 36216[1], 36221[1], 36222[1], 36223[1], 36224[1], 36225[1], 36226[1], 36228[1], 36245[1], 36246[1], 36400[1], 36405[1], 36406[1], 36410[1], 36420[1], 36425[1], 36430[1], 36440[1], 36591[0], 36592[0], 36600[1], 36620[1], 36625[1], 36640[1], 36800[1], 36810[1], 36815[1], 36821[1], 36825[1], 36830[1], 36831[1], 36832[1], 36833[1], 36835[1], 36860[1], 36861[1], 37200[1], 37214[1], 43752[1], 51701[1], 51702[1], 51703[1], 62320[0], 62321[0], 62322[0], 62323[0], 62324[0], 62325[0], 62326[0], 62327[0], 64400[0], 64405[0], 64408[0], 64415[0], 64416[0], 64417[0], 64418[0], 64420[0], 64421[0], 64425[0], 64430[0], 64435[0], 64445[0], 64446[0], 64447[0], 64448[0], 64449[0], 64450[0], 64451[0], 64454[0], 64479[0], 64483[0], 64486[0], 64487[0], 64488[0], 64489[0], 64490[0], 64493[0], 64505[0], 64510[0], 64517[0], 64520[0], 64530[0], 69990[0], 75600[1], 75605[1], 75625[1], 75630[1], 75635[1], 75705[1], 75710[1], 75716[1], 75726[1], 75731[1], 75733[1], 75736[1], 75741[1], 75743[1], 75746[1], 75756[1], 75774[1], 75810[1], 75820[1], 75822[1], 75825[1], 75827[1], 75831[1], 75833[1], 75840[1], 75842[1], 75860[1], 75870[1], 75872[1], 75880[1], 75885[1], 75887[1], 75889[1], 75891[1], 75893[1], 75898[1], 76000[1], 76380[1], 76942[1], 76970[1], 76998[1], 77001[1], 77002[1], 77012[1], 77021[1], 92012[1], 92014[1], 92585[0], 93000[1], 93005[1], 93010[1], 93040[1], 93041[1], 93042[1], 93318[1], 93355[1], 94002[1], 94200[1], 94250[1], 94680[1], 94681[1], 94690[1], 94770[1], 95812[1], 95813[1], 95816[1], 95819[1], 95822[1], 95829[1], 95860[0], 95861[0], 95863[0], 95864[0], 95865[0], 95866[0], 95867[0], 95868[0], 95869[0], 95870[0], 95907[0], 95908[0], 95909[0], 95910[0], 95911[0], 95912[0], 95913[0], 95925[0], 95926[0], 95927[0], 95928[0], 95929[0], 95930[0], 95933[0], 95937[0], 95938[0], 95939[0], 95940[0], 95941[0], 95955[1], 96360[1], 96365[1], 96372[1], 96373[1], 96374[1], 96375[1], 96376[1], 96377[1], 96420[1], 96422[1], 96423[1], 96425[1], 96523[0], 99155[0], 99156[0], 99157[0], 99211[1], 99212[1], 99213[1], 99214[1], 99215[1], 99217[1], 99218[1], 99219[1], 99220[1], 99221[1], 99222[1], 99223[1], 99231[1], 99232[1], 99233[1], 99234[1], 99235[1], 99236[1], 99238[1], 99239[1], 99241[1], 99242[1], 99243[1], 99244[1], 99245[1], 99251[1], 99252[1], 99253[1], 99254[1], 99255[1], 99291[1], 99292[1], 99304[1], 99305[1], 99306[1], 99307[1], 99308[1], 99309[1], 99310[1], 99315[1], 99316[1], 99334[1], 99335[1], 99336[1], 99337[1], 99347[1], 99348[1], 99349[1], 99350[1], 99374[1], 99375[1], 99377[1], 99378[1], 99446[0], 99447[0], 99448[0], 99449[0], 99451[0], 99452[0], 99495[1], 99496[1], G0453[0], G0463[1], G0471[1]
61680	0213T[0], 0216T[0], 0228T[0], 0230T[0], 0333T[0], 0464T[0], 12001[1], 12002[1], 12004[1], 12005[1], 12006[1], 12007[1], 12011[1], 12013[1], 12014[1], 12015[1], 12016[1], 12017[1], 12018[1], 12020[1], 12021[1], 12031[1], 12032[1], 12034[1], 12035[1], 12036[1], 12037[1], 12041[1], 12042[1], 12044[1], 12045[1], 12046[1], 12047[1], 12051[1], 12052[1], 12053[1], 12054[1], 12055[1], 12056[1], 12057[1], 13100[1], 13101[1], 13102[1], 13120[1], 13121[1], 13122[1], 13131[1], 13132[1], 13133[1], 13151[1], 13152[1], 13153[1], 36000[1], 36400[1], 36405[1], 36406[1], 36410[1], 36420[1], 36425[1], 36430[1], 36440[1], 36591[0], 36592[0], 36600[1], 36640[1], 43752[1], 51701[1], 51702[1], 51703[1], 61304[1], 61312[1], 61313[1], 61340[1], 62320[0], 62321[0], 62322[0], 62323[0], 62324[0], 62325[0], 62326[0], 62327[0], 64400[0], 64405[0], 64408[0], 64415[0], 64416[0], 64417[0], 64418[0], 64420[0], 64421[0], 64425[0], 64430[0], 64435[0], 64445[0], 64446[0], 64447[0], 64448[0], 64449[0], 64450[0], 64451[0], 64454[0], 64461[0], 64462[0], 64463[0], 64479[0], 64480[0], 64483[0], 64484[0], 64486[0], 64487[0], 64488[0], 64489[0], 64490[0], 64491[0], 64492[0], 64493[0], 64494[0], 64495[0], 64505[0], 64510[0], 64517[0], 64520[0], 64530[0], 92012[1], 92014[1], 92585[0], 93000[1], 93005[1], 93010[1], 93040[1], 93041[1], 93042[1], 93318[1], 93355[1], 94002[1], 94200[1], 94250[1], 94680[1], 94681[1], 94690[1], 94770[1], 95812[1], 95813[1], 95816[1], 95819[1], 95822[0], 95829[1], 95860[0], 95861[0], 95863[0], 95864[0], 95865[0], 95866[0], 95867[0], 95868[0], 95869[0], 95870[0], 95907[0], 95908[0], 95909[0], 95910[0], 95911[0], 95912[0], 95913[0], 95925[0], 95926[0], 95927[0], 95928[0], 95929[0], 95930[0], 95933[0], 95937[0], 95938[0], 95939[0], 95940[0], 95955[1], 96360[1], 96361[1], 96365[1], 96366[1], 96367[1], 96368[1], 96372[1], 96374[1], 96375[1], 96376[1], 96377[1], 96523[0], 99155[0], 99156[0], 99157[0], 99211[1], 99212[1], 99213[1], 99214[1], 99215[1], 99217[1], 99218[1], 99219[1], 99220[1], 99221[1], 99222[1], 99223[1], 99231[1], 99232[1], 99233[1], 99234[1], 99235[1], 99236[1], 99238[1], 99239[1], 99241[1], 99242[1], 99243[1], 99244[1], 99245[1], 99251[1], 99252[1], 99253[1], 99254[1], 99255[1], 99291[1], 99292[1], 99304[1], 99305[1], 99306[1], 99307[1], 99308[1], 99309[1], 99310[1], 99315[1], 99316[1], 99334[1], 99335[1], 99336[1], 99337[1], 99347[1], 99348[1], 99349[1], 99350[1], 99374[1], 99375[1], 99377[1], 99378[1], 99446[0], 99447[0], 99448[0], 99449[0], 99451[0], 99452[0], 99495[0], 99496[0], G0453[0], G0463[1], G0471[1]
61682	0213T[0], 0216T[0], 0228T[0], 0230T[0], 0333T[0], 0464T[0], 12001[1], 12002[1], 12004[1], 12005[1], 12006[1], 12007[1], 12011[1], 12013[1], 12014[1], 12015[1], 12016[1], 12017[1], 12018[1], 12020[1], 12021[1], 12031[1], 12032[1], 12034[1], 12035[1], 12036[1], 12037[1], 12041[1], 12042[1], 12044[1], 12045[1], 12046[1], 12047[1], 12051[1], 12052[1], 12053[1], 12054[1], 12055[1], 12056[1], 12057[1], 13100[1], 13101[1], 13102[1], 13120[1], 13121[1], 13122[1], 13131[1], 13132[1], 13133[1], 13151[1], 13152[1], 13153[1], 36000[1], 36400[1], 36405[1], 36406[1], 36410[1], 36420[1], 36425[1], 36430[1], 36440[1], 36591[0], 36592[0], 36600[1], 36640[1], 43752[1], 51701[1], 51702[1], 51703[1], 61304[1], 61312[1], 61313[1], 61340[1], 61680[1], 62320[0], 62321[0], 62322[0], 62323[0], 62324[0], 62325[0], 62326[0], 62327[0], 64400[0], 64405[0], 64408[0], 64415[0], 64416[0], 64417[0], 64418[0], 64420[0], 64421[0], 64425[0], 64430[0], 64435[0], 64445[0], 64446[0], 64447[0], 64448[0], 64449[0], 64450[0], 64451[0], 64454[0], 64461[0], 64462[0], 64463[0], 64479[0], 64480[0], 64483[0], 64484[0], 64486[0], 64487[0], 64488[0], 64489[0], 64490[0], 64491[0], 64492[0], 64493[0], 64494[0], 64495[0], 64505[0], 64510[0], 64517[0], 64520[0], 64530[0], 92012[1], 92014[1], 92585[0], 93000[1], 93005[1], 93010[1], 93040[1], 93041[1], 93042[1], 93318[1], 93355[1], 94002[1], 94200[1], 94250[1], 94680[1], 94681[1], 94690[1], 94770[1], 95812[1], 95813[1], 95816[1], 95819[1], 95822[0], 95829[1], 95860[0], 95861[0], 95863[0], 95864[0], 95865[0], 95866[0], 95867[0], 95868[0], 95869[0], 95870[0], 95907[0], 95908[0], 95909[0], 95910[0], 95911[0], 95912[0], 95913[0], 95925[0], 95926[0], 95927[0], 95928[0], 95929[0], 95930[0], 95933[0], 95937[0], 95938[0], 95939[0], 95940[0], 95955[1], 96360[1], 96361[1], 96365[1], 96366[1], 96367[1], 96368[1], 96372[1], 96374[1], 96375[1], 96376[1], 96377[1], 96523[0], 99155[0], 99156[0], 99157[0], 99211[1], 99212[1], 99213[1], 99214[1], 99215[1], 99217[1], 99218[1], 99219[1], 99220[1], 99221[1], 99222[1], 99223[1], 99231[1], 99232[1], 99233[1], 99234[1], 99235[1], 99236[1], 99238[1], 99239[1], 99241[1], 99242[1], 99243[1], 99244[1], 99245[1], 99251[1], 99252[1], 99253[1], 99254[1], 99255[1], 99291[1], 99292[1], 99304[1], 99305[1], 99306[1], 99307[1], 99308[1], 99309[1], 99310[1], 99315[1], 99316[1], 99334[1], 99335[1], 99336[1], 99337[1], 99347[1], 99348[1], 99349[1], 99350[1], 99374[1], 99375[1], 99377[1], 99378[1], 99446[0], 99447[0], 99448[0], 99449[0], 99451[0], 99452[0], 99495[0], 99496[0], G0453[0], G0463[1], G0471[1]
61684	0213T[0], 0216T[0], 0228T[0], 0230T[0], 0333T[0], 0464T[0], 12001[1], 12002[1], 12004[1], 12005[1], 12006[1], 12007[1], 12011[1], 12013[1], 12014[1], 12015[1], 12016[1], 12017[1], 12018[1], 12020[1], 12021[1], 12031[1], 12032[1], 12034[1], 12035[1], 12036[1], 12037[1], 12041[1], 12042[1], 12044[1], 12045[1], 12046[1], 12047[1], 12051[1], 12052[1], 12053[1], 12054[1], 12055[1], 12056[1], 12057[1], 13100[1], 13101[1], 13102[1], 13120[1], 13121[1], 13122[1], 13131[1], 13132[1], 13133[1], 13151[1], 13152[1], 13153[1], 36000[1], 36400[1], 36405[1], 36406[1], 36410[1], 36420[1], 36425[1], 36430[1], 36440[1], 36591[0], 36592[0], 36600[1], 36640[1], 43752[1], 51701[1], 51702[1], 51703[1], 61305[1], 61314[1], 61315[1], 61345[1], 62320[0], 62321[0], 62322[0], 62323[0], 62324[0], 62325[0], 62326[0], 62327[0], 64400[0], 64405[0], 64408[0], 64415[0], 64416[0], 64417[0], 64418[0], 64420[0], 64421[0], 64425[0], 64430[0], 64435[0], 64445[0], 64446[0], 64447[0], 64448[0], 64449[0], 64450[0], 64451[0], 64454[0], 64461[0], 64462[0], 64463[0], 64479[0], 64480[0], 64483[0], 64484[0], 64486[0], 64487[0], 64488[0], 64489[0], 64490[0], 64491[0], 64492[0], 64493[0], 64494[0], 64495[0], 64505[0], 64510[0], 64517[0], 64520[0], 64530[0], 92012[1], 92014[1], 92585[0], 93000[1], 93005[1], 93010[1], 93040[1], 93041[1], 93042[1], 93318[1], 93355[1], 94002[1], 94200[1], 94250[1], 94680[1], 94681[1], 94690[1], 94770[1], 95812[1], 95813[1], 95816[1], 95819[1], 95822[0], 95829[1], 95860[0], 95861[0], 95863[0], 95864[0], 95865[0], 95866[0], 95867[0], 95868[0], 95869[0], 95870[0], 95907[0], 95908[0], 95909[0], 95910[0], 95911[0], 95912[0], 95913[0], 95925[0], 95926[0], 95927[0], 95928[0], 95929[0], 95930[0], 95933[0], 95937[0], 95938[0], 95939[0], 95940[0], 95955[1], 96360[1], 96361[1], 96365[1], 96366[1], 96367[1], 96368[1], 96372[1], 96374[1], 96375[1], 96376[1], 96377[1], 96523[0], 99155[0], 99156[0], 99157[0], 99211[1], 99212[1], 99213[1], 99214[1], 99215[1], 99217[1], 99218[1], 99219[1], 99220[1], 99221[1], 99222[1], 99223[1], 99231[1], 99232[1], 99233[1], 99234[1], 99235[1], 99236[1], 99238[1], 99239[1], 99241[1], 99242[1], 99243[1], 99244[1], 99245[1], 99251[1], 99252[1], 99253[1], 99254[1], 99255[1], 99291[1], 99292[1], 99304[1], 99305[1], 99306[1], 99307[1], 99308[1], 99309[1], 99310[1], 99315[1], 99316[1], 99334[1], 99335[1], 99336[1], 99337[1], 99347[1], 99348[1], 99349[1], 99350[1], 99374[1], 99375[1], 99377[1], 99378[1], 99446[0], 99447[0], 99448[0], 99449[0], 99451[0], 99452[0], 99495[0], 99496[0], G0453[0], G0463[1], G0471[1]
61686	0213T[0], 0216T[0], 0228T[0], 0230T[0], 0333T[0], 0464T[0], 12001[1], 12002[1], 12004[1], 12005[1], 12006[1], 12007[1], 12011[1], 12013[1], 12014[1], 12015[1], 12016[1], 12017[1], 12018[1], 12020[1], 12021[1], 12031[1], 12032[1], 12034[1], 12035[1], 12036[1], 12037[1], 12041[1], 12042[1], 12044[1], 12045[1], 12046[1], 12047[1], 12051[1], 12052[1], 12053[1], 12054[1], 12055[1], 12056[1], 12057[1], 13100[1], 13101[1], 13102[1], 13120[1], 13121[1], 13122[1], 13131[1], 13132[1], 13133[1], 13151[1], 13152[1], 13153[1], 36000[1], 36400[1], 36405[1], 36406[1], 36410[1], 36420[1], 36425[1], 36430[1], 36440[1], 36591[0], 36592[0], 36600[1], 36640[1], 43752[1], 51701[1], 51702[1], 51703[1], 61305[1], 61314[1], 61315[1], 61345[1], 61684[1], 62320[0], 62321[0], 62322[0], 62323[0], 62324[0], 62325[0], 62326[0], 62327[0], 64400[0], 64405[0], 64408[0], 64415[0], 64416[0], 64417[0], 64418[0], 64420[0], 64421[0], 64425[0], 64430[0], 64435[0], 64445[0], 64446[0], 64447[0], 64448[0], 64449[0], 64450[0], 64451[0], 64454[0], 64461[0], 64462[0], 64463[0], 64479[0], 64480[0], 64483[0], 64484[0], 64486[0], 64487[0], 64488[0], 64489[0], 64490[0], 64491[0], 64492[0], 64493[0], 64494[0], 64495[0], 64505[0], 64510[0], 64517[0], 64520[0], 64530[0], 92012[1], 92014[1], 92585[0], 93000[1], 93005[1], 93010[1], 93040[1], 93041[1], 93042[1], 93318[1], 93355[1], 94002[1], 94200[1], 94250[1], 94680[1], 94681[1], 94690[1], 94770[1], 95812[1], 95813[1], 95816[1], 95819[1], 95822[0], 95829[1], 95860[0], 95861[0], 95863[0], 95864[0], 95865[0], 95866[0], 95867[0], 95868[0], 95869[0], 95870[0], 95907[0], 95908[0], 95909[0], 95910[0], 95911[0], 95912[0], 95913[0], 95925[0], 95926[0], 95927[0], 95928[0], 95929[0], 95930[0], 95933[0], 95937[0], 95938[0], 95939[0], 95940[0], 95955[1], 96360[1], 96361[1], 96365[1], 96366[1], 96367[1], 96368[1], 96372[1], 96374[1], 96375[1], 96376[1], 96377[1], 96523[0], 99155[0], 99156[0], 99157[0], 99211[1], 99212[1], 99213[1], 99214[1], 99215[1], 99217[1], 99218[1], 99219[1], 99220[1], 99221[1], 99222[1], 99223[1], 99231[1], 99232[1], 99233[1], 99234[1], 99235[1], 99236[1],

0 = Modifier usage not allowed or inappropriate 1 = Modifier usage allowed

Code 1	Code 2
	99238^1, 99239^1, 99241^1, 99242^1, 99243^1, 99244^1, 99245^1, 99251^1, 99252^1, 99253^1, 99254^1, 99255^1, 99291^1, 99292^1, 99304^1, 99305^1, 99306^1, 99307^1, 99308^1, 99309^1, 99310^1, 99315^1, 99316^1, 99334^1, 99335^1, 99336^1, 99337^1, 99347^1, 99348^1, 99349^1, 99350^1, 99374^1, 99375^1, 99377^1, 99378^1, 99446^0, 99447^0, 99448^0, 99449^0, 99451^0, 99452^0, 99495^0, 99496^0, G0453^0, G0463^1, G0471^1
61690	0213T^0, 0216T^0, 0228T^0, 0230T^0, 0333T^0, 0464T^0, 12001^1, 12002^1, 12004^1, 12005^1, 12006^1, 12007^1, 12011^1, 12013^1, 12014^1, 12015^1, 12016^1, 12017^1, 12018^1, 12020^1, 12021^1, 12031^1, 12032^1, 12034^1, 12035^1, 12036^1, 12037^1, 12041^1, 12042^1, 12044^1, 12045^1, 12046^1, 12047^1, 12051^1, 12052^1, 12053^1, 12054^1, 12055^1, 12056^1, 12057^1, 13100^1, 13101^1, 13102^1, 13120^1, 13121^1, 13122^1, 13131^1, 13132^1, 13133^1, 13151^1, 13152^1, 13153^1, 36000^1, 36400^1, 36405^1, 36406^1, 36410^1, 36420^1, 36425^1, 36430^1, 36440^1, 36591^0, 36592^0, 36600^1, 36640^1, 43752^1, 51701^1, 51702^1, 51703^1, 61304^1, 61305^1, 61312^1, 61314^1, 61340^1, 61345^1, 62320^0, 62321^0, 62322^0, 62323^0, 62324^0, 62325^0, 62326^0, 62327^0, 64400^0, 64405^0, 64408^0, 64415^0, 64416^0, 64417^0, 64418^0, 64420^0, 64421^0, 64425^0, 64430^0, 64435^0, 64445^0, 64446^0, 64447^0, 64448^0, 64449^0, 64450^0, 64451^0, 64454^0, 64461^0, 64462^0, 64463^0, 64479^0, 64480^0, 64483^0, 64484^0, 64486^0, 64487^0, 64488^0, 64489^0, 64490^0, 64491^0, 64492^0, 64493^0, 64494^0, 64495^0, 64505^0, 64510^0, 64517^0, 64520^0, 64530^0, 92012^1, 92014^1, 92585^0, 93000^1, 93005^1, 93010^1, 93040^1, 93041^1, 93042^1, 93318^1, 93355^1, 94002^1, 94200^1, 94250^1, 94680^1, 94681^1, 94690^1, 94770^1, 95812^1, 95813^1, 95816^1, 95819^1, 95822^0, 95829^1, 95860^0, 95861^0, 95863^0, 95864^0, 95865^0, 95866^0, 95867^0, 95868^0, 95869^0, 95870^0, 95907^0, 95908^0, 95909^0, 95910^0, 95911^0, 95912^0, 95913^0, 95925^0, 95926^0, 95927^0, 95928^0, 95929^0, 95930^0, 95933^0, 95937^0, 95938^0, 95939^0, 95940^0, 95955^1, 96360^1, 96361^1, 96365^1, 96366^1, 96367^1, 96368^1, 96372^1, 96374^1, 96375^1, 96376^1, 96377^1, 96523^0, 99155^0, 99156^0, 99157^0, 99211^1, 99212^1, 99213^1, 99214^1, 99215^1, 99217^1, 99218^1, 99219^1, 99220^1, 99221^1, 99222^1, 99223^1, 99231^1, 99232^1, 99233^1, 99234^1, 99235^1, 99236^1, 99238^1, 99239^1, 99241^1, 99242^1, 99243^1, 99244^1, 99245^1, 99251^1, 99252^1, 99253^1, 99254^1, 99255^1, 99291^1, 99292^1, 99304^1, 99305^1, 99306^1, 99307^1, 99308^1, 99309^1, 99310^1, 99315^1, 99316^1, 99334^1, 99335^1, 99336^1, 99337^1, 99347^1, 99348^1, 99349^1, 99350^1, 99374^1, 99375^1, 99377^1, 99378^1, 99446^0, 99447^0, 99448^0, 99449^0, 99451^0, 99452^0, 99495^0, 99496^0, G0453^0, G0463^1, G0471^1
61692	0213T^0, 0216T^0, 0228T^0, 0230T^0, 0333T^0, 0464T^0, 12001^1, 12002^1, 12004^1, 12005^1, 12006^1, 12007^1, 12011^1, 12013^1, 12014^1, 12015^1, 12016^1, 12017^1, 12018^1, 12020^1, 12021^1, 12031^1, 12032^1, 12034^1, 12035^1, 12036^1, 12037^1, 12041^1, 12042^1, 12044^1, 12045^1, 12046^1, 12047^1, 12051^1, 12052^1, 12053^1, 12054^1, 12055^1, 12056^1, 12057^1, 13100^1, 13101^1, 13102^1, 13120^1, 13121^1, 13122^1, 13131^1, 13132^1, 13133^1, 13151^1, 13152^1, 13153^1, 36000^1, 36400^1, 36405^1, 36406^1, 36410^1, 36420^1, 36425^1, 36430^1, 36440^1, 36591^0, 36592^0, 36600^1, 36640^1, 43752^1, 51701^1, 51702^1, 51703^1, 61304^1, 61305^1, 61312^1, 61314^1, 61340^1, 61345^1, 61690^1, 62320^0, 62321^0, 62322^0, 62323^0, 62324^0, 62325^0, 62326^0, 62327^0, 64400^0, 64405^0, 64408^0, 64415^0, 64416^0, 64417^0, 64418^0, 64420^0, 64421^0, 64425^0, 64430^0, 64435^0, 64445^0, 64446^0, 64447^0, 64448^0, 64449^0, 64450^0, 64451^0, 64454^0, 64461^0, 64462^0, 64463^0, 64479^0, 64480^0, 64483^0, 64484^0, 64486^0, 64487^0, 64488^0, 64489^0, 64490^0, 64491^0, 64492^0, 64493^0, 64494^0, 64495^0, 64505^0, 64510^0, 64517^0, 64520^0, 64530^0, 92012^1, 92014^1, 92585^0, 93000^1, 93005^1, 93010^1, 93040^1, 93041^1, 93042^1, 93318^1, 93355^1, 94002^1, 94200^1, 94250^1, 94680^1, 94681^1, 94690^1, 94770^1, 95812^1, 95813^1, 95816^1, 95819^1, 95822^0, 95829^1, 95860^0, 95861^0, 95863^0, 95864^0, 95865^0, 95866^0, 95867^0, 95868^0, 95869^0, 95870^0, 95907^0, 95908^0, 95909^0, 95910^0, 95911^0, 95912^0, 95913^0, 95925^0, 95926^0, 95927^0, 95928^0, 95929^0, 95930^0, 95933^0, 95937^0, 95938^0, 95939^0, 95940^0, 95955^1, 96360^1, 96361^1, 96365^1, 96366^1, 96367^1, 96368^1, 96372^1, 96374^1, 96375^1, 96376^1, 96377^1, 96523^0, 99155^0, 99156^0, 99157^0, 99211^1, 99212^1, 99213^1, 99214^1, 99215^1, 99217^1, 99218^1, 99219^1, 99220^1, 99221^1, 99222^1, 99223^1, 99231^1, 99232^1, 99233^1, 99234^1, 99235^1, 99236^1, 99238^1, 99239^1, 99241^1, 99242^1, 99243^1, 99244^1, 99245^1, 99251^1, 99252^1, 99253^1, 99254^1, 99255^1, 99291^1, 99292^1, 99304^1, 99305^1, 99306^1, 99307^1, 99308^1, 99309^1, 99310^1, 99315^1, 99316^1, 99334^1, 99335^1, 99336^1, 99337^1, 99347^1, 99348^1, 99349^1, 99350^1, 99374^1, 99375^1, 99377^1, 99378^1, 99446^0, 99447^0, 99448^0, 99449^0, 99451^0, 99452^0, 99495^0, 99496^0, G0453^0, G0463^1, G0471^1
61697	0213T^0, 0216T^0, 0228T^0, 0230T^0, 0333T^0, 0464T^0, 12001^1, 12002^1, 12004^1, 12005^1, 12006^1, 12007^1, 12011^1, 12013^1, 12014^1, 12015^1, 12016^1, 12017^1, 12018^1, 12020^1, 12021^1, 12031^1, 12032^1, 12034^1, 12035^1, 12036^1, 12037^1, 12041^1, 12042^1, 12044^1, 12045^1, 12046^1, 12047^1, 12051^1, 12052^1, 12053^1, 12054^1, 12055^1, 12056^1, 12057^1, 13100^1, 13101^1, 13102^1, 13120^1, 13121^1, 13122^1, 13131^1, 13132^1, 13133^1, 13151^1, 13152^1, 13153^1, 35701^1, 35702^1, 35703^1, 36000^1, 36400^1, 36405^1, 36406^1, 36410^1, 36420^1, 36425^1, 36430^1, 36440^1, 36591^0, 36592^0, 36600^1, 36640^1, 43752^1, 51701^1, 51702^1, 51703^1, 61304^1, 61312^1, 61313^1, 61340^1, 61700^0, 61781^1, 61782^1, 61783^1, 62320^0, 62321^0, 62322^0, 62323^0, 62324^0, 62325^0, 62326^0, 62327^0, 64400^0, 64405^0, 64408^0, 64415^0, 64416^0, 64417^0, 64418^0, 64420^0, 64421^0, 64425^0, 64430^0, 64435^0, 64445^0, 64446^0, 64447^0, 64448^0, 64449^0, 64450^0, 64451^0, 64454^0, 64461^0, 64462^0, 64463^0, 64479^0, 64480^0, 64483^0, 64484^0, 64486^0, 64487^0, 64488^0, 64489^0, 64490^0, 64491^0, 64492^0, 64493^0, 64494^0, 64495^0, 64505^0, 64510^0, 64517^0, 64520^0, 64530^0, 92012^1, 92014^1, 92585^0, 93000^1, 93005^1, 93010^1, 93040^1, 93041^1, 93042^1, 93318^1, 93355^1, 94002^1, 94200^1, 94250^1, 94680^1, 94681^1, 94690^1, 94770^1, 95812^1, 95813^1, 95816^1, 95819^1, 95822^0, 95829^1, 95860^0, 95861^0, 95863^0, 95864^0, 95865^0, 95866^0, 95867^0, 95868^0, 95869^0, 95870^0, 95907^0, 95908^0, 95909^0, 95910^0, 95911^0, 95912^0, 95913^0, 95925^0, 95926^0, 95927^0, 95928^0, 95929^0, 95930^0, 95933^0, 95937^0, 95938^0, 95939^0, 95940^0, 95955^1, 96360^1, 96361^1, 96365^1, 96366^1, 96367^1, 96368^1, 96372^1, 96374^1, 96375^1, 96376^1, 96377^1, 96523^0, 99155^0, 99156^0, 99157^0, 99211^1, 99212^1, 99213^1, 99214^1, 99215^1, 99217^1, 99218^1, 99219^1, 99220^1, 99221^1, 99222^1, 99223^1, 99231^1, 99232^1, 99233^1, 99234^1, 99235^1, 99236^1, 99238^1, 99239^1, 99241^1, 99242^1, 99243^1, 99244^1, 99245^1, 99251^1, 99252^1, 99253^1, 99254^1, 99255^1, 99291^1, 99292^1, 99304^1, 99305^1, 99306^1, 99307^1, 99308^1, 99309^1, 99310^1, 99315^1, 99316^1, 99334^1, 99335^1, 99336^1, 99337^1, 99347^1, 99348^1, 99349^1, 99350^1, 99374^1, 99375^1, 99377^1, 99378^1, 99446^0, 99447^0, 99448^0, 99449^0, 99451^0, 99452^0, 99495^0, 99496^0, G0453^0, G0463^1, G0471^1
61698	0213T^0, 0216T^0, 0228T^0, 0230T^0, 0333T^0, 0464T^0, 12001^1, 12002^1, 12004^1, 12005^1, 12006^1, 12007^1, 12011^1, 12013^1, 12014^1, 12015^1, 12016^1, 12017^1, 12018^1, 12020^1, 12021^1, 12031^1, 12032^1, 12034^1, 12035^1, 12036^1, 12037^1, 12041^1, 12042^1, 12044^1, 12045^1, 12046^1, 12047^1, 12051^1, 12052^1, 12053^1, 12054^1, 12055^1, 12056^1, 12057^1, 13100^1, 13101^1, 13102^1, 13120^1, 13121^1, 13122^1, 13131^1, 13132^1, 13133^1, 13151^1, 13152^1, 13153^1, 35702^1, 35703^1, 36000^1, 36400^1, 36405^1, 36406^1, 36410^1, 36420^1, 36425^1, 36430^1, 36440^1, 36591^0, 36592^0, 36600^1, 36640^1, 43752^1, 51701^1, 51702^1, 51703^1, 61304^1, 61312^1, 61313^1, 61340^1, 61702^0, 61781^1, 61782^1, 61783^1, 62320^0, 62321^0, 62322^0, 62323^0, 62324^0, 62325^0, 62326^0, 62327^0, 64400^0, 64405^0, 64408^0, 64415^0, 64416^0, 64417^0, 64418^0, 64420^0, 64421^0, 64425^0, 64430^0, 64435^0, 64445^0, 64446^0, 64447^0, 64448^0, 64449^0, 64450^0, 64451^0, 64454^0, 64461^0, 64462^0, 64463^0, 64479^0, 64480^0, 64483^0, 64484^0, 64486^0, 64487^0, 64488^0, 64489^0, 64490^0, 64491^0, 64492^0, 64493^0, 64494^0, 64495^0, 64505^0, 64510^0, 64517^0, 64520^0, 64530^0, 92012^1, 92014^1, 92585^0, 93000^1, 93005^1, 93010^1, 93040^1, 93041^1, 93042^1, 93318^1, 93355^1, 94002^1, 94200^1, 94250^1, 94680^1, 94681^1, 94690^1, 94770^1, 95812^1, 95813^1, 95816^1, 95819^1, 95822^0, 95829^1, 95860^0, 95861^0, 95863^0, 95864^0, 95865^0, 95866^0, 95867^0, 95868^0, 95869^0, 95870^0, 95907^0, 95908^0, 95909^0, 95910^0, 95911^0, 95912^0, 95913^0, 95925^0, 95926^0, 95927^0, 95928^0, 95929^0, 95930^0, 95933^0, 95937^0, 95938^0, 95939^0, 95940^0, 95955^1, 96360^1, 96361^1, 96365^1, 96366^1, 96367^1, 96368^1, 96372^1, 96374^1, 96375^1, 96376^1, 96377^1, 96523^0, 99155^0, 99156^0, 99157^0, 99211^1, 99212^1, 99213^1, 99214^1, 99215^1, 99217^1, 99218^1, 99219^1, 99220^1, 99221^1, 99222^1, 99223^1, 99231^1, 99232^1, 99233^1, 99234^1, 99235^1, 99236^1, 99238^1, 99239^1, 99241^1, 99242^1, 99243^1, 99244^1, 99245^1, 99251^1, 99252^1, 99253^1, 99254^1, 99255^1, 99291^1, 99292^1, 99304^1, 99305^1, 99306^1, 99307^1, 99308^1, 99309^1, 99310^1, 99315^1, 99316^1, 99334^1, 99335^1, 99336^1, 99337^1, 99347^1, 99348^1, 99349^1, 99350^1, 99374^1, 99375^1, 99377^1, 99378^1, 99446^0, 99447^0, 99448^0, 99449^0, 99451^0, 99452^0, 99495^0, 99496^0, G0453^0, G0463^1, G0471^1
61700	0213T^0, 0216T^0, 0228T^0, 0230T^0, 0333T^0, 0464T^0, 12001^1, 12002^1, 12004^1, 12005^1, 12006^1, 12007^1, 12011^1, 12013^1, 12014^1, 12015^1, 12016^1, 12017^1, 12018^1, 12020^1, 12021^1, 12031^1, 12032^1, 12034^1, 12035^1, 12036^1, 12037^1, 12041^1, 12042^1, 12044^1, 12045^1, 12046^1, 12047^1, 12051^1, 12052^1, 12053^1, 12054^1, 12055^1, 12056^1, 12057^1, 13100^1, 13101^1, 13102^1, 13120^1, 13121^1, 13122^1, 13131^1, 13132^1, 13133^1, 13151^1, 13152^1, 13153^1, 35701^1, 35702^1, 35703^1, 36000^1, 36400^1, 36405^1, 36406^1, 36410^1, 36420^1, 36425^1, 36430^1, 36440^1, 36591^0, 36592^0, 36600^1, 36640^1, 43752^1, 51701^1, 51702^1, 51703^1, 61304^1, 61312^1, 61313^1, 62320^0, 62321^0, 62322^0, 62323^0, 62324^0, 62325^0, 62326^0, 62327^0, 64400^0, 64405^0, 64408^0, 64415^0, 64416^0, 64417^0, 64418^0, 64420^0, 64421^0, 64425^0, 64430^0, 64435^0, 64445^0, 64446^0, 64447^0, 64448^0, 64449^0, 64450^0, 64451^0, 64454^0, 64461^0, 64462^0, 64463^0, 64479^0, 64480^0, 64483^0, 64484^0, 64486^0, 64487^0, 64488^0, 64489^0, 64490^0, 64491^0, 64492^0, 64493^0, 64494^0, 64495^0, 64505^0, 64510^0, 64517^0, 64520^0, 64530^0, 92012^1, 92014^1, 92585^0, 93000^1, 93005^1, 93010^1, 93040^1, 93041^1, 93042^1, 93318^1, 93355^1, 94002^1, 94200^1, 94250^1, 94680^1, 94681^1, 94690^1, 94770^1, 95812^1, 95813^1, 95816^1, 95819^1, 95822^0, 95829^1, 95860^0, 95861^0, 95863^0, 95864^0, 95865^0, 95866^0, 95867^0, 95868^0, 95869^0, 95870^0, 95907^0, 95908^0, 95909^0, 95910^0, 95911^0, 95912^0, 95913^0, 95925^0, 95926^0, 95927^0, 95928^0, 95929^0, 95930^0, 95933^0, 95937^0, 95938^0, 95939^0, 95940^0, 95955^1, 96360^1, 96361^1, 96365^1, 96366^1, 96367^1, 96368^1, 96372^1, 96374^1, 96375^1, 96376^1, 96377^1, 96523^0, 99155^0, 99156^0, 99157^0, 99211^1, 99212^1, 99213^1, 99214^1, 99215^1, 99217^1, 99218^1,

0 = Modifier usage not allowed or inappropriate 1 = Modifier usage allowed

Code 1	Code 2
	99219[1], 99220[1], 99221[1], 99222[1], 99223[1], 99231[1], 99232[1], 99233[1], 99234[1], 99235[1], 99236[1], 99238[1], 99239[1], 99241[1], 99242[1], 99243[1], 99244[1], 99245[1], 99251[1], 99252[1], 99253[1], 99254[1], 99255[1], 99291[1], 99292[1], 99304[1], 99305[1], 99306[1], 99307[1], 99308[1], 99309[1], 99310[1], 99315[1], 99316[1], 99334[1], 99335[1], 99336[1], 99337[1], 99347[1], 99348[1], 99349[1], 99350[1], 99374[1], 99375[1], 99377[1], 99378[1], 99446[0], 99447[0], 99448[0], 99449[0], 99451[0], 99452[0], 99495[0], 99496[0], G0453[0], G0463[1], G0471[1]
61702	0213T[0], 0216T[0], 0228T[0], 0230T[0], 0333T[0], 0464T[0], 12001[1], 12002[1], 12004[1], 12005[1], 12006[1], 12007[1], 12011[1], 12013[1], 12014[1], 12015[1], 12016[1], 12017[1], 12018[1], 12020[1], 12021[1], 12031[1], 12032[1], 12034[1], 12035[1], 12036[1], 12037[1], 12041[1], 12042[1], 12044[1], 12045[1], 12046[1], 12047[1], 12051[1], 12052[1], 12053[1], 12054[1], 12055[1], 12056[1], 12057[1], 13100[1], 13101[1], 13102[1], 13120[1], 13121[1], 13122[1], 13131[1], 13132[1], 13133[1], 13151[1], 13152[1], 13153[1], 35702[1], 35703[1], 36000[1], 36400[1], 36405[1], 36406[1], 36410[1], 36420[1], 36425[1], 36430[1], 36440[1], 36591[0], 36592[0], 36600[1], 36640[1], 43752[1], 51701[1], 51702[1], 51703[1], 61304[1], 61312[1], 61313[1], 61340[1], 62320[0], 62321[0], 62322[0], 62323[0], 62324[0], 62325[0], 62326[0], 62327[0], 64400[0], 64405[0], 64408[0], 64415[0], 64416[0], 64417[0], 64418[0], 64420[0], 64421[0], 64425[0], 64430[0], 64435[0], 64445[0], 64446[0], 64447[0], 64448[0], 64449[0], 64450[0], 64451[0], 64454[0], 64461[0], 64462[0], 64463[0], 64479[0], 64480[0], 64483[0], 64484[0], 64486[0], 64487[0], 64488[0], 64489[0], 64490[0], 64491[0], 64492[0], 64493[0], 64494[0], 64495[0], 64505[0], 64510[0], 64517[0], 64520[0], 64530[0], 92012[1], 92014[1], 92585[0], 93000[1], 93005[1], 93010[1], 93040[1], 93041[1], 93042[1], 93318[1], 93355[1], 94002[1], 94200[1], 94250[1], 94680[1], 94681[1], 94690[1], 94770[1], 95812[1], 95813[1], 95816[1], 95819[1], 95822[0], 95829[1], 95860[0], 95861[0], 95863[0], 95864[0], 95865[0], 95866[0], 95867[0], 95868[0], 95869[0], 95870[0], 95907[0], 95908[0], 95909[0], 95910[0], 95911[0], 95912[0], 95913[0], 95925[0], 95926[0], 95927[0], 95928[0], 95929[0], 95930[0], 95933[0], 95937[0], 95938[0], 95939[0], 95940[0], 95955[1], 96360[1], 96361[1], 96365[1], 96366[1], 96367[1], 96368[1], 96372[1], 96374[1], 96375[1], 96376[1], 96377[1], 96523[0], 99155[0], 99156[0], 99157[0], 99211[1], 99212[1], 99213[1], 99214[1], 99215[1], 99217[1], 99218[1], 99219[1], 99220[1], 99221[1], 99222[1], 99223[1], 99231[1], 99232[1], 99233[1], 99234[1], 99235[1], 99236[1], 99238[1], 99239[1], 99241[1], 99242[1], 99243[1], 99244[1], 99245[1], 99251[1], 99252[1], 99253[1], 99254[1], 99255[1], 99291[1], 99292[1], 99304[1], 99305[1], 99306[1], 99307[1], 99308[1], 99309[1], 99310[1], 99315[1], 99316[1], 99334[1], 99335[1], 99336[1], 99337[1], 99347[1], 99348[1], 99349[1], 99350[1], 99374[1], 99375[1], 99377[1], 99378[1], 99446[0], 99447[0], 99448[0], 99449[0], 99451[0], 99452[0], 99495[0], 99496[0], G0453[0], G0463[1], G0471[1]
61703	0213T[0], 0216T[0], 0228T[0], 0230T[0], 0333T[0], 0464T[0], 12001[1], 12002[1], 12004[1], 12005[1], 12006[1], 12007[1], 12011[1], 12013[1], 12014[1], 12015[1], 12016[1], 12017[1], 12018[1], 12020[1], 12021[1], 12031[1], 12032[1], 12034[1], 12035[1], 12036[1], 12037[1], 12041[1], 12042[1], 12044[1], 12045[1], 12046[1], 12047[1], 12051[1], 12052[1], 12053[1], 12054[1], 12055[1], 12056[1], 12057[1], 13100[1], 13101[1], 13102[1], 13120[1], 13121[1], 13122[1], 13131[1], 13132[1], 13133[1], 13151[1], 13152[1], 13153[1], 35701[1], 35702[1], 35703[1], 36000[1], 36400[1], 36405[1], 36406[1], 36410[1], 36420[1], 36425[1], 36430[1], 36440[1], 36591[0], 36592[0], 36600[1], 36640[1], 43752[1], 51701[1], 51702[1], 51703[1], 61705[1], 61710[1], 62320[0], 62321[0], 62322[0], 62323[0], 62324[0], 62325[0], 62326[0], 62327[0], 64400[0], 64405[0], 64408[0], 64415[0], 64416[0], 64417[0], 64418[0], 64420[0], 64421[0], 64425[0], 64430[0], 64435[0], 64445[0], 64446[0], 64447[0], 64448[0], 64449[0], 64450[0], 64451[0], 64454[0], 64461[0], 64462[0], 64463[0], 64479[0], 64480[0], 64483[0], 64484[0], 64486[0], 64487[0], 64488[0], 64489[0], 64490[0], 64491[0], 64492[0], 64493[0], 64494[0], 64495[0], 64505[0], 64510[0], 64517[0], 64520[0], 64530[0], 92012[1], 92014[1], 92585[0], 93000[1], 93005[1], 93010[1], 93040[1], 93041[1], 93042[1], 93318[1], 93355[1], 94002[1], 94200[1], 94250[1], 94680[1], 94681[1], 94690[1], 94770[1], 95812[1], 95813[1], 95816[1], 95819[1], 95822[0], 95829[1], 95860[0], 95861[0], 95863[0], 95864[0], 95865[0], 95866[0], 95867[0], 95868[0], 95869[0], 95870[0], 95907[0], 95908[0], 95909[0], 95910[0], 95911[0], 95912[0], 95913[0], 95925[0], 95926[0], 95927[0], 95928[0], 95929[0], 95930[0], 95933[0], 95937[0], 95938[0], 95939[0], 95940[0], 95955[1], 96360[1], 96361[1], 96365[1], 96366[1], 96367[1], 96368[1], 96372[1], 96374[1], 96375[1], 96376[1], 96377[1], 96523[0], 99155[0], 99156[0], 99157[0], 99211[1], 99212[1], 99213[1], 99214[1], 99215[1], 99217[1], 99218[1], 99219[1], 99220[1], 99221[1], 99222[1], 99223[1], 99231[1], 99232[1], 99233[1], 99234[1], 99235[1], 99236[1], 99238[1], 99239[1], 99241[1], 99242[1], 99243[1], 99244[1], 99245[1], 99251[1], 99252[1], 99253[1], 99254[1], 99255[1], 99291[1], 99292[1], 99304[1], 99305[1], 99306[1], 99307[1], 99308[1], 99309[1], 99310[1], 99315[1], 99316[1], 99334[1], 99335[1], 99336[1], 99337[1], 99347[1], 99348[1], 99349[1], 99350[1], 99374[1], 99375[1], 99377[1], 99378[1], 99446[0], 99447[0], 99448[0], 99449[0], 99451[0], 99452[0], 99495[0], 99496[0], G0453[0], G0463[1], G0471[1]
61705	0213T[0], 0216T[0], 0228T[0], 0230T[0], 0333T[0], 0464T[0], 12001[1], 12002[1], 12004[1], 12005[1], 12006[1], 12007[1], 12011[1], 12013[1], 12014[1], 12015[1], 12016[1], 12017[1], 12018[1], 12020[1], 12021[1], 12031[1], 12032[1], 12034[1], 12035[1], 12036[1], 12037[1], 12041[1], 12042[1], 12044[1], 12045[1], 12046[1], 12047[1], 12051[1], 12052[1], 12053[1], 12054[1], 12055[1], 12056[1], 12057[1], 13100[1], 13101[1], 13102[1], 13120[1], 13121[1], 13122[1], 13131[1], 13132[1], 13133[1], 13151[1], 13152[1], 13153[1], 35701[1], 35702[1], 35703[1], 36000[1], 36400[1], 36405[1], 36406[1], 36410[1], 36420[1], 36425[1], 36430[1], 36440[1], 36591[0], 36592[0], 36600[1], 36640[1], 43752[1], 51701[1], 51702[1], 51703[1], 61304[1], 61312[1], 61313[1], 61340[1], 62320[0], 62321[0], 62322[0], 62323[0], 62324[0], 62325[0], 62326[0], 62327[0], 64400[0], 64405[0], 64408[0], 64415[0], 64416[0], 64417[0], 64418[0], 64420[0], 64421[0], 64425[0], 64430[0], 64435[0], 64445[0], 64446[0], 64447[0], 64448[0], 64449[0], 64450[0], 64451[0], 64454[0], 64461[0], 64462[0], 64463[0], 64479[0], 64480[0], 64483[0], 64484[0], 64486[0], 64487[0], 64488[0], 64489[0], 64490[0], 64491[0], 64492[0], 64493[0], 64494[0], 64495[0], 64505[0], 64510[0], 64517[0], 64520[0], 64530[0], 92012[1], 92014[1], 92585[0], 93000[1], 93005[1], 93010[1], 93040[1], 93041[1], 93042[1], 93318[1], 93355[1], 94002[1], 94200[1], 94250[1], 94680[1], 94681[1], 94690[1], 94770[1], 95812[1], 95813[1], 95816[1], 95819[1], 95822[0], 95829[1], 95860[0], 95861[0], 95863[0], 95864[0], 95865[0], 95866[0], 95867[0], 95868[0], 95869[0], 95870[0], 95907[0], 95908[0], 95909[0], 95910[0], 95911[0], 95912[0], 95913[0], 95925[0], 95926[0], 95927[0], 95928[0], 95929[0], 95930[0], 95933[0], 95937[0], 95938[0], 95939[0], 95940[0], 95955[1], 96360[1], 96361[1], 96365[1], 96366[1], 96367[1], 96368[1], 96372[1], 96374[1], 96375[1], 96376[1], 96377[1], 96523[0], 99155[0], 99156[0], 99157[0], 99211[1], 99212[1], 99213[1], 99214[1], 99215[1], 99217[1], 99218[1], 99219[1], 99220[1], 99221[1], 99222[1], 99223[1], 99231[1], 99232[1], 99233[1], 99234[1], 99235[1], 99236[1], 99238[1], 99239[1], 99241[1], 99242[1], 99243[1], 99244[1], 99245[1], 99251[1], 99252[1], 99253[1], 99254[1], 99255[1], 99291[1], 99292[1], 99304[1], 99305[1], 99306[1], 99307[1], 99308[1], 99309[1], 99310[1], 99315[1], 99316[1], 99334[1], 99335[1], 99336[1], 99337[1], 99347[1], 99348[1], 99349[1], 99350[1], 99374[1], 99375[1], 99377[1], 99378[1], 99446[0], 99447[0], 99448[0], 99449[0], 99451[0], 99452[0], 99495[0], 99496[0], G0453[0], G0463[1], G0471[1]
61708	0213T[0], 0216T[0], 0228T[0], 0230T[0], 0333T[0], 0464T[0], 12001[1], 12002[1], 12004[1], 12005[1], 12006[1], 12007[1], 12011[1], 12013[1], 12014[1], 12015[1], 12016[1], 12017[1], 12018[1], 12020[1], 12021[1], 12031[1], 12032[1], 12034[1], 12035[1], 12036[1], 12037[1], 12041[1], 12042[1], 12044[1], 12045[1], 12046[1], 12047[1], 12051[1], 12052[1], 12053[1], 12054[1], 12055[1], 12056[1], 12057[1], 13100[1], 13101[1], 13102[1], 13120[1], 13121[1], 13122[1], 13131[1], 13132[1], 13133[1], 13151[1], 13152[1], 13153[1], 35702[1], 35703[1], 36000[1], 36400[1], 36405[1], 36406[1], 36410[1], 36420[1], 36425[1], 36430[1], 36440[1], 36591[0], 36592[0], 36600[1], 36640[1], 43752[1], 51701[1], 51702[1], 51703[1], 61304[1], 61312[1], 61313[1], 61340[1], 61705[1], 62320[0], 62321[0], 62322[0], 62323[0], 62324[0], 62325[0], 62326[0], 62327[0], 64400[0], 64405[0], 64408[0], 64415[0], 64416[0], 64417[0], 64418[0], 64420[0], 64421[0], 64425[0], 64430[0], 64435[0], 64445[0], 64446[0], 64447[0], 64448[0], 64449[0], 64450[0], 64451[0], 64454[0], 64461[0], 64462[0], 64463[0], 64479[0], 64480[0], 64483[0], 64484[0], 64486[0], 64487[0], 64488[0], 64489[0], 64490[0], 64491[0], 64492[0], 64493[0], 64494[0], 64495[0], 64505[0], 64510[0], 64517[0], 64520[0], 64530[0], 92012[1], 92014[1], 92585[0], 93000[1], 93005[1], 93010[1], 93040[1], 93041[1], 93042[1], 93318[1], 93355[1], 94002[1], 94200[1], 94250[1], 94680[1], 94681[1], 94690[1], 94770[1], 95812[1], 95813[1], 95816[1], 95819[1], 95822[0], 95829[1], 95860[0], 95861[0], 95863[0], 95864[0], 95865[0], 95866[0], 95867[0], 95868[0], 95869[0], 95870[0], 95907[0], 95908[0], 95909[0], 95910[0], 95911[0], 95912[0], 95913[0], 95925[0], 95926[0], 95927[0], 95928[0], 95929[0], 95930[0], 95933[0], 95937[0], 95938[0], 95939[0], 95940[0], 95955[1], 96360[1], 96361[1], 96365[1], 96366[1], 96367[1], 96368[1], 96372[1], 96374[1], 96375[1], 96376[1], 96377[1], 96523[0], 99155[0], 99156[0], 99157[0], 99211[1], 99212[1], 99213[1], 99214[1], 99215[1], 99217[1], 99218[1], 99219[1], 99220[1], 99221[1], 99222[1], 99223[1], 99231[1], 99232[1], 99233[1], 99234[1], 99235[1], 99236[1], 99238[1], 99239[1], 99241[1], 99242[1], 99243[1], 99244[1], 99245[1], 99251[1], 99252[1], 99253[1], 99254[1], 99255[1], 99291[1], 99292[1], 99304[1], 99305[1], 99306[1], 99307[1], 99308[1], 99309[1], 99310[1], 99315[1], 99316[1], 99334[1], 99335[1], 99336[1], 99337[1], 99347[1], 99348[1], 99349[1], 99350[1], 99374[1], 99375[1], 99377[1], 99378[1], 99446[0], 99447[0], 99448[0], 99449[0], 99451[0], 99452[0], 99495[0], 99496[0], G0453[0], G0463[1], G0471[1]
61710	0213T[0], 0216T[0], 0228T[0], 0230T[0], 0333T[0], 0464T[0], 12001[1], 12002[1], 12004[1], 12005[1], 12006[1], 12007[1], 12011[1], 12013[1], 12014[1], 12015[1], 12016[1], 12017[1], 12018[1], 12020[1], 12021[1], 12031[1], 12032[1], 12034[1], 12035[1], 12036[1], 12037[1], 12041[1], 12042[1], 12044[1], 12045[1], 12046[1], 12047[1], 12051[1], 12052[1], 12053[1], 12054[1], 12055[1], 12056[1], 12057[1], 13100[1], 13101[1], 13102[1], 13120[1], 13121[1], 13122[1], 13131[1], 13132[1], 13133[1], 13151[1], 13152[1], 13153[1], 36000[1], 36400[1], 36405[1], 36406[1], 36410[1], 36420[1], 36425[1], 36430[1], 36440[1], 36591[0], 36592[0], 36600[1], 36640[1], 37241[1], 37242[1], 37244[1], 43752[1], 51701[1], 51702[1], 51703[1], 61304[1], 61312[1], 61313[1], 61340[1], 61705[1], 61708[1], 62320[0], 62321[0], 62322[0], 62323[0], 62324[0], 62325[0], 62326[0], 62327[0], 64400[0], 64405[0], 64408[0], 64415[0], 64416[0], 64417[0], 64418[0], 64420[0], 64421[0], 64425[0], 64430[0], 64435[0], 64445[0], 64446[0], 64447[0], 64448[0], 64449[0], 64450[0], 64451[0], 64454[0], 64461[0], 64462[0], 64463[0], 64479[0], 64480[0], 64483[0], 64484[0], 64486[0], 64487[0], 64488[0], 64489[0], 64490[0], 64491[0], 64492[0], 64493[0], 64494[0], 64495[0], 64505[0], 64510[0], 64517[0], 64520[0], 64530[0], 92012[1], 92014[1], 92585[0], 93000[1], 93005[1], 93010[1], 93040[1], 93041[1], 93042[1], 93318[1], 93355[1], 94002[1], 94200[1], 94250[1], 94680[1], 94681[1], 94690[1], 94770[1], 95812[1], 95813[1], 95816[1], 95819[1], 95822[0], 95829[1], 95860[0], 95861[0], 95863[0], 95864[0], 95865[0], 95866[0], 95867[0], 95868[0], 95869[0], 95870[0], 95907[0], 95908[0], 95909[0], 95910[0], 95911[0], 95912[0], 95913[0], 95925[0], 95926[0], 95927[0], 95928[0], 95929[0], 95930[0], 95933[0], 95937[0], 95938[0], 95939[0], 95940[0], 95955[1], 96360[1], 96361[1], 96365[1], 96366[1], 96367[1], 96368[1], 96372[1], 96374[1], 96375[1], 96376[1], 96377[1], 96523[0], 99155[0], 99156[0], 99157[0], 99211[1], 99212[1], 99213[1], 99214[1], 99215[1], 99217[1], 99218[1], 99219[1], 99220[1], 99221[1], 99222[1], 99223[1], 99231[1], 99232[1],

0 = Modifier usage not allowed or inappropriate 1 = Modifier usage allowed

Code 1	Code 2
	99233[1], 99234[1], 99235[1], 99236[1], 99238[1], 99239[1], 99241[1], 99242[1], 99243[1], 99244[1], 99245[1], 99251[1], 99252[1], 99253[1], 99254[1], 99255[1], 99291[1], 99292[1], 99304[1], 99305[1], 99306[1], 99307[1], 99308[1], 99309[1], 99310[1], 99315[1], 99316[1], 99334[1], 99335[1], 99336[1], 99337[1], 99347[1], 99348[1], 99349[1], 99350[1], 99374[1], 99375[1], 99377[1], 99378[1], 99446[0], 99447[0], 99448[0], 99449[0], 99451[0], 99452[0], 99495[0], 99496[0], G0453[0], G0463[1], G0471[1]
61711	0213T[0], 0216T[0], 0228T[0], 0230T[0], 0333T[0], 0464T[0], 12001[1], 12002[1], 12004[1], 12005[1], 12006[1], 12007[1], 12011[1], 12013[1], 12014[1], 12015[1], 12016[1], 12017[1], 12018[1], 12020[1], 12021[1], 12031[1], 12032[1], 12034[1], 12035[1], 12036[1], 12037[1], 12041[1], 12042[1], 12044[1], 12045[1], 12046[1], 12047[1], 12051[1], 12052[1], 12053[1], 12054[1], 12055[1], 12056[1], 12057[1], 13100[1], 13101[1], 13102[1], 13120[1], 13121[1], 13122[1], 13131[1], 13132[1], 13133[1], 13151[1], 13152[1], 13153[1], 35702[1], 35703[1], 36000[1], 36400[1], 36405[1], 36406[1], 36410[1], 36420[1], 36425[1], 36430[1], 36440[1], 36591[0], 36592[0], 36600[1], 36640[1], 43752[1], 51701[1], 51702[1], 51703[1], 61304[1], 61312[1], 61313[1], 61340[1], 62320[0], 62321[0], 62322[0], 62323[0], 62324[0], 62325[0], 62326[0], 62327[0], 64400[0], 64405[0], 64408[0], 64415[0], 64416[0], 64417[0], 64418[0], 64420[0], 64421[0], 64425[0], 64430[0], 64435[0], 64445[0], 64446[0], 64447[0], 64448[0], 64449[0], 64450[0], 64451[0], 64454[0], 64461[0], 64462[0], 64463[0], 64479[0], 64480[0], 64483[0], 64484[0], 64486[0], 64487[0], 64488[0], 64489[0], 64490[0], 64491[0], 64492[0], 64493[0], 64494[0], 64495[0], 64505[0], 64510[0], 64517[0], 64520[0], 64530[0], 92012[1], 92014[1], 92585[0], 93000[1], 93005[1], 93010[1], 93040[1], 93041[1], 93042[1], 93318[1], 93355[1], 94002[1], 94200[1], 94250[1], 94680[1], 94681[1], 94690[1], 94770[1], 95812[1], 95813[1], 95816[1], 95819[1], 95822[0], 95829[1], 95860[0], 95861[0], 95863[0], 95864[0], 95865[0], 95866[0], 95867[0], 95868[0], 95869[0], 95870[0], 95907[0], 95908[0], 95909[0], 95910[0], 95911[0], 95912[0], 95913[0], 95925[0], 95926[0], 95927[0], 95928[0], 95929[0], 95930[0], 95933[0], 95937[0], 95938[0], 95939[0], 95940[0], 95955[1], 96360[1], 96361[1], 96365[1], 96366[1], 96367[1], 96368[1], 96372[1], 96374[1], 96375[1], 96376[1], 96377[1], 96523[0], 99155[0], 99156[0], 99157[0], 99211[1], 99212[1], 99213[1], 99214[1], 99215[1], 99217[1], 99218[1], 99219[1], 99220[1], 99221[1], 99222[1], 99223[1], 99231[1], 99232[1], 99233[1], 99234[1], 99235[1], 99236[1], 99238[1], 99239[1], 99241[1], 99242[1], 99243[1], 99244[1], 99245[1], 99251[1], 99252[1], 99253[1], 99254[1], 99255[1], 99291[1], 99292[1], 99304[1], 99305[1], 99306[1], 99307[1], 99308[1], 99309[1], 99310[1], 99315[1], 99316[1], 99334[1], 99335[1], 99336[1], 99337[1], 99347[1], 99348[1], 99349[1], 99350[1], 99374[1], 99375[1], 99377[1], 99378[1], 99446[0], 99447[0], 99448[0], 99449[0], 99451[0], 99452[0], 99495[0], 99496[0], G0453[0], G0463[1], G0471[1]
61720	0213T[0], 0216T[0], 0228T[0], 0230T[0], 0333T[0], 0464T[0], 12001[1], 12002[1], 12004[1], 12005[1], 12006[1], 12007[1], 12011[1], 12013[1], 12014[1], 12015[1], 12016[1], 12017[1], 12018[1], 12020[1], 12021[1], 12031[1], 12032[1], 12034[1], 12035[1], 12036[1], 12037[1], 12041[1], 12042[1], 12044[1], 12045[1], 12046[1], 12047[1], 12051[1], 12052[1], 12053[1], 12054[1], 12055[1], 12056[1], 12057[1], 13100[1], 13101[1], 13102[1], 13120[1], 13121[1], 13122[1], 13131[1], 13132[1], 13133[1], 13151[1], 13152[1], 13153[1], 20660[0], 20661[1], 36000[1], 36400[1], 36405[1], 36406[1], 36410[1], 36420[1], 36425[1], 36430[1], 36440[1], 36591[0], 36592[0], 36600[1], 36640[1], 43752[1], 51701[1], 51702[1], 51703[1], 61531[1], 61533[1], 61535[1], 61735[1], 61781[1], 61782[1], 61783[0], 61796[1], 61797[1], 61798[1], 61799[1], 61863[0], 62100[1], 62320[0], 62321[0], 62322[0], 62323[0], 62324[0], 62325[0], 62326[0], 62327[0], 63620[1], 64400[0], 64405[0], 64408[0], 64415[0], 64416[0], 64417[0], 64418[0], 64420[0], 64421[0], 64425[0], 64430[0], 64435[0], 64445[0], 64446[0], 64447[0], 64448[0], 64449[0], 64450[0], 64451[0], 64454[0], 64461[0], 64462[0], 64463[0], 64479[0], 64480[0], 64483[0], 64484[0], 64486[0], 64487[0], 64488[0], 64489[0], 64490[0], 64491[0], 64492[0], 64493[0], 64494[0], 64495[0], 64505[0], 64510[0], 64517[0], 64520[0], 64530[0], 69990[0], 77372[1], 92012[1], 92014[1], 92585[0], 93000[1], 93005[1], 93010[1], 93040[1], 93041[1], 93042[1], 93318[1], 93355[1], 94002[1], 94200[1], 94250[1], 94680[1], 94681[1], 94690[1], 94770[1], 95812[1], 95813[1], 95816[1], 95819[1], 95822[0], 95829[1], 95860[0], 95861[0], 95863[0], 95864[0], 95865[0], 95866[0], 95867[0], 95868[0], 95869[0], 95870[0], 95907[0], 95908[0], 95909[0], 95910[0], 95911[0], 95912[0], 95913[0], 95925[0], 95926[0], 95927[0], 95928[0], 95929[0], 95930[0], 95933[0], 95937[0], 95938[0], 95939[0], 95940[0], 95955[1], 96360[1], 96361[1], 96365[1], 96366[1], 96367[1], 96368[1], 96372[1], 96374[1], 96375[1], 96376[1], 96377[1], 96523[0], 99155[0], 99156[0], 99157[0], 99211[1], 99212[1], 99213[1], 99214[1], 99215[1], 99217[1], 99218[1], 99219[1], 99220[1], 99221[1], 99222[1], 99223[1], 99231[1], 99232[1], 99233[1], 99234[1], 99235[1], 99236[1], 99238[1], 99239[1], 99241[1], 99242[1], 99243[1], 99244[1], 99245[1], 99251[1], 99252[1], 99253[1], 99254[1], 99255[1], 99291[1], 99292[1], 99304[1], 99305[1], 99306[1], 99307[1], 99308[1], 99309[1], 99310[1], 99315[1], 99316[1], 99334[1], 99335[1], 99336[1], 99337[1], 99347[1], 99348[1], 99349[1], 99350[1], 99374[1], 99375[1], 99377[1], 99378[1], 99446[0], 99447[0], 99448[0], 99449[0], 99451[0], 99452[0], 99495[0], 99496[0], G0339[1], G0340[1], G0453[0], G0463[1], G0471[1]
61735	0213T[0], 0216T[0], 0228T[0], 0230T[0], 0333T[0], 0464T[0], 12001[1], 12002[1], 12004[1], 12005[1], 12006[1], 12007[1], 12011[1], 12013[1], 12014[1], 12015[1], 12016[1], 12017[1], 12018[1], 12020[1], 12021[1], 12031[1], 12032[1], 12034[1], 12035[1], 12036[1], 12037[1], 12041[1], 12042[1], 12044[1], 12045[1], 12046[1], 12047[1], 12051[1], 12052[1], 12053[1], 12054[1], 12055[1], 12056[1], 12057[1], 13100[1], 13101[1], 13102[1], 13120[1], 13121[1], 13122[1], 13131[1], 13132[1], 13133[1], 13151[1], 13152[1], 13153[1], 20660[0], 20661[1], 36000[1], 36400[1], 36405[1], 36406[1], 36410[1], 36420[1], 36425[1], 36430[1], 36440[1], 36591[0], 36592[0], 36600[1], 36640[1], 43752[1], 51701[1], 51702[1], 51703[1], 61531[1], 61533[1], 61535[1], 61781[1], 61782[1], 61783[0], 61796[1], 61797[1], 61798[1], 61799[1], 61863[0], 62100[1], 62320[0], 62321[0], 62322[0], 62323[0], 62324[0], 62325[0], 62326[0], 62327[0], 64400[0], 64405[0], 64408[0], 64415[0], 64416[0], 64417[0], 64418[0], 64420[0], 64421[0], 64425[0], 64430[0], 64435[0], 64445[0], 64446[0], 64447[0], 64448[0], 64449[0], 64450[0], 64451[0], 64454[0], 64461[0], 64462[0], 64463[0], 64479[0], 64480[0], 64483[0], 64484[0], 64486[0], 64487[0], 64488[0], 64489[0], 64490[0], 64491[0], 64492[0], 64493[0], 64494[0], 64495[0], 64505[0], 64510[0], 64517[0], 64520[0], 64530[0], 69990[0], 77371[1], 77372[1], 92012[1], 92014[1], 92585[0], 93000[1], 93005[1], 93010[1], 93040[1], 93041[1], 93042[1], 93318[1], 93355[1], 94002[1], 94200[1], 94250[1], 94680[1], 94681[1], 94690[1], 94770[1], 95812[1], 95813[1], 95816[1], 95819[1], 95822[0], 95829[1], 95860[0], 95861[0], 95863[0], 95864[0], 95865[0], 95866[0], 95867[0], 95868[0], 95869[0], 95870[0], 95907[0], 95908[0], 95909[0], 95910[0], 95911[0], 95912[0], 95913[0], 95925[0], 95926[0], 95927[0], 95928[0], 95929[0], 95930[0], 95933[0], 95937[0], 95938[0], 95939[0], 95940[0], 95955[1], 96360[1], 96361[1], 96365[1], 96366[1], 96367[1], 96368[1], 96372[1], 96374[1], 96375[1], 96376[1], 96377[1], 96523[0], 99155[0], 99156[0], 99157[0], 99211[1], 99212[1], 99213[1], 99214[1], 99215[1], 99217[1], 99218[1], 99219[1], 99220[1], 99221[1], 99222[1], 99223[1], 99231[1], 99232[1], 99233[1], 99234[1], 99235[1], 99236[1], 99238[1], 99239[1], 99241[1], 99242[1], 99243[1], 99244[1], 99245[1], 99251[1], 99252[1], 99253[1], 99254[1], 99255[1], 99291[1], 99292[1], 99304[1], 99305[1], 99306[1], 99307[1], 99308[1], 99309[1], 99310[1], 99315[1], 99316[1], 99334[1], 99335[1], 99336[1], 99337[1], 99347[1], 99348[1], 99349[1], 99350[1], 99374[1], 99375[1], 99377[1], 99378[1], 99446[0], 99447[0], 99448[0], 99449[0], 99451[0], 99452[0], 99495[0], 99496[0], G0453[0], G0463[1], G0471[1]
61750	0213T[0], 0216T[0], 0228T[0], 0230T[0], 0333T[0], 0464T[0], 10005[1], 10007[1], 10009[1], 10011[1], 10021[1], 11000[1], 11001[1], 11004[1], 11005[1], 11006[1], 11042[1], 11043[1], 11044[1], 11045[1], 11046[1], 11047[1], 12001[1], 12002[1], 12004[1], 12005[1], 12006[1], 12007[1], 12011[1], 12013[1], 12014[1], 12015[1], 12016[1], 12017[1], 12018[1], 12020[1], 12021[1], 12031[1], 12032[1], 12034[1], 12035[1], 12036[1], 12037[1], 12041[1], 12042[1], 12044[1], 12045[1], 12046[1], 12047[1], 12051[1], 12052[1], 12053[1], 12054[1], 12055[1], 12056[1], 12057[1], 13100[1], 13101[1], 13102[1], 13120[1], 13121[1], 13122[1], 13131[1], 13132[1], 13133[1], 13151[1], 13152[1], 13153[1], 20660[0], 20661[1], 36000[1], 36400[1], 36405[1], 36406[1], 36410[1], 36420[1], 36425[1], 36430[1], 36440[1], 36591[0], 36592[0], 36600[1], 36640[1], 43752[1], 51701[1], 51702[1], 51703[1], 61140[0], 61156[0], 61531[1], 61533[1], 61534[1], 61535[1], 61536[1], 61537[1], 61538[1], 61539[1], 61540[1], 61541[1], 61543[1], 61544[1], 61545[1], 61566[1], 61567[1], 61781[1], 61782[1], 61783[0], 61796[1], 61798[1], 61863[0], 62100[1], 62320[0], 62321[0], 62322[0], 62323[0], 62324[0], 62325[0], 62326[0], 62327[0], 63620[1], 64400[0], 64405[0], 64408[0], 64415[0], 64416[0], 64417[0], 64418[0], 64420[0], 64421[0], 64425[0], 64430[0], 64435[0], 64445[0], 64446[0], 64447[0], 64448[0], 64449[0], 64450[0], 64451[0], 64454[0], 64461[0], 64462[0], 64463[0], 64479[0], 64480[0], 64483[0], 64484[0], 64486[0], 64487[0], 64488[0], 64489[0], 64490[0], 64491[0], 64492[0], 64493[0], 64494[0], 64495[0], 64505[0], 64510[0], 64517[0], 64520[0], 64530[0], 69990[0], 77371[1], 77372[1], 77373[1], 92012[1], 92014[1], 92585[0], 93000[1], 93005[1], 93010[1], 93040[1], 93041[1], 93042[1], 93318[1], 93355[1], 94002[1], 94200[1], 94250[1], 94680[1], 94681[1], 94690[1], 94770[1], 95812[1], 95813[1], 95816[1], 95819[1], 95822[0], 95829[1], 95860[0], 95861[0], 95863[0], 95864[0], 95865[0], 95866[0], 95867[0], 95868[0], 95869[0], 95870[0], 95907[0], 95908[0], 95909[0], 95910[0], 95911[0], 95912[0], 95913[0], 95925[0], 95926[0], 95927[0], 95928[0], 95929[0], 95930[0], 95933[0], 95937[0], 95938[0], 95939[0], 95940[0], 95955[1], 96360[1], 96361[1], 96365[1], 96366[1], 96367[1], 96368[1], 96372[1], 96374[1], 96375[1], 96376[1], 96377[1], 96523[0], 97597[1], 97598[1], 97602[1], 99155[0], 99156[0], 99157[0], 99211[1], 99212[1], 99213[1], 99214[1], 99215[1], 99217[1], 99218[1], 99219[1], 99220[1], 99221[1], 99222[1], 99223[1], 99231[1], 99232[1], 99233[1], 99234[1], 99235[1], 99236[1], 99238[1], 99239[1], 99241[1], 99242[1], 99243[1], 99244[1], 99245[1], 99251[1], 99252[1], 99253[1], 99254[1], 99255[1], 99291[1], 99292[1], 99304[1], 99305[1], 99306[1], 99307[1], 99308[1], 99309[1], 99310[1], 99315[1], 99316[1], 99334[1], 99335[1], 99336[1], 99337[1], 99347[1], 99348[1], 99349[1], 99350[1], 99374[1], 99375[1], 99377[1], 99378[1], 99446[0], 99447[0], 99448[0], 99449[0], 99451[0], 99452[0], 99495[0], 99496[0], G0339[1], G0340[1], G0453[0], G0463[1], G0471[1]
61751	0213T[0], 0216T[0], 0228T[0], 0230T[0], 0333T[0], 0464T[0], 10005[1], 10007[1], 10009[1], 10011[1], 10021[1], 11000[1], 11001[1], 11004[1], 11005[1], 11006[1], 11042[1], 11043[1], 11044[1], 11045[1], 11046[1], 11047[1], 12001[1], 12002[1], 12004[1], 12005[1], 12006[1], 12007[1], 12011[1], 12013[1], 12014[1], 12015[1], 12016[1], 12017[1], 12018[1], 12020[1], 12021[1], 12031[1], 12032[1], 12034[1], 12035[1], 12036[1], 12037[1], 12041[1], 12042[1], 12044[1], 12045[1], 12046[1], 12047[1], 12051[1], 12052[1], 12053[1], 12054[1], 12055[1], 12056[1], 12057[1], 13100[1], 13101[1], 13102[1], 13120[1], 13121[1], 13122[1], 13131[1], 13132[1], 13133[1], 13151[1], 13152[1], 13153[1], 20660[0], 20661[1], 36000[1], 36400[1], 36405[1], 36406[1], 36410[1], 36420[1], 36425[1], 36430[1], 36440[1], 36591[0], 36592[0], 36600[1], 36640[1], 43752[1], 51701[1], 51702[1], 51703[1], 61140[0], 61156[0], 61531[1], 61533[1], 61534[1], 61535[1], 61536[1], 61537[1], 61538[1], 61539[1], 61540[1], 61541[1], 61543[1], 61544[1], 61545[1], 61566[1], 61567[1], 61750[1], 61781[1], 61782[1], 61783[0], 61796[1], 61798[1], 61863[0], 62100[1], 62320[0], 62321[0], 62322[0], 62323[0], 62324[0], 62325[0], 62326[0], 62327[0], 63620[1], 64400[0], 64405[0], 64408[0], 64415[0], 64416[0], 64417[0], 64418[0], 64420[0], 64421[0], 64425[0], 64430[0], 64435[0], 64445[0], 64446[0], 64447[0], 64448[0], 64449[0], 64450[0], 64451[0],

0 = Modifier usage not allowed or inappropriate 1 = Modifier usage allowed

Appendix A: NCCI - CPT Codes

Code 1	Code 2
	64454[0], 64461[0], 64462[0], 64463[0], 64479[0], 64480[0], 64483[0], 64484[0], 64486[0], 64487[0], 64488[0], 64489[0], 64490[0], 64491[0], 64492[0], 64493[0], 64494[0], 64495[0], 64505[0], 64510[0], 64517[0], 64520[0], 64530[0], 69990[0], 77011[1], 77371[1], 77372[1], 77373[1], 92012[1], 92014[1], 92585[0], 93000[1], 93005[1], 93010[1], 93040[1], 93041[1], 93042[1], 93318[1], 93355[1], 94002[1], 94200[1], 94250[1], 94680[1], 94681[1], 94690[1], 94770[1], 95812[1], 95813[1], 95816[1], 95819[1], 95822[0], 95829[1], 95860[0], 95861[0], 95863[0], 95864[0], 95865[0], 95866[0], 95867[0], 95868[0], 95869[0], 95870[0], 95907[0], 95908[0], 95909[0], 95910[0], 95911[0], 95912[0], 95913[0], 95925[0], 95926[0], 95927[0], 95928[0], 95929[0], 95930[0], 95933[0], 95937[0], 95938[0], 95939[0], 95940[0], 95955[1], 96360[1], 96361[1], 96365[1], 96366[1], 96367[1], 96368[1], 96372[1], 96374[1], 96375[1], 96376[1], 96377[1], 96523[0], 97597[1], 97598[1], 97602[1], 99155[0], 99156[0], 99157[0], 99211[1], 99212[1], 99213[1], 99214[1], 99215[1], 99217[1], 99218[1], 99219[1], 99220[1], 99221[1], 99222[1], 99223[1], 99231[1], 99232[1], 99233[1], 99234[1], 99235[1], 99236[1], 99238[1], 99239[1], 99241[1], 99242[1], 99243[1], 99244[1], 99245[1], 99251[1], 99252[1], 99253[1], 99254[1], 99255[1], 99291[1], 99292[1], 99304[1], 99305[1], 99306[1], 99307[1], 99308[1], 99309[1], 99310[1], 99315[1], 99316[1], 99334[1], 99335[1], 99336[1], 99337[1], 99347[1], 99348[1], 99349[1], 99350[1], 99374[1], 99375[1], 99377[1], 99378[1], 99446[0], 99447[0], 99448[0], 99449[0], 99451[0], 99452[0], 99495[0], 99496[0], G0339[1], G0340[1], G0453[0], G0463[1], G0471[1]
61760	0213T[0], 0216T[0], 0228T[0], 0230T[0], 0333T[0], 0464T[0], 12001[1], 12002[1], 12004[1], 12005[1], 12006[1], 12007[1], 12011[1], 12013[1], 12014[1], 12015[1], 12016[1], 12017[1], 12018[1], 12020[1], 12021[1], 12031[1], 12032[1], 12034[1], 12035[1], 12036[1], 12037[1], 12041[1], 12042[1], 12044[1], 12045[1], 12046[1], 12047[1], 12051[1], 12052[1], 12053[1], 12054[1], 12055[1], 12056[1], 12057[1], 13100[1], 13101[1], 13102[1], 13120[1], 13121[1], 13122[1], 13131[1], 13132[1], 13133[1], 13151[1], 13152[1], 13153[1], 20660[0], 20661[1], 36000[1], 36400[1], 36405[1], 36406[1], 36410[1], 36420[1], 36425[1], 36430[1], 36440[1], 36591[0], 36592[0], 36600[1], 36640[1], 43752[1], 51701[1], 51702[1], 51703[1], 61531[1], 61533[1], 61535[1], 61781[1], 61782[1], 61783[0], 61796[1], 61798[1], 61863[0], 62320[0], 62321[0], 62322[0], 62323[0], 62324[0], 62325[0], 62326[0], 62327[0], 63620[1], 64400[0], 64405[0], 64408[0], 64415[0], 64416[0], 64417[0], 64418[0], 64420[0], 64421[0], 64425[0], 64430[0], 64435[0], 64445[0], 64446[0], 64447[0], 64448[0], 64449[0], 64450[0], 64451[0], 64454[0], 64461[0], 64462[0], 64463[0], 64479[0], 64480[0], 64483[0], 64484[0], 64486[0], 64487[0], 64488[0], 64489[0], 64490[0], 64491[0], 64492[0], 64493[0], 64494[0], 64495[0], 64505[0], 64510[0], 64517[0], 64520[0], 64530[0], 69990[0], 77371[1], 77372[1], 77373[1], 92012[1], 92014[1], 92585[0], 93000[1], 93005[1], 93010[1], 93040[1], 93041[1], 93042[1], 93318[1], 93355[1], 94002[1], 94200[1], 94250[1], 94680[1], 94681[1], 94690[1], 94770[1], 95812[1], 95813[1], 95816[1], 95819[1], 95822[0], 95829[1], 95860[0], 95861[0], 95863[0], 95864[0], 95865[0], 95866[0], 95867[0], 95868[0], 95869[0], 95870[0], 95907[0], 95908[0], 95909[0], 95910[0], 95911[0], 95912[0], 95913[0], 95925[0], 95926[0], 95927[0], 95928[0], 95929[0], 95930[0], 95933[0], 95937[0], 95938[0], 95939[0], 95940[0], 95955[1], 96360[1], 96361[1], 96365[1], 96366[1], 96367[1], 96368[1], 96372[1], 96374[1], 96375[1], 96376[1], 96377[1], 96523[0], 99155[0], 99156[0], 99157[0], 99211[1], 99212[1], 99213[1], 99214[1], 99215[1], 99217[1], 99218[1], 99219[1], 99220[1], 99221[1], 99222[1], 99223[1], 99231[1], 99232[1], 99233[1], 99234[1], 99235[1], 99236[1], 99238[1], 99239[1], 99241[1], 99242[1], 99243[1], 99244[1], 99245[1], 99251[1], 99252[1], 99253[1], 99254[1], 99255[1], 99291[1], 99292[1], 99304[1], 99305[1], 99306[1], 99307[1], 99308[1], 99309[1], 99310[1], 99315[1], 99316[1], 99334[1], 99335[1], 99336[1], 99337[1], 99347[1], 99348[1], 99349[1], 99350[1], 99374[1], 99375[1], 99377[1], 99378[1], 99446[0], 99447[0], 99448[0], 99449[0], 99451[0], 99452[0], 99495[0], 99496[0], G0339[1], G0340[1], G0453[0], G0463[1], G0471[1]
61781	0054T[1], 0055T[1], 0333T[0], 0464T[0], 20660[0], 20661[0], 20985[1], 36591[0], 36592[0], 61782[0], 61783[1], 69990[1], 70557[1], 70558[1], 70559[1], 76380[1], 77012[1], 77021[1], 92585[0], 95822[0], 95860[0], 95861[0], 95863[0], 95864[0], 95865[0], 95866[0], 95867[0], 95868[0], 95869[0], 95870[0], 95907[0], 95908[0], 95909[0], 95910[0], 95911[0], 95912[0], 95913[0], 95925[0], 95926[0], 95927[0], 95928[0], 95929[0], 95930[0], 95933[0], 95937[0], 95938[0], 95939[0], 95940[0], 96523[0], G0453[0]
61782	0054T[1], 0055T[1], 0333T[0], 0464T[0], 20660[0], 20661[0], 20985[1], 36591[0], 36592[0], 69990[1], 70557[1], 70558[1], 70559[1], 76380[1], 77012[1], 77021[1], 92585[0], 95822[0], 95860[0], 95861[0], 95863[0], 95864[0], 95865[0], 95866[0], 95867[0], 95868[0], 95869[0], 95870[0], 95907[0], 95908[0], 95909[0], 95910[0], 95911[0], 95912[0], 95913[0], 95925[0], 95926[0], 95927[0], 95928[0], 95929[0], 95930[0], 95933[0], 95937[0], 95938[0], 95939[0], 95940[0], 96523[0], G0453[0]
61783	0054T[1], 0055T[1], 0333T[0], 0464T[0], 20660[0], 20661[0], 20985[1], 36591[0], 36592[0], 69990[1], 70557[1], 70558[1], 70559[1], 76380[1], 77012[1], 77021[1], 92585[0], 95822[0], 95860[0], 95861[0], 95863[0], 95864[0], 95865[0], 95866[0], 95867[0], 95868[0], 95869[0], 95870[0], 95907[0], 95908[0], 95909[0], 95910[0], 95911[0], 95912[0], 95913[0], 95925[0], 95926[0], 95927[0], 95928[0], 95929[0], 95930[0], 95933[0], 95937[0], 95938[0], 95939[0], 95940[0], 96523[0], G0453[0]
61790	00222[0], 0213T[0], 0216T[0], 0228T[0], 0230T[0], 0333T[0], 0464T[0], 12001[1], 12002[1], 12004[1], 12005[1], 12006[1], 12007[1], 12011[1], 12013[1], 12014[1], 12015[1], 12016[1], 12017[1], 12018[1], 12020[1], 12021[1], 12031[1], 12032[1], 12034[1], 12035[1], 12036[1], 12037[1], 12041[1], 12042[1], 12044[1], 12045[1], 12046[1], 12047[1], 12051[1], 12052[1], 12053[1], 12054[1], 12055[1], 12056[1], 12057[1], 13100[1], 13101[1], 13102[1], 13120[1], 13121[1], 13122[1], 13131[1], 13132[1], 13133[1], 13151[1], 13152[1], 13153[1], 20660[0], 20661[1], 36000[1], 36400[1], 36405[1], 36406[1], 36410[1], 36420[1], 36425[1], 36430[1], 36440[1], 36591[0], 36592[0], 36600[1], 36640[1], 43752[1], 51701[1], 51702[1], 51703[1], 61781[1], 61782[1], 61783[0], 61796[1], 61797[1], 61798[1], 61799[1], 62320[0], 62321[0], 62322[0], 62323[0], 62324[0], 62325[0], 62326[0], 62327[0], 63620[1], 64400[0], 64405[0], 64408[0], 64415[0], 64416[0], 64417[0], 64418[0], 64420[0], 64421[0], 64425[0], 64430[0], 64435[0], 64445[0], 64446[0], 64447[0], 64448[0], 64449[0], 64450[0], 64451[0], 64454[0], 64461[0], 64462[0], 64463[0], 64479[0], 64480[0], 64483[0], 64484[0], 64486[0], 64487[0], 64488[0], 64489[0], 64490[0], 64491[0], 64492[0], 64493[0], 64494[0], 64495[0], 64505[0], 64510[0], 64517[0], 64520[0], 64530[0], 69990[0], 92012[1], 92014[1], 92585[0], 93000[1], 93005[1], 93010[1], 93040[1], 93041[1], 93042[1], 93318[1], 93355[1], 94002[1], 94200[1], 94250[1], 94680[1], 94681[1], 94690[1], 94770[1], 95812[1], 95813[1], 95816[1], 95819[1], 95822[0], 95829[1], 95860[0], 95861[0], 95863[0], 95864[0], 95865[0], 95866[0], 95867[0], 95868[0], 95869[0], 95870[0], 95907[0], 95908[0], 95909[0], 95910[0], 95911[0], 95912[0], 95913[0], 95925[0], 95926[0], 95927[0], 95928[0], 95929[0], 95930[0], 95933[0], 95937[0], 95938[0], 95939[0], 95940[0], 95955[1], 96360[1], 96361[1], 96365[1], 96366[1], 96367[1], 96368[1], 96372[1], 96374[1], 96375[1], 96376[1], 96377[1], 96523[0], 99155[0], 99156[0], 99157[0], 99211[1], 99212[1], 99213[1], 99214[1], 99215[1], 99217[1], 99218[1], 99219[1], 99220[1], 99221[1], 99222[1], 99223[1], 99231[1], 99232[1], 99233[1], 99234[1], 99235[1], 99236[1], 99238[1], 99239[1], 99241[1], 99242[1], 99243[1], 99244[1], 99245[1], 99251[1], 99252[1], 99253[1], 99254[1], 99255[1], 99291[1], 99292[1], 99304[1], 99305[1], 99306[1], 99307[1], 99308[1], 99309[1], 99310[1], 99315[1], 99316[1], 99334[1], 99335[1], 99336[1], 99337[1], 99347[1], 99348[1], 99349[1], 99350[1], 99374[1], 99375[1], 99377[1], 99378[1], 99446[0], 99447[0], 99448[0], 99449[0], 99451[0], 99452[0], 99495[0], 99496[0], G0339[1], G0340[1], G0453[0], G0463[1], G0471[1]
61791	00222[0], 0213T[0], 0216T[0], 0228T[0], 0230T[0], 0333T[0], 0464T[0], 12001[1], 12002[1], 12004[1], 12005[1], 12006[1], 12007[1], 12011[1], 12013[1], 12014[1], 12015[1], 12016[1], 12017[1], 12018[1], 12020[1], 12021[1], 12031[1], 12032[1], 12034[1], 12035[1], 12036[1], 12037[1], 12041[1], 12042[1], 12044[1], 12045[1], 12046[1], 12047[1], 12051[1], 12052[1], 12053[1], 12054[1], 12055[1], 12056[1], 12057[1], 13100[1], 13101[1], 13102[1], 13120[1], 13121[1], 13122[1], 13131[1], 13132[1], 13133[1], 13151[1], 13152[1], 13153[1], 20660[0], 20661[1], 36000[1], 36400[1], 36405[1], 36406[1], 36410[1], 36420[1], 36425[1], 36430[1], 36440[1], 36591[0], 36592[0], 36600[1], 36640[1], 43752[1], 51701[1], 51702[1], 51703[1], 61781[1], 61782[1], 61783[0], 61796[1], 61798[1], 61863[0], 62320[0], 62321[0], 62322[0], 62323[0], 62324[0], 62325[0], 62326[0], 62327[0], 63620[1], 64400[0], 64405[0], 64408[0], 64415[0], 64416[0], 64417[0], 64418[0], 64420[0], 64421[0], 64425[0], 64430[0], 64435[0], 64445[0], 64446[0], 64447[0], 64448[0], 64449[0], 64450[0], 64451[0], 64454[0], 64461[0], 64462[0], 64463[0], 64479[0], 64480[0], 64483[0], 64484[0], 64486[0], 64487[0], 64488[0], 64489[0], 64490[0], 64491[0], 64492[0], 64493[0], 64494[0], 64495[0], 64505[0], 64510[0], 64517[0], 64520[0], 64530[0], 69990[0], 77372[1], 92012[1], 92014[1], 92585[0], 93000[1], 93005[1], 93010[1], 93040[1], 93041[1], 93042[1], 93318[1], 93355[1], 94002[1], 94200[1], 94250[1], 94680[1], 94681[1], 94690[1], 94770[1], 95812[1], 95813[1], 95816[1], 95819[1], 95822[0], 95829[1], 95860[0], 95861[0], 95863[0], 95864[0], 95865[0], 95866[0], 95867[0], 95868[0], 95869[0], 95870[0], 95907[0], 95908[0], 95909[0], 95910[0], 95911[0], 95912[0], 95913[0], 95925[0], 95926[0], 95927[0], 95928[0], 95929[0], 95930[0], 95933[0], 95937[0], 95938[0], 95939[0], 95940[0], 95955[1], 96360[1], 96361[1], 96365[1], 96366[1], 96367[1], 96368[1], 96372[1], 96374[1], 96375[1], 96376[1], 96377[1], 96523[0], 99155[0], 99156[0], 99157[0], 99211[1], 99212[1], 99213[1], 99214[1], 99215[1], 99217[1], 99218[1], 99219[1], 99220[1], 99221[1], 99222[1], 99223[1], 99231[1], 99232[1], 99233[1], 99234[1], 99235[1], 99236[1], 99238[1], 99239[1], 99241[1], 99242[1], 99243[1], 99244[1], 99245[1], 99251[1], 99252[1], 99253[1], 99254[1], 99255[1], 99291[1], 99292[1], 99304[1], 99305[1], 99306[1], 99307[1], 99308[1], 99309[1], 99310[1], 99315[1], 99316[1], 99334[1], 99335[1], 99336[1], 99337[1], 99347[1], 99348[1], 99349[1], 99350[1], 99374[1], 99375[1], 99377[1], 99378[1], 99446[0], 99447[0], 99448[0], 99449[0], 99451[0], 99452[0], 99495[0], 99496[0], G0339[1], G0340[1], G0453[0], G0463[1], G0471[1]
61796	0213T[1], 0216T[1], 0333T[0], 0398T[1], 0464T[0], 12001[1], 12002[1], 12004[1], 12005[1], 12006[1], 12007[1], 12011[1], 12013[1], 12014[1], 12015[1], 12016[1], 12017[1], 12018[1], 12020[1], 12021[1], 12031[1], 12032[1], 12034[1], 12035[1], 12036[1], 12037[1], 12041[1], 12042[1], 12044[1], 12045[1], 12046[1], 12047[1], 12051[1], 12052[1], 12053[1], 12054[1], 12055[1], 12056[1], 12057[1], 13100[1], 13101[1], 13102[1], 13120[1], 13121[1], 13122[1], 13131[1], 13132[1], 13133[1], 13151[1], 13152[1], 13153[1], 20660[0], 20661[1], 20693[1], 20694[1], 36000[1], 36400[1], 36405[1], 36406[1], 36410[1], 36420[1], 36425[1], 36430[1], 36440[1], 36591[0], 36592[0], 36600[1], 36640[1], 43752[1], 51701[1], 51702[1], 51703[1], 61781[0], 61782[0], 61783[0], 61799[0], 62320[0], 62321[0], 62322[0], 62323[0], 62324[0], 62325[0], 62326[0], 62327[0], 64400[0], 64405[0], 64408[0], 64415[1], 64416[1], 64417[1], 64418[0], 64420[0], 64421[0], 64425[0], 64430[0], 64435[0], 64445[0], 64446[0], 64447[0], 64448[0], 64449[0], 64450[1], 64451[0], 64454[1], 64461[0], 64462[0], 64463[0], 64479[0], 64480[0], 64483[0], 64484[0], 64486[0], 64487[0], 64488[0], 64489[0], 64490[1], 64491[0], 64492[0], 64493[1], 64494[0], 64495[0], 64505[0], 64510[0], 64517[0], 64520[0], 64530[0], 69990[0], 77261[0], 77262[0], 77263[0], 77280[0], 77285[0], 77290[0], 77295[0], 77300[0], 77301[0], 77306[0], 77307[0], 77316[0], 77317[0], 77318[0], 77321[0], 77331[0], 77332[0], 77333[0], 77334[0], 77336[0], 77338[0], 77370[0], 77371[0], 77372[0], 77373[0], 77401[0], 77402[0], 77407[0], 77412[0], 77417[0], 77427[0], 77431[0], 77432[0], 77435[0], 77469[0], 77470[0], 92012[1], 92014[1], 92585[0], 93000[1], 93005[1], 93010[1], 93040[1], 93041[1], 93042[1], 93318[1], 93355[1], 94002[1], 94200[1], 94250[1], 94680[1], 94681[1], 94690[1],

0 = Modifier usage not allowed or inappropriate 1 = Modifier usage allowed

Appendix A: NCCI - CPT Codes

Code 1	Code 2
	94770[1], 95812[1], 95813[1], 95816[1], 95819[1], 95822[0], 95829[1], 95860[0], 95861[0], 95863[0], 95864[0], 95865[0], 95866[0], 95867[0], 95868[0], 95869[0], 95870[0], 95907[0], 95908[0], 95909[0], 95910[0], 95911[0], 95912[0], 95913[0], 95925[0], 95926[0], 95927[0], 95928[0], 95929[0], 95930[0], 95933[0], 95937[0], 95938[0], 95939[0], 95940[0], 95955[1], 96360[1], 96361[1], 96365[1], 96366[1], 96367[1], 96368[1], 96372[1], 96374[1], 96375[1], 96376[1], 96377[1], 96523[0], 99155[0], 99156[0], 99157[0], 99211[1], 99212[1], 99213[1], 99214[1], 99215[1], 99217[1], 99218[1], 99219[1], 99220[1], 99221[1], 99222[1], 99223[1], 99231[1], 99232[1], 99233[1], 99234[1], 99235[1], 99236[1], 99238[1], 99239[1], 99241[1], 99242[1], 99243[1], 99244[1], 99245[1], 99251[1], 99252[1], 99253[1], 99254[1], 99255[1], 99291[1], 99292[1], 99304[1], 99305[1], 99306[1], 99307[1], 99308[1], 99309[1], 99310[1], 99315[1], 99316[1], 99334[1], 99335[1], 99336[1], 99337[1], 99347[1], 99348[1], 99349[1], 99350[1], 99374[1], 99375[1], 99377[1], 99378[1], 99446[0], 99447[0], 99448[0], 99449[0], 99451[0], 99452[0], 99495[0], 99496[0], G0339[0], G0340[0], G0453[0], G0463[1], G0471[1], G6002[0], G6003[0], G6004[0], G6005[0], G6006[0], G6007[0], G6008[0], G6009[0], G6010[0], G6011[0], G6012[0], G6013[0], G6014[0], G6015[0], G6016[0], G6017[1]
61797	36591[0], 36592[0], 61781[1], 61782[1], 95863[0], 95864[0], 95865[0], 95866[0], 95869[0], 96523[0]
61798	0213T[1], 0216T[1], 0333T[0], 0398T[1], 0464T[0], 12001[1], 12002[1], 12004[1], 12005[1], 12006[1], 12007[1], 12011[1], 12013[1], 12014[1], 12015[1], 12016[1], 12017[1], 12018[1], 12020[1], 12021[1], 12031[1], 12032[1], 12034[1], 12035[1], 12036[1], 12037[1], 12041[1], 12042[1], 12044[1], 12045[1], 12046[1], 12047[1], 12051[1], 12052[1], 12053[1], 12054[1], 12055[1], 12056[1], 12057[1], 13100[1], 13101[1], 13102[1], 13120[1], 13121[1], 13122[1], 13131[1], 13132[1], 13133[1], 13151[1], 13152[1], 13153[1], 20660[0], 20661[1], 20693[1], 20694[1], 36000[1], 36400[1], 36405[1], 36406[1], 36410[1], 36420[1], 36425[1], 36430[1], 36440[1], 36591[0], 36592[0], 36600[1], 36640[1], 43752[1], 51701[1], 51702[1], 51703[1], 61781[1], 61782[1], 61783[0], 61796[0], 62320[0], 62321[0], 62322[0], 62323[0], 62324[0], 62325[0], 62326[0], 62327[0], 64400[0], 64405[0], 64408[0], 64415[1], 64416[1], 64417[1], 64418[0], 64420[0], 64421[0], 64425[0], 64430[0], 64435[0], 64445[0], 64446[0], 64447[0], 64448[0], 64449[0], 64450[1], 64451[0], 64454[1], 64461[0], 64462[0], 64463[0], 64479[0], 64480[0], 64483[0], 64484[0], 64486[0], 64487[0], 64488[0], 64489[0], 64490[1], 64491[0], 64492[0], 64493[1], 64494[0], 64495[0], 64505[0], 64510[0], 64517[0], 64520[0], 64530[0], 69990[0], 77261[0], 77262[0], 77263[0], 77280[0], 77285[0], 77290[0], 77295[0], 77300[0], 77301[0], 77306[0], 77307[0], 77316[0], 77317[0], 77318[0], 77321[0], 77331[0], 77332[0], 77333[0], 77334[0], 77336[0], 77338[0], 77370[0], 77371[0], 77372[0], 77373[0], 77401[0], 77402[0], 77407[0], 77412[0], 77417[0], 77427[0], 77431[0], 77432[0], 77435[0], 77469[0], 77470[0], 92012[1], 92014[1], 92585[0], 93000[1], 93005[1], 93010[1], 93040[1], 93041[1], 93042[1], 93318[1], 93355[1], 94002[1], 94200[1], 94250[1], 94680[1], 94681[1], 94690[1], 94770[1], 95812[1], 95813[1], 95816[1], 95819[1], 95822[0], 95829[1], 95860[0], 95861[0], 95863[0], 95864[0], 95865[0], 95866[0], 95867[0], 95868[0], 95869[0], 95870[0], 95907[0], 95908[0], 95909[0], 95910[0], 95911[0], 95912[0], 95913[0], 95925[0], 95926[0], 95927[0], 95928[0], 95929[0], 95930[0], 95933[0], 95937[0], 95938[0], 95939[0], 95940[0], 95955[1], 96360[1], 96361[1], 96365[1], 96366[1], 96367[1], 96368[1], 96372[1], 96374[1], 96375[1], 96376[1], 96377[1], 96523[0], 99155[0], 99156[0], 99157[0], 99211[1], 99212[1], 99213[1], 99214[1], 99215[1], 99217[1], 99218[1], 99219[1], 99220[1], 99221[1], 99222[1], 99223[1], 99231[1], 99232[1], 99233[1], 99234[1], 99235[1], 99236[1], 99238[1], 99239[1], 99241[1], 99242[1], 99243[1], 99244[1], 99245[1], 99251[1], 99252[1], 99253[1], 99254[1], 99255[1], 99291[1], 99292[1], 99304[1], 99305[1], 99306[1], 99307[1], 99308[1], 99309[1], 99310[1], 99315[1], 99316[1], 99334[1], 99335[1], 99336[1], 99337[1], 99347[1], 99348[1], 99349[1], 99350[1], 99374[1], 99375[1], 99377[1], 99378[1], 99446[0], 99447[0], 99448[0], 99449[0], 99451[0], 99452[0], 99495[0], 99496[0], G0339[0], G0340[0], G0453[0], G0463[1], G0471[1], G6002[0], G6003[0], G6004[0], G6005[0], G6006[0], G6007[0], G6008[0], G6009[0], G6010[0], G6011[0], G6012[0], G6013[0], G6014[0], G6015[0], G6016[0], G6017[1]
61799	36591[0], 36592[0], 61781[1], 61782[1], 95863[0], 95864[0], 95865[0], 95866[0], 95869[0], 96523[0]
61800	20660[0], 36591[0], 36592[0], 61781[0], 95863[0], 95864[0], 95865[0], 95866[0], 95869[0], 96523[0]
61863	0213T[0], 0216T[0], 0228T[0], 0230T[0], 0333T[0], 0398T[0], 0464T[0], 0589T[0], 0590T[0], 11000[1], 11001[1], 11004[1], 11005[1], 11006[1], 11042[1], 11043[1], 11044[1], 11045[1], 11046[1], 11047[1], 12001[1], 12002[1], 12004[1], 12005[1], 12006[1], 12007[1], 12011[1], 12013[1], 12014[1], 12015[1], 12016[1], 12017[1], 12018[1], 12020[1], 12021[1], 12031[1], 12032[1], 12034[1], 12035[1], 12036[1], 12037[1], 12041[1], 12042[1], 12044[1], 12045[1], 12046[1], 12047[1], 12051[1], 12052[1], 12053[1], 12054[1], 12055[1], 12056[1], 12057[1], 13100[1], 13101[1], 13102[1], 13120[1], 13121[1], 13122[1], 13131[1], 13132[1], 13133[1], 13151[1], 13152[1], 13153[1], 20660[0], 36000[1], 36400[1], 36405[1], 36406[1], 36410[1], 36420[1], 36425[1], 36430[1], 36440[1], 36591[0], 36592[0], 36600[1], 36640[1], 43752[1], 51701[1], 51702[1], 51703[1], 61781[1], 61782[1], 61783[0], 61790[0], 61796[0], 61798[0], 61850[0], 61880[0], 62100[1], 62320[0], 62321[0], 62322[0], 62323[0], 62324[0], 62325[0], 62326[0], 62327[0], 64400[0], 64405[0], 64408[0], 64415[0], 64416[0], 64417[0], 64418[0], 64420[0], 64421[0], 64425[0], 64430[0], 64435[0], 64445[0], 64446[0], 64447[0], 64448[0], 64449[0], 64450[0], 64451[0], 64454[0], 64461[0], 64462[0], 64463[0], 64479[0], 64480[0], 64483[0], 64484[0], 64486[0], 64487[0], 64488[0], 64489[0], 64490[0], 64491[0], 64492[0], 64493[0], 64494[0], 64495[0], 64505[0], 64510[0], 64517[0], 64520[0], 64530[0], 64553[0], 64555[0], 64575[0], 64580[0], 69990[0], 76000[1], 77002[1], 92012[1], 92014[1], 92585[0], 93000[1], 93005[1], 93010[1], 93040[1], 93041[1], 93042[1], 93318[1], 93355[1], 94002[1], 94200[1], 94250[1], 94680[1], 94681[1], 94690[1], 94770[1], 95812[1], 95813[1], 95816[1], 95819[1], 95822[0], 95829[1], 95860[0], 95861[0], 95863[0], 95864[0], 95865[0], 95866[0], 95867[0], 95868[0], 95869[0], 95870[0], 95907[0], 95908[0], 95909[0], 95910[0], 95911[0], 95912[0], 95913[0], 95925[0], 95926[0], 95927[0], 95928[0], 95929[0], 95930[0], 95933[0], 95937[0], 95938[0], 95939[0], 95940[0], 95955[1], 95961[0], 95970[1], 95983[1], 95984[1], 96360[1], 96361[1], 96365[1], 96366[1], 96367[1], 96368[1], 96372[1], 96374[1], 96375[1], 96376[1], 96377[1], 96523[0], 97597[1], 97598[1], 97602[1], 99155[0], 99156[0], 99157[0], 99211[1], 99212[1], 99213[1], 99214[1], 99215[1], 99217[1], 99218[1], 99219[1], 99220[1], 99221[1], 99222[1], 99223[1], 99231[1], 99232[1], 99233[1], 99234[1], 99235[1], 99236[1], 99238[1], 99239[1], 99241[1], 99242[1], 99243[1], 99244[1], 99245[1], 99251[1], 99252[1], 99253[1], 99254[1], 99255[1], 99291[1], 99292[1], 99304[1], 99305[1], 99306[1], 99307[1], 99308[1], 99309[1], 99310[1], 99315[1], 99316[1], 99334[1], 99335[1], 99336[1], 99337[1], 99347[1], 99348[1], 99349[1], 99350[1], 99374[1], 99375[1], 99377[1], 99378[1], 99446[0], 99447[0], 99448[0], 99449[0], 99451[0], 99452[0], 99495[0], 99496[0], G0339[0], G0340[0], G0453[0], G0463[1], G0471[1]
61864	0333T[0], 0464T[0], 0589T[0], 0590T[0], 11000[1], 11001[1], 11004[1], 11005[1], 11006[1], 11042[1], 11043[1], 11044[1], 11045[1], 11046[1], 11047[1], 20660[0], 36591[0], 36592[0], 61781[1], 61782[1], 62100[1], 76000[1], 77002[1], 92585[0], 95822[0], 95860[0], 95861[0], 95863[0], 95864[0], 95865[0], 95866[0], 95867[0], 95868[0], 95869[0], 95907[0], 95908[0], 95909[0], 95910[0], 95911[0], 95912[0], 95913[0], 95925[0], 95926[0], 95927[0], 95930[0], 95933[0], 95937[0], 95938[0], 95939[0], 95940[0], 95970[1], 95983[1], 95984[1], 96523[0], 97597[1], 97598[1], 97602[1], G0453[0]
61867	0213T[0], 0216T[0], 0228T[0], 0230T[0], 0333T[0], 0398T[0], 0464T[0], 0589T[0], 0590T[0], 11000[1], 11001[1], 11004[1], 11005[1], 11006[1], 11042[1], 11043[1], 11044[1], 11045[1], 11046[1], 11047[1], 12001[1], 12002[1], 12004[1], 12005[1], 12006[1], 12007[1], 12011[1], 12013[1], 12014[1], 12015[1], 12016[1], 12017[1], 12018[1], 12020[1], 12021[1], 12031[1], 12032[1], 12034[1], 12035[1], 12036[1], 12037[1], 12041[1], 12042[1], 12044[1], 12045[1], 12046[1], 12047[1], 12051[1], 12052[1], 12053[1], 12054[1], 12055[1], 12056[1], 12057[1], 13100[1], 13101[1], 13102[1], 13120[1], 13121[1], 13122[1], 13131[1], 13132[1], 13133[1], 13151[1], 13152[1], 13153[1], 20660[0], 36000[1], 36400[1], 36405[1], 36406[1], 36410[1], 36420[1], 36425[1], 36430[1], 36440[1], 36591[0], 36592[0], 36600[1], 36640[1], 43752[1], 51701[1], 51702[1], 51703[1], 61720[0], 61735[0], 61750[0], 61751[0], 61760[0], 61770[0], 61781[1], 61782[1], 61783[0], 61790[0], 61791[0], 61796[0], 61798[0], 61850[0], 61860[0], 61863[0], 61870[0], 61880[0], 62100[1], 62320[0], 62321[0], 62322[0], 62323[0], 62324[0], 62325[0], 62326[0], 62327[0], 63620[0], 64400[0], 64405[0], 64408[0], 64415[0], 64416[0], 64417[0], 64418[0], 64420[0], 64421[0], 64425[0], 64430[0], 64435[0], 64445[0], 64446[0], 64447[0], 64448[0], 64449[0], 64450[0], 64451[0], 64454[0], 64461[0], 64462[0], 64463[0], 64479[0], 64480[0], 64483[0], 64484[0], 64486[0], 64487[0], 64488[0], 64489[0], 64490[0], 64491[0], 64492[0], 64493[0], 64494[0], 64495[0], 64505[0], 64510[0], 64517[0], 64520[0], 64530[0], 64553[0], 64555[0], 64575[0], 64580[0], 69990[0], 76000[1], 77002[1], 92012[1], 92014[1], 92585[0], 93000[1], 93005[1], 93010[1], 93040[1], 93041[1], 93042[1], 93318[1], 93355[1], 94002[1], 94200[1], 94250[1], 94680[1], 94681[1], 94690[1], 94770[1], 95812[1], 95813[1], 95816[1], 95819[1], 95822[0], 95829[1], 95860[0], 95861[0], 95863[0], 95864[0], 95865[0], 95866[0], 95867[0], 95868[0], 95869[0], 95870[0], 95907[0], 95908[0], 95909[0], 95910[0], 95911[0], 95912[0], 95913[0], 95925[0], 95926[0], 95927[0], 95928[0], 95929[0], 95930[0], 95933[0], 95937[0], 95938[0], 95939[0], 95940[0], 95955[1], 95961[0], 95970[1], 95983[1], 95984[1], 96360[1], 96361[1], 96365[1], 96366[1], 96367[1], 96368[1], 96372[1], 96374[1], 96375[1], 96376[1], 96377[1], 96523[0], 97597[1], 97598[1], 97602[1], 99155[0], 99156[0], 99157[0], 99211[1], 99212[1], 99213[1], 99214[1], 99215[1], 99217[1], 99218[1], 99219[1], 99220[1], 99221[1], 99222[1], 99223[1], 99231[1], 99232[1], 99233[1], 99234[1], 99235[1], 99236[1], 99238[1], 99239[1], 99241[1], 99242[1], 99243[1], 99244[1], 99245[1], 99251[1], 99252[1], 99253[1], 99254[1], 99255[1], 99291[1], 99292[1], 99304[1], 99305[1], 99306[1], 99307[1], 99308[1], 99309[1], 99310[1], 99315[1], 99316[1], 99334[1], 99335[1], 99336[1], 99337[1], 99347[1], 99348[1], 99349[1], 99350[1], 99374[1], 99375[1], 99377[1], 99378[1], 99446[0], 99447[0], 99448[0], 99449[0], 99451[0], 99452[0], 99495[0], 99496[0], G0339[0], G0340[0], G0453[0], G0463[1], G0471[1]
61868	0333T[0], 0464T[0], 0589T[0], 0590T[0], 11000[1], 11001[1], 11004[1], 11005[1], 11006[1], 11042[1], 11043[1], 11044[1], 11045[1], 11046[1], 11047[1], 20660[0], 36591[0], 36592[0], 61781[1], 61782[1], 62100[1], 76000[1], 77002[1], 92585[0], 95822[0], 95860[0], 95861[0], 95863[0], 95864[0], 95865[0], 95866[0], 95867[0], 95868[0], 95869[0], 95907[0], 95908[0], 95909[0], 95910[0], 95911[0], 95912[0], 95913[0], 95925[0], 95926[0], 95927[0], 95930[0], 95933[0], 95937[0], 95938[0], 95939[0], 95940[0], 95970[1], 95983[1], 95984[1], 96523[0], 97597[1], 97598[1], 97602[1], G0453[0]
61880	0213T[0], 0216T[0], 0228T[0], 0230T[0], 0333T[0], 0464T[0], 0589T[0], 0590T[0], 11000[1], 11001[1], 11004[1], 11005[1], 11006[1], 11042[1], 11043[1], 11044[1], 11045[1], 11046[1], 11047[1], 12001[1], 12002[1], 12004[1], 12005[1], 12006[1], 12007[1], 12011[1], 12013[1], 12014[1], 12015[1], 12016[1], 12017[1], 12018[1], 12020[1], 12021[1], 12031[1], 12032[1], 12034[1], 12035[1], 12036[1], 12037[1], 12041[1], 12042[1], 12044[1], 12045[1], 12046[1], 12047[1], 12051[1], 12052[1], 12053[1], 12054[1], 12055[1], 12056[1], 12057[1], 13100[1], 13101[1], 13102[1], 13120[1], 13121[1], 13122[1], 13131[1], 13132[1], 13133[1], 13151[1], 13152[1], 13153[1], 20660[0], 36000[1], 36400[1], 36405[1], 36406[1], 36410[1], 36420[1], 36425[1], 36430[1], 36440[1], 36591[0], 36592[0], 36600[1], 36640[1], 43752[1],

0 = Modifier usage not allowed or inappropriate 1 = Modifier usage allowed

Code 1	Code 2
	51701[1], 51702[1], 51703[1], 61535[1], 61850[0], 61860[0], 61870[0], 62320[0], 62321[0], 62322[0], 62323[0], 62324[0], 62325[0], 62326[0], 62327[0], 64400[0], 64405[0], 64408[0], 64415[0], 64416[0], 64417[0], 64418[0], 64420[0], 64421[0], 64425[0], 64430[0], 64435[0], 64445[0], 64446[0], 64447[0], 64448[0], 64449[0], 64450[0], 64451[0], 64454[0], 64461[0], 64462[0], 64463[0], 64479[0], 64480[0], 64483[0], 64484[0], 64486[0], 64487[0], 64488[0], 64489[0], 64490[0], 64491[0], 64492[0], 64493[0], 64494[0], 64495[0], 64505[0], 64510[0], 64517[0], 64520[0], 64530[0], 69990[0], 92012[1], 92014[1], 92585[0], 93000[1], 93005[1], 93010[1], 93040[1], 93041[1], 93042[1], 93318[1], 93355[1], 94002[1], 94200[1], 94250[1], 94680[1], 94681[1], 94690[1], 94770[1], 95812[1], 95813[1], 95816[1], 95819[1], 95822[0], 95829[1], 95860[0], 95861[0], 95863[0], 95864[0], 95865[0], 95866[0], 95867[0], 95868[0], 95869[0], 95870[0], 95907[0], 95908[0], 95909[0], 95910[0], 95911[0], 95912[0], 95913[0], 95925[0], 95926[0], 95927[0], 95928[0], 95929[0], 95930[0], 95933[0], 95937[0], 95938[0], 95939[0], 95940[0], 95955[1], 95970[1], 95983[1], 95984[1], 96360[1], 96361[1], 96365[1], 96366[1], 96367[1], 96368[1], 96372[1], 96374[1], 96375[1], 96376[1], 96377[1], 96523[0], 97597[1], 97598[1], 97602[1], 99155[0], 99156[0], 99157[0], 99211[1], 99212[1], 99213[1], 99214[1], 99215[1], 99217[1], 99218[1], 99219[1], 99220[1], 99221[1], 99222[1], 99223[1], 99231[1], 99232[1], 99233[1], 99234[1], 99235[1], 99236[1], 99238[1], 99239[1], 99241[1], 99242[1], 99243[1], 99244[1], 99245[1], 99251[1], 99252[1], 99253[1], 99254[1], 99255[1], 99291[1], 99292[1], 99304[1], 99305[1], 99306[1], 99307[1], 99308[1], 99309[1], 99310[1], 99315[1], 99316[1], 99334[1], 99335[1], 99336[1], 99337[1], 99347[1], 99348[1], 99349[1], 99350[1], 99374[1], 99375[1], 99377[1], 99378[1], 99446[0], 99447[0], 99448[0], 99449[0], 99451[0], 99452[0], 99495[0], 99496[0], G0453[0], G0463[1], G0471[1]
61885	0213T[0], 0216T[0], 0228T[0], 0230T[0], 0333T[0], 0464T[0], 0589T[0], 0590T[0], 11000[1], 11001[1], 11004[1], 11005[1], 11006[1], 11042[1], 11043[1], 11044[1], 11045[1], 11046[1], 11047[1], 12001[1], 12002[1], 12004[1], 12005[1], 12006[1], 12007[1], 12011[1], 12013[1], 12014[1], 12015[1], 12016[1], 12017[1], 12018[1], 12020[1], 12021[1], 12031[1], 12032[1], 12034[1], 12035[1], 12036[1], 12037[1], 12041[1], 12042[1], 12044[1], 12045[1], 12046[1], 12047[1], 12051[1], 12052[1], 12053[1], 12054[1], 12055[1], 12056[1], 12057[1], 13100[1], 13101[1], 13102[1], 13120[1], 13121[1], 13122[1], 13131[1], 13132[1], 13133[1], 13151[1], 13152[1], 13153[1], 36000[1], 36400[1], 36405[1], 36406[1], 36410[1], 36420[1], 36425[1], 36430[1], 36440[1], 36591[0], 36592[0], 36600[1], 36640[1], 43752[1], 51701[1], 51702[1], 51703[1], 61886[1], 61888[1], 62320[0], 62321[0], 62322[0], 62323[0], 62324[0], 62325[0], 62326[0], 62327[0], 64400[0], 64405[0], 64408[0], 64415[0], 64416[0], 64417[0], 64418[0], 64420[0], 64421[0], 64425[0], 64430[0], 64435[0], 64445[0], 64446[0], 64447[0], 64448[0], 64449[0], 64450[0], 64451[0], 64454[0], 64461[0], 64462[0], 64463[0], 64479[0], 64480[0], 64483[0], 64484[0], 64486[0], 64487[0], 64488[0], 64489[0], 64490[0], 64491[0], 64492[0], 64493[0], 64494[0], 64495[0], 64505[0], 64510[0], 64517[0], 64520[0], 64530[0], 69990[0], 92012[1], 92014[1], 92585[0], 93000[1], 93005[1], 93010[1], 93040[1], 93041[1], 93042[1], 93318[1], 93355[1], 94002[1], 94200[1], 94250[1], 94680[1], 94681[1], 94690[1], 94770[1], 95812[1], 95813[1], 95816[1], 95819[1], 95822[0], 95829[1], 95860[0], 95861[0], 95863[0], 95864[0], 95865[0], 95866[0], 95867[0], 95868[0], 95869[0], 95870[0], 95907[0], 95908[0], 95909[0], 95910[0], 95911[0], 95912[0], 95913[0], 95925[0], 95926[0], 95927[0], 95928[0], 95929[0], 95930[0], 95933[0], 95937[0], 95938[0], 95939[0], 95940[0], 95955[1], 95970[1], 95983[1], 95984[1], 96360[1], 96361[1], 96365[1], 96366[1], 96367[1], 96368[1], 96372[1], 96374[1], 96375[1], 96376[1], 96377[1], 96523[0], 97597[1], 97598[1], 97602[1], 99155[0], 99156[0], 99157[0], 99211[1], 99212[1], 99213[1], 99214[1], 99215[1], 99217[1], 99218[1], 99219[1], 99220[1], 99221[1], 99222[1], 99223[1], 99231[1], 99232[1], 99233[1], 99234[1], 99235[1], 99236[1], 99238[1], 99239[1], 99241[1], 99242[1], 99243[1], 99244[1], 99245[1], 99251[1], 99252[1], 99253[1], 99254[1], 99255[1], 99291[1], 99292[1], 99304[1], 99305[1], 99306[1], 99307[1], 99308[1], 99309[1], 99310[1], 99315[1], 99316[1], 99334[1], 99335[1], 99336[1], 99337[1], 99347[1], 99348[1], 99349[1], 99350[1], 99374[1], 99375[1], 99377[1], 99378[1], 99446[0], 99447[0], 99448[0], 99449[0], 99451[0], 99452[0], 99495[0], 99496[0], G0453[0], G0463[1], G0471[1]
61886	0213T[0], 0216T[0], 0228T[0], 0230T[0], 0333T[0], 0464T[0], 0466T[1], 0589T[0], 0590T[0], 11000[1], 11001[1], 11004[1], 11005[1], 11006[1], 11042[1], 11043[1], 11044[1], 11045[1], 11046[1], 11047[1], 12001[1], 12002[1], 12004[1], 12005[1], 12006[1], 12007[1], 12011[1], 12013[1], 12014[1], 12015[1], 12016[1], 12017[1], 12018[1], 12020[1], 12021[1], 12031[1], 12032[1], 12034[1], 12035[1], 12036[1], 12037[1], 12041[1], 12042[1], 12044[1], 12045[1], 12046[1], 12047[1], 12051[1], 12052[1], 12053[1], 12054[1], 12055[1], 12056[1], 12057[1], 13100[1], 13101[1], 13102[1], 13120[1], 13121[1], 13122[1], 13131[1], 13132[1], 13133[1], 13151[1], 13152[1], 13153[1], 36000[1], 36400[1], 36405[1], 36406[1], 36410[1], 36420[1], 36425[1], 36430[1], 36440[1], 36591[0], 36592[0], 36600[1], 36640[1], 43752[1], 51701[1], 51702[1], 51703[1], 61888[1], 62320[0], 62321[0], 62322[0], 62323[0], 62324[0], 62325[0], 62326[0], 62327[0], 64400[0], 64405[0], 64408[0], 64415[0], 64416[0], 64417[0], 64418[0], 64420[0], 64421[0], 64425[0], 64430[0], 64435[0], 64445[0], 64446[0], 64447[0], 64448[0], 64449[0], 64450[0], 64451[0], 64454[0], 64461[0], 64462[0], 64463[0], 64479[0], 64480[0], 64483[0], 64484[0], 64486[0], 64487[0], 64488[0], 64489[0], 64490[0], 64491[0], 64492[0], 64493[0], 64494[0], 64495[0], 64505[0], 64510[0], 64517[0], 64520[0], 64530[0], 64568[1], 69990[0], 92012[1], 92014[1], 92585[0], 93000[1], 93005[1], 93010[1], 93040[1], 93041[1], 93042[1], 93318[1], 93355[1], 94002[1], 94200[1], 94250[1], 94680[1], 94681[1], 94690[1], 94770[1], 95812[1], 95813[1], 95816[1], 95819[1], 95822[0], 95829[1], 95860[0], 95861[0], 95863[0], 95864[0], 95865[0], 95866[0], 95867[0], 95868[0], 95869[0], 95870[0], 95907[0], 95908[0], 95909[0], 95910[0], 95911[0], 95912[0], 95913[0], 95925[0], 95926[0], 95927[0], 95928[0], 95929[0], 95930[0], 95933[0], 95937[0], 95938[0], 95939[0], 95940[0], 95955[1], 95970[1], 95983[1], 95984[1], 96360[1], 96361[1], 96365[1], 96366[1], 96367[1], 96368[1], 96372[1], 96374[1], 96375[1], 96376[1], 96377[1], 96523[0], 97597[1], 97598[1], 97602[1], 99155[0], 99156[0], 99157[0], 99211[1], 99212[1], 99213[1], 99214[1], 99215[1], 99217[1], 99218[1], 99219[1], 99220[1], 99221[1], 99222[1], 99223[1], 99231[1], 99232[1], 99233[1], 99234[1], 99235[1], 99236[1], 99238[1], 99239[1], 99241[1], 99242[1], 99243[1], 99244[1], 99245[1], 99251[1], 99252[1], 99253[1], 99254[1], 99255[1], 99291[1], 99292[1], 99304[1], 99305[1], 99306[1], 99307[1], 99308[1], 99309[1], 99310[1], 99315[1], 99316[1], 99334[1], 99335[1], 99336[1], 99337[1], 99347[1], 99348[1], 99349[1], 99350[1], 99374[1], 99375[1], 99377[1], 99378[1], 99446[0], 99447[0], 99448[0], 99449[0], 99451[0], 99452[0], 99495[0], 99496[0], G0453[0], G0463[1], G0471[1]
61888	0213T[0], 0216T[0], 0228T[0], 0230T[0], 0333T[0], 0464T[0], 0589T[0], 0590T[0], 11000[1], 11001[1], 11004[1], 11005[1], 11006[1], 11042[1], 11043[1], 11044[1], 11045[1], 11046[1], 11047[1], 12001[1], 12002[1], 12004[1], 12005[1], 12006[1], 12007[1], 12011[1], 12013[1], 12014[1], 12015[1], 12016[1], 12017[1], 12018[1], 12020[1], 12021[1], 12031[1], 12032[1], 12034[1], 12035[1], 12036[1], 12037[1], 12041[1], 12042[1], 12044[1], 12045[1], 12046[1], 12047[1], 12051[1], 12052[1], 12053[1], 12054[1], 12055[1], 12056[1], 12057[1], 13100[1], 13101[1], 13102[1], 13120[1], 13121[1], 13122[1], 13131[1], 13132[1], 13133[1], 13151[1], 13152[1], 13153[1], 36000[1], 36400[1], 36405[1], 36406[1], 36410[1], 36420[1], 36425[1], 36430[1], 36440[1], 36591[0], 36592[0], 36600[1], 36640[1], 43752[1], 51701[1], 51702[1], 51703[1], 62320[0], 62321[0], 62322[0], 62323[0], 62324[0], 62325[0], 62326[0], 62327[0], 64400[0], 64405[0], 64408[0], 64415[0], 64416[0], 64417[0], 64418[0], 64420[0], 64421[0], 64425[0], 64430[0], 64435[0], 64445[0], 64446[0], 64447[0], 64448[0], 64449[0], 64450[0], 64451[0], 64454[0], 64461[0], 64462[0], 64463[0], 64479[0], 64480[0], 64483[0], 64484[0], 64486[0], 64487[0], 64488[0], 64489[0], 64490[0], 64491[0], 64492[0], 64493[0], 64494[0], 64495[0], 64505[0], 64510[0], 64517[0], 64520[0], 64530[0], 69990[0], 92012[1], 92014[1], 92585[0], 93000[1], 93005[1], 93010[1], 93040[1], 93041[1], 93042[1], 93318[1], 93355[1], 94002[1], 94200[1], 94250[1], 94680[1], 94681[1], 94690[1], 94770[1], 95812[1], 95813[1], 95816[1], 95819[1], 95822[0], 95829[1], 95860[0], 95861[0], 95863[0], 95864[0], 95865[0], 95866[0], 95867[0], 95868[0], 95869[0], 95870[0], 95907[0], 95908[0], 95909[0], 95910[0], 95911[0], 95912[0], 95913[0], 95925[0], 95926[0], 95927[0], 95928[0], 95929[0], 95930[0], 95933[0], 95937[0], 95938[0], 95939[0], 95940[0], 95955[1], 95970[1], 95983[1], 95984[1], 96360[1], 96361[1], 96365[1], 96366[1], 96367[1], 96368[1], 96372[1], 96374[1], 96375[1], 96376[1], 96377[1], 96523[0], 97597[1], 97598[1], 97602[1], 99155[0], 99156[0], 99157[0], 99211[1], 99212[1], 99213[1], 99214[1], 99215[1], 99217[1], 99218[1], 99219[1], 99220[1], 99221[1], 99222[1], 99223[1], 99231[1], 99232[1], 99233[1], 99234[1], 99235[1], 99236[1], 99238[1], 99239[1], 99241[1], 99242[1], 99243[1], 99244[1], 99245[1], 99251[1], 99252[1], 99253[1], 99254[1], 99255[1], 99291[1], 99292[1], 99304[1], 99305[1], 99306[1], 99307[1], 99308[1], 99309[1], 99310[1], 99315[1], 99316[1], 99334[1], 99335[1], 99336[1], 99337[1], 99347[1], 99348[1], 99349[1], 99350[1], 99374[1], 99375[1], 99377[1], 99378[1], 99446[0], 99447[0], 99448[0], 99449[0], 99451[0], 99452[0], 99495[0], 99496[0], G0453[0], G0463[1], G0471[1]
62000	0213T[0], 0216T[0], 0228T[0], 0230T[0], 0333T[0], 0464T[0], 12001[1], 12002[1], 12004[1], 12005[1], 12006[1], 12007[1], 12011[1], 12013[1], 12014[1], 12015[1], 12016[1], 12017[1], 12018[1], 12020[1], 12021[1], 12031[1], 12032[1], 12034[1], 12035[1], 12036[1], 12037[1], 12041[1], 12042[1], 12044[1], 12045[1], 12046[1], 12047[1], 12051[1], 12052[1], 12053[1], 12054[1], 12055[1], 12056[1], 12057[1], 13100[1], 13101[1], 13102[1], 13120[1], 13121[1], 13122[1], 13131[1], 13132[1], 13133[1], 13151[1], 13152[1], 13153[1], 36000[1], 36400[1], 36405[1], 36406[1], 36410[1], 36420[1], 36425[1], 36430[1], 36440[1], 36591[0], 36592[0], 36600[1], 36640[1], 43752[1], 51701[1], 51702[1], 51703[1], 62320[0], 62321[0], 62322[0], 62323[0], 62324[0], 62325[0], 62326[0], 62327[0], 64400[0], 64405[0], 64408[0], 64415[0], 64416[0], 64417[0], 64418[0], 64420[0], 64421[0], 64425[0], 64430[0], 64435[0], 64445[0], 64446[0], 64447[0], 64448[0], 64449[0], 64450[0], 64451[0], 64454[0], 64461[0], 64462[0], 64463[0], 64479[0], 64480[0], 64483[0], 64484[0], 64486[0], 64487[0], 64488[0], 64489[0], 64490[0], 64491[0], 64492[0], 64493[0], 64494[0], 64495[0], 64505[0], 64510[0], 64517[0], 64520[0], 64530[0], 69990[1], 92012[1], 92014[1], 92585[0], 93000[1], 93005[1], 93010[1], 93040[1], 93041[1], 93042[1], 93318[1], 93355[1], 94002[1], 94200[1], 94250[1], 94680[1], 94681[1], 94690[1], 94770[1], 95812[1], 95813[1], 95816[1], 95819[1], 95822[0], 95829[1], 95860[0], 95861[0], 95863[0], 95864[0], 95865[0], 95866[0], 95867[0], 95868[0], 95869[0], 95870[0], 95907[0], 95908[0], 95909[0], 95910[0], 95911[0], 95912[0], 95913[0], 95925[0], 95926[0], 95927[0], 95928[0], 95929[0], 95930[0], 95933[0], 95937[0], 95938[0], 95939[0], 95940[0], 95955[1], 96360[1], 96361[1], 96365[1], 96366[1], 96367[1], 96368[1], 96372[1], 96374[1], 96375[1], 96376[1], 96377[1], 96523[0], 99155[0], 99156[0], 99157[0], 99211[1], 99212[1], 99213[1], 99214[1], 99215[1], 99217[1], 99218[1], 99219[1], 99220[1], 99221[1], 99222[1], 99223[1], 99231[1], 99232[1], 99233[1], 99234[1], 99235[1], 99236[1], 99238[1], 99239[1], 99241[1], 99242[1], 99243[1], 99244[1], 99245[1], 99251[1], 99252[1], 99253[1], 99254[1], 99255[1], 99291[1], 99292[1], 99304[1], 99305[1], 99306[1], 99307[1], 99308[1], 99309[1], 99310[1], 99315[1], 99316[1], 99334[1], 99335[1], 99336[1], 99337[1], 99347[1], 99348[1], 99349[1], 99350[1], 99374[1], 99375[1], 99377[1], 99378[1], 99446[0], 99447[0], 99448[0], 99449[0], 99451[0], 99452[0], 99495[0], 99496[0], G0453[0], G0463[1], G0471[1]

0 = Modifier usage not allowed or inappropriate 1 = Modifier usage allowed

Code 1	Code 2
62005	0213T[0], 0216T[0], 0228T[0], 0230T[0], 0333T[0], 0464T[0], 12001[1], 12002[1], 12004[1], 12005[1], 12006[1], 12007[1], 12011[1], 12013[1], 12014[1], 12015[1], 12016[1], 12017[1], 12018[1], 12020[1], 12021[1], 12031[1], 12032[1], 12034[1], 12035[1], 12036[1], 12037[1], 12041[1], 12042[1], 12044[1], 12045[1], 12046[1], 12047[1], 12051[1], 12052[1], 12053[1], 12054[1], 12055[1], 12056[1], 12057[1], 13100[1], 13101[1], 13102[1], 13120[1], 13121[1], 13122[1], 13131[1], 13132[1], 13133[1], 13151[1], 13152[1], 13153[1], 36000[1], 36400[1], 36405[1], 36406[1], 36410[1], 36420[1], 36425[1], 36430[1], 36440[1], 36591[0], 36592[0], 36600[1], 36640[1], 43752[1], 51701[1], 51702[1], 51703[1], 62000[1], 62320[0], 62321[0], 62322[0], 62323[0], 62324[0], 62325[0], 62326[0], 62327[0], 64400[0], 64405[0], 64408[0], 64415[0], 64416[0], 64417[0], 64418[0], 64420[0], 64421[0], 64425[0], 64430[0], 64435[0], 64445[0], 64446[0], 64447[0], 64448[0], 64449[0], 64450[0], 64451[0], 64454[0], 64461[0], 64462[0], 64463[0], 64479[0], 64480[0], 64483[0], 64484[0], 64486[0], 64487[0], 64488[0], 64489[0], 64490[0], 64491[0], 64492[0], 64493[0], 64494[0], 64495[0], 64505[0], 64510[0], 64517[0], 64520[0], 64530[0], 69990[1], 92012[1], 92014[1], 92585[0], 93000[1], 93005[1], 93010[1], 93040[1], 93041[1], 93042[1], 93318[1], 93355[1], 94002[1], 94200[1], 94250[1], 94680[1], 94681[1], 94690[1], 94770[1], 95812[1], 95813[1], 95816[1], 95819[1], 95822[0], 95829[1], 95860[0], 95861[0], 95863[0], 95864[0], 95865[0], 95866[0], 95867[0], 95868[0], 95869[0], 95870[0], 95907[0], 95908[0], 95909[0], 95910[0], 95911[0], 95912[0], 95913[0], 95925[0], 95926[0], 95927[0], 95928[0], 95929[0], 95930[0], 95933[0], 95937[0], 95938[0], 95939[0], 95940[0], 95955[1], 96360[1], 96361[1], 96365[1], 96366[1], 96367[1], 96368[1], 96372[1], 96374[1], 96375[1], 96376[1], 96377[1], 96523[0], 99155[0], 99156[0], 99157[0], 99211[1], 99212[1], 99213[1], 99214[1], 99215[1], 99217[1], 99218[1], 99219[1], 99220[1], 99221[1], 99222[1], 99223[1], 99231[1], 99232[1], 99233[1], 99234[1], 99235[1], 99236[1], 99238[1], 99239[1], 99241[1], 99242[1], 99243[1], 99244[1], 99245[1], 99251[1], 99252[1], 99253[1], 99254[1], 99255[1], 99291[1], 99292[1], 99304[1], 99305[1], 99306[1], 99307[1], 99308[1], 99309[1], 99310[1], 99315[1], 99316[1], 99334[1], 99335[1], 99336[1], 99337[1], 99347[1], 99348[1], 99349[1], 99350[1], 99374[1], 99375[1], 99377[1], 99378[1], 99446[0], 99447[0], 99448[0], 99449[0], 99451[0], 99452[0], 99495[0], 99496[0], G0453[0], G0463[1], G0471[1]
62010	0213T[0], 0216T[0], 0228T[0], 0230T[0], 0333T[0], 0464T[0], 12001[1], 12002[1], 12004[1], 12005[1], 12006[1], 12007[1], 12011[1], 12013[1], 12014[1], 12015[1], 12016[1], 12017[1], 12018[1], 12020[1], 12021[1], 12031[1], 12032[1], 12034[1], 12035[1], 12036[1], 12037[1], 12041[1], 12042[1], 12044[1], 12045[1], 12046[1], 12047[1], 12051[1], 12052[1], 12053[1], 12054[1], 12055[1], 12056[1], 12057[1], 13100[1], 13101[1], 13102[1], 13120[1], 13121[1], 13122[1], 13131[1], 13132[1], 13133[1], 13151[1], 13152[1], 13153[1], 36000[1], 36400[1], 36405[1], 36406[1], 36410[1], 36420[1], 36425[1], 36430[1], 36440[1], 36591[0], 36592[0], 36600[1], 36640[1], 43752[1], 51701[1], 51702[1], 51703[1], 62000[1], 62005[1], 62320[0], 62321[0], 62322[0], 62323[0], 62324[0], 62325[0], 62326[0], 62327[0], 64400[0], 64405[0], 64408[0], 64415[0], 64416[0], 64417[0], 64418[0], 64420[0], 64421[0], 64425[0], 64430[0], 64435[0], 64445[0], 64446[0], 64447[0], 64448[0], 64449[0], 64450[0], 64451[0], 64454[0], 64461[0], 64462[0], 64463[0], 64479[0], 64480[0], 64483[0], 64484[0], 64486[0], 64487[0], 64488[0], 64489[0], 64490[0], 64491[0], 64492[0], 64493[0], 64494[0], 64495[0], 64505[0], 64510[0], 64517[0], 64520[0], 64530[0], 92012[1], 92014[1], 92585[0], 93000[1], 93005[1], 93010[1], 93040[1], 93041[1], 93042[1], 93318[1], 93355[1], 94002[1], 94200[1], 94250[1], 94680[1], 94681[1], 94690[1], 94770[1], 95812[1], 95813[1], 95816[1], 95819[1], 95822[0], 95829[1], 95860[0], 95861[0], 95863[0], 95864[0], 95865[0], 95866[0], 95867[0], 95868[0], 95869[0], 95870[0], 95907[0], 95908[0], 95909[0], 95910[0], 95911[0], 95912[0], 95913[0], 95925[0], 95926[0], 95927[0], 95928[0], 95929[0], 95930[0], 95933[0], 95937[0], 95938[0], 95939[0], 95940[0], 95955[1], 96360[1], 96361[1], 96365[1], 96366[1], 96367[1], 96368[1], 96372[1], 96374[1], 96375[1], 96376[1], 96377[1], 96523[0], 99155[0], 99156[0], 99157[0], 99211[1], 99212[1], 99213[1], 99214[1], 99215[1], 99217[1], 99218[1], 99219[1], 99220[1], 99221[1], 99222[1], 99223[1], 99231[1], 99232[1], 99233[1], 99234[1], 99235[1], 99236[1], 99238[1], 99239[1], 99241[1], 99242[1], 99243[1], 99244[1], 99245[1], 99251[1], 99252[1], 99253[1], 99254[1], 99255[1], 99291[1], 99292[1], 99304[1], 99305[1], 99306[1], 99307[1], 99308[1], 99309[1], 99310[1], 99315[1], 99316[1], 99334[1], 99335[1], 99336[1], 99337[1], 99347[1], 99348[1], 99349[1], 99350[1], 99374[1], 99375[1], 99377[1], 99378[1], 99446[0], 99447[0], 99448[0], 99449[0], 99451[0], 99452[0], 99495[0], 99496[0], G0453[0], G0463[1], G0471[1]
62100	0213T[0], 0216T[0], 0228T[0], 0230T[0], 0333T[0], 0464T[0], 11000[1], 11001[1], 11004[1], 11005[1], 11006[1], 11042[1], 11043[1], 11044[1], 11045[1], 11046[1], 11047[1], 12001[1], 12002[1], 12004[1], 12005[1], 12006[1], 12007[1], 12011[1], 12013[1], 12014[1], 12015[1], 12016[1], 12017[1], 12018[1], 12020[1], 12021[1], 12031[1], 12032[1], 12034[1], 12035[1], 12036[1], 12037[1], 12041[1], 12042[1], 12044[1], 12045[1], 12046[1], 12047[1], 12051[1], 12052[1], 12053[1], 12054[1], 12055[1], 12056[1], 12057[1], 13100[1], 13101[1], 13102[1], 13120[1], 13121[1], 13122[1], 13131[1], 13132[1], 13133[1], 13151[1], 13152[1], 13153[1], 36000[1], 36400[1], 36405[1], 36406[1], 36410[1], 36420[1], 36425[1], 36430[1], 36440[1], 36591[0], 36592[0], 36600[1], 36640[1], 43752[1], 51701[1], 51702[1], 51703[1], 62320[0], 62321[0], 62322[0], 62323[0], 62324[0], 62325[0], 62326[0], 62327[0], 64400[0], 64405[0], 64408[0], 64415[0], 64416[0], 64417[0], 64418[0], 64420[0], 64421[0], 64425[0], 64430[0], 64435[0], 64445[0], 64446[0], 64447[0], 64448[0], 64449[0], 64450[0], 64451[0], 64454[0], 64461[0], 64462[0], 64463[0], 64479[0], 64480[0], 64483[0], 64484[0], 64486[0], 64487[0], 64488[0], 64489[0], 64490[0], 64491[0], 64492[0], 64493[0], 64494[0], 64495[0], 64505[0], 64510[0], 64517[0], 64520[0], 64530[0], 92012[1], 92014[1], 92585[0], 93000[1], 93005[1], 93010[1], 93040[1], 93041[1], 93042[1], 93318[1], 93355[1], 94002[1], 94200[1], 94250[1], 94680[1], 94681[1], 94690[1], 94770[1], 95812[1], 95813[1], 95816[1], 95819[1], 95822[0], 95829[1], 95860[0], 95861[0], 95863[0], 95864[0], 95865[0], 95866[0], 95867[0], 95868[0], 95869[0], 95870[0], 95907[0], 95908[0], 95909[0], 95910[0], 95911[0], 95912[0], 95913[0], 95925[0], 95926[0], 95927[0], 95928[0], 95929[0], 95930[0], 95933[0], 95937[0], 95938[0], 95939[0], 95940[0], 95955[1], 96360[1], 96361[1], 96365[1], 96366[1], 96367[1], 96368[1], 96372[1], 96374[1], 96375[1], 96376[1], 96377[1], 96523[0], 97597[1], 97598[1], 97602[1], 99155[0], 99156[0], 99157[0], 99211[1], 99212[1], 99213[1], 99214[1], 99215[1], 99217[1], 99218[1], 99219[1], 99220[1], 99221[1], 99222[1], 99223[1], 99231[1], 99232[1], 99233[1], 99234[1], 99235[1], 99236[1], 99238[1], 99239[1], 99241[1], 99242[1], 99243[1], 99244[1], 99245[1], 99251[1], 99252[1], 99253[1], 99254[1], 99255[1], 99291[1], 99292[1], 99304[1], 99305[1], 99306[1], 99307[1], 99308[1], 99309[1], 99310[1], 99315[1], 99316[1], 99334[1], 99335[1], 99336[1], 99337[1], 99347[1], 99348[1], 99349[1], 99350[1], 99374[1], 99375[1], 99377[1], 99378[1], 99446[0], 99447[0], 99448[0], 99449[0], 99451[0], 99452[0], 99495[0], 99496[0], G0453[0], G0463[1], G0471[1]
62120	0213T[0], 0216T[0], 0228T[0], 0230T[0], 0333T[0], 0464T[0], 11000[1], 11001[1], 11004[1], 11005[1], 11006[1], 11042[1], 11043[1], 11044[1], 11045[1], 11046[1], 11047[1], 12001[1], 12002[1], 12004[1], 12005[1], 12006[1], 12007[1], 12011[1], 12013[1], 12014[1], 12015[1], 12016[1], 12017[1], 12018[1], 12020[1], 12021[1], 12031[1], 12032[1], 12034[1], 12035[1], 12036[1], 12037[1], 12041[1], 12042[1], 12044[1], 12045[1], 12046[1], 12047[1], 12051[1], 12052[1], 12053[1], 12054[1], 12055[1], 12056[1], 12057[1], 13100[1], 13101[1], 13102[1], 13120[1], 13121[1], 13122[1], 13131[1], 13132[1], 13133[1], 13151[1], 13152[1], 13153[1], 36000[1], 36400[1], 36405[1], 36406[1], 36410[1], 36420[1], 36425[1], 36430[1], 36440[1], 36591[0], 36592[0], 36600[1], 36640[1], 43752[1], 51701[1], 51702[1], 51703[1], 62117[1], 62140[1], 62141[1], 62320[0], 62321[0], 62322[0], 62323[0], 62324[0], 62325[0], 62326[0], 62327[0], 64400[0], 64405[0], 64408[0], 64415[0], 64416[0], 64417[0], 64418[0], 64420[0], 64421[0], 64425[0], 64430[0], 64435[0], 64445[0], 64446[0], 64447[0], 64448[0], 64449[0], 64450[0], 64451[0], 64454[0], 64461[0], 64462[0], 64463[0], 64479[0], 64480[0], 64483[0], 64484[0], 64486[0], 64487[0], 64488[0], 64489[0], 64490[0], 64491[0], 64492[0], 64493[0], 64494[0], 64495[0], 64505[0], 64510[0], 64517[0], 64520[0], 64530[0], 69990[1], 92012[1], 92014[1], 92585[0], 93000[1], 93005[1], 93010[1], 93040[1], 93041[1], 93042[1], 93318[1], 93355[1], 94002[1], 94200[1], 94250[1], 94680[1], 94681[1], 94690[1], 94770[1], 95812[1], 95813[1], 95816[1], 95819[1], 95822[0], 95829[1], 95860[0], 95861[0], 95863[0], 95864[0], 95865[0], 95866[0], 95867[0], 95868[0], 95869[0], 95870[0], 95907[0], 95908[0], 95909[0], 95910[0], 95911[0], 95912[0], 95913[0], 95925[0], 95926[0], 95927[0], 95928[0], 95929[0], 95930[0], 95933[0], 95937[0], 95938[0], 95939[0], 95940[0], 95955[1], 96360[1], 96361[1], 96365[1], 96366[1], 96367[1], 96368[1], 96372[1], 96374[1], 96375[1], 96376[1], 96377[1], 96523[0], 97597[1], 97598[1], 97602[1], 99155[0], 99156[0], 99157[0], 99211[1], 99212[1], 99213[1], 99214[1], 99215[1], 99217[1], 99218[1], 99219[1], 99220[1], 99221[1], 99222[1], 99223[1], 99231[1], 99232[1], 99233[1], 99234[1], 99235[1], 99236[1], 99238[1], 99239[1], 99241[1], 99242[1], 99243[1], 99244[1], 99245[1], 99251[1], 99252[1], 99253[1], 99254[1], 99255[1], 99291[1], 99292[1], 99304[1], 99305[1], 99306[1], 99307[1], 99308[1], 99309[1], 99310[1], 99315[1], 99316[1], 99334[1], 99335[1], 99336[1], 99337[1], 99347[1], 99348[1], 99349[1], 99350[1], 99374[1], 99375[1], 99377[1], 99378[1], 99446[0], 99447[0], 99448[0], 99449[0], 99451[0], 99452[0], 99495[0], 99496[0], G0453[0], G0463[1], G0471[1]
62121	0213T[0], 0216T[0], 0228T[0], 0230T[0], 0333T[0], 0464T[0], 11000[1], 11001[1], 11004[1], 11005[1], 11006[1], 11042[1], 11043[1], 11044[1], 11045[1], 11046[1], 11047[1], 12001[1], 12002[1], 12004[1], 12005[1], 12006[1], 12007[1], 12011[1], 12013[1], 12014[1], 12015[1], 12016[1], 12017[1], 12018[1], 12020[1], 12021[1], 12031[1], 12032[1], 12034[1], 12035[1], 12036[1], 12037[1], 12041[1], 12042[1], 12044[1], 12045[1], 12046[1], 12047[1], 12051[1], 12052[1], 12053[1], 12054[1], 12055[1], 12056[1], 12057[1], 13100[1], 13101[1], 13102[1], 13120[1], 13121[1], 13122[1], 13131[1], 13132[1], 13133[1], 13151[1], 13152[1], 13153[1], 36000[1], 36400[1], 36405[1], 36406[1], 36410[1], 36420[1], 36425[1], 36430[1], 36440[1], 36591[0], 36592[0], 36600[1], 36640[1], 43752[1], 51701[1], 51702[1], 51703[1], 62100[1], 62320[0], 62321[0], 62322[0], 62323[0], 62324[0], 62325[0], 62326[0], 62327[0], 64400[0], 64405[0], 64408[0], 64415[0], 64416[0], 64417[0], 64418[0], 64420[0], 64421[0], 64425[0], 64430[0], 64435[0], 64445[0], 64446[0], 64447[0], 64448[0], 64449[0], 64450[0], 64451[0], 64454[0], 64461[0], 64462[0], 64463[0], 64479[0], 64480[0], 64483[0], 64484[0], 64486[0], 64487[0], 64488[0], 64489[0], 64490[0], 64491[0], 64492[0], 64493[0], 64494[0], 64495[0], 64505[0], 64510[0], 64517[0], 64520[0], 64530[0], 69990[1], 92012[1], 92014[1], 92585[0], 93000[1], 93005[1], 93010[1], 93040[1], 93041[1], 93042[1], 93318[1], 93355[1], 94002[1], 94200[1], 94250[1], 94680[1], 94681[1], 94690[1], 94770[1], 95812[1], 95813[1], 95816[1], 95819[1], 95822[0], 95829[1], 95860[0], 95861[0], 95863[0], 95864[0], 95865[0], 95866[0], 95867[0], 95868[0], 95869[0], 95870[0], 95907[0], 95908[0], 95909[0], 95910[0], 95911[0], 95912[0], 95913[0], 95925[0], 95926[0], 95927[0], 95928[0], 95929[0], 95930[0], 95933[0], 95937[0], 95938[0], 95939[0], 95940[0], 95955[1], 96360[1], 96361[1], 96365[1], 96366[1], 96367[1], 96368[1], 96372[1], 96374[1], 96375[1], 96376[1], 96377[1], 96523[0], 97597[1], 97598[1], 97602[1], 99155[0], 99156[0], 99157[0], 99211[1], 99212[1], 99213[1], 99214[1], 99215[1], 99217[1], 99218[1], 99219[1], 99220[1], 99221[1], 99222[1], 99223[1], 99231[1], 99232[1], 99233[1], 99234[1], 99235[1], 99236[1], 99238[1], 99239[1], 99241[1], 99242[1], 99243[1], 99244[1], 99245[1], 99251[1], 99252[1], 99253[1], 99254[1], 99255[1], 99291[1], 99292[1], 99304[1], 99305[1], 99306[1], 99307[1], 99308[1], 99309[1], 99310[1], 99315[1], 99316[1], 99334[1], 99335[1], 99336[1], 99337[1], 99347[1], 99348[1],

0 = Modifier usage not allowed or inappropriate 1 = Modifier usage allowed

Code 1	Code 2
	99349[1], 99350[1], 99374[1], 99375[1], 99377[1], 99378[1], 99446[0], 99447[0], 99448[0], 99449[0], 99451[0], 99452[0], 99495[0], 99496[0], G0453[0], G0463[1], G0471[1]
62140	0213T[0], 0216T[0], 0228T[0], 0230T[0], 0333T[0], 0464T[0], 11000[1], 11001[1], 11004[1], 11005[1], 11006[1], 11042[1], 11043[1], 11044[1], 11045[1], 11046[1], 11047[1], 12001[1], 12002[1], 12004[1], 12005[1], 12006[1], 12007[1], 12011[1], 12013[1], 12014[1], 12015[1], 12016[1], 12017[1], 12018[1], 12020[1], 12021[1], 12031[1], 12032[1], 12034[1], 12035[1], 12036[1], 12037[1], 12041[1], 12042[1], 12044[1], 12045[1], 12046[1], 12047[1], 12051[1], 12052[1], 12053[1], 12054[1], 12055[1], 12056[1], 12057[1], 13100[1], 13101[1], 13102[1], 13120[1], 13121[1], 13122[1], 13131[1], 13132[1], 13133[1], 13151[1], 13152[1], 13153[1], 36000[1], 36400[1], 36405[1], 36406[1], 36410[1], 36420[1], 36425[1], 36430[1], 36440[1], 36591[0], 36592[0], 36600[1], 36640[1], 43752[1], 51701[1], 51702[1], 51703[1], 62141[1], 62320[0], 62321[0], 62322[0], 62323[0], 62324[0], 62325[0], 62326[0], 62327[0], 64400[0], 64405[0], 64408[0], 64415[0], 64416[0], 64417[0], 64418[0], 64420[0], 64421[0], 64425[0], 64430[0], 64435[0], 64445[0], 64446[0], 64447[0], 64448[0], 64449[0], 64450[0], 64451[0], 64454[0], 64461[0], 64462[0], 64463[0], 64479[0], 64480[0], 64483[0], 64484[0], 64486[0], 64487[0], 64488[0], 64489[0], 64490[0], 64491[0], 64492[0], 64493[0], 64494[0], 64495[0], 64505[0], 64510[0], 64517[0], 64520[0], 64530[0], 69990[1], 92012[1], 92014[1], 92585[0], 93000[1], 93005[1], 93010[1], 93040[1], 93041[1], 93042[1], 93318[1], 93355[1], 94002[1], 94200[1], 94250[1], 94680[1], 94681[1], 94690[1], 94770[1], 95812[1], 95813[1], 95816[1], 95819[1], 95822[0], 95829[1], 95860[0], 95861[0], 95863[0], 95864[0], 95865[0], 95866[0], 95867[0], 95868[0], 95869[0], 95870[0], 95907[0], 95908[0], 95909[0], 95910[0], 95911[0], 95912[0], 95913[0], 95925[0], 95926[0], 95927[0], 95928[0], 95929[0], 95930[0], 95933[0], 95937[0], 95938[0], 95939[0], 95940[0], 95955[1], 96360[1], 96361[1], 96365[1], 96366[1], 96367[1], 96368[1], 96372[1], 96374[1], 96375[1], 96376[1], 96377[1], 96523[0], 97597[1], 97598[1], 97602[1], 99155[0], 99156[0], 99157[0], 99211[1], 99212[1], 99213[1], 99214[1], 99215[1], 99217[1], 99218[1], 99219[1], 99220[1], 99221[1], 99222[1], 99223[1], 99231[1], 99232[1], 99233[1], 99234[1], 99235[1], 99236[1], 99238[1], 99239[1], 99241[1], 99242[1], 99243[1], 99244[1], 99245[1], 99251[1], 99252[1], 99253[1], 99254[1], 99255[1], 99291[1], 99292[1], 99304[1], 99305[1], 99306[1], 99307[1], 99308[1], 99309[1], 99310[1], 99315[1], 99316[1], 99334[1], 99335[1], 99336[1], 99337[1], 99347[1], 99348[1], 99349[1], 99350[1], 99374[1], 99375[1], 99377[1], 99378[1], 99446[0], 99447[0], 99448[0], 99449[0], 99451[0], 99452[0], 99495[0], 99496[0], G0453[0], G0463[1], G0471[1]
62141	0213T[0], 0216T[0], 0228T[0], 0230T[0], 0333T[0], 0464T[0], 11000[1], 11001[1], 11004[1], 11005[1], 11006[1], 11042[1], 11043[1], 11044[1], 11045[1], 11046[1], 11047[1], 12001[1], 12002[1], 12004[1], 12005[1], 12006[1], 12007[1], 12011[1], 12013[1], 12014[1], 12015[1], 12016[1], 12017[1], 12018[1], 12020[1], 12021[1], 12031[1], 12032[1], 12034[1], 12035[1], 12036[1], 12037[1], 12041[1], 12042[1], 12044[1], 12045[1], 12046[1], 12047[1], 12051[1], 12052[1], 12053[1], 12054[1], 12055[1], 12056[1], 12057[1], 13100[1], 13101[1], 13102[1], 13120[1], 13121[1], 13122[1], 13131[1], 13132[1], 13133[1], 13151[1], 13152[1], 13153[1], 36000[1], 36400[1], 36405[1], 36406[1], 36410[1], 36420[1], 36425[1], 36430[1], 36440[1], 36591[0], 36592[0], 36600[1], 36640[1], 43752[1], 51701[1], 51702[1], 51703[1], 62320[0], 62321[0], 62322[0], 62323[0], 62324[0], 62325[0], 62326[0], 62327[0], 64400[0], 64405[0], 64408[0], 64415[0], 64416[0], 64417[0], 64418[0], 64420[0], 64421[0], 64425[0], 64430[0], 64435[0], 64445[0], 64446[0], 64447[0], 64448[0], 64449[0], 64450[0], 64451[0], 64454[0], 64461[0], 64462[0], 64463[0], 64479[0], 64480[0], 64483[0], 64484[0], 64486[0], 64487[0], 64488[0], 64489[0], 64490[0], 64491[0], 64492[0], 64493[0], 64494[0], 64495[0], 64505[0], 64510[0], 64517[0], 64520[0], 64530[0], 69990[1], 92012[1], 92014[1], 92585[0], 93000[1], 93005[1], 93010[1], 93040[1], 93041[1], 93042[1], 93318[1], 93355[1], 94002[1], 94200[1], 94250[1], 94680[1], 94681[1], 94690[1], 94770[1], 95812[1], 95813[1], 95816[1], 95819[1], 95822[0], 95829[1], 95860[0], 95861[0], 95863[0], 95864[0], 95865[0], 95866[0], 95867[0], 95868[0], 95869[0], 95870[0], 95907[0], 95908[0], 95909[0], 95910[0], 95911[0], 95912[0], 95913[0], 95925[0], 95926[0], 95927[0], 95928[0], 95929[0], 95930[0], 95933[0], 95937[0], 95938[0], 95939[0], 95940[0], 95955[1], 96360[1], 96361[1], 96365[1], 96366[1], 96367[1], 96368[1], 96372[1], 96374[1], 96375[1], 96376[1], 96377[1], 96523[0], 97597[1], 97598[1], 97602[1], 99155[0], 99156[0], 99157[0], 99211[1], 99212[1], 99213[1], 99214[1], 99215[1], 99217[1], 99218[1], 99219[1], 99220[1], 99221[1], 99222[1], 99223[1], 99231[1], 99232[1], 99233[1], 99234[1], 99235[1], 99236[1], 99238[1], 99239[1], 99241[1], 99242[1], 99243[1], 99244[1], 99245[1], 99251[1], 99252[1], 99253[1], 99254[1], 99255[1], 99291[1], 99292[1], 99304[1], 99305[1], 99306[1], 99307[1], 99308[1], 99309[1], 99310[1], 99315[1], 99316[1], 99334[1], 99335[1], 99336[1], 99337[1], 99347[1], 99348[1], 99349[1], 99350[1], 99374[1], 99375[1], 99377[1], 99378[1], 99446[0], 99447[0], 99448[0], 99449[0], 99451[0], 99452[0], 99495[0], 99496[0], G0453[0], G0463[1], G0471[1]
62142	0213T[0], 0216T[0], 0228T[0], 0230T[0], 0333T[0], 0464T[0], 11000[1], 11001[1], 11004[1], 11005[1], 11006[1], 11042[1], 11043[1], 11044[1], 11045[1], 11046[1], 11047[1], 12001[1], 12002[1], 12004[1], 12005[1], 12006[1], 12007[1], 12011[1], 12013[1], 12014[1], 12015[1], 12016[1], 12017[1], 12018[1], 12020[1], 12021[1], 12031[1], 12032[1], 12034[1], 12035[1], 12036[1], 12037[1], 12041[1], 12042[1], 12044[1], 12045[1], 12046[1], 12047[1], 12051[1], 12052[1], 12053[1], 12054[1], 12055[1], 12056[1], 12057[1], 13100[1], 13101[1], 13102[1], 13120[1], 13121[1], 13122[1], 13131[1], 13132[1], 13133[1], 13151[1], 13152[1], 13153[1], 36000[1], 36400[1], 36405[1], 36406[1], 36410[1], 36420[1], 36425[1], 36430[1], 36440[1], 36591[0], 36592[0], 36600[1], 36640[1], 43752[1], 51701[1], 51702[1], 51703[1], 62320[0], 62321[0], 62322[0], 62323[0], 62324[0], 62325[0], 62326[0], 62327[0], 64400[0], 64405[0], 64408[0], 64415[0], 64416[0], 64417[0], 64418[0], 64420[0], 64421[0], 64425[0], 64430[0], 64435[0], 64445[0], 64446[0], 64447[0], 64448[0], 64449[0], 64450[0], 64451[0], 64454[0], 64461[0], 64462[0], 64463[0], 64479[0], 64480[0], 64483[0], 64484[0], 64486[0], 64487[0], 64488[0], 64489[0], 64490[0], 64491[0], 64492[0], 64493[0], 64494[0], 64495[0], 64505[0], 64510[0], 64517[0], 64520[0], 64530[0], 69990[1], 92012[1], 92014[1], 92585[0], 93000[1], 93005[1], 93010[1], 93040[1], 93041[1], 93042[1], 93318[1], 93355[1], 94002[1], 94200[1], 94250[1], 94680[1], 94681[1], 94690[1], 94770[1], 95812[1], 95813[1], 95816[1], 95819[1], 95822[0], 95829[1], 95860[0], 95861[0], 95863[0], 95864[0], 95865[0], 95866[0], 95867[0], 95868[0], 95869[0], 95870[0], 95907[0], 95908[0], 95909[0], 95910[0], 95911[0], 95912[0], 95913[0], 95925[0], 95926[0], 95927[0], 95928[0], 95929[0], 95930[0], 95933[0], 95937[0], 95938[0], 95939[0], 95940[0], 95955[1], 96360[1], 96361[1], 96365[1], 96366[1], 96367[1], 96368[1], 96372[1], 96374[1], 96375[1], 96376[1], 96377[1], 96523[0], 97597[1], 97598[1], 97602[1], 99155[0], 99156[0], 99157[0], 99211[1], 99212[1], 99213[1], 99214[1], 99215[1], 99217[1], 99218[1], 99219[1], 99220[1], 99221[1], 99222[1], 99223[1], 99231[1], 99232[1], 99233[1], 99234[1], 99235[1], 99236[1], 99238[1], 99239[1], 99241[1], 99242[1], 99243[1], 99244[1], 99245[1], 99251[1], 99252[1], 99253[1], 99254[1], 99255[1], 99291[1], 99292[1], 99304[1], 99305[1], 99306[1], 99307[1], 99308[1], 99309[1], 99310[1], 99315[1], 99316[1], 99334[1], 99335[1], 99336[1], 99337[1], 99347[1], 99348[1], 99349[1], 99350[1], 99374[1], 99375[1], 99377[1], 99378[1], 99446[0], 99447[0], 99448[0], 99449[0], 99451[0], 99452[0], 99495[0], 99496[0], G0453[0], G0463[1], G0471[1]
62143	0213T[0], 0216T[0], 0228T[0], 0230T[0], 0333T[0], 0464T[0], 11000[1], 11001[1], 11004[1], 11005[1], 11006[1], 11042[1], 11043[1], 11044[1], 11045[1], 11046[1], 11047[1], 12001[1], 12002[1], 12004[1], 12005[1], 12006[1], 12007[1], 12011[1], 12013[1], 12014[1], 12015[1], 12016[1], 12017[1], 12018[1], 12020[1], 12021[1], 12031[1], 12032[1], 12034[1], 12035[1], 12036[1], 12037[1], 12041[1], 12042[1], 12044[1], 12045[1], 12046[1], 12047[1], 12051[1], 12052[1], 12053[1], 12054[1], 12055[1], 12056[1], 12057[1], 13100[1], 13101[1], 13102[1], 13120[1], 13121[1], 13122[1], 13131[1], 13132[1], 13133[1], 13151[1], 13152[1], 13153[1], 36000[1], 36400[1], 36405[1], 36406[1], 36410[1], 36420[1], 36425[1], 36430[1], 36440[1], 36591[0], 36592[0], 36600[1], 36640[1], 43752[1], 51701[1], 51702[1], 51703[1], 62320[0], 62321[0], 62322[0], 62323[0], 62324[0], 62325[0], 62326[0], 62327[0], 64400[0], 64405[0], 64408[0], 64415[0], 64416[0], 64417[0], 64418[0], 64420[0], 64421[0], 64425[0], 64430[0], 64435[0], 64445[0], 64446[0], 64447[0], 64448[0], 64449[0], 64450[0], 64451[0], 64454[0], 64461[0], 64462[0], 64463[0], 64479[0], 64480[0], 64483[0], 64484[0], 64486[0], 64487[0], 64488[0], 64489[0], 64490[0], 64491[0], 64492[0], 64493[0], 64494[0], 64495[0], 64505[0], 64510[0], 64517[0], 64520[0], 64530[0], 69990[1], 92012[1], 92014[1], 92585[0], 93000[1], 93005[1], 93010[1], 93040[1], 93041[1], 93042[1], 93318[1], 93355[1], 94002[1], 94200[1], 94250[1], 94680[1], 94681[1], 94690[1], 94770[1], 95812[1], 95813[1], 95816[1], 95819[1], 95822[0], 95829[1], 95860[0], 95861[0], 95863[0], 95864[0], 95865[0], 95866[0], 95867[0], 95868[0], 95869[0], 95870[0], 95907[0], 95908[0], 95909[0], 95910[0], 95911[0], 95912[0], 95913[0], 95925[0], 95926[0], 95927[0], 95928[0], 95929[0], 95930[0], 95933[0], 95937[0], 95938[0], 95939[0], 95940[0], 95955[1], 96360[1], 96361[1], 96365[1], 96366[1], 96367[1], 96368[1], 96372[1], 96374[1], 96375[1], 96376[1], 96377[1], 96523[0], 97597[1], 97598[1], 97602[1], 99155[0], 99156[0], 99157[0], 99211[1], 99212[1], 99213[1], 99214[1], 99215[1], 99217[1], 99218[1], 99219[1], 99220[1], 99221[1], 99222[1], 99223[1], 99231[1], 99232[1], 99233[1], 99234[1], 99235[1], 99236[1], 99238[1], 99239[1], 99241[1], 99242[1], 99243[1], 99244[1], 99245[1], 99251[1], 99252[1], 99253[1], 99254[1], 99255[1], 99291[1], 99292[1], 99304[1], 99305[1], 99306[1], 99307[1], 99308[1], 99309[1], 99310[1], 99315[1], 99316[1], 99334[1], 99335[1], 99336[1], 99337[1], 99347[1], 99348[1], 99349[1], 99350[1], 99374[1], 99375[1], 99377[1], 99378[1], 99446[0], 99447[0], 99448[0], 99449[0], 99451[0], 99452[0], 99495[0], 99496[0], G0453[0], G0463[1], G0471[1]
62145	0213T[0], 0216T[0], 0228T[0], 0230T[0], 0333T[0], 0464T[0], 11000[1], 11001[1], 11004[1], 11005[1], 11006[1], 11042[1], 11043[1], 11044[1], 11045[1], 11046[1], 11047[1], 12001[1], 12002[1], 12004[1], 12005[1], 12006[1], 12007[1], 12011[1], 12013[1], 12014[1], 12015[1], 12016[1], 12017[1], 12018[1], 12020[1], 12021[1], 12031[1], 12032[1], 12034[1], 12035[1], 12036[1], 12037[1], 12041[1], 12042[1], 12044[1], 12045[1], 12046[1], 12047[1], 12051[1], 12052[1], 12053[1], 12054[1], 12055[1], 12056[1], 12057[1], 13100[1], 13101[1], 13102[1], 13120[1], 13121[1], 13122[1], 13131[1], 13132[1], 13133[1], 13151[1], 13152[1], 13153[1], 36000[1], 36400[1], 36405[1], 36406[1], 36410[1], 36420[1], 36425[1], 36430[1], 36440[1], 36591[0], 36592[0], 36600[1], 36640[1], 43752[1], 51701[1], 51702[1], 51703[1], 62140[1], 62141[1], 62147[1], 62320[0], 62321[0], 62322[0], 62323[0], 62324[0], 62325[0], 62326[0], 62327[0], 64400[0], 64405[0], 64408[0], 64415[0], 64416[0], 64417[0], 64418[0], 64420[0], 64421[0], 64425[0], 64430[0], 64435[0], 64445[0], 64446[0], 64447[0], 64448[0], 64449[0], 64450[0], 64451[0], 64454[0], 64461[0], 64462[0], 64463[0], 64479[0], 64480[0], 64483[0], 64484[0], 64486[0], 64487[0], 64488[0], 64489[0], 64490[0], 64491[0], 64492[0], 64493[0], 64494[0], 64495[0], 64505[0], 64510[0], 64517[0], 64520[0], 64530[0], 69990[1], 92012[1], 92014[1], 92585[0], 93000[1], 93005[1], 93010[1], 93040[1], 93041[1], 93042[1], 93318[1], 93355[1], 94002[1], 94200[1], 94250[1], 94680[1], 94681[1], 94690[1], 94770[1], 95812[1], 95813[1], 95816[1], 95819[1], 95822[0], 95829[1], 95860[0], 95861[0], 95863[0], 95864[0], 95865[0], 95866[0], 95867[0], 95868[0], 95869[0], 95870[0], 95907[0], 95908[0], 95909[0], 95910[0], 95911[0], 95912[0], 95913[0], 95925[0], 95926[0], 95927[0], 95928[0], 95929[0], 95930[0], 95933[0], 95937[0], 95938[0], 95939[0], 95940[0], 95955[1], 96360[1], 96361[1], 96365[1], 96366[1], 96367[1], 96368[1], 96372[1], 96374[1], 96375[1], 96376[1], 96377[1], 96523[0], 97597[1], 97598[1], 97602[1], 99155[0], 99156[0], 99157[0], 99211[1], 99212[1], 99213[1], 99214[1], 99215[1],

0 = Modifier usage not allowed or inappropriate   1 = Modifier usage allowed

Code 1	Code 2
	99217[1], 99218[1], 99219[1], 99220[1], 99221[1], 99222[1], 99223[1], 99231[1], 99232[1], 99233[1], 99234[1], 99235[1], 99236[1], 99238[1], 99239[1], 99241[1], 99242[1], 99243[1], 99244[1], 99245[1], 99251[1], 99252[1], 99253[1], 99254[1], 99255[1], 99291[1], 99292[1], 99304[1], 99305[1], 99306[1], 99307[1], 99308[1], 99309[1], 99310[1], 99315[1], 99316[1], 99334[1], 99335[1], 99336[1], 99337[1], 99347[1], 99348[1], 99349[1], 99350[1], 99374[1], 99375[1], 99377[1], 99378[1], 99446[0], 99447[0], 99448[0], 99449[0], 99451[0], 99452[0], 99495[0], 99496[0], G0453[0], G0463[1], G0471[1]
62146	0213T[0], 0216T[0], 0228T[0], 0230T[0], 0333T[0], 0464T[0], 11000[1], 11001[1], 11004[1], 11005[1], 11006[1], 11042[1], 11043[1], 11044[1], 11045[1], 11046[1], 11047[1], 12001[1], 12002[1], 12004[1], 12005[1], 12006[1], 12007[1], 12011[1], 12013[1], 12014[1], 12015[1], 12016[1], 12017[1], 12018[1], 12020[1], 12021[1], 12031[1], 12032[1], 12034[1], 12035[1], 12036[1], 12037[1], 12041[1], 12042[1], 12044[1], 12045[1], 12046[1], 12047[1], 12051[1], 12052[1], 12053[1], 12054[1], 12055[1], 12056[1], 12057[1], 13100[1], 13101[1], 13102[1], 13120[1], 13121[1], 13122[1], 13131[1], 13132[1], 13133[1], 13151[1], 13152[1], 13153[1], 36000[1], 36400[1], 36405[1], 36406[1], 36410[1], 36420[1], 36425[1], 36430[1], 36440[1], 36591[0], 36592[0], 36600[1], 36640[1], 43752[1], 51701[1], 51702[1], 51703[1], 62117[1], 62140[1], 62141[1], 62145[1], 62320[0], 62321[0], 62322[0], 62323[0], 62324[0], 62325[0], 62326[0], 62327[0], 64400[0], 64405[0], 64408[0], 64415[0], 64416[0], 64417[0], 64418[0], 64420[0], 64421[0], 64425[0], 64430[0], 64435[0], 64445[0], 64446[0], 64447[0], 64448[0], 64449[0], 64450[0], 64451[0], 64454[0], 64461[0], 64462[0], 64463[0], 64479[0], 64480[0], 64483[0], 64484[0], 64486[0], 64487[0], 64488[0], 64489[0], 64490[0], 64491[0], 64492[0], 64493[0], 64494[0], 64495[0], 64505[0], 64510[0], 64517[0], 64520[0], 64530[0], 69990[1], 92012[1], 92014[1], 92585[0], 93000[1], 93005[1], 93010[1], 93040[1], 93041[1], 93042[1], 93318[1], 93355[1], 94002[1], 94200[1], 94250[1], 94680[1], 94681[1], 94690[1], 94770[1], 95812[1], 95813[1], 95816[1], 95819[1], 95822[0], 95829[1], 95860[0], 95861[0], 95863[0], 95864[0], 95865[0], 95866[0], 95867[0], 95868[0], 95869[0], 95870[0], 95907[0], 95908[0], 95909[0], 95910[0], 95911[0], 95912[0], 95913[0], 95925[0], 95926[0], 95927[0], 95928[0], 95929[0], 95930[0], 95933[0], 95937[0], 95938[0], 95939[0], 95940[0], 95955[1], 96360[1], 96361[1], 96365[1], 96366[1], 96367[1], 96368[1], 96372[1], 96374[1], 96375[1], 96376[1], 96377[1], 96523[0], 97597[1], 97598[1], 97602[1], 99155[0], 99156[0], 99157[0], 99211[1], 99212[1], 99213[1], 99214[1], 99215[1], 99217[1], 99218[1], 99219[1], 99220[1], 99221[1], 99222[1], 99223[1], 99231[1], 99232[1], 99233[1], 99234[1], 99235[1], 99236[1], 99238[1], 99239[1], 99241[1], 99242[1], 99243[1], 99244[1], 99245[1], 99251[1], 99252[1], 99253[1], 99254[1], 99255[1], 99291[1], 99292[1], 99304[1], 99305[1], 99306[1], 99307[1], 99308[1], 99309[1], 99310[1], 99315[1], 99316[1], 99334[1], 99335[1], 99336[1], 99337[1], 99347[1], 99348[1], 99349[1], 99350[1], 99374[1], 99375[1], 99377[1], 99378[1], 99446[0], 99447[0], 99448[0], 99449[0], 99451[0], 99452[0], 99495[0], 99496[0], G0453[0], G0463[1], G0471[1]
62147	0213T[0], 0216T[0], 0228T[0], 0230T[0], 0333T[0], 0464T[0], 11000[1], 11001[1], 11004[1], 11005[1], 11006[1], 11042[1], 11043[1], 11044[1], 11045[1], 11046[1], 11047[1], 12001[1], 12002[1], 12004[1], 12005[1], 12006[1], 12007[1], 12011[1], 12013[1], 12014[1], 12015[1], 12016[1], 12017[1], 12018[1], 12020[1], 12021[1], 12031[1], 12032[1], 12034[1], 12035[1], 12036[1], 12037[1], 12041[1], 12042[1], 12044[1], 12045[1], 12046[1], 12047[1], 12051[1], 12052[1], 12053[1], 12054[1], 12055[1], 12056[1], 12057[1], 13100[1], 13101[1], 13102[1], 13120[1], 13121[1], 13122[1], 13131[1], 13132[1], 13133[1], 13151[1], 13152[1], 13153[1], 36000[1], 36400[1], 36405[1], 36406[1], 36410[1], 36420[1], 36425[1], 36430[1], 36440[1], 36591[0], 36592[0], 36600[1], 36640[1], 43752[1], 51701[1], 51702[1], 51703[1], 62117[1], 62140[1], 62141[1], 62146[1], 62320[0], 62321[0], 62322[0], 62323[0], 62324[0], 62325[0], 62326[0], 62327[0], 64400[0], 64405[0], 64408[0], 64415[0], 64416[0], 64417[0], 64418[0], 64420[0], 64421[0], 64425[0], 64430[0], 64435[0], 64445[0], 64446[0], 64447[0], 64448[0], 64449[0], 64450[0], 64451[0], 64454[0], 64461[0], 64462[0], 64463[0], 64479[0], 64480[0], 64483[0], 64484[0], 64486[0], 64487[0], 64488[0], 64489[0], 64490[0], 64491[0], 64492[0], 64493[0], 64494[0], 64495[0], 64505[0], 64510[0], 64517[0], 64520[0], 64530[0], 69990[1], 92012[1], 92014[1], 92585[0], 93000[1], 93005[1], 93010[1], 93040[1], 93041[1], 93042[1], 93318[1], 93355[1], 94002[1], 94200[1], 94250[1], 94680[1], 94681[1], 94690[1], 94770[1], 95812[1], 95813[1], 95816[1], 95819[1], 95822[0], 95829[1], 95860[0], 95861[0], 95863[0], 95864[0], 95865[0], 95866[0], 95867[0], 95868[0], 95869[0], 95870[0], 95907[0], 95908[0], 95909[0], 95910[0], 95911[0], 95912[0], 95913[0], 95925[0], 95926[0], 95927[0], 95928[0], 95929[0], 95930[0], 95933[0], 95937[0], 95938[0], 95939[0], 95940[0], 95955[1], 96360[1], 96361[1], 96365[1], 96366[1], 96367[1], 96368[1], 96372[1], 96374[1], 96375[1], 96376[1], 96377[1], 96523[0], 97597[1], 97598[1], 97602[1], 99155[0], 99156[0], 99157[0], 99211[1], 99212[1], 99213[1], 99214[1], 99215[1], 99217[1], 99218[1], 99219[1], 99220[1], 99221[1], 99222[1], 99223[1], 99231[1], 99232[1], 99233[1], 99234[1], 99235[1], 99236[1], 99238[1], 99239[1], 99241[1], 99242[1], 99243[1], 99244[1], 99245[1], 99251[1], 99252[1], 99253[1], 99254[1], 99255[1], 99291[1], 99292[1], 99304[1], 99305[1], 99306[1], 99307[1], 99308[1], 99309[1], 99310[1], 99315[1], 99316[1], 99334[1], 99335[1], 99336[1], 99337[1], 99347[1], 99348[1], 99349[1], 99350[1], 99374[1], 99375[1], 99377[1], 99378[1], 99446[0], 99447[0], 99448[0], 99449[0], 99451[0], 99452[0], 99495[0], 99496[0], G0453[0], G0463[1], G0471[1]
62148	0213T[1], 0216T[1], 0333T[0], 0464T[0], 11000[1], 11001[1], 11004[1], 11005[1], 11006[1], 11042[1], 11043[1], 11044[1], 11045[1], 11046[1], 11047[1], 36000[1], 36410[1], 36591[0], 36592[0], 61650[1], 62324[0], 62325[0], 62326[0], 62327[0], 64415[1], 64417[1], 64450[1], 64454[1], 64486[1], 64487[1], 64488[1], 64489[1], 64490[1], 64493[1], 92585[0], 95822[0], 95860[0], 95861[0], 95863[0], 95864[0], 95865[0], 95866[0], 95867[0], 95868[0], 95869[0], 95907[0], 95908[0], 95909[0], 95910[0], 95911[0], 95912[0], 95913[0], 95925[0], 95926[0], 95927[0], 95930[0], 95933[0], 95937[0], 95938[0], 95939[0], 95940[0], 96523[0], 97597[1], 97598[1], 97602[1], G0453[0]
62160	0213T[1], 0216T[1], 0333T[0], 0464T[0], 11000[1], 11001[1], 11004[1], 11005[1], 11006[1], 11042[1], 11043[1], 11044[1], 11045[1], 11046[1], 11047[1], 36000[1], 36410[1], 36591[0], 36592[0], 61650[1], 62324[0], 62325[0], 62326[0], 62327[0], 64415[1], 64417[1], 64450[1], 64454[1], 64486[1], 64487[1], 64488[1], 64489[1], 64490[1], 64493[1], 69990[1], 92585[0], 95822[0], 95860[0], 95861[0], 95863[0], 95864[0], 95865[0], 95866[0], 95867[0], 95868[0], 95869[0], 95907[0], 95908[0], 95909[0], 95910[0], 95911[0], 95912[0], 95913[0], 95925[0], 95926[0], 95927[0], 95930[0], 95933[0], 95937[0], 95938[0], 95939[0], 95940[0], 96523[0], 97597[1], 97598[1], 97602[1], G0453[0]
62161	0213T[0], 0216T[0], 0228T[0], 0230T[0], 0333T[0], 0464T[0], 11000[1], 11001[1], 11004[1], 11005[1], 11006[1], 11042[1], 11043[1], 11044[1], 11045[1], 11046[1], 11047[1], 12001[1], 12002[1], 12004[1], 12005[1], 12006[1], 12007[1], 12011[1], 12013[1], 12014[1], 12015[1], 12016[1], 12017[1], 12018[1], 12020[1], 12021[1], 12031[1], 12032[1], 12034[1], 12035[1], 12036[1], 12037[1], 12041[1], 12042[1], 12044[1], 12045[1], 12046[1], 12047[1], 12051[1], 12052[1], 12053[1], 12054[1], 12055[1], 12056[1], 12057[1], 13100[1], 13101[1], 13102[1], 13120[1], 13121[1], 13122[1], 13131[1], 13132[1], 13133[1], 13151[1], 13152[1], 13153[1], 36000[1], 36400[1], 36405[1], 36406[1], 36410[1], 36420[1], 36425[1], 36430[1], 36440[1], 36591[0], 36592[0], 36600[1], 36640[1], 43752[1], 51701[1], 51702[1], 51703[1], 61105[1], 61107[0], 61108[1], 61120[1], 61140[1], 61150[1], 61151[1], 61154[1], 61156[1], 61210[1], 61215[1], 61250[1], 61253[1], 62160[1], 62201[1], 62220[1], 62223[1], 62225[1], 62230[1], 62256[1], 62258[1], 62320[0], 62321[0], 62322[0], 62323[0], 62324[0], 62325[0], 62326[0], 62327[0], 64400[0], 64405[0], 64408[0], 64415[0], 64416[0], 64417[0], 64418[0], 64420[0], 64421[0], 64425[0], 64430[0], 64435[0], 64445[0], 64446[0], 64447[0], 64448[0], 64449[0], 64450[0], 64451[0], 64454[0], 64461[0], 64462[0], 64463[0], 64479[0], 64480[0], 64483[0], 64484[0], 64486[0], 64487[0], 64488[0], 64489[0], 64490[0], 64491[0], 64492[0], 64493[0], 64494[0], 64495[0], 64505[0], 64510[0], 64517[0], 64520[0], 64530[0], 69990[0], 76000[1], 77001[1], 77002[1], 92012[1], 92014[1], 92585[0], 93000[1], 93005[1], 93010[1], 93040[1], 93041[1], 93042[1], 93318[1], 93355[1], 94002[1], 94200[1], 94250[1], 94680[1], 94681[1], 94690[1], 94770[1], 95812[1], 95813[1], 95816[1], 95819[1], 95822[0], 95829[1], 95860[0], 95861[0], 95863[0], 95864[0], 95865[0], 95866[0], 95867[0], 95868[0], 95869[0], 95870[0], 95907[0], 95908[0], 95909[0], 95910[0], 95911[0], 95912[0], 95913[0], 95925[0], 95926[0], 95927[0], 95928[0], 95929[0], 95930[0], 95933[0], 95937[0], 95938[0], 95939[0], 95940[0], 95955[1], 96360[1], 96361[1], 96365[1], 96366[1], 96367[1], 96368[1], 96372[1], 96374[1], 96375[1], 96376[1], 96377[1], 96523[0], 97597[1], 97598[1], 97602[1], 99155[0], 99156[0], 99157[0], 99211[1], 99212[1], 99213[1], 99214[1], 99215[1], 99217[1], 99218[1], 99219[1], 99220[1], 99221[1], 99222[1], 99223[1], 99231[1], 99232[1], 99233[1], 99234[1], 99235[1], 99236[1], 99238[1], 99239[1], 99241[1], 99242[1], 99243[1], 99244[1], 99245[1], 99251[1], 99252[1], 99253[1], 99254[1], 99255[1], 99291[1], 99292[1], 99304[1], 99305[1], 99306[1], 99307[1], 99308[1], 99309[1], 99310[1], 99315[1], 99316[1], 99334[1], 99335[1], 99336[1], 99337[1], 99347[1], 99348[1], 99349[1], 99350[1], 99374[1], 99375[1], 99377[1], 99378[1], 99446[0], 99447[0], 99448[0], 99449[0], 99451[0], 99452[0], 99495[0], 99496[0], G0453[0], G0463[1], G0471[1]
62162	0213T[0], 0216T[0], 0228T[0], 0230T[0], 0333T[0], 0464T[0], 11000[1], 11001[1], 11004[1], 11005[1], 11006[1], 11042[1], 11043[1], 11044[1], 11045[1], 11046[1], 11047[1], 12001[1], 12002[1], 12004[1], 12005[1], 12006[1], 12007[1], 12011[1], 12013[1], 12014[1], 12015[1], 12016[1], 12017[1], 12018[1], 12020[1], 12021[1], 12031[1], 12032[1], 12034[1], 12035[1], 12036[1], 12037[1], 12041[1], 12042[1], 12044[1], 12045[1], 12046[1], 12047[1], 12051[1], 12052[1], 12053[1], 12054[1], 12055[1], 12056[1], 12057[1], 13100[1], 13101[1], 13102[1], 13120[1], 13121[1], 13122[1], 13131[1], 13132[1], 13133[1], 13151[1], 13152[1], 13153[1], 36000[1], 36400[1], 36405[1], 36406[1], 36410[1], 36420[1], 36425[1], 36430[1], 36440[1], 36591[0], 36592[0], 36600[1], 36640[1], 43752[1], 51701[1], 51702[1], 51703[1], 61105[1], 61107[1], 61108[1], 61120[1], 61140[1], 61150[1], 61151[1], 61154[1], 61156[1], 61210[1], 61215[1], 61250[1], 61253[1], 61516[1], 62160[1], 62201[1], 62220[1], 62223[1], 62320[0], 62321[0], 62322[0], 62323[0], 62324[0], 62325[0], 62326[0], 62327[0], 64400[0], 64405[0], 64408[0], 64415[0], 64416[0], 64417[0], 64418[0], 64420[0], 64421[0], 64425[0], 64430[0], 64435[0], 64445[0], 64446[0], 64447[0], 64448[0], 64449[0], 64450[0], 64451[0], 64454[0], 64461[0], 64462[0], 64463[0], 64479[0], 64480[0], 64483[0], 64484[0], 64486[0], 64487[0], 64488[0], 64489[0], 64490[0], 64491[0], 64492[0], 64493[0], 64494[0], 64495[0], 64505[0], 64510[0], 64517[0], 64520[0], 64530[0], 69990[0], 76000[1], 77001[1], 77002[1], 92012[1], 92014[1], 92585[0], 93000[1], 93005[1], 93010[1], 93040[1], 93041[1], 93042[1], 93318[1], 93355[1], 94002[1], 94200[1], 94250[1], 94680[1], 94681[1], 94690[1], 94770[1], 95812[1], 95813[1], 95816[1], 95819[1], 95822[0], 95829[1], 95860[0], 95861[0], 95863[0], 95864[0], 95865[0], 95866[0], 95867[0], 95868[0], 95869[0], 95870[0], 95907[0], 95908[0], 95909[0], 95910[0], 95911[0], 95912[0], 95913[0], 95925[0], 95926[0], 95927[0], 95928[0], 95929[0], 95930[0], 95933[0], 95937[0], 95938[0], 95939[0], 95940[0], 95955[1], 96360[1], 96361[1], 96365[1], 96366[1], 96367[1], 96368[1], 96372[1], 96374[1], 96375[1], 96376[1], 96377[1], 96523[0], 97597[1], 97598[1], 97602[1], 99155[0], 99156[0], 99157[0], 99211[1], 99212[1], 99213[1], 99214[1], 99215[1], 99217[1], 99218[1], 99219[1], 99220[1], 99221[1], 99222[1], 99223[1], 99231[1], 99232[1], 99233[1], 99234[1], 99235[1], 99236[1], 99238[1], 99239[1], 99241[1], 99242[1], 99243[1], 99244[1], 99245[1], 99251[1], 99252[1], 99253[1], 99254[1], 99255[1], 99291[1], 99292[1], 99304[1], 99305[1], 99306[1], 99307[1], 99308[1], 99309[1], 99310[1], 99315[1], 99316[1], 99334[1], 99335[1], 99336[1], 99337[1], 99347[1], 99348[1],

0 = Modifier usage not allowed or inappropriate 1 = Modifier usage allowed

Code 1	Code 2
	99349[1], 99350[1], 99374[1], 99375[1], 99377[1], 99378[1], 99446[0], 99447[0], 99448[0], 99449[0], 99451[0], 99452[0], 99495[0], 99496[0], G0453[0], G0463[1], G0471[1]
62164	0213T[0], 0216T[0], 0228T[0], 0230T[0], 0333T[0], 0464T[0], 11000[1], 11001[1], 11004[1], 11005[1], 11006[1], 11042[1], 11043[1], 11044[1], 11045[1], 11046[1], 11047[1], 12001[1], 12002[1], 12004[1], 12005[1], 12006[1], 12007[1], 12011[1], 12013[1], 12014[1], 12015[1], 12016[1], 12017[1], 12018[1], 12020[1], 12021[1], 12031[1], 12032[1], 12034[1], 12035[1], 12036[1], 12037[1], 12041[1], 12042[1], 12044[1], 12045[1], 12046[1], 12047[1], 12051[1], 12052[1], 12053[1], 12054[1], 12055[1], 12056[1], 12057[1], 13100[1], 13101[1], 13102[1], 13120[1], 13121[1], 13122[1], 13131[1], 13132[1], 13133[1], 13151[1], 13152[1], 13153[1], 36000[1], 36400[1], 36405[1], 36406[1], 36410[1], 36420[1], 36425[1], 36430[1], 36440[1], 36591[0], 36592[0], 36600[1], 36640[1], 43752[1], 51701[1], 51702[1], 51703[1], 61105[1], 61107[1], 61108[1], 61120[1], 61140[1], 61150[1], 61151[1], 61154[1], 61156[1], 61210[1], 61215[1], 61250[1], 61253[1], 61600[1], 61605[1], 62160[1], 62201[1], 62220[1], 62223[1], 62320[0], 62321[0], 62322[0], 62323[0], 62324[0], 62325[0], 62326[0], 62327[0], 64400[0], 64405[0], 64408[0], 64415[0], 64416[0], 64417[0], 64418[0], 64420[0], 64421[0], 64425[0], 64430[0], 64435[0], 64445[0], 64446[0], 64447[0], 64448[0], 64449[0], 64450[0], 64451[0], 64454[0], 64461[0], 64462[0], 64463[0], 64479[0], 64480[0], 64483[0], 64484[0], 64486[0], 64487[0], 64488[0], 64489[0], 64490[0], 64491[0], 64492[0], 64493[0], 64494[0], 64495[0], 64505[0], 64510[0], 64517[0], 64520[0], 64530[0], 69990[0], 76000[1], 77001[1], 77002[1], 92012[1], 92014[1], 92585[0], 93000[1], 93005[1], 93010[1], 93040[1], 93041[1], 93042[1], 93318[1], 93355[1], 94002[1], 94200[1], 94250[1], 94680[1], 94681[1], 94690[1], 94770[1], 95812[1], 95813[1], 95816[1], 95819[1], 95822[0], 95829[1], 95860[0], 95861[0], 95863[0], 95864[0], 95865[0], 95866[0], 95867[0], 95868[0], 95869[0], 95870[0], 95907[0], 95908[0], 95909[0], 95910[0], 95911[0], 95912[0], 95913[0], 95925[0], 95926[0], 95927[0], 95928[0], 95929[0], 95930[0], 95933[0], 95937[0], 95938[0], 95939[0], 95940[0], 95955[1], 96360[1], 96361[1], 96365[1], 96366[1], 96367[1], 96368[1], 96372[1], 96374[1], 96375[1], 96376[1], 96377[1], 96523[0], 97597[1], 97598[1], 97602[1], 99155[0], 99156[0], 99157[0], 99211[1], 99212[1], 99213[1], 99214[1], 99215[1], 99217[1], 99218[1], 99219[1], 99220[1], 99221[1], 99222[1], 99223[1], 99231[1], 99232[1], 99233[1], 99234[1], 99235[1], 99236[1], 99238[1], 99239[1], 99241[1], 99242[1], 99243[1], 99244[1], 99245[1], 99251[1], 99252[1], 99253[1], 99254[1], 99255[1], 99291[1], 99292[1], 99304[1], 99305[1], 99306[1], 99307[1], 99308[1], 99309[1], 99310[1], 99315[1], 99316[1], 99334[1], 99335[1], 99336[1], 99337[1], 99347[1], 99348[1], 99349[1], 99350[1], 99374[1], 99375[1], 99377[1], 99378[1], 99446[0], 99447[0], 99448[0], 99449[0], 99451[0], 99452[0], 99495[0], 99496[0], G0453[0], G0463[1], G0471[1]
62165	0213T[0], 0216T[0], 0228T[0], 0230T[0], 0333T[0], 0464T[0], 11000[1], 11001[1], 11004[1], 11005[1], 11006[1], 11042[1], 11043[1], 11044[1], 11045[1], 11046[1], 11047[1], 12001[1], 12002[1], 12004[1], 12005[1], 12006[1], 12007[1], 12011[1], 12013[1], 12014[1], 12015[1], 12016[1], 12017[1], 12018[1], 12020[1], 12021[1], 12031[1], 12032[1], 12034[1], 12035[1], 12036[1], 12037[1], 12041[1], 12042[1], 12044[1], 12045[1], 12046[1], 12047[1], 12051[1], 12052[1], 12053[1], 12054[1], 12055[1], 12056[1], 12057[1], 13100[1], 13101[1], 13102[1], 13120[1], 13121[1], 13122[1], 13131[1], 13132[1], 13133[1], 13151[1], 13152[1], 13153[1], 30520[0], 30930[0], 36000[1], 36400[1], 36405[1], 36406[1], 36410[1], 36420[1], 36425[1], 36430[1], 36440[1], 36591[0], 36592[0], 36600[1], 36640[1], 43752[1], 51701[1], 51702[1], 51703[1], 61105[1], 61107[1], 61108[1], 61120[1], 61140[1], 61150[1], 61151[1], 61154[1], 61156[1], 61210[1], 61215[1], 61250[1], 61253[1], 61548[0], 62160[1], 62201[1], 62320[0], 62321[0], 62322[0], 62323[0], 62324[0], 62325[0], 62326[0], 62327[0], 64400[0], 64405[0], 64408[0], 64415[0], 64416[0], 64417[0], 64418[0], 64420[0], 64421[0], 64425[0], 64430[0], 64435[0], 64445[0], 64446[0], 64447[0], 64448[0], 64449[0], 64450[0], 64451[0], 64454[0], 64461[0], 64462[0], 64463[0], 64479[0], 64480[0], 64483[0], 64484[0], 64486[0], 64487[0], 64488[0], 64489[0], 64490[0], 64491[0], 64492[0], 64493[0], 64494[0], 64495[0], 64505[0], 64510[0], 64517[0], 64520[0], 64530[0], 69990[0], 76000[1], 77001[1], 77002[1], 92012[1], 92014[1], 92585[0], 93000[1], 93005[1], 93010[1], 93040[1], 93041[1], 93042[1], 93318[1], 93355[1], 94002[1], 94200[1], 94250[1], 94680[1], 94681[1], 94690[1], 94770[1], 95812[1], 95813[1], 95816[1], 95819[1], 95822[0], 95829[1], 95860[0], 95861[0], 95863[0], 95864[0], 95865[0], 95866[0], 95867[0], 95868[0], 95869[0], 95870[0], 95907[0], 95908[0], 95909[0], 95910[0], 95911[0], 95912[0], 95913[0], 95925[0], 95926[0], 95927[0], 95928[0], 95929[0], 95930[0], 95933[0], 95937[0], 95938[0], 95939[0], 95940[0], 95955[1], 96360[1], 96361[1], 96365[1], 96366[1], 96367[1], 96368[1], 96372[1], 96374[1], 96375[1], 96376[1], 96377[1], 96523[0], 97597[1], 97598[1], 97602[1], 99155[0], 99156[0], 99157[0], 99211[1], 99212[1], 99213[1], 99214[1], 99215[1], 99217[1], 99218[1], 99219[1], 99220[1], 99221[1], 99222[1], 99223[1], 99231[1], 99232[1], 99233[1], 99234[1], 99235[1], 99236[1], 99238[1], 99239[1], 99241[1], 99242[1], 99243[1], 99244[1], 99245[1], 99251[1], 99252[1], 99253[1], 99254[1], 99255[1], 99291[1], 99292[1], 99304[1], 99305[1], 99306[1], 99307[1], 99308[1], 99309[1], 99310[1], 99315[1], 99316[1], 99334[1], 99335[1], 99336[1], 99337[1], 99347[1], 99348[1], 99349[1], 99350[1], 99374[1], 99375[1], 99377[1], 99378[1], 99446[0], 99447[0], 99448[0], 99449[0], 99451[0], 99452[0], 99495[0], 99496[0], G0453[0], G0463[1], G0471[1]
62190	0213T[0], 0216T[0], 0228T[0], 0230T[0], 0333T[0], 0464T[0], 12001[1], 12002[1], 12004[1], 12005[1], 12006[1], 12007[1], 12011[1], 12013[1], 12014[1], 12015[1], 12016[1], 12017[1], 12018[1], 12020[1], 12021[1], 12031[1], 12032[1], 12034[1], 12035[1], 12036[1], 12037[1], 12041[1], 12042[1], 12044[1], 12045[1], 12046[1], 12047[1], 12051[1], 12052[1], 12053[1], 12054[1], 12055[1], 12056[1], 12057[1], 13100[1], 13101[1], 13102[1], 13120[1], 13121[1], 13122[1], 13131[1], 13132[1], 13133[1], 13151[1], 13152[1], 13153[1], 36000[1], 36400[1], 36405[1], 36406[1], 36410[1], 36420[1], 36425[1], 36430[1], 36440[1], 36591[0], 36592[0], 36600[1], 36640[1], 43752[1], 51701[1], 51702[1], 51703[1], 61070[1], 62180[1], 62252[1], 62320[0], 62321[0], 62322[0], 62323[0], 62324[0], 62325[0], 62326[0], 62327[0], 64400[0], 64405[0], 64408[0], 64415[0], 64416[0], 64417[0], 64418[0], 64420[0], 64421[0], 64425[0], 64430[0], 64435[0], 64445[0], 64446[0], 64447[0], 64448[0], 64449[0], 64450[0], 64451[0], 64454[0], 64461[0], 64462[0], 64463[0], 64479[0], 64480[0], 64483[0], 64484[0], 64486[0], 64487[0], 64488[0], 64489[0], 64490[0], 64491[0], 64492[0], 64493[0], 64494[0], 64495[0], 64505[0], 64510[0], 64517[0], 64520[0], 64530[0], 69990[0], 92012[1], 92014[1], 92585[0], 93000[1], 93005[1], 93010[1], 93040[1], 93041[1], 93042[1], 93318[1], 93355[1], 94002[1], 94200[1], 94250[1], 94680[1], 94681[1], 94690[1], 94770[1], 95812[1], 95813[1], 95816[1], 95819[1], 95822[0], 95829[1], 95860[0], 95861[0], 95863[0], 95864[0], 95865[0], 95866[0], 95867[0], 95868[0], 95869[0], 95870[0], 95907[0], 95908[0], 95909[0], 95910[0], 95911[0], 95912[0], 95913[0], 95925[0], 95926[0], 95927[0], 95928[0], 95929[0], 95930[0], 95933[0], 95937[0], 95938[0], 95939[0], 95940[0], 95955[1], 96360[1], 96361[1], 96365[1], 96366[1], 96367[1], 96368[1], 96372[1], 96374[1], 96375[1], 96376[1], 96377[1], 96523[0], 99155[0], 99156[0], 99157[0], 99211[1], 99212[1], 99213[1], 99214[1], 99215[1], 99217[1], 99218[1], 99219[1], 99220[1], 99221[1], 99222[1], 99223[1], 99231[1], 99232[1], 99233[1], 99234[1], 99235[1], 99236[1], 99238[1], 99239[1], 99241[1], 99242[1], 99243[1], 99244[1], 99245[1], 99251[1], 99252[1], 99253[1], 99254[1], 99255[1], 99291[1], 99292[1], 99304[1], 99305[1], 99306[1], 99307[1], 99308[1], 99309[1], 99310[1], 99315[1], 99316[1], 99334[1], 99335[1], 99336[1], 99337[1], 99347[1], 99348[1], 99349[1], 99350[1], 99374[1], 99375[1], 99377[1], 99378[1], 99446[0], 99447[0], 99448[0], 99449[0], 99451[0], 99452[0], 99495[0], 99496[0], G0453[0], G0463[1], G0471[1]
62192	0213T[0], 0216T[0], 0228T[0], 0230T[0], 0333T[0], 0464T[0], 12001[1], 12002[1], 12004[1], 12005[1], 12006[1], 12007[1], 12011[1], 12013[1], 12014[1], 12015[1], 12016[1], 12017[1], 12018[1], 12020[1], 12021[1], 12031[1], 12032[1], 12034[1], 12035[1], 12036[1], 12037[1], 12041[1], 12042[1], 12044[1], 12045[1], 12046[1], 12047[1], 12051[1], 12052[1], 12053[1], 12054[1], 12055[1], 12056[1], 12057[1], 13100[1], 13101[1], 13102[1], 13120[1], 13121[1], 13122[1], 13131[1], 13132[1], 13133[1], 13151[1], 13152[1], 13153[1], 36000[1], 36400[1], 36405[1], 36406[1], 36410[1], 36420[1], 36425[1], 36430[1], 36440[1], 36591[0], 36592[0], 36600[1], 36640[1], 43752[1], 51701[1], 51702[1], 51703[1], 61070[1], 62180[1], 62252[1], 62320[0], 62321[0], 62322[0], 62323[0], 62324[0], 62325[0], 62326[0], 62327[0], 64400[0], 64405[0], 64408[0], 64415[0], 64416[0], 64417[0], 64418[0], 64420[0], 64421[0], 64425[0], 64430[0], 64435[0], 64445[0], 64446[0], 64447[0], 64448[0], 64449[0], 64450[0], 64451[0], 64454[0], 64461[0], 64462[0], 64463[0], 64479[0], 64480[0], 64483[0], 64484[0], 64486[0], 64487[0], 64488[0], 64489[0], 64490[0], 64491[0], 64492[0], 64493[0], 64494[0], 64495[0], 64505[0], 64510[0], 64517[0], 64520[0], 64530[0], 69990[0], 92012[1], 92014[1], 92585[0], 93000[1], 93005[1], 93010[1], 93040[1], 93041[1], 93042[1], 93318[1], 93355[1], 94002[1], 94200[1], 94250[1], 94680[1], 94681[1], 94690[1], 94770[1], 95812[1], 95813[1], 95816[1], 95819[1], 95822[0], 95829[1], 95860[0], 95861[0], 95863[0], 95864[0], 95865[0], 95866[0], 95867[0], 95868[0], 95869[0], 95870[0], 95907[0], 95908[0], 95909[0], 95910[0], 95911[0], 95912[0], 95913[0], 95925[0], 95926[0], 95927[0], 95928[0], 95929[0], 95930[0], 95933[0], 95937[0], 95938[0], 95939[0], 95940[0], 95955[1], 96360[1], 96361[1], 96365[1], 96366[1], 96367[1], 96368[1], 96372[1], 96374[1], 96375[1], 96376[1], 96377[1], 96523[0], 99155[0], 99156[0], 99157[0], 99211[1], 99212[1], 99213[1], 99214[1], 99215[1], 99217[1], 99218[1], 99219[1], 99220[1], 99221[1], 99222[1], 99223[1], 99231[1], 99232[1], 99233[1], 99234[1], 99235[1], 99236[1], 99238[1], 99239[1], 99241[1], 99242[1], 99243[1], 99244[1], 99245[1], 99251[1], 99252[1], 99253[1], 99254[1], 99255[1], 99291[1], 99292[1], 99304[1], 99305[1], 99306[1], 99307[1], 99308[1], 99309[1], 99310[1], 99315[1], 99316[1], 99334[1], 99335[1], 99336[1], 99337[1], 99347[1], 99348[1], 99349[1], 99350[1], 99374[1], 99375[1], 99377[1], 99378[1], 99446[0], 99447[0], 99448[0], 99449[0], 99451[0], 99452[0], 99495[0], 99496[0], G0453[0], G0463[1], G0471[1]
62194	0213T[0], 0216T[0], 0228T[0], 0230T[0], 0333T[0], 0464T[0], 11000[1], 11001[1], 11004[1], 11005[1], 11006[1], 11042[1], 11043[1], 11044[1], 11045[1], 11046[1], 11047[1], 12001[1], 12002[1], 12004[1], 12005[1], 12006[1], 12007[1], 12011[1], 12013[1], 12014[1], 12015[1], 12016[1], 12017[1], 12018[1], 12020[1], 12021[1], 12031[1], 12032[1], 12034[1], 12035[1], 12036[1], 12037[1], 12041[1], 12042[1], 12044[1], 12045[1], 12046[1], 12047[1], 12051[1], 12052[1], 12053[1], 12054[1], 12055[1], 12056[1], 12057[1], 13100[1], 13101[1], 13102[1], 13120[1], 13121[1], 13122[1], 13131[1], 13132[1], 13133[1], 13151[1], 13152[1], 13153[1], 36000[1], 36400[1], 36405[1], 36406[1], 36410[1], 36420[1], 36425[1], 36430[1], 36440[1], 36591[0], 36592[0], 36600[1], 36640[1], 43752[1], 51701[1], 51702[1], 51703[1], 61070[1], 62180[1], 62190[1], 62192[1], 62320[0], 62321[0], 62322[0], 62323[0], 62324[0], 62325[0], 62326[0], 62327[0], 64400[0], 64405[0], 64408[0], 64415[0], 64416[0], 64417[0], 64418[0], 64420[0], 64421[0], 64425[0], 64430[0], 64435[0], 64445[0], 64446[0], 64447[0], 64448[0], 64449[0], 64450[0], 64451[0], 64454[0], 64461[0], 64462[0], 64463[0], 64479[0], 64480[0], 64483[0], 64484[0], 64486[0], 64487[0], 64488[0], 64489[0], 64490[0], 64491[0], 64492[0], 64493[0], 64494[0], 64495[0], 64505[0], 64510[0], 64517[0], 64520[0], 64530[0], 69990[0], 92012[1], 92014[1], 92585[0], 93000[1], 93005[1], 93010[1], 93040[1], 93041[1], 93042[1], 93318[1], 93355[1], 94002[1], 94200[1], 94250[1], 94680[1], 94681[1], 94690[1], 94770[1], 95812[1], 95813[1], 95816[1], 95819[1], 95822[0], 95829[1], 95860[0], 95861[0], 95863[0], 95864[0], 95865[0], 95866[0], 95867[0], 95868[0], 95869[0], 95870[0], 95907[0], 95908[0], 95909[0], 95910[0], 95911[0], 95912[0], 95913[0], 95925[0], 95926[0], 95927[0], 95928[0], 95929[0], 95930[0], 95933[0], 95937[0], 95938[0], 95939[0], 95940[0], 95955[1], 96360[1], 96361[1],

0 = Modifier usage not allowed or inappropriate 1 = Modifier usage allowed

Code 1	Code 2
	96365[1], 96366[1], 96367[1], 96368[1], 96372[1], 96374[1], 96375[1], 96376[1], 96377[1], 96523[0], 97597[1], 97598[1], 97602[1], 99155[0], 99156[0], 99157[0], 99211[1], 99212[1], 99213[1], 99214[1], 99215[1], 99217[1], 99218[1], 99219[1], 99220[1], 99221[1], 99222[1], 99223[1], 99231[1], 99232[1], 99233[1], 99234[1], 99235[1], 99236[1], 99238[1], 99239[1], 99241[1], 99242[1], 99243[1], 99244[1], 99245[1], 99251[1], 99252[1], 99253[1], 99254[1], 99255[1], 99291[1], 99292[1], 99304[1], 99305[1], 99306[1], 99307[1], 99308[1], 99309[1], 99310[1], 99315[1], 99316[1], 99334[1], 99335[1], 99336[1], 99337[1], 99347[1], 99348[1], 99349[1], 99350[1], 99374[1], 99375[1], 99377[1], 99378[1], 99446[0], 99447[0], 99448[0], 99449[0], 99451[0], 99452[0], 99495[0], 99496[0], G0453[0], G0463[1], G0471[1]
62200	0213T[0], 0216T[0], 0228T[0], 0230T[0], 0333T[0], 0464T[0], 12001[1], 12002[1], 12004[1], 12005[1], 12006[1], 12007[1], 12011[1], 12013[1], 12014[1], 12015[1], 12016[1], 12017[1], 12018[1], 12020[1], 12021[1], 12031[1], 12032[1], 12034[1], 12035[1], 12036[1], 12037[1], 12041[1], 12042[1], 12044[1], 12045[1], 12046[1], 12047[1], 12051[1], 12052[1], 12053[1], 12054[1], 12055[1], 12056[1], 12057[1], 13100[1], 13101[1], 13102[1], 13120[1], 13121[1], 13122[1], 13131[1], 13132[1], 13133[1], 13151[1], 13152[1], 13153[1], 36000[1], 36400[1], 36405[1], 36406[1], 36410[1], 36420[1], 36425[1], 36430[1], 36440[1], 36591[0], 36592[0], 36600[1], 36640[1], 43752[1], 51701[1], 51702[1], 51703[1], 62320[0], 62321[0], 62322[0], 62323[0], 62324[0], 62325[0], 62326[0], 62327[0], 64400[0], 64405[0], 64408[0], 64415[0], 64416[0], 64417[0], 64418[0], 64420[0], 64421[0], 64425[0], 64430[0], 64435[0], 64445[0], 64446[0], 64447[0], 64448[0], 64449[0], 64450[0], 64451[0], 64454[0], 64461[0], 64462[0], 64463[0], 64479[0], 64480[0], 64483[0], 64484[0], 64486[0], 64487[0], 64488[0], 64489[0], 64490[0], 64491[0], 64492[0], 64493[0], 64494[0], 64495[0], 64505[0], 64510[0], 64517[0], 64520[0], 64530[0], 69990[0], 92012[1], 92014[1], 92585[0], 93000[1], 93005[1], 93010[1], 93040[1], 93041[1], 93042[1], 93318[1], 93355[1], 94002[1], 94200[1], 94250[1], 94680[1], 94681[1], 94690[1], 94770[1], 95812[1], 95813[1], 95816[1], 95819[1], 95822[0], 95829[1], 95860[0], 95861[0], 95863[0], 95864[0], 95865[0], 95866[0], 95867[0], 95868[0], 95869[0], 95870[0], 95907[0], 95908[0], 95909[0], 95910[0], 95911[0], 95912[0], 95913[0], 95925[0], 95926[0], 95927[0], 95928[0], 95929[0], 95930[0], 95933[0], 95937[0], 95938[0], 95939[0], 95940[0], 95955[1], 96360[1], 96361[1], 96365[1], 96366[1], 96367[1], 96368[1], 96372[1], 96374[1], 96375[1], 96376[1], 96377[1], 96523[0], 99155[0], 99156[0], 99157[0], 99211[1], 99212[1], 99213[1], 99214[1], 99215[1], 99217[1], 99218[1], 99219[1], 99220[1], 99221[1], 99222[1], 99223[1], 99231[1], 99232[1], 99233[1], 99234[1], 99235[1], 99236[1], 99238[1], 99239[1], 99241[1], 99242[1], 99243[1], 99244[1], 99245[1], 99251[1], 99252[1], 99253[1], 99254[1], 99255[1], 99291[1], 99292[1], 99304[1], 99305[1], 99306[1], 99307[1], 99308[1], 99309[1], 99310[1], 99315[1], 99316[1], 99334[1], 99335[1], 99336[1], 99337[1], 99347[1], 99348[1], 99349[1], 99350[1], 99374[1], 99375[1], 99377[1], 99378[1], 99446[0], 99447[0], 99448[0], 99449[0], 99451[0], 99452[0], 99495[0], 99496[0], G0453[0], G0463[1], G0471[1]
62201	0213T[0], 0216T[0], 0228T[0], 0230T[0], 0333T[0], 0464T[0], 12001[1], 12002[1], 12004[1], 12005[1], 12006[1], 12007[1], 12011[1], 12013[1], 12014[1], 12015[1], 12016[1], 12017[1], 12018[1], 12020[1], 12021[1], 12031[1], 12032[1], 12034[1], 12035[1], 12036[1], 12037[1], 12041[1], 12042[1], 12044[1], 12045[1], 12046[1], 12047[1], 12051[1], 12052[1], 12053[1], 12054[1], 12055[1], 12056[1], 12057[1], 13100[1], 13101[1], 13102[1], 13120[1], 13121[1], 13122[1], 13131[1], 13132[1], 13133[1], 13151[1], 13152[1], 13153[1], 36000[1], 36400[1], 36405[1], 36406[1], 36410[1], 36420[1], 36425[1], 36430[1], 36440[1], 36591[0], 36592[0], 36600[1], 36640[1], 43752[1], 51701[1], 51702[1], 51703[1], 61781[1], 61782[1], 61783[0], 62160[0], 62180[1], 62200[1], 62320[0], 62321[0], 62322[0], 62323[0], 62324[0], 62325[0], 62326[0], 62327[0], 64400[0], 64405[0], 64408[0], 64415[0], 64416[0], 64417[0], 64418[0], 64420[0], 64421[0], 64425[0], 64430[0], 64435[0], 64445[0], 64446[0], 64447[0], 64448[0], 64449[0], 64450[0], 64451[0], 64454[0], 64461[0], 64462[0], 64463[0], 64479[0], 64480[0], 64483[0], 64484[0], 64486[0], 64487[0], 64488[0], 64489[0], 64490[0], 64491[0], 64492[0], 64493[0], 64494[0], 64495[0], 64505[0], 64510[0], 64517[0], 64520[0], 64530[0], 69990[0], 92012[1], 92014[1], 92585[0], 93000[1], 93005[1], 93010[1], 93040[1], 93041[1], 93042[1], 93318[1], 93355[1], 94002[1], 94200[1], 94250[1], 94680[1], 94681[1], 94690[1], 94770[1], 95812[1], 95813[1], 95816[1], 95819[1], 95822[0], 95829[1], 95860[0], 95861[0], 95863[0], 95864[0], 95865[0], 95866[0], 95867[0], 95868[0], 95869[0], 95870[0], 95907[0], 95908[0], 95909[0], 95910[0], 95911[0], 95912[0], 95913[0], 95925[0], 95926[0], 95927[0], 95928[0], 95929[0], 95930[0], 95933[0], 95937[0], 95938[0], 95939[0], 95940[0], 95955[1], 96360[1], 96361[1], 96365[1], 96366[1], 96367[1], 96368[1], 96372[1], 96374[1], 96375[1], 96376[1], 96377[1], 96523[0], 99155[0], 99156[0], 99157[0], 99211[1], 99212[1], 99213[1], 99214[1], 99215[1], 99217[1], 99218[1], 99219[1], 99220[1], 99221[1], 99222[1], 99223[1], 99231[1], 99232[1], 99233[1], 99234[1], 99235[1], 99236[1], 99238[1], 99239[1], 99241[1], 99242[1], 99243[1], 99244[1], 99245[1], 99251[1], 99252[1], 99253[1], 99254[1], 99255[1], 99291[1], 99292[1], 99304[1], 99305[1], 99306[1], 99307[1], 99308[1], 99309[1], 99310[1], 99315[1], 99316[1], 99334[1], 99335[1], 99336[1], 99337[1], 99347[1], 99348[1], 99349[1], 99350[1], 99374[1], 99375[1], 99377[1], 99378[1], 99446[0], 99447[0], 99448[0], 99449[0], 99451[0], 99452[0], 99495[0], 99496[0], G0453[0], G0463[1], G0471[1]
62220	0213T[0], 0216T[0], 0228T[0], 0230T[0], 0333T[0], 0464T[0], 12001[1], 12002[1], 12004[1], 12005[1], 12006[1], 12007[1], 12011[1], 12013[1], 12014[1], 12015[1], 12016[1], 12017[1], 12018[1], 12020[1], 12021[1], 12031[1], 12032[1], 12034[1], 12035[1], 12036[1], 12037[1], 12041[1], 12042[1], 12044[1], 12045[1], 12046[1], 12047[1], 12051[1], 12052[1], 12053[1], 12054[1], 12055[1], 12056[1], 12057[1], 13100[1], 13101[1], 13102[1], 13120[1], 13121[1], 13122[1], 13131[1], 13132[1], 13133[1], 13151[1], 13152[1], 13153[1], 36000[1], 36400[1], 36405[1], 36406[1], 36410[1], 36420[1], 36425[1], 36430[1], 36440[1], 36591[0], 36592[0], 36600[1], 36640[1], 43752[1], 51701[1], 51702[1], 51703[1], 61070[1], 62180[1], 62252[1], 62320[0], 62321[0], 62322[0], 62323[0], 62324[0], 62325[0], 62326[0], 62327[0], 64400[0], 64405[0], 64408[0], 64415[0], 64416[0], 64417[0], 64418[0], 64420[0], 64421[0], 64425[0], 64430[0], 64435[0], 64445[0], 64446[0], 64447[0], 64448[0], 64449[0], 64450[0], 64451[0], 64454[0], 64461[0], 64462[0], 64463[0], 64479[0], 64480[0], 64483[0], 64484[0], 64486[0], 64487[0], 64488[0], 64489[0], 64490[0], 64491[0], 64492[0], 64493[0], 64494[0], 64495[0], 64505[0], 64510[0], 64517[0], 64520[0], 64530[0], 69990[0], 92012[1], 92014[1], 92585[0], 93000[1], 93005[1], 93010[1], 93040[1], 93041[1], 93042[1], 93318[1], 93355[1], 94002[1], 94200[1], 94250[1], 94680[1], 94681[1], 94690[1], 94770[1], 95812[1], 95813[1], 95816[1], 95819[1], 95822[0], 95829[1], 95860[0], 95861[0], 95863[0], 95864[0], 95865[0], 95866[0], 95867[0], 95868[0], 95869[0], 95870[0], 95907[0], 95908[0], 95909[0], 95910[0], 95911[0], 95912[0], 95913[0], 95925[0], 95926[0], 95927[0], 95928[0], 95929[0], 95930[0], 95933[0], 95937[0], 95938[0], 95939[0], 95940[0], 95955[1], 96360[1], 96361[1], 96365[1], 96366[1], 96367[1], 96368[1], 96372[1], 96374[1], 96375[1], 96376[1], 96377[1], 96523[0], 99155[0], 99156[0], 99157[0], 99211[1], 99212[1], 99213[1], 99214[1], 99215[1], 99217[1], 99218[1], 99219[1], 99220[1], 99221[1], 99222[1], 99223[1], 99231[1], 99232[1], 99233[1], 99234[1], 99235[1], 99236[1], 99238[1], 99239[1], 99241[1], 99242[1], 99243[1], 99244[1], 99245[1], 99251[1], 99252[1], 99253[1], 99254[1], 99255[1], 99291[1], 99292[1], 99304[1], 99305[1], 99306[1], 99307[1], 99308[1], 99309[1], 99310[1], 99315[1], 99316[1], 99334[1], 99335[1], 99336[1], 99337[1], 99347[1], 99348[1], 99349[1], 99350[1], 99374[1], 99375[1], 99377[1], 99378[1], 99446[0], 99447[0], 99448[0], 99449[0], 99451[0], 99452[0], 99495[0], 99496[0], G0453[0], G0463[1], G0471[1]
62223	0213T[0], 0216T[0], 0228T[0], 0230T[0], 0333T[0], 0464T[0], 12001[1], 12002[1], 12004[1], 12005[1], 12006[1], 12007[1], 12011[1], 12013[1], 12014[1], 12015[1], 12016[1], 12017[1], 12018[1], 12020[1], 12021[1], 12031[1], 12032[1], 12034[1], 12035[1], 12036[1], 12037[1], 12041[1], 12042[1], 12044[1], 12045[1], 12046[1], 12047[1], 12051[1], 12052[1], 12053[1], 12054[1], 12055[1], 12056[1], 12057[1], 13100[1], 13101[1], 13102[1], 13120[1], 13121[1], 13122[1], 13131[1], 13132[1], 13133[1], 13151[1], 13152[1], 13153[1], 36000[1], 36400[1], 36405[1], 36406[1], 36410[1], 36420[1], 36425[1], 36430[1], 36440[1], 36591[0], 36592[0], 36600[1], 36640[1], 43752[1], 51701[1], 51702[1], 51703[1], 61070[1], 62252[0], 62320[0], 62321[0], 62322[0], 62323[0], 62324[0], 62325[0], 62326[0], 62327[0], 64400[0], 64405[0], 64408[0], 64415[0], 64416[0], 64417[0], 64418[0], 64420[0], 64421[0], 64425[0], 64430[0], 64435[0], 64445[0], 64446[0], 64447[0], 64448[0], 64449[0], 64450[0], 64451[0], 64454[0], 64461[0], 64462[0], 64463[0], 64479[0], 64480[0], 64483[0], 64484[0], 64486[0], 64487[0], 64488[0], 64489[0], 64490[0], 64491[0], 64492[0], 64493[0], 64494[0], 64495[0], 64505[0], 64510[0], 64517[0], 64520[0], 64530[0], 69990[0], 92012[1], 92014[1], 92585[0], 93000[1], 93005[1], 93010[1], 93040[1], 93041[1], 93042[1], 93318[1], 93355[1], 94002[1], 94200[1], 94250[1], 94680[1], 94681[1], 94690[1], 94770[1], 95812[1], 95813[1], 95816[1], 95819[1], 95822[0], 95829[1], 95860[0], 95861[0], 95863[0], 95864[0], 95865[0], 95866[0], 95867[0], 95868[0], 95869[0], 95870[0], 95907[0], 95908[0], 95909[0], 95910[0], 95911[0], 95912[0], 95913[0], 95925[0], 95926[0], 95927[0], 95928[0], 95929[0], 95930[0], 95933[0], 95937[0], 95938[0], 95939[0], 95940[0], 95955[1], 96360[1], 96361[1], 96365[1], 96366[1], 96367[1], 96368[1], 96372[1], 96374[1], 96375[1], 96376[1], 96377[1], 96523[0], 99155[0], 99156[0], 99157[0], 99211[1], 99212[1], 99213[1], 99214[1], 99215[1], 99217[1], 99218[1], 99219[1], 99220[1], 99221[1], 99222[1], 99223[1], 99231[1], 99232[1], 99233[1], 99234[1], 99235[1], 99236[1], 99238[1], 99239[1], 99241[1], 99242[1], 99243[1], 99244[1], 99245[1], 99251[1], 99252[1], 99253[1], 99254[1], 99255[1], 99291[1], 99292[1], 99304[1], 99305[1], 99306[1], 99307[1], 99308[1], 99309[1], 99310[1], 99315[1], 99316[1], 99334[1], 99335[1], 99336[1], 99337[1], 99347[1], 99348[1], 99349[1], 99350[1], 99374[1], 99375[1], 99377[1], 99378[1], 99446[0], 99447[0], 99448[0], 99449[0], 99451[0], 99452[0], 99495[0], 99496[0], G0453[0], G0463[1], G0471[1]
62225	0213T[0], 0216T[0], 0228T[0], 0230T[0], 0333T[0], 0464T[0], 11000[1], 11001[1], 11004[1], 11005[1], 11006[1], 11042[1], 11043[1], 11044[1], 11045[1], 11046[1], 11047[1], 12001[1], 12002[1], 12004[1], 12005[1], 12006[1], 12007[1], 12011[1], 12013[1], 12014[1], 12015[1], 12016[1], 12017[1], 12018[1], 12020[1], 12021[1], 12031[1], 12032[1], 12034[1], 12035[1], 12036[1], 12037[1], 12041[1], 12042[1], 12044[1], 12045[1], 12046[1], 12047[1], 12051[1], 12052[1], 12053[1], 12054[1], 12055[1], 12056[1], 12057[1], 13100[1], 13101[1], 13102[1], 13120[1], 13121[1], 13122[1], 13131[1], 13132[1], 13133[1], 13151[1], 13152[1], 13153[1], 36000[1], 36400[1], 36405[1], 36406[1], 36410[1], 36420[1], 36425[1], 36430[1], 36440[1], 36591[0], 36592[0], 36600[1], 36640[1], 43752[1], 51701[1], 51702[1], 51703[1], 61070[1], 62180[1], 62220[1], 62320[0], 62321[0], 62322[0], 62323[0], 62324[0], 62325[0], 62326[0], 62327[0], 64400[0], 64405[0], 64408[0], 64415[0], 64416[0], 64417[0], 64418[0], 64420[0], 64421[0], 64425[0], 64430[0], 64435[0], 64445[0], 64446[0], 64447[0], 64448[0], 64449[0], 64450[0], 64451[0], 64454[0], 64461[0], 64462[0], 64463[0], 64479[0], 64480[0], 64483[0], 64484[0], 64486[0], 64487[0], 64488[0], 64489[0], 64490[0], 64491[0], 64492[0], 64493[0], 64494[0], 64495[0], 64505[0], 64510[0], 64517[0], 64520[0], 64530[0], 69990[0], 92012[1], 92014[1], 92585[0], 93000[1], 93005[1], 93010[1], 93040[1], 93041[1], 93042[1], 93318[1], 93355[1], 94002[1], 94200[1], 94250[1], 94680[1], 94681[1], 94690[1], 94770[1], 95812[1], 95813[1], 95816[1], 95819[1], 95822[0], 95829[1], 95860[0], 95861[0], 95863[0], 95864[0], 95865[0], 95866[0], 95867[0], 95868[0], 95869[0], 95870[0], 95907[0], 95908[0], 95909[0], 95910[0], 95911[0], 95912[0], 95913[0], 95925[0], 95926[0], 95927[0], 95928[0], 95929[0], 95930[0], 95933[0], 95937[0], 95938[0], 95939[0], 95940[0], 95955[1], 96360[1], 96361[1], 96365[1],

0 = Modifier usage not allowed or inappropriate 1 = Modifier usage allowed

Code 1	Code 2
	96366[1], 96367[1], 96368[1], 96372[1], 96374[1], 96375[1], 96376[1], 96377[1], 96523[0], 97597[1], 97598[1], 97602[1], 99155[0], 99156[0], 99157[0], 99211[1], 99212[1], 99213[1], 99214[1], 99215[1], 99217[1], 99218[1], 99219[1], 99220[1], 99221[1], 99222[1], 99223[1], 99231[1], 99232[1], 99233[1], 99234[1], 99235[1], 99236[1], 99238[1], 99239[1], 99241[1], 99242[1], 99243[1], 99244[1], 99245[1], 99251[1], 99252[1], 99253[1], 99254[1], 99255[1], 99291[1], 99292[1], 99304[1], 99305[1], 99306[1], 99307[1], 99308[1], 99309[1], 99310[1], 99315[1], 99316[1], 99334[1], 99335[1], 99336[1], 99337[1], 99347[1], 99348[1], 99349[1], 99350[1], 99374[1], 99375[1], 99377[1], 99378[1], 99446[0], 99447[0], 99448[0], 99449[0], 99451[0], 99452[0], 99495[0], 99496[0], G0453[0], G0463[1], G0471[1]
62230	0213T[0], 0216T[0], 0228T[0], 0230T[0], 0333T[0], 0464T[0], 11000[1], 11001[1], 11004[1], 11005[1], 11006[1], 11042[1], 11043[1], 11044[1], 11045[1], 11046[1], 11047[1], 12001[1], 12002[1], 12004[1], 12005[1], 12006[1], 12007[1], 12011[1], 12013[1], 12014[1], 12015[1], 12016[1], 12017[1], 12018[1], 12020[1], 12021[1], 12031[1], 12032[1], 12034[1], 12035[1], 12036[1], 12037[1], 12041[1], 12042[1], 12044[1], 12045[1], 12046[1], 12047[1], 12051[1], 12052[1], 12053[1], 12054[1], 12055[1], 12056[1], 12057[1], 13100[1], 13101[1], 13102[1], 13120[1], 13121[1], 13122[1], 13131[1], 13132[1], 13133[1], 13151[1], 13152[1], 13153[1], 36000[1], 36400[1], 36405[1], 36406[1], 36410[1], 36420[1], 36425[1], 36430[1], 36440[1], 36591[0], 36592[0], 36600[1], 36640[1], 43752[1], 51701[1], 51702[1], 51703[1], 61070[1], 62180[1], 62252[0], 62320[0], 62321[0], 62322[0], 62323[0], 62324[0], 62325[0], 62326[0], 62327[0], 64400[0], 64405[0], 64408[0], 64415[0], 64416[0], 64417[0], 64418[0], 64420[0], 64421[0], 64425[0], 64430[0], 64435[0], 64445[0], 64446[0], 64447[0], 64448[0], 64449[0], 64450[0], 64451[0], 64454[0], 64461[0], 64462[0], 64463[0], 64479[0], 64480[0], 64483[0], 64484[0], 64486[0], 64487[0], 64488[0], 64489[0], 64490[0], 64491[0], 64492[0], 64493[0], 64494[0], 64495[0], 64505[0], 64510[0], 64517[0], 64520[0], 64530[0], 69990[0], 92012[1], 92014[1], 92585[0], 93000[1], 93005[1], 93010[1], 93040[1], 93041[1], 93042[1], 93318[1], 93355[1], 94002[1], 94200[1], 94250[1], 94680[1], 94681[1], 94690[1], 94770[1], 95812[1], 95813[1], 95816[1], 95819[1], 95822[0], 95829[1], 95860[0], 95861[0], 95863[0], 95864[0], 95865[0], 95866[0], 95867[0], 95868[0], 95869[0], 95870[0], 95907[0], 95908[0], 95909[0], 95910[0], 95911[0], 95912[0], 95913[0], 95925[0], 95926[0], 95927[0], 95928[0], 95929[0], 95930[0], 95933[0], 95937[0], 95938[0], 95939[0], 95940[0], 95955[1], 96360[1], 96361[1], 96365[1], 96366[1], 96367[1], 96368[1], 96372[1], 96374[1], 96375[1], 96376[1], 96377[1], 96523[0], 97597[1], 97598[1], 97602[1], 99155[0], 99156[0], 99157[0], 99211[1], 99212[1], 99213[1], 99214[1], 99215[1], 99217[1], 99218[1], 99219[1], 99220[1], 99221[1], 99222[1], 99223[1], 99231[1], 99232[1], 99233[1], 99234[1], 99235[1], 99236[1], 99238[1], 99239[1], 99241[1], 99242[1], 99243[1], 99244[1], 99245[1], 99251[1], 99252[1], 99253[1], 99254[1], 99255[1], 99291[1], 99292[1], 99304[1], 99305[1], 99306[1], 99307[1], 99308[1], 99309[1], 99310[1], 99315[1], 99316[1], 99334[1], 99335[1], 99336[1], 99337[1], 99347[1], 99348[1], 99349[1], 99350[1], 99374[1], 99375[1], 99377[1], 99378[1], 99446[0], 99447[0], 99448[0], 99449[0], 99451[0], 99452[0], 99495[0], 99496[0], G0453[0], G0463[1], G0471[1]
62252	0213T[1], 0216T[1], 0333T[0], 0464T[0], 36000[1], 36410[1], 36591[0], 36592[0], 61650[1], 62324[1], 62325[1], 62326[1], 62327[1], 64415[1], 64416[1], 64417[1], 64450[1], 64454[1], 64486[1], 64487[1], 64488[1], 64489[1], 64490[1], 64493[1], 92585[0], 95822[0], 95860[0], 95861[0], 95863[0], 95864[0], 95865[0], 95866[0], 95867[0], 95868[0], 95869[0], 95870[0], 95907[0], 95908[0], 95909[0], 95910[0], 95911[0], 95912[0], 95913[0], 95925[0], 95926[0], 95927[0], 95928[0], 95929[0], 95930[0], 95933[0], 95937[0], 95938[0], 95939[0], 95940[0], 96360[1], 96365[1], 96372[1], 96374[1], 96375[1], 96376[1], 96377[1], 96523[0], G0453[0]
62256	0213T[0], 0216T[0], 0228T[0], 0230T[0], 0333T[0], 0464T[0], 11000[1], 11001[1], 11004[1], 11005[1], 11006[1], 11042[1], 11043[1], 11044[1], 11045[1], 11046[1], 11047[1], 12001[1], 12002[1], 12004[1], 12005[1], 12006[1], 12007[1], 12011[1], 12013[1], 12014[1], 12015[1], 12016[1], 12017[1], 12018[1], 12020[1], 12021[1], 12031[1], 12032[1], 12034[1], 12035[1], 12036[1], 12037[1], 12041[1], 12042[1], 12044[1], 12045[1], 12046[1], 12047[1], 12051[1], 12052[1], 12053[1], 12054[1], 12055[1], 12056[1], 12057[1], 13100[1], 13101[1], 13102[1], 13120[1], 13121[1], 13122[1], 13131[1], 13132[1], 13133[1], 13151[1], 13152[1], 13153[1], 36000[1], 36400[1], 36405[1], 36406[1], 36410[1], 36420[1], 36425[1], 36430[1], 36440[1], 36591[0], 36592[0], 36600[1], 36640[1], 43752[1], 51701[1], 51702[1], 51703[1], 61070[1], 62180[1], 62320[0], 62321[0], 62322[0], 62323[0], 62324[0], 62325[0], 62326[0], 62327[0], 64400[0], 64405[0], 64408[0], 64415[0], 64416[0], 64417[0], 64418[0], 64420[0], 64421[0], 64425[0], 64430[0], 64435[0], 64445[0], 64446[0], 64447[0], 64448[0], 64449[0], 64450[0], 64451[0], 64454[0], 64461[0], 64462[0], 64463[0], 64479[0], 64480[0], 64483[0], 64484[0], 64486[0], 64487[0], 64488[0], 64489[0], 64490[0], 64491[0], 64492[0], 64493[0], 64494[0], 64495[0], 64505[0], 64510[0], 64517[0], 64520[0], 64530[0], 69990[0], 92012[1], 92014[1], 92585[0], 93000[1], 93005[1], 93010[1], 93040[1], 93041[1], 93042[1], 93318[1], 93355[1], 94002[1], 94200[1], 94250[1], 94680[1], 94681[1], 94690[1], 94770[1], 95812[1], 95813[1], 95816[1], 95819[1], 95822[0], 95829[1], 95860[0], 95861[0], 95863[0], 95864[0], 95865[0], 95866[0], 95867[0], 95868[0], 95869[0], 95870[0], 95907[0], 95908[0], 95909[0], 95910[0], 95911[0], 95912[0], 95913[0], 95925[0], 95926[0], 95927[0], 95928[0], 95929[0], 95930[0], 95933[0], 95937[0], 95938[0], 95939[0], 95940[0], 95955[1], 96360[1], 96361[1], 96365[1], 96366[1], 96367[1], 96368[1], 96372[1], 96374[1], 96375[1], 96376[1], 96377[1], 96523[0], 97597[1], 97598[1], 97602[1], 99155[0], 99156[0], 99157[0], 99211[1], 99212[1], 99213[1], 99214[1], 99215[1], 99217[1], 99218[1], 99219[1], 99220[1], 99221[1], 99222[1], 99223[1], 99231[1], 99232[1], 99233[1], 99234[1], 99235[1], 99236[1], 99238[1], 99239[1], 99241[1], 99242[1], 99243[1], 99244[1], 99245[1], 99251[1], 99252[1], 99253[1], 99254[1], 99255[1], 99291[1], 99292[1], 99304[1], 99305[1], 99306[1], 99307[1], 99308[1], 99309[1], 99310[1], 99315[1], 99316[1], 99334[1], 99335[1], 99336[1], 99337[1], 99347[1], 99348[1], 99349[1], 99350[1], 99374[1], 99375[1], 99377[1], 99378[1], 99446[0], 99447[0], 99448[0], 99449[0], 99451[0], 99452[0], 99495[0], 99496[0], G0453[0], G0463[1], G0471[1]
62258	0213T[0], 0216T[0], 0228T[0], 0230T[0], 0333T[0], 0464T[0], 11000[1], 11001[1], 11004[1], 11005[1], 11006[1], 11042[1], 11043[1], 11044[1], 11045[1], 11046[1], 11047[1], 12001[1], 12002[1], 12004[1], 12005[1], 12006[1], 12007[1], 12011[1], 12013[1], 12014[1], 12015[1], 12016[1], 12017[1], 12018[1], 12020[1], 12021[1], 12031[1], 12032[1], 12034[1], 12035[1], 12036[1], 12037[1], 12041[1], 12042[1], 12044[1], 12045[1], 12046[1], 12047[1], 12051[1], 12052[1], 12053[1], 12054[1], 12055[1], 12056[1], 12057[1], 13100[1], 13101[1], 13102[1], 13120[1], 13121[1], 13122[1], 13131[1], 13132[1], 13133[1], 13151[1], 13152[1], 13153[1], 36000[1], 36400[1], 36405[1], 36406[1], 36410[1], 36420[1], 36425[1], 36430[1], 36440[1], 36591[0], 36592[0], 36600[1], 36640[1], 43752[1], 51701[1], 51702[1], 51703[1], 61070[1], 62252[1], 62256[1], 62320[0], 62321[0], 62322[0], 62323[0], 62324[0], 62325[0], 62326[0], 62327[0], 64400[0], 64405[0], 64408[0], 64415[0], 64416[0], 64417[0], 64418[0], 64420[0], 64421[0], 64425[0], 64430[0], 64435[0], 64445[0], 64446[0], 64447[0], 64448[0], 64449[0], 64450[0], 64451[0], 64454[0], 64461[0], 64462[0], 64463[0], 64479[0], 64480[0], 64483[0], 64484[0], 64486[0], 64487[0], 64488[0], 64489[0], 64490[0], 64491[0], 64492[0], 64493[0], 64494[0], 64495[0], 64505[0], 64510[0], 64517[0], 64520[0], 64530[0], 69990[0], 92012[1], 92014[1], 92585[0], 93000[1], 93005[1], 93010[1], 93040[1], 93041[1], 93042[1], 93318[1], 93355[1], 94002[1], 94200[1], 94250[1], 94680[1], 94681[1], 94690[1], 94770[1], 95812[1], 95813[1], 95816[1], 95819[1], 95822[0], 95829[1], 95860[0], 95861[0], 95863[0], 95864[0], 95865[0], 95866[0], 95867[0], 95868[0], 95869[0], 95870[0], 95907[0], 95908[0], 95909[0], 95910[0], 95911[0], 95912[0], 95913[0], 95925[0], 95926[0], 95927[0], 95928[0], 95929[0], 95930[0], 95933[0], 95937[0], 95938[0], 95939[0], 95940[0], 95955[1], 96360[1], 96361[1], 96365[1], 96366[1], 96367[1], 96368[1], 96372[1], 96374[1], 96375[1], 96376[1], 96377[1], 96523[0], 97597[1], 97598[1], 97602[1], 99155[0], 99156[0], 99157[0], 99211[1], 99212[1], 99213[1], 99214[1], 99215[1], 99217[1], 99218[1], 99219[1], 99220[1], 99221[1], 99222[1], 99223[1], 99231[1], 99232[1], 99233[1], 99234[1], 99235[1], 99236[1], 99238[1], 99239[1], 99241[1], 99242[1], 99243[1], 99244[1], 99245[1], 99251[1], 99252[1], 99253[1], 99254[1], 99255[1], 99291[1], 99292[1], 99304[1], 99305[1], 99306[1], 99307[1], 99308[1], 99309[1], 99310[1], 99315[1], 99316[1], 99334[1], 99335[1], 99336[1], 99337[1], 99347[1], 99348[1], 99349[1], 99350[1], 99374[1], 99375[1], 99377[1], 99378[1], 99446[0], 99447[0], 99448[0], 99449[0], 99451[0], 99452[0], 99495[0], 99496[0], G0453[0], G0463[1], G0471[1]
62263	00600[0], 00604[0], 00620[0], 00625[0], 00626[0], 00630[0], 00670[0], 01935[0], 01936[0], 0230T[0], 0333T[0], 0464T[0], 12001[1], 12002[1], 12004[1], 12005[1], 12006[1], 12007[1], 12011[1], 12013[1], 12014[1], 12015[1], 12016[1], 12017[1], 12018[1], 12020[1], 12021[1], 12031[1], 12032[1], 12034[1], 12035[1], 12036[1], 12037[1], 12041[1], 12042[1], 12044[1], 12045[1], 12046[1], 12047[1], 12051[1], 12052[1], 12053[1], 12054[1], 12055[1], 12056[1], 12057[1], 13100[1], 13101[1], 13102[1], 13120[1], 13121[1], 13122[1], 13131[1], 13132[1], 13133[1], 13151[1], 13152[1], 13153[1], 36000[1], 36400[1], 36405[1], 36406[1], 36410[1], 36420[1], 36425[1], 36430[1], 36440[1], 36591[0], 36592[0], 36600[1], 36640[1], 43752[1], 51701[1], 51702[1], 51703[1], 62264[0], 62282[1], 62284[1], 62322[0], 62323[0], 62326[0], 62327[0], 64400[0], 64405[0], 64408[0], 64415[0], 64416[0], 64417[0], 64418[0], 64420[0], 64421[0], 64425[0], 64430[0], 64435[0], 64445[0], 64446[0], 64447[0], 64448[0], 64449[0], 64450[0], 64451[0], 64454[0], 64461[0], 64462[0], 64463[0], 64483[0], 64484[0], 64486[0], 64487[0], 64488[0], 64489[0], 64505[0], 64510[0], 64517[0], 64520[0], 64530[0], 64722[1], 69990[0], 72265[1], 72275[0], 76000[1], 77001[1], 77002[1], 77003[1], 92012[1], 92014[1], 92585[0], 93000[1], 93005[1], 93010[1], 93040[1], 93041[1], 93042[1], 93318[1], 93355[1], 94002[1], 94200[1], 94250[1], 94680[1], 94681[1], 94690[1], 94770[1], 95812[1], 95813[1], 95816[1], 95819[1], 95822[0], 95829[1], 95860[0], 95861[0], 95863[0], 95864[0], 95865[0], 95866[0], 95867[0], 95868[0], 95869[0], 95870[0], 95907[0], 95908[0], 95909[0], 95910[0], 95911[0], 95912[0], 95913[0], 95925[0], 95926[0], 95927[0], 95928[0], 95929[0], 95930[0], 95933[0], 95937[0], 95938[0], 95939[0], 95940[0], 95955[1], 96360[1], 96361[1], 96365[1], 96366[1], 96367[1], 96368[1], 96372[1], 96374[1], 96375[1], 96376[1], 96377[1], 96523[0], 99155[0], 99156[0], 99157[0], 99211[1], 99212[1], 99213[1], 99214[1], 99215[1], 99217[1], 99218[1], 99219[1], 99220[1], 99221[1], 99222[1], 99223[1], 99231[1], 99232[1], 99233[1], 99234[1], 99235[1], 99236[1], 99238[1], 99239[1], 99241[1], 99242[1], 99243[1], 99244[1], 99245[1], 99251[1], 99252[1], 99253[1], 99254[1], 99255[1], 99291[1], 99292[1], 99304[1], 99305[1], 99306[1], 99307[1], 99308[1], 99309[1], 99310[1], 99315[1], 99316[1], 99334[1], 99335[1], 99336[1], 99337[1], 99347[1], 99348[1], 99349[1], 99350[1], 99374[1], 99375[1], 99377[1], 99378[1], 99446[0], 99447[0], 99448[0], 99449[0], 99451[0], 99452[0], 99495[0], 99496[0], G0453[0], G0463[1], G0471[1], J2001[1]
62264	00600[0], 00604[0], 00620[0], 00625[0], 00626[0], 00630[0], 00670[0], 01935[0], 01936[0], 0230T[0], 0333T[0], 0464T[0], 12001[1], 12002[1], 12004[1], 12005[1], 12006[1], 12007[1], 12011[1], 12013[1], 12014[1], 12015[1], 12016[1], 12017[1], 12018[1], 12020[1], 12021[1], 12031[1], 12032[1], 12034[1], 12035[1], 12036[1], 12037[1], 12041[1], 12042[1], 12044[1], 12045[1], 12046[1], 12047[1], 12051[1], 12052[1], 12053[1], 12054[1], 12055[1], 12056[1], 12057[1], 13100[1], 13101[1], 13102[1], 13120[1], 13121[1], 13122[1], 13131[1], 13132[1], 13133[1], 13151[1], 13152[1], 13153[1], 36000[1], 36400[1], 36405[1], 36406[1], 36410[1], 36420[1], 36425[1], 36430[1], 36440[1], 36591[0], 36592[0], 36600[1], 36640[1], 43752[1], 51701[1], 51702[1], 51703[1], 62282[0], 62284[1], 62322[0], 62323[0], 62326[0],

Code 1	Code 2
	62327[0], 64400[0], 64405[0], 64408[0], 64415[0], 64416[0], 64417[0], 64418[0], 64420[0], 64421[0], 64425[0], 64430[0], 64435[0], 64445[0], 64446[0], 64447[0], 64448[0], 64449[0], 64450[0], 64451[0], 64454[0], 64461[0], 64462[0], 64463[0], 64483[0], 64484[0], 64486[0], 64487[0], 64488[0], 64489[0], 64505[0], 64510[0], 64517[0], 64520[0], 64530[0], 64722[1], 69990[0], 72265[1], 72275[0], 76000[1], 77001[1], 77002[1], 77003[1], 92012[1], 92014[1], 92585[0], 93000[1], 93005[1], 93010[1], 93040[1], 93041[1], 93042[1], 93318[1], 93355[1], 94002[1], 94200[1], 94250[1], 94680[1], 94681[1], 94690[1], 94770[1], 95812[1], 95813[1], 95816[1], 95819[1], 95822[0], 95829[1], 95860[0], 95861[0], 95863[0], 95864[0], 95865[0], 95866[0], 95867[0], 95868[0], 95869[0], 95870[0], 95907[0], 95908[0], 95909[0], 95910[0], 95911[0], 95912[0], 95913[0], 95925[0], 95926[0], 95927[0], 95928[0], 95929[0], 95930[0], 95933[0], 95937[0], 95938[0], 95939[0], 95940[0], 95955[1], 96360[1], 96361[1], 96365[1], 96366[1], 96367[1], 96368[1], 96372[1], 96374[1], 96375[1], 96376[1], 96377[1], 96523[0], 99155[0], 99156[0], 99157[0], 99211[1], 99212[1], 99213[1], 99214[1], 99215[1], 99217[1], 99218[1], 99219[1], 99220[1], 99221[1], 99222[1], 99223[1], 99231[1], 99232[1], 99233[1], 99234[1], 99235[1], 99236[1], 99238[1], 99239[1], 99241[1], 99242[1], 99243[1], 99244[1], 99245[1], 99251[1], 99252[1], 99253[1], 99254[1], 99255[1], 99291[1], 99292[1], 99304[1], 99305[1], 99306[1], 99307[1], 99308[1], 99309[1], 99310[1], 99315[1], 99316[1], 99334[1], 99335[1], 99336[1], 99337[1], 99347[1], 99348[1], 99349[1], 99350[1], 99374[1], 99375[1], 99377[1], 99378[1], 99446[0], 99447[0], 99448[0], 99449[0], 99451[0], 99452[0], 99495[0], 99496[0], G0453[0], G0463[1], G0471[1]
62267	01935[0], 01936[0], 0213T[0], 0216T[0], 0228T[0], 0230T[0], 0333T[0], 0464T[0], 10005[1], 10006[1], 10007[1], 10008[1], 10009[1], 10010[1], 10011[1], 10012[1], 10021[1], 12001[1], 12002[1], 12004[1], 12005[1], 12006[1], 12007[1], 12011[1], 12013[1], 12014[1], 12015[1], 12016[1], 12017[1], 12018[1], 12020[1], 12021[1], 12031[1], 12032[1], 12034[1], 12035[1], 12036[1], 12037[1], 12041[1], 12042[1], 12044[1], 12045[1], 12046[1], 12047[1], 12051[1], 12052[1], 12053[1], 12054[1], 12055[1], 12056[1], 12057[1], 13100[1], 13101[1], 13102[1], 13120[1], 13121[1], 13122[1], 13131[1], 13132[1], 13133[1], 13151[1], 13152[1], 13153[1], 20220[1], 20225[1], 20240[1], 20245[1], 20250[1], 20251[1], 36000[1], 36400[1], 36405[1], 36406[1], 36410[1], 36420[1], 36425[1], 36430[1], 36440[1], 36591[0], 36592[0], 36600[1], 36640[1], 43752[1], 51701[1], 51702[1], 51703[1], 62291[1], 62320[0], 62321[0], 62322[0], 62323[0], 62324[0], 62325[0], 62326[0], 62327[0], 62380[1], 64400[0], 64405[0], 64408[0], 64415[1], 64416[1], 64417[1], 64418[0], 64420[0], 64421[0], 64425[0], 64430[0], 64435[0], 64445[0], 64446[0], 64447[0], 64448[0], 64449[0], 64450[1], 64451[0], 64454[1], 64455[0], 64461[0], 64462[0], 64463[0], 64479[1], 64480[0], 64483[1], 64484[0], 64486[0], 64487[0], 64488[0], 64489[0], 64490[1], 64491[0], 64492[0], 64493[1], 64494[0], 64495[0], 64505[0], 64510[0], 64517[0], 64520[0], 64530[0], 69990[0], 76000[1], 77001[1], 77002[1], 92012[1], 92014[1], 92585[0], 93000[1], 93005[1], 93010[1], 93040[1], 93041[1], 93042[1], 93318[1], 93355[1], 94002[1], 94200[1], 94250[1], 94680[1], 94681[1], 94690[1], 94770[1], 95812[1], 95813[1], 95816[1], 95819[1], 95822[0], 95829[1], 95860[0], 95861[0], 95863[0], 95864[0], 95865[0], 95866[0], 95867[0], 95868[0], 95869[0], 95870[0], 95907[0], 95908[0], 95909[0], 95910[0], 95911[0], 95912[0], 95913[0], 95925[0], 95926[0], 95927[0], 95928[0], 95929[0], 95930[0], 95933[0], 95937[0], 95938[0], 95939[0], 95940[0], 95955[1], 96360[1], 96361[1], 96365[1], 96366[1], 96367[1], 96368[1], 96372[1], 96374[1], 96375[1], 96376[1], 96377[1], 96523[0], 99155[0], 99156[0], 99157[0], 99211[1], 99212[1], 99213[1], 99214[1], 99215[1], 99217[1], 99218[1], 99219[1], 99220[1], 99221[1], 99222[1], 99223[1], 99231[1], 99232[1], 99233[1], 99234[1], 99235[1], 99236[1], 99238[1], 99239[1], 99241[1], 99242[1], 99243[1], 99244[1], 99245[1], 99251[1], 99252[1], 99253[1], 99254[1], 99255[1], 99291[1], 99292[1], 99304[1], 99305[1], 99306[1], 99307[1], 99308[1], 99309[1], 99310[1], 99315[1], 99316[1], 99334[1], 99335[1], 99336[1], 99337[1], 99347[1], 99348[1], 99349[1], 99350[1], 99374[1], 99375[1], 99377[1], 99378[1], 99446[0], 99447[0], 99448[0], 99449[0], 99451[0], 99452[0], 99495[1], 99496[1], G0453[0], G0463[1], G0471[1]
62270	00635[0], 01935[0], 01936[0], 0213T[0], 0216T[0], 0228T[0], 0230T[0], 12001[1], 12002[1], 12004[1], 12005[1], 12006[1], 12007[1], 12011[1], 12013[1], 12014[1], 12015[1], 12016[1], 12017[1], 12018[1], 12020[1], 12021[1], 12031[1], 12032[1], 12034[1], 12035[1], 12036[1], 12037[1], 12041[1], 12042[1], 12044[1], 12045[1], 12046[1], 12047[1], 12051[1], 12052[1], 12053[1], 12054[1], 12055[1], 12056[1], 12057[1], 13100[1], 13101[1], 13102[1], 13120[1], 13121[1], 13122[1], 13131[1], 13132[1], 13133[1], 13151[1], 13152[1], 13153[1], 36000[1], 36400[1], 36405[1], 36406[1], 36410[1], 36420[1], 36425[1], 36430[1], 36440[1], 36591[0], 36592[0], 36600[1], 36640[1], 43752[1], 51701[1], 51702[1], 51703[1], 62273[1], 62320[1], 62321[1], 62322[0], 62323[0], 64400[0], 64405[0], 64408[0], 64415[0], 64416[0], 64417[0], 64418[0], 64420[0], 64421[0], 64425[0], 64430[0], 64435[0], 64445[0], 64446[0], 64447[0], 64448[0], 64449[0], 64450[0], 64451[0], 64454[0], 64461[0], 64462[0], 64463[0], 64479[0], 64480[0], 64483[0], 64484[0], 64486[0], 64487[0], 64488[0], 64489[0], 64490[0], 64491[0], 64492[0], 64493[0], 64494[0], 64495[0], 64505[0], 64510[0], 64517[0], 64520[0], 64530[0], 69990[0], 76000[1], 76380[1], 76970[1], 76998[1], 77001[1], 77002[1], 77012[1], 92012[1], 92014[1], 93000[1], 93005[1], 93010[1], 93040[1], 93041[1], 93042[1], 93318[1], 93355[1], 94002[1], 94200[1], 94250[1], 94680[1], 94681[1], 94690[1], 94770[1], 95812[1], 95813[1], 95816[1], 95819[1], 95822[0], 95829[1], 95955[1], 96360[1], 96361[1], 96365[1], 96366[1], 96367[1], 96368[1], 96372[1], 96374[1], 96375[1], 96376[1], 96377[1], 96523[0], 99155[0], 99156[0], 99157[0], 99211[1], 99212[1], 99213[1], 99214[1], 99215[1], 99217[1], 99218[1], 99219[1], 99220[1], 99221[1], 99222[1], 99223[1], 99231[1], 99232[1], 99233[1], 99234[1], 99235[1], 99236[1], 99238[1], 99239[1], 99241[1], 99242[1], 99243[1], 99244[1], 99245[1], 99251[1], 99252[1], 99253[1], 99254[1], 99255[1], 99291[1], 99292[1], 99304[1], 99305[1], 99306[1], 99307[1], 99308[1], 99309[1], 99310[1], 99315[1], 99316[1], 99334[1], 99335[1], 99336[1], 99337[1], 99347[1], 99348[1], 99349[1], 99350[1], 99374[1], 99375[1], 99377[1], 99378[1], 99446[0], 99447[0], 99448[0], 99449[0], 99451[0], 99452[0], 99495[1], 99496[1], G0453[0], G0463[1], G0471[1]
62272	00635[0], 01935[0], 01936[0], 0213T[0], 0216T[0], 0228T[0], 0230T[0], 12001[1], 12002[1], 12004[1], 12005[1], 12006[1], 12007[1], 12011[1], 12013[1], 12014[1], 12015[1], 12016[1], 12017[1], 12018[1], 12020[1], 12021[1], 12031[1], 12032[1], 12034[1], 12035[1], 12036[1], 12037[1], 12041[1], 12042[1], 12044[1], 12045[1], 12046[1], 12047[1], 12051[1], 12052[1], 12053[1], 12054[1], 12055[1], 12056[1], 12057[1], 13100[1], 13101[1], 13102[1], 13120[1], 13121[1], 13122[1], 13131[1], 13132[1], 13133[1], 13151[1], 13152[1], 13153[1], 36000[1], 36400[1], 36405[1], 36406[1], 36410[1], 36420[1], 36425[1], 36430[1], 36440[1], 36591[0], 36592[0], 36600[1], 36640[1], 43752[1], 51701[1], 51702[1], 51703[1], 62270[1], 62273[1], 62320[0], 62321[0], 62322[0], 62323[0], 62328[1], 64400[0], 64405[0], 64408[0], 64415[0], 64416[0], 64417[0], 64418[0], 64420[0], 64421[0], 64425[0], 64430[0], 64435[0], 64445[0], 64446[0], 64447[0], 64448[0], 64449[0], 64450[0], 64451[0], 64454[0], 64461[0], 64462[0], 64463[0], 64479[0], 64480[0], 64483[0], 64484[0], 64486[0], 64487[0], 64488[0], 64489[0], 64490[0], 64491[0], 64492[0], 64493[0], 64494[0], 64495[0], 64505[0], 64510[0], 64517[0], 64520[0], 64530[0], 76000[1], 76380[1], 76970[1], 76998[1], 77001[1], 77002[1], 77012[1], 92012[1], 92014[1], 93000[1], 93005[1], 93010[1], 93040[1], 93041[1], 93042[1], 93318[1], 93355[1], 94002[1], 94200[1], 94250[1], 94680[1], 94681[1], 94690[1], 94770[1], 95812[1], 95813[1], 95816[1], 95819[1], 95822[0], 95829[1], 95955[1], 96360[1], 96361[1], 96365[1], 96366[1], 96367[1], 96368[1], 96372[1], 96374[1], 96375[1], 96376[1], 96377[1], 96523[0], 99155[0], 99156[0], 99157[0], 99211[1], 99212[1], 99213[1], 99214[1], 99215[1], 99217[1], 99218[1], 99219[1], 99220[1], 99221[1], 99222[1], 99223[1], 99231[1], 99232[1], 99233[1], 99234[1], 99235[1], 99236[1], 99238[1], 99239[1], 99241[1], 99242[1], 99243[1], 99244[1], 99245[1], 99251[1], 99252[1], 99253[1], 99254[1], 99255[1], 99291[1], 99292[1], 99304[1], 99305[1], 99306[1], 99307[1], 99308[1], 99309[1], 99310[1], 99315[1], 99316[1], 99334[1], 99335[1], 99336[1], 99337[1], 99347[1], 99348[1], 99349[1], 99350[1], 99374[1], 99375[1], 99377[1], 99378[1], 99446[0], 99447[0], 99448[0], 99449[0], 99451[0], 99452[0], 99495[1], 99496[1], G0453[0], G0463[1], G0471[1], J0670[1], J2001[1]
62273	01935[0], 01936[0], 0213T[0], 0216T[0], 0228T[0], 0230T[0], 0333T[0], 0464T[0], 12001[1], 12002[1], 12004[1], 12005[1], 12006[1], 12007[1], 12011[1], 12013[1], 12014[1], 12015[1], 12016[1], 12017[1], 12018[1], 12020[1], 12021[1], 12031[1], 12032[1], 12034[1], 12035[1], 12036[1], 12037[1], 12041[1], 12042[1], 12044[1], 12045[1], 12046[1], 12047[1], 12051[1], 12052[1], 12053[1], 12054[1], 12055[1], 12056[1], 12057[1], 13100[1], 13101[1], 13102[1], 13120[1], 13121[1], 13122[1], 13131[1], 13132[1], 13133[1], 13151[1], 13152[1], 13153[1], 36000[1], 36140[1], 36400[1], 36405[1], 36406[1], 36410[1], 36420[1], 36425[1], 36430[1], 36440[1], 36591[0], 36592[0], 36600[1], 36640[1], 43752[1], 51701[1], 51702[1], 51703[1], 62320[0], 62321[0], 62322[0], 62323[0], 62324[0], 62326[0], 62327[0], 64400[0], 64405[0], 64408[0], 64415[0], 64416[0], 64417[0], 64418[0], 64420[0], 64421[0], 64425[0], 64430[0], 64435[0], 64445[0], 64446[0], 64447[0], 64448[0], 64449[0], 64450[0], 64451[0], 64454[0], 64461[0], 64462[0], 64463[0], 64479[0], 64480[0], 64483[0], 64484[0], 64486[0], 64487[0], 64488[0], 64489[0], 64490[0], 64491[0], 64492[0], 64493[0], 64494[0], 64495[0], 64505[0], 64510[0], 64517[0], 64520[0], 64530[0], 69990[0], 76000[1], 77001[1], 77002[1], 92012[1], 92014[1], 92585[0], 93000[1], 93005[1], 93010[1], 93040[1], 93041[1], 93042[1], 93318[1], 93355[1], 94002[1], 94200[1], 94250[1], 94680[1], 94681[1], 94690[1], 94770[1], 95812[1], 95813[1], 95816[1], 95819[1], 95822[0], 95829[1], 95860[0], 95861[0], 95863[0], 95864[0], 95865[0], 95866[0], 95867[0], 95868[0], 95869[0], 95870[0], 95907[0], 95908[0], 95909[0], 95910[0], 95911[0], 95912[0], 95913[0], 95925[0], 95926[0], 95927[0], 95928[0], 95929[0], 95930[0], 95933[0], 95937[0], 95938[0], 95939[0], 95940[0], 95955[1], 96360[1], 96361[1], 96365[1], 96366[1], 96367[1], 96368[1], 96372[1], 96374[1], 96375[1], 96376[1], 96377[1], 96523[0], 99155[0], 99156[0], 99157[0], 99211[1], 99212[1], 99213[1], 99214[1], 99215[1], 99217[1], 99218[1], 99219[1], 99220[1], 99221[1], 99222[1], 99223[1], 99231[1], 99232[1], 99233[1], 99234[1], 99235[1], 99236[1], 99238[1], 99239[1], 99241[1], 99242[1], 99243[1], 99244[1], 99245[1], 99251[1], 99252[1], 99253[1], 99254[1], 99255[1], 99291[1], 99292[1], 99304[1], 99305[1], 99306[1], 99307[1], 99308[1], 99309[1], 99310[1], 99315[1], 99316[1], 99334[1], 99335[1], 99336[1], 99337[1], 99347[1], 99348[1], 99349[1], 99350[1], 99374[1], 99375[1], 99377[1], 99378[1], 99446[0], 99447[0], 99448[0], 99449[0], 99451[0], 99452[0], 99495[1], 99496[1], G0453[0], G0463[1], G0471[1], J0670[1], J2001[1]
62280	01935[0], 01936[0], 0213T[0], 0216T[0], 0228T[0], 0230T[0], 0333T[0], 0464T[0], 12001[1], 12002[1], 12004[1], 12005[1], 12006[1], 12007[1], 12011[1], 12013[1], 12014[1], 12015[1], 12016[1], 12017[1], 12018[1], 12020[1], 12021[1], 12031[1], 12032[1], 12034[1], 12035[1], 12036[1], 12037[1], 12041[1], 12042[1], 12044[1], 12045[1], 12046[1], 12047[1], 12051[1], 12052[1], 12053[1], 12054[1], 12055[1], 12056[1], 12057[1], 13100[1], 13101[1], 13102[1], 13120[1], 13121[1], 13122[1], 13131[1], 13132[1], 13133[1], 13151[1], 13152[1], 13153[1], 36000[1], 36400[1], 36405[1], 36406[1], 36410[1], 36420[1], 36425[1], 36430[1], 36440[1], 36591[0], 36592[0], 36600[1], 36640[1], 43752[1], 51701[1], 51702[1], 51703[1], 62270[1], 62272[1], 62273[1], 62284[1], 62320[0], 62321[0], 62322[0], 62323[0], 62324[0], 62325[0], 62326[0], 62327[0], 62328[1], 62329[1], 64400[0], 64405[0], 64408[0], 64415[0], 64416[0], 64417[0], 64418[0], 64420[0], 64421[0], 64425[0], 64430[0], 64435[0], 64445[0], 64446[0], 64447[0], 64448[0], 64449[0], 64450[0], 64451[0], 64454[0], 64461[0], 64462[0], 64463[0], 64479[0], 64480[0], 64483[0], 64484[0], 64486[0], 64487[0], 64488[0], 64489[0], 64490[0], 64491[0], 64492[0], 64493[0],

0 = Modifier usage not allowed or inappropriate   1 = Modifier usage allowed

Code 1	Code 2
	64494^0, 64495^0, 64505^0, 64510^0, 64517^0, 64520^0, 64530^0, 69990^0, 76000^1, 77001^1, 77002^1, 92012^1, 92014^1, 92585^0, 93000^1, 93005^1, 93010^1, 93040^1, 93041^1, 93042^1, 93318^1, 93355^1, 94002^1, 94200^1, 94250^1, 94680^1, 94681^1, 94690^1, 94770^1, 95812^1, 95813^1, 95816^1, 95819^1, 95822^0, 95829^1, 95860^0, 95861^0, 95863^0, 95864^0, 95865^0, 95866^0, 95867^0, 95868^0, 95869^0, 95870^0, 95907^0, 95908^0, 95909^0, 95910^0, 95911^0, 95912^0, 95913^0, 95925^0, 95926^0, 95927^0, 95928^0, 95929^0, 95930^0, 95933^0, 95937^0, 95938^0, 95939^0, 95940^0, 95955^1, 96360^1, 96361^1, 96365^1, 96366^1, 96367^1, 96368^1, 96372^1, 96374^1, 96375^1, 96376^1, 96377^1, 96523^0, 99155^0, 99156^0, 99157^0, 99211^1, 99212^1, 99213^1, 99214^1, 99215^1, 99217^1, 99218^1, 99219^1, 99220^1, 99221^1, 99222^1, 99223^1, 99231^1, 99232^1, 99233^1, 99234^1, 99235^1, 99236^1, 99238^1, 99239^1, 99241^1, 99242^1, 99243^1, 99244^1, 99245^1, 99251^1, 99252^1, 99253^1, 99254^1, 99255^1, 99291^1, 99292^1, 99304^1, 99305^1, 99306^1, 99307^1, 99308^1, 99309^1, 99310^1, 99315^1, 99316^1, 99334^1, 99335^1, 99336^1, 99337^1, 99347^1, 99348^1, 99349^1, 99350^1, 99374^1, 99375^1, 99377^1, 99378^1, 99446^0, 99447^0, 99448^0, 99449^0, 99451^0, 99452^0, 99495^0, 99496^0, G0453^0, G0463^1, G0471^1
62281	01935^0, 01936^0, 0213T^0, 0228T^0, 0230T^0, 0333T^0, 0464T^0, 12001^1, 12002^1, 12004^1, 12005^1, 12006^1, 12007^1, 12011^1, 12013^1, 12014^1, 12015^1, 12016^1, 12017^1, 12018^1, 12020^1, 12021^1, 12031^1, 12032^1, 12034^1, 12035^1, 12036^1, 12037^1, 12041^1, 12042^1, 12044^1, 12045^1, 12046^1, 12047^1, 12051^1, 12052^1, 12053^1, 12054^1, 12055^1, 12056^1, 12057^1, 13100^1, 13101^1, 13102^1, 13120^1, 13121^1, 13122^1, 13131^1, 13132^1, 13133^1, 13151^1, 13152^1, 13153^1, 36000^1, 36400^1, 36405^1, 36406^1, 36410^1, 36420^1, 36425^1, 36430^1, 36440^1, 36591^0, 36592^0, 36600^1, 36640^1, 43752^1, 51701^1, 51702^1, 51703^1, 62270^1, 62272^1, 62273^1, 62284^1, 62320^0, 62321^0, 62322^0, 62323^0, 62324^0, 62325^0, 62328^1, 62329^1, 64400^0, 64405^0, 64408^0, 64415^0, 64416^0, 64417^0, 64418^0, 64420^0, 64421^0, 64425^0, 64430^0, 64435^0, 64445^0, 64446^0, 64447^0, 64448^0, 64449^0, 64450^0, 64451^0, 64454^0, 64461^0, 64462^0, 64463^0, 64479^0, 64480^0, 64483^0, 64484^0, 64486^0, 64487^0, 64488^0, 64489^0, 64490^0, 64491^0, 64492^0, 64505^0, 64510^0, 64517^0, 64520^0, 64530^0, 69990^0, 72275^1, 76000^1, 77001^1, 77002^1, 92012^1, 92014^1, 92585^0, 93000^1, 93005^1, 93010^1, 93040^1, 93041^1, 93042^1, 93318^1, 93355^1, 94002^1, 94200^1, 94250^1, 94680^1, 94681^1, 94690^1, 94770^1, 95812^1, 95813^1, 95816^1, 95819^1, 95822^0, 95829^1, 95860^0, 95861^0, 95863^0, 95864^0, 95865^0, 95866^0, 95867^0, 95868^0, 95869^0, 95870^0, 95907^0, 95908^0, 95909^0, 95910^0, 95911^0, 95912^0, 95913^0, 95925^0, 95926^0, 95927^0, 95928^0, 95929^0, 95930^0, 95933^0, 95937^0, 95938^0, 95939^0, 95940^0, 95955^1, 96360^1, 96361^1, 96365^1, 96366^1, 96367^1, 96368^1, 96372^1, 96374^1, 96375^1, 96376^1, 96377^1, 96523^0, 99155^0, 99156^0, 99157^0, 99211^1, 99212^1, 99213^1, 99214^1, 99215^1, 99217^1, 99218^1, 99219^1, 99220^1, 99221^1, 99222^1, 99223^1, 99231^1, 99232^1, 99233^1, 99234^1, 99235^1, 99236^1, 99238^1, 99239^1, 99241^1, 99242^1, 99243^1, 99244^1, 99245^1, 99251^1, 99252^1, 99253^1, 99254^1, 99255^1, 99291^1, 99292^1, 99304^1, 99305^1, 99306^1, 99307^1, 99308^1, 99309^1, 99310^1, 99315^1, 99316^1, 99334^1, 99335^1, 99336^1, 99337^1, 99347^1, 99348^1, 99349^1, 99350^1, 99374^1, 99375^1, 99377^1, 99378^1, 99446^0, 99447^0, 99448^0, 99449^0, 99451^0, 99452^0, 99495^0, 99496^0, G0453^0, G0463^1, G0471^1, J2001^1
62282	01935^0, 01936^0, 0216T^0, 0228T^0, 0230T^0, 0333T^0, 0464T^0, 12001^1, 12002^1, 12004^1, 12005^1, 12006^1, 12007^1, 12011^1, 12013^1, 12014^1, 12015^1, 12016^1, 12017^1, 12018^1, 12020^1, 12021^1, 12031^1, 12032^1, 12034^1, 12035^1, 12036^1, 12037^1, 12041^1, 12042^1, 12044^1, 12045^1, 12046^1, 12047^1, 12051^1, 12052^1, 12053^1, 12054^1, 12055^1, 12056^1, 12057^1, 13100^1, 13101^1, 13102^1, 13120^1, 13121^1, 13122^1, 13131^1, 13132^1, 13133^1, 13151^1, 13152^1, 13153^1, 36000^1, 36400^1, 36405^1, 36406^1, 36410^1, 36420^1, 36425^1, 36430^1, 36440^1, 36591^0, 36592^0, 36600^1, 36640^1, 43752^1, 51701^1, 51702^1, 51703^1, 62270^1, 62272^1, 62273^1, 62320^0, 62321^0, 62322^0, 62323^0, 62326^0, 62327^0, 62328^1, 62329^1, 64400^0, 64405^0, 64408^0, 64415^0, 64416^0, 64417^0, 64418^0, 64420^0, 64421^0, 64425^0, 64430^0, 64435^0, 64445^0, 64446^0, 64447^0, 64448^0, 64449^0, 64450^0, 64451^0, 64454^0, 64461^0, 64462^0, 64463^0, 64479^0, 64480^0, 64483^0, 64484^0, 64486^0, 64487^0, 64488^0, 64489^0, 64493^0, 64494^0, 64495^0, 64505^0, 64510^0, 64517^0, 64520^0, 64530^0, 69990^0, 72275^1, 76000^1, 77001^1, 77002^1, 92012^1, 92014^1, 92585^0, 93000^1, 93005^1, 93010^1, 93040^1, 93041^1, 93042^1, 93318^1, 93355^1, 94002^1, 94200^1, 94250^1, 94680^1, 94681^1, 94690^1, 94770^1, 95812^1, 95813^1, 95816^1, 95819^1, 95822^0, 95829^1, 95860^0, 95861^0, 95863^0, 95864^0, 95865^0, 95866^0, 95867^0, 95868^0, 95869^0, 95870^0, 95907^0, 95908^0, 95909^0, 95910^0, 95911^0, 95912^0, 95913^0, 95925^0, 95926^0, 95927^0, 95928^0, 95929^0, 95930^0, 95933^0, 95937^0, 95938^0, 95939^0, 95940^0, 95955^1, 96360^1, 96361^1, 96365^1, 96366^1, 96367^1, 96368^1, 96372^1, 96374^1, 96375^1, 96376^1, 96377^1, 96523^0, 99155^0, 99156^0, 99157^0, 99211^1, 99212^1, 99213^1, 99214^1, 99215^1, 99217^1, 99218^1, 99219^1, 99220^1, 99221^1, 99222^1, 99223^1, 99231^1, 99232^1, 99233^1, 99234^1, 99235^1, 99236^1, 99238^1, 99239^1, 99241^1, 99242^1, 99243^1, 99244^1, 99245^1, 99251^1, 99252^1, 99253^1, 99254^1, 99255^1, 99291^1, 99292^1, 99304^1, 99305^1, 99306^1, 99307^1, 99308^1, 99309^1, 99310^1, 99315^1, 99316^1, 99334^1, 99335^1, 99336^1, 99337^1, 99347^1, 99348^1, 99349^1, 99350^1, 99374^1, 99375^1, 99377^1, 99378^1, 99446^0, 99447^0, 99448^0, 99449^0, 99451^0, 99452^0, 99495^0, 99496^0, G0453^0, G0463^1, G0471^1, J2001^1
62284	01935^0, 01936^0, 0213T^0, 0216T^0, 0228T^0, 0230T^0, 0333T^0, 0464T^0, 12001^1, 12002^1, 12004^1, 12005^1, 12006^1, 12007^1, 12011^1, 12013^1, 12014^1, 12015^1, 12016^1, 12017^1, 12018^1, 12020^1, 12021^1, 12031^1, 12032^1, 12034^1, 12035^1, 12036^1, 12037^1, 12041^1, 12042^1, 12044^1, 12045^1, 12046^1, 12047^1, 12051^1, 12052^1, 12053^1, 12054^1, 12055^1, 12056^1, 12057^1, 13100^1, 13101^1, 13102^1, 13120^1, 13121^1, 13122^1, 13131^1, 13132^1, 13133^1, 13151^1, 13152^1, 13153^1, 36000^1, 36400^1, 36405^1, 36406^1, 36410^1, 36420^1, 36425^1, 36430^1, 36440^1, 36591^0, 36592^0, 36600^1, 36640^1, 43752^1, 51701^1, 51702^1, 51703^1, 62270^1, 62272^1, 62273^1, 62282^1, 62328^1, 62329^1, 64400^0, 64405^0, 64408^0, 64415^0, 64416^0, 64417^0, 64418^0, 64420^0, 64421^0, 64425^0, 64430^0, 64435^0, 64445^0, 64446^0, 64447^0, 64448^0, 64449^0, 64450^0, 64451^0, 64454^0, 64461^0, 64462^0, 64463^0, 64479^0, 64480^0, 64483^0, 64484^0, 64486^0, 64487^0, 64488^0, 64489^0, 64490^0, 64491^0, 64492^0, 64493^0, 64494^0, 64495^0, 64505^0, 64510^0, 64517^0, 64520^0, 64530^0, 69990^0, 76000^1, 77001^1, 77002^1, 92012^1, 92014^1, 92585^0, 93000^1, 93005^1, 93010^1, 93040^1, 93041^1, 93042^1, 93318^1, 93355^1, 94002^1, 94200^1, 94250^1, 94680^1, 94681^1, 94690^1, 94770^1, 95812^1, 95813^1, 95816^1, 95819^1, 95822^0, 95829^1, 95860^0, 95861^0, 95863^0, 95864^0, 95865^0, 95866^0, 95867^0, 95868^0, 95869^0, 95870^0, 95907^0, 95908^0, 95909^0, 95910^0, 95911^0, 95912^0, 95913^0, 95925^0, 95926^0, 95927^0, 95928^0, 95929^0, 95930^0, 95933^0, 95937^0, 95938^0, 95939^0, 95940^0, 95955^1, 96360^1, 96361^1, 96365^1, 96366^1, 96367^1, 96368^1, 96372^1, 96374^1, 96375^1, 96376^1, 96377^1, 96523^0, 99155^0, 99156^0, 99157^0, 99211^1, 99212^1, 99213^1, 99214^1, 99215^1, 99217^1, 99218^1, 99219^1, 99220^1, 99221^1, 99222^1, 99223^1, 99231^1, 99232^1, 99233^1, 99234^1, 99235^1, 99236^1, 99238^1, 99239^1, 99241^1, 99242^1, 99243^1, 99244^1, 99245^1, 99251^1, 99252^1, 99253^1, 99254^1, 99255^1, 99291^1, 99292^1, 99304^1, 99305^1, 99306^1, 99307^1, 99308^1, 99309^1, 99310^1, 99315^1, 99316^1, 99334^1, 99335^1, 99336^1, 99337^1, 99347^1, 99348^1, 99349^1, 99350^1, 99374^1, 99375^1, 99377^1, 99378^1, 99446^0, 99447^0, 99448^0, 99449^0, 99451^0, 99452^0, 99495^1, 99496^1, G0453^0, G0463^1, G0471^1
62287	01935^0, 01936^0, 0202T^1, 0216T^0, 0228T^1, 0230T^0, 0275T^1, 0333T^0, 0464T^0, 0565T^1, 12001^1, 12002^1, 12004^1, 12005^1, 12006^1, 12007^1, 12011^1, 12013^1, 12014^1, 12015^1, 12016^1, 12017^1, 12018^1, 12020^1, 12021^1, 12031^1, 12032^1, 12034^1, 12035^1, 12036^1, 12037^1, 12041^1, 12042^1, 12044^1, 12045^1, 12046^1, 12047^1, 12051^1, 12052^1, 12053^1, 12054^1, 12055^1, 12056^1, 12057^1, 13100^1, 13101^1, 13102^1, 13120^1, 13121^1, 13122^1, 13131^1, 13132^1, 13133^1, 13151^1, 13152^1, 13153^1, 15769^1, 22102^1, 22224^1, 22558^1, 36000^1, 36400^1, 36405^1, 36406^1, 36410^1, 36420^1, 36425^1, 36430^1, 36440^1, 36591^0, 36592^0, 36600^1, 36640^1, 43752^1, 51701^1, 51702^1, 51703^1, 62267^1, 62290^0, 62322^0, 62323^0, 62326^0, 62327^0, 62380^1, 63005^1, 63017^1, 63030^1, 63042^1, 63056^1, 64400^0, 64405^0, 64408^0, 64415^0, 64416^0, 64417^0, 64418^0, 64420^0, 64421^0, 64425^0, 64430^0, 64435^0, 64445^0, 64446^0, 64447^0, 64448^0, 64449^0, 64450^0, 64451^0, 64454^0, 64455^0, 64461^0, 64462^0, 64463^0, 64479^0, 64480^0, 64483^0, 64484^0, 64486^0, 64487^0, 64488^0, 64489^0, 64490^0, 64493^0, 64494^0, 64495^0, 64505^0, 64510^0, 64517^0, 64520^0, 64530^0, 69990^0, 72295^0, 76000^1, 76380^1, 76942^1, 76970^1, 76998^1, 77001^1, 77002^1, 77003^1, 77012^1, 77021^1, 92012^1, 92014^1, 92585^0, 93000^1, 93005^1, 93010^1, 93040^1, 93041^1, 93042^1, 93318^1, 93355^1, 94002^1, 94200^1, 94250^1, 94680^1, 94681^1, 94690^1, 94770^1, 95812^1, 95813^1, 95816^1, 95819^1, 95822^0, 95829^1, 95860^0, 95861^0, 95863^0, 95864^0, 95865^0, 95866^0, 95867^0, 95868^0, 95869^0, 95870^0, 95907^0, 95908^0, 95909^0, 95910^0, 95911^0, 95912^0, 95913^0, 95925^0, 95926^0, 95927^0, 95928^0, 95929^0, 95930^0, 95933^0, 95937^0, 95938^0, 95939^0, 95940^0, 95955^1, 96360^1, 96361^1, 96365^1, 96366^1, 96367^1, 96368^1, 96372^1, 96374^1, 96375^1, 96376^1, 96377^1, 96523^0, 99155^0, 99156^0, 99157^0, 99211^1, 99212^1, 99213^1, 99214^1, 99215^1, 99217^1, 99218^1, 99219^1, 99220^1, 99221^1, 99222^1, 99223^1, 99231^1, 99232^1, 99233^1, 99234^1, 99235^1, 99236^1, 99238^1, 99239^1, 99241^1, 99242^1, 99243^1, 99244^1, 99245^1, 99251^1, 99252^1, 99253^1, 99254^1, 99255^1, 99291^1, 99292^1, 99304^1, 99305^1, 99306^1, 99307^1, 99308^1, 99309^1, 99310^1, 99315^1, 99316^1, 99334^1, 99335^1, 99336^1, 99337^1, 99347^1, 99348^1, 99349^1, 99350^1, 99374^1, 99375^1, 99377^1, 99378^1, 99446^0, 99447^0, 99448^0, 99449^0, 99451^0, 99452^0, 99495^0, 99496^0, G0276^1, G0453^0, G0463^1, G0471^1
62290	01935^0, 01936^0, 0228T^0, 0333T^0, 0464T^0, 12001^1, 12002^1, 12004^1, 12005^1, 12006^1, 12007^1, 12011^1, 12013^1, 12014^1, 12015^1, 12016^1, 12017^1, 12018^1, 12020^1, 12021^1, 12031^1, 12032^1, 12034^1, 12035^1, 12036^1, 12037^1, 12041^1, 12042^1, 12044^1, 12045^1, 12046^1, 12047^1, 12051^1, 12052^1, 12053^1, 12054^1, 12055^1, 12056^1, 12057^1, 13100^1, 13101^1, 13102^1, 13120^1, 13121^1, 13122^1, 13131^1, 13132^1, 13133^1, 13151^1, 13152^1, 13153^1, 36000^1, 36400^1, 36405^1, 36406^1, 36410^1, 36420^1, 36425^1, 36430^1, 36440^1, 36591^0, 36592^0, 36600^1, 36640^1, 43752^1, 51701^1, 51702^1, 51703^1, 62267^1, 62322^0, 62323^0, 62326^0, 62327^0, 64415^0, 64416^0, 64417^0, 64425^0, 64430^0, 64435^0, 64445^0, 64446^0, 64447^0, 64448^0, 64449^0, 64450^0, 64451^0, 64454^0, 64461^0, 64462^0, 64463^0,

Appendix A: NCCI - CPT Codes

Code 1	Code 2
	64479[0], 64480[0], 64483[0], 64484[0], 64486[0], 64487[0], 64488[0], 64489[0], 64493[0], 64494[0], 64495[0], 64505[0], 64510[0], 64517[0], 64520[0], 64530[0], 69990[0], 76000[1], 76800[1], 76942[1], 76970[1], 76998[1], 77001[1], 77002[1], 77003[1], 92012[1], 92014[1], 92585[0], 93000[1], 93005[1], 93010[1], 93040[1], 93041[1], 93042[1], 93318[1], 93355[1], 94002[1], 94200[1], 94250[1], 94680[1], 94681[1], 94690[1], 94770[1], 95812[1], 95813[1], 95816[1], 95819[1], 95822[0], 95829[1], 95860[0], 95861[0], 95863[0], 95864[0], 95865[0], 95866[0], 95867[0], 95868[0], 95869[0], 95870[0], 95907[0], 95908[0], 95909[0], 95910[0], 95911[0], 95912[0], 95913[0], 95925[0], 95926[0], 95927[0], 95928[0], 95929[0], 95930[0], 95933[0], 95937[0], 95938[0], 95939[0], 95940[0], 95955[1], 96360[1], 96361[1], 96365[1], 96366[1], 96367[1], 96368[1], 96372[1], 96374[1], 96375[1], 96376[1], 96377[1], 96523[0], 99155[0], 99156[0], 99157[0], 99211[1], 99212[1], 99213[1], 99214[1], 99215[1], 99217[1], 99218[1], 99219[1], 99220[1], 99221[1], 99222[1], 99223[1], 99231[1], 99232[1], 99233[1], 99234[1], 99235[1], 99236[1], 99238[1], 99239[1], 99241[1], 99242[1], 99243[1], 99244[1], 99245[1], 99251[1], 99252[1], 99253[1], 99254[1], 99255[1], 99291[1], 99292[1], 99304[1], 99305[1], 99306[1], 99307[1], 99308[1], 99309[1], 99310[1], 99315[1], 99316[1], 99334[1], 99335[1], 99336[1], 99337[1], 99347[1], 99348[1], 99349[1], 99350[1], 99374[1], 99375[1], 99377[1], 99378[1], 99446[0], 99447[0], 99448[0], 99449[0], 99451[0], 99452[0], 99495[1], 99496[1], G0453[0], G0463[1], G0471[1]
62291	01935[0], 01936[0], 0213T[0], 0216T[0], 0228T[0], 0230T[0], 0333T[0], 0464T[0], 12001[1], 12002[1], 12004[1], 12005[1], 12006[1], 12007[1], 12011[1], 12013[1], 12014[1], 12015[1], 12016[1], 12017[1], 12018[1], 12020[1], 12021[1], 12031[1], 12032[1], 12034[1], 12035[1], 12036[1], 12037[1], 12041[1], 12042[1], 12044[1], 12045[1], 12046[1], 12047[1], 12051[1], 12052[1], 12053[1], 12054[1], 12055[1], 12056[1], 12057[1], 13100[1], 13101[1], 13102[1], 13120[1], 13121[1], 13122[1], 13131[1], 13132[1], 13133[1], 13151[1], 13152[1], 13153[1], 36000[1], 36400[1], 36405[1], 36406[1], 36410[1], 36420[1], 36425[1], 36430[1], 36440[1], 36591[0], 36592[0], 36600[1], 36640[1], 43752[1], 51701[1], 51702[1], 51703[1], 62320[0], 62321[0], 62324[0], 62325[0], 64400[0], 64405[0], 64408[0], 64415[0], 64416[0], 64417[0], 64418[0], 64420[0], 64421[0], 64425[0], 64430[0], 64435[0], 64445[0], 64446[0], 64447[0], 64448[0], 64450[1], 64451[0], 64454[1], 64461[0], 64462[0], 64463[0], 64479[0], 64480[0], 64486[0], 64487[0], 64488[0], 64489[0], 64490[0], 64491[0], 64492[0], 64505[0], 64510[0], 64517[0], 64520[0], 64530[0], 69990[0], 76000[1], 76800[1], 76942[1], 76970[1], 76998[1], 77001[1], 77002[1], 77003[1], 92012[1], 92014[1], 92585[0], 93000[1], 93005[1], 93010[1], 93040[1], 93041[1], 93042[1], 93318[1], 93355[1], 94002[1], 94200[1], 94250[1], 94680[1], 94681[1], 94690[1], 94770[1], 95812[1], 95813[1], 95816[1], 95819[1], 95822[0], 95829[1], 95860[0], 95861[0], 95863[0], 95864[0], 95865[0], 95866[0], 95867[0], 95868[0], 95869[0], 95870[0], 95907[0], 95908[0], 95909[0], 95910[0], 95911[0], 95912[0], 95913[0], 95925[0], 95926[0], 95927[0], 95928[0], 95929[0], 95930[0], 95933[0], 95937[0], 95938[0], 95939[0], 95940[0], 95955[1], 96360[1], 96361[1], 96365[1], 96366[1], 96367[1], 96368[1], 96372[1], 96374[1], 96375[1], 96376[1], 96377[1], 96523[0], 99155[0], 99156[0], 99157[0], 99211[1], 99212[1], 99213[1], 99214[1], 99215[1], 99217[1], 99218[1], 99219[1], 99220[1], 99221[1], 99222[1], 99223[1], 99231[1], 99232[1], 99233[1], 99234[1], 99235[1], 99236[1], 99238[1], 99239[1], 99241[1], 99242[1], 99243[1], 99244[1], 99245[1], 99251[1], 99252[1], 99253[1], 99254[1], 99255[1], 99291[1], 99292[1], 99304[1], 99305[1], 99306[1], 99307[1], 99308[1], 99309[1], 99310[1], 99315[1], 99316[1], 99334[1], 99335[1], 99336[1], 99337[1], 99347[1], 99348[1], 99349[1], 99350[1], 99374[1], 99375[1], 99377[1], 99378[1], 99446[0], 99447[0], 99448[0], 99449[0], 99451[0], 99452[0], 99495[1], 99496[1], G0453[0], G0463[1], G0471[1]
62292	01935[0], 01936[0], 0213T[0], 0216T[0], 0228T[0], 0230T[0], 0333T[0], 0464T[0], 12001[1], 12002[1], 12004[1], 12005[1], 12006[1], 12007[1], 12011[1], 12013[1], 12014[1], 12015[1], 12016[1], 12017[1], 12018[1], 12020[1], 12021[1], 12031[1], 12032[1], 12034[1], 12035[1], 12036[1], 12037[1], 12041[1], 12042[1], 12044[1], 12045[1], 12046[1], 12047[1], 12051[1], 12052[1], 12053[1], 12054[1], 12055[1], 12056[1], 12057[1], 13100[1], 13101[1], 13102[1], 13120[1], 13121[1], 13122[1], 13131[1], 13132[1], 13133[1], 13151[1], 13152[1], 13153[1], 36000[1], 36400[1], 36405[1], 36406[1], 36410[1], 36420[1], 36425[1], 36430[1], 36440[1], 36591[0], 36592[0], 36600[1], 36640[1], 43752[1], 51701[1], 51702[1], 51703[1], 62290[1], 62320[0], 62321[0], 62322[0], 62323[0], 62324[0], 62325[0], 62326[0], 62327[0], 64400[0], 64405[0], 64408[0], 64415[0], 64416[0], 64417[0], 64418[0], 64420[0], 64421[0], 64425[0], 64430[0], 64435[0], 64445[0], 64446[0], 64447[0], 64448[0], 64449[0], 64450[0], 64451[0], 64454[0], 64461[0], 64462[0], 64463[0], 64479[0], 64480[0], 64483[0], 64484[0], 64486[0], 64487[0], 64488[0], 64489[0], 64490[0], 64491[0], 64492[0], 64493[0], 64494[0], 64495[0], 64505[0], 64510[0], 64517[0], 64520[0], 64530[0], 69990[0], 76000[1], 77001[1], 77002[1], 77003[1], 92012[1], 92014[1], 92585[0], 93000[1], 93005[1], 93010[1], 93040[1], 93041[1], 93042[1], 93318[1], 93355[1], 94002[1], 94200[1], 94250[1], 94680[1], 94681[1], 94690[1], 94770[1], 95812[1], 95813[1], 95816[1], 95819[1], 95822[0], 95829[1], 95860[0], 95861[0], 95863[0], 95864[0], 95865[0], 95866[0], 95867[0], 95868[0], 95869[0], 95870[0], 95907[0], 95908[0], 95909[0], 95910[0], 95911[0], 95912[0], 95913[0], 95925[0], 95926[0], 95927[0], 95928[0], 95929[0], 95930[0], 95933[0], 95937[0], 95938[0], 95939[0], 95940[0], 95955[1], 96360[1], 96361[1], 96365[1], 96366[1], 96367[1], 96368[1], 96372[1], 96374[1], 96375[1], 96376[1], 96377[1], 96523[0], 99155[0], 99156[0], 99157[0], 99211[1], 99212[1], 99213[1], 99214[1], 99215[1], 99217[1], 99218[1], 99219[1], 99220[1], 99221[1], 99222[1], 99223[1], 99231[1], 99232[1], 99233[1], 99234[1], 99235[1], 99236[1], 99238[1], 99239[1], 99241[1], 99242[1], 99243[1], 99244[1], 99245[1], 99251[1], 99252[1], 99253[1], 99254[1], 99255[1], 99291[1], 99292[1], 99304[1], 99305[1], 99306[1], 99307[1], 99308[1], 99309[1], 99310[1], 99315[1], 99316[1], 99334[1], 99335[1], 99336[1], 99337[1], 99347[1], 99348[1], 99349[1], 99350[1], 99374[1], 99375[1], 99377[1], 99378[1], 99446[0], 99447[0], 99448[0], 99449[0], 99451[0], 99452[0], 99495[0], 99496[0], G0453[0], G0463[1], G0471[1]
62302	00600[0], 01935[0], 01936[0], 0213T[0], 0216T[0], 0228T[0], 0230T[0], 12001[1], 12002[1], 12004[1], 12005[1], 12006[1], 12007[1], 12011[1], 12013[1], 12014[1], 12015[1], 12016[1], 12017[1], 12018[1], 12020[1], 12021[1], 12031[1], 12032[1], 12034[1], 12035[1], 12036[1], 12037[1], 12041[1], 12042[1], 12044[1], 12045[1], 12046[1], 12047[1], 12051[1], 12052[1], 12053[1], 12054[1], 12055[1], 12056[1], 12057[1], 13100[1], 13101[1], 13102[1], 13120[1], 13121[1], 13122[1], 13131[1], 13132[1], 13133[1], 13151[1], 13152[1], 13153[1], 36000[1], 36400[1], 36405[1], 36406[1], 36410[1], 36420[1], 36425[1], 36430[1], 36440[1], 36591[0], 36592[0], 36600[1], 36640[1], 43752[1], 51701[1], 51702[1], 51703[1], 61055[1], 62270[1], 62272[1], 62273[1], 62282[1], 62284[1], 62304[0], 62320[0], 62321[0], 62322[0], 62323[0], 62324[0], 62325[0], 62326[0], 62327[0], 62328[1], 62329[1], 64400[0], 64405[0], 64408[0], 64415[0], 64416[0], 64417[0], 64418[0], 64420[0], 64421[0], 64425[0], 64430[0], 64435[0], 64445[0], 64446[0], 64447[0], 64448[0], 64449[0], 64450[0], 64451[0], 64454[0], 64461[0], 64462[0], 64463[0], 64479[0], 64480[0], 64483[0], 64484[0], 64486[0], 64487[0], 64488[0], 64489[0], 64490[0], 64491[0], 64492[0], 64493[0], 64494[0], 64495[0], 64505[0], 64510[0], 64517[0], 64520[0], 64530[0], 69990[0], 72240[1], 72255[1], 72265[1], 72270[1], 76000[1], 77002[1], 77003[1], 92012[1], 92014[1], 92585[0], 93000[1], 93005[1], 93010[1], 93040[1], 93041[1], 93042[1], 93318[1], 93355[1], 94002[1], 94200[1], 94250[1], 94680[1], 94681[1], 94690[1], 94770[1], 95812[1], 95813[1], 95816[1], 95819[1], 95822[0], 95829[1], 95860[0], 95861[0], 95863[0], 95864[0], 95865[0], 95866[0], 95867[0], 95868[0], 95869[0], 95870[0], 95907[0], 95908[0], 95909[0], 95910[0], 95911[0], 95912[0], 95913[0], 95925[0], 95926[0], 95927[0], 95928[0], 95929[0], 95930[0], 95933[0], 95937[0], 95938[0], 95939[0], 95940[0], 95941[0], 95955[1], 96360[1], 96361[1], 96365[1], 96366[1], 96367[1], 96368[1], 96372[1], 96374[1], 96375[1], 96376[1], 96377[1], 96523[0], 99155[0], 99156[0], 99157[0], 99211[1], 99212[1], 99213[1], 99214[1], 99215[1], 99217[1], 99218[1], 99219[1], 99220[1], 99221[1], 99222[1], 99223[1], 99231[1], 99232[1], 99233[1], 99234[1], 99235[1], 99236[1], 99238[1], 99239[1], 99241[1], 99242[1], 99243[1], 99244[1], 99245[1], 99251[1], 99252[1], 99253[1], 99254[1], 99255[1], 99291[1], 99292[1], 99304[1], 99305[1], 99306[1], 99307[1], 99308[1], 99309[1], 99310[1], 99315[1], 99316[1], 99334[1], 99335[1], 99336[1], 99337[1], 99347[1], 99348[1], 99349[1], 99350[1], 99374[1], 99375[1], 99377[1], 99378[1], G0453[0], G0471[1]
62303	00620[0], 01935[0], 01936[0], 0213T[0], 0216T[0], 0228T[0], 0230T[0], 12001[1], 12002[1], 12004[1], 12005[1], 12006[1], 12007[1], 12011[1], 12013[1], 12014[1], 12015[1], 12016[1], 12017[1], 12018[1], 12020[1], 12021[1], 12031[1], 12032[1], 12034[1], 12035[1], 12036[1], 12037[1], 12041[1], 12042[1], 12044[1], 12045[1], 12046[1], 12047[1], 12051[1], 12052[1], 12053[1], 12054[1], 12055[1], 12056[1], 12057[1], 13100[1], 13101[1], 13102[1], 13120[1], 13121[1], 13122[1], 13131[1], 13132[1], 13133[1], 13151[1], 13152[1], 13153[1], 36000[1], 36400[1], 36405[1], 36406[1], 36410[1], 36420[1], 36425[1], 36430[1], 36440[1], 36591[0], 36592[0], 36600[1], 36640[1], 43752[1], 51701[1], 51702[1], 51703[1], 61055[1], 62270[1], 62272[1], 62273[1], 62282[1], 62284[1], 62302[0], 62304[0], 62320[0], 62321[0], 62322[0], 62323[0], 62324[0], 62325[0], 62326[0], 62327[0], 62328[1], 62329[1], 64400[0], 64405[0], 64408[0], 64415[0], 64416[0], 64417[0], 64418[0], 64420[0], 64421[0], 64425[0], 64430[0], 64435[0], 64445[0], 64446[0], 64447[0], 64448[0], 64449[0], 64450[0], 64451[0], 64454[0], 64461[0], 64462[0], 64463[0], 64479[0], 64480[0], 64483[0], 64484[0], 64486[0], 64487[0], 64488[0], 64489[0], 64490[0], 64491[0], 64492[0], 64493[0], 64494[0], 64495[0], 64505[0], 64510[0], 64517[0], 64520[0], 64530[0], 69990[0], 72240[1], 72255[1], 72265[1], 72270[1], 76000[1], 77002[1], 77003[1], 92012[1], 92014[1], 92585[0], 93000[1], 93005[1], 93010[1], 93040[1], 93041[1], 93042[1], 93318[1], 93355[1], 94002[1], 94200[1], 94250[1], 94680[1], 94681[1], 94690[1], 94770[1], 95812[1], 95813[1], 95816[1], 95819[1], 95822[0], 95829[1], 95860[0], 95861[0], 95863[0], 95864[0], 95865[0], 95866[0], 95867[0], 95868[0], 95869[0], 95870[0], 95907[0], 95908[0], 95909[0], 95910[0], 95911[0], 95912[0], 95913[0], 95925[0], 95926[0], 95927[0], 95928[0], 95929[0], 95930[0], 95933[0], 95937[0], 95938[0], 95939[0], 95940[0], 95941[0], 95955[1], 96360[1], 96361[1], 96365[1], 96366[1], 96367[1], 96368[1], 96372[1], 96374[1], 96375[1], 96376[1], 96377[1], 96523[0], 99155[0], 99156[0], 99157[0], 99211[1], 99212[1], 99213[1], 99214[1], 99215[1], 99217[1], 99218[1], 99219[1], 99220[1], 99221[1], 99222[1], 99223[1], 99231[1], 99232[1], 99233[1], 99234[1], 99235[1], 99236[1], 99238[1], 99239[1], 99241[1], 99242[1], 99243[1], 99244[1], 99245[1], 99251[1], 99252[1], 99253[1], 99254[1], 99255[1], 99291[1], 99292[1], 99304[1], 99305[1], 99306[1], 99307[1], 99308[1], 99309[1], 99310[1], 99315[1], 99316[1], 99334[1], 99335[1], 99336[1], 99337[1], 99347[1], 99348[1], 99349[1], 99350[1], 99374[1], 99375[1], 99377[1], 99378[1], G0453[0], G0471[1]
62304	00630[0], 01935[0], 01936[0], 0213T[0], 0216T[0], 0228T[0], 0230T[0], 12001[1], 12002[1], 12004[1], 12005[1], 12006[1], 12007[1], 12011[1], 12013[1], 12014[1], 12015[1], 12016[1], 12017[1], 12018[1], 12020[1], 12021[1], 12031[1], 12032[1], 12034[1], 12035[1], 12036[1], 12037[1], 12041[1], 12042[1], 12044[1], 12045[1], 12046[1], 12047[1], 12051[1], 12052[1], 12053[1], 12054[1], 12055[1], 12056[1], 12057[1], 13100[1], 13101[1], 13102[1], 13120[1], 13121[1], 13122[1], 13131[1], 13132[1], 13133[1], 13151[1], 13152[1], 13153[1], 36000[1], 36400[1], 36405[1], 36406[1], 36410[1], 36420[1], 36425[1], 36430[1], 36440[1], 36591[0], 36592[0], 36600[1], 36640[1], 43752[1], 51701[1], 51702[1], 51703[1], 61055[1], 62270[1], 62272[1], 62273[1], 62282[1], 62284[1], 62320[0], 62321[0], 62322[0], 62323[0], 62324[0], 62325[0], 62326[0], 62327[0], 62328[1], 62329[1], 64400[0], 64405[0], 64408[0], 64415[0],

0 = Modifier usage not allowed or inappropriate 1 = Modifier usage allowed

Code 1	Code 2
	64416^0, 64417^0, 64418^0, 64420^0, 64421^0, 64425^0, 64430^0, 64435^0, 64445^0, 64446^0, 64447^0, 64448^0, 64449^0, 64450^0, 64451^0, 64454^0, 64461^0, 64462^0, 64463^0, 64479^0, 64480^0, 64483^0, 64484^0, 64486^0, 64487^0, 64488^0, 64489^0, 64490^0, 64491^0, 64492^0, 64493^0, 64494^0, 64495^0, 64505^0, 64510^0, 64517^0, 64520^0, 64530^0, 69990^0, 72240^1, 72255^1, 72265^1, 72270^1, 76000^1, 77002^1, 77003^1, 92012^1, 92014^1, 92585^0, 93000^1, 93005^1, 93010^1, 93040^1, 93041^1, 93042^1, 93318^1, 93355^1, 94002^1, 94200^1, 94250^1, 94680^1, 94681^1, 94690^1, 94770^1, 95812^1, 95813^1, 95816^1, 95819^1, 95822^0, 95829^1, 95860^0, 95861^0, 95863^0, 95864^0, 95865^0, 95866^0, 95867^0, 95868^0, 95869^0, 95870^0, 95907^0, 95908^0, 95909^0, 95910^0, 95911^0, 95912^0, 95913^0, 95925^0, 95926^0, 95927^0, 95928^0, 95929^0, 95930^0, 95933^0, 95937^0, 95938^0, 95939^0, 95940^0, 95941^0, 95955^1, 96360^1, 96361^1, 96365^1, 96366^1, 96367^1, 96368^1, 96372^1, 96374^1, 96375^1, 96376^1, 96377^1, 96523^0, 99155^0, 99156^0, 99157^0, 99211^1, 99212^1, 99213^1, 99214^1, 99215^1, 99217^1, 99218^1, 99219^1, 99220^1, 99221^1, 99222^1, 99223^1, 99231^1, 99232^1, 99233^1, 99234^1, 99235^1, 99236^1, 99238^1, 99239^1, 99241^1, 99242^1, 99243^1, 99244^1, 99245^1, 99251^1, 99252^1, 99253^1, 99254^1, 99255^1, 99291^1, 99292^1, 99304^1, 99305^1, 99306^1, 99307^1, 99308^1, 99309^1, 99310^1, 99315^1, 99316^1, 99334^1, 99335^1, 99336^1, 99337^1, 99347^1, 99348^1, 99349^1, 99350^1, 99374^1, 99375^1, 99377^1, 99378^1, G0453^0, G0471^1
62305	00600^0, 00620^0, 00630^0, 01935^0, 01936^0, 0213T^0, 0216T^0, 0228T^0, 0230T^0, 12001^1, 12002^1, 12004^1, 12005^1, 12006^1, 12007^1, 12011^1, 12013^1, 12014^1, 12015^1, 12016^1, 12017^1, 12018^1, 12020^1, 12021^1, 12031^1, 12032^1, 12034^1, 12035^1, 12036^1, 12037^1, 12041^1, 12042^1, 12044^1, 12045^1, 12046^1, 12047^1, 12051^1, 12052^1, 12053^1, 12054^1, 12055^1, 12056^1, 12057^1, 13100^1, 13101^1, 13102^1, 13120^1, 13121^1, 13122^1, 13131^1, 13132^1, 13133^1, 13151^1, 13152^1, 13153^1, 36000^1, 36400^1, 36405^1, 36406^1, 36410^1, 36420^1, 36425^1, 36430^1, 36440^1, 36591^0, 36592^0, 36600^1, 36640^1, 43752^1, 51701^1, 51702^1, 51703^1, 61055^1, 62270^1, 62272^1, 62273^1, 62282^1, 62284^1, 62302^0, 62303^0, 62304^0, 62320^0, 62321^0, 62322^0, 62323^0, 62324^0, 62325^0, 62326^0, 62327^0, 62328^1, 62329^1, 64400^0, 64405^0, 64408^0, 64415^0, 64416^0, 64417^0, 64418^0, 64420^0, 64421^0, 64425^0, 64430^0, 64435^0, 64445^0, 64446^0, 64447^0, 64448^0, 64449^0, 64450^0, 64451^0, 64454^0, 64461^0, 64462^0, 64463^0, 64479^0, 64480^0, 64483^0, 64484^0, 64486^0, 64487^0, 64488^0, 64489^0, 64490^0, 64491^0, 64492^0, 64493^0, 64494^0, 64495^0, 64505^0, 64510^0, 64517^0, 64520^0, 64530^0, 69990^0, 72240^1, 72255^1, 72265^1, 72270^1, 76000^1, 77002^1, 77003^1, 92012^1, 92014^1, 92585^0, 93000^1, 93005^1, 93010^1, 93040^1, 93041^1, 93042^1, 93318^1, 93355^1, 94002^1, 94200^1, 94250^1, 94680^1, 94681^1, 94690^1, 94770^1, 95812^1, 95813^1, 95816^1, 95819^1, 95822^0, 95829^1, 95860^0, 95861^0, 95863^0, 95864^0, 95865^0, 95866^0, 95867^0, 95868^0, 95869^0, 95870^0, 95907^0, 95908^0, 95909^0, 95910^0, 95911^0, 95912^0, 95913^0, 95925^0, 95926^0, 95927^0, 95928^0, 95929^0, 95930^0, 95933^0, 95937^0, 95938^0, 95939^0, 95940^0, 95941^0, 95955^1, 96360^1, 96361^1, 96365^1, 96366^1, 96367^1, 96368^1, 96372^1, 96374^1, 96375^1, 96376^1, 96377^1, 96523^0, 99155^0, 99156^0, 99157^0, 99211^1, 99212^1, 99213^1, 99214^1, 99215^1, 99217^1, 99218^1, 99219^1, 99220^1, 99221^1, 99222^1, 99223^1, 99231^1, 99232^1, 99233^1, 99234^1, 99235^1, 99236^1, 99238^1, 99239^1, 99241^1, 99242^1, 99243^1, 99244^1, 99245^1, 99251^1, 99252^1, 99253^1, 99254^1, 99255^1, 99291^1, 99292^1, 99304^1, 99305^1, 99306^1, 99307^1, 99308^1, 99309^1, 99310^1, 99315^1, 99316^1, 99334^1, 99335^1, 99336^1, 99337^1, 99347^1, 99348^1, 99349^1, 99350^1, 99374^1, 99375^1, 99377^1, 99378^1, G0453^0, G0471^1
62320	01991^0, 01992^0, 0228T^1, 0333T^0, 0464T^0, 0543T^0, 0544T^0, 0548T^0, 0567T^0, 0568T^0, 0569T^0, 0570T^0, 0571T^0, 0572T^0, 0573T^0, 0574T^0, 0580T^0, 0581T^0, 0582T^0, 12001^1, 12002^1, 12004^1, 12005^1, 12006^1, 12007^1, 12011^1, 12013^1, 12014^1, 12015^1, 12016^1, 12017^1, 12018^1, 12020^1, 12021^1, 12031^1, 12032^1, 12034^1, 12035^1, 12036^1, 12037^1, 12041^1, 12042^1, 12044^1, 12045^1, 12046^1, 12047^1, 12051^1, 12052^1, 12053^1, 12054^1, 12055^1, 12056^1, 12057^1, 13100^1, 13101^1, 13102^1, 13120^1, 13121^1, 13122^1, 13131^1, 13132^1, 13133^1, 13151^1, 13152^1, 13153^1, 20560^0, 20561^0, 20605^1, 20610^1, 20700^0, 20701^0, 36000^1, 36140^1, 36400^1, 36405^1, 36406^1, 36410^1, 36420^1, 36425^1, 36430^1, 36440^1, 36591^0, 36592^0, 36600^1, 36640^1, 43752^1, 51701^0, 51702^0, 51703^0, 62284^0, 64451^0, 64462^0, 64479^1, 64480^0, 66987^0, 66988^0, 69990^0, 72275^1, 76000^1, 76800^1, 76942^1, 76970^1, 76998^1, 77001^1, 77002^1, 77003^1, 77012^1, 92012^1, 92014^1, 92585^0, 93000^1, 93005^1, 93010^1, 93040^1, 93041^1, 93042^1, 93318^1, 93355^1, 94002^1, 94200^1, 94250^1, 94680^1, 94681^1, 94690^1, 94770^1, 95812^1, 95813^1, 95816^1, 95819^1, 95822^0, 95829^1, 95860^0, 95861^0, 95863^0, 95864^0, 95865^0, 95866^0, 95867^0, 95868^0, 95869^0, 95870^0, 95907^0, 95908^0, 95909^0, 95910^0, 95911^0, 95912^0, 95913^0, 95925^0, 95926^0, 95927^0, 95928^0, 95929^0, 95930^0, 95933^0, 95937^0, 95938^0, 95939^0, 95940^0, 95941^0, 95955^1, 96360^1, 96361^1, 96365^1, 96366^1, 96367^1, 96368^1, 96372^1, 96374^1, 96375^1, 96376^1, 96377^1, 96523^0, 99155^0, 99156^0, 99157^0, 99211^1, 99212^1, 99213^1, 99214^1, 99215^1, 99217^1, 99218^1, 99219^1, 99220^1, 99221^1, 99222^1, 99223^1, 99231^1, 99232^1, 99233^1, 99234^1, 99235^1, 99236^1, 99238^1, 99239^1, 99241^1, 99242^1, 99243^1, 99244^1, 99245^1, 99251^1, 99252^1, 99253^1, 99254^1, 99255^1, 99291^1, 99292^1, 99304^1, 99305^1, 99306^1, 99307^1, 99308^1, 99309^1, 99310^1, 99315^1, 99316^1, 99334^1, 99335^1, 99336^1, 99337^1, 99347^1, 99348^1, 99349^1, 99350^1, 99374^1, 99375^1, 99377^1, 99378^1, 99446^0, 99447^0, 99448^0, 99449^0, 99451^0, 99452^0, 99495^1, 99496^1, G0453^0, G0459^1, G0463^1, G0471^0, J2001^1
62321	01991^0, 01992^0, 0228T^1, 0333T^0, 0464T^0, 0543T^0, 0544T^0, 0548T^0, 0567T^0, 0568T^0, 0569T^0, 0570T^0, 0571T^0, 0572T^0, 0573T^0, 0574T^0, 0580T^0, 0581T^0, 0582T^0, 12001^1, 12002^1, 12004^1, 12005^1, 12006^1, 12007^1, 12011^1, 12013^1, 12014^1, 12015^1, 12016^1, 12017^1, 12018^1, 12020^1, 12021^1, 12031^1, 12032^1, 12034^1, 12035^1, 12036^1, 12037^1, 12041^1, 12042^1, 12044^1, 12045^1, 12046^1, 12047^1, 12051^1, 12052^1, 12053^1, 12054^1, 12055^1, 12056^1, 12057^1, 13100^1, 13101^1, 13102^1, 13120^1, 13121^1, 13122^1, 13131^1, 13132^1, 13133^1, 13151^1, 13152^1, 13153^1, 20560^0, 20561^0, 20605^1, 20610^1, 20700^0, 20701^0, 36000^1, 36140^1, 36400^1, 36405^1, 36406^1, 36410^1, 36420^1, 36425^1, 36430^1, 36440^1, 36591^0, 36592^0, 36600^1, 36640^1, 43752^1, 51701^0, 51702^0, 51703^0, 62284^0, 62320^0, 64451^0, 64462^0, 64479^1, 64480^0, 66987^0, 66988^0, 69990^0, 72275^1, 76000^1, 76800^1, 76942^1, 76970^1, 76998^1, 77001^1, 77002^1, 77003^1, 77012^1, 92012^1, 92014^1, 92585^0, 93000^1, 93005^1, 93010^1, 93040^1, 93041^1, 93042^1, 93318^1, 93355^1, 94002^1, 94200^1, 94250^1, 94680^1, 94681^1, 94690^1, 94770^1, 95812^1, 95813^1, 95816^1, 95819^1, 95822^0, 95829^1, 95860^0, 95861^0, 95863^0, 95864^0, 95865^0, 95866^0, 95867^0, 95868^0, 95869^0, 95870^0, 95907^0, 95908^0, 95909^0, 95910^0, 95911^0, 95912^0, 95913^0, 95925^0, 95926^0, 95927^0, 95928^0, 95929^0, 95930^0, 95933^0, 95937^0, 95938^0, 95939^0, 95940^0, 95941^0, 95955^1, 96360^1, 96361^1, 96365^1, 96366^1, 96367^1, 96368^1, 96372^1, 96374^1, 96375^1, 96376^1, 96377^1, 96523^0, 99155^0, 99156^0, 99157^0, 99211^1, 99212^1, 99213^1, 99214^1, 99215^1, 99217^1, 99218^1, 99219^1, 99220^1, 99221^1, 99222^1, 99223^1, 99231^1, 99232^1, 99233^1, 99234^1, 99235^1, 99236^1, 99238^1, 99239^1, 99241^1, 99242^1, 99243^1, 99244^1, 99245^1, 99251^1, 99252^1, 99253^1, 99254^1, 99255^1, 99291^1, 99292^1, 99304^1, 99305^1, 99306^1, 99307^1, 99308^1, 99309^1, 99310^1, 99315^1, 99316^1, 99334^1, 99335^1, 99336^1, 99337^1, 99347^1, 99348^1, 99349^1, 99350^1, 99374^1, 99375^1, 99377^1, 99378^1, 99446^0, 99447^0, 99448^0, 99449^0, 99451^0, 99452^0, 99495^1, 99496^1, G0453^0, G0459^1, G0463^1, G0471^0, J2001^1
62322	01991^0, 01992^0, 0230T^1, 0333T^0, 0464T^0, 0543T^0, 0544T^0, 0548T^0, 0567T^0, 0568T^0, 0569T^0, 0570T^0, 0571T^0, 0572T^0, 0573T^0, 0574T^0, 0580T^0, 0581T^0, 0582T^0, 12001^1, 12002^1, 12004^1, 12005^1, 12006^1, 12007^1, 12011^1, 12013^1, 12014^1, 12015^1, 12016^1, 12017^1, 12018^1, 12020^1, 12021^1, 12031^1, 12032^1, 12034^1, 12035^1, 12036^1, 12037^1, 12041^1, 12042^1, 12044^1, 12045^1, 12046^1, 12047^1, 12051^1, 12052^1, 12053^1, 12054^1, 12055^1, 12056^1, 12057^1, 13100^1, 13101^1, 13102^1, 13120^1, 13121^1, 13122^1, 13131^1, 13132^1, 13133^1, 13151^1, 13152^1, 13153^1, 20560^0, 20561^0, 20605^1, 20610^1, 20700^0, 20701^0, 36000^1, 36140^1, 36400^1, 36405^1, 36406^1, 36410^1, 36420^1, 36425^1, 36430^1, 36440^1, 36591^0, 36592^0, 36600^1, 36640^1, 43752^1, 51701^0, 51702^0, 51703^0, 62284^0, 64451^0, 64483^1, 64484^0, 66987^0, 66988^0, 69990^0, 72275^1, 76000^1, 76800^1, 76942^1, 76970^1, 76998^1, 77001^1, 77002^1, 77003^1, 77012^1, 92012^1, 92014^1, 92585^0, 93000^1, 93005^1, 93010^1, 93040^1, 93041^1, 93042^1, 93318^1, 93355^1, 94002^1, 94200^1, 94250^1, 94680^1, 94681^1, 94690^1, 94770^1, 95812^1, 95813^1, 95816^1, 95819^1, 95822^0, 95829^1, 95860^0, 95861^0, 95863^0, 95864^0, 95865^0, 95866^0, 95867^0, 95868^0, 95869^0, 95870^0, 95907^0, 95908^0, 95909^0, 95910^0, 95911^0, 95912^0, 95913^0, 95925^0, 95926^0, 95927^0, 95928^0, 95929^0, 95930^0, 95933^0, 95937^0, 95938^0, 95939^0, 95940^0, 95941^0, 95955^1, 96360^1, 96361^1, 96365^1, 96366^1, 96367^1, 96368^1, 96372^1, 96374^1, 96375^1, 96376^1, 96377^1, 96523^0, 99155^0, 99156^0, 99157^0, 99211^1, 99212^1, 99213^1, 99214^1, 99215^1, 99217^1, 99218^1, 99219^1, 99220^1, 99221^1, 99222^1, 99223^1, 99231^1, 99232^1, 99233^1, 99234^1, 99235^1, 99236^1, 99238^1, 99239^1, 99241^1, 99242^1, 99243^1, 99244^1, 99245^1, 99251^1, 99252^1, 99253^1, 99254^1, 99255^1, 99291^1, 99292^1, 99304^1, 99305^1, 99306^1, 99307^1, 99308^1, 99309^1, 99310^1, 99315^1, 99316^1, 99334^1, 99335^1, 99336^1, 99337^1, 99347^1, 99348^1, 99349^1, 99350^1, 99374^1, 99375^1, 99377^1, 99378^1, 99446^0, 99447^0, 99448^0, 99449^0, 99451^0, 99452^0, 99495^1, 99496^1, G0453^0, G0459^1, G0463^1, G0471^0, J2001^1
62323	01991^0, 01992^0, 0230T^1, 0333T^0, 0464T^0, 0543T^0, 0544T^0, 0548T^0, 0567T^0, 0568T^0, 0569T^0, 0570T^0, 0571T^0, 0572T^0, 0573T^0, 0574T^0, 0580T^0, 0581T^0, 0582T^0, 12001^1, 12002^1, 12004^1, 12005^1, 12006^1, 12007^1, 12011^1, 12013^1, 12014^1, 12015^1, 12016^1, 12017^1, 12018^1, 12020^1, 12021^1, 12031^1, 12032^1, 12034^1, 12035^1, 12036^1, 12037^1, 12041^1, 12042^1, 12044^1, 12045^1, 12046^1, 12047^1, 12051^1, 12052^1, 12053^1, 12054^1, 12055^1, 12056^1, 12057^1, 13100^1, 13101^1, 13102^1, 13120^1, 13121^1, 13122^1, 13131^1, 13132^1, 13133^1, 13151^1, 13152^1, 13153^1, 20560^0, 20561^0, 20605^1, 20610^1, 20700^0, 20701^0, 36000^1, 36140^1, 36400^1, 36405^1, 36406^1, 36410^1, 36420^1, 36425^1, 36430^1, 36440^1, 36591^0, 36592^0, 36600^1, 36640^1, 43752^1, 51701^0, 51702^0, 51703^0, 62284^0, 62322^0, 64451^0, 64483^1, 64484^1, 66987^0, 66988^0, 69990^0, 72275^1, 76000^1, 76800^1, 76942^1, 76970^1, 76998^1, 77001^1, 77002^1, 77003^1, 77012^1, 92012^1, 92014^1, 92585^0, 93000^1, 93005^1, 93010^1, 93040^1, 93041^1, 93042^1, 93318^1, 93355^1, 94002^1, 94200^1,

0 = Modifier usage not allowed or inappropriate 1 = Modifier usage allowed

Code 1	Code 2
	94250[1], 94680[1], 94681[1], 94690[1], 94770[1], 95812[1], 95813[1], 95816[1], 95819[1], 95822[0], 95829[1], 95860[0], 95861[0], 95863[0], 95864[0], 95865[0], 95866[0], 95867[0], 95868[0], 95869[0], 95870[0], 95907[0], 95908[0], 95909[0], 95910[0], 95911[0], 95912[0], 95913[0], 95925[0], 95926[0], 95927[0], 95928[0], 95929[0], 95930[0], 95933[0], 95937[0], 95938[0], 95939[0], 95940[0], 95941[0], 95955[1], 96360[1], 96361[1], 96365[1], 96366[1], 96367[1], 96368[1], 96372[1], 96374[1], 96375[1], 96376[1], 96377[1], 96523[0], 99155[0], 99156[0], 99157[0], 99211[1], 99212[1], 99213[1], 99214[1], 99215[1], 99217[1], 99218[1], 99219[1], 99220[1], 99221[1], 99222[1], 99223[1], 99231[1], 99232[1], 99233[1], 99234[1], 99235[1], 99236[1], 99238[1], 99239[1], 99241[1], 99242[1], 99243[1], 99244[1], 99245[1], 99251[1], 99252[1], 99253[1], 99254[1], 99255[1], 99291[1], 99292[1], 99304[1], 99305[1], 99306[1], 99307[1], 99308[1], 99309[1], 99310[1], 99315[1], 99316[1], 99334[1], 99335[1], 99336[1], 99337[1], 99347[1], 99348[1], 99349[1], 99350[1], 99374[1], 99375[1], 99377[1], 99378[1], 99446[0], 99447[0], 99448[0], 99449[0], 99451[0], 99452[0], 99495[1], 99496[1], G0453[0], G0459[1], G0463[1], G0471[0], J2001[1]
62324	01991[0], 01992[0], 01996[0], 0228T[1], 0333T[0], 0464T[0], 0543T[0], 0544T[0], 0548T[0], 0567T[0], 0568T[0], 0569T[0], 0570T[0], 0571T[0], 0572T[0], 0573T[0], 0574T[0], 0580T[0], 0581T[0], 0582T[0], 12001[1], 12002[1], 12004[1], 12005[1], 12006[1], 12007[1], 12011[1], 12013[1], 12014[1], 12015[1], 12016[1], 12017[1], 12018[1], 12020[1], 12021[1], 12031[1], 12032[1], 12034[1], 12035[1], 12036[1], 12037[1], 12041[1], 12042[1], 12044[1], 12045[1], 12046[1], 12047[1], 12051[1], 12052[1], 12053[1], 12054[1], 12055[1], 12056[1], 12057[1], 13100[1], 13101[1], 13102[1], 13120[1], 13121[1], 13122[1], 13131[1], 13132[1], 13133[1], 13151[1], 13152[1], 13153[1], 20560[0], 20561[0], 20605[1], 20610[1], 20700[0], 20701[0], 36000[1], 36140[1], 36400[1], 36405[1], 36406[1], 36410[1], 36420[1], 36425[1], 36430[1], 36440[1], 36591[0], 36592[0], 36600[1], 36640[1], 43752[1], 51701[0], 51702[0], 51703[1], 62270[0], 62272[0], 62284[0], 62320[1], 62321[1], 64451[0], 64462[0], 64479[1], 64480[0], 66987[0], 66988[0], 69990[0], 72275[1], 76000[1], 76800[1], 76942[1], 76970[1], 76998[1], 77001[1], 77002[1], 77003[1], 77012[1], 92012[1], 92014[1], 92585[0], 93000[1], 93005[1], 93010[1], 93040[1], 93041[1], 93042[1], 93318[1], 93355[1], 94002[1], 94200[1], 94250[1], 94680[1], 94681[1], 94690[1], 94770[1], 95812[1], 95813[1], 95816[1], 95819[1], 95822[0], 95829[1], 95860[0], 95861[0], 95863[0], 95864[0], 95865[0], 95866[0], 95867[0], 95868[0], 95869[0], 95870[0], 95907[0], 95908[0], 95909[0], 95910[0], 95911[0], 95912[0], 95913[0], 95925[0], 95926[0], 95927[0], 95928[0], 95929[0], 95930[0], 95933[0], 95937[0], 95938[0], 95939[0], 95940[0], 95941[0], 95955[1], 96360[1], 96361[1], 96365[1], 96366[1], 96367[1], 96368[1], 96372[1], 96374[1], 96375[1], 96376[1], 96377[1], 96522[1], 96523[0], 99155[0], 99156[0], 99157[0], 99211[1], 99212[1], 99213[1], 99214[1], 99215[1], 99217[1], 99218[1], 99219[1], 99220[1], 99221[1], 99222[1], 99223[1], 99231[1], 99232[1], 99233[1], 99234[1], 99235[1], 99236[1], 99238[1], 99239[1], 99241[1], 99242[1], 99243[1], 99244[1], 99245[1], 99251[1], 99252[1], 99253[1], 99254[1], 99255[1], 99291[1], 99292[1], 99304[1], 99305[1], 99306[1], 99307[1], 99308[1], 99309[1], 99310[1], 99315[1], 99316[1], 99334[1], 99335[1], 99336[1], 99337[1], 99347[1], 99348[1], 99349[1], 99350[1], 99374[1], 99375[1], 99377[1], 99378[1], 99446[0], 99447[0], 99448[0], 99449[0], 99451[0], 99452[0], 99495[1], 99496[1], G0453[0], G0459[1], G0463[1], G0471[0], J2001[1]
62325	01991[0], 01992[0], 01996[0], 0228T[1], 0333T[0], 0464T[0], 0543T[0], 0544T[0], 0548T[0], 0567T[0], 0568T[0], 0569T[0], 0570T[0], 0571T[0], 0572T[0], 0573T[0], 0574T[0], 0580T[0], 0581T[0], 0582T[0], 12001[1], 12002[1], 12004[1], 12005[1], 12006[1], 12007[1], 12011[1], 12013[1], 12014[1], 12015[1], 12016[1], 12017[1], 12018[1], 12020[1], 12021[1], 12031[1], 12032[1], 12034[1], 12035[1], 12036[1], 12037[1], 12041[1], 12042[1], 12044[1], 12045[1], 12046[1], 12047[1], 12051[1], 12052[1], 12053[1], 12054[1], 12055[1], 12056[1], 12057[1], 13100[1], 13101[1], 13102[1], 13120[1], 13121[1], 13122[1], 13131[1], 13132[1], 13133[1], 13151[1], 13152[1], 13153[1], 20560[0], 20561[0], 20605[1], 20610[1], 20700[0], 20701[0], 36000[1], 36140[1], 36400[1], 36405[1], 36406[1], 36410[1], 36420[1], 36425[1], 36430[1], 36440[1], 36591[0], 36592[0], 36600[1], 36640[1], 43752[1], 51701[0], 51702[0], 51703[1], 62270[0], 62272[0], 62273[0], 62284[0], 62320[1], 62321[1], 62323[0], 62329[0], 64451[0], 64462[0], 64479[1], 64480[0], 66987[0], 66988[0], 69990[0], 72275[1], 76000[1], 76800[1], 76942[1], 76970[1], 76998[1], 77001[1], 77002[1], 77003[1], 77012[1], 92012[1], 92014[1], 92585[0], 93000[1], 93005[1], 93010[1], 93040[1], 93041[1], 93042[1], 93318[1], 93355[1], 94002[1], 94200[1], 94250[1], 94680[1], 94681[1], 94690[1], 94770[1], 95812[1], 95813[1], 95816[1], 95819[1], 95822[0], 95829[1], 95860[0], 95861[0], 95863[0], 95864[0], 95865[0], 95866[0], 95867[0], 95868[0], 95869[0], 95870[0], 95907[0], 95908[0], 95909[0], 95910[0], 95911[0], 95912[0], 95913[0], 95925[0], 95926[0], 95927[0], 95928[0], 95929[0], 95930[0], 95933[0], 95937[0], 95938[0], 95939[0], 95940[0], 95941[0], 95955[1], 96360[1], 96361[1], 96365[1], 96366[1], 96367[1], 96368[1], 96372[1], 96374[1], 96375[1], 96376[1], 96377[1], 96522[1], 96523[0], 99155[0], 99156[0], 99157[0], 99211[1], 99212[1], 99213[1], 99214[1], 99215[1], 99217[1], 99218[1], 99219[1], 99220[1], 99221[1], 99222[1], 99223[1], 99231[1], 99232[1], 99233[1], 99234[1], 99235[1], 99236[1], 99238[1], 99239[1], 99241[1], 99242[1], 99243[1], 99244[1], 99245[1], 99251[1], 99252[1], 99253[1], 99254[1], 99255[1], 99291[1], 99292[1], 99304[1], 99305[1], 99306[1], 99307[1], 99308[1], 99309[1], 99310[1], 99315[1], 99316[1], 99334[1], 99335[1], 99336[1], 99337[1], 99347[1], 99348[1], 99349[1], 99350[1], 99374[1], 99375[1], 99377[1], 99378[1], 99446[0], 99447[0], 99448[0], 99449[0], 99451[0], 99452[0], 99495[1], 99496[1], G0453[0], G0459[1], G0463[1], G0471[0], J2001[1]
62326	01991[0], 01992[0], 01996[0], 0230T[1], 0333T[0], 0464T[0], 0543T[0], 0544T[0], 0548T[0], 0567T[0], 0568T[0], 0569T[0], 0570T[0], 0571T[0], 0572T[0], 0573T[0], 0574T[0], 0580T[0], 0581T[0], 0582T[0], 12001[1], 12002[1], 12004[1], 12005[1], 12006[1], 12007[1], 12011[1], 12013[1], 12014[1], 12015[1], 12016[1], 12017[1], 12018[1], 12020[1], 12021[1], 12031[1], 12032[1], 12034[1], 12035[1], 12036[1], 12037[1], 12041[1], 12042[1], 12044[1], 12045[1], 12046[1], 12047[1], 12051[1], 12052[1], 12053[1], 12054[1], 12055[1], 12056[1], 12057[1], 13100[1], 13101[1], 13102[1], 13120[1], 13121[1], 13122[1], 13131[1], 13132[1], 13133[1], 13151[1], 13152[1], 13153[1], 20560[0], 20561[0], 20605[1], 20610[1], 20700[0], 20701[0], 36000[1], 36140[1], 36400[1], 36405[1], 36406[1], 36410[1], 36420[1], 36425[1], 36430[1], 36440[1], 36591[0], 36592[0], 36600[1], 36640[1], 43752[1], 51701[0], 51702[0], 51703[1], 62270[0], 62272[0], 62284[0], 62322[1], 62323[1], 64451[0], 64483[1], 64484[0], 66987[0], 66988[0], 69990[0], 72275[1], 76000[1], 76800[1], 76942[1], 76970[1], 76998[1], 77001[1], 77002[1], 77003[1], 77012[1], 92012[1], 92014[1], 92585[0], 93000[1], 93005[1], 93010[1], 93040[1], 93041[1], 93042[1], 93318[1], 93355[1], 94002[1], 94200[1], 94250[1], 94680[1], 94681[1], 94690[1], 94770[1], 95812[1], 95813[1], 95816[1], 95819[1], 95822[0], 95829[1], 95860[0], 95861[0], 95863[0], 95864[0], 95865[0], 95866[0], 95867[0], 95868[0], 95869[0], 95870[0], 95907[0], 95908[0], 95909[0], 95910[0], 95911[0], 95912[0], 95913[0], 95925[0], 95926[0], 95927[0], 95928[0], 95929[0], 95930[0], 95933[0], 95937[0], 95938[0], 95939[0], 95940[0], 95941[0], 95955[1], 96360[1], 96361[1], 96365[1], 96366[1], 96367[1], 96368[1], 96372[1], 96374[1], 96375[1], 96376[1], 96377[1], 96522[1], 96523[0], 99155[0], 99156[0], 99157[0], 99211[1], 99212[1], 99213[1], 99214[1], 99215[1], 99217[1], 99218[1], 99219[1], 99220[1], 99221[1], 99222[1], 99223[1], 99231[1], 99232[1], 99233[1], 99234[1], 99235[1], 99236[1], 99238[1], 99239[1], 99241[1], 99242[1], 99243[1], 99244[1], 99245[1], 99251[1], 99252[1], 99253[1], 99254[1], 99255[1], 99291[1], 99292[1], 99304[1], 99305[1], 99306[1], 99307[1], 99308[1], 99309[1], 99310[1], 99315[1], 99316[1], 99334[1], 99335[1], 99336[1], 99337[1], 99347[1], 99348[1], 99349[1], 99350[1], 99374[1], 99375[1], 99377[1], 99378[1], 99446[0], 99447[0], 99448[0], 99449[0], 99451[0], 99452[0], 99495[1], 99496[1], G0453[0], G0459[1], G0463[1], G0471[0], J2001[1]
62327	01991[0], 01992[0], 01996[0], 0230T[1], 0333T[0], 0464T[0], 0543T[0], 0544T[0], 0548T[0], 0567T[0], 0568T[0], 0569T[0], 0570T[0], 0571T[0], 0572T[0], 0573T[0], 0574T[0], 0580T[0], 0581T[0], 0582T[0], 12001[1], 12002[1], 12004[1], 12005[1], 12006[1], 12007[1], 12011[1], 12013[1], 12014[1], 12015[1], 12016[1], 12017[1], 12018[1], 12020[1], 12021[1], 12031[1], 12032[1], 12034[1], 12035[1], 12036[1], 12037[1], 12041[1], 12042[1], 12044[1], 12045[1], 12046[1], 12047[1], 12051[1], 12052[1], 12053[1], 12054[1], 12055[1], 12056[1], 12057[1], 13100[1], 13101[1], 13102[1], 13120[1], 13121[1], 13122[1], 13131[1], 13132[1], 13133[1], 13151[1], 13152[1], 13153[1], 20560[0], 20561[0], 20605[1], 20610[1], 20700[0], 20701[0], 36000[1], 36140[1], 36400[1], 36405[1], 36406[1], 36410[1], 36420[1], 36425[1], 36430[1], 36440[1], 36591[0], 36592[0], 36600[1], 36640[1], 43752[1], 51701[0], 51702[0], 51703[1], 62270[0], 62272[0], 62284[0], 62322[1], 62323[1], 62326[0], 64451[0], 64483[1], 64484[0], 66987[0], 66988[0], 69990[0], 72275[1], 76000[1], 76800[1], 76942[1], 76970[1], 76998[1], 77001[1], 77002[1], 77003[1], 77012[1], 92012[1], 92014[1], 92585[0], 93000[1], 93005[1], 93010[1], 93040[1], 93041[1], 93042[1], 93318[1], 93355[1], 94002[1], 94200[1], 94250[1], 94680[1], 94681[1], 94690[1], 94770[1], 95812[1], 95813[1], 95816[1], 95819[1], 95822[0], 95829[1], 95860[0], 95861[0], 95863[0], 95864[0], 95865[0], 95866[0], 95867[0], 95868[0], 95869[0], 95870[0], 95907[0], 95908[0], 95909[0], 95910[0], 95911[0], 95912[0], 95913[0], 95925[0], 95926[0], 95927[0], 95928[0], 95929[0], 95930[0], 95933[0], 95937[0], 95938[0], 95939[0], 95940[0], 95941[0], 95955[1], 96360[1], 96361[1], 96365[1], 96366[1], 96367[1], 96368[1], 96372[1], 96374[1], 96375[1], 96376[1], 96377[1], 96522[1], 96523[0], 99155[0], 99156[0], 99157[0], 99211[1], 99212[1], 99213[1], 99214[1], 99215[1], 99217[1], 99218[1], 99219[1], 99220[1], 99221[1], 99222[1], 99223[1], 99231[1], 99232[1], 99233[1], 99234[1], 99235[1], 99236[1], 99238[1], 99239[1], 99241[1], 99242[1], 99243[1], 99244[1], 99245[1], 99251[1], 99252[1], 99253[1], 99254[1], 99255[1], 99291[1], 99292[1], 99304[1], 99305[1], 99306[1], 99307[1], 99308[1], 99309[1], 99310[1], 99315[1], 99316[1], 99334[1], 99335[1], 99336[1], 99337[1], 99347[1], 99348[1], 99349[1], 99350[1], 99374[1], 99375[1], 99377[1], 99378[1], 99446[0], 99447[0], 99448[0], 99449[0], 99451[0], 99452[0], 99495[1], 99496[1], G0453[0], G0459[1], G0463[1], G0471[0], J2001[1]
62328	00635[0], 01935[0], 01936[0], 0213T[0], 0216T[0], 0228T[0], 0230T[0], 12001[1], 12002[1], 12004[1], 12005[1], 12006[1], 12007[1], 12011[1], 12013[1], 12014[1], 12015[1], 12016[1], 12017[1], 12018[1], 12020[1], 12021[1], 12031[1], 12032[1], 12034[1], 12035[1], 12036[1], 12037[1], 12041[1], 12042[1], 12044[1], 12045[1], 12046[1], 12047[1], 12051[1], 12052[1], 12053[1], 12054[1], 12055[1], 12056[1], 12057[1], 13100[1], 13101[1], 13102[1], 13120[1], 13121[1], 13122[1], 13131[1], 13132[1], 13133[1], 13151[1], 13152[1], 13153[1], 36000[1], 36400[1], 36405[1], 36406[1], 36410[1], 36420[1], 36425[1], 36430[1], 36440[1], 36591[0], 36592[0], 36600[1], 36640[1], 43752[1], 51701[1], 51702[1], 51703[1], 62270[1], 62273[1], 62320[0], 62321[0], 62322[0], 62323[0], 62324[0], 62325[0], 62326[0], 62327[0], 64400[0], 64405[0], 64408[0], 64415[0], 64416[0], 64417[0], 64418[0], 64420[0], 64421[0], 64425[0], 64430[0], 64435[0], 64445[0], 64446[0], 64447[0], 64448[0], 64449[0], 64461[0], 64462[0], 64463[0], 64479[0], 64480[0], 64483[0], 64484[0], 64486[0], 64487[0], 64488[0], 64489[0], 64490[0], 64491[0], 64492[0], 64493[0], 64494[0], 64495[0], 64505[0], 64510[0], 64517[0], 64520[0], 64530[0], 69990[0], 76000[1], 76380[1], 76942[1], 76970[1], 76998[1], 77001[1], 77002[1], 77003[1], 77012[1], 77021[1], 92012[1], 92014[1], 93000[1], 93005[1], 93010[1], 93040[1], 93041[1], 93042[1], 93318[1], 93355[1], 94002[1], 94200[1], 94250[1], 94680[1], 94681[1], 94690[1], 94770[1], 95812[1], 95813[1], 95816[1], 95819[1], 95822[1], 95829[1], 95955[1], 96360[1], 96361[1], 96365[1], 96366[1], 96367[1], 96368[1],

0 = Modifier usage not allowed or inappropriate   1 = Modifier usage allowed

Code 1	Code 2
	96372[1], 96374[1], 96375[1], 96376[1], 96377[1], 96523[0], 99155[0], 99156[0], 99157[0], 99211[1], 99212[1], 99213[1], 99214[1], 99215[1], 99217[1], 99218[1], 99219[1], 99220[1], 99221[1], 99222[1], 99223[1], 99231[1], 99232[1], 99233[1], 99234[1], 99235[1], 99236[1], 99238[1], 99239[1], 99241[1], 99242[1], 99243[1], 99244[1], 99245[1], 99251[1], 99252[1], 99253[1], 99254[1], 99255[1], 99291[1], 99292[1], 99304[1], 99305[1], 99306[1], 99307[1], 99308[1], 99309[1], 99310[1], 99315[1], 99316[1], 99334[1], 99335[1], 99336[1], 99337[1], 99347[1], 99348[1], 99349[1], 99350[1], 99374[1], 99375[1], 99377[1], 99378[1], 99446[0], 99447[0], 99448[0], 99449[0], 99451[0], 99452[0], 99495[1], 99496[1], G0453[0], G0463[1], G0471[1]
62329	00635[0], 01935[0], 01936[0], 0213T[0], 0216T[0], 0228T[0], 0230T[0], 12001[1], 12002[1], 12004[1], 12005[1], 12006[1], 12007[1], 12011[1], 12013[1], 12014[1], 12015[1], 12016[1], 12017[1], 12018[1], 12020[1], 12021[1], 12031[1], 12032[1], 12034[1], 12035[1], 12036[1], 12037[1], 12041[1], 12042[1], 12044[1], 12045[1], 12046[1], 12047[1], 12051[1], 12052[1], 12053[1], 12054[1], 12055[1], 12056[1], 12057[1], 13100[1], 13101[1], 13102[1], 13120[1], 13121[1], 13122[1], 13131[1], 13132[1], 13133[1], 13151[1], 13152[1], 13153[1], 36000[1], 36400[1], 36405[1], 36406[1], 36410[1], 36420[1], 36425[1], 36430[1], 36440[1], 36591[0], 36592[0], 36600[1], 43752[1], 51701[1], 51702[1], 51703[1], 62270[1], 62272[1], 62273[1], 62320[0], 62321[0], 62322[0], 62323[0], 62324[0], 62326[0], 62327[0], 64400[0], 64405[0], 64408[0], 64415[0], 64416[0], 64417[0], 64418[0], 64420[0], 64421[0], 64425[0], 64430[0], 64435[0], 64445[0], 64446[0], 64447[0], 64448[0], 64449[0], 64461[0], 64462[0], 64463[0], 64480[0], 64483[0], 64484[0], 64486[0], 64487[0], 64488[0], 64489[0], 64490[0], 64491[0], 64492[0], 64493[0], 64494[0], 64495[0], 64505[0], 64510[0], 64520[0], 64530[0], 76000[1], 76380[1], 76942[1], 76970[1], 76998[1], 77001[1], 77002[1], 77003[1], 77012[1], 77021[1], 92012[1], 92014[1], 93000[1], 93005[1], 93010[1], 93040[1], 93041[1], 93042[1], 93318[1], 93355[1], 94002[1], 94200[1], 94250[1], 94680[1], 94681[1], 94690[1], 94770[1], 95812[1], 95813[1], 95816[1], 95819[1], 95822[1], 95955[1], 96360[1], 96361[1], 96365[1], 96366[1], 96367[1], 96368[1], 96372[1], 96374[1], 96375[1], 96376[1], 96377[1], 96523[0], 99155[0], 99156[0], 99157[0], 99211[1], 99212[1], 99213[1], 99214[1], 99217[1], 99218[1], 99219[1], 99221[1], 99231[1], 99232[1], 99233[1], 99238[1], 99239[1], 99241[1], 99242[1], 99243[1], 99251[1], 99252[1], 99304[1], 99307[1], 99308[1], 99309[1], 99315[1], 99316[1], 99334[1], 99335[1], 99347[1], 99348[1], 99374[1], 99375[1], 99377[1], 99378[1], 99446[0], 99447[0], 99448[0], 99449[0], 99451[0], 99452[0], 99495[1], 99496[1], G0453[0], G0463[1], G0471[1], J0670[1], J2001[1]
62350	0213T[0], 0216T[0], 0228T[0], 0230T[0], 0333T[0], 0464T[0], 11000[1], 11001[1], 11004[1], 11005[1], 11006[1], 11042[1], 11043[1], 11044[1], 11045[1], 11046[1], 11047[1], 12001[1], 12002[1], 12004[1], 12005[1], 12006[1], 12007[1], 12011[1], 12013[1], 12014[1], 12015[1], 12016[1], 12017[1], 12018[1], 12020[1], 12021[1], 12031[1], 12032[1], 12034[1], 12035[1], 12036[1], 12037[1], 12041[1], 12042[1], 12044[1], 12045[1], 12046[1], 12047[1], 12051[1], 12052[1], 12053[1], 12054[1], 12055[1], 12056[1], 12057[1], 13100[1], 13101[1], 13102[1], 13120[1], 13121[1], 13122[1], 13131[1], 13132[1], 13133[1], 13151[1], 13152[1], 13153[1], 36000[1], 36400[1], 36405[1], 36406[1], 36410[1], 36420[1], 36425[1], 36430[1], 36440[1], 36591[0], 36592[0], 36600[1], 36640[1], 43752[1], 51701[1], 51702[1], 51703[1], 62270[1], 62272[1], 62273[1], 62280[1], 62281[1], 62282[1], 62320[0], 62321[0], 62322[0], 62323[0], 62324[0], 62325[0], 62326[0], 62327[0], 62328[1], 62329[1], 64400[0], 64405[0], 64408[0], 64415[0], 64416[0], 64417[0], 64418[0], 64420[0], 64421[0], 64425[0], 64430[0], 64435[0], 64445[0], 64446[0], 64447[0], 64448[0], 64449[0], 64450[0], 64451[0], 64454[0], 64461[0], 64462[0], 64463[0], 64479[0], 64480[0], 64483[0], 64484[0], 64486[0], 64487[0], 64488[0], 64489[0], 64490[0], 64491[0], 64492[0], 64493[0], 64494[0], 64495[0], 64505[0], 64510[0], 64517[0], 64520[0], 64530[0], 69990[0], 76000[1], 77001[1], 77002[1], 77003[1], 92012[1], 92014[1], 92585[0], 93000[1], 93005[1], 93010[1], 93040[1], 93041[1], 93042[1], 93318[1], 93355[1], 94002[1], 94200[1], 94250[1], 94680[1], 94681[1], 94690[1], 94770[1], 95812[1], 95813[1], 95816[1], 95819[1], 95822[0], 95829[1], 95860[0], 95861[0], 95863[0], 95864[0], 95865[0], 95866[0], 95867[0], 95868[0], 95869[0], 95870[0], 95907[0], 95908[0], 95909[0], 95910[0], 95911[0], 95912[0], 95913[0], 95925[0], 95926[0], 95927[0], 95928[0], 95929[0], 95930[0], 95933[0], 95937[0], 95938[0], 95939[0], 95940[0], 95955[1], 95990[1], 95991[1], 96360[1], 96361[1], 96365[1], 96366[1], 96367[1], 96368[1], 96372[1], 96374[1], 96375[1], 96376[1], 96377[1], 96521[1], 96522[1], 96523[0], 97597[1], 97598[1], 97602[1], 99155[0], 99156[0], 99157[0], 99211[1], 99212[1], 99213[1], 99214[1], 99215[1], 99217[1], 99218[1], 99219[1], 99220[1], 99221[1], 99222[1], 99223[1], 99231[1], 99232[1], 99233[1], 99234[1], 99235[1], 99236[1], 99238[1], 99239[1], 99241[1], 99242[1], 99243[1], 99244[1], 99245[1], 99251[1], 99252[1], 99253[1], 99254[1], 99255[1], 99291[1], 99292[1], 99304[1], 99305[1], 99306[1], 99307[1], 99308[1], 99309[1], 99310[1], 99315[1], 99316[1], 99334[1], 99335[1], 99336[1], 99337[1], 99347[1], 99348[1], 99349[1], 99350[1], 99374[1], 99375[1], 99377[1], 99378[1], 99446[0], 99447[0], 99448[0], 99449[0], 99451[0], 99452[0], 99495[0], 99496[0], G0453[0], G0463[1], G0471[1]
62351	0213T[0], 0216T[0], 0228T[0], 0230T[0], 0333T[0], 0464T[0], 11000[1], 11001[1], 11004[1], 11005[1], 11006[1], 11042[1], 11043[1], 11044[1], 11045[1], 11046[1], 11047[1], 12001[1], 12002[1], 12004[1], 12005[1], 12006[1], 12007[1], 12011[1], 12013[1], 12014[1], 12015[1], 12016[1], 12017[1], 12018[1], 12020[1], 12021[1], 12031[1], 12032[1], 12034[1], 12035[1], 12036[1], 12037[1], 12041[1], 12042[1], 12044[1], 12045[1], 12046[1], 12047[1], 12051[1], 12052[1], 12053[1], 12054[1], 12055[1], 12056[1], 12057[1], 13100[1], 13101[1], 13102[1], 13120[1], 13121[1], 13122[1], 13131[1], 13132[1], 13133[1], 13151[1], 13152[1], 13153[1], 36000[1], 36400[1], 36405[1], 36406[1], 36410[1], 36420[1], 36425[1], 36430[1], 36440[1], 36591[0], 36592[0], 36600[1], 36640[1], 43752[1], 51701[1], 51702[1], 51703[1], 62280[1], 62281[1], 62282[1], 62320[0], 62321[0], 62322[0], 62323[0], 62324[0], 62325[0], 62326[0], 62327[0], 62350[1], 63707[1], 63709[1], 64400[0], 64405[0], 64408[0], 64415[0], 64416[0], 64417[0], 64418[0], 64420[0], 64421[0], 64425[0], 64430[0], 64435[0], 64445[0], 64446[0], 64447[0], 64448[0], 64449[0], 64450[0], 64451[0], 64454[0], 64461[0], 64462[0], 64463[0], 64479[0], 64480[0], 64483[0], 64484[0], 64486[0], 64487[0], 64488[0], 64489[0], 64490[0], 64491[0], 64492[0], 64493[0], 64494[0], 64495[0], 64505[0], 64510[0], 64517[0], 64520[0], 64530[0], 69990[0], 76000[1], 77001[1], 77002[1], 77003[1], 92012[1], 92014[1], 92585[0], 93000[1], 93005[1], 93010[1], 93040[1], 93041[1], 93042[1], 93318[1], 93355[1], 94002[1], 94200[1], 94250[1], 94680[1], 94681[1], 94690[1], 94770[1], 95812[1], 95813[1], 95816[1], 95819[1], 95822[0], 95829[1], 95860[0], 95861[0], 95863[0], 95864[0], 95865[0], 95866[0], 95867[0], 95868[0], 95869[0], 95870[0], 95907[0], 95908[0], 95909[0], 95910[0], 95911[0], 95912[0], 95913[0], 95925[0], 95926[0], 95927[0], 95928[0], 95929[0], 95930[0], 95933[0], 95937[0], 95938[0], 95939[0], 95940[0], 95955[1], 95990[1], 95991[1], 96360[1], 96361[1], 96365[1], 96366[1], 96367[1], 96368[1], 96372[1], 96374[1], 96375[1], 96376[1], 96377[1], 96522[1], 96523[0], 97597[1], 97598[1], 97602[1], 99155[0], 99156[0], 99157[0], 99211[1], 99212[1], 99213[1], 99214[1], 99215[1], 99217[1], 99218[1], 99219[1], 99220[1], 99221[1], 99222[1], 99223[1], 99231[1], 99232[1], 99233[1], 99234[1], 99235[1], 99236[1], 99238[1], 99239[1], 99241[1], 99242[1], 99243[1], 99244[1], 99245[1], 99251[1], 99252[1], 99253[1], 99254[1], 99255[1], 99291[1], 99292[1], 99304[1], 99305[1], 99306[1], 99307[1], 99308[1], 99309[1], 99310[1], 99315[1], 99316[1], 99334[1], 99335[1], 99336[1], 99337[1], 99347[1], 99348[1], 99349[1], 99350[1], 99374[1], 99375[1], 99377[1], 99378[1], 99446[0], 99447[0], 99448[0], 99449[0], 99451[0], 99452[0], 99495[0], 99496[0], G0453[0], G0463[1], G0471[1]
62355	0213T[0], 0216T[0], 0228T[0], 0230T[0], 0333T[0], 0464T[0], 11000[1], 11001[1], 11004[1], 11005[1], 11006[1], 11042[1], 11043[1], 11044[1], 11045[1], 11046[1], 11047[1], 12001[1], 12002[1], 12004[1], 12005[1], 12006[1], 12007[1], 12011[1], 12013[1], 12014[1], 12015[1], 12016[1], 12017[1], 12018[1], 12020[1], 12021[1], 12031[1], 12032[1], 12034[1], 12035[1], 12036[1], 12037[1], 12041[1], 12042[1], 12044[1], 12045[1], 12046[1], 12047[1], 12051[1], 12052[1], 12053[1], 12054[1], 12055[1], 12056[1], 12057[1], 13100[1], 13101[1], 13102[1], 13120[1], 13121[1], 13122[1], 13131[1], 13132[1], 13133[1], 13151[1], 13152[1], 13153[1], 36000[1], 36400[1], 36405[1], 36406[1], 36410[1], 36420[1], 36425[1], 36430[1], 36440[1], 36591[0], 36592[0], 36600[1], 36640[1], 43752[1], 51701[1], 51702[1], 51703[1], 62270[1], 62272[1], 62320[0], 62321[0], 62322[0], 62323[0], 62324[0], 62325[0], 62326[0], 62327[0], 62328[1], 62329[1], 62350[1], 62351[1], 64400[0], 64405[0], 64408[0], 64415[0], 64416[0], 64417[0], 64418[0], 64420[0], 64421[0], 64425[0], 64430[0], 64435[0], 64445[0], 64446[0], 64447[0], 64448[0], 64449[0], 64450[0], 64451[0], 64454[0], 64461[0], 64462[0], 64463[0], 64479[0], 64480[0], 64483[0], 64484[0], 64486[0], 64487[0], 64488[0], 64489[0], 64490[0], 64491[0], 64492[0], 64493[0], 64494[0], 64495[0], 64505[0], 64510[0], 64517[0], 64520[0], 64530[0], 69990[0], 76000[1], 77001[1], 77002[1], 77003[1], 92012[1], 92014[1], 92585[0], 93000[1], 93005[1], 93010[1], 93040[1], 93041[1], 93042[1], 93318[1], 93355[1], 94002[1], 94200[1], 94250[1], 94680[1], 94681[1], 94690[1], 94770[1], 95812[1], 95813[1], 95816[1], 95819[1], 95822[0], 95829[1], 95860[0], 95861[0], 95863[0], 95864[0], 95865[0], 95866[0], 95867[0], 95868[0], 95869[0], 95870[0], 95907[0], 95908[0], 95909[0], 95910[0], 95911[0], 95912[0], 95913[0], 95925[0], 95926[0], 95927[0], 95928[0], 95929[0], 95930[0], 95933[0], 95937[0], 95938[0], 95939[0], 95940[0], 95955[1], 96360[1], 96361[1], 96365[1], 96366[1], 96367[1], 96368[1], 96372[1], 96374[1], 96375[1], 96376[1], 96377[1], 96523[0], 97597[1], 97598[1], 97602[1], 99155[0], 99156[0], 99157[0], 99211[1], 99212[1], 99213[1], 99214[1], 99215[1], 99217[1], 99218[1], 99219[1], 99220[1], 99221[1], 99222[1], 99223[1], 99231[1], 99232[1], 99233[1], 99234[1], 99235[1], 99236[1], 99238[1], 99239[1], 99241[1], 99242[1], 99243[1], 99244[1], 99245[1], 99251[1], 99252[1], 99253[1], 99254[1], 99255[1], 99291[1], 99292[1], 99304[1], 99305[1], 99306[1], 99307[1], 99308[1], 99309[1], 99310[1], 99315[1], 99316[1], 99334[1], 99335[1], 99336[1], 99337[1], 99347[1], 99348[1], 99349[1], 99350[1], 99374[1], 99375[1], 99377[1], 99378[1], 99446[0], 99447[0], 99448[0], 99449[0], 99451[0], 99452[0], 99495[0], 99496[0], G0453[0], G0463[1], G0471[1]
62360	0213T[0], 0216T[0], 0228T[0], 0230T[0], 0333T[0], 0464T[0], 11000[1], 11001[1], 11004[1], 11005[1], 11006[1], 11042[1], 11043[1], 11044[1], 11045[1], 11046[1], 11047[1], 12001[1], 12002[1], 12004[1], 12005[1], 12006[1], 12007[1], 12011[1], 12013[1], 12014[1], 12015[1], 12016[1], 12017[1], 12018[1], 12020[1], 12021[1], 12031[1], 12032[1], 12034[1], 12035[1], 12036[1], 12037[1], 12041[1], 12042[1], 12044[1], 12045[1], 12046[1], 12047[1], 12051[1], 12052[1], 12053[1], 12054[1], 12055[1], 12056[1], 12057[1], 13100[1], 13101[1], 13102[1], 13120[1], 13121[1], 13122[1], 13131[1], 13132[1], 13133[1], 13151[1], 13152[1], 13153[1], 36000[1], 36400[1], 36405[1], 36406[1], 36410[1], 36420[1], 36425[1], 36430[1], 36440[1], 36591[0], 36592[0], 36600[1], 36640[1], 43752[1], 51701[1], 51702[1], 51703[1], 62270[1], 62272[1], 62273[1], 62280[1], 62281[1], 62282[1], 62320[0], 62321[0], 62322[0], 62323[0], 62324[0], 62325[0], 62326[0], 62327[0], 62328[1], 62329[1], 62362[1], 62365[0], 62367[1], 62368[1], 62369[1], 62370[1], 64400[0], 64405[0], 64408[0], 64415[0], 64416[0], 64417[0], 64418[0], 64420[0], 64421[0], 64425[0], 64430[0], 64435[0], 64445[0], 64446[0], 64447[0], 64448[0], 64449[0], 64450[0], 64451[0], 64454[0], 64461[0], 64462[0], 64463[0], 64479[0], 64480[0], 64483[0], 64484[0], 64486[0], 64487[0], 64488[0], 64489[0], 64490[0], 64491[0], 64492[0], 64493[0], 64494[0], 64495[0], 64505[0], 64510[0], 64517[0], 64520[0], 64530[0], 69990[0], 76000[1], 77001[1], 77002[1], 92012[1], 92014[1], 92585[0], 93000[1], 93005[1], 93010[1], 93040[1], 93041[1], 93042[1], 93318[1], 93355[1], 94002[1], 94200[1], 94250[1], 94680[1], 94681[1], 94690[1], 94770[1], 95812[1], 95813[1], 95816[1], 95819[1],

0 = Modifier usage not allowed or inappropriate 1 = Modifier usage allowed

Code 1	Code 2
	95822[0], 95829[1], 95860[0], 95861[0], 95863[0], 95864[0], 95865[0], 95866[0], 95867[0], 95868[0], 95869[0], 95870[0], 95907[0], 95908[0], 95909[0], 95910[0], 95911[0], 95912[0], 95913[0], 95925[0], 95926[0], 95927[0], 95928[0], 95929[0], 95930[0], 95933[0], 95937[0], 95938[0], 95939[0], 95940[0], 95955[1], 95990[0], 95991[1], 96360[1], 96361[1], 96365[1], 96366[1], 96367[1], 96368[1], 96372[1], 96374[1], 96375[1], 96376[1], 96377[1], 96522[1], 96523[0], 97597[1], 97598[1], 97602[1], 99155[0], 99156[0], 99157[0], 99211[1], 99212[1], 99213[1], 99214[1], 99215[1], 99217[1], 99218[1], 99219[1], 99220[1], 99221[1], 99222[1], 99223[1], 99231[1], 99232[1], 99233[1], 99234[1], 99235[1], 99236[1], 99238[1], 99239[1], 99241[1], 99242[1], 99243[1], 99244[1], 99245[1], 99251[1], 99252[1], 99253[1], 99254[1], 99255[1], 99291[1], 99292[1], 99304[1], 99305[1], 99306[1], 99307[1], 99308[1], 99309[1], 99310[1], 99315[1], 99316[1], 99334[1], 99335[1], 99336[1], 99337[1], 99347[1], 99348[1], 99349[1], 99350[1], 99374[1], 99375[1], 99377[1], 99378[1], 99446[0], 99447[0], 99448[0], 99449[0], 99451[0], 99452[0], 99495[0], 99496[0], G0453[0], G0463[1], G0471[1]
62361	0213T[0], 0216T[0], 0228T[0], 0230T[0], 0333T[0], 0464T[0], 11000[1], 11001[1], 11004[1], 11005[1], 11006[1], 11042[1], 11043[1], 11044[1], 11045[1], 11046[1], 11047[1], 12001[1], 12002[1], 12004[1], 12005[1], 12006[1], 12007[1], 12011[1], 12013[1], 12014[1], 12015[1], 12016[1], 12017[1], 12018[1], 12020[1], 12021[1], 12031[1], 12032[1], 12034[1], 12035[1], 12036[1], 12037[1], 12041[1], 12042[1], 12044[1], 12045[1], 12046[1], 12047[1], 12051[1], 12052[1], 12053[1], 12054[1], 12055[1], 12056[1], 12057[1], 13100[1], 13101[1], 13102[1], 13120[1], 13121[1], 13122[1], 13131[1], 13132[1], 13133[1], 13151[1], 13152[1], 13153[1], 36000[1], 36400[1], 36405[1], 36406[1], 36410[1], 36420[1], 36425[1], 36430[1], 36440[1], 36591[0], 36592[0], 36600[1], 36640[1], 43752[1], 51701[1], 51702[1], 51703[1], 62270[1], 62272[1], 62273[1], 62280[1], 62281[1], 62282[1], 62320[0], 62321[0], 62322[0], 62323[0], 62324[0], 62325[0], 62326[0], 62327[0], 62328[1], 62329[1], 62360[1], 62365[0], 62367[1], 62368[1], 62369[1], 62370[1], 64400[0], 64405[0], 64408[0], 64415[0], 64416[0], 64417[0], 64418[0], 64420[0], 64421[0], 64425[0], 64430[0], 64435[0], 64445[0], 64446[0], 64447[0], 64448[0], 64449[0], 64450[0], 64451[0], 64454[0], 64461[0], 64462[0], 64463[0], 64479[0], 64480[0], 64483[0], 64484[0], 64486[0], 64487[0], 64488[0], 64489[0], 64490[0], 64491[0], 64492[0], 64493[0], 64494[0], 64495[0], 64505[0], 64510[0], 64517[0], 64520[0], 64530[0], 69990[0], 76000[1], 77001[1], 77002[1], 92012[1], 92014[1], 92585[0], 93000[1], 93005[1], 93010[1], 93040[1], 93041[1], 93042[1], 93318[1], 93355[1], 94002[1], 94200[1], 94250[1], 94680[1], 94681[1], 94690[1], 94770[1], 95812[1], 95813[1], 95816[1], 95819[1], 95822[0], 95829[1], 95860[0], 95861[0], 95863[0], 95864[0], 95865[0], 95866[0], 95867[0], 95868[0], 95869[0], 95870[0], 95907[0], 95908[0], 95909[0], 95910[0], 95911[0], 95912[0], 95913[0], 95925[0], 95926[0], 95927[0], 95928[0], 95929[0], 95930[0], 95933[0], 95937[0], 95938[0], 95939[0], 95940[0], 95955[1], 95990[1], 95991[1], 96360[1], 96361[1], 96365[1], 96366[1], 96367[1], 96368[1], 96372[1], 96374[1], 96375[1], 96376[1], 96377[1], 96522[1], 96523[0], 97597[1], 97598[1], 97602[1], 99155[0], 99156[0], 99157[0], 99211[1], 99212[1], 99213[1], 99214[1], 99215[1], 99217[1], 99218[1], 99219[1], 99220[1], 99221[1], 99222[1], 99223[1], 99231[1], 99232[1], 99233[1], 99234[1], 99235[1], 99236[1], 99238[1], 99239[1], 99241[1], 99242[1], 99243[1], 99244[1], 99245[1], 99251[1], 99252[1], 99253[1], 99254[1], 99255[1], 99291[1], 99292[1], 99304[1], 99305[1], 99306[1], 99307[1], 99308[1], 99309[1], 99310[1], 99315[1], 99316[1], 99334[1], 99335[1], 99336[1], 99337[1], 99347[1], 99348[1], 99349[1], 99350[1], 99374[1], 99375[1], 99377[1], 99378[1], 99446[0], 99447[0], 99448[0], 99449[0], 99451[0], 99452[0], 99495[0], 99496[0], G0453[0], G0463[1], G0471[1]
62362	0213T[0], 0216T[0], 0228T[0], 0230T[0], 0333T[0], 0464T[0], 11000[1], 11001[1], 11004[1], 11005[1], 11006[1], 11042[1], 11043[1], 11044[1], 11045[1], 11046[1], 11047[1], 12001[1], 12002[1], 12004[1], 12005[1], 12006[1], 12007[1], 12011[1], 12013[1], 12014[1], 12015[1], 12016[1], 12017[1], 12018[1], 12020[1], 12021[1], 12031[1], 12032[1], 12034[1], 12035[1], 12036[1], 12037[1], 12041[1], 12042[1], 12044[1], 12045[1], 12046[1], 12047[1], 12051[1], 12052[1], 12053[1], 12054[1], 12055[1], 12056[1], 12057[1], 13100[1], 13101[1], 13102[1], 13120[1], 13121[1], 13122[1], 13131[1], 13132[1], 13133[1], 13151[1], 13152[1], 13153[1], 36000[1], 36400[1], 36405[1], 36406[1], 36410[1], 36420[1], 36425[1], 36430[1], 36440[1], 36591[0], 36592[0], 36600[1], 36640[1], 43752[1], 51701[1], 51702[1], 51703[1], 62270[1], 62272[1], 62273[1], 62280[1], 62281[1], 62282[1], 62320[0], 62321[0], 62322[0], 62323[0], 62324[0], 62325[0], 62326[0], 62327[0], 62328[1], 62329[1], 62361[1], 62365[0], 62367[1], 62368[1], 62369[1], 62370[1], 64400[0], 64405[0], 64408[0], 64415[0], 64416[0], 64417[0], 64418[0], 64420[0], 64421[0], 64425[0], 64430[0], 64435[0], 64445[0], 64446[0], 64447[0], 64448[0], 64449[0], 64450[0], 64451[0], 64454[0], 64461[0], 64462[0], 64463[0], 64479[0], 64480[0], 64483[0], 64484[0], 64486[0], 64487[0], 64488[0], 64489[0], 64490[0], 64491[0], 64492[0], 64493[0], 64494[0], 64495[0], 64505[0], 64510[0], 64517[0], 64520[0], 64530[0], 69990[0], 76000[1], 77001[1], 77002[1], 92012[1], 92014[1], 92585[0], 93000[1], 93005[1], 93010[1], 93040[1], 93041[1], 93042[1], 93318[1], 93355[1], 94002[1], 94200[1], 94250[1], 94680[1], 94681[1], 94690[1], 94770[1], 95812[1], 95813[1], 95816[1], 95819[1], 95822[0], 95829[1], 95860[0], 95861[0], 95863[0], 95864[0], 95865[0], 95866[0], 95867[0], 95868[0], 95869[0], 95870[0], 95907[0], 95908[0], 95909[0], 95910[0], 95911[0], 95912[0], 95913[0], 95925[0], 95926[0], 95927[0], 95928[0], 95929[0], 95930[0], 95933[0], 95937[0], 95938[0], 95939[0], 95940[0], 95955[1], 95990[0], 95991[1], 96360[1], 96361[1], 96365[1], 96366[1], 96367[1], 96368[1], 96372[1], 96374[1], 96375[1], 96376[1], 96377[1], 96522[1], 96523[0], 97597[1], 97598[1], 97602[1], 99155[0], 99156[0], 99157[0], 99211[1], 99212[1], 99213[1], 99214[1], 99215[1], 99217[1], 99218[1], 99219[1], 99220[1], 99221[1], 99222[1], 99223[1], 99231[1], 99232[1], 99233[1], 99234[1], 99235[1], 99236[1], 99238[1], 99239[1], 99241[1], 99242[1], 99243[1], 99244[1], 99245[1], 99251[1], 99252[1], 99253[1], 99254[1], 99255[1], 99291[1], 99292[1], 99304[1], 99305[1], 99306[1], 99307[1], 99308[1], 99309[1], 99310[1], 99315[1], 99316[1], 99334[1], 99335[1], 99336[1], 99337[1], 99347[1], 99348[1], 99349[1], 99350[1], 99374[1], 99375[1], 99377[1], 99378[1], 99446[0], 99447[0], 99448[0], 99449[0], 99451[0], 99452[0], 99495[0], 99496[0], G0453[0], G0463[1], G0471[1]
62365	0213T[0], 0216T[0], 0228T[0], 0230T[0], 0333T[0], 0464T[0], 11000[1], 11001[1], 11004[1], 11005[1], 11006[1], 11042[1], 11043[1], 11044[1], 11045[1], 11046[1], 11047[1], 12001[1], 12002[1], 12004[1], 12005[1], 12006[1], 12007[1], 12011[1], 12013[1], 12014[1], 12015[1], 12016[1], 12017[1], 12018[1], 12020[1], 12021[1], 12031[1], 12032[1], 12034[1], 12035[1], 12036[1], 12037[1], 12041[1], 12042[1], 12044[1], 12045[1], 12046[1], 12047[1], 12051[1], 12052[1], 12053[1], 12054[1], 12055[1], 12056[1], 12057[1], 13100[1], 13101[1], 13102[1], 13120[1], 13121[1], 13122[1], 13131[1], 13132[1], 13133[1], 13151[1], 13152[1], 13153[1], 36000[1], 36400[1], 36405[1], 36406[1], 36410[1], 36420[1], 36425[1], 36430[1], 36440[1], 36591[0], 36592[0], 36600[1], 36640[1], 43752[1], 51701[1], 51702[1], 51703[1], 62320[0], 62321[0], 62322[0], 62323[0], 62324[0], 62325[0], 62326[0], 62327[0], 62367[1], 62368[1], 62369[1], 62370[1], 64400[0], 64405[0], 64408[0], 64415[0], 64416[0], 64417[0], 64418[0], 64420[0], 64421[0], 64425[0], 64430[0], 64435[0], 64445[0], 64446[0], 64447[0], 64448[0], 64449[0], 64450[0], 64451[0], 64454[0], 64461[0], 64462[0], 64463[0], 64479[0], 64480[0], 64483[0], 64484[0], 64486[0], 64487[0], 64488[0], 64489[0], 64490[0], 64491[0], 64492[0], 64493[0], 64494[0], 64495[0], 64505[0], 64510[0], 64517[0], 64520[0], 64530[0], 69990[0], 76000[1], 77001[1], 77002[1], 92012[1], 92014[1], 92585[0], 93000[1], 93005[1], 93010[1], 93040[1], 93041[1], 93042[1], 93318[1], 93355[1], 94002[1], 94200[1], 94250[1], 94680[1], 94681[1], 94690[1], 94770[1], 95812[1], 95813[1], 95816[1], 95819[1], 95822[0], 95829[1], 95860[0], 95861[0], 95863[0], 95864[0], 95865[0], 95866[0], 95867[0], 95868[0], 95869[0], 95870[0], 95907[0], 95908[0], 95909[0], 95910[0], 95911[0], 95912[0], 95913[0], 95925[0], 95926[0], 95927[0], 95928[0], 95929[0], 95930[0], 95933[0], 95937[0], 95938[0], 95939[0], 95940[0], 95955[1], 96360[1], 96361[1], 96365[1], 96366[1], 96367[1], 96368[1], 96372[1], 96374[1], 96375[1], 96376[1], 96377[1], 96521[1], 96523[0], 97597[1], 97598[1], 97602[1], 99155[0], 99156[0], 99157[0], 99211[1], 99212[1], 99213[1], 99214[1], 99215[1], 99217[1], 99218[1], 99219[1], 99220[1], 99221[1], 99222[1], 99223[1], 99231[1], 99232[1], 99233[1], 99234[1], 99235[1], 99236[1], 99238[1], 99239[1], 99241[1], 99242[1], 99243[1], 99244[1], 99245[1], 99251[1], 99252[1], 99253[1], 99254[1], 99255[1], 99291[1], 99292[1], 99304[1], 99305[1], 99306[1], 99307[1], 99308[1], 99309[1], 99310[1], 99315[1], 99316[1], 99334[1], 99335[1], 99336[1], 99337[1], 99347[1], 99348[1], 99349[1], 99350[1], 99374[1], 99375[1], 99377[1], 99378[1], 99446[0], 99447[0], 99448[0], 99449[0], 99451[0], 99452[0], 99495[0], 99496[0], G0453[0], G0463[1], G0471[1]
62367	0213T[1], 0216T[1], 0333T[0], 0464T[0], 36000[1], 36410[1], 36591[0], 36592[0], 61650[1], 62324[1], 62325[1], 62326[1], 62327[1], 64415[1], 64416[1], 64417[1], 64450[1], 64454[1], 64486[1], 64487[1], 64488[1], 64489[1], 64490[1], 69990[0], 92585[0], 95822[0], 95860[0], 95861[0], 95863[0], 95864[0], 95865[0], 95866[0], 95867[0], 95868[0], 95869[0], 95870[0], 95907[0], 95908[0], 95909[0], 95910[0], 95911[0], 95912[0], 95913[0], 95925[0], 95926[0], 95927[0], 95928[0], 95929[0], 95930[0], 95933[0], 95937[0], 95938[0], 95939[0], 95940[0], 96360[1], 96365[1], 96522[1], 96523[0], G0453[0]
62368	0213T[1], 0216T[1], 0333T[0], 0464T[0], 36000[1], 36410[1], 36591[0], 36592[0], 61650[1], 62324[1], 62325[1], 62326[1], 62327[1], 62367[0], 64415[1], 64416[1], 64417[1], 64450[1], 64454[1], 64486[1], 64487[1], 64488[1], 64489[1], 64490[1], 69990[0], 92585[0], 95822[0], 95860[0], 95861[0], 95863[0], 95864[0], 95865[0], 95866[0], 95867[0], 95868[0], 95869[0], 95870[0], 95907[0], 95908[0], 95909[0], 95910[0], 95911[0], 95912[0], 95913[0], 95925[0], 95926[0], 95927[0], 95928[0], 95929[0], 95930[0], 95933[0], 95937[0], 95938[0], 95939[0], 95940[0], 96360[1], 96365[1], 96522[1], 96523[0], G0453[0]
62369	0213T[1], 0216T[1], 0333T[0], 0464T[0], 36000[1], 36410[1], 36591[0], 36592[0], 61650[1], 62324[1], 62325[1], 62326[1], 62327[1], 62367[0], 62368[0], 64415[1], 64416[1], 64417[1], 64450[1], 64454[1], 64486[1], 64487[1], 64488[1], 64489[1], 64490[1], 69990[0], 92585[0], 95822[0], 95860[0], 95861[0], 95863[0], 95864[0], 95865[0], 95866[0], 95867[0], 95868[0], 95869[0], 95870[0], 95907[0], 95908[0], 95909[0], 95910[0], 95911[0], 95912[0], 95913[0], 95925[0], 95926[0], 95927[0], 95928[0], 95929[0], 95930[0], 95933[0], 95937[0], 95938[0], 95939[0], 95940[0], 95990[0], 95991[0], 96360[1], 96365[1], 96523[0], A4220[0], G0453[0]
62370	0213T[1], 0216T[1], 0333T[0], 0464T[0], 36000[1], 36410[1], 36591[0], 36592[0], 61650[1], 62324[1], 62325[1], 62326[1], 62327[1], 62367[0], 62368[0], 62369[0], 64415[1], 64416[1], 64417[1], 64450[1], 64454[1], 64486[1], 64487[1], 64488[1], 64489[1], 64490[1], 69990[0], 92585[0], 95822[0], 95860[0], 95861[0], 95863[0], 95864[0], 95865[0], 95866[0], 95867[0], 95868[0], 95869[0], 95870[0], 95907[0], 95908[0], 95909[0], 95910[0], 95911[0], 95912[0], 95913[0], 95925[0], 95926[0], 95927[0], 95928[0], 95929[0], 95930[0], 95933[0], 95937[0], 95938[0], 95939[0], 95940[0], 95990[0], 95991[0], 96360[1], 96365[1], 96522[1], 96523[0], A4220[0], G0453[0]
62380	0202T[1], 0213T[0], 0216T[0], 0228T[0], 0230T[0], 0275T[1], 0333T[0], 0464T[0], 0565T[1], 11000[1], 11001[1], 11004[1], 11005[1], 11006[1], 11042[1], 11043[1], 11044[1], 11045[1], 11046[1], 11047[1], 12001[1], 12002[1], 12004[1], 12005[1], 12006[1], 12007[1], 12011[1], 12013[1], 12014[1], 12015[1], 12016[1], 12017[1], 12018[1], 12020[1], 12021[1], 12031[1], 12032[1], 12034[1], 12035[1], 12036[1], 12037[1], 12041[1], 12042[1], 12044[1], 12045[1], 12046[1], 12047[1], 12051[1], 12052[1], 12053[1], 12054[1], 12055[1], 12056[1], 12057[1], 13100[1], 13101[1], 13102[1], 13120[1], 13121[1], 13122[1], 13131[1], 13132[1], 13133[1], 13151[1], 13152[1], 13153[1], 15769[1], 20251[1], 22102[1], 22208[1],

0 = Modifier usage not allowed or inappropriate 1 = Modifier usage allowed

Code 1	Code 2
	22505[0], 36000[1], 36400[1], 36405[1], 36406[1], 36410[1], 36420[1], 36425[1], 36430[1], 36440[1], 36591[0], 36592[0], 36600[1], 36640[1], 38220[0], 38222[0], 38230[0], 38232[0], 43752[1], 51701[1], 51702[1], 51703[1], 61783[1], 62284[1], 62290[0], 62320[0], 62321[0], 62322[0], 62323[0], 62324[0], 62325[0], 62326[0], 62327[0], 63707[1], 63709[1], 64400[0], 64405[0], 64408[0], 64415[0], 64416[0], 64417[0], 64418[0], 64420[0], 64421[0], 64425[0], 64430[0], 64435[0], 64445[0], 64446[0], 64447[0], 64448[0], 64449[0], 64450[0], 64451[0], 64454[0], 64461[0], 64462[0], 64463[0], 64479[0], 64480[0], 64483[0], 64484[0], 64486[0], 64487[0], 64488[0], 64489[0], 64490[0], 64491[0], 64492[0], 64493[0], 64494[0], 64495[0], 64505[0], 64510[0], 64517[0], 64520[0], 64530[0], 64722[1], 69990[0], 72295[0], 76000[1], 77001[1], 77002[1], 77003[1], 92012[1], 92014[1], 92585[0], 93000[1], 93005[1], 93010[1], 93040[1], 93041[1], 93042[1], 93318[1], 93355[1], 94002[1], 94200[1], 94250[1], 94680[1], 94681[1], 94690[1], 94770[1], 95812[1], 95813[1], 95816[1], 95819[1], 95822[0], 95829[1], 95860[0], 95861[0], 95863[0], 95864[0], 95865[0], 95866[0], 95867[0], 95868[0], 95869[0], 95870[0], 95907[0], 95908[0], 95909[0], 95910[0], 95911[0], 95912[0], 95913[0], 95925[0], 95926[0], 95927[0], 95928[0], 95929[0], 95930[0], 95933[0], 95937[0], 95938[0], 95939[0], 95940[0], 95941[0], 95955[1], 96360[1], 96361[1], 96365[1], 96366[1], 96367[1], 96368[1], 96372[1], 96374[1], 96375[1], 96376[1], 96377[1], 96523[0], 97597[1], 97598[1], 97602[1], 99155[0], 99156[0], 99157[0], 99211[1], 99212[1], 99213[1], 99214[1], 99215[1], 99217[1], 99218[1], 99219[1], 99220[1], 99221[1], 99222[1], 99223[1], 99231[1], 99232[1], 99233[1], 99234[1], 99235[1], 99236[1], 99238[1], 99239[1], 99241[1], 99242[1], 99243[1], 99244[1], 99245[1], 99251[1], 99252[1], 99253[1], 99254[1], 99255[1], 99291[1], 99292[1], 99304[1], 99305[1], 99306[1], 99307[1], 99308[1], 99309[1], 99310[1], 99315[1], 99316[1], 99334[1], 99335[1], 99336[1], 99337[1], 99347[1], 99348[1], 99349[1], 99350[1], 99374[1], 99375[1], 99377[1], 99378[1], 99446[0], 99447[0], 99448[0], 99449[0], 99451[0], 99452[0], 99495[0], 99496[0], G0276[0], G0453[0], G0463[1], G0471[1]
63001	0213T[0], 0216T[0], 0228T[0], 0230T[0], 0274T[1], 0275T[1], 0333T[0], 0464T[0], 0565T[1], 11000[1], 11001[1], 11004[1], 11005[1], 11006[1], 11042[1], 11043[1], 11044[1], 11045[1], 11046[1], 11047[1], 12001[1], 12002[1], 12004[1], 12005[1], 12006[1], 12007[1], 12011[1], 12013[1], 12014[1], 12015[1], 12016[1], 12017[1], 12018[1], 12020[1], 12021[1], 12031[1], 12032[1], 12034[1], 12035[1], 12036[1], 12037[1], 12041[1], 12042[1], 12044[1], 12045[1], 12046[1], 12047[1], 12051[1], 12052[1], 12053[1], 12054[1], 12055[1], 12056[1], 12057[1], 13100[1], 13101[1], 13102[1], 13120[1], 13121[1], 13122[1], 13131[1], 13132[1], 13133[1], 13151[1], 13152[1], 13153[1], 15769[1], 20660[0], 22100[1], 22208[1], 22505[0], 36000[1], 36400[1], 36405[1], 36406[1], 36410[1], 36420[1], 36425[1], 36430[1], 36440[1], 36591[0], 36592[0], 36600[1], 36640[1], 38220[0], 38222[0], 38230[0], 38232[0], 43752[1], 51701[1], 51702[1], 51703[1], 61783[1], 62291[1], 62320[0], 62321[0], 62322[0], 62323[0], 62324[0], 62325[0], 62326[0], 62327[0], 62380[1], 63020[1], 63030[1], 63707[1], 63709[1], 64400[0], 64405[0], 64408[0], 64415[0], 64416[0], 64417[0], 64418[0], 64420[0], 64421[0], 64425[0], 64430[0], 64435[0], 64445[0], 64446[0], 64447[0], 64448[0], 64449[0], 64450[0], 64451[0], 64454[0], 64461[0], 64462[0], 64463[0], 64479[0], 64480[0], 64483[0], 64484[0], 64486[0], 64487[0], 64488[0], 64489[0], 64490[0], 64491[0], 64492[0], 64493[0], 64494[0], 64495[0], 64505[0], 64510[0], 64517[0], 64520[0], 64530[0], 69990[0], 72285[1], 76000[1], 77001[1], 77002[1], 92012[1], 92014[1], 92585[0], 93000[1], 93005[1], 93010[1], 93040[1], 93041[1], 93042[1], 93318[1], 93355[1], 94002[1], 94200[1], 94250[1], 94680[1], 94681[1], 94690[1], 94770[1], 95812[1], 95813[1], 95816[1], 95819[1], 95822[0], 95829[1], 95860[0], 95861[0], 95863[0], 95864[0], 95865[0], 95866[0], 95867[0], 95868[0], 95869[0], 95870[0], 95907[0], 95908[0], 95909[0], 95910[0], 95911[0], 95912[0], 95913[0], 95925[0], 95926[0], 95927[0], 95928[0], 95929[0], 95930[0], 95933[0], 95937[0], 95938[0], 95939[0], 95940[0], 95955[1], 96360[1], 96361[1], 96365[1], 96366[1], 96367[1], 96368[1], 96372[1], 96374[1], 96375[1], 96376[1], 96377[1], 96523[0], 97597[1], 97598[1], 97602[1], 99155[0], 99156[0], 99157[0], 99211[1], 99212[1], 99213[1], 99214[1], 99215[1], 99217[1], 99218[1], 99219[1], 99220[1], 99221[1], 99222[1], 99223[1], 99231[1], 99232[1], 99233[1], 99234[1], 99235[1], 99236[1], 99238[1], 99239[1], 99241[1], 99242[1], 99243[1], 99244[1], 99245[1], 99251[1], 99252[1], 99253[1], 99254[1], 99255[1], 99291[1], 99292[1], 99304[1], 99305[1], 99306[1], 99307[1], 99308[1], 99309[1], 99310[1], 99315[1], 99316[1], 99334[1], 99335[1], 99336[1], 99337[1], 99347[1], 99348[1], 99349[1], 99350[1], 99374[1], 99375[1], 99377[1], 99378[1], 99446[0], 99447[0], 99448[0], 99449[0], 99451[0], 99452[0], 99495[0], 99496[0], G0276[1], G0453[0], G0463[1], G0471[1]
63003	0213T[0], 0216T[0], 0228T[0], 0230T[0], 0333T[0], 0464T[0], 0565T[1], 11000[1], 11001[1], 11004[1], 11005[1], 11006[1], 11042[1], 11043[1], 11044[1], 11045[1], 11046[1], 11047[1], 12001[1], 12002[1], 12004[1], 12005[1], 12006[1], 12007[1], 12011[1], 12013[1], 12014[1], 12015[1], 12016[1], 12017[1], 12018[1], 12020[1], 12021[1], 12031[1], 12032[1], 12034[1], 12035[1], 12036[1], 12037[1], 12041[1], 12042[1], 12044[1], 12045[1], 12046[1], 12047[1], 12051[1], 12052[1], 12053[1], 12054[1], 12055[1], 12056[1], 12057[1], 13100[1], 13101[1], 13102[1], 13120[1], 13121[1], 13122[1], 13131[1], 13132[1], 13133[1], 13151[1], 13152[1], 13153[1], 15769[1], 20650[1], 22101[1], 22208[1], 22505[0], 36000[1], 36400[1], 36405[1], 36406[1], 36410[1], 36420[1], 36425[1], 36430[1], 36440[1], 36591[0], 36592[0], 36600[1], 36640[1], 38220[0], 38222[0], 38230[0], 38232[0], 43752[1], 51701[1], 51702[1], 51703[1], 61783[1], 62291[1], 62320[0], 62321[0], 62322[0], 62323[0], 62324[0], 62325[0], 62326[0], 62327[0], 63046[1], 63707[1], 63709[1], 64400[0], 64405[0], 64408[0], 64415[0], 64416[0], 64417[0], 64418[0], 64420[0], 64421[0], 64425[0], 64430[0], 64435[0], 64445[0], 64446[0], 64447[0], 64448[0], 64449[0], 64450[0], 64451[0], 64454[0], 64461[0], 64462[0], 64463[0], 64479[0], 64480[0], 64483[0], 64484[0], 64486[0], 64487[0], 64488[0], 64489[0], 64490[0], 64491[0], 64492[0], 64493[0], 64494[0], 64495[0], 64505[0], 64510[0], 64517[0], 64520[0], 64530[0], 69990[0], 72285[1], 76000[1], 77001[1], 77002[1], 92012[1], 92014[1], 92585[0], 93000[1], 93005[1], 93010[1], 93040[1], 93041[1], 93042[1], 93318[1], 93355[1], 94002[1], 94200[1], 94250[1], 94680[1], 94681[1], 94690[1], 94770[1], 95812[1], 95813[1], 95816[1], 95819[1], 95822[0], 95829[1], 95860[0], 95861[0], 95863[0], 95864[0], 95865[0], 95866[0], 95867[0], 95868[0], 95869[0], 95870[0], 95907[0], 95908[0], 95909[0], 95910[0], 95911[0], 95912[0], 95913[0], 95925[0], 95926[0], 95927[0], 95928[0], 95929[0], 95930[0], 95933[0], 95937[0], 95938[0], 95939[0], 95940[0], 95955[1], 96360[1], 96361[1], 96365[1], 96366[1], 96367[1], 96368[1], 96372[1], 96374[1], 96375[1], 96376[1], 96377[1], 96523[0], 97597[1], 97598[1], 97602[1], 99155[0], 99156[0], 99157[0], 99211[1], 99212[1], 99213[1], 99214[1], 99215[1], 99217[1], 99218[1], 99219[1], 99220[1], 99221[1], 99222[1], 99223[1], 99231[1], 99232[1], 99233[1], 99234[1], 99235[1], 99236[1], 99238[1], 99239[1], 99241[1], 99242[1], 99243[1], 99244[1], 99245[1], 99251[1], 99252[1], 99253[1], 99254[1], 99255[1], 99291[1], 99292[1], 99304[1], 99305[1], 99306[1], 99307[1], 99308[1], 99309[1], 99310[1], 99315[1], 99316[1], 99334[1], 99335[1], 99336[1], 99337[1], 99347[1], 99348[1], 99349[1], 99350[1], 99374[1], 99375[1], 99377[1], 99378[1], 99446[0], 99447[0], 99448[0], 99449[0], 99451[0], 99452[0], 99495[0], 99496[0], G0453[0], G0463[1], G0471[1]
63005	0202T[1], 0213T[0], 0216T[0], 0228T[0], 0230T[0], 0274T[1], 0275T[1], 0333T[0], 0464T[0], 0565T[1], 11000[1], 11001[1], 11004[1], 11005[1], 11006[1], 11042[1], 11043[1], 11044[1], 11045[1], 11046[1], 11047[1], 12001[1], 12002[1], 12004[1], 12005[1], 12006[1], 12007[1], 12011[1], 12013[1], 12014[1], 12015[1], 12016[1], 12017[1], 12018[1], 12020[1], 12021[1], 12031[1], 12032[1], 12034[1], 12035[1], 12036[1], 12037[1], 12041[1], 12042[1], 12044[1], 12045[1], 12046[1], 12047[1], 12051[1], 12052[1], 12053[1], 12054[1], 12055[1], 12056[1], 12057[1], 13100[1], 13101[1], 13102[1], 13120[1], 13121[1], 13122[1], 13131[1], 13132[1], 13133[1], 13151[1], 13152[1], 13153[1], 15769[1], 20660[0], 22102[1], 22208[1], 22505[0], 22867[1], 22868[1], 22869[1], 22870[1], 36000[1], 36400[1], 36405[1], 36406[1], 36410[1], 36420[1], 36425[1], 36430[1], 36440[1], 36591[0], 36592[0], 36600[1], 36640[1], 38220[0], 38222[0], 38230[0], 38232[0], 43752[1], 51701[1], 51702[1], 51703[1], 61783[1], 62267[1], 62284[1], 62290[0], 62320[0], 62321[0], 62322[0], 62323[0], 62324[0], 62325[0], 62326[0], 62327[0], 62380[1], 63020[1], 63030[1], 63056[1], 63707[1], 63709[1], 64400[0], 64405[0], 64408[0], 64415[0], 64416[0], 64417[0], 64418[0], 64420[0], 64421[0], 64425[0], 64430[0], 64435[0], 64445[0], 64446[0], 64447[0], 64448[0], 64449[0], 64450[0], 64451[0], 64454[0], 64461[0], 64462[0], 64463[0], 64479[0], 64480[0], 64483[0], 64484[0], 64486[0], 64487[0], 64488[0], 64489[0], 64490[0], 64491[0], 64492[0], 64493[0], 64494[0], 64495[0], 64505[0], 64510[0], 64517[0], 64520[0], 64530[0], 64722[1], 64831[1], 64834[1], 64835[1], 64836[1], 64840[1], 64856[1], 64857[1], 64858[1], 64861[1], 64862[1], 64864[1], 64865[1], 64866[1], 64868[1], 64885[1], 64886[1], 64890[1], 64891[1], 64892[1], 64893[1], 64895[1], 64896[1], 64897[1], 64898[1], 64905[1], 64907[1], 64912[1], 64913[1], 69990[0], 72295[1], 76000[1], 77001[1], 77002[1], 92012[1], 92014[1], 92585[0], 93000[1], 93005[1], 93010[1], 93040[1], 93041[1], 93042[1], 93318[1], 93355[1], 94002[1], 94200[1], 94250[1], 94680[1], 94681[1], 94690[1], 94770[1], 95812[1], 95813[1], 95816[1], 95819[1], 95822[0], 95829[1], 95860[0], 95861[0], 95863[0], 95864[0], 95865[0], 95866[0], 95867[0], 95868[0], 95869[0], 95870[0], 95907[0], 95908[0], 95909[0], 95910[0], 95911[0], 95912[0], 95913[0], 95925[0], 95926[0], 95927[0], 95928[0], 95929[0], 95930[0], 95933[0], 95937[0], 95938[0], 95939[0], 95940[0], 95955[1], 96360[1], 96361[1], 96365[1], 96366[1], 96367[1], 96368[1], 96372[1], 96374[1], 96375[1], 96376[1], 96377[1], 96523[0], 97597[1], 97598[1], 97602[1], 99155[0], 99156[0], 99157[0], 99211[1], 99212[1], 99213[1], 99214[1], 99215[1], 99217[1], 99218[1], 99219[1], 99220[1], 99221[1], 99222[1], 99223[1], 99231[1], 99232[1], 99233[1], 99234[1], 99235[1], 99236[1], 99238[1], 99239[1], 99241[1], 99242[1], 99243[1], 99244[1], 99245[1], 99251[1], 99252[1], 99253[1], 99254[1], 99255[1], 99291[1], 99292[1], 99304[1], 99305[1], 99306[1], 99307[1], 99308[1], 99309[1], 99310[1], 99315[1], 99316[1], 99334[1], 99335[1], 99336[1], 99337[1], 99347[1], 99348[1], 99349[1], 99350[1], 99374[1], 99375[1], 99377[1], 99378[1], 99446[0], 99447[0], 99448[0], 99449[0], 99451[0], 99452[0], 99495[0], 99496[0], G0276[1], G0453[0], G0463[1], G0471[1]
63011	0213T[0], 0216T[0], 0228T[0], 0230T[0], 0333T[0], 0464T[0], 0565T[1], 11000[1], 11001[1], 11004[1], 11005[1], 11006[1], 11042[1], 11043[1], 11044[1], 11045[1], 11046[1], 11047[1], 12001[1], 12002[1], 12004[1], 12005[1], 12006[1], 12007[1], 12011[1], 12013[1], 12014[1], 12015[1], 12016[1], 12017[1], 12018[1], 12020[1], 12021[1], 12031[1], 12032[1], 12034[1], 12035[1], 12036[1], 12037[1], 12041[1], 12042[1], 12044[1], 12045[1], 12046[1], 12047[1], 12051[1], 12052[1], 12053[1], 12054[1], 12055[1], 12056[1], 12057[1], 13100[1], 13101[1], 13102[1], 13120[1], 13121[1], 13122[1], 13131[1], 13132[1], 13133[1], 13151[1], 13152[1], 13153[1], 15769[1], 20660[0], 22102[1], 22208[1], 22505[0], 36000[1], 36400[1], 36405[1], 36406[1], 36410[1], 36420[1], 36425[1], 36430[1], 36440[1], 36591[0], 36592[0], 36600[1], 36640[1], 38220[0], 38222[0], 38230[0], 38232[0], 43752[1], 51701[1], 51702[1], 51703[1], 61783[1], 62320[0], 62321[0], 62322[0], 62323[0], 62324[0], 62325[0], 62326[0], 62327[0], 63707[1], 63709[1], 64400[0], 64405[0], 64408[0], 64415[0], 64416[0], 64417[0], 64418[0], 64420[0], 64421[0], 64425[0], 64430[0], 64435[0], 64445[0], 64446[0], 64447[0], 64448[0], 64449[0], 64450[0], 64451[0], 64454[0], 64461[0], 64462[0], 64463[0], 64479[0], 64480[0], 64483[0], 64484[0], 64486[0], 64487[0], 64488[0], 64489[0], 64490[0], 64491[0], 64492[0], 64493[0], 64494[0], 64495[0], 64505[0], 64510[0], 64517[0], 64520[0], 64530[0], 64714[1], 69990[0], 76000[1], 77001[1], 77002[1], 92012[1], 92014[1], 92585[0], 93000[1], 93005[1], 93010[1], 93040[1], 93041[1], 93042[1], 93318[1], 93355[1], 94002[1], 94200[1], 94250[1], 94680[1], 94681[1], 94690[1], 94770[1], 95812[1], 95813[1], 95816[1], 95819[1], 95822[0], 95829[1], 95860[0], 95861[0], 95863[0], 95864[0], 95865[0], 95866[0], 95867[0], 95868[0],

0 = Modifier usage not allowed or inappropriate 1 = Modifier usage allowed

Code 1	Code 2
	95869^0, 95870^0, 95907^0, 95908^0, 95909^0, 95910^0, 95911^0, 95912^0, 95913^0, 95925^0, 95926^0, 95927^0, 95928^0, 95929^0, 95930^0, 95933^0, 95937^0, 95938^0, 95939^0, 95940^0, 95955^1, 96360^1, 96361^1, 96365^1, 96366^1, 96367^1, 96368^1, 96372^1, 96374^1, 96375^1, 96376^1, 96377^1, 96523^0, 97597^1, 97598^1, 97602^1, 99155^0, 99156^0, 99157^0, 99211^1, 99212^1, 99213^1, 99214^1, 99215^1, 99217^1, 99218^1, 99219^1, 99220^1, 99221^1, 99222^1, 99223^1, 99231^1, 99232^1, 99233^1, 99234^1, 99235^1, 99236^1, 99238^1, 99239^1, 99241^1, 99242^1, 99243^1, 99244^1, 99245^1, 99251^1, 99252^1, 99253^1, 99254^1, 99255^1, 99291^1, 99292^1, 99304^1, 99305^1, 99306^1, 99307^1, 99308^1, 99309^1, 99310^1, 99315^1, 99316^1, 99334^1, 99335^1, 99336^1, 99337^1, 99347^1, 99348^1, 99349^1, 99350^1, 99374^1, 99375^1, 99377^1, 99378^1, 99446^0, 99447^0, 99448^0, 99449^0, 99451^0, 99452^0, 99495^0, 99496^0, G0453^0, G0463^1, G0471^1
63012	0202T^1, 0213T^0, 0216T^0, 0228T^0, 0230T^0, 0275T^1, 0333T^0, 0464T^0, 0565T^1, 11000^1, 11001^1, 11004^1, 11005^1, 11006^1, 11042^1, 11043^1, 11044^1, 11045^1, 11046^1, 11047^1, 12001^1, 12002^1, 12004^1, 12005^1, 12006^1, 12007^1, 12011^1, 12013^1, 12014^1, 12015^1, 12016^1, 12017^1, 12018^1, 12020^1, 12021^1, 12031^1, 12032^1, 12034^1, 12035^1, 12036^1, 12037^1, 12041^1, 12042^1, 12044^1, 12045^1, 12046^1, 12047^1, 12051^1, 12052^1, 12053^1, 12054^1, 12055^1, 12056^1, 12057^1, 13100^1, 13101^1, 13102^1, 13120^1, 13121^1, 13122^1, 13131^1, 13132^1, 13133^1, 13151^1, 13152^1, 13153^1, 15769^1, 20660^0, 22102^1, 22208^1, 22505^0, 22867^1, 22868^1, 22869^1, 22870^1, 36000^1, 36400^1, 36405^1, 36406^1, 36410^1, 36420^1, 36425^1, 36430^1, 36440^1, 36591^0, 36592^0, 36600^1, 36640^1, 38220^0, 38222^0, 38230^0, 38232^0, 43752^1, 51701^1, 51702^1, 51703^1, 61783^1, 62287^1, 62320^0, 62321^0, 62322^0, 62323^0, 62324^0, 62325^0, 62326^0, 62327^0, 62380^1, 63005^1, 63030^1, 63042^1, 63045^1, 63046^1, 63056^1, 63275^1, 63707^1, 63709^1, 64400^0, 64405^0, 64408^0, 64415^0, 64416^0, 64417^0, 64418^0, 64420^0, 64421^0, 64425^0, 64430^0, 64435^0, 64445^0, 64446^0, 64447^0, 64448^0, 64449^0, 64450^0, 64451^0, 64454^0, 64461^0, 64462^0, 64463^0, 64479^0, 64480^0, 64483^0, 64484^0, 64486^0, 64487^0, 64488^0, 64489^0, 64490^0, 64491^0, 64492^0, 64493^0, 64494^0, 64495^0, 64505^0, 64510^0, 64517^0, 64520^0, 64530^0, 64714^1, 64722^1, 64831^1, 64834^1, 64835^1, 64836^1, 64840^1, 64856^1, 64857^1, 64858^1, 64861^1, 64862^1, 64864^1, 64865^1, 64866^1, 64868^1, 64885^1, 64886^1, 64890^1, 64891^1, 64892^1, 64893^1, 64895^1, 64896^1, 64897^1, 64898^1, 64905^1, 64907^1, 64912^1, 64913^1, 69990^0, 76000^1, 77001^1, 77002^1, 92012^1, 92014^1, 92585^0, 93000^1, 93005^1, 93010^1, 93040^1, 93041^1, 93042^1, 93318^1, 93355^1, 94002^1, 94200^1, 94250^1, 94680^1, 94681^1, 94690^1, 94770^1, 95812^1, 95813^1, 95816^1, 95819^1, 95822^0, 95829^1, 95860^0, 95861^0, 95863^0, 95864^0, 95865^0, 95866^0, 95867^0, 95868^0, 95869^0, 95870^0, 95907^0, 95908^0, 95909^0, 95910^0, 95911^0, 95912^0, 95913^0, 95925^0, 95926^0, 95927^0, 95928^0, 95929^0, 95930^0, 95933^0, 95937^0, 95938^0, 95939^0, 95940^0, 95955^1, 96360^1, 96361^1, 96365^1, 96366^1, 96367^1, 96368^1, 96372^1, 96374^1, 96375^1, 96376^1, 96377^1, 96523^0, 97597^1, 97598^1, 97602^1, 99155^0, 99156^0, 99157^0, 99211^1, 99212^1, 99213^1, 99214^1, 99215^1, 99217^1, 99218^1, 99219^1, 99220^1, 99221^1, 99222^1, 99223^1, 99231^1, 99232^1, 99233^1, 99234^1, 99235^1, 99236^1, 99238^1, 99239^1, 99241^1, 99242^1, 99243^1, 99244^1, 99245^1, 99251^1, 99252^1, 99253^1, 99254^1, 99255^1, 99291^1, 99292^1, 99304^1, 99305^1, 99306^1, 99307^1, 99308^1, 99309^1, 99310^1, 99315^1, 99316^1, 99334^1, 99335^1, 99336^1, 99337^1, 99347^1, 99348^1, 99349^1, 99350^1, 99374^1, 99375^1, 99377^1, 99378^1, 99446^0, 99447^0, 99448^0, 99449^0, 99451^0, 99452^0, 99495^0, 99496^0, G0276^1, G0453^0, G0463^1, G0471^1
63015	0213T^0, 0216T^0, 0228T^0, 0230T^0, 0274T^1, 0275T^1, 0333T^0, 0464T^0, 0565T^1, 11000^1, 11001^1, 11004^1, 11005^1, 11006^1, 11042^1, 11043^1, 11044^1, 11045^1, 11046^1, 11047^1, 12001^1, 12002^1, 12004^1, 12005^1, 12006^1, 12007^1, 12011^1, 12013^1, 12014^1, 12015^1, 12016^1, 12017^1, 12018^1, 12020^1, 12021^1, 12031^1, 12032^1, 12034^1, 12035^1, 12036^1, 12037^1, 12041^1, 12042^1, 12044^1, 12045^1, 12046^1, 12047^1, 12051^1, 12052^1, 12053^1, 12054^1, 12055^1, 12056^1, 12057^1, 13100^1, 13101^1, 13102^1, 13120^1, 13121^1, 13122^1, 13131^1, 13132^1, 13133^1, 13151^1, 13152^1, 13153^1, 15769^1, 20660^0, 22100^1, 22208^1, 22505^0, 36000^1, 36400^1, 36405^1, 36406^1, 36410^1, 36420^1, 36425^1, 36430^1, 36440^1, 36591^0, 36592^0, 36600^1, 36640^1, 38220^0, 38222^0, 38230^0, 38232^0, 43752^1, 51701^1, 51702^1, 51703^1, 61783^1, 62291^1, 62320^0, 62321^0, 62322^0, 62323^0, 62324^0, 62325^0, 62326^0, 62327^0, 62380^1, 63001^1, 63020^1, 63030^1, 63040^1, 63707^1, 63709^1, 64400^0, 64405^0, 64408^0, 64415^0, 64416^0, 64417^0, 64418^0, 64420^0, 64421^0, 64425^0, 64430^0, 64435^0, 64445^0, 64446^0, 64447^0, 64448^0, 64449^0, 64450^0, 64451^0, 64454^0, 64461^0, 64462^0, 64463^0, 64479^0, 64480^0, 64483^0, 64484^0, 64486^0, 64487^0, 64488^0, 64489^0, 64490^0, 64491^0, 64492^0, 64493^0, 64494^0, 64495^0, 64505^0, 64510^0, 64517^0, 64520^0, 64530^0, 69990^0, 72285^1, 76000^1, 77001^1, 77002^1, 92012^1, 92014^1, 92585^0, 93000^1, 93005^1, 93010^1, 93040^1, 93041^1, 93042^1, 93318^1, 93355^1, 94002^1, 94200^1, 94250^1, 94680^1, 94681^1, 94690^1, 94770^1, 95812^1, 95813^1, 95816^1, 95819^1, 95822^0, 95829^1, 95860^0, 95861^0, 95863^0, 95864^0, 95865^0, 95866^0, 95867^0, 95868^0, 95869^0, 95870^0, 95907^0, 95908^0, 95909^0, 95910^0, 95911^0, 95912^0, 95913^0, 95925^0, 95926^0, 95927^0, 95928^0, 95929^0, 95930^0, 95933^0, 95937^0, 95938^0, 95939^0, 95940^0, 95955^1, 96360^1, 96361^1, 96365^1, 96366^1, 96367^1, 96368^1, 96372^1, 96374^1, 96375^1, 96376^1, 96377^1, 96523^0, 97597^1, 97598^1, 97602^1, 99155^0, 99156^0, 99157^0, 99211^1, 99212^1, 99213^1, 99214^1, 99215^1, 99217^1, 99218^1, 99219^1, 99220^1, 99221^1, 99222^1, 99223^1, 99231^1, 99232^1, 99233^1, 99234^1, 99235^1, 99236^1, 99238^1, 99239^1, 99241^1, 99242^1, 99243^1, 99244^1, 99245^1, 99251^1, 99252^1, 99253^1, 99254^1, 99255^1, 99291^1, 99292^1, 99304^1, 99305^1, 99306^1, 99307^1, 99308^1, 99309^1, 99310^1, 99315^1, 99316^1, 99334^1, 99335^1, 99336^1, 99337^1, 99347^1, 99348^1, 99349^1, 99350^1, 99374^1, 99375^1, 99377^1, 99378^1, 99446^0, 99447^0, 99448^0, 99449^0, 99451^0, 99452^0, 99495^0, 99496^0, G0276^1, G0453^0, G0463^1, G0471^1
63016	0213T^0, 0216T^0, 0228T^0, 0230T^0, 0333T^0, 0464T^0, 0565T^1, 11000^1, 11001^1, 11004^1, 11005^1, 11006^1, 11042^1, 11043^1, 11044^1, 11045^1, 11046^1, 11047^1, 12001^1, 12002^1, 12004^1, 12005^1, 12006^1, 12007^1, 12011^1, 12013^1, 12014^1, 12015^1, 12016^1, 12017^1, 12018^1, 12020^1, 12021^1, 12031^1, 12032^1, 12034^1, 12035^1, 12036^1, 12037^1, 12041^1, 12042^1, 12044^1, 12045^1, 12046^1, 12047^1, 12051^1, 12052^1, 12053^1, 12054^1, 12055^1, 12056^1, 12057^1, 13100^1, 13101^1, 13102^1, 13120^1, 13121^1, 13122^1, 13131^1, 13132^1, 13133^1, 13151^1, 13152^1, 13153^1, 15769^1, 22101^1, 22208^1, 22505^0, 36000^1, 36400^1, 36405^1, 36406^1, 36410^1, 36420^1, 36425^1, 36430^1, 36440^1, 36591^0, 36592^0, 36600^1, 36640^1, 38220^0, 38222^0, 38230^0, 38232^0, 43752^1, 51701^1, 51702^1, 51703^1, 61783^1, 62291^1, 62320^0, 62321^0, 62322^0, 62323^0, 62324^0, 62325^0, 62326^0, 62327^0, 63003^1, 63046^1, 63707^1, 63709^1, 64400^0, 64405^0, 64408^0, 64415^0, 64416^0, 64417^0, 64418^0, 64420^0, 64421^0, 64425^0, 64430^0, 64435^0, 64445^0, 64446^0, 64447^0, 64448^0, 64449^0, 64450^0, 64451^0, 64454^0, 64461^0, 64462^0, 64463^0, 64479^0, 64480^0, 64483^0, 64484^0, 64486^0, 64487^0, 64488^0, 64489^0, 64490^0, 64491^0, 64492^0, 64493^0, 64494^0, 64495^0, 64505^0, 64510^0, 64517^0, 64520^0, 64530^0, 69990^0, 72285^1, 76000^1, 77001^1, 77002^1, 92012^1, 92014^1, 92585^0, 93000^1, 93005^1, 93010^1, 93040^1, 93041^1, 93042^1, 93318^1, 93355^1, 94002^1, 94200^1, 94250^1, 94680^1, 94681^1, 94690^1, 94770^1, 95812^1, 95813^1, 95816^1, 95819^1, 95822^0, 95829^1, 95860^0, 95861^0, 95863^0, 95864^0, 95865^0, 95866^0, 95867^0, 95868^0, 95869^0, 95870^0, 95907^0, 95908^0, 95909^0, 95910^0, 95911^0, 95912^0, 95913^0, 95925^0, 95926^0, 95927^0, 95928^0, 95929^0, 95930^0, 95933^0, 95937^0, 95938^0, 95939^0, 95940^0, 95955^1, 96360^1, 96361^1, 96365^1, 96366^1, 96367^1, 96368^1, 96372^1, 96374^1, 96375^1, 96376^1, 96377^1, 96523^0, 97597^1, 97598^1, 97602^1, 99155^0, 99156^0, 99157^0, 99211^1, 99212^1, 99213^1, 99214^1, 99215^1, 99217^1, 99218^1, 99219^1, 99220^1, 99221^1, 99222^1, 99223^1, 99231^1, 99232^1, 99233^1, 99234^1, 99235^1, 99236^1, 99238^1, 99239^1, 99241^1, 99242^1, 99243^1, 99244^1, 99245^1, 99251^1, 99252^1, 99253^1, 99254^1, 99255^1, 99291^1, 99292^1, 99304^1, 99305^1, 99306^1, 99307^1, 99308^1, 99309^1, 99310^1, 99315^1, 99316^1, 99334^1, 99335^1, 99336^1, 99337^1, 99347^1, 99348^1, 99349^1, 99350^1, 99374^1, 99375^1, 99377^1, 99378^1, 99446^0, 99447^0, 99448^0, 99449^0, 99451^0, 99452^0, 99495^0, 99496^0, G0453^0, G0463^1, G0471^1
63017	0202T^1, 0213T^0, 0216T^0, 0228T^0, 0230T^0, 0274T^1, 0275T^1, 0333T^0, 0464T^0, 0565T^1, 11000^1, 11001^1, 11004^1, 11005^1, 11006^1, 11042^1, 11043^1, 11044^1, 11045^1, 11046^1, 11047^1, 12001^1, 12002^1, 12004^1, 12005^1, 12006^1, 12007^1, 12011^1, 12013^1, 12014^1, 12015^1, 12016^1, 12017^1, 12018^1, 12020^1, 12021^1, 12031^1, 12032^1, 12034^1, 12035^1, 12036^1, 12037^1, 12041^1, 12042^1, 12044^1, 12045^1, 12046^1, 12047^1, 12051^1, 12052^1, 12053^1, 12054^1, 12055^1, 12056^1, 12057^1, 13100^1, 13101^1, 13102^1, 13120^1, 13121^1, 13122^1, 13131^1, 13132^1, 13133^1, 13151^1, 13152^1, 13153^1, 15769^1, 22102^1, 22208^1, 22505^0, 22867^1, 22868^1, 22869^1, 22870^1, 36000^1, 36400^1, 36405^1, 36406^1, 36410^1, 36420^1, 36425^1, 36430^1, 36440^1, 36591^0, 36592^0, 36600^1, 36640^1, 38220^0, 38222^0, 38230^0, 38232^0, 43752^1, 51701^1, 51702^1, 51703^1, 61783^1, 62267^1, 62290^1, 62320^0, 62321^0, 62322^0, 62323^0, 62324^0, 62325^0, 62326^0, 62327^0, 62380^1, 63005^1, 63012^1, 63020^1, 63030^1, 63056^1, 63707^1, 63709^1, 64400^0, 64405^0, 64408^0, 64415^0, 64416^0, 64417^0, 64418^0, 64420^0, 64421^0, 64425^0, 64430^0, 64435^0, 64445^0, 64446^0, 64447^0, 64448^0, 64449^0, 64450^0, 64451^0, 64454^0, 64461^0, 64462^0, 64463^0, 64479^0, 64480^0, 64483^0, 64484^0, 64486^0, 64487^0, 64488^0, 64489^0, 64490^0, 64491^0, 64492^0, 64493^0, 64494^0, 64495^0, 64505^0, 64510^0, 64517^0, 64520^0, 64530^0, 64712^1, 64722^1, 64831^1, 64834^1, 64835^1, 64836^1, 64840^1, 64856^1, 64857^1, 64858^1, 64861^1, 64862^1, 64864^1, 64865^1, 64866^1, 64868^1, 64885^1, 64886^1, 64890^1, 64891^1, 64892^1, 64893^1, 64895^1, 64896^1, 64897^1, 64898^1, 64905^1, 64907^1, 64912^1, 64913^1, 69990^0, 72295^1, 76000^1, 77001^1, 77002^1, 92012^1, 92014^1, 92585^0, 93000^1, 93005^1, 93010^1, 93040^1, 93041^1, 93042^1, 93318^1, 93355^1, 94002^1, 94200^1, 94250^1, 94680^1, 94681^1, 94690^1, 94770^1, 95812^1, 95813^1, 95816^1, 95819^1, 95822^0, 95829^1, 95860^0, 95861^0, 95863^0, 95864^0, 95865^0, 95866^0, 95867^0, 95868^0, 95869^0, 95870^0, 95907^0, 95908^0, 95909^0, 95910^0, 95911^0, 95912^0, 95913^0, 95925^0, 95926^0, 95927^0, 95928^0, 95929^0, 95930^0, 95933^0, 95937^0, 95938^0, 95939^0, 95940^0, 95955^1, 96360^1, 96361^1, 96365^1, 96366^1, 96367^1, 96368^1, 96372^1, 96374^1, 96375^1, 96376^1, 96377^1, 96523^0, 97597^1, 97598^1, 97602^1, 99155^0, 99156^0, 99157^0, 99211^1, 99212^1, 99213^1, 99214^1, 99215^1, 99217^1, 99218^1, 99219^1, 99220^1, 99221^1, 99222^1, 99223^1, 99231^1, 99232^1, 99233^1, 99234^1, 99235^1, 99236^1, 99238^1, 99239^1, 99241^1, 99242^1, 99243^1, 99244^1, 99245^1, 99251^1, 99252^1,

0 = Modifier usage not allowed or inappropriate 1 = Modifier usage allowed

Code 1	Code 2
	99253[1], 99254[1], 99255[1], 99291[1], 99292[1], 99304[1], 99305[1], 99306[1], 99307[1], 99308[1], 99309[1], 99310[1], 99315[1], 99316[1], 99334[1], 99335[1], 99336[1], 99337[1], 99347[1], 99348[1], 99349[1], 99350[1], 99374[1], 99375[1], 99377[1], 99378[1], 99446[0], 99447[0], 99448[0], 99449[0], 99451[0], 99452[0], 99495[0], 99496[0], G0276[1], G0453[0], G0463[1], G0471[1]
63020	0213T[0], 0216T[0], 0228T[0], 0230T[0], 0274T[1], 0333T[0], 0464T[0], 0565T[1], 11000[1], 11001[1], 11004[1], 11005[1], 11006[1], 11042[1], 11043[1], 11044[1], 11045[1], 11046[1], 11047[1], 12001[1], 12002[1], 12004[1], 12005[1], 12006[1], 12007[1], 12011[1], 12013[1], 12014[1], 12015[1], 12016[1], 12017[1], 12018[1], 12020[1], 12021[1], 12031[1], 12032[1], 12034[1], 12035[1], 12036[1], 12037[1], 12041[1], 12042[1], 12044[1], 12045[1], 12046[1], 12047[1], 12051[1], 12052[1], 12053[1], 12054[1], 12055[1], 12056[1], 12057[1], 13100[1], 13101[1], 13102[1], 13120[1], 13121[1], 13122[1], 13131[1], 13132[1], 13133[1], 13151[1], 13152[1], 13153[1], 15769[1], 20251[1], 22100[1], 22102[1], 22208[1], 22505[0], 36000[1], 36400[1], 36405[1], 36406[1], 36410[1], 36420[1], 36425[1], 36430[1], 36440[1], 36591[0], 36592[0], 36600[1], 36640[1], 38220[0], 38222[0], 38230[0], 38232[0], 43752[1], 51701[1], 51702[1], 51703[1], 61783[1], 62291[0], 62320[0], 62321[0], 62322[0], 62323[0], 62324[0], 62325[0], 62326[0], 62327[0], 63042[1], 63707[1], 63709[1], 64400[0], 64405[0], 64408[0], 64415[0], 64416[0], 64417[0], 64418[0], 64420[0], 64421[0], 64425[0], 64430[0], 64435[0], 64445[0], 64446[0], 64447[0], 64448[0], 64449[0], 64450[0], 64451[0], 64454[0], 64461[0], 64462[0], 64463[0], 64479[0], 64480[0], 64483[0], 64484[0], 64486[0], 64487[0], 64488[0], 64489[0], 64490[0], 64491[0], 64492[0], 64493[0], 64494[0], 64495[0], 64505[0], 64510[0], 64517[0], 64520[0], 64530[0], 64722[1], 69990[0], 72285[0], 76000[1], 77001[1], 77002[1], 92012[1], 92014[1], 92585[0], 93000[1], 93005[1], 93010[1], 93040[1], 93041[1], 93042[1], 93318[1], 93355[1], 94002[1], 94200[1], 94250[1], 94680[1], 94681[1], 94690[1], 94770[1], 95812[1], 95813[1], 95816[1], 95819[1], 95822[0], 95829[1], 95860[0], 95861[0], 95863[0], 95864[0], 95865[0], 95866[0], 95867[0], 95868[0], 95869[0], 95870[0], 95907[0], 95908[0], 95909[0], 95910[0], 95911[0], 95912[0], 95913[0], 95925[0], 95926[0], 95927[0], 95928[0], 95929[0], 95930[0], 95933[0], 95937[0], 95938[0], 95939[0], 95940[0], 95955[1], 96360[1], 96361[1], 96365[1], 96366[1], 96367[1], 96368[1], 96372[1], 96374[1], 96375[1], 96376[1], 96377[1], 96523[0], 97597[1], 97598[1], 97602[1], 99155[0], 99156[0], 99157[0], 99211[1], 99212[1], 99213[1], 99214[1], 99215[1], 99217[1], 99218[1], 99219[1], 99220[1], 99221[1], 99222[1], 99223[1], 99231[1], 99232[1], 99233[1], 99234[1], 99235[1], 99236[1], 99238[1], 99239[1], 99241[1], 99242[1], 99243[1], 99244[1], 99245[1], 99251[1], 99252[1], 99253[1], 99254[1], 99255[1], 99291[1], 99292[1], 99304[1], 99305[1], 99306[1], 99307[1], 99308[1], 99309[1], 99310[1], 99315[1], 99316[1], 99334[1], 99335[1], 99336[1], 99337[1], 99347[1], 99348[1], 99349[1], 99350[1], 99374[1], 99375[1], 99377[1], 99378[1], 99446[0], 99447[0], 99448[0], 99449[0], 99451[0], 99452[0], 99495[0], 99496[0], G0453[0], G0463[1], G0471[1]
63030	0202T[1], 0213T[0], 0216T[0], 0228T[0], 0230T[0], 0275T[1], 0333T[0], 0464T[0], 0565T[1], 11000[1], 11001[1], 11004[1], 11005[1], 11006[1], 11042[1], 11043[1], 11044[1], 11045[1], 11046[1], 11047[1], 12001[1], 12002[1], 12004[1], 12005[1], 12006[1], 12007[1], 12011[1], 12013[1], 12014[1], 12015[1], 12016[1], 12017[1], 12018[1], 12020[1], 12021[1], 12031[1], 12032[1], 12034[1], 12035[1], 12036[1], 12037[1], 12041[1], 12042[1], 12044[1], 12045[1], 12046[1], 12047[1], 12051[1], 12052[1], 12053[1], 12054[1], 12055[1], 12056[1], 12057[1], 13100[1], 13101[1], 13102[1], 13120[1], 13121[1], 13122[1], 13131[1], 13132[1], 13133[1], 13151[1], 13152[1], 13153[1], 15769[1], 20251[1], 22102[1], 22208[1], 22505[0], 22869[1], 22870[1], 36000[1], 36400[1], 36405[1], 36406[1], 36410[1], 36420[1], 36425[1], 36430[1], 36440[1], 36591[0], 36592[0], 36600[1], 36640[1], 38220[0], 38222[0], 38230[0], 38232[0], 43752[1], 51701[1], 51702[1], 51703[1], 61783[1], 62267[1], 62284[1], 62290[0], 62320[0], 62321[0], 62322[0], 62323[0], 62324[0], 62325[0], 62326[0], 62327[0], 62380[1], 63042[1], 63056[1], 63707[1], 63709[1], 64400[0], 64405[0], 64408[0], 64415[0], 64416[0], 64417[0], 64418[0], 64420[0], 64421[0], 64425[0], 64430[0], 64435[0], 64445[0], 64446[0], 64447[0], 64448[0], 64449[0], 64450[0], 64451[0], 64454[0], 64461[0], 64462[0], 64463[0], 64479[0], 64480[0], 64483[0], 64484[0], 64486[0], 64487[0], 64488[0], 64489[0], 64490[0], 64491[0], 64492[0], 64493[0], 64494[0], 64495[0], 64505[0], 64510[0], 64517[0], 64520[0], 64530[0], 64722[1], 69990[0], 72295[0], 76000[1], 77001[1], 77002[1], 77003[1], 92012[1], 92014[1], 92585[0], 93000[1], 93005[1], 93010[1], 93040[1], 93041[1], 93042[1], 93318[1], 93355[1], 94002[1], 94200[1], 94250[1], 94680[1], 94681[1], 94690[1], 94770[1], 95812[1], 95813[1], 95816[1], 95819[1], 95822[0], 95829[1], 95860[0], 95861[0], 95863[0], 95864[0], 95865[0], 95866[0], 95867[0], 95868[0], 95869[0], 95870[0], 95907[0], 95908[0], 95909[0], 95910[0], 95911[0], 95912[0], 95913[0], 95925[0], 95926[0], 95927[0], 95928[0], 95929[0], 95930[0], 95933[0], 95937[0], 95938[0], 95939[0], 95940[0], 95955[1], 96360[1], 96361[1], 96365[1], 96366[1], 96367[1], 96368[1], 96372[1], 96374[1], 96375[1], 96376[1], 96377[1], 96523[0], 97597[1], 97598[1], 97602[1], 99155[0], 99156[0], 99157[0], 99211[1], 99212[1], 99213[1], 99214[1], 99215[1], 99217[1], 99218[1], 99219[1], 99220[1], 99221[1], 99222[1], 99223[1], 99231[1], 99232[1], 99233[1], 99234[1], 99235[1], 99236[1], 99238[1], 99239[1], 99241[1], 99242[1], 99243[1], 99244[1], 99245[1], 99251[1], 99252[1], 99253[1], 99254[1], 99255[1], 99291[1], 99292[1], 99304[1], 99305[1], 99306[1], 99307[1], 99308[1], 99309[1], 99310[1], 99315[1], 99316[1], 99334[1], 99335[1], 99336[1], 99337[1], 99347[1], 99348[1], 99349[1], 99350[1], 99374[1], 99375[1], 99377[1], 99378[1], 99446[0], 99447[0], 99448[0], 99449[0], 99451[0], 99452[0], 99495[0], 99496[0], G0276[0], G0453[0], G0463[1], G0471[1]
63035	0333T[0], 0464T[0], 11000[1], 11001[1], 11004[1], 11005[1], 11006[1], 11042[1], 11043[1], 11044[1], 11045[1], 11046[1], 11047[1], 22100[1], 22869[1], 22870[1], 36591[0], 36592[0], 38220[0], 38222[0], 38230[0], 38232[0], 63707[1], 63709[1], 92585[0], 95822[0], 95860[0], 95861[0], 95863[0], 95864[0], 95865[0], 95866[0], 95867[0], 95868[0], 95869[0], 95907[0], 95908[0], 95909[0], 95910[0], 95911[0], 95912[0], 95913[0], 95925[0], 95926[0], 95927[0], 95930[0], 95933[0], 95937[0], 95938[0], 95939[0], 95940[0], 96523[0], 97597[1], 97598[1], 97602[1], G0453[0]
63040	0213T[0], 0216T[0], 0228T[0], 0230T[0], 0274T[1], 0333T[0], 0464T[0], 0565T[1], 11000[1], 11001[1], 11004[1], 11005[1], 11006[1], 11042[1], 11043[1], 11044[1], 11045[1], 11046[1], 11047[1], 12001[1], 12002[1], 12004[1], 12005[1], 12006[1], 12007[1], 12011[1], 12013[1], 12014[1], 12015[1], 12016[1], 12017[1], 12018[1], 12020[1], 12021[1], 12031[1], 12032[1], 12034[1], 12035[1], 12036[1], 12037[1], 12041[1], 12042[1], 12044[1], 12045[1], 12046[1], 12047[1], 12051[1], 12052[1], 12053[1], 12054[1], 12055[1], 12056[1], 12057[1], 13100[1], 13101[1], 13102[1], 13120[1], 13121[1], 13122[1], 13131[1], 13132[1], 13133[1], 13151[1], 13152[1], 13153[1], 15769[1], 20251[1], 22100[1], 22208[1], 22505[0], 36000[1], 36400[1], 36405[1], 36406[1], 36410[1], 36420[1], 36425[1], 36430[1], 36440[1], 36591[0], 36592[0], 36600[1], 36640[1], 38220[0], 38222[0], 38230[0], 38232[0], 43752[1], 51701[1], 51702[1], 51703[1], 61783[1], 62291[0], 62320[0], 62321[0], 62322[0], 62323[0], 62324[0], 62325[0], 62326[0], 62327[0], 63001[1], 63020[1], 63707[1], 63709[1], 64400[0], 64405[0], 64408[0], 64415[0], 64416[0], 64417[0], 64418[0], 64420[0], 64421[0], 64425[0], 64430[0], 64435[0], 64445[0], 64446[0], 64447[0], 64448[0], 64449[0], 64450[0], 64451[0], 64454[0], 64461[0], 64462[0], 64463[0], 64479[0], 64480[0], 64483[0], 64484[0], 64486[0], 64487[0], 64488[0], 64489[0], 64490[0], 64491[0], 64492[0], 64493[0], 64494[0], 64495[0], 64505[0], 64510[0], 64517[0], 64520[0], 64530[0], 64722[1], 69990[0], 72285[0], 76000[1], 77001[1], 77002[1], 92012[1], 92014[1], 92585[0], 93000[1], 93005[1], 93010[1], 93040[1], 93041[1], 93042[1], 93318[1], 93355[1], 94002[1], 94200[1], 94250[1], 94680[1], 94681[1], 94690[1], 94770[1], 95812[1], 95813[1], 95816[1], 95819[1], 95822[0], 95829[1], 95860[0], 95861[0], 95863[0], 95864[0], 95865[0], 95866[0], 95867[0], 95868[0], 95869[0], 95870[0], 95907[0], 95908[0], 95909[0], 95910[0], 95911[0], 95912[0], 95913[0], 95925[0], 95926[0], 95927[0], 95928[0], 95929[0], 95930[0], 95933[0], 95937[0], 95938[0], 95939[0], 95940[0], 95955[1], 96360[1], 96361[1], 96365[1], 96366[1], 96367[1], 96368[1], 96372[1], 96374[1], 96375[1], 96376[1], 96377[1], 96523[0], 97597[1], 97598[1], 97602[1], 99155[0], 99156[0], 99157[0], 99211[1], 99212[1], 99213[1], 99214[1], 99215[1], 99217[1], 99218[1], 99219[1], 99220[1], 99221[1], 99222[1], 99223[1], 99231[1], 99232[1], 99233[1], 99234[1], 99235[1], 99236[1], 99238[1], 99239[1], 99241[1], 99242[1], 99243[1], 99244[1], 99245[1], 99251[1], 99252[1], 99253[1], 99254[1], 99255[1], 99291[1], 99292[1], 99304[1], 99305[1], 99306[1], 99307[1], 99308[1], 99309[1], 99310[1], 99315[1], 99316[1], 99334[1], 99335[1], 99336[1], 99337[1], 99347[1], 99348[1], 99349[1], 99350[1], 99374[1], 99375[1], 99377[1], 99378[1], 99446[0], 99447[0], 99448[0], 99449[0], 99451[0], 99452[0], 99495[0], 99496[0], G0453[0], G0463[1], G0471[1]
63042	0202T[1], 0213T[0], 0216T[0], 0228T[0], 0230T[0], 0333T[0], 0464T[0], 0565T[1], 11000[1], 11001[1], 11004[1], 11005[1], 11006[1], 11042[1], 11043[1], 11044[1], 11045[1], 11046[1], 11047[1], 12001[1], 12002[1], 12004[1], 12005[1], 12006[1], 12007[1], 12011[1], 12013[1], 12014[1], 12015[1], 12016[1], 12017[1], 12018[1], 12020[1], 12021[1], 12031[1], 12032[1], 12034[1], 12035[1], 12036[1], 12037[1], 12041[1], 12042[1], 12044[1], 12045[1], 12046[1], 12047[1], 12051[1], 12052[1], 12053[1], 12054[1], 12055[1], 12056[1], 12057[1], 13100[1], 13101[1], 13102[1], 13120[1], 13121[1], 13122[1], 13131[1], 13132[1], 13133[1], 13151[1], 13152[1], 13153[1], 15769[1], 20251[1], 22102[1], 22114[1], 22208[1], 22505[0], 22867[1], 22868[1], 22869[1], 22870[1], 36000[1], 36400[1], 36405[1], 36406[1], 36410[1], 36420[1], 36425[1], 36430[1], 36440[1], 36591[0], 36592[0], 36600[1], 36640[1], 38220[0], 38222[0], 38230[0], 38232[0], 43752[1], 51701[1], 51702[1], 51703[1], 61783[1], 62267[1], 62290[0], 62320[0], 62321[0], 62322[0], 62323[0], 62324[0], 62325[0], 62326[0], 62327[0], 62380[1], 63005[1], 63017[1], 63056[1], 63267[1], 63707[1], 63709[1], 64400[0], 64405[0], 64408[0], 64415[0], 64416[0], 64417[0], 64418[0], 64420[0], 64421[0], 64425[0], 64430[0], 64435[0], 64445[0], 64446[0], 64447[0], 64448[0], 64449[0], 64450[0], 64451[0], 64454[0], 64461[0], 64462[0], 64463[0], 64479[0], 64480[0], 64483[0], 64484[0], 64486[0], 64487[0], 64488[0], 64489[0], 64490[0], 64491[0], 64492[0], 64493[0], 64494[0], 64495[0], 64505[0], 64510[0], 64517[0], 64520[0], 64530[0], 64714[1], 64722[1], 64831[1], 64834[1], 64835[1], 64836[1], 64840[1], 64856[1], 64857[1], 64858[1], 64861[1], 64862[1], 64864[1], 64865[1], 64866[1], 64868[1], 64885[1], 64886[1], 64890[1], 64891[1], 64892[1], 64893[1], 64895[1], 64896[1], 64897[1], 64898[1], 64905[1], 64907[1], 64912[1], 64913[1], 69990[0], 72295[0], 76000[1], 77001[1], 77002[1], 77003[1], 92012[1], 92014[1], 92585[0], 93000[1], 93005[1], 93010[1], 93040[1], 93041[1], 93042[1], 93318[1], 93355[1], 94002[1], 94200[1], 94250[1], 94680[1], 94681[1], 94690[1], 94770[1], 95812[1], 95813[1], 95816[1], 95819[1], 95822[0], 95829[1], 95860[0], 95861[0], 95863[0], 95864[0], 95865[0], 95866[0], 95867[0], 95868[0], 95869[0], 95870[0], 95907[0], 95908[0], 95909[0], 95910[0], 95911[0], 95912[0], 95913[0], 95925[0], 95926[0], 95927[0], 95928[0], 95929[0], 95930[0], 95933[0], 95937[0], 95938[0], 95939[0], 95940[0], 95955[1], 96360[1], 96361[1], 96365[1], 96366[1], 96367[1], 96368[1], 96372[1], 96374[1], 96375[1], 96376[1], 96377[1], 96523[0], 97597[1], 97598[1], 97602[1], 99155[0], 99156[0], 99157[0], 99211[1], 99212[1], 99213[1], 99214[1], 99215[1], 99217[1], 99218[1], 99219[1], 99220[1], 99221[1], 99222[1], 99223[1], 99231[1], 99232[1], 99233[1], 99234[1], 99235[1], 99236[1], 99238[1], 99239[1], 99241[1], 99242[1], 99243[1], 99244[1], 99245[1], 99251[1], 99252[1], 99253[1], 99254[1], 99255[1], 99291[1], 99292[1], 99304[1], 99305[1], 99306[1], 99307[1], 99308[1], 99309[1], 99310[1], 99315[1], 99316[1], 99334[1], 99335[1], 99336[1], 99337[1], 99347[1], 99348[1], 99349[1], 99350[1], 99374[1], 99375[1], 99377[1], 99378[1], 99446[0], 99447[0], 99448[0], 99449[0], 99451[0], 99452[0], 99495[0], 99496[0], G0453[0], G0463[1], G0471[1]

0 = Modifier usage not allowed or inappropriate 1 = Modifier usage allowed

Code 1	Code 2
63043	0333T[0], 0464T[0], 11000[1], 11001[1], 11004[1], 11005[1], 11006[1], 11042[1], 11043[1], 11044[1], 11045[1], 11046[1], 11047[1], 36591[0], 36592[0], 38220[0], 38222[0], 38230[0], 38232[0], 63707[1], 63709[1], 92585[0], 95822[0], 95860[0], 95861[0], 95863[0], 95864[0], 95865[0], 95866[0], 95867[0], 95868[0], 95869[0], 95907[0], 95908[0], 95909[0], 95910[0], 95911[0], 95912[0], 95913[0], 95925[0], 95926[0], 95927[0], 95930[0], 95933[0], 95937[0], 95938[0], 95939[0], 95940[0], 96523[0], 97597[1], 97598[1], 97602[1], G0453[0]
63044	0333T[0], 0464T[0], 11000[1], 11001[1], 11004[1], 11005[1], 11006[1], 11042[1], 11043[1], 11044[1], 11045[1], 11046[1], 11047[1], 22867[1], 22868[1], 22869[1], 22870[1], 36591[0], 36592[0], 38220[0], 38222[0], 38230[0], 38232[0], 63707[1], 63709[1], 92585[0], 95822[0], 95860[0], 95861[0], 95863[0], 95864[0], 95865[0], 95866[0], 95867[0], 95868[0], 95869[0], 95907[0], 95908[0], 95909[0], 95910[0], 95911[0], 95912[0], 95913[0], 95925[0], 95926[0], 95927[0], 95930[0], 95933[0], 95937[0], 95938[0], 95939[0], 95940[0], 96523[0], 97597[1], 97598[1], 97602[1], G0453[0]
63045	0213T[0], 0216T[0], 0228T[0], 0230T[0], 0274T[1], 0333T[0], 0464T[0], 0565T[1], 11000[1], 11001[1], 11004[1], 11005[1], 11006[1], 11042[1], 11043[1], 11044[1], 11045[1], 11046[1], 11047[1], 12001[1], 12002[1], 12004[1], 12005[1], 12006[1], 12007[1], 12011[1], 12013[1], 12014[1], 12015[1], 12016[1], 12017[1], 12018[1], 12020[1], 12021[1], 12031[1], 12032[1], 12034[1], 12035[1], 12036[1], 12037[1], 12041[1], 12042[1], 12044[1], 12045[1], 12046[1], 12047[1], 12051[1], 12052[1], 12053[1], 12054[1], 12055[1], 12056[1], 12057[1], 13100[1], 13101[1], 13102[1], 13120[1], 13121[1], 13122[1], 13131[1], 13132[1], 13133[1], 13151[1], 13152[1], 13153[1], 15769[1], 20660[1], 22100[1], 22208[1], 22505[0], 36000[1], 36400[1], 36405[1], 36406[1], 36410[1], 36420[1], 36425[1], 36430[1], 36440[1], 36591[0], 36592[0], 36600[1], 36640[1], 38220[0], 38222[0], 38230[0], 38232[0], 43752[1], 51701[1], 51702[1], 51703[1], 61783[1], 62320[0], 62321[0], 62322[0], 62323[0], 62324[0], 62325[0], 62326[0], 62327[0], 63001[1], 63015[1], 63017[1], 63020[1], 63040[1], 63046[1], 63707[1], 63709[1], 64400[0], 64405[0], 64408[0], 64415[0], 64416[0], 64417[0], 64418[0], 64420[0], 64421[0], 64425[0], 64430[0], 64435[0], 64445[0], 64446[0], 64447[0], 64448[0], 64449[0], 64450[0], 64451[0], 64454[0], 64461[0], 64462[0], 64463[0], 64479[0], 64480[0], 64483[0], 64484[0], 64486[0], 64487[0], 64488[0], 64489[0], 64490[0], 64491[0], 64492[0], 64493[0], 64494[0], 64495[0], 64505[0], 64510[0], 64517[0], 64520[0], 64530[0], 69990[0], 76000[1], 77001[1], 77002[1], 92012[1], 92014[1], 92585[0], 93000[1], 93005[1], 93010[1], 93040[1], 93041[1], 93042[1], 93318[1], 93355[1], 94002[1], 94200[1], 94250[1], 94680[1], 94681[1], 94690[1], 94770[1], 95812[1], 95813[1], 95816[1], 95819[1], 95822[0], 95829[1], 95860[0], 95861[0], 95863[0], 95864[0], 95865[0], 95866[0], 95867[0], 95868[0], 95869[0], 95870[0], 95907[0], 95908[0], 95909[0], 95910[0], 95911[0], 95912[0], 95913[0], 95925[0], 95926[0], 95927[0], 95928[0], 95929[0], 95930[0], 95933[0], 95937[0], 95938[0], 95939[0], 95940[0], 95955[1], 96360[1], 96361[1], 96365[1], 96366[1], 96367[1], 96368[1], 96372[1], 96374[1], 96375[1], 96376[1], 96377[1], 96523[0], 97597[1], 97598[1], 97602[1], 99155[0], 99156[0], 99157[0], 99211[1], 99212[1], 99213[1], 99214[1], 99215[1], 99217[1], 99218[1], 99219[1], 99220[1], 99221[1], 99222[1], 99223[1], 99231[1], 99232[1], 99233[1], 99234[1], 99235[1], 99236[1], 99238[1], 99239[1], 99241[1], 99242[1], 99243[1], 99244[1], 99245[1], 99251[1], 99252[1], 99253[1], 99254[1], 99255[1], 99291[1], 99292[1], 99304[1], 99305[1], 99306[1], 99307[1], 99308[1], 99309[1], 99310[1], 99315[1], 99316[1], 99334[1], 99335[1], 99336[1], 99337[1], 99347[1], 99348[1], 99349[1], 99350[1], 99374[1], 99375[1], 99377[1], 99378[1], 99446[0], 99447[0], 99448[0], 99449[0], 99451[0], 99452[0], 99495[0], 99496[0], G0453[0], G0463[1], G0471[1]
63046	0213T[0], 0216T[0], 0228T[0], 0230T[0], 0333T[0], 0464T[0], 0565T[1], 11000[1], 11001[1], 11004[1], 11005[1], 11006[1], 11042[1], 11043[1], 11044[1], 11045[1], 11046[1], 11047[1], 12001[1], 12002[1], 12004[1], 12005[1], 12006[1], 12007[1], 12011[1], 12013[1], 12014[1], 12015[1], 12016[1], 12017[1], 12018[1], 12020[1], 12021[1], 12031[1], 12032[1], 12034[1], 12035[1], 12036[1], 12037[1], 12041[1], 12042[1], 12044[1], 12045[1], 12046[1], 12047[1], 12051[1], 12052[1], 12053[1], 12054[1], 12055[1], 12056[1], 12057[1], 13100[1], 13101[1], 13102[1], 13120[1], 13121[1], 13122[1], 13131[1], 13132[1], 13133[1], 13151[1], 13152[1], 13153[1], 15769[1], 22101[1], 22208[1], 22212[1], 22505[0], 36000[1], 36400[1], 36405[1], 36406[1], 36410[1], 36420[1], 36425[1], 36430[1], 36440[1], 36591[0], 36592[0], 36600[1], 36640[1], 38220[0], 38222[0], 38230[0], 38232[0], 43752[1], 51701[1], 51702[1], 51703[1], 61783[1], 62320[0], 62321[0], 62322[0], 62323[0], 62324[0], 62325[0], 62326[0], 62327[0], 63015[1], 63017[1], 63047[1], 63707[1], 63709[1], 64400[0], 64405[0], 64408[0], 64415[0], 64416[0], 64417[0], 64418[0], 64420[0], 64421[0], 64425[0], 64430[0], 64435[0], 64445[0], 64446[0], 64447[0], 64448[0], 64449[0], 64450[0], 64451[0], 64454[0], 64461[0], 64462[0], 64463[0], 64479[0], 64480[0], 64483[0], 64484[0], 64486[0], 64487[0], 64488[0], 64489[0], 64490[0], 64491[0], 64492[0], 64493[0], 64494[0], 64495[0], 64505[0], 64510[0], 64517[0], 64520[0], 64530[0], 69990[0], 76000[1], 77001[1], 77002[1], 92012[1], 92014[1], 92585[0], 93000[1], 93005[1], 93010[1], 93040[1], 93041[1], 93042[1], 93318[1], 93355[1], 94002[1], 94200[1], 94250[1], 94680[1], 94681[1], 94690[1], 94770[1], 95812[1], 95813[1], 95816[1], 95819[1], 95822[0], 95829[1], 95860[0], 95861[0], 95863[0], 95864[0], 95865[0], 95866[0], 95867[0], 95868[0], 95869[0], 95870[0], 95907[0], 95908[0], 95909[0], 95910[0], 95911[0], 95912[0], 95913[0], 95925[0], 95926[0], 95927[0], 95928[0], 95929[0], 95930[0], 95933[0], 95937[0], 95938[0], 95939[0], 95940[0], 95955[1], 96360[1], 96361[1], 96365[1], 96366[1], 96367[1], 96368[1], 96372[1], 96374[1], 96375[1], 96376[1], 96377[1], 96523[0], 97597[1], 97598[1], 97602[1], 99155[0], 99156[0], 99157[0], 99211[1], 99212[1], 99213[1], 99214[1], 99215[1], 99217[1], 99218[1], 99219[1], 99220[1], 99221[1], 99222[1], 99223[1], 99231[1], 99232[1], 99233[1], 99234[1], 99235[1], 99236[1], 99238[1], 99239[1], 99241[1], 99242[1], 99243[1], 99244[1], 99245[1], 99251[1], 99252[1], 99253[1], 99254[1], 99255[1], 99291[1], 99292[1], 99304[1], 99305[1], 99306[1], 99307[1], 99308[1], 99309[1], 99310[1], 99315[1], 99316[1], 99334[1], 99335[1], 99336[1], 99337[1], 99347[1], 99348[1], 99349[1], 99350[1], 99374[1], 99375[1], 99377[1], 99378[1], 99446[0], 99447[0], 99448[0], 99449[0], 99451[0], 99452[0], 99495[0], 99496[0], G0453[0], G0463[1], G0471[1]
63047	0202T[1], 0213T[0], 0216T[0], 0228T[0], 0230T[0], 0274T[1], 0275T[1], 0333T[0], 0464T[0], 0565T[1], 11000[1], 11001[1], 11004[1], 11005[1], 11006[1], 11042[1], 11043[1], 11044[1], 11045[1], 11046[1], 11047[1], 12001[1], 12002[1], 12004[1], 12005[1], 12006[1], 12007[1], 12011[1], 12013[1], 12014[1], 12015[1], 12016[1], 12017[1], 12018[1], 12020[1], 12021[1], 12031[1], 12032[1], 12034[1], 12035[1], 12036[1], 12037[1], 12041[1], 12042[1], 12044[1], 12045[1], 12046[1], 12047[1], 12051[1], 12052[1], 12053[1], 12054[1], 12055[1], 12056[1], 12057[1], 13100[1], 13101[1], 13102[1], 13120[1], 13121[1], 13122[1], 13131[1], 13132[1], 13133[1], 13151[1], 13152[1], 13153[1], 15769[1], 22102[1], 22208[1], 22325[1], 22505[0], 22852[1], 22867[1], 22868[1], 22869[1], 22870[1], 32100[1], 36000[1], 36400[1], 36405[1], 36406[1], 36410[1], 36420[1], 36425[1], 36430[1], 36440[1], 36591[0], 36592[0], 36600[1], 36640[1], 38220[0], 38222[0], 38230[0], 38232[0], 43752[1], 51701[1], 51702[1], 51703[1], 61783[1], 62284[1], 62287[1], 62320[0], 62321[0], 62322[0], 62323[0], 62324[0], 62325[0], 62326[0], 62327[0], 62380[1], 63005[1], 63012[1], 63015[1], 63017[1], 63020[1], 63030[1], 63042[1], 63056[1], 63707[1], 63709[1], 63710[1], 64400[0], 64405[0], 64408[0], 64415[0], 64416[0], 64417[0], 64418[0], 64420[0], 64421[0], 64425[0], 64430[0], 64435[0], 64445[0], 64446[0], 64447[0], 64448[0], 64449[0], 64450[0], 64451[0], 64454[0], 64461[0], 64462[0], 64463[0], 64479[0], 64480[0], 64483[0], 64484[0], 64486[0], 64487[0], 64488[0], 64489[0], 64490[0], 64491[0], 64492[0], 64493[0], 64494[0], 64495[0], 64505[0], 64510[0], 64517[0], 64520[0], 64530[0], 64722[1], 64831[1], 64834[1], 64835[1], 64836[1], 64840[1], 64856[1], 64857[1], 64858[1], 64861[1], 64862[1], 64864[1], 64865[1], 64866[1], 64868[1], 64885[1], 64886[1], 64890[1], 64891[1], 64892[1], 64893[1], 64895[1], 64896[1], 64897[1], 64898[1], 64905[1], 64907[1], 64912[1], 64913[1], 69990[0], 76000[1], 77001[1], 77002[1], 92012[1], 92014[1], 92585[0], 93000[1], 93005[1], 93010[1], 93040[1], 93041[1], 93042[1], 93318[1], 93355[1], 94002[1], 94200[1], 94250[1], 94680[1], 94681[1], 94690[1], 94770[1], 95812[1], 95813[1], 95816[1], 95819[1], 95822[0], 95829[1], 95860[0], 95861[0], 95863[0], 95864[0], 95865[0], 95866[0], 95867[0], 95868[0], 95869[0], 95870[0], 95907[0], 95908[0], 95909[0], 95910[0], 95911[0], 95912[0], 95913[0], 95925[0], 95926[0], 95927[0], 95928[0], 95929[0], 95930[0], 95933[0], 95937[0], 95938[0], 95939[0], 95940[0], 95955[1], 96360[1], 96361[1], 96365[1], 96366[1], 96367[1], 96368[1], 96372[1], 96374[1], 96375[1], 96376[1], 96377[1], 96523[0], 97597[1], 97598[1], 97602[1], 99155[0], 99156[0], 99157[0], 99211[1], 99212[1], 99213[1], 99214[1], 99215[1], 99217[1], 99218[1], 99219[1], 99220[1], 99221[1], 99222[1], 99223[1], 99231[1], 99232[1], 99233[1], 99234[1], 99235[1], 99236[1], 99238[1], 99239[1], 99241[1], 99242[1], 99243[1], 99244[1], 99245[1], 99251[1], 99252[1], 99253[1], 99254[1], 99255[1], 99291[1], 99292[1], 99304[1], 99305[1], 99306[1], 99307[1], 99308[1], 99309[1], 99310[1], 99315[1], 99316[1], 99334[1], 99335[1], 99336[1], 99337[1], 99347[1], 99348[1], 99349[1], 99350[1], 99374[1], 99375[1], 99377[1], 99378[1], 99446[0], 99447[0], 99448[0], 99449[0], 99451[0], 99452[0], 99495[0], 99496[0], G0276[1], G0453[0], G0463[1], G0471[1]
63048	0333T[0], 0464T[0], 11000[1], 11001[1], 11004[1], 11005[1], 11006[1], 11042[1], 11043[1], 11044[1], 11045[1], 11046[1], 11047[1], 22867[1], 22868[1], 22869[1], 22870[1], 36591[0], 36592[0], 38220[0], 38222[0], 38230[0], 38232[0], 63707[1], 63709[1], 92585[0], 95822[0], 95860[0], 95861[0], 95863[0], 95864[0], 95865[0], 95866[0], 95867[0], 95868[0], 95869[0], 95907[0], 95908[0], 95909[0], 95910[0], 95911[0], 95912[0], 95913[0], 95925[0], 95926[0], 95927[0], 95930[0], 95933[0], 95937[0], 95938[0], 95939[0], 95940[0], 96523[0], 97597[1], 97598[1], 97602[1], G0453[0]
63050	0213T[0], 0216T[0], 0228T[0], 0230T[0], 0274T[1], 0333T[0], 0464T[0], 0565T[1], 11000[1], 11001[1], 11004[1], 11005[1], 11006[1], 11042[1], 11043[1], 11044[1], 11045[1], 11046[1], 11047[1], 12001[1], 12002[1], 12004[1], 12005[1], 12006[1], 12007[1], 12011[1], 12013[1], 12014[1], 12015[1], 12016[1], 12017[1], 12018[1], 12020[1], 12021[1], 12031[1], 12032[1], 12034[1], 12035[1], 12036[1], 12037[1], 12041[1], 12042[1], 12044[1], 12045[1], 12046[1], 12047[1], 12051[1], 12052[1], 12053[1], 12054[1], 12055[1], 12056[1], 12057[1], 13100[1], 13101[1], 13102[1], 13120[1], 13121[1], 13122[1], 13131[1], 13132[1], 13133[1], 13151[1], 13152[1], 13153[1], 15769[1], 22100[1], 22505[0], 22600[1], 22614[1], 36000[1], 36400[1], 36405[1], 36406[1], 36410[1], 36420[1], 36425[1], 36430[1], 36440[1], 36591[0], 36592[0], 36600[1], 36640[1], 38220[0], 38222[0], 38230[0], 38232[0], 43752[1], 51701[1], 51702[1], 51703[1], 61783[1], 62320[0], 62321[0], 62322[0], 62323[0], 62324[0], 62325[0], 62326[0], 62327[0], 63001[1], 63015[1], 63020[1], 63040[1], 63045[1], 63048[1], 63295[1], 63707[1], 63709[1], 64400[0], 64405[0], 64408[0], 64415[0], 64416[0], 64417[0], 64418[0], 64420[0], 64421[0], 64425[0], 64430[0], 64435[0], 64445[0], 64446[0], 64447[0], 64448[0], 64449[0], 64450[0], 64451[0], 64454[0], 64461[0], 64462[0], 64463[0], 64479[0], 64480[0], 64483[0], 64484[0], 64486[0], 64487[0], 64488[0], 64489[0], 64490[0], 64491[0], 64492[0], 64493[0], 64494[0], 64495[0], 64505[0], 64510[0], 64517[0], 64520[0], 64530[0], 69990[0], 76000[1], 77001[1], 77002[1], 92012[1], 92014[1], 92585[0], 93000[1], 93005[1], 93010[1], 93040[1], 93041[1], 93042[1], 93318[1], 93355[1], 94002[1], 94200[1], 94250[1], 94680[1], 94681[1], 94690[1], 94770[1], 95812[1], 95813[1], 95816[1], 95819[1], 95822[0], 95829[1], 95860[0], 95861[0], 95863[0], 95864[0], 95865[0], 95866[0], 95867[0], 95868[0], 95869[0], 95870[0], 95907[0], 95908[0], 95909[0], 95910[0], 95911[0], 95912[0], 95913[0], 95925[0], 95926[0], 95927[0], 95928[0],

0 = Modifier usage not allowed or inappropriate 1 = Modifier usage allowed

Code 1	Code 2
	95929^0, 95930^0, 95933^0, 95937^0, 95938^0, 95939^0, 95940^0, 95955^1, 96360^1, 96361^1, 96365^1, 96366^1, 96367^1, 96368^1, 96372^1, 96374^1, 96375^1, 96376^1, 96377^1, 96523^0, 97597^1, 97598^1, 97602^1, 99155^0, 99156^0, 99157^0, 99211^1, 99212^1, 99213^1, 99214^1, 99215^1, 99217^1, 99218^1, 99219^1, 99220^1, 99221^1, 99222^1, 99223^1, 99231^1, 99232^1, 99233^1, 99234^1, 99235^1, 99236^1, 99238^1, 99239^1, 99241^1, 99242^1, 99243^1, 99244^1, 99245^1, 99251^1, 99252^1, 99253^1, 99254^1, 99255^1, 99291^1, 99292^1, 99304^1, 99305^1, 99306^1, 99307^1, 99308^1, 99309^1, 99310^1, 99315^1, 99316^1, 99334^1, 99335^1, 99336^1, 99337^1, 99347^1, 99348^1, 99349^1, 99350^1, 99374^1, 99375^1, 99377^1, 99378^1, 99446^0, 99447^0, 99448^0, 99449^0, 99451^0, 99452^0, 99495^0, 99496^0, G0453^0, G0463^1, G0471^1
63051	0213T^0, 0216T^0, 0228T^0, 0230T^0, 0274T^1, 0333T^0, 0464T^0, 0565T^1, 11000^1, 11001^1, 11004^1, 11005^1, 11006^1, 11042^1, 11043^1, 11044^1, 11045^1, 11046^1, 11047^1, 12001^1, 12002^1, 12004^1, 12005^1, 12006^1, 12007^1, 12011^1, 12013^1, 12014^1, 12015^1, 12016^1, 12017^1, 12018^1, 12020^1, 12021^1, 12031^1, 12032^1, 12034^1, 12035^1, 12036^1, 12037^1, 12041^1, 12042^1, 12044^1, 12045^1, 12046^1, 12047^1, 12051^1, 12052^1, 12053^1, 12054^1, 12055^1, 12056^1, 12057^1, 13100^1, 13101^1, 13102^1, 13120^1, 13121^1, 13122^1, 13131^1, 13132^1, 13133^1, 13151^1, 13152^1, 13153^1, 15769^1, 22100^1, 22505^0, 22600^1, 22614^1, 36000^1, 36400^1, 36405^1, 36406^1, 36410^1, 36420^1, 36425^1, 36430^1, 36440^1, 36591^0, 36592^0, 36600^1, 36640^1, 38220^0, 38222^0, 38230^0, 38232^0, 43752^1, 51701^1, 51702^1, 51703^1, 61783^1, 62320^0, 62321^0, 62322^0, 62323^0, 62324^0, 62325^0, 62326^0, 62327^0, 63001^1, 63015^1, 63020^1, 63040^1, 63045^1, 63048^1, 63050^1, 63055^1, 63265^1, 63295^1, 63707^1, 63709^1, 64400^0, 64405^0, 64408^0, 64415^0, 64416^0, 64417^0, 64418^0, 64420^0, 64421^0, 64425^0, 64430^0, 64435^0, 64445^0, 64446^0, 64447^0, 64448^0, 64449^0, 64450^0, 64451^0, 64454^0, 64461^0, 64462^0, 64463^0, 64479^0, 64480^0, 64483^0, 64484^0, 64486^0, 64487^0, 64488^0, 64489^0, 64490^0, 64491^0, 64492^0, 64493^0, 64494^0, 64495^0, 64505^0, 64510^0, 64517^0, 64520^0, 64530^0, 69990^0, 76000^1, 77001^1, 77002^1, 92012^1, 92014^1, 92585^0, 93000^1, 93005^1, 93010^1, 93040^1, 93041^1, 93042^1, 93318^1, 93355^1, 94002^1, 94200^1, 94250^1, 94680^1, 94681^1, 94690^1, 94770^1, 95812^1, 95813^1, 95816^1, 95819^1, 95822^0, 95829^1, 95860^0, 95861^0, 95863^0, 95864^0, 95865^0, 95866^0, 95867^0, 95868^0, 95869^0, 95870^0, 95907^0, 95908^0, 95909^0, 95910^0, 95911^0, 95912^0, 95913^0, 95925^0, 95926^0, 95927^0, 95928^0, 95929^0, 95930^0, 95933^0, 95937^0, 95938^0, 95939^0, 95940^0, 95955^1, 96360^1, 96361^1, 96365^1, 96366^1, 96367^1, 96368^1, 96372^1, 96374^1, 96375^1, 96376^1, 96377^1, 96523^0, 97597^1, 97598^1, 97602^1, 99155^0, 99156^0, 99157^0, 99211^1, 99212^1, 99213^1, 99214^1, 99215^1, 99217^1, 99218^1, 99219^1, 99220^1, 99221^1, 99222^1, 99223^1, 99231^1, 99232^1, 99233^1, 99234^1, 99235^1, 99236^1, 99238^1, 99239^1, 99241^1, 99242^1, 99243^1, 99244^1, 99245^1, 99251^1, 99252^1, 99253^1, 99254^1, 99255^1, 99291^1, 99292^1, 99304^1, 99305^1, 99306^1, 99307^1, 99308^1, 99309^1, 99310^1, 99315^1, 99316^1, 99334^1, 99335^1, 99336^1, 99337^1, 99347^1, 99348^1, 99349^1, 99350^1, 99374^1, 99375^1, 99377^1, 99378^1, 99446^0, 99447^0, 99448^0, 99449^0, 99451^0, 99452^0, 99495^0, 99496^0, G0453^0, G0463^1, G0471^1
63055	0213T^0, 0216T^0, 0228T^0, 0230T^0, 0274T^1, 0333T^0, 0464T^0, 12001^1, 12002^1, 12004^1, 12005^1, 12006^1, 12007^1, 12011^1, 12013^1, 12014^1, 12015^1, 12016^1, 12017^1, 12018^1, 12020^1, 12021^1, 12031^1, 12032^1, 12034^1, 12035^1, 12036^1, 12037^1, 12041^1, 12042^1, 12044^1, 12045^1, 12046^1, 12047^1, 12051^1, 12052^1, 12053^1, 12054^1, 12055^1, 12056^1, 12057^1, 13100^1, 13101^1, 13102^1, 13120^1, 13121^1, 13122^1, 13131^1, 13132^1, 13133^1, 13151^1, 13152^1, 13153^1, 22101^1, 22208^1, 22212^1, 22222^1, 22505^0, 36000^1, 36400^1, 36405^1, 36406^1, 36410^1, 36420^1, 36425^1, 36430^1, 36440^1, 36591^0, 36592^0, 36600^1, 36640^1, 38220^0, 38222^0, 38230^0, 38232^0, 43752^1, 51701^1, 51702^1, 51703^1, 62291^1, 62320^0, 62321^0, 62322^0, 62323^0, 62324^0, 62325^0, 62326^0, 62327^0, 63001^1, 63003^1, 63015^1, 63016^1, 63020^1, 63040^1, 63045^1, 63046^1, 63050^1, 63056^1, 63075^1, 63707^1, 63709^1, 64400^0, 64405^0, 64408^0, 64415^0, 64416^0, 64417^0, 64418^0, 64420^0, 64421^0, 64425^0, 64430^0, 64435^0, 64445^0, 64446^0, 64447^0, 64448^0, 64449^0, 64450^0, 64451^0, 64454^0, 64461^0, 64462^0, 64463^0, 64479^0, 64480^0, 64483^0, 64484^0, 64486^0, 64487^0, 64488^0, 64489^0, 64490^0, 64491^0, 64492^0, 64493^0, 64494^0, 64495^0, 64505^0, 64510^0, 64517^0, 64520^0, 64530^0, 69990^0, 72285^1, 76000^1, 77001^1, 77002^1, 92012^1, 92014^1, 92585^0, 93000^1, 93005^1, 93010^1, 93040^1, 93041^1, 93042^1, 93318^1, 93355^1, 94002^1, 94200^1, 94250^1, 94680^1, 94681^1, 94690^1, 94770^1, 95812^1, 95813^1, 95816^1, 95819^1, 95822^0, 95829^1, 95860^0, 95861^0, 95863^0, 95864^0, 95865^0, 95866^0, 95867^0, 95868^0, 95869^0, 95870^0, 95907^0, 95908^0, 95909^0, 95910^0, 95911^0, 95912^0, 95913^0, 95925^0, 95926^0, 95927^0, 95928^0, 95929^0, 95930^0, 95933^0, 95937^0, 95938^0, 95939^0, 95940^0, 95955^1, 96360^1, 96361^1, 96365^1, 96366^1, 96367^1, 96368^1, 96372^1, 96374^1, 96375^1, 96376^1, 96377^1, 96523^0, 99155^0, 99156^0, 99157^0, 99211^1, 99212^1, 99213^1, 99214^1, 99215^1, 99217^1, 99218^1, 99219^1, 99220^1, 99221^1, 99222^1, 99223^1, 99231^1, 99232^1, 99233^1, 99234^1, 99235^1, 99236^1, 99238^1, 99239^1, 99241^1, 99242^1, 99243^1, 99244^1, 99245^1, 99251^1, 99252^1, 99253^1, 99254^1, 99255^1, 99291^1, 99292^1, 99304^1, 99305^1, 99306^1, 99307^1, 99308^1, 99309^1, 99310^1, 99315^1, 99316^1, 99334^1, 99335^1, 99336^1, 99337^1, 99347^1, 99348^1, 99349^1, 99350^1, 99374^1, 99375^1, 99377^1, 99378^1, 99446^0, 99447^0, 99448^0, 99449^0, 99451^0, 99452^0, 99495^0, 99496^0, G0453^0, G0463^1, G0471^1
63056	0202T^1, 0213T^0, 0216T^0, 0228T^0, 0230T^0, 0275T^1, 0333T^0, 0464T^0, 12001^1, 12002^1, 12004^1, 12005^1, 12006^1, 12007^1, 12011^1, 12013^1, 12014^1, 12015^1, 12016^1, 12017^1, 12018^1, 12020^1, 12021^1, 12031^1, 12032^1, 12034^1, 12035^1, 12036^1, 12037^1, 12041^1, 12042^1, 12044^1, 12045^1, 12046^1, 12047^1, 12051^1, 12052^1, 12053^1, 12054^1, 12055^1, 12056^1, 12057^1, 13100^1, 13101^1, 13102^1, 13120^1, 13121^1, 13122^1, 13131^1, 13132^1, 13133^1, 13151^1, 13152^1, 13153^1, 22102^1, 22208^1, 22214^1, 22224^1, 22505^0, 22867^1, 22868^1, 22869^1, 22870^1, 36000^1, 36400^1, 36405^1, 36406^1, 36410^1, 36420^1, 36425^1, 36430^1, 36440^1, 36591^0, 36592^0, 36600^1, 36640^1, 38220^0, 38222^0, 38230^0, 38232^0, 43752^1, 51701^1, 51702^1, 51703^1, 62267^1, 62290^1, 62320^0, 62321^0, 62322^0, 62323^0, 62324^0, 62325^0, 62326^0, 62327^0, 62380^1, 63087^1, 63090^1, 63707^1, 63709^1, 64400^0, 64405^0, 64408^0, 64415^0, 64416^0, 64417^0, 64418^0, 64420^0, 64421^0, 64425^0, 64430^0, 64435^0, 64445^0, 64446^0, 64447^0, 64448^0, 64449^0, 64450^0, 64451^0, 64454^0, 64461^0, 64462^0, 64463^0, 64479^0, 64480^0, 64483^0, 64484^0, 64486^0, 64487^0, 64488^0, 64489^0, 64490^0, 64491^0, 64492^0, 64493^0, 64494^0, 64495^0, 64505^0, 64510^0, 64517^0, 64520^0, 64530^0, 69990^0, 72295^1, 76000^1, 77001^1, 77002^1, 92012^1, 92014^1, 92585^0, 93000^1, 93005^1, 93010^1, 93040^1, 93041^1, 93042^1, 93318^1, 93355^1, 94002^1, 94200^1, 94250^1, 94680^1, 94681^1, 94690^1, 94770^1, 95812^1, 95813^1, 95816^1, 95819^1, 95822^0, 95829^1, 95860^0, 95861^0, 95863^0, 95864^0, 95865^0, 95866^0, 95867^0, 95868^0, 95869^0, 95870^0, 95907^0, 95908^0, 95909^0, 95910^0, 95911^0, 95912^0, 95913^0, 95925^0, 95926^0, 95927^0, 95928^0, 95929^0, 95930^0, 95933^0, 95937^0, 95938^0, 95939^0, 95940^0, 95955^1, 96360^1, 96361^1, 96365^1, 96366^1, 96367^1, 96368^1, 96372^1, 96374^1, 96375^1, 96376^1, 96377^1, 96523^0, 99155^0, 99156^0, 99157^0, 99211^1, 99212^1, 99213^1, 99214^1, 99215^1, 99217^1, 99218^1, 99219^1, 99220^1, 99221^1, 99222^1, 99223^1, 99231^1, 99232^1, 99233^1, 99234^1, 99235^1, 99236^1, 99238^1, 99239^1, 99241^1, 99242^1, 99243^1, 99244^1, 99245^1, 99251^1, 99252^1, 99253^1, 99254^1, 99255^1, 99291^1, 99292^1, 99304^1, 99305^1, 99306^1, 99307^1, 99308^1, 99309^1, 99310^1, 99315^1, 99316^1, 99334^1, 99335^1, 99336^1, 99337^1, 99347^1, 99348^1, 99349^1, 99350^1, 99374^1, 99375^1, 99377^1, 99378^1, 99446^0, 99447^0, 99448^0, 99449^0, 99451^0, 99452^0, 99495^0, 99496^0, G0453^0, G0463^1, G0471^1
63057	0333T^0, 0464T^0, 22867^1, 22868^1, 22869^1, 22870^1, 36591^0, 36592^0, 38220^0, 38222^0, 38230^0, 38232^0, 63707^1, 63709^1, 92585^0, 95822^0, 95860^0, 95861^0, 95863^0, 95864^0, 95865^0, 95866^0, 95867^0, 95868^0, 95869^0, 95907^0, 95908^0, 95909^0, 95910^0, 95911^0, 95912^0, 95913^0, 95925^0, 95926^0, 95927^0, 95930^0, 95933^0, 95937^0, 95938^0, 95939^0, 95940^0, 96523^0, G0453^0
63064	0213T^0, 0216T^0, 0228T^0, 0230T^0, 0333T^0, 0464T^0, 12001^1, 12002^1, 12004^1, 12005^1, 12006^1, 12007^1, 12011^1, 12013^1, 12014^1, 12015^1, 12016^1, 12017^1, 12018^1, 12020^1, 12021^1, 12031^1, 12032^1, 12034^1, 12035^1, 12036^1, 12037^1, 12041^1, 12042^1, 12044^1, 12045^1, 12046^1, 12047^1, 12051^1, 12052^1, 12053^1, 12054^1, 12055^1, 12056^1, 12057^1, 13100^1, 13101^1, 13102^1, 13120^1, 13121^1, 13122^1, 13131^1, 13132^1, 13133^1, 13151^1, 13152^1, 13153^1, 22208^1, 22505^0, 36000^1, 36400^1, 36405^1, 36406^1, 36410^1, 36420^1, 36425^1, 36430^1, 36440^1, 36591^0, 36592^0, 36600^1, 36640^1, 38220^0, 38222^0, 38230^0, 38232^0, 43752^1, 51701^1, 51702^1, 51703^1, 62291^1, 62320^0, 62321^0, 62322^0, 62323^0, 62324^0, 62325^0, 62326^0, 62327^0, 63003^1, 63055^1, 63707^1, 63709^1, 64400^0, 64405^0, 64408^0, 64415^0, 64416^0, 64417^0, 64418^0, 64420^0, 64421^0, 64425^0, 64430^0, 64435^0, 64445^0, 64446^0, 64447^0, 64448^0, 64449^0, 64450^0, 64451^0, 64454^0, 64461^0, 64462^0, 64463^0, 64479^0, 64480^0, 64483^0, 64484^0, 64486^0, 64487^0, 64488^0, 64489^0, 64490^0, 64491^0, 64492^0, 64493^0, 64494^0, 64495^0, 64505^0, 64510^0, 64517^0, 64520^0, 64530^0, 69990^0, 72285^1, 76000^1, 77001^1, 77002^1, 92012^1, 92014^1, 92585^0, 93000^1, 93005^1, 93010^1, 93040^1, 93041^1, 93042^1, 93318^1, 93355^1, 94002^1, 94200^1, 94250^1, 94680^1, 94681^1, 94690^1, 94770^1, 95812^1, 95813^1, 95816^1, 95819^1, 95822^0, 95829^1, 95860^0, 95861^0, 95863^0, 95864^0, 95865^0, 95866^0, 95867^0, 95868^0, 95869^0, 95870^0, 95907^0, 95908^0, 95909^0, 95910^0, 95911^0, 95912^0, 95913^0, 95925^0, 95926^0, 95927^0, 95928^0, 95929^0, 95930^0, 95933^0, 95937^0, 95938^0, 95939^0, 95940^0, 95955^1, 96360^1, 96361^1, 96365^1, 96366^1, 96367^1, 96368^1, 96372^1, 96374^1, 96375^1, 96376^1, 96377^1, 96523^0, 99155^0, 99156^0, 99157^0, 99211^1, 99212^1, 99213^1, 99214^1, 99215^1, 99217^1, 99218^1, 99219^1, 99220^1, 99221^1, 99222^1, 99223^1, 99231^1, 99232^1, 99233^1, 99234^1, 99235^1, 99236^1, 99238^1, 99239^1, 99241^1, 99242^1, 99243^1, 99244^1, 99245^1, 99251^1, 99252^1, 99253^1, 99254^1, 99255^1, 99291^1, 99292^1, 99304^1, 99305^1, 99306^1, 99307^1, 99308^1, 99309^1, 99310^1, 99315^1, 99316^1, 99334^1, 99335^1, 99336^1, 99337^1, 99347^1, 99348^1, 99349^1, 99350^1, 99374^1, 99375^1, 99377^1, 99378^1, 99446^0, 99447^0, 99448^0, 99449^0, 99451^0, 99452^0, 99495^0, 99496^0, G0453^0, G0463^1, G0471^1
63066	0333T^0, 0464T^0, 36591^0, 36592^0, 38220^0, 38222^0, 38230^0, 38232^0, 63707^1, 63709^1, 92585^0, 95822^0, 95860^0, 95861^0, 95863^0, 95864^0, 95865^0, 95866^0, 95867^0, 95868^0,

0 = Modifier usage not allowed or inappropriate   1 = Modifier usage allowed

Code 1	Code 2
	95869[0], 95907[0], 95908[0], 95909[0], 95910[0], 95911[0], 95912[0], 95913[0], 95925[0], 95926[0], 95927[0], 95930[0], 95933[0], 95937[0], 95938[0], 95939[0], 95940[0], 96523[0], G0453[0]
63075	0213T[0], 0216T[0], 0228T[0], 0230T[0], 0333T[0], 0464T[0], 11000[1], 11001[1], 11004[1], 11005[1], 11006[1], 11042[1], 11043[1], 11044[1], 11045[1], 11046[1], 11047[1], 12001[1], 12002[1], 12004[1], 12005[1], 12006[1], 12007[1], 12011[1], 12013[1], 12014[1], 12015[1], 12016[1], 12017[1], 12018[1], 12020[1], 12021[1], 12031[1], 12032[1], 12034[1], 12035[1], 12036[1], 12037[1], 12041[1], 12042[1], 12044[1], 12045[1], 12046[1], 12047[1], 12051[1], 12052[1], 12053[1], 12054[1], 12055[1], 12056[1], 12057[1], 13100[1], 13101[1], 13102[1], 13120[1], 13121[1], 13122[1], 13131[1], 13132[1], 13133[1], 13151[1], 13152[1], 13153[1], 22208[1], 22505[0], 22552[1], 22554[1], 22585[1], 36000[1], 36400[1], 36405[1], 36406[1], 36410[1], 36420[1], 36425[1], 36430[1], 36440[1], 36591[0], 36592[0], 36600[1], 36640[1], 38220[0], 38222[0], 38230[0], 38232[0], 43752[1], 51701[1], 51702[1], 51703[1], 62291[1], 62320[0], 62321[0], 62322[0], 62323[0], 62324[0], 62325[0], 62326[0], 62327[0], 63077[1], 63707[1], 63709[1], 64400[0], 64405[0], 64408[0], 64415[0], 64416[0], 64417[0], 64418[0], 64420[0], 64421[0], 64425[0], 64430[0], 64435[0], 64445[0], 64446[0], 64447[0], 64448[0], 64449[0], 64450[0], 64451[0], 64454[0], 64461[0], 64462[0], 64463[0], 64479[0], 64480[0], 64483[0], 64484[0], 64486[0], 64487[0], 64488[0], 64489[0], 64490[0], 64491[0], 64492[0], 64493[0], 64494[0], 64495[0], 64505[0], 64510[0], 64517[0], 64520[0], 64530[0], 69990[0], 72285[1], 76000[1], 77001[1], 77002[1], 92012[1], 92014[1], 92585[0], 93000[1], 93005[1], 93010[1], 93040[1], 93041[1], 93042[1], 93318[1], 93355[1], 94002[1], 94200[1], 94250[1], 94680[1], 94681[1], 94690[1], 94770[1], 95812[1], 95813[1], 95816[1], 95819[1], 95822[0], 95829[1], 95860[0], 95861[0], 95863[0], 95864[0], 95865[0], 95866[0], 95867[0], 95868[0], 95869[0], 95870[0], 95907[0], 95908[0], 95909[0], 95910[0], 95911[0], 95912[0], 95913[0], 95925[0], 95926[0], 95927[0], 95928[0], 95929[0], 95930[0], 95933[0], 95937[0], 95938[0], 95939[0], 95940[0], 95955[1], 96360[1], 96361[1], 96365[1], 96366[1], 96367[1], 96368[1], 96372[1], 96374[1], 96375[1], 96376[1], 96377[1], 96523[0], 97597[1], 97598[1], 97602[1], 99155[0], 99156[0], 99157[0], 99211[1], 99212[1], 99213[1], 99214[1], 99215[1], 99217[1], 99218[1], 99219[1], 99220[1], 99221[1], 99222[1], 99223[1], 99231[1], 99232[1], 99233[1], 99234[1], 99235[1], 99236[1], 99238[1], 99239[1], 99241[1], 99242[1], 99243[1], 99244[1], 99245[1], 99251[1], 99252[1], 99253[1], 99254[1], 99255[1], 99291[1], 99292[1], 99304[1], 99305[1], 99306[1], 99307[1], 99308[1], 99309[1], 99310[1], 99315[1], 99316[1], 99334[1], 99335[1], 99336[1], 99337[1], 99347[1], 99348[1], 99349[1], 99350[1], 99374[1], 99375[1], 99377[1], 99378[1], 99446[0], 99447[0], 99448[0], 99449[0], 99451[0], 99452[0], 99495[0], 99496[0], G0453[0], G0463[1], G0471[1]
63076	0333T[0], 0464T[0], 11000[1], 11001[1], 11004[1], 11005[1], 11006[1], 11042[1], 11043[1], 11044[1], 11045[1], 11046[1], 11047[1], 36591[0], 36592[0], 38220[0], 38222[0], 38230[0], 38232[0], 63707[1], 63709[1], 69990[0], 92585[0], 95822[0], 95860[0], 95861[0], 95863[0], 95864[0], 95865[0], 95866[0], 95867[0], 95868[0], 95869[0], 95907[0], 95908[0], 95909[0], 95910[0], 95911[0], 95912[0], 95913[0], 95925[0], 95926[0], 95927[0], 95930[0], 95933[0], 95937[0], 95938[0], 95939[0], 95940[0], 96523[0], 97597[1], 97598[1], 97602[1], G0453[0]
63077	0213T[0], 0216T[0], 0228T[0], 0230T[0], 0333T[0], 0464T[0], 11000[1], 11001[1], 11004[1], 11005[1], 11006[1], 11042[1], 11043[1], 11044[1], 11045[1], 11046[1], 11047[1], 12001[1], 12002[1], 12004[1], 12005[1], 12006[1], 12007[1], 12011[1], 12013[1], 12014[1], 12015[1], 12016[1], 12017[1], 12018[1], 12020[1], 12021[1], 12031[1], 12032[1], 12034[1], 12035[1], 12036[1], 12037[1], 12041[1], 12042[1], 12044[1], 12045[1], 12046[1], 12047[1], 12051[1], 12052[1], 12053[1], 12054[1], 12055[1], 12056[1], 12057[1], 13100[1], 13101[1], 13102[1], 13120[1], 13121[1], 13122[1], 13131[1], 13132[1], 13133[1], 13151[1], 13152[1], 13153[1], 22208[1], 22505[0], 32100[1], 36000[1], 36400[1], 36405[1], 36406[1], 36410[1], 36420[1], 36425[1], 36430[1], 36440[1], 36591[0], 36592[0], 36600[1], 36640[1], 38220[0], 38222[0], 38230[0], 38232[0], 43752[1], 51701[1], 51702[1], 51703[1], 62291[1], 62320[0], 62321[0], 62322[0], 62323[0], 62324[0], 62325[0], 62326[0], 62327[0], 63003[1], 63707[1], 63709[1], 64400[0], 64405[0], 64408[0], 64415[0], 64416[0], 64417[0], 64418[0], 64420[0], 64421[0], 64425[0], 64430[0], 64435[0], 64445[0], 64446[0], 64447[0], 64448[0], 64449[0], 64450[0], 64451[0], 64454[0], 64461[0], 64462[0], 64463[0], 64479[0], 64480[0], 64483[0], 64484[0], 64486[0], 64487[0], 64488[0], 64489[0], 64490[0], 64491[0], 64492[0], 64493[0], 64494[0], 64495[0], 64505[0], 64510[0], 64517[0], 64520[0], 64530[0], 69990[0], 72285[1], 76000[1], 77001[1], 77002[1], 92012[1], 92014[1], 92585[0], 93000[1], 93005[1], 93010[1], 93040[1], 93041[1], 93042[1], 93318[1], 93355[1], 94002[1], 94200[1], 94250[1], 94680[1], 94681[1], 94690[1], 94770[1], 95812[1], 95813[1], 95816[1], 95819[1], 95822[0], 95829[1], 95860[0], 95861[0], 95863[0], 95864[0], 95865[0], 95866[0], 95867[0], 95868[0], 95869[0], 95870[0], 95907[0], 95908[0], 95909[0], 95910[0], 95911[0], 95912[0], 95913[0], 95925[0], 95926[0], 95927[0], 95928[0], 95929[0], 95930[0], 95933[0], 95937[0], 95938[0], 95939[0], 95940[0], 95955[1], 96360[1], 96361[1], 96365[1], 96366[1], 96367[1], 96368[1], 96372[1], 96374[1], 96375[1], 96376[1], 96377[1], 96523[0], 97597[1], 97598[1], 97602[1], 99155[0], 99156[0], 99157[0], 99211[1], 99212[1], 99213[1], 99214[1], 99215[1], 99217[1], 99218[1], 99219[1], 99220[1], 99221[1], 99222[1], 99223[1], 99231[1], 99232[1], 99233[1], 99234[1], 99235[1], 99236[1], 99238[1], 99239[1], 99241[1], 99242[1], 99243[1], 99244[1], 99245[1], 99251[1], 99252[1], 99253[1], 99254[1], 99255[1], 99291[1], 99292[1], 99304[1], 99305[1], 99306[1], 99307[1], 99308[1], 99309[1], 99310[1], 99315[1], 99316[1], 99334[1], 99335[1], 99336[1], 99337[1], 99347[1], 99348[1], 99349[1], 99350[1], 99374[1], 99375[1], 99377[1], 99378[1], 99446[0], 99447[0], 99448[0], 99449[0], 99451[0], 99452[0], 99495[0], 99496[0], G0453[0], G0463[1], G0471[1]
63078	0333T[0], 0464T[0], 11000[1], 11001[1], 11004[1], 11005[1], 11006[1], 11042[1], 11043[1], 11044[1], 11045[1], 11046[1], 11047[1], 36591[0], 36592[0], 38220[0], 38222[0], 38230[0], 38232[0], 63707[1], 63709[1], 69990[0], 92585[0], 95822[0], 95860[0], 95861[0], 95863[0], 95864[0], 95865[0], 95866[0], 95867[0], 95868[0], 95869[0], 95907[0], 95908[0], 95909[0], 95910[0], 95911[0], 95912[0], 95913[0], 95925[0], 95926[0], 95927[0], 95930[0], 95933[0], 95937[0], 95938[0], 95939[0], 95940[0], 96523[0], 97597[1], 97598[1], 97602[1], G0453[0]
63081	0213T[0], 0216T[0], 0228T[0], 0230T[0], 0333T[0], 0464T[0], 11000[1], 11001[1], 11004[1], 11005[1], 11006[1], 11042[1], 11043[1], 11044[1], 11045[1], 11046[1], 11047[1], 12001[1], 12002[1], 12004[1], 12005[1], 12006[1], 12007[1], 12011[1], 12013[1], 12014[1], 12015[1], 12016[1], 12017[1], 12018[1], 12020[1], 12021[1], 12031[1], 12032[1], 12034[1], 12035[1], 12036[1], 12037[1], 12041[1], 12042[1], 12044[1], 12045[1], 12046[1], 12047[1], 12051[1], 12052[1], 12053[1], 12054[1], 12055[1], 12056[1], 12057[1], 13100[1], 13101[1], 13102[1], 13120[1], 13121[1], 13122[1], 13131[1], 13132[1], 13133[1], 13151[1], 13152[1], 13153[1], 22100[1], 22101[1], 22102[1], 22110[1], 22112[1], 22114[1], 22208[1], 22505[0], 22551[1], 36000[1], 36400[1], 36405[1], 36406[1], 36410[1], 36420[1], 36425[1], 36430[1], 36440[1], 36591[0], 36592[0], 36600[1], 36640[1], 38220[0], 38221[1], 38222[0], 38230[0], 38232[0], 43752[1], 51701[1], 51702[1], 51703[1], 62320[0], 62321[0], 62322[0], 62323[0], 62324[0], 62325[0], 62326[0], 62327[0], 63055[1], 63075[1], 63076[1], 63707[1], 63709[1], 64400[0], 64405[0], 64408[0], 64415[0], 64416[0], 64417[0], 64418[0], 64420[0], 64421[0], 64425[0], 64430[0], 64435[0], 64445[0], 64446[0], 64447[0], 64448[0], 64449[0], 64450[0], 64451[0], 64454[0], 64461[0], 64462[0], 64463[0], 64479[0], 64480[0], 64483[0], 64484[0], 64486[0], 64487[0], 64488[0], 64489[0], 64490[0], 64491[0], 64492[0], 64493[0], 64494[0], 64495[0], 64505[0], 64510[0], 64517[0], 64520[0], 64530[0], 76000[1], 77001[1], 77002[1], 92012[1], 92014[1], 92585[0], 93000[1], 93005[1], 93010[1], 93040[1], 93041[1], 93042[1], 93318[1], 93355[1], 94002[1], 94200[1], 94250[1], 94680[1], 94681[1], 94690[1], 94770[1], 95812[1], 95813[1], 95816[1], 95819[1], 95822[0], 95829[1], 95860[0], 95861[0], 95863[0], 95864[0], 95865[0], 95866[0], 95867[0], 95868[0], 95869[0], 95870[0], 95907[0], 95908[0], 95909[0], 95910[0], 95911[0], 95912[0], 95913[0], 95925[0], 95926[0], 95927[0], 95928[0], 95929[0], 95930[0], 95933[0], 95937[0], 95938[0], 95939[0], 95940[0], 95955[1], 96360[1], 96361[1], 96365[1], 96366[1], 96367[1], 96368[1], 96372[1], 96374[1], 96375[1], 96376[1], 96377[1], 96523[0], 97597[1], 97598[1], 97602[1], 99155[0], 99156[0], 99157[0], 99211[1], 99212[1], 99213[1], 99214[1], 99215[1], 99217[1], 99218[1], 99219[1], 99220[1], 99221[1], 99222[1], 99223[1], 99231[1], 99232[1], 99233[1], 99234[1], 99235[1], 99236[1], 99238[1], 99239[1], 99241[1], 99242[1], 99243[1], 99244[1], 99245[1], 99251[1], 99252[1], 99253[1], 99254[1], 99255[1], 99291[1], 99292[1], 99304[1], 99305[1], 99306[1], 99307[1], 99308[1], 99309[1], 99310[1], 99315[1], 99316[1], 99334[1], 99335[1], 99336[1], 99337[1], 99347[1], 99348[1], 99349[1], 99350[1], 99374[1], 99375[1], 99377[1], 99378[1], 99446[0], 99447[0], 99448[0], 99449[0], 99451[0], 99452[0], 99495[0], 99496[0], G0453[0], G0463[1], G0471[1]
63082	0333T[0], 0464T[0], 11000[1], 11001[1], 11004[1], 11005[1], 11006[1], 11042[1], 11043[1], 11044[1], 11045[1], 11046[1], 11047[1], 36591[0], 36592[0], 38220[0], 38221[1], 38222[0], 38230[0], 38232[0], 63075[1], 63707[1], 63709[1], 92585[0], 95822[0], 95860[0], 95861[0], 95863[0], 95864[0], 95865[0], 95866[0], 95867[0], 95868[0], 95869[0], 95907[0], 95908[0], 95909[0], 95910[0], 95911[0], 95912[0], 95913[0], 95925[0], 95926[0], 95927[0], 95930[0], 95933[0], 95937[0], 95938[0], 95939[0], 95940[0], 96523[0], 97597[1], 97598[1], 97602[1], G0453[0]
63085	0213T[0], 0216T[0], 0228T[0], 0230T[0], 0333T[0], 0464T[0], 11000[1], 11001[1], 11004[1], 11005[1], 11006[1], 11042[1], 11043[1], 11044[1], 11045[1], 11046[1], 11047[1], 12001[1], 12002[1], 12004[1], 12005[1], 12006[1], 12007[1], 12011[1], 12013[1], 12014[1], 12015[1], 12016[1], 12017[1], 12018[1], 12020[1], 12021[1], 12031[1], 12032[1], 12034[1], 12035[1], 12036[1], 12037[1], 12041[1], 12042[1], 12044[1], 12045[1], 12046[1], 12047[1], 12051[1], 12052[1], 12053[1], 12054[1], 12055[1], 12056[1], 12057[1], 13100[1], 13101[1], 13102[1], 13120[1], 13121[1], 13122[1], 13131[1], 13132[1], 13133[1], 13151[1], 13152[1], 13153[1], 22100[1], 22101[1], 22102[1], 22110[1], 22112[1], 22114[1], 22208[1], 22505[0], 22551[1], 32100[1], 36000[1], 36400[1], 36405[1], 36406[1], 36410[1], 36420[1], 36425[1], 36430[1], 36440[1], 36591[0], 36592[0], 36600[1], 36640[1], 38220[0], 38221[1], 38222[0], 38230[0], 38232[0], 39540[0], 43752[1], 49000[0], 51701[1], 51702[1], 51703[1], 62320[0], 62321[0], 62322[0], 62323[0], 62324[0], 62325[0], 62326[0], 62327[0], 63003[1], 63075[1], 63077[1], 63078[1], 63707[1], 63709[1], 64400[0], 64405[0], 64408[0], 64415[0], 64416[0], 64417[0], 64418[0], 64420[0], 64421[0], 64425[0], 64430[0], 64435[0], 64445[0], 64446[0], 64447[0], 64448[0], 64449[0], 64450[0], 64451[0], 64454[0], 64461[0], 64462[0], 64463[0], 64479[0], 64480[0], 64483[0], 64484[0], 64486[0], 64487[0], 64488[0], 64489[0], 64490[0], 64491[0], 64492[0], 64493[0], 64494[0], 64495[0], 64505[0], 64510[0], 64517[0], 64520[0], 64530[0], 76000[1], 77001[1], 77002[1], 92012[1], 92014[1], 92585[0], 93000[1], 93005[1], 93010[1], 93040[1], 93041[1], 93042[1], 93318[1], 93355[1], 94002[1], 94200[1], 94250[1], 94680[1], 94681[1], 94690[1], 94770[1], 95812[1], 95813[1], 95816[1], 95819[1], 95822[0], 95829[1], 95860[0], 95861[0], 95863[0], 95864[0], 95865[0], 95866[0], 95867[0], 95868[0], 95869[0], 95870[0], 95907[0], 95908[0], 95909[0], 95910[0], 95911[0], 95912[0], 95913[0], 95925[0], 95926[0], 95927[0], 95928[0], 95929[0], 95930[0], 95933[0], 95937[0], 95938[0], 95939[0], 95940[0], 95955[1], 96360[1], 96361[1], 96365[1], 96366[1], 96367[1], 96368[1], 96372[1], 96374[1], 96375[1], 96376[1], 96377[1],

0 = Modifier usage not allowed or inappropriate 1 = Modifier usage allowed

Code 1	Code 2
	96523[0], 97597[1], 97598[1], 97602[1], 99155[0], 99156[0], 99157[0], 99211[1], 99212[1], 99213[1], 99214[1], 99215[1], 99217[1], 99218[1], 99219[1], 99220[1], 99221[1], 99222[1], 99223[1], 99231[1], 99232[1], 99233[1], 99234[1], 99235[1], 99236[1], 99238[1], 99239[1], 99241[1], 99242[1], 99243[1], 99244[1], 99245[1], 99251[1], 99252[1], 99253[1], 99254[1], 99255[1], 99291[1], 99292[1], 99304[1], 99305[1], 99306[1], 99307[1], 99308[1], 99309[1], 99310[1], 99315[1], 99316[1], 99334[1], 99335[1], 99336[1], 99337[1], 99347[1], 99348[1], 99349[1], 99350[1], 99374[1], 99375[1], 99377[1], 99378[1], 99446[0], 99447[0], 99448[0], 99449[0], 99451[0], 99452[0], 99495[0], 99496[0], G0453[0], G0463[1], G0471[1]
63086	0333T[0], 0464T[0], 11000[1], 11001[1], 11004[1], 11005[1], 11006[1], 11042[1], 11043[1], 11044[1], 11045[1], 11046[1], 11047[1], 36591[0], 36592[0], 38220[0], 38221[1], 38222[0], 38230[0], 38232[0], 63707[1], 63709[1], 92585[0], 95822[0], 95860[0], 95861[0], 95863[0], 95864[0], 95865[0], 95866[0], 95867[0], 95868[0], 95869[0], 95907[0], 95908[0], 95909[0], 95910[0], 95911[0], 95912[0], 95913[0], 95925[0], 95926[0], 95927[0], 95930[0], 95933[0], 95937[0], 95938[0], 95939[0], 95940[0], 96523[0], 97597[1], 97598[1], 97602[1], G0453[0]
63087	0213T[0], 0216T[0], 0228T[0], 0230T[0], 0275T[1], 0333T[0], 0464T[0], 11000[1], 11001[1], 11004[1], 11005[1], 11006[1], 11042[1], 11043[1], 11044[1], 11045[1], 11046[1], 11047[1], 12001[1], 12002[1], 12004[1], 12005[1], 12006[1], 12007[1], 12011[1], 12013[1], 12014[1], 12015[1], 12016[1], 12017[1], 12018[1], 12020[1], 12021[1], 12031[1], 12032[1], 12034[1], 12035[1], 12036[1], 12037[1], 12041[1], 12042[1], 12044[1], 12045[1], 12046[1], 12047[1], 12051[1], 12052[1], 12053[1], 12054[1], 12055[1], 12056[1], 12057[1], 13100[1], 13101[1], 13102[1], 13120[1], 13121[1], 13122[1], 13131[1], 13132[1], 13133[1], 13151[1], 13152[1], 13153[1], 22100[1], 22101[1], 22102[1], 22110[1], 22112[1], 22114[1], 22208[1], 22505[0], 22551[1], 22857[1], 22862[1], 22865[1], 22867[1], 22868[1], 22869[1], 22870[1], 32096[1], 32097[1], 32098[1], 32100[1], 36000[1], 36400[1], 36405[1], 36406[1], 36410[1], 36420[1], 36425[1], 36430[1], 36440[1], 36591[0], 36592[0], 36600[1], 36640[1], 38220[0], 38221[1], 38222[0], 38230[0], 38232[0], 39540[0], 43336[0], 43337[0], 43752[1], 49000[0], 49002[1], 49010[0], 51701[1], 51702[1], 51703[1], 62287[1], 62320[0], 62321[0], 62322[0], 62323[0], 62324[0], 62325[0], 62326[0], 62327[0], 62380[1], 63003[1], 63075[1], 63077[1], 63078[1], 63085[1], 63090[1], 63101[1], 63102[1], 63707[1], 63709[1], 64400[0], 64405[0], 64408[0], 64415[0], 64416[0], 64417[0], 64418[0], 64420[0], 64421[0], 64425[0], 64430[0], 64435[0], 64445[0], 64446[0], 64447[0], 64448[0], 64449[0], 64450[0], 64451[0], 64454[0], 64461[0], 64462[0], 64463[0], 64479[0], 64480[0], 64483[0], 64484[0], 64486[0], 64487[0], 64488[0], 64489[0], 64490[0], 64491[0], 64492[0], 64493[0], 64494[0], 64495[0], 64505[0], 64510[0], 64517[0], 64520[0], 64530[0], 76000[1], 77001[1], 77002[1], 92012[1], 92014[1], 92585[0], 93000[1], 93005[1], 93010[1], 93040[1], 93041[1], 93042[1], 93318[1], 93355[1], 94002[1], 94200[1], 94250[1], 94680[1], 94681[1], 94690[1], 94770[1], 95812[1], 95813[1], 95816[1], 95819[1], 95822[0], 95829[1], 95860[0], 95861[0], 95863[0], 95864[0], 95865[0], 95866[0], 95867[0], 95868[0], 95869[0], 95870[0], 95907[0], 95908[0], 95909[0], 95910[0], 95911[0], 95912[0], 95913[0], 95925[0], 95926[0], 95927[0], 95928[0], 95929[0], 95930[0], 95933[0], 95937[0], 95938[0], 95939[0], 95940[0], 95955[1], 96360[1], 96361[1], 96365[1], 96366[1], 96367[1], 96368[1], 96372[1], 96374[1], 96375[1], 96376[1], 96377[1], 96523[0], 97597[1], 97598[1], 97602[1], 99155[0], 99156[0], 99157[0], 99211[1], 99212[1], 99213[1], 99214[1], 99215[1], 99217[1], 99218[1], 99219[1], 99220[1], 99221[1], 99222[1], 99223[1], 99231[1], 99232[1], 99233[1], 99234[1], 99235[1], 99236[1], 99238[1], 99239[1], 99241[1], 99242[1], 99243[1], 99244[1], 99245[1], 99251[1], 99252[1], 99253[1], 99254[1], 99255[1], 99291[1], 99292[1], 99304[1], 99305[1], 99306[1], 99307[1], 99308[1], 99309[1], 99310[1], 99315[1], 99316[1], 99334[1], 99335[1], 99336[1], 99337[1], 99347[1], 99348[1], 99349[1], 99350[1], 99374[1], 99375[1], 99377[1], 99378[1], 99446[0], 99447[0], 99448[0], 99449[0], 99451[0], 99452[0], 99495[0], 99496[0], G0453[0], G0463[1], G0471[1]
63088	0333T[0], 0464T[0], 11000[1], 11001[1], 11004[1], 11005[1], 11006[1], 11042[1], 11043[1], 11044[1], 11045[1], 11046[1], 11047[1], 22867[1], 22868[1], 22869[1], 22870[1], 36591[0], 36592[0], 38220[0], 38221[1], 38222[0], 38230[0], 38232[0], 63707[1], 63709[1], 92585[0], 95822[0], 95860[0], 95861[0], 95863[0], 95864[0], 95865[0], 95866[0], 95867[0], 95868[0], 95869[0], 95907[0], 95908[0], 95909[0], 95910[0], 95911[0], 95912[0], 95913[0], 95925[0], 95926[0], 95927[0], 95930[0], 95933[0], 95937[0], 95938[0], 95939[0], 95940[0], 96523[0], 97597[1], 97598[1], 97602[1], G0453[0]
63090	0213T[0], 0216T[0], 0228T[0], 0230T[0], 0275T[1], 0333T[0], 0464T[0], 11000[1], 11001[1], 11004[1], 11005[1], 11006[1], 11042[1], 11043[1], 11044[1], 11045[1], 11046[1], 11047[1], 12001[1], 12002[1], 12004[1], 12005[1], 12006[1], 12007[1], 12011[1], 12013[1], 12014[1], 12015[1], 12016[1], 12017[1], 12018[1], 12020[1], 12021[1], 12031[1], 12032[1], 12034[1], 12035[1], 12036[1], 12037[1], 12041[1], 12042[1], 12044[1], 12045[1], 12046[1], 12047[1], 12051[1], 12052[1], 12053[1], 12054[1], 12055[1], 12056[1], 12057[1], 13100[1], 13101[1], 13102[1], 13120[1], 13121[1], 13122[1], 13131[1], 13132[1], 13133[1], 13151[1], 13152[1], 13153[1], 22208[1], 22505[0], 22551[1], 22857[1], 22862[1], 22865[1], 22867[1], 22868[1], 22869[1], 22870[1], 32100[1], 36000[1], 36400[1], 36405[1], 36406[1], 36410[1], 36420[1], 36425[1], 36430[1], 36440[1], 36591[0], 36592[0], 36600[1], 36640[1], 38220[0], 38221[1], 38222[0], 38230[0], 38232[0], 39540[0], 43752[1], 49000[0], 49002[1], 51701[1], 51702[1], 51703[1], 62287[1], 62320[0], 62321[0], 62322[0], 62323[0], 62324[0], 62325[0], 62326[0], 62327[0], 62380[1], 63003[1], 63064[1], 63075[1], 63077[1], 63078[1], 63085[1], 63170[1], 63707[1], 63709[1], 64400[0], 64405[0], 64408[0], 64415[0], 64416[0], 64417[0], 64418[0], 64420[0], 64421[0], 64425[0], 64430[0], 64435[0], 64445[0], 64446[0], 64447[0], 64448[0], 64449[0], 64450[0], 64451[0], 64454[0], 64461[0], 64462[0], 64463[0], 64479[0], 64480[0], 64483[0], 64484[0], 64486[0], 64487[0], 64488[0], 64489[0], 64490[0], 64491[0], 64492[0], 64493[0], 64494[0], 64495[0], 64505[0], 64510[0], 64517[0], 64520[0], 64530[0], 76000[1], 77001[1], 77002[1], 92012[1], 92014[1], 92585[0], 93000[1], 93005[1], 93010[1], 93040[1], 93041[1], 93042[1], 93318[1], 93355[1], 94002[1], 94200[1], 94250[1], 94680[1], 94681[1], 94690[1], 94770[1], 95812[1], 95813[1], 95816[1], 95819[1], 95822[0], 95829[1], 95860[0], 95861[0], 95863[0], 95864[0], 95865[0], 95866[0], 95867[0], 95868[0], 95869[0], 95870[0], 95907[0], 95908[0], 95909[0], 95910[0], 95911[0], 95912[0], 95913[0], 95925[0], 95926[0], 95927[0], 95928[0], 95929[0], 95930[0], 95933[0], 95937[0], 95938[0], 95939[0], 95940[0], 95955[1], 96360[1], 96361[1], 96365[1], 96366[1], 96367[1], 96368[1], 96372[1], 96374[1], 96375[1], 96376[1], 96377[1], 96523[0], 97597[1], 97598[1], 97602[1], 99155[0], 99156[0], 99157[0], 99211[1], 99212[1], 99213[1], 99214[1], 99215[1], 99217[1], 99218[1], 99219[1], 99220[1], 99221[1], 99222[1], 99223[1], 99231[1], 99232[1], 99233[1], 99234[1], 99235[1], 99236[1], 99238[1], 99239[1], 99241[1], 99242[1], 99243[1], 99244[1], 99245[1], 99251[1], 99252[1], 99253[1], 99254[1], 99255[1], 99291[1], 99292[1], 99304[1], 99305[1], 99306[1], 99307[1], 99308[1], 99309[1], 99310[1], 99315[1], 99316[1], 99334[1], 99335[1], 99336[1], 99337[1], 99347[1], 99348[1], 99349[1], 99350[1], 99374[1], 99375[1], 99377[1], 99378[1], 99446[0], 99447[0], 99448[0], 99449[0], 99451[0], 99452[0], 99495[0], 99496[0], G0453[0], G0463[1], G0471[1]
63091	0333T[0], 0464T[0], 11000[1], 11001[1], 11004[1], 11005[1], 11006[1], 11042[1], 11043[1], 11044[1], 11045[1], 11046[1], 11047[1], 22867[1], 22868[1], 22869[1], 22870[1], 36591[0], 36592[0], 38220[0], 38221[1], 38222[0], 38230[0], 38232[0], 63707[1], 63709[1], 92585[0], 95822[0], 95860[0], 95861[0], 95863[0], 95864[0], 95865[0], 95866[0], 95867[0], 95868[0], 95869[0], 95907[0], 95908[0], 95909[0], 95910[0], 95911[0], 95912[0], 95913[0], 95925[0], 95926[0], 95927[0], 95930[0], 95933[0], 95937[0], 95938[0], 95939[0], 95940[0], 96523[0], 97597[1], 97598[1], 97602[1], G0453[0]
63101	0213T[0], 0216T[0], 0228T[0], 0230T[0], 0333T[0], 0464T[0], 11000[1], 11001[1], 11004[1], 11005[1], 11006[1], 11042[1], 11043[1], 11044[1], 11045[1], 11046[1], 11047[1], 12001[1], 12002[1], 12004[1], 12005[1], 12006[1], 12007[1], 12011[1], 12013[1], 12014[1], 12015[1], 12016[1], 12017[1], 12018[1], 12020[1], 12021[1], 12031[1], 12032[1], 12034[1], 12035[1], 12036[1], 12037[1], 12041[1], 12042[1], 12044[1], 12045[1], 12046[1], 12047[1], 12051[1], 12052[1], 12053[1], 12054[1], 12055[1], 12056[1], 12057[1], 13100[1], 13101[1], 13102[1], 13120[1], 13121[1], 13122[1], 13131[1], 13132[1], 13133[1], 13151[1], 13152[1], 13153[1], 22112[1], 22208[1], 22505[0], 36000[1], 36400[1], 36405[1], 36406[1], 36410[1], 36420[1], 36425[1], 36430[1], 36440[1], 36591[0], 36592[0], 36600[1], 36640[1], 38220[0], 38221[1], 38222[0], 38230[0], 38232[0], 43752[1], 51701[1], 51702[1], 51703[1], 62320[0], 62321[0], 62322[0], 62323[0], 62324[0], 62325[0], 62326[0], 62327[0], 63003[1], 63055[1], 63064[1], 63077[1], 63085[1], 63090[1], 63301[1], 63302[1], 63707[1], 63709[1], 64400[0], 64405[0], 64408[0], 64415[0], 64416[0], 64417[0], 64418[0], 64420[0], 64421[0], 64425[0], 64430[0], 64435[0], 64445[0], 64446[0], 64447[0], 64448[0], 64449[0], 64450[0], 64451[0], 64454[0], 64461[0], 64462[0], 64463[0], 64479[0], 64480[0], 64483[0], 64484[0], 64486[0], 64487[0], 64488[0], 64489[0], 64490[0], 64491[0], 64492[0], 64493[0], 64494[0], 64495[0], 64505[0], 64510[0], 64517[0], 64520[0], 64530[0], 76000[1], 77001[1], 77002[1], 92012[1], 92014[1], 92585[0], 93000[1], 93005[1], 93010[1], 93040[1], 93041[1], 93042[1], 93318[1], 93355[1], 94002[1], 94200[1], 94250[1], 94680[1], 94681[1], 94690[1], 94770[1], 95812[1], 95813[1], 95816[1], 95819[1], 95822[0], 95829[1], 95860[0], 95861[0], 95863[0], 95864[0], 95865[0], 95866[0], 95867[0], 95868[0], 95869[0], 95870[0], 95907[0], 95908[0], 95909[0], 95910[0], 95911[0], 95912[0], 95913[0], 95925[0], 95926[0], 95927[0], 95928[0], 95929[0], 95930[0], 95933[0], 95937[0], 95938[0], 95939[0], 95940[0], 95955[1], 96360[1], 96361[1], 96365[1], 96366[1], 96367[1], 96368[1], 96372[1], 96374[1], 96375[1], 96376[1], 96377[1], 96523[0], 97597[1], 97598[1], 97602[1], 99155[0], 99156[0], 99157[0], 99211[1], 99212[1], 99213[1], 99214[1], 99215[1], 99217[1], 99218[1], 99219[1], 99220[1], 99221[1], 99222[1], 99223[1], 99231[1], 99232[1], 99233[1], 99234[1], 99235[1], 99236[1], 99238[1], 99239[1], 99241[1], 99242[1], 99243[1], 99244[1], 99245[1], 99251[1], 99252[1], 99253[1], 99254[1], 99255[1], 99291[1], 99292[1], 99304[1], 99305[1], 99306[1], 99307[1], 99308[1], 99309[1], 99310[1], 99315[1], 99316[1], 99334[1], 99335[1], 99336[1], 99337[1], 99347[1], 99348[1], 99349[1], 99350[1], 99374[1], 99375[1], 99377[1], 99378[1], 99446[0], 99447[0], 99448[0], 99449[0], 99451[0], 99452[0], 99495[0], 99496[0], G0453[0], G0463[1], G0471[1]
63102	0213T[0], 0216T[0], 0228T[0], 0230T[0], 0275T[1], 0333T[0], 0464T[0], 11000[1], 11001[1], 11004[1], 11005[1], 11006[1], 11042[1], 11043[1], 11044[1], 11045[1], 11046[1], 11047[1], 12001[1], 12002[1], 12004[1], 12005[1], 12006[1], 12007[1], 12011[1], 12013[1], 12014[1], 12015[1], 12016[1], 12017[1], 12018[1], 12020[1], 12021[1], 12031[1], 12032[1], 12034[1], 12035[1], 12036[1], 12037[1], 12041[1], 12042[1], 12044[1], 12045[1], 12046[1], 12047[1], 12051[1], 12052[1], 12053[1], 12054[1], 12055[1], 12056[1], 12057[1], 13100[1], 13101[1], 13102[1], 13120[1], 13121[1], 13122[1], 13131[1], 13132[1], 13133[1], 13151[1], 13152[1], 13153[1], 22114[1], 22208[1], 22505[0], 22630[1], 22633[1], 22867[1], 22868[1], 22869[1], 22870[1], 36000[1], 36400[1], 36405[1], 36406[1], 36410[1], 36420[1], 36425[1], 36430[1], 36440[1], 36591[0], 36592[0], 36600[1], 36640[1], 38220[0], 38221[1], 38222[0], 38230[0], 38232[0], 43752[1], 51701[1], 51702[1], 51703[1], 62287[1], 62320[0], 62321[0], 62322[0], 62323[0], 62324[0], 62325[0], 62326[0], 62327[0], 62380[1], 63056[1], 63090[1], 63303[1], 63307[1], 63707[1], 63709[1], 64400[0], 64405[0], 64408[0], 64415[0], 64416[0], 64417[0], 64418[0], 64420[0], 64421[0], 64425[0], 64430[0], 64435[0], 64445[0], 64446[0], 64447[0], 64448[0], 64449[0], 64450[0], 64451[0],

0 = Modifier usage not allowed or inappropriate 1 = Modifier usage allowed

Code 1	Code 2
	64454[0], 64461[0], 64462[0], 64463[0], 64479[0], 64480[0], 64483[0], 64484[0], 64486[0], 64487[0], 64488[0], 64489[0], 64490[0], 64491[0], 64492[0], 64493[0], 64494[0], 64495[0], 64505[0], 64510[0], 64517[0], 64520[0], 64530[0], 76000[1], 77001[1], 77002[1], 92012[1], 92014[1], 92585[0], 93000[1], 93005[1], 93010[1], 93040[1], 93041[1], 93042[1], 93318[1], 93355[1], 94002[1], 94200[1], 94250[1], 94680[1], 94681[1], 94690[1], 94770[1], 95812[1], 95813[1], 95816[1], 95819[1], 95822[0], 95829[1], 95860[0], 95861[0], 95863[0], 95864[0], 95865[0], 95866[0], 95867[0], 95868[0], 95869[0], 95870[0], 95907[0], 95908[0], 95909[0], 95910[0], 95911[0], 95912[0], 95913[0], 95925[0], 95926[0], 95927[0], 95928[0], 95929[0], 95930[0], 95933[0], 95937[0], 95938[0], 95939[0], 95940[0], 95955[1], 96360[1], 96361[1], 96365[1], 96366[1], 96367[1], 96368[1], 96372[1], 96374[1], 96375[1], 96376[1], 96377[1], 96523[0], 97597[1], 97598[1], 97602[1], 99155[0], 99156[0], 99157[0], 99211[1], 99212[1], 99213[1], 99214[1], 99215[1], 99217[1], 99218[1], 99219[1], 99220[1], 99221[1], 99222[1], 99223[1], 99231[1], 99232[1], 99233[1], 99234[1], 99235[1], 99236[1], 99238[1], 99239[1], 99241[1], 99242[1], 99243[1], 99244[1], 99245[1], 99251[1], 99252[1], 99253[1], 99254[1], 99255[1], 99291[1], 99292[1], 99304[1], 99305[1], 99306[1], 99307[1], 99308[1], 99309[1], 99310[1], 99315[1], 99316[1], 99334[1], 99335[1], 99336[1], 99337[1], 99347[1], 99348[1], 99349[1], 99350[1], 99374[1], 99375[1], 99377[1], 99378[1], 99446[0], 99447[0], 99448[0], 99449[0], 99451[0], 99452[0], 99495[0], 99496[0], G0453[0], G0463[1], G0471[1]
63103	0333T[0], 0464T[0], 11000[1], 11001[1], 11004[1], 11005[1], 11006[1], 11042[1], 11043[1], 11044[1], 11045[1], 11046[1], 11047[1], 22867[1], 22868[1], 22869[1], 22870[1], 36591[0], 36592[0], 38220[0], 38221[1], 38222[0], 38230[0], 38232[0], 63707[1], 63709[1], 92585[0], 95822[0], 95860[0], 95861[0], 95863[0], 95864[0], 95865[0], 95866[0], 95867[0], 95868[0], 95869[0], 95907[0], 95908[0], 95909[0], 95910[0], 95911[0], 95912[0], 95913[0], 95925[0], 95926[0], 95927[0], 95930[0], 95933[0], 95937[0], 95938[0], 95939[0], 95940[0], 96523[0], 97597[1], 97598[1], 97602[1], G0453[0]
63172	0213T[0], 0216T[0], 0228T[0], 0230T[0], 0333T[0], 0464T[0], 0565T[1], 11000[1], 11001[1], 11004[1], 11005[1], 11006[1], 11042[1], 11043[1], 11044[1], 11045[1], 11046[1], 11047[1], 12001[1], 12002[1], 12004[1], 12005[1], 12006[1], 12007[1], 12011[1], 12013[1], 12014[1], 12015[1], 12016[1], 12017[1], 12018[1], 12020[1], 12021[1], 12031[1], 12032[1], 12034[1], 12035[1], 12036[1], 12037[1], 12041[1], 12042[1], 12044[1], 12045[1], 12046[1], 12047[1], 12051[1], 12052[1], 12053[1], 12054[1], 12055[1], 12056[1], 12057[1], 13100[1], 13101[1], 13102[1], 13120[1], 13121[1], 13122[1], 13131[1], 13132[1], 13133[1], 13151[1], 13152[1], 13153[1], 15769[1], 22505[0], 36000[1], 36400[1], 36405[1], 36406[1], 36410[1], 36420[1], 36425[1], 36430[1], 36440[1], 36591[0], 36592[0], 36600[1], 36640[1], 38220[0], 38222[0], 38230[0], 38232[0], 43752[1], 49000[0], 49002[1], 51701[1], 51702[1], 51703[1], 62320[0], 62321[0], 62322[0], 62323[0], 62324[0], 62325[0], 62326[0], 62327[0], 63173[1], 63707[1], 63709[1], 64400[0], 64405[0], 64408[0], 64415[0], 64416[0], 64417[0], 64418[0], 64420[0], 64421[0], 64425[0], 64430[0], 64435[0], 64445[0], 64446[0], 64447[0], 64448[0], 64449[0], 64450[0], 64451[0], 64454[0], 64461[0], 64462[0], 64463[0], 64479[0], 64480[0], 64483[0], 64484[0], 64486[0], 64487[0], 64488[0], 64489[0], 64490[0], 64491[0], 64492[0], 64493[0], 64494[0], 64495[0], 64505[0], 64510[0], 64517[0], 64520[0], 64530[0], 76000[1], 77001[1], 77002[1], 92012[1], 92014[1], 92585[0], 93000[1], 93005[1], 93010[1], 93040[1], 93041[1], 93042[1], 93318[1], 93355[1], 94002[1], 94200[1], 94250[1], 94680[1], 94681[1], 94690[1], 94770[1], 95812[1], 95813[1], 95816[1], 95819[1], 95822[0], 95829[1], 95860[0], 95861[0], 95863[0], 95864[0], 95865[0], 95866[0], 95867[0], 95868[0], 95869[0], 95870[0], 95907[0], 95908[0], 95909[0], 95910[0], 95911[0], 95912[0], 95913[0], 95925[0], 95926[0], 95927[0], 95928[0], 95929[0], 95930[0], 95933[0], 95937[0], 95938[0], 95939[0], 95940[0], 95955[1], 96360[1], 96361[1], 96365[1], 96366[1], 96367[1], 96368[1], 96372[1], 96374[1], 96375[1], 96376[1], 96377[1], 96523[0], 97597[1], 97598[1], 97602[1], 99155[0], 99156[0], 99157[0], 99211[1], 99212[1], 99213[1], 99214[1], 99215[1], 99217[1], 99218[1], 99219[1], 99220[1], 99221[1], 99222[1], 99223[1], 99231[1], 99232[1], 99233[1], 99234[1], 99235[1], 99236[1], 99238[1], 99239[1], 99241[1], 99242[1], 99243[1], 99244[1], 99245[1], 99251[1], 99252[1], 99253[1], 99254[1], 99255[1], 99291[1], 99292[1], 99304[1], 99305[1], 99306[1], 99307[1], 99308[1], 99309[1], 99310[1], 99315[1], 99316[1], 99334[1], 99335[1], 99336[1], 99337[1], 99347[1], 99348[1], 99349[1], 99350[1], 99374[1], 99375[1], 99377[1], 99378[1], 99446[0], 99447[0], 99448[0], 99449[0], 99451[0], 99452[0], 99495[0], 99496[0], G0453[0], G0463[1], G0471[1]
63173	0213T[0], 0216T[0], 0228T[0], 0230T[0], 0333T[0], 0464T[0], 0565T[1], 11000[1], 11001[1], 11004[1], 11005[1], 11006[1], 11042[1], 11043[1], 11044[1], 11045[1], 11046[1], 11047[1], 12001[1], 12002[1], 12004[1], 12005[1], 12006[1], 12007[1], 12011[1], 12013[1], 12014[1], 12015[1], 12016[1], 12017[1], 12018[1], 12020[1], 12021[1], 12031[1], 12032[1], 12034[1], 12035[1], 12036[1], 12037[1], 12041[1], 12042[1], 12044[1], 12045[1], 12046[1], 12047[1], 12051[1], 12052[1], 12053[1], 12054[1], 12055[1], 12056[1], 12057[1], 13100[1], 13101[1], 13102[1], 13120[1], 13121[1], 13122[1], 13131[1], 13132[1], 13133[1], 13151[1], 13152[1], 13153[1], 15769[1], 22505[0], 32096[1], 32097[1], 32098[1], 32100[1], 32551[1], 32554[1], 32555[1], 32556[1], 32557[1], 36000[1], 36400[1], 36405[1], 36406[1], 36410[1], 36420[1], 36425[1], 36430[1], 36440[1], 36591[0], 36592[0], 36600[1], 36640[1], 38220[0], 38222[0], 38230[0], 38232[0], 43752[1], 49000[0], 49002[1], 51701[1], 51702[1], 51703[1], 62320[0], 62321[0], 62322[0], 62323[0], 62324[0], 62325[0], 62326[0], 62327[0], 63707[1], 63709[1], 64400[0], 64405[0], 64408[0], 64415[0], 64416[0], 64417[0], 64418[0], 64420[0], 64421[0], 64425[0], 64430[0], 64435[0], 64445[0], 64446[0], 64447[0], 64448[0], 64449[0], 64450[0], 64451[0], 64454[0], 64461[0], 64462[0], 64463[0], 64479[0], 64480[0], 64483[0], 64484[0], 64486[0], 64487[0], 64488[0], 64489[0], 64490[0], 64491[0], 64492[0], 64493[0], 64494[0], 64495[0], 64505[0], 64510[0], 64517[0], 64520[0], 64530[0], 76000[1], 77001[1], 77002[1], 92012[1], 92014[1], 92585[0], 93000[1], 93005[1], 93010[1], 93040[1], 93041[1], 93042[1], 93318[1], 93355[1], 94002[1], 94200[1], 94250[1], 94680[1], 94681[1], 94690[1], 94770[1], 95812[1], 95813[1], 95816[1], 95819[1], 95822[0], 95829[1], 95860[0], 95861[0], 95863[0], 95864[0], 95865[0], 95866[0], 95867[0], 95868[0], 95869[0], 95870[0], 95907[0], 95908[0], 95909[0], 95910[0], 95911[0], 95912[0], 95913[0], 95925[0], 95926[0], 95927[0], 95928[0], 95929[0], 95930[0], 95933[0], 95937[0], 95938[0], 95939[0], 95940[0], 95955[1], 96360[1], 96361[1], 96365[1], 96366[1], 96367[1], 96368[1], 96372[1], 96374[1], 96375[1], 96376[1], 96377[1], 96523[0], 97597[1], 97598[1], 97602[1], 99155[0], 99156[0], 99157[0], 99211[1], 99212[1], 99213[1], 99214[1], 99215[1], 99217[1], 99218[1], 99219[1], 99220[1], 99221[1], 99222[1], 99223[1], 99231[1], 99232[1], 99233[1], 99234[1], 99235[1], 99236[1], 99238[1], 99239[1], 99241[1], 99242[1], 99243[1], 99244[1], 99245[1], 99251[1], 99252[1], 99253[1], 99254[1], 99255[1], 99291[1], 99292[1], 99304[1], 99305[1], 99306[1], 99307[1], 99308[1], 99309[1], 99310[1], 99315[1], 99316[1], 99334[1], 99335[1], 99336[1], 99337[1], 99347[1], 99348[1], 99349[1], 99350[1], 99374[1], 99375[1], 99377[1], 99378[1], 99446[0], 99447[0], 99448[0], 99449[0], 99451[0], 99452[0], 99495[0], 99496[0], G0453[0], G0463[1], G0471[1]
63185	0213T[0], 0216T[0], 0228T[0], 0230T[0], 0333T[0], 0464T[0], 0565T[1], 11000[1], 11001[1], 11004[1], 11005[1], 11006[1], 11042[1], 11043[1], 11044[1], 11045[1], 11046[1], 11047[1], 12001[1], 12002[1], 12004[1], 12005[1], 12006[1], 12007[1], 12011[1], 12013[1], 12014[1], 12015[1], 12016[1], 12017[1], 12018[1], 12020[1], 12021[1], 12031[1], 12032[1], 12034[1], 12035[1], 12036[1], 12037[1], 12041[1], 12042[1], 12044[1], 12045[1], 12046[1], 12047[1], 12051[1], 12052[1], 12053[1], 12054[1], 12055[1], 12056[1], 12057[1], 13100[1], 13101[1], 13102[1], 13120[1], 13121[1], 13122[1], 13131[1], 13132[1], 13133[1], 13151[1], 13152[1], 13153[1], 15769[1], 22505[0], 22867[1], 22868[1], 22869[1], 22870[1], 36000[1], 36400[1], 36405[1], 36406[1], 36410[1], 36420[1], 36425[1], 36430[1], 36440[1], 36591[0], 36592[0], 36600[1], 36640[1], 38220[0], 38222[0], 38230[0], 38232[0], 43752[1], 49000[0], 49002[1], 51701[1], 51702[1], 51703[1], 62320[0], 62321[0], 62322[0], 62323[0], 62324[0], 62325[0], 62326[0], 62327[0], 63190[1], 63707[1], 63709[1], 64400[0], 64405[0], 64408[0], 64415[0], 64416[0], 64417[0], 64418[0], 64420[0], 64421[0], 64425[0], 64430[0], 64435[0], 64445[0], 64446[0], 64447[0], 64448[0], 64449[0], 64450[0], 64451[0], 64454[0], 64461[0], 64462[0], 64463[0], 64479[0], 64480[0], 64483[0], 64484[0], 64486[0], 64487[0], 64488[0], 64489[0], 64490[0], 64491[0], 64492[0], 64493[0], 64494[0], 64495[0], 64505[0], 64510[0], 64517[0], 64520[0], 64530[0], 76000[1], 77001[1], 77002[1], 92012[1], 92014[1], 92585[0], 93000[1], 93005[1], 93010[1], 93040[1], 93041[1], 93042[1], 93318[1], 93355[1], 94002[1], 94200[1], 94250[1], 94680[1], 94681[1], 94690[1], 94770[1], 95812[1], 95813[1], 95816[1], 95819[1], 95822[0], 95829[1], 95860[0], 95861[0], 95863[0], 95864[0], 95865[0], 95866[0], 95867[0], 95868[0], 95869[0], 95870[0], 95907[0], 95908[0], 95909[0], 95910[0], 95911[0], 95912[0], 95913[0], 95925[0], 95926[0], 95927[0], 95928[0], 95929[0], 95930[0], 95933[0], 95937[0], 95938[0], 95939[0], 95940[0], 95955[1], 96360[1], 96361[1], 96365[1], 96366[1], 96367[1], 96368[1], 96372[1], 96374[1], 96375[1], 96376[1], 96377[1], 96523[0], 97597[1], 97598[1], 97602[1], 99155[0], 99156[0], 99157[0], 99211[1], 99212[1], 99213[1], 99214[1], 99215[1], 99217[1], 99218[1], 99219[1], 99220[1], 99221[1], 99222[1], 99223[1], 99231[1], 99232[1], 99233[1], 99234[1], 99235[1], 99236[1], 99238[1], 99239[1], 99241[1], 99242[1], 99243[1], 99244[1], 99245[1], 99251[1], 99252[1], 99253[1], 99254[1], 99255[1], 99291[1], 99292[1], 99304[1], 99305[1], 99306[1], 99307[1], 99308[1], 99309[1], 99310[1], 99315[1], 99316[1], 99334[1], 99335[1], 99336[1], 99337[1], 99347[1], 99348[1], 99349[1], 99350[1], 99374[1], 99375[1], 99377[1], 99378[1], 99446[0], 99447[0], 99448[0], 99449[0], 99451[0], 99452[0], 99495[0], 99496[0], G0453[0], G0463[1], G0471[1]
63190	0213T[0], 0216T[0], 0228T[0], 0230T[0], 0333T[0], 0464T[0], 0565T[1], 11000[1], 11001[1], 11004[1], 11005[1], 11006[1], 11042[1], 11043[1], 11044[1], 11045[1], 11046[1], 11047[1], 12001[1], 12002[1], 12004[1], 12005[1], 12006[1], 12007[1], 12011[1], 12013[1], 12014[1], 12015[1], 12016[1], 12017[1], 12018[1], 12020[1], 12021[1], 12031[1], 12032[1], 12034[1], 12035[1], 12036[1], 12037[1], 12041[1], 12042[1], 12044[1], 12045[1], 12046[1], 12047[1], 12051[1], 12052[1], 12053[1], 12054[1], 12055[1], 12056[1], 12057[1], 13100[1], 13101[1], 13102[1], 13120[1], 13121[1], 13122[1], 13131[1], 13132[1], 13133[1], 13151[1], 13152[1], 13153[1], 15769[1], 22505[0], 22867[1], 22868[1], 22869[1], 22870[1], 36000[1], 36400[1], 36405[1], 36406[1], 36410[1], 36420[1], 36425[1], 36430[1], 36440[1], 36591[0], 36592[0], 36600[1], 36640[1], 38220[0], 38222[0], 38230[0], 38232[0], 43752[1], 49000[0], 49002[1], 51701[1], 51702[1], 51703[1], 62320[0], 62321[0], 62322[0], 62323[0], 62324[0], 62325[0], 62326[0], 62327[0], 63707[1], 63709[1], 64400[0], 64405[0], 64408[0], 64415[0], 64416[0], 64417[0], 64418[0], 64420[0], 64421[0], 64425[0], 64430[0], 64435[0], 64445[0], 64446[0], 64447[0], 64448[0], 64449[0], 64450[0], 64451[0], 64454[0], 64461[0], 64462[0], 64463[0], 64479[0], 64480[0], 64483[0], 64484[0], 64486[0], 64487[0], 64488[0], 64489[0], 64490[0], 64491[0], 64492[0], 64493[0], 64494[0], 64495[0], 64505[0], 64510[0], 64517[0], 64520[0], 64530[0], 76000[1], 77001[1], 77002[1], 92012[1], 92014[1], 92585[0], 93000[1], 93005[1], 93010[1], 93040[1], 93041[1], 93042[1], 93318[1], 93355[1], 94002[1], 94200[1], 94250[1], 94680[1], 94681[1], 94690[1], 94770[1], 95812[1], 95813[1], 95816[1], 95819[1], 95822[0], 95829[1], 95860[0], 95861[0], 95863[0], 95864[0], 95865[0], 95866[0], 95867[0], 95868[0], 95869[0], 95870[0], 95907[0], 95908[0], 95909[0], 95910[0], 95911[0], 95912[0], 95913[0], 95925[0], 95926[0], 95927[0], 95928[0], 95929[0], 95930[0], 95933[0], 95937[0], 95938[0], 95939[0], 95940[0], 95955[1], 96360[1], 96361[1], 96365[1], 96366[1], 96367[1], 96368[1], 96372[1], 96374[1], 96375[1], 96376[1], 96377[1], 96523[0], 97597[1], 97598[1], 97602[1], 99155[0], 99156[0], 99157[0], 99211[1],

0 = Modifier usage not allowed or inappropriate 1 = Modifier usage allowed

Code 1	Code 2
	99212[1], 99213[1], 99214[1], 99215[1], 99217[1], 99218[1], 99219[1], 99220[1], 99221[1], 99222[1], 99223[1], 99231[1], 99232[1], 99233[1], 99234[1], 99235[1], 99236[1], 99238[1], 99239[1], 99241[1], 99242[1], 99243[1], 99244[1], 99245[1], 99251[1], 99252[1], 99253[1], 99254[1], 99255[1], 99291[1], 99292[1], 99304[1], 99305[1], 99306[1], 99307[1], 99308[1], 99309[1], 99310[1], 99315[1], 99316[1], 99334[1], 99335[1], 99336[1], 99337[1], 99347[1], 99348[1], 99349[1], 99350[1], 99374[1], 99375[1], 99377[1], 99378[1], 99446[0], 99447[0], 99448[0], 99449[0], 99451[0], 99452[0], 99495[0], 99496[0], G0453[0], G0463[1], G0471[1]
63198	0213T[0], 0216T[0], 0228T[0], 0230T[0], 0333T[0], 0464T[0], 0565T[1], 11000[1], 11001[1], 11004[1], 11005[1], 11006[1], 11042[1], 11043[1], 11044[1], 11045[1], 11046[1], 11047[1], 12001[1], 12002[1], 12004[1], 12005[1], 12006[1], 12007[1], 12011[1], 12013[1], 12014[1], 12015[1], 12016[1], 12017[1], 12018[1], 12020[1], 12021[1], 12031[1], 12032[1], 12034[1], 12035[1], 12036[1], 12037[1], 12041[1], 12042[1], 12044[1], 12045[1], 12046[1], 12047[1], 12051[1], 12052[1], 12053[1], 12054[1], 12055[1], 12056[1], 12057[1], 13100[1], 13101[1], 13102[1], 13120[1], 13121[1], 13122[1], 13131[1], 13132[1], 13133[1], 13151[1], 13152[1], 13153[1], 15769[1], 22505[0], 36000[1], 36400[1], 36405[1], 36406[1], 36410[1], 36420[1], 36425[1], 36430[1], 36440[1], 36591[0], 36592[0], 36600[1], 36640[1], 38220[0], 38222[0], 38230[0], 38232[0], 43752[1], 51701[1], 51702[1], 51703[1], 62320[0], 62321[0], 62322[0], 62323[0], 62324[0], 62325[0], 62326[0], 62327[0], 63194[1], 63196[1], 63707[1], 63709[1], 64400[0], 64405[0], 64408[0], 64415[0], 64416[0], 64417[0], 64418[0], 64420[0], 64421[0], 64425[0], 64430[0], 64435[0], 64445[0], 64446[0], 64447[0], 64448[0], 64449[0], 64450[0], 64451[0], 64454[0], 64461[0], 64462[0], 64463[0], 64479[0], 64480[0], 64483[0], 64484[0], 64486[0], 64487[0], 64488[0], 64489[0], 64490[0], 64491[0], 64492[0], 64493[0], 64494[0], 64495[0], 64505[0], 64510[0], 64517[0], 64520[0], 64530[0], 76000[1], 77001[1], 77002[1], 92012[1], 92014[1], 92585[0], 93000[1], 93005[1], 93010[1], 93040[1], 93041[1], 93042[1], 93318[1], 93355[1], 94002[1], 94200[1], 94250[1], 94680[1], 94681[1], 94690[1], 94770[1], 95812[1], 95813[1], 95816[1], 95819[1], 95822[0], 95829[1], 95860[0], 95861[0], 95863[0], 95864[0], 95865[0], 95866[0], 95867[0], 95868[0], 95869[0], 95870[0], 95907[0], 95908[0], 95909[0], 95910[0], 95911[0], 95912[0], 95913[0], 95925[0], 95926[0], 95927[0], 95928[0], 95929[0], 95930[0], 95933[0], 95937[0], 95938[0], 95939[0], 95940[0], 95955[1], 96360[1], 96361[1], 96365[1], 96366[1], 96367[1], 96368[1], 96372[1], 96374[1], 96375[1], 96376[1], 96377[1], 96523[0], 97597[1], 97598[1], 97602[1], 99155[0], 99156[0], 99157[0], 99211[1], 99212[1], 99213[1], 99214[1], 99215[1], 99217[1], 99218[1], 99219[1], 99220[1], 99221[1], 99222[1], 99223[1], 99231[1], 99232[1], 99233[1], 99234[1], 99235[1], 99236[1], 99238[1], 99239[1], 99241[1], 99242[1], 99243[1], 99244[1], 99245[1], 99251[1], 99252[1], 99253[1], 99254[1], 99255[1], 99291[1], 99292[1], 99304[1], 99305[1], 99306[1], 99307[1], 99308[1], 99309[1], 99310[1], 99315[1], 99316[1], 99334[1], 99335[1], 99336[1], 99337[1], 99347[1], 99348[1], 99349[1], 99350[1], 99374[1], 99375[1], 99377[1], 99378[1], 99446[0], 99447[0], 99448[0], 99449[0], 99451[0], 99452[0], 99495[0], 99496[0], G0453[0], G0463[1], G0471[1]
63199	0213T[0], 0216T[0], 0228T[0], 0230T[0], 0333T[0], 0464T[0], 0565T[1], 11000[1], 11001[1], 11004[1], 11005[1], 11006[1], 11042[1], 11043[1], 11044[1], 11045[1], 11046[1], 11047[1], 12001[1], 12002[1], 12004[1], 12005[1], 12006[1], 12007[1], 12011[1], 12013[1], 12014[1], 12015[1], 12016[1], 12017[1], 12018[1], 12020[1], 12021[1], 12031[1], 12032[1], 12034[1], 12035[1], 12036[1], 12037[1], 12041[1], 12042[1], 12044[1], 12045[1], 12046[1], 12047[1], 12051[1], 12052[1], 12053[1], 12054[1], 12055[1], 12056[1], 12057[1], 13100[1], 13101[1], 13102[1], 13120[1], 13121[1], 13122[1], 13131[1], 13132[1], 13133[1], 13151[1], 13152[1], 13153[1], 15769[1], 22505[0], 36000[1], 36400[1], 36405[1], 36406[1], 36410[1], 36420[1], 36425[1], 36430[1], 36440[1], 36591[0], 36592[0], 36600[1], 36640[1], 38220[0], 38222[0], 38230[0], 38232[0], 43752[1], 51701[1], 51702[1], 51703[1], 62320[0], 62321[0], 62322[0], 62323[0], 62324[0], 62325[0], 62326[0], 62327[0], 63195[1], 63197[1], 63707[1], 63709[1], 64400[0], 64405[0], 64408[0], 64415[0], 64416[0], 64417[0], 64418[0], 64420[0], 64421[0], 64425[0], 64430[0], 64435[0], 64445[0], 64446[0], 64447[0], 64448[0], 64449[0], 64450[0], 64451[0], 64454[0], 64461[0], 64462[0], 64463[0], 64479[0], 64480[0], 64483[0], 64484[0], 64486[0], 64487[0], 64488[0], 64489[0], 64490[0], 64491[0], 64492[0], 64493[0], 64494[0], 64495[0], 64505[0], 64510[0], 64517[0], 64520[0], 64530[0], 76000[1], 77001[1], 77002[1], 92012[1], 92014[1], 92585[0], 93000[1], 93005[1], 93010[1], 93040[1], 93041[1], 93042[1], 93318[1], 93355[1], 94002[1], 94200[1], 94250[1], 94680[1], 94681[1], 94690[1], 94770[1], 95812[1], 95813[1], 95816[1], 95819[1], 95822[0], 95829[1], 95860[0], 95861[0], 95863[0], 95864[0], 95865[0], 95866[0], 95867[0], 95868[0], 95869[0], 95870[0], 95907[0], 95908[0], 95909[0], 95910[0], 95911[0], 95912[0], 95913[0], 95925[0], 95926[0], 95927[0], 95928[0], 95929[0], 95930[0], 95933[0], 95937[0], 95938[0], 95939[0], 95940[0], 95955[1], 96360[1], 96361[1], 96365[1], 96366[1], 96367[1], 96368[1], 96372[1], 96374[1], 96375[1], 96376[1], 96377[1], 96523[0], 97597[1], 97598[1], 97602[1], 99155[0], 99156[0], 99157[0], 99211[1], 99212[1], 99213[1], 99214[1], 99215[1], 99217[1], 99218[1], 99219[1], 99220[1], 99221[1], 99222[1], 99223[1], 99231[1], 99232[1], 99233[1], 99234[1], 99235[1], 99236[1], 99238[1], 99239[1], 99241[1], 99242[1], 99243[1], 99244[1], 99245[1], 99251[1], 99252[1], 99253[1], 99254[1], 99255[1], 99291[1], 99292[1], 99304[1], 99305[1], 99306[1], 99307[1], 99308[1], 99309[1], 99310[1], 99315[1], 99316[1], 99334[1], 99335[1], 99336[1], 99337[1], 99347[1], 99348[1], 99349[1], 99350[1], 99374[1], 99375[1], 99377[1], 99378[1], 99446[0], 99447[0], 99448[0], 99449[0], 99451[0], 99452[0], 99495[0], 99496[0], G0453[0], G0463[1], G0471[1]
63200	0213T[0], 0216T[0], 0228T[0], 0230T[0], 0333T[0], 0464T[0], 0565T[1], 11000[1], 11001[1], 11004[1], 11005[1], 11006[1], 11042[1], 11043[1], 11044[1], 11045[1], 11046[1], 11047[1], 12001[1], 12002[1], 12004[1], 12005[1], 12006[1], 12007[1], 12011[1], 12013[1], 12014[1], 12015[1], 12016[1], 12017[1], 12018[1], 12020[1], 12021[1], 12031[1], 12032[1], 12034[1], 12035[1], 12036[1], 12037[1], 12041[1], 12042[1], 12044[1], 12045[1], 12046[1], 12047[1], 12051[1], 12052[1], 12053[1], 12054[1], 12055[1], 12056[1], 12057[1], 13100[1], 13101[1], 13102[1], 13120[1], 13121[1], 13122[1], 13131[1], 13132[1], 13133[1], 13151[1], 13152[1], 13153[1], 15769[1], 22102[1], 22505[0], 22867[1], 22868[1], 22869[1], 22870[1], 36000[1], 36400[1], 36405[1], 36406[1], 36410[1], 36420[1], 36425[1], 36430[1], 36440[1], 36591[0], 36592[0], 36600[1], 36640[1], 38220[0], 38222[0], 38230[0], 38232[0], 43752[1], 49000[0], 49002[1], 51701[1], 51702[1], 51703[1], 62320[0], 62321[0], 62322[0], 62323[0], 62324[0], 62325[0], 62326[0], 62327[0], 63047[1], 63707[1], 63709[1], 64400[0], 64405[0], 64408[0], 64415[0], 64416[0], 64417[0], 64418[0], 64420[0], 64421[0], 64425[0], 64430[0], 64435[0], 64445[0], 64446[0], 64447[0], 64448[0], 64449[0], 64450[0], 64451[0], 64454[0], 64461[0], 64462[0], 64463[0], 64479[0], 64480[0], 64483[0], 64484[0], 64486[0], 64487[0], 64488[0], 64489[0], 64490[0], 64491[0], 64492[0], 64493[0], 64494[0], 64495[0], 64505[0], 64510[0], 64517[0], 64520[0], 64530[0], 76000[1], 77001[1], 77002[1], 92012[1], 92014[1], 92585[0], 93000[1], 93005[1], 93010[1], 93040[1], 93041[1], 93042[1], 93318[1], 93355[1], 94002[1], 94200[1], 94250[1], 94680[1], 94681[1], 94690[1], 94770[1], 95812[1], 95813[1], 95816[1], 95819[1], 95822[0], 95829[1], 95860[0], 95861[0], 95863[0], 95864[0], 95865[0], 95866[0], 95867[0], 95868[0], 95869[0], 95870[0], 95907[0], 95908[0], 95909[0], 95910[0], 95911[0], 95912[0], 95913[0], 95925[0], 95926[0], 95927[0], 95928[0], 95929[0], 95930[0], 95933[0], 95937[0], 95938[0], 95939[0], 95940[0], 95955[1], 96360[1], 96361[1], 96365[1], 96366[1], 96367[1], 96368[1], 96372[1], 96374[1], 96375[1], 96376[1], 96377[1], 96523[0], 97597[1], 97598[1], 97602[1], 99155[0], 99156[0], 99157[0], 99211[1], 99212[1], 99213[1], 99214[1], 99215[1], 99217[1], 99218[1], 99219[1], 99220[1], 99221[1], 99222[1], 99223[1], 99231[1], 99232[1], 99233[1], 99234[1], 99235[1], 99236[1], 99238[1], 99239[1], 99241[1], 99242[1], 99243[1], 99244[1], 99245[1], 99251[1], 99252[1], 99253[1], 99254[1], 99255[1], 99291[1], 99292[1], 99304[1], 99305[1], 99306[1], 99307[1], 99308[1], 99309[1], 99310[1], 99315[1], 99316[1], 99334[1], 99335[1], 99336[1], 99337[1], 99347[1], 99348[1], 99349[1], 99350[1], 99374[1], 99375[1], 99377[1], 99378[1], 99446[0], 99447[0], 99448[0], 99449[0], 99451[0], 99452[0], 99495[0], 99496[0], G0453[0], G0463[1], G0471[1]
63250	0213T[0], 0216T[0], 0228T[0], 0230T[0], 0274T[1], 0333T[0], 0464T[0], 0565T[1], 11000[1], 11001[1], 11004[1], 11005[1], 11006[1], 11042[1], 11043[1], 11044[1], 11045[1], 11046[1], 11047[1], 12001[1], 12002[1], 12004[1], 12005[1], 12006[1], 12007[1], 12011[1], 12013[1], 12014[1], 12015[1], 12016[1], 12017[1], 12018[1], 12020[1], 12021[1], 12031[1], 12032[1], 12034[1], 12035[1], 12036[1], 12037[1], 12041[1], 12042[1], 12044[1], 12045[1], 12046[1], 12047[1], 12051[1], 12052[1], 12053[1], 12054[1], 12055[1], 12056[1], 12057[1], 13100[1], 13101[1], 13102[1], 13120[1], 13121[1], 13122[1], 13131[1], 13132[1], 13133[1], 13151[1], 13152[1], 13153[1], 15769[1], 22100[1], 22206[1], 22207[1], 22505[0], 36000[1], 36400[1], 36405[1], 36406[1], 36410[1], 36420[1], 36425[1], 36430[1], 36440[1], 36591[0], 36592[0], 36600[1], 36640[1], 38220[0], 38222[0], 38230[0], 38232[0], 43752[1], 51701[1], 51702[1], 51703[1], 62320[0], 62321[0], 62322[0], 62323[0], 62324[0], 62325[0], 62326[0], 62327[0], 63001[1], 63015[1], 63020[1], 63040[1], 63045[1], 63050[1], 63051[1], 63251[1], 63252[1], 63707[1], 63709[1], 64400[0], 64405[0], 64408[0], 64415[0], 64416[0], 64417[0], 64418[0], 64420[0], 64421[0], 64425[0], 64430[0], 64435[0], 64445[0], 64446[0], 64447[0], 64448[0], 64449[0], 64450[0], 64451[0], 64454[0], 64461[0], 64462[0], 64463[0], 64479[0], 64480[0], 64483[0], 64484[0], 64486[0], 64487[0], 64488[0], 64489[0], 64490[0], 64491[0], 64492[0], 64493[0], 64494[0], 64495[0], 64505[0], 64510[0], 64517[0], 64520[0], 64530[0], 76000[1], 77001[1], 77002[1], 92012[1], 92014[1], 92585[0], 93000[1], 93005[1], 93010[1], 93040[1], 93041[1], 93042[1], 93318[1], 93355[1], 94002[1], 94200[1], 94250[1], 94680[1], 94681[1], 94690[1], 94770[1], 95812[1], 95813[1], 95816[1], 95819[1], 95822[0], 95829[1], 95860[0], 95861[0], 95863[0], 95864[0], 95865[0], 95866[0], 95867[0], 95868[0], 95869[0], 95870[0], 95907[0], 95908[0], 95909[0], 95910[0], 95911[0], 95912[0], 95913[0], 95925[0], 95926[0], 95927[0], 95928[0], 95929[0], 95930[0], 95933[0], 95937[0], 95938[0], 95939[0], 95940[0], 95955[1], 96360[1], 96361[1], 96365[1], 96366[1], 96367[1], 96368[1], 96372[1], 96374[1], 96375[1], 96376[1], 96377[1], 96523[0], 97597[1], 97598[1], 97602[1], 99155[0], 99156[0], 99157[0], 99211[1], 99212[1], 99213[1], 99214[1], 99215[1], 99217[1], 99218[1], 99219[1], 99220[1], 99221[1], 99222[1], 99223[1], 99231[1], 99232[1], 99233[1], 99234[1], 99235[1], 99236[1], 99238[1], 99239[1], 99241[1], 99242[1], 99243[1], 99244[1], 99245[1], 99251[1], 99252[1], 99253[1], 99254[1], 99255[1], 99291[1], 99292[1], 99304[1], 99305[1], 99306[1], 99307[1], 99308[1], 99309[1], 99310[1], 99315[1], 99316[1], 99334[1], 99335[1], 99336[1], 99337[1], 99347[1], 99348[1], 99349[1], 99350[1], 99374[1], 99375[1], 99377[1], 99378[1], 99446[0], 99447[0], 99448[0], 99449[0], 99451[0], 99452[0], 99495[0], 99496[0], G0453[0], G0463[1], G0471[1]
63251	0213T[0], 0216T[0], 0228T[0], 0230T[0], 0333T[0], 0464T[0], 0565T[1], 11000[1], 11001[1], 11004[1], 11005[1], 11006[1], 11042[1], 11043[1], 11044[1], 11045[1], 11046[1], 11047[1], 12001[1], 12002[1], 12004[1], 12005[1], 12006[1], 12007[1], 12011[1], 12013[1], 12014[1], 12015[1], 12016[1], 12017[1], 12018[1], 12020[1], 12021[1], 12031[1], 12032[1], 12034[1], 12035[1], 12036[1], 12037[1], 12041[1], 12042[1], 12044[1], 12045[1], 12046[1], 12047[1], 12051[1], 12052[1], 12053[1], 12054[1], 12055[1], 12056[1], 12057[1], 13100[1], 13101[1], 13102[1], 13120[1], 13121[1], 13122[1], 13131[1], 13132[1], 13133[1], 13151[1], 13152[1], 13153[1], 15769[1], 22101[1], 22206[1], 22207[1], 22505[0], 36000[1], 36400[1], 36405[1], 36406[1], 36410[1], 36420[1], 36425[1], 36430[1], 36440[1], 36591[0], 36592[0], 36600[1], 36640[1], 38220[0], 38222[0], 38230[0], 38232[0], 43752[1], 51701[1], 51702[1], 51703[1], 62320[0], 62321[0], 62322[0], 62323[0], 62324[0], 62325[0], 62326[0], 62327[0], 63003[1], 63016[1],

Appendix A: NCCI - CPT Codes

0 = Modifier usage not allowed or inappropriate 1 = Modifier usage allowed

Code 1	Code 2
	63046^1, 63707^1, 63709^1, 64400^0, 64405^0, 64408^0, 64415^0, 64416^0, 64417^0, 64418^0, 64420^0, 64421^0, 64425^0, 64430^0, 64435^0, 64445^0, 64446^0, 64447^0, 64448^0, 64449^0, 64450^0, 64451^0, 64454^0, 64461^0, 64462^0, 64463^0, 64479^0, 64480^0, 64483^0, 64484^0, 64486^0, 64487^0, 64488^0, 64489^0, 64490^0, 64491^0, 64492^0, 64493^0, 64494^0, 64495^0, 64505^0, 64510^0, 64517^0, 64520^0, 64530^0, 76000^1, 77001^1, 77002^1, 92012^1, 92014^1, 92585^0, 93000^1, 93005^1, 93010^1, 93040^1, 93041^1, 93042^1, 93318^1, 93355^1, 94002^1, 94200^1, 94250^1, 94680^1, 94681^1, 94690^1, 94770^1, 95812^1, 95813^1, 95816^1, 95819^1, 95822^0, 95829^1, 95860^0, 95861^0, 95863^0, 95864^0, 95865^0, 95866^0, 95867^0, 95868^0, 95869^0, 95870^0, 95907^0, 95908^0, 95909^0, 95910^0, 95911^0, 95912^0, 95913^0, 95925^0, 95926^0, 95927^0, 95928^0, 95929^0, 95930^0, 95933^0, 95937^0, 95938^0, 95939^0, 95940^0, 95955^1, 96360^1, 96361^1, 96365^1, 96366^1, 96367^1, 96368^1, 96372^1, 96374^1, 96375^1, 96376^1, 96377^1, 96523^0, 97597^1, 97598^1, 97602^1, 99155^0, 99156^0, 99157^0, 99211^1, 99212^1, 99213^1, 99214^1, 99215^1, 99217^1, 99218^1, 99219^1, 99220^1, 99221^1, 99222^1, 99223^1, 99231^1, 99232^1, 99233^1, 99234^1, 99235^1, 99236^1, 99238^1, 99239^1, 99241^1, 99242^1, 99243^1, 99244^1, 99245^1, 99251^1, 99252^1, 99253^1, 99254^1, 99255^1, 99291^1, 99292^1, 99304^1, 99305^1, 99306^1, 99307^1, 99308^1, 99309^1, 99310^1, 99315^1, 99316^1, 99334^1, 99335^1, 99336^1, 99337^1, 99347^1, 99348^1, 99349^1, 99350^1, 99374^1, 99375^1, 99377^1, 99378^1, 99446^0, 99447^0, 99448^0, 99449^0, 99451^0, 99452^0, 99495^0, 99496^0, G0453^0, G0463^1, G0471^1
63252	0202T^1, 0213T^0, 0216T^0, 0228T^0, 0230T^0, 0275T^1, 0333T^0, 0464T^0, 0565T^1, 11000^1, 11001^1, 11004^1, 11005^1, 11006^1, 11042^1, 11043^1, 11044^1, 11045^1, 11046^1, 11047^1, 12001^1, 12002^1, 12004^1, 12005^1, 12006^1, 12007^1, 12011^1, 12013^1, 12014^1, 12015^1, 12016^1, 12017^1, 12018^1, 12020^1, 12021^1, 12031^1, 12032^1, 12034^1, 12035^1, 12036^1, 12037^1, 12041^1, 12042^1, 12044^1, 12045^1, 12046^1, 12047^1, 12051^1, 12052^1, 12053^1, 12054^1, 12055^1, 12056^1, 12057^1, 13100^1, 13101^1, 13102^1, 13120^1, 13121^1, 13122^1, 13131^1, 13132^1, 13133^1, 13151^1, 13152^1, 13153^1, 15769^1, 22102^1, 22206^1, 22207^1, 22505^0, 22630^1, 22633^1, 22867^1, 22868^1, 22869^1, 22870^1, 36000^1, 36400^1, 36405^1, 36406^1, 36410^1, 36420^1, 36425^1, 36430^1, 36440^1, 36591^0, 36592^0, 36600^1, 36640^1, 38220^0, 38222^0, 38230^0, 38232^0, 43752^1, 49000^0, 49002^1, 51701^1, 51702^1, 51703^1, 62320^0, 62321^0, 62322^0, 62323^0, 62324^0, 62325^0, 62326^0, 62327^0, 62380^1, 63003^1, 63005^1, 63012^1, 63016^1, 63017^1, 63030^1, 63042^1, 63046^1, 63047^1, 63251^1, 63707^1, 63709^1, 64400^0, 64405^0, 64408^0, 64415^0, 64416^0, 64417^0, 64418^0, 64420^0, 64421^0, 64425^0, 64430^0, 64435^0, 64445^0, 64446^0, 64447^0, 64448^0, 64449^0, 64450^0, 64451^0, 64454^0, 64461^0, 64462^0, 64463^0, 64479^0, 64480^0, 64483^0, 64484^0, 64486^0, 64487^0, 64488^0, 64489^0, 64490^0, 64491^0, 64492^0, 64493^0, 64494^0, 64495^0, 64505^0, 64510^0, 64517^0, 64520^0, 64530^0, 76000^1, 77001^1, 77002^1, 92012^1, 92014^1, 92585^0, 93000^1, 93005^1, 93010^1, 93040^1, 93041^1, 93042^1, 93318^1, 93355^1, 94002^1, 94200^1, 94250^1, 94680^1, 94681^1, 94690^1, 94770^1, 95812^1, 95813^1, 95816^1, 95819^1, 95822^0, 95829^1, 95860^0, 95861^0, 95863^0, 95864^0, 95865^0, 95866^0, 95867^0, 95868^0, 95869^0, 95870^0, 95907^0, 95908^0, 95909^0, 95910^0, 95911^0, 95912^0, 95913^0, 95925^0, 95926^0, 95927^0, 95928^0, 95929^0, 95930^0, 95933^0, 95937^0, 95938^0, 95939^0, 95940^0, 95955^1, 96360^1, 96361^1, 96365^1, 96366^1, 96367^1, 96368^1, 96372^1, 96374^1, 96375^1, 96376^1, 96377^1, 96523^0, 97597^1, 97598^1, 97602^1, 99155^0, 99156^0, 99157^0, 99211^1, 99212^1, 99213^1, 99214^1, 99215^1, 99217^1, 99218^1, 99219^1, 99220^1, 99221^1, 99222^1, 99223^1, 99231^1, 99232^1, 99233^1, 99234^1, 99235^1, 99236^1, 99238^1, 99239^1, 99241^1, 99242^1, 99243^1, 99244^1, 99245^1, 99251^1, 99252^1, 99253^1, 99254^1, 99255^1, 99291^1, 99292^1, 99304^1, 99305^1, 99306^1, 99307^1, 99308^1, 99309^1, 99310^1, 99315^1, 99316^1, 99334^1, 99335^1, 99336^1, 99337^1, 99347^1, 99348^1, 99349^1, 99350^1, 99374^1, 99375^1, 99377^1, 99378^1, 99446^0, 99447^0, 99448^0, 99449^0, 99451^0, 99452^0, 99495^0, 99496^0, G0276^1, G0453^0, G0463^1, G0471^1
63265	0213T^0, 0216T^0, 0228T^0, 0230T^0, 0274T^1, 0333T^0, 0464T^0, 0565T^1, 11000^1, 11001^1, 11004^1, 11005^1, 11006^1, 11042^1, 11043^1, 11044^1, 11045^1, 11046^1, 11047^1, 12001^1, 12002^1, 12004^1, 12005^1, 12006^1, 12007^1, 12011^1, 12013^1, 12014^1, 12015^1, 12016^1, 12017^1, 12018^1, 12020^1, 12021^1, 12031^1, 12032^1, 12034^1, 12035^1, 12036^1, 12037^1, 12041^1, 12042^1, 12044^1, 12045^1, 12046^1, 12047^1, 12051^1, 12052^1, 12053^1, 12054^1, 12055^1, 12056^1, 12057^1, 13100^1, 13101^1, 13102^1, 13120^1, 13121^1, 13122^1, 13131^1, 13132^1, 13133^1, 13151^1, 13152^1, 13153^1, 15769^1, 22100^1, 22505^0, 36000^1, 36400^1, 36405^1, 36406^1, 36410^1, 36420^1, 36425^1, 36430^1, 36440^1, 36591^0, 36592^0, 36600^1, 36640^1, 38220^0, 38221^1, 38222^0, 38230^0, 38232^0, 43752^1, 51701^1, 51702^1, 51703^1, 62320^0, 62321^0, 62322^0, 62323^0, 62324^0, 62325^0, 62326^0, 62327^0, 63001^1, 63015^1, 63020^1, 63040^1, 63045^1, 63050^1, 63707^1, 63709^1, 64400^0, 64405^0, 64408^0, 64415^0, 64416^0, 64417^0, 64418^0, 64420^0, 64421^0, 64425^0, 64430^0, 64435^0, 64445^0, 64446^0, 64447^0, 64448^0, 64449^0, 64450^0, 64451^0, 64454^0, 64461^0, 64462^0, 64463^0, 64479^0, 64480^0, 64483^0, 64484^0, 64486^0, 64487^0, 64488^0, 64489^0, 64490^0, 64491^0, 64492^0, 64493^0, 64494^0, 64495^0, 64505^0, 64510^0, 64517^0, 64520^0, 64530^0, 76000^1, 77001^1, 77002^1, 92012^1, 92014^1, 92585^0, 93000^1, 93005^1, 93010^1, 93040^1, 93041^1, 93042^1, 93318^1, 93355^1, 94002^1, 94200^1, 94250^1, 94680^1, 94681^1, 94690^1, 94770^1, 95812^1, 95813^1, 95816^1, 95819^1, 95822^0, 95829^1, 95860^0, 95861^0, 95863^0, 95864^0, 95865^0, 95866^0, 95867^0, 95868^0, 95869^0, 95870^0, 95907^0, 95908^0, 95909^0, 95910^0, 95911^0, 95912^0, 95913^0, 95925^0, 95926^0, 95927^0, 95928^0, 95929^0, 95930^0, 95933^0, 95937^0, 95938^0, 95939^0, 95940^0, 95955^1, 96360^1, 96361^1, 96365^1, 96366^1, 96367^1, 96368^1, 96372^1, 96374^1, 96375^1, 96376^1, 96377^1, 96523^0, 97597^1, 97598^1, 97602^1, 99155^0, 99156^0, 99157^0, 99211^1, 99212^1, 99213^1, 99214^1, 99215^1, 99217^1, 99218^1, 99219^1, 99220^1, 99221^1, 99222^1, 99223^1, 99231^1, 99232^1, 99233^1, 99234^1, 99235^1, 99236^1, 99238^1, 99239^1, 99241^1, 99242^1, 99243^1, 99244^1, 99245^1, 99251^1, 99252^1, 99253^1, 99254^1, 99255^1, 99291^1, 99292^1, 99304^1, 99305^1, 99306^1, 99307^1, 99308^1, 99309^1, 99310^1, 99315^1, 99316^1, 99334^1, 99335^1, 99336^1, 99337^1, 99347^1, 99348^1, 99349^1, 99350^1, 99374^1, 99375^1, 99377^1, 99378^1, 99446^0, 99447^0, 99448^0, 99449^0, 99451^0, 99452^0, 99495^0, 99496^0, G0453^0, G0463^1, G0471^1
63266	0213T^0, 0216T^0, 0228T^0, 0230T^0, 0333T^0, 0464T^0, 0565T^1, 11000^1, 11001^1, 11004^1, 11005^1, 11006^1, 11042^1, 11043^1, 11044^1, 11045^1, 11046^1, 11047^1, 12001^1, 12002^1, 12004^1, 12005^1, 12006^1, 12007^1, 12011^1, 12013^1, 12014^1, 12015^1, 12016^1, 12017^1, 12018^1, 12020^1, 12021^1, 12031^1, 12032^1, 12034^1, 12035^1, 12036^1, 12037^1, 12041^1, 12042^1, 12044^1, 12045^1, 12046^1, 12047^1, 12051^1, 12052^1, 12053^1, 12054^1, 12055^1, 12056^1, 12057^1, 13100^1, 13101^1, 13102^1, 13120^1, 13121^1, 13122^1, 13131^1, 13132^1, 13133^1, 13151^1, 13152^1, 13153^1, 15769^1, 22101^1, 22505^0, 36000^1, 36400^1, 36405^1, 36406^1, 36410^1, 36420^1, 36425^1, 36430^1, 36440^1, 36591^0, 36592^0, 36600^1, 36640^1, 38220^0, 38221^1, 38222^0, 38230^0, 38232^0, 43752^1, 51701^1, 51702^1, 51703^1, 62320^0, 62321^0, 62322^0, 62323^0, 62324^0, 62325^0, 62326^0, 62327^0, 63003^1, 63016^1, 63046^1, 63707^1, 63709^1, 64400^0, 64405^0, 64408^0, 64415^0, 64416^0, 64417^0, 64418^0, 64420^0, 64421^0, 64425^0, 64430^0, 64435^0, 64445^0, 64446^0, 64447^0, 64448^0, 64449^0, 64450^0, 64451^0, 64454^0, 64461^0, 64462^0, 64463^0, 64479^0, 64480^0, 64483^0, 64484^0, 64486^0, 64487^0, 64488^0, 64489^0, 64490^0, 64491^0, 64492^0, 64493^0, 64494^0, 64495^0, 64505^0, 64510^0, 64517^0, 64520^0, 64530^0, 76000^1, 77001^1, 77002^1, 92012^1, 92014^1, 92585^0, 93000^1, 93005^1, 93010^1, 93040^1, 93041^1, 93042^1, 93318^1, 93355^1, 94002^1, 94200^1, 94250^1, 94680^1, 94681^1, 94690^1, 94770^1, 95812^1, 95813^1, 95816^1, 95819^1, 95822^0, 95829^1, 95860^0, 95861^0, 95863^0, 95864^0, 95865^0, 95866^0, 95867^0, 95868^0, 95869^0, 95870^0, 95907^0, 95908^0, 95909^0, 95910^0, 95911^0, 95912^0, 95913^0, 95925^0, 95926^0, 95927^0, 95928^0, 95929^0, 95930^0, 95933^0, 95937^0, 95938^0, 95939^0, 95940^0, 95955^1, 96360^1, 96361^1, 96365^1, 96366^1, 96367^1, 96368^1, 96372^1, 96374^1, 96375^1, 96376^1, 96377^1, 96523^0, 97597^1, 97598^1, 97602^1, 99155^0, 99156^0, 99157^0, 99211^1, 99212^1, 99213^1, 99214^1, 99215^1, 99217^1, 99218^1, 99219^1, 99220^1, 99221^1, 99222^1, 99223^1, 99231^1, 99232^1, 99233^1, 99234^1, 99235^1, 99236^1, 99238^1, 99239^1, 99241^1, 99242^1, 99243^1, 99244^1, 99245^1, 99251^1, 99252^1, 99253^1, 99254^1, 99255^1, 99291^1, 99292^1, 99304^1, 99305^1, 99306^1, 99307^1, 99308^1, 99309^1, 99310^1, 99315^1, 99316^1, 99334^1, 99335^1, 99336^1, 99337^1, 99347^1, 99348^1, 99349^1, 99350^1, 99374^1, 99375^1, 99377^1, 99378^1, 99446^0, 99447^0, 99448^0, 99449^0, 99451^0, 99452^0, 99495^0, 99496^0, G0453^0, G0463^1, G0471^1
63267	0202T^1, 0213T^0, 0216T^0, 0228T^0, 0230T^0, 0275T^1, 0333T^0, 0464T^0, 0565T^1, 11000^1, 11001^1, 11004^1, 11005^1, 11006^1, 11042^1, 11043^1, 11044^1, 11045^1, 11046^1, 11047^1, 12001^1, 12002^1, 12004^1, 12005^1, 12006^1, 12007^1, 12011^1, 12013^1, 12014^1, 12015^1, 12016^1, 12017^1, 12018^1, 12020^1, 12021^1, 12031^1, 12032^1, 12034^1, 12035^1, 12036^1, 12037^1, 12041^1, 12042^1, 12044^1, 12045^1, 12046^1, 12047^1, 12051^1, 12052^1, 12053^1, 12054^1, 12055^1, 12056^1, 12057^1, 13100^1, 13101^1, 13102^1, 13120^1, 13121^1, 13122^1, 13131^1, 13132^1, 13133^1, 13151^1, 13152^1, 13153^1, 15769^1, 22102^1, 22505^0, 22867^1, 22868^1, 22869^1, 22870^1, 36000^1, 36400^1, 36405^1, 36406^1, 36410^1, 36420^1, 36425^1, 36430^1, 36440^1, 36591^0, 36592^0, 36600^1, 36640^1, 38220^0, 38221^1, 38222^0, 38230^0, 38232^0, 43752^1, 49000^0, 49002^1, 51701^1, 51702^1, 51703^1, 62320^0, 62321^0, 62322^0, 62323^0, 62324^0, 62325^0, 62326^0, 62327^0, 62380^1, 63005^1, 63012^1, 63017^1, 63030^1, 63047^1, 63707^1, 63709^1, 64400^0, 64405^0, 64408^0, 64415^0, 64416^0, 64417^0, 64418^0, 64420^0, 64421^0, 64425^0, 64430^0, 64435^0, 64445^0, 64446^0, 64447^0, 64448^0, 64449^0, 64450^0, 64451^0, 64454^0, 64461^0, 64462^0, 64463^0, 64479^0, 64480^0, 64483^0, 64484^0, 64486^0, 64487^0, 64488^0, 64489^0, 64490^0, 64491^0, 64492^0, 64493^0, 64494^0, 64495^0, 64505^0, 64510^0, 64517^0, 64520^0, 64530^0, 76000^1, 77001^1, 77002^1, 92012^1, 92014^1, 92585^0, 93000^1, 93005^1, 93010^1, 93040^1, 93041^1, 93042^1, 93318^1, 93355^1, 94002^1, 94200^1, 94250^1, 94680^1, 94681^1, 94690^1, 94770^1, 95812^1, 95813^1, 95816^1, 95819^1, 95822^0, 95829^1, 95860^0, 95861^0, 95863^0, 95864^0, 95865^0, 95866^0, 95867^0, 95868^0, 95869^0, 95870^0, 95907^0, 95908^0, 95909^0, 95910^0, 95911^0, 95912^0, 95913^0, 95925^0, 95926^0, 95927^0, 95928^0, 95929^0, 95930^0, 95933^0, 95937^0, 95938^0, 95939^0, 95940^0, 95955^1, 96360^1, 96361^1, 96365^1, 96366^1, 96367^1, 96368^1, 96372^1, 96374^1, 96375^1, 96376^1, 96377^1, 96523^0, 97597^1, 97598^1, 97602^1, 99155^0, 99156^0, 99157^0, 99211^1, 99212^1, 99213^1, 99214^1, 99215^1, 99217^1, 99218^1, 99219^1, 99220^1, 99221^1, 99222^1,

0 = Modifier usage not allowed or inappropriate 1 = Modifier usage allowed

Code 1	Code 2
	99223[1], 99231[1], 99232[1], 99233[1], 99234[1], 99235[1], 99236[1], 99238[1], 99239[1], 99241[1], 99242[1], 99243[1], 99244[1], 99245[1], 99251[1], 99252[1], 99253[1], 99254[1], 99255[1], 99291[1], 99292[1], 99304[1], 99305[1], 99306[1], 99307[1], 99308[1], 99309[1], 99310[1], 99315[1], 99316[1], 99334[1], 99335[1], 99336[1], 99337[1], 99347[1], 99348[1], 99349[1], 99350[1], 99374[1], 99375[1], 99377[1], 99378[1], 99446[0], 99447[0], 99448[0], 99449[0], 99451[0], 99452[0], 99495[0], 99496[0], G0276[1], G0453[0], G0463[1], G0471[1]
63268	0213T[0], 0216T[0], 0228T[0], 0230T[0], 0333T[0], 0464T[0], 0565T[1], 11000[1], 11001[1], 11004[1], 11005[1], 11006[1], 11042[1], 11043[1], 11044[1], 11045[1], 11046[1], 11047[1], 12001[1], 12002[1], 12004[1], 12005[1], 12006[1], 12007[1], 12011[1], 12013[1], 12014[1], 12015[1], 12016[1], 12017[1], 12018[1], 12020[1], 12021[1], 12031[1], 12032[1], 12034[1], 12035[1], 12036[1], 12037[1], 12041[1], 12042[1], 12044[1], 12045[1], 12046[1], 12047[1], 12051[1], 12052[1], 12053[1], 12054[1], 12055[1], 12056[1], 12057[1], 13100[1], 13101[1], 13102[1], 13120[1], 13121[1], 13122[1], 13131[1], 13132[1], 13133[1], 13151[1], 13152[1], 13153[1], 15769[1], 22102[1], 22505[0], 36000[1], 36400[1], 36405[1], 36406[1], 36410[1], 36420[1], 36425[1], 36430[1], 36440[1], 36591[0], 36592[0], 36600[1], 36640[1], 38220[0], 38221[1], 38222[0], 38230[0], 38232[0], 43752[1], 49000[0], 49002[1], 51701[1], 51702[1], 51703[1], 62320[0], 62321[0], 62322[0], 62323[0], 62324[0], 62325[0], 62326[0], 62327[0], 63011[1], 63047[1], 63707[1], 63709[1], 64400[0], 64405[0], 64408[0], 64415[0], 64416[0], 64417[0], 64418[0], 64420[0], 64421[0], 64425[0], 64430[0], 64435[0], 64445[0], 64446[0], 64447[0], 64448[0], 64449[0], 64450[0], 64451[0], 64454[0], 64461[0], 64462[0], 64463[0], 64479[0], 64480[0], 64483[0], 64484[0], 64486[0], 64487[0], 64488[0], 64489[0], 64490[0], 64491[0], 64492[0], 64493[0], 64494[0], 64495[0], 64505[0], 64510[0], 64517[0], 64520[0], 64530[0], 76000[1], 77001[1], 77002[1], 92012[1], 92014[1], 92585[0], 93000[1], 93005[1], 93010[1], 93040[1], 93041[1], 93042[1], 93318[1], 93355[1], 94002[1], 94200[1], 94250[1], 94680[1], 94681[1], 94690[1], 94770[1], 95812[1], 95813[1], 95816[1], 95819[1], 95822[0], 95829[1], 95860[0], 95861[0], 95863[0], 95864[0], 95865[0], 95866[0], 95867[0], 95868[0], 95869[0], 95870[0], 95907[0], 95908[0], 95909[0], 95910[0], 95911[0], 95912[0], 95913[0], 95925[0], 95926[0], 95927[0], 95928[0], 95929[0], 95930[0], 95933[0], 95937[0], 95938[0], 95939[0], 95940[0], 95955[1], 96360[1], 96361[1], 96365[1], 96366[1], 96367[1], 96368[1], 96372[1], 96374[1], 96375[1], 96376[1], 96377[1], 96523[0], 97597[1], 97598[1], 97602[1], 99155[0], 99156[0], 99157[0], 99211[1], 99212[1], 99213[1], 99214[1], 99215[1], 99217[1], 99218[1], 99219[1], 99220[1], 99221[1], 99222[1], 99223[1], 99231[1], 99232[1], 99233[1], 99234[1], 99235[1], 99236[1], 99238[1], 99239[1], 99241[1], 99242[1], 99243[1], 99244[1], 99245[1], 99251[1], 99252[1], 99253[1], 99254[1], 99255[1], 99291[1], 99292[1], 99304[1], 99305[1], 99306[1], 99307[1], 99308[1], 99309[1], 99310[1], 99315[1], 99316[1], 99334[1], 99335[1], 99336[1], 99337[1], 99347[1], 99348[1], 99349[1], 99350[1], 99374[1], 99375[1], 99377[1], 99378[1], 99446[0], 99447[0], 99448[0], 99449[0], 99451[0], 99452[0], 99495[0], 99496[0], G0453[0], G0463[1], G0471[1]
63270	0213T[0], 0216T[0], 0228T[0], 0230T[0], 0274T[1], 0333T[0], 0464T[0], 0565T[1], 11000[1], 11001[1], 11004[1], 11005[1], 11006[1], 11042[1], 11043[1], 11044[1], 11045[1], 11046[1], 11047[1], 12001[1], 12002[1], 12004[1], 12005[1], 12006[1], 12007[1], 12011[1], 12013[1], 12014[1], 12015[1], 12016[1], 12017[1], 12018[1], 12020[1], 12021[1], 12031[1], 12032[1], 12034[1], 12035[1], 12036[1], 12037[1], 12041[1], 12042[1], 12044[1], 12045[1], 12046[1], 12047[1], 12051[1], 12052[1], 12053[1], 12054[1], 12055[1], 12056[1], 12057[1], 13100[1], 13101[1], 13102[1], 13120[1], 13121[1], 13122[1], 13131[1], 13132[1], 13133[1], 13151[1], 13152[1], 13153[1], 15769[1], 22100[1], 22505[0], 36000[1], 36400[1], 36405[1], 36406[1], 36410[1], 36420[1], 36425[1], 36430[1], 36440[1], 36591[0], 36592[0], 36600[1], 36640[1], 38220[0], 38221[1], 38222[0], 38230[0], 38232[0], 43752[1], 51701[1], 51702[1], 51703[1], 62320[0], 62321[0], 62322[0], 62323[0], 62324[0], 62325[0], 62326[0], 62327[0], 63001[1], 63015[1], 63020[1], 63040[1], 63045[1], 63050[1], 63051[1], 63265[1], 63707[1], 63709[1], 64400[0], 64405[0], 64408[0], 64415[0], 64416[0], 64417[0], 64418[0], 64420[0], 64421[0], 64425[0], 64430[0], 64435[0], 64445[0], 64446[0], 64447[0], 64448[0], 64449[0], 64450[0], 64451[0], 64454[0], 64461[0], 64462[0], 64463[0], 64479[0], 64480[0], 64483[0], 64484[0], 64486[0], 64487[0], 64488[0], 64489[0], 64490[0], 64491[0], 64492[0], 64493[0], 64494[0], 64495[0], 64505[0], 64510[0], 64517[0], 64520[0], 64530[0], 76000[1], 77001[1], 77002[1], 92012[1], 92014[1], 92585[0], 93000[1], 93005[1], 93010[1], 93040[1], 93041[1], 93042[1], 93318[1], 93355[1], 94002[1], 94200[1], 94250[1], 94680[1], 94681[1], 94690[1], 94770[1], 95812[1], 95813[1], 95816[1], 95819[1], 95822[0], 95829[1], 95860[0], 95861[0], 95863[0], 95864[0], 95865[0], 95866[0], 95867[0], 95868[0], 95869[0], 95870[0], 95907[0], 95908[0], 95909[0], 95910[0], 95911[0], 95912[0], 95913[0], 95925[0], 95926[0], 95927[0], 95928[0], 95929[0], 95930[0], 95933[0], 95937[0], 95938[0], 95939[0], 95940[0], 95955[1], 96360[1], 96361[1], 96365[1], 96366[1], 96367[1], 96368[1], 96372[1], 96374[1], 96375[1], 96376[1], 96377[1], 96523[0], 97597[1], 97598[1], 97602[1], 99155[0], 99156[0], 99157[0], 99211[1], 99212[1], 99213[1], 99214[1], 99215[1], 99217[1], 99218[1], 99219[1], 99220[1], 99221[1], 99222[1], 99223[1], 99231[1], 99232[1], 99233[1], 99234[1], 99235[1], 99236[1], 99238[1], 99239[1], 99241[1], 99242[1], 99243[1], 99244[1], 99245[1], 99251[1], 99252[1], 99253[1], 99254[1], 99255[1], 99291[1], 99292[1], 99304[1], 99305[1], 99306[1], 99307[1], 99308[1], 99309[1], 99310[1], 99315[1], 99316[1], 99334[1], 99335[1], 99336[1], 99337[1], 99347[1], 99348[1], 99349[1], 99350[1], 99374[1], 99375[1], 99377[1], 99378[1], 99446[0], 99447[0], 99448[0], 99449[0], 99451[0], 99452[0], 99495[0], 99496[0], G0453[0], G0463[1], G0471[1]
63271	0213T[0], 0216T[0], 0228T[0], 0230T[0], 0333T[0], 0464T[0], 0565T[1], 11000[1], 11001[1], 11004[1], 11005[1], 11006[1], 11042[1], 11043[1], 11044[1], 11045[1], 11046[1], 11047[1], 12001[1], 12002[1], 12004[1], 12005[1], 12006[1], 12007[1], 12011[1], 12013[1], 12014[1], 12015[1], 12016[1], 12017[1], 12018[1], 12020[1], 12021[1], 12031[1], 12032[1], 12034[1], 12035[1], 12036[1], 12037[1], 12041[1], 12042[1], 12044[1], 12045[1], 12046[1], 12047[1], 12051[1], 12052[1], 12053[1], 12054[1], 12055[1], 12056[1], 12057[1], 13100[1], 13101[1], 13102[1], 13120[1], 13121[1], 13122[1], 13131[1], 13132[1], 13133[1], 13151[1], 13152[1], 13153[1], 15769[1], 22101[1], 22505[0], 36000[1], 36400[1], 36405[1], 36406[1], 36410[1], 36420[1], 36425[1], 36430[1], 36440[1], 36591[0], 36592[0], 36600[1], 36640[1], 38220[0], 38221[1], 38222[0], 38230[0], 38232[0], 43752[1], 51701[1], 51702[1], 51703[1], 62320[0], 62321[0], 62322[0], 62323[0], 62324[0], 62325[0], 62326[0], 62327[0], 63003[1], 63016[1], 63046[1], 63266[1], 63707[1], 63709[1], 64400[0], 64405[0], 64408[0], 64415[0], 64416[0], 64417[0], 64418[0], 64420[0], 64421[0], 64425[0], 64430[0], 64435[0], 64445[0], 64446[0], 64447[0], 64448[0], 64449[0], 64450[0], 64451[0], 64454[0], 64461[0], 64462[0], 64463[0], 64479[0], 64480[0], 64483[0], 64484[0], 64486[0], 64487[0], 64488[0], 64489[0], 64490[0], 64491[0], 64492[0], 64493[0], 64494[0], 64495[0], 64505[0], 64510[0], 64517[0], 64520[0], 64530[0], 76000[1], 77001[1], 77002[1], 92012[1], 92014[1], 92585[0], 93000[1], 93005[1], 93010[1], 93040[1], 93041[1], 93042[1], 93318[1], 93355[1], 94002[1], 94200[1], 94250[1], 94680[1], 94681[1], 94690[1], 94770[1], 95812[1], 95813[1], 95816[1], 95819[1], 95822[0], 95829[1], 95860[0], 95861[0], 95863[0], 95864[0], 95865[0], 95866[0], 95867[0], 95868[0], 95869[0], 95870[0], 95907[0], 95908[0], 95909[0], 95910[0], 95911[0], 95912[0], 95913[0], 95925[0], 95926[0], 95927[0], 95928[0], 95929[0], 95930[0], 95933[0], 95937[0], 95938[0], 95939[0], 95940[0], 95955[1], 96360[1], 96361[1], 96365[1], 96366[1], 96367[1], 96368[1], 96372[1], 96374[1], 96375[1], 96376[1], 96377[1], 96523[0], 97597[1], 97598[1], 97602[1], 99155[0], 99156[0], 99157[0], 99211[1], 99212[1], 99213[1], 99214[1], 99215[1], 99217[1], 99218[1], 99219[1], 99220[1], 99221[1], 99222[1], 99223[1], 99231[1], 99232[1], 99233[1], 99234[1], 99235[1], 99236[1], 99238[1], 99239[1], 99241[1], 99242[1], 99243[1], 99244[1], 99245[1], 99251[1], 99252[1], 99253[1], 99254[1], 99255[1], 99291[1], 99292[1], 99304[1], 99305[1], 99306[1], 99307[1], 99308[1], 99309[1], 99310[1], 99315[1], 99316[1], 99334[1], 99335[1], 99336[1], 99337[1], 99347[1], 99348[1], 99349[1], 99350[1], 99374[1], 99375[1], 99377[1], 99378[1], 99446[0], 99447[0], 99448[0], 99449[0], 99451[0], 99452[0], 99495[0], 99496[0], G0453[0], G0463[1], G0471[1]
63272	0202T[1], 0213T[0], 0216T[0], 0228T[0], 0230T[0], 0275T[1], 0333T[0], 0464T[0], 0565T[1], 11000[1], 11001[1], 11004[1], 11005[1], 11006[1], 11042[1], 11043[1], 11044[1], 11045[1], 11046[1], 11047[1], 12001[1], 12002[1], 12004[1], 12005[1], 12006[1], 12007[1], 12011[1], 12013[1], 12014[1], 12015[1], 12016[1], 12017[1], 12018[1], 12020[1], 12021[1], 12031[1], 12032[1], 12034[1], 12035[1], 12036[1], 12037[1], 12041[1], 12042[1], 12044[1], 12045[1], 12046[1], 12047[1], 12051[1], 12052[1], 12053[1], 12054[1], 12055[1], 12056[1], 12057[1], 13100[1], 13101[1], 13102[1], 13120[1], 13121[1], 13122[1], 13131[1], 13132[1], 13133[1], 13151[1], 13152[1], 13153[1], 15769[1], 22102[1], 22505[0], 22630[1], 22633[1], 22867[1], 22868[1], 22869[1], 22870[1], 36000[1], 36400[1], 36405[1], 36406[1], 36410[1], 36420[1], 36425[1], 36430[1], 36440[1], 36591[0], 36592[0], 36600[1], 36640[1], 38220[0], 38221[1], 38222[0], 38230[0], 38232[0], 43752[1], 49000[0], 49002[1], 51701[1], 51702[1], 51703[1], 62320[0], 62321[0], 62322[0], 62323[0], 62324[0], 62325[0], 62326[0], 62327[0], 62380[1], 63005[1], 63012[1], 63017[1], 63030[1], 63042[1], 63047[1], 63267[1], 63707[1], 63709[1], 64400[0], 64405[0], 64408[0], 64415[0], 64416[0], 64417[0], 64418[0], 64420[0], 64421[0], 64425[0], 64430[0], 64435[0], 64445[0], 64446[0], 64447[0], 64448[0], 64449[0], 64450[0], 64451[0], 64454[0], 64461[0], 64462[0], 64463[0], 64479[0], 64480[0], 64483[0], 64484[0], 64486[0], 64487[0], 64488[0], 64489[0], 64490[0], 64491[0], 64492[0], 64493[0], 64494[0], 64495[0], 64505[0], 64510[0], 64517[0], 64520[0], 64530[0], 76000[1], 77001[1], 77002[1], 92012[1], 92014[1], 92585[0], 93000[1], 93005[1], 93010[1], 93040[1], 93041[1], 93042[1], 93318[1], 93355[1], 94002[1], 94200[1], 94250[1], 94680[1], 94681[1], 94690[1], 94770[1], 95812[1], 95813[1], 95816[1], 95819[1], 95822[0], 95829[1], 95860[0], 95861[0], 95863[0], 95864[0], 95865[0], 95866[0], 95867[0], 95868[0], 95869[0], 95870[0], 95907[0], 95908[0], 95909[0], 95910[0], 95911[0], 95912[0], 95913[0], 95925[0], 95926[0], 95927[0], 95928[0], 95929[0], 95930[0], 95933[0], 95937[0], 95938[0], 95939[0], 95940[0], 95955[1], 96360[1], 96361[1], 96365[1], 96366[1], 96367[1], 96368[1], 96372[1], 96374[1], 96375[1], 96376[1], 96377[1], 96523[0], 97597[1], 97598[1], 97602[1], 99155[0], 99156[0], 99157[0], 99211[1], 99212[1], 99213[1], 99214[1], 99215[1], 99217[1], 99218[1], 99219[1], 99220[1], 99221[1], 99222[1], 99223[1], 99231[1], 99232[1], 99233[1], 99234[1], 99235[1], 99236[1], 99238[1], 99239[1], 99241[1], 99242[1], 99243[1], 99244[1], 99245[1], 99251[1], 99252[1], 99253[1], 99254[1], 99255[1], 99291[1], 99292[1], 99304[1], 99305[1], 99306[1], 99307[1], 99308[1], 99309[1], 99310[1], 99315[1], 99316[1], 99334[1], 99335[1], 99336[1], 99337[1], 99347[1], 99348[1], 99349[1], 99350[1], 99374[1], 99375[1], 99377[1], 99378[1], 99446[0], 99447[0], 99448[0], 99449[0], 99451[0], 99452[0], 99495[0], 99496[0], G0276[1], G0453[0], G0463[1], G0471[1]
63273	0213T[0], 0216T[0], 0228T[0], 0230T[0], 0333T[0], 0464T[0], 0565T[1], 11000[1], 11001[1], 11004[1], 11005[1], 11006[1], 11042[1], 11043[1], 11044[1], 11045[1], 11046[1], 11047[1], 12001[1], 12002[1], 12004[1], 12005[1], 12006[1], 12007[1], 12011[1], 12013[1], 12014[1], 12015[1], 12016[1], 12017[1], 12018[1], 12020[1], 12021[1], 12031[1], 12032[1], 12034[1], 12035[1], 12036[1], 12037[1], 12041[1], 12042[1], 12044[1], 12045[1], 12046[1], 12047[1], 12051[1], 12052[1], 12053[1], 12054[1], 12055[1], 12056[1], 12057[1], 13100[1], 13101[1], 13102[1], 13120[1], 13121[1], 13122[1], 13131[1], 13132[1], 13133[1], 13151[1], 13152[1], 13153[1], 15769[1], 22102[1], 22505[0], 36000[1], 36400[1], 36405[1],

0 = Modifier usage not allowed or inappropriate 1 = Modifier usage allowed

Code 1	Code 2
	36406[1], 36410[1], 36420[1], 36425[1], 36430[1], 36440[1], 36591[0], 36592[0], 36600[1], 36640[1], 38220[0], 38221[1], 38222[0], 38230[0], 38232[0], 43752[1], 49000[0], 49002[1], 51701[1], 51702[1], 51703[1], 62320[0], 62321[0], 62322[0], 62323[0], 62324[0], 62325[0], 62326[0], 62327[0], 63011[1], 63047[1], 63268[1], 63707[1], 63709[1], 64400[0], 64405[0], 64408[0], 64415[0], 64416[0], 64417[0], 64418[0], 64420[0], 64421[0], 64425[0], 64430[0], 64435[0], 64445[0], 64446[0], 64447[0], 64448[0], 64449[0], 64450[0], 64451[0], 64454[0], 64461[0], 64462[0], 64463[0], 64479[0], 64480[0], 64483[0], 64484[0], 64486[0], 64487[0], 64488[0], 64489[0], 64490[0], 64491[0], 64492[0], 64493[0], 64494[0], 64495[0], 64505[0], 64510[0], 64517[0], 64520[0], 64530[0], 76000[1], 77001[1], 77002[1], 92012[1], 92014[1], 92585[0], 93000[1], 93005[1], 93010[1], 93040[1], 93041[1], 93042[1], 93318[1], 93355[1], 94002[1], 94200[1], 94250[1], 94680[1], 94681[1], 94690[1], 94770[1], 95812[1], 95813[1], 95816[1], 95819[1], 95822[0], 95829[1], 95860[0], 95861[0], 95863[0], 95864[0], 95865[0], 95866[0], 95867[0], 95868[0], 95869[0], 95870[0], 95907[0], 95908[0], 95909[0], 95910[0], 95911[0], 95912[0], 95913[0], 95925[0], 95926[0], 95927[0], 95928[0], 95929[0], 95930[0], 95933[0], 95937[0], 95938[0], 95939[0], 95940[0], 95955[1], 96360[1], 96361[1], 96365[1], 96366[1], 96367[1], 96368[1], 96372[1], 96374[1], 96375[1], 96376[1], 96377[1], 96523[0], 97597[1], 97598[1], 97602[1], 99155[0], 99156[0], 99157[0], 99211[1], 99212[1], 99213[1], 99214[1], 99215[1], 99217[1], 99218[1], 99219[1], 99220[1], 99221[1], 99222[1], 99223[1], 99231[1], 99232[1], 99233[1], 99234[1], 99235[1], 99236[1], 99238[1], 99239[1], 99241[1], 99242[1], 99243[1], 99244[1], 99245[1], 99251[1], 99252[1], 99253[1], 99254[1], 99255[1], 99291[1], 99292[1], 99304[1], 99305[1], 99306[1], 99307[1], 99308[1], 99309[1], 99310[1], 99315[1], 99316[1], 99334[1], 99335[1], 99336[1], 99337[1], 99347[1], 99348[1], 99349[1], 99350[1], 99374[1], 99375[1], 99377[1], 99378[1], 99446[0], 99447[0], 99448[0], 99449[0], 99451[0], 99452[0], 99495[0], 99496[0], G0453[0], G0463[1], G0471[1]
63275	0213T[0], 0216T[0], 0228T[0], 0230T[0], 0274T[1], 0333T[0], 0464T[0], 0565T[1], 10005[1], 10007[1], 10009[1], 10011[1], 10021[1], 11000[1], 11001[1], 11004[1], 11005[1], 11006[1], 11042[1], 11043[1], 11044[1], 11045[1], 11046[1], 11047[1], 12001[1], 12002[1], 12004[1], 12005[1], 12006[1], 12007[1], 12011[1], 12013[1], 12014[1], 12015[1], 12016[1], 12017[1], 12018[1], 12020[1], 12021[1], 12031[1], 12032[1], 12034[1], 12035[1], 12036[1], 12037[1], 12041[1], 12042[1], 12044[1], 12045[1], 12046[1], 12047[1], 12051[1], 12052[1], 12053[1], 12054[1], 12055[1], 12056[1], 12057[1], 13100[1], 13101[1], 13102[1], 13120[1], 13121[1], 13122[1], 13131[1], 13132[1], 13133[1], 13151[1], 13152[1], 13153[1], 15769[1], 22100[1], 22505[0], 36000[1], 36400[1], 36405[1], 36406[1], 36410[1], 36420[1], 36425[1], 36430[1], 36440[1], 36591[0], 36592[0], 36600[1], 36640[1], 38220[0], 38221[1], 38222[0], 38230[0], 38232[0], 43752[1], 51701[1], 51702[1], 51703[1], 62320[0], 62321[0], 62322[0], 62323[0], 62324[0], 62325[0], 62326[0], 62327[0], 63001[1], 63015[1], 63020[1], 63040[1], 63045[1], 63050[1], 63051[1], 63707[1], 63709[1], 64400[0], 64405[0], 64408[0], 64415[0], 64416[0], 64417[0], 64418[0], 64420[0], 64421[0], 64425[0], 64430[0], 64435[0], 64445[0], 64446[0], 64447[0], 64448[0], 64449[0], 64450[0], 64451[0], 64454[0], 64461[0], 64462[0], 64463[0], 64479[0], 64480[0], 64483[0], 64484[0], 64486[0], 64487[0], 64488[0], 64489[0], 64490[0], 64491[0], 64492[0], 64493[0], 64494[0], 64495[0], 64505[0], 64510[0], 64517[0], 64520[0], 64530[0], 76000[1], 77001[1], 77002[1], 92012[1], 92014[1], 92585[0], 93000[1], 93005[1], 93010[1], 93040[1], 93041[1], 93042[1], 93318[1], 93355[1], 94002[1], 94200[1], 94250[1], 94680[1], 94681[1], 94690[1], 94770[1], 95812[1], 95813[1], 95816[1], 95819[1], 95822[0], 95829[1], 95860[0], 95861[0], 95863[0], 95864[0], 95865[0], 95866[0], 95867[0], 95868[0], 95869[0], 95870[0], 95907[0], 95908[0], 95909[0], 95910[0], 95911[0], 95912[0], 95913[0], 95925[0], 95926[0], 95927[0], 95928[0], 95929[0], 95930[0], 95933[0], 95937[0], 95938[0], 95939[0], 95940[0], 95955[1], 96360[1], 96361[1], 96365[1], 96366[1], 96367[1], 96368[1], 96372[1], 96374[1], 96375[1], 96376[1], 96377[1], 96523[0], 97597[1], 97598[1], 97602[1], 99155[0], 99156[0], 99157[0], 99211[1], 99212[1], 99213[1], 99214[1], 99215[1], 99217[1], 99218[1], 99219[1], 99220[1], 99221[1], 99222[1], 99223[1], 99231[1], 99232[1], 99233[1], 99234[1], 99235[1], 99236[1], 99238[1], 99239[1], 99241[1], 99242[1], 99243[1], 99244[1], 99245[1], 99251[1], 99252[1], 99253[1], 99254[1], 99255[1], 99291[1], 99292[1], 99304[1], 99305[1], 99306[1], 99307[1], 99308[1], 99309[1], 99310[1], 99315[1], 99316[1], 99334[1], 99335[1], 99336[1], 99337[1], 99347[1], 99348[1], 99349[1], 99350[1], 99374[1], 99375[1], 99377[1], 99378[1], 99446[0], 99447[0], 99448[0], 99449[0], 99451[0], 99452[0], 99495[0], 99496[0], G0453[0], G0463[1], G0471[1]
63276	0213T[0], 0216T[0], 0228T[0], 0230T[0], 0333T[0], 0464T[0], 0565T[1], 10005[1], 10007[1], 10009[1], 10011[1], 10021[1], 11000[1], 11001[1], 11004[1], 11005[1], 11006[1], 11042[1], 11043[1], 11044[1], 11045[1], 11046[1], 11047[1], 12001[1], 12002[1], 12004[1], 12005[1], 12006[1], 12007[1], 12011[1], 12013[1], 12014[1], 12015[1], 12016[1], 12017[1], 12018[1], 12020[1], 12021[1], 12031[1], 12032[1], 12034[1], 12035[1], 12036[1], 12037[1], 12041[1], 12042[1], 12044[1], 12045[1], 12046[1], 12047[1], 12051[1], 12052[1], 12053[1], 12054[1], 12055[1], 12056[1], 12057[1], 13100[1], 13101[1], 13102[1], 13120[1], 13121[1], 13122[1], 13131[1], 13132[1], 13133[1], 13151[1], 13152[1], 13153[1], 15769[1], 22101[1], 22505[0], 36000[1], 36400[1], 36405[1], 36406[1], 36410[1], 36420[1], 36425[1], 36430[1], 36440[1], 36591[0], 36592[0], 36600[1], 36640[1], 38220[0], 38221[1], 38222[0], 38230[0], 38232[0], 43752[1], 51701[1], 51702[1], 51703[1], 62320[0], 62321[0], 62322[0], 62323[0], 62324[0], 62325[0], 62326[0], 62327[0], 63003[1], 63016[1], 63046[1], 63707[1], 63709[1], 64400[0], 64405[0], 64408[0], 64415[0], 64416[0], 64417[0], 64418[0], 64420[0], 64421[0], 64425[0], 64430[0], 64435[0], 64445[0], 64446[0], 64447[0], 64448[0], 64449[0], 64450[0], 64451[0], 64454[0], 64461[0], 64462[0], 64463[0], 64479[0], 64480[0], 64483[0], 64484[0], 64486[0], 64487[0], 64488[0], 64489[0], 64490[0], 64491[0], 64492[0], 64493[0], 64494[0], 64495[0], 64505[0], 64510[0], 64517[0], 64520[0], 64530[0], 76000[1], 77001[1], 77002[1], 92012[1], 92014[1], 92585[0], 93000[1], 93005[1], 93010[1], 93040[1], 93041[1], 93042[1], 93318[1], 93355[1], 94002[1], 94200[1], 94250[1], 94680[1], 94681[1], 94690[1], 94770[1], 95812[1], 95813[1], 95816[1], 95819[1], 95822[0], 95829[1], 95860[0], 95861[0], 95863[0], 95864[0], 95865[0], 95866[0], 95867[0], 95868[0], 95869[0], 95870[0], 95907[0], 95908[0], 95909[0], 95910[0], 95911[0], 95912[0], 95913[0], 95925[0], 95926[0], 95927[0], 95928[0], 95929[0], 95930[0], 95933[0], 95937[0], 95938[0], 95939[0], 95940[0], 95955[1], 96360[1], 96361[1], 96365[1], 96366[1], 96367[1], 96368[1], 96372[1], 96374[1], 96375[1], 96376[1], 96377[1], 96523[0], 97597[1], 97598[1], 97602[1], 99155[0], 99156[0], 99157[0], 99211[1], 99212[1], 99213[1], 99214[1], 99215[1], 99217[1], 99218[1], 99219[1], 99220[1], 99221[1], 99222[1], 99223[1], 99231[1], 99232[1], 99233[1], 99234[1], 99235[1], 99236[1], 99238[1], 99239[1], 99241[1], 99242[1], 99243[1], 99244[1], 99245[1], 99251[1], 99252[1], 99253[1], 99254[1], 99255[1], 99291[1], 99292[1], 99304[1], 99305[1], 99306[1], 99307[1], 99308[1], 99309[1], 99310[1], 99315[1], 99316[1], 99334[1], 99335[1], 99336[1], 99337[1], 99347[1], 99348[1], 99349[1], 99350[1], 99374[1], 99375[1], 99377[1], 99378[1], 99446[0], 99447[0], 99448[0], 99449[0], 99451[0], 99452[0], 99495[0], 99496[0], G0453[0], G0463[1], G0471[1]
63277	0202T[1], 0213T[0], 0216T[0], 0228T[0], 0230T[0], 0275T[1], 0333T[0], 0464T[0], 0565T[1], 10005[1], 10007[1], 10009[1], 10011[1], 10021[1], 11000[1], 11001[1], 11004[1], 11005[1], 11006[1], 11042[1], 11043[1], 11044[1], 11045[1], 11046[1], 11047[1], 12001[1], 12002[1], 12004[1], 12005[1], 12006[1], 12007[1], 12011[1], 12013[1], 12014[1], 12015[1], 12016[1], 12017[1], 12018[1], 12020[1], 12021[1], 12031[1], 12032[1], 12034[1], 12035[1], 12036[1], 12037[1], 12041[1], 12042[1], 12044[1], 12045[1], 12046[1], 12047[1], 12051[1], 12052[1], 12053[1], 12054[1], 12055[1], 12056[1], 12057[1], 13100[1], 13101[1], 13102[1], 13120[1], 13121[1], 13122[1], 13131[1], 13132[1], 13133[1], 13151[1], 13152[1], 13153[1], 15769[1], 22102[1], 22505[0], 22867[1], 22868[1], 22869[1], 22870[1], 36000[1], 36400[1], 36405[1], 36406[1], 36410[1], 36420[1], 36425[1], 36430[1], 36440[1], 36591[0], 36592[0], 36600[1], 36640[1], 38220[0], 38221[1], 38222[0], 38230[0], 38232[0], 43752[1], 49000[0], 49002[1], 51701[1], 51702[1], 51703[1], 62320[0], 62321[0], 62322[0], 62323[0], 62324[0], 62325[0], 62326[0], 62327[0], 62380[1], 63005[1], 63012[1], 63017[1], 63030[1], 63042[1], 63047[1], 63707[1], 63709[1], 64400[0], 64405[0], 64408[0], 64415[0], 64416[0], 64417[0], 64418[0], 64420[0], 64421[0], 64425[0], 64430[0], 64435[0], 64445[0], 64446[0], 64447[0], 64448[0], 64449[0], 64450[0], 64451[0], 64454[0], 64461[0], 64462[0], 64463[0], 64479[0], 64480[0], 64483[0], 64484[0], 64486[0], 64487[0], 64488[0], 64489[0], 64490[0], 64491[0], 64492[0], 64493[0], 64494[0], 64495[0], 64505[0], 64510[0], 64517[0], 64520[0], 64530[0], 76000[1], 77001[1], 77002[1], 92012[1], 92014[1], 92585[0], 93000[1], 93005[1], 93010[1], 93040[1], 93041[1], 93042[1], 93318[1], 93355[1], 94002[1], 94200[1], 94250[1], 94680[1], 94681[1], 94690[1], 94770[1], 95812[1], 95813[1], 95816[1], 95819[1], 95822[0], 95829[1], 95860[0], 95861[0], 95863[0], 95864[0], 95865[0], 95866[0], 95867[0], 95868[0], 95869[0], 95870[0], 95907[0], 95908[0], 95909[0], 95910[0], 95911[0], 95912[0], 95913[0], 95925[0], 95926[0], 95927[0], 95928[0], 95929[0], 95930[0], 95933[0], 95937[0], 95938[0], 95939[0], 95940[0], 95955[1], 96360[1], 96361[1], 96365[1], 96366[1], 96367[1], 96368[1], 96372[1], 96374[1], 96375[1], 96376[1], 96377[1], 96523[0], 97597[1], 97598[1], 97602[1], 99155[0], 99156[0], 99157[0], 99211[1], 99212[1], 99213[1], 99214[1], 99215[1], 99217[1], 99218[1], 99219[1], 99220[1], 99221[1], 99222[1], 99223[1], 99231[1], 99232[1], 99233[1], 99234[1], 99235[1], 99236[1], 99238[1], 99239[1], 99241[1], 99242[1], 99243[1], 99244[1], 99245[1], 99251[1], 99252[1], 99253[1], 99254[1], 99255[1], 99291[1], 99292[1], 99304[1], 99305[1], 99306[1], 99307[1], 99308[1], 99309[1], 99310[1], 99315[1], 99316[1], 99334[1], 99335[1], 99336[1], 99337[1], 99347[1], 99348[1], 99349[1], 99350[1], 99374[1], 99375[1], 99377[1], 99378[1], 99446[0], 99447[0], 99448[0], 99449[0], 99451[0], 99452[0], 99495[0], 99496[0], G0276[1], G0453[0], G0463[1], G0471[1]
63278	0213T[0], 0216T[0], 0228T[0], 0230T[0], 0333T[0], 0464T[0], 0565T[1], 10005[1], 10007[1], 10009[1], 10011[1], 10021[1], 11000[1], 11001[1], 11004[1], 11005[1], 11006[1], 11042[1], 11043[1], 11044[1], 11045[1], 11046[1], 11047[1], 12001[1], 12002[1], 12004[1], 12005[1], 12006[1], 12007[1], 12011[1], 12013[1], 12014[1], 12015[1], 12016[1], 12017[1], 12018[1], 12020[1], 12021[1], 12031[1], 12032[1], 12034[1], 12035[1], 12036[1], 12037[1], 12041[1], 12042[1], 12044[1], 12045[1], 12046[1], 12047[1], 12051[1], 12052[1], 12053[1], 12054[1], 12055[1], 12056[1], 12057[1], 13100[1], 13101[1], 13102[1], 13120[1], 13121[1], 13122[1], 13131[1], 13132[1], 13133[1], 13151[1], 13152[1], 13153[1], 15769[1], 22102[1], 22505[0], 36000[1], 36400[1], 36405[1], 36406[1], 36410[1], 36420[1], 36425[1], 36430[1], 36440[1], 36591[0], 36592[0], 36600[1], 36640[1], 38220[0], 38221[1], 38222[0], 38230[0], 38232[0], 43752[1], 51701[1], 51702[1], 51703[1], 62320[0], 62321[0], 62322[0], 62323[0], 62324[0], 62325[0], 62326[0], 62327[0], 63011[1], 63707[1], 63709[1], 64400[0], 64405[0], 64408[0], 64415[0], 64416[0], 64417[0], 64418[0], 64420[0], 64421[0], 64425[0], 64430[0], 64435[0], 64445[0], 64446[0], 64447[0], 64448[0], 64449[0], 64450[0], 64451[0], 64454[0], 64461[0], 64462[0], 64463[0], 64479[0], 64480[0], 64483[0], 64484[0], 64486[0], 64487[0], 64488[0], 64489[0], 64490[0], 64491[0], 64492[0], 64493[0], 64494[0], 64495[0], 64505[0], 64510[0], 64517[0], 64520[0], 64530[0], 76000[1], 77001[1], 77002[1], 92012[1], 92014[1], 92585[0], 93000[1], 93005[1], 93010[1], 93040[1], 93041[1], 93042[1], 93318[1], 93355[1], 94002[1], 94200[1], 94250[1], 94680[1], 94681[1], 94690[1], 94770[1], 95812[1], 95813[1], 95816[1], 95819[1], 95822[0], 95829[1], 95860[0], 95861[0], 95863[0], 95864[0], 95865[0], 95866[0], 95867[0], 95868[0], 95869[0], 95870[0], 95907[0], 95908[0], 95909[0], 95910[0], 95911[0], 95912[0], 95913[0], 95925[0], 95926[0], 95927[0], 95928[0], 95929[0], 95930[0], 95933[0], 95937[0], 95938[0], 95939[0], 95940[0], 95955[1], 96360[1], 96361[1], 96365[1], 96366[1], 96367[1], 96368[1], 96372[1],

0 = Modifier usage not allowed or inappropriate 1 = Modifier usage allowed

Code 1	Code 2
	96374[1], 96375[1], 96376[1], 96377[1], 96523[0], 97597[1], 97598[1], 97602[1], 99155[0], 99156[0], 99157[0], 99211[1], 99212[1], 99213[1], 99214[1], 99215[1], 99217[1], 99218[1], 99219[1], 99220[1], 99221[1], 99222[1], 99223[1], 99231[1], 99232[1], 99233[1], 99234[1], 99235[1], 99236[1], 99238[1], 99239[1], 99241[1], 99242[1], 99243[1], 99244[1], 99245[1], 99251[1], 99252[1], 99253[1], 99254[1], 99255[1], 99291[1], 99292[1], 99304[1], 99305[1], 99306[1], 99307[1], 99308[1], 99309[1], 99310[1], 99315[1], 99316[1], 99334[1], 99335[1], 99336[1], 99337[1], 99347[1], 99348[1], 99349[1], 99350[1], 99374[1], 99375[1], 99377[1], 99378[1], 99446[0], 99447[0], 99448[0], 99449[0], 99451[0], 99452[0], 99495[0], 99496[0], G0453[0], G0463[1], G0471[1]
63280	0213T[0], 0216T[0], 0228T[0], 0230T[0], 0274T[1], 0333T[0], 0464T[0], 0565T[1], 10005[1], 10007[1], 10009[1], 10011[1], 10021[1], 11000[1], 11001[1], 11004[1], 11005[1], 11006[1], 11042[1], 11043[1], 11044[1], 11045[1], 11046[1], 11047[1], 12001[1], 12002[1], 12004[1], 12005[1], 12006[1], 12007[1], 12011[1], 12013[1], 12014[1], 12015[1], 12016[1], 12017[1], 12018[1], 12020[1], 12021[1], 12031[1], 12032[1], 12034[1], 12035[1], 12036[1], 12037[1], 12041[1], 12042[1], 12044[1], 12045[1], 12046[1], 12047[1], 12051[1], 12052[1], 12053[1], 12054[1], 12055[1], 12056[1], 12057[1], 13100[1], 13101[1], 13102[1], 13120[1], 13121[1], 13122[1], 13131[1], 13132[1], 13133[1], 13151[1], 13152[1], 13153[1], 15769[1], 22100[1], 22505[0], 36000[1], 36400[1], 36405[1], 36406[1], 36410[1], 36420[1], 36425[1], 36430[1], 36440[1], 36591[0], 36592[0], 36600[1], 36640[1], 38220[0], 38221[1], 38222[0], 38230[0], 38232[0], 43752[1], 49000[0], 49002[1], 51701[1], 51702[1], 51703[1], 62320[0], 62321[0], 62322[0], 62323[0], 62324[0], 62325[0], 62326[0], 62327[0], 63001[1], 63015[1], 63020[1], 63040[1], 63045[1], 63050[1], 63051[1], 63275[1], 63707[1], 63709[1], 64400[0], 64405[0], 64408[0], 64415[0], 64416[0], 64417[0], 64418[0], 64420[0], 64421[0], 64425[0], 64430[0], 64435[0], 64445[0], 64446[0], 64447[0], 64448[0], 64449[0], 64450[0], 64451[0], 64454[0], 64461[0], 64462[0], 64463[0], 64479[0], 64480[0], 64483[0], 64484[0], 64486[0], 64487[0], 64488[0], 64489[0], 64490[0], 64491[0], 64492[0], 64493[0], 64494[0], 64495[0], 64505[0], 64510[0], 64517[0], 64520[0], 64530[0], 76000[1], 77001[1], 77002[1], 92012[1], 92014[1], 92585[0], 93000[1], 93005[1], 93010[1], 93040[1], 93041[1], 93042[1], 93318[1], 93355[1], 94002[1], 94200[1], 94250[1], 94680[1], 94681[1], 94690[1], 94770[1], 95812[1], 95813[1], 95816[1], 95819[1], 95822[0], 95829[1], 95860[0], 95861[0], 95863[0], 95864[0], 95865[0], 95866[0], 95867[0], 95868[0], 95869[0], 95870[0], 95907[0], 95908[0], 95909[0], 95910[0], 95911[0], 95912[0], 95913[0], 95925[0], 95926[0], 95927[0], 95928[0], 95929[0], 95930[0], 95933[0], 95937[0], 95938[0], 95939[0], 95940[0], 95955[1], 96360[1], 96361[1], 96365[1], 96366[1], 96367[1], 96368[1], 96372[1], 96374[1], 96375[1], 96376[1], 96377[1], 96523[0], 97597[1], 97598[1], 97602[1], 99155[0], 99156[0], 99157[0], 99211[1], 99212[1], 99213[1], 99214[1], 99215[1], 99217[1], 99218[1], 99219[1], 99220[1], 99221[1], 99222[1], 99223[1], 99231[1], 99232[1], 99233[1], 99234[1], 99235[1], 99236[1], 99238[1], 99239[1], 99241[1], 99242[1], 99243[1], 99244[1], 99245[1], 99251[1], 99252[1], 99253[1], 99254[1], 99255[1], 99291[1], 99292[1], 99304[1], 99305[1], 99306[1], 99307[1], 99308[1], 99309[1], 99310[1], 99315[1], 99316[1], 99334[1], 99335[1], 99336[1], 99337[1], 99347[1], 99348[1], 99349[1], 99350[1], 99374[1], 99375[1], 99377[1], 99378[1], 99446[0], 99447[0], 99448[0], 99449[0], 99451[0], 99452[0], 99495[0], 99496[0], G0453[0], G0463[1], G0471[1]
63281	0213T[0], 0216T[0], 0228T[0], 0230T[0], 0333T[0], 0464T[0], 0565T[1], 10005[1], 10007[1], 10009[1], 10011[1], 10021[1], 11000[1], 11001[1], 11004[1], 11005[1], 11006[1], 11042[1], 11043[1], 11044[1], 11045[1], 11046[1], 11047[1], 12001[1], 12002[1], 12004[1], 12005[1], 12006[1], 12007[1], 12011[1], 12013[1], 12014[1], 12015[1], 12016[1], 12017[1], 12018[1], 12020[1], 12021[1], 12031[1], 12032[1], 12034[1], 12035[1], 12036[1], 12037[1], 12041[1], 12042[1], 12044[1], 12045[1], 12046[1], 12047[1], 12051[1], 12052[1], 12053[1], 12054[1], 12055[1], 12056[1], 12057[1], 13100[1], 13101[1], 13102[1], 13120[1], 13121[1], 13122[1], 13131[1], 13132[1], 13133[1], 13151[1], 13152[1], 13153[1], 15769[1], 22101[1], 22505[0], 36000[1], 36400[1], 36405[1], 36406[1], 36410[1], 36420[1], 36425[1], 36430[1], 36440[1], 36591[0], 36592[0], 36600[1], 36640[1], 38220[0], 38221[1], 38222[0], 38230[0], 38232[0], 43752[1], 51701[1], 51702[1], 51703[1], 62320[0], 62321[0], 62322[0], 62323[0], 62324[0], 62325[0], 62326[0], 62327[0], 63003[1], 63016[1], 63046[1], 63276[1], 63282[1], 63707[1], 63709[1], 64400[0], 64405[0], 64408[0], 64415[0], 64416[0], 64417[0], 64418[0], 64420[0], 64421[0], 64425[0], 64430[0], 64435[0], 64445[0], 64446[0], 64447[0], 64448[0], 64449[0], 64450[0], 64451[0], 64454[0], 64461[0], 64462[0], 64463[0], 64479[0], 64480[0], 64483[0], 64484[0], 64486[0], 64487[0], 64488[0], 64489[0], 64490[0], 64491[0], 64492[0], 64493[0], 64494[0], 64495[0], 64505[0], 64510[0], 64517[0], 64520[0], 64530[0], 76000[1], 77001[1], 77002[1], 92012[1], 92014[1], 92585[0], 93000[1], 93005[1], 93010[1], 93040[1], 93041[1], 93042[1], 93318[1], 93355[1], 94002[1], 94200[1], 94250[1], 94680[1], 94681[1], 94690[1], 94770[1], 95812[1], 95813[1], 95816[1], 95819[1], 95822[0], 95829[1], 95860[0], 95861[0], 95863[0], 95864[0], 95865[0], 95866[0], 95867[0], 95868[0], 95869[0], 95870[0], 95907[0], 95908[0], 95909[0], 95910[0], 95911[0], 95912[0], 95913[0], 95925[0], 95926[0], 95927[0], 95928[0], 95929[0], 95930[0], 95933[0], 95937[0], 95938[0], 95939[0], 95940[0], 95955[1], 96360[1], 96361[1], 96365[1], 96366[1], 96367[1], 96368[1], 96372[1], 96374[1], 96375[1], 96376[1], 96377[1], 96523[0], 97597[1], 97598[1], 97602[1], 99155[0], 99156[0], 99157[0], 99211[1], 99212[1], 99213[1], 99214[1], 99215[1], 99217[1], 99218[1], 99219[1], 99220[1], 99221[1], 99222[1], 99223[1], 99231[1], 99232[1], 99233[1], 99234[1], 99235[1], 99236[1], 99238[1], 99239[1], 99241[1], 99242[1], 99243[1], 99244[1], 99245[1], 99251[1], 99252[1], 99253[1], 99254[1], 99255[1], 99291[1], 99292[1], 99304[1], 99305[1], 99306[1], 99307[1], 99308[1], 99309[1], 99310[1], 99315[1], 99316[1], 99334[1], 99335[1], 99336[1], 99337[1], 99347[1], 99348[1], 99349[1], 99350[1], 99374[1], 99375[1], 99377[1], 99378[1], 99446[0], 99447[0], 99448[0], 99449[0], 99451[0], 99452[0], 99495[0], 99496[0], G0453[0], G0463[1], G0471[1]
63282	0202T[1], 0213T[0], 0216T[0], 0228T[0], 0230T[0], 0275T[1], 0333T[0], 0464T[0], 0565T[1], 10005[1], 10007[1], 10009[1], 10011[1], 10021[1], 11000[1], 11001[1], 11004[1], 11005[1], 11006[1], 11042[1], 11043[1], 11044[1], 11045[1], 11046[1], 11047[1], 12001[1], 12002[1], 12004[1], 12005[1], 12006[1], 12007[1], 12011[1], 12013[1], 12014[1], 12015[1], 12016[1], 12017[1], 12018[1], 12020[1], 12021[1], 12031[1], 12032[1], 12034[1], 12035[1], 12036[1], 12037[1], 12041[1], 12042[1], 12044[1], 12045[1], 12046[1], 12047[1], 12051[1], 12052[1], 12053[1], 12054[1], 12055[1], 12056[1], 12057[1], 13100[1], 13101[1], 13102[1], 13120[1], 13121[1], 13122[1], 13131[1], 13132[1], 13133[1], 13151[1], 13152[1], 13153[1], 15769[1], 22102[1], 22505[0], 22630[1], 22633[1], 22867[1], 22868[1], 22869[1], 22870[1], 36000[1], 36400[1], 36405[1], 36406[1], 36410[1], 36420[1], 36425[1], 36430[1], 36440[1], 36591[0], 36592[0], 36600[1], 36640[1], 38220[0], 38221[1], 38222[0], 38230[0], 38232[0], 43752[1], 49000[0], 49002[1], 51701[1], 51702[1], 51703[1], 62320[0], 62321[0], 62322[0], 62323[0], 62324[0], 62325[0], 62326[0], 62327[0], 62380[1], 63005[1], 63012[1], 63017[1], 63030[1], 63042[1], 63047[1], 63277[1], 63707[1], 63709[1], 64400[0], 64405[0], 64408[0], 64415[0], 64416[0], 64417[0], 64418[0], 64420[0], 64421[0], 64425[0], 64430[0], 64435[0], 64445[0], 64446[0], 64447[0], 64448[0], 64449[0], 64450[0], 64451[0], 64454[0], 64461[0], 64462[0], 64463[0], 64479[0], 64480[0], 64483[0], 64484[0], 64486[0], 64487[0], 64488[0], 64489[0], 64490[0], 64491[0], 64492[0], 64493[0], 64494[0], 64495[0], 64505[0], 64510[0], 64517[0], 64520[0], 64530[0], 76000[1], 77001[1], 77002[1], 92012[1], 92014[1], 92585[0], 93000[1], 93005[1], 93010[1], 93040[1], 93041[1], 93042[1], 93318[1], 93355[1], 94002[1], 94200[1], 94250[1], 94680[1], 94681[1], 94690[1], 94770[1], 95812[1], 95813[1], 95816[1], 95819[1], 95822[0], 95829[1], 95860[0], 95861[0], 95863[0], 95864[0], 95865[0], 95866[0], 95867[0], 95868[0], 95869[0], 95870[0], 95907[0], 95908[0], 95909[0], 95910[0], 95911[0], 95912[0], 95913[0], 95925[0], 95926[0], 95927[0], 95928[0], 95929[0], 95930[0], 95933[0], 95937[0], 95938[0], 95939[0], 95940[0], 95955[1], 96360[1], 96361[1], 96365[1], 96366[1], 96367[1], 96368[1], 96372[1], 96374[1], 96375[1], 96376[1], 96377[1], 96523[0], 97597[1], 97598[1], 97602[1], 99155[0], 99156[0], 99157[0], 99211[1], 99212[1], 99213[1], 99214[1], 99215[1], 99217[1], 99218[1], 99219[1], 99220[1], 99221[1], 99222[1], 99223[1], 99231[1], 99232[1], 99233[1], 99234[1], 99235[1], 99236[1], 99238[1], 99239[1], 99241[1], 99242[1], 99243[1], 99244[1], 99245[1], 99251[1], 99252[1], 99253[1], 99254[1], 99255[1], 99291[1], 99292[1], 99304[1], 99305[1], 99306[1], 99307[1], 99308[1], 99309[1], 99310[1], 99315[1], 99316[1], 99334[1], 99335[1], 99336[1], 99337[1], 99347[1], 99348[1], 99349[1], 99350[1], 99374[1], 99375[1], 99377[1], 99378[1], 99446[0], 99447[0], 99448[0], 99449[0], 99451[0], 99452[0], 99495[0], 99496[0], G0276[1], G0453[0], G0463[1], G0471[1]
63283	0213T[0], 0216T[0], 0228T[0], 0230T[0], 0333T[0], 0464T[0], 0565T[1], 10005[1], 10007[1], 10009[1], 10011[1], 10021[1], 11000[1], 11001[1], 11004[1], 11005[1], 11006[1], 11042[1], 11043[1], 11044[1], 11045[1], 11046[1], 11047[1], 12001[1], 12002[1], 12004[1], 12005[1], 12006[1], 12007[1], 12011[1], 12013[1], 12014[1], 12015[1], 12016[1], 12017[1], 12018[1], 12020[1], 12021[1], 12031[1], 12032[1], 12034[1], 12035[1], 12036[1], 12037[1], 12041[1], 12042[1], 12044[1], 12045[1], 12046[1], 12047[1], 12051[1], 12052[1], 12053[1], 12054[1], 12055[1], 12056[1], 12057[1], 13100[1], 13101[1], 13102[1], 13120[1], 13121[1], 13122[1], 13131[1], 13132[1], 13133[1], 13151[1], 13152[1], 13153[1], 15769[1], 22102[1], 22505[0], 36000[1], 36400[1], 36405[1], 36406[1], 36410[1], 36420[1], 36425[1], 36430[1], 36440[1], 36591[0], 36592[0], 36600[1], 36640[1], 38220[0], 38221[1], 38222[0], 38230[0], 38232[0], 43752[1], 49000[0], 49002[1], 51701[1], 51702[1], 51703[1], 62320[0], 62321[0], 62322[0], 62323[0], 62324[0], 62325[0], 62326[0], 62327[0], 63011[1], 63278[1], 63707[1], 63709[1], 64400[0], 64405[0], 64408[0], 64415[0], 64416[0], 64417[0], 64418[0], 64420[0], 64421[0], 64425[0], 64430[0], 64435[0], 64445[0], 64446[0], 64447[0], 64448[0], 64449[0], 64450[0], 64451[0], 64454[0], 64461[0], 64462[0], 64463[0], 64479[0], 64480[0], 64483[0], 64484[0], 64486[0], 64487[0], 64488[0], 64489[0], 64490[0], 64491[0], 64492[0], 64493[0], 64494[0], 64495[0], 64505[0], 64510[0], 64517[0], 64520[0], 64530[0], 76000[1], 77001[1], 77002[1], 92012[1], 92014[1], 92585[0], 93000[1], 93005[1], 93010[1], 93040[1], 93041[1], 93042[1], 93318[1], 93355[1], 94002[1], 94200[1], 94250[1], 94680[1], 94681[1], 94690[1], 94770[1], 95812[1], 95813[1], 95816[1], 95819[1], 95822[0], 95829[1], 95860[0], 95861[0], 95863[0], 95864[0], 95865[0], 95866[0], 95867[0], 95868[0], 95869[0], 95870[0], 95907[0], 95908[0], 95909[0], 95910[0], 95911[0], 95912[0], 95913[0], 95925[0], 95926[0], 95927[0], 95928[0], 95929[0], 95930[0], 95933[0], 95937[0], 95938[0], 95939[0], 95940[0], 95955[1], 96360[1], 96361[1], 96365[1], 96366[1], 96367[1], 96368[1], 96372[1], 96374[1], 96375[1], 96376[1], 96377[1], 96523[0], 97597[1], 97598[1], 97602[1], 99155[0], 99156[0], 99157[0], 99211[1], 99212[1], 99213[1], 99214[1], 99215[1], 99217[1], 99218[1], 99219[1], 99220[1], 99221[1], 99222[1], 99223[1], 99231[1], 99232[1], 99233[1], 99234[1], 99235[1], 99236[1], 99238[1], 99239[1], 99241[1], 99242[1], 99243[1], 99244[1], 99245[1], 99251[1], 99252[1], 99253[1], 99254[1], 99255[1], 99291[1], 99292[1], 99304[1], 99305[1], 99306[1], 99307[1], 99308[1], 99309[1], 99310[1], 99315[1], 99316[1], 99334[1], 99335[1], 99336[1], 99337[1], 99347[1], 99348[1], 99349[1], 99350[1], 99374[1], 99375[1], 99377[1], 99378[1], 99446[0], 99447[0], 99448[0], 99449[0], 99451[0], 99452[0], 99495[0], 99496[0], G0453[0], G0463[1], G0471[1]
63285	0213T[0], 0216T[0], 0228T[0], 0230T[0], 0274T[1], 0333T[0], 0464T[0], 0565T[1], 10005[1], 10007[1], 10009[1], 10011[1], 10021[1], 11000[1], 11001[1], 11004[1], 11005[1], 11006[1], 11042[1], 11043[1], 11044[1], 11045[1], 11046[1], 11047[1], 12001[1], 12002[1], 12004[1], 12005[1], 12006[1], 12007[1],

0 = Modifier usage not allowed or inappropriate 1 = Modifier usage allowed

Code 1	Code 2
	12011[1], 12013[1], 12014[1], 12015[1], 12016[1], 12017[1], 12018[1], 12020[1], 12021[1], 12031[1], 12032[1], 12034[1], 12035[1], 12036[1], 12037[1], 12041[1], 12042[1], 12044[1], 12045[1], 12046[1], 12047[1], 12051[1], 12052[1], 12053[1], 12054[1], 12055[1], 12056[1], 12057[1], 13100[1], 13101[1], 13102[1], 13120[1], 13121[1], 13122[1], 13131[1], 13132[1], 13133[1], 13151[1], 13152[1], 13153[1], 15769[1], 22100[1], 22206[1], 22207[1], 22505[0], 36000[1], 36400[1], 36405[1], 36406[1], 36410[1], 36420[1], 36425[1], 36430[1], 36440[1], 36591[0], 36592[0], 36600[1], 36640[1], 38220[0], 38221[1], 38222[0], 38230[0], 38232[0], 43752[1], 51701[1], 51702[1], 51703[1], 62320[0], 62321[0], 62322[0], 62323[0], 62324[0], 62325[0], 62326[0], 62327[0], 63001[1], 63015[1], 63020[1], 63040[1], 63045[1], 63050[1], 63051[1], 63275[1], 63280[1], 63707[1], 63709[1], 64400[0], 64405[0], 64408[0], 64415[0], 64416[0], 64417[0], 64418[0], 64420[0], 64421[0], 64425[0], 64430[0], 64435[0], 64445[0], 64446[0], 64447[0], 64448[0], 64449[0], 64450[0], 64451[0], 64454[0], 64461[0], 64462[0], 64463[0], 64479[0], 64480[0], 64483[0], 64484[0], 64486[0], 64487[0], 64488[0], 64489[0], 64490[0], 64491[0], 64492[0], 64493[0], 64494[0], 64495[0], 64505[0], 64510[0], 64517[0], 64520[0], 64530[0], 76000[1], 77001[1], 77002[1], 92012[1], 92014[1], 92585[0], 93000[1], 93005[1], 93010[1], 93040[1], 93041[1], 93042[1], 93318[1], 93355[1], 94002[1], 94200[1], 94250[1], 94680[1], 94681[1], 94690[1], 94770[1], 95812[1], 95813[1], 95816[1], 95819[1], 95822[0], 95829[1], 95860[0], 95861[0], 95863[0], 95864[0], 95865[0], 95866[0], 95867[0], 95868[0], 95869[0], 95870[0], 95907[0], 95908[0], 95909[0], 95910[0], 95911[0], 95912[0], 95913[0], 95925[0], 95926[0], 95927[0], 95928[0], 95929[0], 95930[0], 95933[0], 95937[0], 95938[0], 95939[0], 95940[0], 95955[1], 96360[1], 96361[1], 96365[1], 96366[1], 96367[1], 96368[1], 96372[1], 96374[1], 96375[1], 96376[1], 96377[1], 96523[0], 97597[1], 97598[1], 97602[1], 99155[0], 99156[0], 99157[0], 99211[1], 99212[1], 99213[1], 99214[1], 99215[1], 99217[1], 99218[1], 99219[1], 99220[1], 99221[1], 99222[1], 99223[1], 99231[1], 99232[1], 99233[1], 99234[1], 99235[1], 99236[1], 99238[1], 99239[1], 99241[1], 99242[1], 99243[1], 99244[1], 99245[1], 99251[1], 99252[1], 99253[1], 99254[1], 99255[1], 99291[1], 99292[1], 99304[1], 99305[1], 99306[1], 99307[1], 99308[1], 99309[1], 99310[1], 99315[1], 99316[1], 99334[1], 99335[1], 99336[1], 99337[1], 99347[1], 99348[1], 99349[1], 99350[1], 99374[1], 99375[1], 99377[1], 99378[1], 99446[0], 99447[0], 99448[0], 99449[0], 99451[0], 99452[0], 99495[0], 99496[0], G0453[0], G0463[1], G0471[1]
63286	0213T[0], 0216T[0], 0228T[0], 0230T[0], 0333T[0], 0464T[0], 0565T[1], 10005[1], 10007[1], 10009[1], 10011[1], 10021[1], 11000[1], 11001[1], 11004[1], 11005[1], 11006[1], 11042[1], 11043[1], 11044[1], 11045[1], 11046[1], 11047[1], 12001[1], 12002[1], 12004[1], 12005[1], 12006[1], 12007[1], 12011[1], 12013[1], 12014[1], 12015[1], 12016[1], 12017[1], 12018[1], 12020[1], 12021[1], 12031[1], 12032[1], 12034[1], 12035[1], 12036[1], 12037[1], 12041[1], 12042[1], 12044[1], 12045[1], 12046[1], 12047[1], 12051[1], 12052[1], 12053[1], 12054[1], 12055[1], 12056[1], 12057[1], 13100[1], 13101[1], 13102[1], 13120[1], 13121[1], 13122[1], 13131[1], 13132[1], 13133[1], 13151[1], 13152[1], 13153[1], 15769[1], 22101[1], 22206[1], 22207[1], 22505[0], 36000[1], 36400[1], 36405[1], 36406[1], 36410[1], 36420[1], 36425[1], 36430[1], 36440[1], 36591[0], 36592[0], 36600[1], 36640[1], 38220[0], 38221[1], 38222[0], 38230[0], 38232[0], 43752[1], 51701[1], 51702[1], 51703[1], 62320[0], 62321[0], 62322[0], 62323[0], 62324[0], 62325[0], 62326[0], 62327[0], 63003[1], 63016[1], 63046[1], 63276[1], 63281[1], 63707[1], 63709[1], 64400[0], 64405[0], 64408[0], 64415[0], 64416[0], 64417[0], 64418[0], 64420[0], 64421[0], 64425[0], 64430[0], 64435[0], 64445[0], 64446[0], 64447[0], 64448[0], 64449[0], 64450[0], 64451[0], 64454[0], 64461[0], 64462[0], 64463[0], 64479[0], 64480[0], 64483[0], 64484[0], 64486[0], 64487[0], 64488[0], 64489[0], 64490[0], 64491[0], 64492[0], 64493[0], 64494[0], 64495[0], 64505[0], 64510[0], 64517[0], 64520[0], 64530[0], 76000[1], 77001[1], 77002[1], 92012[1], 92014[1], 92585[0], 93000[1], 93005[1], 93010[1], 93040[1], 93041[1], 93042[1], 93318[1], 93355[1], 94002[1], 94200[1], 94250[1], 94680[1], 94681[1], 94690[1], 94770[1], 95812[1], 95813[1], 95816[1], 95819[1], 95822[0], 95829[1], 95860[0], 95861[0], 95863[0], 95864[0], 95865[0], 95866[0], 95867[0], 95868[0], 95869[0], 95870[0], 95907[0], 95908[0], 95909[0], 95910[0], 95911[0], 95912[0], 95913[0], 95925[0], 95926[0], 95927[0], 95928[0], 95929[0], 95930[0], 95933[0], 95937[0], 95938[0], 95939[0], 95940[0], 95955[1], 96360[1], 96361[1], 96365[1], 96366[1], 96367[1], 96368[1], 96372[1], 96374[1], 96375[1], 96376[1], 96377[1], 96523[0], 97597[1], 97598[1], 97602[1], 99155[0], 99156[0], 99157[0], 99211[1], 99212[1], 99213[1], 99214[1], 99215[1], 99217[1], 99218[1], 99219[1], 99220[1], 99221[1], 99222[1], 99223[1], 99231[1], 99232[1], 99233[1], 99234[1], 99235[1], 99236[1], 99238[1], 99239[1], 99241[1], 99242[1], 99243[1], 99244[1], 99245[1], 99251[1], 99252[1], 99253[1], 99254[1], 99255[1], 99291[1], 99292[1], 99304[1], 99305[1], 99306[1], 99307[1], 99308[1], 99309[1], 99310[1], 99315[1], 99316[1], 99334[1], 99335[1], 99336[1], 99337[1], 99347[1], 99348[1], 99349[1], 99350[1], 99374[1], 99375[1], 99377[1], 99378[1], 99446[0], 99447[0], 99448[0], 99449[0], 99451[0], 99452[0], 99495[0], 99496[0], G0453[0], G0463[1], G0471[1]
63287	0202T[1], 0213T[0], 0216T[0], 0228T[0], 0230T[0], 0275T[1], 0333T[0], 0464T[0], 0565T[1], 10005[1], 10007[1], 10009[1], 10011[1], 10021[1], 11000[1], 11001[1], 11004[1], 11005[1], 11006[1], 11042[1], 11043[1], 11044[1], 11045[1], 11046[1], 11047[1], 12001[1], 12002[1], 12004[1], 12005[1], 12006[1], 12007[1], 12011[1], 12013[1], 12014[1], 12015[1], 12016[1], 12017[1], 12018[1], 12020[1], 12021[1], 12031[1], 12032[1], 12034[1], 12035[1], 12036[1], 12037[1], 12041[1], 12042[1], 12044[1], 12045[1], 12046[1], 12047[1], 12051[1], 12052[1], 12053[1], 12054[1], 12055[1], 12056[1], 12057[1], 13100[1], 13101[1], 13102[1], 13120[1], 13121[1], 13122[1], 13131[1], 13132[1], 13133[1], 13151[1], 13152[1], 13153[1], 15769[1], 22101[1], 22102[1], 22206[1], 22207[1], 22505[0], 22630[1], 22633[1], 22867[1], 22868[1], 22869[1], 22870[1], 36000[1], 36400[1], 36405[1], 36406[1], 36410[1], 36420[1], 36425[1], 36430[1], 36440[1], 36591[0], 36592[0], 36600[1], 36640[1], 38220[0], 38221[1], 38222[0], 38230[0], 38232[0], 43752[1], 49000[0], 49002[1], 51701[1], 51702[1], 51703[1], 62320[0], 62321[0], 62322[0], 62323[0], 62324[0], 62325[0], 62326[0], 62327[0], 62380[1], 63003[1], 63005[1], 63012[1], 63016[1], 63017[1], 63030[1], 63042[1], 63046[1], 63047[1], 63276[1], 63277[1], 63281[1], 63282[1], 63286[1], 63707[1], 63709[1], 64400[0], 64405[0], 64408[0], 64415[0], 64416[0], 64417[0], 64418[0], 64420[0], 64421[0], 64425[0], 64430[0], 64435[0], 64445[0], 64446[0], 64447[0], 64448[0], 64449[0], 64450[0], 64451[0], 64454[0], 64461[0], 64462[0], 64463[0], 64479[0], 64480[0], 64483[0], 64484[0], 64486[0], 64487[0], 64488[0], 64489[0], 64490[0], 64491[0], 64492[0], 64493[0], 64494[0], 64495[0], 64505[0], 64510[0], 64517[0], 64520[0], 64530[0], 76000[1], 77001[1], 77002[1], 92012[1], 92014[1], 92585[0], 93000[1], 93005[1], 93010[1], 93040[1], 93041[1], 93042[1], 93318[1], 93355[1], 94002[1], 94200[1], 94250[1], 94680[1], 94681[1], 94690[1], 94770[1], 95812[1], 95813[1], 95816[1], 95819[1], 95822[0], 95829[1], 95860[0], 95861[0], 95863[0], 95864[0], 95865[0], 95866[0], 95867[0], 95868[0], 95869[0], 95870[0], 95907[0], 95908[0], 95909[0], 95910[0], 95911[0], 95912[0], 95913[0], 95925[0], 95926[0], 95927[0], 95928[0], 95929[0], 95930[0], 95933[0], 95937[0], 95938[0], 95939[0], 95940[0], 95955[1], 96360[1], 96361[1], 96365[1], 96366[1], 96367[1], 96368[1], 96372[1], 96374[1], 96375[1], 96376[1], 96377[1], 96523[0], 97597[1], 97598[1], 97602[1], 99155[0], 99156[0], 99157[0], 99211[1], 99212[1], 99213[1], 99214[1], 99215[1], 99217[1], 99218[1], 99219[1], 99220[1], 99221[1], 99222[1], 99223[1], 99231[1], 99232[1], 99233[1], 99234[1], 99235[1], 99236[1], 99238[1], 99239[1], 99241[1], 99242[1], 99243[1], 99244[1], 99245[1], 99251[1], 99252[1], 99253[1], 99254[1], 99255[1], 99291[1], 99292[1], 99304[1], 99305[1], 99306[1], 99307[1], 99308[1], 99309[1], 99310[1], 99315[1], 99316[1], 99334[1], 99335[1], 99336[1], 99337[1], 99347[1], 99348[1], 99349[1], 99350[1], 99374[1], 99375[1], 99377[1], 99378[1], 99446[0], 99447[0], 99448[0], 99449[0], 99451[0], 99452[0], 99495[0], 99496[0], G0276[1], G0453[0], G0463[1], G0471[1]
63290	0202T[1], 0213T[0], 0216T[0], 0228T[0], 0230T[0], 0274T[1], 0275T[1], 0333T[0], 0464T[0], 0565T[1], 10005[1], 10007[1], 10009[1], 10011[1], 10021[1], 11000[1], 11001[1], 11004[1], 11005[1], 11006[1], 11042[1], 11043[1], 11044[1], 11045[1], 11046[1], 11047[1], 12001[1], 12002[1], 12004[1], 12005[1], 12006[1], 12007[1], 12011[1], 12013[1], 12014[1], 12015[1], 12016[1], 12017[1], 12018[1], 12020[1], 12021[1], 12031[1], 12032[1], 12034[1], 12035[1], 12036[1], 12037[1], 12041[1], 12042[1], 12044[1], 12045[1], 12046[1], 12047[1], 12051[1], 12052[1], 12053[1], 12054[1], 12055[1], 12056[1], 12057[1], 13100[1], 13101[1], 13102[1], 13120[1], 13121[1], 13122[1], 13131[1], 13132[1], 13133[1], 13151[1], 13152[1], 13153[1], 15769[1], 22100[1], 22101[1], 22102[1], 22206[1], 22207[1], 22505[0], 22630[1], 22633[1], 22867[1], 22868[1], 22869[1], 22870[1], 36000[1], 36400[1], 36405[1], 36406[1], 36410[1], 36420[1], 36425[1], 36430[1], 36440[1], 36591[0], 36592[0], 36600[1], 36640[1], 38220[0], 38221[1], 38222[0], 38230[0], 38232[0], 43752[1], 49000[0], 49002[1], 51701[1], 51702[1], 51703[1], 62320[0], 62321[0], 62322[0], 62323[0], 62324[0], 62325[0], 62326[0], 62327[0], 62380[1], 63001[1], 63003[1], 63005[1], 63011[1], 63012[1], 63015[1], 63016[1], 63017[1], 63020[1], 63030[1], 63040[1], 63042[1], 63045[1], 63046[1], 63047[1], 63050[1], 63051[1], 63275[1], 63276[1], 63277[1], 63278[1], 63280[1], 63281[1], 63282[1], 63283[1], 63285[1], 63286[1], 63287[1], 63707[1], 63709[1], 64400[0], 64405[0], 64408[0], 64415[0], 64416[0], 64417[0], 64418[0], 64420[0], 64421[0], 64425[0], 64430[0], 64435[0], 64445[0], 64446[0], 64447[0], 64448[0], 64449[0], 64450[0], 64451[0], 64454[0], 64461[0], 64462[0], 64463[0], 64479[0], 64480[0], 64483[0], 64484[0], 64486[0], 64487[0], 64488[0], 64489[0], 64490[0], 64491[0], 64492[0], 64493[0], 64494[0], 64495[0], 64505[0], 64510[0], 64517[0], 64520[0], 64530[0], 76000[1], 77001[1], 77002[1], 92012[1], 92014[1], 92585[0], 93000[1], 93005[1], 93010[1], 93040[1], 93041[1], 93042[1], 93318[1], 93355[1], 94002[1], 94200[1], 94250[1], 94680[1], 94681[1], 94690[1], 94770[1], 95812[1], 95813[1], 95816[1], 95819[1], 95822[0], 95829[1], 95860[0], 95861[0], 95863[0], 95864[0], 95865[0], 95866[0], 95867[0], 95868[0], 95869[0], 95870[0], 95907[0], 95908[0], 95909[0], 95910[0], 95911[0], 95912[0], 95913[0], 95925[0], 95926[0], 95927[0], 95928[0], 95929[0], 95930[0], 95933[0], 95937[0], 95938[0], 95939[0], 95940[0], 95955[1], 96360[1], 96361[1], 96365[1], 96366[1], 96367[1], 96368[1], 96372[1], 96374[1], 96375[1], 96376[1], 96377[1], 96523[0], 97597[1], 97598[1], 97602[1], 99155[0], 99156[0], 99157[0], 99211[1], 99212[1], 99213[1], 99214[1], 99215[1], 99217[1], 99218[1], 99219[1], 99220[1], 99221[1], 99222[1], 99223[1], 99231[1], 99232[1], 99233[1], 99234[1], 99235[1], 99236[1], 99238[1], 99239[1], 99241[1], 99242[1], 99243[1], 99244[1], 99245[1], 99251[1], 99252[1], 99253[1], 99254[1], 99255[1], 99291[1], 99292[1], 99304[1], 99305[1], 99306[1], 99307[1], 99308[1], 99309[1], 99310[1], 99315[1], 99316[1], 99334[1], 99335[1], 99336[1], 99337[1], 99347[1], 99348[1], 99349[1], 99350[1], 99374[1], 99375[1], 99377[1], 99378[1], 99446[0], 99447[0], 99448[0], 99449[0], 99451[0], 99452[0], 99495[0], 99496[0], G0276[1], G0453[0], G0463[1], G0471[1]
63300	0213T[0], 0216T[0], 0228T[0], 0230T[0], 0333T[0], 0464T[0], 0565T[1], 11000[1], 11001[1], 11004[1], 11005[1], 11006[1], 11042[1], 11043[1], 11044[1], 11045[1], 11046[1], 11047[1], 12001[1], 12002[1], 12004[1], 12005[1], 12006[1], 12007[1], 12011[1], 12013[1], 12014[1], 12015[1], 12016[1], 12017[1], 12018[1], 12020[1], 12021[1], 12031[1], 12032[1], 12034[1], 12035[1], 12036[1], 12037[1], 12041[1], 12042[1], 12044[1], 12045[1], 12046[1], 12047[1], 12051[1], 12052[1], 12053[1], 12054[1], 12055[1], 12056[1], 12057[1], 13100[1], 13101[1], 13102[1], 13120[1], 13121[1], 13122[1], 13131[1], 13132[1], 13133[1], 13151[1], 13152[1], 13153[1], 15769[1], 22505[0], 36000[1], 36400[1], 36405[1], 36406[1], 36410[1], 36420[1], 36425[1], 36430[1], 36440[1], 36591[0], 36592[0], 36600[1], 36640[1], 38220[0], 38221[1], 38222[0], 38230[0], 38232[0], 43752[1], 49000[0], 49002[1], 51701[1], 51702[1], 51703[1], 62320[0], 62321[0], 62322[0], 62323[0], 62324[0], 62325[0], 62326[0], 62327[0], 63075[1], 63707[1],

0 = Modifier usage not allowed or inappropriate 1 = Modifier usage allowed

Appendix A: NCCI - CPT Codes

Code 1	Code 2
	63709[1], 64400[0], 64405[0], 64408[0], 64415[0], 64416[0], 64417[0], 64418[0], 64420[0], 64421[0], 64425[0], 64430[0], 64435[0], 64445[0], 64446[0], 64447[0], 64448[0], 64449[0], 64450[0], 64451[0], 64454[0], 64461[0], 64462[0], 64463[0], 64479[0], 64480[0], 64483[0], 64484[0], 64486[0], 64487[0], 64488[0], 64489[0], 64490[0], 64491[0], 64492[0], 64493[0], 64494[0], 64495[0], 64505[0], 64510[0], 64517[0], 64520[0], 64530[0], 76000[1], 77001[1], 77002[1], 92012[1], 92014[1], 92585[0], 93000[1], 93005[1], 93010[1], 93040[1], 93041[1], 93042[1], 93318[1], 93355[1], 94002[1], 94200[1], 94250[1], 94680[1], 94681[1], 94690[1], 94770[1], 95812[1], 95813[1], 95816[1], 95819[1], 95822[0], 95829[1], 95860[0], 95861[0], 95863[0], 95864[0], 95865[0], 95866[0], 95867[0], 95868[0], 95869[0], 95870[0], 95907[0], 95908[0], 95909[0], 95910[0], 95911[0], 95912[0], 95913[0], 95925[0], 95926[0], 95927[0], 95928[0], 95929[0], 95930[0], 95933[0], 95937[0], 95938[0], 95939[0], 95940[0], 95955[1], 96360[1], 96361[1], 96365[1], 96366[1], 96367[1], 96368[1], 96372[1], 96374[1], 96375[1], 96376[1], 96377[1], 96523[0], 97597[1], 97598[1], 97602[1], 99155[0], 99156[0], 99157[0], 99211[1], 99212[1], 99213[1], 99214[1], 99215[1], 99217[1], 99218[1], 99219[1], 99220[1], 99221[1], 99222[1], 99223[1], 99231[1], 99232[1], 99233[1], 99234[1], 99235[1], 99236[1], 99238[1], 99239[1], 99241[1], 99242[1], 99243[1], 99244[1], 99245[1], 99251[1], 99252[1], 99253[1], 99254[1], 99255[1], 99291[1], 99292[1], 99304[1], 99305[1], 99306[1], 99307[1], 99308[1], 99309[1], 99310[1], 99315[1], 99316[1], 99334[1], 99335[1], 99336[1], 99337[1], 99347[1], 99348[1], 99349[1], 99350[1], 99374[1], 99375[1], 99377[1], 99378[1], 99446[0], 99447[0], 99448[0], 99449[0], 99451[0], 99452[0], 99495[0], 99496[0], G0453[0], G0463[1], G0471[1]
63301	0213T[0], 0216T[0], 0228T[0], 0230T[0], 0333T[0], 0464T[0], 0565T[1], 11000[1], 11001[1], 11004[1], 11005[1], 11006[1], 11042[1], 11043[1], 11044[1], 11045[1], 11046[1], 11047[1], 12001[1], 12002[1], 12004[1], 12005[1], 12006[1], 12007[1], 12011[1], 12013[1], 12014[1], 12015[1], 12016[1], 12017[1], 12018[1], 12020[1], 12021[1], 12031[1], 12032[1], 12034[1], 12035[1], 12036[1], 12037[1], 12041[1], 12042[1], 12044[1], 12045[1], 12046[1], 12047[1], 12051[1], 12052[1], 12053[1], 12054[1], 12055[1], 12056[1], 12057[1], 13100[1], 13101[1], 13102[1], 13120[1], 13121[1], 13122[1], 13131[1], 13132[1], 13133[1], 13151[1], 13152[1], 13153[1], 15769[1], 22505[0], 32100[1], 32110[1], 32150[1], 32160[1], 36000[1], 36400[1], 36405[1], 36406[1], 36410[1], 36420[1], 36425[1], 36430[1], 36440[1], 36591[0], 36592[0], 36600[1], 36640[1], 38220[0], 38221[1], 38222[0], 38230[0], 38232[0], 43336[1], 43337[1], 43752[1], 49000[0], 49002[1], 51701[1], 51702[1], 51703[1], 62320[0], 62321[0], 62322[0], 62323[0], 62324[0], 62325[0], 62326[0], 62327[0], 63077[1], 63707[1], 63709[1], 64400[0], 64405[0], 64408[0], 64415[0], 64416[0], 64417[0], 64418[0], 64420[0], 64421[0], 64425[0], 64430[0], 64435[0], 64445[0], 64446[0], 64447[0], 64448[0], 64449[0], 64450[0], 64451[0], 64454[0], 64461[0], 64462[0], 64463[0], 64479[0], 64480[0], 64483[0], 64484[0], 64486[0], 64487[0], 64488[0], 64489[0], 64490[0], 64491[0], 64492[0], 64493[0], 64494[0], 64495[0], 64505[0], 64510[0], 64517[0], 64520[0], 64530[0], 76000[1], 77001[1], 77002[1], 92012[1], 92014[1], 92585[0], 93000[1], 93005[1], 93010[1], 93040[1], 93041[1], 93042[1], 93318[1], 93355[1], 94002[1], 94200[1], 94250[1], 94680[1], 94681[1], 94690[1], 94770[1], 95812[1], 95813[1], 95816[1], 95819[1], 95822[0], 95829[1], 95860[0], 95861[0], 95863[0], 95864[0], 95865[0], 95866[0], 95867[0], 95868[0], 95869[0], 95870[0], 95907[0], 95908[0], 95909[0], 95910[0], 95911[0], 95912[0], 95913[0], 95925[0], 95926[0], 95927[0], 95928[0], 95929[0], 95930[0], 95933[0], 95937[0], 95938[0], 95939[0], 95940[0], 95955[1], 96360[1], 96361[1], 96365[1], 96366[1], 96367[1], 96368[1], 96372[1], 96374[1], 96375[1], 96376[1], 96377[1], 96523[0], 97597[1], 97598[1], 97602[1], 99155[0], 99156[0], 99157[0], 99211[1], 99212[1], 99213[1], 99214[1], 99215[1], 99217[1], 99218[1], 99219[1], 99220[1], 99221[1], 99222[1], 99223[1], 99231[1], 99232[1], 99233[1], 99234[1], 99235[1], 99236[1], 99238[1], 99239[1], 99241[1], 99242[1], 99243[1], 99244[1], 99245[1], 99251[1], 99252[1], 99253[1], 99254[1], 99255[1], 99291[1], 99292[1], 99304[1], 99305[1], 99306[1], 99307[1], 99308[1], 99309[1], 99310[1], 99315[1], 99316[1], 99334[1], 99335[1], 99336[1], 99337[1], 99347[1], 99348[1], 99349[1], 99350[1], 99374[1], 99375[1], 99377[1], 99378[1], 99446[0], 99447[0], 99448[0], 99449[0], 99451[0], 99452[0], 99495[0], 99496[0], G0453[0], G0463[1], G0471[1]
63302	0213T[0], 0216T[0], 0228T[0], 0230T[0], 0333T[0], 0464T[0], 0565T[1], 11000[1], 11001[1], 11004[1], 11005[1], 11006[1], 11042[1], 11043[1], 11044[1], 11045[1], 11046[1], 11047[1], 12001[1], 12002[1], 12004[1], 12005[1], 12006[1], 12007[1], 12011[1], 12013[1], 12014[1], 12015[1], 12016[1], 12017[1], 12018[1], 12020[1], 12021[1], 12031[1], 12032[1], 12034[1], 12035[1], 12036[1], 12037[1], 12041[1], 12042[1], 12044[1], 12045[1], 12046[1], 12047[1], 12051[1], 12052[1], 12053[1], 12054[1], 12055[1], 12056[1], 12057[1], 13100[1], 13101[1], 13102[1], 13120[1], 13121[1], 13122[1], 13131[1], 13132[1], 13133[1], 13151[1], 13152[1], 13153[1], 15769[1], 22505[0], 32100[1], 32110[1], 32150[1], 32160[1], 36000[1], 36400[1], 36405[1], 36406[1], 36410[1], 36420[1], 36425[1], 36430[1], 36440[1], 36591[0], 36592[0], 36600[1], 36640[1], 38220[0], 38221[1], 38222[0], 38230[0], 38232[0], 43336[1], 43337[1], 43752[1], 49000[0], 49002[1], 49010[0], 51701[1], 51702[1], 51703[1], 62320[0], 62321[0], 62322[0], 62323[0], 62324[0], 62325[0], 62326[0], 62327[0], 63077[1], 63707[1], 63709[1], 64400[0], 64405[0], 64408[0], 64415[0], 64416[0], 64417[0], 64418[0], 64420[0], 64421[0], 64425[0], 64430[0], 64435[0], 64445[0], 64446[0], 64447[0], 64448[0], 64449[0], 64450[0], 64451[0], 64454[0], 64461[0], 64462[0], 64463[0], 64479[0], 64480[0], 64483[0], 64484[0], 64486[0], 64487[0], 64488[0], 64489[0], 64490[0], 64491[0], 64492[0], 64493[0], 64494[0], 64495[0], 64505[0], 64510[0], 64517[0], 64520[0], 64530[0], 76000[1], 77001[1], 77002[1], 92012[1], 92014[1], 92585[0], 93000[1], 93005[1], 93010[1], 93040[1], 93041[1], 93042[1], 93318[1], 93355[1], 94002[1], 94200[1], 94250[1], 94680[1], 94681[1], 94690[1], 94770[1], 95812[1], 95813[1], 95816[1], 95819[1], 95822[0], 95829[1], 95860[0], 95861[0], 95863[0], 95864[0], 95865[0], 95866[0], 95867[0], 95868[0], 95869[0], 95870[0], 95907[0], 95908[0], 95909[0], 95910[0], 95911[0], 95912[0], 95913[0], 95925[0], 95926[0], 95927[0], 95928[0], 95929[0], 95930[0], 95933[0], 95937[0], 95938[0], 95939[0], 95940[0], 95955[1], 96360[1], 96361[1], 96365[1], 96366[1], 96367[1], 96368[1], 96372[1], 96374[1], 96375[1], 96376[1], 96377[1], 96523[0], 97597[1], 97598[1], 97602[1], 99155[0], 99156[0], 99157[0], 99211[1], 99212[1], 99213[1], 99214[1], 99215[1], 99217[1], 99218[1], 99219[1], 99220[1], 99221[1], 99222[1], 99223[1], 99231[1], 99232[1], 99233[1], 99234[1], 99235[1], 99236[1], 99238[1], 99239[1], 99241[1], 99242[1], 99243[1], 99244[1], 99245[1], 99251[1], 99252[1], 99253[1], 99254[1], 99255[1], 99291[1], 99292[1], 99304[1], 99305[1], 99306[1], 99307[1], 99308[1], 99309[1], 99310[1], 99315[1], 99316[1], 99334[1], 99335[1], 99336[1], 99337[1], 99347[1], 99348[1], 99349[1], 99350[1], 99374[1], 99375[1], 99377[1], 99378[1], 99446[0], 99447[0], 99448[0], 99449[0], 99451[0], 99452[0], 99495[0], 99496[0], G0453[0], G0463[1], G0471[1]
63303	0213T[0], 0216T[0], 0228T[0], 0230T[0], 0333T[0], 0464T[0], 0565T[1], 11000[1], 11001[1], 11004[1], 11005[1], 11006[1], 11042[1], 11043[1], 11044[1], 11045[1], 11046[1], 11047[1], 12001[1], 12002[1], 12004[1], 12005[1], 12006[1], 12007[1], 12011[1], 12013[1], 12014[1], 12015[1], 12016[1], 12017[1], 12018[1], 12020[1], 12021[1], 12031[1], 12032[1], 12034[1], 12035[1], 12036[1], 12037[1], 12041[1], 12042[1], 12044[1], 12045[1], 12046[1], 12047[1], 12051[1], 12052[1], 12053[1], 12054[1], 12055[1], 12056[1], 12057[1], 13100[1], 13101[1], 13102[1], 13120[1], 13121[1], 13122[1], 13131[1], 13132[1], 13133[1], 13151[1], 13152[1], 13153[1], 15769[1], 22505[0], 36000[1], 36400[1], 36405[1], 36406[1], 36410[1], 36420[1], 36425[1], 36430[1], 36440[1], 36591[0], 36592[0], 36600[1], 36640[1], 38220[0], 38221[1], 38222[0], 38230[0], 38232[0], 43752[1], 44005[0], 44180[0], 44820[0], 44850[0], 49000[0], 49002[1], 49010[0], 49255[0], 51701[1], 51702[1], 51703[1], 62320[0], 62321[0], 62322[0], 62323[0], 62324[0], 62325[0], 62326[0], 62327[0], 63707[1], 63709[1], 64400[0], 64405[0], 64408[0], 64415[0], 64416[0], 64417[0], 64418[0], 64420[0], 64421[0], 64425[0], 64430[0], 64435[0], 64445[0], 64446[0], 64447[0], 64448[0], 64449[0], 64450[0], 64451[0], 64454[0], 64461[0], 64462[0], 64463[0], 64479[0], 64480[0], 64483[0], 64484[0], 64486[0], 64487[0], 64488[0], 64489[0], 64490[0], 64491[0], 64492[0], 64493[0], 64494[0], 64495[0], 64505[0], 64510[0], 64517[0], 64520[0], 64530[0], 76000[1], 77001[1], 77002[1], 92012[1], 92014[1], 92585[0], 93000[1], 93005[1], 93010[1], 93040[1], 93041[1], 93042[1], 93318[1], 93355[1], 94002[1], 94200[1], 94250[1], 94680[1], 94681[1], 94690[1], 94770[1], 95812[1], 95813[1], 95816[1], 95819[1], 95822[0], 95829[1], 95860[0], 95861[0], 95863[0], 95864[0], 95865[0], 95866[0], 95867[0], 95868[0], 95869[0], 95870[0], 95907[0], 95908[0], 95909[0], 95910[0], 95911[0], 95912[0], 95913[0], 95925[0], 95926[0], 95927[0], 95928[0], 95929[0], 95930[0], 95933[0], 95937[0], 95938[0], 95939[0], 95940[0], 95955[1], 96360[1], 96361[1], 96365[1], 96366[1], 96367[1], 96368[1], 96372[1], 96374[1], 96375[1], 96376[1], 96377[1], 96523[0], 97597[1], 97598[1], 97602[1], 99155[0], 99156[0], 99157[0], 99211[1], 99212[1], 99213[1], 99214[1], 99215[1], 99217[1], 99218[1], 99219[1], 99220[1], 99221[1], 99222[1], 99223[1], 99231[1], 99232[1], 99233[1], 99234[1], 99235[1], 99236[1], 99238[1], 99239[1], 99241[1], 99242[1], 99243[1], 99244[1], 99245[1], 99251[1], 99252[1], 99253[1], 99254[1], 99255[1], 99291[1], 99292[1], 99304[1], 99305[1], 99306[1], 99307[1], 99308[1], 99309[1], 99310[1], 99315[1], 99316[1], 99334[1], 99335[1], 99336[1], 99337[1], 99347[1], 99348[1], 99349[1], 99350[1], 99374[1], 99375[1], 99377[1], 99378[1], 99446[0], 99447[0], 99448[0], 99449[0], 99451[0], 99452[0], 99495[0], 99496[0], G0453[0], G0463[1], G0471[1]
63304	0213T[0], 0216T[0], 0228T[0], 0230T[0], 0333T[0], 0464T[0], 0565T[1], 11000[1], 11001[1], 11004[1], 11005[1], 11006[1], 11042[1], 11043[1], 11044[1], 11045[1], 11046[1], 11047[1], 12001[1], 12002[1], 12004[1], 12005[1], 12006[1], 12007[1], 12011[1], 12013[1], 12014[1], 12015[1], 12016[1], 12017[1], 12018[1], 12020[1], 12021[1], 12031[1], 12032[1], 12034[1], 12035[1], 12036[1], 12037[1], 12041[1], 12042[1], 12044[1], 12045[1], 12046[1], 12047[1], 12051[1], 12052[1], 12053[1], 12054[1], 12055[1], 12056[1], 12057[1], 13100[1], 13101[1], 13102[1], 13120[1], 13121[1], 13122[1], 13131[1], 13132[1], 13133[1], 13151[1], 13152[1], 13153[1], 15769[1], 22505[0], 36000[1], 36400[1], 36405[1], 36406[1], 36410[1], 36420[1], 36425[1], 36430[1], 36440[1], 36591[0], 36592[0], 36600[1], 36640[1], 38220[0], 38221[1], 38222[0], 38230[0], 38232[0], 43752[1], 51701[1], 51702[1], 51703[1], 62320[0], 62321[0], 62322[0], 62323[0], 62324[0], 62325[0], 62326[0], 62327[0], 63075[1], 63300[1], 63707[1], 63709[1], 64400[0], 64405[0], 64408[0], 64415[0], 64416[0], 64417[0], 64418[0], 64420[0], 64421[0], 64425[0], 64430[0], 64435[0], 64445[0], 64446[0], 64447[0], 64448[0], 64449[0], 64450[0], 64451[0], 64454[0], 64461[0], 64462[0], 64463[0], 64479[0], 64480[0], 64483[0], 64484[0], 64486[0], 64487[0], 64488[0], 64489[0], 64490[0], 64491[0], 64492[0], 64493[0], 64494[0], 64495[0], 64505[0], 64510[0], 64517[0], 64520[0], 64530[0], 76000[1], 77001[1], 77002[1], 92012[1], 92014[1], 92585[0], 93000[1], 93005[1], 93010[1], 93040[1], 93041[1], 93042[1], 93318[1], 93355[1], 94002[1], 94200[1], 94250[1], 94680[1], 94681[1], 94690[1], 94770[1], 95812[1], 95813[1], 95816[1], 95819[1], 95822[0], 95829[1], 95860[0], 95861[0], 95863[0], 95864[0], 95865[0], 95866[0], 95867[0], 95868[0], 95869[0], 95870[0], 95907[0], 95908[0], 95909[0], 95910[0], 95911[0], 95912[0], 95913[0], 95925[0], 95926[0], 95927[0], 95928[0], 95929[0], 95930[0], 95933[0], 95937[0], 95938[0], 95939[0], 95940[0], 95955[1], 96360[1], 96361[1], 96365[1], 96366[1], 96367[1], 96368[1], 96372[1], 96374[1], 96375[1], 96376[1], 96377[1], 96523[0], 97597[1], 97598[1], 97602[1], 99155[0], 99156[0], 99157[0], 99211[1], 99212[1], 99213[1], 99214[1], 99215[1], 99217[1], 99218[1], 99219[1], 99220[1], 99221[1], 99222[1], 99223[1], 99231[1], 99232[1], 99233[1], 99234[1], 99235[1], 99236[1], 99238[1], 99239[1], 99241[1], 99242[1], 99243[1], 99244[1], 99245[1], 99251[1], 99252[1], 99253[1], 99254[1], 99255[1], 99291[1], 99292[1], 99304[1], 99305[1], 99306[1], 99307[1], 99308[1], 99309[1], 99310[1], 99315[1], 99316[1], 99334[1], 99335[1], 99336[1],

0 = Modifier usage not allowed or inappropriate 1 = Modifier usage allowed

Code 1	Code 2
	99337[1], 99347[1], 99348[1], 99349[1], 99350[1], 99374[1], 99375[1], 99377[1], 99378[1], 99446[0], 99447[0], 99448[0], 99449[0], 99451[0], 99452[0], 99495[0], 99496[0], G0453[0], G0463[1], G0471[1]
63305	0213T[0], 0216T[0], 0228T[0], 0230T[0], 0333T[0], 0464T[0], 0565T[1], 11000[1], 11001[1], 11004[1], 11005[1], 11006[1], 11042[1], 11043[1], 11044[1], 11045[1], 11046[1], 11047[1], 12001[1], 12002[1], 12004[1], 12005[1], 12006[1], 12007[1], 12011[1], 12013[1], 12014[1], 12015[1], 12016[1], 12017[1], 12018[1], 12020[1], 12021[1], 12031[1], 12032[1], 12034[1], 12035[1], 12036[1], 12037[1], 12041[1], 12042[1], 12044[1], 12045[1], 12046[1], 12047[1], 12051[1], 12052[1], 12053[1], 12054[1], 12055[1], 12056[1], 12057[1], 13100[1], 13101[1], 13102[1], 13120[1], 13121[1], 13122[1], 13131[1], 13132[1], 13133[1], 13151[1], 13152[1], 13153[1], 15769[1], 22505[0], 32100[1], 32110[1], 32150[1], 32160[1], 36000[1], 36400[1], 36405[1], 36406[1], 36410[1], 36420[1], 36425[1], 36430[1], 36440[1], 36591[0], 36592[0], 36600[1], 36640[1], 38220[0], 38221[1], 38222[0], 38230[0], 38232[0], 43336[1], 43337[1], 43752[1], 49000[0], 49002[1], 51701[1], 51702[1], 51703[1], 62320[0], 62321[0], 62322[0], 62323[0], 62324[0], 62325[0], 62326[0], 62327[0], 63077[1], 63101[1], 63301[1], 63707[1], 63709[1], 64400[0], 64405[0], 64408[0], 64415[0], 64416[0], 64417[0], 64418[0], 64420[0], 64421[0], 64425[0], 64430[0], 64435[0], 64445[0], 64446[0], 64447[0], 64448[0], 64449[0], 64450[0], 64451[0], 64454[0], 64461[0], 64462[0], 64463[0], 64479[0], 64480[0], 64483[0], 64484[0], 64486[0], 64487[0], 64488[0], 64489[0], 64490[0], 64491[0], 64492[0], 64493[0], 64494[0], 64495[0], 64505[0], 64510[0], 64517[0], 64520[0], 64530[0], 76000[1], 77001[1], 77002[1], 92012[1], 92014[1], 92585[0], 93000[1], 93005[1], 93010[1], 93040[1], 93041[1], 93042[1], 93318[1], 93355[1], 94002[1], 94200[1], 94250[1], 94680[1], 94681[1], 94690[1], 94770[1], 95812[1], 95813[1], 95816[1], 95819[1], 95822[0], 95829[1], 95860[0], 95861[0], 95863[0], 95864[0], 95865[0], 95866[0], 95867[0], 95868[0], 95869[0], 95870[0], 95907[0], 95908[0], 95909[0], 95910[0], 95911[0], 95912[0], 95913[0], 95925[0], 95926[0], 95927[0], 95928[0], 95929[0], 95930[0], 95933[0], 95937[0], 95938[0], 95939[0], 95940[0], 95955[1], 96360[1], 96361[1], 96365[1], 96366[1], 96367[1], 96368[1], 96372[1], 96374[1], 96375[1], 96376[1], 96377[1], 96523[0], 97597[1], 97598[1], 97602[1], 99155[0], 99156[0], 99157[0], 99211[1], 99212[1], 99213[1], 99214[1], 99215[1], 99217[1], 99218[1], 99219[1], 99220[1], 99221[1], 99222[1], 99223[1], 99231[1], 99232[1], 99233[1], 99234[1], 99235[1], 99236[1], 99238[1], 99239[1], 99241[1], 99242[1], 99243[1], 99244[1], 99245[1], 99251[1], 99252[1], 99253[1], 99254[1], 99255[1], 99291[1], 99292[1], 99304[1], 99305[1], 99306[1], 99307[1], 99308[1], 99309[1], 99310[1], 99315[1], 99316[1], 99334[1], 99335[1], 99336[1], 99337[1], 99347[1], 99348[1], 99349[1], 99350[1], 99374[1], 99375[1], 99377[1], 99378[1], 99446[0], 99447[0], 99448[0], 99449[0], 99451[0], 99452[0], 99495[0], 99496[0], G0453[0], G0463[1], G0471[1]
63306	0213T[0], 0216T[0], 0228T[0], 0230T[0], 0333T[0], 0464T[0], 0565T[1], 11000[1], 11001[1], 11004[1], 11005[1], 11006[1], 11042[1], 11043[1], 11044[1], 11045[1], 11046[1], 11047[1], 12001[1], 12002[1], 12004[1], 12005[1], 12006[1], 12007[1], 12011[1], 12013[1], 12014[1], 12015[1], 12016[1], 12017[1], 12018[1], 12020[1], 12021[1], 12031[1], 12032[1], 12034[1], 12035[1], 12036[1], 12037[1], 12041[1], 12042[1], 12044[1], 12045[1], 12046[1], 12047[1], 12051[1], 12052[1], 12053[1], 12054[1], 12055[1], 12056[1], 12057[1], 13100[1], 13101[1], 13102[1], 13120[1], 13121[1], 13122[1], 13131[1], 13132[1], 13133[1], 13151[1], 13152[1], 13153[1], 15769[1], 22206[1], 22505[0], 32100[1], 32110[1], 32150[1], 32160[1], 36000[1], 36400[1], 36405[1], 36406[1], 36410[1], 36420[1], 36425[1], 36430[1], 36440[1], 36591[0], 36592[0], 36600[1], 36640[1], 38220[0], 38221[1], 38222[0], 38230[0], 38232[0], 43336[1], 43337[1], 43752[1], 49000[0], 49002[1], 49010[0], 51701[1], 51702[1], 51703[1], 62320[0], 62321[0], 62322[0], 62323[0], 62324[0], 62325[0], 62326[0], 62327[0], 63077[1], 63101[1], 63302[1], 63707[1], 63709[1], 64400[0], 64405[0], 64408[0], 64415[0], 64416[0], 64417[0], 64418[0], 64420[0], 64421[0], 64425[0], 64430[0], 64435[0], 64445[0], 64446[0], 64447[0], 64448[0], 64449[0], 64450[0], 64451[0], 64454[0], 64461[0], 64462[0], 64463[0], 64479[0], 64480[0], 64483[0], 64484[0], 64486[0], 64487[0], 64488[0], 64489[0], 64490[0], 64491[0], 64492[0], 64493[0], 64494[0], 64495[0], 64505[0], 64510[0], 64517[0], 64520[0], 64530[0], 76000[1], 77001[1], 77002[1], 92012[1], 92014[1], 92585[0], 93000[1], 93005[1], 93010[1], 93040[1], 93041[1], 93042[1], 93318[1], 93355[1], 94002[1], 94200[1], 94250[1], 94680[1], 94681[1], 94690[1], 94770[1], 95812[1], 95813[1], 95816[1], 95819[1], 95822[0], 95829[1], 95860[0], 95861[0], 95863[0], 95864[0], 95865[0], 95866[0], 95867[0], 95868[0], 95869[0], 95870[0], 95907[0], 95908[0], 95909[0], 95910[0], 95911[0], 95912[0], 95913[0], 95925[0], 95926[0], 95927[0], 95928[0], 95929[0], 95930[0], 95933[0], 95937[0], 95938[0], 95939[0], 95940[0], 95955[1], 96360[1], 96361[1], 96365[1], 96366[1], 96367[1], 96368[1], 96372[1], 96374[1], 96375[1], 96376[1], 96377[1], 96523[0], 97597[1], 97598[1], 97602[1], 99155[0], 99156[0], 99157[0], 99211[1], 99212[1], 99213[1], 99214[1], 99215[1], 99217[1], 99218[1], 99219[1], 99220[1], 99221[1], 99222[1], 99223[1], 99231[1], 99232[1], 99233[1], 99234[1], 99235[1], 99236[1], 99238[1], 99239[1], 99241[1], 99242[1], 99243[1], 99244[1], 99245[1], 99251[1], 99252[1], 99253[1], 99254[1], 99255[1], 99291[1], 99292[1], 99304[1], 99305[1], 99306[1], 99307[1], 99308[1], 99309[1], 99310[1], 99315[1], 99316[1], 99334[1], 99335[1], 99336[1], 99337[1], 99347[1], 99348[1], 99349[1], 99350[1], 99374[1], 99375[1], 99377[1], 99378[1], 99446[0], 99447[0], 99448[0], 99449[0], 99451[0], 99452[0], 99495[0], 99496[0], G0453[0], G0463[1], G0471[1]
63307	0213T[0], 0216T[0], 0228T[0], 0230T[0], 0333T[0], 0464T[0], 0565T[1], 11000[1], 11001[1], 11004[1], 11005[1], 11006[1], 11042[1], 11043[1], 11044[1], 11045[1], 11046[1], 11047[1], 12001[1], 12002[1], 12004[1], 12005[1], 12006[1], 12007[1], 12011[1], 12013[1], 12014[1], 12015[1], 12016[1], 12017[1], 12018[1], 12020[1], 12021[1], 12031[1], 12032[1], 12034[1], 12035[1], 12036[1], 12037[1], 12041[1], 12042[1], 12044[1], 12045[1], 12046[1], 12047[1], 12051[1], 12052[1], 12053[1], 12054[1], 12055[1], 12056[1], 12057[1], 13100[1], 13101[1], 13102[1], 13120[1], 13121[1], 13122[1], 13131[1], 13132[1], 13133[1], 13151[1], 13152[1], 13153[1], 15769[1], 22505[0], 36000[1], 36400[1], 36405[1], 36406[1], 36410[1], 36420[1], 36425[1], 36430[1], 36440[1], 36591[0], 36592[0], 36600[1], 36640[1], 38220[0], 38221[1], 38222[0], 38230[0], 38232[0], 43752[1], 44005[0], 44180[0], 44820[0], 44850[0], 49000[0], 49002[1], 49010[0], 49255[0], 51701[1], 51702[1], 51703[1], 62320[0], 62321[0], 62322[0], 62323[0], 62324[0], 62325[0], 62326[0], 62327[0], 63303[1], 63707[1], 63709[1], 64400[0], 64405[0], 64408[0], 64415[0], 64416[0], 64417[0], 64418[0], 64420[0], 64421[0], 64425[0], 64430[0], 64435[0], 64445[0], 64446[0], 64447[0], 64448[0], 64449[0], 64450[0], 64451[0], 64454[0], 64461[0], 64462[0], 64463[0], 64479[0], 64480[0], 64483[0], 64484[0], 64486[0], 64487[0], 64488[0], 64489[0], 64490[0], 64491[0], 64492[0], 64493[0], 64494[0], 64495[0], 64505[0], 64510[0], 64517[0], 64520[0], 64530[0], 76000[1], 77001[1], 77002[1], 92012[1], 92014[1], 92585[0], 93000[1], 93005[1], 93010[1], 93040[1], 93041[1], 93042[1], 93318[1], 93355[1], 94002[1], 94200[1], 94250[1], 94680[1], 94681[1], 94690[1], 94770[1], 95812[1], 95813[1], 95816[1], 95819[1], 95822[0], 95829[1], 95860[0], 95861[0], 95863[0], 95864[0], 95865[0], 95866[0], 95867[0], 95868[0], 95869[0], 95870[0], 95907[0], 95908[0], 95909[0], 95910[0], 95911[0], 95912[0], 95913[0], 95925[0], 95926[0], 95927[0], 95928[0], 95929[0], 95930[0], 95933[0], 95937[0], 95938[0], 95939[0], 95940[0], 95955[1], 96360[1], 96361[1], 96365[1], 96366[1], 96367[1], 96368[1], 96372[1], 96374[1], 96375[1], 96376[1], 96377[1], 96523[0], 97597[1], 97598[1], 97602[1], 99155[0], 99156[0], 99157[0], 99211[1], 99212[1], 99213[1], 99214[1], 99215[1], 99217[1], 99218[1], 99219[1], 99220[1], 99221[1], 99222[1], 99223[1], 99231[1], 99232[1], 99233[1], 99234[1], 99235[1], 99236[1], 99238[1], 99239[1], 99241[1], 99242[1], 99243[1], 99244[1], 99245[1], 99251[1], 99252[1], 99253[1], 99254[1], 99255[1], 99291[1], 99292[1], 99304[1], 99305[1], 99306[1], 99307[1], 99308[1], 99309[1], 99310[1], 99315[1], 99316[1], 99334[1], 99335[1], 99336[1], 99337[1], 99347[1], 99348[1], 99349[1], 99350[1], 99374[1], 99375[1], 99377[1], 99378[1], 99446[0], 99447[0], 99448[0], 99449[0], 99451[0], 99452[0], 99495[0], 99496[0], G0453[0], G0463[1], G0471[1]
63308	0333T[0], 0464T[0], 11000[1], 11001[1], 11004[1], 11005[1], 11006[1], 11042[1], 11043[1], 11044[1], 11045[1], 11046[1], 11047[1], 36591[0], 36592[0], 38220[0], 38221[1], 38222[0], 38230[0], 38232[0], 63707[1], 63709[1], 92585[0], 95822[0], 95860[0], 95861[0], 95863[0], 95864[0], 95865[0], 95866[0], 95867[0], 95868[0], 95869[0], 95907[0], 95908[0], 95909[0], 95910[0], 95911[0], 95912[0], 95913[0], 95925[0], 95926[0], 95927[0], 95930[0], 95933[0], 95937[0], 95938[0], 95939[0], 95940[0], 96523[0], 97597[1], 97598[1], 97602[1], G0453[0]
63620	0213T[1], 0216T[1], 0333T[0], 0398T[1], 0464T[0], 12001[1], 12002[1], 12004[1], 12005[1], 12006[1], 12007[1], 12011[1], 12013[1], 12014[1], 12015[1], 12016[1], 12017[1], 12018[1], 12020[1], 12021[1], 12031[1], 12032[1], 12034[1], 12035[1], 12036[1], 12037[1], 12041[1], 12042[1], 12044[1], 12045[1], 12046[1], 12047[1], 12051[1], 12052[1], 12053[1], 12054[1], 12055[1], 12056[1], 12057[1], 13100[1], 13101[1], 13102[1], 13120[1], 13121[1], 13122[1], 13131[1], 13132[1], 13133[1], 13151[1], 13152[1], 13153[1], 20661[1], 20693[1], 20694[1], 22505[0], 36000[1], 36400[1], 36405[1], 36406[1], 36410[1], 36420[1], 36425[1], 36430[1], 36440[1], 36591[0], 36592[0], 36600[1], 36640[1], 43752[1], 51701[1], 51702[1], 51703[1], 61304[1], 61305[1], 61312[1], 61313[1], 61314[1], 61315[1], 61320[1], 61321[1], 61330[1], 61333[1], 61450[1], 61458[1], 61460[1], 61500[1], 61510[1], 61512[1], 61514[1], 61516[1], 61518[1], 61519[1], 61520[1], 61521[1], 61522[1], 61524[1], 61526[1], 61530[1], 61563[1], 61564[1], 61735[1], 61781[1], 61782[1], 61783[1], 61863[0], 62324[0], 62325[0], 62326[0], 62327[0], 64415[1], 64416[1], 64417[1], 64450[1], 64454[1], 64461[0], 64462[0], 64463[0], 64486[0], 64487[0], 64488[0], 64489[0], 64490[1], 64491[0], 64492[0], 64493[1], 64494[0], 64495[0], 69990[0], 76000[1], 77001[1], 77002[1], 77261[0], 77262[0], 77263[0], 77280[0], 77285[0], 77290[0], 77295[0], 77300[0], 77301[0], 77306[1], 77307[1], 77316[1], 77317[1], 77318[1], 77321[0], 77331[0], 77332[1], 77333[1], 77334[1], 77336[0], 77338[0], 77370[0], 77371[1], 77372[1], 77373[1], 77401[0], 77402[0], 77407[0], 77412[0], 77417[0], 77427[0], 77431[1], 77432[0], 77435[1], 77469[1], 77470[1], 92012[1], 92014[1], 92585[0], 93000[1], 93005[1], 93010[1], 93040[1], 93041[1], 93042[1], 93318[1], 93355[1], 94002[1], 94200[1], 94250[1], 94680[1], 94681[1], 94690[1], 94770[1], 95812[1], 95813[1], 95816[1], 95819[1], 95822[0], 95829[1], 95860[0], 95861[0], 95863[0], 95864[0], 95865[0], 95866[0], 95867[0], 95868[0], 95869[0], 95870[0], 95907[0], 95908[0], 95909[0], 95910[0], 95911[0], 95912[0], 95913[0], 95925[0], 95926[0], 95927[0], 95928[0], 95929[0], 95930[0], 95933[0], 95937[0], 95938[0], 95939[0], 95940[0], 95955[1], 96360[1], 96361[1], 96365[1], 96366[1], 96367[1], 96368[1], 96372[1], 96374[1], 96375[1], 96376[1], 96377[1], 96523[0], 99155[0], 99156[0], 99157[0], 99211[1], 99212[1], 99213[1], 99214[1], 99215[1], 99217[1], 99218[1], 99219[1], 99220[1], 99221[1], 99222[1], 99223[1], 99231[1], 99232[1], 99233[1], 99234[1], 99235[1], 99236[1], 99238[1], 99239[1], 99241[1], 99242[1], 99243[1], 99244[1], 99245[1], 99251[1], 99252[1], 99253[1], 99254[1], 99255[1], 99291[1], 99292[1], 99304[1], 99305[1], 99306[1], 99307[1], 99308[1], 99309[1], 99310[1], 99315[1], 99316[1], 99334[1], 99335[1], 99336[1], 99337[1], 99347[1], 99348[1], 99349[1], 99350[1], 99374[1], 99375[1], 99377[1], 99378[1], 99446[0], 99447[0], 99448[0], 99449[0], 99451[0], 99452[0], 99495[0], 99496[0], G0339[1], G0340[1], G0453[0], G0463[1], G0471[1], G6002[0], G6003[0], G6004[0], G6005[0], G6006[0], G6007[0], G6008[0], G6009[0], G6010[0], G6011[0], G6012[0], G6013[0], G6014[0], G6015[0], G6016[0], G6017[1]
63621	36591[0], 36592[0], 61783[1], 95863[0], 95864[0], 95865[0], 95866[0], 95869[0], 96523[0]

0 = Modifier usage not allowed or inappropriate 1 = Modifier usage allowed

Code 1	Code 2
63650	01935[0], 01936[0], 0213T[0], 0216T[0], 0228T[0], 0230T[0], 0333T[0], 0464T[0], 0589T[1], 0590T[1], 12001[1], 12002[1], 12004[1], 12005[1], 12006[1], 12007[1], 12011[1], 12013[1], 12014[1], 12015[1], 12016[1], 12017[1], 12018[1], 12020[1], 12021[1], 12031[1], 12032[1], 12034[1], 12035[1], 12036[1], 12037[1], 12041[1], 12042[1], 12044[1], 12045[1], 12046[1], 12047[1], 12051[1], 12052[1], 12053[1], 12054[1], 12055[1], 12056[1], 12057[1], 13100[1], 13101[1], 13102[1], 13120[1], 13121[1], 13122[1], 13131[1], 13132[1], 13133[1], 13151[1], 13152[1], 13153[1], 22505[0], 36000[1], 36400[1], 36405[1], 36406[1], 36410[1], 36420[1], 36425[1], 36430[1], 36440[1], 36591[0], 36592[0], 36600[1], 36640[1], 43752[1], 51701[1], 51702[1], 51703[1], 62320[0], 62321[0], 62322[0], 62323[0], 62324[0], 62325[0], 62326[0], 62327[0], 63610[0], 63655[1], 63661[0], 64400[0], 64405[0], 64408[0], 64415[0], 64416[0], 64417[0], 64418[0], 64420[0], 64421[0], 64425[0], 64430[0], 64435[0], 64445[0], 64446[0], 64447[0], 64448[0], 64449[0], 64450[0], 64451[0], 64454[0], 64461[0], 64462[0], 64463[0], 64479[0], 64480[0], 64483[0], 64484[0], 64486[0], 64487[0], 64488[0], 64489[0], 64490[0], 64491[0], 64492[0], 64493[0], 64494[0], 64495[0], 64505[0], 64510[0], 64517[0], 64520[0], 64530[0], 69990[0], 76000[1], 77001[1], 77002[1], 77003[1], 92012[1], 92014[1], 92585[0], 93000[1], 93005[1], 93010[1], 93040[1], 93041[1], 93042[1], 93318[1], 93355[1], 94002[1], 94200[1], 94250[1], 94680[1], 94681[1], 94690[1], 94770[1], 95812[1], 95813[1], 95816[1], 95819[1], 95822[0], 95829[1], 95860[0], 95861[0], 95863[0], 95864[0], 95865[0], 95866[0], 95867[0], 95868[0], 95869[0], 95870[0], 95907[0], 95908[0], 95909[0], 95910[0], 95911[0], 95912[0], 95913[0], 95925[0], 95926[0], 95927[0], 95928[0], 95929[0], 95930[0], 95933[0], 95937[0], 95938[0], 95939[0], 95940[0], 95955[1], 95970[1], 95971[1], 95972[1], 96360[1], 96361[1], 96365[1], 96366[1], 96367[1], 96368[1], 96372[1], 96374[1], 96375[1], 96376[1], 96377[1], 96523[0], 99155[0], 99156[0], 99157[0], 99211[1], 99212[1], 99213[1], 99214[1], 99215[1], 99217[1], 99218[1], 99219[1], 99220[1], 99221[1], 99222[1], 99223[1], 99231[1], 99232[1], 99233[1], 99234[1], 99235[1], 99236[1], 99238[1], 99239[1], 99241[1], 99242[1], 99243[1], 99244[1], 99245[1], 99251[1], 99252[1], 99253[1], 99254[1], 99255[1], 99291[1], 99292[1], 99304[1], 99305[1], 99306[1], 99307[1], 99308[1], 99309[1], 99310[1], 99315[1], 99316[1], 99334[1], 99335[1], 99336[1], 99337[1], 99347[1], 99348[1], 99349[1], 99350[1], 99374[1], 99375[1], 99377[1], 99378[1], 99446[0], 99447[0], 99448[0], 99449[0], 99451[0], 99452[0], 99495[0], 99496[0], G0453[0], G0463[1], G0471[1]
63655	0213T[0], 0216T[0], 0228T[0], 0230T[0], 0333T[0], 0464T[0], 0565T[1], 0589T[1], 0590T[1], 11000[1], 11001[1], 11004[1], 11005[1], 11006[1], 11042[1], 11043[1], 11044[1], 11045[1], 11046[1], 11047[1], 12001[1], 12002[1], 12004[1], 12005[1], 12006[1], 12007[1], 12011[1], 12013[1], 12014[1], 12015[1], 12016[1], 12017[1], 12018[1], 12020[1], 12021[1], 12031[1], 12032[1], 12034[1], 12035[1], 12036[1], 12037[1], 12041[1], 12042[1], 12044[1], 12045[1], 12046[1], 12047[1], 12051[1], 12052[1], 12053[1], 12054[1], 12055[1], 12056[1], 12057[1], 13100[1], 13101[1], 13102[1], 13120[1], 13121[1], 13122[1], 13131[1], 13132[1], 13133[1], 13151[1], 13152[1], 13153[1], 15769[1], 22505[0], 36000[1], 36400[1], 36405[1], 36406[1], 36410[1], 36420[1], 36425[1], 36430[1], 36440[1], 36591[0], 36592[0], 36600[1], 36640[1], 43752[1], 51701[1], 51702[1], 51703[1], 62320[0], 62321[0], 62322[0], 62323[0], 62324[0], 62325[0], 62326[0], 62327[0], 63610[0], 63662[0], 63663[0], 63707[1], 63709[1], 64400[0], 64405[0], 64408[0], 64415[0], 64416[0], 64417[0], 64418[0], 64420[0], 64421[0], 64425[0], 64430[0], 64435[0], 64445[0], 64446[0], 64447[0], 64448[0], 64449[0], 64450[0], 64451[0], 64454[0], 64461[0], 64462[0], 64463[0], 64479[0], 64480[0], 64483[0], 64484[0], 64486[0], 64487[0], 64488[0], 64489[0], 64490[0], 64491[0], 64492[0], 64493[0], 64494[0], 64495[0], 64505[0], 64510[0], 64517[0], 64520[0], 64530[0], 69990[0], 76000[1], 77001[1], 77002[1], 77003[1], 92012[1], 92014[1], 92585[0], 93000[1], 93005[1], 93010[1], 93040[1], 93041[1], 93042[1], 93318[1], 93355[1], 94002[1], 94200[1], 94250[1], 94680[1], 94681[1], 94690[1], 94770[1], 95812[1], 95813[1], 95816[1], 95819[1], 95822[0], 95829[1], 95860[0], 95861[0], 95863[0], 95864[0], 95865[0], 95866[0], 95867[0], 95868[0], 95869[0], 95870[0], 95907[0], 95908[0], 95909[0], 95910[0], 95911[0], 95912[0], 95913[0], 95925[0], 95926[0], 95927[0], 95928[0], 95929[0], 95930[0], 95933[0], 95937[0], 95938[0], 95939[0], 95940[0], 95955[1], 95970[1], 95971[1], 95972[1], 96360[1], 96361[1], 96365[1], 96366[1], 96367[1], 96368[1], 96372[1], 96374[1], 96375[1], 96376[1], 96377[1], 96523[0], 97597[1], 97598[1], 97602[1], 99155[0], 99156[0], 99157[0], 99211[1], 99212[1], 99213[1], 99214[1], 99215[1], 99217[1], 99218[1], 99219[1], 99220[1], 99221[1], 99222[1], 99223[1], 99231[1], 99232[1], 99233[1], 99234[1], 99235[1], 99236[1], 99238[1], 99239[1], 99241[1], 99242[1], 99243[1], 99244[1], 99245[1], 99251[1], 99252[1], 99253[1], 99254[1], 99255[1], 99291[1], 99292[1], 99304[1], 99305[1], 99306[1], 99307[1], 99308[1], 99309[1], 99310[1], 99315[1], 99316[1], 99334[1], 99335[1], 99336[1], 99337[1], 99347[1], 99348[1], 99349[1], 99350[1], 99374[1], 99375[1], 99377[1], 99378[1], 99446[0], 99447[0], 99448[0], 99449[0], 99451[0], 99452[0], 99495[0], 99496[0], G0453[0], G0463[1], G0471[1]
63661	01935[0], 01936[0], 0213T[0], 0216T[0], 0228T[0], 0230T[0], 0333T[0], 0464T[0], 0589T[0], 0590T[0], 11000[1], 11001[1], 11004[1], 11005[1], 11006[1], 11042[1], 11043[1], 11044[1], 11045[1], 11046[1], 11047[1], 12001[1], 12002[1], 12004[1], 12005[1], 12006[1], 12007[1], 12011[1], 12013[1], 12014[1], 12015[1], 12016[1], 12017[1], 12018[1], 12020[1], 12021[1], 12031[1], 12032[1], 12034[1], 12035[1], 12036[1], 12037[1], 12041[1], 12042[1], 12044[1], 12045[1], 12046[1], 12047[1], 12051[1], 12052[1], 12053[1], 12054[1], 12055[1], 12056[1], 12057[1], 13100[1], 13101[1], 13102[1], 13120[1], 13121[1], 13122[1], 13131[1], 13132[1], 13133[1], 13151[1], 13152[1], 13153[1], 22505[0], 36000[1], 36400[1], 36405[1], 36406[1], 36410[1], 36420[1], 36425[1], 36430[1], 36440[1], 36591[0], 36592[0], 36600[1], 36640[1], 43752[1], 51701[1], 51702[1], 51703[1], 62273[1], 62320[0], 62321[0], 62322[0], 62323[0], 62324[0], 62325[0], 62326[0], 62327[0], 63610[0], 64400[0], 64405[0], 64408[0], 64415[0], 64416[0], 64417[0], 64418[0], 64420[0], 64421[0], 64425[0], 64430[0], 64435[0], 64445[0], 64446[0], 64447[0], 64448[0], 64449[0], 64450[0], 64451[0], 64454[0], 64461[0], 64462[0], 64463[0], 64479[0], 64480[0], 64483[0], 64484[0], 64486[0], 64487[0], 64488[0], 64489[0], 64490[0], 64491[0], 64492[0], 64493[0], 64494[0], 64495[0], 64505[0], 64510[0], 64517[0], 64520[0], 64530[0], 69990[0], 76000[1], 77001[1], 77002[1], 77003[1], 92012[1], 92014[1], 92585[0], 93000[1], 93005[1], 93010[1], 93040[1], 93041[1], 93042[1], 93318[1], 93355[1], 94002[1], 94200[1], 94250[1], 94680[1], 94681[1], 94690[1], 94770[1], 95812[1], 95813[1], 95816[1], 95819[1], 95822[0], 95829[1], 95860[0], 95861[0], 95863[0], 95864[0], 95865[0], 95866[0], 95867[0], 95868[0], 95869[0], 95870[0], 95907[0], 95908[0], 95909[0], 95910[0], 95911[0], 95912[0], 95913[0], 95925[0], 95926[0], 95927[0], 95928[0], 95929[0], 95930[0], 95933[0], 95937[0], 95938[0], 95939[0], 95940[0], 95955[1], 95970[1], 95971[1], 95972[1], 96360[1], 96361[1], 96365[1], 96366[1], 96367[1], 96368[1], 96372[1], 96374[1], 96375[1], 96376[1], 96377[1], 96523[0], 97597[1], 97598[1], 97602[1], 99155[0], 99156[0], 99157[0], 99211[1], 99212[1], 99213[1], 99214[1], 99215[1], 99217[1], 99218[1], 99219[1], 99220[1], 99221[1], 99222[1], 99223[1], 99231[1], 99232[1], 99233[1], 99234[1], 99235[1], 99236[1], 99238[1], 99239[1], 99241[1], 99242[1], 99243[1], 99244[1], 99245[1], 99251[1], 99252[1], 99253[1], 99254[1], 99255[1], 99291[1], 99292[1], 99304[1], 99305[1], 99306[1], 99307[1], 99308[1], 99309[1], 99310[1], 99315[1], 99316[1], 99334[1], 99335[1], 99336[1], 99337[1], 99347[1], 99348[1], 99349[1], 99350[1], 99374[1], 99375[1], 99377[1], 99378[1], 99446[0], 99447[0], 99448[0], 99449[0], 99451[0], 99452[0], 99495[0], 99496[0], G0453[0], G0463[1], G0471[1]
63662	0213T[0], 0216T[0], 0228T[0], 0230T[0], 0333T[0], 0464T[0], 0589T[0], 0590T[0], 11000[1], 11001[1], 11004[1], 11005[1], 11006[1], 11042[1], 11043[1], 11044[1], 11045[1], 11046[1], 11047[1], 12001[1], 12002[1], 12004[1], 12005[1], 12006[1], 12007[1], 12011[1], 12013[1], 12014[1], 12015[1], 12016[1], 12017[1], 12018[1], 12020[1], 12021[1], 12031[1], 12032[1], 12034[1], 12035[1], 12036[1], 12037[1], 12041[1], 12042[1], 12044[1], 12045[1], 12046[1], 12047[1], 12051[1], 12052[1], 12053[1], 12054[1], 12055[1], 12056[1], 12057[1], 13100[1], 13101[1], 13102[1], 13120[1], 13121[1], 13122[1], 13131[1], 13132[1], 13133[1], 13151[1], 13152[1], 13153[1], 22505[0], 36000[1], 36400[1], 36405[1], 36406[1], 36410[1], 36420[1], 36425[1], 36430[1], 36440[1], 36591[0], 36592[0], 36600[1], 36640[1], 43752[1], 51701[1], 51702[1], 51703[1], 62263[1], 62273[1], 62320[0], 62321[0], 62322[0], 62323[0], 62324[0], 62325[0], 62326[0], 62327[0], 63610[0], 63650[1], 63661[1], 63663[1], 63707[1], 63709[1], 64400[0], 64405[0], 64408[0], 64415[0], 64416[0], 64417[0], 64418[0], 64420[0], 64421[0], 64425[0], 64430[0], 64435[0], 64445[0], 64446[0], 64447[0], 64448[0], 64449[0], 64450[0], 64451[0], 64454[0], 64461[0], 64462[0], 64463[0], 64479[0], 64480[0], 64483[0], 64484[0], 64486[0], 64487[0], 64488[0], 64489[0], 64490[0], 64491[0], 64492[0], 64493[0], 64494[0], 64495[0], 64505[0], 64510[0], 64517[0], 64520[0], 64530[0], 69990[0], 76000[1], 77001[1], 77002[1], 77003[1], 92012[1], 92014[1], 92585[0], 93000[1], 93005[1], 93010[1], 93040[1], 93041[1], 93042[1], 93318[1], 93355[1], 94002[1], 94200[1], 94250[1], 94680[1], 94681[1], 94690[1], 94770[1], 95812[1], 95813[1], 95816[1], 95819[1], 95822[0], 95829[1], 95860[0], 95861[0], 95863[0], 95864[0], 95865[0], 95866[0], 95867[0], 95868[0], 95869[0], 95870[0], 95907[0], 95908[0], 95909[0], 95910[0], 95911[0], 95912[0], 95913[0], 95925[0], 95926[0], 95927[0], 95928[0], 95929[0], 95930[0], 95933[0], 95937[0], 95938[0], 95939[0], 95940[0], 95955[1], 95970[1], 95971[1], 95972[1], 96360[1], 96361[1], 96365[1], 96366[1], 96367[1], 96368[1], 96372[1], 96374[1], 96375[1], 96376[1], 96377[1], 96523[0], 97597[1], 97598[1], 97602[1], 99155[0], 99156[0], 99157[0], 99211[1], 99212[1], 99213[1], 99214[1], 99215[1], 99217[1], 99218[1], 99219[1], 99220[1], 99221[1], 99222[1], 99223[1], 99231[1], 99232[1], 99233[1], 99234[1], 99235[1], 99236[1], 99238[1], 99239[1], 99241[1], 99242[1], 99243[1], 99244[1], 99245[1], 99251[1], 99252[1], 99253[1], 99254[1], 99255[1], 99291[1], 99292[1], 99304[1], 99305[1], 99306[1], 99307[1], 99308[1], 99309[1], 99310[1], 99315[1], 99316[1], 99334[1], 99335[1], 99336[1], 99337[1], 99347[1], 99348[1], 99349[1], 99350[1], 99374[1], 99375[1], 99377[1], 99378[1], 99446[0], 99447[0], 99448[0], 99449[0], 99451[0], 99452[0], 99495[0], 99496[0], G0453[0], G0463[1], G0471[1]
63663	01935[0], 01936[0], 0213T[0], 0216T[0], 0228T[0], 0230T[0], 0333T[0], 0464T[0], 0589T[0], 0590T[0], 11000[1], 11001[1], 11004[1], 11005[1], 11006[1], 11042[1], 11043[1], 11044[1], 11045[1], 11046[1], 11047[1], 12001[1], 12002[1], 12004[1], 12005[1], 12006[1], 12007[1], 12011[1], 12013[1], 12014[1], 12015[1], 12016[1], 12017[1], 12018[1], 12020[1], 12021[1], 12031[1], 12032[1], 12034[1], 12035[1], 12036[1], 12037[1], 12041[1], 12042[1], 12044[1], 12045[1], 12046[1], 12047[1], 12051[1], 12052[1], 12053[1], 12054[1], 12055[1], 12056[1], 12057[1], 13100[1], 13101[1], 13102[1], 13120[1], 13121[1], 13122[1], 13131[1], 13132[1], 13133[1], 13151[1], 13152[1], 13153[1], 22505[0], 36000[1], 36400[1], 36405[1], 36406[1], 36410[1], 36420[1], 36425[1], 36430[1], 36440[1], 36591[0], 36592[0], 36600[1], 36640[1], 43752[1], 51701[1], 51702[1], 51703[1], 62273[1], 62320[0], 62321[0], 62322[0], 62323[0], 62324[0], 62325[0], 62326[0], 62327[0], 63610[0], 63650[0], 63661[0], 64400[0], 64405[0], 64408[0], 64415[0], 64416[0], 64417[0], 64418[0], 64420[0], 64421[0], 64425[0], 64430[0], 64435[0], 64445[0], 64446[0], 64447[0], 64448[0], 64449[0], 64450[0], 64451[0], 64454[0], 64461[0], 64462[0], 64463[0], 64479[0], 64480[0], 64483[0], 64484[0], 64486[0], 64487[0], 64488[0], 64489[0], 64490[0], 64491[0], 64492[0], 64493[0], 64494[0], 64495[0], 64505[0], 64510[0], 64517[0], 64520[0], 64530[0], 69990[0], 76000[1], 77001[1], 77002[1], 77003[1], 92012[1], 92014[1], 92585[0], 93000[1], 93005[1], 93010[1], 93040[1], 93041[1], 93042[1], 93318[1], 93355[1], 94002[1], 94200[1], 94250[1], 94680[1], 94681[1], 94690[1], 94770[1], 95812[1], 95813[1], 95816[1], 95819[1], 95822[0], 95829[1], 95860[0], 95861[0], 95863[0], 95864[0], 95865[0], 95866[0], 95867[0], 95868[0], 95869[0], 95870[0], 95907[0], 95908[0], 95909[0], 95910[0], 95911[0], 95912[0], 95913[0], 95925[0], 95926[0], 95927[0], 95928[0], 95929[0],

0 = Modifier usage not allowed or inappropriate 1 = Modifier usage allowed

Code 1	Code 2
	95930[0], 95933[0], 95937[0], 95938[0], 95939[0], 95940[0], 95955[1], 95970[1], 95971[1], 95972[1], 96360[1], 96361[1], 96365[1], 96366[1], 96367[1], 96368[1], 96372[1], 96374[1], 96375[1], 96376[1], 96377[1], 96523[0], 97597[1], 97598[1], 97602[1], 99155[0], 99156[0], 99157[0], 99211[1], 99212[1], 99213[1], 99214[1], 99215[1], 99217[1], 99218[1], 99219[1], 99220[1], 99221[1], 99222[1], 99223[1], 99231[1], 99232[1], 99233[1], 99234[1], 99235[1], 99236[1], 99238[1], 99239[1], 99241[1], 99242[1], 99243[1], 99244[1], 99245[1], 99251[1], 99252[1], 99253[1], 99254[1], 99255[1], 99291[1], 99292[1], 99304[1], 99305[1], 99306[1], 99307[1], 99308[1], 99309[1], 99310[1], 99315[1], 99316[1], 99334[1], 99335[1], 99336[1], 99337[1], 99347[1], 99348[1], 99349[1], 99350[1], 99374[1], 99375[1], 99377[1], 99378[1], 99446[0], 99447[0], 99448[0], 99449[0], 99451[0], 99452[0], 99495[0], 99496[0], G0453[0], G0463[1], G0471[1]
63664	0213T[0], 0216T[0], 0228T[0], 0230T[0], 0333T[0], 0464T[0], 0589T[0], 0590T[0], 11000[1], 11001[1], 11004[1], 11005[1], 11006[1], 11042[1], 11043[1], 11044[1], 11045[1], 11046[1], 11047[1], 12001[1], 12002[1], 12004[1], 12005[1], 12006[1], 12007[1], 12011[1], 12013[1], 12014[1], 12015[1], 12016[1], 12017[1], 12018[1], 12020[1], 12021[1], 12031[1], 12032[1], 12034[1], 12035[1], 12036[1], 12037[1], 12041[1], 12042[1], 12044[1], 12045[1], 12046[1], 12047[1], 12051[1], 12052[1], 12053[1], 12054[1], 12055[1], 12056[1], 12057[1], 13100[1], 13101[1], 13102[1], 13120[1], 13121[1], 13122[1], 13131[1], 13132[1], 13133[1], 13151[1], 13152[1], 13153[1], 22505[0], 36000[1], 36400[1], 36405[1], 36406[1], 36410[1], 36420[1], 36425[1], 36430[1], 36440[1], 36591[0], 36592[0], 36600[1], 36640[1], 43752[1], 51701[1], 51702[1], 51703[1], 62263[1], 62273[1], 62320[0], 62321[0], 62322[0], 62323[0], 62324[0], 62325[0], 62326[0], 62327[0], 63610[0], 63650[0], 63655[0], 63661[0], 63662[1], 63663[0], 63707[1], 63709[1], 64400[0], 64405[0], 64408[0], 64415[0], 64416[0], 64417[0], 64418[0], 64420[0], 64421[0], 64425[0], 64430[0], 64435[0], 64445[0], 64446[0], 64447[0], 64448[0], 64449[0], 64450[0], 64451[0], 64454[0], 64461[0], 64462[0], 64463[0], 64479[0], 64480[0], 64483[0], 64484[0], 64486[0], 64487[0], 64488[0], 64489[0], 64490[0], 64491[0], 64492[0], 64493[0], 64494[0], 64495[0], 64505[0], 64510[0], 64517[0], 64520[0], 64530[0], 69990[0], 76000[1], 77001[1], 77002[1], 77003[1], 92012[1], 92014[1], 92585[0], 93000[1], 93005[1], 93010[1], 93040[1], 93041[1], 93042[1], 93318[1], 93355[1], 94002[1], 94200[1], 94250[1], 94680[1], 94681[1], 94690[1], 94770[1], 95812[1], 95813[1], 95816[1], 95819[1], 95822[0], 95829[1], 95860[0], 95861[0], 95863[0], 95864[0], 95865[0], 95866[0], 95867[0], 95868[0], 95869[0], 95870[0], 95907[0], 95908[0], 95909[0], 95910[0], 95911[0], 95912[0], 95913[0], 95925[0], 95926[0], 95927[0], 95928[0], 95929[0], 95930[0], 95933[0], 95937[0], 95938[0], 95939[0], 95940[0], 95955[1], 95970[1], 95971[1], 95972[1], 96360[1], 96361[1], 96365[1], 96366[1], 96367[1], 96368[1], 96372[1], 96374[1], 96375[1], 96376[1], 96377[1], 96523[0], 97597[1], 97598[1], 97602[1], 99155[0], 99156[0], 99157[0], 99211[1], 99212[1], 99213[1], 99214[1], 99215[1], 99217[1], 99218[1], 99219[1], 99220[1], 99221[1], 99222[1], 99223[1], 99231[1], 99232[1], 99233[1], 99234[1], 99235[1], 99236[1], 99238[1], 99239[1], 99241[1], 99242[1], 99243[1], 99244[1], 99245[1], 99251[1], 99252[1], 99253[1], 99254[1], 99255[1], 99291[1], 99292[1], 99304[1], 99305[1], 99306[1], 99307[1], 99308[1], 99309[1], 99310[1], 99315[1], 99316[1], 99334[1], 99335[1], 99336[1], 99337[1], 99347[1], 99348[1], 99349[1], 99350[1], 99374[1], 99375[1], 99377[1], 99378[1], 99446[0], 99447[0], 99448[0], 99449[0], 99451[0], 99452[0], 99495[0], 99496[0], G0453[0], G0463[1], G0471[1]
63685	01935[0], 01936[0], 0213T[0], 0216T[0], 0228T[0], 0230T[0], 0333T[0], 0424T[1], 0427T[1], 0428T[1], 0431T[1], 0446T[1], 0448T[1], 0464T[0], 0589T[0], 0590T[0], 11000[1], 11001[1], 11004[1], 11005[1], 11006[1], 11042[1], 11043[1], 11044[1], 11045[1], 11046[1], 11047[1], 12001[1], 12002[1], 12004[1], 12005[1], 12006[1], 12007[1], 12011[1], 12013[1], 12014[1], 12015[1], 12016[1], 12017[1], 12018[1], 12020[1], 12021[1], 12031[1], 12032[1], 12034[1], 12035[1], 12036[1], 12037[1], 12041[1], 12042[1], 12044[1], 12045[1], 12046[1], 12047[1], 12051[1], 12052[1], 12053[1], 12054[1], 12055[1], 12056[1], 12057[1], 13100[1], 13101[1], 13102[1], 13120[1], 13121[1], 13122[1], 13131[1], 13132[1], 13133[1], 13151[1], 13152[1], 13153[1], 36000[1], 36400[1], 36405[1], 36406[1], 36410[1], 36420[1], 36425[1], 36430[1], 36440[1], 36591[0], 36592[0], 36600[1], 36640[1], 43752[1], 51701[1], 51702[1], 51703[1], 62320[0], 62321[0], 62322[0], 62323[0], 62324[0], 62325[0], 62326[0], 62327[0], 63610[0], 63688[1], 64400[0], 64405[0], 64408[0], 64415[0], 64416[0], 64417[0], 64418[0], 64420[0], 64421[0], 64425[0], 64430[0], 64435[0], 64445[0], 64446[0], 64447[0], 64448[0], 64449[0], 64450[0], 64451[0], 64454[0], 64461[0], 64462[0], 64463[0], 64479[0], 64480[0], 64483[0], 64484[0], 64486[0], 64487[0], 64488[0], 64489[0], 64490[0], 64491[0], 64492[0], 64493[0], 64494[0], 64495[0], 64505[0], 64510[0], 64517[0], 64520[0], 64530[0], 69990[0], 76000[1], 77001[1], 77002[1], 77003[1], 92012[1], 92014[1], 92585[0], 93000[1], 93005[1], 93010[1], 93040[1], 93041[1], 93042[1], 93318[1], 93355[1], 94002[1], 94200[1], 94250[1], 94680[1], 94681[1], 94690[1], 94770[1], 95812[1], 95813[1], 95816[1], 95819[1], 95822[0], 95829[1], 95860[0], 95861[0], 95863[0], 95864[0], 95865[0], 95866[0], 95867[0], 95868[0], 95869[0], 95870[0], 95907[0], 95908[0], 95909[0], 95910[0], 95911[0], 95912[0], 95913[0], 95925[0], 95926[0], 95927[0], 95928[0], 95929[0], 95930[0], 95933[0], 95937[0], 95938[0], 95939[0], 95940[0], 95955[1], 95970[1], 95971[1], 95972[1], 95976[1], 95977[1], 96360[1], 96361[1], 96365[1], 96366[1], 96367[1], 96368[1], 96372[1], 96374[1], 96375[1], 96376[1], 96377[1], 96523[0], 97597[1], 97598[1], 97602[1], 99155[0], 99156[0], 99157[0], 99211[1], 99212[1], 99213[1], 99214[1], 99215[1], 99217[1], 99218[1], 99219[1], 99220[1], 99221[1], 99222[1], 99223[1], 99231[1], 99232[1], 99233[1], 99234[1], 99235[1], 99236[1], 99238[1], 99239[1], 99241[1], 99242[1], 99243[1], 99244[1], 99245[1], 99251[1], 99252[1], 99253[1], 99254[1], 99255[1], 99291[1], 99292[1], 99304[1], 99305[1], 99306[1], 99307[1], 99308[1], 99309[1], 99310[1], 99315[1], 99316[1], 99334[1], 99335[1], 99336[1], 99337[1], 99347[1], 99348[1], 99349[1], 99350[1], 99374[1], 99375[1], 99377[1], 99378[1], 99446[0], 99447[0], 99448[0], 99449[0], 99451[0], 99452[0], 99495[0], 99496[0], G0453[0], G0463[1], G0471[1]
63688	01935[0], 01936[0], 0213T[0], 0216T[0], 0228T[0], 0230T[0], 0333T[0], 0447T[1], 0448T[1], 0464T[0], 0589T[0], 0590T[0], 11000[1], 11001[1], 11004[1], 11005[1], 11006[1], 11042[1], 11043[1], 11044[1], 11045[1], 11046[1], 11047[1], 12001[1], 12002[1], 12004[1], 12005[1], 12006[1], 12007[1], 12011[1], 12013[1], 12014[1], 12015[1], 12016[1], 12017[1], 12018[1], 12020[1], 12021[1], 12031[1], 12032[1], 12034[1], 12035[1], 12036[1], 12037[1], 12041[1], 12042[1], 12044[1], 12045[1], 12046[1], 12047[1], 12051[1], 12052[1], 12053[1], 12054[1], 12055[1], 12056[1], 12057[1], 13100[1], 13101[1], 13102[1], 13120[1], 13121[1], 13122[1], 13131[1], 13132[1], 13133[1], 13151[1], 13152[1], 13153[1], 36000[1], 36400[1], 36405[1], 36406[1], 36410[1], 36420[1], 36425[1], 36430[1], 36440[1], 36591[0], 36592[0], 36600[1], 36640[1], 43752[1], 51701[1], 51702[1], 51703[1], 62320[0], 62321[0], 62322[0], 62323[0], 62324[0], 62325[0], 62326[0], 62327[0], 63610[0], 64400[0], 64405[0], 64408[0], 64415[0], 64416[0], 64417[0], 64418[0], 64420[0], 64421[0], 64425[0], 64430[0], 64435[0], 64445[0], 64446[0], 64447[0], 64448[0], 64449[0], 64450[0], 64451[0], 64454[0], 64461[0], 64462[0], 64463[0], 64479[0], 64480[0], 64483[0], 64484[0], 64486[0], 64487[0], 64488[0], 64489[0], 64490[0], 64491[0], 64492[0], 64493[0], 64494[0], 64495[0], 64505[0], 64510[0], 64517[0], 64520[0], 64530[0], 69990[0], 76000[1], 77001[1], 77002[1], 92012[1], 92014[1], 92585[0], 93000[1], 93005[1], 93010[1], 93040[1], 93041[1], 93042[1], 93318[1], 93355[1], 94002[1], 94200[1], 94250[1], 94680[1], 94681[1], 94690[1], 94770[1], 95812[1], 95813[1], 95816[1], 95819[1], 95822[0], 95829[1], 95860[0], 95861[0], 95863[0], 95864[0], 95865[0], 95866[0], 95867[0], 95868[0], 95869[0], 95870[0], 95907[0], 95908[0], 95909[0], 95910[0], 95911[0], 95912[0], 95913[0], 95925[0], 95926[0], 95927[0], 95928[0], 95929[0], 95930[0], 95933[0], 95937[0], 95938[0], 95939[0], 95940[0], 95955[1], 95970[1], 95971[1], 95972[1], 95976[1], 95977[1], 96360[1], 96361[1], 96365[1], 96366[1], 96367[1], 96368[1], 96372[1], 96374[1], 96375[1], 96376[1], 96377[1], 96523[0], 97597[1], 97598[1], 97602[1], 99155[0], 99156[0], 99157[0], 99211[1], 99212[1], 99213[1], 99214[1], 99215[1], 99217[1], 99218[1], 99219[1], 99220[1], 99221[1], 99222[1], 99223[1], 99231[1], 99232[1], 99233[1], 99234[1], 99235[1], 99236[1], 99238[1], 99239[1], 99241[1], 99242[1], 99243[1], 99244[1], 99245[1], 99251[1], 99252[1], 99253[1], 99254[1], 99255[1], 99291[1], 99292[1], 99304[1], 99305[1], 99306[1], 99307[1], 99308[1], 99309[1], 99310[1], 99315[1], 99316[1], 99334[1], 99335[1], 99336[1], 99337[1], 99347[1], 99348[1], 99349[1], 99350[1], 99374[1], 99375[1], 99377[1], 99378[1], 99446[0], 99447[0], 99448[0], 99449[0], 99451[0], 99452[0], 99495[0], 99496[0], G0453[0], G0463[1], G0471[1]
63707	0213T[0], 0216T[0], 0228T[0], 0230T[0], 0333T[0], 0464T[0], 0565T[1], 11000[1], 11001[1], 11004[1], 11005[1], 11006[1], 11042[1], 11043[1], 11044[1], 11045[1], 11046[1], 11047[1], 12001[1], 12002[1], 12004[1], 12005[1], 12006[1], 12007[1], 12011[1], 12013[1], 12014[1], 12015[1], 12016[1], 12017[1], 12018[1], 12020[1], 12021[1], 12031[1], 12032[1], 12034[1], 12035[1], 12036[1], 12037[1], 12041[1], 12042[1], 12044[1], 12045[1], 12046[1], 12047[1], 12051[1], 12052[1], 12053[1], 12054[1], 12055[1], 12056[1], 12057[1], 13100[1], 13101[1], 13102[1], 13120[1], 13121[1], 13122[1], 13131[1], 13132[1], 13133[1], 13151[1], 13152[1], 13153[1], 15769[1], 22505[0], 36000[1], 36400[1], 36405[1], 36406[1], 36410[1], 36420[1], 36425[1], 36430[1], 36440[1], 36591[0], 36592[0], 36600[1], 36640[1], 43752[1], 51701[1], 51702[1], 51703[1], 62320[0], 62321[0], 62322[0], 62323[0], 62324[0], 62325[0], 62326[0], 62327[0], 63700[1], 63702[1], 63704[1], 63706[1], 64400[0], 64405[0], 64408[0], 64415[0], 64416[0], 64417[0], 64418[0], 64420[0], 64421[0], 64425[0], 64430[0], 64435[0], 64445[0], 64446[0], 64447[0], 64448[0], 64449[0], 64450[0], 64451[0], 64454[0], 64461[0], 64462[0], 64463[0], 64479[0], 64480[0], 64483[0], 64484[0], 64486[0], 64487[0], 64488[0], 64489[0], 64490[0], 64491[0], 64492[0], 64493[0], 64494[0], 64495[0], 64505[0], 64510[0], 64517[0], 64520[0], 64530[0], 76000[1], 77001[1], 77002[1], 92012[1], 92014[1], 92585[0], 93000[1], 93005[1], 93010[1], 93040[1], 93041[1], 93042[1], 93318[1], 93355[1], 94002[1], 94200[1], 94250[1], 94680[1], 94681[1], 94690[1], 94770[1], 95812[1], 95813[1], 95816[1], 95819[1], 95822[0], 95829[1], 95860[0], 95861[0], 95863[0], 95864[0], 95865[0], 95866[0], 95867[0], 95868[0], 95869[0], 95870[0], 95907[0], 95908[0], 95909[0], 95910[0], 95911[0], 95912[0], 95913[0], 95925[0], 95926[0], 95927[0], 95928[0], 95929[0], 95930[0], 95933[0], 95937[0], 95938[0], 95939[0], 95940[0], 95955[1], 96360[1], 96361[1], 96365[1], 96366[1], 96367[1], 96368[1], 96372[1], 96374[1], 96375[1], 96376[1], 96377[1], 96523[0], 97597[1], 97598[1], 97602[1], 99155[0], 99156[0], 99157[0], 99211[1], 99212[1], 99213[1], 99214[1], 99215[1], 99217[1], 99218[1], 99219[1], 99220[1], 99221[1], 99222[1], 99223[1], 99231[1], 99232[1], 99233[1], 99234[1], 99235[1], 99236[1], 99238[1], 99239[1], 99241[1], 99242[1], 99243[1], 99244[1], 99245[1], 99251[1], 99252[1], 99253[1], 99254[1], 99255[1], 99291[1], 99292[1], 99304[1], 99305[1], 99306[1], 99307[1], 99308[1], 99309[1], 99310[1], 99315[1], 99316[1], 99334[1], 99335[1], 99336[1], 99337[1], 99347[1], 99348[1], 99349[1], 99350[1], 99374[1], 99375[1], 99377[1], 99378[1], 99446[0], 99447[0], 99448[0], 99449[0], 99451[0], 99452[0], 99495[0], 99496[0], G0453[0], G0463[1], G0471[1]
63709	0213T[0], 0216T[0], 0228T[0], 0230T[0], 0333T[0], 0464T[0], 0565T[1], 11000[1], 11001[1], 11004[1], 11005[1], 11006[1], 11042[1], 11043[1], 11044[1], 11045[1], 11046[1], 11047[1], 12001[1], 12002[1], 12004[1], 12005[1], 12006[1], 12007[1], 12011[1], 12013[1], 12014[1], 12015[1], 12016[1], 12017[1], 12018[1], 12020[1], 12021[1], 12031[1], 12032[1], 12034[1], 12035[1], 12036[1], 12037[1], 12041[1], 12042[1], 12044[1], 12045[1], 12046[1], 12047[1], 12051[1], 12052[1], 12053[1], 12054[1], 12055[1], 12056[1], 12057[1], 13100[1], 13101[1], 13102[1], 13120[1], 13121[1], 13122[1], 13131[1], 13132[1],

0 = Modifier usage not allowed or inappropriate 1 = Modifier usage allowed

Code 1	Code 2
	13133[1], 13151[1], 13152[1], 13153[1], 15769[1], 22505[0], 36000[1], 36400[1], 36405[1], 36406[1], 36410[1], 36420[1], 36425[1], 36430[1], 36440[1], 36591[0], 36592[0], 36600[1], 36640[1], 43752[1], 51701[1], 51702[1], 51703[1], 62320[0], 62321[0], 62322[0], 62323[0], 62324[0], 62325[0], 62326[0], 62327[0], 63700[1], 63702[1], 63704[1], 63706[1], 63707[0], 64400[0], 64405[0], 64408[0], 64415[0], 64416[0], 64417[0], 64418[0], 64420[0], 64421[0], 64425[0], 64430[0], 64435[0], 64445[0], 64446[0], 64447[0], 64448[0], 64449[0], 64450[0], 64451[0], 64454[0], 64461[0], 64462[0], 64463[0], 64479[0], 64480[0], 64483[0], 64484[0], 64486[0], 64487[0], 64488[0], 64489[0], 64490[0], 64491[0], 64492[0], 64493[0], 64494[0], 64495[0], 64505[0], 64510[0], 64517[0], 64520[0], 64530[0], 76000[1], 77001[1], 77002[1], 92012[1], 92014[1], 92585[0], 93000[1], 93005[1], 93010[1], 93040[1], 93041[1], 93042[1], 93318[1], 93355[1], 94002[1], 94200[1], 94250[1], 94680[1], 94681[1], 94690[1], 94770[1], 95812[1], 95813[1], 95816[1], 95819[1], 95822[0], 95829[1], 95860[0], 95861[0], 95863[0], 95864[0], 95865[0], 95866[0], 95867[0], 95868[0], 95869[0], 95870[0], 95907[0], 95908[0], 95909[0], 95910[0], 95911[0], 95912[0], 95913[0], 95925[0], 95926[0], 95927[0], 95928[0], 95929[0], 95930[0], 95933[0], 95937[0], 95938[0], 95939[0], 95940[0], 95955[1], 96360[1], 96361[1], 96365[1], 96366[1], 96367[1], 96368[1], 96372[1], 96374[1], 96375[1], 96376[1], 96377[1], 96523[0], 97597[1], 97598[1], 97602[1], 99155[0], 99156[0], 99157[0], 99211[1], 99212[1], 99213[1], 99214[1], 99215[1], 99217[1], 99218[1], 99219[1], 99220[1], 99221[1], 99222[1], 99223[1], 99231[1], 99232[1], 99233[1], 99234[1], 99235[1], 99236[1], 99238[1], 99239[1], 99241[1], 99242[1], 99243[1], 99244[1], 99245[1], 99251[1], 99252[1], 99253[1], 99254[1], 99255[1], 99291[1], 99292[1], 99304[1], 99305[1], 99306[1], 99307[1], 99308[1], 99309[1], 99310[1], 99315[1], 99316[1], 99334[1], 99335[1], 99336[1], 99337[1], 99347[1], 99348[1], 99349[1], 99350[1], 99374[1], 99375[1], 99377[1], 99378[1], 99446[0], 99447[0], 99448[0], 99449[0], 99451[0], 99452[0], 99495[0], 99496[0], G0453[0], G0463[1], G0471[1]
63710	0213T[0], 0216T[0], 0228T[0], 0230T[0], 0333T[0], 0464T[0], 0565T[1], 12001[1], 12002[1], 12004[1], 12005[1], 12006[1], 12007[1], 12011[1], 12013[1], 12014[1], 12015[1], 12016[1], 12017[1], 12018[1], 12020[1], 12021[1], 12031[1], 12032[1], 12034[1], 12035[1], 12036[1], 12037[1], 12041[1], 12042[1], 12044[1], 12045[1], 12046[1], 12047[1], 12051[1], 12052[1], 12053[1], 12054[1], 12055[1], 12056[1], 12057[1], 13100[1], 13101[1], 13102[1], 13120[1], 13121[1], 13122[1], 13131[1], 13132[1], 13133[1], 13151[1], 13152[1], 13153[1], 15769[1], 22100[1], 22102[1], 22505[0], 36000[1], 36400[1], 36405[1], 36406[1], 36410[1], 36420[1], 36425[1], 36430[1], 36440[1], 36591[0], 36592[0], 36600[1], 36640[1], 43752[1], 51701[1], 51702[1], 51703[1], 62320[0], 62321[0], 62322[0], 62323[0], 62324[0], 62325[0], 62326[0], 62327[0], 63707[1], 63709[1], 64400[0], 64405[0], 64408[0], 64415[0], 64416[0], 64417[0], 64418[0], 64420[0], 64421[0], 64425[0], 64430[0], 64435[0], 64445[0], 64446[0], 64447[0], 64448[0], 64449[0], 64450[0], 64451[0], 64454[0], 64461[0], 64462[0], 64463[0], 64479[0], 64480[0], 64483[0], 64484[0], 64486[0], 64487[0], 64488[0], 64489[0], 64490[0], 64491[0], 64492[0], 64493[0], 64494[0], 64495[0], 64505[0], 64510[0], 64517[0], 64520[0], 64530[0], 76000[1], 77001[1], 77002[1], 92012[1], 92014[1], 92585[0], 93000[1], 93005[1], 93010[1], 93040[1], 93041[1], 93042[1], 93318[1], 93355[1], 94002[1], 94200[1], 94250[1], 94680[1], 94681[1], 94690[1], 94770[1], 95812[1], 95813[1], 95816[1], 95819[1], 95822[0], 95829[1], 95860[0], 95861[0], 95863[0], 95864[0], 95865[0], 95866[0], 95867[0], 95868[0], 95869[0], 95870[0], 95907[0], 95908[0], 95909[0], 95910[0], 95911[0], 95912[0], 95913[0], 95925[0], 95926[0], 95927[0], 95928[0], 95929[0], 95930[0], 95933[0], 95937[0], 95938[0], 95939[0], 95940[0], 95955[1], 96360[1], 96361[1], 96365[1], 96366[1], 96367[1], 96368[1], 96372[1], 96374[1], 96375[1], 96376[1], 96377[1], 96523[0], 99155[0], 99156[0], 99157[0], 99211[1], 99212[1], 99213[1], 99214[1], 99215[1], 99217[1], 99218[1], 99219[1], 99220[1], 99221[1], 99222[1], 99223[1], 99231[1], 99232[1], 99233[1], 99234[1], 99235[1], 99236[1], 99238[1], 99239[1], 99241[1], 99242[1], 99243[1], 99244[1], 99245[1], 99251[1], 99252[1], 99253[1], 99254[1], 99255[1], 99291[1], 99292[1], 99304[1], 99305[1], 99306[1], 99307[1], 99308[1], 99309[1], 99310[1], 99315[1], 99316[1], 99334[1], 99335[1], 99336[1], 99337[1], 99347[1], 99348[1], 99349[1], 99350[1], 99374[1], 99375[1], 99377[1], 99378[1], 99446[0], 99447[0], 99448[0], 99449[0], 99451[0], 99452[0], 99495[0], 99496[0], G0453[0], G0463[1], G0471[1]
63740	0213T[0], 0216T[0], 0228T[0], 0230T[0], 0333T[0], 0464T[0], 11000[1], 11001[1], 11004[1], 11005[1], 11006[1], 11042[1], 11043[1], 11044[1], 11045[1], 11046[1], 11047[1], 12001[1], 12002[1], 12004[1], 12005[1], 12006[1], 12007[1], 12011[1], 12013[1], 12014[1], 12015[1], 12016[1], 12017[1], 12018[1], 12020[1], 12021[1], 12031[1], 12032[1], 12034[1], 12035[1], 12036[1], 12037[1], 12041[1], 12042[1], 12044[1], 12045[1], 12046[1], 12047[1], 12051[1], 12052[1], 12053[1], 12054[1], 12055[1], 12056[1], 12057[1], 13100[1], 13101[1], 13102[1], 13120[1], 13121[1], 13122[1], 13131[1], 13132[1], 13133[1], 13151[1], 13152[1], 13153[1], 22505[0], 36000[1], 36400[1], 36405[1], 36406[1], 36410[1], 36420[1], 36425[1], 36430[1], 36440[1], 36591[0], 36592[0], 36600[1], 36640[1], 43752[1], 44005[0], 44180[0], 44820[0], 44850[0], 49000[0], 49002[1], 49010[0], 49255[0], 51701[1], 51702[1], 51703[1], 62320[0], 62321[0], 62322[0], 62323[0], 62324[0], 62325[0], 62326[0], 62327[0], 63707[1], 63709[1], 63741[1], 64400[0], 64405[0], 64408[0], 64415[0], 64416[0], 64417[0], 64418[0], 64420[0], 64421[0], 64425[0], 64430[0], 64435[0], 64445[0], 64446[0], 64447[0], 64448[0], 64449[0], 64450[0], 64451[0], 64454[0], 64461[0], 64462[0], 64463[0], 64479[0], 64480[0], 64483[0], 64484[0], 64486[0], 64487[0], 64488[0], 64489[0], 64490[0], 64491[0], 64492[0], 64493[0], 64494[0], 64495[0], 64505[0], 64510[0], 64517[0], 64520[0], 64530[0], 69990[0], 76000[1], 77001[1], 77002[1], 92012[1], 92014[1], 92585[0], 93000[1], 93005[1], 93010[1], 93040[1], 93041[1], 93042[1], 93318[1], 93355[1], 94002[1], 94200[1], 94250[1], 94680[1], 94681[1], 94690[1], 94770[1], 95812[1], 95813[1], 95816[1], 95819[1], 95822[0], 95829[1], 95860[0], 95861[0], 95863[0], 95864[0], 95865[0], 95866[0], 95867[0], 95868[0], 95869[0], 95870[0], 95907[0], 95908[0], 95909[0], 95910[0], 95911[0], 95912[0], 95913[0], 95925[0], 95926[0], 95927[0], 95928[0], 95929[0], 95930[0], 95933[0], 95937[0], 95938[0], 95939[0], 95940[0], 95955[1], 96360[1], 96361[1], 96365[1], 96366[1], 96367[1], 96368[1], 96372[1], 96374[1], 96375[1], 96376[1], 96377[1], 96523[0], 97597[1], 97598[1], 97602[1], 99155[0], 99156[0], 99157[0], 99211[1], 99212[1], 99213[1], 99214[1], 99215[1], 99217[1], 99218[1], 99219[1], 99220[1], 99221[1], 99222[1], 99223[1], 99231[1], 99232[1], 99233[1], 99234[1], 99235[1], 99236[1], 99238[1], 99239[1], 99241[1], 99242[1], 99243[1], 99244[1], 99245[1], 99251[1], 99252[1], 99253[1], 99254[1], 99255[1], 99291[1], 99292[1], 99304[1], 99305[1], 99306[1], 99307[1], 99308[1], 99309[1], 99310[1], 99315[1], 99316[1], 99334[1], 99335[1], 99336[1], 99337[1], 99347[1], 99348[1], 99349[1], 99350[1], 99374[1], 99375[1], 99377[1], 99378[1], 99446[0], 99447[0], 99448[0], 99449[0], 99451[0], 99452[0], 99495[0], 99496[0], G0453[0], G0463[1], G0471[1]
63741	01935[0], 01936[0], 0213T[0], 0216T[0], 0228T[0], 0230T[0], 0333T[0], 0464T[0], 11000[1], 11001[1], 11004[1], 11005[1], 11006[1], 11042[1], 11043[1], 11044[1], 11045[1], 11046[1], 11047[1], 12001[1], 12002[1], 12004[1], 12005[1], 12006[1], 12007[1], 12011[1], 12013[1], 12014[1], 12015[1], 12016[1], 12017[1], 12018[1], 12020[1], 12021[1], 12031[1], 12032[1], 12034[1], 12035[1], 12036[1], 12037[1], 12041[1], 12042[1], 12044[1], 12045[1], 12046[1], 12047[1], 12051[1], 12052[1], 12053[1], 12054[1], 12055[1], 12056[1], 12057[1], 13100[1], 13101[1], 13102[1], 13120[1], 13121[1], 13122[1], 13131[1], 13132[1], 13133[1], 13151[1], 13152[1], 13153[1], 22505[0], 36000[1], 36400[1], 36405[1], 36406[1], 36410[1], 36420[1], 36425[1], 36430[1], 36440[1], 36591[0], 36592[0], 36600[1], 36640[1], 43752[1], 51701[1], 51702[1], 51703[1], 62320[0], 62321[0], 62322[0], 62323[0], 62324[0], 62325[0], 62326[0], 62327[0], 64400[0], 64405[0], 64408[0], 64415[0], 64416[0], 64417[0], 64418[0], 64420[0], 64421[0], 64425[0], 64430[0], 64435[0], 64445[0], 64446[0], 64447[0], 64448[0], 64449[0], 64450[0], 64451[0], 64454[0], 64461[0], 64462[0], 64463[0], 64479[0], 64480[0], 64483[0], 64484[0], 64486[0], 64487[0], 64488[0], 64489[0], 64490[0], 64491[0], 64492[0], 64493[0], 64494[0], 64495[0], 64505[0], 64510[0], 64517[0], 64520[0], 64530[0], 69990[0], 76000[1], 77001[1], 77002[1], 77003[1], 92012[1], 92014[1], 92585[0], 93000[1], 93005[1], 93010[1], 93040[1], 93041[1], 93042[1], 93318[1], 93355[1], 94002[1], 94200[1], 94250[1], 94680[1], 94681[1], 94690[1], 94770[1], 95812[1], 95813[1], 95816[1], 95819[1], 95822[0], 95829[1], 95860[0], 95861[0], 95863[0], 95864[0], 95865[0], 95866[0], 95867[0], 95868[0], 95869[0], 95870[0], 95907[0], 95908[0], 95909[0], 95910[0], 95911[0], 95912[0], 95913[0], 95925[0], 95926[0], 95927[0], 95928[0], 95929[0], 95930[0], 95933[0], 95937[0], 95938[0], 95939[0], 95940[0], 95955[1], 96360[1], 96361[1], 96365[1], 96366[1], 96367[1], 96368[1], 96372[1], 96374[1], 96375[1], 96376[1], 96377[1], 96523[0], 97597[1], 97598[1], 97602[1], 99155[0], 99156[0], 99157[0], 99211[1], 99212[1], 99213[1], 99214[1], 99215[1], 99217[1], 99218[1], 99219[1], 99220[1], 99221[1], 99222[1], 99223[1], 99231[1], 99232[1], 99233[1], 99234[1], 99235[1], 99236[1], 99238[1], 99239[1], 99241[1], 99242[1], 99243[1], 99244[1], 99245[1], 99251[1], 99252[1], 99253[1], 99254[1], 99255[1], 99291[1], 99292[1], 99304[1], 99305[1], 99306[1], 99307[1], 99308[1], 99309[1], 99310[1], 99315[1], 99316[1], 99334[1], 99335[1], 99336[1], 99337[1], 99347[1], 99348[1], 99349[1], 99350[1], 99374[1], 99375[1], 99377[1], 99378[1], 99446[0], 99447[0], 99448[0], 99449[0], 99451[0], 99452[0], 99495[0], 99496[0], G0453[0], G0463[1], G0471[1]
63744	01935[0], 01936[0], 0213T[0], 0216T[0], 0228T[0], 0230T[0], 0333T[0], 0464T[0], 11000[1], 11001[1], 11004[1], 11005[1], 11006[1], 11042[1], 11043[1], 11044[1], 11045[1], 11046[1], 11047[1], 12001[1], 12002[1], 12004[1], 12005[1], 12006[1], 12007[1], 12011[1], 12013[1], 12014[1], 12015[1], 12016[1], 12017[1], 12018[1], 12020[1], 12021[1], 12031[1], 12032[1], 12034[1], 12035[1], 12036[1], 12037[1], 12041[1], 12042[1], 12044[1], 12045[1], 12046[1], 12047[1], 12051[1], 12052[1], 12053[1], 12054[1], 12055[1], 12056[1], 12057[1], 13100[1], 13101[1], 13102[1], 13120[1], 13121[1], 13122[1], 13131[1], 13132[1], 13133[1], 13151[1], 13152[1], 13153[1], 22505[0], 36000[1], 36400[1], 36405[1], 36406[1], 36410[1], 36420[1], 36425[1], 36430[1], 36440[1], 36591[0], 36592[0], 36600[1], 36640[1], 43752[1], 51701[1], 51702[1], 51703[1], 62320[0], 62321[0], 62322[0], 62323[0], 62324[0], 62325[0], 62326[0], 62327[0], 64400[0], 64405[0], 64408[0], 64415[0], 64416[0], 64417[0], 64418[0], 64420[0], 64421[0], 64425[0], 64430[0], 64435[0], 64445[0], 64446[0], 64447[0], 64448[0], 64449[0], 64450[0], 64451[0], 64454[0], 64461[0], 64462[0], 64463[0], 64479[0], 64480[0], 64483[0], 64484[0], 64486[0], 64487[0], 64488[0], 64489[0], 64490[0], 64491[0], 64492[0], 64493[0], 64494[0], 64495[0], 64505[0], 64510[0], 64517[0], 64520[0], 64530[0], 69990[0], 76000[1], 77001[1], 77002[1], 92012[1], 92014[1], 92585[0], 93000[1], 93005[1], 93010[1], 93040[1], 93041[1], 93042[1], 93318[1], 93355[1], 94002[1], 94200[1], 94250[1], 94680[1], 94681[1], 94690[1], 94770[1], 95812[1], 95813[1], 95816[1], 95819[1], 95822[0], 95829[1], 95860[0], 95861[0], 95863[0], 95864[0], 95865[0], 95866[0], 95867[0], 95868[0], 95869[0], 95870[0], 95907[0], 95908[0], 95909[0], 95910[0], 95911[0], 95912[0], 95913[0], 95925[0], 95926[0], 95927[0], 95928[0], 95929[0], 95930[0], 95933[0], 95937[0], 95938[0], 95939[0], 95940[0], 95955[1], 96360[1], 96361[1], 96365[1], 96366[1], 96367[1], 96368[1], 96372[1], 96374[1], 96375[1], 96376[1], 96377[1], 96523[0], 97597[1], 97598[1], 97602[1], 99155[0], 99156[0], 99157[0], 99211[1], 99212[1], 99213[1], 99214[1], 99215[1], 99217[1], 99218[1], 99219[1], 99220[1], 99221[1], 99222[1], 99223[1], 99231[1], 99232[1], 99233[1], 99234[1], 99235[1], 99236[1], 99238[1], 99239[1], 99241[1], 99242[1], 99243[1], 99244[1], 99245[1], 99251[1], 99252[1], 99253[1], 99254[1], 99255[1], 99291[1], 99292[1], 99304[1], 99305[1], 99306[1], 99307[1], 99308[1], 99309[1], 99310[1], 99315[1], 99316[1], 99334[1], 99335[1], 99336[1], 99337[1], 99347[1], 99348[1], 99349[1], 99350[1], 99374[1], 99375[1], 99377[1],

0 = Modifier usage not allowed or inappropriate 1 = Modifier usage allowed

Code 1	Code 2
	99378[1], 99446[0], 99447[0], 99448[0], 99449[0], 99451[0], 99452[0], 99495[0], 99496[0], G0453[0], G0463[1], G0471[1]
63746	01935[0], 01936[0], 0213T[0], 0216T[0], 0228T[0], 0230T[0], 0333T[0], 0464T[0], 11000[1], 11001[1], 11004[1], 11005[1], 11006[1], 11042[1], 11043[1], 11044[1], 11045[1], 11046[1], 11047[1], 12001[1], 12002[1], 12004[1], 12005[1], 12006[1], 12007[1], 12011[1], 12013[1], 12014[1], 12015[1], 12016[1], 12017[1], 12018[1], 12020[1], 12021[1], 12031[1], 12032[1], 12034[1], 12035[1], 12036[1], 12037[1], 12041[1], 12042[1], 12044[1], 12045[1], 12046[1], 12047[1], 12051[1], 12052[1], 12053[1], 12054[1], 12055[1], 12056[1], 12057[1], 13100[1], 13101[1], 13102[1], 13120[1], 13121[1], 13122[1], 13131[1], 13132[1], 13133[1], 13151[1], 13152[1], 13153[1], 22505[0], 36000[1], 36400[1], 36405[1], 36406[1], 36410[1], 36420[1], 36425[1], 36430[1], 36440[1], 36591[0], 36592[0], 36600[1], 36640[1], 43752[1], 51701[1], 51702[1], 51703[1], 62320[0], 62321[0], 62322[0], 62323[0], 62324[0], 62325[0], 62326[0], 62327[0], 63740[1], 63741[1], 63744[1], 64400[0], 64405[0], 64408[0], 64415[0], 64416[0], 64417[0], 64418[0], 64420[0], 64421[0], 64425[0], 64430[0], 64435[0], 64445[0], 64446[0], 64447[0], 64448[0], 64449[0], 64450[0], 64451[0], 64454[0], 64461[0], 64462[0], 64463[0], 64479[0], 64480[0], 64483[0], 64484[0], 64486[0], 64487[0], 64488[0], 64489[0], 64490[0], 64491[0], 64492[0], 64493[0], 64494[0], 64495[0], 64505[0], 64510[0], 64517[0], 64520[0], 64530[0], 69990[0], 76000[1], 77001[1], 77002[1], 92012[1], 92014[1], 92585[0], 93000[1], 93005[1], 93010[1], 93040[1], 93041[1], 93042[1], 93318[1], 93355[1], 94002[1], 94200[1], 94250[1], 94680[1], 94681[1], 94690[1], 94770[1], 95812[1], 95813[1], 95816[1], 95819[1], 95822[0], 95829[1], 95860[0], 95861[0], 95863[0], 95864[0], 95865[0], 95866[0], 95867[0], 95868[0], 95869[0], 95870[0], 95907[0], 95908[0], 95909[0], 95910[0], 95911[0], 95912[0], 95913[0], 95925[0], 95926[0], 95927[0], 95928[0], 95929[0], 95930[0], 95933[0], 95937[0], 95938[0], 95939[0], 95940[0], 95955[1], 96360[1], 96361[1], 96365[1], 96366[1], 96367[1], 96368[1], 96372[1], 96374[1], 96375[1], 96376[1], 96377[1], 96523[0], 97597[1], 97598[1], 97602[1], 99155[0], 99156[0], 99157[0], 99211[1], 99212[1], 99213[1], 99214[1], 99215[1], 99217[1], 99218[1], 99219[1], 99220[1], 99221[1], 99222[1], 99223[1], 99231[1], 99232[1], 99233[1], 99234[1], 99235[1], 99236[1], 99238[1], 99239[1], 99241[1], 99242[1], 99243[1], 99244[1], 99245[1], 99251[1], 99252[1], 99253[1], 99254[1], 99255[1], 99291[1], 99292[1], 99304[1], 99305[1], 99306[1], 99307[1], 99308[1], 99309[1], 99310[1], 99315[1], 99316[1], 99334[1], 99335[1], 99336[1], 99337[1], 99347[1], 99348[1], 99349[1], 99350[1], 99374[1], 99375[1], 99377[1], 99378[1], 99446[0], 99447[0], 99448[0], 99449[0], 99451[0], 99452[0], 99495[0], 99496[0], G0453[0], G0463[1], G0471[1]
64400	01991[0], 01992[0], 0333T[0], 0464T[0], 0543T[0], 0544T[0], 0548T[0], 0567T[0], 0568T[0], 0569T[0], 0570T[0], 0571T[0], 0572T[0], 0573T[0], 0574T[0], 0580T[0], 0581T[0], 0582T[0], 20550[1], 20551[1], 20560[0], 20561[0], 36000[1], 36400[1], 36405[1], 36406[1], 36410[1], 36420[1], 36425[1], 36430[1], 36440[1], 36591[0], 36592[0], 36600[1], 51701[0], 51702[0], 51703[0], 66987[0], 66988[0], 69990[0], 76000[1], 76970[1], 76998[1], 77001[1], 77002[1], 92012[1], 92014[1], 92585[0], 93000[1], 93005[1], 93010[1], 93040[1], 93041[1], 93042[1], 93318[1], 93355[1], 94002[1], 94200[1], 94250[1], 94680[1], 94681[1], 94690[1], 94770[1], 95812[1], 95813[1], 95816[1], 95819[1], 95822[0], 95829[1], 95860[1], 95861[1], 95863[1], 95864[1], 95865[1], 95866[1], 95867[1], 95868[1], 95869[1], 95870[1], 95907[1], 95908[1], 95909[1], 95910[1], 95911[1], 95912[1], 95913[1], 95925[0], 95926[0], 95927[0], 95928[0], 95929[0], 95930[0], 95933[0], 95937[0], 95938[0], 95939[0], 95940[0], 95955[1], 96360[1], 96361[1], 96365[1], 96366[1], 96367[1], 96368[1], 96372[1], 96374[1], 96375[1], 96376[1], 96377[1], 96523[0], 99155[0], 99156[0], 99157[0], 99211[1], 99212[1], 99213[1], 99214[1], 99215[1], 99217[1], 99218[1], 99219[1], 99220[1], 99221[1], 99222[1], 99223[1], 99231[1], 99232[1], 99233[1], 99234[1], 99235[1], 99236[1], 99238[1], 99239[1], 99241[1], 99242[1], 99243[1], 99244[1], 99245[1], 99251[1], 99252[1], 99253[1], 99254[1], 99255[1], 99291[1], 99292[1], 99304[1], 99305[1], 99306[1], 99307[1], 99308[1], 99309[1], 99310[1], 99315[1], 99316[1], 99334[1], 99335[1], 99336[1], 99337[1], 99347[1], 99348[1], 99349[1], 99350[1], 99374[1], 99375[1], 99377[1], 99378[1], 99446[0], 99447[0], 99448[0], 99449[0], 99451[0], 99452[0], 99495[1], 99496[1], G0453[0], G0459[1], G0463[1], G0471[0], J0670[1], J2001[1]
64405	01991[0], 01992[0], 0333T[0], 0464T[0], 0543T[0], 0544T[0], 0548T[0], 0567T[0], 0568T[0], 0569T[0], 0570T[0], 0571T[0], 0572T[0], 0573T[0], 0574T[0], 0580T[0], 0581T[0], 0582T[0], 20550[1], 20551[1], 20560[0], 20561[0], 36000[1], 36400[1], 36405[1], 36406[1], 36410[1], 36420[1], 36425[1], 36430[1], 36440[1], 36591[0], 36592[0], 36600[1], 51701[0], 51702[0], 51703[0], 66987[0], 66988[0], 69990[0], 76000[1], 76970[1], 76998[1], 77001[1], 77002[1], 92012[1], 92014[1], 92585[0], 93000[1], 93005[1], 93010[1], 93040[1], 93041[1], 93042[1], 93318[1], 93355[1], 94002[1], 94200[1], 94250[1], 94680[1], 94681[1], 94690[1], 94770[1], 95812[1], 95813[1], 95816[1], 95819[1], 95822[0], 95829[1], 95860[1], 95861[1], 95863[1], 95864[1], 95865[1], 95866[1], 95867[1], 95868[1], 95869[1], 95870[1], 95907[1], 95908[1], 95909[1], 95910[1], 95911[1], 95912[1], 95913[1], 95925[0], 95926[0], 95927[0], 95928[0], 95929[0], 95930[0], 95933[0], 95937[0], 95938[0], 95939[0], 95940[0], 95955[1], 96360[1], 96361[1], 96365[1], 96366[1], 96367[1], 96368[1], 96372[1], 96374[1], 96375[1], 96376[1], 96377[1], 96523[0], 99155[0], 99156[0], 99157[0], 99211[1], 99212[1], 99213[1], 99214[1], 99215[1], 99217[1], 99218[1], 99219[1], 99220[1], 99221[1], 99222[1], 99223[1], 99231[1], 99232[1], 99233[1], 99234[1], 99235[1], 99236[1], 99238[1], 99239[1], 99241[1], 99242[1], 99243[1], 99244[1], 99245[1], 99251[1], 99252[1], 99253[1], 99254[1], 99255[1], 99291[1], 99292[1], 99304[1], 99305[1], 99306[1], 99307[1], 99308[1], 99309[1], 99310[1], 99315[1], 99316[1], 99334[1], 99335[1], 99336[1], 99337[1], 99347[1], 99348[1], 99349[1], 99350[1], 99374[1], 99375[1], 99377[1], 99378[1], 99446[0], 99447[0], 99448[0], 99449[0], 99451[0], 99452[0], 99495[1], 99496[1], G0453[0], G0459[1], G0463[1], G0471[0], J0670[1], J2001[1]
64415	01991[0], 01992[0], 0333T[0], 0464T[0], 0543T[0], 0544T[0], 0548T[0], 0567T[0], 0568T[0], 0569T[0], 0570T[0], 0571T[0], 0572T[0], 0573T[0], 0574T[0], 0580T[0], 0581T[0], 0582T[0], 20550[1], 20551[1], 20560[0], 20561[0], 20701[0], 36591[0], 36592[0], 51701[0], 51702[0], 66987[0], 66988[0], 69990[0], 76000[1], 76970[1], 76998[1], 77001[1], 77002[1], 92012[1], 92014[1], 92585[0], 93000[1], 93005[1], 93010[1], 93040[1], 93041[1], 93042[1], 93318[1], 93355[1], 94002[1], 94200[1], 94250[1], 94680[1], 94681[1], 94690[1], 94770[1], 95812[1], 95813[1], 95816[1], 95819[1], 95822[0], 95829[1], 95860[1], 95861[1], 95863[1], 95864[1], 95865[1], 95866[1], 95867[1], 95868[1], 95869[1], 95870[1], 95907[1], 95908[1], 95909[1], 95910[1], 95911[1], 95912[1], 95913[1], 95925[0], 95926[0], 95927[0], 95928[0], 95929[0], 95930[0], 95933[0], 95937[0], 95938[0], 95939[0], 95940[0], 95955[1], 96360[1], 96361[1], 96365[1], 96366[1], 96367[1], 96368[1], 96372[1], 96374[1], 96375[1], 96376[1], 96377[1], 96523[0], 99155[0], 99156[0], 99157[0], 99211[1], 99212[1], 99213[1], 99214[1], 99215[1], 99217[1], 99218[1], 99219[1], 99220[1], 99221[1], 99222[1], 99223[1], 99231[1], 99232[1], 99233[1], 99234[1], 99235[1], 99236[1], 99238[1], 99239[1], 99241[1], 99242[1], 99243[1], 99244[1], 99245[1], 99251[1], 99252[1], 99253[1], 99254[1], 99255[1], 99291[1], 99292[1], 99304[1], 99305[1], 99306[1], 99307[1], 99308[1], 99309[1], 99310[1], 99315[1], 99316[1], 99334[1], 99335[1], 99336[1], 99337[1], 99347[1], 99348[1], 99349[1], 99350[1], 99374[1], 99375[1], 99377[1], 99378[1], 99446[0], 99447[0], 99448[0], 99449[0], 99451[0], 99452[0], 99495[1], 99496[1], G0453[0], G0459[1], G0463[1], G0471[0], J0670[1], J2001[1]
64416	01991[0], 01992[0], 01996[0], 0333T[0], 0464T[0], 0543T[0], 0544T[0], 0548T[0], 0567T[0], 0568T[0], 0569T[0], 0570T[0], 0571T[0], 0572T[0], 0573T[0], 0574T[0], 0580T[0], 0581T[0], 0582T[0], 20550[1], 20551[1], 20560[0], 20561[0], 20701[0], 36000[1], 36410[1], 36591[0], 36592[0], 51701[0], 51702[0], 51703[0], 66987[0], 66988[0], 69990[0], 76000[1], 76970[1], 76998[1], 77001[1], 77002[1], 92012[1], 92014[1], 92585[0], 93000[1], 93005[1], 93010[1], 93040[1], 93041[1], 93042[1], 93318[1], 93355[1], 94002[1], 94200[1], 94250[1], 94680[1], 94681[1], 94690[1], 94770[1], 95812[1], 95813[1], 95816[1], 95819[1], 95822[0], 95829[1], 95860[1], 95861[1], 95863[1], 95864[1], 95865[1], 95866[1], 95867[1], 95868[1], 95869[1], 95870[1], 95907[1], 95908[1], 95909[1], 95910[1], 95911[1], 95912[1], 95913[1], 95925[0], 95926[0], 95927[0], 95928[0], 95929[0], 95930[0], 95933[0], 95937[0], 95938[0], 95939[0], 95940[0], 95955[1], 96360[1], 96361[1], 96365[1], 96366[1], 96367[1], 96368[1], 96372[1], 96374[1], 96375[1], 96376[1], 96377[1], 96523[0], 99155[0], 99156[0], 99157[0], 99211[1], 99212[1], 99213[1], 99214[1], 99215[1], 99217[1], 99218[1], 99219[1], 99220[1], 99221[1], 99222[1], 99223[1], 99231[1], 99232[1], 99233[1], 99234[1], 99235[1], 99236[1], 99238[1], 99239[1], 99241[1], 99242[1], 99243[1], 99244[1], 99245[1], 99251[1], 99252[1], 99253[1], 99254[1], 99255[1], 99291[1], 99292[1], 99304[1], 99305[1], 99306[1], 99307[1], 99308[1], 99309[1], 99310[1], 99315[1], 99316[1], 99334[1], 99335[1], 99336[1], 99337[1], 99347[1], 99348[1], 99349[1], 99350[1], 99374[1], 99375[1], 99377[1], 99378[1], 99446[0], 99447[0], 99448[0], 99449[0], 99451[0], 99452[0], 99495[1], 99496[1], G0453[0], G0459[1], G0463[1], G0471[0], J2001[1]
64417	01991[0], 01992[0], 0333T[0], 0464T[0], 0543T[0], 0544T[0], 0548T[0], 0567T[0], 0568T[0], 0569T[0], 0570T[0], 0571T[0], 0572T[0], 0573T[0], 0574T[0], 0580T[0], 0581T[0], 0582T[0], 20550[1], 20551[1], 20560[0], 20561[0], 20701[0], 36591[0], 36592[0], 51701[0], 51702[0], 66987[0], 66988[0], 69990[0], 76000[1], 76970[1], 76998[1], 77001[1], 77002[1], 92012[1], 92014[1], 92585[0], 93000[1], 93005[1], 93010[1], 93040[1], 93041[1], 93042[1], 93318[1], 93355[1], 94002[1], 94200[1], 94250[1], 94680[1], 94681[1], 94690[1], 94770[1], 95812[1], 95813[1], 95816[1], 95819[1], 95822[0], 95829[1], 95860[1], 95861[1], 95863[1], 95864[1], 95865[1], 95866[1], 95867[1], 95868[1], 95869[1], 95870[1], 95907[1], 95908[1], 95909[1], 95910[1], 95911[1], 95912[1], 95913[1], 95925[0], 95926[0], 95927[0], 95928[0], 95929[0], 95930[0], 95933[0], 95937[0], 95938[0], 95939[0], 95940[0], 95955[1], 96360[1], 96361[1], 96365[1], 96366[1], 96367[1], 96368[1], 96372[1], 96374[1], 96375[1], 96376[1], 96377[1], 96523[0], 99155[0], 99156[0], 99157[0], 99211[1], 99212[1], 99213[1], 99214[1], 99215[1], 99217[1], 99218[1], 99219[1], 99220[1], 99221[1], 99222[1], 99223[1], 99231[1], 99232[1], 99233[1], 99234[1], 99235[1], 99236[1], 99238[1], 99239[1], 99241[1], 99242[1], 99243[1], 99244[1], 99245[1], 99251[1], 99252[1], 99253[1], 99254[1], 99255[1], 99291[1], 99292[1], 99304[1], 99305[1], 99306[1], 99307[1], 99308[1], 99309[1], 99310[1], 99315[1], 99316[1], 99334[1], 99335[1], 99336[1], 99337[1], 99347[1], 99348[1], 99349[1], 99350[1], 99374[1], 99375[1], 99377[1], 99378[1], 99446[0], 99447[0], 99448[0], 99449[0], 99451[0], 99452[0], 99495[1], 99496[1], G0453[0], G0459[1], G0463[1], G0471[0], J0670[1], J2001[1]
64418	01991[0], 01992[0], 0333T[0], 0464T[0], 0543T[0], 0544T[0], 0548T[0], 0567T[0], 0568T[0], 0569T[0], 0570T[0], 0571T[0], 0572T[0], 0573T[0], 0574T[0], 0580T[0], 0581T[0], 0582T[0], 20550[1], 20551[1], 20560[0], 20561[0], 36000[1], 36400[1], 36405[1], 36406[1], 36410[1], 36420[1], 36425[1], 36430[1], 36440[1], 36591[0], 36592[0], 36600[1], 51701[0], 51702[0], 51703[0], 66987[0], 66988[0], 69990[0], 76000[1], 76970[1], 76998[1], 77001[1], 77002[1], 92012[1], 92014[1], 92585[0], 93000[1], 93005[1], 93010[1], 93040[1], 93041[1], 93042[1], 93318[1], 93355[1], 94002[1], 94200[1], 94250[1], 94680[1], 94681[1], 94690[1], 94770[1], 95812[1], 95813[1], 95816[1], 95819[1], 95822[0], 95829[1], 95860[1], 95861[1], 95863[1], 95864[1], 95865[1], 95866[1], 95867[1], 95868[1], 95869[1], 95870[1], 95907[1], 95908[1], 95909[1], 95910[1], 95911[1], 95912[1], 95913[1], 95925[0], 95926[0], 95927[0], 95928[0], 95929[0], 95930[0], 95933[0], 95937[0], 95938[0], 95939[0], 95940[0], 95955[1], 96360[1], 96361[1], 96365[1], 96366[1], 96367[1], 96368[1], 96372[1], 96374[1], 96375[1], 96376[1], 96377[1], 96523[0],

0 = Modifier usage not allowed or inappropriate 1 = Modifier usage allowed

Code 1	Code 2
	99155^0, 99156^0, 99157^0, 99211^1, 99212^1, 99213^1, 99214^1, 99215^1, 99217^1, 99218^1, 99219^1, 99220^1, 99221^1, 99222^1, 99223^1, 99231^1, 99232^1, 99233^1, 99234^1, 99235^1, 99236^1, 99238^1, 99239^1, 99241^1, 99242^1, 99243^1, 99244^1, 99245^1, 99251^1, 99252^1, 99253^1, 99254^1, 99255^1, 99291^1, 99292^1, 99304^1, 99305^1, 99306^1, 99307^1, 99308^1, 99309^1, 99310^1, 99315^1, 99316^1, 99334^1, 99335^1, 99336^1, 99337^1, 99347^1, 99348^1, 99349^1, 99350^1, 99374^1, 99375^1, 99377^1, 99378^1, 99446^0, 99447^0, 99448^0, 99449^0, 99451^0, 99452^0, 99495^1, 99496^1, G0453^0, G0459^1, G0463^1, G0471^0, J0670^1, J2001^1
64420	01991^0, 01992^0, 0333T^0, 0464T^0, 0543T^0, 0544T^0, 0548T^0, 0567T^0, 0568T^0, 0569T^0, 0570T^0, 0571T^0, 0572T^0, 0573T^0, 0574T^0, 0580T^0, 0581T^0, 0582T^0, 20550^1, 20551^1, 20560^0, 20561^0, 36000^1, 36400^1, 36405^1, 36406^1, 36410^1, 36420^1, 36425^1, 36430^1, 36440^1, 36591^0, 36592^0, 36600^1, 51701^0, 51702^0, 51703^0, 66987^0, 66988^0, 69990^0, 76000^1, 76970^1, 76998^1, 77001^1, 77002^1, 92012^1, 92014^1, 92585^0, 93000^1, 93005^1, 93010^1, 93040^1, 93041^1, 93042^1, 93318^1, 93355^1, 94002^1, 94200^1, 94250^1, 94680^1, 94681^1, 94690^1, 94770^1, 95812^1, 95813^1, 95816^1, 95819^1, 95822^0, 95829^1, 95860^1, 95861^1, 95863^1, 95864^1, 95865^1, 95866^1, 95867^1, 95868^1, 95869^1, 95870^1, 95907^1, 95908^1, 95909^1, 95910^1, 95911^1, 95912^1, 95913^1, 95925^0, 95926^0, 95927^0, 95928^0, 95929^0, 95930^0, 95933^0, 95937^0, 95938^0, 95939^0, 95940^0, 95955^1, 96360^1, 96361^1, 96365^1, 96366^1, 96367^1, 96368^1, 96372^1, 96374^1, 96375^1, 96376^1, 96377^1, 96523^0, 99155^0, 99156^0, 99157^0, 99211^1, 99212^1, 99213^1, 99214^1, 99215^1, 99217^1, 99218^1, 99219^1, 99220^1, 99221^1, 99222^1, 99223^1, 99231^1, 99232^1, 99233^1, 99234^1, 99235^1, 99236^1, 99238^1, 99239^1, 99241^1, 99242^1, 99243^1, 99244^1, 99245^1, 99251^1, 99252^1, 99253^1, 99254^1, 99255^1, 99291^1, 99292^1, 99304^1, 99305^1, 99306^1, 99307^1, 99308^1, 99309^1, 99310^1, 99315^1, 99316^1, 99334^1, 99335^1, 99336^1, 99337^1, 99347^1, 99348^1, 99349^1, 99350^1, 99374^1, 99375^1, 99377^1, 99378^1, 99446^0, 99447^0, 99448^0, 99449^0, 99451^0, 99452^0, 99495^1, 99496^1, G0453^0, G0459^1, G0463^1, G0471^0, J0670^1, J2001^1
64421	01991^0, 01992^0, 0333T^0, 0464T^0, 0543T^0, 0544T^0, 0548T^0, 0567T^0, 0568T^0, 0569T^0, 0570T^0, 0571T^0, 0572T^0, 0573T^0, 0574T^0, 0580T^0, 0581T^0, 0582T^0, 20550^1, 20551^1, 20560^0, 20561^0, 36000^1, 36400^1, 36405^1, 36406^1, 36410^1, 36420^1, 36425^1, 36430^1, 36440^1, 36591^0, 36592^0, 36600^1, 51701^0, 51702^0, 51703^0, 64420^1, 66987^0, 66988^0, 69990^0, 76000^1, 76970^1, 76998^1, 77001^1, 77002^1, 92012^1, 92014^1, 92585^0, 93000^1, 93005^1, 93010^1, 93040^1, 93041^1, 93042^1, 93318^1, 93355^1, 94002^1, 94200^1, 94250^1, 94680^1, 94681^1, 94690^1, 94770^1, 95812^1, 95813^1, 95816^1, 95819^1, 95822^0, 95829^1, 95860^1, 95861^1, 95863^1, 95864^1, 95865^1, 95866^1, 95867^1, 95868^1, 95869^1, 95870^1, 95907^1, 95908^1, 95909^1, 95910^1, 95911^1, 95912^1, 95913^1, 95925^0, 95926^0, 95927^0, 95928^0, 95929^0, 95930^0, 95933^0, 95937^0, 95938^0, 95939^0, 95940^0, 95955^1, 96360^1, 96361^1, 96365^1, 96366^1, 96367^1, 96368^1, 96372^1, 96374^1, 96375^1, 96376^1, 96377^1, 96523^0, 99155^0, 99156^0, 99157^0, 99211^1, 99212^1, 99213^1, 99214^1, 99215^1, 99217^1, 99218^1, 99219^1, 99220^1, 99221^1, 99222^1, 99223^1, 99231^1, 99232^1, 99233^1, 99234^1, 99235^1, 99236^1, 99238^1, 99239^1, 99241^1, 99242^1, 99243^1, 99244^1, 99245^1, 99251^1, 99252^1, 99253^1, 99254^1, 99255^1, 99291^1, 99292^1, 99304^1, 99305^1, 99306^1, 99307^1, 99308^1, 99309^1, 99310^1, 99315^1, 99316^1, 99334^1, 99335^1, 99336^1, 99337^1, 99347^1, 99348^1, 99349^1, 99350^1, 99374^1, 99375^1, 99377^1, 99378^1, 99446^0, 99447^0, 99448^0, 99449^0, 99451^0, 99452^0, 99495^1, 99496^1, G0453^0, G0459^1, G0463^1, G0471^0, J0670^1, J2001^1
64425	01991^0, 01992^0, 0333T^0, 0464T^0, 0543T^0, 0544T^0, 0548T^0, 0567T^0, 0568T^0, 0569T^0, 0570T^0, 0571T^0, 0572T^0, 0573T^0, 0574T^0, 0580T^0, 0581T^0, 0582T^0, 20550^1, 20551^1, 20560^0, 20561^0, 36000^1, 36400^1, 36405^1, 36406^1, 36410^1, 36420^1, 36425^1, 36430^1, 36440^1, 36591^0, 36592^0, 36600^1, 51701^0, 51702^0, 51703^0, 66987^0, 66988^0, 69990^0, 76000^1, 76970^1, 76998^1, 77001^1, 77002^1, 92012^1, 92014^1, 92585^0, 93000^1, 93005^1, 93010^1, 93040^1, 93041^1, 93042^1, 93318^1, 93355^1, 94002^1, 94200^1, 94250^1, 94680^1, 94681^1, 94690^1, 94770^1, 95812^1, 95813^1, 95816^1, 95819^1, 95822^0, 95829^1, 95860^1, 95861^1, 95863^1, 95864^1, 95865^1, 95866^1, 95867^1, 95868^1, 95869^1, 95870^1, 95907^1, 95908^1, 95909^1, 95910^1, 95911^1, 95912^1, 95913^1, 95925^0, 95926^0, 95927^0, 95928^0, 95929^0, 95930^0, 95933^0, 95937^0, 95938^0, 95939^0, 95940^0, 95955^1, 96360^1, 96361^1, 96365^1, 96366^1, 96367^1, 96368^1, 96372^1, 96374^1, 96375^1, 96376^1, 96377^1, 96523^0, 99155^0, 99156^0, 99157^0, 99211^1, 99212^1, 99213^1, 99214^1, 99215^1, 99217^1, 99218^1, 99219^1, 99220^1, 99221^1, 99222^1, 99223^1, 99231^1, 99232^1, 99233^1, 99234^1, 99235^1, 99236^1, 99238^1, 99239^1, 99241^1, 99242^1, 99243^1, 99244^1, 99245^1, 99251^1, 99252^1, 99253^1, 99254^1, 99255^1, 99291^1, 99292^1, 99304^1, 99305^1, 99306^1, 99307^1, 99308^1, 99309^1, 99310^1, 99315^1, 99316^1, 99334^1, 99335^1, 99336^1, 99337^1, 99347^1, 99348^1, 99349^1, 99350^1, 99374^1, 99375^1, 99377^1, 99378^1, 99446^0, 99447^0, 99448^0, 99449^0, 99451^0, 99452^0, 99495^1, 99496^1, G0453^0, G0459^1, G0463^1, G0471^0, J0670^1, J2001^1
64445	01991^0, 01992^0, 0333T^0, 0464T^0, 0543T^0, 0544T^0, 0548T^0, 0567T^0, 0568T^0, 0569T^0, 0570T^0, 0571T^0, 0572T^0, 0573T^0, 0574T^0, 0580T^0, 0581T^0, 0582T^0, 20550^1, 20551^1, 20560^0, 20561^0, 36000^1, 36400^1, 36405^1, 36406^1, 36410^1, 36420^1, 36425^1, 36430^1, 36440^1, 36591^0, 36592^0, 36600^1, 51701^0, 51702^0, 51703^0, 66987^0, 66988^0, 69990^0, 76000^1, 76800^1, 76970^1, 76998^1, 77001^1, 77002^1, 92012^1, 92014^1, 92585^0, 93000^1, 93005^1, 93010^1, 93040^1, 93041^1, 93042^1, 93318^1, 93355^1, 94002^1, 94200^1, 94250^1, 94680^1, 94681^1, 94690^1, 94770^1, 95812^1, 95813^1, 95816^1, 95819^1, 95822^0, 95829^1, 95860^1, 95861^1, 95863^1, 95864^1, 95865^1, 95866^1, 95867^1, 95868^1, 95869^1, 95870^1, 95907^1, 95908^1, 95909^1, 95910^1, 95911^1, 95912^1, 95913^1, 95925^0, 95926^0, 95927^0, 95928^0, 95929^0, 95930^0, 95933^0, 95937^0, 95938^0, 95939^0, 95940^0, 95955^1, 96360^1, 96361^1, 96365^1, 96366^1, 96367^1, 96368^1, 96372^1, 96374^1, 96375^1, 96376^1, 96377^1, 96523^0, 99155^0, 99156^0, 99157^0, 99211^1, 99212^1, 99213^1, 99214^1, 99215^1, 99217^1, 99218^1, 99219^1, 99220^1, 99221^1, 99222^1, 99223^1, 99231^1, 99232^1, 99233^1, 99234^1, 99235^1, 99236^1, 99238^1, 99239^1, 99241^1, 99242^1, 99243^1, 99244^1, 99245^1, 99251^1, 99252^1, 99253^1, 99254^1, 99255^1, 99291^1, 99292^1, 99304^1, 99305^1, 99306^1, 99307^1, 99308^1, 99309^1, 99310^1, 99315^1, 99316^1, 99334^1, 99335^1, 99336^1, 99337^1, 99347^1, 99348^1, 99349^1, 99350^1, 99374^1, 99375^1, 99377^1, 99378^1, 99446^0, 99447^0, 99448^0, 99449^0, 99451^0, 99452^0, 99495^1, 99496^1, G0453^0, G0459^1, G0463^1, G0471^0, J0670^1, J2001^1
64446	01991^0, 01992^0, 01996^0, 0333T^0, 0464T^0, 0543T^0, 0544T^0, 0548T^0, 0567T^0, 0568T^0, 0569T^0, 0570T^0, 0571T^0, 0572T^0, 0573T^0, 0574T^0, 0580T^0, 0581T^0, 0582T^0, 20550^1, 20551^1, 20560^0, 20561^0, 20701^0, 36000^1, 36400^1, 36405^1, 36406^1, 36410^1, 36420^1, 36425^1, 36430^1, 36440^1, 36591^0, 36592^0, 36600^1, 51701^0, 51702^0, 51703^0, 66987^0, 66988^0, 69990^0, 76000^1, 76800^1, 76970^1, 76998^1, 77001^1, 77002^1, 92012^1, 92014^1, 92585^0, 93000^1, 93005^1, 93010^1, 93040^1, 93041^1, 93042^1, 93318^1, 93355^1, 94002^1, 94200^1, 94250^1, 94680^1, 94681^1, 94690^1, 94770^1, 95812^1, 95813^1, 95816^1, 95819^1, 95822^0, 95829^1, 95860^1, 95861^1, 95863^1, 95864^1, 95865^1, 95866^1, 95867^1, 95868^1, 95869^1, 95870^1, 95907^1, 95908^1, 95909^1, 95910^1, 95911^1, 95912^1, 95913^1, 95925^0, 95926^0, 95927^0, 95928^0, 95929^0, 95930^0, 95933^0, 95937^0, 95938^0, 95939^0, 95940^0, 95955^1, 96360^1, 96361^1, 96365^1, 96366^1, 96367^1, 96368^1, 96372^1, 96374^1, 96375^1, 96376^1, 96377^1, 96523^0, 99155^0, 99156^0, 99157^0, 99211^1, 99212^1, 99213^1, 99214^1, 99215^1, 99217^1, 99218^1, 99219^1, 99220^1, 99221^1, 99222^1, 99223^1, 99231^1, 99232^1, 99233^1, 99234^1, 99235^1, 99236^1, 99238^1, 99239^1, 99241^1, 99242^1, 99243^1, 99244^1, 99245^1, 99251^1, 99252^1, 99253^1, 99254^1, 99255^1, 99291^1, 99292^1, 99304^1, 99305^1, 99306^1, 99307^1, 99308^1, 99309^1, 99310^1, 99315^1, 99316^1, 99334^1, 99335^1, 99336^1, 99337^1, 99347^1, 99348^1, 99349^1, 99350^1, 99374^1, 99375^1, 99377^1, 99378^1, 99446^0, 99447^0, 99448^0, 99449^0, 99451^0, 99452^0, 99495^1, 99496^1, G0453^0, G0459^1, G0463^1, G0471^0, J2001^1
64447	01991^0, 01992^0, 01996^0, 0333T^0, 0464T^0, 0543T^0, 0544T^0, 0548T^0, 0567T^0, 0568T^0, 0569T^0, 0570T^0, 0571T^0, 0572T^0, 0573T^0, 0574T^0, 0580T^0, 0581T^0, 0582T^0, 20550^1, 20551^1, 20560^0, 20561^0, 36000^1, 36400^1, 36405^1, 36406^1, 36410^1, 36420^1, 36425^1, 36430^1, 36440^1, 36591^0, 36592^0, 36600^1, 51701^0, 51702^0, 51703^0, 66987^0, 66988^0, 69990^0, 76000^1, 76970^1, 76998^1, 77001^1, 77002^1, 92012^1, 92014^1, 92585^0, 93000^1, 93005^1, 93010^1, 93040^1, 93041^1, 93042^1, 93318^1, 93355^1, 94002^1, 94200^1, 94250^1, 94680^1, 94681^1, 94690^1, 94770^1, 95812^1, 95813^1, 95816^1, 95819^1, 95822^0, 95829^1, 95860^1, 95861^1, 95863^1, 95864^1, 95865^1, 95866^1, 95867^1, 95868^1, 95869^1, 95870^1, 95907^1, 95908^1, 95909^1, 95910^1, 95911^1, 95912^1, 95913^1, 95925^0, 95926^0, 95927^0, 95928^0, 95929^0, 95930^0, 95933^0, 95937^0, 95938^0, 95939^0, 95940^0, 95955^1, 96360^1, 96361^1, 96365^1, 96366^1, 96367^1, 96368^1, 96372^1, 96374^1, 96375^1, 96376^1, 96377^1, 96523^0, 99155^0, 99156^0, 99157^0, 99211^1, 99212^1, 99213^1, 99214^1, 99215^1, 99217^1, 99218^1, 99219^1, 99220^1, 99221^1, 99222^1, 99223^1, 99231^1, 99232^1, 99233^1, 99234^1, 99235^1, 99236^1, 99238^1, 99239^1, 99241^1, 99242^1, 99243^1, 99244^1, 99245^1, 99251^1, 99252^1, 99253^1, 99254^1, 99255^1, 99291^1, 99292^1, 99304^1, 99305^1, 99306^1, 99307^1, 99308^1, 99309^1, 99310^1, 99315^1, 99316^1, 99334^1, 99335^1, 99336^1, 99337^1, 99347^1, 99348^1, 99349^1, 99350^1, 99374^1, 99375^1, 99377^1, 99378^1, 99446^0, 99447^0, 99448^0, 99449^0, 99451^0, 99452^0, 99495^1, 99496^1, G0453^0, G0459^1, G0463^1, G0471^0, J0670^1, J2001^1
64448	01991^0, 01992^0, 01996^0, 0333T^0, 0464T^0, 0543T^0, 0544T^0, 0548T^0, 0567T^0, 0568T^0, 0569T^0, 0570T^0, 0571T^0, 0572T^0, 0573T^0, 0574T^0, 0580T^0, 0581T^0, 0582T^0, 20550^1, 20551^1, 20560^0, 20561^0, 20701^0, 36000^1, 36400^1, 36405^1, 36406^1, 36410^1, 36420^1, 36425^1, 36430^1, 36440^1, 36591^0, 36592^0, 36600^1, 51701^0, 51702^0, 51703^0, 66987^0, 66988^0, 69990^0, 76000^1, 76970^1, 76998^1, 77001^1, 77002^1, 92012^1, 92014^1, 92585^0, 93000^1, 93005^1, 93010^1, 93040^1, 93041^1, 93042^1, 93318^1, 93355^1, 94002^1, 94200^1, 94250^1, 94680^1, 94681^1, 94690^1, 94770^1, 95812^1, 95813^1, 95816^1, 95819^1, 95822^0, 95829^1, 95860^1, 95861^1, 95863^1, 95864^1, 95865^1, 95866^1, 95867^1, 95868^1, 95869^1, 95870^1, 95907^1, 95908^1, 95909^1, 95910^1, 95911^1, 95912^1, 95913^1, 95925^0, 95926^0, 95927^0, 95928^0, 95929^0, 95930^0, 95933^0, 95937^0, 95938^0, 95939^0, 95940^0, 95955^1, 96360^1, 96361^1, 96365^1, 96366^1, 96367^1, 96368^1, 96372^1, 96374^1, 96375^1, 96376^1,

0 = Modifier usage not allowed or inappropriate 1 = Modifier usage allowed

Code 1	Code 2
	96377[1], 96523[0], 99155[0], 99156[0], 99157[0], 99211[1], 99212[1], 99213[1], 99214[1], 99215[1], 99217[1], 99218[1], 99219[1], 99220[1], 99221[1], 99222[1], 99223[1], 99231[1], 99232[1], 99233[1], 99234[1], 99235[1], 99236[1], 99238[1], 99239[1], 99241[1], 99242[1], 99243[1], 99244[1], 99245[1], 99251[1], 99252[1], 99253[1], 99254[1], 99255[1], 99291[1], 99292[1], 99304[1], 99305[1], 99306[1], 99307[1], 99308[1], 99309[1], 99310[1], 99315[1], 99316[1], 99334[1], 99335[1], 99336[1], 99337[1], 99347[1], 99348[1], 99349[1], 99350[1], 99374[1], 99375[1], 99377[1], 99378[1], 99446[0], 99447[0], 99448[0], 99449[0], 99451[0], 99452[0], 99495[1], 99496[1], G0453[0], G0459[1], G0463[1], G0471[0], J2001[1]
64449	01991[0], 01992[0], 01996[0], 0333T[0], 0464T[0], 0543T[0], 0544T[0], 0548T[0], 0567T[0], 0568T[0], 0569T[0], 0570T[0], 0571T[0], 0572T[0], 0573T[0], 0574T[0], 0580T[0], 0581T[0], 0582T[0], 20550[1], 20551[1], 20560[0], 20561[0], 20701[0], 36000[1], 36400[1], 36405[1], 36406[1], 36410[1], 36420[1], 36425[1], 36430[1], 36440[1], 36591[0], 36592[0], 36600[1], 51701[0], 51702[0], 51703[0], 66987[0], 66988[0], 69990[0], 76000[1], 76800[1], 76970[1], 76998[1], 77001[1], 77002[1], 92012[1], 92014[1], 92585[0], 93000[1], 93005[1], 93010[1], 93040[1], 93041[1], 93042[1], 93318[1], 93355[1], 94002[1], 94200[1], 94250[1], 94680[1], 94681[1], 94690[1], 94770[1], 95812[1], 95813[1], 95816[1], 95819[1], 95822[0], 95829[1], 95860[1], 95861[1], 95863[1], 95864[1], 95865[1], 95866[1], 95867[1], 95868[1], 95869[1], 95870[1], 95907[1], 95908[1], 95909[1], 95910[1], 95911[1], 95912[1], 95913[1], 95925[0], 95926[0], 95927[0], 95928[0], 95929[0], 95930[0], 95933[0], 95937[0], 95938[0], 95939[0], 95940[0], 95955[1], 96360[1], 96361[1], 96365[1], 96366[1], 96367[1], 96368[1], 96372[1], 96374[1], 96375[1], 96376[1], 96377[1], 96523[0], 97033[1], 99155[0], 99156[0], 99157[0], 99211[1], 99212[1], 99213[1], 99214[1], 99215[1], 99217[1], 99218[1], 99219[1], 99220[1], 99221[1], 99222[1], 99223[1], 99231[1], 99232[1], 99233[1], 99234[1], 99235[1], 99236[1], 99238[1], 99239[1], 99241[1], 99242[1], 99243[1], 99244[1], 99245[1], 99251[1], 99252[1], 99253[1], 99254[1], 99255[1], 99291[1], 99292[1], 99304[1], 99305[1], 99306[1], 99307[1], 99308[1], 99309[1], 99310[1], 99315[1], 99316[1], 99334[1], 99335[1], 99336[1], 99337[1], 99347[1], 99348[1], 99349[1], 99350[1], 99374[1], 99375[1], 99377[1], 99378[1], 99446[0], 99447[0], 99448[0], 99449[0], 99451[0], 99452[0], 99495[1], 99496[1], G0453[0], G0459[1], G0463[1], G0471[0], J2001[1]
64450	01991[0], 01992[0], 0333T[0], 0464T[0], 20526[1], 20550[1], 20551[1], 29515[0], 29540[0], 29580[0], 36591[0], 36592[0], 51701[0], 51702[0], 64455[1], 69990[0], 76000[1], 76970[1], 76998[1], 77001[1], 77002[1], 92012[1], 92014[1], 92585[0], 93000[1], 93005[1], 93010[1], 93040[1], 93041[1], 93042[1], 93318[1], 93355[1], 94002[1], 94200[1], 94250[1], 94680[1], 94681[1], 94690[1], 94770[1], 95812[1], 95813[1], 95816[1], 95819[1], 95822[0], 95829[1], 95860[1], 95861[1], 95863[1], 95864[1], 95865[1], 95866[1], 95867[1], 95868[1], 95869[1], 95870[1], 95907[1], 95908[1], 95909[1], 95910[1], 95911[1], 95912[1], 95913[1], 95925[0], 95926[0], 95927[0], 95928[0], 95929[0], 95930[0], 95933[0], 95937[0], 95938[0], 95939[0], 95940[0], 95955[1], 96361[1], 96366[1], 96367[1], 96368[1], 96372[1], 96374[1], 96375[1], 96376[1], 96377[1], 96523[0], 99155[0], 99156[0], 99157[0], 99211[1], 99212[1], 99213[1], 99214[1], 99215[1], 99217[1], 99218[1], 99219[1], 99220[1], 99221[1], 99222[1], 99223[1], 99231[1], 99232[1], 99233[1], 99234[1], 99235[1], 99236[1], 99238[1], 99239[1], 99241[1], 99242[1], 99243[1], 99244[1], 99245[1], 99251[1], 99252[1], 99253[1], 99254[1], 99255[1], 99291[1], 99292[1], 99304[1], 99305[1], 99306[1], 99307[1], 99308[1], 99309[1], 99310[1], 99315[1], 99316[1], 99334[1], 99335[1], 99336[1], 99337[1], 99347[1], 99348[1], 99349[1], 99350[1], 99374[1], 99375[1], 99377[1], 99378[1], 99446[0], 99447[0], 99448[0], 99449[0], 99451[0], 99452[0], 99495[1], 99496[1], G0453[0], G0459[1], G0463[1], G0471[0], J0670[1], J2001[1]
64451	01991[0], 01992[0], 0213T[0], 0216T[0], 0228T[0], 0230T[0], 0333T[0], 0464T[0], 12001[1], 12002[1], 12004[1], 12011[1], 12013[1], 13102[1], 13122[1], 20526[1], 20550[1], 20551[1], 29515[0], 29540[0], 29580[0], 36000[1], 36400[1], 36405[1], 36406[1], 36410[1], 36420[1], 36425[1], 36430[1], 36440[1], 36591[0], 36592[0], 36600[1], 36640[1], 43752[1], 51701[1], 51702[1], 51703[1], 64400[0], 64405[0], 64408[0], 64415[0], 64416[0], 64417[0], 64418[0], 64420[0], 64421[0], 64425[0], 64430[0], 64435[0], 64446[0], 64447[0], 64448[0], 64449[0], 64455[1], 64462[0], 64480[0], 64484[0], 64486[0], 64487[0], 64491[0], 64492[0], 64505[0], 64510[0], 64520[0], 64530[0], 76000[1], 76380[1], 76800[1], 76970[1], 76998[1], 77001[1], 77002[1], 77003[1], 77012[1], 92012[1], 92014[1], 92585[0], 93000[1], 93005[1], 93010[1], 93040[1], 93041[1], 93042[1], 93318[1], 93355[1], 94200[1], 94250[1], 94680[1], 94681[1], 94690[1], 94770[1], 95812[1], 95816[1], 95819[1], 95822[1], 95860[1], 95861[1], 95863[1], 95864[1], 95865[1], 95866[1], 95867[1], 95868[1], 95869[1], 95870[1], 95873[1], 95874[1], 95907[1], 95908[1], 95909[1], 95910[1], 95911[1], 95912[1], 95913[1], 95925[0], 95926[0], 95927[0], 95928[0], 95929[0], 95930[0], 95933[0], 95937[0], 95938[0], 95939[0], 95940[0], 95955[1], 96360[1], 96361[1], 96365[1], 96366[1], 96367[1], 96368[1], 96372[1], 96374[1], 96375[1], 96376[1], 96377[1], 96523[0], 99157[0], 99211[1], 99212[1], 99213[1], 99214[1], 99215[1], 99217[1], 99218[1], 99219[1], 99220[1], 99221[1], 99222[1], 99223[1], 99231[1], 99232[1], 99233[1], 99234[1], 99235[1], 99236[1], 99238[1], 99239[1], 99241[1], 99242[1], 99243[1], 99244[1], 99245[1], 99251[1], 99252[1], 99253[1], 99254[1], 99255[1], 99291[1], 99292[1], 99304[1], 99305[1], 99306[1], 99307[1], 99308[1], 99309[1], 99310[1], 99315[1], 99316[1], 99334[1], 99335[1], 99336[1], 99337[1], 99347[1], 99348[1], 99349[1], 99350[1], 99374[1], 99375[1], 99377[1], 99378[1], 99446[0], 99447[0], 99448[0], 99449[0], 99451[0], 99452[0], 99495[1], 99496[1], G0453[0], G0459[1], G0463[1], G0471[0], J0670[1], J2001[1]
64479	01991[0], 01992[0], 0228T[0], 0229T[1], 0333T[0], 0464T[0], 0543T[0], 0544T[0], 0548T[0], 0567T[0], 0568T[0], 0569T[0], 0570T[0], 0571T[0], 0572T[0], 0573T[0], 0574T[0], 0580T[0], 0581T[0], 0582T[0], 20550[1], 20551[1], 20560[0], 20561[0], 20605[1], 20610[1], 20700[0], 20701[0], 36000[1], 36140[1], 36400[1], 36405[1], 36406[1], 36410[1], 36420[1], 36425[1], 36430[1], 36440[1], 36591[0], 36592[0], 36600[1], 51701[0], 51702[0], 51703[0], 62329[0], 64451[0], 66987[0], 66988[0], 69990[0], 72275[1], 76000[1], 76380[1], 76800[1], 76942[1], 76970[1], 76998[1], 77001[1], 77002[1], 77003[1], 77012[1], 92012[1], 92014[1], 92585[0], 93000[1], 93005[1], 93010[1], 93040[1], 93041[1], 93042[1], 93318[1], 93355[1], 94002[1], 94200[1], 94250[1], 94680[1], 94681[1], 94690[1], 94770[1], 95812[1], 95813[1], 95816[1], 95819[1], 95822[0], 95829[1], 95860[1], 95861[1], 95863[1], 95864[1], 95865[1], 95866[1], 95869[1], 95870[1], 95907[1], 95908[1], 95909[1], 95910[1], 95911[1], 95912[1], 95913[1], 95925[0], 95926[0], 95927[0], 95928[0], 95929[0], 95930[0], 95933[0], 95937[0], 95938[0], 95939[0], 95940[0], 95955[1], 96360[1], 96361[1], 96365[1], 96366[1], 96367[1], 96368[1], 96372[1], 96374[1], 96375[1], 96376[1], 96377[1], 96523[0], 99155[0], 99156[0], 99157[0], 99211[1], 99212[1], 99213[1], 99214[1], 99215[1], 99217[1], 99218[1], 99219[1], 99220[1], 99221[1], 99222[1], 99223[1], 99231[1], 99232[1], 99233[1], 99234[1], 99235[1], 99236[1], 99238[1], 99239[1], 99241[1], 99242[1], 99243[1], 99244[1], 99245[1], 99251[1], 99252[1], 99253[1], 99254[1], 99255[1], 99291[1], 99292[1], 99304[1], 99305[1], 99306[1], 99307[1], 99308[1], 99309[1], 99310[1], 99315[1], 99316[1], 99334[1], 99335[1], 99336[1], 99337[1], 99347[1], 99348[1], 99349[1], 99350[1], 99374[1], 99375[1], 99377[1], 99378[1], 99446[0], 99447[0], 99448[0], 99449[0], 99451[0], 99452[0], 99495[1], 99496[1], G0453[0], G0459[1], G0463[1], G0471[0], J2001[1]
64480	01991[0], 01992[0], 0229T[0], 0333T[0], 0464T[0], 0543T[0], 0544T[0], 0548T[0], 0567T[0], 0568T[0], 0569T[0], 0570T[0], 0571T[0], 0572T[0], 0573T[0], 0574T[0], 0580T[0], 0581T[0], 0582T[0], 20560[0], 20561[0], 20701[0], 36591[0], 36592[0], 66987[0], 66988[0], 69990[0], 76000[1], 76380[1], 76800[1], 76942[1], 76970[1], 76998[1], 77002[1], 77003[1], 77012[1], 92585[0], 93000[1], 93005[1], 93010[1], 93040[1], 93041[1], 93042[1], 95822[0], 95860[1], 95861[1], 95863[1], 95864[1], 95865[1], 95866[1], 95869[1], 95907[1], 95908[1], 95909[1], 95910[1], 95911[1], 95912[1], 95913[1], 95925[0], 95926[0], 95927[0], 95930[0], 95933[0], 95937[0], 95938[0], 95939[0], 95940[0], 96523[0], G0453[0], G0459[1]
64483	01991[0], 01992[0], 0230T[0], 0231T[1], 0333T[0], 0464T[0], 0543T[0], 0544T[0], 0548T[0], 0567T[0], 0568T[0], 0569T[0], 0570T[0], 0571T[0], 0572T[0], 0573T[0], 0574T[0], 0580T[0], 0581T[0], 0582T[0], 20550[1], 20551[1], 20560[0], 20561[0], 20605[1], 20610[1], 20700[0], 20701[0], 36000[1], 36140[1], 36400[1], 36405[1], 36406[1], 36410[1], 36420[1], 36425[1], 36430[1], 36440[1], 36591[0], 36592[0], 36600[1], 51701[0], 51702[0], 51703[0], 64451[0], 66987[0], 66988[0], 72275[1], 76000[1], 76380[1], 76800[1], 76942[1], 76970[1], 76998[1], 77001[1], 77002[1], 77003[1], 77012[1], 92012[1], 92014[1], 92585[0], 93000[1], 93005[1], 93010[1], 93040[1], 93041[1], 93042[1], 93318[1], 93355[1], 94002[1], 94200[1], 94250[1], 94680[1], 94681[1], 94690[1], 94770[1], 95812[1], 95813[1], 95816[1], 95819[1], 95822[0], 95829[1], 95860[1], 95861[1], 95863[1], 95864[1], 95865[1], 95866[1], 95869[1], 95870[1], 95907[1], 95908[1], 95909[1], 95910[1], 95911[1], 95912[1], 95913[1], 95925[0], 95926[0], 95927[0], 95928[0], 95929[0], 95930[0], 95933[0], 95937[0], 95938[0], 95939[0], 95940[0], 95955[1], 96360[1], 96361[1], 96365[1], 96366[1], 96367[1], 96368[1], 96372[1], 96374[1], 96375[1], 96376[1], 96377[1], 96523[0], 99155[0], 99156[0], 99157[0], 99211[1], 99212[1], 99213[1], 99214[1], 99215[1], 99217[1], 99218[1], 99219[1], 99220[1], 99221[1], 99222[1], 99223[1], 99231[1], 99232[1], 99233[1], 99234[1], 99235[1], 99236[1], 99238[1], 99239[1], 99241[1], 99242[1], 99243[1], 99244[1], 99245[1], 99251[1], 99252[1], 99253[1], 99254[1], 99255[1], 99291[1], 99292[1], 99304[1], 99305[1], 99306[1], 99307[1], 99308[1], 99309[1], 99310[1], 99315[1], 99316[1], 99334[1], 99335[1], 99336[1], 99337[1], 99347[1], 99348[1], 99349[1], 99350[1], 99374[1], 99375[1], 99377[1], 99378[1], 99446[0], 99447[0], 99448[0], 99449[0], 99451[0], 99452[0], 99495[1], 99496[1], G0453[0], G0459[1], G0463[1], G0471[0], J2001[1]
64484	01991[0], 01992[0], 0231T[0], 0333T[0], 0464T[0], 0543T[0], 0544T[0], 0548T[0], 0567T[0], 0568T[0], 0569T[0], 0570T[0], 0571T[0], 0572T[0], 0573T[0], 0574T[0], 0580T[0], 0581T[0], 0582T[0], 20560[0], 20561[0], 36591[0], 36592[0], 66987[0], 66988[0], 76000[1], 76380[1], 76800[1], 76942[1], 76970[1], 76998[1], 77002[1], 77003[1], 77012[1], 92585[0], 93000[1], 93005[1], 93010[1], 93040[1], 93041[1], 93042[1], 95822[0], 95860[1], 95861[1], 95863[1], 95864[1], 95865[1], 95866[1], 95869[1], 95907[1], 95908[1], 95909[1], 95910[1], 95911[1], 95912[1], 95913[1], 95925[0], 95926[0], 95927[0], 95930[0], 95933[0], 95937[0], 95938[0], 95939[0], 95940[0], 96523[0], G0453[0], G0459[1]
64490	01991[0], 01992[0], 0213T[0], 0214T[0], 0215T[0], 0216T[0], 0217T[0], 0218T[0], 0333T[0], 0464T[0], 0543T[0], 0544T[0], 0548T[0], 0567T[0], 0568T[0], 0569T[0], 0570T[0], 0571T[0], 0572T[0], 0573T[0], 0574T[0], 0580T[0], 0581T[0], 0582T[0], 20550[1], 20551[1], 20560[0], 20561[0], 20600[1], 20605[1], 20610[1], 20700[0], 20701[0], 36140[1], 36410[1], 36591[0], 36592[0], 51701[1], 51702[1], 51703[1], 64451[0], 66987[0], 66988[0], 69990[0], 72275[1], 76000[1], 76380[1], 76800[1], 76942[1], 76970[1], 76998[1], 77001[1], 77002[1], 77003[1], 77012[1], 77021[1], 92012[1], 92014[1], 92585[0], 93000[1], 93005[1], 93010[1], 93040[1], 93041[1], 93042[1], 93318[1], 93355[1], 94002[1], 94200[1], 94250[1], 94680[1], 94681[1], 94690[1], 94770[1], 95812[1], 95813[1], 95816[1], 95819[1], 95822[0], 95829[1], 95860[1], 95861[1], 95863[1], 95864[1], 95865[1], 95866[1], 95867[1], 95868[1], 95869[1], 95870[1], 95907[1], 95908[1], 95909[1], 95910[1], 95911[1], 95912[1], 95913[1], 95925[0], 95926[0], 95927[0], 95928[0], 95929[0], 95930[0], 95933[0], 95937[0], 95938[0], 95939[0], 95940[0], 95955[1], 96360[1], 96361[1], 96365[1], 96366[1], 96367[1], 96368[1], 96372[1], 96374[1], 96375[1], 96376[1], 96377[1],

0 = Modifier usage not allowed or inappropriate 1 = Modifier usage allowed

Code 1	Code 2
	96523[0], 99155[0], 99156[0], 99157[0], 99211[1], 99212[1], 99213[1], 99214[1], 99215[1], 99217[1], 99218[1], 99219[1], 99220[1], 99221[1], 99222[1], 99223[1], 99231[1], 99232[1], 99233[1], 99234[1], 99235[1], 99236[1], 99238[1], 99239[1], 99241[1], 99242[1], 99243[1], 99244[1], 99245[1], 99251[1], 99252[1], 99253[1], 99254[1], 99255[1], 99291[1], 99292[1], 99304[1], 99305[1], 99306[1], 99307[1], 99308[1], 99309[1], 99310[1], 99315[1], 99316[1], 99334[1], 99335[1], 99336[1], 99337[1], 99347[1], 99348[1], 99349[1], 99350[1], 99374[1], 99375[1], 99377[1], 99378[1], 99446[0], 99447[0], 99448[0], 99449[0], 99451[0], 99452[0], 99495[1], 99496[1], G0453[0], G0459[1], G0463[1], G0471[1], J0670[1], J2001[1]
64491	0213T[0], 0214T[0], 0215T[0], 0216T[0], 0217T[0], 0218T[0], 0333T[0], 0464T[0], 0543T[0], 0544T[0], 0548T[0], 0567T[0], 0568T[0], 0569T[0], 0570T[0], 0571T[0], 0572T[0], 0573T[0], 0574T[0], 0580T[0], 0581T[0], 0582T[0], 20560[0], 20561[0], 20701[0], 36591[0], 36592[0], 51701[1], 51702[1], 51703[1], 66987[0], 66988[0], 69990[0], 76000[1], 76380[1], 76800[1], 76942[1], 76970[1], 76998[1], 77001[1], 77002[1], 77003[1], 77012[1], 77021[1], 92585[0], 95822[0], 95860[1], 95861[1], 95863[1], 95864[1], 95865[1], 95866[1], 95867[1], 95868[1], 95869[1], 95870[1], 95907[1], 95908[1], 95909[1], 95910[1], 95911[1], 95912[1], 95913[1], 95925[0], 95926[0], 95927[0], 95928[0], 95929[0], 95930[0], 95933[0], 95937[0], 95938[0], 95939[0], 95940[0], 96523[0], G0453[0], G0471[1], J0670[1], J2001[1]
64492	0213T[0], 0214T[0], 0215T[0], 0216T[0], 0217T[0], 0218T[0], 0333T[0], 0464T[0], 0543T[0], 0544T[0], 0548T[0], 0567T[0], 0568T[0], 0569T[0], 0570T[0], 0571T[0], 0572T[0], 0573T[0], 0574T[0], 0580T[0], 0581T[0], 0582T[0], 20560[0], 20561[0], 20701[0], 36591[0], 36592[0], 51701[1], 51702[1], 51703[1], 66987[0], 66988[0], 69990[0], 76000[1], 76380[1], 76800[1], 76942[1], 76970[1], 76998[1], 77001[1], 77002[1], 77003[1], 77012[1], 77021[1], 92585[0], 95822[0], 95860[1], 95861[1], 95863[1], 95864[1], 95865[1], 95866[1], 95867[1], 95868[1], 95869[1], 95870[1], 95907[1], 95908[1], 95909[1], 95910[1], 95911[1], 95912[1], 95913[1], 95925[0], 95926[0], 95927[0], 95928[0], 95929[0], 95930[0], 95933[0], 95937[0], 95938[0], 95939[0], 95940[0], 96523[0], G0453[0], G0471[1], J0670[1], J2001[1]
64493	01991[0], 01992[0], 0213T[0], 0214T[0], 0215T[0], 0216T[0], 0217T[0], 0218T[0], 0333T[0], 0464T[0], 0543T[0], 0544T[0], 0548T[0], 0567T[0], 0568T[0], 0569T[0], 0570T[0], 0571T[0], 0572T[0], 0573T[0], 0574T[0], 0580T[0], 0581T[0], 0582T[0], 20550[1], 20551[1], 20560[0], 20561[0], 20600[1], 20605[1], 20610[1], 20700[0], 20701[0], 36140[1], 36591[0], 36592[0], 51701[1], 51702[1], 51703[1], 66987[0], 66988[0], 69990[0], 72275[1], 76000[1], 76380[1], 76800[1], 76942[1], 76970[1], 76998[1], 77001[1], 77002[1], 77003[1], 77012[1], 77021[1], 92012[1], 92014[1], 92585[0], 93000[1], 93005[1], 93010[1], 93040[1], 93041[1], 93042[1], 93318[1], 93355[1], 94002[1], 94200[1], 94250[1], 94680[1], 94681[1], 94690[1], 94770[1], 95812[1], 95813[1], 95816[1], 95819[1], 95822[0], 95829[1], 95860[1], 95861[1], 95863[1], 95864[1], 95865[1], 95866[1], 95867[1], 95868[1], 95869[1], 95870[1], 95907[1], 95908[1], 95909[1], 95910[1], 95911[1], 95912[1], 95913[1], 95925[0], 95926[0], 95927[0], 95928[0], 95929[0], 95930[0], 95933[0], 95937[0], 95938[0], 95939[0], 95940[0], 95955[1], 96360[1], 96361[1], 96365[1], 96366[1], 96367[1], 96368[1], 96372[1], 96374[1], 96375[1], 96376[1], 96377[1], 96523[0], 99155[0], 99156[0], 99157[0], 99211[1], 99212[1], 99213[1], 99214[1], 99215[1], 99217[1], 99218[1], 99219[1], 99220[1], 99221[1], 99222[1], 99223[1], 99231[1], 99232[1], 99233[1], 99234[1], 99235[1], 99236[1], 99238[1], 99239[1], 99241[1], 99242[1], 99243[1], 99244[1], 99245[1], 99251[1], 99252[1], 99253[1], 99254[1], 99255[1], 99291[1], 99292[1], 99304[1], 99305[1], 99306[1], 99307[1], 99308[1], 99309[1], 99310[1], 99315[1], 99316[1], 99334[1], 99335[1], 99336[1], 99337[1], 99347[1], 99348[1], 99349[1], 99350[1], 99374[1], 99375[1], 99377[1], 99378[1], 99446[0], 99447[0], 99448[0], 99449[0], 99451[0], 99452[0], 99495[1], 99496[1], G0453[0], G0459[1], G0463[1], G0471[1], J0670[1], J2001[1]
64494	0213T[0], 0214T[0], 0215T[0], 0216T[0], 0217T[0], 0218T[0], 0333T[0], 0464T[0], 0543T[0], 0544T[0], 0548T[0], 0567T[0], 0568T[0], 0569T[0], 0570T[0], 0571T[0], 0572T[0], 0573T[0], 0574T[0], 0580T[0], 0581T[0], 0582T[0], 20560[0], 20561[0], 36591[0], 36592[0], 51701[1], 51702[1], 51703[1], 66987[0], 66988[0], 69990[0], 76000[1], 76380[1], 76800[1], 76942[1], 76970[1], 76998[1], 77001[1], 77002[1], 77003[1], 77012[1], 77021[1], 92585[0], 95822[0], 95860[1], 95861[1], 95863[1], 95864[1], 95865[1], 95866[1], 95867[1], 95868[1], 95869[1], 95870[1], 95907[1], 95908[1], 95909[1], 95910[1], 95911[1], 95912[1], 95913[1], 95925[0], 95926[0], 95927[0], 95928[0], 95929[0], 95930[0], 95933[0], 95937[0], 95938[0], 95939[0], 95940[0], 96523[0], G0453[0], G0471[1], J0670[1], J2001[1]
64495	0213T[0], 0214T[0], 0215T[0], 0216T[0], 0217T[0], 0218T[0], 0333T[0], 0464T[0], 0543T[0], 0544T[0], 0548T[0], 0567T[0], 0568T[0], 0569T[0], 0570T[0], 0571T[0], 0572T[0], 0573T[0], 0574T[0], 0580T[0], 0581T[0], 0582T[0], 20560[0], 20561[0], 36591[0], 36592[0], 51701[1], 51702[1], 51703[1], 66987[0], 66988[0], 69990[0], 76000[1], 76380[1], 76800[1], 76942[1], 76970[1], 76998[1], 77001[1], 77002[1], 77003[1], 77012[1], 77021[1], 92585[0], 95822[0], 95860[1], 95861[1], 95863[1], 95864[1], 95865[1], 95866[1], 95867[1], 95868[1], 95869[1], 95870[1], 95907[1], 95908[1], 95909[1], 95910[1], 95911[1], 95912[1], 95913[1], 95925[0], 95926[0], 95927[0], 95928[0], 95929[0], 95930[0], 95933[0], 95937[0], 95938[0], 95939[0], 95940[0], 96523[0], G0453[0], G0471[1], J0670[1], J2001[1]
64505	01991[0], 01992[0], 0333T[0], 0464T[0], 0543T[0], 0544T[0], 0548T[0], 0567T[0], 0568T[0], 0569T[0], 0570T[0], 0571T[0], 0572T[0], 0573T[0], 0574T[0], 0580T[0], 0581T[0], 0582T[0], 20560[0], 20561[0], 20701[0], 36000[1], 36400[1], 36405[1], 36406[1], 36410[1], 36420[1], 36425[1], 36430[1], 36440[1], 36591[0], 36592[0], 36600[1], 51701[0], 51702[0], 51703[0], 66987[0], 66988[0], 69990[0], 76000[1], 76970[1], 76998[1], 77001[1], 92012[1], 92014[1], 92585[0], 93000[1], 93005[1], 93010[1], 93040[1], 93041[1], 93042[1], 93318[1], 93355[1], 94002[1], 94200[1], 94250[1], 94680[1], 94681[1], 94690[1], 94770[1], 95812[1], 95813[1], 95816[1], 95819[1], 95822[0], 95829[1], 95860[1], 95861[1], 95863[1], 95864[1], 95865[1], 95866[1], 95867[1], 95868[1], 95869[1], 95870[1], 95907[1], 95908[1], 95909[1], 95910[1], 95911[1], 95912[1], 95913[1], 95925[0], 95926[0], 95927[0], 95928[0], 95929[0], 95930[0], 95933[0], 95937[0], 95938[0], 95939[0], 95940[0], 95955[1], 96360[1], 96361[1], 96365[1], 96366[1], 96367[1], 96368[1], 96372[1], 96374[1], 96375[1], 96376[1], 96377[1], 96523[0], 99155[0], 99156[0], 99157[0], 99211[1], 99212[1], 99213[1], 99214[1], 99215[1], 99217[1], 99218[1], 99219[1], 99220[1], 99221[1], 99222[1], 99223[1], 99231[1], 99232[1], 99233[1], 99234[1], 99235[1], 99236[1], 99238[1], 99239[1], 99241[1], 99242[1], 99243[1], 99244[1], 99245[1], 99251[1], 99252[1], 99253[1], 99254[1], 99255[1], 99291[1], 99292[1], 99304[1], 99305[1], 99306[1], 99307[1], 99308[1], 99309[1], 99310[1], 99315[1], 99316[1], 99334[1], 99335[1], 99336[1], 99337[1], 99347[1], 99348[1], 99349[1], 99350[1], 99374[1], 99375[1], 99377[1], 99378[1], 99446[0], 99447[0], 99448[0], 99449[0], 99451[0], 99452[0], 99495[1], 99496[1], G0453[0], G0459[1], G0463[1], G0471[0], J0670[1], J2001[1]
64520	01991[0], 01992[0], 0333T[0], 0464T[0], 0543T[0], 0544T[0], 0548T[0], 0567T[0], 0568T[0], 0569T[0], 0570T[0], 0571T[0], 0572T[0], 0573T[0], 0574T[0], 0580T[0], 0581T[0], 0582T[0], 20560[0], 20561[0], 20701[0], 36000[1], 36400[1], 36405[1], 36406[1], 36410[1], 36420[1], 36425[1], 36430[1], 36440[1], 36591[0], 36592[0], 36600[1], 51701[0], 51702[0], 51703[0], 66987[0], 66988[0], 69990[0], 76000[1], 76800[1], 76970[1], 76998[1], 77001[1], 77002[1], 92012[1], 92014[1], 92585[0], 93000[1], 93005[1], 93010[1], 93040[1], 93041[1], 93042[1], 93318[1], 93355[1], 94002[1], 94200[1], 94250[1], 94680[1], 94681[1], 94690[1], 94770[1], 95812[1], 95813[1], 95816[1], 95819[1], 95822[0], 95829[1], 95860[1], 95861[1], 95863[1], 95864[1], 95865[1], 95866[1], 95867[1], 95868[1], 95869[1], 95870[1], 95907[1], 95908[1], 95909[1], 95910[1], 95911[1], 95912[1], 95913[1], 95925[0], 95926[0], 95927[0], 95928[0], 95929[0], 95930[0], 95933[0], 95937[0], 95938[0], 95939[0], 95940[0], 95955[1], 96360[1], 96361[1], 96365[1], 96366[1], 96367[1], 96368[1], 96372[1], 96374[1], 96375[1], 96376[1], 96377[1], 96523[0], 99155[0], 99156[0], 99157[0], 99211[1], 99212[1], 99213[1], 99214[1], 99215[1], 99217[1], 99218[1], 99219[1], 99220[1], 99221[1], 99222[1], 99223[1], 99231[1], 99232[1], 99233[1], 99234[1], 99235[1], 99236[1], 99238[1], 99239[1], 99241[1], 99242[1], 99243[1], 99244[1], 99245[1], 99251[1], 99252[1], 99253[1], 99254[1], 99255[1], 99291[1], 99292[1], 99304[1], 99305[1], 99306[1], 99307[1], 99308[1], 99309[1], 99310[1], 99315[1], 99316[1], 99334[1], 99335[1], 99336[1], 99337[1], 99347[1], 99348[1], 99349[1], 99350[1], 99374[1], 99375[1], 99377[1], 99378[1], 99446[0], 99447[0], 99448[0], 99449[0], 99451[0], 99452[0], 99495[1], 99496[1], G0453[0], G0459[1], G0463[1], G0471[0], J0670[1], J2001[1]
64553	0213T[0], 0216T[0], 0228T[0], 0230T[0], 0333T[0], 0464T[0], 0589T[0], 0590T[0], 12001[1], 12002[1], 12004[1], 12005[1], 12006[1], 12007[1], 12011[1], 12013[1], 12014[1], 12015[1], 12016[1], 12017[1], 12018[1], 12020[1], 12021[1], 12031[1], 12032[1], 12034[1], 12035[1], 12036[1], 12037[1], 12041[1], 12042[1], 12044[1], 12045[1], 12046[1], 12047[1], 12051[1], 12052[1], 12053[1], 12054[1], 12055[1], 12056[1], 12057[1], 13100[1], 13101[1], 13102[1], 13120[1], 13121[1], 13122[1], 13131[1], 13132[1], 13133[1], 13151[1], 13152[1], 13153[1], 36000[1], 36400[1], 36405[1], 36406[1], 36410[1], 36420[1], 36425[1], 36430[1], 36440[1], 36591[0], 36592[0], 36600[1], 36640[1], 43752[1], 51701[1], 51702[1], 51703[1], 61850[0], 61860[0], 61870[0], 61880[0], 62320[0], 62321[0], 62322[0], 62323[0], 62324[0], 62325[0], 62326[0], 62327[0], 63685[1], 64400[0], 64405[0], 64408[0], 64415[0], 64416[0], 64417[0], 64418[0], 64420[0], 64421[0], 64425[0], 64430[0], 64435[0], 64445[0], 64446[0], 64447[0], 64448[0], 64449[0], 64450[0], 64451[0], 64454[0], 64461[0], 64462[0], 64463[0], 64479[0], 64480[0], 64483[0], 64484[0], 64486[0], 64487[0], 64488[0], 64489[0], 64490[0], 64491[0], 64492[0], 64493[0], 64494[0], 64495[0], 64505[0], 64510[0], 64517[0], 64520[0], 64530[0], 64561[1], 64575[0], 64580[0], 64581[1], 69990[0], 92012[1], 92014[1], 92585[0], 93000[1], 93005[1], 93010[1], 93040[1], 93041[1], 93042[1], 93318[1], 93355[1], 94002[1], 94200[1], 94250[1], 94680[1], 94681[1], 94690[1], 94770[1], 95812[1], 95813[1], 95816[1], 95819[1], 95822[0], 95829[1], 95860[0], 95861[0], 95863[0], 95864[0], 95865[0], 95866[0], 95867[0], 95868[0], 95869[0], 95870[0], 95907[0], 95908[0], 95909[0], 95910[0], 95911[0], 95912[0], 95913[0], 95925[0], 95926[0], 95927[0], 95928[0], 95929[0], 95930[0], 95933[0], 95937[0], 95938[0], 95939[0], 95940[0], 95955[1], 95970[1], 95976[1], 95977[1], 96360[1], 96361[1], 96365[1], 96366[1], 96367[1], 96368[1], 96372[1], 96374[1], 96375[1], 96376[1], 96377[1], 96523[0], 99155[0], 99156[0], 99157[0], 99211[1], 99212[1], 99213[1], 99214[1], 99215[1], 99217[1], 99218[1], 99219[1], 99220[1], 99221[1], 99222[1], 99223[1], 99231[1], 99232[1], 99233[1], 99234[1], 99235[1], 99236[1], 99238[1], 99239[1], 99241[1], 99242[1], 99243[1], 99244[1], 99245[1], 99251[1], 99252[1], 99253[1], 99254[1], 99255[1], 99291[1], 99292[1], 99304[1], 99305[1], 99306[1], 99307[1], 99308[1], 99309[1], 99310[1], 99315[1], 99316[1], 99334[1], 99335[1], 99336[1], 99337[1], 99347[1], 99348[1], 99349[1], 99350[1], 99374[1], 99375[1], 99377[1], 99378[1], 99446[0], 99447[0], 99448[0], 99449[0], 99451[0], 99452[0], 99495[0], 99496[0], G0453[0], G0463[1], G0471[1]
64555	0213T[0], 0216T[0], 0228T[0], 0230T[0], 0333T[0], 0464T[0], 0587T[0], 0588T[0], 0589T[0], 0590T[0], 12001[1], 12002[1], 12004[1], 12005[1], 12006[1], 12007[1], 12011[1], 12013[1], 12014[1], 12015[1], 12016[1], 12017[1], 12018[1], 12020[1], 12021[1], 12031[1], 12032[1], 12034[1], 12035[1], 12036[1], 12037[1], 12041[1], 12042[1], 12044[1], 12045[1], 12046[1], 12047[1], 12051[1], 12052[1], 12053[1], 12054[1], 12055[1], 12056[1], 12057[1], 13100[1], 13101[1], 13102[1], 13120[1], 13121[1], 13122[1], 13131[1], 13132[1], 13133[1], 13151[1], 13152[1], 13153[1], 36000[1], 36400[1], 36405[1], 36406[1], 36410[1], 36420[1], 36425[1], 36430[1], 36440[1], 36591[0], 36592[0], 36600[1], 36640[1], 43752[1], 51701[1], 51702[1], 51703[1], 61850[0], 61860[0], 61870[0], 61880[0], 61885[0], 61886[0], 62320[0],

Appendix A: NCCI - CPT Codes

Code 1	Code 2
	62321[0], 62322[0], 62323[0], 62324[0], 62325[0], 62326[0], 62327[0], 64400[0], 64405[0], 64408[0], 64415[0], 64416[0], 64417[0], 64418[0], 64420[0], 64421[0], 64425[0], 64430[0], 64435[0], 64445[0], 64446[0], 64447[0], 64448[0], 64449[0], 64450[0], 64451[0], 64454[0], 64461[0], 64462[0], 64463[0], 64479[0], 64480[0], 64483[0], 64484[0], 64486[0], 64487[0], 64488[0], 64489[0], 64490[0], 64491[0], 64492[0], 64493[0], 64494[0], 64495[0], 64505[0], 64510[0], 64517[0], 64520[0], 64530[0], 64553[1], 64561[1], 64566[1], 64575[1], 64580[0], 64581[0], 69990[0], 76000[1], 77001[1], 77002[1], 92012[1], 92014[1], 92585[0], 93000[1], 93005[1], 93010[1], 93040[1], 93041[1], 93042[1], 93318[1], 93355[1], 94002[1], 94200[1], 94250[1], 94680[1], 94681[1], 94690[1], 94770[1], 95812[1], 95813[1], 95816[1], 95819[1], 95822[0], 95829[1], 95860[0], 95861[0], 95863[0], 95864[0], 95865[0], 95866[0], 95867[0], 95868[0], 95869[0], 95870[0], 95907[0], 95908[0], 95909[0], 95910[0], 95911[0], 95912[0], 95913[0], 95925[0], 95926[0], 95927[0], 95928[0], 95929[0], 95930[0], 95933[0], 95937[0], 95938[0], 95939[0], 95940[0], 95955[1], 95970[1], 95971[1], 95972[1], 96360[1], 96361[1], 96365[1], 96366[1], 96367[1], 96368[1], 96372[1], 96374[1], 96375[1], 96376[1], 96377[1], 96523[0], 99155[0], 99156[0], 99157[0], 99211[1], 99212[1], 99213[1], 99214[1], 99215[1], 99217[1], 99218[1], 99219[1], 99220[1], 99221[1], 99222[1], 99223[1], 99231[1], 99232[1], 99233[1], 99234[1], 99235[1], 99236[1], 99238[1], 99239[1], 99241[1], 99242[1], 99243[1], 99244[1], 99245[1], 99251[1], 99252[1], 99253[1], 99254[1], 99255[1], 99291[1], 99292[1], 99304[1], 99305[1], 99306[1], 99307[1], 99308[1], 99309[1], 99310[1], 99315[1], 99316[1], 99334[1], 99335[1], 99336[1], 99337[1], 99347[1], 99348[1], 99349[1], 99350[1], 99374[1], 99375[1], 99377[1], 99378[1], 99446[0], 99447[0], 99448[0], 99449[0], 99451[0], 99452[0], 99495[0], 99496[0], G0453[0], G0463[1], G0471[1]
64566	0333T[0], 0464T[0], 0588T[1], 0589T[0], 0590T[0], 12001[1], 12002[1], 12004[1], 12005[1], 12006[1], 12007[1], 12011[1], 12013[1], 12014[1], 12015[1], 12016[1], 12017[1], 12018[1], 12020[1], 12021[1], 12031[1], 12032[1], 12034[1], 12035[1], 12036[1], 12037[1], 12041[1], 12042[1], 12044[1], 12045[1], 12046[1], 12047[1], 12051[1], 12052[1], 12053[1], 12054[1], 12055[1], 12056[1], 12057[1], 13100[1], 13101[1], 13102[1], 13120[1], 13121[1], 13122[1], 13131[1], 13132[1], 13133[1], 13151[1], 13152[1], 13153[1], 36000[1], 36400[1], 36405[1], 36406[1], 36410[1], 36420[1], 36425[1], 36430[1], 36440[1], 36591[0], 36592[0], 36600[1], 36640[1], 43752[1], 51701[1], 51702[1], 51703[1], 62320[0], 62321[0], 62322[0], 62323[0], 62324[0], 62325[0], 62326[0], 62327[0], 64400[0], 64405[0], 64408[0], 64415[0], 64416[0], 64417[0], 64418[0], 64420[0], 64421[0], 64425[0], 64430[0], 64435[0], 64445[0], 64446[0], 64447[0], 64448[0], 64449[0], 64450[0], 64451[0], 64454[0], 64461[0], 64462[0], 64463[0], 64479[0], 64480[0], 64483[0], 64484[0], 64486[0], 64487[0], 64488[0], 64489[0], 64490[0], 64491[0], 64492[0], 64493[0], 64494[0], 64495[0], 64505[0], 64510[0], 64517[0], 64520[0], 64530[0], 64585[1], 69990[0], 76000[1], 76942[1], 76970[1], 76998[1], 77002[1], 92012[1], 92014[1], 92585[0], 93000[1], 93005[1], 93010[1], 93040[1], 93041[1], 93042[1], 93318[1], 93355[1], 94002[1], 94200[1], 94250[1], 94680[1], 94681[1], 94690[1], 94770[1], 95812[1], 95813[1], 95816[1], 95819[1], 95822[0], 95829[1], 95860[0], 95861[0], 95863[0], 95864[0], 95865[0], 95866[0], 95867[0], 95868[0], 95869[0], 95870[0], 95907[0], 95908[0], 95909[0], 95910[0], 95911[0], 95912[0], 95913[0], 95925[0], 95926[0], 95927[0], 95928[0], 95929[0], 95930[0], 95933[0], 95937[0], 95938[0], 95939[0], 95940[0], 95955[1], 95970[1], 95971[1], 95972[1], 96360[1], 96361[1], 96365[1], 96366[1], 96367[1], 96368[1], 96372[1], 96374[1], 96375[1], 96376[1], 96377[1], 96523[0], 99155[0], 99156[0], 99157[0], 99211[1], 99212[1], 99213[1], 99214[1], 99215[1], 99217[1], 99218[1], 99219[1], 99220[1], 99221[1], 99222[1], 99223[1], 99231[1], 99232[1], 99233[1], 99234[1], 99235[1], 99236[1], 99238[1], 99239[1], 99241[1], 99242[1], 99243[1], 99244[1], 99245[1], 99251[1], 99252[1], 99253[1], 99254[1], 99255[1], 99291[1], 99292[1], 99304[1], 99305[1], 99306[1], 99307[1], 99308[1], 99309[1], 99310[1], 99315[1], 99316[1], 99334[1], 99335[1], 99336[1], 99337[1], 99347[1], 99348[1], 99349[1], 99350[1], 99374[1], 99375[1], 99377[1], 99378[1], 99446[0], 99447[0], 99448[0], 99449[0], 99451[0], 99452[0], 99495[1], 99496[1], G0453[0], G0463[1], G0471[1], J0670[1], J2001[1]
64568	0333T[0], 0464T[0], 0589T[0], 0590T[0], 12001[1], 12002[1], 12004[1], 12005[1], 12006[1], 12007[1], 12011[1], 12013[1], 12014[1], 12015[1], 12016[1], 12017[1], 12018[1], 12020[1], 12021[1], 12031[1], 12032[1], 12034[1], 12035[1], 12036[1], 12037[1], 12041[1], 12042[1], 12044[1], 12045[1], 12046[1], 12047[1], 12051[1], 12052[1], 12053[1], 12054[1], 12055[1], 12056[1], 12057[1], 13100[1], 13101[1], 13102[1], 13120[1], 13121[1], 13122[1], 13131[1], 13132[1], 13133[1], 13151[1], 13152[1], 13153[1], 36000[1], 36400[1], 36405[1], 36406[1], 36410[1], 36420[1], 36425[1], 36430[1], 36440[1], 36591[0], 36592[0], 36600[1], 36640[1], 43752[1], 51701[1], 51702[1], 51703[1], 61885[1], 61888[1], 62320[0], 62321[0], 62322[0], 62323[0], 62324[0], 62325[0], 62326[0], 62327[0], 64400[0], 64405[0], 64408[0], 64415[0], 64416[0], 64417[0], 64418[0], 64420[0], 64421[0], 64425[0], 64430[0], 64435[0], 64445[0], 64446[0], 64447[0], 64448[0], 64449[0], 64450[0], 64451[0], 64454[0], 64461[0], 64462[0], 64463[0], 64479[0], 64480[0], 64483[0], 64484[0], 64486[0], 64487[0], 64488[0], 64489[0], 64490[0], 64491[0], 64492[0], 64493[0], 64494[0], 64495[0], 64505[0], 64510[0], 64517[0], 64520[0], 64530[0], 69990[0], 92012[1], 92014[1], 92585[0], 93000[1], 93005[1], 93010[1], 93040[1], 93041[1], 93042[1], 93318[1], 93355[1], 94002[1], 94200[1], 94250[1], 94680[1], 94681[1], 94690[1], 94770[1], 95812[1], 95813[1], 95816[1], 95819[1], 95822[0], 95829[1], 95860[0], 95861[0], 95863[0], 95864[0], 95865[0], 95866[0], 95867[0], 95868[0], 95869[0], 95870[0], 95907[0], 95908[0], 95909[0], 95910[0], 95911[0], 95912[0], 95913[0], 95925[0], 95926[0], 95927[0], 95928[0], 95929[0], 95930[0], 95933[0], 95937[0], 95938[0], 95939[0], 95940[0], 95955[1], 95970[1], 95971[1], 95972[1], 95976[1], 95977[1], 96360[1], 96361[1], 96365[1], 96366[1], 96367[1], 96368[1], 96372[1], 96374[1], 96375[1], 96376[1], 96377[1], 96523[0], 99155[0], 99156[0], 99157[0], 99211[1], 99212[1], 99213[1], 99214[1], 99215[1], 99217[1], 99218[1], 99219[1], 99220[1], 99221[1], 99222[1], 99223[1], 99231[1], 99232[1], 99233[1], 99234[1], 99235[1], 99236[1], 99238[1], 99239[1], 99241[1], 99242[1], 99243[1], 99244[1], 99245[1], 99251[1], 99252[1], 99253[1], 99254[1], 99255[1], 99291[1], 99292[1], 99304[1], 99305[1], 99306[1], 99307[1], 99308[1], 99309[1], 99310[1], 99315[1], 99316[1], 99334[1], 99335[1], 99336[1], 99337[1], 99347[1], 99348[1], 99349[1], 99350[1], 99374[1], 99375[1], 99377[1], 99378[1], 99446[0], 99447[0], 99448[0], 99449[0], 99451[0], 99452[0], 99495[0], 99496[0], G0453[0], G0463[1], G0471[1]
64569	0333T[0], 0464T[0], 0466T[1], 0468T[1], 0589T[0], 0590T[0], 11000[1], 11001[1], 11004[1], 11005[1], 11006[1], 11042[1], 11043[1], 11044[1], 11045[1], 11046[1], 11047[1], 12001[1], 12002[1], 12004[1], 12005[1], 12006[1], 12007[1], 12011[1], 12013[1], 12014[1], 12015[1], 12016[1], 12017[1], 12018[1], 12020[1], 12021[1], 12031[1], 12032[1], 12034[1], 12035[1], 12036[1], 12037[1], 12041[1], 12042[1], 12044[1], 12045[1], 12046[1], 12047[1], 12051[1], 12052[1], 12053[1], 12054[1], 12055[1], 12056[1], 12057[1], 13100[1], 13101[1], 13102[1], 13120[1], 13121[1], 13122[1], 13131[1], 13132[1], 13133[1], 13151[1], 13152[1], 13153[1], 36000[1], 36400[1], 36405[1], 36406[1], 36410[1], 36420[1], 36425[1], 36430[1], 36440[1], 36591[0], 36592[0], 36600[1], 36640[1], 43752[1], 51701[1], 51702[1], 51703[1], 61888[1], 62320[0], 62321[0], 62322[0], 62323[0], 62324[0], 62325[0], 62326[0], 62327[0], 64400[0], 64405[0], 64408[0], 64415[0], 64416[0], 64417[0], 64418[0], 64420[0], 64421[0], 64425[0], 64430[0], 64435[0], 64445[0], 64446[0], 64447[0], 64448[0], 64449[0], 64450[0], 64451[0], 64454[0], 64461[0], 64462[0], 64463[0], 64479[0], 64480[0], 64483[0], 64484[0], 64486[0], 64487[0], 64488[0], 64489[0], 64490[0], 64491[0], 64492[0], 64493[0], 64494[0], 64495[0], 64505[0], 64510[0], 64517[0], 64520[0], 64530[0], 64568[1], 64570[1], 69990[0], 92012[1], 92014[1], 92585[0], 93000[1], 93005[1], 93010[1], 93040[1], 93041[1], 93042[1], 93318[1], 93355[1], 94002[1], 94200[1], 94250[1], 94680[1], 94681[1], 94690[1], 94770[1], 95812[1], 95813[1], 95816[1], 95819[1], 95822[0], 95829[1], 95860[0], 95861[0], 95863[0], 95864[0], 95865[0], 95866[0], 95867[0], 95868[0], 95869[0], 95870[0], 95907[0], 95908[0], 95909[0], 95910[0], 95911[0], 95912[0], 95913[0], 95925[0], 95926[0], 95927[0], 95928[0], 95929[0], 95930[0], 95933[0], 95937[0], 95938[0], 95939[0], 95940[0], 95955[1], 95970[1], 95976[1], 95977[1], 96360[1], 96361[1], 96365[1], 96366[1], 96367[1], 96368[1], 96372[1], 96374[1], 96375[1], 96376[1], 96377[1], 96523[0], 97597[1], 97598[1], 97602[1], 99155[0], 99156[0], 99157[0], 99211[1], 99212[1], 99213[1], 99214[1], 99215[1], 99217[1], 99218[1], 99219[1], 99220[1], 99221[1], 99222[1], 99223[1], 99231[1], 99232[1], 99233[1], 99234[1], 99235[1], 99236[1], 99238[1], 99239[1], 99241[1], 99242[1], 99243[1], 99244[1], 99245[1], 99251[1], 99252[1], 99253[1], 99254[1], 99255[1], 99291[1], 99292[1], 99304[1], 99305[1], 99306[1], 99307[1], 99308[1], 99309[1], 99310[1], 99315[1], 99316[1], 99334[1], 99335[1], 99336[1], 99337[1], 99347[1], 99348[1], 99349[1], 99350[1], 99374[1], 99375[1], 99377[1], 99378[1], 99446[0], 99447[0], 99448[0], 99449[0], 99451[0], 99452[0], 99495[0], 99496[0], G0453[0], G0463[1], G0471[1]
64570	0333T[0], 0464T[0], 0466T[1], 0589T[0], 0590T[0], 11000[1], 11001[1], 11004[1], 11005[1], 11006[1], 11042[1], 11043[1], 11044[1], 11045[1], 11046[1], 11047[1], 12001[1], 12002[1], 12004[1], 12005[1], 12006[1], 12007[1], 12011[1], 12013[1], 12014[1], 12015[1], 12016[1], 12017[1], 12018[1], 12020[1], 12021[1], 12031[1], 12032[1], 12034[1], 12035[1], 12036[1], 12037[1], 12041[1], 12042[1], 12044[1], 12045[1], 12046[1], 12047[1], 12051[1], 12052[1], 12053[1], 12054[1], 12055[1], 12056[1], 12057[1], 13100[1], 13101[1], 13102[1], 13120[1], 13121[1], 13122[1], 13131[1], 13132[1], 13133[1], 13151[1], 13152[1], 13153[1], 36000[1], 36400[1], 36405[1], 36406[1], 36410[1], 36420[1], 36425[1], 36430[1], 36440[1], 36591[0], 36592[0], 36600[1], 36640[1], 43752[1], 51701[1], 51702[1], 51703[1], 61888[1], 62320[0], 62321[0], 62322[0], 62323[0], 62324[0], 62325[0], 62326[0], 62327[0], 64400[0], 64405[0], 64408[0], 64415[0], 64416[0], 64417[0], 64418[0], 64420[0], 64421[0], 64425[0], 64430[0], 64435[0], 64445[0], 64446[0], 64447[0], 64448[0], 64449[0], 64450[0], 64451[0], 64454[0], 64461[0], 64462[0], 64463[0], 64479[0], 64480[0], 64483[0], 64484[0], 64486[0], 64487[0], 64488[0], 64489[0], 64490[0], 64491[0], 64492[0], 64493[0], 64494[0], 64495[0], 64505[0], 64510[0], 64517[0], 64520[0], 64530[0], 64568[1], 69990[0], 92012[1], 92014[1], 92585[0], 93000[1], 93005[1], 93010[1], 93040[1], 93041[1], 93042[1], 93318[1], 93355[1], 94002[1], 94200[1], 94250[1], 94680[1], 94681[1], 94690[1], 94770[1], 95812[1], 95813[1], 95816[1], 95819[1], 95822[0], 95829[1], 95860[0], 95861[0], 95863[0], 95864[0], 95865[0], 95866[0], 95867[0], 95868[0], 95869[0], 95870[0], 95907[0], 95908[0], 95909[0], 95910[0], 95911[0], 95912[0], 95913[0], 95925[0], 95926[0], 95927[0], 95928[0], 95929[0], 95930[0], 95933[0], 95937[0], 95938[0], 95939[0], 95940[0], 95955[1], 95970[1], 95976[1], 95977[1], 96360[1], 96361[1], 96365[1], 96366[1], 96367[1], 96368[1], 96372[1], 96374[1], 96375[1], 96376[1], 96377[1], 96523[0], 97597[1], 97598[1], 97602[1], 99155[0], 99156[0], 99157[0], 99211[1], 99212[1], 99213[1], 99214[1], 99215[1], 99217[1], 99218[1], 99219[1], 99220[1], 99221[1], 99222[1], 99223[1], 99231[1], 99232[1], 99233[1], 99234[1], 99235[1], 99236[1], 99238[1], 99239[1], 99241[1], 99242[1], 99243[1], 99244[1], 99245[1], 99251[1], 99252[1], 99253[1], 99254[1], 99255[1], 99291[1], 99292[1], 99304[1], 99305[1], 99306[1], 99307[1], 99308[1], 99309[1], 99310[1], 99315[1], 99316[1], 99334[1], 99335[1], 99336[1], 99337[1], 99347[1], 99348[1], 99349[1], 99350[1], 99374[1], 99375[1], 99377[1], 99378[1], 99446[0], 99447[0], 99448[0], 99449[0], 99451[0], 99452[0], 99495[0], 99496[0], G0453[0], G0463[1], G0471[1]
64575	0213T[0], 0216T[0], 0228T[0], 0230T[0], 0333T[0], 0464T[0], 0587T[0], 0588T[0], 0589T[0], 0590T[0], 12001[1], 12002[1], 12004[1], 12005[1], 12006[1], 12007[1], 12011[1], 12013[1], 12014[1], 12015[1], 12016[1], 12017[1], 12018[1], 12020[1], 12021[1], 12031[1], 12032[1], 12034[1], 12035[1], 12036[1],

0 = Modifier usage not allowed or inappropriate 1 = Modifier usage allowed

Code 1	Code 2
	12037[1], 12041[1], 12042[1], 12044[1], 12045[1], 12046[1], 12047[1], 12051[1], 12052[1], 12053[1], 12054[1], 12055[1], 12056[1], 12057[1], 13100[1], 13101[1], 13102[1], 13120[1], 13121[1], 13122[1], 13131[1], 13132[1], 13133[1], 13151[1], 13152[1], 13153[1], 36000[1], 36400[1], 36405[1], 36406[1], 36410[1], 36420[1], 36425[1], 36430[1], 36440[1], 36591[0], 36592[0], 36600[1], 36640[1], 43752[1], 51701[1], 51702[1], 51703[1], 61850[0], 61860[0], 61870[0], 61880[0], 61885[0], 61886[1], 62320[0], 62321[0], 62322[0], 62323[0], 62324[0], 62325[0], 62326[0], 62327[0], 64400[0], 64405[0], 64408[0], 64415[0], 64416[0], 64417[0], 64418[0], 64420[0], 64421[0], 64425[0], 64430[0], 64435[0], 64445[0], 64446[0], 64447[0], 64448[0], 64449[0], 64450[0], 64451[0], 64454[0], 64461[0], 64462[0], 64463[0], 64479[0], 64480[0], 64483[0], 64484[0], 64486[0], 64487[0], 64488[0], 64489[0], 64490[0], 64491[0], 64492[0], 64493[0], 64494[0], 64495[0], 64505[0], 64510[0], 64517[0], 64520[0], 64530[0], 64561[1], 64566[1], 64581[0], 69990[0], 92012[1], 92014[1], 92585[0], 93000[1], 93005[1], 93010[1], 93040[1], 93041[1], 93042[1], 93318[1], 93355[1], 94002[1], 94200[1], 94250[1], 94680[1], 94681[1], 94690[1], 94770[1], 95812[1], 95813[1], 95816[1], 95819[1], 95822[0], 95829[1], 95860[0], 95861[0], 95863[0], 95864[0], 95865[0], 95866[0], 95867[0], 95868[0], 95869[0], 95870[0], 95907[0], 95908[0], 95909[0], 95910[0], 95911[0], 95912[0], 95913[0], 95925[0], 95926[0], 95927[0], 95928[0], 95929[0], 95930[0], 95933[0], 95937[0], 95938[0], 95939[0], 95940[0], 95955[1], 95970[1], 96360[1], 96361[1], 96365[1], 96366[1], 96367[1], 96368[1], 96372[1], 96374[1], 96375[1], 96376[1], 96377[1], 96523[0], 99155[0], 99156[0], 99157[0], 99211[1], 99212[1], 99213[1], 99214[1], 99215[1], 99217[1], 99218[1], 99219[1], 99220[1], 99221[1], 99222[1], 99223[1], 99231[1], 99232[1], 99233[1], 99234[1], 99235[1], 99236[1], 99238[1], 99239[1], 99241[1], 99242[1], 99243[1], 99244[1], 99245[1], 99251[1], 99252[1], 99253[1], 99254[1], 99255[1], 99291[1], 99292[1], 99304[1], 99305[1], 99306[1], 99307[1], 99308[1], 99309[1], 99310[1], 99315[1], 99316[1], 99334[1], 99335[1], 99336[1], 99337[1], 99347[1], 99348[1], 99349[1], 99350[1], 99374[1], 99375[1], 99377[1], 99378[1], 99446[0], 99447[0], 99448[0], 99449[0], 99451[0], 99452[0], 99495[0], 99496[0], G0453[0], G0463[1], G0471[1]
64585	0213T[0], 0216T[0], 0228T[0], 0230T[0], 0333T[0], 0464T[0], 0588T[0], 0589T[0], 0590T[0], 11000[1], 11001[1], 11004[1], 11005[1], 11006[1], 11042[1], 11043[1], 11044[1], 11045[1], 11046[1], 11047[1], 12001[1], 12002[1], 12004[1], 12005[1], 12006[1], 12007[1], 12011[1], 12013[1], 12014[1], 12015[1], 12016[1], 12017[1], 12018[1], 12020[1], 12021[1], 12031[1], 12032[1], 12034[1], 12035[1], 12036[1], 12037[1], 12041[1], 12042[1], 12044[1], 12045[1], 12046[1], 12047[1], 12051[1], 12052[1], 12053[1], 12054[1], 12055[1], 12056[1], 12057[1], 13100[1], 13101[1], 13102[1], 13120[1], 13121[1], 13122[1], 13131[1], 13132[1], 13133[1], 13151[1], 13152[1], 13153[1], 36000[1], 36400[1], 36405[1], 36406[1], 36410[1], 36420[1], 36425[1], 36430[1], 36440[1], 36591[0], 36592[0], 36600[1], 36640[1], 43752[1], 51701[1], 51702[1], 51703[1], 61886[1], 62320[0], 62321[0], 62322[0], 62323[0], 62324[0], 62325[0], 62326[0], 62327[0], 63688[1], 64400[0], 64405[0], 64408[0], 64415[0], 64416[0], 64417[0], 64418[0], 64420[0], 64421[0], 64425[0], 64430[0], 64435[0], 64445[0], 64446[0], 64447[0], 64448[0], 64449[0], 64450[0], 64451[0], 64454[0], 64461[0], 64462[0], 64463[0], 64479[0], 64480[0], 64483[0], 64484[0], 64486[0], 64487[0], 64488[0], 64489[0], 64490[0], 64491[0], 64492[0], 64493[0], 64494[0], 64495[0], 64505[0], 64510[0], 64517[0], 64520[0], 64530[0], 64553[1], 64555[1], 64561[1], 64575[1], 64580[1], 64581[0], 69990[0], 92012[1], 92014[1], 92585[0], 93000[1], 93005[1], 93010[1], 93040[1], 93041[1], 93042[1], 93318[1], 93355[1], 94002[1], 94200[1], 94250[1], 94680[1], 94681[1], 94690[1], 94770[1], 95812[1], 95813[1], 95816[1], 95819[1], 95822[0], 95829[1], 95860[0], 95861[0], 95863[0], 95864[0], 95865[0], 95866[0], 95867[0], 95868[0], 95869[0], 95870[0], 95907[0], 95908[0], 95909[0], 95910[0], 95911[0], 95912[0], 95913[0], 95925[0], 95926[0], 95927[0], 95928[0], 95929[0], 95930[0], 95933[0], 95937[0], 95938[0], 95939[0], 95940[0], 95955[1], 95970[1], 96360[1], 96361[1], 96365[1], 96366[1], 96367[1], 96368[1], 96372[1], 96374[1], 96375[1], 96376[1], 96377[1], 96523[0], 97597[1], 97598[1], 97602[1], 99155[0], 99156[0], 99157[0], 99211[1], 99212[1], 99213[1], 99214[1], 99215[1], 99217[1], 99218[1], 99219[1], 99220[1], 99221[1], 99222[1], 99223[1], 99231[1], 99232[1], 99233[1], 99234[1], 99235[1], 99236[1], 99238[1], 99239[1], 99241[1], 99242[1], 99243[1], 99244[1], 99245[1], 99251[1], 99252[1], 99253[1], 99254[1], 99255[1], 99291[1], 99292[1], 99304[1], 99305[1], 99306[1], 99307[1], 99308[1], 99309[1], 99310[1], 99315[1], 99316[1], 99334[1], 99335[1], 99336[1], 99337[1], 99347[1], 99348[1], 99349[1], 99350[1], 99374[1], 99375[1], 99377[1], 99378[1], 99446[0], 99447[0], 99448[0], 99449[0], 99451[0], 99452[0], 99495[0], 99496[0], G0453[0], G0463[1], G0471[1], J0670[1], J2001[1]
64590	0213T[0], 0216T[0], 0228T[0], 0230T[0], 0333T[0], 0424T[0], 0427T[0], 0428T[0], 0431T[0], 0464T[0], 0587T[0], 0588T[0], 0589T[0], 0590T[0], 11000[1], 11001[1], 11004[1], 11005[1], 11006[1], 11042[1], 11043[1], 11044[1], 11045[1], 11046[1], 11047[1], 12001[1], 12002[1], 12004[1], 12005[1], 12006[1], 12007[1], 12011[1], 12013[1], 12014[1], 12015[1], 12016[1], 12017[1], 12018[1], 12020[1], 12021[1], 12031[1], 12032[1], 12034[1], 12035[1], 12036[1], 12037[1], 12041[1], 12042[1], 12044[1], 12045[1], 12046[1], 12047[1], 12051[1], 12052[1], 12053[1], 12054[1], 12055[1], 12056[1], 12057[1], 13100[1], 13101[1], 13102[1], 13120[1], 13121[1], 13122[1], 13131[1], 13132[1], 13133[1], 13151[1], 13152[1], 13153[1], 36000[1], 36400[1], 36405[1], 36406[1], 36410[1], 36420[1], 36425[1], 36430[1], 36440[1], 36591[0], 36592[0], 36600[1], 36640[1], 43752[1], 51701[1], 51702[1], 51703[1], 61885[0], 61886[0], 62320[0], 62321[0], 62322[0], 62323[0], 62324[0], 62325[0], 62326[0], 62327[0], 63685[1], 64400[0], 64405[0], 64408[0], 64415[0], 64416[0], 64417[0], 64418[0], 64420[0], 64421[0], 64425[0], 64430[0], 64435[0], 64445[0], 64446[0], 64447[0], 64448[0], 64449[0], 64450[0], 64451[0], 64454[0], 64461[0], 64462[0], 64463[0], 64479[0], 64480[0], 64483[0], 64484[0], 64486[0], 64487[0], 64488[0], 64489[0], 64490[0], 64491[0], 64492[0], 64493[0], 64494[0], 64495[0], 64505[0], 64510[0], 64517[0], 64520[0], 64530[0], 64595[1], 69990[0], 92012[1], 92014[1], 92585[0], 93000[1], 93005[1], 93010[1], 93040[1], 93041[1], 93042[1], 93318[1], 93355[1], 94002[1], 94200[1], 94250[1], 94680[1], 94681[1], 94690[1], 94770[1], 95812[1], 95813[1], 95816[1], 95819[1], 95822[0], 95829[1], 95860[0], 95861[0], 95863[0], 95864[0], 95865[0], 95866[0], 95867[0], 95868[0], 95869[0], 95870[0], 95907[0], 95908[0], 95909[0], 95910[0], 95911[0], 95912[0], 95913[0], 95925[0], 95926[0], 95927[0], 95928[0], 95929[0], 95930[0], 95933[0], 95937[0], 95938[0], 95939[0], 95940[0], 95955[1], 95970[1], 95976[1], 95977[1], 95981[1], 95982[1], 96360[1], 96361[1], 96365[1], 96366[1], 96367[1], 96368[1], 96372[1], 96374[1], 96375[1], 96376[1], 96377[1], 96523[0], 97597[1], 97598[1], 97602[1], 99155[0], 99156[0], 99157[0], 99211[1], 99212[1], 99213[1], 99214[1], 99215[1], 99217[1], 99218[1], 99219[1], 99220[1], 99221[1], 99222[1], 99223[1], 99231[1], 99232[1], 99233[1], 99234[1], 99235[1], 99236[1], 99238[1], 99239[1], 99241[1], 99242[1], 99243[1], 99244[1], 99245[1], 99251[1], 99252[1], 99253[1], 99254[1], 99255[1], 99291[1], 99292[1], 99304[1], 99305[1], 99306[1], 99307[1], 99308[1], 99309[1], 99310[1], 99315[1], 99316[1], 99334[1], 99335[1], 99336[1], 99337[1], 99347[1], 99348[1], 99349[1], 99350[1], 99374[1], 99375[1], 99377[1], 99378[1], 99446[0], 99447[0], 99448[0], 99449[0], 99451[0], 99452[0], 99495[0], 99496[0], G0453[0], G0463[1], G0471[1], J0670[1], J2001[1]
64595	0213T[0], 0216T[0], 0228T[0], 0230T[0], 0333T[0], 0464T[0], 0588T[0], 0589T[0], 0590T[0], 11000[1], 11001[1], 11004[1], 11005[1], 11006[1], 11042[1], 11043[1], 11044[1], 11045[1], 11046[1], 11047[1], 12001[1], 12002[1], 12004[1], 12005[1], 12006[1], 12007[1], 12011[1], 12013[1], 12014[1], 12015[1], 12016[1], 12017[1], 12018[1], 12020[1], 12021[1], 12031[1], 12032[1], 12034[1], 12035[1], 12036[1], 12037[1], 12041[1], 12042[1], 12044[1], 12045[1], 12046[1], 12047[1], 12051[1], 12052[1], 12053[1], 12054[1], 12055[1], 12056[1], 12057[1], 13100[1], 13101[1], 13102[1], 13120[1], 13121[1], 13122[1], 13131[1], 13132[1], 13133[1], 13151[1], 13152[1], 13153[1], 36000[1], 36400[1], 36405[1], 36406[1], 36410[1], 36420[1], 36425[1], 36430[1], 36440[1], 36591[0], 36592[0], 36600[1], 36640[1], 43752[1], 51701[1], 51702[1], 51703[1], 62320[0], 62321[0], 62322[0], 62323[0], 62324[0], 62325[0], 62326[0], 62327[0], 63688[1], 64400[0], 64405[0], 64408[0], 64415[0], 64416[0], 64417[0], 64418[0], 64420[0], 64421[0], 64425[0], 64430[0], 64435[0], 64445[0], 64446[0], 64447[0], 64448[0], 64449[0], 64450[0], 64451[0], 64454[0], 64461[0], 64462[0], 64463[0], 64479[0], 64480[0], 64483[0], 64484[0], 64486[0], 64487[0], 64488[0], 64489[0], 64490[0], 64491[0], 64492[0], 64493[0], 64494[0], 64495[0], 64505[0], 64510[0], 64517[0], 64520[0], 64530[0], 69990[0], 92012[1], 92014[1], 92585[0], 93000[1], 93005[1], 93010[1], 93040[1], 93041[1], 93042[1], 93318[1], 93355[1], 94002[1], 94200[1], 94250[1], 94680[1], 94681[1], 94690[1], 94770[1], 95812[1], 95813[1], 95816[1], 95819[1], 95822[0], 95829[1], 95860[0], 95861[0], 95863[0], 95864[0], 95865[0], 95866[0], 95867[0], 95868[0], 95869[0], 95870[0], 95907[0], 95908[0], 95909[0], 95910[0], 95911[0], 95912[0], 95913[0], 95925[0], 95926[0], 95927[0], 95928[0], 95929[0], 95930[0], 95933[0], 95937[0], 95938[0], 95939[0], 95940[0], 95955[1], 95970[1], 95976[1], 95977[1], 95981[1], 95982[1], 96360[1], 96361[1], 96365[1], 96366[1], 96367[1], 96368[1], 96372[1], 96374[1], 96375[1], 96376[1], 96377[1], 96523[0], 97597[1], 97598[1], 97602[1], 99155[0], 99156[0], 99157[0], 99211[1], 99212[1], 99213[1], 99214[1], 99215[1], 99217[1], 99218[1], 99219[1], 99220[1], 99221[1], 99222[1], 99223[1], 99231[1], 99232[1], 99233[1], 99234[1], 99235[1], 99236[1], 99238[1], 99239[1], 99241[1], 99242[1], 99243[1], 99244[1], 99245[1], 99251[1], 99252[1], 99253[1], 99254[1], 99255[1], 99291[1], 99292[1], 99304[1], 99305[1], 99306[1], 99307[1], 99308[1], 99309[1], 99310[1], 99315[1], 99316[1], 99334[1], 99335[1], 99336[1], 99337[1], 99347[1], 99348[1], 99349[1], 99350[1], 99374[1], 99375[1], 99377[1], 99378[1], 99446[0], 99447[0], 99448[0], 99449[0], 99451[0], 99452[0], 99495[0], 99496[0], G0453[0], G0463[1], G0471[1], J0670[1], J2001[1]
64600	0213T[0], 0216T[0], 0228T[0], 0230T[0], 0333T[0], 0464T[0], 12001[1], 12002[1], 12004[1], 12005[1], 12006[1], 12007[1], 12011[1], 12013[1], 12014[1], 12015[1], 12016[1], 12017[1], 12018[1], 12020[1], 12021[1], 12031[1], 12032[1], 12034[1], 12035[1], 12036[1], 12037[1], 12041[1], 12042[1], 12044[1], 12045[1], 12046[1], 12047[1], 12051[1], 12052[1], 12053[1], 12054[1], 12055[1], 12056[1], 12057[1], 13100[1], 13101[1], 13102[1], 13120[1], 13121[1], 13122[1], 13131[1], 13132[1], 13133[1], 13151[1], 13152[1], 13153[1], 20550[1], 20551[1], 20552[1], 20553[1], 20560[1], 20561[1], 36000[1], 36400[1], 36405[1], 36406[1], 36410[1], 36420[1], 36425[1], 36430[1], 36440[1], 36591[0], 36592[0], 36600[1], 36640[1], 43752[1], 51701[1], 51702[1], 51703[1], 62320[1], 62321[1], 62322[1], 62323[1], 62324[1], 62325[1], 62326[1], 62327[1], 64400[1], 64405[1], 64408[1], 64415[1], 64416[1], 64417[1], 64418[1], 64420[1], 64421[1], 64425[1], 64430[1], 64435[1], 64445[1], 64446[1], 64447[1], 64448[1], 64449[1], 64450[1], 64451[1], 64454[1], 64461[0], 64462[0], 64463[0], 64479[1], 64480[0], 64483[1], 64484[0], 64486[0], 64487[0], 64488[0], 64489[0], 64490[1], 64491[0], 64492[0], 64493[1], 64494[0], 64495[0], 64505[1], 64510[1], 64517[1], 64520[1], 64530[1], 69990[0], 76000[1], 77001[1], 92012[1], 92014[1], 92585[0], 93000[1], 93005[1], 93010[1], 93040[1], 93041[1], 93042[1], 93318[1], 93355[1], 94002[1], 94200[1], 94250[1], 94680[1], 94681[1], 94690[1], 94770[1], 95812[1], 95813[1], 95816[1], 95819[1], 95822[0], 95829[1], 95860[0], 95861[0], 95863[0], 95864[0], 95865[0], 95866[0], 95867[0], 95868[0], 95869[0], 95870[0], 95907[0], 95908[0], 95909[0], 95910[0], 95911[0], 95912[0], 95913[0], 95925[0], 95926[0], 95927[0], 95928[0], 95929[0], 95930[0], 95933[0], 95937[0], 95938[0], 95939[0], 95940[0], 95955[1], 96360[1], 96361[1], 96365[1], 96366[1], 96367[1], 96368[1], 96372[1], 96374[1], 96375[1], 96376[1], 96377[1], 96523[0], 99155[0], 99156[0], 99157[0], 99211[1], 99212[1], 99213[1], 99214[1], 99215[1], 99217[1], 99218[1], 99219[1], 99220[1], 99221[1], 99222[1], 99223[1], 99231[1], 99232[1], 99233[1], 99234[1], 99235[1], 99236[1], 99238[1], 99239[1], 99241[1], 99242[1], 99243[1], 99244[1], 99245[1], 99251[1], 99252[1], 99253[1], 99254[1], 99255[1], 99291[1], 99292[1], 99304[1], 99305[1],

0 = Modifier usage not allowed or inappropriate 1 = Modifier usage allowed

Code 1	Code 2
	99306[1], 99307[1], 99308[1], 99309[1], 99310[1], 99315[1], 99316[1], 99334[1], 99335[1], 99336[1], 99337[1], 99347[1], 99348[1], 99349[1], 99350[1], 99374[1], 99375[1], 99377[1], 99378[1], 99446[0], 99447[0], 99448[0], 99449[0], 99451[0], 99452[0], 99495[0], 99496[0], G0453[0], G0463[1], G0471[1], J2001[1]
64605	0213T[0], 0216T[0], 0228T[0], 0230T[0], 0333T[0], 0464T[0], 12001[1], 12002[1], 12004[1], 12005[1], 12006[1], 12007[1], 12011[1], 12013[1], 12014[1], 12015[1], 12016[1], 12017[1], 12018[1], 12020[1], 12021[1], 12031[1], 12032[1], 12034[1], 12035[1], 12036[1], 12037[1], 12041[1], 12042[1], 12044[1], 12045[1], 12046[1], 12047[1], 12051[1], 12052[1], 12053[1], 12054[1], 12055[1], 12056[1], 12057[1], 13100[1], 13101[1], 13102[1], 13120[1], 13121[1], 13122[1], 13131[1], 13132[1], 13133[1], 13151[1], 13152[1], 13153[1], 20550[1], 20551[1], 20552[1], 20553[1], 20560[1], 20561[1], 36000[1], 36400[1], 36405[1], 36406[1], 36410[1], 36420[1], 36425[1], 36430[1], 36440[1], 36591[0], 36592[0], 36600[1], 36640[1], 43752[1], 51701[1], 51702[1], 51703[1], 62320[1], 62321[1], 62322[1], 62323[1], 62324[1], 62325[1], 62326[1], 62327[1], 64400[1], 64405[1], 64408[1], 64415[1], 64416[1], 64417[1], 64418[1], 64420[1], 64421[1], 64425[1], 64430[1], 64435[1], 64445[1], 64446[1], 64447[1], 64448[1], 64449[1], 64450[1], 64451[1], 64454[1], 64461[0], 64462[0], 64463[0], 64479[1], 64480[0], 64483[1], 64484[0], 64486[0], 64487[0], 64488[0], 64489[0], 64490[1], 64491[0], 64492[0], 64493[1], 64494[0], 64495[0], 64505[1], 64510[1], 64517[1], 64520[1], 64530[1], 69990[0], 76000[1], 77001[1], 92012[1], 92014[1], 92585[0], 93000[1], 93005[1], 93010[1], 93040[1], 93041[1], 93042[1], 93318[1], 93355[1], 94002[1], 94200[1], 94250[1], 94680[1], 94681[1], 94690[1], 94770[1], 95812[1], 95813[1], 95816[1], 95819[1], 95822[0], 95829[1], 95860[0], 95861[0], 95863[0], 95864[0], 95865[0], 95866[0], 95867[0], 95868[0], 95869[0], 95870[0], 95907[0], 95908[0], 95909[0], 95910[0], 95911[0], 95912[0], 95913[0], 95925[0], 95926[0], 95927[0], 95928[0], 95929[0], 95930[0], 95933[0], 95937[0], 95938[0], 95939[0], 95940[0], 95955[1], 96360[1], 96361[1], 96365[1], 96366[1], 96367[1], 96368[1], 96372[1], 96374[1], 96375[1], 96376[1], 96377[1], 96523[0], 99155[0], 99156[0], 99157[0], 99211[1], 99212[1], 99213[1], 99214[1], 99215[1], 99217[1], 99218[1], 99219[1], 99220[1], 99221[1], 99222[1], 99223[1], 99231[1], 99232[1], 99233[1], 99234[1], 99235[1], 99236[1], 99238[1], 99239[1], 99241[1], 99242[1], 99243[1], 99244[1], 99245[1], 99251[1], 99252[1], 99253[1], 99254[1], 99255[1], 99291[1], 99292[1], 99304[1], 99305[1], 99306[1], 99307[1], 99308[1], 99309[1], 99310[1], 99315[1], 99316[1], 99334[1], 99335[1], 99336[1], 99337[1], 99347[1], 99348[1], 99349[1], 99350[1], 99374[1], 99375[1], 99377[1], 99378[1], 99446[0], 99447[0], 99448[0], 99449[0], 99451[0], 99452[0], 99495[0], 99496[0], G0453[0], G0463[1], G0471[1], J2001[1]
64610	0213T[0], 0216T[0], 0228T[0], 0230T[0], 0333T[0], 0464T[0], 12001[1], 12002[1], 12004[1], 12005[1], 12006[1], 12007[1], 12011[1], 12013[1], 12014[1], 12015[1], 12016[1], 12017[1], 12018[1], 12020[1], 12021[1], 12031[1], 12032[1], 12034[1], 12035[1], 12036[1], 12037[1], 12041[1], 12042[1], 12044[1], 12045[1], 12046[1], 12047[1], 12051[1], 12052[1], 12053[1], 12054[1], 12055[1], 12056[1], 12057[1], 13100[1], 13101[1], 13102[1], 13120[1], 13121[1], 13122[1], 13131[1], 13132[1], 13133[1], 13151[1], 13152[1], 13153[1], 20550[1], 20551[1], 20552[1], 20553[1], 20560[1], 20561[1], 36000[1], 36400[1], 36405[1], 36406[1], 36410[1], 36420[1], 36425[1], 36430[1], 36440[1], 36591[0], 36592[0], 36600[1], 36640[1], 43752[1], 51701[1], 51702[1], 51703[1], 62320[1], 62321[1], 62322[1], 62323[1], 62324[1], 62325[1], 62326[1], 62327[1], 64400[1], 64405[1], 64408[1], 64415[1], 64416[1], 64417[1], 64418[1], 64420[1], 64421[1], 64425[1], 64430[1], 64435[1], 64445[1], 64446[1], 64447[1], 64448[1], 64449[1], 64450[1], 64451[1], 64454[1], 64461[0], 64462[0], 64463[0], 64479[1], 64480[0], 64483[1], 64484[0], 64486[0], 64487[0], 64488[0], 64489[0], 64490[1], 64491[0], 64492[0], 64493[1], 64494[0], 64495[0], 64505[1], 64510[1], 64517[1], 64520[1], 64530[1], 64605[1], 69990[0], 76000[1], 77001[1], 77002[1], 92012[1], 92014[1], 92585[0], 93000[1], 93005[1], 93010[1], 93040[1], 93041[1], 93042[1], 93318[1], 93355[1], 94002[1], 94200[1], 94250[1], 94680[1], 94681[1], 94690[1], 94770[1], 95812[1], 95813[1], 95816[1], 95819[1], 95822[0], 95829[1], 95860[0], 95861[0], 95863[0], 95864[0], 95865[0], 95866[0], 95867[0], 95868[0], 95869[0], 95870[0], 95907[0], 95908[0], 95909[0], 95910[0], 95911[0], 95912[0], 95913[0], 95925[0], 95926[0], 95927[0], 95928[0], 95929[0], 95930[0], 95933[0], 95937[0], 95938[0], 95939[0], 95940[0], 95955[1], 96360[1], 96361[1], 96365[1], 96366[1], 96367[1], 96368[1], 96372[1], 96374[1], 96375[1], 96376[1], 96377[1], 96523[0], 99155[0], 99156[0], 99157[0], 99211[1], 99212[1], 99213[1], 99214[1], 99215[1], 99217[1], 99218[1], 99219[1], 99220[1], 99221[1], 99222[1], 99223[1], 99231[1], 99232[1], 99233[1], 99234[1], 99235[1], 99236[1], 99238[1], 99239[1], 99241[1], 99242[1], 99243[1], 99244[1], 99245[1], 99251[1], 99252[1], 99253[1], 99254[1], 99255[1], 99291[1], 99292[1], 99304[1], 99305[1], 99306[1], 99307[1], 99308[1], 99309[1], 99310[1], 99315[1], 99316[1], 99334[1], 99335[1], 99336[1], 99337[1], 99347[1], 99348[1], 99349[1], 99350[1], 99374[1], 99375[1], 99377[1], 99378[1], 99446[0], 99447[0], 99448[0], 99449[0], 99451[0], 99452[0], 99495[0], 99496[0], G0453[0], G0463[1], G0471[1]
64611	00100[0], 0333T[0], 0464T[0], 12001[1], 12002[1], 12004[1], 12005[1], 12006[1], 12007[1], 12011[1], 12013[1], 12014[1], 12015[1], 12016[1], 12017[1], 12018[1], 12020[1], 12021[1], 12031[1], 12032[1], 12034[1], 12035[1], 12036[1], 12037[1], 12041[1], 12042[1], 12044[1], 12045[1], 12046[1], 12047[1], 12051[1], 12052[1], 12053[1], 12054[1], 12055[1], 12056[1], 12057[1], 13100[1], 13101[1], 13102[1], 13120[1], 13121[1], 13122[1], 13131[1], 13132[1], 13133[1], 13151[1], 13152[1], 13153[1], 20550[1], 20551[1], 20552[1], 20553[1], 20560[1], 20561[1], 36000[1], 36400[1], 36405[1], 36406[1], 36410[1], 36420[1], 36425[1], 36430[1], 36440[1], 36591[0], 36592[0], 36600[1], 36640[1], 43752[1], 51701[1], 51702[1], 51703[1], 62320[1], 62321[1], 62322[1], 62323[1], 62324[1], 62325[1], 62326[1], 62327[1], 64400[1], 64405[1], 64408[1], 64415[1], 64416[1], 64417[1], 64418[1], 64420[1], 64421[1], 64425[1], 64430[1], 64435[1], 64445[1], 64446[1], 64447[1], 64448[1], 64449[1], 64450[1], 64451[1], 64454[1], 64461[0], 64462[0], 64463[0], 64479[1], 64480[0], 64483[1], 64484[0], 64486[0], 64487[0], 64488[0], 64489[0], 64490[1], 64491[0], 64492[0], 64493[1], 64494[0], 64495[0], 64505[1], 64510[1], 64517[1], 64520[1], 64530[1], 69990[0], 92012[1], 92014[1], 92585[0], 93000[1], 93005[1], 93010[1], 93040[1], 93041[1], 93042[1], 93318[1], 93355[1], 94002[1], 94200[1], 94250[1], 94680[1], 94681[1], 94690[1], 94770[1], 95812[1], 95813[1], 95816[1], 95819[1], 95822[0], 95829[1], 95860[0], 95861[0], 95863[0], 95864[0], 95865[0], 95866[0], 95867[0], 95868[0], 95870[0], 95907[0], 95908[0], 95909[0], 95910[0], 95911[0], 95912[0], 95913[0], 95925[0], 95926[0], 95927[0], 95928[0], 95929[0], 95930[0], 95933[0], 95937[0], 95938[0], 95939[0], 95940[0], 95955[1], 96360[1], 96361[1], 96365[1], 96366[1], 96367[1], 96368[1], 96372[1], 96374[1], 96375[1], 96376[1], 96377[1], 96523[0], 99155[0], 99156[0], 99157[0], 99211[1], 99212[1], 99213[1], 99214[1], 99215[1], 99217[1], 99218[1], 99219[1], 99220[1], 99221[1], 99222[1], 99223[1], 99231[1], 99232[1], 99233[1], 99234[1], 99235[1], 99236[1], 99238[1], 99239[1], 99241[1], 99242[1], 99243[1], 99244[1], 99245[1], 99251[1], 99252[1], 99253[1], 99254[1], 99255[1], 99291[1], 99292[1], 99304[1], 99305[1], 99306[1], 99307[1], 99308[1], 99309[1], 99310[1], 99315[1], 99316[1], 99334[1], 99335[1], 99336[1], 99337[1], 99347[1], 99348[1], 99349[1], 99350[1], 99374[1], 99375[1], 99377[1], 99378[1], 99446[0], 99447[0], 99448[0], 99449[0], 99451[0], 99452[0], 99495[0], 99496[0], G0453[0], G0463[1], G0471[1]
64612	0213T[0], 0216T[0], 0228T[0], 0230T[0], 0333T[0], 0464T[0], 12001[1], 12002[1], 12004[1], 12005[1], 12006[1], 12007[1], 12011[1], 12013[1], 12014[1], 12015[1], 12016[1], 12017[1], 12018[1], 12020[1], 12021[1], 12031[1], 12032[1], 12034[1], 12035[1], 12036[1], 12037[1], 12041[1], 12042[1], 12044[1], 12045[1], 12046[1], 12047[1], 12051[1], 12052[1], 12053[1], 12054[1], 12055[1], 12056[1], 12057[1], 13100[1], 13101[1], 13102[1], 13120[1], 13121[1], 13122[1], 13131[1], 13132[1], 13133[1], 13151[1], 13152[1], 13153[1], 20550[1], 20551[1], 20552[1], 20553[1], 20560[1], 20561[1], 36000[1], 36400[1], 36405[1], 36406[1], 36410[1], 36420[1], 36425[1], 36430[1], 36440[1], 36591[0], 36592[0], 36600[1], 36640[1], 43752[1], 51701[1], 51702[1], 51703[1], 62320[1], 62321[1], 62322[1], 62323[1], 62324[1], 62325[1], 62326[1], 62327[1], 64400[1], 64405[1], 64408[1], 64415[1], 64416[1], 64417[1], 64418[1], 64420[1], 64421[1], 64425[1], 64430[1], 64435[1], 64445[1], 64446[1], 64447[1], 64448[1], 64449[1], 64450[1], 64451[1], 64454[1], 64461[0], 64462[0], 64463[0], 64479[1], 64480[0], 64483[1], 64484[0], 64486[0], 64487[0], 64488[0], 64489[0], 64490[1], 64491[0], 64492[0], 64493[1], 64494[0], 64495[0], 64505[1], 64510[1], 64517[1], 64520[1], 64530[1], 69990[0], 92012[1], 92014[1], 92585[0], 93000[1], 93005[1], 93010[1], 93040[1], 93041[1], 93042[1], 93318[1], 93355[1], 94002[1], 94200[1], 94250[1], 94680[1], 94681[1], 94690[1], 94770[1], 95812[1], 95813[1], 95816[1], 95819[1], 95822[0], 95829[1], 95860[0], 95861[0], 95863[0], 95864[0], 95865[0], 95866[0], 95867[0], 95868[0], 95870[0], 95907[0], 95908[0], 95909[0], 95910[0], 95911[0], 95912[0], 95913[0], 95925[0], 95926[0], 95927[0], 95928[0], 95929[0], 95930[0], 95933[0], 95937[0], 95938[0], 95939[0], 95940[0], 95955[1], 96360[1], 96361[1], 96365[1], 96366[1], 96367[1], 96368[1], 96372[1], 96374[1], 96375[1], 96376[1], 96377[1], 96523[0], 99155[0], 99156[0], 99157[0], 99211[1], 99212[1], 99213[1], 99214[1], 99215[1], 99217[1], 99218[1], 99219[1], 99220[1], 99221[1], 99222[1], 99223[1], 99231[1], 99232[1], 99233[1], 99234[1], 99235[1], 99236[1], 99238[1], 99239[1], 99241[1], 99242[1], 99243[1], 99244[1], 99245[1], 99251[1], 99252[1], 99253[1], 99254[1], 99255[1], 99291[1], 99292[1], 99304[1], 99305[1], 99306[1], 99307[1], 99308[1], 99309[1], 99310[1], 99315[1], 99316[1], 99334[1], 99335[1], 99336[1], 99337[1], 99347[1], 99348[1], 99349[1], 99350[1], 99374[1], 99375[1], 99377[1], 99378[1], 99446[0], 99447[0], 99448[0], 99449[0], 99451[0], 99452[0], 99495[0], 99496[0], G0453[0], G0463[1], G0471[1], J2001[1]
64615	0213T[0], 0216T[0], 0228T[0], 0230T[0], 0333T[1], 0464T[1], 12001[1], 12002[1], 12004[1], 12005[1], 12006[1], 12007[1], 12011[1], 12013[1], 12014[1], 12015[1], 12016[1], 12017[1], 12018[1], 12020[1], 12021[1], 12031[1], 12032[1], 12034[1], 12035[1], 12036[1], 12037[1], 12041[1], 12042[1], 12044[1], 12045[1], 12046[1], 12047[1], 12051[1], 12052[1], 12053[1], 12054[1], 12055[1], 12056[1], 12057[1], 13100[1], 13101[1], 13102[1], 13120[1], 13121[1], 13122[1], 13131[1], 13132[1], 13133[1], 13151[1], 13152[1], 13153[1], 20550[1], 20551[1], 20552[1], 20553[1], 20560[1], 20561[1], 36000[1], 36400[1], 36405[1], 36406[1], 36410[1], 36420[1], 36425[1], 36430[1], 36440[1], 36591[0], 36592[0], 36600[1], 36640[1], 43752[1], 51701[1], 51702[1], 51703[1], 62320[1], 62321[1], 62322[1], 62323[1], 62324[1], 62325[1], 62326[1], 62327[1], 64400[1], 64405[1], 64408[1], 64415[1], 64416[1], 64417[1], 64418[1], 64420[1], 64421[1], 64425[1], 64430[1], 64435[1], 64445[1], 64446[1], 64447[1], 64448[1], 64449[1], 64450[1], 64451[1], 64454[1], 64461[0], 64462[0], 64463[0], 64479[1], 64480[0], 64483[1], 64484[0], 64486[0], 64487[0], 64488[0], 64489[0], 64490[1], 64491[0], 64492[0], 64493[1], 64494[0], 64495[0], 64505[1], 64510[1], 64517[1], 64520[1], 64530[1], 64612[0], 64616[0], 64642[1], 64643[1], 64644[1], 64645[1], 64646[1], 69990[0], 92012[1], 92014[1], 92585[1], 93000[1], 93005[1], 93010[1], 93040[1], 93041[1], 93042[1], 93318[1], 93355[1], 94002[1], 94200[1], 94250[1], 94680[1], 94681[1], 94690[1], 94770[1], 95812[1], 95813[1], 95816[1], 95819[1], 95822[1], 95829[1], 95860[1], 95861[1], 95863[1], 95864[1], 95865[1], 95866[1], 95867[1], 95868[1], 95870[1], 95907[1], 95908[1], 95909[1], 95910[1], 95911[1], 95912[1], 95913[1], 95925[1], 95926[1], 95927[1], 95928[1], 95929[1], 95930[1], 95933[1], 95937[1], 95938[1], 95939[1], 95940[1], 95955[1], 96360[1], 96361[1], 96365[1], 96366[1], 96367[1], 96368[1], 96372[1], 96374[1], 96375[1], 96376[1], 96377[1], 96523[0], 99155[0], 99156[0], 99157[0], 99211[1], 99212[1], 99213[1], 99214[1], 99215[1], 99217[1], 99218[1], 99219[1], 99220[1], 99221[1],

0 = Modifier usage not allowed or inappropriate 1 = Modifier usage allowed

Code 1	Code 2
	99222[1], 99223[1], 99231[1], 99232[1], 99233[1], 99234[1], 99235[1], 99236[1], 99238[1], 99239[1], 99241[1], 99242[1], 99243[1], 99244[1], 99245[1], 99251[1], 99252[1], 99253[1], 99254[1], 99255[1], 99291[1], 99292[1], 99304[1], 99305[1], 99306[1], 99307[1], 99308[1], 99309[1], 99310[1], 99315[1], 99316[1], 99334[1], 99335[1], 99336[1], 99337[1], 99347[1], 99348[1], 99349[1], 99350[1], 99374[1], 99375[1], 99377[1], 99378[1], 99446[0], 99447[0], 99448[0], 99449[0], 99451[0], 99452[0], 99495[0], 99496[0], G0453[0], G0463[1], G0471[1], J2001[1]
64616	0213T[1], 0216T[1], 0228T[1], 0230T[1], 0333T[0], 0464T[0], 12001[1], 12002[1], 12004[1], 12005[1], 12006[1], 12007[1], 12011[1], 12013[1], 12014[1], 12015[1], 12016[1], 12017[1], 12018[1], 12020[1], 12021[1], 12031[1], 12032[1], 12034[1], 12035[1], 12036[1], 12037[1], 12041[1], 12042[1], 12044[1], 12045[1], 12046[1], 12047[1], 12051[1], 12052[1], 12053[1], 12054[1], 12055[1], 12056[1], 12057[1], 13100[1], 13101[1], 13102[1], 13120[1], 13121[1], 13122[1], 13131[1], 13132[1], 13133[1], 13151[1], 13152[1], 13153[1], 20550[1], 20551[1], 20552[1], 20553[1], 20560[1], 20561[1], 36000[1], 36400[1], 36405[1], 36406[1], 36410[1], 36420[1], 36425[1], 36430[1], 36440[1], 36591[0], 36592[0], 36600[1], 36640[1], 43752[1], 51701[1], 51702[1], 51703[1], 62320[1], 62321[1], 62322[1], 62323[1], 62324[1], 62325[1], 62326[1], 62327[1], 64400[1], 64405[1], 64408[1], 64415[1], 64416[1], 64417[1], 64418[1], 64420[1], 64421[1], 64425[1], 64430[1], 64435[1], 64445[1], 64446[1], 64447[1], 64448[1], 64449[1], 64450[1], 64451[1], 64454[1], 64461[0], 64462[0], 64463[0], 64479[1], 64480[0], 64483[1], 64484[0], 64486[0], 64487[0], 64488[0], 64489[0], 64490[1], 64491[0], 64492[0], 64493[1], 64494[0], 64495[0], 64505[1], 64510[1], 64517[1], 64520[1], 64530[1], 69990[0], 92012[1], 92014[1], 93000[1], 93005[1], 93010[1], 93040[1], 93041[1], 93042[1], 93318[1], 93355[1], 94002[1], 94200[1], 94250[1], 94680[1], 94681[1], 94690[1], 94770[1], 95812[1], 95813[1], 95816[1], 95819[1], 95829[1], 95860[1], 95861[1], 95863[1], 95864[1], 95865[1], 95866[1], 95867[1], 95868[1], 95869[1], 95870[1], 95930[0], 95933[0], 95937[0], 95940[0], 95941[0], 95955[1], 96360[1], 96361[1], 96365[1], 96366[1], 96367[1], 96368[1], 96372[1], 96374[1], 96375[1], 96376[1], 96377[1], 96523[0], 99155[0], 99156[0], 99157[0], 99211[1], 99212[1], 99213[1], 99214[1], 99215[1], 99217[1], 99218[1], 99219[1], 99220[1], 99221[1], 99222[1], 99223[1], 99231[1], 99232[1], 99233[1], 99234[1], 99235[1], 99236[1], 99238[1], 99239[1], 99241[1], 99242[1], 99243[1], 99244[1], 99245[1], 99251[1], 99252[1], 99253[1], 99254[1], 99255[1], 99291[1], 99292[1], 99304[1], 99305[1], 99306[1], 99307[1], 99308[1], 99309[1], 99310[1], 99315[1], 99316[1], 99334[1], 99335[1], 99336[1], 99337[1], 99347[1], 99348[1], 99349[1], 99350[1], 99374[1], 99375[1], 99377[1], 99378[1], 99446[0], 99447[0], 99448[0], 99449[0], 99451[0], 99452[0], G0453[0], G0463[1], G0471[1], J2001[1]
64617	0213T[0], 0216T[0], 0228T[0], 0230T[0], 0333T[0], 0464T[0], 12001[1], 12002[1], 12004[1], 12005[1], 12006[1], 12007[1], 12011[1], 12013[1], 12014[1], 12015[1], 12016[1], 12017[1], 12018[1], 12020[1], 12021[1], 12031[1], 12032[1], 12034[1], 12035[1], 12036[1], 12037[1], 12041[1], 12042[1], 12044[1], 12045[1], 12046[1], 12047[1], 12051[1], 12052[1], 12053[1], 12054[1], 12055[1], 12056[1], 12057[1], 13100[1], 13101[1], 13102[1], 13120[1], 13121[1], 13122[1], 13131[1], 13132[1], 13133[1], 13151[1], 13152[1], 13153[1], 20550[1], 20551[1], 20552[1], 20553[1], 20560[1], 20561[1], 36000[1], 36400[1], 36405[1], 36406[1], 36410[1], 36420[1], 36425[1], 36430[1], 36440[1], 36591[0], 36592[0], 36600[1], 36640[1], 43752[1], 51701[1], 51702[1], 51703[1], 62320[0], 62321[0], 62322[0], 62323[0], 62324[0], 62325[0], 62326[0], 62327[0], 64400[0], 64405[0], 64408[0], 64415[0], 64416[0], 64417[0], 64418[0], 64420[0], 64421[0], 64425[0], 64430[0], 64435[0], 64445[0], 64446[0], 64447[0], 64448[0], 64449[0], 64450[0], 64451[0], 64454[0], 64461[0], 64462[0], 64463[0], 64479[0], 64480[0], 64483[0], 64484[0], 64486[0], 64487[0], 64488[0], 64489[0], 64490[0], 64491[0], 64492[0], 64493[0], 64494[0], 64495[0], 64505[0], 64510[0], 64517[0], 64520[0], 64530[0], 64615[1], 69990[0], 92012[1], 92014[1], 93000[1], 93005[1], 93010[1], 93040[1], 93041[1], 93042[1], 93318[1], 93355[1], 94002[1], 94200[1], 94250[1], 94680[1], 94681[1], 94690[1], 94770[1], 95812[1], 95813[1], 95816[1], 95819[1], 95829[1], 95865[1], 95873[0], 95874[0], 95930[0], 95933[0], 95937[0], 95940[0], 95941[0], 95955[1], 96360[1], 96361[1], 96365[1], 96366[1], 96367[1], 96368[1], 96372[1], 96374[1], 96375[1], 96376[1], 96377[1], 96523[0], 99155[0], 99156[0], 99157[0], 99211[1], 99212[1], 99213[1], 99214[1], 99215[1], 99217[1], 99218[1], 99219[1], 99220[1], 99221[1], 99222[1], 99223[1], 99231[1], 99232[1], 99233[1], 99234[1], 99235[1], 99236[1], 99238[1], 99239[1], 99241[1], 99242[1], 99243[1], 99244[1], 99245[1], 99251[1], 99252[1], 99253[1], 99254[1], 99255[1], 99291[1], 99292[1], 99304[1], 99305[1], 99306[1], 99307[1], 99308[1], 99309[1], 99310[1], 99315[1], 99316[1], 99334[1], 99335[1], 99336[1], 99337[1], 99347[1], 99348[1], 99349[1], 99350[1], 99374[1], 99375[1], 99377[1], 99378[1], 99446[0], 99447[0], 99448[0], 99449[0], 99451[0], 99452[0], G0453[0], G0463[1], G0471[1], J2001[1]
64625	0213T[0], 0216T[0], 0228T[0], 0230T[0], 0333T[0], 0464T[0], 12001[1], 12002[1], 12004[1], 12005[1], 12006[1], 12007[1], 12011[1], 12013[1], 12014[1], 12015[1], 12016[1], 12017[1], 12020[1], 12021[1], 12031[1], 12032[1], 12034[1], 12041[1], 12042[1], 12044[1], 12051[1], 12052[1], 12053[1], 13100[1], 13102[1], 13120[1], 13122[1], 13133[1], 13153[1], 20550[1], 20551[1], 20552[1], 20553[1], 36000[1], 36400[1], 36405[1], 36406[1], 36410[1], 36420[1], 36425[1], 36430[1], 36440[1], 36591[0], 36592[0], 36600[1], 36640[1], 43752[1], 51701[1], 51702[1], 51703[1], 62320[0], 62321[0], 62322[0], 62323[0], 62324[0], 62325[0], 62326[0], 62327[0], 64400[0], 64405[0], 64408[0], 64415[0], 64416[0], 64417[0], 64418[0], 64420[0], 64421[0], 64425[0], 64430[0], 64435[0], 64445[0], 64446[0], 64447[0], 64448[0], 64449[0], 64455[1], 64461[0], 64462[0], 64463[0], 64479[0], 64480[0], 64483[0], 64484[0], 64486[0], 64487[0], 64488[0], 64489[0], 64490[0], 64491[0], 64492[0], 64493[0], 64494[0], 64495[0], 64505[0], 64510[0], 64517[0], 64520[0], 64530[0], 64632[1], 64636[1], 76000[1], 76380[1], 76942[1], 76970[1], 76998[1], 77002[1], 77003[1], 77012[1], 77021[1], 92012[1], 92014[1], 92585[0], 93000[1], 93005[1], 93010[1], 93040[1], 93041[1], 93042[1], 93318[1], 93355[1], 94002[1], 94200[1], 94250[1], 94680[1], 94681[1], 94690[1], 94770[1], 95812[1], 95813[1], 95816[1], 95819[1], 95822[1], 95829[1], 95860[0], 95861[0], 95863[0], 95864[0], 95865[0], 95866[0], 95867[0], 95868[0], 95869[0], 95870[0], 95873[1], 95874[1], 95907[0], 95908[0], 95909[0], 95910[0], 95911[0], 95912[0], 95913[0], 95925[0], 95926[0], 95927[0], 95928[0], 95929[0], 95930[0], 95933[0], 95937[0], 95938[0], 95939[0], 95940[0], 95955[1], 96360[1], 96361[1], 96365[1], 96366[1], 96367[1], 96368[1], 96372[1], 96374[1], 96375[1], 96376[1], 96377[1], 96523[0], 99155[0], 99156[0], 99157[0], 99211[1], 99212[1], 99213[1], 99214[1], 99215[1], 99217[1], 99218[1], 99219[1], 99220[1], 99221[1], 99222[1], 99223[1], 99231[1], 99232[1], 99233[1], 99234[1], 99235[1], 99236[1], 99238[1], 99239[1], 99241[1], 99242[1], 99243[1], 99244[1], 99245[1], 99251[1], 99252[1], 99253[1], 99254[1], 99255[1], 99291[1], 99292[1], 99304[1], 99305[1], 99306[1], 99307[1], 99308[1], 99309[1], 99310[1], 99315[1], 99316[1], 99334[1], 99335[1], 99336[1], 99337[1], 99347[1], 99348[1], 99349[1], 99350[1], 99374[1], 99375[1], 99377[1], 99378[1], 99446[0], 99447[0], 99448[0], 99449[0], 99451[0], 99452[0], 99495[0], 99496[0], G0453[0], G0463[1], G0471[1], J0670[1], J2001[1]
64633	0213T[0], 0216T[0], 0228T[0], 0230T[0], 0333T[0], 0464T[0], 12001[1], 12002[1], 12004[1], 12005[1], 12006[1], 12007[1], 12011[1], 12013[1], 12014[1], 12015[1], 12016[1], 12017[1], 12018[1], 12020[1], 12021[1], 12031[1], 12032[1], 12034[1], 12035[1], 12036[1], 12037[1], 12041[1], 12042[1], 12044[1], 12045[1], 12046[1], 12047[1], 12051[1], 12052[1], 12053[1], 12054[1], 12055[1], 12056[1], 12057[1], 13100[1], 13101[1], 13102[1], 13120[1], 13121[1], 13122[1], 13131[1], 13132[1], 13133[1], 13151[1], 13152[1], 13153[1], 20550[1], 20551[1], 20552[1], 20553[1], 20560[1], 20561[1], 36000[1], 36400[1], 36405[1], 36406[1], 36410[1], 36420[1], 36425[1], 36430[1], 36440[1], 36591[0], 36592[0], 36600[1], 36640[1], 43752[1], 51701[1], 51702[1], 51703[1], 62320[1], 62321[1], 62322[1], 62323[1], 62324[1], 62325[1], 62326[1], 62327[1], 64400[1], 64405[1], 64408[1], 64415[1], 64416[1], 64417[1], 64418[1], 64420[1], 64421[1], 64425[1], 64430[1], 64435[1], 64445[1], 64446[1], 64447[1], 64448[1], 64449[1], 64450[1], 64451[1], 64454[1], 64461[0], 64462[0], 64463[0], 64479[1], 64480[0], 64483[1], 64484[1], 64486[0], 64487[0], 64488[0], 64489[0], 64490[1], 64491[1], 64492[1], 64493[1], 64494[1], 64495[1], 64505[1], 64510[1], 64517[1], 64520[1], 64530[1], 69990[0], 76000[1], 76380[1], 77001[1], 77002[1], 77003[1], 77012[1], 92012[1], 92014[1], 92585[0], 93000[1], 93005[1], 93010[1], 93040[1], 93041[1], 93042[1], 93318[1], 93355[1], 94002[1], 94200[1], 94250[1], 94680[1], 94681[1], 94690[1], 94770[1], 95812[1], 95813[1], 95816[1], 95819[1], 95822[0], 95829[1], 95860[0], 95861[0], 95863[0], 95864[0], 95865[0], 95866[0], 95867[0], 95868[0], 95869[0], 95870[0], 95907[0], 95908[0], 95909[0], 95910[0], 95911[0], 95912[0], 95913[0], 95925[0], 95926[0], 95927[0], 95928[0], 95929[0], 95930[0], 95933[0], 95937[0], 95938[0], 95939[0], 95940[0], 95955[1], 96360[1], 96361[1], 96365[1], 96366[1], 96367[1], 96368[1], 96372[1], 96374[1], 96375[1], 96376[1], 96377[1], 96523[0], 99155[0], 99156[0], 99157[0], 99211[1], 99212[1], 99213[1], 99214[1], 99215[1], 99217[1], 99218[1], 99219[1], 99220[1], 99221[1], 99222[1], 99223[1], 99231[1], 99232[1], 99233[1], 99234[1], 99235[1], 99236[1], 99238[1], 99239[1], 99241[1], 99242[1], 99243[1], 99244[1], 99245[1], 99251[1], 99252[1], 99253[1], 99254[1], 99255[1], 99291[1], 99292[1], 99304[1], 99305[1], 99306[1], 99307[1], 99308[1], 99309[1], 99310[1], 99315[1], 99316[1], 99334[1], 99335[1], 99336[1], 99337[1], 99347[1], 99348[1], 99349[1], 99350[1], 99374[1], 99375[1], 99377[1], 99378[1], 99446[0], 99447[0], 99448[0], 99449[0], 99451[0], 99452[0], 99495[0], 99496[0], G0453[0], G0463[1], G0471[1], J0670[1], J2001[1]
64634	0213T[0], 0216T[0], 0228T[0], 0230T[0], 0333T[0], 0464T[0], 20550[1], 20551[1], 20552[1], 20553[1], 20560[1], 20561[1], 36000[1], 36400[1], 36405[1], 36406[1], 36410[1], 36420[1], 36425[1], 36430[1], 36440[1], 36591[0], 36592[0], 36600[1], 36640[1], 43752[1], 51701[1], 51702[1], 51703[1], 61650[1], 62320[1], 62321[1], 62322[1], 62323[1], 62324[1], 62325[1], 62326[1], 62327[1], 64400[1], 64405[1], 64408[1], 64415[1], 64416[1], 64417[1], 64418[1], 64420[1], 64421[1], 64425[1], 64430[1], 64435[1], 64445[1], 64446[1], 64447[1], 64448[1], 64449[1], 64450[1], 64451[1], 64454[1], 64461[1], 64463[1], 64479[1], 64483[1], 64486[1], 64487[1], 64488[1], 64489[1], 64490[1], 64493[1], 64505[1], 64510[1], 64517[1], 64520[1], 64530[1], 69990[0], 76000[1], 76380[1], 77002[1], 77003[1], 77012[1], 92585[0], 93000[1], 93005[1], 93010[1], 93040[1], 93041[1], 93042[1], 93318[1], 93355[1], 94002[1], 94200[1], 94250[1], 94680[1], 94681[1], 94690[1], 94770[1], 95812[1], 95813[1], 95816[1], 95819[1], 95822[0], 95829[1], 95860[0], 95861[0], 95863[0], 95864[0], 95865[0], 95866[0], 95867[0], 95868[0], 95869[0], 95870[0], 95907[0], 95908[0], 95909[0], 95910[0], 95911[0], 95912[0], 95913[0], 95925[0], 95926[0], 95927[0], 95928[0], 95929[0], 95930[0], 95933[0], 95937[0], 95938[0], 95939[0], 95940[0], 95955[1], 96360[1], 96365[1], 96372[1], 96374[1], 96375[1], 96376[1], 96377[1], 96523[0], 99155[0], 99156[0], 99157[0], G0453[0], G0471[1], J0670[1], J2001[1]
64635	0213T[0], 0216T[0], 0228T[0], 0230T[0], 0333T[0], 0464T[0], 12001[1], 12002[1], 12004[1], 12005[1], 12006[1], 12007[1], 12011[1], 12013[1], 12014[1], 12015[1], 12016[1], 12017[1], 12018[1], 12020[1], 12021[1], 12031[1], 12032[1], 12034[1], 12035[1], 12036[1], 12037[1], 12041[1], 12042[1], 12044[1], 12045[1], 12046[1], 12047[1], 12051[1], 12052[1], 12053[1], 12054[1], 12055[1], 12056[1], 12057[1], 13100[1], 13101[1], 13102[1], 13120[1], 13121[1], 13122[1], 13131[1], 13132[1], 13133[1], 13151[1], 13152[1], 13153[1], 20550[1], 20551[1], 20552[1], 20553[1], 20560[1], 20561[1], 36000[1], 36400[1], 36405[1], 36406[1], 36410[1], 36420[1], 36425[1], 36430[1], 36440[1], 36591[0], 36592[0], 36600[1],

0 = Modifier usage not allowed or inappropriate 1 = Modifier usage allowed

Code 1	Code 2
	36640[1], 43752[1], 51701[1], 51702[1], 51703[1], 62320[1], 62321[1], 62322[1], 62323[1], 62324[1], 62325[1], 62326[1], 62327[1], 64400[1], 64405[1], 64408[1], 64415[1], 64416[1], 64417[1], 64418[1], 64420[1], 64421[1], 64425[1], 64430[1], 64435[1], 64445[1], 64446[1], 64447[1], 64448[1], 64449[1], 64450[1], 64451[1], 64454[1], 64461[0], 64462[0], 64463[0], 64479[1], 64480[0], 64483[1], 64484[1], 64486[0], 64487[0], 64488[0], 64489[0], 64490[1], 64491[1], 64492[1], 64493[1], 64494[1], 64495[1], 64505[1], 64510[1], 64517[1], 64520[1], 64530[1], 64625[1], 69990[0], 76000[1], 76380[1], 77001[1], 77002[1], 77003[1], 77012[1], 92012[1], 92014[1], 92585[0], 93000[1], 93005[1], 93010[1], 93040[1], 93041[1], 93042[1], 93318[1], 93355[1], 94002[1], 94200[1], 94250[1], 94680[1], 94681[1], 94690[1], 94770[1], 95812[1], 95813[1], 95816[1], 95819[1], 95822[0], 95829[1], 95860[0], 95861[0], 95863[0], 95864[0], 95865[0], 95866[0], 95867[0], 95868[0], 95869[0], 95870[0], 95907[0], 95908[0], 95909[0], 95910[0], 95911[0], 95912[0], 95913[0], 95925[0], 95926[0], 95927[0], 95928[0], 95929[0], 95930[0], 95933[0], 95937[0], 95938[0], 95939[0], 95940[0], 95955[1], 96360[1], 96361[1], 96365[1], 96366[1], 96367[1], 96368[1], 96372[1], 96374[1], 96375[1], 96376[1], 96377[1], 96523[0], 99155[0], 99156[0], 99157[0], 99211[1], 99212[1], 99213[1], 99214[1], 99215[1], 99217[1], 99218[1], 99219[1], 99220[1], 99221[1], 99222[1], 99223[1], 99231[1], 99232[1], 99233[1], 99234[1], 99235[1], 99236[1], 99238[1], 99239[1], 99241[1], 99242[1], 99243[1], 99244[1], 99245[1], 99251[1], 99252[1], 99253[1], 99254[1], 99255[1], 99291[1], 99292[1], 99304[1], 99305[1], 99306[1], 99307[1], 99308[1], 99309[1], 99310[1], 99315[1], 99316[1], 99334[1], 99335[1], 99336[1], 99337[1], 99347[1], 99348[1], 99349[1], 99350[1], 99374[1], 99375[1], 99377[1], 99378[1], 99446[0], 99447[0], 99448[0], 99449[0], 99451[0], 99452[0], 99495[0], 99496[0], G0453[0], G0463[1], G0471[1], J0670[1], J2001[1]
64636	0213T[0], 0216T[0], 0228T[0], 0230T[0], 0333T[0], 0464T[0], 20550[1], 20551[1], 20552[1], 20553[1], 20560[1], 20561[1], 36000[1], 36400[1], 36405[1], 36406[1], 36410[1], 36420[1], 36425[1], 36430[1], 36440[1], 36591[0], 36592[0], 36600[1], 36640[1], 43752[1], 51701[1], 51702[1], 51703[1], 61650[1], 62320[1], 62321[1], 62322[1], 62323[1], 62324[1], 62325[1], 62326[1], 62327[1], 64400[1], 64405[1], 64408[1], 64415[1], 64416[1], 64417[1], 64418[1], 64420[1], 64421[1], 64425[1], 64430[1], 64435[1], 64445[1], 64446[1], 64447[1], 64448[1], 64449[1], 64450[1], 64451[1], 64454[1], 64461[1], 64463[1], 64479[1], 64483[1], 64486[1], 64487[1], 64488[1], 64489[1], 64490[1], 64493[1], 64505[1], 64510[1], 64517[1], 64520[1], 64530[1], 69990[0], 76000[1], 76380[1], 77002[1], 77003[1], 77012[1], 92585[0], 93000[1], 93005[1], 93010[1], 93040[1], 93041[1], 93042[1], 93318[1], 93355[1], 94002[1], 94200[1], 94250[1], 94680[1], 94681[1], 94690[1], 94770[1], 95812[1], 95813[1], 95816[1], 95819[1], 95822[0], 95829[1], 95860[0], 95861[0], 95863[0], 95864[0], 95865[0], 95866[0], 95867[0], 95868[0], 95869[0], 95870[0], 95907[0], 95908[0], 95909[0], 95910[0], 95911[0], 95912[0], 95913[0], 95925[0], 95926[0], 95927[0], 95928[0], 95929[0], 95930[0], 95933[0], 95937[0], 95938[0], 95939[0], 95940[0], 95955[1], 96360[1], 96365[1], 96372[1], 96374[1], 96375[1], 96376[1], 96377[1], 96523[0], 99155[0], 99156[0], 99157[0], G0453[0], G0471[1], J0670[1], J2001[1]
64640	0213T[0], 0216T[0], 0228T[0], 0230T[0], 0333T[0], 0464T[0], 12001[1], 12002[1], 12004[1], 12005[1], 12006[1], 12007[1], 12011[1], 12013[1], 12014[1], 12015[1], 12016[1], 12017[1], 12018[1], 12020[1], 12021[1], 12031[1], 12032[1], 12034[1], 12035[1], 12036[1], 12037[1], 12041[1], 12042[1], 12044[1], 12045[1], 12046[1], 12047[1], 12051[1], 12052[1], 12053[1], 12054[1], 12055[1], 12056[1], 12057[1], 13100[1], 13101[1], 13102[1], 13120[1], 13121[1], 13122[1], 13131[1], 13132[1], 13133[1], 13151[1], 13152[1], 13153[1], 20550[1], 20551[1], 20552[1], 20553[1], 20560[1], 20561[1], 36000[1], 36400[1], 36405[1], 36406[1], 36410[1], 36420[1], 36425[1], 36430[1], 36440[1], 36591[0], 36592[0], 36600[1], 36640[1], 43752[1], 51701[1], 51702[1], 51703[1], 62320[1], 62321[1], 62322[1], 62323[1], 62324[1], 62325[1], 62326[1], 62327[1], 64400[1], 64405[1], 64408[1], 64415[1], 64416[1], 64417[1], 64418[1], 64420[1], 64421[1], 64425[1], 64430[1], 64435[1], 64445[1], 64446[1], 64447[1], 64448[1], 64449[1], 64450[1], 64451[1], 64454[1], 64455[1], 64461[0], 64462[0], 64463[0], 64479[1], 64480[0], 64483[1], 64484[0], 64486[0], 64487[0], 64488[0], 64489[0], 64490[1], 64491[0], 64492[0], 64493[1], 64494[0], 64495[0], 64505[1], 64510[1], 64517[1], 64520[1], 64530[1], 64632[1], 69990[0], 92012[1], 92014[1], 92585[0], 93000[1], 93005[1], 93010[1], 93040[1], 93041[1], 93042[1], 93318[1], 93355[1], 94002[1], 94200[1], 94250[1], 94680[1], 94681[1], 94690[1], 94770[1], 95812[1], 95813[1], 95816[1], 95819[1], 95822[0], 95829[1], 95860[0], 95861[0], 95863[0], 95864[0], 95865[0], 95866[0], 95867[0], 95868[0], 95869[0], 95870[0], 95907[0], 95908[0], 95909[0], 95910[0], 95911[0], 95912[0], 95913[0], 95925[0], 95926[0], 95927[0], 95928[0], 95929[0], 95930[0], 95933[0], 95937[0], 95938[0], 95939[0], 95940[0], 95955[1], 96360[1], 96361[1], 96365[1], 96366[1], 96367[1], 96368[1], 96372[1], 96374[1], 96375[1], 96376[1], 96377[1], 96523[0], 99155[0], 99156[0], 99157[0], 99211[1], 99212[1], 99213[1], 99214[1], 99215[1], 99217[1], 99218[1], 99219[1], 99220[1], 99221[1], 99222[1], 99223[1], 99231[1], 99232[1], 99233[1], 99234[1], 99235[1], 99236[1], 99238[1], 99239[1], 99241[1], 99242[1], 99243[1], 99244[1], 99245[1], 99251[1], 99252[1], 99253[1], 99254[1], 99255[1], 99291[1], 99292[1], 99304[1], 99305[1], 99306[1], 99307[1], 99308[1], 99309[1], 99310[1], 99315[1], 99316[1], 99334[1], 99335[1], 99336[1], 99337[1], 99347[1], 99348[1], 99349[1], 99350[1], 99374[1], 99375[1], 99377[1], 99378[1], 99446[0], 99447[0], 99448[0], 99449[0], 99451[0], 99452[0], 99495[0], 99496[0], G0453[0], G0463[1], G0471[1], J0670[1], J2001[1]
64642	0213T[0], 0216T[0], 0228T[0], 0230T[0], 0333T[0], 0440T[1], 0441T[1], 0464T[0], 12001[1], 12002[1], 12004[1], 12005[1], 12006[1], 12007[1], 12011[1], 12013[1], 12014[1], 12015[1], 12016[1], 12017[1], 12018[1], 12020[1], 12021[1], 12031[1], 12032[1], 12034[1], 12035[1], 12036[1], 12037[1], 12041[1], 12042[1], 12044[1], 12045[1], 12046[1], 12047[1], 12051[1], 12052[1], 12053[1], 12054[1], 12055[1], 12056[1], 12057[1], 13100[1], 13101[1], 13102[1], 13120[1], 13121[1], 13122[1], 13131[1], 13132[1], 13133[1], 13151[1], 13152[1], 13153[1], 20550[1], 20551[1], 20552[1], 20553[1], 20560[1], 20561[1], 36000[1], 36400[1], 36405[1], 36406[1], 36410[1], 36420[1], 36425[1], 36430[1], 36440[1], 36591[0], 36592[0], 36600[1], 36640[1], 43752[1], 51701[1], 51702[1], 51703[1], 62320[0], 62321[0], 62322[0], 62323[0], 62324[0], 62325[0], 62326[0], 62327[0], 64400[0], 64405[0], 64408[0], 64415[0], 64416[0], 64417[0], 64418[0], 64420[0], 64421[0], 64425[0], 64430[0], 64435[0], 64445[0], 64446[0], 64447[0], 64448[0], 64449[0], 64450[0], 64451[0], 64454[0], 64461[0], 64462[0], 64463[0], 64479[0], 64480[0], 64483[0], 64484[0], 64486[0], 64487[0], 64488[0], 64489[0], 64490[0], 64491[0], 64492[0], 64493[0], 64494[0], 64495[0], 64505[0], 64510[0], 64517[0], 64520[0], 64530[0], 69990[0], 92012[1], 92014[1], 93000[1], 93005[1], 93010[1], 93040[1], 93041[1], 93042[1], 93318[1], 93355[1], 94002[1], 94200[1], 94250[1], 94680[1], 94681[1], 94690[1], 94770[1], 95812[1], 95813[1], 95816[1], 95819[1], 95829[1], 95930[0], 95933[0], 95937[0], 95940[0], 95941[0], 95955[1], 96360[1], 96361[1], 96365[1], 96366[1], 96367[1], 96368[1], 96372[1], 96374[1], 96375[1], 96376[1], 96377[1], 96523[0], 99155[0], 99156[0], 99157[0], 99211[1], 99212[1], 99213[1], 99214[1], 99215[1], 99217[1], 99218[1], 99219[1], 99220[1], 99221[1], 99222[1], 99223[1], 99231[1], 99232[1], 99233[1], 99234[1], 99235[1], 99236[1], 99238[1], 99239[1], 99241[1], 99242[1], 99243[1], 99244[1], 99245[1], 99251[1], 99252[1], 99253[1], 99254[1], 99255[1], 99291[1], 99292[1], 99304[1], 99305[1], 99306[1], 99307[1], 99308[1], 99309[1], 99310[1], 99315[1], 99316[1], 99334[1], 99335[1], 99336[1], 99337[1], 99347[1], 99348[1], 99349[1], 99350[1], 99374[1], 99375[1], 99377[1], 99378[1], 99446[0], 99447[0], 99448[0], 99449[0], 99451[0], 99452[0], G0453[0], G0463[1], G0471[1]
64643	0213T[0], 0216T[0], 0228T[0], 0230T[0], 0333T[0], 0440T[1], 0441T[1], 0464T[0], 12001[1], 12002[1], 12004[1], 12005[1], 12006[1], 12007[1], 12011[1], 12013[1], 12014[1], 12015[1], 12016[1], 12017[1], 12018[1], 12020[1], 12021[1], 12031[1], 12032[1], 12034[1], 12035[1], 12036[1], 12037[1], 12041[1], 12042[1], 12044[1], 12045[1], 12046[1], 12047[1], 12051[1], 12052[1], 12053[1], 12054[1], 12055[1], 12056[1], 12057[1], 13100[1], 13101[1], 13102[1], 13120[1], 13121[1], 13122[1], 13131[1], 13132[1], 13133[1], 13151[1], 13152[1], 13153[1], 20550[1], 20551[1], 20552[1], 20553[1], 20560[1], 20561[1], 36000[1], 36400[1], 36405[1], 36406[1], 36410[1], 36420[1], 36425[1], 36430[1], 36440[1], 36591[0], 36592[0], 36600[1], 36640[1], 43752[1], 51701[1], 51702[1], 51703[1], 61650[1], 62320[1], 62321[1], 62322[1], 62323[1], 62324[1], 62325[1], 62326[1], 62327[1], 64400[1], 64405[1], 64408[1], 64415[1], 64416[1], 64417[1], 64418[1], 64420[1], 64421[1], 64425[1], 64430[1], 64435[1], 64445[1], 64446[1], 64447[1], 64448[1], 64449[1], 64450[1], 64451[1], 64454[1], 64461[1], 64463[1], 64479[1], 64483[1], 64486[1], 64487[1], 64488[1], 64489[1], 64490[1], 64493[1], 64505[1], 64510[1], 64517[1], 64520[1], 64530[1], 69990[0], 93000[1], 93005[1], 93010[1], 93040[1], 93041[1], 93042[1], 93318[1], 93355[1], 94002[1], 94200[1], 94250[1], 94680[1], 94681[1], 94690[1], 94770[1], 95812[1], 95813[1], 95816[1], 95819[1], 95829[1], 95930[0], 95933[0], 95937[0], 95940[0], 95941[0], 95955[1], 96360[1], 96365[1], 96372[1], 96374[1], 96375[1], 96376[1], 96377[1], 96523[0], 99155[0], 99156[0], 99157[0], 99211[1], 99212[1], 99213[1], 99214[1], 99215[1], 99217[1], 99218[1], 99219[1], 99220[1], 99221[1], 99222[1], 99223[1], 99231[1], 99232[1], 99233[1], 99234[1], 99235[1], 99236[1], 99238[1], 99239[1], 99241[1], 99242[1], 99243[1], 99244[1], 99245[1], 99251[1], 99252[1], 99253[1], 99254[1], 99255[1], 99291[1], 99292[1], 99304[1], 99305[1], 99306[1], 99307[1], 99308[1], 99309[1], 99310[1], 99315[1], 99316[1], 99334[1], 99335[1], 99336[1], 99337[1], 99347[1], 99348[1], 99349[1], 99350[1], 99374[1], 99375[1], 99377[1], 99378[1], 99446[0], 99447[0], 99448[0], 99449[0], 99451[0], 99452[0], G0453[0], G0463[1], G0471[1]
64644	0213T[0], 0216T[0], 0228T[0], 0230T[0], 0333T[0], 0440T[1], 0441T[1], 0464T[0], 12001[1], 12002[1], 12004[1], 12005[1], 12006[1], 12007[1], 12011[1], 12013[1], 12014[1], 12015[1], 12016[1], 12017[1], 12018[1], 12020[1], 12021[1], 12031[1], 12032[1], 12034[1], 12035[1], 12036[1], 12037[1], 12041[1], 12042[1], 12044[1], 12045[1], 12046[1], 12047[1], 12051[1], 12052[1], 12053[1], 12054[1], 12055[1], 12056[1], 12057[1], 13100[1], 13101[1], 13102[1], 13120[1], 13121[1], 13122[1], 13131[1], 13132[1], 13133[1], 13151[1], 13152[1], 13153[1], 20550[1], 20551[1], 20552[1], 20553[1], 20560[1], 20561[1], 36000[1], 36400[1], 36405[1], 36406[1], 36410[1], 36420[1], 36425[1], 36430[1], 36440[1], 36591[0], 36592[0], 36600[1], 36640[1], 43752[1], 51701[1], 51702[1], 51703[1], 62320[0], 62321[0], 62322[0], 62323[0], 62324[0], 62325[0], 62326[0], 62327[0], 64400[0], 64405[0], 64408[0], 64415[0], 64416[0], 64417[0], 64418[0], 64420[0], 64421[0], 64425[0], 64430[0], 64435[0], 64445[0], 64446[0], 64447[0], 64448[0], 64449[0], 64450[0], 64451[0], 64454[0], 64461[0], 64462[0], 64463[0], 64479[0], 64480[0], 64483[0], 64484[0], 64486[0], 64487[0], 64488[0], 64489[0], 64490[0], 64491[0], 64492[0], 64493[0], 64494[0], 64495[0], 64505[0], 64510[0], 64517[0], 64520[0], 64530[0], 64642[0], 69990[0], 92012[1], 92014[1], 93000[1], 93005[1], 93010[1], 93040[1], 93041[1], 93042[1], 93318[1], 93355[1], 94002[1], 94200[1], 94250[1], 94680[1], 94681[1], 94690[1], 94770[1], 95812[1], 95813[1], 95816[1], 95819[1], 95829[1], 95930[0], 95933[0], 95937[0], 95940[0], 95941[0], 95955[1], 96360[1], 96361[1], 96365[1], 96366[1], 96367[1], 96368[1], 96372[1], 96374[1], 96375[1], 96376[1], 96377[1], 96523[0], 99155[0], 99156[0], 99157[0], 99211[1], 99212[1], 99213[1], 99214[1], 99215[1], 99217[1], 99218[1], 99219[1], 99220[1], 99221[1], 99222[1], 99223[1], 99231[1], 99232[1], 99233[1], 99234[1], 99235[1], 99236[1], 99238[1], 99239[1], 99241[1], 99242[1], 99243[1], 99244[1], 99245[1], 99251[1], 99252[1], 99253[1], 99254[1], 99255[1], 99291[1], 99292[1], 99304[1], 99305[1], 99306[1], 99307[1], 99308[1], 99309[1], 99310[1], 99315[1], 99316[1], 99334[1], 99335[1], 99336[1], 99337[1], 99347[1], 99348[1], 99349[1],

Appendix A: NCCI - CPT Codes

0 = Modifier usage not allowed or inappropriate 1 = Modifier usage allowed

Code 1	Code 2
	99350[1], 99374[1], 99375[1], 99377[1], 99378[1], 99446[0], 99447[0], 99448[0], 99449[0], 99451[0], 99452[0], G0453[0], G0463[1], G0471[1]
64645	0213T[0], 0216T[0], 0228T[0], 0230T[0], 0333T[0], 0440T[1], 0441T[1], 0464T[0], 12001[1], 12002[1], 12004[1], 12005[1], 12006[1], 12007[1], 12011[1], 12013[1], 12014[1], 12015[1], 12016[1], 12017[1], 12018[1], 12020[1], 12021[1], 12031[1], 12032[1], 12034[1], 12035[1], 12036[1], 12037[1], 12041[1], 12042[1], 12044[1], 12045[1], 12046[1], 12047[1], 12051[1], 12052[1], 12053[1], 12054[1], 12055[1], 12056[1], 12057[1], 13100[1], 13101[1], 13102[1], 13120[1], 13121[1], 13122[1], 13131[1], 13132[1], 13133[1], 13151[1], 13152[1], 13153[1], 20550[1], 20551[1], 20552[1], 20553[1], 20560[1], 20561[1], 36000[1], 36400[1], 36405[1], 36406[1], 36410[1], 36420[1], 36425[1], 36430[1], 36440[1], 36591[0], 36592[0], 36600[1], 36640[1], 43752[1], 51701[1], 51702[1], 51703[1], 61650[1], 62320[1], 62321[1], 62322[1], 62323[1], 62324[1], 62325[1], 62326[1], 62327[1], 64400[1], 64405[1], 64408[1], 64415[1], 64416[1], 64417[1], 64418[1], 64420[1], 64421[1], 64425[1], 64430[1], 64435[1], 64445[1], 64446[1], 64447[1], 64448[1], 64449[1], 64450[1], 64451[1], 64454[1], 64461[1], 64463[1], 64479[1], 64483[1], 64486[1], 64487[1], 64488[1], 64489[1], 64490[1], 64493[1], 64505[1], 64510[1], 64517[1], 64520[1], 64530[1], 69990[0], 93000[1], 93005[1], 93010[1], 93040[1], 93041[1], 93042[1], 93318[1], 93355[1], 94002[1], 94200[1], 94250[1], 94680[1], 94681[1], 94690[1], 94770[1], 95812[1], 95813[1], 95816[1], 95819[1], 95829[1], 95930[0], 95933[0], 95937[0], 95940[0], 95941[0], 95955[1], 96360[1], 96365[1], 96372[1], 96374[1], 96375[1], 96376[1], 96377[1], 96523[0], 99155[0], 99156[0], 99157[0], 99211[1], 99212[1], 99213[1], 99214[1], 99215[1], 99217[1], 99218[1], 99219[1], 99220[1], 99221[1], 99222[1], 99223[1], 99231[1], 99232[1], 99233[1], 99234[1], 99235[1], 99236[1], 99238[1], 99239[1], 99241[1], 99242[1], 99243[1], 99244[1], 99245[1], 99251[1], 99252[1], 99253[1], 99254[1], 99255[1], 99291[1], 99292[1], 99304[1], 99305[1], 99306[1], 99307[1], 99308[1], 99309[1], 99310[1], 99315[1], 99316[1], 99334[1], 99335[1], 99336[1], 99337[1], 99347[1], 99348[1], 99349[1], 99350[1], 99374[1], 99375[1], 99377[1], 99378[1], 99446[0], 99447[0], 99448[0], 99449[0], 99451[0], 99452[0], G0453[0], G0463[1], G0471[1]
64646	0213T[0], 0216T[0], 0228T[0], 0230T[0], 0333T[0], 0442T[1], 0464T[0], 12001[1], 12002[1], 12004[1], 12005[1], 12006[1], 12007[1], 12011[1], 12013[1], 12014[1], 12015[1], 12016[1], 12017[1], 12018[1], 12020[1], 12021[1], 12031[1], 12032[1], 12034[1], 12035[1], 12036[1], 12037[1], 12041[1], 12042[1], 12044[1], 12045[1], 12046[1], 12047[1], 12051[1], 12052[1], 12053[1], 12054[1], 12055[1], 12056[1], 12057[1], 13100[1], 13101[1], 13102[1], 13120[1], 13121[1], 13122[1], 13131[1], 13132[1], 13133[1], 13151[1], 13152[1], 13153[1], 20550[1], 20551[1], 20552[1], 20553[1], 20560[1], 20561[1], 36000[1], 36400[1], 36405[1], 36406[1], 36410[1], 36420[1], 36425[1], 36430[1], 36440[1], 36591[0], 36592[0], 36600[1], 36640[1], 43752[1], 51701[1], 51702[1], 51703[1], 62320[0], 62321[0], 62322[0], 62323[0], 62324[0], 62325[0], 62326[0], 62327[0], 64400[0], 64405[0], 64408[0], 64415[0], 64416[0], 64417[0], 64418[0], 64420[0], 64421[0], 64425[0], 64430[0], 64435[0], 64445[0], 64446[0], 64447[0], 64448[0], 64449[0], 64450[0], 64451[0], 64454[0], 64461[0], 64462[0], 64463[0], 64479[0], 64480[0], 64483[0], 64484[0], 64486[0], 64487[0], 64488[0], 64489[0], 64490[0], 64491[0], 64492[0], 64493[0], 64494[0], 64495[0], 64505[0], 64510[0], 64517[0], 64520[0], 64530[0], 69990[0], 92012[1], 92014[1], 93000[1], 93005[1], 93010[1], 93040[1], 93041[1], 93042[1], 93318[1], 93355[1], 94002[1], 94200[1], 94250[1], 94680[1], 94681[1], 94690[1], 94770[1], 95812[1], 95813[1], 95816[1], 95819[1], 95829[1], 95930[0], 95933[0], 95937[0], 95940[0], 95941[0], 95955[1], 96360[1], 96361[1], 96365[1], 96366[1], 96367[1], 96368[1], 96372[1], 96374[1], 96375[1], 96376[1], 96377[1], 96523[0], 99155[0], 99156[0], 99157[0], 99211[1], 99212[1], 99213[1], 99214[1], 99215[1], 99217[1], 99218[1], 99219[1], 99220[1], 99221[1], 99222[1], 99223[1], 99231[1], 99232[1], 99233[1], 99234[1], 99235[1], 99236[1], 99238[1], 99239[1], 99241[1], 99242[1], 99243[1], 99244[1], 99245[1], 99251[1], 99252[1], 99253[1], 99254[1], 99255[1], 99291[1], 99292[1], 99304[1], 99305[1], 99306[1], 99307[1], 99308[1], 99309[1], 99310[1], 99315[1], 99316[1], 99334[1], 99335[1], 99336[1], 99337[1], 99347[1], 99348[1], 99349[1], 99350[1], 99374[1], 99375[1], 99377[1], 99378[1], 99446[0], 99447[0], 99448[0], 99449[0], 99451[0], 99452[0], G0453[0], G0463[1], G0471[1]
64647	0213T[0], 0216T[0], 0228T[0], 0230T[0], 0333T[0], 0442T[1], 0464T[0], 12001[1], 12002[1], 12004[1], 12005[1], 12006[1], 12007[1], 12011[1], 12013[1], 12014[1], 12015[1], 12016[1], 12017[1], 12018[1], 12020[1], 12021[1], 12031[1], 12032[1], 12034[1], 12035[1], 12036[1], 12037[1], 12041[1], 12042[1], 12044[1], 12045[1], 12046[1], 12047[1], 12051[1], 12052[1], 12053[1], 12054[1], 12055[1], 12056[1], 12057[1], 13100[1], 13101[1], 13102[1], 13120[1], 13121[1], 13122[1], 13131[1], 13132[1], 13133[1], 13151[1], 13152[1], 13153[1], 20550[1], 20551[1], 20552[1], 20553[1], 20560[1], 20561[1], 36000[1], 36400[1], 36405[1], 36406[1], 36410[1], 36420[1], 36425[1], 36430[1], 36440[1], 36591[0], 36592[0], 36600[1], 36640[1], 43752[1], 51701[1], 51702[1], 51703[1], 62320[0], 62321[0], 62322[0], 62323[0], 62324[0], 62325[0], 62326[0], 62327[0], 64400[0], 64405[0], 64408[0], 64415[0], 64416[0], 64417[0], 64418[0], 64420[0], 64421[0], 64425[0], 64430[0], 64435[0], 64445[0], 64446[0], 64447[0], 64448[0], 64449[0], 64450[0], 64451[0], 64454[0], 64461[0], 64462[0], 64463[0], 64479[0], 64480[0], 64483[0], 64484[0], 64486[0], 64487[0], 64488[0], 64489[0], 64490[0], 64491[0], 64492[0], 64493[0], 64494[0], 64495[0], 64505[0], 64510[0], 64517[0], 64520[0], 64530[0], 64615[1], 64646[0], 69990[0], 92012[1], 92014[1], 93000[1], 93005[1], 93010[1], 93040[1], 93041[1], 93042[1], 93318[1], 93355[1], 94002[1], 94200[1], 94250[1], 94680[1], 94681[1], 94690[1], 94770[1], 95812[1], 95813[1], 95816[1], 95819[1], 95829[1], 95930[0], 95933[0], 95937[0], 95940[0], 95941[0], 95955[1], 96360[1], 96361[1], 96365[1], 96366[1], 96367[1], 96368[1], 96372[1], 96374[1], 96375[1], 96376[1], 96377[1], 96523[0], 99155[0], 99156[0], 99157[0], 99211[1], 99212[1], 99213[1], 99214[1], 99215[1], 99217[1], 99218[1], 99219[1], 99220[1], 99221[1], 99222[1], 99223[1], 99231[1], 99232[1], 99233[1], 99234[1], 99235[1], 99236[1], 99238[1], 99239[1], 99241[1], 99242[1], 99243[1], 99244[1], 99245[1], 99251[1], 99252[1], 99253[1], 99254[1], 99255[1], 99291[1], 99292[1], 99304[1], 99305[1], 99306[1], 99307[1], 99308[1], 99309[1], 99310[1], 99315[1], 99316[1], 99334[1], 99335[1], 99336[1], 99337[1], 99347[1], 99348[1], 99349[1], 99350[1], 99374[1], 99375[1], 99377[1], 99378[1], 99446[0], 99447[0], 99448[0], 99449[0], 99451[0], 99452[0], G0453[0], G0463[1], G0471[1]
64650	00400[0], 01610[0], 01710[0], 01991[0], 0213T[0], 0216T[0], 0228T[0], 0230T[0], 0333T[0], 0464T[0], 12001[1], 12002[1], 12004[1], 12005[1], 12006[1], 12007[1], 12011[1], 12013[1], 12014[1], 12015[1], 12016[1], 12017[1], 12018[1], 12020[1], 12021[1], 12031[1], 12032[1], 12034[1], 12035[1], 12036[1], 12037[1], 12041[1], 12042[1], 12044[1], 12045[1], 12046[1], 12047[1], 12051[1], 12052[1], 12053[1], 12054[1], 12055[1], 12056[1], 12057[1], 13100[1], 13101[1], 13102[1], 13120[1], 13121[1], 13122[1], 13131[1], 13132[1], 13133[1], 13151[1], 13152[1], 13153[1], 20550[1], 20551[1], 20552[1], 20553[1], 20560[1], 20561[1], 36000[1], 36400[1], 36405[1], 36406[1], 36410[1], 36420[1], 36425[1], 36430[1], 36440[1], 36591[0], 36592[0], 36600[1], 36640[1], 43752[1], 51701[1], 51702[1], 51703[1], 62320[1], 62321[1], 62322[1], 62323[1], 62324[1], 62325[1], 62326[1], 62327[1], 64400[1], 64405[1], 64408[1], 64415[1], 64416[1], 64417[1], 64418[1], 64420[1], 64421[1], 64425[1], 64430[1], 64435[1], 64445[1], 64446[1], 64447[1], 64448[1], 64449[1], 64450[1], 64451[1], 64454[1], 64461[0], 64462[0], 64463[0], 64479[1], 64480[0], 64483[1], 64484[0], 64486[0], 64487[0], 64488[0], 64489[0], 64490[1], 64491[0], 64492[0], 64493[1], 64494[0], 64495[0], 64505[1], 64510[1], 64517[1], 64520[1], 64530[1], 92012[1], 92014[1], 92585[0], 93000[1], 93005[1], 93010[1], 93040[1], 93041[1], 93042[1], 93318[1], 93355[1], 94002[1], 94200[1], 94250[1], 94680[1], 94681[1], 94690[1], 94770[1], 95812[1], 95813[1], 95816[1], 95819[1], 95822[0], 95829[1], 95860[0], 95861[0], 95863[0], 95864[0], 95865[0], 95866[0], 95867[0], 95868[0], 95869[0], 95870[0], 95907[0], 95908[0], 95909[0], 95910[0], 95911[0], 95912[0], 95913[0], 95925[0], 95926[0], 95927[0], 95928[0], 95929[0], 95930[0], 95933[0], 95937[0], 95938[0], 95939[0], 95940[0], 95955[1], 96360[1], 96361[1], 96365[1], 96366[1], 96367[1], 96368[1], 96372[1], 96374[1], 96375[1], 96376[1], 96377[1], 96523[0], 99155[0], 99156[0], 99157[0], 99211[1], 99212[1], 99213[1], 99214[1], 99215[1], 99217[1], 99218[1], 99219[1], 99220[1], 99221[1], 99222[1], 99223[1], 99231[1], 99232[1], 99233[1], 99234[1], 99235[1], 99236[1], 99238[1], 99239[1], 99241[1], 99242[1], 99243[1], 99244[1], 99245[1], 99251[1], 99252[1], 99253[1], 99254[1], 99255[1], 99291[1], 99292[1], 99304[1], 99305[1], 99306[1], 99307[1], 99308[1], 99309[1], 99310[1], 99315[1], 99316[1], 99334[1], 99335[1], 99336[1], 99337[1], 99347[1], 99348[1], 99349[1], 99350[1], 99374[1], 99375[1], 99377[1], 99378[1], 99446[0], 99447[0], 99448[0], 99449[0], 99451[0], 99452[0], 99495[1], 99496[1], G0453[0], G0463[1], G0471[1], J2001[1]
64653	00160[0], 00218[0], 00300[0], 00400[0], 01320[0], 01470[0], 01610[0], 01710[0], 01810[0], 01991[0], 0213T[0], 0216T[0], 0228T[0], 0230T[0], 0333T[0], 0464T[0], 12001[1], 12002[1], 12004[1], 12005[1], 12006[1], 12007[1], 12011[1], 12013[1], 12014[1], 12015[1], 12016[1], 12017[1], 12018[1], 12020[1], 12021[1], 12031[1], 12032[1], 12034[1], 12035[1], 12036[1], 12037[1], 12041[1], 12042[1], 12044[1], 12045[1], 12046[1], 12047[1], 12051[1], 12052[1], 12053[1], 12054[1], 12055[1], 12056[1], 12057[1], 13100[1], 13101[1], 13102[1], 13120[1], 13121[1], 13122[1], 13131[1], 13132[1], 13133[1], 13151[1], 13152[1], 13153[1], 20550[1], 20551[1], 20552[1], 20553[1], 20560[1], 20561[1], 36000[1], 36400[1], 36405[1], 36406[1], 36410[1], 36420[1], 36425[1], 36430[1], 36440[1], 36591[0], 36592[0], 36600[1], 36640[1], 43752[1], 51701[1], 51702[1], 51703[1], 62320[1], 62321[1], 62322[1], 62323[1], 62324[1], 62325[1], 62326[1], 62327[1], 64400[1], 64405[1], 64408[1], 64415[1], 64416[1], 64417[1], 64418[1], 64420[1], 64421[1], 64425[1], 64430[1], 64435[1], 64445[1], 64446[1], 64447[1], 64448[1], 64449[1], 64450[1], 64451[1], 64454[1], 64461[0], 64462[0], 64463[0], 64479[1], 64480[0], 64483[1], 64484[0], 64486[0], 64487[0], 64488[0], 64489[0], 64490[1], 64491[0], 64492[0], 64493[1], 64494[0], 64495[0], 64505[1], 64510[1], 64517[1], 64520[1], 64530[1], 92012[1], 92014[1], 92585[0], 93000[1], 93005[1], 93010[1], 93040[1], 93041[1], 93042[1], 93318[1], 93355[1], 94002[1], 94200[1], 94250[1], 94680[1], 94681[1], 94690[1], 94770[1], 95812[1], 95813[1], 95816[1], 95819[1], 95822[0], 95829[1], 95860[0], 95861[0], 95863[0], 95864[0], 95865[0], 95866[0], 95867[0], 95868[0], 95869[0], 95870[0], 95907[0], 95908[0], 95909[0], 95910[0], 95911[0], 95912[0], 95913[0], 95925[0], 95926[0], 95927[0], 95928[0], 95929[0], 95930[0], 95933[0], 95937[0], 95938[0], 95939[0], 95940[0], 95955[1], 96360[1], 96361[1], 96365[1], 96366[1], 96367[1], 96368[1], 96372[1], 96374[1], 96375[1], 96376[1], 96377[1], 96523[0], 99155[0], 99156[0], 99157[0], 99211[1], 99212[1], 99213[1], 99214[1], 99215[1], 99217[1], 99218[1], 99219[1], 99220[1], 99221[1], 99222[1], 99223[1], 99231[1], 99232[1], 99233[1], 99234[1], 99235[1], 99236[1], 99238[1], 99239[1], 99241[1], 99242[1], 99243[1], 99244[1], 99245[1], 99251[1], 99252[1], 99253[1], 99254[1], 99255[1], 99291[1], 99292[1], 99304[1], 99305[1], 99306[1], 99307[1], 99308[1], 99309[1], 99310[1], 99315[1], 99316[1], 99334[1], 99335[1], 99336[1], 99337[1], 99347[1], 99348[1], 99349[1], 99350[1], 99374[1], 99375[1], 99377[1], 99378[1], 99446[0], 99447[0], 99448[0], 99449[0], 99451[0], 99452[0], 99495[1], 99496[1], G0453[0], G0463[1], G0471[1], J2001[1]
64681	0216T[0], 0228T[0], 0230T[0], 0333T[0], 0464T[0], 12001[1], 12002[1], 12004[1], 12005[1], 12006[1], 12007[1], 12011[1], 12013[1], 12014[1], 12015[1], 12016[1], 12017[1], 12018[1], 12020[1], 12021[1], 12031[1], 12032[1], 12034[1], 12035[1], 12036[1], 12037[1], 12041[1], 12042[1], 12044[1], 12045[1],

0 = Modifier usage not allowed or inappropriate 1 = Modifier usage allowed

Code 1	Code 2
	12046[1], 12047[1], 12051[1], 12052[1], 12053[1], 12054[1], 12055[1], 12056[1], 12057[1], 13100[1], 13101[1], 13102[1], 13120[1], 13121[1], 13122[1], 13131[1], 13132[1], 13133[1], 13151[1], 13152[1], 13153[1], 20550[1], 20551[1], 20552[1], 20553[1], 20560[1], 20561[1], 36000[1], 36400[1], 36405[1], 36406[1], 36410[1], 36420[1], 36425[1], 36430[1], 36440[1], 36591[0], 36592[0], 36600[1], 36640[1], 43752[1], 51701[1], 51702[1], 51703[1], 62320[1], 62321[1], 62322[1], 62323[1], 62324[1], 62325[1], 62326[1], 62327[1], 64400[1], 64405[1], 64408[1], 64415[1], 64416[1], 64417[1], 64418[1], 64420[1], 64421[1], 64425[1], 64430[1], 64435[1], 64445[1], 64446[1], 64447[1], 64448[1], 64449[1], 64450[1], 64451[1], 64454[1], 64461[0], 64462[0], 64463[0], 64479[1], 64480[0], 64483[1], 64484[0], 64486[0], 64487[0], 64488[0], 64489[0], 64493[1], 64494[0], 64495[0], 64505[1], 64510[1], 64517[1], 64520[1], 64530[1], 69990[0], 76000[1], 77001[1], 77002[1], 77003[1], 92012[1], 92014[1], 92585[0], 93000[1], 93005[1], 93010[1], 93040[1], 93041[1], 93042[1], 93318[1], 93355[1], 94002[1], 94200[1], 94250[1], 94680[1], 94681[1], 94690[1], 94770[1], 95812[1], 95813[1], 95816[1], 95819[1], 95822[0], 95829[1], 95860[0], 95861[0], 95863[0], 95864[0], 95865[0], 95866[0], 95867[0], 95868[0], 95869[0], 95870[0], 95907[0], 95908[0], 95909[0], 95910[0], 95911[0], 95912[0], 95913[0], 95925[0], 95926[0], 95927[0], 95928[0], 95929[0], 95930[0], 95933[0], 95937[0], 95938[0], 95939[0], 95940[0], 95955[1], 96360[1], 96361[1], 96365[1], 96366[1], 96367[1], 96368[1], 96372[1], 96374[1], 96375[1], 96376[1], 96377[1], 96523[0], 99155[0], 99156[0], 99157[0], 99211[1], 99212[1], 99213[1], 99214[1], 99215[1], 99217[1], 99218[1], 99219[1], 99220[1], 99221[1], 99222[1], 99223[1], 99231[1], 99232[1], 99233[1], 99234[1], 99235[1], 99236[1], 99238[1], 99239[1], 99241[1], 99242[1], 99243[1], 99244[1], 99245[1], 99251[1], 99252[1], 99253[1], 99254[1], 99255[1], 99291[1], 99292[1], 99304[1], 99305[1], 99306[1], 99307[1], 99308[1], 99309[1], 99310[1], 99315[1], 99316[1], 99334[1], 99335[1], 99336[1], 99337[1], 99347[1], 99348[1], 99349[1], 99350[1], 99374[1], 99375[1], 99377[1], 99378[1], 99446[0], 99447[0], 99448[0], 99449[0], 99451[0], 99452[0], 99495[0], 99496[0], G0453[0], G0463[1], G0471[1]
64708	01250[0], 01320[0], 01470[0], 01610[0], 01710[0], 01782[0], 01810[0], 0213T[0], 0216T[0], 0228T[0], 0230T[0], 0333T[0], 0464T[0], 11000[1], 11001[1], 11004[1], 11005[1], 11006[1], 11042[1], 11043[1], 11044[1], 11045[1], 11046[1], 11047[1], 12001[1], 12002[1], 12004[1], 12005[1], 12006[1], 12007[1], 12011[1], 12013[1], 12014[1], 12015[1], 12016[1], 12017[1], 12018[1], 12020[1], 12021[1], 12031[1], 12032[1], 12034[1], 12035[1], 12036[1], 12037[1], 12041[1], 12042[1], 12044[1], 12045[1], 12046[1], 12047[1], 12051[1], 12052[1], 12053[1], 12054[1], 12055[1], 12056[1], 12057[1], 13100[1], 13101[1], 13102[1], 13120[1], 13121[1], 13122[1], 13131[1], 13132[1], 13133[1], 13151[1], 13152[1], 13153[1], 24332[1], 25000[1], 28070[1], 28086[1], 28088[1], 28090[1], 29125[1], 36000[1], 36400[1], 36405[1], 36406[1], 36410[1], 36420[1], 36425[1], 36430[1], 36440[1], 36591[0], 36592[0], 36600[1], 36640[1], 43752[1], 51701[1], 51702[1], 51703[1], 62320[0], 62321[0], 62322[0], 62323[0], 62324[0], 62325[0], 62326[0], 62327[0], 64400[0], 64405[0], 64408[0], 64415[0], 64416[0], 64417[0], 64418[0], 64420[0], 64421[0], 64425[0], 64430[0], 64435[0], 64445[0], 64446[0], 64447[0], 64448[0], 64449[0], 64450[0], 64451[0], 64454[0], 64461[0], 64462[0], 64463[0], 64479[0], 64480[0], 64483[0], 64484[0], 64486[0], 64487[0], 64488[0], 64489[0], 64490[0], 64491[0], 64492[0], 64493[0], 64494[0], 64495[0], 64505[0], 64510[0], 64517[0], 64520[0], 64530[0], 64718[1], 64719[1], 64721[1], 64722[1], 64795[1], 64856[1], 64857[1], 69990[0], 92012[1], 92014[1], 92585[0], 93000[1], 93005[1], 93010[1], 93040[1], 93041[1], 93042[1], 93318[1], 93355[1], 94002[1], 94200[1], 94250[1], 94680[1], 94681[1], 94690[1], 94770[1], 95812[1], 95813[1], 95816[1], 95819[1], 95822[0], 95829[1], 95860[0], 95861[0], 95863[0], 95864[0], 95865[0], 95866[0], 95867[0], 95868[0], 95869[0], 95870[0], 95907[0], 95908[0], 95909[0], 95910[0], 95911[0], 95912[0], 95913[0], 95925[0], 95926[0], 95927[0], 95928[0], 95929[0], 95930[0], 95933[0], 95937[0], 95938[0], 95939[0], 95940[0], 95955[1], 96360[1], 96361[1], 96365[1], 96366[1], 96367[1], 96368[1], 96372[1], 96374[1], 96375[1], 96376[1], 96377[1], 96523[0], 97597[1], 97598[1], 97602[1], 97605[1], 97606[1], 97607[1], 97608[1], 99155[0], 99156[0], 99157[0], 99211[1], 99212[1], 99213[1], 99214[1], 99215[1], 99217[1], 99218[1], 99219[1], 99220[1], 99221[1], 99222[1], 99223[1], 99231[1], 99232[1], 99233[1], 99234[1], 99235[1], 99236[1], 99238[1], 99239[1], 99241[1], 99242[1], 99243[1], 99244[1], 99245[1], 99251[1], 99252[1], 99253[1], 99254[1], 99255[1], 99291[1], 99292[1], 99304[1], 99305[1], 99306[1], 99307[1], 99308[1], 99309[1], 99310[1], 99315[1], 99316[1], 99334[1], 99335[1], 99336[1], 99337[1], 99347[1], 99348[1], 99349[1], 99350[1], 99374[1], 99375[1], 99377[1], 99378[1], 99446[0], 99447[0], 99448[0], 99449[0], 99451[0], 99452[0], 99495[0], 99496[0], G0453[0], G0463[1], G0471[1]
64712	01250[0], 01320[0], 01470[0], 01610[0], 01710[0], 01782[0], 01810[0], 0213T[0], 0216T[0], 0228T[0], 0230T[0], 0333T[0], 0464T[0], 11000[1], 11001[1], 11004[1], 11005[1], 11006[1], 11042[1], 11043[1], 11044[1], 11045[1], 11046[1], 11047[1], 12001[1], 12002[1], 12004[1], 12005[1], 12006[1], 12007[1], 12011[1], 12013[1], 12014[1], 12015[1], 12016[1], 12017[1], 12018[1], 12020[1], 12021[1], 12031[1], 12032[1], 12034[1], 12035[1], 12036[1], 12037[1], 12041[1], 12042[1], 12044[1], 12045[1], 12046[1], 12047[1], 12051[1], 12052[1], 12053[1], 12054[1], 12055[1], 12056[1], 12057[1], 13100[1], 13101[1], 13102[1], 13120[1], 13121[1], 13122[1], 13131[1], 13132[1], 13133[1], 13151[1], 13152[1], 13153[1], 27305[1], 27345[1], 27496[1], 27600[1], 27601[1], 27630[1], 36000[1], 36400[1], 36405[1], 36406[1], 36410[1], 36420[1], 36425[1], 36430[1], 36440[1], 36591[0], 36592[0], 36600[1], 36640[1], 43752[1], 51701[1], 51702[1], 51703[1], 62320[0], 62321[0], 62322[0], 62323[0], 62324[0], 62325[0], 62326[0], 62327[0], 64400[0], 64405[0], 64408[0], 64415[0], 64416[0], 64417[0], 64418[0], 64420[0], 64421[0], 64425[0], 64430[0], 64435[0], 64445[0], 64446[0], 64447[0], 64448[0], 64449[0], 64450[0], 64451[0], 64454[0], 64461[0], 64462[0], 64463[0], 64479[0], 64480[0], 64483[0], 64484[0], 64486[0], 64487[0], 64488[0], 64489[0], 64490[0], 64491[0], 64492[0], 64493[0], 64494[0], 64495[0], 64505[0], 64510[0], 64517[0], 64520[0], 64530[0], 64722[1], 64795[1], 64858[1], 69990[0], 92012[1], 92014[1], 92585[0], 93000[1], 93005[1], 93010[1], 93040[1], 93041[1], 93042[1], 93318[1], 93355[1], 94002[1], 94200[1], 94250[1], 94680[1], 94681[1], 94690[1], 94770[1], 95812[1], 95813[1], 95816[1], 95819[1], 95822[0], 95829[1], 95860[0], 95861[0], 95863[0], 95864[0], 95865[0], 95866[0], 95867[0], 95868[0], 95869[0], 95870[0], 95907[0], 95908[0], 95909[0], 95910[0], 95911[0], 95912[0], 95913[0], 95925[0], 95926[0], 95927[0], 95928[0], 95929[0], 95930[0], 95933[0], 95937[0], 95938[0], 95939[0], 95940[0], 95955[1], 96360[1], 96361[1], 96365[1], 96366[1], 96367[1], 96368[1], 96372[1], 96374[1], 96375[1], 96376[1], 96377[1], 96523[0], 97597[1], 97598[1], 97602[1], 97605[1], 97606[1], 97607[1], 97608[1], 99155[0], 99156[0], 99157[0], 99211[1], 99212[1], 99213[1], 99214[1], 99215[1], 99217[1], 99218[1], 99219[1], 99220[1], 99221[1], 99222[1], 99223[1], 99231[1], 99232[1], 99233[1], 99234[1], 99235[1], 99236[1], 99238[1], 99239[1], 99241[1], 99242[1], 99243[1], 99244[1], 99245[1], 99251[1], 99252[1], 99253[1], 99254[1], 99255[1], 99291[1], 99292[1], 99304[1], 99305[1], 99306[1], 99307[1], 99308[1], 99309[1], 99310[1], 99315[1], 99316[1], 99334[1], 99335[1], 99336[1], 99337[1], 99347[1], 99348[1], 99349[1], 99350[1], 99374[1], 99375[1], 99377[1], 99378[1], 99446[0], 99447[0], 99448[0], 99449[0], 99451[0], 99452[0], 99495[0], 99496[0], G0453[0], G0463[1], G0471[1]
64713	0213T[0], 0216T[0], 0228T[0], 0230T[0], 0333T[0], 0464T[0], 11000[1], 11001[1], 11004[1], 11005[1], 11006[1], 11042[1], 11043[1], 11044[1], 11045[1], 11046[1], 11047[1], 12001[1], 12002[1], 12004[1], 12005[1], 12006[1], 12007[1], 12011[1], 12013[1], 12014[1], 12015[1], 12016[1], 12017[1], 12018[1], 12020[1], 12021[1], 12031[1], 12032[1], 12034[1], 12035[1], 12036[1], 12037[1], 12041[1], 12042[1], 12044[1], 12045[1], 12046[1], 12047[1], 12051[1], 12052[1], 12053[1], 12054[1], 12055[1], 12056[1], 12057[1], 13100[1], 13101[1], 13102[1], 13120[1], 13121[1], 13122[1], 13131[1], 13132[1], 13133[1], 13151[1], 13152[1], 13153[1], 21700[0], 21705[0], 36000[1], 36400[1], 36405[1], 36406[1], 36410[1], 36420[1], 36425[1], 36430[1], 36440[1], 36591[0], 36592[0], 36600[1], 36640[1], 43752[1], 51701[1], 51702[1], 51703[1], 62320[0], 62321[0], 62322[0], 62323[0], 62324[0], 62325[0], 62326[0], 62327[0], 64400[0], 64405[0], 64408[0], 64415[0], 64416[0], 64417[0], 64418[0], 64420[0], 64421[0], 64425[0], 64430[0], 64435[0], 64445[0], 64446[0], 64447[0], 64448[0], 64449[0], 64450[0], 64451[0], 64454[0], 64461[0], 64462[0], 64463[0], 64479[0], 64480[0], 64483[0], 64484[0], 64486[0], 64487[0], 64488[0], 64489[0], 64490[0], 64491[0], 64492[0], 64493[0], 64494[0], 64495[0], 64505[0], 64510[0], 64517[0], 64520[0], 64530[0], 64722[1], 64795[1], 64861[1], 69990[0], 92012[1], 92014[1], 92585[0], 93000[1], 93005[1], 93010[1], 93040[1], 93041[1], 93042[1], 93318[1], 93355[1], 94002[1], 94200[1], 94250[1], 94680[1], 94681[1], 94690[1], 94770[1], 95812[1], 95813[1], 95816[1], 95819[1], 95822[0], 95829[1], 95860[0], 95861[0], 95863[0], 95864[0], 95865[0], 95866[0], 95867[0], 95868[0], 95869[0], 95870[0], 95907[0], 95908[0], 95909[0], 95910[0], 95911[0], 95912[0], 95913[0], 95925[0], 95926[0], 95927[0], 95928[0], 95929[0], 95930[0], 95933[0], 95937[0], 95938[0], 95939[0], 95940[0], 95955[1], 96360[1], 96361[1], 96365[1], 96366[1], 96367[1], 96368[1], 96372[1], 96374[1], 96375[1], 96376[1], 96377[1], 96523[0], 97597[1], 97598[1], 97602[1], 97605[1], 97606[1], 97607[1], 97608[1], 99155[0], 99156[0], 99157[0], 99211[1], 99212[1], 99213[1], 99214[1], 99215[1], 99217[1], 99218[1], 99219[1], 99220[1], 99221[1], 99222[1], 99223[1], 99231[1], 99232[1], 99233[1], 99234[1], 99235[1], 99236[1], 99238[1], 99239[1], 99241[1], 99242[1], 99243[1], 99244[1], 99245[1], 99251[1], 99252[1], 99253[1], 99254[1], 99255[1], 99291[1], 99292[1], 99304[1], 99305[1], 99306[1], 99307[1], 99308[1], 99309[1], 99310[1], 99315[1], 99316[1], 99334[1], 99335[1], 99336[1], 99337[1], 99347[1], 99348[1], 99349[1], 99350[1], 99374[1], 99375[1], 99377[1], 99378[1], 99446[0], 99447[0], 99448[0], 99449[0], 99451[0], 99452[0], 99495[0], 99496[0], G0453[0], G0463[1], G0471[1]
64714	0213T[0], 0216T[0], 0228T[0], 0230T[0], 0333T[0], 0464T[0], 11000[1], 11001[1], 11004[1], 11005[1], 11006[1], 11042[1], 11043[1], 11044[1], 11045[1], 11046[1], 11047[1], 12001[1], 12002[1], 12004[1], 12005[1], 12006[1], 12007[1], 12011[1], 12013[1], 12014[1], 12015[1], 12016[1], 12017[1], 12018[1], 12020[1], 12021[1], 12031[1], 12032[1], 12034[1], 12035[1], 12036[1], 12037[1], 12041[1], 12042[1], 12044[1], 12045[1], 12046[1], 12047[1], 12051[1], 12052[1], 12053[1], 12054[1], 12055[1], 12056[1], 12057[1], 13100[1], 13101[1], 13102[1], 13120[1], 13121[1], 13122[1], 13131[1], 13132[1], 13133[1], 13151[1], 13152[1], 13153[1], 20551[1], 20552[1], 20553[1], 20560[1], 20561[1], 27305[1], 27345[1], 27496[1], 27600[1], 27601[1], 27630[1], 36000[1], 36400[1], 36405[1], 36406[1], 36410[1], 36420[1], 36425[1], 36430[1], 36440[1], 36591[0], 36592[0], 36600[1], 36640[1], 43752[1], 51701[1], 51702[1], 51703[1], 62320[0], 62321[0], 62322[0], 62323[0], 62324[0], 62325[0], 62326[0], 62327[0], 64400[0], 64405[0], 64408[0], 64415[0], 64416[0], 64417[0], 64418[0], 64420[0], 64421[0], 64425[0], 64430[0], 64435[0], 64445[0], 64446[0], 64447[0], 64448[0], 64449[0], 64450[0], 64451[0], 64454[0], 64461[0], 64462[0], 64463[0], 64479[0], 64480[0], 64483[0], 64484[0], 64486[0], 64487[0], 64488[0], 64489[0], 64490[0], 64491[0], 64492[0], 64493[0], 64494[0], 64495[0], 64505[0], 64510[0], 64517[0], 64520[0], 64530[0], 64722[1], 64795[1], 64862[1], 69990[0], 92012[1], 92014[1], 92585[0], 93000[1], 93005[1], 93010[1], 93040[1], 93041[1], 93042[1], 93318[1], 93355[1], 94002[1], 94200[1], 94250[1], 94680[1], 94681[1], 94690[1], 94770[1], 95812[1], 95813[1], 95816[1], 95819[1], 95822[0], 95829[1], 95860[0], 95861[0], 95863[0], 95864[0], 95865[0], 95866[0], 95867[0], 95868[0], 95869[0], 95870[0], 95907[0], 95908[0], 95909[0], 95910[0], 95911[0], 95912[0], 95913[0], 95925[0], 95926[0], 95927[0], 95928[0], 95929[0], 95930[0], 95933[0], 95937[0], 95938[0], 95939[0], 95940[0], 95955[1], 96360[1], 96361[1], 96365[1], 96366[1], 96367[1], 96368[1], 96372[1], 96374[1], 96375[1], 96376[1], 96377[1], 96523[0], 97597[1], 97598[1], 97602[1], 97605[1], 97606[1], 97607[1], 97608[1], 99155[0], 99156[0], 99157[0],

0 = Modifier usage not allowed or inappropriate 1 = Modifier usage allowed

Code 1	Code 2
	99211[1], 99212[1], 99213[1], 99214[1], 99215[1], 99217[1], 99218[1], 99219[1], 99220[1], 99221[1], 99222[1], 99223[1], 99231[1], 99232[1], 99233[1], 99234[1], 99235[1], 99236[1], 99238[1], 99239[1], 99241[1], 99242[1], 99243[1], 99244[1], 99245[1], 99251[1], 99252[1], 99253[1], 99254[1], 99255[1], 99291[1], 99292[1], 99304[1], 99305[1], 99306[1], 99307[1], 99308[1], 99309[1], 99310[1], 99315[1], 99316[1], 99334[1], 99335[1], 99336[1], 99337[1], 99347[1], 99348[1], 99349[1], 99350[1], 99374[1], 99375[1], 99377[1], 99378[1], 99446[0], 99447[0], 99448[0], 99449[0], 99451[0], 99452[0], 99495[0], 99496[0], G0453[0], G0463[1], G0471[1]
64718	01250[0], 01320[0], 01470[0], 01610[0], 01710[0], 01782[0], 01810[0], 0213T[0], 0216T[0], 0228T[0], 0230T[0], 0333T[0], 0464T[0], 11000[1], 11001[1], 11004[1], 11005[1], 11006[1], 11042[1], 11043[1], 11044[1], 11045[1], 11046[1], 11047[1], 12001[1], 12002[1], 12004[1], 12005[1], 12006[1], 12007[1], 12011[1], 12013[1], 12014[1], 12015[1], 12016[1], 12017[1], 12018[1], 12020[1], 12021[1], 12031[1], 12032[1], 12034[1], 12035[1], 12036[1], 12037[1], 12041[1], 12042[1], 12044[1], 12045[1], 12046[1], 12047[1], 12051[1], 12052[1], 12053[1], 12054[1], 12055[1], 12056[1], 12057[1], 13100[1], 13101[1], 13102[1], 13120[1], 13121[1], 13122[1], 13131[1], 13132[1], 13133[1], 13151[1], 13152[1], 13153[1], 24310[1], 24332[1], 24357[1], 24358[1], 25290[1], 29105[1], 36000[1], 36400[1], 36405[1], 36406[1], 36410[1], 36420[1], 36425[1], 36430[1], 36440[1], 36591[0], 36592[0], 36600[1], 36640[1], 43752[1], 51701[1], 51702[1], 51703[1], 62320[0], 62321[0], 62322[0], 62323[0], 62324[0], 62325[0], 62326[0], 62327[0], 64400[0], 64405[0], 64408[0], 64415[0], 64416[0], 64417[0], 64418[0], 64420[0], 64421[0], 64425[0], 64430[0], 64435[0], 64445[0], 64446[0], 64447[0], 64448[0], 64449[0], 64450[0], 64451[0], 64454[0], 64461[0], 64462[0], 64463[0], 64479[0], 64480[0], 64483[0], 64484[0], 64486[0], 64487[0], 64488[0], 64489[0], 64490[0], 64491[0], 64492[0], 64493[0], 64494[0], 64495[0], 64505[0], 64510[0], 64517[0], 64520[0], 64530[0], 64722[1], 64795[1], 64836[1], 69990[0], 92012[1], 92014[1], 92585[0], 93000[1], 93005[1], 93010[1], 93040[1], 93041[1], 93042[1], 93318[1], 93355[1], 94002[1], 94200[1], 94250[1], 94680[1], 94681[1], 94690[1], 94770[1], 95812[1], 95813[1], 95816[1], 95819[1], 95822[0], 95829[1], 95860[0], 95861[0], 95863[0], 95864[0], 95865[0], 95866[0], 95867[0], 95868[0], 95869[0], 95870[0], 95907[0], 95908[0], 95909[0], 95910[0], 95911[0], 95912[0], 95913[0], 95925[0], 95926[0], 95927[0], 95928[0], 95929[0], 95930[0], 95933[0], 95937[0], 95938[0], 95939[0], 95940[0], 95955[1], 96360[1], 96361[1], 96365[1], 96366[1], 96367[1], 96368[1], 96372[1], 96374[1], 96375[1], 96376[1], 96377[1], 96523[0], 97597[1], 97598[1], 97602[1], 97605[1], 97606[1], 97607[1], 97608[1], 99155[0], 99156[0], 99157[0], 99211[1], 99212[1], 99213[1], 99214[1], 99215[1], 99217[1], 99218[1], 99219[1], 99220[1], 99221[1], 99222[1], 99223[1], 99231[1], 99232[1], 99233[1], 99234[1], 99235[1], 99236[1], 99238[1], 99239[1], 99241[1], 99242[1], 99243[1], 99244[1], 99245[1], 99251[1], 99252[1], 99253[1], 99254[1], 99255[1], 99291[1], 99292[1], 99304[1], 99305[1], 99306[1], 99307[1], 99308[1], 99309[1], 99310[1], 99315[1], 99316[1], 99334[1], 99335[1], 99336[1], 99337[1], 99347[1], 99348[1], 99349[1], 99350[1], 99374[1], 99375[1], 99377[1], 99378[1], 99446[0], 99447[0], 99448[0], 99449[0], 99451[0], 99452[0], 99495[0], 99496[0], G0453[0], G0463[1], G0471[1]
64719	01250[0], 01320[0], 01470[0], 01610[0], 01710[0], 01782[0], 01810[0], 0213T[0], 0216T[0], 0228T[0], 0230T[0], 0333T[0], 0464T[0], 11000[1], 11001[1], 11004[1], 11005[1], 11006[1], 11042[1], 11043[1], 11044[1], 11045[1], 11046[1], 11047[1], 12001[1], 12002[1], 12004[1], 12005[1], 12006[1], 12007[1], 12011[1], 12013[1], 12014[1], 12015[1], 12016[1], 12017[1], 12018[1], 12020[1], 12021[1], 12031[1], 12032[1], 12034[1], 12035[1], 12036[1], 12037[1], 12041[1], 12042[1], 12044[1], 12045[1], 12046[1], 12047[1], 12051[1], 12052[1], 12053[1], 12054[1], 12055[1], 12056[1], 12057[1], 13100[1], 13101[1], 13102[1], 13120[1], 13121[1], 13122[1], 13131[1], 13132[1], 13133[1], 13151[1], 13152[1], 13153[1], 25000[1], 25001[1], 25020[1], 25024[1], 25025[1], 25110[1], 25111[1], 25118[1], 29125[1], 35702[1], 35703[1], 36000[1], 36400[1], 36405[1], 36406[1], 36410[1], 36420[1], 36425[1], 36430[1], 36440[1], 36591[0], 36592[0], 36600[1], 36640[1], 43752[1], 51701[1], 51702[1], 51703[1], 62320[0], 62321[0], 62322[0], 62323[0], 62324[0], 62325[0], 62326[0], 62327[0], 64400[0], 64405[0], 64408[0], 64415[0], 64416[0], 64417[0], 64418[0], 64420[0], 64421[0], 64425[0], 64430[0], 64435[0], 64445[0], 64446[0], 64447[0], 64448[0], 64449[0], 64450[0], 64451[0], 64454[0], 64461[0], 64462[0], 64463[0], 64479[0], 64480[0], 64483[0], 64484[0], 64486[0], 64487[0], 64488[0], 64489[0], 64490[0], 64491[0], 64492[0], 64493[0], 64494[0], 64495[0], 64505[0], 64510[0], 64517[0], 64520[0], 64530[0], 64722[1], 64795[1], 64836[1], 69990[0], 92012[1], 92014[1], 92585[0], 93000[1], 93005[1], 93010[1], 93040[1], 93041[1], 93042[1], 93318[1], 93355[1], 94002[1], 94200[1], 94250[1], 94680[1], 94681[1], 94690[1], 94770[1], 95812[1], 95813[1], 95816[1], 95819[1], 95822[0], 95829[1], 95860[0], 95861[0], 95863[0], 95864[0], 95865[0], 95866[0], 95867[0], 95868[0], 95869[0], 95870[0], 95907[0], 95908[0], 95909[0], 95910[0], 95911[0], 95912[0], 95913[0], 95925[0], 95926[0], 95927[0], 95928[0], 95929[0], 95930[0], 95933[0], 95937[0], 95938[0], 95939[0], 95940[0], 95955[1], 96360[1], 96361[1], 96365[1], 96366[1], 96367[1], 96368[1], 96372[1], 96374[1], 96375[1], 96376[1], 96377[1], 96523[0], 97597[1], 97598[1], 97602[1], 97605[1], 97606[1], 97607[1], 97608[1], 99155[0], 99156[0], 99157[0], 99211[1], 99212[1], 99213[1], 99214[1], 99215[1], 99217[1], 99218[1], 99219[1], 99220[1], 99221[1], 99222[1], 99223[1], 99231[1], 99232[1], 99233[1], 99234[1], 99235[1], 99236[1], 99238[1], 99239[1], 99241[1], 99242[1], 99243[1], 99244[1], 99245[1], 99251[1], 99252[1], 99253[1], 99254[1], 99255[1], 99291[1], 99292[1], 99304[1], 99305[1], 99306[1], 99307[1], 99308[1], 99309[1], 99310[1], 99315[1], 99316[1], 99334[1], 99335[1], 99336[1], 99337[1], 99347[1], 99348[1], 99349[1], 99350[1], 99374[1], 99375[1], 99377[1], 99378[1], 99446[0], 99447[0], 99448[0], 99449[0], 99451[0], 99452[0], 99495[0], 99496[0], G0453[0], G0463[1], G0471[1]
64721	01250[0], 01320[0], 01470[0], 01610[0], 01710[0], 01782[0], 01810[0], 0213T[0], 0216T[0], 0228T[0], 0230T[0], 0333T[0], 0464T[0], 0490T[1], 11000[1], 11001[1], 11004[1], 11005[1], 11006[1], 11042[1], 11043[1], 11044[1], 11045[1], 11046[1], 11047[1], 11900[1], 12001[1], 12002[1], 12004[1], 12005[1], 12006[1], 12007[1], 12011[1], 12013[1], 12014[1], 12015[1], 12016[1], 12017[1], 12018[1], 12020[1], 12021[1], 12031[1], 12032[1], 12034[1], 12035[1], 12036[1], 12037[1], 12041[1], 12042[1], 12044[1], 12045[1], 12046[1], 12047[1], 12051[1], 12052[1], 12053[1], 12054[1], 12055[1], 12056[1], 12057[1], 13100[1], 13101[1], 13102[1], 13120[1], 13121[1], 13122[1], 13131[1], 13132[1], 13133[1], 13151[1], 13152[1], 13153[1], 20526[1], 20527[1], 20550[1], 20551[1], 20552[1], 20553[1], 20560[1], 20561[1], 25001[1], 25071[1], 25110[1], 25111[1], 25295[1], 29075[1], 29125[1], 29584[1], 29843[1], 29844[1], 29845[1], 29848[1], 36000[1], 36400[1], 36405[1], 36406[1], 36410[1], 36420[1], 36425[1], 36430[1], 36440[1], 36591[0], 36592[0], 36600[1], 36640[1], 43752[1], 51701[1], 51702[1], 51703[1], 62320[0], 62321[0], 62322[0], 62323[0], 62324[0], 62325[0], 62326[0], 62327[0], 64400[0], 64405[0], 64408[0], 64415[0], 64416[0], 64417[0], 64418[0], 64420[0], 64421[0], 64425[0], 64430[0], 64435[0], 64445[0], 64446[0], 64447[0], 64448[0], 64449[0], 64450[1], 64451[0], 64454[1], 64461[0], 64462[0], 64463[0], 64479[0], 64480[0], 64483[0], 64484[0], 64486[0], 64487[0], 64488[0], 64489[0], 64490[0], 64491[0], 64492[0], 64493[0], 64494[0], 64495[0], 64505[0], 64510[0], 64517[0], 64520[0], 64530[0], 64712[1], 64719[1], 64722[1], 69990[0], 92012[1], 92014[1], 92585[0], 93000[1], 93005[1], 93010[1], 93040[1], 93041[1], 93042[1], 93318[1], 93355[1], 94002[1], 94200[1], 94250[1], 94680[1], 94681[1], 94690[1], 94770[1], 95812[1], 95813[1], 95816[1], 95819[1], 95822[0], 95829[1], 95860[0], 95861[0], 95863[0], 95864[0], 95865[0], 95866[0], 95867[0], 95868[0], 95869[0], 95870[0], 95907[0], 95908[0], 95909[0], 95910[0], 95911[0], 95912[0], 95913[0], 95925[0], 95926[0], 95927[0], 95928[0], 95929[0], 95930[0], 95933[0], 95937[0], 95938[0], 95939[0], 95940[0], 95955[1], 96360[1], 96361[1], 96365[1], 96366[1], 96367[1], 96368[1], 96372[1], 96374[1], 96375[1], 96376[1], 96377[1], 96523[0], 97597[1], 97598[1], 97602[1], 97605[1], 97606[1], 97607[1], 97608[1], 99155[0], 99156[0], 99157[0], 99211[1], 99212[1], 99213[1], 99214[1], 99215[1], 99217[1], 99218[1], 99219[1], 99220[1], 99221[1], 99222[1], 99223[1], 99231[1], 99232[1], 99233[1], 99234[1], 99235[1], 99236[1], 99238[1], 99239[1], 99241[1], 99242[1], 99243[1], 99244[1], 99245[1], 99251[1], 99252[1], 99253[1], 99254[1], 99255[1], 99291[1], 99292[1], 99304[1], 99305[1], 99306[1], 99307[1], 99308[1], 99309[1], 99310[1], 99315[1], 99316[1], 99334[1], 99335[1], 99336[1], 99337[1], 99347[1], 99348[1], 99349[1], 99350[1], 99374[1], 99375[1], 99377[1], 99378[1], 99446[0], 99447[0], 99448[0], 99449[0], 99451[0], 99452[0], 99495[0], 99496[0], G0453[0], G0463[1], G0471[1]
64722	01250[0], 01320[0], 01470[0], 01610[0], 01710[0], 01782[0], 01810[0], 0213T[0], 0216T[0], 0228T[0], 0230T[0], 0333T[0], 0464T[0], 12001[1], 12002[1], 12004[1], 12005[1], 12006[1], 12007[1], 12011[1], 12013[1], 12014[1], 12015[1], 12016[1], 12017[1], 12018[1], 12020[1], 12021[1], 12031[1], 12032[1], 12034[1], 12035[1], 12036[1], 12037[1], 12041[1], 12042[1], 12044[1], 12045[1], 12046[1], 12047[1], 12051[1], 12052[1], 12053[1], 12054[1], 12055[1], 12056[1], 12057[1], 13100[1], 13101[1], 13102[1], 13120[1], 13121[1], 13122[1], 13131[1], 13132[1], 13133[1], 13151[1], 13152[1], 13153[1], 27325[1], 27326[1], 28055[1], 36000[1], 36400[1], 36405[1], 36406[1], 36410[1], 36420[1], 36425[1], 36430[1], 36440[1], 36591[0], 36592[0], 36600[1], 36640[1], 43752[1], 51701[1], 51702[1], 51703[1], 62320[0], 62321[0], 62322[0], 62323[0], 62324[0], 62325[0], 62326[0], 62327[0], 64400[0], 64405[0], 64408[0], 64415[0], 64416[0], 64417[0], 64418[0], 64420[0], 64421[0], 64425[0], 64430[0], 64435[0], 64445[0], 64446[0], 64447[0], 64448[0], 64449[0], 64450[0], 64451[0], 64454[0], 64461[0], 64462[0], 64463[0], 64479[0], 64480[0], 64483[0], 64484[0], 64486[0], 64487[0], 64488[0], 64489[0], 64490[0], 64491[0], 64492[0], 64493[0], 64494[0], 64495[0], 64505[0], 64510[0], 64517[0], 64520[0], 64530[0], 69990[0], 76000[1], 77001[1], 77002[1], 92012[1], 92014[1], 92585[0], 93000[1], 93005[1], 93010[1], 93040[1], 93041[1], 93042[1], 93318[1], 93355[1], 94002[1], 94200[1], 94250[1], 94680[1], 94681[1], 94690[1], 94770[1], 95812[1], 95813[1], 95816[1], 95819[1], 95822[0], 95829[1], 95860[0], 95861[0], 95863[0], 95864[0], 95865[0], 95866[0], 95867[0], 95868[0], 95869[0], 95870[0], 95907[0], 95908[0], 95909[0], 95910[0], 95911[0], 95912[0], 95913[0], 95925[0], 95926[0], 95927[0], 95928[0], 95929[0], 95930[0], 95933[0], 95937[0], 95938[0], 95939[0], 95940[0], 95955[1], 96360[1], 96361[1], 96365[1], 96366[1], 96367[1], 96368[1], 96372[1], 96374[1], 96375[1], 96376[1], 96377[1], 96523[0], 99155[0], 99156[0], 99157[0], 99211[1], 99212[1], 99213[1], 99214[1], 99215[1], 99217[1], 99218[1], 99219[1], 99220[1], 99221[1], 99222[1], 99223[1], 99231[1], 99232[1], 99233[1], 99234[1], 99235[1], 99236[1], 99238[1], 99239[1], 99241[1], 99242[1], 99243[1], 99244[1], 99245[1], 99251[1], 99252[1], 99253[1], 99254[1], 99255[1], 99291[1], 99292[1], 99304[1], 99305[1], 99306[1], 99307[1], 99308[1], 99309[1], 99310[1], 99315[1], 99316[1], 99334[1], 99335[1], 99336[1], 99337[1], 99347[1], 99348[1], 99349[1], 99350[1], 99374[1], 99375[1], 99377[1], 99378[1], 99446[0], 99447[0], 99448[0], 99449[0], 99451[0], 99452[0], 99495[0], 99496[0], G0453[0], G0463[1], G0471[1]
64727	0333T[0], 0464T[0], 11000[1], 11001[1], 11004[1], 11005[1], 11006[1], 11042[1], 11043[1], 11044[1], 11045[1], 11046[1], 11047[1], 36591[0], 36592[0], 62320[0], 62321[0], 62322[0], 62323[0], 69990[0], 92585[0], 95822[0], 95860[0], 95861[0], 95863[0], 95864[0], 95865[0], 95866[0], 95867[0], 95868[0], 95869[0], 95870[0], 95907[0], 95908[0], 95909[0], 95910[0], 95911[0], 95912[0], 95913[0], 95925[0], 95926[0], 95927[0], 95928[0], 95929[0], 95930[0], 95933[0], 95937[0], 95938[0], 95939[0], 95940[0], 96523[0], 97597[1], 97598[1], 97602[1], G0453[0]

0 = Modifier usage not allowed or inappropriate 1 = Modifier usage allowed

Code 1	Code 2
64771	0213T[0], 0216T[0], 0228T[0], 0230T[0], 0333T[0], 0464T[0], 12001[1], 12002[1], 12004[1], 12005[1], 12006[1], 12007[1], 12011[1], 12013[1], 12014[1], 12015[1], 12016[1], 12017[1], 12018[1], 12020[1], 12021[1], 12031[1], 12032[1], 12034[1], 12035[1], 12036[1], 12037[1], 12041[1], 12042[1], 12044[1], 12045[1], 12046[1], 12047[1], 12051[1], 12052[1], 12053[1], 12054[1], 12055[1], 12056[1], 12057[1], 13100[1], 13101[1], 13102[1], 13120[1], 13121[1], 13122[1], 13131[1], 13132[1], 13133[1], 13151[1], 13152[1], 13153[1], 36000[1], 36400[1], 36405[1], 36406[1], 36410[1], 36420[1], 36425[1], 36430[1], 36440[1], 36591[0], 36592[0], 36600[1], 36640[1], 43752[1], 51701[1], 51702[1], 51703[1], 62320[0], 62321[0], 62322[0], 62323[0], 62324[0], 62325[0], 62326[0], 62327[0], 64400[0], 64405[0], 64408[0], 64415[0], 64416[0], 64417[0], 64418[0], 64420[0], 64421[0], 64425[0], 64430[0], 64435[0], 64445[0], 64446[0], 64447[0], 64448[0], 64449[0], 64450[0], 64451[0], 64454[0], 64461[0], 64462[0], 64463[0], 64479[0], 64480[0], 64483[0], 64484[0], 64486[0], 64487[0], 64488[0], 64489[0], 64490[0], 64491[0], 64492[0], 64493[0], 64494[0], 64495[0], 64505[0], 64510[0], 64517[0], 64520[0], 64530[0], 69990[0], 92012[1], 92014[1], 92585[0], 93000[1], 93005[1], 93010[1], 93040[1], 93041[1], 93042[1], 93318[1], 93355[1], 94002[1], 94200[1], 94250[1], 94680[1], 94681[1], 94690[1], 94770[1], 95812[1], 95813[1], 95816[1], 95819[1], 95822[0], 95829[1], 95860[0], 95861[0], 95863[0], 95864[0], 95865[0], 95866[0], 95867[0], 95868[0], 95869[0], 95870[0], 95907[0], 95908[0], 95909[0], 95910[0], 95911[0], 95912[0], 95913[0], 95925[0], 95926[0], 95927[0], 95928[0], 95929[0], 95930[0], 95933[0], 95937[0], 95938[0], 95939[0], 95940[0], 95955[1], 96360[1], 96361[1], 96365[1], 96366[1], 96367[1], 96368[1], 96372[1], 96374[1], 96375[1], 96376[1], 96377[1], 96523[0], 99155[0], 99156[0], 99157[0], 99211[1], 99212[1], 99213[1], 99214[1], 99215[1], 99217[1], 99218[1], 99219[1], 99220[1], 99221[1], 99222[1], 99223[1], 99231[1], 99232[1], 99233[1], 99234[1], 99235[1], 99236[1], 99238[1], 99239[1], 99241[1], 99242[1], 99243[1], 99244[1], 99245[1], 99251[1], 99252[1], 99253[1], 99254[1], 99255[1], 99291[1], 99292[1], 99304[1], 99305[1], 99306[1], 99307[1], 99308[1], 99309[1], 99310[1], 99315[1], 99316[1], 99334[1], 99335[1], 99336[1], 99337[1], 99347[1], 99348[1], 99349[1], 99350[1], 99374[1], 99375[1], 99377[1], 99378[1], 99446[0], 99447[0], 99448[0], 99449[0], 99451[0], 99452[0], 99495[0], 99496[0], G0453[0], G0463[1], G0471[1]
64772	0213T[0], 0216T[0], 0228T[0], 0230T[0], 0333T[0], 0464T[0], 12001[1], 12002[1], 12004[1], 12005[1], 12006[1], 12007[1], 12011[1], 12013[1], 12014[1], 12015[1], 12016[1], 12017[1], 12018[1], 12020[1], 12021[1], 12031[1], 12032[1], 12034[1], 12035[1], 12036[1], 12037[1], 12041[1], 12042[1], 12044[1], 12045[1], 12046[1], 12047[1], 12051[1], 12052[1], 12053[1], 12054[1], 12055[1], 12056[1], 12057[1], 13100[1], 13101[1], 13102[1], 13120[1], 13121[1], 13122[1], 13131[1], 13132[1], 13133[1], 13151[1], 13152[1], 13153[1], 36000[1], 36400[1], 36405[1], 36406[1], 36410[1], 36420[1], 36425[1], 36430[1], 36440[1], 36591[0], 36592[0], 36600[1], 36640[1], 43752[1], 51701[1], 51702[1], 51703[1], 62320[0], 62321[0], 62322[0], 62323[0], 62324[0], 62325[0], 62326[0], 62327[0], 64400[0], 64405[0], 64408[0], 64415[0], 64416[0], 64417[0], 64418[0], 64420[0], 64421[0], 64425[0], 64430[0], 64435[0], 64445[0], 64446[0], 64447[0], 64448[0], 64449[0], 64450[0], 64451[0], 64454[0], 64461[0], 64462[0], 64463[0], 64479[0], 64480[0], 64483[0], 64484[0], 64486[0], 64487[0], 64488[0], 64489[0], 64490[0], 64491[0], 64492[0], 64493[0], 64494[0], 64495[0], 64505[0], 64510[0], 64517[0], 64520[0], 64530[0], 69990[0], 92012[1], 92014[1], 92585[0], 93000[1], 93005[1], 93010[1], 93040[1], 93041[1], 93042[1], 93318[1], 93355[1], 94002[1], 94200[1], 94250[1], 94680[1], 94681[1], 94690[1], 94770[1], 95812[1], 95813[1], 95816[1], 95819[1], 95822[0], 95829[1], 95860[0], 95861[0], 95863[0], 95864[0], 95865[0], 95866[0], 95867[0], 95868[0], 95869[0], 95870[0], 95907[0], 95908[0], 95909[0], 95910[0], 95911[0], 95912[0], 95913[0], 95925[0], 95926[0], 95927[0], 95928[0], 95929[0], 95930[0], 95933[0], 95937[0], 95938[0], 95939[0], 95940[0], 95955[1], 96360[1], 96361[1], 96365[1], 96366[1], 96367[1], 96368[1], 96372[1], 96374[1], 96375[1], 96376[1], 96377[1], 96523[0], 99155[0], 99156[0], 99157[0], 99211[1], 99212[1], 99213[1], 99214[1], 99215[1], 99217[1], 99218[1], 99219[1], 99220[1], 99221[1], 99222[1], 99223[1], 99231[1], 99232[1], 99233[1], 99234[1], 99235[1], 99236[1], 99238[1], 99239[1], 99241[1], 99242[1], 99243[1], 99244[1], 99245[1], 99251[1], 99252[1], 99253[1], 99254[1], 99255[1], 99291[1], 99292[1], 99304[1], 99305[1], 99306[1], 99307[1], 99308[1], 99309[1], 99310[1], 99315[1], 99316[1], 99334[1], 99335[1], 99336[1], 99337[1], 99347[1], 99348[1], 99349[1], 99350[1], 99374[1], 99375[1], 99377[1], 99378[1], 99446[0], 99447[0], 99448[0], 99449[0], 99451[0], 99452[0], 99495[0], 99496[0], G0453[0], G0463[1], G0471[1]
64788	01250[0], 01320[0], 01470[0], 01610[0], 01710[0], 01782[0], 01810[0], 0213T[0], 0216T[0], 0228T[0], 0230T[0], 0333T[0], 0464T[0], 11000[1], 11001[1], 11004[1], 11005[1], 11006[1], 11042[1], 11043[1], 11044[1], 11045[1], 11046[1], 11047[1], 12001[1], 12002[1], 12004[1], 12005[1], 12006[1], 12007[1], 12011[1], 12013[1], 12014[1], 12015[1], 12016[1], 12017[1], 12018[1], 12020[1], 12021[1], 12031[1], 12032[1], 12034[1], 12035[1], 12036[1], 12037[1], 12041[1], 12042[1], 12044[1], 12045[1], 12046[1], 12047[1], 12051[1], 12052[1], 12053[1], 12054[1], 12055[1], 12056[1], 12057[1], 13100[1], 13101[1], 13102[1], 13120[1], 13121[1], 13122[1], 13131[1], 13132[1], 13133[1], 13151[1], 13152[1], 13153[1], 36000[1], 36400[1], 36405[1], 36406[1], 36410[1], 36420[1], 36425[1], 36430[1], 36440[1], 36591[0], 36592[0], 36600[1], 36640[1], 43752[1], 51701[1], 51702[1], 51703[1], 62320[0], 62321[0], 62322[0], 62323[0], 62324[0], 62325[0], 62326[0], 62327[0], 64400[0], 64405[0], 64408[0], 64415[0], 64416[0], 64417[0], 64418[0], 64420[0], 64421[0], 64425[0], 64430[0], 64435[0], 64445[0], 64446[0], 64447[0], 64448[0], 64449[0], 64450[0], 64451[0], 64454[0], 64455[1], 64461[0], 64462[0], 64463[0], 64479[0], 64480[0], 64483[0], 64484[0], 64486[0], 64487[0], 64488[0], 64489[0], 64490[0], 64491[0], 64492[0], 64493[0], 64494[0], 64495[0], 64505[0], 64510[0], 64517[0], 64520[0], 64530[0], 64702[1], 64704[1], 64722[1], 64726[1], 64795[1], 69990[0], 92012[1], 92014[1], 92585[0], 93000[1], 93005[1], 93010[1], 93040[1], 93041[1], 93042[1], 93318[1], 93355[1], 94002[1], 94200[1], 94250[1], 94680[1], 94681[1], 94690[1], 94770[1], 95812[1], 95813[1], 95816[1], 95819[1], 95822[0], 95829[1], 95860[0], 95861[0], 95863[0], 95864[0], 95865[0], 95866[0], 95867[0], 95868[0], 95869[0], 95870[0], 95907[0], 95908[0], 95909[0], 95910[0], 95911[0], 95912[0], 95913[0], 95925[0], 95926[0], 95927[0], 95928[0], 95929[0], 95930[0], 95933[0], 95937[0], 95938[0], 95939[0], 95940[0], 95955[1], 96360[1], 96361[1], 96365[1], 96366[1], 96367[1], 96368[1], 96372[1], 96374[1], 96375[1], 96376[1], 96377[1], 96523[0], 97597[1], 97598[1], 97602[1], 99155[0], 99156[0], 99157[0], 99211[1], 99212[1], 99213[1], 99214[1], 99215[1], 99217[1], 99218[1], 99219[1], 99220[1], 99221[1], 99222[1], 99223[1], 99231[1], 99232[1], 99233[1], 99234[1], 99235[1], 99236[1], 99238[1], 99239[1], 99241[1], 99242[1], 99243[1], 99244[1], 99245[1], 99251[1], 99252[1], 99253[1], 99254[1], 99255[1], 99291[1], 99292[1], 99304[1], 99305[1], 99306[1], 99307[1], 99308[1], 99309[1], 99310[1], 99315[1], 99316[1], 99334[1], 99335[1], 99336[1], 99337[1], 99347[1], 99348[1], 99349[1], 99350[1], 99374[1], 99375[1], 99377[1], 99378[1], 99446[0], 99447[0], 99448[0], 99449[0], 99451[0], 99452[0], 99495[0], 99496[0], G0453[0], G0463[1], G0471[1]
64790	01250[0], 01320[0], 01470[0], 01610[0], 01710[0], 01782[0], 01810[0], 0213T[0], 0216T[0], 0228T[0], 0230T[0], 0333T[0], 0464T[0], 11000[1], 11001[1], 11004[1], 11005[1], 11006[1], 11042[1], 11043[1], 11044[1], 11045[1], 11046[1], 11047[1], 12001[1], 12002[1], 12004[1], 12005[1], 12006[1], 12007[1], 12011[1], 12013[1], 12014[1], 12015[1], 12016[1], 12017[1], 12018[1], 12020[1], 12021[1], 12031[1], 12032[1], 12034[1], 12035[1], 12036[1], 12037[1], 12041[1], 12042[1], 12044[1], 12045[1], 12046[1], 12047[1], 12051[1], 12052[1], 12053[1], 12054[1], 12055[1], 12056[1], 12057[1], 13100[1], 13101[1], 13102[1], 13120[1], 13121[1], 13122[1], 13131[1], 13132[1], 13133[1], 13151[1], 13152[1], 13153[1], 29125[1], 36000[1], 36400[1], 36405[1], 36406[1], 36410[1], 36420[1], 36425[1], 36430[1], 36440[1], 36591[0], 36592[0], 36600[1], 36640[1], 43752[1], 51701[1], 51702[1], 51703[1], 62320[0], 62321[0], 62322[0], 62323[0], 62324[0], 62325[0], 62326[0], 62327[0], 64400[0], 64405[0], 64408[0], 64415[0], 64416[0], 64417[0], 64418[0], 64420[0], 64421[0], 64425[0], 64430[0], 64435[0], 64445[0], 64446[0], 64447[0], 64448[0], 64449[0], 64450[0], 64451[0], 64454[0], 64461[0], 64462[0], 64463[0], 64479[0], 64480[0], 64483[0], 64484[0], 64486[0], 64487[0], 64488[0], 64489[0], 64490[0], 64491[0], 64492[0], 64493[0], 64494[0], 64495[0], 64505[0], 64510[0], 64517[0], 64520[0], 64530[0], 64702[1], 64704[1], 64708[1], 64712[1], 64713[1], 64714[1], 64716[1], 64718[1], 64719[1], 64721[1], 64722[1], 64726[1], 64795[1], 69990[0], 92012[1], 92014[1], 92585[0], 93000[1], 93005[1], 93010[1], 93040[1], 93041[1], 93042[1], 93318[1], 93355[1], 94002[1], 94200[1], 94250[1], 94680[1], 94681[1], 94690[1], 94770[1], 95812[1], 95813[1], 95816[1], 95819[1], 95822[0], 95829[1], 95860[0], 95861[0], 95863[0], 95864[0], 95865[0], 95866[0], 95867[0], 95868[0], 95869[0], 95870[0], 95907[0], 95908[0], 95909[0], 95910[0], 95911[0], 95912[0], 95913[0], 95925[0], 95926[0], 95927[0], 95928[0], 95929[0], 95930[0], 95933[0], 95937[0], 95938[0], 95939[0], 95940[0], 95955[1], 96360[1], 96361[1], 96365[1], 96366[1], 96367[1], 96368[1], 96372[1], 96374[1], 96375[1], 96376[1], 96377[1], 96523[0], 97597[1], 97598[1], 97602[1], 99155[0], 99156[0], 99157[0], 99211[1], 99212[1], 99213[1], 99214[1], 99215[1], 99217[1], 99218[1], 99219[1], 99220[1], 99221[1], 99222[1], 99223[1], 99231[1], 99232[1], 99233[1], 99234[1], 99235[1], 99236[1], 99238[1], 99239[1], 99241[1], 99242[1], 99243[1], 99244[1], 99245[1], 99251[1], 99252[1], 99253[1], 99254[1], 99255[1], 99291[1], 99292[1], 99304[1], 99305[1], 99306[1], 99307[1], 99308[1], 99309[1], 99310[1], 99315[1], 99316[1], 99334[1], 99335[1], 99336[1], 99337[1], 99347[1], 99348[1], 99349[1], 99350[1], 99374[1], 99375[1], 99377[1], 99378[1], 99446[0], 99447[0], 99448[0], 99449[0], 99451[0], 99452[0], 99495[0], 99496[0], G0453[0], G0463[1], G0471[1]
64792	01250[0], 01320[0], 01470[0], 01610[0], 01710[0], 01782[0], 01810[0], 0213T[0], 0216T[0], 0228T[0], 0230T[0], 0333T[0], 0464T[0], 11000[1], 11001[1], 11004[1], 11005[1], 11006[1], 11042[1], 11043[1], 11044[1], 11045[1], 11046[1], 11047[1], 12001[1], 12002[1], 12004[1], 12005[1], 12006[1], 12007[1], 12011[1], 12013[1], 12014[1], 12015[1], 12016[1], 12017[1], 12018[1], 12020[1], 12021[1], 12031[1], 12032[1], 12034[1], 12035[1], 12036[1], 12037[1], 12041[1], 12042[1], 12044[1], 12045[1], 12046[1], 12047[1], 12051[1], 12052[1], 12053[1], 12054[1], 12055[1], 12056[1], 12057[1], 13100[1], 13101[1], 13102[1], 13120[1], 13121[1], 13122[1], 13131[1], 13132[1], 13133[1], 13151[1], 13152[1], 13153[1], 36000[1], 36400[1], 36405[1], 36406[1], 36410[1], 36420[1], 36425[1], 36430[1], 36440[1], 36591[0], 36592[0], 36600[1], 36640[1], 43752[1], 51701[1], 51702[1], 51703[1], 62320[0], 62321[0], 62322[0], 62323[0], 62324[0], 62325[0], 62326[0], 62327[0], 64400[0], 64405[0], 64408[0], 64415[0], 64416[0], 64417[0], 64418[0], 64420[0], 64421[0], 64425[0], 64430[0], 64435[0], 64445[0], 64446[0], 64447[0], 64448[0], 64449[0], 64450[0], 64451[0], 64454[0], 64461[0], 64462[0], 64463[0], 64479[0], 64480[0], 64483[0], 64484[0], 64486[0], 64487[0], 64488[0], 64489[0], 64490[0], 64491[0], 64492[0], 64493[0], 64494[0], 64495[0], 64505[0], 64510[0], 64517[0], 64520[0], 64530[0], 64702[1], 64704[1], 64708[1], 64712[1], 64713[1], 64714[1], 64716[1], 64718[1], 64719[1], 64721[1], 64722[1], 64726[1], 64795[1], 69990[0], 92012[1], 92014[1], 92585[0], 93000[1], 93005[1], 93010[1], 93040[1], 93041[1], 93042[1], 93318[1], 93355[1], 94002[1], 94200[1], 94250[1], 94680[1], 94681[1], 94690[1], 94770[1], 95812[1], 95813[1], 95816[1], 95819[1], 95822[0], 95829[1], 95860[0], 95861[0], 95863[0], 95864[0], 95865[0], 95866[0], 95867[0], 95868[0], 95869[0], 95870[0], 95907[0], 95908[0], 95909[0], 95910[0], 95911[0], 95912[0], 95913[0], 95925[0], 95926[0], 95927[0], 95928[0], 95929[0], 95930[0], 95933[0], 95937[0], 95938[0], 95939[0], 95940[0], 95955[1], 96360[1], 96361[1], 96365[1], 96366[1], 96367[1], 96368[1], 96372[1], 96374[1], 96375[1], 96376[1], 96377[1], 96523[0], 97597[1], 97598[1], 97602[1], 99155[0], 99156[0], 99157[0], 99211[1], 99212[1], 99213[1], 99214[1], 99215[1], 99217[1], 99218[1], 99219[1],

0 = Modifier usage not allowed or inappropriate 1 = Modifier usage allowed

Code 1	Code 2
	99220[1], 99221[1], 99222[1], 99223[1], 99231[1], 99232[1], 99233[1], 99234[1], 99235[1], 99236[1], 99238[1], 99239[1], 99241[1], 99242[1], 99243[1], 99244[1], 99245[1], 99251[1], 99252[1], 99253[1], 99254[1], 99255[1], 99291[1], 99292[1], 99304[1], 99305[1], 99306[1], 99307[1], 99308[1], 99309[1], 99310[1], 99315[1], 99316[1], 99334[1], 99335[1], 99336[1], 99337[1], 99347[1], 99348[1], 99349[1], 99350[1], 99374[1], 99375[1], 99377[1], 99378[1], 99446[0], 99447[0], 99448[0], 99449[0], 99451[0], 99452[0], 99495[0], 99496[0], G0453[0], G0463[1], G0471[1]
64795	01250[0], 01320[0], 01470[0], 01610[0], 01710[0], 01782[0], 01810[0], 0213T[0], 0216T[0], 0228T[0], 0230T[0], 0333T[0], 0464T[0], 10005[1], 10007[1], 10009[1], 10011[1], 10021[1], 12001[1], 12002[1], 12004[1], 12005[1], 12006[1], 12007[1], 12011[1], 12013[1], 12014[1], 12015[1], 12016[1], 12017[1], 12018[1], 12020[1], 12021[1], 12031[1], 12032[1], 12034[1], 12035[1], 12036[1], 12037[1], 12041[1], 12042[1], 12044[1], 12045[1], 12046[1], 12047[1], 12051[1], 12052[1], 12053[1], 12054[1], 12055[1], 12056[1], 12057[1], 13100[1], 13101[1], 13102[1], 13120[1], 13121[1], 13122[1], 13131[1], 13132[1], 13133[1], 13151[1], 13152[1], 13153[1], 20205[1], 36000[1], 36400[1], 36405[1], 36406[1], 36410[1], 36420[1], 36425[1], 36430[1], 36440[1], 36591[0], 36592[0], 36600[1], 36640[1], 43752[1], 51701[1], 51702[1], 51703[1], 62320[0], 62321[0], 62322[0], 62323[0], 62324[0], 62325[0], 62326[0], 62327[0], 64400[0], 64405[0], 64408[0], 64415[0], 64416[0], 64417[0], 64418[0], 64420[0], 64421[0], 64425[0], 64430[0], 64435[0], 64445[0], 64446[0], 64447[0], 64448[0], 64449[0], 64450[0], 64451[0], 64454[0], 64455[1], 64461[0], 64462[0], 64463[0], 64479[0], 64480[0], 64483[0], 64484[0], 64486[0], 64487[0], 64488[0], 64489[0], 64490[0], 64491[0], 64492[0], 64493[0], 64494[0], 64495[0], 64505[0], 64510[0], 64517[0], 64520[0], 64530[0], 64721[1], 64726[1], 69990[0], 92012[1], 92014[1], 92585[0], 93000[1], 93005[1], 93010[1], 93040[1], 93041[1], 93042[1], 93318[1], 93355[1], 94002[1], 94200[1], 94250[1], 94680[1], 94681[1], 94690[1], 94770[1], 95812[1], 95813[1], 95816[1], 95819[1], 95822[0], 95829[1], 95860[0], 95861[0], 95863[0], 95864[0], 95865[0], 95866[0], 95867[0], 95868[0], 95869[0], 95870[0], 95907[0], 95908[0], 95909[0], 95910[0], 95911[0], 95912[0], 95913[0], 95925[0], 95926[0], 95927[0], 95928[0], 95929[0], 95930[0], 95933[0], 95937[0], 95938[0], 95939[0], 95940[0], 95955[1], 96360[1], 96361[1], 96365[1], 96366[1], 96367[1], 96368[1], 96372[1], 96374[1], 96375[1], 96376[1], 96377[1], 96523[0], 99155[0], 99156[0], 99157[0], 99211[1], 99212[1], 99213[1], 99214[1], 99215[1], 99217[1], 99218[1], 99219[1], 99220[1], 99221[1], 99222[1], 99223[1], 99231[1], 99232[1], 99233[1], 99234[1], 99235[1], 99236[1], 99238[1], 99239[1], 99241[1], 99242[1], 99243[1], 99244[1], 99245[1], 99251[1], 99252[1], 99253[1], 99254[1], 99255[1], 99291[1], 99292[1], 99304[1], 99305[1], 99306[1], 99307[1], 99308[1], 99309[1], 99310[1], 99315[1], 99316[1], 99334[1], 99335[1], 99336[1], 99337[1], 99347[1], 99348[1], 99349[1], 99350[1], 99374[1], 99375[1], 99377[1], 99378[1], 99446[0], 99447[0], 99448[0], 99449[0], 99451[0], 99452[0], 99495[1], 99496[1], G0453[0], G0463[1], G0471[1]
64910	01250[0], 01320[0], 01470[0], 01610[0], 01710[0], 01810[0], 0213T[0], 0216T[0], 0228T[0], 0230T[0], 0333T[0], 0464T[0], 0565T[1], 12001[1], 12002[1], 12004[1], 12005[1], 12006[1], 12007[1], 12011[1], 12013[1], 12014[1], 12015[1], 12016[1], 12017[1], 12018[1], 12020[1], 12021[1], 12031[1], 12032[1], 12034[1], 12035[1], 12036[1], 12037[1], 12041[1], 12042[1], 12044[1], 12045[1], 12046[1], 12047[1], 12051[1], 12052[1], 12053[1], 12054[1], 12055[1], 12056[1], 12057[1], 13100[1], 13101[1], 13102[1], 13120[1], 13121[1], 13122[1], 13131[1], 13132[1], 13133[1], 13151[1], 13152[1], 13153[1], 15769[1], 36000[1], 36400[1], 36405[1], 36406[1], 36410[1], 36420[1], 36425[1], 36430[1], 36440[1], 36591[0], 36592[0], 36600[1], 36640[1], 43752[1], 51701[1], 51702[1], 51703[1], 62320[0], 62321[0], 62322[0], 62323[0], 62324[0], 62325[0], 62326[0], 62327[0], 64400[0], 64405[0], 64408[0], 64415[0], 64416[0], 64417[0], 64418[0], 64420[0], 64421[0], 64425[0], 64430[0], 64435[0], 64445[0], 64446[0], 64447[0], 64448[0], 64449[0], 64450[0], 64451[0], 64454[0], 64455[1], 64461[0], 64462[0], 64463[0], 64479[0], 64480[0], 64483[0], 64484[0], 64486[0], 64487[0], 64488[0], 64489[0], 64490[0], 64491[0], 64492[0], 64493[0], 64494[0], 64495[0], 64505[0], 64510[0], 64517[0], 64520[0], 64530[0], 64702[1], 64704[1], 64708[1], 64712[1], 64713[1], 64714[1], 64716[1], 64718[1], 64719[1], 64721[1], 64722[1], 64726[1], 64727[1], 64774[1], 64776[1], 64782[1], 64784[1], 64831[1], 64834[1], 64835[1], 64836[1], 64840[1], 64856[1], 64857[1], 64858[1], 64861[1], 64862[1], 64864[1], 64865[1], 64866[1], 64868[1], 64912[1], 64913[1], 69990[0], 92012[1], 92014[1], 92585[0], 93000[1], 93005[1], 93010[1], 93040[1], 93041[1], 93042[1], 93318[1], 93355[1], 94002[1], 94200[1], 94250[1], 94680[1], 94681[1], 94690[1], 94770[1], 95812[1], 95813[1], 95816[1], 95819[1], 95822[0], 95829[1], 95860[0], 95861[0], 95863[0], 95864[0], 95865[0], 95866[0], 95867[0], 95868[0], 95869[0], 95870[0], 95907[0], 95908[0], 95909[0], 95910[0], 95911[0], 95912[0], 95913[0], 95925[0], 95926[0], 95927[0], 95928[0], 95929[0], 95930[0], 95933[0], 95937[0], 95938[0], 95939[0], 95940[0], 95955[1], 96360[1], 96361[1], 96365[1], 96366[1], 96367[1], 96368[1], 96372[1], 96374[1], 96375[1], 96376[1], 96377[1], 96523[0], 99155[0], 99156[0], 99157[0], 99211[1], 99212[1], 99213[1], 99214[1], 99215[1], 99217[1], 99218[1], 99219[1], 99220[1], 99221[1], 99222[1], 99223[1], 99231[1], 99232[1], 99233[1], 99234[1], 99235[1], 99236[1], 99238[1], 99239[1], 99241[1], 99242[1], 99243[1], 99244[1], 99245[1], 99251[1], 99252[1], 99253[1], 99254[1], 99255[1], 99291[1], 99292[1], 99304[1], 99305[1], 99306[1], 99307[1], 99308[1], 99309[1], 99310[1], 99315[1], 99316[1], 99334[1], 99335[1], 99336[1], 99337[1], 99347[1], 99348[1], 99349[1], 99350[1], 99374[1], 99375[1], 99377[1], 99378[1], 99446[0], 99447[0], 99448[0], 99449[0], 99451[0], 99452[0], 99495[0], 99496[0], G0453[0], G0463[1], G0471[1]
64911	01250[0], 01320[0], 01470[0], 01610[0], 01710[0], 01810[0], 0213T[0], 0216T[0], 0228T[0], 0230T[0], 0333T[0], 0464T[0], 0565T[1], 12001[1], 12002[1], 12004[1], 12005[1], 12006[1], 12007[1], 12011[1], 12013[1], 12014[1], 12015[1], 12016[1], 12017[1], 12018[1], 12020[1], 12021[1], 12031[1], 12032[1], 12034[1], 12035[1], 12036[1], 12037[1], 12041[1], 12042[1], 12044[1], 12045[1], 12046[1], 12047[1], 12051[1], 12052[1], 12053[1], 12054[1], 12055[1], 12056[1], 12057[1], 13100[1], 13101[1], 13102[1], 13120[1], 13121[1], 13122[1], 13131[1], 13132[1], 13133[1], 13151[1], 13152[1], 13153[1], 15769[1], 36000[1], 36400[1], 36405[1], 36406[1], 36410[1], 36420[1], 36425[1], 36430[1], 36440[1], 36591[0], 36592[0], 36600[1], 36640[1], 43752[1], 51701[1], 51702[1], 51703[1], 62320[0], 62321[0], 62322[0], 62323[0], 62324[0], 62325[0], 62326[0], 62327[0], 64400[0], 64405[0], 64408[0], 64415[0], 64416[0], 64417[0], 64418[0], 64420[0], 64421[0], 64425[0], 64430[0], 64435[0], 64445[0], 64446[0], 64447[0], 64448[0], 64449[0], 64450[0], 64451[0], 64454[0], 64455[1], 64461[0], 64462[0], 64463[0], 64479[0], 64480[0], 64483[0], 64484[0], 64486[0], 64487[0], 64488[0], 64489[0], 64490[0], 64491[0], 64492[0], 64493[0], 64494[0], 64495[0], 64505[0], 64510[0], 64517[0], 64520[0], 64530[0], 64702[1], 64704[1], 64708[1], 64712[1], 64713[1], 64714[1], 64716[1], 64718[1], 64719[1], 64721[1], 64722[1], 64726[1], 64727[1], 64774[1], 64776[1], 64782[1], 64784[1], 64831[1], 64834[1], 64835[1], 64836[1], 64840[1], 64856[1], 64857[1], 64858[1], 64861[1], 64862[1], 64864[1], 64865[1], 64866[1], 64868[1], 64910[1], 64912[1], 64913[1], 69990[0], 92012[1], 92014[1], 92585[0], 93000[1], 93005[1], 93010[1], 93040[1], 93041[1], 93042[1], 93318[1], 93355[1], 94002[1], 94200[1], 94250[1], 94680[1], 94681[1], 94690[1], 94770[1], 95812[1], 95813[1], 95816[1], 95819[1], 95822[0], 95829[1], 95860[0], 95861[0], 95863[0], 95864[0], 95865[0], 95866[0], 95867[0], 95868[0], 95869[0], 95870[0], 95907[0], 95908[0], 95909[0], 95910[0], 95911[0], 95912[0], 95913[0], 95925[0], 95926[0], 95927[0], 95928[0], 95929[0], 95930[0], 95933[0], 95937[0], 95938[0], 95939[0], 95940[0], 95955[1], 96360[1], 96361[1], 96365[1], 96366[1], 96367[1], 96368[1], 96372[1], 96374[1], 96375[1], 96376[1], 96377[1], 96523[0], 99155[0], 99156[0], 99157[0], 99211[1], 99212[1], 99213[1], 99214[1], 99215[1], 99217[1], 99218[1], 99219[1], 99220[1], 99221[1], 99222[1], 99223[1], 99231[1], 99232[1], 99233[1], 99234[1], 99235[1], 99236[1], 99238[1], 99239[1], 99241[1], 99242[1], 99243[1], 99244[1], 99245[1], 99251[1], 99252[1], 99253[1], 99254[1], 99255[1], 99291[1], 99292[1], 99304[1], 99305[1], 99306[1], 99307[1], 99308[1], 99309[1], 99310[1], 99315[1], 99316[1], 99334[1], 99335[1], 99336[1], 99337[1], 99347[1], 99348[1], 99349[1], 99350[1], 99374[1], 99375[1], 99377[1], 99378[1], 99446[0], 99447[0], 99448[0], 99449[0], 99451[0], 99452[0], 99495[0], 99496[0], G0453[0], G0463[1], G0471[1]
69990	0543T[0], 0544T[0], 0548T[0], 0567T[0], 0568T[0], 0569T[0], 0570T[0], 0571T[0], 0572T[0], 0573T[0], 0574T[0], 0580T[0], 0581T[0], 0582T[0], 0583T[0], 15772[0], 15774[0], 20560[0], 20561[0], 20700[0], 20701[0], 36591[0], 36592[0], 62329[0], 64451[0], 64625[0], 66987[0], 66988[0], 96523[0]

0 = Modifier usage not allowed or inappropriate 1 = Modifier usage allowed

Code 1	Code 2
G0453	36591[0], 36592[0], 95872[1], 95875[1], 95941[0], 96523[0]
Q9967	Q9951[0], Q9959[0], Q9964[0], Q9965[1], Q9966[1]

0 = Modifier usage not allowed or inappropriate 1 = Modifier usage allowed

Clinical Documentation Checklists

Introduction

Appendix B provides checklists for common diagnoses and other conditions which are designed to be used for review of current records to help identify any documentation deficiencies. The checklists begin with the applicable ICD-10-CM categories, subcategories, and/or codes being covered. Definitions and other information pertinent to coding the condition are then provided. This is followed by a checklist that identifies each element needed for assignment of the most specific code. If one or more of the required elements are not documented, this information should be shared with the physician and a corrective action plan initiated to ensure that the necessary information is captured in the future.

Similar documentation and coding checklists for conditions not addressed in this book can be created using the checklists provided as a template. There are a few different formats and styles of checklists so users can determine which style works best for their practice and then create additional checklists using that format and style.

Burns, Corrosions, and Frostbite

ICD-10-CM Categories

Burns and corrosions are classified in the following ICD-10-CM categories:

T20	Burn and corrosion of head, face and neck
T21	Burn and corrosion of trunk
T22	Burn and corrosion of shoulder and upper limb, except wrist and hand
T23	Burn and corrosion of wrist and hand
T24	Burn and corrosion of lower limb, except ankle and foot
T25	Burn and corrosion of ankle and foot
T26	Burn and corrosion confined to eye and adnexa
T27	Burn and corrosion of respiratory tract
T28	Burn and corrosion of internal organ
T30	Burn and corrosion, body region unspecified
T31	Burns classified according to extent of body surface involved
T33	Superficial frostbite

ICD-10-CM Definitions

Burn – A thermal injury due to a heat source such as fire, a hot appliance, friction, hot objects, hot air, hot water, electricity, lightning, and radiation. Burns due to exposure to the sun are not considered burns in ICD-10-CM.

Corrosion – A thermal injury due to chemicals.

Episode of Care – There are three (3) possible 7th character values for burns and corrosions. The 7th character defines the stage of treatment and residual effects related to the initial injury.

A Initial encounter. The period when the patient is receiving active treatment for the injury, poisoning, or other consequences of an external cause. An 'A' may be assigned on more than one claim.

D Subsequent encounter. Encounter after the active phase of treatment and when the patient is receiving routine care for the injury during the period of healing or recovery.

S Sequela. Encounter for complications or conditions that arise as a direct result of an injury.

Extent of body surface – The amount of body surface burned is governed by the rule of nines. These percentages may be modified for infants and children or adults with large buttocks, thighs, and abdomens when those regions are burned.

Head and neck – 9%

Each arm – 9%

Each leg – 18%

Anterior trunk – 18%

Posterior trunk – 18%

Genitalia – 1%

Levels of Burns:

First Degree – Affects only the epidermis causing pain, redness, and swelling.

Second Degree – Affects both the dermis and epidermis causing pain, redness, white or blotchy skin, and swelling. Blistering may occur and pain can be intense. Scarring can develop.

Third Degree – Affects the fat or subcutaneous layer of the skin. The skin will appear white or charred black or may look leathery. Third degree burns can destroy nerves resulting in numbness.

Note: Burns noted as non-healing are coded as acute burns and necrosis of burned skin should be coded as a non-healing burn.

Checklist

1. Identify the type of thermal injury:
   - ☐ Burn
   - ☐ Corrosion
   - ☐ Frostbite (Proceed to #9)
2. Identify the body region:
   - ☐ Eye
   - ☐ Internal organs
   - ☐ Skin (external body surface)
   - ☐ Multiple areas
   - ☐ Unspecified body region

Note: Codes from category T30 Burn and corrosion, body region unspecified, is extremely vague and should rarely be used.

3. Identify the body area
   - ☐ Eye and adnexa
     - ☐ Eyelid and periocular area
     - ☐ Cornea and conjunctival sac
     - ☐ With resulting rupture and destruction of eyeball
     - ☐ Unspecified site – review medical record/query physician
   - ☐ External body surface
     - ☐ Head, face and neck
       - ☐ Scalp
       - ☐ Forehead and cheek
       - ☐ Ear
       - ☐ Nose
       - ☐ Lips
       - ☐ Chin
       - ☐ Neck
       - ☐ Multiple sites of head, face, and neck
       - ☐ Unspecified site – review medical record/query physician
       - ☐ Trunk
         - ☐ Chest wall
         - ☐ Abdominal wall
       - ☐ Upper back
       - ☐ Lower back
       - ☐ Buttocks
       - ☐ Genital region
         - ☐ Female

- ☐ Male
- ☐ Other site
- ☐ Unspecified site – review medical record/query physician
- ☐ Shoulder and upper limb (excluding wrist and hand)
  - ☐ Scapula
  - ☐ Shoulder
  - ☐ Axilla
  - ☐ Upper arm
  - ☐ Elbow
  - ☐ Forearm
  - ☐ Multiple sites shoulder and upper limb (excluding wrist and hand)
  - ☐ Unspecified site – review medical record/query physician
- ☐ Wrist and hand
  - ☐ Wrist
  - ☐ Hand
    - ☐ Back of hand
    - ☐ Palm
    - ☐ Finger
      - ☐ Multiple fingers not including thumb
      - ☐ Multiple fingers including thumb
      - ☐ Single except thumb
      - ☐ Thumb
      - ☐ Unspecified site hand – review medical record/query physician
    - ☐ Multiple sites of wrist and hand
- ☐ Lower limb except ankle and foot
  - ☐ Thigh
  - ☐ Knee
  - ☐ Lower leg
  - ☐ Multiple sites of lower limb
  - ☐ Unspecified site lower limb – review medical record/query physician
- ☐ Ankle and foot
  - ☐ Ankle
  - ☐ Foot
  - ☐ Toe(s)
  - ☐ Multiple sites of ankle and foot
  - ☐ Unspecified site ankle or foot – review medical record/query physician
- ☐ Internal Organs
  - ☐ Ear drum
  - ☐ Esophagus
  - ☐ Genitourinary organs, internal
  - ☐ Mouth and pharynx
  - ☐ Other parts of alimentary tract
  - ☐ Respiratory tract
    - ☐ Larynx and trachea
    - ☐ Larynx and trachea with lung
    - ☐ Other parts of respiratory tract (thoracic cavity)
    - ☐ Unspecified site respiratory tract- review medical record/query physician
  - ☐ Other internal organ
  - ☐ Unspecified internal organ

4. Identify degree of burn:
   - ☐ First degree
   - ☐ Second degree
   - ☐ Third degree
   - ☐ Unspecified degree – review medical record/query physician
5. Identify laterality:
   - ☐ Left
   - ☐ Right
   - ☐ Unspecified – review medical record/query physician

Note: Laterality only applies to burns and corrosions involving the extremities, ears, and eyes.

6. Identify episode of care/stage of healing/complication
   - ☐ A Initial encounter
   - ☐ D Subsequent encounter
   - ☐ S Sequela
7. Identify extent of body surface involved and percent of third degree burns, if over 10% of body surface:
   - ☐ Less than 10% of body surface
   - ☐ 10-19% of body surface
     - ☐ 0% to 9% of third degree burns
     - ☐ 10-19% of third degree burns
   - ☐ 20-29% of body surface
     - ☐ 0% to 9% of third degree burns
     - ☐ 10-19% of third degree burns
     - ☐ 20-29% of third degree burns
   - ☐ 30-39% of body surface
     - ☐ 0% to 9% of third degree burns
     - ☐ 10-19% of third degree burns
     - ☐ 20-29% of third degree burns
     - ☐ 30-39% of third degree burns
   - ☐ 40-49% of body surface
     - ☐ 0% to 9% of third degree burns
     - ☐ 10-19% of third degree burns
     - ☐ 20-29% of third degree burns
     - ☐ 30-39% of third degree burns
     - ☐ 40-49% of third degree burns
   - ☐ 50-59% of body surface
     - ☐ 0% to 9% of third degree burns
     - ☐ 10-19% of third degree burns
     - ☐ 20-29% of third degree burns
     - ☐ 30-39% of third degree burns
     - ☐ 40-49% of third degree burns
     - ☐ 50-59% of third degree burns
   - ☐ 60-69% of body surface
     - ☐ 0% to 9% of third degree burns
     - ☐ 10-19% of third degree burns
     - ☐ 20-29% of third degree burns
     - ☐ 30-39% of third degree burns
     - ☐ 40-49% of third degree burns
     - ☐ 50-59% of third degree burns
     - ☐ 60-69% of third degree burns

- ☐ 70-79% of body surface
  - ☐ Ø% to 9% of third degree burns
  - ☐ 1Ø-19% of third degree burns
  - ☐ 2Ø-29% of third degree burns
  - ☐ 3Ø-39% of third degree burns
  - ☐ 4Ø-49% of third degree burns
  - ☐ 5Ø-59% of third degree burns
  - ☐ 6Ø-69% of third degree burns
  - ☐ 7Ø-79% of third degree burns
- ☐ 8Ø-89% of body surface
  - ☐ Ø% to 9% of third degree burns
  - ☐ 1Ø-19% of third degree burns
  - ☐ 2Ø-29% of third degree burns
  - ☐ 3Ø-39% of third degree burns
  - ☐ 4Ø-49% of third degree burns
  - ☐ 5Ø-59% of third degree burns
  - ☐ 6Ø-69% of third degree burns
  - ☐ 7Ø-79% of third degree burns
  - ☐ 8Ø-89% of third degree burns
- ☐ 9Ø% or more of body surface
  - ☐ Ø% to 9% of third degree burns
  - ☐ 1Ø-19% of third degree burns
  - ☐ 2Ø-29% of third degree burns
  - ☐ 3Ø-39% of third degree burns
  - ☐ 4Ø-49% of third degree burns
  - ☐ 5Ø-59% of third degree burns
  - ☐ 6Ø-69% of third degree burns
  - ☐ 7Ø-79% third degree burns
  - ☐ 8Ø-89% third degree burns
  - ☐ 9Ø% or more third degree burns

Note: Extent of body surface is to be coded as a supplementary code for burns of an external body surface when the site is specified. It should only be used as the primary code when the site of the burn is unspecified.

8. Identify the external cause source/chemical agent, intent and place:
   - ☐ If burn, identify the source and intent XØØ-X19, X75-X77, X96-X98
   - ☐ If corrosion, code first the chemical agent and intent (T51-T65)
   - ☐ Place Y92
9. For frostbite, identify extent of tissue involvement:
   - ☐ Superficial
   - ☐ With tissue necrosis
10. For frostbite, identify body area:
    - ☐ Head
      - ☐ Ear
      - ☐ Nose
      - ☐ Other part of head
    - ☐ Neck
    - ☐ Thorax
    - ☐ Abdominal wall, lower back and pelvis
    - ☐ Arm
    - ☐ Wrist, hand, and fingers
      - ☐ Wrist
      - ☐ Hand
      - ☐ Finger(s)
    - ☐ Hip and thigh
    - ☐ Knee and lower leg
    - ☐ Ankle, foot, and toes
      - ☐ Ankle
      - ☐ Foot
      - ☐ Toe(s)
    - ☐ Other sites
    - ☐ Unspecified site
11. Identify laterality (excluding nose, neck, thorax, abdominal wall, lower back and pelvis):
    - ☐ Left
    - ☐ Right
    - ☐ Unspecified – review medical record/query physician
12. For sequencing of multiple burns and/or burns with related conditions:
    - Multiple external burns only. When more than one external burn is present, the first listed diagnosis code is the code that reflects the highest degree burn
    - Internal and external burns. The circumstances of the admission or encounter govern the selection of the principle or first-listed diagnosis
    - Burn injuries and other related conditions such as smoke inhalation or respiratory failure. The circumstances of the admission or encounter govern the selection of the principal or first-listed diagnosis.
    - Assign separate codes for each burn site
    - Classify burns of the same local site (three-digit category level) but of different degrees to the subcategory identifying the highest degree recorded in the diagnosis.

Cholecystitis, Cholelithiasis, Choledocholithiasis, and Cholangitis

ICD-10-CM Categories/Codes

K80	Cholelithiasis
K81	Cholecystitis
K83.0	Cholangitis

ICD-10-CM Definitions

Cholangitis – Inflammation of the bile ducts most often caused by the presence of stones or calculi in the bile ducts.

Cholecystitis – Inflammation of the gallbladder most often caused by the presence of calculi or sludge that blocks the flow of bile. Cholecystitis may be acute or chronic and chronic cases may be complicated by an acute inflammation.

Choledocholithiasis – Calculi in the bile ducts that may also cause inflammation of the bile ducts, referred to as cholangitis. A complication of calculi in the bile ducts is obstruction of the flow of bile.

Cholelithiasis – The presence of stones or calculi in the gallbladder. Cholelithiasis may occur alone or with cholecystitis. A complication of calculi in the gallbladder is obstruction of the flow of bile.

Checklist

1. Cholecystitis
   - ☐ With cholelithiasis or choledocholithiasis – Proceed to 3
   - ☐ Without cholelithiasis or choledocholithiasis
     - ☐ Acute (K81.Ø)
     - ☐ Acute with chronic (K81.2)
     - ☐ Chronic (K81.1)
     - ☐ Unspecified (K81.9) – review medical record/query physician
2. Cholangitis
   - ☐ With choledocholithiasis – Proceed to 3
   - ☐ Without choledocholithiasis (K83.Ø)
3. Cholelithiasis – Identify site of calculus:
   - ☐ Bile duct only – Proceed to 5
   - ☐ Gallbladder only – Proceed to 4
   - ☐ Gallbladder and bile duct – Proceed to 6
   - ☐ Other
     - ☐ With obstruction (K8Ø.81)
     - ☐ Without obstruction (K8Ø.8Ø)
4. Calculus of gallbladder only
   - ☐ With cholecystitis
     - ☐ Acute
       - ☐ With obstruction (K8Ø.Ø1)
       - ☐ Without obstruction (K8Ø.ØØ)
     - ☐ Acute and chronic

- With obstruction (K8Ø.13)
- Without obstruction (K8Ø.12)

     - ☐ Chronic

- With obstruction (K8Ø.11)
- Without obstruction (K8Ø.1Ø)

     - ☐ Other
       - ☐ With obstruction (K8Ø.19)
       - ☐ Without obstruction (K8Ø.18)
   - ☐ Without cholecystitis
     - ☐ With obstruction (K8Ø.21)
     - ☐ Without obstruction (K8Ø.2Ø)
5. Calculus of bile duct only
   - ☐ With cholangitis
     - ☐ Acute
       - ☐ With obstruction (K8Ø.33)
       - ☐ Without obstruction (K8Ø.32)
     - ☐ Acute and chronic
       - ☐ With obstruction (K8Ø.37)
       - ☐ Without obstruction (K8Ø.36)
     - ☐ Chronic
       - ☐ With obstruction (K8Ø.35)
       - ☐ Without obstruction (K8Ø.34)
     - ☐ Unspecified
       - ☐ With obstruction (K8Ø.31) – review medical record/query physician
       - ☐ Without obstruction (K8Ø.3Ø) – review medical record/query physician
   - ☐ With cholecystitis (includes cholangitis if present)
     - ☐ Acute
       - ☐ With obstruction (K8Ø.43)
       - ☐ Without obstruction (K8Ø.42)
     - ☐ Acute and chronic
       - ☐ With obstruction (K8Ø.47)
       - ☐ Without obstruction (K8Ø.46)
     - ☐ Chronic
       - ☐ With obstruction (K8Ø.45)
       - ☐ Without obstruction (K8Ø.44)
     - ☐ Unspecified
       - ☐ With obstruction (K8Ø.41) – review medical record/query physician
       - ☐ Without obstruction (K8Ø.4Ø) – review medical record/query physician
   - ☐ Without cholangitis or cholecystitis
     - ☐ With obstruction (K8Ø.51)
     - ☐ Without obstruction (K8Ø.5Ø)
6. For calculus of gallbladder and bile duct, identify:
   - ☐ With cholecystitis
     - ☐ Acute
       - ☐ With obstruction (K8Ø.63)
       - ☐ Without obstruction (K8Ø.62)
     - ☐ Acute and chronic
       - ☐ With obstruction (K8Ø.67)
       - ☐ Without obstruction (K8Ø.66)
     - ☐ Chronic
       - ☐ With obstruction (K8Ø.65)
       - ☐ Without obstruction (K8Ø.64)
     - ☐ Unspecified
       - ☐ With obstruction (K8Ø.61) – review medical record/query physician
       - ☐ Without obstruction (K8Ø.6Ø) – review medical record/query physician
   - ☐ Without cholecystitis
     - ☐ With obstruction (K8Ø.71)
     - ☐ Without obstruction (K8Ø.7Ø)

Diabetes Mellitus

ICD-10-CM Categories

E08	Diabetes mellitus due to underlying condition
E09	Drug or chemical induced diabetes mellitus
E10	Type 1 diabetes mellitus
E11	Type 2 diabetes mellitus
E13	Other specified diabetes mellitus

ICD-10-CM Definitions

Codes for diabetes mellitus are combination codes that reflect the type of diabetes, the body system affected, and any specific complications/manifestations affecting that body system.

Other specified diabetes (E13) includes secondary diabetes specified as:

- Due to genetic defects of beta-cell function
- Due to genetic defects in insulin action
- Postpancreatectomy
- Postprocedural
- Secondary diabetes not elsewhere classified

Checklist

1. Identify the type of diabetes mellitus:
   - ☐ Type 1
   - ☐ Type 2 (includes unspecified)
   - ☐ Secondary diabetes
     - ☐ Drug or chemical induced
     - ☐ Due to underlying condition
     - ☐ Other specified diabetes mellitus
2. Identify the body system affected and any manifestations/complications:
   - ☐ No complications
   - ☐ Arthropathy
     - ☐ Neuropathic
     - ☐ Other arthropathy
   - ☐ Circulatory complications
     - ☐ Peripheral angiopathy
       - ☐ With gangrene
       - ☐ Without gangrene
     - ☐ Other circulatory complication
   - ☐ Hyperglycemia
   - ☐ Hyperosmolarity (except type 1)
     - ☐ With coma
     - ☐ Without coma
   - ☐ Hypoglycemia
     - ☐ With coma
     - ☐ Without coma
   - ☐ Ketoacidosis
     - ☐ With coma
     - ☐ Without coma
   - ☐ Kidney complications
     - ☐ Nephropathy
     - ☐ Chronic kidney disease – Use additional code (N18.1-N18.6) for stage of CKD
     - ☐ Other diabetic kidney complication
   - ☐ Neurological complications
     - ☐ Amyotrophy
     - ☐ Autonomic (poly)neuropathy
     - ☐ Mononeuropathy
     - ☐ Polyneuropathy
     - ☐ Other diabetic neurological complication
     - ☐ Unspecified diabetic neuropathy
   - ☐ Ophthalmic complications
     - ☐ Diabetic retinopathy
       - ☐ Mild nonproliferative
         - ☐ With macular edema
         - ☐ Without macular edema
       - ☐ Moderate nonproliferative
         - ☐ With macular edema
         - ☐ Without macular edema
       - ☐ Severe nonproliferative
         - ☐ With macular edema
         - ☐ Without macular edema
       - ☐ Proliferative
         - ☐ With traction retinal detachment involving the macula
         - ☐ With traction retinal detachment not involving the macula
         - ☐ With combined traction retinal detachment and rhegmatogenous retinal detachment
         - ☐ With macular edema
         - ☐ Without macular edema
       - ☐ Unspecified
         - ☐ With macular edema
         - ☐ Without macular edema
       - ☐ Identify laterality (*except with diabetic cataract, unspecified diabetic retinopathy, and other diabetic ophthalmic complication*)
         - ☐ Right eye
         - ☐ Left eye
         - ☐ Bilateral
         - ☐ Unspecified eye
     - ☐ Diabetic cataract
     - ☐ Diabetic macular edema, resolved following treatment
     - ☐ Other diabetic ophthalmic complication
   - ☐ Oral complications
     - ☐ Periodontal disease
     - ☐ Other oral complications
   - ☐ Skin complications
     - ☐ Dermatitis
     - ☐ Foot ulcer – Use additional code (L97.4-, L97.5-) to identify site of ulcer

- ☐ Other skin ulcer – Use additional code (L97.1-L97.9, L98.41-L98.49) to identify site of ulcer
- ☐ Other skin complication

☐ Other specified complication – Use additional code to identify complication

☐ Unspecified complication

For Type II (E11) and secondary diabetes types (E08, E09, E13), use additional code to identify any long-term insulin use (Z79.4).

For diabetes due to underlying disease (E08), code first the underlying condition.

For diabetes due to drugs or chemicals (E09):

- Code first poisoning due to drug or toxin (T36-T65 with 5th or 6th character 1-4 or 6) – OR-
- Use additional code for adverse effect, if applicable, to identify drug (T36-T5Ø with 5th or 6th character 5)

For other specified diabetes mellitus (E13) documented as due to pancreatectomy:

- Assign first code E89.1 Postprocedural hypoinsulinemia
- Assign the applicable codes from category E13
- Assign a code from Z9Ø.41- Acquired absence of pancreas
- Use additional code (Z79.4, Z79.84) to identify type of control

Gout

ICD-10-CM Categories

Gout is classified in two categories in Chapter 13 as a disease of the musculoskeletal system and connective tissue:

M1A	Chronic gout
M10	Gout

ICD-10-CM Definitions

Chronic gout – Long term gout that develops in cases where uric acid levels remain consistently high over a number of years, resulting in more frequent attacks and pain that may remain constant.

Gout – A complex type of arthritis characterized by the accumulation of uric acid crystals within the joints, causing severe pain, redness, swelling, and stiffness, particularly in the big toe. The needle-like crystal deposits in a joint cause sudden attacks or flares of severe pain and inflammation that intensify before subsiding.

Uric acid – A chemical compound of ions and salts formed by the metabolic breakdown of purines, found in foods such as meats and shellfish, and in cells of the body.

Checklist

1. Identify type of gout:
   - ☐ Acute (attack) (flare)
   - ☐ Chronic
   - ☐ Unspecified
2. Identify cause:
   - ☐ Drug-induced
     - ☐ Use additional code to identify drug and adverse effect, if applicable
   - ☐ Due to renal impairment
     - ☐ Code first causative renal disease
   - ☐ Idiopathic (primary)
   - ☐ Lead-induced
     - ☐ Code first toxic effects of lead and lead compounds
   - ☐ Secondary
     - ☐ Code first associated condition
   - ☐ Unspecified
3. Identify site:
   - ☐ Lower extremity
     - ☐ Ankle/foot
     - ☐ Hip
     - ☐ Knee
   - ☐ Upper extremity
     - ☐ Elbow
     - ☐ Hand
     - ☐ Shoulder
     - ☐ Wrist
   - ☐ Vertebrae
   - ☐ Multiple sites
   - ☐ Unspecified site
4. Identify laterality for extremities:
   - ☐ Left
   - ☐ Right
   - ☐ Unspecified
5. For chronic gout, identify presence/absence of tophi:
   - ☐ With tophi
   - ☐ Without tophi
6. For all types of gout, identify any accompanying conditions with the underlying gout:
   - ☐ Autonomic neuropathy
   - ☐ Cardiomyopathy
   - ☐ Disorders of external ear, iris, or ciliary body
   - ☐ Glomerular disorders
   - ☐ Urinary calculus

Lymphoma – Follicular

ICD-10-CM Category

C82 Follicular lymphoma

ICD-10-CM Definitions

Follicular lymphoma – Lymphoma is a cancer of the lymph system. Follicular lymphoma is an indolent (slow growing), non-Hodgkin lymphoma (NHL) that arises from B-lymphocytes, which means that it is a B-cell lymphoma.

Follicular lymphoma is subdivided into several different types with some types being further differentiated by grade. The grading system used in ICD-10-CM was developed by the Revised European-American Classification of Lymphoid Neoplasms (REAL) which has also been adopted by the World Health Organization (WHO). The REAL/WHO classification grades follicular lymphoma based on the number of centroblasts per high-power field (hpf). The grades are as follows:

- Grade I (1) Ø-5 centroblasts per hpf with a predominance of small centrocytes
- Grade II (2) 6-15 centroblasts per hpf with centrocytes present
- Grade III (3) >15 centroblasts per hpf with a decreased number or no centrocytes present
  - Grade IIIa (3A) >15 centroblasts per hpf with centrocytes still present
  - Grade IIIb (3B) >15 centroblasts per hpf presenting as solid sheets with no centrocytes present

The REAL/WHO classification also recognizes 2 variants of follicular lymphoma—cutaneous follicle center lymphoma and diffuse follicle center lymphoma, which have specific ICD-10-CM codes.

Checklist

1. Review notes and/or pathology report and identify the non-Hodgkin follicular lymphoma:
   - ☐ Follicular lymphoma
     - ☐ Grade I
     - ☐ Grade II
     - ☐ Grade IIIa
     - ☐ Grade IIIb
     - ☐ Grade III, unspecified – review medical record/query physician
   - ☐ Diffuse follicle center lymphoma
   - ☐ Cutaneous follicle center lymphoma
   - ☐ Other types of follicular lymphoma
   - ☐ Unspecified follicular lymphoma – review medical record/query physician
2. Identify site or sites:
   - ☐ Lymph nodes
     - ☐ Head/face/neck
     - ☐ Intrathoracic
     - ☐ Intra-abdominal
     - ☐ Axilla and upper limb
     - ☐ Inguinal region and lower limb
     - ☐ Intrapelvic
     - ☐ Multiple lymph node sites
   - ☐ Spleen
   - ☐ Extranodal/solid organ sites
   - ☐ Unspecified site – review medical record/query physician

Melanoma/Melanoma In Situ

ICD-10-CM Categories

C43	Malignant melanoma of skin
D03	Melanoma in situ

ICD-10-CM Definitions

Melanoma in situ – Malignant neoplasm of the melanin (brown pigment producing) cells that is documented as in situ, which includes melanoma that is described as:

- Stage Ø
- TIS (tumor in situ)
- Epidermal layer only

Melanoma – Malignant neoplasm of the melanin (brown pigment producing) cells that is described as having invaded the dermis or as one of the following stages:

- Stage I – localized
  - Stage IA - less than 1.Ø mm thick, no ulceration, no lymph node involvement, no distant metastases
  - Stage 1B – less than 1.Ø mm thick with ulceration or less than 2.Ø mm thick without ulceration, no lymph node involvement, no distant metastases
- Stage II – localized
  - Stage IIA - 1.Ø1-2.ØØ mm thick with ulceration, no lymph node involvement, no distant metastases
  - Stage IIB - 2.Ø1-4.ØØ mm thick without ulceration, no lymph node involvement, no distant metastases
  - Stage IIC - greater than 4.ØØ mm thick with ulceration, no lymph node involvement, no distant metastases
- Stage III – tumor spread to regional lymph nodes or development of in transit metastases or satellites without spread to distant sites. Three substages IIIA, IIIB, IIIC.
- Stage IV – tumor spread beyond regional lymph nodes with metastases to distant sites

Checklist

1. Review physician notes and/or pathology report and identify as:
   - ☐ Melanoma In Situ (see category DØ3)
   - ☐ Malignant melanoma (see category C43)
2. Identify site:
   - ☐ Head and Neck
     - ☐ Lip
     - ☐ Eyelid/canthus
       - ☐ Right
       - ☐ Left
       - ☐ Unspecified side – review medical record/query physician
     - ☐ Ear/external auricular canal
       - ☐ Right
       - ☐ Left
       - ☐ Unspecified side – review medical record/query physician
     - ☐ Nose (C43.31)
     - ☐ Other parts of face (includes nose for melanoma in situ)
     - ☐ Unspecified part of face – review medical record/query physician
     - ☐ Scalp/neck
   - ☐ Trunk
     - ☐ Anal skin
     - ☐ Skin of breast
     - ☐ Other parts of trunk
   - ☐ Extremities
     - ☐ Upper limb, including shoulder
       - ☐ Right
       - ☐ Left
       - ☐ Unspecified side – review medical record/query physician
     - ☐ Lower limb, including hip
       - ☐ Right
       - ☐ Left
       - ☐ Unspecified side – review medical record/query physician
   - ☐ Other sites (DØ3.8)
   - ☐ Overlapping sites of skin (C43.8)
   - ☐ Unspecified site – review medical record/query physician

   Note: Overlapping sites of skin applies only to malignant melanoma.

   Other sites apply only to melanoma in situ.

   Reference the Alphabetic Index carefully as there are other identified body sites listed under Melanoma (malignant), skin, but they are not coded to C43. These include male and female external genital organs.

Open Wound

ICD-10-CM Categories

Open wound codes are used for wounds caused by trauma. Do not assign a code for "open wound" unless the etiology of the wound is related to trauma. Open wounds are classified in the following ICD-10-CM categories:

S01	Open wound of head
S11	Open wound of neck
S21	Open wound of thorax
S31	Open wound of abdomen, lower back, pelvis, and external genitalia
S41	Open wound of shoulder and upper arm
S51	Open wound of elbow and forearm
S61	Open wound of wrist, hand, and fingers
S71	Open wound of hip and thigh
S81	Open wound of knee and lower leg
S91	Open wound of ankle, foot, and toes

ICD-10-CM Definitions

Episode of Care – There are three (3) possible 7th character values to select from for open wounds. The 7th character defines the stage of treatment and residual effects related to the initial injury.

A **Initial encounter.** The period when the patient is receiving active treatment for the injury, poisoning, or other consequences of an external cause. An 'A' may be assigned on more than one claim.

D **Subsequent encounter.** Encounter after the active phase of treatment and when the patient is receiving routine care for the injury during the period of healing or recovery.

S **Sequela.** Encounter for complications or conditions that arise as a direct result of an injury.

Laceration – A tear, cut or gash caused by a sharp object producing edges that may be jagged or straight.

Puncture wound – A wound caused by an object that pierces the skin or an organ, creating a small hole.

Checklist

1. Identify the type of open wound:
   - ☐ Bite
   - ☐ Laceration
     - ☐ With foreign body
     - ☐ Without foreign body
   - ☐ Puncture wound
     - ☐ With foreign body
     - ☐ Without foreign body
   - ☐ Unspecified open wound – review medical record/query physician
2. Identify the body area:
   - ☐ Head
     - ☐ Scalp
     - ☐ Eyelid and periocular area
     - ☐ Ear
     - ☐ Nose
     - ☐ Cheek and temporomandibular area
     - ☐ Lip and oral cavity
     - ☐ Other parts of head
     - ☐ Unspecified part of head – review medical record/query physician
   - ☐ Neck
     - ☐ Larynx
     - ☐ Trachea
     - ☐ Vocal cord
     - ☐ Thyroid gland
     - ☐ Pharynx and cervical esophagus
     - ☐ Other specified parts of neck
     - ☐ Unspecified part of neck – review medical record/query physician
   - ☐ Thorax
     - ☐ Front wall of thorax
       - ☐ With penetration into thoracic cavity
       - ☐ Without penetration into thoracic cavity
     - ☐ Back wall of thorax
       - ☐ With penetration into thoracic cavity
       - ☐ Without penetration into thoracic cavity
     - ☐ Unspecified part of thorax – review medical record/query physician
   - ☐ Abdomen, lower back, pelvis, and external genitalia
     - ☐ Abdominal wall
       - ☐ Upper quadrant
         - ☐ With penetration into peritoneal cavity
         - ☐ Without penetration into peritoneal cavity
       - ☐ Epigastric region
         - ☐ With penetration into peritoneal cavity
         - ☐ Without penetration into peritoneal cavity
       - ☐ Lower quadrant
         - ☐ With penetration into peritoneal cavity
         - ☐ Without penetration into peritoneal cavity
     - ☐ Penis
     - ☐ Scrotum and testis
     - ☐ Vagina and vulva
     - ☐ Unspecified external genital organs – review medical record/query physician
     - ☐ Lower back and pelvis
       - ☐ With penetration into retroperitoneum
       - ☐ Without penetration into retroperitoneum
     - ☐ Buttock
     - ☐ Anus
   - ☐ Shoulder and upper arm
     - ☐ Shoulder
     - ☐ Upper arm
   - ☐ Elbow and forearm
     - ☐ Elbow
     - ☐ Forearm
   - ☐ Wrist, hand, and fingers
     - ☐ Wrist
     - ☐ Hand

- ☐ Thumb
  - ☐ With damage to nail
  - ☐ Without damage to nail
- ☐ Other finger
  - ☐ Index finger
    - ☐ With damage to nail
    - ☐ Without damage to nail
  - ☐ Middle finger
    - ☐ With damage to nail
    - ☐ Without damage to nail
  - ☐ Ring finger
    - ☐ With damage to nail
    - ☐ Without damage to nail
  - ☐ Little finger
    - ☐ With damage to nail
    - ☐ Without damage to nail

☐ Hip and thigh
- ☐ Hip
- ☐ Thigh

☐ Knee and lower leg
- ☐ Knee
- ☐ Lower leg

☐ Ankle, foot, and toes
- ☐ Ankle
- ☐ Foot
- ☐ Toe
  - ☐ Great toe
    - ☐ With damage to nail
    - ☐ Without damage to nail
  - ☐ Lesser toe
    - ☐ With damage to nail
    - ☐ Without damage to nail

3. Identify laterality:
   - ☐ Left
   - ☐ Right
   - ☐ Unspecified – review medical record/query physician

Note: Not all codes require laterality. Laterality is pertinent whenever there are two sides for the same structure, such as but not limited to eyelids, cheeks, extremities, buttocks, upper and lower abdominal quadrants, breasts, and chest wall.

4. Identify episode of care/stage of healing/complication:
   - ☐ A Initial encounter
   - ☐ D Subsequent encounter
   - ☐ S Sequela
5. Code also any associated wound infection
6. Identify any associated injury and report with additional codes
   - ☐ Open wound of head
     - ☐ Cranial nerve injury (SØ4)
     - ☐ Intracranial injury (SØ6)
     - ☐ Muscle and tendon of head (SØ9.1-)
   - ☐ Open wound of neck
     - ☐ Associated spinal cord injury (S14.Ø–S14.1-)
     - ☐ Blood vessel injury (S15)
     - ☐ Dislocation and subluxation (S13)
   - ☐ Open wound of thorax
     - ☐ Blood vessel injury (S25)
     - ☐ Dislocation and subluxation (S23)
     - ☐ Injury of heart (S26)
     - ☐ Injury of intrathoracic organs (S27)
     - ☐ Injury of muscle and tendon of thorax (S29)
     - ☐ Rib fracture (S22.3-, S22.4-)
     - ☐ Spinal cord injury (S24.Ø, S24.1-)
     - ☐ Traumatic hemopneumothorax (S27.32)
     - ☐ Traumatic hemothorax (S27.1)
     - ☐ Traumatic pneumothorax (S27.Ø)
   - ☐ Open wound of abdomen, lower back, pelvis, and external genitalia
     - ☐ Associated spinal cord injury (S24.Ø, S24.1-, S34.Ø-, S34.1-)
     - ☐ Blood vessel injury (S35)
     - ☐ Dislocation and subluxation of lumbar vertebra (S33)
     - ☐ Injury of intra-abdominal organ (S36)
     - ☐ Injury of muscle, fascia, and tendon of abdomen, lower back and pelvis (S39)
     - ☐ Injury of urinary and pelvic organs (S37)
   - ☐ Open wound of shoulder and upper arm
     - ☐ Blood vessel injury (S45)
     - ☐ Dislocation and subluxation (S43)
     - ☐ Muscle, fascia, and tendon injury (S46)
     - ☐ Nerve injury (S44)
   - ☐ Open wound of elbow and forearm
     - ☐ Blood vessel injury (S55)
     - ☐ Dislocation and subluxation (S53)
     - ☐ Muscle, fascia, and tendon injury (S56)
     - ☐ Nerve injury (S54)
   - ☐ Open wound of wrist, hand, and fingers
     - ☐ Blood vessel injury (S65)
     - ☐ Dislocation and subluxation (S63)
     - ☐ Muscle, fascia, and tendon injury (S66)
     - ☐ Nerve injury (S64)
   - ☐ Open wound of hip and thigh
     - ☐ Blood vessel injury (S75)
     - ☐ Dislocation and subluxation (S73)
     - ☐ Muscle, fascia, and tendon injury (S76)
     - ☐ Nerve injury (S74)
   - ☐ Open wound of knee and lower leg
     - ☐ Blood vessel injury (S85)
     - ☐ Dislocation and subluxation (S83)
     - ☐ Muscle, fascia, and tendon injury (S86)
     - ☐ Nerve injury (S84)
   - ☐ Open wound of foot, ankle, and toes
     - ☐ Blood vessel injury (S95)
     - ☐ Dislocation and subluxation (S93)
     - ☐ Muscle, fascia, and tendon injury (S96)
     - ☐ Nerve injury (S94)
7. Identify the external cause, intent, activity, place and status where applicable.

Pharyngitis/Tonsillitis, Acute

ICD-10-CM Categories

J02	Acute pharyngitis
J03	Acute tonsillitis

ICD-10-CM Definitions

Acute Pharyngitis – Acute inflammation of the throat including the mucous membrane and underlying part of the pharynx. Additional terms used to describe acute pharyngitis include: gangrenous pharyngitis, infective pharyngitis, sore throat, suppurative pharyngitis, ulcerative pharyngitis.

Acute Tonsillitis – Acute inflammation of the palatine tonsils. Tonsillitis may be a single acute inflammation or may occur repeatedly in which case it is classified as acute recurrent. Additional terms used to describe acute tonsillitis include: follicular tonsillitis, gangrenous tonsillitis, infective tonsillitis, ulcerative tonsillitis.

Streptococcal Pharyngitis – Acute inflammation of the throat including the mucous membrane and underlying part of the pharynx due to Group A, beta-hemolytic streptococcus (GABHS) infection. Additional terms used to describe streptococcal pharyngitis include: septic pharyngitis, streptococcal sore throat.

Streptococcal Tonsillitis – Acute inflammation of the palatine tonsils due to Group A, beta-hemolytic streptococcus (GABHS) infection. Streptococcal tonsillitis may be a single acute infection or may occur repeatedly in which case it is classified as acute recurrent.

Checklist

1. Identify as acute pharyngitis/tonsillitis
   - ☐ Acute Pharyngitis
   - ☐ Acute Tonsillitis
2. Identify organism
   - ☐ Streptococcus
   - ☐ Assign additional code to identify organism (B95-B97)

     ____
   - ☐ Unspecified organism
3. For acute tonsillitis, identify as:
   - ☐ Acute (single episode)
   - ☐ Acute recurrent (multiple repeat episodes)

Pneumonia

ICD-10-CM Categories/Subcategories

Codes for pneumonia are located across multiple categories, found mainly in Chapter 10 Diseases of the Respiratory System with some codes listed in Chapter 1 Certain Infectious and Parasitic Diseases. Congenital pneumonia is coded in Chapter 17 Congenital Malformations, Deformations, and Chromosomal Abnormalities.

Coding pneumonia may require more than one code to capture the type of pneumonia, infecting organism, associated or underlying conditions, and any related abscess. Follow all coding instructions carefully for sequencing and assigning pneumonia codes for the specific type of organism, and all other related conditions or factors.

The main categories and some specific codes for pneumonia are listed below, although the list is not all inclusive of codes that report pneumonia or conditions occurring with pneumonia:

A15.0	Tuberculous pneumonia
B01.2	Varicella pneumonia
J12	Viral pneumonia, not elsewhere classified
J13	Pneumonia due to Streptococcus pneumoniae
J14	Pneumonia due to Hemophilus influenzae
J15	Bacterial pneumonia, not elsewhere classified
J16	Pneumonia due to infectious organisms, not elsewhere classified
J17	Pneumonia in diseases classified elsewhere
J18	Pneumonia, unspecific organism
J69	Pneumonitis due to solids and liquids
J84.11	Idiopathic interstitial pneumonia
J95.851	Ventilator associated pneumonia
P23	Congenital pneumonia
P24.01	Meconium aspiration pneumonia

ICD-10-CM Definitions

Pneumonia – An inflammation or infection of the lung(s) caused by microorganisms such as bacteria, viruses, or fungi; aspiration of foreign material; or inhalation of chemicals or hazardous materials, causing an accumulation of fluid, inflammatory cells, and fibrin that impairs the exchange of oxygen and carbon dioxide in the alveoli.

Checklist

1. Identify the type of pneumonia:
   - ☐ Aspiration/Inhalation – Proceed to #2
   - ☐ Bacterial – Proceed to #3
   - ☐ Congenital – Proceed to #4
   - ☐ Fungal – Proceed to #5
   - ☐ Interstitial – Proceed to #6
   - ☐ Other specified types – Proceed to #7
   - ☐ Viral – Proceed to #8
2. Aspiration/Inhalation pneumonia
   a. Identify causative aspirate:
      - ☐ Anesthesia
        - ☐ During labor and delivery (O74.Ø)
        - ☐ During pregnancy (O29.Ø1-)
        - ☐ During puerperium (O89.Ø1)
        - ☐ Postprocedural, chemical (J95.4)
      - ☐ Fumes, Vapors, Gases (J68.Ø)
      - ☐ Solids and liquids
        - ☐ Blood (J69.8)
        - ☐ Detergent (J69.8)
        - ☐ Food (J69.Ø)
        - ☐ Gastric Secretions (J69.Ø)
        - ☐ Oils and Essences (J69.1)
        - ☐ Other Solids and Liquids (J69.8)
        - ☐ Vomit (J69.Ø)
      - ☐ Unspecified (J69.Ø)
3. Bacterial pneumonia
   a. Identify causative bacteria:
      - ☐ Actinomyces (A42.Ø)
      - ☐ Bacillus anthracis (A22.1)
      - ☐ Bacteroides (J15.8)
      - ☐ Bordetella
        - ☐ Other (A37.81)
        - ☐ Parapertussis (A37.11)
        - ☐ Pertussis (A37.Ø1)
      - ☐ Burkholderia pseudomallei (A24.1)
      - ☐ Butyrivibrio fibriosolvens (J15.8)
      - ☐ Chlamydia (J16.Ø)
        - ☐ Psittaci (A7Ø)
      - ☐ Clostridium (J15.8)
      - ☐ Eaton's agent (J15.7)
      - ☐ Enterobacter (J15.6)
      - ☐ Escherichia coli (J15.5)
      - ☐ Friedlander's bacillus (J15.Ø)
      - ☐ Fusobacterium nucleatum (J15.8)
      - ☐ Gram-negative, other (J15.6)
      - ☐ Gram-positive (J15.9)
      - ☐ Hemophilus influenzae (J14)
      - ☐ Klebsiella pneumoniae (J15.Ø)
      - ☐ Melioidosis (A24.1)
      - ☐ Mycoplasma pneumoniae (J15.7)
      - ☐ Neisseria gonorrhoeae (A54.84)
      - ☐ Nocardia asteroides (A43.Ø)
      - ☐ Other specified (J15.8)
      - ☐ Proteus (J15.6)
      - ☐ Pseudomonas (J15.1)
      - ☐ Salmonella (AØ2.22)
        - ☐ typhi (AØ1.Ø3)
      - ☐ Serratia marcescens (J15.6)
      - ☐ Staphylococcus
        - ☐ Aureus, Methicillin resistant (J15.212)
        - ☐ Aureus, Methicillin susceptible (J15.211)
        - ☐ Other (J15.29)
        - ☐ Unspecified staphylococcus (J15.2Ø)

- ☐ Streptococcus
  - ☐ Group B (J15.3)
  - ☐ Other (J15.4)
  - ☐ S. pneumoniae (J13)
- ☐ Tuberculosis (A15.Ø)
- ☐ Unspecified bacteria (J15.9)

4. Congenital pneumonia
   a. Identify causative source:
   - ☐ Aspiration
     - ☐ Amniotic fluid and mucus (P24.11)
     - ☐ Blood (P24.21)
     - ☐ Meconium (P24.Ø1)
     - ☐ Milk and regurgitated food (P24.31)
     - ☐ Other/Unspecified (P24.81)
   - ☐ Infectious Agent
     - ☐ Chlamydia (P23.1)
     - ☐ Escherichia coli (P23.4)
     - ☐ Francisella tularensis (A21.2)
     - ☐ Hemophilus influenzae (P23.6)
     - ☐ Klebsiella pneumoniae (P23.6)
     - ☐ Mycoplasma (P23.6)
     - ☐ Other bacterial agent (P23.6)
     - ☐ Other organisms (P23.8)
     - ☐ Pseudomonas (P23.5)
     - ☐ Rubella (P35.Ø)
     - ☐ Staphylococcus (P23.2)
     - ☐ Streptococcus
       - ☐ Group B (P23.3)
       - ☐ Other (P23.6)
     - ☐ Syphilitic, early (A5Ø.Ø4)
     - ☐ Viral agent (P23.Ø)
     - ☐ Unspecified (P23.9)

5. Fungal pneumonia
   a. Identify causative type:
   - ☐ Aspergillosis
     - ☐ Invasive (B44.Ø)
     - ☐ Other (B44.1)
   - ☐ Blastomycosis
     - ☐ Acute (B4Ø.Ø)
     - ☐ Chronic (B4Ø.1)
     - ☐ Unspecified (B4Ø.2)
   - ☐ Candidiasis (B37.1)
   - ☐ Coccidioidomycosis
     - ☐ Acute (B38.Ø)
     - ☐ Chronic (B38.1)
     - ☐ Unspecified (B38.2)
   - ☐ Cryptococcosis (B45.Ø)
   - ☐ Histoplasmosis
     - ☐ Acute (B39.Ø)
     - ☐ Chronic (B39.1)
     - ☐ Unspecified (B39.2)
   - ☐ Paracoccidioidomycosis (B41.Ø)
   - ☐ Pneumocystosis (B59)
   - ☐ Sporotrichosis (B42.Ø)

6. Interstitial pneumonia
   a. Identify type:
   - ☐ Idiopathic
     - ☐ Acute (J84.114)
     - ☐ Cryptogenic organizing (J84.116)
     - ☐ Desquamative (J84.117)
     - ☐ Fibrosing (J84.112)
     - ☐ Hamman-Rich (J84.114)
     - ☐ Nonspecific (J84.113)
     - ☐ Not otherwise specified (J84.111)
     - ☐ Respiratory bronchiolitis (J84.115)
   - ☐ In diseases classified elsewhere (J84.17)
   - ☐ Lymphoid (J84.2)

7. Other specified types
   a. Identify type, other causative agent, or site:
   - ☐ Allergic/eosinophilic (J82)
   - ☐ Ascariasis (B77.81)
   - ☐ Bronchopneumonia (J18.Ø)
   - ☐ Due to other specified infectious organism (J16.8)
   - ☐ Hypostatic (J18.2)
   - ☐ In diseases classified elsewhere (J17)
   - ☐ Lobar (J18.1)
   - ☐ Other (J18.8)
   - ☐ Passive (J18.2)
   - ☐ Toxoplasma gondii (B58.3)
   - ☐ Ventilator associated (J95.851)

8. Viral pneumonia
   a. Identify causative virus:
   - ☐ Adenoviral (J12.Ø)
   - ☐ Human metapneumovirus (J12.3)
   - ☐ Other virus (J12.89)
   - ☐ Parainfluenza (J12.2)
   - ☐ Postmeasles (BØ5.2)
   - ☐ Respiratory syncytial virus (J12.1)
   - ☐ Rubella (BØ6.81)
   - ☐ SARS-associated coronavirus (J12.81)
   - ☐ Varicella (BØ1.2)
   - ☐ Unspecified (J12.9)

9. Unspecified pneumonia (J18.9)

Seizures

ICD-10-CM Categories/Subcategories

Codes for seizures are located across multiple categories in different chapters. Epileptic seizures are the only group classified to Chapter 6 Diseases of the Nervous System. Other types of nonepileptic seizures such as new onset, febrile, or hysterical seizure are classified to other chapters.

F44.5	Conversion disorder with seizures or convulsions
G40	Epilepsy and recurrent seizures
P90	Convulsions of newborn
R56	Convulsions, not elsewhere classified

ICD-10-CM Definitions

Absence seizure – A type of seizure common in children that appears as brief, sudden lapses in attention or vacant staring spells during which the child is unresponsive; often accompanied by other signs such as lip smacking, chewing motions, eyelid fluttering, and small finger or hand movements; formerly called petit mal seizure.

Epilepsy – Disorder of the central nervous system characterized by long-term predisposition to recurring episodes of sudden onset seizures, muscle contractions, sensory disturbance, and loss of consciousness caused by excessive neuronal activity in the brain and resulting in cognitive, psychological, and neurobiological consequences.

Generalized tonic clonic seizure – A type of seizure involving the entire body that usually begins on both sides of the brain and manifests with loss of consciousness, muscle stiffness, and convulsive, jerking movements; also called grand mal seizure.

Juvenile myoclonic epilepsy – A form of generalized epilepsy manifesting in mid or late childhood typically emerging first as absence seizures, then the presence of myoclonic jerks upon awakening from sleep in another 1-9 years as its hallmark feature, followed by generalized tonic clonic seizures some months later in nearly all cases.

Lennox-Gastaut syndrome – Severe form of epilepsy characterized by multiple different seizure types that are hard to control that may be absence, tonic (muscle stiffening), atonic (muscle drop), myoclonic, tonic clonic (grand mal); usually beginning before age 4 and associated with impaired intellectual functioning, developmental delay, and behavioral disturbances.

Localization-related epilepsy – Focal epilepsy generating seizures from one localized area of the brain where excessive or abnormal electrical discharges begin; synonymous with partial epilepsy.

Myoclonic jerks – Irregular, shock-like movements in the arms or legs that occur upon awakening, usually seen affecting both arms but sometimes restricted to the fingers, and may occur unilaterally, typically occurring in clusters and often a warning sign before generalized tonic clonic seizure.

Seizure – A transient occurrence of abnormal or uncontrolled electrical discharges in the brain resulting in an event of physical convulsions, thought and sensory disturbances, other minor physical signs, and possible loss of consciousness.

Checklist

1. Identify type of seizure(s):
   - ☐ Epileptic – Proceed to #2
   - ☐ Other (nonepileptic) type – Proceed to #3
2. Epilepsy and recurrent seizures
   a. Identify type of epilepsy or epileptic syndrome:
      - ☐ Absence epileptic syndrome (G4Ø.A-)
      - ☐ Epileptic spasms (G4Ø.82-)
      - ☐ Generalized
        - ☐ Idiopathic (G4Ø.3-)
        - ☐ Other (G4Ø.4-)
      - ☐ Juvenile myoclonic epilepsy (G4Ø.B-)
      - ☐ Lennox-Gastaut syndrome (G4Ø.81-)
      - ☐ Localization-related (focal) (partial)
        - ☐ Idiopathic (G4Ø.Ø-)
        - ☐ Symptomatic
          - ☐ With complex partial seizures (G4Ø.2-)
          - ☐ With simple partial seizures (G4Ø.1-)
      - ☐ Other epilepsy (G4Ø.8Ø-)
      - ☐ Other seizures (G4Ø.89)
      - ☐ Related to external causes (G4Ø.5-)
      - ☐ Unspecified epilepsy (G4Ø.9-)

   b. Determine intractability status:
      - ☐ Intractable
      - ☐ Not intractable

   Note: Intractable status does not apply to other seizures or to epileptic seizures related to external causes.

   c. Determine status epilepticus:
      - ☐ With status epilepticus
      - ☐ Without status epilepticus

   Note: Status epilepticus does not apply to other seizures.
3. Other (nonepileptic) type seizures
   a. Identify type of other nonepileptic seizure:
      - ☐ Febrile
        - ☐ Complex (R56.Ø1)
        - ☐ Simple (R56.ØØ)
      - ☐ Hysterical (F44.5)
      - ☐ Newborn (P9Ø)
      - ☐ Post-traumatic (R56.1)
      - ☐ Unspecified (R56.9)

Documentation Guidelines for Evaluation and Management (E/M) Services

I. Introduction

What is documentation and why is it important?

Medical record documentation is required to record pertinent facts, findings, and observations about an individual's health history including past and present illnesses, examinations, tests, treatments, and outcomes. The medical record chronologically documents the care of the patient and is an important element contributing to high-quality care. The medical record facilitates:

- the ability of the physician and other health care professionals to evaluate and plan the patient's immediate treatment, and to monitor his/her health care over time;
- communication and continuity of care among physicians and other health care professionals involved in the patient's care;
- accurate and timely claims review and payment;
- appropriate utilization review and quality of care evaluations; and
- collection of data that may be useful for research and education.

An appropriately documented medical record can reduce many of the "hassles" associated with claims processing and may serve as a legal document to verify the care provided, if necessary.

What do payers want and why?

Because payers have a contractual obligation to enrollees, they may require reasonable documentation that services are consistent with the insurance coverage provided. They may request information to validate:

- the site of service;
- the medical necessity and appropriateness of the diagnostic and/or therapeutic services provided; and/or
- that services provided have been accurately reported.

II. General Principles of Medical Record Documentation

The principles of documentation listed below are applicable to all types of medical and surgical services in all settings. For Evaluation and Management (E/M) services, the nature and amount of physician work and documentation varies by type of service, place of service and the patient's status. The general principles listed below may be modified to account for these variable circumstances in providing E/M services.

1. The medical record should be complete and legible.
2. The documentation of each patient encounter should include:
   - reason for the encounter and relevant history, physical examination findings and prior diagnostic test results;
   - assessment, clinical impression or diagnosis;
   - plan for care; and
   - date and legible identity of the observer.
3. If not documented, the rationale for ordering diagnostic and other ancillary services should be easily inferred.
4. Past and present diagnoses should be accessible to the treating and/or consulting physician.
5. Appropriate health risk factors should be identified.
6. The patient's progress, response to and changes in treatment, and revision of diagnosis should be documented.
7. The CPT® and ICD-10-CM codes reported on the health insurance claim form or billing statement should be supported by the documentation in the medical record.

III. Documentation of E/M Services

This publication provides definitions and documentation guidelines for the three *key* components of E/M services and for visits which consist predominately of counseling or coordination of care. The three key components — history, examination, and medical decision-making — appear in the descriptors for office and other outpatient services, hospital observation services, hospital inpatient services, consultations, emergency department services, nursing facility services, domiciliary care services and home services. While some of the text of CPT® has been repeated in this publication, the reader should refer to CPT® for the complete descriptors for E/M services and instructions for selecting a level of service.

Documentation Guidelines are identified by the symbol • *DG.*

The descriptors for the levels of E/M services recognize seven components which are used in defining the levels of E/M services. These components are:

- history;
- examination;
- medical decision-making;
- counseling;
- coordination of care;
- nature of presenting problem; and
- time.

The first three of these components (i.e., history, examination and medical decision-making) are the key components in selecting the level of E/M services. In the case of visits which consist predominantly of counseling or coordination of care, time is the key or controlling factor to qualify for a particular level of E/M service.

Because the level of E/M service is dependent on two or three *key* components, performance and documentation of one component (e.g., examination) at the highest level does not necessarily mean that the encounter in its entirety qualifies for the highest level of E/M service.

These documentation guidelines for E/M services reflect the needs of the typical adult population. For certain groups of patients, the recorded information may vary slightly from that described here. Specifically, the medical records of infants, children, adolescents and pregnant women may have additional or modified information recorded in each history and examination area.

As an example, newborn records may include under history of the present illness (HPI) the details of mother's pregnancy and the infant's status at birth; social history will focus on family structure; family history will focus on congenital anomalies and hereditary disorders in the family. In addition, the content of a pediatric examination will vary with the age and development of the child. Although not specifically defined in these documentation guidelines, these patient group variations on history and examination are appropriate.

A. Documentation of History

The levels of E/M services are based on four types of history (Problem Focused, Expanded Problem Focused, Detailed and Comprehensive). Each type of history includes some or all of the following elements:

- Chief complaint (CC);
- History of present illness (HPI);
- Review of systems (ROS); and
- Past, family and/or social history (PFSH).

The extent of history of present illness, review of systems and past, family and/or social history that is obtained and documented is dependent upon clinical judgment and the nature of the presenting problem(s).

The chart below shows the progression of the elements required for each type of history. To qualify for a given type of history all three elements in the table must be met. (A chief complaint is indicated at all levels.)

History of Present Illness (HPI)	Review of Systems (ROS)	Past, Family, and/or Social History (PFSH)	Type of History
Brief	N/A	N/A	Problem Focused
Brief	Problem Pertinent	Problem Pertinent	Expanded Problem Focused
Extended	Extended	Pertinent	Detailed
Extended	Complete	Complete	Comprehensive

• ***DG:*** *The CC, ROS and PFSH may be listed as separate elements of history, or they may be included in the description of the history of the present illness.*

• ***DG:*** *A ROS and/or a PFSH obtained during an earlier encounter does not need to be re-recorded if there is evidence that the physician reviewed and updated the previous information. This may occur when a physician updates his or her own record or in an institutional setting or group practice where many physicians use a common record. The review and update may be documented by:*

- *describing any new ROS and/or PFSH information or noting there has been no change in the information; and*
- *noting the date and location of the earlier ROS and/or PFSH.*

• ***DG:*** *The ROS and/or PFSH may be recorded by ancillary staff or on a form completed by the patient. To document that the physician reviewed the information, there must be a notation supplementing or confirming the information recorded by others.*

• ***DG:*** *If the physician is unable to obtain a history from the patient or other source, the record should describe the patient's condition or other circumstance which precludes obtaining a history.*

Definitions and specific documentation guidelines for each of the elements of history are listed below.

Chief Complaint (CC)

The CC is a concise statement describing the symptom, problem, condition, diagnosis, physician recommended return, or other factor that is the reason for the encounter, usually stated in the patient's words.

• *DG: The medical record should clearly reflect the chief complaint.*

History of Present Illness (HPI)

The HPI is a chronological description of the development of the patient's present illness from the first sign and/or symptom or from the previous encounter to the present. It includes the following elements:

- location,
- quality,
- severity,
- duration,
- timing,
- context,
- modifying factors, and
- associated signs and symptoms.

Brief and ***extended*** HPIs are distinguished by the amount of detail needed to accurately characterize the clinical problem(s).

A brief HPI consists of one to three elements of the HPI.

• *DG: The medical record should describe one to three elements of the present illness (HPI).*

An ***extended*** HPI consists of at least four elements of the HPI or the status of at least three chronic or inactive conditions.

• *DG: The medical record should describe at least four elements of the present illness (HPI), or the status of at least three chronic or inactive conditions.*

Review of Systems (ROS)

A ROS is an inventory of body systems obtained through a series of questions seeking to identify signs and/or symptoms which the patient may be experiencing or has experienced.

For purposes of ROS, the following systems are recognized:

- Constitutional symptoms (e.g., fever, weight loss)
- Eyes
- Ears, Nose, Mouth, Throat
- Cardiovascular
- Respiratory
- Gastrointestinal
- Genitourinary
- Musculoskeletal
- Integumentary (skin and/or breast)
- Neurological
- Psychiatric
- Endocrine
- Hematologic/Lymphatic
- Allergic/Immunologic

A ***problem*** pertinent ROS inquires about the system directly related to the problem(s) identified in the HPI.

• *DG: The patient's positive responses and pertinent negatives for the system related to the problem should be documented.*

An ***extended*** ROS inquires about the system directly related to the problem(s) identified in the HPI and a

limited number of additional systems.

• *DG: The patient's positive responses and pertinent negatives for two to nine systems should be documented.*

A ***complete*** ROS inquires about the system(s) directly related to the problem(s) identified in the HPI plus all additional body systems.

• *DG: At least 10 organ systems must be reviewed. Those systems with positive or pertinent negative responses must be individually documented. For the remaining systems, a notation indicating all other systems are negative is permissible. In the absence of such a notation, at least 10 systems must be individually documented.*

Past, Family and/or Social History (PFSH)

The PFSH consists of a review of three areas: past history (the patient's past experiences with illnesses, operations, injuries and treatments); family history (a review of medical events in the patient's family, including diseases which may be hereditary or place the patient at risk); and social history (an age-appropriate review of past and current activities).

For certain categories of E/M services that include only an interval history, it is not necessary to record information about the PFSH. Those categories are subsequent hospital care, follow-up inpatient consultations and subsequent nursing facility care.

A ***pertinent*** PFSH is a review of the history area(s) directly related to the problem(s) identified in the HPI.

• *DG: At least one specific item from any of the three history areas must be documented for a pertinent PFSH.*

A ***complete*** PFSH is of a review of two or all three of the PFSH history areas, depending on the category of the E/M service. A review of all three history areas is required for services that by their nature include a comprehensive assessment or reassessment of the patient. A review of two of the three history areas is sufficient for other services.

• *DG: At least one specific item from two of the three history areas must be documented for a complete PFSH for the following categories of E/M services: office or other outpatient services, established patient; emergency department; domiciliary care, established patient; and home care, established patient.*

• *DG: At least one specific item from each of the three history areas must be documented for a complete PFSH for the following categories of E/M services: office or other outpatient services, new patient; hospital observation services; hospital inpatient services, initial care; consultations; comprehensive nursing facility assessments; domiciliary care, new patient; and home care, new patient.*

B. Documentation of Examination

The levels of E/M services are based on four types of examination:

- ***Problem Focused*** — a limited examination of the affected body area or organ system.
- ***Expanded Problem Focused*** — a limited examination of the affected body area or organ system and any other symptomatic or related body area(s) or organ system(s).

Appendix C: E/M Documentation

- ***Detailed*** — an extended examination of the affected body area(s) or organ system(s) and any other symptomatic or related body area(s) or organ system(s).
- ***Comprehensive*** — a general multi-system examination, or complete examination of a single organ system and other symptomatic or related body area(s) or organ system(s).

These types of examinations have been defined for general multi-system and the following single organ systems:

- Cardiovascular
- Ears, Nose, Mouth and Throat
- Eyes
- Genitourinary (Female)
- Genitourinary (Male)
- Hematologic/Lymphatic/Immunologic
- Musculoskeletal
- Neurological
- Psychiatric
- Respiratory
- Skin

A general multi-system examination or a single organ system examination may be performed by any physician regardless of specialty. The type (general multi-system or single organ system) and content of examination are selected by the examining physician and are based upon clinical judgment, the patient's history, and the nature of the presenting problem(s).

The content and documentation requirements for each type and level of examination are summarized below and described in detail in tables. In the tables, organ systems and body areas recognized by CPT® for purposes of describing examinations are shown in the left column. The content, or individual elements, of the examination pertaining to that body area or organ system are identified by bullets (•) in the right column.

Parenthetical examples, "(e.g., ...)", have been used for clarification and to provide guidance regarding documentation. Documentation for each element must satisfy any numeric requirements (such as "Measurement of any three of the following seven ... ") included in the description of the element. Elements with multiple components but with no specific numeric requirement (such as "Examination of liver and spleen") require documentation of at least one component. It is possible for a given examination to be expanded beyond what is defined here. When that occurs, findings related to the additional systems and/or areas should be documented.

• *DG: Specific abnormal and relevant negative findings of the examination of the affected or symptomatic body area(s) or organ system(s) should be documented. A notation of "abnormal" without elaboration is insufficient.*

• *DG: Abnormal or unexpected findings of the examination of any asymptomatic body area(s) or organ system(s) should be described.*

• *DG: A brief statement or notation indicating "negative" or "normal" is sufficient to document normal findings related to unaffected area(s) or asymptomatic organ system(s).*

General Multi-System Examinations

General multi-system examinations are described in detail below. To qualify for a given level of multi-system examination, the following content and documentation requirements should be met:

- ***Problem Focused Examination*** — should include performance and documentation of one to five elements identified by a bullet (•) in one or more organ system(s) or body area(s).
- ***Expanded Problem Focused Examination*** — should include performance and documentation of at least six elements identified by a bullet (•) in one or more organ system(s) or body area(s).
- ***Detailed Examination*** — should include at least six organ systems or body areas. For each system/area selected, performance and documentation of at least two elements identified by a bullet (•) is expected. Alternatively, a detailed examination may include performance and documentation of at least 12 elements identified by a bullet (•) in two or more organ systems or body areas.
- ***Comprehensive Examination*** — should include at least nine organ systems or body areas. For each system/area selected, all elements of the examination identified by a bullet (•) should be performed, unless specific directions limit the content of the examination. For each area/system, documentation of at least two elements identified by a bullet is expected.

Single Organ System Examinations

The single organ system examinations recognized by CPT® are described in detail previously. Variations among these examinations in the organ systems and body areas identified in the left columns and in the elements of the examinations described in the right columns reflect differing emphases among specialties. To qualify for a given level of single organ system examination, the following content and documentation requirements should be met:

- ***Problem Focused Examination*** — should include performance and documentation of one to five elements identified by a bullet (•), whether in a box with a shaded or unshaded border.
- ***Expanded Problem Focused Examination*** — should include performance and documentation of at least six elements identified by a bullet (•), whether in a box with a shaded or unshaded border.
- ***Detailed Examination*** — examinations other than the eye and psychiatric examinations should include performance and documentation of at least 12 elements identified by a bullet (•), whether in box with a shaded or unshaded border.

Eye and psychiatric examinations should include the performance and documentation of at least nine elements identified by a bullet (•), whether in a box with a shaded or unshaded border.

- *Comprehensive Examination* — should include performance of all elements identified by a bullet (•), whether in a shaded or unshaded box. Documentation of every element in each box with a shaded border and at least one element in each box with an unshaded border is expected.

General Multi-System Examination

System/Body Area	Elements of Examination
Constitutional	Measurement of **any three of the following seven** vital signs: 1) sitting or standing blood pressure, 2) supine blood pressure, 3) pulse rate and regularity, 4) respiration, 5) temperature, 6) height, 7) weight (May be measured and recorded by ancillary staff) General appearance of patient (e.g., development, nutrition, body habitus, deformities, attention to grooming)
Eyes	Inspection of conjunctivae and lids Examination of pupils and irises (e.g., reaction to light and accommodation, size and symmetry) Ophthalmoscopic examination of optic discs (e.g., size, C/D ratio, appearance) and posterior segments (e.g., vessel changes, exudates, hemorrhages)
Ears, Nose, Mouth, and Throat	External inspection of ears and nose (e.g., overall appearance, scars, lesions, masses) Otoscopic examination of external auditory canals and tympanic membranes Assessment of hearing (e.g., whispered voice, finger rub, tuning fork) Inspection of nasal mucosa, septum and turbinates Inspection of lips, teeth and gums Examination of oropharynx: oral mucosa, salivary glands, hard and soft palates, tongue, tonsils and posterior pharynx
Neck	Examination of neck (e.g., masses, overall appearance, symmetry, tracheal position, crepitus Examination of thyroid (e.g., enlargement, tenderness, mass)
Respiratory	Assessment of respiratory effort (e.g., intercostal retractions, use of accessory muscles, diaphragmatic movement) Percussion of chest (e.g., dullness, flatness, hyperresonance) Palpation of chest (e.g., tactile fremitus) Auscultation of lungs (e.g., breath sounds, adventitious sounds, rubs)
Cardiovascular	Palpation of heart (e.g., location, size, thrills) Auscultation of heart with notation of abnormal sounds and murmurs Examination of: Carotid arteries (e.g., pulse amplitude, bruits) Abdominal aorta (e.g., size, bruits) Femoral arteries (e.g., pulse amplitude, bruits) Pedal pulses (e.g., pulse amplitude) Extremities for edema and/or varicosities
Chest (Breasts)	Inspection of breasts (e.g., symmetry, nipple discharge) Palpation of breasts and axillae (e.g., masses or lumps, tenderness)
Gastrointestinal (Abdomen)	Examination of abdomen with notation of presence of masses or tenderness Examination of liver and spleen Examination for presence or absence of hernia Examination (when indicated) of anus, perineum and rectum, including sphincter tone, presence of hemorrhoids, rectal masses Obtain stool sample for occult blood test when indicated
Genitourinary	Male: Examination of the scrotal contents (e.g., hydrocele, spermatocele, tenderness of cord, testicular mass) Examination of the penis Digital rectal examination of prostate gland (e.g., size, symmetry, nodularity, tenderness) Female: Pelvic examination (with or without specimen collection for smears and cultures), including: Examination of external genitalia (e.g., general appearance, hair distribution, lesions) and vagina (e.g., general appearance, estrogen effect, discharge, lesions, pelvic support, cystocele, rectocele) Examination of urethra (e.g., masses, tenderness, scarring) Examination of bladder (e.g., fullness, masses, tenderness) Cervix (e.g., general appearance, lesions, discharge) Uterus (e.g., size, contour, position, mobility, tenderness, consistency, descent or support) Adnexa/parametria (e.g., masses, tenderness, organomegaly, nodularity)
Lymphatic	Palpation of lymph nodes in **two or more** areas: Neck Axillae Groin Other

System/Body Area	Elements of Examination
Musculoskeletal	Examination of gait and station Inspection and/or palpation of digits and nails (e.g., clubbing, cyanosis, inflammatory conditions, petechiae, ischemia, infections, nodes) Examination of joints, bones and muscles of **one or more of the following six** areas: 1) head and neck; 2) spine, ribs and pelvis; 3) right upper extremity; 4) left upper extremity; 5) right lower extremity; and 6) left lower extremity. The examination of a given area includes: Inspection and/or palpation with notation of presence of any misalignment, asymmetry, crepitation, defects, tenderness, masses, effusions Assessment of range of motion with notation of any pain, crepitation or contracture Assessment of stability with notation of any dislocation (luxation), subluxation or laxity Assessment of muscle strength and tone (e.g., flaccid, cog wheel, spastic) with notation of any atrophy or abnormal movements
Skin	Inspection of skin and subcutaneous tissue (e.g., rashes, lesions, ulcers) Palpation of skin and subcutaneous tissue (e.g., induration, subcutaneous nodules, tightening)
Neurologic	Test cranial nerves with notation of any deficits Examination of deep tendon reflexes with notation of pathological reflexes (e.g., Babinski) Examination of sensation (e.g., by touch, pin, vibration, proprioception)
Psychiatric	Description of patient's judgment and insight Brief assessment of mental status including: Orientation to time, place and person Recent and remote memory Mood and affect (e.g., depression, anxiety, agitation)

General Multi-System Examination Content and Documentation Requirements

Level of Exam	Perform and Document
Problem Focused	**One to five** elements identified by a bullet
Expanded Problem Focused	**At least six** elements identified by a bullet
Detailed	**At least two** elements identified by a bullet **from each of six areas/systems** OR **at least 12** elements identified by a bullet **in two or more areas/systems.**
Comprehensive	Perform **all elements** identified by a bullet in **at least nine** organ systems or body areas and document **at least two** elements identified by a bullet **from each of nine areas/systems.**

Cardiovascular Examination

System/Body Area	Elements of Examination
Constitutional	Measurement of **any three of the following seven** vital signs: 1) sitting or standing blood pressure, 2) supine blood pressure, 3) pulse rate and regularity, 4) respiration, 5) temperature, 6) height, 7) weight (May be measured and recorded by ancillary staff) General appearance of patient (e.g., development, nutrition, body habitus, deformities, attention to grooming)
Eyes	Inspection of conjunctivae and lids (e.g., xanthelasma)
Ears, Nose, Mouth, and Throat	Inspection of teeth, gums and palate Inspection of oral mucosa with notation of presence of pallor or cyanosis
Neck	Examination of jugular veins (e.g., distension; a, v or cannon a waves) Examination of thyroid (e.g., enlargement, tenderness, mass)
Respiratory	Assessment of respiratory effort (e.g., intercostal retractions, use of accessory muscles, diaphragmatic movement) Auscultation of lungs (e.g., breath sounds, adventitious sounds, rubs)
Cardiovascular	Palpation of heart (e.g., location, size and forcefulness of the point of maximal impact; thrills; lifts; palpable S3 or S4) Auscultation of heart including sounds, abnormal sounds and murmurs Measurement of blood pressure in two or more extremities when indicated (e.g., aortic dissection, coarctation) Examination of: Carotid arteries (e.g., waveform, pulse amplitude, bruits, apical-carotid delay) Abdominal aorta (e.g., size, bruits) Femoral arteries (e.g., pulse amplitude, bruits) Pedal pulses (e.g., pulse amplitude) Extremities for peripheral edema and/or varicosities
Gastrointestinal (Abdomen)	Examination of abdomen with notation of presence of masses or tenderness Examination of liver and spleen Obtain stool sample for occult blood from patients who are being considered for thrombolytic or anticoagulant therapy
Musculoskeletal	Examination of the back with notation of kyphosis or scoliosis Examination of gait with notation of ability to undergo exercise testing and/or participation in exercise programs Assessment of muscle strength and tone (e.g., flaccid, cog wheel, spastic) with notation of any atrophy and abnormal movements
Extremities	Inspection and palpation of digits and nails (e.g., clubbing, cyanosis, inflammation, petechiae, ischemia, infections, Osler's nodes)

System/Body Area	Elements of Examination
Skin	Inspection and/or palpation of skin and subcutaneous tissue (e.g., stasis dermatitis, ulcers, scars, xanthomas)
Neurological/ Psychiatric	Brief assessment of mental status including: Orientation to time, place and person, Mood and affect (e.g., depression, anxiety, agitation)

Cardiovascular Examination Content and Documentation Requirements

Level of Exam	Perform and Document
Problem Focused	**One to five** elements identified by a bullet
Expanded Problem Focused	**At least six** elements identified by a bullet
Detailed	**At least 12** elements identified by a bullet
Comprehensive	Perform all elements identified by a bullet; document every element in each box with a shaded border and at least one element in each box with an unshaded border.

C. Documentation of the Complexity of Medical Decision-Making

The levels of E/M services recognize four types of medical decision-making (Straightforward, Low Complexity, Moderate Complexity and High Complexity). Medical decision-making refers to the complexity of establishing a diagnosis and/or selecting a management option as measured by:

- the number of possible diagnoses and/or the number of management options that must be considered;
- the amount and/or complexity of medical records, diagnostic tests, and/or other information that must be obtained, reviewed and analyzed; and
- the risk of significant complications, morbidity and/or mortality, as well as comorbidities associated with the patient's presenting problem(s), the diagnostic procedure(s) and/or the possible management options.

The chart below shows the progression of the elements required for each level of medical decision-making. To qualify for a given type of decision-making, two of the three elements in the table must be either met or exceeded.

Number of diagnoses or management options	Amount and/or complexity of data	Risk of complications and/or morbidity or mortality	Type of decision-making
Minimal	Minimal or None	Minimal	**Straightforward**
Limited	Limited	Low	**Low Complexity**
Multiple	Moderate	Moderate	**Moderate Complexity**
Extensive	Extensive	High	**High Complexity**

The following is a description of elements of medical decision-making.

Number of Diagnoses of Management Options

The number of possible diagnoses and/or the number of management options that must be considered is based on the number and types of problems addressed during the encounter, the complexity of establishing a diagnosis and the management decisions that are made by the physician.

Generally, decision-making with respect to a diagnosed problem is easier than that for an identified but undiagnosed problem. The number and type of diagnostic tests employed may be an indicator of the number of possible diagnoses. Problems which are improving or resolving are less complex than those which are worsening or failing to change as expected. The need to seek advice from others is another indicator of complexity of diagnostic or management problems.

• *DG: For each encounter, an assessment, clinical impression, or diagnosis should be documented. It may be explicitly stated or implied in documented decisions regarding management plans and/or further evaluation.*

- For a presenting problem with an established diagnosis the record should reflect whether the problem is: a) improved, well controlled, resolving or resolved; or, b) inadequately controlled, worsening, or failing to change as expected.
- For a presenting problem without an established diagnosis, the assessment or clinical impression may be stated in the form of differential diagnoses or as a "possible," "probable," or "rule out" (R/O) diagnosis.

• *DG: The initiation of, or changes in, treatment should be documented. Treatment includes a wide range of management options including patient instructions, nursing instructions, therapies, and medications.*

• *DG: If referrals are made, consultations requested or advice sought, the record should indicate to whom or where the referral or consultation is made or from whom the advice is requested.*

Amount and/or Complexity of Data to be Reviewed

The amount and complexity of data to be reviewed is based on the types of diagnostic testing ordered or reviewed. A decision to obtain and review old medical records and/or obtain history from sources other than the patient increases the amount and complexity of data to be reviewed.

Discussion of contradictory or unexpected test results with the physician who performed or interpreted the test is an indication of the complexity of data being reviewed. On occasion the physician who ordered a test may personally review the image, tracing or specimen to supplement information from the physician who prepared the test report or interpretation; this is another indication of the complexity of data being reviewed.

• *DG: If a diagnostic service (test or procedure) is ordered, planned, scheduled, or performed at the time of the E/M encounter, the type of service, e.g., lab or X-ray, should be documented.*

• *DG: The review of lab, radiology and/or other diagnostic tests should be documented. A simple notation such as "WB elevated" or "chest X-ray unremarkable" is acceptable. Alternatively, the review may be documented by initialing and dating the report containing the test results.*

- *DG: A decision to obtain old records or decision to obtain additional history from the family, caretaker or other source to supplement that obtained from the patient should be documented.*
- *DG: Relevant findings from the review of old records, and/or the receipt of additional history from the family, caretaker or other source to supplement that obtained from the patient should be documented. If there is no relevant information beyond that already obtained, that fact should be documented. A notation of "old records reviewed" or "additional history obtained from family" without elaboration is insufficient.*
- *DG: The results of discussion of laboratory, radiology or other diagnostic tests with the physician who performed or interpreted the study should be documented.*
- *DG: The direct visualization and independent interpretation of an image, tracing or specimen previously or subsequently interpreted by another physician should be documented.*

Risk of Significant Complications, Morbidity and/or Mortality

The risk of significant complications, morbidity and/or mortality is based on the risks associated with the presenting problem(s), the diagnostic procedure(s) and the possible management options.

- *DG: Comorbidities/underlying diseases or other factors that increase the complexity of medical decision-making by increasing the risk of complications, morbidity, and/or mortality should be documented.*
- *DG: If a surgical or invasive diagnostic procedure is ordered, planned or scheduled at the time of the E/M encounter, the type of procedure, e.g., laparoscopy, should be documented.*
- *DG: If a surgical or invasive diagnostic procedure is performed at the time of the E/M encounter, the specific procedure should be documented.*
- *DG: The referral for or decision to perform a surgical or invasive diagnostic procedure on an urgent basis should be documented or implied.*

The following table may be used to help determine whether the risk of significant complications, morbidity and/or mortality is minimal, low, moderate or high. Because the determination of risk is complex and not readily quantifiable, the table includes common clinical examples rather than absolute measures of risk. The assessment of risk of the presenting problem(s) is based on the risk related to the disease process anticipated between the present encounter and the next one. The assessment of risk of selecting diagnostic procedures and management options is based on the risk during and immediately following any procedures or treatment. **The highest level of risk in any one category (presenting problem(s), diagnostic procedure(s) or management options) determines the overall risk.**

D. Documentation of an Encounter Dominated by Counseling or Coordination of Care

In the case where counseling and/or coordination of care dominates (more than 50%) of the physician/patient and/or family encounter (face-to-face time in the office or other or outpatient setting, floor/unit time in the hospital or nursing facility), time is considered the key or controlling factor to qualify for a particular level of E/M services.

- *DG: If the physician elects to report the level of service based on counseling and/or coordination of care, the total length of time of the encounter (face-to-face or floor time, as appropriate) should be documented and the record should describe the counseling and/or activities to coordinate care.*

Table of Risk

Level of Risk	Presenting Problem(s)	Diagnostic Procedure(s) Ordered	Management Options Selected
Minimal	One self-limited or minor problem, e.g., cold, insect bite, tinea corporis	Laboratory tests requiring venipuncture Chest X-rays EKG/EEG Urinalysis Ultrasound, e.g., echocardiography KOH prep	Rest Gargles Elastic bandages Superficial dressings
Low	Two or more self-limited or minor problems One stable chronic illness, e.g., well controlled hypertension, non-insulin dependent diabetes, cataract, BPH Acute uncomplicated illness or injury, e.g., cystitis, allergic rhinitis, simple sprain	Physiologic tests not under stress, e.g., pulmonary function test Non-cardiovascular imaging studies with contrast, e.g., barium enema Superficial needle biopsies Clinical laboratory tests requiring arterial puncture Skin biopsies	Over-the-counter drugs Minor surgery with no identified risk factors Physical therapy Occupational therapy IV fluids without additives
Moderate	One or more chronic illnesses with mild exacerbation, progression, or side effects of treatment Two or more stable chronic illnesses Undiagnosed new problem with uncertain prognosis, e.g., lump in breast Acute illness with systemic symptoms, e.g., pyelonephritis, pneumonitis, colitis Acute complicated injury, e.g., head injury with brief loss of consciousness	Physiologic tests under stress, e.g., cardio stress test, fetal contraction stress test Diagnostic endoscopies with no identified risk factors Deep needle or incisional biopsy Cardiovascular imaging studies with contrast and no identified risk factors, e.g., arteriogram, cardiac catheterization Obtain fluid from body cavity, e.g. lumbar puncture, thoracentesis, culdocentesis	Minor surgery with identified risk factors Elective major surgery (open, percutaneous or endoscopic) with no identified risk factors Prescription drug management Therapeutic nuclear medicine IV fluids with additives Closed treatment of fracture or dislocation without manipulation
High	One or more chronic illnesses with severe exacerbation, progression, or side effects of treatment Acute or chronic illnesses or injuries that pose a threat to life or bodily function, e.g., multiple trauma, acute MI, pulmonary embolus, severe respiratory distress, progressive severe rheumatoid arthritis, psychiatric illness with potential threat to self or others, peritonitis, acute renal failure An abrupt change in neurologic status, e.g., seizure, TIA, weakness, sensory loss	Cardiovascular imaging studies with contrast with identified risk factors Cardiac electrophysiological tests Diagnostic endoscopies with identified risk factors Discography	Elective major surgery (open, percutaneous or endoscopic) with identified risk factors Emergency major surgery (open, percutaneous or endoscopic) Parenteral controlled substances Drug therapy requiring intensive monitoring for toxicity Decision not to resuscitate or to deescalate care because of poor prognosis

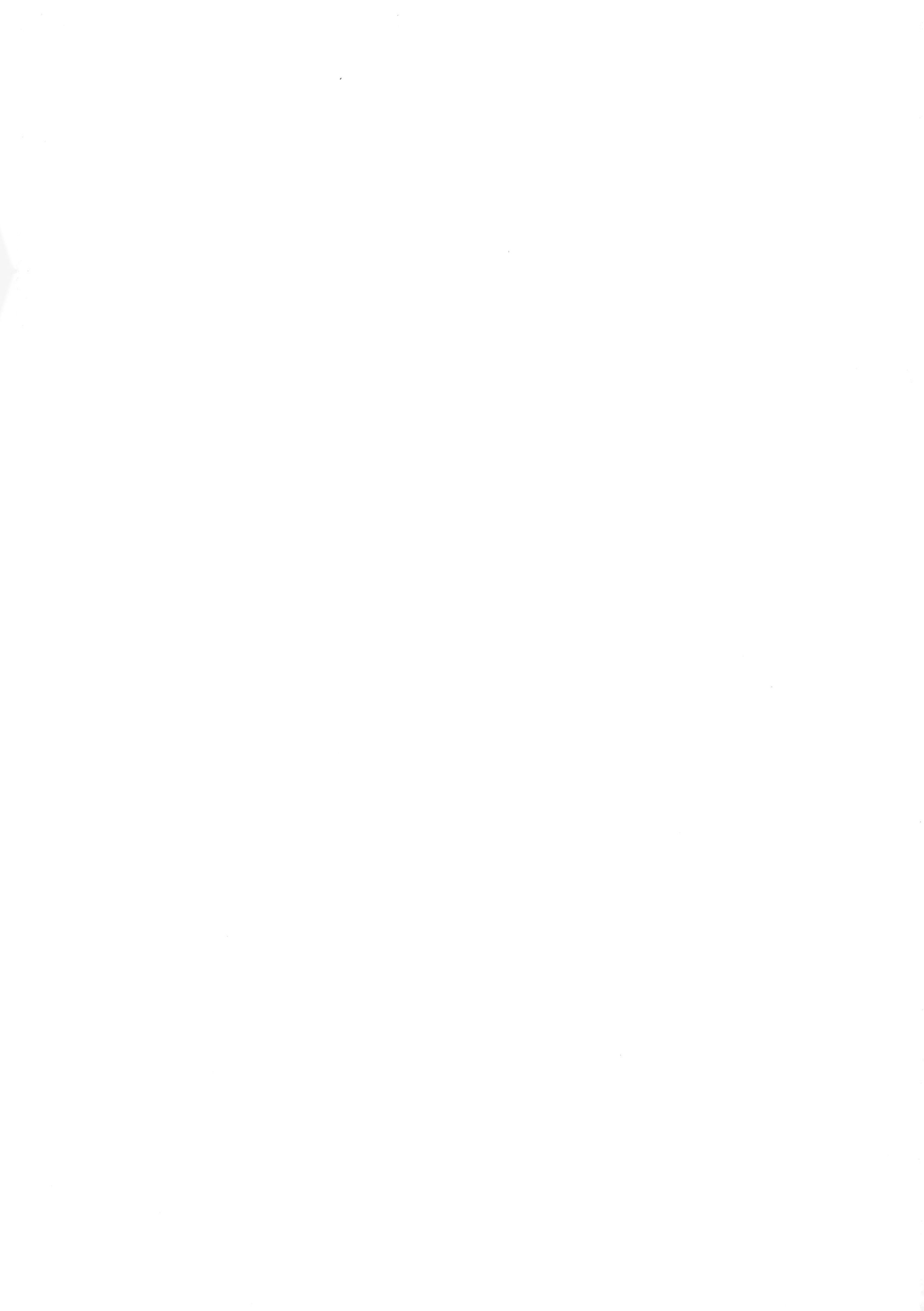